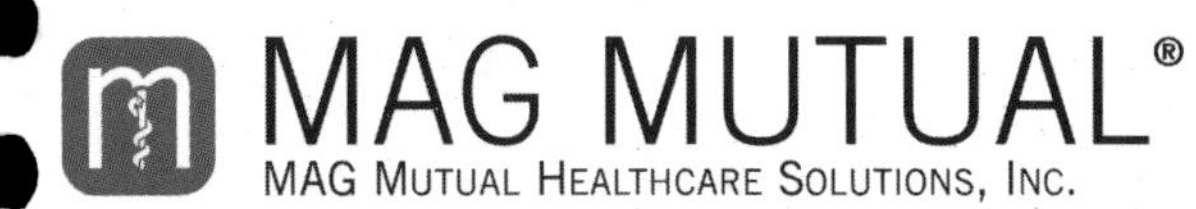

7 Piedmont Center, Suite 601
3525 Piedmont Rd | Atlanta, GA 30305
ph 800.253.4945 | fax 888.676.4222
www.coderscentral.com

Who We Are

MAG Mutual Healthcare Solutions, Inc. (MMHSI) is a subsidiary of physician-led and physician-owned MAG Mutual Insurance Company (MMIC). MMIC is dedicated to helping physicians and others in the medical community focus on providing quality patient care. Working together, our companies develop and provide innovative business, financial and insurance solutions to help those we serve meet their professional, business, and personal goals. MMHSI's mission is to protect physicians through financial services and practice management solutions that increase revenues and save time and resources.

MMIC was founded in 1982 by physicians to provide medical professional liability insurance and now serves about 17,000 policyholders as the largest insurer in the Southeast, in premium volume. MMIC is the eighth-largest medical malpractice insurer in the US with assets exceeding $1.4 billion, according to the A.M. Best 200 ratings. In 1996, MMIC purchased HealthCare Consultants of America (HCCA). In 2002, the operations of HCCA were integrated into MMHSI, which also provided other physician support services such as medical billing, consulting, tax and accounting, IT and provider enrollment.

Why We Are Different

Unlike some of our competitors, MMHSI is not owned by a large healthcare insurer or consortium of private investors and/or venture capitalists; we are physician-owned. This is critical because it means that there is nothing more important to us that helping our customers overcome their challenges. Through our physician-led Board of Directors, our customers' biggest challenges are passed down as our company's strategic goals. This translates to our publications and software directly in that they are developed to be accurate, cutting-edge, easy to incorporate into your workflow, and unabashedly pro-physician.

In the past year, MMHSI has relocated to the MMIC corporate offices to allow us to better support our physicians. All warehousing and fulfillment of MMHSI's products are handled in our own facilities. This results in faster turn-around on orders (commonly same-day) and more accurate delivery.

Because we are more interested in maintaining our valued relationships with customers than simply growing the top line, our sales and marketing efforts are also unique in the industry. We do not use outsourced telemarketers, choosing to employ Account Representatives who are trained to solve your problems, not simply haggle with you over pricing. **The average tenure of our Account Reps is approximately than 6 years!** As such, our customer service is unparalleled in this industry.

Thank you for reading this far, and if you have any needs or concerns, please let us know.

Sincerely,

David Miller
President, MMHSI

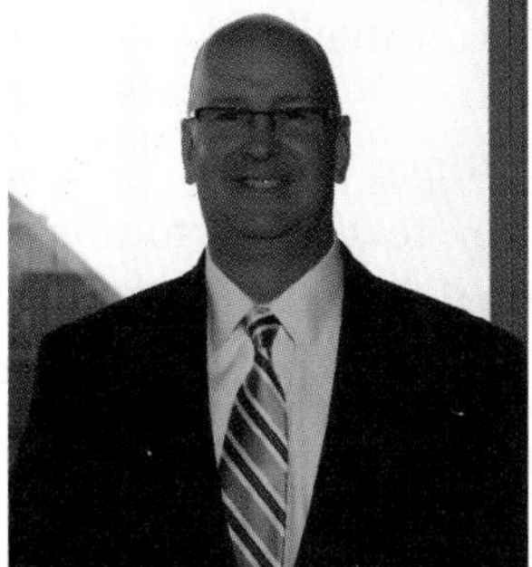

MAG Mutual Healthcare Solutions, Inc.

Renewable♻Renewal Program

Our Commitment

MAG Mutual Healthcare Solutions, Inc. (MMHSI) is dedicated to the preservation of our environment. Forest management has been shown to be more fundamentally important than even the recycling of paper products to responsibly meet today's demands for paper. We proudly back the mission of the Forest Stewardship Council to support environmentally appropriate, socially beneficial, and economically viable management of the world's forests. In turn, we strive to minimize the environmental impact of all of our products.

To that end, this book was produced with material from well-managed forests, controlled sources and recycled wood or fiber by a print vendor with a current and valid FSC certificate.

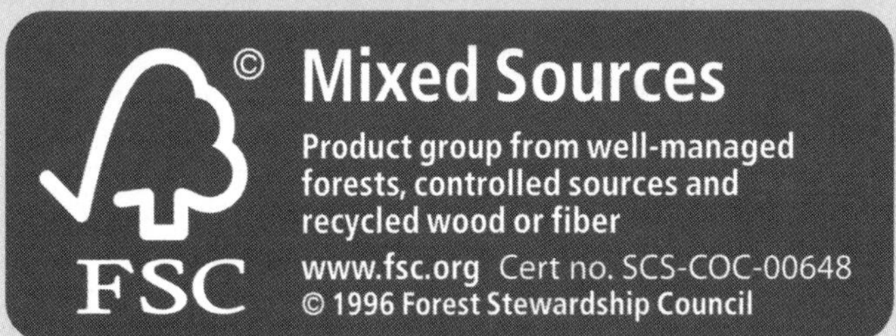

Our Goal

It is our goal to recycle 15% of all published copies of this book within 18 months of its publication. While we understand that many organizations will archive past edition years' code books for auditing purposes, we are also aware that a large quantity of code books are thrown in the trash upon release of the new edition year's book.

Saving the World's Forests Saves You Money

To encourage you to help us with our commitment to environmentally responsible products, MMHSI has launched the **Renewable♻Renewal Program**. We want to save as many of these books from landfills as possible by incentivizing organizations to return unused books to us. We will then ensure they are properly recycled. **Therefore, MMHSI will not only pay return postage to have your obsolete copies shipped to us for processing, but will also apply a $25 credit toward your purchase of the 2011 edition of this book.** The $25 credit may not be combined with any other offers or discounts; however, each returned copy is valid for one $25 credit towards the purchase of a 2011 edition (i.e., if you return 5 copies of the 2010 edition, you will receive 5 credits, each redeemable for $25 off of a MAG Mutual *2011 ICD-9-CM Professional*).

It is our hope that through the use of FSC-certified paper and the creation of the **Renewable♻Renewal Program** that we will make a small contribution to a better tomorrow. We hope you join us and welcome your feedback on our efforts to reach the highest attainable social and environmental standards possible. For more information and to begin saving today, contact an MMHSI Account Representative at 800-253-4549.

The FSC logo and trademark are ® FSC Forest Stewardship Council, A.C. All rights reserved. FSR-SECR-0002
We encourage you to learn more about responsible forestry and its environmental and social ramifications at www.fsc.org

2010 ICD-9-CM
Volumes 1 & 2
Professional Edition for Physicians

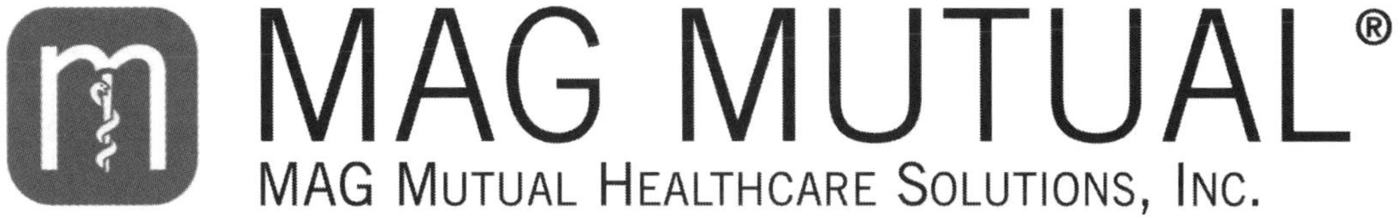

MAG Mutual Healthcare Solutions, Inc.
7 Piedmont Center, Suite 601
3525 Piedmont Road
Atlanta, GA 30305
phone: 800-253-4945
www.coderscentral.com

2010 ICD-9-CM Volumes 1&2 - Professional Edition for Physicians

© 2009 MAG Mutual Healthcare Solutions, Inc. All rights reserved.
ISBN 978-1-60099-021-2 (softbound edition) or 978-1-60099-022-9 (spiral edition)
Printed in the United States of America: August 2009.

MAG Mutual Healthcare Solutions, Inc.
7 Piedmont Center, Suite 601
3525 Piedmont Road
Atlanta, GA 30305
(800) 253-4945
www.coderscentral.com

CPT® codes © 2008 American Medical Association. All rights reserved. CPT is a registered trademark of the American Medical Association

See page 45 of the PQRI Coding Guidance chapter for copyright attribution for individual PQRI measures.

Anatomical illustrations © 2008 Fairman Studios, LLC unless otherwise noted. All rights reserved.

Additional illustrations © 2006 Anatomical Chart Company and © Icon Learning Systems where attributed.

Disclaimers

MAG Mutual Healthcare Solutions, Inc. provides this resource guide to help physicians and managers in the rapidly changing medical practice environment. The information presented is based upon the sixth edition of the International Classification of Diseases, 9th revision, Clinical Modification (ICD-9-CM) published by the United States Government.

This sixth edition of the International Classification of Diseases, 9th Revision, Clinical Modification (ICD-9-CM) is published by the United States Government in recognition of its responsibility to promulgate this classification throughout the United States for morbidity coding. The International Classification of Diseases, 9th Revision (ICD-9), published by the World Health Organization (WHO) is the foundation of the ICD-9-CM and continues to be the classification employed in cause-of-death coding in the United States. The ICD-9-CM is completely comparable with the ICD-9. The WHO Collaborating Center for Classification of Diseases in North America serves as liaison between the international obligations for comparable classifications and the national health data needs of the United States.

The ICD-9-CM is recommended for use in all clinical settings but is required for reporting diagnoses and diseases to all U.S. Public Health Service and the Centers for Medicare & Medicaid Services (formerly the Health Care Financing Administration) programs.

ICD-9-CM extensions, interpretations, modifications, addenda, or errata other than those approved by the U.S. Public Health Service and the Centers for Medicare & Medicaid Services are not to be considered official and should not be utilized. Continuous maintenance of the ICD-9-CM is the responsibility of the Federal Government. However, because the ICD-9-CM represents the best in contemporary thinking of clinicians, nosologists, epidemiologists, and statisticians from both public and private sectors, no future modifications will be considered without extensive advice from the appropriate representatives of all major users.

The authors, publisher, distributors, and corporations involved in the writing and/or production of this book do not accept responsibility or liability for any adverse outcome from using this guide for any reason including undetected errors or the user's misunderstanding or misapplication of the information contained within or otherwise. As this is a coding reference, no guarantee is made regarding the clinical accuracy of the content (including anatomical illustrations and labels as well as the code set) contained herein.

2010 ICD-9-CM Volumes 1 & 2

Professional edition, valid for use October 1, 2009-September 30, 2010

Table of Contents

We Appreciate Your Interest In Our Publications

David A. Miller, President
David has 25 years experience in sales, marketing, insurance and physicians practice management. David has been in the Heath Care Sector for the last 15 years. He is currently the President of MAG Mutual Healthcare Solutions Inc. (MMHSI) and is responsible for the day to day management and strategic direction for all four of MMHSI's business services to Physicians. Those lines of business are Physician Billing Services, Medical Practice Management Consulting Services, Tax and Accounting for Physicians, and Medical Publications.

Rodney P. Benefield, Director of Publications
Rodney attended Georgia Southwestern College. In addition to practice management and marketing expertise, he has experience in the computer industry as a medical billing software designer, manager, business owner, and consultant. Mr. Benefield served as a senior practice management consultant, and Publications Manager for HealthCare Consultants of America, Inc. from 1993 to October, 2002.

Tony Mistretta, Senior Product Developer
Tony is a graduate of Duke University. He has edited, authored and developed coding and practice management publications since 1997. Mr. Mistretta served in management and VP roles in Product Development and Management for the Medical Management Institute (1997-2006) and Contexo Media (2006-2008) prior to joining MAG Mutual Healthcare Solutions, Inc.

Project Consulting Staff: Steve Adams, CPC; Ed Frankfort, CHBC; Richard Pilson, CHBC; Michael Riddick, CHBC; Alan Stroud, CHBC; Ken Waldron, CHBC; Josh Turbeville, CHBC; Deana Bailey, RN, David Huff, CPA

Special Support: Robin Eubanks

Special thanks to the management team at MAG Mutual and The MAG Mutual Board of Directors

ACKNOWLEDGMENTS

MAG Mutual Healthcare Solutions, Inc. utilizes the services of the following consultants with extensive experience in medical practice management, finance, coding, and reimbursement and medical illustration.

Hoyt W. Torras, MPA, MHA
Hoyt is a graduate of Georgia Tech. Holds two master's degrees including Master's of Health Administration. Experience includes hospital administration; healthcare consulting; research; government health programs; Individual Practice Associations; medical societies consulting; and Associate Director, Medical Association of Georgia (1984-1988). Mr. Torras was a founding member and served as Vice President, HealthCare Consultants of America, Inc. from 1989 to July, 2002.

Jennifer Fairman, MA, CMI
Fairman Studios is an award-willing board certified biomedical communications studio specializing in medical illustration, scientific and biological illustration, medical animation, interactive design, web publication and graphic design for the Biomedical, Scientific and Healthcare industries.

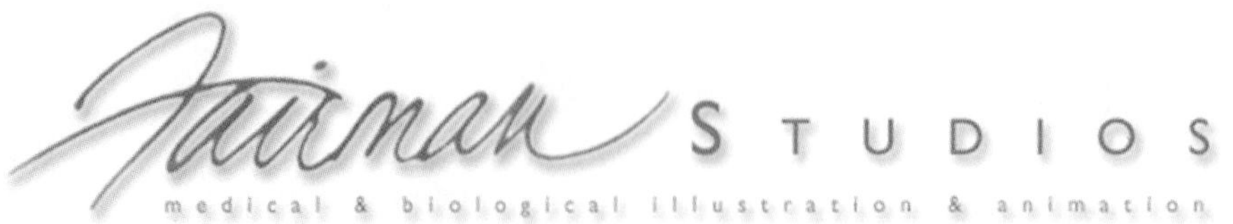

Introduction

INTRODUCTION

The *International Classification of Diseases, 9th Revision, Clinical Modification* (*ICD-9-CM*) is based on the official version of the World Health Organization's *9th Revision, International Classification of Diseases* (*ICD-9*). *ICD-9* is designed for the classification of morbidity and mortality information for statistical purposes, and for the indexing of hospital records by disease and operations, for data storage and retrieval. The historical background of the International Classification of Diseases may be found in the Introduction to ICD-9 (*Manual of the International Classification of Diseases, Injuries, and Causes of Death, World Health Organization*, Geneva, Switzerland, 1977).

ICD-9-CM is a clinical modification of the World Health Organization's *International Classification of Diseases, 9th Revision* (*ICD-9*). The term "clinical" is used to emphasize the modification's intent: to serve as a useful tool in the area of classification of morbidity data for indexing of medical records, medical care review, and ambulatory and other medical care programs, as well as for basic health statistics. To describe the clinical picture of the patient, the codes must be more precise than those needed only for statistical groupings and trend analysis.

THE ICD-9-CM COORDINATION AND MAINTENANCE COMMITTEE

Annual modifications are made to the ICD-9-CM through the ICD-9-CM Coordination and Maintenance Committee (C&M). The Committee is made up of representatives from two Federal Government agencies, the National Center for Health Statistics and the Centers for Medicare & Medicaid Services (formerly the Health Care Financing Administration). The Committee holds meetings twice a year which are open to the public. Modification proposals submitted to the Committee for consideration are presented at the meetings for public discussion. Those modification proposals which are approved are incorporated into the official government version of the *ICD-9-CM* and become effective for use the October 1 of the year following their presentation.

CHARACTERISTICS OF ICD-9-CM

ICD-9-CM far exceeds its predecessors in the number of codes provided. The disease classification has been expanded to include health-related conditions and to provide greater specificity at the fifth-digit level of detail. These fifth digits are not optional; they are intended for use in recording the information substantiated in the clinical record.

Volume I of *ICD-9-CM* contains four appendices:

Appendix A	Morphology of Neoplasms
Appendix C	Classification of Drugs by American Hospital Formulary Service List Number and Their ICD-9-CM Equivalents
Appendix D	Classification of Industrial Accidents According to Agency
Appendix E	List of Three-Digit Categories
Appendix B	(the Glossary of Mental Disorders) was deleted effective October 1, 2004.

These appendices are included as a reference to the user in order to provide further information about the patient's clinical picture, to further define a diagnostic statement, to aid in classifying new drugs, or to reference three-digit categories.

Volume 2 of *ICD-9-CM* contains many diagnostic terms which do not appear in Volume 1 since the index includes most diagnostic terms currently in use.

© 2009 MAG Mutual Healthcare Solutions, Inc.

GUIDANCE IN THE USE OF ICD-9-CM

To code accurately, it is necessary to have a working knowledge of medical terminology and to understand the characteristics, terminology, and conventions of the *ICD-9-CM*. Transforming verbal descriptions of diseases, injuries, conditions, and procedures into numerical designations (coding) is a complex activity and should not be undertaken without proper training.

Originally coding was accomplished to provide access to medical records by diagnoses and operations through retrieval for medical research, education, and administration. Medical codes today are utilized to facilitate payment of health services, to evaluate utilization patterns, and to study the appropriateness of health care costs. Coding provides the bases for epidemiological studies and research into the quality of health care.

Coding must be performed correctly and consistently to produce meaningful statistics to aid in the planning for the health needs of the Nation.

Basic Steps in Coding Diagnoses/Diseases

1. Always consult Volume 2, Alphabetic Index to ICD-9-CM first.

   Locate the main entry term. The Alphabetic Index is arranged by condition. Conditions may be expressed as nouns, adjectives, and eponyms. Some conditions have multiple entries under their synonyms. Select the appropriate code.

2. Refer to Volume 1 of the *ICD-9-CM* locating the selected code.

   Be guided by any exclusion notes or other instructions that would direct the use of a different code from that selected in the Index for a particular diagnosis, condition, or disease.

3. Read and be guided by the conventions used in the Tabular List (Volume 1, *ICD-9-CM*).

   As reference for use by researchers and to maintain comparability with its parent, the ICD-9, a list of three-digit ICD-9-CM categories is given in Appendix E. While these categories form natural statistical groupings, they cannot substitute for the required five-digit ICD-9-CM code.

CONVENTIONS USED IN THE ICD-9-CM

The ICD-9-CM Tabular List and Alphabetic Index both make use of certain abbreviations, punctuation, and other conventions which need to be clearly understood. The conventions on the following pages apply to both the Tabular and Alphabetic sections unless otherwise stated:

Abbreviations:

NEC Not elsewhere classifiable. The category number for the term including NEC is to be used only when the coder lacks the information necessary to code the term to a more specific category. e.g.,

755.22 Longitudinal deficiency of upper limb, NEC

NOS Not otherwise specified. This abbreviation is the equivalent of "unspecified." e.g.,

921.0 Black eye, NOS

Punctuation:

[ ] Brackets are used to enclose synonyms, alternative wordings, or explanatory phrases. (Red brackets beneath codes in the Tabular List have a different meaning which is explained on the next page) e.g,

4th 891 Open wound of knee, leg [except thigh], and ankle

[ ] Italicized brackets are found only in the Alphabetic Index and signify the need to submit a manifestation code secondary to the principal diagnosis. e.g,

Arthritis, arthritic
ankylosing (crippling) (spine) 720.0 *[713.2]*

( ) Parentheses are used to enclose supplementary words which may be present or absent in the statement of a disease or procedure without affecting the code number to which it is assigned. e.g.,

477.2 Due to animal (cat) (dog) hair and dander

: Colons are used in the Tabular List after an incomplete term which needs one or more of the modifiers which follow in order to make it assignable to a given category. e.g.,

379.21 Vitreous degeneration
Vitreous:
cavitation
detachment
liquefaction

© 2009 MAG Mutual Healthcare Solutions, Inc.

Other Conventions

ICD-9-CM uses an indented format for ease in reference.

Instructional Notations:

Includes This note appears immediately under a three-digit code title to further define, or give example of, the contents of the category. e.g.,

4th 582 **Chronic glomerulonephritis**
Includes chronic nephritis

Excludes Terms following the word "excludes" are to be coded elsewhere. The term excludes means "DO NOT CODE HERE". e.g.,

5th 478.1 **Other diseases of nasal cavity and sinuses**
Excludes *varicose ulcer of nasal septum (456.8)*

Use additional code:

This instruction is placed in the Tabular List in those categories where the user will need to add further information (by using an additional code) to give a more complete picture of the diagnosis or procedure. e.g.,

5th 525.4 **Complete edentulism**
Use additional code to identify cause of edentulism (525.10-525.19)

Code first underlying disease:

This instructional note is used for those codes not intended to be used as a principal diagnosis, or not to be sequenced before the underlying disease. The note requires that the underlying disease (etiology) be recorded first and the particular manifestation recorded secondarily. This note appears only in the Tabular List. e.g.,

590.81 **Pyelitis or pyelonephritis in diseases classified elsewhere**
Code first underlying disease, as:
tuberculosis (016.0)

Value-Added Conventions

MAG Mutual Healthcare Solutions, Inc. (MMHSI) has developed and included several additional conventions to facilitate correct coding selection:

Update Conventions:

● In the Tabular List, a bullet denotes a new category, subcategory or code. In other sections, the bullet denotes a completely new line of text. e.g.,

● 416.2 **Chronic pulmonary embolism**

▲ In the Tabular List, a delta denotes a revised category, subcategory or code. In other sections, the delta denotes a revised line of text. e.g.,

▲ 584.5 **Acute kidney failure with lesion of tubular necrosis**

text (underlined) In all sections of the ICD-9-CM, underlined text highlights newly added text. e.g.,

5th V54.2 **Aftercare for healing pathologic fracture**
Excludes *aftercare following joint replacement (V54.81)* (underlined)

~~text~~ In all sections of the ICD-9-CM, strikethrough text highlights newly deleted text. e.g.,

5th 789.0 **Abdominal pain**
[0-7,9] ~~Colic:~~
~~NOS~~
~~infantile~~
Cramps, abdominal
~~Excludes *renal colic (788.0)*~~

Additional Digit Specificity Needed:

In both the Alphabetic Index and Tabular List, the following symbols alert the user to the need for a more specific code:

4th Denotes the need for 4th digit specificity. e.g.,

4th 427 **Cardiac dysrhythmias**

5th Denotes the need for 5th digit specificity. e.g.,

5th 012.0 **Tuberculous pleurisy**

[#-#] In the Tabular List, some categories and subcategories have common 4th or 5th digits for all subsets. To save space, these common description suffixes are often printed once (in red text) at the beginning of that section, rather than repeated a number of times. The red bracketed digit, range or comma-separated list provides the only applicable 4th or 5th digits for that category or subcategory. e.g.,

5th 250.0 **Diabetes mellitus without mention of complication**
[0-3]

© 2009 MAG Mutual Healthcare Solutions, Inc.

Diagnosis Code-Specific Color Highlights:

Code Manifestation codes are backed by blue highlights and describe the manifestation of an underlying disease, not the disease. Do not use them as principal diagnoses. e.g.,

376.13 *Parasitic infestation of orbit*

Code "Other specified" (NEC) codes are backed by green highlighting and are catch-all codes where there is no more specific code. e.g.,

733.19 Pathologic fracture of other specified site

Code "Unspecified" (NOS) codes are backed by gold highlighting and should only be used when it is not possible to assign a more specific code as they can result in denied claims or requests for additional documentation. e.g.,

590.9 Infection of kidney, unspecified

Medicare Age Conflict Edits:

The Medicare Outpatient Code Editor detects inconsistencies between a patient's age and any diagnosis on the patient's record. For example, a five-year-old patient with benign prostatic hypertrophy. MMHSI flags codes to which these edits apply using orange symbols:

N Newborn - Age of 0 years; a subset of diagnoses intended only for newborns and neonates. e.g.,

762.0 Placenta previa N

P Pediatric - Age range is 0–17 years inclusive. e.g.,

331.81 Reye's syndrome P

M Maternity - Age range is 12–55 years inclusive. e.g.,

5th 644.2 Early onset of delivery M

A Adult - Age range is 15–124 years inclusive. e.g.,

290.0 Senile dementia, uncomplicated A

Medicare Sex Conflict Edits:

Medicare Outpatient Code Editor detects inconsistencies between a patient's sex and any diagnosis or procedure on the patient's record (e.g., a male patient with cervical cancer). MMHSI flags codes to which these edits apply using color-coded gender symbols:

♀ Female only diagnosis e.g.,

622.11 Mild dysplasia of cervix ♀

♂ Male only diagnosis e.g.,

608.0 Seminal vesiculitis ♂

Medicare PQRI Coding Indicators:

ICD-9-CM codes implicated by at least one Medicare PQRI measure are flagged with purple references. See the PQRI Coding Specification Summary section at the end of this Introduction for more instruction on the appropriate use of these indicators.

1 . . . 186 PQRI Measure(s) referenced. e.g.,

365.11 Primary open angle glaucoma 12, 141

Principal vs. Secondary Only Diagnosis Edits:

Certain V codes may only be used as first listed (principal), others only as secondary codes. All V codes without a maroon flag can be used as either a first listed or secondary code, depending on the circumstances of the encounter.

1 Principal (1st listed) Diagnosis only. e.g.,

V22.0 Supervision of normal first pregnancy ♀ 1

2 Secondary Diagnosis only. e.g.,

V46.11 Dependence on respirator, status 2

ICD-9-CM Official Guidelines References:

The section starting on page 15 of this Introduction presents the "ICD-9-CM Official Guidelines for Coding and Reporting" as developed and maintained by CMS and the NCHS. The chapter-specific guidelines are reprinted in blue italicized text throughout the Tabular List next to the applicable code(s) for easy referencing. e.g.,

362.11 Hypertensive retinopathy

ICD-9-CM Official Guidelines (Chapter 7a):

6) ***Hypertensive Retinopathy***

Two codes are necessary to identify the condition. First assign the code from subcategory 362.11, Hypertensive retinopathy, then the appropriate code from categories 401-405 to indicate the type of hypertension.

ICD-10-CM Crosswalks:

To begin to familiarize coders with the ICD-10-CM code set and its relationship to ICD-9-CM, the top 500 utilized ICD-9 codes have their ICD-10-CM equivalents crosswalked beneath them in white text on a salmon-colored background. e.g.,

466.0 Acute bronchitis

J20.9 Acute bronchitis, unspecified

Lay Descriptions:

Another new feature for 2010 is the inclusion of lay descriptions for many confusing codes. e.g.,

272.0 Pure hypercholesterolemia

Layman's: *Raised total cholesterol, exhibiting significantly high LDL, but HDL and triglycerides at normal levels.*

© 2009 MAG Mutual Healthcare Solutions, Inc.

2010 Tabular List Updates

- 008.63 Inclusion term added
- ▲ **008.65 Calicivirus**
- 035 Excludes note term revised
- 037 Excludes note term revised
- ▲ **041.3 Klebsiella pneumoniae ~~Friedländer's bacillus~~**
  Inclusion term deleted
- ▲ **041.86 Heliobacter pylori [H. pylori]**
- 046.1 Use additional code note terms added
- 078.89 Inclusion term deleted
- 190 Excludes note terms added
- 196 Excludes note term added
- 197 Excludes note terms added
- 198 Excludes note term added
- 199 Excludes note terms added, revised
- 199.2 Use additional code note term revised
- 202.0 Inclusion note term revised
- 202.1 Excludes note added
- 209.30 Excludes note added
- ● **209.31 Merkel cell carcinoma of the face**
- ● **209.32 Merkel cell carcinoma of the scalp and neck**
- ● **209.33 Merkel cell carcinoma of the upper limb**
- ● **209.34 Merkel cell carcinoma of the lower limb**
- ● **209.35 Merkel cell carcinoma of the trunk**
- ● **209.36 Merkel cell carcinoma of other sites**
- ● **209.7 Secondary neuroendocrine tumors**
- ● **209.70 Secondary neuroendocrine tumor, unspecified site**
- ● **209.71 Secondary neuroendocrine tumor of distant lymph nodes**
- ● **209.72 Secondary neuroendocrine tumor of liver**
- ● **209.73 Secondary neuroendocrine tumor of bone**
- ● **209.74 Secondary neuroendocrine tumor of peritoneum**
- ● **209.75 Secondary Merkel cell carcinoma**
- ● **209.79 Secondary neuroendocrine tumor of other sites**
- 238.72 Inclusion term added
- 238.83 Inclusion term deleted
- ● **239.81 Neoplasm of unspecified nature of retina and choroid**
- ● **239.89 Neoplasm of unspecified nature of other specified sites**
- 251.3 Use additional code note terms added
  Excludes note terms added
- 269.8 Excludes note term revised
- 270 Excludes note term revised
- 272.2 Inclusion terms added
- 272.4 Inclusion term deleted
- ● **274.00 Gouty arthropathy, unspecified**
- ● **274.01 Acute gouty arthropathy**
- ● **274.02 Chronic gouty arthropathy without mention of tophus (tophi)**
- ● **274.03 Chronic gouty arthropathy with tophus (tophi)**
- 274.82 Excludes note added
- 277.2 Excludes note term revised
- ● **277.88 Tumor lysis syndrome**
- 279.4 Inclusion term deleted
- ● **279.41 Autoimmune lymphoproliferative syndrome**
- ● **279.49 Autoimmune disease, not elsewhere classified**
- 279.5 Code first note terms revised
- 285.2 Inclusion term revised
- 285.22 Excludes note added
- ● **285.3 Antineoplastic chemotherapy induced anemia**
- 290.0 Excludes note term revised
- 294.1 Code first note term revised
- 294.8 Excludes note term revised
- 307.0 Excludes note terms added, revised
- 310.1 Excludes note terms added, deleted
- 310.8 Excludes note added
- 331.7 Excludes note term revised
- 331.83 Excludes note term added
- 333.2 Inclusion terms added, deleted
  Excludes note added
- 345.01 Inclusion terms added
  Excludes note added
- 345.1 Inclusion terms added
- 345.11 Inclusion terms added
  Excludes note added
- 345.41 Inclusion terms added
  Excludes note added
- 345.51 Inclusion terms added
  Excludes note added
- 345.61 Inclusion terms added
  Excludes note added
- 345.71 Inclusion terms added
  Excludes note added
- 345.81 Inclusion terms added
  Excludes note added
- 345.91 Inclusion terms added
  Excludes note added
- 348.8 Inclusion terms deleted
- ● **348.81 Temporal sclerosis**
- ● **348.89 Other conditions of brain**
- 359.22 Inclusion term added
- 359.29 Inclusion term deleted
- ● **359.7 Inflammatory and immune myopathies, NEC**
- ● **359.71 Inclusion body myositis**
- ● **359.79 Other inflammatory and immune myopathies, NEC**
- ● **372.06 Acute chemical conjunctivitis**
- 372.34 Excludes note added
- 372.51 Excludes note added
- 403 Excludes note term revised
- 413.9 Inclusion term added
  Use additional code note added
- 415.1 Excludes note terms added
- ● **416.2 Chronic pulmonary embolism**
- ● **438.13 Dysarthria**
- ● **438.14 Fluency disorder**
- 445.81 Use additional code note revised
- 453 Excludes note term deleted
- ▲ **453.2 Other venous embolism and thrombosis of inferior vena cava**
- ▲ **453.4 Acute venous embolism and thrombosis or deep vessels of lower extremity**
- ▲ **453.40 Acute venous embolism and thrombosis of unspecified deep vessels of lower extremity**
- ▲ **453.41 Acute venous embolism and thrombosis of deep vessels of proximal lower extremity**

▲ 453.42 **Acute venous embolism and thrombosis of deep vessels of distal lower extremity**

● 453.5 **Chronic venous embolism and thrombosis of deep vessels of lower extremity**

● 453.50 **Chronic venous embolism and thrombosis of unspecified deep vessels of lower extremity**

● 453.51 **Chronic venous embolism and thrombosis of deep vessels of proximal lower extremity**

● 453.52 **Chronic venous embolism and thrombosis of deep vessels of distal lower extremity**

● 453.6 **Venous embolism and thrombosis of superficial vessels of lower extremity**

● 453.7 **Chronic venous embolism and thrombosis of other specified vessels**

● 453.71 **Chronic venous embolism and thrombosis of superficial veins of upper extremity**

● 453.72 **Chronic venous embolism and thrombosis of deep veins of upper extremity**

● 453.73 **Chronic venous embolism and thrombosis of upper extremity, unspecified**

● 453.74 **Chronic venous embolism and thrombosis of axillary veins**

● 453.75 **Chronic venous embolism and thrombosis of subclavian veins**

● 453.76 **Chronic venous embolism and thrombosis of internal jugular veins**

● 453.77 **Chronic venous embolism and thrombosis of other thoracic veins**

● 453.79 **Chronic venous embolism and thrombosis of other specified veins**

▲ 453.8 **Acute venous embolism and thrombosis of other specified veins**

● 453.81 **Acute venous embolism and thrombosis of superficial veins of upper extremity**

● 453.82 **Acute venous embolism and thrombosis of deep veins of upper extremity**

● 453.83 **Acute venous embolism and thrombosis of upper extremity, unspecified**

● 453.84 **Acute venous embolism and thrombosis of axillary veins**

● 453.85 **Acute venous embolism and thrombosis of subclavian veins**

● 453.86 **Acute venous embolism and thrombosis of internal jugular veins**

● 453.87 **Acute venous embolism and thrombosis of other thoracic veins**

● 453.89 **Acute venous embolism and thrombosis of other specified veins**

487 Inclusion term added
Excludes note terms added, revised

▲ 488 **Influenza due to certain identified ~~avian~~ influenza viruses**
Note deleted
Excludes note term revised

● 488.0 **Influenza due to identified avian influenza virus**

● 488.1 **Influenza due to identified novel H1N1 influenza virus**

536.2 Excludes note terms added

567 Excludes note term revised

● 569.7 **Complications of intestinal pouch**

● 569.71 **Pouchitis**

● 569.79 **Other complications of intestinal pouch**

● 569.87 **Vomiting of fecal matter**

▲ 572.2 **Hepatic encephalopathy ~~coma~~**
Inclusion terms added, deleted

▲ 584 **Acute kidney ~~renal~~ failure**
Includes note added

▲ 584.5 **Acute kidney ~~renal~~ failure with lesion of tubular necrosis**

▲ 584.6 **Acute kidney ~~renal~~ failure with lesion of renal cortical necrosis**

▲ 584.7 **Acute kidney ~~renal~~ failure with lesion of renal medullary [papillary] necrosis**

▲ 584.8 **Acute kidney ~~renal~~ failure with other specified pathological lesion in kidney**

▲ 584.9 **Acute kidney ~~renal~~ failure, with unspecified type of lesion**

587 Includes note added
Inclusion term deleted

611.82 Excludes note term added

614 Excludes note term revised

615 Excludes note terms revised

621.3 Inclusion terms deleted

621.30 Inclusion terms added

621.31 Excludes note added

621.32 Excludes note added

621.33 Excludes note added

● 621.34 **Benign endometrial hyperplasia**

● 621.35 **Endometrial intraepithelial neoplasia [EIN]**

624 Excludes note term revised

▲ 639.3 **Kidney ~~renal~~ failure following abortion and ectopic and molar pregnancies**
Inclusion term revised

646.6 Excludes note term revised

649.3 Includes note term revised
Use additional code note revised

▲ 669.3 **Acute kidney ~~renal~~ failure following labor and delivery**

670 Inclusion terms deleted

▲ 670.0 **Major puerperal infection, unspecified**

▲ 670.00 **Major puerperal infection, unspecified, unspecified as to episode of care or not applicable**

▲ 670.02 **Major puerperal infection, unspecified, delivered, with mention of postpartum complcation**

▲ 670.04 **Major puerperal infection, unspecified, postpartum condition or complication**

● 670.1 **Puerperal endometritis**

 © 2009 MAG Mutual Healthcare Solutions, Inc.

● **670.10 Puerperal endometritis, unspecified as to episode of care or not applicable**
● **670.12 Puerperal endometritis, delivered, with mention of postpartum complcation**
● **670.14 Puerperal endometritis, postpartum condition or complication**
● **670.2 Puerperal sepsis**
● **670.20 Puerperal sepsis, unspecified as to episode of care or not applicable**
● **670.22 Puerperal sepsis, delivered, with mention of postpartum complcation**
● **670.24 Puerperal sepsis, postpartum condition or complication**
● **670.3 Puerperal septic thrombophlebitis**
● **670.30 Puerperal septic thrombophlebitis, unspecified as to episode of care or not applicable**
● **670.32 Puerperal septic thrombophlebitis, delivered, with mention of postpartum complcation**
● **670.34 Puerperal septic thrombophlebitis, postpartum condition or complication**
● **670.8 Other major puerperal infection**
● **670.80 Other major puerperal infection, unspecified as to episode of care or not applicable**
● **670.82 Other major puerperal infection, delivered, with mention of postpartum complcation**
● **670.84 Other major puerperal infection, postpartum condition or complication**
671 Excludes note terms added
671.2 Inclusion terms added
671.3 Use additional code notes added
671.4 Use additional code notes added
671.9 Inclusion terms deleted
707.03 Inclusion term added
712 Excludes note term revised
713.0 Excludes note term revised
727.01 Excludes note term revised
733.1 Inclusion term added
● **756.72 Omphalocele**
● **756.73 Gastroschisis**
● **756.79 Other congenital anomalies of abdominal wall**
▲ 757.6 **Specified congenital anomalies of breast**
Inclusion term revised
762.3 Use additional code note revised
768.5 Excludes note term revised
768.6 Excludes note term revised
● **768.70 Hypoxic-ischemic encephalopathy, unspecified**
● **768.71 Mild hypoxic-ischemic encephalopathy**
● **768.72 Moderate hypoxic-ischemic encephalopathy**
● **768.73 Severe hypoxic-ischemic encephalopathy**
772 Excludes note term added
▲ 772.0 **Fetal blood loss affecting newborn**
776 Includes note term revised
▲ 776.9 **Unspecified hematological disorder specific to ~~fetus or~~ newborn**
777.5 Inclusion term deleted
777.51 Inclusion term added
▲ 779.3 **Disorder of stomach function and feeding problems in newborn**
Inclusion terms deleted
● **779.31 Feeding problems in newborn**
● **779.32 Bilious vomiting in newborn**
● **779.33 Other vomiting in newborn**
● **779.34 Failure to thrive in newborn**
780.0 Excludes note terms added
780.93 Excludes note terms added, revised
783.3 Excludes note term revised
783.41 Excludes note added
▲ 784.4 **Voice ~~disturbance~~ and resonance disorders**
▲ 784.40 **Voice ~~disturbance~~ and resonance disorder, unspecified**
● **784.42 Dysphonia**
● **784.43 Hypernasality**
● **784.44 Hyponasality**
▲ 784.49 **Other voice and resonance disorders**
Inclusion terms deleted
784.5 Inclusion terms deleted
Excludes note term added
● **784.51 Dysarthria**
● **784.59 Other speech disturbance**
787.0 Excludes note terms added, revised
● **787.04 Bilious emesis**
789.0 Inclusion terms deleted
Excludes note deleted
● **789.7 Colic**
790.01 Inclusion term added
▲ 793 **Nonspecific (abnormal) findings on radiological and other examination of body structure**
▲ 793.0 **Nonspecific (abnormal) findings on radiological and other examination of skull and head**
▲ 793.1 **Nonspecific (abnormal) findings on radiological and other examination of lung field**
▲ 793.2 **Nonspecific (abnormal) findings on radiological and other examination of other intrathoracic organ**
▲ 793.3 **Nonspecific (abnormal) findings on radiological and other examination of biliary tract**
▲ 793.4 **Nonspecific (abnormal) findings on radiological and other examination of gastrointestinal tract**
▲ 793.5 **Nonspecific (abnormal) findings on radiological and other examination of genitourinary organs**
▲ 793.6 **Nonspecific (abnormal) findings on radiological and other examination of abdominal area, including retroperitoneum**
▲ 793.7 **Nonspecific (abnormal) findings on radiological and other examination of musculoskeletal system**
▲ 793.8 **Nonspecific (abnormal) findings on radiological and other examination of breast**

- ● **793.82 Inconclusive mammogram**
- ▲ **793.89 Other (abnormal) findings on radiological examination of breast**
- ▲ **793.99 Other nonspecific (abnormal) findings on radiological examination of breast**
- 795.0 Excludes note term revised
- 795.39 Excludes note added
- 796.7 Excludes note term revised
- ▲ **799.2 Signs and symptoms involving emotional state ~~nervousness~~**
  Inclusion term deleted
  Excludes note added
- ● **799.21 Nervousness**
- ● **799.22 Irritability**
- ● **799.23 Impulsiveness**
- ● **799.24 Emotional lability**
- ● **799.25 Demoralization and apathy**
- ● **799.29 Other signs and symptoms involving emotional state**
- ● **799.82 Apparent life threatening event in infant**
- ▲ **813.45 Torus fracture of radius (alone)**
  Excludes note added
- ● **813.46 Torus fracture of ulna (alone)**
- ● **813.47 Torus fracture of radius and ulna**
- ● **832.2 Nursemaid's elbow**
- 854 Includes note terms added, revised
- 969.0 Inclusion terms deleted
- ● **969.00 Antidepressant, unspecified**
- ● **969.01 Monoamine oxidase inhibitors**
- ● **969.02 Selective serotonin and norepinephrine reuptake**
- ● **969.03 Selective serotonin reuptake inhibitors**
- ● **969.04 Tetracyclic antidepressants**
- ● **969.05 Tricyclic antidepressants**
- ● **969.09 Other antidepressants**
- 969.7 Inclusion terms deleted
- ● **969.70 Psychostimulant, unspecified**
- ● **969.71 Caffeine**
- ● **969.72 Amphetamines**
- ● **969.73 Methylphenidate**
- ● **969.79 Other psychostimulants**
- 974.1 Excludes note term revised
- ● **995.24 Failed moderate sedation during procedure**
- 995.92 Use additional code note revised
- 995.94 Use additional code note revised
- ▲ **996.43 Broken prosthetic joint implant ~~failure~~**
- 996.47 Inclusion term added
- 997.31 Inclusion term added
- 997.4 Excludes note terms added
- 997.5 Inclusion term revised
- 999.6 Excludes note added
- V07.52 Inclusion term revised
- V10 Code first note deleted
- V10.0 Excludes note added
- V10.1 Excludes note added
- V10.8 Excludes note added
- ▲ **V10.9 Other and unspecified personal history of malignant neoplasm**
- ● **V10.90 Personal history of unspecified malignant neoplasm**
- ● **V10.91 Personal history of malignant neuroendocrine tumor**
- V12.54 Excludes note term added
- ▲ **V15.06 Personal history of allergy to insects and arachnids**
- ● **V15.52 History of traumatic brain injury**
- ● **V15.80 History of failed moderate sedation**
- ● **V15.83 Underimmunization status**
- ▲ **V15.84 Contact with and (suspected) exposure to asbestos**
- ▲ **V15.85 Contact with and (suspected) exposure to potentially hazardous body fluids**
- ● **V15.86 Contact with and (suspected) exposure to lead**
- V20.2 Inclusion terms added, deleted
  Excludes note terms added
- ● **V20.3 Newborn health supervision**
- ● **V20.31 Health supervision for newborn under 8 days old**
- ● **V20.32 Health supervision for newborn 8 to 28 days old**
- V23.86 Excludes note term revised
- ● **V26.42 Encounter for fertility preservation counseling**
- ● **V26.82 Encounter for fertility preservation procedure**
- V45.71 Excludes note added
- ▲ **V53.5 Other gastrointestinal appliance and device**
- ● **V53.50 Fitting and adjustment of intestinal appliance and device**
- ● **V53.51 Fitting and adjustment of gastric lap band**
- ● **V53.59 Fitting and adjustment of other gastrointestinal appliance and device**
- V54.1 Excludes note term added
- V54.2 Excludes note added
- ▲ **V57.3 Encounted for care involving speech-language therapy**
- ● **V60.81 Foster care (status)**
- ● **V60.89 Other specified housing or economic circumstances**
- V61.01 Excludes note added
- ● **V61.07 Family disruption due to death of family member**
- ● **V61.08 Family disruption due to other extended absence of family member**
- ● **V61.23 Counseling for parent-biological child problem**
- ● **V61.24 Counseling for parent-adopted child problem**
- ● **V61.25 Counseling for parent (guardian)-foster child problem**
- ▲ **V61.29 Other parent-child problems**
  Inclusion term deleted
- ● **V61.42 Substance abuse in family**
- V62.82 Excludes note term added
- ▲ **V65.11 Encounter for pediatric pre-birth visit for expectant ~~mother~~ parent(s)**
  Inclusion term added
- V70.0 Excludes note terms added, revised
- V72 Excludes note terms added, revised
- V72.5 Excludes note terms added, deleted
- V72.6 Excludes note term deleted
- ● **V72.60 Laboratory examination, unspecified**

© 2009 MAG Mutual Healthcare Solutions, Inc.

- ● V72.61 Antibody response examination
- ● V72.62 Laboratory examination ordered as part of a routine general medical examination
- ● V72.63 Pre-procedural laboratory examination
- ● V72.69 Other laboratory examination
- V72.8 Excludes note added
- V72.83 Inclusion term added
- ● V80.01 Traumatic brain injury
- ● V80.09 Other neurological conditions
- ● V87.32 Contact with and (suspected) exposure to algae bloom
- ● V87.43 Personal history of estrogen therapy
- ● V87.44 Personal history of inhaled steroid therapy
- ● V87.45 Personal history of systemic steroid therapy
- ● V87.46 Personal history of immunosuppression therapy
- ● E000 External cause status
- ● E000.0 Civilian activity done for income or pay
- ● E000.1 Military activity
- ● E000.8 Other external cause status
- ● E000.9 Unspecified external cause status
- ● E001 Activities involving walking and running
- ● E001.0 Walking, marching and hiking
- ● E001.1 Running
- ● E002 Activities involving water and water craft
- ● E002.0 Swimming
- ● E002.1 Springboard and platform diving
- ● E002.2 Water polo
- ● E002.3 Water aerobics and water exercise
- ● E002.4 Underwater diving and snorkeling
- ● E002.5 Rowing, canoeing, kayaking, rafting and tubing
- ● E002.6 Water skiing and wake boarding
- ● E002.7 Surfing, windsurfing and boogie boarding
- ● E002.8 Water sliding
- ● E002.9 Other activity involving water and watercraft
- ● E003 Activities involving ice and snow
- ● E003.0 Ice skating
- ● E003.1 Ice hockey
- ● E003.2 Snow (alpine) (downhill) skiing, snow boarding, sledding, tobogganing and snow tubing
- ● E003.3 Cross country skiing
- ● E003.9 Other activity involving ice and snow
- ● E004 Activities involving climbing, rappelling and jumping off
- ● E004.0 Mountain climbing, rock climbing and wall climbing
- ● E004.1 Rappelling
- ● E004.2 BASE jumping
- ● E004.3 Bungee jumping
- ● E004.4 Hang gliding
- ● E004.9 Other activity involving climbing, rappelling and jumping off
- ● E005 Activities involving dancing and other rhythmic movement
- ● E005.0 Dancing
- ● E005.1 Yoga
- ● E005.2 Gymnastics
- ● E005.3 Trampoline
- ● E005.4 Cheerleading
- ● E005.9 Other activity involving dancing and other rhythmic movements
- ● E006 Activities involving other sports and athletics played individually
- ● E006.0 Roller skating (inline) and skateboarding
- ● E006.1 Horseback riding
- ● E006.2 Golf
- ● E006.3 Bowling
- ● E006.4 Bike riding
- ● E006.5 Jumping rope
- ● E006.6 Non-running track and field events
- ● E006.9 Other activity involving other sports and athletics played individually
- ● E007 Activities involving other sports and athletics played as a team or group
- ● E007.0 American tackle football
- ● E007.1 American flag or touch football
- ● E007.2 Rugby
- ● E007.3 Baseball
- ● E007.4 Lacrosse and field hockey
- ● E007.5 Soccer
- ● E007.6 Basketball
- ● E007.7 Volleyball (beach) (court)
- ● E007.8 Physical games generally associated with school recess, summer camp and children
- ● E007.9 Other activity involving other sports and athletics played as a team or group
- ● E008 Activities involving other specified sports and athletics
- ● E008.0 Boxing
- ● E008.1 Wrestling
- ● E008.2 Racquet and hand sports
- ● E008.3 Frisbee
- ● E008.4 Martial arts
- ● E008.9 Other specified sports and athletics activity
- ● E009 Activity involving other cardiorespiratory exercise
- ● E009.0 Exercise machines primarily for cardiorespiratory
- ● E009.1 Calisthenics
- ● E009.2 Aerobic and step exercise
- ● E009.3 Circuit training
- ● E009.4 Obstacle course
- ● E009.5 Grass drills
- ● E009.9 Other activity involving other cardiorespiratory exercise
- ● E010 Activity involving other muscle strengthening exercises
- ● E010.0 Exercise machines primarily for muscle strengthening
- ● E010.1 Push-ups, pull-ups, sit-ups
- ● E010.2 Free weights
- ● E010.3 Pilates
- ● E010.9 Other activity involving other muscle strengthening exercises

- ● E011 Activities involving computer technology and electronic devices
- ● E011.0 Computer keyboarding
- ● E011.1 Hand held interactive electronic device
- ● E011.9 Other activity involving computer technology and electronic devices
- ● E012 Activities involving arts and handcrafts
- ● E012.0 Knitting and crocheting
- ● E012.1 Sewing
- ● E012.2 Furniture building and finishing
- ● E012.9 Activity involving other arts and handcrafts
- ● E013 Activities involving personal hygiene and household maintenance
- ● E013.0 Personal bathing and showering
- ● E013.1 Laundry
- ● E013.2 Vacuuming
- ● E013.3 Ironing
- ● E013.4 Floor mopping and cleaning
- ● E013.5 Residential relocation
- ● E013.8 Other personal hygiene activity
- ● E013.9 Other household maintenance
- ● E014 Activities involving person providing caregiving
- ● E014.0 Caregiving involving bathing
- ● E014.1 Caregiving involving lifting
- ● E014.9 Other activity involving person providing caregiving
- ● E015 Activities involving food preparation, cooking and grilling
- ● E015.0 Food preparation and clean up
- ● E015.1 Grilling and smoking food
- ● E015.2 Cooking and baking
- ● E015.9 Other activity involving cooking and grilling
- ● E016 Activities involving property and land maintenance, building and construction
- ● E016.0 Digging, shoveling and raking
- ● E016.1 Gardening and landscaping
- ● E016.2 Building and construction
- ● E016.9 Other activity involving property and land maintenance, building and construction
- ● E017 Activities involving roller coasters and other types of external motion
- ● E017.0 Rollercoaster riding
- ● E017.9 Other activity involving external motion
- ● E018 Activities involving playing musical instrument
- ● E018.0 Piano playing
- ● E018.1 Drum and other percussion instrument playing
- ● E018.2 String instrument playing
- ● E018.3 Wind and brass instrument playing
- ● E019 Activities involving animal care
- ● E019.0 Walking an animal
- ● E019.1 Milking an animal
- ● E019.2 Grooming and shearing an animal
- ● E019.9 Other activity involving animal care
- ● E029 Other activity
- ● E029.0 Refereeing a sports activity
- ● E029.1 Spectator at an event
- ● E029.2 Rough housing and horseplay
- ● E029.9 Other activity
- ● E030 Unspecified activity
- ● E830.7 Accident to watercraft causing submersion injuring occupant of military watercraft, any type
- ● E831.7 Accident to watercraft causing other injury to to occupant of military watercraft, any type
- ● E832.7 Other accidental submersion or drowning in water transport accident injuring occupant of military watercraft, any type
- ● E833.7 Fall on stairs or ladders in water transport injuring occupant of military watercraft, any type
- ● E834.7 Other fall from one level to another in water transport injuring occupant of military watercraft, any type
- ● E835.7 Other and unspecified fall in water transport injuring occupant of military watercraft, any type
- ● E836.7 Machinery accident in water transport injuring occupant of military watercraft, any type
- ● E837.7 Explosion fire or burning in watercraft injuring occupant of military watercraft, any type
- ● E838.7 Other and unspecified water transport accident injuring occupant of military watercraft, any type
- ▲ E876.5 Performance of inappropriate ~~wrong~~ operation (procedure) on correct patient
  - Inclusion term added
  - Excludes note added
- ● E876.6 Performance of operation (procedure) on patient not scheduled for surgery
- ● E876.7 Performance of correct operation (procedure) on wrong side/body part
- E918 Excludes note term added
- E919 Excludes note term added
- E920 Excludes note term added
- E922 Excludes note term added
- E923 Excludes note term added
- E927 Use additional code note added
- ● E928.7 Accident caused by mechanism or component of firearm and air gun
- E990.0 Inclusion term added
- ● E990.1 Injury due to war operations from flamethrower
- ● E990.2 Injury due to war operations from incendiary bullet
- ● E990.3 Injury due to war operations from fire caused indirectly from conventional weapon
- E991 Excludes note added

 © 2009 MAG Mutual Healthcare Solutions, Inc.

- ● E991.4 Injury due to war operations by fragments from munitions
- ● E991.5 Injury due to war operations by fragments from person-borne improvised explosive device [IED]
- ● E991.6 Injury due to war operations by fragments from vehicle-borne improvised explosive device [IED]
- ● E991.7 Injury due to war operations by fragments from other improvised explosive device [IED]
- ● E991.8 Injury due to war operations by fragments from weapons
- E991.9 Inclusion terms deleted, revised
- E992 Inclusion terms deleted
- ● E992.0 Injury due to war operations by explosion of torpedo
- ● E992.1 Injury due to war operations by explosion of depth charge
- ● E992.2 Injury due to war operations by explosion of marine mines
- ● E992.3 Injury due to war operations by explosion of sea-based artillery shell
- ● E992.8 Injury due to war operations by other explosion by other marine weapons
- ● E992.9 Injury due to war operations by explosion of unspecified marine weapon
- E993 Inclusion terms added, deleted
  Excludes note added
- ● E993.0 Injury due to war operations by aerial bomb
- ● E993.1 Injury due to war operations by guided missile
- ● E993.2 Injury due to war operations by mortar
- ● E993.3 Injury due to war operations by person-borne improvised explosive device [IED]
- ● E993.4 Injury due to war operations by vehicle-borne improvised explosive device [IED]
- ● E993.5 Injury due to war operations by other improvised explosive device [IED]
- ● E993.6 Injury due to war operations by unintentional detonation of own munitions
- ● E993.7 Injury due to war operations by unintentional discharge of own munitions launch
- ● E993.8 Injury due to war operations by other specified explosion
- ● E993.9 Injury due to war operations by unspecified explosion
- E994 Inclusion terms deleted
- ● E994.0 Injury due to war operations by destruction of aircraft due to enemy fire or explosives
- ● E994.1 Injury due to war operations by unintentional destruction of aircraft due to own onboard explosives
- ● E994.2 Injury due to war operations by destruction of aircraft due to collision with other aircraft
- ● E994.3 Injury due to war operations by destruction of aircraft due to onboard fire
- ● E994.8 Injury due to war operations by other destruction of aircraft
- ● E994.9 Injury due to war operations by unspecified destruction of aircraft
- E995 Inclusion terms deleted
- ● E995.0 Injury due to war operations by unarmed hand-to-hand combat
- ● E995.1 Injury due to war operations, struck by blunt object
- ● E995.2 Injury due to war operations by piercing object
- ● E995.3 Injury due to war operations by intentional restriction of air and airway
- ● E995.4 Injury due to war operations by unintentional drowning due to inability to surface or obtain air
- ● E995.8 Injury due to war operations by other forms of conventional warfare
- ● E995.9 Injury due to war operations by unspecified form of conventional warfare
- E996 Inclusion terms deleted
  Excludes note added
- ● E996.0 Injury due to war operations by direct blast effect of nuclear weapon
- ● E996.1 Injury due to war operations by indirect blast effect of nuclear weapon
- ● E996.2 Injury due to war operations by thermal radiation effect of nuclear weapon
- ● E996.3 Injury due to war operations by nuclear radiation effects
- ● E996.8 Injury due to war operations by other effects of nuclear weapons
- ● E996.9 Injury due to war operations by unspecified effect of nuclear weapon
- ● E997.3 Injury due to war operations by weapon of mass destruction [WMD], unspecified
- ● E998.0 Injury due to war operations by explosion of mines
- ● E998.1 Injury due to war operations by explosion of bombs
- ● E998.8 Injury due to other war operations but occurring after cessation of hostilities
- ● E998.9 Injury due to unspecified war operations but occurring after cessation of hostilities

ICD-9-CM Official Guidelines for Coding and Reporting

Effective October 1, 2009. Underlined text has been added or moved since the October 2008 update.

The Centers for Medicare and Medicaid Services (CMS) and the National Center for Health Statistics (NCHS), two departments within the U.S. Federal Government's Department of Health and Human Services (DHHS) provide the following guidelines for coding and reporting using the International Classification of Diseases, 9th Revision, Clinical Modification (ICD-9-CM). These guidelines have been approved by the four organizations that make up the Cooperating Parties for the ICD-9-CM: the American Hospital Association (AHA), the American Health Information Management Association (AHIMA), CMS, and NCHS. The instructions and conventions of the classification take precedence over guidelines. These guidelines are included on the official government version of the ICD-9-CM, and also appear in "Coding Clinic for ICD-9-CM" published by the AHA.

These guidelines are a set of rules that have been developed to accompany and complement the official conventions and instructions provided within the ICD-9-CM itself. These guidelines are based on the coding and sequencing instructions in Volumes I, II and III of ICD-9-CM, but provide additional instruction. Adherence to these guidelines when assigning ICD-9-CM diagnosis and procedure codes is required under the Health Insurance Portability and Accountability Act (HIPAA). The diagnosis codes (Volumes 1-2) have been adopted under HIPAA for all healthcare settings. Volume 3 procedure codes have been adopted for inpatient procedures reported by hospitals. A joint effort between the healthcare provider and the coder is essential to achieve complete and accurate documentation, code assignment, and reporting of diagnoses and procedures. These guidelines have been developed to assist both the healthcare provider and the coder in identifying those diagnoses and procedures that are to be reported. The importance of consistent, complete documentation in the medical record cannot be overemphasized. Without such documentation accurate coding cannot be achieved. The entire record should be reviewed to determine the specific reason for the encounter and the conditions treated.

The term encounter is used for all settings, including hospital admissions. In the context of these guidelines, the term provider is used throughout the guidelines to mean physician or any qualified health care practitioner who is legally accountable for establishing the patient's diagnosis. Only this set of guidelines, approved by the Cooperating Parties, is official.

The guidelines are organized into sections. Section I includes the structure and conventions of the classification and general guidelines that apply to the entire classification, and chapter-specific guidelines that correspond to the chapters as they are arranged in the classification. Section II includes guidelines for selection of principal diagnosis for non-outpatient settings. Section III includes guidelines for reporting additional diagnoses in non-outpatient settings. Section IV is for outpatient coding and reporting.

Section I. Conventions, general coding guidelines and chapter specific guidelines

The conventions, general guidelines and chapter-specific guidelines are applicable to all health care settings unless otherwise indicated. The conventions and instructions of the classification take precedence over guidelines.

A. Conventions for the ICD-9-CM

The conventions for the ICD-9-CM are the general rules for use of the classification independent of the guidelines. These conventions are incorporated within the index and tabular of the ICD-9-CM as instructional notes. The conventions are as follows:

1. Format:

The ICD-9-CM uses an indented format for ease in reference

2. Abbreviations

a. Index abbreviations

NEC "Not elsewhere classifiable" This abbreviation in the index represents "other specified" when a specific code is not available for a condition the index directs the coder to the "other specified" code in the tabular.

b. Tabular abbreviations

NEC "Not elsewhere classifiable" This abbreviation in the tabular represents "other specified". When a specific code is not available for a condition the tabular includes an NEC entry under a code to identify the code as the "other specified" code.

(See Section I.A.5.a. "Other" codes").

NOS "Not otherwise specified" This abbreviation is the equivalent of unspecified.

(See Section I.A.5.b., "Unspecified" codes)

3. Punctuation

[ ] Brackets are used in the tabular list to enclose synonyms, alternative wording or explanatory phrases. Brackets are used in the index to identify manifestation codes.

(See Section I.A.6. "Etiology/manifestations")

( ) Parentheses are used in both the index and tabular to enclose supplementary words that may be present or absent in the statement of a disease or procedure without affecting the code number to which it is assigned. The terms within the parentheses are referred to as nonessential modifiers.

: Colons are used in the Tabular list after an incomplete term which needs one or more of the modifiers following the colon to make it assignable to a given category.

4. Includes and Excludes Notes and Inclusion terms

Includes: This note appears immediately under a three-digit code title to further define, or give examples of, the content of the category.

Excludes: An excludes note under a code indicates that the terms excluded from the code are to be coded elsewhere. In some cases the codes for the excluded terms should not be used in conjunction with the code from which it is excluded. An example of this is a congenital condition excluded from an acquired form of the same condition. The congenital and acquired codes should not be used together. In other cases, the excluded terms may be used together with an excluded code. An example of this is when fractures of different bones are coded to different codes. Both codes may be used together if both types of fractures are present.

Inclusion terms: List of terms is included under certain four and five digit codes. These terms are the conditions for which that code number is to be used. The terms may be synonyms of the code title, or, in the case of "other specified" codes, the terms are a list of the various conditions assigned to that code. The inclusion terms are not necessarily exhaustive. Additional terms found only in the index may also be assigned to a code.

5. Other and Unspecified codes

a. "Other" codes

Codes titled "other" or "other specified" (usually a code with a 4th digit 8 or 5th digit 9 for diagnosis codes) are for use when the information in the medical record provides detail for which a specific code does not exist. Index entries with NEC in the line designate "other" codes in the tabular. These index entries represent specific disease entities for which no specific code exists so the term is included within an "other" code.

b. "Unspecified" codes

Codes (usually a code with a 4th digit 9 or 5th digit 0 for diagnosis codes) titled "unspecified" are for use when the information in the medical record is insufficient to assign a more specific code.

6. Etiology/manifestation convention ("code first", "use additional code" and "in diseases classified elsewhere" notes)

Certain conditions have both an underlying etiology and multiple body system manifestations due to the underlying etiology. For such conditions, the ICD-9-CM has a coding convention that requires the underlying condition be sequenced first followed by the manifestation. Wherever such a combination exists, there is a "use additional code" note at the etiology code, and a "code first" note at the manifestation code. These instructional notes indicate the proper sequencing order of the codes, etiology followed by manifestation.

In most cases the manifestation codes will have in the code title, "in diseases classified elsewhere." Codes with this title are a component of the etiology/manifestation convention. The code title indicates that it is a manifestation code. "In diseases classified elsewhere" codes are never permitted to be used as first listed or principal diagnosis codes. They must be used in conjunction with an underlying condition code and they must be listed following the underlying condition.

There are manifestation codes that do not have "in diseases classified elsewhere" in the title. For such codes a "use additional code" note will still be present and the rules for sequencing apply.

In addition to the notes in the tabular, these conditions also have a specific index entry structure. In the index both conditions are listed together with the etiology code first followed by the manifestation codes in brackets. The code in brackets is always to be sequenced second.

The most commonly used etiology/manifestation combinations are the codes for Diabetes mellitus, category 250. For each code under category 250 there is a use additional code note for the manifestation that is specific for that particular diabetic manifestation. Should a patient have more than one manifestation of diabetes, more than one code from category 250 may be used with as many manifestation codes as are needed to fully describe the patient's complete diabetic condition. The category 250 diabetes codes should be sequenced first, followed by the manifestation codes.

"Code first" and "Use additional code" notes are also used as sequencing rules in the classification for certain codes that are not part of an etiology/ manifestation combination.

See - Section I.B.9. "Multiple coding for a single condition".

7. "And"

The word "and" should be interpreted to mean either "and" or "or" when it appears in a title.

8. "With"

The word "with" in the alphabetic index is sequenced immediately following the main term, not in alphabetical order.

9. "See" and "See Also"

The "see" instruction following a main term in the index indicates that another term should be referenced. It is necessary to go to the main term referenced with the "see" note to locate the correct code.

A "see also" instruction following a main term in the index instructs that there is another main term that may also be referenced that may provide additional index entries that may be useful. It is not necessary to follow the "see also" note when the original main term provides the necessary code.

B. General Coding Guidelines

1. Use of Both Alphabetic Index and Tabular List

Use both the Alphabetic Index and the Tabular List when locating and assigning a code. Reliance on only the Alphabetic Index or the Tabular List leads to errors in code assignments and less specificity in code selection.

2. Locate each term in the Alphabetic Index

Locate each term in the Alphabetic Index and verify the code selected in the Tabular List. Read and be guided by instructional notations that appear in both the Alphabetic Index and the Tabular List.

3. Level of Detail in Coding

Diagnosis and procedure codes are to be used at their highest number of digits available.

ICD-9-CM diagnosis codes are composed of codes with 3, 4, or 5 digits. Codes with three digits are included in ICD-9-CM as the heading of a category of codes that may be further subdivided by the use of fourth and/or fifth digits, which provide greater detail.

A three-digit code is to be used only if it is not further subdivided. Where fourth-digit subcategories and/or fifth-digit subclassifications are provided, they must be assigned. A code is invalid if it has not been coded to the full number of digits required for that code. For example, Acute myocardial infarction, code 410, has fourth digits that describe the location of the infarction (e.g., 410.2, Of inferolateral wall), and fifth digits that identify the episode of care. It would be incorrect to report a code in category 410 without a fourth and fifth digit.

4. Code or codes from 001.0 through V89.09

The appropriate code or codes from 001.0 through V89.09 must be used to identify diagnoses, symptoms, conditions, problems, complaints or other reason(s) for the encounter/visit.

5. Selection of codes 001.0 through 999.9

The selection of codes 001.0 through 999.9 will frequently be used to describe the reason for the admission/encounter. These codes are from the section of ICD-9-CM for the classification of diseases and injuries (e.g., infectious and parasitic diseases; neoplasms; symptoms, signs, and ill-defined conditions, etc.).

6. Signs and symptoms

Codes that describe symptoms and signs, as opposed to diagnoses, are acceptable for reporting purposes when a related definitive diagnosis has not been established (confirmed) by the provider. Chapter 16 of ICD-9-CM, Symptoms, Signs, and Ill-defined conditions (codes 780.0 - 799.9) contain many, but not all codes for symptoms.

7. Conditions that are an integral part of a disease process

Signs and symptoms that are associated routinely with a disease process should not be assigned as additional codes, unless otherwise instructed by the classification.

8. Conditions that are not an integral part of a disease process

Additional signs and symptoms that may not be associated routinely with a disease process should be coded when present.

9. Multiple coding for a single condition

In addition to the etiology/manifestation convention that requires two codes to fully describe a single condition that affects multiple body systems, there are other single conditions that also require more than one code. "Use additional code" notes are found in the tabular at codes that are not part of an etiology/ manifestation pair where a secondary code is useful to fully describe a condition. The sequencing rule is the same as the etiology/manifestation pair - , "use additional code" indicates that a secondary code should be added.

For example, for infections that are not included in chapter 1, a secondary code from category 041, Bacterial infection in conditions classified elsewhere and of unspecified site, may be required to identify the bacterial organism causing the infection. A "use additional code" note will normally be found at the infectious disease code, indicating a need for the organism code to be added as a secondary code.

"Code first" notes are also under certain codes that are not specifically manifestation codes but may be due to an underlying cause. When a "code first" note is present and an underlying condition is present the underlying condition should be sequenced first.

"Code, if applicable, any causal condition first", notes indicate that this code may be assigned as a principal diagnosis when the causal condition is unknown or not applicable. If a causal condition is known, then the code for that condition should be sequenced as the principal or first-listed diagnosis.

Multiple codes may be needed for late effects, complication codes and obstetric codes to more fully describe a condition. See the specific guidelines for these conditions for further instruction.

10. Acute and Chronic Conditions

If the same condition is described as both acute (subacute) and chronic, and separate subentries exist in the Alphabetic Index at the same indentation level, code both and sequence the acute (subacute) code first.

11. Combination Code

A combination code is a single code used to classify:

- Two diagnoses, or
- A diagnosis with an associated secondary process (manifestation)
- A diagnosis with an associated complication

Combination codes are identified by referring to subterm entries in the Alphabetic Index and by reading the inclusion and exclusion notes in the Tabular List.

Assign only the combination code when that code fully identifies the diagnostic conditions involved or when the Alphabetic Index so directs. Multiple coding should not be used when the classification provides a combination code that clearly identifies all of the elements documented in the diagnosis. When the combination code lacks necessary specificity in describing the manifestation or complication, an additional code should be used as a secondary code.

12. Late Effects

A late effect is the residual effect (condition produced) after the acute phase of an illness or injury has terminated. There is no time limit on when a late effect code can be used. The residual may be apparent early, such as in cerebrovascular accident cases, or it may occur months or years later, such as that due to a previous injury. Coding of late effects generally requires two codes sequenced in the following order: The condition or nature of the late effect is sequenced first. The late effect code is sequenced second.

An exception to the above guidelines are those instances where the code for late effect is followed by a manifestation code identified in the Tabular List and title, or the late effect code has been expanded (at the fourth and fifth-digit levels) to include the manifestation(s). The code for the acute phase of an illness or injury that led to the late effect is never used with a code for the late effect.

13. Impending or Threatened Condition

Code any condition described at the time of discharge as "impending" or "threatened" as follows: If it did occur, code as confirmed diagnosis. If it did not occur, reference the Alphabetic Index to determine if the condition has a subentry term for "impending" or "threatened" and also reference main term entries for "Impending" and for "Threatened." If the subterms are listed, assign the given code. If the subterms are not listed, code the existing underlying condition(s) and not the condition described as impending or threatened.

14. Reporting Same Diagnosis Code More than Once

Each unique ICD-9-CM diagnosis code may be reported only once for an encounter. This applies to bilateral conditions or two different conditions classified to the same ICD-9-CM diagnosis code.

15. Admissions/Encounters for Rehabilitation

When the purpose for the admission/encounter is rehabilitation, sequence the appropriate V code from category V57, Care involving use of rehabilitation procedures, as the principal/first-listed diagnosis. The code for the condition for which the service is being performed should be reported as an additional diagnosis.

Only one code from category V57 is required. Code V57.89, Other specified rehabilitation procedures, should be assigned if more than one type of rehabilitation is performed during a single encounter. A procedure code should be reported to identify each type of rehabilitation therapy actually performed.

16. Documentation for BMI and Pressure Ulcer Stages

For the Body Mass Index (BMI) and pressure ulcer stage codes, code assignment may be based on medical record documentation from clinicians who are not the patient's provider (i.e., physician or other qualified healthcare practitioner legally accountable for establishing the patient's diagnosis), since this information is typically documented by other clinicians involved in the care of the patient (e.g., a dietitian often documents the BMI and nurses often documents the pressure ulcer stages). However, the associated diagnosis (such as overweight, obesity, or pressure ulcer) must be documented by the patient's provider. If there is conflicting medical record documentation, either from the same clinician or different clinicians, the patient's attending provider should be queried for clarification.

The BMI and pressure ulcer stage codes should only be reported as secondary diagnoses. As with all other secondary diagnosis codes, the BMI and pressure ulcer stage codes should only be assigned when they meet the definition of a reportable additional diagnosis (see Section III, Reporting Additional Diagnoses).

17. Syndromes

Follow the Alphabetic Index guidance when coding syndromes. In the absence of index guidance, assign codes for the documented manifestations of the syndrome.

C. Chapter-Specific Coding Guidelines

In addition to general coding guidelines, there are guidelines for specific diagnoses and/or conditions in the classification. Unless otherwise indicated, these guidelines apply to all health care settings. Please refer to Section II for guidelines on the selection of principal diagnosis.

1. Chapter 1: Infectious and Parasitic Diseases (001-139)

a. Human Immunodeficiency Virus (HIV) Infections

1) Code only confirmed cases

Code only confirmed cases of HIV infection/illness. This is an exception to the hospital inpatient guideline Section II, H.

In this context, "confirmation" does not require documentation of positive serology or culture for HIV; the provider's diagnostic statement that the patient is HIV positive, or has an HIV-related illness is sufficient.

2) Selection and sequencing of HIV codes

(a) Patient admitted for HIV-related condition

If a patient is admitted for an HIV-related condition, the principal diagnosis should be 042, followed by additional diagnosis codes for all reported HIV-related conditions.

(b) Patient with HIV disease admitted for unrelated condition

If a patient with HIV disease is admitted for an unrelated condition (such as a traumatic injury), the code for the unrelated condition (e.g., the nature of injury code) should be the principal diagnosis. Other diagnoses would be 042 followed by additional diagnosis codes for all reported HIV-related conditions.

(c) Whether the patient is newly diagnosed

Whether the patient is newly diagnosed or has had previous admissions/encounters for HIV conditions is irrelevant to the sequencing decision.

(d) Asymptomatic human immunodeficiency virus

V08 Asymptomatic human immunodeficiency virus [HIV] infection, is to be applied when the patient without any documentation of symptoms is listed as being "HIV positive," "known HIV," "HIV test positive," or similar terminology. Do not use this code if the term "AIDS" is used or if the patient is treated for any HIV-related illness or is described as having any condition(s) resulting from his/her HIV positive status; use 042 in these cases.

(e) Patients with inconclusive HIV serology

Patients with inconclusive HIV serology, but no definitive diagnosis or manifestations of the illness, may be assigned code 795.71, Inconclusive serologic test for Human Immunodeficiency Virus [HIV].

(f) Previously diagnosed HIV-related illness

Patients with any known prior diagnosis of an HIV-related illness should be coded to 042. Once a patient has developed an HIV-related illness, the patient should always be assigned code 042 on every subsequent admission/encounter. Patients previously diagnosed with any HIV illness (042) should never be assigned to 795.71 or V08.

(g) HIV Infection in Pregnancy, Childbirth and the Puerperium

During pregnancy, childbirth or the puerperium, a patient admitted (or presenting for a health care encounter) because of an HIV-related illness should receive a principal diagnosis code of 647.6X, Other specified infectious and parasitic diseases in the mother classifiable elsewhere, but complicating the pregnancy, childbirth or the puerperium, followed by 042 and the code(s) for the HIV-related illness(es). Codes from Chapter 15 always take sequencing priority.

Patients with asymptomatic HIV infection status admitted (or presenting for a health care encounter) during pregnancy, childbirth, or the puerperium should receive codes of 647.6X and V08.

(h) Encounters for testing for HIV

If a patient is being seen to determine his/her HIV status, use code V73.89, Screening for other specified viral disease. Use code V69.8, Other problems related to lifestyle, as a secondary code if an asymptomatic patient is in a known high risk group for HIV. Should a patient with signs or symptoms or illness, or a confirmed HIV related diagnosis be tested for HIV, code the signs and symptoms or the diagnosis. An additional counseling code V65.44 may be used if counseling is provided during the encounter for the test.

When a patient returns to be informed of his/her HIV test results use code V65.44, HIV counseling, if the results of the test are negative.

If the results are positive but the patient is asymptomatic use code V08, Asymptomatic HIV infection. If the results are positive and the patient is symptomatic use code 042, HIV infection, with codes for the HIV related symptoms or diagnosis. The HIV counseling code may also be used if counseling is provided for patients with positive test results.

b. Septicemia, Systemic Inflammatory Response Syndrome (SIRS), Sepsis, Severe Sepsis, and Septic Shock

1) SIRS, Septicemia, and Sepsis

(a) The terms *septicemia* and *sepsis* are often used interchangeably by providers, however they are not considered synonymous terms. The following descriptions are provided for reference but do not preclude querying the provider for clarification about terms used in the documentation:

(i) Septicemia generally refers to a systemic disease associated with the presence of pathological microorganisms or toxins in the blood, which can include bacteria, viruses, fungi or other organisms.

(ii) Systemic inflammatory response syndrome (SIRS) generally refers to the systemic response to infection, trauma/burns, or other insult (such as cancer) with symptoms including fever, tachycardia, tachypnea, and leukocytosis.

(iii) Sepsis generally refers to SIRS due to infection.

(iv) Severe sepsis generally refers to sepsis with associated acute organ dysfunction.

(b) The Coding of SIRS, sepsis and severe sepsis

The coding of SIRS, sepsis and severe sepsis requires a minimum of 2 codes: a code for the underlying cause (such as infection or trauma) and a code from subcategory 995.9 Systemic inflammatory response syndrome (SIRS).

(i) The code for the underlying cause (such as infection or trauma) must be sequenced before the code from subcategory 995.9 Systemic inflammatory response syndrome (SIRS).

(ii) Sepsis and severe sepsis require a code for the systemic infection (038.xx, 112.5, etc.) and either code 995.91, Sepsis, or 995.92, Severe sepsis. If the causal organism is not documented, assign code 038.9, Unspecified septicemia.

(iii) Severe sepsis requires additional code(s) for the associated acute organ dysfunction(s).

(iv) If a patient has sepsis with multiple organ dysfunctions, follow the instructions for coding severe sepsis.

(v) Either the term sepsis or SIRS must be documented to assign a code from subcategory 995.9.

See Section I.C.17.g), Injury and poisoning, for information regarding systemic inflammatory response syndrome (SIRS) due to trauma/burns and other non-infectious processes.

(c) Due to the complex nature of sepsis and severe sepsis, some cases may require querying the provider prior to assignment of the codes.

2) Sequencing sepsis and severe sepsis

(a) Sepsis and severe sepsis as principal diagnosis

If sepsis or severe sepsis is present on admission, and meets the definition of principal diagnosis, the systemic infection code (e.g., 038.xx, 112.5, etc) should be assigned as the principal diagnosis, followed by code 995.91, Sepsis, or 995.92, Severe sepsis, as required by the sequencing rules in the Tabular List. Codes from subcategory 995.9 can never be assigned as a principal diagnosis. A code should also be assigned for any localized infection, if present.

If the sepsis or severe sepsis is due to a postprocedural infection, see Section I.C.1.b.10 for guidelines related to sepsis due to postprocedural infection.

(b) Sepsis and severe sepsis as secondary diagnoses

When sepsis or severe sepsis develops during the encounter (it was not present on admission), the systemic infection code and code 995.91 or 995.92 should be assigned as secondary diagnoses.

(c) Documentation unclear as to whether sepsis or severe sepsis is present on admission

Sepsis or severe sepsis may be present on admission but the diagnosis may not be confirmed until sometime after admission. If the documentation is not clear whether the sepsis or severe sepsis was present on admission, the provider should be queried.

3) Sepsis/SIRS with Localized Infection

If the reason for admission is both sepsis, severe sepsis, or SIRS and a localized infection, such as pneumonia or cellulitis, a code for the systemic infection (038.xx, 112.5, etc) should be assigned first, then code 995.91 or 995.92, followed by the code for the localized infection. If the patient is admitted with a localized infection, such as pneumonia, and sepsis/SIRS doesn't develop until after admission, see guideline I.C.1.b.2.b).

If the localized infection is postprocedural, see Section I.C.1.b.10 for guidelines related to sepsis due to postprocedural infection.

Note: The term urosepsis is a nonspecific term. If that is the only term documented then only code 599.0 should be assigned based on the default for the term in the ICD-9-CM index, in addition to the code for the causal organism if known.

4) Bacterial Sepsis and Septicemia

In most cases, it will be a code from category 038, Septicemia, that will be used in conjunction with a code from subcategory 995.9 such as the following:

(a) Streptococcal sepsis

If the documentation in the record states streptococcal sepsis, codes 038.0, Streptococcal septicemia, and code 995.91 should be used, in that sequence.

(b) Streptococcal septicemia

If the documentation states streptococcal septicemia, only code 038.0 should be assigned, however, the provider should be queried whether the patient has sepsis, an infection with SIRS.

5) Acute organ dysfunction that is not clearly associated with the sepsis

If a patient has sepsis and an acute organ dysfunction, but the medical record documentation indicates that the acute organ dysfunction is related to a medical condition other than the sepsis, do not assign code 995.92, Severe sepsis. An acute organ dysfunction must be associated with the sepsis in order to assign the severe sepsis code. If the documentation is not clear as to whether an acute organ dysfunction is related to the sepsis or another medical condition, query the provider.

6) Septic shock

(a) Sequencing of septic shock

Septic shock generally refers to circulatory failure associated with severe sepsis, and, therefore, it represents a type of acute organ dysfunction.

For all cases of septic shock, the code for the systemic infection should be sequenced first, followed by codes 995.92 and 785.52. Any additional codes for other acute organ dysfunctions should also be assigned. As noted in the sequencing instructions in the Tabular List, the code for septic shock cannot be assigned as a principal diagnosis.

(b) Septic Shock without documentation of severe sepsis

Septic shock indicates the presence of severe sepsis.

Code 995.92, Severe sepsis, must be assigned with code 785.52, Septic shock, even if the term severe sepsis is not documented in the record. The "use additional code" note and the "code first" note in the tabular support this guideline.

7) Sepsis and septic shock complicating abortion and pregnancy

Sepsis and septic shock complicating abortion, ectopic pregnancy, and molar pregnancy are classified to category codes in Chapter 11 (630-639).

See section I.C.11.i.7. for information on the coding of puerperal sepsis.

8) Negative or inconclusive blood cultures

Negative or inconclusive blood cultures do not preclude a diagnosis of septicemia or sepsis in patients with clinical evidence of the condition, however, the provider should be queried.

9) Newborn sepsis

See Section I.C.15.j for information on the coding of newborn sepsis.

10) Sepsis due to a Postprocedural Infection

(a) Documentation of causal relationship

As with all postprocedural complications, code assignment is based on the provider's documentation of the relationship between the infection and the procedure.

(b) Sepsis due to postprocedural infection

In cases of postprocedural sepsis, the complication code, such as code 998.59, Other postoperative infection, or 674.3x, Other complications of obstetrical surgical wounds should be coded first followed by the appropriate sepsis codes (systemic infection code and either code 995.91or 995.92). An additional code(s) for any acute organ dysfunction should also be assigned for cases of severe sepsis.

11) External cause of injury codes with SIRS

Refer to Section I.C.19.a.7 for instruction on the use of external cause of injury codes with codes for SIRS resulting from trauma.

12) Sepsis and Severe Sepsis Associated with Non-infectious Process

In some cases, a non-infectious process, such as trauma, may lead to an infection which can result in sepsis or severe sepsis. If sepsis or severe sepsis is documented as associated with a non-infectious condition, such as a burn or serious injury, and this condition meets the definition for principal diagnosis, the code for the non-infectious condition should be sequenced first, followed by the code for the systemic infection and either code 995.91, Sepsis, or 995.92, Severe sepsis. Additional codes for any associated acute organ dysfunction(s) should also be assigned for cases of severe sepsis. If the sepsis or severe sepsis meets the definition of principal diagnosis, the systemic infection and sepsis codes should be sequenced before the non-infectious condition. When both the associated non-infectious condition and the sepsis or severe sepsis meet the definition of principal diagnosis, either may be assigned as principal diagnosis.

See Section I.C.1.b.2.a. for guidelines pertaining to sepsis or severe sepsis as the principal diagnosis.

Only one code from subcategory 995.9 should be assigned. Therefore, when a non-infectious condition leads to an infection resulting in sepsis or severe sepsis, assign either code 995.91 or 995.92. Do not additionally assign code 995.93, Systemic inflammatory response syndrome due to non-infectious process without acute organ dysfunction, or 995.94, Systemic inflammatory response syndrome with acute organ dysfunction.

See Section I.C.17.g for information on the coding of SIRS due to trauma/burns or other non-infectious disease processes.

c. **Methicillin Resistant *Staphylococcus aureus* (MRSA) Conditions**

1) Selection and sequencing of MRSA codes

(a) Combination codes for MRSA infection

When a patient is diagnosed with an infection that is due to methicillin resistant *Staphylococcus aureus* (MRSA), and that infection has a combination code that includes the causal organism (e.g., septicemia, pneumonia) assign the appropriate code for the condition (e.g., code 038.12, Methicillin resistant Staphylococcus aureus septicemia or code 482.42, Methicillin resistant pneumonia due to Staphylococcus aureus). Do not assign code 041.12, Methicillin resistant Staphylococcus aureus, as an additional code because the code includes the type of infection and the MRSA organism. Do not assign a code from subcategory V09.0, Infection with microorganisms resistant to penicillins, as an additional diagnosis.

See Section C.1.b.1 for instructions on coding and sequencing of septicemia.

(b) Other codes for MRSA infection

When there is documentation of a current infection (e.g., wound infection, stitch abscess, urinary tract infection) due to MRSA, and that infection does not have a combination code that includes the causal organism, select the appropriate code to identify the condition along with code 041.12, Methicillin resistant Staphylococcus aureus, for the MRSA infection. Do not assign a code from subcategory V09.0, Infection with microorganisms resistant to penicillins.

(c) Methicillin susceptible *Staphylococcus aureus* (MSSA) and MRSA colonization

The condition or state of being colonized or carrying MSSA or MRSA is called colonization or carriage, while an individual person is described as being colonized or being a carrier. Colonization means that MSSA or MSRA is present on or in the body without necessarily causing illness. A positive MRSA colonization test might be documented by the provider as "MRSA screen positive" or "MRSA nasal swab positive".

Assign code V02.54, Carrier or suspected carrier, Methicillin resistant Staphylococcus aureus, for patients documented as having MRSA colonization. Assign code V02.53, Carrier or suspected carrier, Methicillin susceptible Staphylococcus aureus, for patient documented as having MSSA colonization. Colonization is not necessarily indicative of a disease process or as the cause of a specific condition the patient may have unless documented as such by the provider.

Code V02.59, Other specified bacterial diseases, should be assigned for other types of staphylococcal colonization (e.g., *S. epidermidis, S. saprophyticus*). Code V02.59 should not be assigned for colonization with any type of *Staphylococcus aureus* (MRSA, MSSA).

(d) MRSA colonization and infection

If a patient is documented as having both MRSA colonization and infection during a hospital admission, code V02.54, Carrier or suspected carrier, Methicillin resistant Staphylococcus aureus, and a code for the MRSA infection may both be assigned.

2. Chapter 2: Neoplasms (140-239)

General guidelines

Chapter 2 of the ICD-9-CM contains the codes for most benign and all malignant neoplasms. Certain benign neoplasms, such as prostatic adenomas, may be found in the specific body system chapters. To properly code a neoplasm it is necessary to determine from the record if the neoplasm is benign, in-situ, malignant, or of uncertain histologic behavior. If malignant, any secondary (metastatic) sites should also be determined.

The neoplasm table in the Alphabetic Index should be referenced first. However, if the histological term is documented, that term should be referenced first, rather than going immediately to the Neoplasm Table, in order to determine which column in the Neoplasm Table is appropriate. For example, if the documentation indicates "adenoma," refer to the term in the Alphabetic Index to review the entries under this term and the instructional note to "see also neoplasm, by site, benign." The table provides the proper code based on the type of neoplasm and the site. It is important to select the proper column in the table that corresponds to the type of neoplasm. The tabular should then be referenced to verify that the correct code has been selected from the table and that a more specific site code does not exist.

See Section I. C. 18.d.4. for information regarding V codes for genetic susceptibility to cancer.

a. **Treatment directed at the malignancy**

If the treatment is directed at the malignancy, designate the malignancy as the principal diagnosis.

The only exception to this guideline is if a patient admission/encounter is solely for the administration of chemotherapy, immunotherapy or radiation therapy, assign the appropriate V58.x code as the first-listed or principal diagnosis, and the diagnosis or problem for which the service is being performed as a secondary diagnosis.

b. **Treatment of secondary site**

When a patient is admitted because of a primary neoplasm with metastasis and treatment is directed toward the secondary site only, the secondary neoplasm is designated as the principal diagnosis even though the primary malignancy is still present.

c. **Coding and sequencing of complications**

Coding and sequencing of complications associated with the malignancies or with the therapy thereof are subject to the following guidelines:

1) Anemia associated with malignancy

When admission/encounter is for management of an anemia associated with the malignancy, and the treatment is only for anemia, the appropriate anemia code (such as code 285.22, Anemia in neoplastic disease) is designated as the principal diagnosis and is followed by the appropriate code(s) for the malignancy.

Code 285.22 may also be used as a secondary code if the patient suffers from anemia and is being treated for the malignancy.

Code 285.22, Anemia in neoplastic disease, and code 285.3, Antineoplastic chemotherapy induced anemia, may both be assigned if anemia in neoplastic disease and anemia due to antineoplastic chemotherapy are both documented.

2) Anemia associated with chemotherapy, immunotherapy and radiation therapy

When the admission/encounter is for management of an anemia associated with chemotherapy, immunotherapy or radiotherapy and the only treatment is for the anemia, the anemia is sequenced first. The appropriate neoplasm code should be assigned as an additional code.

3) Management of dehydration due to the malignancy

When the admission/encounter is for management of dehydration due to the malignancy or the therapy, or a combination of both, and only the dehydration is being treated (intravenous rehydration), the dehydration is sequenced first, followed by the code(s) for the malignancy.

4) Treatment of a complication resulting from a surgical procedure

When the admission/encounter is for treatment of a complication resulting from a surgical procedure, designate the complication as the principal or first-listed diagnosis if treatment is directed at resolving the complication.

d. Primary malignancy previously excised

When a primary malignancy has been previously excised or eradicated from its site and there is no further treatment directed to that site and there is no evidence of any existing primary malignancy, a code from category V10, Personal history of malignant neoplasm, should be used to indicate the former site of the malignancy. Any mention of extension, invasion, or metastasis to another site is coded as a secondary malignant neoplasm to that site. The secondary site may be the principal or first-listed with the V10 code used as a secondary code.

e. Admissions/Encounters involving chemotherapy, immunotherapy and radiation therapy

1) Episode of care involves surgical removal of neoplasm

When an episode of care involves the surgical removal of a neoplasm, primary or secondary site, followed by adjunct chemotherapy or radiation treatment during the same episode of care, the neoplasm code should be assigned as principal or first-listed diagnosis, using codes in the 140-198 series or where appropriate in the 200-203 series.

2) Patient admission/encounter solely for administration of chemotherapy, immunotherapy and radiation therapy

If a patient admission/encounter is solely for the administration of chemotherapy, immunotherapy or radiation therapy assign code V58.0, Encounter for radiation therapy, or V58.11, Encounter for antineoplastic chemotherapy, or V58.12, Encounter for antineoplastic immunotherapy as the first-listed or principal diagnosis. If a patient receives more than one of these therapies during the same admission more than one of these codes may be assigned, in any sequence.

The malignancy for which the therapy is being administered should be assigned as a secondary diagnosis.

3) Patient admitted for radiotherapy/chemotherapy and immunotherapy and develops complications

When a patient is admitted for the purpose of radiotherapy, immunotherapy or chemotherapy and develops complications such as uncontrolled nausea and vomiting or dehydration, the principal or first-listed diagnosis is V58.0, Encounter for radiotherapy, or V58.11, Encounter for antineoplastic chemotherapy, or V58.12, Encounter for antineoplastic immunotherapy followed by any codes for the complications.

f. Admission/encounter to determine extent of malignancy

When the reason for admission/encounter is to determine the extent of the malignancy, or for a procedure such as paracentesis or thoracentesis, the primary malignancy or appropriate metastatic site is designated as the principal or first-listed diagnosis, even though chemotherapy or radiotherapy is administered.

g. Symptoms, signs, and ill-defined conditions listed in Chapter 16 associated with neoplasms

Symptoms, signs, and ill-defined conditions listed in Chapter 16 characteristic of, or associated with, an existing primary or secondary site malignancy cannot be used to replace the malignancy as principal or first-listed diagnosis, regardless of the number of admissions or encounters for treatment and care of the neoplasm.

h. Admission/encounter for pain control/management

See Section I.C.6.a.5 for information on coding admission/encounter for pain control/management.

i. Malignant neoplasm associated with transplanted organ

A malignant neoplasm of a transplanted organ should be coded as a transplant complication. Assign first the appropriate code from subcategory 996.8, Complications of transplanted organ, followed by code 199.2, Malignant neoplasm associated with transplanted organ. Use an additional code for the specific malignancy.

3. Chapter 3: Endocrine, Nutritional, and Metabolic Diseases and Immunity Disorders (240-279)

a. Diabetes mellitus

Codes under category 250, Diabetes mellitus, identify complications/manifestations associated with diabetes mellitus. A fifth-digit is required for all category 250 codes to identify the type of diabetes mellitus and whether the diabetes is controlled or uncontrolled.

See I.C.3.a.7 for secondary diabetes

1) Fifth-digits for category 250:

The following are the fifth-digits for the codes under category 250:

0 type II or unspecified type, not stated as uncontrolled
1 type I, [juvenile type], not stated as uncontrolled
2 type II or unspecified type, uncontrolled
3 type I, [juvenile type], uncontrolled

The age of a patient is not the sole determining factor, though most type I diabetics develop the condition before reaching puberty. For this reason type I diabetes mellitus is also referred to as juvenile diabetes.

2) Type of diabetes mellitus not documented

If the type of diabetes mellitus is not documented in the medical record the default is type II.

3) Diabetes mellitus and the use of insulin

All type I diabetics must use insulin to replace what their bodies do not produce. However, the use of insulin does not mean that a patient is a type I diabetic. Some patients with type II diabetes mellitus are unable to control their blood sugar through diet and oral medication alone and do require insulin. If the documentation in a medical record does not indicate the type of diabetes but does indicate that the patient uses insulin, the appropriate fifth-digit for type II must be used. For type II patients who routinely use insulin, code V58.67, Long-term (current) use of insulin, should also be assigned to indicate that the patient uses insulin. Code V58.67 should not be assigned if insulin is given temporarily to bring a type II patient's blood sugar under control during an encounter.

4) Assigning and sequencing diabetes codes and associated conditions

When assigning codes for diabetes and its associated conditions, the code(s) from category 250 must be sequenced before the codes for the associated conditions. The diabetes codes and the secondary codes that correspond to them are paired codes that follow the etiology/manifestation convention of the classification (*See Section I.A.6., Etiology/manifestation convention*). Assign as many codes from category 250 as needed to identify all of the associated conditions that the patient has. The corresponding secondary codes are listed under each of the diabetes codes.

(a) Diabetic retinopathy/diabetic macular edema

Diabetic macular edema, code 362.07, is only present with diabetic retinopathy. Another code from subcategory 362.0, Diabetic retinopathy, must be used with code 362.07. Codes under subcategory 362.0 are diabetes manifestation codes, so they must be used following the appropriate diabetes code.

5) Diabetes mellitus in pregnancy and gestational diabetes

(a) For diabetes mellitus complicating pregnancy, *see Section I.C.11.f., Diabetes mellitus in pregnancy.*

(b) For gestational diabetes, *see Section I.C.11, g., Gestational diabetes.*

6) Insulin pump malfunction

(a) Underdose of insulin due insulin pump failure

An underdose of insulin due to an insulin pump failure should be assigned 996.57, Mechanical complication due to insulin pump, as the principal or first listed code, followed by the appropriate diabetes mellitus code based on documentation.

(b) Overdose of insulin due to insulin pump failure

The principal or first listed code for an encounter due to an insulin pump malfunction resulting in an overdose of insulin, should also be 996.57, Mechanical complication due to insulin pump, followed by code 962.3, Poisoning by insulins and antidiabetic agents, and the appropriate diabetes mellitus code based on documentation.

7) Secondary Diabetes Mellitus

Codes under category 249, Secondary diabetes mellitus, identify complications/manifestations associated with secondary diabetes mellitus. Secondary diabetes is always caused by another condition or event (e.g., cystic fibrosis, malignant neoplasm of pancreas, pancreatectomy, adverse effect of drug, or poisoning).

(a) Fifth-digits for category 249:

A fifth-digit is required for all category 249 codes to identify whether the diabetes is controlled or uncontrolled.

(b) Secondary diabetes mellitus and the use of insulin

For patients who routinely use insulin, code V58.67, Long-term (current) use of insulin, should also be assigned. Code V58.67 should not be assigned if insulin is given temporarily to bring a patient's blood sugar under control during an encounter.

(c) Assigning and sequencing secondary diabetes codes and associated conditions

When assigning codes for secondary diabetes and its associated conditions (e.g. renal manifestations), the code(s) from category 249 must be sequenced before the codes for the associated conditions. The secondary diabetes codes and the diabetic manifestation codes that correspond to them are paired codes that follow the etiology/manifestation convention of the classification. Assign as many codes from category 249 as needed to identify all of the associated conditions that the patient has. The corresponding codes for the associated conditions are listed under each of the secondary diabetes codes. For example, secondary diabetes with diabetic nephrosis is assigned to code 249.40, followed by 581.81.

(d) Assigning and sequencing secondary diabetes codes and its causes

The sequencing of the secondary diabetes codes in relationship to codes for the cause of the diabetes is based on the reason for the encounter, applicable ICD-9-CM sequencing conventions, and chapter-specific guidelines.

If a patient is seen for treatment of the secondary diabetes or one of its associated conditions, a code from category 249 is sequenced as the principal or first-listed diagnosis, with the cause of the secondary diabetes (e.g. cystic fibrosis) sequenced as an additional diagnosis.

If, however, the patient is seen for the treatment of the condition causing the secondary diabetes (e.g., malignant neoplasm of pancreas), the code for the cause of the secondary diabetes should be sequenced as the principal or first-listed diagnosis followed by a code from category 249.

(i) Secondary diabetes mellitus due to pancreatectomy

For postpancreatectomy diabetes mellitus (lack of insulin due to the surgical removal of all or part of the pancreas), assign code 251.3, Postsurgical hypoinsulinemia. Assign a code from subcategory 249 and code V45.79, Other acquired absence of organ, as additional codes. Code also any diabetic manifestations (e.g. diabetic nephrosis 581.81).

(ii) Secondary diabetes due to drugs

Secondary diabetes may be caused by an adverse effect of correctly administered medications, poisoning or late effect of poisoning.

See section I.C.17.e for coding of adverse effects and poisoning, and section I.C.19 for E code reporting.

4. Chapter 4: Diseases of Blood and Blood Forming Organs (280-289)

a. Anemia of chronic disease

Subcategory 285.2, Anemia in chronic illness, has codes for anemia in chronic kidney disease, code 285.21; anemia in neoplastic disease, code 285.22; and anemia in other chronic illness, code 285.29. These codes can be used as the principal/first listed code if the reason for the encounter is to treat the anemia. They may also be used as secondary codes if treatment of the anemia is a component of an encounter, but not the primary reason for the encounter. When using a code from subcategory 285 it is also necessary to use the code for the chronic condition causing the anemia.

1) Anemia in chronic kidney disease

When assigning code 285.21, Anemia in chronic kidney disease, it is also necessary to assign a code from category 585, Chronic kidney disease, to indicate the stage of chronic kidney disease.

See I.C.10.a. Chronic kidney disease (CKD).

2) Anemia in neoplastic disease

When assigning code 285.22, Anemia in neoplastic disease, it is also necessary to assign the neoplasm code that is responsible for the anemia. Code 285.22 is for use for anemia that is due to the malignancy, not for anemia due to antineoplastic chemotherapy drugs. Assign code 285.3 for anemia due to antineoplastic chemotherapy.

See I.C.2.c.1 Anemia associated with malignancy.

See I.C.2.c.2 Anemia associated with chemotherapy, immunotherapy and radiation therapy.

5. Chapter 5: Mental Disorders (290-319)

Reserved for future guideline expansion

6. Chapter 6: Diseases of Nervous System and Sense Organs (320-389)

a. Pain - Category 338

1) General coding information

Codes in category 338 may be used in conjunction with codes from other categories and chapters to provide more detail about acute or chronic pain and neoplasm-related pain, unless otherwise indicated below.

If the pain is not specified as acute or chronic, do not assign codes from category 338, except for post-thoracotomy pain, postoperative pain, neoplasm related pain, or central pain syndrome.

A code from subcategories 338.1 and 338.2 should not be assigned if the underlying (definitive) diagnosis is known, unless the reason for the encounter is pain control/ management and not management of the underlying condition.

(a) Category 338 Codes as Principal or First-Listed Diagnosis

Category 338 codes are acceptable as principal diagnosis or the first-listed code:

- When pain control or pain management is the reason for the admission/encounter (e.g., a patient with displaced intervertebral disc, nerve impingement and severe back pain presents for injection of steroid into the spinal canal). The underlying cause of the pain should be reported as an additional diagnosis, if known.
- When an admission or encounter is for a procedure aimed at treating the underlying condition (e.g., spinal fusion, kyphoplasty), a code for the underlying condition (e.g., vertebral fracture, spinal stenosis) should be assigned as the principal diagnosis. No code from category 338 should be assigned.
- When a patient is admitted for the insertion of a neurostimulator for pain control, assign the appropriate pain code as the principal or first listed diagnosis. When an admission or encounter is for a procedure aimed at treating the underlying condition and a neurostimulator is inserted for pain control during the same admission/ encounter, a code for the underlying condition should be assigned as the principal diagnosis and the appropriate pain code should be assigned as a secondary diagnosis.

(b) Use of Category 338 Codes in Conjunction with Site Specific Pain Codes

(i) Assigning Category 338 Codes and Site-Specific Pain Codes

Codes from category 338 may be used in conjunction with codes that identify the site of pain (including codes from chapter 16) if the category 338 code provides additional information. For example, if the code describes the site of the pain, but does not fully describe whether the pain is acute or chronic, then both codes should be assigned.

(ii) Sequencing of Category 338 Codes with Site-Specific Pain Codes

The sequencing of category 338 codes with site-specific pain codes (including chapter 16 codes), is dependent on the circumstances of the encounter/admission as follows:

- If the encounter is for pain control or pain management, assign the code from category 338 followed by the code identifying the specific site of pain (e.g., encounter for pain management for acute neck pain from trauma is assigned code 338.11, Acute pain due to trauma, followed by code 723.1, Cervicalgia, to identify the site of pain).
- If the encounter is for any other reason except pain control or pain management, and a related definitive diagnosis has not been established (confirmed) by the provider, assign the code for the specific site of pain first, followed by the appropriate code from category 338.

2) Pain due to devices, implants and grafts
Pain associated with devices, implants or grafts left in a surgical site (for example painful hip prosthesis) is assigned to the appropriate code(s) found in Chapter 17, Injury and Poisoning. Use additional code(s) from category 338 to identify acute or chronic pain due to presence of the device, implant or graft (338.18-338.19 or 338.28-338.29).

3) Postoperative Pain
Post-thoracotomy pain and other postoperative pain are classified to subcategories 338.1 and 338.2, depending on whether the pain is acute or chronic. The default for post-thoracotomy and other postoperative pain not specified as acute or chronic is the code for the acute form.
Routine or expected postoperative pain immediately after surgery should not be coded.

(a) Postoperative pain not associated with specific postoperative complication
Postoperative pain not associated with a specific postoperative complication is assigned to the appropriate postoperative pain code in category 338.

(b) Postoperative pain associated with specific postoperative complication
Postoperative pain associated with a specific postoperative complication (such as painful wire sutures) is assigned to the appropriate code(s) found in Chapter 17, Injury and Poisoning. If appropriate, use additional code(s) from category 338 to identify acute or chronic pain (338.18 or 338.28). If pain control/management is the reason for the encounter, a code from category 338 should be assigned as the principal or first-listed diagnosis in accordance with *Section I.C.6.a.1.a above.*

(c) Postoperative pain as principal or first-listed diagnosis
Postoperative pain may be reported as the principal or first-listed diagnosis when the stated reason for the admission/encounter is documented as postoperative pain control/management.

(d) Postoperative pain as secondary diagnosis
Postoperative pain may be reported as a secondary diagnosis code when a patient presents for outpatient surgery and develops an unusual or inordinate amount of postoperative pain.
The provider's documentation should be used to guide the coding of postoperative pain, as well as *Section III. Reporting Additional Diagnoses and Section IV. Diagnostic Coding and Reporting in the Outpatient Setting.*
See Section II.I.2 for information on sequencing of diagnoses for patients admitted to hospital inpatient care following post-operative observation.
See Section II.J for information on sequencing of diagnoses for patients admitted to hospital inpatient care from outpatient surgery.
See Section IV.A.2 for information on sequencing of diagnoses for patients admitted for observation.

4) Chronic pain
Chronic pain is classified to subcategory 338.2. There is no time frame defining when pain becomes chronic pain. The provider's documentation should be used to guide use of these codes.

5) Neoplasm Related Pain
Code 338.3 is assigned to pain documented as being related, associated or due to cancer, primary or secondary malignancy, or tumor. This code is assigned regardless of whether the pain is acute or chronic.
This code may be assigned as the principal or first-listed code when the stated reason for the admission/encounter is documented as pain control/pain management. The underlying neoplasm should be reported as an additional diagnosis.
When the reason for the admission/encounter is management of the neoplasm and the pain associated with the neoplasm is also documented, code 338.3 may be assigned as an additional diagnosis.
See Section I.C.2 for instructions on the sequencing of neoplasms for all other stated reasons for the admission/encounter (except for pain control/pain management).

6) Chronic pain syndrome
This condition is different than the term "chronic pain," and therefore this code should only be used when the provider has specifically documented this condition.

7. Chapter 7: Diseases of Circulatory System (390-459)

a. Hypertension

Hypertension Table
The Hypertension Table, found under the main term, "Hypertension", in the Alphabetic Index, contains a complete listing of all conditions due to or associated with hypertension and classifies them according to malignant, benign, and unspecified.

1) Hypertension, Essential, or NOS
Assign hypertension (arterial) (essential) (primary) (systemic) (NOS) to category code 401 with the appropriate fourth digit to indicate malignant (.0), benign (.1), or unspecified (.9). Do not use either .0 malignant or .1 benign unless medical record documentation supports such a designation.

2) Hypertension with Heart Disease
Heart conditions (425.8, 429.0-429.3, 429.8, 429.9) are assigned to a code from category 402 when a causal relationship is stated (due to hypertension) or implied (hypertensive). Use an additional code from category 428 to identify the type of heart failure in those patients with heart failure. More than one code from category 428 may be assigned if the patient has systolic or diastolic failure and congestive heart failure.
The same heart conditions (425.8, 429.0-429.3, 429.8, 429.9) with hypertension, but without a stated causal relationship, are coded separately. Sequence according to the circumstances of the admission/encounter.

3) Hypertensive Chronic Kidney Disease
Assign codes from category 403, Hypertensive chronic kidney disease, when conditions classified to category 585 are present. Unlike hypertension with heart disease, ICD-9-CM presumes a cause-and-effect relationship and classifies chronic kidney disease (CKD) with hypertension as hypertensive chronic kidney disease.
Fifth digits for category 403 should be assigned as follows:

- 0 with CKD stage I through stage IV, or unspecified.
- 1 with CKD stage V or end stage renal disease.
  The appropriate code from category 585, Chronic kidney disease, should be used as a secondary code with a code from category 403 to identify the stage of chronic kidney disease.

See Section I.C.10.a for information on the coding of chronic kidney disease.

4) Hypertensive Heart and Chronic Kidney Disease
Assign codes from combination category 404, Hypertensive heart and chronic kidney disease, when both hypertensive kidney disease and hypertensive heart disease are stated in the diagnosis. Assume a relationship between the hypertension and the chronic kidney disease, whether or not the condition is so designated. Assign an additional code from category 428, to identify the type of heart failure. More than one code from category 428 may be assigned if the patient has systolic or diastolic failure and congestive heart failure.
Fifth digits for category 404 should be assigned as follows:

- 0 without heart failure and with chronic kidney disease (CKD) stage I through stage IV, or unspecified
- 1 with heart failure and with CKD stage I through stage IV, or unspecified
- 2 without heart failure and with CKD stage V or end stage renal disease
- 3 with heart failure and with CKD stage V or end stage renal disease

The appropriate code from category 585, Chronic kidney disease, should be used as a secondary code with a code from category 404 to identify the stage of kidney disease.
See Section I.C.10.a for information on the coding of chronic kidney disease.

5) Hypertensive Cerebrovascular Disease
First assign codes from 430-438, Cerebrovascular disease, then the appropriate hypertension code from categories 401-405.

6) Hypertensive Retinopathy

Two codes are necessary to identify the condition. First assign the code from subcategory 362.11, Hypertensive retinopathy, then the appropriate code from categories 401-405 to indicate the type of hypertension.

7) Hypertension, Secondary
Two codes are required: one to identify the underlying etiology and one from category 405 to identify the hypertension. Sequencing of codes is determined by the reason for admission/encounter.

8) Hypertension, Transient
Assign code 796.2, Elevated blood pressure reading without diagnosis of hypertension, unless patient has an established diagnosis of hypertension. Assign code 642.3x for transient hypertension of pregnancy.

9) Hypertension, Controlled
Assign appropriate code from categories 401-405. This diagnostic statement usually refers to an existing state of hypertension under control by therapy.

10) Hypertension, Uncontrolled
Uncontrolled hypertension may refer to untreated hypertension or hypertension not responding to current therapeutic regimen. In either case, assign the appropriate code from categories 401-405 to designate the stage and type of hypertension. Code to the type of hypertension.

11) Elevated Blood Pressure
For a statement of elevated blood pressure without further specificity, assign code 796.2, Elevated blood pressure reading without diagnosis of hypertension, rather than a code from category 401.

b. Cerebral infarction/stroke/cerebrovascular accident (CVA)

The terms stroke and CVA are often used interchangeably to refer to a cerebral infarction. The terms stroke, CVA, and cerebral infarction NOS are all indexed to the default code 434.91, Cerebral artery occlusion, unspecified, with infarction. Code 436, Acute, but ill-defined, cerebrovascular disease, should not be used when the documentation states stroke or CVA.

See Section I.C.18.d.3 for information on coding status post administration of tPA in a different facility within the last 24 hours.

c. Postoperative cerebrovascular accident

A cerebrovascular hemorrhage or infarction that occurs as a result of medical intervention is coded to 997.02, Iatrogenic cerebrovascular infarction or hemorrhage. Medical record documentation should clearly specify the cause- and-effect relationship between the medical intervention and the cerebrovascular accident in order to assign this code. A secondary code from the code range 430-432 or from a code from subcategories 433 or 434 with a fifth digit of "1" should also be used to identify the type of hemorrhage or infarct.

This guideline conforms to the use additional code note instruction at category 997. Code 436, Acute, but ill-defined, cerebrovascular disease, should not be used as a secondary code with code 997.02.

d. Late Effects of Cerebrovascular Disease

1) Category 438, Late Effects of Cerebrovascular disease
Category 438 is used to indicate conditions classifiable to categories 430-437 as the causes of late effects (neurologic deficits), themselves classified elsewhere. These "late effects" include neurologic deficits that persist after initial onset of conditions classifiable to 430-437. The neurologic deficits caused by cerebrovascular disease may be present from the onset or may arise at any time after the onset of the condition classifiable to 430-437.

2) Codes from category 438 with codes from 430-437
Codes from category 438 may be assigned on a health care record with codes from 430-437, if the patient has a current cerebrovascular accident (CVA) and deficits from an old CVA.

3) Code V12.54
Assign code V12.54, Transient ischemic attack (TIA), and cerebral infarction without residual deficits (and not a code from category 438) as an additional code for history of cerebrovascular disease when no neurologic deficits are present.

e. Acute myocardial infarction (AMI)

1) ST elevation myocardial infarction (STEMI) and non ST elevation myocardial infarction (NSTEMI)
The ICD-9-CM codes for acute myocardial infarction (AMI) identify the site, such as anterolateral wall or true posterior wall. Subcategories 410.0-410.6 and 410.8 are used for ST elevation myocardial infarction (STEMI). Subcategory 410.7, Subendocardial infarction, is used for non ST elevation myocardial infarction (NSTEMI) and nontransmural MIs.

2) Acute myocardial infarction, unspecified
Subcategory 410.9 is the default for the unspecified term acute myocardial infarction. If only STEMI or transmural MI without the site is documented, query the provider as to the site, or assign a code from subcategory 410.9.

3) AMI documented as nontransmural or subendocardial but site provided
If an AMI is documented as nontransmural or subendocardial, but the site is provided, it is still coded as a subendocardial AMI. If NSTEMI evolves to STEMI, assign the STEMI code. If STEMI converts to NSTEMI due to thrombolytic therapy, it is still coded as STEMI.
See Section I.C.18.d.3 for information on coding status post administration of tPA in a different facility within the last 24 hours.

8. Chapter 8: Diseases of Respiratory System (460-519)

See I.C.17.f. for ventilator-associated pneumonia.

a. Chronic Obstructive Pulmonary Disease [COPD] and Asthma

1) Conditions that comprise COPD and Asthma
The conditions that comprise COPD are obstructive chronic bronchitis, subcategory 491.2, and emphysema, category 492. All asthma codes are under category 493, Asthma. Code 496, Chronic airway obstruction, not elsewhere classified, is a nonspecific code that should only be used when the documentation in a medical record does not specify the type of COPD being treated.

2) Acute exacerbation of chronic obstructive bronchitis and asthma
The codes for chronic obstructive bronchitis and asthma distinguish between uncomplicated cases and those in acute exacerbation. An acute exacerbation is a worsening or a decompensation of a chronic condition. An acute exacerbation is not equivalent to an infection superimposed on a chronic condition, though an exacerbation may be triggered by an infection.

3) Overlapping nature of the conditions that comprise COPD and asthma
Due to the overlapping nature of the conditions that make up COPD and asthma, there are many variations in the way these conditions are documented. Code selection must be based on the terms as documented. When selecting the correct code for the documented type of COPD and asthma, it is essential to first review the index, and then verify the code in the tabular list. There are many instructional notes under the different COPD subcategories and codes. It is important that all such notes be reviewed to assure correct code assignment.

4) Acute exacerbation of asthma and status asthmaticus
An acute exacerbation of asthma is an increased severity of the asthma symptoms, such as wheezing and shortness of breath. Status asthmaticus refers to a patient's failure to respond to therapy administered during an asthmatic episode and is a life threatening complication that requires emergency care. If status asthmaticus is documented by the provider with any type of COPD or with acute bronchitis, the status asthmaticus should be sequenced first. It supersedes any type of COPD including that with acute exacerbation or acute bronchitis. It is inappropriate to assign an asthma code with 5th digit 2, with acute exacerbation, together with an asthma code with 5th digit 1, with status asthmatics. Only the 5th digit 1 should be assigned.

b. Chronic Obstructive Pulmonary Disease [COPD] and Bronchitis

1) Acute bronchitis with COPD
Acute bronchitis, code 466.0, is due to an infectious organism. When acute bronchitis is documented with COPD, code 491.22, Obstructive chronic bronchitis with acute bronchitis, should be assigned. It is not necessary to also assign code 466.0. If a medical record documents acute bronchitis with COPD with acute exacerbation, only code 491.22 should be assigned. The acute bronchitis included in code 491.22 supersedes the acute exacerbation. If a medical record documents COPD with acute exacerbation without mention of acute bronchitis, only code 491.21 should be assigned.

c. **Acute Respiratory Failure**

1) Acute respiratory failure as principal diagnosis

Code 518.81, Acute respiratory failure, may be assigned as a principal diagnosis when it is the condition established after study to be chiefly responsible for occasioning the admission to the hospital, and the selection is supported by the Alphabetic Index and Tabular List. However, chapter-specific coding guidelines (such as obstetrics, poisoning, HIV, newborn) that provide sequencing direction take precedence.

2) Acute respiratory failure as secondary diagnosis

Respiratory failure may be listed as a secondary diagnosis if it occurs after admission, or if it is present on admission, but does not meet the definition of principal diagnosis.

3) Sequencing of acute respiratory failure and another acute condition

When a patient is admitted with respiratory failure and another acute condition, (e.g., myocardial infarction, cerebrovascular accident, aspiration pneumonia), the principal diagnosis will not be the same in every situation. This applies whether the other acute condition is a respiratory or nonrespiratory condition. Selection of the principal diagnosis will be dependent on the circumstances of admission. If both the respiratory failure and the other acute condition are equally responsible for occasioning the admission to the hospital, and there are no chapter-specific sequencing rules, the guideline regarding two or more diagnoses that equally meet the definition for principal diagnosis (*Section II, C.*) may be applied in these situations.

If the documentation is not clear as to whether acute respiratory failure and another condition are equally responsible for occasioning the admission, query the provider for clarification.

d. **Influenza due to certain identified viruses**

Code only confirmed cases of avian influenza (code 488.0, Influenza due to identified avian influenza virus) or novel H1N1 influenza virus (H1N1 or swine flu, code 488.1). This is an exception to the hospital inpatient guideline Section II, H. (Uncertain Diagnosis).

In this context, "confirmation" does not require documentation of positive laboratory testing specific for avian or novel H1N1 influenza. However, coding should be based on the provider's diagnostic statement that the patient has avian or novel H1N1 (H1N1 or swine flu) influenza.

If the provider records "suspected or possible or probable avian or novel H1N1 influenza (H1N1 or swine flu)," the appropriate influenza code from category 487 should be assigned. A code from category 488, Influenza due to certain identified influenza viruses, should not be assigned.

9. Chapter 9: Diseases of Digestive System (520-579)

Reserved for future guideline expansion

10. Chapter 10: Diseases of Genitourinary System (580-629)

a. **Chronic kidney disease**

1) Stages of chronic kidney disease (CKD)

The ICD-9-CM classifies CKD based on severity. The severity of CKD is designated by stages I-V. Stage II, code 585.2, equates to mild CKD; stage III, code 585.3, equates to moderate CKD; and stage IV, code 585.4, equates to severe CKD. Code 585.6, End stage renal disease (ESRD), is assigned when the provider has documented end-stage-renal disease (ESRD).

If both a stage of CKD and ESRD are documented, assign code 585.6 only.

2) Chronic kidney disease and kidney transplant status

Patients who have undergone kidney transplant may still have some form of CKD, because the kidney transplant may not fully restore kidney function. Therefore, the presence of CKD alone does not constitute a transplant complication. Assign the appropriate 585 code for the patient's stage of CKD and code V42.0. If a transplant complication such as failure or rejection is documented, *see section I.C.17.f.2.b* for information on coding complications of a kidney transplant. If the documentation is unclear as to whether the patient has a complication of the transplant, query the provider.

3) Chronic kidney disease with other conditions

Patients with CKD may also suffer from other serious conditions, most commonly diabetes mellitus and hypertension. The sequencing of the CKD code in relationship to codes for other contributing conditions is based on the conventions in the tabular list.

See I.C.3.a.4 for sequencing instructions for diabetes. See I.C.4.a.1 for anemia in CKD. See I.C.7.a.3 for hypertensive chronic kidney disease. See I.C.17.f.2.b, Kidney transplant complications, for instructions on coding of documented rejection or failure.

11. Chapter 11: Complications of Pregnancy, Childbirth, and the Puerperium (630-679)

a. **General Rules for Obstetric Cases**

1) Codes from chapter 11 and sequencing priority

Obstetric cases require codes from chapter 11, codes in the range 630-679, Complications of Pregnancy, Childbirth, and the Puerperium. Chapter 11 codes have sequencing priority over codes from other chapters. Additional codes from other chapters may be used in conjunction with chapter 11 codes to further specify conditions. Should the provider document that the pregnancy is incidental to the encounter, then code V22.2 should be used in place of any chapter 11 codes. It is the provider's responsibility to state that the condition being treated is not affecting the pregnancy.

2) Chapter 11 codes used only on the maternal record

Chapter 11 codes are to be used only on the maternal record, never on the record of the newborn.

3) Chapter 11 fifth-digits

Categories 640-648, 651-676 have required fifth-digits, which indicate whether the encounter is antepartum, postpartum and whether a delivery has also occurred.

4) Fifth-digits, appropriate for each code

The fifth-digits, which are appropriate for each code number, are listed in brackets under each code. The fifth-digits on each code should all be consistent with each other. That is, should a delivery occur all of the fifth-digits should indicate the delivery.

b. **Selection of OB Principal or First-listed Diagnosis**

1) Routine outpatient prenatal visits

For routine outpatient prenatal visits when no complications are present codes V22.0, Supervision of normal first pregnancy, and V22.1, Supervision of other normal pregnancy, should be used as the first-listed diagnoses. These codes should not be used in conjunction with chapter 11 codes.

2) Prenatal outpatient visits for high-risk patients

For routine prenatal outpatient visits for patients with high-risk pregnancies, a code from category V23, Supervision of high-risk pregnancy, should be used as the first-listed diagnosis. Secondary chapter 11 codes may be used in conjunction with these codes if appropriate.

3) Episodes when no delivery occurs

In episodes when no delivery occurs, the principal diagnosis should correspond to the principal complication of the pregnancy, which necessitated the encounter. Should more than one complication exist, all of which are treated or monitored, any of the complications codes may be sequenced first.

4) When a delivery occurs

When a delivery occurs, the principal diagnosis should correspond to the main circumstances or complication of the delivery. In cases of cesarean delivery, the selection of the principal diagnosis should be the condition established after study that was responsible for the patient's admission. If the patient was admitted with a condition that resulted in the performance of a cesarean procedure, that condition should be selected as the principal diagnosis. If the reason for the admission/encounter was unrelated to the condition resulting in the cesarean delivery, the condition related to the reason for the admission/encounter should be selected as the principal diagnosis, even if a cesarean was performed.

5) Outcome of delivery

An outcome of delivery code, V27.0-V27.9, should be included on every maternal record when a delivery has occurred. These codes are not to be used on subsequent records or on the newborn record.

c. **Fetal Conditions Affecting the Management of the Mother**

1) Codes from category 655

Known or suspected fetal abnormality affecting management of the mother, and category 656, Other fetal and placental problems affecting the management of the mother, are assigned only when the fetal condition is actually responsible for modifying the management of the mother, i.e., by requiring diagnostic studies, additional observation, special care, or termination of pregnancy.

The fact that the fetal condition exists does not justify assigning a code from this series to the mother's record.

See I.C.18.d. for suspected maternal and fetal conditions not found

2) In utero surgery

In cases when surgery is performed on the fetus, a diagnosis code from category 655, Known or suspected fetal abnormalities affecting management of the mother, should be assigned identifying the fetal condition. Procedure code 75.36, Correction of fetal defect, should be assigned on the hospital inpatient record.

No code from Chapter 15, the perinatal codes, should be used on the mother's record to identify fetal conditions. Surgery performed in utero on a fetus is still to be coded as an obstetric encounter.

d. HIV Infection in Pregnancy, Childbirth and the Puerperium

During pregnancy, childbirth or the puerperium, a patient admitted because of an HIV-related illness should receive a principal diagnosis of 647.6X, Other specified infectious and parasitic diseases in the mother classifiable elsewhere, but complicating the pregnancy, childbirth or the puerperium, followed by 042 and the code(s) for the HIV-related illness(es).

Patients with asymptomatic HIV infection status admitted during pregnancy, childbirth, or the puerperium should receive codes of 647.6X and V08.

e. Current Conditions Complicating Pregnancy

Assign a code from subcategory 648.x for patients that have current conditions when the condition affects the management of the pregnancy, childbirth, or the puerperium. Use additional secondary codes from other chapters to identify the conditions, as appropriate.

f. Diabetes mellitus in pregnancy

Diabetes mellitus is a significant complicating factor in pregnancy. Pregnant women who are diabetic should be assigned code 648.0x, Diabetes mellitus complicating pregnancy, and a secondary code from category 250, Diabetes mellitus, or category 249, Secondary diabetes to identify the type of diabetes.

Code V58.67, Long-term (current) use of insulin, should also be assigned if the diabetes mellitus is being treated with insulin.

g. Gestational diabetes

Gestational diabetes can occur during the second and third trimester of pregnancy in women who were not diabetic prior to pregnancy. Gestational diabetes can cause complications in the pregnancy similar to those of pre-existing diabetes mellitus. It also puts the woman at greater risk of developing diabetes after the pregnancy. Gestational diabetes is coded to 648.8x, Abnormal glucose tolerance. Codes 648.0x and 648.8x should never be used together on the same record.

Code V58.67, Long-term (current) use of insulin, should also be assigned if the gestational diabetes is being treated with insulin.

h. Normal Delivery, Code 650

1) Normal delivery

Code 650 is for use in cases when a woman is admitted for a full-term normal delivery and delivers a single, healthy infant without any complications antepartum, during the delivery, or postpartum during the delivery episode. Code 650 is always a principal diagnosis. It is not to be used if any other code from chapter 11 is needed to describe a current complication of the antenatal, delivery, or perinatal period. Additional codes from other chapters may be used with code 650 if they are not related to or are in any way complicating the pregnancy.

2) Normal delivery with resolved antepartum complication

Code 650 may be used if the patient had a complication at some point during her pregnancy, but the complication is not present at the time of the admission for delivery.

3) V27.0, Single liveborn, outcome of delivery

V27.0, Single liveborn, is the only outcome of delivery code appropriate for use with 650.

i. The Postpartum and Peripartum Periods

1) Postpartum and peripartum periods

The postpartum period begins immediately after delivery and continues for six weeks following delivery. The peripartum period is defined as the last month of pregnancy to five months postpartum.

2) Postpartum complication

A postpartum complication is any complication occurring within the six-week period.

3) Pregnancy-related complications after 6 week period

Chapter 11 codes may also be used to describe pregnancy-related complications after the six-week period should the provider document that a condition is pregnancy related.

4) Postpartum complications occurring during the same admission as delivery

Postpartum complications that occur during the same admission as the delivery are identified with a fifth digit of "2." Subsequent admissions/encounters for postpartum complications should be identified with a fifth digit of "4."

5) Admission for routine postpartum care following delivery outside hospital

When the mother delivers outside the hospital prior to admission and is admitted for routine postpartum care and no complications are noted, code V24.0, Postpartum care and examination immediately after delivery, should be assigned as the principal diagnosis.

6) Admission following delivery outside hospital with postpartum conditions

A delivery diagnosis code should not be used for a woman who has delivered prior to admission to the hospital. Any postpartum conditions and/or postpartum procedures should be coded.

7) Puerperal sepsis

Code 670.2x, Puerperal sepsis, should be assigned with a secondary code to identify the causal organism (e.g., for a bacterial infection, assign a code from category 041, Bacterial infections in conditions classified elsewhere and of unspecified site). A code from category 038, Septicemia, should not be used for puerperal sepsis. Do not assign code 995.91, Sepsis, as code 670.2x describes the sepsis. If applicable, use additional codes to identify severe sepsis (995.92) and any associated acute organ dysfunction.

j. Code 677, Late effect of complication of pregnancy

1) Code 677

Code 677, Late effect of complication of pregnancy, childbirth, and the puerperium is for use in those cases when an initial complication of a pregnancy develops a sequelae requiring care or treatment at a future date.

2) After the initial postpartum period

This code may be used at any time after the initial postpartum period.

3) Sequencing of Code 677

This code, like all late effect codes, is to be sequenced following the code describing the sequelae of the complication.

k. Abortions

1) Fifth-digits required for abortion categories

Fifth-digits are required for abortion categories 634-637. Fifth digit assignment is based on the status of the patient at the beginning (or start) of the encounter. Fifth-digit 1, incomplete, indicates that all of the products of conception have not been expelled from the uterus. Fifth-digit 2, complete, indicates that all products of conception have been expelled from the uterus.

2) Code from categories 640-648 and 651-659

A code from categories 640-648 and 651-659 may be used as additional codes with an abortion code to indicate the complication leading to the abortion.

Fifth digit 3 is assigned with codes from these categories when used with an abortion code because the other fifth digits will not apply. Codes from the 660-669 series are not to be used for complications of abortion.

3) Code 639 for complications

Code 639 is to be used for all complications following abortion. Code 639 cannot be assigned with codes from categories 634-638.

4) Abortion with Liveborn Fetus

When an attempted termination of pregnancy results in a liveborn fetus assign code 644.21, Early onset of delivery, with an appropriate code from category V27, Outcome of Delivery. The procedure code for the attempted termination of pregnancy should also be assigned.

5) Retained Products of Conception following an abortion

Subsequent admissions for retained products of conception following a spontaneous or legally induced abortion are assigned the appropriate code from category 634, Spontaneous abortion, or 635 Legally induced abortion, with a fifth digit of "1" (incomplete).

This advice is appropriate even when the patient was discharged previously with a discharge diagnosis of complete abortion.

12. Chapter 12: Diseases Skin & Subcutaneous Tissue (680-709)

a. Pressure ulcer stage codes

1) Pressure ulcer stages

Two codes are needed to completely describe a pressure ulcer: A code from subcategory 707.0, Pressure ulcer, to identify the site of the pressure ulcer and a code from subcategory 707.2, Pressure ulcer stages.

The codes in subcategory 707.2, Pressure ulcer stages, are to be used as an additional diagnosis with a code(s) from subcategory 707.0, Pressure Ulcer. Codes from 707.2, Pressure ulcer stages, may not be assigned as a principal or first-listed diagnosis. The pressure ulcer stage codes should only be used with pressure ulcers and not with other types of ulcers (e.g., stasis ulcer).

The ICD-9-CM classifies pressure ulcer stages based on severity, which is designated by stages I-IV and unstageable.

2) Unstageable pressure ulcers

Assignment of code 707.25, Pressure ulcer, unstageable, should be based on the clinical documentation. Code 707.25 is used for pressure ulcers whose stage cannot be clinically determined (e.g., the ulcer is covered by eschar or has been treated with a skin or muscle graft) and pressure ulcers that are documented as deep tissue injury but not documented as due to trauma. This code should not be confused with code 707.20, Pressure ulcer, stage unspecified. Code 707.20 should be assigned when there is no documentation regarding the stage of the pressure ulcer.

3) Documented pressure ulcer stage

Assignment of the pressure ulcer stage code should be guided by clinical documentation of the stage or documentation of the terms found in the index. For clinical terms describing the stage that are not found in the index, and there is no documentation of the stage, the provider should be queried.

4) Bilateral pressure ulcers with same stage

When a patient has bilateral pressure ulcers (e.g., both buttocks) and both pressure ulcers are documented as being the same stage, only the code for the site and one code for the stage should be reported.

5) Bilateral pressure ulcers with different stages

When a patient has bilateral pressure ulcers at the same site (e.g., both buttocks) and each pressure ulcer is documented as being at a different stage, assign one code for the site and the appropriate codes for the pressure ulcer stage.

6) Multiple pressure ulcers of different sites and stages

When a patient has multiple pressure ulcers at different sites (e.g., buttock, heel, shoulder) and each pressure ulcer is documented as being at different stages (e.g., stage 3 and stage 4), assign the appropriate codes for each different site and a code for each different pressure ulcer stage.

7) Patients admitted with pressure ulcers documented as healed

No code is assigned if the documentation states that the pressure ulcer is completely healed.

8) Patients admitted with pressure ulcers documented as healing

Pressure ulcers described as healing should be assigned the appropriate pressure ulcer stage code based on the documentation in the medical record. If the documentation does not provide information about the stage of the healing pressure ulcer, assign code 707.20, Pressure ulcer stage, unspecified.

If the documentation is unclear as to whether the patient has a current (new) pressure ulcer or if the patient is being treated for a healing pressure ulcer, query the provider.

9) Patient admitted with pressure ulcer evolving into another stage during the admission

If a patient is admitted with a pressure ulcer at one stage and it progresses to a higher stage, assign the code for highest stage reported for that site.

13. Chapter 13: Diseases of Musculoskeletal and Connective Tissue (710-739)

a. Coding of Pathologic Fractures

1) Acute Fractures vs. Aftercare

Pathologic fractures are reported using subcategory 733.1, when the fracture is newly diagnosed. Subcategory 733.1 may be used while the patient is receiving active treatment for the fracture. Examples of active treatment are: surgical treatment, emergency department encounter, evaluation and treatment by a new physician.

Fractures are coded using the aftercare codes (subcategories V54.0, V54.2, V54.8 or V54.9) for encounters after the patient has completed active treatment of the fracture and is receiving routine care for the fracture during the healing or recovery phase. Examples of fracture aftercare are: cast change or removal, removal of external or internal fixation device, medication adjustment, and follow up visits following fracture treatment.

Care for complications of surgical treatment for fracture repairs during the healing or recovery phase should be coded with the appropriate complication codes.

Care of complications of fractures, such as malunion and nonunion, should be reported with the appropriate codes.

See Section I. C. 17.b for information on the coding of traumatic fractures.

14. Chapter 14: Congenital Anomalies (740-759)

a. Codes in categories 740-759, Congenital Anomalies

Assign an appropriate code(s) from categories 740-759, Congenital Anomalies, when an anomaly is documented. A congenital anomaly may be the principal/first listed diagnosis on a record or a secondary diagnosis.

When a congenital anomaly does not have a unique code assignment, assign additional code(s) for any manifestations that may be present.

When the code assignment specifically identifies the congenital anomaly, manifestations that are an inherent component of the anomaly should not be coded separately. Additional codes should be assigned for manifestations that are not an inherent component.

Codes from Chapter 14 may be used throughout the life of the patient. If a congenital anomaly has been corrected, a personal history code should be used to identify the history of the anomaly. Although present at birth, a congenital anomaly may not be identified until later in life. Whenever the condition is diagnosed by the physician, it is appropriate to assign a code from codes 740-759.

For the birth admission, the appropriate code from category V30, Liveborn infants, according to type of birth should be sequenced as the principal diagnosis, followed by any congenital anomaly codes, 740-759.

15. Chapter 15: Newborn (Perinatal) Guidelines (760-779)

For coding and reporting purposes the perinatal period is defined as before birth through the 28th day following birth. The following guidelines are provided for reporting purposes. Hospitals may record other diagnoses as needed for internal data use.

a. General Perinatal Rules

1) Chapter 15 Codes

They are never for use on the maternal record. Codes from Chapter 11, the obstetric chapter, are never permitted on the newborn record. Chapter 15 code may be used throughout the life of the patient if the condition is still present.

2) Sequencing of perinatal codes

Generally, codes from Chapter 15 should be sequenced as the principal/first-listed diagnosis on the newborn record, with the exception of the appropriate V30 code for the birth episode, followed by codes from any other chapter that provide additional detail. The "use additional code" note at the beginning of the chapter supports this guideline. If the index does not provide a specific code for a perinatal condition, assign code 779.89, Other specified conditions originating in the perinatal period, followed by the code from another chapter that specifies the condition. Codes for signs and symptoms may be assigned when a definitive diagnosis has not been established.

3) Birth process or community acquired conditions

If a newborn has a condition that may be either due to the birth process or community acquired and the documentation does not indicate which it is, the default is due to the birth process and the code from Chapter 15 should be used. If the condition is community-acquired, a code from Chapter 15 should not be assigned.

4) Code all clinically significant conditions

All clinically significant conditions noted on routine newborn examination should be coded. A condition is clinically significant if it requires:

- clinical evaluation; or
- therapeutic treatment; or
- diagnostic procedures; or
- extended length of hospital stay; or

- increased nursing care and/or monitoring; or
- has implications for future health care needs

Note: The perinatal guidelines listed above are the same as the general coding guidelines for "additional diagnoses", except for the final point regarding implications for future health care needs. Codes should be assigned for conditions that have been specified by the provider as having implications for future health care needs. Codes from the perinatal chapter should not be assigned unless the provider has established a definitive diagnosis.

b. Use of codes V30-V39

When coding the birth of an infant, assign a code from categories V30-V39, according to the type of birth. A code from this series is assigned as a principal diagnosis, and assigned only once to a newborn at the time of birth.

c. Newborn transfers

If the newborn is transferred to another institution, the V30 series is not used at the receiving hospital.

d. Use of category V29

1) Assigning a code from category V29

Assign a code from category V29, Observation and evaluation of newborns and infants for suspected conditions not found, to identify those instances when a healthy newborn is evaluated for a suspected condition that is determined after study not to be present. Do not use a code from category V29 when the patient has identified signs or symptoms of a suspected problem; in such cases, code the sign or symptom.

A code from category V29 may also be assigned as a principal code for readmissions or encounters when the V30 code no longer applies. Codes from category V29 are for use only for healthy newborns and infants for which no condition after study is found to be present.

2) V29 code on a birth record

A V29 code is to be used as a secondary code after the V30, Outcome of delivery, code.

e. Use of other V codes on perinatal records

V codes other than V30 and V29 may be assigned on a perinatal or newborn record code. The codes may be used as a principal or first-listed diagnosis for specific types of encounters or for readmissions or encounters when the V30 code no longer applies.

See Section I.C.18 for information regarding the assignment of V codes.

f. Maternal Causes of Perinatal Morbidity

Codes from categories 760-763, Maternal causes of perinatal morbidity and mortality, are assigned only when the maternal condition has actually affected the fetus or newborn. The fact that the mother has an associated medical condition or experiences some complication of pregnancy, labor or delivery does not justify the routine assignment of codes from these categories to the newborn record.

g. Congenital Anomalies in Newborns

For the birth admission, the appropriate code from category V30, Liveborn infants according to type of birth, should be used, followed by any congenital anomaly codes, categories 740-759. Use additional secondary codes from other chapters to specify conditions associated with the anomaly, if applicable.

Also, see Section I.C.14 for information on the coding of congenital anomalies.

h. Coding Additional Perinatal Diagnoses

1) Assigning codes for conditions that require treatment

Assign codes for conditions that require treatment or further investigation, prolong the length of stay, or require resource utilization.

2) Codes for conditions specified as having implications for future health care needs

Assign codes for conditions that have been specified by the provider as having implications for future health care needs.

Note: This guideline should not be used for adult patients.

3) Codes for newborn conditions originating in the perinatal period

Assign a code for newborn conditions originating in the perinatal period (categories 760-779), as well as complications arising during the current episode of care classified in other chapters, only if the diagnoses have been documented by the responsible provider at the time of transfer or discharge as having affected the fetus or newborn.

i. Prematurity and Fetal Growth Retardation

Providers utilize different criteria in determining prematurity. A code for prematurity should not be assigned unless it is documented. The 5th digit assignment for codes from category 764 and subcategories 765.0 and 765.1 should be based on the recorded birth weight and estimated gestational age. A code from subcategory 765.2, Weeks of gestation, should be assigned as an additional code with category 764 and codes from 765.0 and 765.1 to specify weeks of gestation as documented by the provider in the record.

j. Newborn sepsis

Code 771.81, Septicemia [sepsis] of newborn, should be assigned with a secondary code from category 041, Bacterial infections in conditions classified elsewhere and of unspecified site, to identify the organism. A code from category 038, Septicemia, should not be used on a newborn record. Do not assign code 995.91, Sepsis, as code 771.81 describes the sepsis. If applicable, use additional codes to identify severe sepsis (995.92) and any associated acute organ dysfunction.

16. Chapter 16: Signs, Symptoms and Ill-Defined Conditions (780-799)

Reserved for future guideline expansion

17. Chapter 17: Injury and Poisoning (800-999)

a. Coding of Injuries

When coding injuries, assign separate codes for each injury unless a combination code is provided, in which case the combination code is assigned. Multiple injury codes are provided in ICD-9-CM, but should not be assigned unless information for a more specific code is not available. These traumatic injury codes are not to be used for normal, healing surgical wounds or to identify complications of surgical wounds.

The code for the most serious injury, as determined by the provider and the focus of treatment, is sequenced first.

1) Superficial injuries

Superficial injuries such as abrasions or contusions are not coded when associated with more severe injuries of the same site.

2) Primary injury with damage to nerves/blood vessels

When a primary injury results in minor damage to peripheral nerves or blood vessels, the primary injury is sequenced first with additional code(s) from categories 950-957, Injury to nerves and spinal cord, and/or 900-904, Injury to blood vessels. When the primary injury is to the blood vessels or nerves, that injury should be sequenced first.

b. Coding of Traumatic Fractures

The principles of multiple coding of injuries should be followed in coding fractures. Fractures of specified sites are coded individually by site in accordance with both the provisions within categories 800-829 and the level of detail furnished by medical record content. Combination categories for multiple fractures are provided for use when there is insufficient detail in the medical record (such as trauma cases transferred to another hospital), when the reporting form limits the number of codes that can be used in reporting pertinent clinical data, or when there is insufficient specificity at the fourth-digit or fifth-digit level. More specific guidelines are as follows:

1) Acute Fractures vs. Aftercare

Traumatic fractures are coded using the acute fracture codes (800-829) while the patient is receiving active treatment for the fracture. Examples of active treatment are: surgical treatment, emergency department encounter, and evaluation and treatment by a new physician.

Fractures are coded using the aftercare codes (subcategories V54.0, V54.1, V54.8, or V54.9) for encounters after the patient has completed active treatment of the fracture and is receiving routine care for the fracture during the healing or recovery phase. Examples of fracture aftercare are: cast change or removal, removal of external or internal fixation device, medication adjustment, and follow up visits following fracture treatment.

Care for complications of surgical treatment for fracture repairs during the healing or recovery phase should be coded with the appropriate complication codes.

Care of complications of fractures, such as malunion and nonunion, should be reported with the appropriate codes.

Pathologic fractures are not coded in the 800-829 range, but instead are assigned to subcategory 733.1. *See Section I.C.13.a for additional information.*

2) Multiple fractures of same limb

Multiple fractures of same limb classifiable to the same three-digit or four-digit category are coded to that category.

3) Multiple unilateral or bilateral fractures of same bone

Multiple unilateral or bilateral fractures of same bone(s) but classified to different fourth-digit subdivisions (bone part) within the same three-digit category are coded individually by site.

4) Multiple fracture categories 819 and 828

Multiple fracture categories 819 and 828 classify bilateral fractures of both upper limbs (819) and both lower limbs (828), but without any detail at the fourth-digit level other than open and closed type of fractures.

5) Multiple fractures sequencing

Multiple fractures are sequenced in accordance with the severity of the fracture. The provider should be asked to list the fracture diagnoses in the order of severity.

c. Coding of Burns

Current burns (940-948) are classified by depth, extent and by agent (E code). Burns are classified by depth as first degree (erythema), second degree (blistering), and third degree (full-thickness involvement).

1) Sequencing of burn and related condition codes

Sequence first the code that reflects the highest degree of burn when more than one burn is present.

a. When the reason for the admission or encounter is for treatment of external multiple burns, sequence first the code that reflects the burn of the highest degree.

b. When a patient has both internal and external burns, the circumstances of admission govern the selection of the principal diagnosis or first-listed diagnosis.

c. When a patient is admitted for burn injuries and other related conditions such as smoke inhalation and/or respiratory failure, the circumstances of admission govern the selection of the principal or first-listed diagnosis.

2) Burns of the same local site

Classify burns of the same local site (three-digit category level, 940-947) but of different degrees to the subcategory identifying the highest degree recorded in the diagnosis.

3) Non-healing burns

Non-healing burns are coded as acute burns.

Necrosis of burned skin should be coded as a non-healed burn.

4) Code 958.3, Posttraumatic wound infection

Assign code 958.3, Posttraumatic wound infection, not elsewhere classified, as an additional code for any documented infected burn site.

5) Assign separate codes for each burn site

When coding burns, assign separate codes for each burn site. Category 946 Burns of Multiple specified sites, should only be used if the location of the burns are not documented.

Category 949, Burn, unspecified, is extremely vague and should rarely be used.

6) Assign codes from category 948, Burns

Burns classified according to extent of body surface involved, when the site of the burn is not specified or when there is a need for additional data. It is advisable to use category 948 as additional coding when needed to provide data for evaluating burn mortality, such as that needed by burn units. It is also advisable to use category 948 as an additional code for reporting purposes when there is mention of a third-degree burn involving 20 percent or more of the body surface.

In assigning a code from category 948:

Fourth-digit codes are used to identify the percentage of total body surface involved in a burn (all degree).

Fifth-digits are assigned to identify the percentage of body surface involved in third-degree burn.

Fifth-digit zero (0) is assigned when less than 10 percent or when no body surface is involved in a third-degree burn.

Category 948 is based on the classic "rule of nines" in estimating body surface involved: head and neck are assigned nine percent, each arm nine percent, each leg 18 percent, the anterior trunk 18 percent, posterior trunk 18 percent, and genitalia one percent. Providers may change these percentage assignments where necessary to accommodate infants and children who have proportionately larger heads than adults and patients who have large buttocks, thighs, or abdomen that involve burns.

7) Encounters for treatment of late effects of burns

Encounters for the treatment of the late effects of burns (i.e., scars or joint contractures) should be coded to the residual condition (sequelae) followed by the appropriate late effect code (906.5-906.9). A late effect E code may also be used, if desired.

8) Sequelae with a late effect code and current burn

When appropriate, both a sequelae with a late effect code, and a current burn code may be assigned on the same record (when both a current burn and sequelae of an old burn exist).

d. Coding of Debridement of Wound, Infection, or Burn

Excisional debridement involves surgical removal or cutting away, as opposed to a mechanical (brushing, scrubbing, washing) debridement. For coding purposes, excisional debridement is assigned to code 86.22. Nonexcisional debridement is assigned to code 86.28.

e. Adverse Effects, Poisoning and Toxic Effects

The properties of certain drugs, medicinal and biological substances or combinations of such substances, may cause toxic reactions. The occurrence of drug toxicity is classified in ICD-9-CM as follows:

1) Adverse Effect

When the drug was correctly prescribed and properly administered, code the reaction plus the appropriate code from the E930-E949 series. Codes from the E930-E949 series must be used to identify the causative substance for an adverse effect of drug, medicinal and biological substances, correctly prescribed and properly administered. The effect, such as tachycardia, delirium, gastrointestinal hemorrhaging, vomiting, hypokalemia, hepatitis, renal failure, or respiratory failure, is coded and followed by the appropriate code from the E930-E949 series.

Adverse effects of therapeutic substances correctly prescribed and properly administered (toxicity, synergistic reaction, side effect, and idiosyncratic reaction) may be due to (1) differences among patients, such as age, sex, disease, and genetic factors, and (2) drug-related factors, such as type of drug, route of administration, duration of therapy, dosage, and bioavailability.

2) Poisoning

(a) Error was made in drug prescription

Errors made in drug prescription or in the administration of the drug by provider, nurse, patient, or other person, use the appropriate poisoning code from the 960-979 series.

(b) Overdose of a drug intentionally taken

If an overdose of a drug was intentionally taken or administered and resulted in drug toxicity, it would be coded as a poisoning (960-979 series).

(c) Nonprescribed drug taken with correctly prescribed and properly administered drug

If a nonprescribed drug or medicinal agent was taken in combination with a correctly prescribed and properly administered drug, any drug toxicity or other reaction resulting from the interaction of the two drugs would be classified as a poisoning.

(d) Interaction of drug(s) and alcohol

When a reaction results from the interaction of a drug(s) and alcohol, this would be classified as poisoning.

(e) Sequencing of poisoning

When coding a poisoning or reaction to the improper use of a medication (e.g., wrong dose, wrong substance, wrong route of administration) the poisoning code is sequenced first, followed by a code for the manifestation. If there is also a diagnosis of drug abuse or dependence to the substance, the abuse or dependence is coded as an additional code.

See Section I.C.3.a.6.b. if poisoning is the result of insulin pump malfunctions and Section I.C.19 for general use of E-codes.

3) Toxic Effects

(a) Toxic effect codes

When a harmful substance is ingested or comes in contact with a person, this is classified as a toxic effect. The toxic effect codes are in categories 980-989.

(b) Sequencing toxic effect codes

A toxic effect code should be sequenced first, followed by the code(s) that identify the result of the toxic effect.

(c) External cause codes for toxic effects

An external cause code from categories E860-E869 for accidental exposure, codes E950.6 or E950.7 for intentional self-harm, category E962 for assault, or categories E980-E982, for undetermined, should also be assigned to indicate intent.

f. Complications of care

1) Complications of care

(a) Documentation of complications of care

As with all procedural or postprocedural complications, code assignment is based on the provider's documentation of the relationship between the condition and the procedure.

2) Transplant complications

(a) Transplant complications other than kidney

Codes under subcategory 996.8, Complications of transplanted organ, are for use for both complications and rejection of transplanted organs. A transplant complication code is only assigned if the complication affects the function of the transplanted organ. Two codes are required to fully describe a transplant complication, the appropriate code from subcategory 996.8 and a secondary code that identifies the complication.

Pre-existing conditions or conditions that develop after the transplant are not coded as complications unless they affect the function of the transplanted organs.

See I.C.18.d.3) for transplant organ removal status. See I.C.2.i for malignant neoplasm associated with transplanted organ.

(b) Chronic kidney disease and kidney transplant complications

Patients who have undergone kidney transplant may still have some form of chronic kidney disease (CKD) because the kidney transplant may not fully restore kidney function. Code 996.81 should be assigned for documented complications of a kidney transplant, such as transplant failure or rejection or other transplant complication. Code 996.81 should not be assigned for post kidney transplant patients who have chronic kidney (CKD) unless a transplant complication such as transplant failure or rejection is documented. If the documentation is unclear as to whether the patient has a complication of the transplant, query the provider.

For patients with CKD following a kidney transplant, but who do not have a complication such as failure or rejection, *see section I.C.10.a.2, Chronic kidney disease and kidney transplant status.*

3) Ventilator associated pneumonia

(a) Documentation of Ventilator associated Pneumonia

As with all procedural or postprocedural complications, code assignment is based on the provider's documentation of the relationship between the condition and the procedure.

Code 997.31, Ventilator associated pneumonia, should be assigned only when the provider has documented ventilator associated pneumonia (VAP). An additional code to identify the organism (e.g., Pseudomonas aeruginosa, code 041.7) should also be assigned. Do not assign an additional code from categories 480-484 to identify the type of pneumonia.

Code 997.31 should not be assigned for cases where the patient has pneumonia and is on a mechanical ventilator but the provider has not specifically stated that the pneumonia is ventilator-associated pneumonia.

If the documentation is unclear as to whether the patient has a pneumonia that is a complication attributable to the mechanical ventilator, query the provider.

(b) Patient admitted with pneumonia and develops VAP

A patient may be admitted with one type of pneumonia (e.g., code 481, Pneumococcal pneumonia) and subsequently develop VAP. In this instance, the principal diagnosis would be the appropriate code from categories 480-484 for the pneumonia diagnosed at the time of admission. Code 997.31, Ventilator associated pneumonia, would be assigned as an additional diagnosis when the provider has also documented the presence of ventilator associated pneumonia.

g. SIRS due to Non-infectious Process

The systemic inflammatory response syndrome (SIRS) can develop as a result of certain non-infectious disease processes, such as trauma, malignant neoplasm, or pancreatitis. When SIRS is documented with a noninfectious condition, and no subsequent infection is documented, the code for the underlying condition, such as an injury, should be assigned, followed by code 995.93, Systemic inflammatory response syndrome due to noninfectious process without acute organ dysfunction, or 995.94, Systemic inflammatory response syndrome due to non-infectious process with acute organ dysfunction. If an acute organ dysfunction is documented, the appropriate code(s) for the associated acute organ dysfunction(s) should be assigned in addition to code 995.94. If acute organ dysfunction is documented, but it cannot be determined if the acute organ dysfunction is associated with SIRS or due to another condition (e.g., directly due to the trauma), the provider should be queried.

When the non-infectious condition has led to an infection that results in SIRS, *see Section I.C.1.b.12 for the guideline for sepsis and severe sepsis associated with a non-infectious process.*

18. Classification of Factors Influencing Health Status and Contact with Health Service (Supplemental V01-V89)

Note: The chapter specific guidelines provide additional information about the use of V codes for specified encounters.

a. Introduction

ICD-9-CM provides codes to deal with encounters for circumstances other than a disease or injury. The Supplementary Classification of Factors Influencing Health Status and Contact with Health Services (V01.0 - V89.09) is provided to deal with occasions when circumstances other than a disease or injury (codes 001-999) are recorded as a diagnosis or problem.

There are four primary circumstances for the use of V codes:

1) A person who is not currently sick encounters the health services for some specific reason, such as to act as an organ donor, to receive prophylactic care, such as inoculations or health screenings, or to receive counseling on health related issues.
2) A person with a resolving disease or injury, or a chronic, long-term condition requiring continuous care, encounters the health care system for specific aftercare of that disease or injury (e.g., dialysis for renal disease; chemotherapy for malignancy; cast change). A diagnosis/symptom code should be used whenever a current, acute, diagnosis is being treated or a sign or symptom is being studied.
3) Circumstances or problems influence a person's health status but are not in themselves a current illness or injury.
4) Newborns, to indicate birth status

b. V codes use in any healthcare setting

V codes are for use in any healthcare setting. V codes may be used as either a first listed (principal diagnosis code in the inpatient setting) or secondary code, depending on the circumstances of the encounter. Certain V codes may only be used as first listed, others only as secondary codes.

See Section I.C.18.e, V Codes That May Only be Principal/First-Listed Diagnosis.

c. V Codes indicate a reason for an encounter

They are not procedure codes. A corresponding procedure code must accompany a V code to describe the procedure performed.

d. Categories of V Codes

1) Contact/Exposure

Category V01 indicates contact with or exposure to communicable diseases. These codes are for patients who do not show any sign or symptom of a disease but have been exposed to it by close personal contact with an infected individual or are in an area where a disease is epidemic. These codes may be used as a first listed code to explain an encounter for testing, or, more commonly, as a secondary code to identify a potential risk.

2) Inoculations and vaccinations

Categories V03-V06 are for encounters for inoculations and vaccinations. They indicate that a patient is being seen to receive a prophylactic inoculation against a disease. The injection itself must be represented by the appropriate procedure code. A code from V03-V06 may be used as a secondary code if the inoculation is given as a routine part of preventive health care, such as a well-baby visit.

3) Status

Status codes indicate that a patient is either a carrier of a disease or has the sequelae or residual of a past disease or condition. This includes such things as the presence of prosthetic or mechanical devices resulting from past treatment. A status code is informative, because the status may affect the course of treatment and its outcome. A status code is distinct from a history code. The history code indicates that the patient no longer has the condition.

A status code should not be used with a diagnosis code from one of the body system chapters, if the diagnosis code includes the information provided by the status code. For example, code V42.1, Heart transplant status, should not be used with code 996.83, Complications of transplanted heart. The status code does not provide additional information. The complication code indicates that the patient is a heart transplant patient.

The status V codes/categories are:

V02 Carrier or suspected carrier of infectious diseases
Carrier status indicates that a person harbors the specific organisms of a disease without manifest symptoms and is capable of transmitting the infection.

V07.5x Prophylactic use of agents affecting estrogen receptors and estrogen level
This code indicates when a patient is receiving a drug that affects estrogen receptors and estrogen levels for prevention of cancer.

V08 Asymptomatic HIV infection status
This code indicates that a patient has tested positive for HIV but has manifested no signs or symptoms of the disease.

V09 Infection with drug-resistant microorganisms
This category indicates that a patient has an infection that is resistant to drug treatment. Sequence the infection code first.

V21 Constitutional states in development

V22.2 Pregnant state, incidental
This code is a secondary code only for use when the pregnancy is in no way complicating the reason for visit. Otherwise, a code from the obstetric chapter is required.

V26.5x Sterilization status

V42 Organ or tissue replaced by transplant

V43 Organ or tissue replaced by other means

V44 Artificial opening status

V45 Other postsurgical states
Assign code V45.87, Transplant organ removal status, to indicate that a transplanted organ has been previously removed. This code should not be assigned for the encounter in which the transplanted organ is removed. The complication necessitating removal of the transplant organ should be assigned for that encounter.
See section I.C17.f.2. for information on the coding of organ transplant complications.
Assign code V45.88, Status post administration of tPA (rtPA) in a different facility within the last 24 hours prior to admission to the current facility, as a secondary diagnosis when a patient is received by transfer into a facility and documentation indicates they were administered tissue plasminogen activator (tPA) within the last 24 hours prior to admission to the current facility.
This guideline applies even if the patient is still receiving the tPA at the time they are received into the current facility.
The appropriate code for the condition for which the tPA was administered (such as cerebrovascular disease or myocardial infarction) should be assigned first.
Code V45.88 is only applicable to the receiving facility record and not to the transferring facility record.

V46 Other dependence on machines

V49.6 Upper limb amputation status

V49.7 Lower limb amputation status
Note: Categories V42-V46, and subcategories V49.6, V49.7 are for use only if there are no complications or malfunctions of the organ or tissue replaced, the amputation site or the equipment on which the patient is dependent.

V49.81 Postmenopausal status

V49.82 Dental sealant status

V49.83 Awaiting organ transplant status

V58.6x Long-term (current) drug use
Codes from this subcategory indicate a patient's continuous use of a prescribed drug (including such things as aspirin therapy) for the long-term treatment of a condition or for prophylactic use. It is not for use for patients who have addictions to drugs. This subcategory is not for use of medications for detoxification or maintenance programs to prevent withdrawal symptoms in patients with drug dependence (e.g., methadone maintenance for opiate dependence). Assign the appropriate code for the drug dependence instead.
Assign a code from subcategory V58.6, Long-term (current) drug use, if the patient is receiving a medication for an extended period as a prophylactic measure (such as for the prevention of deep vein thrombosis) or as treatment of a chronic condition (such as arthritis) or a disease requiring a lengthy course of treatment (such as cancer). Do not assign a code from subcategory V58.6 for medication being administered for a brief period of time to treat an acute illness or injury (such as a course of antibiotics to treat acute bronchitis).

V83 Genetic carrier status
Genetic carrier status indicates that a person carries a gene, associated with a particular disease, which may be passed to offspring who may develop that disease. The person does not have the disease and is not at risk of developing the disease.

V84 Genetic susceptibility status
Genetic susceptibility indicates that a person has a gene that increases the risk of that person developing the disease.
Codes from category V84, Genetic susceptibility to disease, should not be used as principal or first-listed codes. If the patient has the condition to which he/she is susceptible, and that condition is the reason for the encounter, the code for the current condition should be sequenced first. If the patient is being seen for follow-up after completed treatment for this condition, and the condition no longer exists, a follow-up code should be sequenced first, followed by the appropriate personal history and genetic susceptibility codes. If the purpose of the encounter is genetic counseling associated with procreative management, a code from subcategory V26.3, Genetic counseling and testing, should be assigned as the first-listed code, followed by a code from category V84. Additional codes should be assigned for any applicable family or personal history.
See Section I.C. 18.d.14 for information on prophylactic organ removal due to a genetic susceptibility.

V85 Body Mass Index (BMI)

V86 Estrogen receptor status

V88 Acquired absence of other organs and tissue

4) History (of)

There are two types of history V codes, personal and family. Personal history codes explain a patient's past medical condition that no longer exists and is not receiving any treatment, but that has the potential for recurrence, and therefore may require continued monitoring. The exceptions to this general rule are category V14, Personal history of allergy to medicinal agents, and subcategory V15.0, Allergy, other than to medicinal agents. A person who has had an allergic episode to a substance or food in the past should always be considered allergic to the substance.

Family history codes are for use when a patient has a family member(s) who has had a particular disease that causes the patient to be at higher risk of also contracting the disease.

Personal history codes may be used in conjunction with follow-up codes and family history codes may be used in conjunction with screening codes to explain the need for a test or procedure. History codes are also acceptable on any medical record regardless of the reason for visit. A history of an illness, even if no longer present, is important information that may alter the type of treatment ordered.

The history V code categories are:

V10 Personal history of malignant neoplasm
V12 Personal history of certain other diseases
V13 Personal history of other diseases
Except: V13.4, Personal history of arthritis, and V13.6, Personal history of congenital malformations. These conditions are life-long so are not true history codes.
V14 Personal history of allergy to medicinal agents
V15 Other personal history presenting hazards to health
Except: V15.7, Personal history of contraception.
V16 Family history of malignant neoplasm
V17 Family history of certain chronic disabling diseases
V18 Family history of certain other specific diseases
V19 Family history of other conditions
V87 Other specified personal exposures and history presenting hazards to health

5) Screening

Screening is the testing for disease or disease precursors in seemingly well individuals so that early detection and treatment can be provided for those who test positive for the disease. Screenings that are recommended for many subgroups in a population include: routine mammograms for women over 40, a fecal occult blood test for everyone over 50, an amniocentesis to rule out a fetal anomaly for pregnant women over 35, because the incidence of breast cancer and colon cancer in these subgroups is higher than in the general population, as is the incidence of Down's syndrome in older mothers.

The testing of a person to rule out or confirm a suspected diagnosis because the patient has some sign or symptom is a diagnostic examination, not a screening. In these cases, the sign or symptom is used to explain the reason for the test.

A screening code may be a first listed code if the reason for the visit is specifically the screening exam. It may also be used as an additional code if the screening is done during an office visit for other health problems. A screening code is not necessary if the screening is inherent to a routine examination, such as a pap smear done during a routine pelvic examination.

Should a condition be discovered during the screening then the code for the condition may be assigned as an additional diagnosis.

The V code indicates that a screening exam is planned. A procedure code is required to confirm that the screening was performed.

The screening V code categories:

V28 Antenatal screening
V73-V82 Special screening examinations

6) Observation

There are three observation V code categories. They are for use in very limited circumstances when a person is being observed for a suspected condition that is ruled out. The observation codes are not for use if an injury or illness or any signs or symptoms related to the suspected condition are present. In such cases the diagnosis/symptom code is used with the corresponding E code to identify any external cause.

The observation codes are to be used as principal diagnosis only. The only exception to this is when the principal diagnosis is required to be a code from the V30, Live born infant, category. Then the V29 observation code is sequenced after the V30 code. Additional codes may be used in addition to the observation code but only if they are unrelated to the suspected condition being observed.

Codes from subcategory V89.0, Suspected maternal and fetal conditions not found, may either be used as a first listed or as an additional code assignment depending on the case. They are for use in very limited circumstances on a maternal record when an encounter is for a suspected maternal or fetal condition that is ruled out during that encounter (for example, a maternal or fetal condition may be suspected due to an abnormal test result). These codes should not be used when the condition is confirmed. In those cases, the confirmed condition should be coded. In addition, these codes are not for use if an illness or any signs or symptoms related to the suspected condition or problem are present. In such cases the diagnosis/symptom code is used.

Additional codes may be used in addition to the code from subcategory V89.0, but only if they are unrelated to the suspected condition being evaluated.

Codes from subcategory V89.0 may not be used for encounters for antenatal screening of mother. *See Section I.C.18.d., Screening).*

For encounters for suspected fetal condition that are inconclusive following testing and evaluation, assign the appropriate code from category 655, 656, 657 or 658.

The observation V code categories:

V29 Observation and evaluation of newborns for suspected condition not found
For the birth encounter, a code from category V30 should be sequenced before the V29 code.
V71 Observation and evaluation for suspected condition not found
V89 Suspected maternal and fetal conditions not found

7) Aftercare

Aftercare visit codes cover situations when the initial treatment of a disease or injury has been performed and the patient requires continued care during the healing or recovery phase, or for the long-term consequences of the disease. The aftercare V code should not be used if treatment is directed at a current, acute disease or injury. The diagnosis code is to be used in these cases. Exceptions to this rule are codes V58.0, Radiotherapy, and codes from subcategory V58.1, Encounter for chemotherapy and immunotherapy for neoplastic conditions. These codes are to be first listed, followed by the diagnosis code when a patient's encounter is solely to receive radiation therapy or chemotherapy for the treatment of a neoplasm. Should a patient receive both chemotherapy and radiation therapy during the same encounter code V58.0 and V58.1 may be used together on a record with either one being sequenced first.

The aftercare codes are generally first listed to explain the specific reason for the encounter. An aftercare code may be used as an additional code when some type of aftercare is provided in addition to the reason for admission and no diagnosis code is applicable. An example of this would be the closure of a colostomy during an encounter for treatment of another condition.

Aftercare codes should be used in conjunction with any other aftercare codes or other diagnosis codes to provide better detail on the specifics of an aftercare encounter visit, unless otherwise directed by the classification. The sequencing of multiple aftercare codes is discretionary.

Certain aftercare V code categories need a secondary diagnosis code to describe the resolving condition or sequelae, for others, the condition is inherent in the code title.

Additional V code aftercare category terms include fitting and adjustment, and attention to artificial openings.

Status V codes may be used with aftercare V codes to indicate the nature of the aftercare. For example code V45.81, Aortocoronary bypass status, may be used with code V58.73, Aftercare following surgery of the circulatory system, NEC, to indicate the surgery for which the aftercare is being performed. Also, a transplant status code may be used following code V58.44, Aftercare following organ transplant, to identify the organ transplanted. A status code should not be used when the aftercare code indicates the type of status, such as using V55.0, Attention to tracheostomy with V44.0, Tracheostomy status.

See Section I. B.16 Admissions/Encounter for Rehabilitation

The aftercare V category/codes:

V51.0 Encounter for breast reconstruction following mastectomy
V52 Fitting and adjustment of prosthetic device and implant

V53 Fitting and adjustment of other device
V54 Other orthopedic aftercare
V55 Attention to artificial openings
V56 Encounter for dialysis and dialysis catheter care
V57 Care involving the use of rehabilitation procedures
V58.0 Radiotherapy
V58.11 Encounter for antineoplastic chemotherapy
V58.12 Encounter for antineoplastic immunotherapy
V58.3x Attention to dressings and sutures
V58.41 Encounter for planned post-operative wound closure
V58.42 Aftercare, surgery, neoplasm
V58.43 Aftercare, surgery, trauma
V58.44 Aftercare involving organ transplant
V58.49 Other specified aftercare following surgery
V58.7x Aftercare following surgery
V58.81 Fitting and adjustment of vascular catheter
V58.82 Fitting and adjustment of non-vascular catheter
V58.83 Monitoring therapeutic drug
V58.89 Other specified aftercare

8) Follow-up

The follow-up codes are used to explain continuing surveillance following completed treatment of a disease, condition, or injury. They imply that the condition has been fully treated and no longer exists. They should not be confused with aftercare codes that explain current treatment for a healing condition or its sequelae. Follow-up codes may be used in conjunction with history codes to provide the full picture of the healed condition and its treatment. The follow-up code is sequenced first, followed by the history code.

A follow-up code may be used to explain repeated visits. Should a condition be found to have recurred on the follow-up visit, then the diagnosis code should be used in place of the follow-up code.

The follow-up V code categories:

V24 Postpartum care and evaluation
V67 Follow-up examination

9) Donor

Category V59 is the donor codes. They are used for living individuals who are donating blood or other body tissue. These codes are only for individuals donating for others, not for self donations. They are not for use to identify cadaveric donations.

10) Counseling

Counseling V codes are used when a patient or family member receives assistance in the aftermath of an illness or injury, or when support is required in coping with family or social problems. They are not necessary for use in conjunction with a diagnosis code when the counseling component of care is considered integral to standard treatment.

The counseling V categories/codes:

V25.0 General counseling and advice for contraceptive management
V26.3 Genetic counseling
V26.4 General counseling and advice for procreative management
V61.X Other family circumstances
V65.1 Person consulted on behalf of another person
V65.3 Dietary surveillance and counseling
V65.4 Other counseling, not elsewhere classified

11) Obstetrics and related conditions

See Section I.C.11., the Obstetrics guidelines for further instruction on the use of these codes.

V codes for pregnancy are for use in those circumstances when none of the problems or complications included in the codes from the Obstetrics chapter exist (a routine prenatal visit or postpartum care). Codes V22.0, Supervision of normal first pregnancy, and V22.1, Supervision of other normal pregnancy, are always first listed and are not to be used with any other code from the OB chapter.

The outcome of delivery, category V27, should be included on all maternal delivery records. It is always a secondary code.

V codes for family planning (contraceptive) or procreative management and counseling should be included on an obstetric record either during the pregnancy or the postpartum stage, if applicable.

Obstetrics and related conditions V code categories:

V22 Normal pregnancy
V23 Supervision of high-risk pregnancy
Except: V23.2, Pregnancy with history of abortion. Code 646.3, Habitual aborter, from the OB chapter is required to indicate a history of abortion during a pregnancy.
V24 Postpartum care and evaluation
V25 Encounter for contraceptive management
Except V25.0x *(See Section I.C.18.d.11, Counseling)*
V26 Procreative management
Except V26.5x, Sterilization status, V26.3 & V26.4 *(See Section I.C.18.d.11., Counseling)*
V27 Outcome of delivery
V28 Antenatal screening
(See Section I.C.18.d.6., Screening)

12) Newborn, infant and child

See Section I.C.15, the Newborn guidelines for further instruction on the use of these codes.

Newborn V code categories:

V20 Health supervision of infant or child
V29 Observation and evaluation of newborns for suspected condition not found
(See Section I.C.18.d.7, Observation)
V30-V39 Liveborn infant according to type of birth

13) Routine and administrative examinations

The V codes allow for the description of encounters for routine examinations, such as, a general check-up, or examinations for administrative purposes, such as a pre-employment physical. The codes are not to be used if the examination is for diagnosis of a suspected condition or for treatment purposes. In such cases the diagnosis code is used. During a routine exam, should a diagnosis or condition be discovered, it should be coded as an additional code. Pre-existing and chronic conditions and history codes may also be included as additional codes as long as the examination is for administrative purposes and not focused on any particular condition.

Pre-operative examination and pre-procedural laboratory examination V codes are for use only in those situations when a patient is being cleared for a procedure or surgery and no treatment is given.

The V codes categories/code for routine and administrative examinations:

V20.2 Routine infant or child health check
Any injections given should have a corresponding procedure code.
V70 General medical examination
V72 Special investigations and examinations
Codes V72.5 and V72.62 may be used if the reason for the patient encounter is for routine laboratory/radiology testing in the absence of any signs, symptoms, or associated diagnosis. If routine testing is performed during the same encounter as a test to evaluate a sign, symptom, or diagnosis, it is appropriate to assign both the V code and the code describing the reason for the non-routine test.

14) Miscellaneous V codes

The miscellaneous V codes capture a number of other health care encounters that do not fall into one of the other categories. Certain of these codes identify the reason for the encounter, others are for use as additional codes that provide useful information on circumstances that may affect a patient's care and treatment.

Prophylactic Organ Removal

For encounters specifically for prophylactic removal of breasts, ovaries, or another organ due to a genetic susceptibility to cancer or a family history of cancer, the principal or first listed code should be a code from subcategory V50.4, Prophylactic organ removal, followed by the appropriate genetic susceptibility code and the appropriate family history code.

If the patient has a malignancy of one site and is having prophylactic removal at another site to prevent either a new primary malignancy or metastatic disease, a code for the malignancy should also be assigned in addition to a code from subcategory V50.4. A V50.4 code should not be assigned if the patient is having organ removal for treatment of a malignancy, such as the removal of the testes for the treatment of prostate cancer.

Miscellaneous V code categories/codes:

V07 Need for isolation and other prophylactic measures
 Except V07.5, Prophylactic use of agents affecting estrogen receptors and estrogen levels
V50 Elective surgery for purposes other than remedying health states
V58.5 Orthodontics
V60 Housing, household, and economic circumstances
V62 Other psychosocial circumstances
V63 Unavailability of other medical facilities for care
V64 Persons encountering health services for specific procedures, not carried out
V66 Convalescence and Palliative Care
V68 Encounters for administrative purposes
V69 Problems related to lifestyle

15) Nonspecific V codes

Certain V codes are so non-specific, or potentially redundant with other codes in the classification, that there can be little justification for their use in the inpatient setting. Their use in the outpatient setting should be limited to those instances when there is no further documentation to permit more precise coding. Otherwise, any sign or symptom or any other reason for visit that is captured in another code should be used.

Nonspecific V code categories/codes:

V11 Personal history of mental disorder
 A code from the mental disorders chapter, with an in remission fifth-digit, should be used.
V13.4 Personal history of arthritis
V13.6 Personal history of congenital malformations
V15.7 Personal history of contraception
V23.2 Pregnancy with history of abortion
V40 Mental and behavioral problems
V41 Problems with special senses and other special functions
V47 Other problems with internal organs
V48 Problems with head, neck, and trunk
V49 Problems with limbs and other problems
 Exceptions:
  V49.6 Upper limb amputation status
  V49.7 Lower limb amputation status
  V49.81 Postmenopausal status
  V49.82 Dental sealant status
  V49.83 Awaiting organ transplant status
V51.8 Other aftercare involving the use of plastic surgery
V58.2 Blood transfusion, without reported diagnosis
V58.9 Unspecified aftercare
 See Section IV.K. and Section IV.L. of the Outpatient guidelines.

e. V Codes That May Only be Principal/First-Listed Diagnosis

The list of V codes/categories below may only be reported as the principal/first-listed diagnosis, except when there are multiple encounters on the same day and the medical records for the encounters are combined or when there is more than one V code that meets the definition of principal diagnosis (e.g., a patient is admitted to home healthcare for both aftercare and rehabilitation and they equally meet the definition of principal diagnosis). These codes should not be reported if they do not meet the definition of principal or first-listed diagnosis.

See Section II and Section IV.A for information on selection of principal and first-listed diagnosis.

See Section II.C for information on two or more diagnoses that equally meet the definition for principal diagnosis.

V20.X Health supervision of infant or child
V22.0 Supervision of normal first pregnancy
V22.1 Supervision of other normal pregnancy
V24.X Postpartum care and examination
V26.81 Encounter for assisted reproductive fertility procedure cycle
V26.82 Encounter for fertility preservation procedure
V30.X Single liveborn
V31.X Twin, mate liveborn
V32.X Twin, mate stillborn
V33.X Twin, unspecified
V34.X Other multiple, mates all liveborn
V35.X Other multiple, mates all stillborn
V36.X Other multiple, mates live- and stillborn
V37.X Other multiple, unspecified
V39.X Unspecified
V46.12 Encounter for respirator dependence during power failure
V46.13 Encounter for weaning from respirator [ventilator]
V51.0 Encounter for breast reconstruction following mastectomy
V56.0 Extracorporeal dialysis
V57.X Care involving use of rehabilitation procedures
V58.0 Radiotherapy
V58.11 Encounter for antineoplastic chemotherapy
V58.12 Encounter for antineoplastic immunotherapy
V59.X Donors
V66.0 Convalescence and palliative care following surgery
V66.1 Convalescence and palliative care following radiotherapy
V66.2 Convalescence and palliative care following chemotherapy
V66.3 Convalescence and palliative care following psychotherapy and other treatment for mental disorder
V66.4 Convalescence and palliative care following treatment of fracture
V66.5 Convalescence and palliative care following other treatment
V66.6 Convalescence and palliative care following combined treatment
V66.9 Unspecified convalescence
V68.X Encounters for administrative purposes
V70.0 Routine general medical examination at a health care facility
V70.1 General psychiatric examination, requested by the authority
V70.2 General psychiatric examination, other and unspecified
V70.3 Other medical examination for administrative purposes
V70.4 Examination for medicolegal reasons
V70.5 Health examination of defined subpopulations
V70.6 Health examination in population surveys
V70.8 Other specified general medical examinations
V70.9 Unspecified general medical examination
V71.X Observation and evaluation for suspected conditions not found

19. Supplemental Classification of External Causes of Injury and Poisoning (E-codes, E800-E999)

Introduction: These guidelines are provided for those who are currently collecting E codes in order that there will be standardization in the process. If your institution plans to begin collecting E codes, these guidelines are to be applied. The use of E codes is supplemental to the application of ICD-9-CM diagnosis codes.

External causes of injury and poisoning codes (categories E000 and E800-E999) are intended to provide data for injury research and evaluation of injury prevention strategies. Activity codes (categories E001-E030) are intended to be used to describe the activity of a person seeking care for injuries as well as other health conditions, when the injury or other health condition resulted from an activity or the activity contributed to a condition. E codes capture how the injury, poisoning, or adverse effect happened (cause), the intent (unintentional or accidental; or intentional, such as suicide or assault), the person's status (e.g. civilian, military), the associated activity and the place where the event occurred.

Some major categories of E codes include:

transport accidents

poisoning and adverse effects of drugs, medicinal substances and biologicals

accidental falls
accidents caused by fire and flames
accidents due to natural and environmental factors
late effects of accidents, assaults or self injury
assaults or purposely inflicted injury
suicide or self inflicted injury

These guidelines apply for the coding and collection of E codes from records in hospitals, outpatient clinics, emergency departments, other ambulatory care settings and provider offices, and nonacute care settings, except when other specific guidelines apply.

a. General E Code Coding Guidelines

1) Used with any code in the range of 001-V89

An E code from categories E800-E999 may be used with any code in the range of 001-V89, which indicates an injury, poisoning, or adverse effect due to an external cause.

An activity E code (categories E001-E030) may be used with any code in the range of 001-V89 that indicates an injury, or other health condition that resulted from an activity, or the activity contributed to a condition.

2) Assign the appropriate E code for all initial treatments

Assign the appropriate E code for the initial encounter of an injury, poisoning, or adverse effect of drugs, not for subsequent treatment.

External cause of injury codes (E-codes) may be assigned while the acute fracture codes are still applicable.

See Section I.C.17.b.1 for coding of acute fractures.

3) Use the full range of E codes

Use the full range of E codes (E800 – E999) to completely describe the cause, the intent and the place of occurrence, if applicable, for all injuries, poisonings, and adverse effects of drugs.

See a.1.), j.), and k.) in this section for information on the use of status and activity E codes.

4) Assign as many E codes as necessary

Assign as many E codes as necessary to fully explain each cause.

5) The selection of the appropriate E code

The selection of the appropriate E code is guided by the Index to External Causes, which is located after the alphabetical index to diseases and by Inclusion and Exclusion notes in the Tabular List.

6) E code can never be a principal diagnosis

An E code can never be a principal (first listed) diagnosis.

7) External cause code(s) with systemic inflammatory response syndrome (SIRS)

An external cause code is not appropriate with a code from subcategory 995.9, unless the patient also has another condition for which an E code would be appropriate (such as an injury, poisoning, or adverse effect of drugs).

8) Multiple Cause E Code Coding Guidelines

More than one E-code is required to fully describe the external cause of an illness, injury or poisoning. The assignment of E-codes should be sequenced in the following priority:

If two or more events cause separate injuries, an E code should be assigned for each cause. The first listed E code will be selected in the following order:

E codes for child and adult abuse take priority over all other E codes.

See Section I.C.19.e., Child and Adult abuse guidelines.

E codes for terrorism events take priority over all other E codes except child and adult abuse.

E codes for cataclysmic events take priority over all other E codes except child and adult abuse and terrorism.

E codes for transport accidents take priority over all other E codes except cataclysmic events, child and adult abuse and terrorism.

Activity and external cause status codes are assigned following all causal (intent) E codes.

The first-listed E code should correspond to the cause of the most serious diagnosis due to an assault, accident, or self-harm, following the order of hierarchy listed above.

9) If the reporting format limits the number of E codes

If the reporting format limits the number of E codes that can be used in reporting clinical data, report the code for the cause/intent most related to the principal diagnosis. If the format permits capture of additional E codes, the cause/intent, including medical misadventures, of the additional events should be reported rather than the codes for place, activity or external status.

b. Place of Occurrence Guideline

Use an additional code from category E849 to indicate the Place of Occurrence. The Place of Occurrence describes the place where the event occurred and not the patient's activity at the time of the event.

Do not use E849.9 if the place of occurrence is not stated.

c. Adverse Effects of Drugs, Medicinal and Biological Substances Guidelines

1) Do not code directly from the Table of Drugs

Do not code directly from the Table of Drugs and Chemicals. Always refer back to the Tabular List.

2) Use as many codes as necessary to describe

Use as many codes as necessary to describe completely all drugs, medicinal or biological substances.

If the reporting format limits the number of E codes, and there are different fourth digit codes in the same three digit category, use the code for "Other specified" of that category of drugs, medicinal or biological substances. If there is no "Other specified" code in that category, use the appropriate "Unspecified" code in that category.

If the reporting format limits the number of E codes, and the codes are in different three digit categories, assign the appropriate E code for other multiple drugs and medicinal substances.

3) If the same E code would describe the causative agent

If the same E code would describe the causative agent for more than one adverse reaction, assign the code only once.

4) If two or more drugs, medicinal or biological substances

If two or more drugs, medicinal or biological substances are reported, code each individually unless the combination code is listed in the Table of Drugs and Chemicals. In that case, assign the E code for the combination.

5) When a reaction results from the interaction of a drug(s)

When a reaction results from the interaction of a drug(s) and alcohol, use poisoning codes and E codes for both.

6) Codes from the E930-E949 series

Codes from the E930-E949 series must be used to identify the causative substance for an adverse effect of drug, medicinal and biological substances, correctly prescribed and properly administered. The effect, such as tachycardia, delirium, gastrointestinal hemorrhaging, vomiting, hypokalemia, hepatitis, renal failure, or respiratory failure, is coded and followed by the appropriate code from the E930-E949 series.

d. Child and Adult Abuse Guideline

1) Intentional injury

When the cause of an injury or neglect is intentional child or adult abuse, the first listed E code should be assigned from categories E960-E968, Homicide and injury purposely inflicted by other persons, (except category E967). An E code from category E967, Child and adult battering and other maltreatment, should be added as an additional code to identify the perpetrator, if known.

2) Accidental intent

In cases of neglect when the intent is determined to be accidental E code E904.0, Abandonment or neglect of infant and helpless person, should be the first listed E code.

e. Unknown or Suspected Intent Guideline

1) If the intent (accident, self-harm, assault) of the cause of an injury or poisoning is unknown

If the intent (accident, self-harm, assault) of the cause of an injury or poisoning is unknown or unspecified, code the intent as undetermined E980-E989.

2) If the intent (accident, self-harm, assault) of the cause of an injury or poisoning is questionable

If the intent (accident, self-harm, assault) of the cause of an injury or poisoning is questionable, probable or suspected, code the intent as undetermined E980-E989.

f. Undetermined Cause

When the intent of an injury or poisoning is known, but the cause is unknown, use codes: E928.9, Unspecified accident, E958.9, Suicide and self-inflicted injury by unspecified means, and E968.9, Assault by unspecified means.

These E codes should rarely be used, as the documentation in the medical record, in both the inpatient outpatient and other settings, should normally provide sufficient detail to determine the cause of the injury.

g. **Late Effects of External Cause Guidelines**

1) Late effect E codes

Late effect E codes exist for injuries and poisonings but not for adverse effects of drugs, misadventures and surgical complications.

2) Late effect E codes (E929, E959, E969, E977, E989, or E999.1)

A late effect E code (E929, E959, E969, E977, E989, or E999.1) should be used with any report of a late effect or sequela resulting from a previous injury or poisoning (905-909).

3) Late effect E code with a related current injury

A late effect E code should never be used with a related current nature of injury code.

4) Use of late effect E codes for subsequent visits

Use a late effect E code for subsequent visits when a late effect of the initial injury or poisoning is being treated. There is no late effect E code for adverse effects of drugs.

Do not use a late effect E code for subsequent visits for follow-up care (e.g., to assess healing, to receive rehabilitative therapy) of the injury or poisoning when no late effect of the injury has been documented.

h. **Misadventures and Complications of Care Guidelines**

1) Code range E870-E876

Assign a code in the range of E870-E876 if misadventures are stated by the provider. When applying the E code guidelines pertaining to sequencing, these E codes are considered causal codes.

2) Code range E878-E879

Assign a code in the range of E878-E879 if the provider attributes an abnormal reaction or later complication to a surgical or medical procedure, but does not mention misadventure at the time of the procedure as the cause of the reaction.

i. **Terrorism Guidelines**

1) Cause of injury identified by the Federal Government (FBI) as terrorism

When the cause of an injury is identified by the Federal Government (FBI) as terrorism, the first-listed E-code should be a code from category E979, Terrorism. The definition of terrorism employed by the FBI is found at the inclusion note at E979. The terrorism E-code is the only E-code that should be assigned. Additional E codes from the assault categories should not be assigned.

2) Cause of an injury is suspected to be the result of terrorism

When the cause of an injury is suspected to be the result of terrorism a code from category E979 should not be assigned. Assign a code in the range of E codes based circumstances on the documentation of intent and mechanism.

3) Code E979.9, Terrorism, secondary effects

Assign code E979.9, Terrorism, secondary effects, for conditions occurring subsequent to the terrorist event. This code should not be assigned for conditions that are due to the initial terrorist act.

4) Statistical tabulation of terrorism codes

For statistical purposes these codes will be tabulated within the category for assault, expanding the current category from E960-E969 to include E979 and E999.1.

j. **Activity Code Guidelines**

Assign a code from category E001-E030 to describe the activity that caused or contributed to the injury or other health condition.

Unlike other E codes, activity E codes may be assigned to indicate a health condition (not just injuries) resulted from an activity, or the activity contributed to the condition.

The activity codes are not applicable to poisonings, adverse effects, misadventures or late effects.

k. **External cause status**

A code from category E000, External cause status, should be assigned whenever any other E code is assigned for an encounter, including an Activity E code, except for the events noted below. Assign a code from category E000, External cause status, to indicate the work status of the person at the time the event occurred. The status code indicates whether the event occurred during military activity, whether a non-military person was at work, whether an individual including a student or volunteer was involved in a non-work activity at the time of the causal event.

A code from E000, External cause status, should be assigned, when applicable, with other external cause codes, such as transport accidents and falls. The external cause status codes are not applicable to poisonings, adverse effects, misadventures or late effects.

Do not assign a code from category E000 if no other E codes (cause, activity) are applicable for the encounter.

Do not assign code E000.9, Unspecified external cause status, if the status is not stated.

Section II. Selection of Principal Diagnosis

The circumstances of inpatient admission always govern the selection of principal diagnosis. The principal diagnosis is defined in the Uniform Hospital Discharge Data Set (UHDDS) as "that condition established after study to be chiefly responsible for occasioning the admission of the patient to the hospital for care."

The UHDDS definitions are used by hospitals to report inpatient data elements in a standardized manner. These data elements and their definitions can be found in the July 31, 1985, Federal Register (Vol. 50, No, 147), pp. 31038-40.

Since that time the application of the UHDDS definitions has been expanded to include all non-outpatient settings (acute care, short term, long term care and psychiatric hospitals; home health agencies; rehab facilities; nursing homes, etc).

In determining principal diagnosis the coding conventions in the ICD-9-CM, Volumes I and II take precedence over these official coding guidelines.

(See Section I.A., Conventions for the ICD-9-CM)

The importance of consistent, complete documentation in the medical record cannot be overemphasized. Without such documentation the application of all coding guidelines is a difficult, if not impossible, task.

A. Codes for symptoms, signs, and ill-defined conditions

Codes for symptoms, signs, and ill-defined conditions from Chapter 16 are not to be used as principal diagnosis when a related definitive diagnosis has been established.

B. Two or more interrelated conditions, each potentially meeting the definition for principal diagnosis.

When there are two or more interrelated conditions (such as diseases in the same ICD-9-CM chapter or manifestations characteristically associated with a certain disease) potentially meeting the definition of principal diagnosis, either condition may be sequenced first, unless the circumstances of the admission, the therapy provided, the Tabular List, or the Alphabetic Index indicate otherwise.

C. Two or more diagnoses that equally meet the definition for principal diagnosis

In the unusual instance when two or more diagnoses equally meet the criteria for principal diagnosis as determined by the circumstances of admission, diagnostic workup and/or therapy provided, and the Alphabetic Index, Tabular List, or another coding guidelines does not provide sequencing direction, any one of the diagnoses may be sequenced first.

D. Two or more comparative or contrasting conditions.

In those rare instances when two or more contrasting or comparative diagnoses are documented as "either/or" (or similar terminology), they are coded as if the diagnoses were confirmed and the diagnoses are sequenced according to the circumstances of the admission. If no further determination can be made as to which diagnosis should be principal, either diagnosis may be sequenced first.

E. A symptom(s) followed by contrasting/comparative diagnoses

When a symptom(s) is followed by contrasting/comparative diagnoses, the symptom code is sequenced first. All the contrasting/comparative diagnoses should be coded as additional diagnoses.

F. Original treatment plan not carried out

Sequence as the principal diagnosis the condition, which after study occasioned the admission to the hospital, even though treatment may not have been carried out due to unforeseen circumstances.

G. Complications of surgery and other medical care

When the admission is for treatment of a complication resulting from surgery or other medical care, the complication code is sequenced as the principal diagnosis. If the complication is classified to the 996-999 series and the code lacks the necessary specificity in describing the complication, an additional code for the specific complication should be assigned.

H. Uncertain Diagnosis

If the diagnosis documented at the time of discharge is qualified as "probable", "suspected", "likely", "questionable", "possible", or "still to be ruled out", or other similar terms indicating uncertainty, code the condition as if it existed or was established. The bases for these guidelines are the diagnostic workup, arrangements for further workup or observation, and initial therapeutic approach that correspond most closely with the established diagnosis.

Note: This guideline is applicable only to inpatient admissions to short-term, acute, long-term care and psychiatric hospitals.

I. Admission from Observation Unit

1. Admission Following Medical Observation

When a patient is admitted to an observation unit for a medical condition, which either worsens or does not improve, and is subsequently admitted as an inpatient of the same hospital for this same medical condition, the principal diagnosis would be the medical condition which led to the hospital admission.

2. Admission Following Post-Operative Observation

When a patient is admitted to an observation unit to monitor a condition (or complication) that develops following outpatient surgery, and then is subsequently admitted as an inpatient of the same hospital, hospitals should apply the Uniform Hospital Discharge Data Set (UHDDS) definition of principal diagnosis as "that condition established after study to be chiefly responsible for occasioning the admission of the patient to the hospital for care."

J. Admission from Outpatient Surgery

When a patient receives surgery in the hospital's outpatient surgery department and is subsequently admitted for continuing inpatient care at the same hospital, the following guidelines should be followed in selecting the principal diagnosis for the inpatient admission:

- If the reason for the inpatient admission is a complication, assign the complication as the principal diagnosis.
- If no complication, or other condition, is documented as the reason for the inpatient admission, assign the reason for the outpatient surgery as the principal diagnosis.
- If the reason for the inpatient admission is another condition unrelated to the surgery, assign the unrelated condition as the principal diagnosis.

Section III. Reporting Additional Diagnoses

GENERAL RULES FOR OTHER (ADDITIONAL) DIAGNOSES

For reporting purposes the definition for "other diagnoses" is interpreted as additional conditions that affect patient care in terms of requiring:

clinical evaluation; or
therapeutic treatment; or
diagnostic procedures; or
extended length of hospital stay; or
increased nursing care and/or monitoring.

The UHDDS item #11-b defines Other Diagnoses as "all conditions that coexist at the time of admission, that develop subsequently, or that affect the treatment received and/or the length of stay. Diagnoses that relate to an earlier episode which have no bearing on the current hospital stay are to be excluded." UHDDS definitions apply to inpatients in acute care, short-term, long term care and psychiatric hospital setting. The UHDDS definitions are used by acute care short-term hospitals to report inpatient data elements in a standardized manner. These data elements and their definitions can be found in the July 31, 1985, Federal Register (Vol. 50, No, 147), pp. 31038-40.

Since that time the application of the UHDDS definitions has been expanded to include all non-outpatient settings (acute care, short term, long term care and psychiatric hospitals; home health agencies; rehab facilities; nursing homes, etc).

The following guidelines are to be applied in designating "other diagnoses" when neither the Alphabetic Index nor the Tabular List in ICD-9-CM provide direction. The listing of the diagnoses in the patient record is the responsibility of the attending provider.

A. Previous conditions

If the provider has included a diagnosis in the final diagnostic statement, such as the discharge summary or the face sheet, it should ordinarily be coded. Some providers include in the diagnostic statement resolved conditions or diagnoses and status-post procedures from previous admission that have no bearing on the current stay. Such conditions are not to be reported and are coded only if required by hospital policy.

However, history codes (V10-V19) may be used as secondary codes if the historical condition or family history has an impact on current care or influences treatment.

B. Abnormal findings

Abnormal findings (laboratory, x-ray, pathologic, and other diagnostic results) are not coded and reported unless the provider indicates their clinical significance. If the findings are outside the normal range and the attending provider has ordered other tests to evaluate the condition or prescribed treatment, it is appropriate to ask the provider whether the abnormal finding should be added.

Please note: This differs from the coding practices in the outpatient setting for coding encounters for diagnostic tests that have been interpreted by a provider.

C. Uncertain Diagnosis

If the diagnosis documented at the time of discharge is qualified as "probable", "suspected", "likely", "questionable", "possible", or "still to be ruled out" or other similar terms indicating uncertainty, code the condition as if it existed or was established. The bases for these guidelines are the diagnostic workup, arrangements for further workup or observation, and initial therapeutic approach that correspond most closely with the established diagnosis.

Note: This guideline is applicable only to inpatient admissions to short-term, acute, long-term care and psychiatric hospitals.

Section IV. Diagnostic Coding and Reporting Guidelines for Outpatient Services

These coding guidelines for outpatient diagnoses have been approved for use by hospitals/ providers in coding and reporting hospital-based outpatient services and provider-based office visits.

Information about the use of certain abbreviations, punctuation, symbols, and other conventions used in the ICD-9-CM Tabular List (code numbers and titles), can be found in Section IA of these guidelines, under "Conventions Used in the Tabular List." Information about the correct sequence to use in finding a code is also described in Section I.

The terms encounter and visit are often used interchangeably in describing outpatient service contacts and, therefore, appear together in these guidelines without distinguishing one from the other.

Though the conventions and general guidelines apply to all settings, coding guidelines for outpatient and provider reporting of diagnoses will vary in a number of instances from those for inpatient diagnoses, recognizing that:

The Uniform Hospital Discharge Data Set (UHDDS) definition of principal diagnosis applies only to inpatients in acute, short-term, long-term care and psychiatric hospitals.

Coding guidelines for inconclusive diagnoses (probable, suspected, rule out, etc.) were developed for inpatient reporting and do not apply to outpatients.

A. Selection of first-listed condition

In the outpatient setting, the term first-listed diagnosis is used in lieu of principal diagnosis.

In determining the first-listed diagnosis the coding conventions of ICD-9-CM, as well as the general and disease specific guidelines take precedence over the outpatient guidelines.

Diagnoses often are not established at the time of the initial encounter/visit. It may take two or more visits before the diagnosis is confirmed.

The most critical rule involves beginning the search for the correct code assignment through the Alphabetic Index. Never begin searching initially in the Tabular List as this will lead to coding errors.

1. Outpatient Surgery

   When a patient presents for outpatient surgery, code the reason for the surgery as the first-listed diagnosis (reason for the encounter), even if the surgery is not performed due to a contraindication.

2. Observation Stay

   When a patient is admitted for observation for a medical condition, assign a code for the medical condition as the first-listed diagnosis.

   When a patient presents for outpatient surgery and develops complications requiring admission to observation, code the reason for the surgery as the first reported diagnosis (reason for the encounter), followed by codes for the complications as secondary diagnoses.

B. Codes from 001.0 through V89

The appropriate code or codes from 001.0 through V89 must be used to identify diagnoses, symptoms, conditions, problems, complaints, or other reason(s) for the encounter/visit.

C. Accurate reporting of ICD-9-CM diagnosis codes

For accurate reporting of ICD-9-CM diagnosis codes, the documentation should describe the patient's condition, using terminology which includes specific diagnoses as well as symptoms, problems, or reasons for the encounter. There are ICD-9-CM codes to describe all of these.

D. Selection of codes 001.0 through 999.9

The selection of codes 001.0 through 999.9 will frequently be used to describe the reason for the encounter. These codes are from the section of ICD-9-CM for the classification of diseases and injuries (e.g. infectious and parasitic diseases; neoplasms; symptoms, signs, and ill-defined conditions, etc.).

E. Codes that describe symptoms and signs

Codes that describe symptoms and signs, as opposed to diagnoses, are acceptable for reporting purposes when a diagnosis has not been established (confirmed) by the provider. Chapter 16 of ICD-9-CM, Symptoms, Signs, and Ill-defined conditions (codes 780.0 - 799.9) contain many, but not all codes for symptoms.

F. Encounters for circumstances other than a disease or injury

ICD-9-CM provides codes to deal with encounters for circumstances other than a disease or injury. The Supplementary Classification of factors Influencing Health Status and Contact with Health Services (V01.0- V89) is provided to deal with occasions when circumstances other than a disease or injury are recorded as diagnosis or problems. *See Section I.C. 18 for information on V-codes.*

G. Level of Detail in Coding

1. ICD-9-CM codes with 3, 4, or 5 digits

ICD-9-CM is composed of codes with either 3, 4, or 5 digits. Codes with three digits are included in ICD-9-CM as the heading of a category of codes that may be further subdivided by the use of fourth and/or fifth digits, which provide greater specificity.

2. Use of full number of digits required for a code

A three-digit code is to be used only if it is not further subdivided. Where fourth-digit subcategories and/or fifth-digit subclassifications are provided, they must be assigned. A code is invalid if it has not been coded to the full number of digits required for that code.

See also discussion under Section I.b.3., General Coding Guidelines, Level of Detail in Coding.

H. ICD-9-CM code for the diagnosis, condition, problem, or other reason for encounter/visit

List first the ICD-9-CM code for the diagnosis, condition, problem, or other reason for encounter/visit shown in the medical record to be chiefly responsible for the services provided. List additional codes that describe any coexisting conditions. In some cases the first-listed diagnosis may be a symptom when a diagnosis has not been established (confirmed) by the physician.

I. Uncertain diagnosis

Do not code diagnoses documented as "probable", "suspected," "questionable," "rule out," or "working diagnosis" or other similar terms indicating uncertainty. Rather, code the condition(s) to the highest degree of certainty for that encounter/visit, such as symptoms, signs, abnormal test results, or other reason for the visit.

Please note: This differs from the coding practices used by short-term, acute care, long-term care and psychiatric hospitals.

J. Chronic diseases

Chronic diseases treated on an ongoing basis may be coded and reported as many times as the patient receives treatment and care for the condition(s)

K. Code all documented conditions that coexist

Code all documented conditions that coexist at the time of the encounter/visit, and require or affect patient care treatment or management. Do not code conditions that were previously treated and no longer exist. However, history codes (V10-V19) may be used as secondary codes if the historical condition or family history has an impact on current care or influences treatment.

L. Patients receiving diagnostic services only

For patients receiving diagnostic services only during an encounter/visit, sequence first the diagnosis, condition, problem, or other reason for encounter/visit shown in the medical record to be chiefly responsible for the outpatient services provided during the encounter/visit. Codes for other diagnoses (e.g., chronic conditions) may be sequenced as additional diagnoses.

For encounters for routine laboratory/radiology testing in the absence of any signs, symptoms, or associated diagnosis, assign V72.5 and a code from subcategory V72.6. If routine testing is performed during the same encounter as a test to evaluate a sign, symptom, or diagnosis, it is appropriate to assign both the V code and the code describing the reason for the non-routine test.

For outpatient encounters for diagnostic tests that have been interpreted by a physician, and the final report is available at the time of coding, code any confirmed or definitive diagnosis(es) documented in the interpretation. Do not code related signs and symptoms as additional diagnoses.

Please note: This differs from the coding practice in the hospital inpatient setting regarding abnormal findings on test results.

M. Patients receiving therapeutic services only

For patients receiving therapeutic services only during an encounter/visit, sequence first the diagnosis, condition, problem, or other reason for encounter/visit shown in the medical record to be chiefly responsible for the outpatient services provided during the encounter/visit. Codes for other diagnoses (e.g., chronic conditions) may be sequenced as additional diagnoses.

The only exception to this rule is that when the primary reason for the admission/encounter is chemotherapy, radiation therapy, or rehabilitation, the appropriate V code for the service is listed first, and the diagnosis or problem for which the service is being performed listed second.

N. Patients receiving preoperative evaluations only

For patients receiving preoperative evaluations only, sequence first a code from category V72.8, Other specified examinations, to describe the pre-op consultations. Assign a code for the condition to describe the reason for the surgery as an additional diagnosis. Code also any findings related to the pre-op evaluation.

O. Ambulatory surgery

For ambulatory surgery, code the diagnosis for which the surgery was performed. If the postoperative diagnosis is known to be different from the preoperative diagnosis at the time the diagnosis is confirmed, select the postoperative diagnosis for coding, since it is the most definitive.

P. Routine outpatient prenatal visits

For routine outpatient prenatal visits when no complications are present, codes V22.0, Supervision of normal first pregnancy, or V22.1, Supervision of other normal pregnancy, should be used as the principal diagnosis. These codes should not be used in conjunction with chapter 11 codes.

Appendix I

Present on Admission Reporting Guidelines

Introduction

These guidelines are to be used as a supplement to the ICD-9-CM Official Guidelines for Coding and Reporting to facilitate the assignment of the Present on Admission (POA) indicator for each diagnosis and external cause of injury code reported on claim forms (UB-04 and 837 Institutional).

These guidelines are not intended to replace any guidelines in the main body of the ICD-9-CM Official Guidelines for Coding and Reporting. The POA guidelines are not intended to provide guidance on when a condition should be coded, but rather, how to apply the POA indicator to the final set of diagnosis codes that have been assigned in accordance with Sections I, II, and III of the official coding guidelines. Subsequent to the assignment of the ICD-9-CM codes, the POA indicator should then be assigned to those conditions that have been coded.

As stated in the Introduction to the ICD-9-CM Official Guidelines for Coding and Reporting, a joint effort between the healthcare provider and the coder is essential to achieve complete and accurate documentation, code assignment, and reporting of diagnoses and procedures. The importance of consistent, complete documentation in the medical record cannot be overemphasized. Medical record documentation from any provider involved in the care and treatment of the patient may be used to support the determination of whether a condition was present on admission or not. In the context of the official coding guidelines, the term "provider" means a physician or any qualified healthcare practitioner who is legally accountable for establishing the patient's diagnosis.

These guidelines are not a substitute for the provider's clinical judgment as to the determination of whether a condition was/was not present on admission. The provider should be queried regarding issues related to the linking of signs/ symptoms, timing of test results, and the timing of findings.

General Reporting Requirements

All claims involving inpatient admissions to general acute care hospitals or other facilities that are subject to a law or regulation mandating collection of present on admission information.

Present on admission is defined as present at the time the order for inpatient admission occurs -- conditions that develop during an outpatient encounter, including emergency department, observation, or outpatient surgery, are considered as present on admission.

POA indicator is assigned to principal and secondary diagnoses (as defined in Section II of the Official Guidelines for Coding and Reporting) and the external cause of injury codes.

Issues related to inconsistent, missing, conflicting or unclear documentation must still be resolved by the provider.

If a condition would not be coded and reported based on UHDDS definitions and current official coding guidelines, then the POA indicator would not be reported.

Reporting Options

Y - Yes

N - No

U - Unknown

W – Clinically undetermined

Unreported/Not used (or "1" for Medicare usage) – (Exempt from POA reporting)

Reporting Definitions

Y = present at the time of inpatient admission

N = not present at the time of inpatient admission

U = documentation is insufficient to determine if condition is present on admission

W = provider is unable to clinically determine whether condition was present on admission or not

Timeframe for POA Identification and Documentation

There is no required timeframe as to when a provider (per the definition of "provider" used in these guidelines) must identify or document a condition to be present on admission. In some clinical situations, it may not be possible for a provider to make a definitive diagnosis (or a condition may not be recognized or reported by the patient) for a period of time after admission. In some cases it may be several days before the provider arrives at a definitive diagnosis. This does not mean that the condition was not present on admission. Determination of whether the condition was present on admission or not will be based on the applicable POA guideline as identified in this document, or on the provider's best clinical judgment.

If at the time of code assignment the documentation is unclear as to whether a condition was present on admission or not, it is appropriate to query the provider for clarification.

Assigning the POA Indicator

Condition is on the "Exempt from Reporting" list

Leave the "present on admission" field blank if the condition is on the list of ICD-9-CM codes for which this field is not applicable. This is the only circumstance in which the field may be left blank.

POA Explicitly Documented

Assign Y for any condition the provider explicitly documents as being present on admission.

Assign N for any condition the provider explicitly documents as not present at the time of admission.

Conditions diagnosed prior to inpatient admission

Assign "Y" for conditions that were diagnosed prior to admission (example: hypertension, diabetes mellitus, asthma)

Conditions diagnosed during the admission but clearly present before admission

Assign "Y" for conditions diagnosed during the admission that were clearly present but not diagnosed until after admission occurred.

Diagnoses subsequently confirmed after admission are considered present on admission if at the time of admission they are documented as suspected, possible, rule out, differential diagnosis, or constitute an underlying cause of a symptom that is present at the time of admission.

Condition develops during outpatient encounter prior to inpatient admission

Assign Y for any condition that develops during an outpatient encounter prior to a written order for inpatient admission.

Documentation does not indicate whether condition was present on admission

Assign "U" when the medical record documentation is unclear as to whether the condition was present on admission. "U" should not be routinely assigned and used only in very limited circumstances. Coders are encouraged to query the providers when the documentation is unclear.

Documentation states that it cannot be determined whether the condition was or was not present on admission

Assign "W" when the medical record documentation indicates that it cannot be clinically determined whether or not the condition was present on admission.

Chronic condition with acute exacerbation during the admission

If the code is a combination code that identifies both the chronic condition and the acute exacerbation, see POA guidelines pertaining to combination codes.

If the combination code only identifies the chronic condition and not the acute exacerbation (e.g., acute exacerbation of CHF), assign "Y."

Conditions documented as possible, probable, suspected, or rule out at the time of discharge

If the final diagnosis contains a possible, probable, suspected, or rule out diagnosis, and this diagnosis was based on signs, symptoms or clinical findings suspected at the time of inpatient admission, assign "Y."

If the final diagnosis contains a possible, probable, suspected, or rule out diagnosis, and this diagnosis was based on signs, symptoms or clinical findings that were not present on admission, assign "N".

Conditions documented as impending or threatened at the time of discharge

If the final diagnosis contains an impending or threatened diagnosis, and this diagnosis is based on symptoms or clinical findings that were present on admission, assign "Y".

If the final diagnosis contains an impending or threatened diagnosis, and this diagnosis is based on symptoms or clinical findings that were not present on admission, assign "N".

Acute and Chronic Conditions

Assign "Y" for acute conditions that are present at time of admission and N for acute conditions that are not present at time of admission.

Assign "Y" for chronic conditions, even though the condition may not be diagnosed until after admission.

If a single code identifies both an acute and chronic condition, see the POA guidelines for combination codes.

Combination Codes

Assign "N" if any part of the combination code was not present on admission (e.g., obstructive chronic bronchitis with acute exacerbation and the exacerbation was not present on admission; gastric ulcer that does not start bleeding until after admission; asthma patient develops status asthmaticus after admission)

Assign "Y" if all parts of the combination code were present on admission (e.g., patient with diabetic nephropathy is admitted with uncontrolled diabetes)

If the final diagnosis includes comparative or contrasting diagnoses, and both were present, or suspected, at the time of admission, assign "Y".

For infection codes that include the causal organism, assign "Y" if the infection (or signs of the infection) was present on admission, even though the culture results may not be known until after admission (e.g., patient is admitted with pneumonia and the provider documents pseudomonas as the causal organism a few days later).

Same Diagnosis Code for Two or More Conditions

When the same ICD-9-CM diagnosis code applies to two or more conditions during the same encounter (e.g. bilateral condition, or two separate conditions classified to the same ICD-9-CM diagnosis code):

Assign "Y" if all conditions represented by the single ICD-9-CM code were present on admission (e.g. bilateral fracture of the same bone, same site, and both fractures were present on admission)

Assign "N" if any of the conditions represented by the single ICD-9-CM code was not present on admission (e.g. dehydration with hyponatremia is assigned to code 276.1, but only one of these conditions was present on admission).

Obstetrical conditions

Whether or not the patient delivers during the current hospitalization does not affect assignment of the POA indicator. The determining factor for POA assignment is whether the pregnancy complication or obstetrical condition described by the code was present at the time of admission or not.

If the pregnancy complication or obstetrical condition was present on admission (e.g., patient admitted in preterm labor), assign "Y".

If the pregnancy complication or obstetrical condition was not present on admission (e.g., 2nd degree laceration during delivery, postpartum hemorrhage that occurred during current hospitalization, fetal distress develops after admission), assign "N".

If the obstetrical code includes more than one diagnosis and any of the diagnoses identified by the code were not present on admission assign "N".

(e.g., Code 642.7, Pre-eclampsia or eclampsia superimposed on pre-existing hypertension).

If the obstetrical code includes information that is not a diagnosis, do not consider that information in the POA determination.

(e.g. Code 652.1x, Breech or other malpresentation successfully converted to cephalic presentation should be reported as present on admission if the fetus was breech on admission but was converted to cephalic presentation after admission (since the conversion to cephalic presentation does not represent a diagnosis, the fact that the conversion occurred after admission has no bearing on the POA determination).

Perinatal conditions

Newborns are not considered to be admitted until after birth. Therefore, any condition present at birth or that developed in utero is considered present at admission and should be assigned "Y". This includes conditions that occur during delivery (e.g., injury during delivery, meconium aspiration, exposure to streptococcus B in the vaginal canal).

Congenital conditions and anomalies

Assign "Y" for congenital conditions and anomalies. Congenital conditions are always considered present on admission.

External cause of injury codes

Assign "Y" for any E code representing an external cause of injury or poisoning that occurred prior to inpatient admission (e.g., patient fell out of bed at home, patient fell out of bed in emergency room prior to admission)

Assign "N" for any E code representing an external cause of injury or poisoning that occurred during inpatient hospitalization (e.g., patient fell out of hospital bed during hospital stay, patient experienced an adverse reaction to a medication administered after inpatient admission)

Categories and Codes Exempt from Diagnosis Present on Admission Requirement

Note: "Diagnosis present on admission" for these code categories are exempt because they represent circumstances regarding the healthcare encounter or factors influencing health status that do not represent a current disease or injury or are always present on admission

137-139	Late effects of infectious and parasitic diseases
268.1	Rickets, late effect
326	Late effects of intracranial abscess or pyogenic infection
412	Old myocardial infarction
438	Late effects of cerebrovascular disease
650	Normal delivery
660.7	Failed forceps or vacuum extractor, unspecified
677	Late effect of complication of pregnancy, childbirth, and the puerperium
905-909	Late effects of injuries, poisonings, toxic effects, and other external causes
V02	Carrier or suspected carrier of infectious diseases
V03	Need for prophylactic vaccination and inoculation against bacterial diseases
V04	Need for prophylactic vaccination and inoculation against certain viral diseases
V05	Need for other prophylactic vaccination and inoculation against single diseases
V06	Need for prophylactic vaccination and inoculation against combinations of diseases
V07	Need for isolation and other prophylactic measures
V10	Personal history of malignant neoplasm
V11	Personal history of mental disorder
V12	Personal history of certain other diseases
V13	Personal history of other diseases
V14	Personal history of allergy to medicinal agents
V15.01-V15.09	Other personal history, Allergy, other than to medicinal agents
V15.1	Other personal history, Surgery to heart and great vessels
V15.2	Other personal history, Surgery to other major organs
V15.3	Other personal history, Irradiation
V15.4	Other personal history, Psychological trauma
V15.5	Other personal history, Injury
V15.6	Other personal history, Poisoning
V15.7	Other personal history, Contraception
V15.80	Other personal history, History of failed moderate sedation
V15.81	Other personal history, Noncompliance with medical treatment
V15.82	Other personal history, History of tobacco use
V15.83	Other personal history, Underimmunization status
V15.84	Other personal history, Contact with and (suspected) exposure to asbestos
V15.85	Other personal history, Contact with and (suspected) exposure to potentially hazardous body fluids
V15.86	Other personal history, Contact with and (suspected) exposure to lead
V15.88	Other personal history, History of fall
V15.89	Other personal history, Other
V15.9	Unspecified personal history presenting hazards to health
V16	Family history of malignant neoplasm
V17	Family history of certain chronic disabling diseases
V18	Family history of certain other specific conditions
V19	Family history of other conditions
V20	Health supervision of infant or child
V21	Constitutional states in development
V22	Normal pregnancy
V23	Supervision of high-risk pregnancy
V24	Postpartum care and examination
V25	Encounter for contraceptive management
V26	Procreative management
V27	Outcome of delivery
V28	Antenatal screening

V29 Observation and evaluation of newborns for suspected condition not found
V30-V39 Liveborn infants according to type of birth
V42 Organ or tissue replaced by transplant
V43 Organ or tissue replaced by other means
V44 Artificial opening status
V45 Other postprocedural states
V46 Other dependence on machines
V49.60-V49.77 Upper and lower limb amputation status
V49.81-V49.84 Other specified conditions influencing health status
V50 Elective surgery for purposes other than remedying health states
V51 Aftercare involving the use of plastic surgery
V52 Fitting and adjustment of prosthetic device and implant
V53 Fitting and adjustment of other device
V54 Other orthopedic aftercare
V55 Attention to artificial openings
V56 Encounter for dialysis and dialysis catheter care
V57 Care involving use of rehabilitation procedures
V58 Encounter for other and unspecified procedures and aftercare
V59 Donors
V60 Housing, household, and economic circumstances
V61 Other family circumstances
V62 Other psychosocial circumstances
V64 Persons encountering health services for specific procedures, not carried out
V65 Other persons seeking consultation
V66 Convalescence and palliative care
V67 Follow-up examination
V68 Encounters for administrative purposes
V69 Problems related to lifestyle
V70 General medical examination
V71 Observation and evaluation for suspected condition not found
V72 Special investigations and examinations
V73 Special screening examination for viral and chlamydial diseases
V74 Special screening examination for bacterial and spirochetal diseases
V75 Special screening examination for other infectious diseases
V76 Special screening for malignant neoplasms
V77 Special screening for endocrine, nutritional, metabolic, and immunity disorders
V78 Special screening for disorders of blood and blood-forming organs
V79 Special screening for mental disorders and developmental handicaps
V80 Special screening for neurological, eye, and ear diseases
V81 Special screening for cardiovascular, respiratory, and genitourinary diseases
V82 Special screening for other conditions
V83 Genetic carrier status
V84 Genetic susceptibility to disease
V85 Body Mass Index
V86 Estrogen receptor status
V87.32 Contact with and (suspected) exposure to algae bloom
V87.4 Personal history of drug therapy
V88 Acquired absence of cervix and uterus
V89, Suspected maternal and fetal conditions not found
E000 External cause status
E001-E030 Activity
E800-E807 Railway accidents
E810-E819 Motor vehicle traffic accidents
E820-E825 Motor vehicle nontraffic accidents
E826-E829 Other road vehicle accidents
E830-E838 Water transport accidents
E840-E845 Air and space transport accidents
E846-E848 Vehicle accidents not elsewhere classifiable
E849.0-E849.6 Place of occurrence
E849.8-E849.9 Place of occurrence
E883.1 Accidental fall into well
E883.2 Accidental fall into storm drain or manhole
E884.0 Fall from playground equipment
E884.1 Fall from cliff
E885.0 Fall from (nonmotorized) scooter
E885.1 Fall from roller skates
E885.2 Fall from skateboard
E885.3 Fall from skis
E885.4 Fall from snowboard
E886.0 Fall on same level from collision, pushing, or shoving, by or with other person, In sports
E890.0-E890.9 Conflagration in private dwelling
E893.0 Accident caused by ignition of clothing, from controlled fire in private dwelling
E893.2 Accident caused by ignition of clothing, from controlled fire not in building or structure
E894 Ignition of highly inflammable material
E895 Accident caused by controlled fire in private dwelling
E897 Accident caused by controlled fire not in building or structure
E898.0-E898.1 Accident caused by other specified fire and flames
E917.0 Striking against or struck accidentally by objects or persons, in sports without subsequent fall
E917.1 Striking against or struck accidentally by objects or persons, caused by a crowd, by collective fear or panic without subsequent fall
E917.2 Striking against or struck accidentally by objects or persons, in running water without subsequent fall
E917.5 Striking against or struck accidentally by objects or persons, object in sports with subsequent fall
E917.6 Striking against or struck accidentally by objects or persons, caused by a crowd, by collective fear or panic with subsequent fall
E919.0-E919.1 Accidents caused by machinery
E919.3-E919.9 Accidents caused by machinery
E921.0-E921.9 Accident caused by explosion of pressure vessel
E922.0-E922.9 Accident caused by firearm and air gun missile
E924.1 Caustic and corrosive substances
E926.2 Visible and ultraviolet light sources
E928.0-E928.8 Other and unspecified environmental and accidental causes
E929.0-E929.9 Late effects of accidental injury
E959 Late effects of self-inflicted injury
E970-E978 Legal intervention
E979 Terrorism
E981.0-E981.8 Poisoning by gases in domestic use, undetermined whether accidentally or purposely inflicted
E982.0-E982.9 Poisoning by other gases, undetermined whether accidentally or purposely inflicted
E985.0-E985.7 Injury by firearms, air guns and explosives, undetermined whether accidentally or purposely inflicted
E987.0 Falling from high place, undetermined whether accidentally or purposely inflicted, residential premises
E987.2 Falling from high place, undetermined whether accidentally or purposely inflicted, natural sites
E989 Late effects of injury, undetermined whether accidentally or purposely inflicted
E990-E999 Injury resulting from operations of war

POA Examples

The POA examples have been removed from the guidelines.

PQRI Coding Specifications Summary

The contents of this section were culled from CMS's release of the specifications for the 153 measures that make up the 2009 Physician Quality Reporting Initiative (PQRI). The complete text of these specifications can be found at:

http://www.cms.hhs.gov/apps/ama/license.asp?file=/PQRI/downloads/2009PQRIQualityMeasureSpecificationsManualAndReleaseNotes.zip

It is important to note that this appendix is abridged and focuses on the coding impact of PQRI not the clinical details. To create an effective PQRI reporting program, it is important to review the full specification and other CMS tools and resources that can be found at: http://www.cms.hhs.gov/PQRI/

Each PQRI measure is assigned a unique number. Measure numbers for 2009 PQRI represent a continuation in numbering from the 2007 PQRI Measures 1 through 74 and the 2008 measures 75 through 134. Gaps in measure numbering reflect those 2007 and/or 2008 PQRI measures that are not included for implementation in 2009 PQRI. In general, the quality measures consist of a numerator and a denominator that permit the calculation of the percentage of a defined patient population that receive a particular process of care or achieve a particular outcome.

The denominator population is defined by certain ICD-9 and CPT Category I codes specified in the measure that are submitted by eligible professionals as part of a claim for covered services under the Medicare Physician Fee Schedule. Some measure coding specifications are adapted as needed for implementation in PQRI in agreement with Medicare's coverage policies. For example, CPT codes for non-covered services such as preventive visits are not included in the denominator. If the specified denominator codes for a measure are not included in the patient's claim as submitted, then the patient does not fall into the denominator population, and the PQRI measure does not apply to the patient.

If the patient does fall into the denominator population, the applicable CPT Category II code (or temporary G-code, where CPT Category II codes are not yet available) that defines the numerator should be submitted.

Where a patient falls in the denominator population but specifications define circumstances in which a patient may be excluded from the measure's denominator population, CPT Category II code modifiers such as 1P, 2P, or 3P are available to describe medical, patient, system, or other reasons for such exclusion. Where the performance exclusion does not apply, a measure-specific CPT Category II modifier 8P or HCPCS G-code may be used to indicate that the process of care was not provided for a reason not otherwise specified.

To successfully report quality data for a measure under the PQRI program, it is necessary in all circumstances to report numerator coding (CPT Category II code and/or G-code), with or without an applicable CPT Category II code modifier (1P, 2P, 3P, or 8P).

Instructions for some measures limit the frequency of reporting necessary in certain circumstances, such as for patients with chronic illness for whom a particular process of care is provided only periodically.

The complete measure specifications are organized to provide the following information:

- Measure title
- Measure description
- Instructions on reporting including frequency, timeframes, and applicability
- Numerator coding
- Definitions of terms
- Coding instructions
- Use of CPT Category II exclusion modifiers, where applicable
- Denominator coding
- Rationale statement for measure
- Clinical recommendations or evidence forming the basis or supporting criteria for the measure

This section has been abridged to include only these elements (see page PQRI – 6 for further description of these elements):

- Measure title
- Measure description
- Instructions on reporting including frequency, timeframes, and applicability (abridged)
- Numerator coding
- Denominator coding (including Category II modifier coding)

PQRI Measure Index

CPT only © 2005-2009 American Medical Association. All rights reserved.

CPT only © 2005-2009 American Medical Association. All rights reserved.

CPT only © 2005-2009 American Medical Association. All rights reserved.

CPT only © 2005-2009 American Medical Association. All rights reserved.

PQRI Coding Specifications

= PQRI measure number as referenced in the preceding index and in the Tabular List

Title = Official CMS title for the corresponding measure

Description = Official CMS brief description of the corresponding PQRI measure

Reporting Requirements = CMS's frequency limits and other demographic requirements that must be met by the encounter to be eligible for PQRI reporting

Numerator Code(s) = CPT Category II and/or HCPCS Level II G codes, code combinations, and modifiers required for numerator reporting under PQRI

Denominator Code(s) = ICD-9, CPT and/or HCPCS Level II codes that must be documented for the encounter to qualify for PQRI denominator reporting

Note: *As this is an ICD-9-CM publication and we have attempted to represent the diagnostic coding implications of the PQRI program in this section and in the PQRI indicators in the Tabular Index, it is important to note that several performance measures are ICD-9 code independent – that is, those measures are not tied to any specific ICD-9 code (as indicated by an "Any" in the ICD-9 portion of the Denominator Code(s) cells) thereby making any diagnosis code acceptable for PQRI reporting. This reference should be used in conjunction with publications or software for CPT and HCPCS Level II coding that include the PQRI codes and guidance relevant to those code sets.*

#	Title	Description	Reporting Requirements	Numerator Code(s)	Denominator Code(s)
1	Diabetes Mellitus: Hemoglobin A1c Poor Control in Diabetes Mellitus	Percentage of patients aged 18 through 75 years with diabetes mellitus who had most recent hemoglobin A1c greater than 9.0%	≥ once per 12 months per diabetic patient seen during reporting period	1 of: 3044F 3045F 3046F 3046F-8P	**ICD-9**: 250.00, 250.01, 250.02, 250.03, 250.10, 250.11, 250.12, 250.13, 250.20, 250.21, 250.22, 250.23, 250.30, 250.31, 250.32, 250.33, 250.40, 250.41, 250.42, 250.43, 250.50, 250.51, 250.52, 250.53, 250.60, 250.61, 250.62, 250.63, 250.70, 250.71, 250.72, 250.73, 250.80, 250.81, 250.82, 250.83, 250.90, 250.91, 250.92, 250.93, 357.2, 362.01, 362.02, 362.03, 362.04, 362.05, 362.06, 362.07, 366.41, 648.00, 648.01, 648.02, 648.03, 648.04 **and** **CPT/HCPCS II**: 97802, 97803, 97804, 99201, 99202, 99203, 99204, 99205, 99212, 99213, 99214, 99215, 99304, 99305, 99306, 99307, 99308, 99309, 99310, 99324, 99325, 99326, 99327, 99328, 99334, 99335, 99336, 99337, 99341, 99342, 99343, 99344, 99345, 99347, 99348, 99349, 99350, G0270, G0271
2	Diabetes Mellitus: Low Density Lipoprotein (LDL-C) Control in Diabetes Mellitus	Percentage of patients aged 18 through 75 years with diabetes mellitus who had most recent LDL-C level in control (less than 100 mg/dl)	≥ once per 12 months per diabetic patient seen during reporting period	1 of: 3048F 3048F-8P 3049F 3050F	**ICD-9**: 250.00, 250.01, 250.02, 250.03, 250.10, 250.11, 250.12, 250.13, 250.20, 250.21, 250.22, 250.23, 250.30, 250.31, 250.32, 250.33, 250.40, 250.41, 250.42, 250.43, 250.50, 250.51, 250.52, 250.53, 250.60, 250.61, 250.62, 250.63, 250.70, 250.71, 250.72, 250.73, 250.80, 250.81, 250.82, 250.83, 250.90, 250.91, 250.92, 250.93, 357.2, 362.01, 362.02, 362.03, 362.04, 362.05, 362.06, 362.07, 366.41, 648.00, 648.01, 648.02, 648.03, 648.04 **and** **CPT/HCPCS II**: 97802, 97803, 97804, 99201, 99202, 99203, 99204, 99205, 99212, 99213, 99214, 99215, 99304, 99305, 99306, 99307, 99308, 99309, 99310, 99324, 99325, 99326, 99327, 99328, 99334, 99335, 99336, 99337, 99341, 99342, 99343, 99344, 99345, 99347, 99348, 99349, 99350, G0270, G0271
3	Diabetes Mellitus: High Blood Pressure Control in Diabetes Mellitus	Percentage of patients aged 18 through 75 years with diabetes mellitus who had most recent blood pressure in control (less than 140/80 mmHg)	≥ once per 12 months per diabetic patient seen during reporting period	1 of: 3074F 3075F 3077F **and** 1 of: 3078F 3079F 3080F **OR** 2000F-8P	**ICD-9**: 250.00, 250.01, 250.02, 250.03, 250.10, 250.11, 250.12, 250.13, 250.20, 250.21, 250.22, 250.23, 250.30, 250.31, 250.32, 250.33, 250.40, 250.41, 250.42, 250.43, 250.50, 250.51, 250.52, 250.53, 250.60, 250.61, 250.62, 250.63, 250.70, 250.71, 250.72, 250.73, 250.80, 250.81, 250.82, 250.83, 250.90, 250.91, 250.92, 250.93, 357.2, 362.01, 362.02, 362.03, 362.04, 362.05, 362.06, 362.07, 366.41, 648.00, 648.01, 648.02, 648.03, 648.04 **and** **CPT/HCPCS II**: 97802, 97803, 97804, 99201, 99202, 99203, 99204, 99205, 99212, 99213, 99214, 99215, 99304, 99305, 99306, 99307, 99308, 99309, 99310, 99324, 99325, 99326, 99327, 99328, 99334, 99335, 99336, 99337, 99341, 99342, 99343, 99344, 99345, 99347, 99348, 99349, 99350, G0270, G0271

CPT only © 2005-2009 American Medical Association. All rights reserved.

#	Title	Description	Reporting Requirements	Numerator Code(s)	Denominator Code(s)
5	Heart Failure: Angiotensin-Converting Enzyme (ACE) Inhibitor or Angiotensin Receptor Blocker (ARB) Therapy for Left Ventricular Systolic Dysfunction (LVSD)	Percentage of patients aged 18 years and older with a diagnosis of heart failure and left ventricular systolic dysfunction (LVSD) who were prescribed ACE inhibitor or ARB therapy	≥ once per reporting period for all heart failure patients seen during the reporting period	3021F **and** 1 of: 4009F 4009F-1P 4009F-2P 4009F-3P 4009F-8P **OR** 3021F-8P **OR** 3022F	**ICD-9**: 402.01, 402.11, 402.91, 404.01, 404.03, 404.11, 404.13, 404.91, 404.93, 428.0, 428.1, 428.20, 428.21, 428.22, 428.23, 428.30, 428.31, 428.32, 428.33, 428.40, 428.41, 428.42, 428.43, 428.9 **and** **CPT**: 99201, 99202, 99203, 99204, 99205, 99212, 99213, 99214, 99215, 99238, 99239, 99241, 99242, 99243, 99244, 99245, 99304, 99305, 99306, 99307, 99308, 99309, 99310, 99324, 99325, 99326, 99327, 99328, 99334, 99335, 99336, 99337, 99341, 99342, 99343, 99344, 99345, 99347, 99348, 99349, 99350
6	Coronary Artery Disease (CAD): Oral Antiplatelet Therapy Prescribed for Patients with CAD	Percentage of patients aged 18 years and older with a diagnosis of coronary artery disease who were prescribed oral antiplatelet therapy	≥ once per reporting period for patients with coronary artery disease seen during the reporting period	1 of: 4011F 4011F-1P 4011F-2P 4011F-3P 4011F-8P	**ICD-9**: 410.00, 410.01, 410.02, 410.10, 410.11, 410.12, 410.20, 410.21, 410.22, 410.30, 410.31, 410.32, 410.40, 410.41, 410.42, 410.50, 410.51, 410.52, 410.60, 410.61, 410.62, 410.70, 410.71, 410.72, 410.80, 410.81, 410.82, 410.90, 410.91, 410.92, 411.0, 411.1, 411.81, 411.89, 412, 413.0, 413.1, 413.9, 414.00, 414.01, 414.02, 414.03, 414.04, 414.05, 414.06, 414.07, 414.8, 414.9, V45.81, V45.82 **and** **CPT**: 99201, 99202, 99203, 99204, 99205, 99212, 99213, 99214, 99215, 99238, 99239, 99241, 99242, 99243, 99244, 99245, 99304, 99305, 99306, 99307, 99308, 99309, 99310, 99324, 99325, 99326, 99327, 99328, 99334, 99335, 99336, 99337, 99341, 99342, 99343, 99344, 99345, 99347, 99348, 99349, 99350
7	Coronary Artery Disease (CAD): Beta-blocker Therapy for CAD Patients with Prior Myocardial Infarction (MI)	Percentage of patients aged 18 years and older with a diagnosis of coronary artery disease and prior myocardial infarction (MI) who were prescribed beta-blocker therapy	≥ once/reponce per reporting period for patients with prior myocardial infarction (MI) seen during the reporting period	Registry only (no codes)	**ICD-9**: 411.0, 411.1, 411.81, 411.89, 413.0, 413.1, 413.9, 414.00, 414.01, 414.02, 414.03, 414.04, 414.05, 414.06, 414.07, 414.8, 414.9, V45.81, V45.82, 410.00*, 410.01*, 410.02*, 410.10*, 410.11*, 410.12*, 410.20*, 410.21*, 410.22*, 410.30*, 410.31*, 410.32*, 410.40*, 410.41*, 410.42*, 410.50*, 410.51*, 410.52*, 410.60*, 410.61*, 410.62*, 410.70, 410.71*, 410.72*, 410.80*, 410.81*, 410.82*, 410.90*, 410.91*, 410.92*, 412* * Denominator inclusion for this measure requires the presence of a prior MI diagnosis **AND** at least one E/M code during the measurement period. Diagnosis codes for Coronary Artery Disease (which include MI diagnosis codes) may also accompany the MI diagnosis code, but are not required for inclusion in the measure. **and** **CPT**: 99201, 99202, 99203, 99204, 99205, 99212, 99213, 99214, 99215, 99238, 99239, 99241, 99242, 99243, 99244, 99245, 99304, 99305, 99306, 99307, 99308, 99309, 99310, 99324, 99325, 99326, 99327, 99328, 99334, 99335, 99336, 99337, 99341, 99342, 99343, 99344, 99345, 99347, 99348, 99349, 99350
8	Heart Failure: Beta-Blocker Therapy for Left Ventricular Systolic Dysfunction (LVSD)	Percentage of patients aged 18 years and older with a diagnosis of heart failure who also have left ventricular systolic dysfunction (LVSD) and who were prescribed beta blocker therapy	≥ once per reporting period for all heart failure patients seen during the reporting period	1 of: G8450 G0451 G0452 G8395 G8396	**ICD-9**: 402.01, 402.11, 402.91, 404.01, 404.03, 404.11, 404.13, 404.91, 404.93, 428.0, 428.1, 428.20, 428.21, 428.22, 428.23, 428.30, 428.31, 428.32, 428.33, 428.40, 428.41, 428.42, 428.43, 428.9 **and** **CPT**: 99201, 99202, 99203, 99204, 99205, 99212, 99213, 99214, 99215, 99241, 99242, 99243, 99244, 99245, 99304, 99305, 99306, 99307, 99308, 99309, 99310, 99324, 99325, 99326, 99327, 99328, 99334, 99335, 99336, 99337, 99341, 99342, 99343, 99344, 99345, 99347, 99348, 99349, 99350

CPT only © 2005-2009 American Medical Association. All rights reserved.

#	Title	Description	Reporting Requirements	Numerator Code(s)	Denominator Code(s)
9	Major Depressive Disorder (MDD): Antidepressant Medication During Acute Phase for Patients with MDD	Percentage of patients aged 18 years and older diagnosed with new episode of major depressive disorder (MDD) and documented as treated with antidepressant medication during the entire 84- day (12 week) acute treatment phase	each occurrence of MDD during the reporting period	1 of: G8126 G8127 G8128	**ICD-9**: 296.20, 296.21, 296.22, 296.23, 296.24, 296.25, 296.30, 296.31, 296.32, 296.33, 296.34, 296.35, 298.0, 300.4, 309.0, 309.1, 311 **and** **CPT**: 90801, 90802, 90804, 90805, 90806, 90807, 90808, 90809, 90810, 90811, 90812, 90813, 90814, 90815, 90821, 90822, 90823, 90824, 90829, 90845, 90849, 90853, 90857, 90862, 99078, 99201, 99202, 99203, 99204, 99205, 99212, 99213, 99214, 99215, 99241, 99242, 99243, 99244, 99245, 99341, 99342, 99343, 99344, 99345, 99347, 99348, 99349, 99350, 99510
10	Stroke and Stroke Rehabilitation: Computed Tomography (CT) or Magnetic Resonance Imaging (MRI) Reports	Percentage of final reports for CT or MRI studies of the brain performed within 24 hours of arrival to the hospital for patients aged 18 years and older with either a diagnosis of ischemic stroke or transient ischemic attack (TIA) or intracranial hemorrhage or at least one documented symptom consistent with ischemic stroke or TIA or intracranial hemorrhage that includes documentation of the presence or absence of each of the following: hemorrhage and mass lesion and acute infarction	each time a CT or MRI is performed in a hospital or outpatient setting during the reporting period for patients with a diagnosis or symptom of ischemic stroke, TIA, or intracranial hemorrhage	3111F **and** 1 of: 3110F 3110F-8P **OR** 3112F	**ICD-9**: 368.12, 368.2, 386.2, 431, 433.01, 433.11, 433.21, 433.31, 433.81, 433.91, 434.01, 434.11, 434.91, 435.0, 435.1, 435.2, 435.3, 435.8, 435.9, 437.7, 780.02, 781.3, 781.4, 781.94, 782.0, 784.3, 784.5 **and** **CPT**: 70450, 70460, 70470, 70551, 70552, 70553, 0042T
11	Stroke and Stroke Rehabilitation: Carotid Imaging Reports	Percentage of final reports for carotid imaging studies (neck MR angiography [MRA], neck CT angiography [CTA], neck duplex ultrasound, carotid angiogram) performed for patients aged 18 years and older with the diagnosis of ischemic stroke or transient ischemic attack (TIA) that include direct or indirect reference to measurements of distal internal carotid diameter as the denominator for stenosis measurement	each time a carotid imaging study is performed during the reporting period for patients with a diagnosis of ischemic stroke or TIA	1 of: 3100F 3100F-1P 3100F-8P	**ICD-9**: 433.01, 433.11, 433.21, 433.31, 433.81, 433.91, 434.01, 434.11, 434.91, 435.0, 435.1, 435.2, 435.3, 435.8, 435.9 **and** **CPT**: 70498, 70547, 70548, 70549, 75660, 75662, 75665, 75671, 75676, 75680, 93880, 93882
12	Primary Open Angle Glaucoma (POAG): Optic Nerve Evaluation	Percentage of patients aged 18 years and older with a diagnosis of primary open-angle glaucoma (POAG) who have an optic nerve head evaluation during one or more office visits within 12 months	≥ once per reporting period for patients seen during the reporting period	1 of: 2027F 2027F-1P 2027F-3P 2027F-8P	**ICD-9**: 365.01, 365.10, 365.11, 365.12, 365.15 **and** **CPT**: 92002, 92004, 92012, 92014, 99201, 99202, 99203, 99204, 99205, 99212, 99213, 99214, 99215, 99241, 99242, 99243, 99244, 99245, 99304, 99305, 99306, 99307, 99308, 99309, 99310, 99324, 99325, 99326, 99327, 99328, 99334, 99335, 99336, 99337
14	Age-Related Macular Degeneration (AMD): Dilated Macular Examination	Percentage of patients aged 50 years and older with a diagnosis of age-related macular degeneration who had a dilated macular examination performed which included documentation of the presence or absence of macular thickening or hemorrhage AND the level of macular degeneration severity during one or more office visits within 12 months	≥ once per reporting period for patients seen during the reporting period	1 of: 2019F 2019F-1P 2019F-2P 2019F-3P 2019F-8P	**ICD-9**: 362.50, 362.51, 362.52 **and** **CPT**: 92002, 92004, 92012, 92014, 99201, 99202, 99203, 99204, 99205, 99212, 99213, 99214, 99215, 99241, 99242, 99243, 99244, 99245, 99304, 99305, 99306, 99307, 99308, 99309, 99310, 99324, 99325, 99326, 99327, 99328, 99334, 99335, 99336, 99337

CPT only © 2005-2009 American Medical Association. All rights reserved.

#	Title	Description	Reporting Requirements	Numerator Code(s)	Denominator Code(s)
18	Diabetic Retinopathy: Documentation of Presence or Absence of Macular Edema and Level of Severity of Retinopathy	Percentage of patients aged 18 years and older with a diagnosis of diabetic retinopathy who had a dilated macular or fundus exam performed which included documentation of the level of severity of retinopathy and the presence or absence of macular edema during one or more office visits within 12 months	≥ once per reporting period for patients seen during the reporting period	1 of: 2021F 2021F-1P 2021F-2P 2021F-3P 2021F-8P	**ICD-9**: 362.01, 362.02, 362.03, 362.04, 362.05, 362.06 **and** **CPT**: 92002, 92004, 92012, 92014, 99201, 99202, 99203, 99204, 99205, 99212, 99213, 99214, 99215, 99241, 99242, 99243, 99244, 99245, 99304, 99305, 99306, 99307, 99308, 99309, 99310, 99324, 99325, 99326, 99327, 99328, 99334, 99335, 99336, 99337
19	Diabetic Retinopathy: Communication with the Physician Managing Ongoing Diabetes Care	Percentage of patients aged 18 years and older with a diagnosis of diabetic retinopathy who had a dilated macular or fundus exam performed with documented communication to the physician who manages the ongoing care of the patient with diabetes mellitus regarding the findings of the macular or fundus exam at least once within 12 months	≥ once per reporting period for all patients with diabetic retinopathy seen during the reporting period	G8397 **and** 1 of: 5010F 5010F-2P 5010F-3P 5010F-8P **OR** G8398	**ICD-9**: 362.01, 362.02, 362.03, 362.04, 362.05, 362.06 **and** **CPT**: 92002, 92004, 92012, 92014, 99201, 99202, 99203, 99204, 99205, 99212, 99213, 99214, 99215, 99241, 99242, 99243, 99244, 99245, 99304, 99305, 99306, 99307, 99308, 99309, 99310, 99324, 99325, 99326, 99327, 99328, 99334, 99335, 99336, 99337
20	Perioperative Care: Timing of Antibiotic Prophylaxis – Ordering Physician	Percentage of surgical patients aged 18 years and older undergoing procedures with the indications for prophylactic parenteral antibiotics, who have an order for prophylactic antibiotic to be given within one hour (if fluoroquinolone or vancomycin, two hours), prior to the surgical incision (or start of procedure when no incision is required)	each time a procedure is performed during the reporting period for patients who undergo surgical procedures with the indications for prophylactic antibiotics	1 of: 4047F 4047F-1P 4047F-8P 4048F	**ICD-9**: Any **and** **CPT**: 15734, 15738, 19260, 19271, 19272, 19301, 19302, 19303, 19304, 19305, 19306, 19307, 19361, 19364, 19366, 19367, 19368, 19369, 21346, 21347, 21348, 21422, 21423, 21432, 21433, 21435, 21436, 21454, 21461, 21462, 21465, 21470, 21627, 21632, 21740, 21750, 21805, 21825, 22325, 22524, 22554, 22558, 22600, 22612, 22630, 22800, 22802, 22804, 27125, 27130, 27132, 27134, 27137, 27138, 27235, 27236, 27244, 27245, 27269, 27440, 27441, 27442, 27443, 27445, 27446, 27447, 27702, 27703, 27704, 27758, 27759, 27766, 27769, 27792, 27814, 27870, 28192, 28193, 28293, 28296, 28299, 28300, 28306, 28307, 28308, 28309, 28310, 28320, 28322, 28415, 28420, 28445, 28465, 28485, 28505, 28525, 28531, 28555, 28585, 28615, 28645, 28675, 28705, 28715, 28725, 28730, 28735, 28737, 28740, 28750, 28755, 28760, 31360, 31365, 31367, 31368, 31370, 31375, 31380, 31382, 31390, 31395, 31760, 31766, 31770, 31775, 31786, 31805, 32095, 32100, 32110, 32120, 32124, 32140, 32141, 32150, 32215, 32220, 32225, 32310, 32320, 32402, 32440, 32442, 32445, 32480, 32482, 32484, 32486, 32488, 32491, 32500, 32501, 32800, 32810, 32815, 32900, 32905, 32906, 32940, 33020, 33025, 33030, 33031, 33050, 33120, 33130, 33140, 33141, 33202, 33203, 33206, 33207, 33208, 33212, 33213, 33214, 33215, 33216, 33217, 33218, 33220, 33222, 33223, 33224, 33225, 33226, 33233, 33234, 33235, 33236, 33237, 33238, 33240, 33241, 33243, 33244, 33249, 33250, 33251, 33254, 33255, 33256, 33261, 33300, 33305, 33310, 33315, 33320, 33321, 33322, 33332, 33335, 33400, 33401, 33403, 33404, 33405, 33406, 33410, 33411, 33413, 33416, 33422, 33425, 33426, 33427, 33430, 33460, 33463, 33464, 33465, 33475, 33496, 33510, 33511, 33512, 33513, 33514, 33516, 33517, 33518, 33519, 33521, 33522, 33523, 33530, 33533, 33534, 33535, 33536, 33542, 33545, 33548, 33572, 33877, 33880, 33881, 33883, 33886, 33891, 34051, 34800, 34802, 34803, 34804, 34805, 34825, 34830, 34831, 34832, 34900, 35021, 35081, 35091, 35102, 35131, 35141, 35151, 35211, 35216, 35241, 35246, 35271, 35276, 35301, 35311, 35481, 35526, 35601, 35606, 35612, 35616, 35621, 35623, 35626, 35631, 35632, 35633, 35634, 35636, 35637, 35638, *continued on the next page*

 CPT only © 2005-2009 American Medical Association. All rights reserved.

#	Title	Description	Reporting Requirements	Numerator Code(s)	Denominator Code(s)
20	*see previous page*	*see previous page*	*see previous page*	*see previous page*	*continued from previous page* 35642, 35645, 35646, 35647, 35650, 35651, 35654, 35656, 35661, 35663, 35665, 35666, 35671, 36830, 37616, 38115, 38381, 38746, 39000, 39010, 39200, 39220, 39545, 39561, 41130, 41135, 41140, 41145, 41150, 41153, 41155, 43045, 43100, 43101, 43107, 43108, 43112, 43113, 43116, 43117, 43118, 43121, 43122, 43123, 43124, 43130, 43135, 43300, 43305, 43310, 43312, 43313, 43320, 43324, 43325, 43326, 43330, 43331, 43340, 43341, 43350, 43351, 43352, 43360, 43361, 43400, 43401, 43405, 43410, 43415, 43420, 43425, 43496, 43500, 43501, 43502, 43510, 43520, 43605, 43610, 43611, 43620, 43621, 43622, 43631, 43632, 43633, 43634, 43640, 43641, 43653, 43800, 43810, 43820, 43825, 43830, 43831, 43832, 43840, 43843, 43845, 43846, 43847, 43848, 43850, 43855, 43860, 43865, 43870, 43880, 44005, 44010, 44020, 44021, 44025, 44050, 44055, 44100, 44110, 44111, 44120, 44125, 44126, 44127, 44130, 44132, 44133, 44135, 44136, 44140, 44141, 44143, 44144, 44145, 44146, 44147, 44150, 44151, 44155, 44156, 44157, 44158, 44160, 44202, 44204, 44205, 44206, 44207, 44208, 44210, 44211, 44212, 44300, 44310, 44312, 44314, 44316, 44320, 44322, 44340, 44345, 44346, 44602, 44603, 44604, 44605, 44615, 44620, 44625, 44626, 44640, 44650, 44660, 44661, 44700, 44950, 45108, 45110, 45111, 45112, 45113, 45114, 45116, 45119, 45120, 45121, 45123, 45126, 45130, 45135, 45136, 45150, 45160, 45170, 45190, 45500, 45505, 45520, 45540, 45541, 45550, 45560, 45562, 45563, 45800, 45805, 45820, 45825, 47133, 47135, 47136, 47140, 47141, 47142, 47420, 47425, 47460, 47480, 47560, 47561, 47570, 47600, 47605, 47610, 47612, 47620, 47700, 47701, 47711, 47712, 47715, 47720, 47721, 47740, 47741, 47760, 47765, 47780, 47785, 47800, 47802, 47900, 48020, 48100, 48120, 48140, 48145, 48146, 48148, 48150, 48152, 48153, 48154, 48155, 48500, 48510, 48511, 48520, 48540, 48545, 48547, 48548, 48550, 48554, 48556, 49215, 49568, 50300, 50320, 50340, 50360, 50365, 50370, 50380, 51550, 51555, 51565, 51570, 51575, 51580, 51585, 51590, 51595, 51596, 51597, 51920, 51925, 52450, 52601, 52630, 52647, 52648, 52649, 54401, 54405, 54406, 54408, 54410, 54415, 54416, 55801, 55810, 55812, 55815, 55821, 55831, 55840, 55842, 55845, 58150, 58152, 58180, 58200, 58210, 58260, 58262, 58263, 58267, 58270, 58275, 58280, 58285, 58290, 58291, 58292, 58293, 58294, 60521, 60522, 61154, 61312, 61313, 61315, 61510, 61512, 61518, 61520, 61526, 61530, 61548, 61591, 61595, 61596, 61598, 61606, 61616, 61618, 61619, 61697, 61700, 61750, 61751, 61867, 62223, 62230, 63015, 63020, 63030, 63042, 63045, 63047, 63056, 63075, 63081, 63267, 63276, 64746, 69720, 69930, 69955, 69960, 69970
21	Perioperative Care: Selection of Prophylactic Antibiotic – First OR Second Generation Cephalosporin	Percentage of surgical patients aged 18 years and older undergoing procedures with the indications for a first OR second generation cephalosporin prophylactic antibiotic, who had an order for cefazolin OR cefuroxime for antimicrobial prophylaxis	each time a procedure is performed during the reporting period for patients who undergo surgical procedures with the indications for a first or second generation cephalosporin prophylactic antibiotic	1 of: 4041F 4041F-1P 4041F-8P	**ICD-9**: Any **and** **CPT**: 15734, 15738, 19260, 19271, 19272, 19301, 19302, 19303, 19304, 19305, 19306, 19307, 19361, 19364, 19366, 19367, 19368, 19369, 21627, 21632, 21740, 21750, 21805, 21825, 22325, 22524, 22554, 22558, 22600, 22612, 22630, 22800, 22802, 22804, 27125, 27130, 27132, 27134, 27137, 27138, 27235, 27236, 27244, 27245, 27269, 27440, 27441, 27442, 27443, 27445, 27446, 27447, 27702, 27703, 27704, 27758, 27759, 27766, 27769, 27792, 27814, 27870, 28192, 28193, 28293, 28296, 28299, 28300, 28306, 28307, 28308, 28309, 28310, 28320, 28322, 28415, 28420, 28445, 28465, 28485, 28505, 28525, 28531, 28555, 28585, 28615, 28645, 28675, 28705, 28715, 28725, 28730, 28735, 28737, 28740, 28750, 28755, 28760, 31760, 31766, 31770, 31775, 31786, 31805, 32095, 32100, 32110, 32120, 32124, 32140, 32141, *continued on the next page*

CPT only © 2005-2009 American Medical Association. All rights reserved.

#	Title	Description	Reporting Requirements	Numerator Code(s)	Denominator Code(s)
21	*see previous page*	*see previous page*	*see previous page*	*see previous page*	*continued from previous page* 32150, 32215, 32220, 32225, 32310, 32320, 32402, 32440, 32442, 32445, 32480, 32482, 32484, 32486, 32488, 32491, 32500, 32501, 32800, 32810, 32815, 32900, 32905, 32906, 32940, 33000, 33020, 33025, 33030, 33031, 33050, 33120, 33130, 33140, 33141, 33202, 33250, 33251, 33256, 33261, 33305, 33310, 33315, 33320, 33321, 33322, 33332, 33335, 33400, 33401, 33403, 33404, 33405, 33406, 33410, 33411, 33413, 33416, 33422, 33425, 33426, 33427, 33430, 33460, 33463, 33464, 33465, 33475, 33496, 33510, 33511, 33512, 33513, 33514, 33516, 33517, 33518, 33519, 33521, 33522, 33523, 33530, 33533, 33534, 33535, 33536, 33542, 33545, 33548, 33572, 33877, 33880, 33881, 33883, 33886, 33891, 34051, 34800, 34802, 34803, 34804, 34805, 34825, 34830, 34831, 34832, 34900, 35021, 35081, 35091, 35102, 35131, 35141, 35151, 35211, 35216, 35241, 35246, 35271, 35276, 35301, 35311, 35481, 35526, 35601, 35606, 35612, 35616, 35621, 35623, 35626, 35631, 35632, 35633, 35634, 35636, 35637, 35638, 35642, 35645, 35646, 35647, 35650, 35651, 35654, 35656, 35661, 35663, 35665, 35666, 35671, 36830, 37616, 38115, 38381, 38746, 39000, 39010, 39200, 39220, 39545, 39561, 43045, 43100, 43101, 43107, 43108, 43112, 43113, 43116, 43117, 43118, 43121, 43122, 43123, 43124, 43130, 43135, 43300, 43305, 43310, 43312, 43313, 43320, 43324, 43325, 43326, 43330, 43331, 43340, 43341, 43350, 43351, 43352, 43360, 43361, 43400, 43401, 43405, 43410, 43415, 43420, 43425, 43496, 43500, 43501, 43502, 43510, 43520, 43605, 43610, 43611, 43620, 43621, 43622, 43631, 43632, 43633, 43634, 43640, 43641, 43653, 43800, 43810, 43820, 43825, 43830, 43831, 43832, 43840, 43843, 43845, 43846, 43847, 43848, 43850, 43855, 43860, 43865, 43870, 44005, 44010, 44020, 44021, 44050, 44055, 44100, 44120, 44125, 44126, 44127, 44130, 44132, 44133, 44135, 44136, 47420, 47425, 47460, 47480, 47560, 47561, 47570, 47600, 47605, 47610, 47612, 47620, 47700, 47701, 47711, 47712, 47715, 47720, 47721, 47740, 47741, 47760, 47765, 47780, 47785, 47800, 47802, 47900, 48020, 48100, 48120, 48140, 48145, 48146, 48148, 48150, 48152, 48153, 48154, 48155, 48500, 48510, 48511, 48520, 48540, 48545, 48547, 48548, 48550, 48554, 48556, 49215, 49568, 50300, 50320, 50340, 50360, 50365, 50370, 50380, 60521, 60522, 61154, 61312, 61313, 61315, 61510, 61512, 61518, 61548, 61697, 61700, 61750, 61751, 61867, 62223, 62230, 63015, 63020, 63030, 63042, 63045, 63047, 63056, 63075, 63081, 63267, 63276, 64746
22	Perioperative Care: Discontinuation of Prophylactic Antibiotics (Non-Cardiac Procedures)	Percentage of non-cardiac surgical patients aged 18 years and older undergoing procedures with the indications for prophylactic antibiotics AND who received a prophylactic antibiotic, who have an order for discontinuation of prophylactic antibiotics within 24 hours of surgical end time	each time a procedure is performed during the reporting period for patients who undergo non-cardiac surgical procedures with the indications for prophylactic antibiotics.	4046F **and** 1 of: 4042F 4049F 4049F-1P 4049F-8P	**ICD-9**: Any **and** **CPT**: 15734, 15738, 19260, 19271, 19272, 19301, 19302, 19303, 19304, 19305, 19306, 19307, 19361, 19364, 19366, 19367, 19368, 19369, 21346, 21347, 21348, 21422, 21423, 21432, 21433, 21435, 21436, 21454, 21461, 21462, 21465, 21470, 21627, 21632, 21740, 21750, 21805, 21825, 22325, 22524, 22554, 22558, 22600, 22612, 22630, 22800, 22802, 22804, 27125, 27130, 27132, 27134, 27137, 27138, 27235, 27236, 27244, 27245, 27269, 27440, 27441, 27442, 27443, 27445, 27446, 27447, 27702, 27703, 27704, 27758, 27759, 27766, 27769, 27792, 27814, 27870, 28192, 28193, 28293,28296, 28299, 28300, 28306, 28307, 28308, 28309, 28310, 28320, 28322, 28415, 28420, 28445, 28465, 28485, 28505, 28525, 28531, 28555, 28585, 28615, 28645, 28675, 28705, 28715, 28725, 28730, 28735, 28737, 28740, 28750, 28755, 28760, 31360, 31365, 31367, 31368, 31370, 31375, *continued on the next page*

 CPT only © 2005-2009 American Medical Association. All rights reserved.

#	Title	Description	Reporting Requirements	Numerator Code(s)	Denominator Code(s)
22	*see previous page*	*see previous page*	*see previous page*	*see previous page*	*continued from previous page* 31380, 31382, 31390, 31395, 31760, 31766, 31770, 31775, 31786, 31805, 32095, 32100, 32110, 32120, 32124, 32140, 32141, 32150, 32215, 32220, 32225, 32310, 32320, 32402, 32440, 32442, 32445, 32480, 32482, 32484, 32486, 32488, 32491, 32500, 32501, 32800, 32810, 32815, 32900, 32905, 32906, 32940, 33020, 33025, 33030, 33031, 33050, 33202, 33203, 33206, 33207, 33208, 33212, 33213, 33214, 33215, 33216, 33217, 33218, 33220, 33222, 33223, 33224, 33225, 33226, 33233, 33234, 33235, 33236, 33237, 33238, 33240, 33241, 33243, 33244, 33249, 33254, 33255, 33300, 33310, 33320, 33321, 33322, 33877, 33880, 33881, 33883, 33886, 33891, 34051, 34800, 34802, 34803, 34804, 34805, 34825, 34830, 34831, 34832, 34900, 35021, 35081, 35091, 35102, 35131, 35141, 35151, 35211, 35216, 35241, 35246, 35271, 35276, 35301, 35311, 35481, 35526, 35601, 35606, 35612, 35616, 35621, 35623, 35626, 35631, 35632, 35633, 35634, 35636, 35637, 35638, 35642, 35645, 35646, 35647, 35650, 35651, 35654, 35656, 35661, 35663, 35665, 35666, 35671, 36830, 37616, 38381, 38746, 39000, 39010, 39200, 39220, 39545, 39561, 41130, 41135, 41140, 41145, 41150, 41153, 41155, 43045, 43100, 43101, 43107, 43108, 43112, 43113, 43116, 43117, 43118, 43121, 43122, 43123, 43124, 43130, 43135, 43300, 43305, 43310, 43312, 43313, 43320, 43324, 43325, 43326, 43330, 43331, 43340, 43341, 43350, 43351, 43352, 43360, 43361, 43400, 43401, 43405, 43410, 43415, 43420, 43425, 43496, 43500, 43501, 43502, 43510, 43520, 43605, 43610, 43611, 43620, 43621, 43622, 43631, 43632, 43633, 43634, 43640, 43641, 43653, 43800, 43810, 43820, 43825, 43830, 43831, 43832, 43840, 43843, 43845, 43846, 43847, 43848, 43850, 43855, 43860, 43865, 43870, 43880, 44005, 44010, 44020, 44021, 44025, 44050, 44055, 44100, 44110, 44111, 44120, 44125, 44126, 44127, 44130, 44132, 44133, 44135, 44136, 44140, 44141, 44143, 44144, 44145, 44146, 44147, 44150, 44151, 44155, 44156, 44157, 44158, 44160, 44202, 44204, 44205, 44206, 44207, 44208, 44210, 44211, 44212, 44300, 44310, 44312, 44314, 44316, 44320, 44322, 44340, 44345, 44346, 44615, 44620, 44625, 44626, 44640, 44650, 44660, 44661, 44700, 44950, 45108, 45110, 45111, 45112, 45113, 45114, 45116, 45119, 45120, 45121, 45123, 45126, 45130, 45135, 45136, 45150, 45160, 45170, 45190, 45500, 45505, 45520, 45540, 45541, 45550, 45560, 45562, 45563, 45800, 45805, 45820, 45825, 47420, 47425, 47460, 47480, 47560, 47561, 47570, 47600, 47605, 47610, 47612, 47620, 47700, 47701, 47711, 47712, 47715, 47720, 47721, 47740, 47741, 47760, 47765, 47780, 47785, 47800, 47802, 47900, 48020, 48100, 48120, 48140, 48145, 48146, 48148, 48150, 48152, 48153, 48154, 48155, 48500, 48510, 48511, 48520, 48540, 48545, 48547, 48548, 48550, 48554, 48556, 49215, 49568, 50300, 50320, 50340, 50360, 50365, 50370, 50380, 51597, 58150, 58152, 58180, 58200, 58210, 58260, 58262, 58263, 58267, 58270, 58275, 58280, 58285, 58290, 58291, 58292, 58293, 58294, 60521, 60522, 61154, 61312, 61313, 61315, 61510, 61512, 61518, 61520, 61526, 61530, 61548, 61591, 61595, 61596, 61598, 61606, 61616, 61618, 61619, 61697, 61700, 61750, 61751, 61867, 62223, 62230, 63015, 63020, 63030, 63042, 63045, 63047, 63056, 63075, 63081, 63267, 63276, 64746, 69720, 69930, 69955, 69960, 69970

CPT only © 2005-2009 American Medical Association. All rights reserved.

#	Title	Description	Reporting Requirements	Numerator Code(s)	Denominator Code(s)
23	Perioperative Care: Venous Thromboembolism (VTE) Prophylaxis (When Indicated in ALL Patients)	Percentage of patients aged 18 years and older undergoing procedures for which VTE prophylaxis is indicated in all patients, who had an order for Low Molecular Weight Heparin (LMWH), Low-Dose Unfractionated Heparin (LDUH), adjusted-dose warfarin, fondaparinux or mechanical prophylaxis to be given within 24 hours prior to incision time or within 24 hours after surgery end time	each time a procedure is performed during the reporting period for all patients who undergo surgical procedures for which VTE prophylaxis is indicated	1 of: 4044F 4044F-1P 4044F-8P	**ICD-9**: Any **and** **CPT**: 19260, 19271, 19272, 19301, 19302, 19303, 19304, 19305, 19306, 19307, 19316, 19318, 19324, 19325, 19328, 19330, 19342, 19350, 19355, 19357, 19361, 19364, 19366, 19367, 19368, 19369, 19370, 19371, 19380, 22558, 22600, 22612, 22630, 27125, 27130, 27132, 27134, 27137, 27138, 27235, 27236, 27244, 27245, 27269, 27440, 27441, 27442, 27443, 27445, 27446, 27447, 38100, 38101, 38115, 38120, 38571, 38572, 38700, 38720, 38724, 38740, 38745, 38747, 38760, 38765, 38770, 38780, 39501, 39502, 39503, 39520, 39530, 39531, 39540, 39541, 39545, 39560, 39561, 43020, 43030, 43045, 43100, 43101, 43107, 43108, 43112, 43113, 43116, 43117, 43118, 43121, 43122, 43123, 43124, 43130, 43135, 43279, 43280, 43300, 43305, 43310, 43312, 43313, 43314, 43320, 43324, 43325, 43326, 43330, 43331, 43340, 43341, 43350, 43351, 43352, 43360, 43361, 43400, 43401, 43405, 43410, 43415, 43420, 43425, 43496, 43500, 43501, 43502, 43510, 43520, 43605, 43610, 43611, 43620, 43621, 43622, 43631, 43632, 43633, 43634, 43640, 43641, 43644, 43645, 43651, 43652, 43653, 43770, 43771, 43772, 43773, 43774, 43800, 43810, 43820, 43825, 43830, 43832, 43840, 43843, 43845, 43846, 43847, 43848, 43850, 43855, 43860, 43865, 43870, 43880, 43886, 43887, 43888, 44005, 44010, 44020, 44021, 44025, 44050, 44055, 44110, 44111, 44120, 44125, 44126, 44127, 44130, 44140, 44141, 44143, 44144, 44145, 44146, 44147, 44150, 44151, 44155, 44156, 44157, 44158, 44160, 44180, 44186, 44187, 44188, 44202, 44204, 44205, 44206, 44207, 44208, 44210, 44211, 44212, 44227, 44300, 44310, 44312, 44314, 44316, 44320, 44322, 44340, 44345, 44346, 44602, 44603, 44604, 44605, 44615, 44620, 44625, 44626, 44640, 44650, 44660, 44661, 44680, 44700, 44800, 44820, 44850, 44900, 44950, 44960, 44970, 45000, 45020, 45100, 45108, 45110, 45111, 45112, 45113, 45114, 45116, 45119, 45120, 45121, 45123, 45126, 45130, 45135, 45136, 45150, 45160, 45170, 45190, 45395, 45397, 45400, 45402, 45500, 45505, 45550, 45560, 45562, 45563, 45800, 45805, 45820, 45825, 46715, 46716, 46730, 46735, 46740, 46742, 46744, 46746, 46748, 46750, 46751, 46753, 46754, 46760, 46761, 46762, 47010, 47100, 47120, 47122, 47125, 47130, 47135, 47136, 47140, 47141, 47142, 47300, 47350, 47360, 47361, 47362, 47370, 47371, 47380, 47381, 47382, 47400, 47420, 47425, 47460, 47480, 47500, 47505, 47560, 47561, 47562, 47563, 47564, 47570, 47600, 47605, 47610, 47612, 47620, 47630, 47700, 47701, 47711, 47712, 47715, 47720, 47721, 47740, 47741, 47760, 47765, 47780, 47785, 47800, 47801, 47802, 47900, 48000, 48001, 48020, 48100, 48105, 48120, 48140, 48145, 48146, 48148, 48150, 48152, 48153, 48154, 48155, 48500, 48510, 48520, 48540, 48545, 48547, 48548, 48554, 48556, 49000, 49002, 49010, 49020, 49040, 49060, 49203, 49204, 49205, 49215, 49220, 49250, 49255, 49320, 49321, 49322, 49323, 49560, 49561, 49565, 49566, 49570, 50020, 50220, 50225, 50230, 50234, 50236, 50240, 50320, 50340, 50360, 50365, 50370, 50380, 50543, 50545, 50546, 50547, 50548, 50715, 50722, 50725, 50727, 50728, 50760, 50770, 50780, 50782, 50783, 50785, 50800, 50810, 50815, 50820, 50947, 50948, 51550, 51555, 51565, 51570, 51575, 51580, 51585, 51590, 51595, 51596, 51597, 51800, 51820, 51900, 51920, 51925, 51960, 55810, 55812, 55815, 55821, 55831, 55840, 55842, 55845, 55866, 56630, 56631, 56632, 56633, 56634, 56637, 56640, 58200, 58210, 58240, 58285, 58951, 58953, 58954, 58956, 60200, 60210, 60212, 60220, 60225, 60240, 60252, 60254, 60260, 60270, 60271, 60280, 60281, 60500, 60502, 60505, 60520, 60521, 60522, 60540, 60545, 60600, 60605, 60650, 61313, 61510, 61512, 61518, 61548, 61697, 61700, 62230, 63015, 63020, 63047, 63056, 63081, 63267, 63276

CPT only © 2005-2009 American Medical Association. All rights reserved.

#	Title	Description	Reporting Requirements	Numerator Code(s)	Denominator Code(s)
24	Osteoporosis: Communication with the Physician Managing Ongoing Care Post-Fracture	Percentage of patients aged 50 years and older treated for a hip, spine, or distal radial fracture with documentation of communication with the physician managing the patient's on-going care that a fracture occurred and that the patient was or should be tested or treated for osteoporosis	each occurrence of a fracture during the reporting period	1 of: 5015F 5015F-1P 5015F-2P 5015F-8P	**ICD-9**: 733.12, 733.13, 733.14, 805.00, 805.01, 805.02, 805.03, 805.04, 805.05, 805.06, 805.07, 805.08, 805.2, 805.4, 805.6, 805.8, 813.40, 813.41, 813.42, 813.44, 813.45, 813.50, 813.51, 813.52, 813.54, 820.00, 820.01, 820.02, 820.03, 820.09, 820.20, 820.21, 820.22, 820.8 **and** **CPT**: 22305, 22310, 22315, 22318, 22319, 22325, 22326, 22327, 22520, 22521, 22523, 22524, 25600, 25605, 25606, 25607, 25608, 25609, 27230, 27232, 27235, 27236, 27238, 27240, 27244, 27245, 27246, 27248, 99201, 99202, 99203, 99204, 99205, 99212, 99213, 99214, 99215, 99241, 99242, 99243, 99244, 99245
28	Aspirin at Arrival for Acute Myocardial Infarction (AMI)	Percentage of patients, regardless of age, with an emergency department discharge diagnosis of AMI who had documentation of receiving aspirin within 24 hours before emergency department arrival or during emergency department stay	each time during the reporting period a patient has been discharged from the emergency department with a diagnosis of AMI	1 of: 4084F 4084F-1P 4084F-2P 4084F-8P	**ICD-9**: 410.01, 410.11, 410.21, 410.31, 410.41, 410.51, 410.61, 410.71, 410.81, 410.91 **and** **CPT**: 99281, 99282, 99283, 99284, 99285, 99291 **and** **POS**: 23
30	Perioperative Care: Timing of Prophylactic Antibiotic – Administering Physician	Percentage of surgical patients aged 18 and older who have an order for a parenteral antibiotic to be given within one hour (if fluoroquinolone or vancomycin, two hours) prior to the surgical incision (or start of procedure when no incision is required) for whom administration of prophylactic antibiotic has been initiated within one hour (if fluoroquinolone or vancomycin, two hours) prior to the surgical incision (or start of procedure when no incision is required)	each time a procedure is performed during the reporting period for patients who undergo surgical procedures with an order for prophylactic antibiotics.	1 of: 4047F-8P 4048F 4048F-8P	**ICD-9**: Any **and** **CPT**: 00100, 00102, 00103, 00120, 00140, 00145, 00147, 00160, 00162, 00164, 00170, 00172, 00174, 00176, 00190, 00192, 00210, 00211, 00212, 00214, 00215, 00216, 00218, 00220, 00222, 00300, 00320, 00322, 00350, 00352, 00400, 00402, 00404, 00406, 00450, 00452, 00454, 00470, 00472, 00474, 00500, 00528, 00529, 00530, 00532, 00534, 00537, 00539, 00540, 00541, 00542, 00546, 00548, 00550, 00560, 00561, 00562, 00563, 00566, 00567, 00580, 00600, 00604, 00620, 00622, 00625, 00626, 00630, 00632, 00634, 00670, 00700, 00730, 00750, 00752, 00754, 00756, 00770, 00790, 00792, 00794, 00796, 00797, 00800, 00802, 00820, 00830, 00832, 00840, 00844, 00846, 00848, 00851, 00860, 00862, 00864, 00865, 00866, 00868, 00870, 00880, 00882, 00902, 00904, 00906, 00908, 00910, 00912, 00914, 00916, 00918, 00920, 00921, 00922, 00924, 00926, 00928, 00930, 00932, 00934, 00936, 00938, 00940, 00942, 00944, 01120, 01140, 01150, 01170, 01173, 01180, 01190, 01202, 01210, 01212, 01214, 01215, 01230, 01232, 01234, 01250, 01260, 01270, 01272, 01274, 01320, 01360, 01382, 01392, 01400, 01402, 01404, 01430, 01432, 01440, 01442, 01444, 01464, 01470, 01472, 01474, 01480, 01482, 01484, 01486, 01500, 01502, 01520, 01522, 01610, 01622, 01630, 01632, 01634, 01636, 01638, 01650, 01652, 01654, 01656, 01670, 01710, 01712, 01714, 01716, 01732, 01740, 01742, 01744, 01756, 01758, 01760, 01770, 01772, 01780, 01782, 01810, 01829, 01830, 01832, 01840, 01842, 01844, 01850, 01852, 01924, 01925, 01926, 01951, 01952, 01953, 01961, 01962, 01963, 01965, 01966, 01968, 01969
31	Stroke and Stroke Rehabilitation: Deep Vein Thrombosis Prophylaxis (DVT) for Ischemic Stroke or Intracranial Hemorrhage	Percentage of patients aged 18 years and older with a diagnosis of ischemic stroke or intracranial hemorrhage who received DVT prophylaxis by end of hospital day two	each hospital stay when a patient is under active treatment for ischemic stroke or intracranial hemorrhage during the reporting period	1 of: 4070F 4070F-1P 4070F-2P 4070F-8P	**ICD-9**: 431, 433.01, 433.11, 433.21, 433.31, 433.81, 433.91, 434.01, 434.11, 434.91 **and** **CPT**: 99221, 99222, 99223, 99251, 99252, 99253, 99254, 99255, 99291

CPT only © 2005-2009 American Medical Association. All rights reserved.

#	Title	Description	Reporting Requirements	Numerator Code(s)	Denominator Code(s)
32	Stroke and Stroke Rehabilitation: Discharged on Antiplatelet Therapy	Percentage of patients aged 18 years and older with a diagnosis of ischemic stroke or transient ischemic attack (TIA) who were prescribed antiplatelet therapy at discharge	for patients under active treatment for ischemic stroke or TIA at discharge from a hospital during the reporting period. Part B claims data will be analyzed to determine the hospital discharge	1 of: 4073F 4073F-1P 4073F-2P 4073F-8P	**ICD-9**: 433.01, 433.11, 433.21, 433.31, 433.81, 433.91, 434.01, 434.11, 434.91, 435.0, 435.1, 435.2, 435.3, 435.8, 435.9 **and** **CPT**: 99238, 99239, 99251, 99252, 99253, 99254, 99255
33	Stroke and Stroke Rehabilitation: Anticoagulant Therapy Prescribed for Atrial Fibrillation at Discharge	Percentage of patients aged 18 years and older with a diagnosis of ischemic stroke or transient ischemic attack (TIA) with documented permanent, persistent, or paroxysmal atrial fibrillation who were prescribed an anticoagulant at discharge	for patients under active treatment for ischemic stroke or TIA with documented atrial fibrillation at discharge from a hospital during the reporting period	Registry only (no codes)	**ICD-9**: 433.01, 433.11, 433.21, 433.31, 433.81, 433.91, 434.01, 434.11, 434.91, 435.0, 435.1, 435.2, 435.3, 435.8, 435.9 **and** **ICD-9**: 427.31 **and** **CPT**: 99238, 99239, 99251, 99252, 99253, 99254, 99255
34	Stroke and Stroke Rehabilitation: Tissue Plasminogen Activator (t-PA) Considered	Percentage of patients aged 18 years and older with a diagnosis of ischemic stroke whose time from symptom onset to arrival is less than 3 hours who were considered for t-PA administration	each hospital stay for all patients under active treatment for ischemic stroke during the reporting period	1065F **and** 1 of: 4077F 4077F-8P **OR** 1066F	**ICD-9**: 433.01, 433.11, 433.21, 433.31, 433.81, 433.91, 434.01, 434.11, 434.91 **and** **CPT**: 99221, 99222, 99223, 99251, 99252, 99253, 99254, 99255, 99291
35	Stroke and Stroke Rehabilitation: Screening for Dysphagia	Percentage of patients aged 18 years and older with a diagnosis of ischemic stroke or intracranial hemorrhage who underwent a dysphagia screening process before taking any foods, fluids or medication by mouth	each hospital stay for all patients under active treatment for ischemic stroke or intracranial hemorrhage during the reporting period	6015F **and** 1 of: 6010F 6010F-1P 6010F-8P **OR** 6020F	**ICD-9**: 431, 433.01, 433.11, 433.21, 433.31, 433.81, 433.91, 434.01, 434.11, 434.91 **and** **CPT**: 99221, 99222, 99223, 99251, 99252, 99253, 99254, 99255
36	Stroke and Stroke Rehabilitation: Consideration of Rehabilitation Services	Percentage of patients aged 18 years and older with a diagnosis of ischemic stroke or intracranial hemorrhage for whom consideration of rehabilitation services is documented	≥ once/ reporting period	1 of: 4079F 4079F-8P	**ICD-9**: 431, 433.01, 433.11, 433.21, 433.31, 433.81, 433.91, 434.01, 434.11, 434.91 **and** **CPT**: 99238, 99239, 99251, 99252, 99253, 99254, 99255
39	Screening or Therapy for Osteoporosis for Women Aged 65 Years and Older	Percentage of female patients aged 65 years and older who have a central dual-energy X-ray absorptiometry (DXA) measurement ordered or performed at least once since age 60 or pharmacologic therapy prescribed within 12 months	≥ once/ reporting period	1 of: G8399 G8400 G8401	**ICD-9**: Any **and** **CPT**: 99201, 99202, 99203, 99204, 99205, 99212, 99213, 99214, 99215

CPT only © 2005-2009 American Medical Association. All rights reserved.

#	Title	Description	Reporting Requirements	Numerator Code(s)	Denominator Code(s)
40	Osteoporosis: Management Following Fracture	Percentage of patients aged 50 years and older with fracture of the hip, spine or distal radius who had a central dual-energy X-ray absorptiometry (DXA) measurement ordered or performed or pharmacologic therapy prescribed	each occurrence of a fracture during the reporting period	1 of: 3095F 3095F-1P 3095F-2P 3095F-3P 3095F-8P 3096F 3096F-1P 3096F-2P 3096F-3P 3096F-8P 4005F 4005F-1P 4005F-2P 4005F-3P 4005F-8P	**ICD-9**: 733.12, 733.13, 733.14, 805.00, 805.01, 805.02, 805.03, 805.04, 805.05, 805.06, 805.07, 805.08, 805.2, 805.4, 805.6, 805.8, 813.40, 813.41, 813.42, 813.44, 813.45, 813.50, 813.51, 813.52, 813.54, 820.00, 820.01, 820.02, 820.03, 820.09, 820.20, 820.21, 820.22, 820.8 **and** **CPT**: 22305, 22310, 22315, 22318, 22319, 22325, 22326, 22327, 22520, 22521, 22523, 22524, 25600, 25605, 25606, 25607, 25608, 25609, 27230, 27232, 27235, 27236, 27238, 27240, 27244, 27245, 27246, 27248, 99201, 99202, 99203, 99204, 99205, 99212, 99213, 99214, 99215, 99241, 99242, 99243, 99244, 99245
41	Osteoporosis: Pharmacologic Therapy	Percentage of patients aged 50 years and older with a diagnosis of osteoporosis who were prescribed pharmacologic therapy within 12 months	≥ once per reporting period for patients seen during the reporting period.	1 of: 4005F 4005F-1P 4005F-2P 4005F-3P 4005F-8P	**ICD-9**: 733.00, 733.01, 733.02, 733.03, 733.09 **and** **CPT**: 99201, 99202, 99203, 99204, 99205, 99212, 99213, 99214, 99215, 99241, 99242, 99243, 99244, 99245
43	Coronary Artery Bypass Graft (CABG): Use of Internal Mammary Artery (IMA) in Patients with Isolated CABG Surgery	Percentage of patients aged 18 years and older undergoing isolated CABG surgery using an IMA graft	each time an isolated CABG procedure is performed during the reporting period	1 of: 4110F 4110F-1P 4110F-8P	**ICD-9**: Any **and** **CPT**: 33510, 33511, 33512, 33513, 33514, 33516, 33517, 33518, 33519, 33521, 33522, 33523, 33533, 33534, 33535, 33536
44	Coronary Artery Bypass Graft (CABG): Preoperative Beta-Blocker in Patients with Isolated CABG Surgery	Percentage of patients aged 18 years and older undergoing isolated CABG surgery who received a beta-blocker within 24 hours prior to surgical incision	each time an isolated CABG procedure is performed during the reporting period	1 of: 4115F 4115F-1P 4115F-8P	**ICD-9**: Any **and** **CPT**: 33510, 33511, 33512, 33513, 33514, 33516, 33517, 33518, 33519, 33521, 33522, 33523, 33533, 33534, 33535, 33536
45	Perioperative Care: Discontinuation of Prophylactic Antibiotics (Cardiac Procedures)	Percentage of cardiac surgical patients aged 18 years and older undergoing procedures with the indications for prophylactic antibiotics AND who received a prophylactic antibiotic, who have an order for discontinuation of prophylactic antibiotics within 48 hours of surgical end time	each time a procedure is performed during the reporting period for patients who undergo cardiac procedures with the indications for prophylactic antibiotics	4046F **and** 1 of: 4043F 4043F-1P 4043F-8P **OR** 4042F	**ICD-9**: Any **and** **CPT**: 33120, 33130, 33140, 33141, 33250, 33251, 33256, 33261, 33305, 33315, 33332, 33335, 33400, 33401, 33403, 33404, 33405, 33406, 33410, 33411, 33413, 33416, 33422, 33425, 33426, 33427, 33430, 33460, 33463, 33464, 33465, 33475, 33496, 33510, 33511, 33512, 33513, 33514, 33516, 33517, 33518, 33519, 33521, 33522, 33523, 33530, 33533, 33534, 33535, 33536, 33542, 33545, 33548, 33572

CPT only © 2005-2009 American Medical Association. All rights reserved.

#	Title	Description	Reporting Requirements	Numerator Code(s)	Denominator Code(s)
46	Medication Reconciliation: Reconciliation After Discharge from an Inpatient Facility	Percentage of patients aged 65 years and older discharged from any inpatient facility (e.g., hospital, skilled nursing facility, or rehabilitation facility) and seen within 60 days following discharge in the office by the physician providing on-going care who had a reconciliation of the discharge medications with the current medication list in the medical record documented	at an office visit occurring within 60 days of each inpatient facility discharge date during the reporting period	Registry only (no codes)	**ICD-9**: Any **and** **CPT**: 99201, 99202, 99203, 99204, 99205, 99212, 99213, 99214, 99215, 99324, 99325, 99326, 99327, 99328, 99334, 99335, 99336, 99337, 99341, 99342, 99343, 99344, 99345, 99347, 99348, 99349, 99350
47	Advance Care Plan	Percentage of patients aged 65 years and older who have an advance care plan or surrogate decision maker documented in the medical record or documentation in the medical record that an advance care plan was discussed but the patient did not wish or was not able to name a surrogate decision maker or provide an advance care plan	≥ once per reporting period for patients seen during the reporting period	1124F **and** 1 of: 1123F 1123F-8P	**ICD-9**: Any **and** **CPT**: 99201, 99202, 99203, 99204, 99205, 99212, 99213, 99214, 99215, 99218, 99219, 99220, 99221, 99222, 99223, 99231, 99232, 99233, 99234, 99235, 99236, 99291*, 99304, 99305, 99306, 99307, 99308, 99309, 99310, 99324, 99325, 99326, 99327, 99328, 99334, 99335, 99336, 99337, 99341, 99342, 99343, 99344, 99345, 99347, 99348, 99349, 99350 * Clinicians indicating the place of service as the emergency department will not be included in this measure.
48	Urinary Incontinence: Assessment of Presence or Absence of Urinary Incontinence in Women Aged 65 Years and Older	Percentage of female patients aged 65 years and older who were assessed for the presence or absence of urinary incontinence within 12 months	≥ once per reporting period for patients seen during the reporting period	1 of: 1090F 1090F-1P 1090F-8P	**ICD-9**: Any **and** **CPT**: 99201, 99202, 99203, 99204, 99205, 99212, 99213, 99214, 99215, 99324, 99325, 99326, 99327, 99328, 99334, 99335, 99336, 99337, 99341, 99342, 99343, 99344, 99345, 99347, 99348, 99349, 99350 **and** **POS**: Ambulatory setting only
49	Urinary Incontinence: Characterization of Urinary Incontinence in Women Aged 65 Years and Older	Percentage of female patients aged 65 years and older with a diagnosis of urinary incontinence whose urinary incontinence was characterized at least once within 12 months	≥ once per reporting period for patients seen during the reporting period	1 of: 1091F 1091F-8P	**ICD-9**: 307.6, 625.6, 788.30, 788.31, 788.33, 788.34, 788.35, 788.36, 788.37, 788.38, 788.39 **and** **CPT**: 99201, 99202, 99203, 99204, 99205, 99212, 99213, 99214, 99215, 99241, 99242, 99243, 99244, 99245, 99324, 99325, 99326, 99327, 99328, 99334, 99335, 99336, 99337, 99341, 99342, 99343, 99344, 99345, 99347, 99348, 99349, 99350 **and** **POS**: Ambulatory setting only
50	Urinary Incontinence: Plan of Care for Urinary Incontinence in Women Aged 65 Years and Older	Percentage of female patients aged 65 years and older with a diagnosis of urinary incontinence with a documented plan of care for urinary incontinence at least once within 12 months	≥ once per reporting period for patients seen during the reporting period	1 of: 0509F 0509F-8P	**ICD-9**: 307.6, 625.6, 788.30, 788.31, 788.33, 788.34, 788.35, 788.36, 788.37, 788.38, 788.39 **and** **CPT**: 99201, 99202, 99203, 99204, 99205, 99212, 99213, 99214, 99215, 99241, 99242, 99243, 99244, 99245, 99324, 99325, 99326, 99327, 99328, 99334, 99335, 99336, 99337, 99341, 99342, 99343, 99344, 99345, 99347, 99348, 99349, 99350 **and** **POS**: Ambulatory setting only

CPT only © 2005-2009 American Medical Association. All rights reserved.

#	Title	Description	Reporting Requirements	Numerator Code(s)	Denominator Code(s)
51	Chronic Obstructive Pulmonary Disease (COPD): Spirometry Evaluation	Percentage of patients aged 18 years and older with a diagnosis of COPD who had spirometry evaluation results documented	≥ once per reporting period using the most recent spirometry results in the patient record for patients seen during the reporting period.	1 of: 3023F 3023F-1P 3023F-2P 3023F-3P 3023F-8P	**ICD-9**: 491.0, 491.1, 491.20, 491.21, 491.22, 491.8, 491.9, 492.0, 492.8, 496 **and** **CPT**: 99201, 99202, 99203, 99204, 99205, 99212, 99213, 99214, 99215, 99241, 99242, 99243, 99244, 99245
52	Chronic Obstructive Pulmonary Disease (COPD): Bronchodilator Therapy	Percentage of patients aged 18 years and older with a diagnosis of COPD and who have an FEV1/FVC less than 70% and have symptoms who were prescribed an inhaled bronchodilator	≥ once per reporting period for all COPD patients seen during the reporting period	3025F **and** 1 of: 4025F 4025F-1P 4025F-2P 4025F-3P 4025F-8P **OR** 3025F-8P **OR** 3027F	**ICD-9**: 491.0, 491.1, 491.20, 491.21, 491.22, 491.8, 491.9, 492.0, 492.8, 496 **and** **CPT**: 99201, 99202, 99203, 99204, 99205, 99212, 99213, 99214, 99215, 99241, 99242, 99243, 99244, 99245
53	Asthma: Pharmacologic Therapy	Percentage of patients aged 5 through 40 years with a diagnosis of mild, moderate, or severe persistent asthma who were prescribed either the preferred long-term control medication (inhaled corticosteroid) or an acceptable alternative treatment	≥ once per reporting period for all asthma patients seen during the reporting period	1038F **and** 1 of: 4015F 4015F-8P **OR** 4015F-2P **and** 1 of: 1038F 1039F	**ICD-9**: 493.00, 493.01, 493.02, 493.10, 493.11, 493.12, 493.20, 493.21, 493.22, 493.81, 493.82, 493.90, 493.91, 493.92 **and** **CPT**: 99201, 99202, 99203, 99204, 99205, 99212, 99213, 99214, 99215, 99241, 99242, 99243, 99244, 99245
54	12-Lead Electrocardiogram (ECG) Performed for Non-Traumatic Chest Pain	Percentage of patients aged 40 years and older with an emergency department discharge diagnosis of non-traumatic chest pain who had a 12-lead electrocardiogram (ECG) performed	each time a patient has been discharged from the emergency department with a discharge diagnosis of non-traumatic chest pain during the reporting period	1 of: 3120F 3120F-1P 3120F-2P 3120F-8P	**ICD-9**: 413.0, 413.1, 413.9, 786.50, 786.51, 786.52, 786.59 **and** **CPT**: 99281, 99282, 99283, 99284, 99285, 99291 **and** **POS**: 23
55	12-Lead Electrocardiogram (ECG) Performed for Syncope	Percentage of patients aged 60 years and older with an emergency department discharge diagnosis of syncope who had a 12-lead ECG performed	each time a patient has been discharged from the emergency department with a discharge diagnosis of syncope during the reporting period.	1 of: 3120F 3120F-1P 3120F-2P 3120F-8P	**ICD-9**: 780.2 **and** **CPT**: 99281, 99282, 99283, 99284, 99285, 99291 **and** POS: 23

CPT only © 2005-2009 American Medical Association. All rights reserved.

#	Title	Description	Reporting Requirements	Numerator Code(s)	Denominator Code(s)
56	Community-Acquired Pneumonia (CAP): Vital Signs	Percentage of patients aged 18 years and older with a diagnosis of community-acquired bacterial pneumonia with vital signs documented and reviewed	once for each occurrence of community-acquired bacterial pneumonia during the reporting period	1 of: 2010F 2010F-8P	**ICD-9**: 481, 482.0, 482.1, 482.2, 482.30, 482.31, 482.32, 482.39, 482.40, 482.41, 482.42, 482.49, 482.81, 482.82, 482.83, 482.84, 482.89, 482.9, 483.0, 483.1, 483.8, 485, 486, 487.0 **and** **CPT**: 99201, 99202, 99203, 99204, 99205, 99212, 99213, 99214, 99215, 99241, 99242, 99243, 99244, 99245, 99281, 99282, 99283, 99284, 99285, 99291*, 99324, 99325, 99326, 99327, 99328, 99334, 99335, 99336, 99337, 99341, 99342, 99343, 99344, 99345, 99347, 99348, 99349, 99350 * Clinicians utilizing the critical care code must indicate the emergency department place-of-service (23) on the Part B claim form in order to report this measure.
57	Community-Acquired Pneumonia (CAP): Assessment of Oxygen Saturation	Percentage of patients aged 18 years and older with a diagnosis of community-acquired bacterial pneumonia with oxygen saturation documented and reviewed	once for each occurrence of community-acquired bacterial pneumonia during the reporting period	1 of: 3028F 3028F-1P 3028F-2P 3028F-3P 3028F-8P	**ICD-9**: 481, 482.0, 482.1, 482.2, 482.30, 482.31, 482.32, 482.39, 482.40, 482.41, 482.42, 482.49, 482.81, 482.82, 482.83, 482.84, 482.89, 482.9, 483.0, 483.1, 483.8, 485, 486, 487.0 **and** **CPT**: 99201, 99202, 99203, 99204, 99205, 99212, 99213, 99214, 99215, 99241, 99242, 99243, 99244, 99245, 99281, 99282, 99283, 99284, 99285, 99291*, 99324, 99325, 99326, 99327, 99328, 99334, 99335, 99336, 99337, 99341, 99342, 99343, 99344, 99345, 99347, 99348, 99349, 99350 * Clinicians utilizing the critical care code must indicate the emergency department place-of-service (23) on the Part B claim form in order to report this measure.
58	Community-Acquired Pneumonia (CAP): Assessment of Mental Status	Percentage of patients aged 18 years and older with a diagnosis of community-acquired bacterial pneumonia with mental status assessed	once for each occurrence of community-acquired bacterial pneumonia during the reporting period	1 of: 2014F 2014F-8P	**ICD-9**: 481, 482.0, 482.1, 482.2, 482.30, 482.31, 482.32, 482.39, 482.40, 482.41, 482.42, 482.49, 482.81, 482.82, 482.83, 482.84, 482.89, 482.9, 483.0, 483.1, 483.8, 485, 486, 487.0 **and** **CPT**: 99201, 99202, 99203, 99204, 99205, 99212, 99213, 99214, 99215, 99241, 99242, 99243, 99244, 99245, 99281, 99282, 99283, 99284, 99285, 99291*, 99324, 99325, 99326, 99327, 99328, 99334, 99335, 99336, 99337, 99341, 99342, 99343, 99344, 99345, 99347, 99348, 99349, 99350 * Clinicians utilizing the critical care code must indicate the emergency department place-of-service (23) on the Part B claim form in order to report this measure.
59	Community-Acquired Pneumonia (CAP): Empiric Antibiotic	Percentage of patients aged 18 years and older with a diagnosis of community-acquired bacterial pneumonia with an appropriate empiric antibiotic prescribed	once for each occurrence of community-acquired bacterial pneumonia during the reporting period	1 of: 4045F 4045F-1P 4045F-2P 4045F-3P 4045F-8P	**ICD-9**: 481, 482.0, 482.1, 482.2, 482.30, 482.31, 482.32, 482.39, 482.40, 482.41, 482.42, 482.49, 482.81, 482.82, 482.83, 482.84, 482.89, 482.9, 483.0, 483.1, 483.8, 485, 486, 487.0 **and** **CPT**: 99201, 99202, 99203, 99204, 99205, 99212, 99213, 99214, 99215, 99241, 99242, 99243, 99244, 99245, 99281, 99282, 99283, 99284, 99285, 99291*, 99324, 99325, 99326, 99327, 99328, 99334, 99335, 99336, 99337, 99341, 99342, 99343, 99344, 99345, 99347, 99348, 99349, 99350 * Clinicians utilizing the critical care code must indicate the emergency department place-of-service (23) on the Part B claim form in order to report this measure.
64	Asthma: Asthma Assessment	Percentage of patients aged 5 through 40 years with a diagnosis of asthma who were evaluated during at least one office visit within 12 months for the frequency (numeric) of daytime and nocturnal asthma symptoms	once per reporting period for patients with asthma seen during the reporting period	1 of: 1005F 1005F-8P	**ICD-9**: 493.00, 493.01, 493.02, 493.10, 493.11, 493.12, 493.20, 493.21, 493.22, 493.81, 493.82, 493.90, 493.91, 493.92 **and** **CPT**: 99201, 99202, 99203, 99204, 99205, 99212, 99213, 99214, 99215, 99241, 99242, 99243, 99244, 99245

CPT only © 2005-2009 American Medical Association. All rights reserved.

#	Title	Description	Reporting Requirements	Numerator Code(s)	Denominator Code(s)
65	Treatment for Children with Upper Respiratory Infection (URI): Avoidance of Inappropriate Use	Percentage of children aged 3 months through 18 years with a diagnosis of upper respiratory infection (URI) who were not prescribed or dispensed an antibiotic prescription on or within 3 days of the initial date of service	once for each occurrence of upper respiratory infection during the reporting period.	1 of: 4120F 4124F 4124F-1P	**ICD-9**:460, 465.0, 465.8, 465.9 **and** **CPT**: 99201, 99202, 99203, 99204, 99205, 99212, 99213, 99214, 99215, 99217, 99218, 99219, 99220, 99241, 99242, 99243, 99244, 99245
66	Appropriate Testing for Children with Pharyngitis	Percentage of children aged 2 through 18 years with a diagnosis of pharyngitis, who were prescribed an antibiotic and who received a group A streptococcus (strep) test for the episode	once for each occurrence of pharyngitis during the reporting period	4120F **and** 1 of: 3210F 3210F-1P 3210F-8P **OR** 4124F **and** 3210F-1P	**ICD-9**: 034.0, 462, 463 **and** **CPT**: 99201, 99202, 99203, 99204, 99205, 99212, 99213, 99214, 99215, 99217, 99218, 99219, 99220, 99241, 99242, 99243, 99244, 99245
67	Myelodysplastic Syndrome (MDS) and Acute Leukemias: Baseline Cytogenetic Testing Performed on Bone Marrow	Percentage of patients aged 18 years and older with a diagnosis of MDS or an acute leukemia who had baseline cytogenetic testing performed on bone marrow	≥ once per reporting period for patients seen during the reporting period, regardless of when the baseline testing is performed	1 of: 3155F 3155F-1P 3155F-2P 3155F-3P 3155F-8P	**ICD-9**: 204.00, 204.02, 205.00, 205.02, 206.00, 206.02, 207.00, 207.02, 207.20, 207.22, 208.00, 208.02, 238.72, 238.73, 238.74, 238.75 **and** **CPT**: 99201, 99202, 99203, 99204, 99205, 99212, 99213, 99214, 99215, 99241, 99242, 99243, 99244, 99245
68	Myelodysplastic Syndrome (MDS): Documentation of Iron Stores in Patients Receiving Erythropoietin Therapy	Percentage of patients aged 18 years and older with a diagnosis of MDS who are receiving erythropoietin therapy with documentation of iron stores prior to initiating erythropoietin therapy	≥ once/ reporting period for all MDS patients seen during the reporting period, regardless of when the documentation of iron stores occurs	4090F **and** 1 of: 3160F 3160F-3P 3160F-8P	**ICD-9**: 238.72, 238.73, 238.74, 238.75 **and** **CPT**: 99201, 99202, 99203, 99204, 99205, 99212, 99213, 99214, 99215, 99241, 99242, 99243, 99244, 99245
69	Multiple Myeloma: Treatment with Bisphosphonates	Percentage of patients aged 18 years and older with a diagnosis of multiple myeloma, not in remission, who were prescribed or received intravenous bisphosphonate therapy within the 12-month reporting period	≥ once per reporting period for patients seen during the reporting period	1 of: 4100F 4100F-1P 4100F-2P 4100F-8P	**ICD-9**: 203.00, 203.02 **and** **CPT**: 99201, 99202, 99203, 99204, 99205, 99212, 99213, 99214, 99215, 99241, 99242, 99243, 99244, 99245
70	Chronic Lymphocytic Leukemia (CLL): Baseline Flow Cytometry	Percentage of patients aged 18 years and older with a diagnosis of CLL who had baseline flow cytometry studies performed	≥ once per reporting period for patients seen during the reporting period, regardless of when the baseline flow cytometry studies are performed	1 of: 3170F 3170F-1P 3170F-2P 3170F-3P 3170F-8P	**ICD-9**: 204.10, 204.12 **and** **CPT**: 99201, 99202, 99203, 99204, 99205, 99212, 99213, 99214, 99215, 99241, 99242, 99243, 99244, 99245

CPT only © 2005-2009 American Medical Association. All rights reserved.

#	Title	Description	Reporting Requirements	Numerator Code(s)	Denominator Code(s)
71	Breast Cancer: Hormonal Therapy for Stage IC - IIIC Estrogen Receptor/ Progesterone Receptor (ER/PR) Positive Breast Cancer	Percentage of female patients aged 18 years and older with Stage IC through IIIC, estrogen receptor (ER) or progesterone receptor (PR) positive breast cancer who were prescribed tamoxifen or aromatase inhibitor (AI) during the 12-month reporting period	≥ once per reporting period for all female patients with breast cancer seen during the reporting period	3315F **and** 1 of: 3374F 3376F 3378F **and** 1 of: 4179F 4179F-1P 4179F-2P 4179F-3P 4179F-8P **OR** 1 of: 3316F 3316F-8P 3370F 3370F-8P 3372F 3380F	**ICD-9**: 174.0, 174.1, 174.2, 174.3, 174.4, 174.5, 174.6, 174.8, 174.9 **and** **CPT**: 99201, 99202, 99203, 99204, 99205, 99212, 99213, 99214, 99215
72	Colon Cancer: Chemotherapy for Stage III Colon Cancer Patients	Percentage of patients aged 18 years and older with Stage IIIA through IIIC colon cancer who are prescribed or who have received adjuvant chemotherapy during the 12-month reporting period	≥ once per reporting period for all patients with colon cancer seen during the reporting period	1 of: 3388F **and** 1 of: 4080F 4080F-1P 4080F-2P 4080F-3P 4080F-8P **OR** 1 of: 3382F 3382F-8P 3384F 3386F 3390F	**ICD-9**: 153.0, 153.1, 153.2, 153.3, 153.4, 153.5, 153.6, 153.7, 153.8, 153.9 **and** **CPT**: 99201, 99202, 99203, 99204, 99205, 99212, 99213, 99214, 99215
76	Prevention of Catheter-Related Bloodstream Infections (CRBSI): Central Venous Catheter (CVC) Insertion Protocol	Percentage of patients, regardless of age, who undergo central venous catheter (CVC) insertion for whom CVC was inserted with all elements of maximal sterile barrier technique [cap AND mask AND sterile gown AND sterile gloves AND a large sterile sheet AND hand hygiene AND 2% chlorhexidine for cutaneous antisepsis (or acceptable alternative antiseptics per current guideline)] followed	each time a CVC insertion is performed during the reporting period	1 of: 6030F 6030F-1P 6030F-8P	**ICD-9**: Any **and** **CPT**: 36555, 36556, 36557, 36558, 36560, 36561, 36563, 36565, 36566, 36568, 36569, 36570, 36571, 36578, 36580, 36581, 36582, 36583, 36584, 36585, 93503
79	End Stage Renal Disease (ESRD): Influenza Immunization in Patients with ESRD	Percentage of patients aged 18 years and older with a diagnosis of ESRD and receiving dialysis who received the influenza immunization during the flu season (September through February)	≥ once per reporting period for ESRD patients receiving dialysis seen during the reporting period	1 of: 4037F 4037F-1P 4037F-2P 4037F-3P 4037F-8P	**ICD-9**: 585.6 **and** **CPT/HCPCS II**: 90935, 90937, 90945, 90947, 90957, 90958, 90959, 90960, 90961, 90962, 90965, 90966, 90969, 90970

CPT only © 2005-2009 American Medical Association. All rights reserved.

#	Title	Description	Reporting Requirements	Numerator Code(s)	Denominator Code(s)
81	End Stage Renal Disease (ESRD): Plan of Care for Inadequate Hemodialysis in ESRD Patients	Percentage of patient calendar months during the 12-month reporting period in which patients aged 18 years and older with a diagnosis of end stage renal disease (ESRD) receiving hemodialysis have a Kt/V ≥ 1.2 OR patients who have a Kt/V < 1.2 with a documented plan of care for inadequate hemodialysis	each calendar month hemodialysis is performed on ESRD patients seen during the reporting period	Registry only (no codes)	**ICD-9**: 585.6 **and** **CPT/HCPCS II**: 90935, 90937, 90957, 90958, 90959, 90960, 90961, 90962
82	End Stage Renal Disease (ESRD): Plan of Care for Inadequate Peritoneal Dialysis	Percentage of patients aged 18 years and older with a diagnosis of end stage renal disease (ESRD) receiving peritoneal dialysis who have a Kt/V ≥ 1.7 OR patients who have a Kt/V < 1.7 with a documented plan of care for inadequate peritoneal dialysis at least three times during the 12-month reporting period	≤ three times per reporting year for ESRD patients receiving peritoneal dialysis during the entire reporting period and seen during the reporting period	Registry only (no codes)	**ICD-9**: 585.6 **and** **CPT/HCPCS II**: 90945, 90947, 90965, 90966, 90969, 90970
83	Hepatitis C: Testing for Chronic Hepatitis C - Confirmation of Hepatitis C Viremia	Percentage of patients aged 18 years and older with a diagnosis of hepatitis C seen for an initial evaluation who had HCV RNA testing ordered or previously performed	first visit occurring during the reporting period for all patients with a diagnosis of hepatitis C seen during the reporting period	1 of: 3265F 3265F-1P 3265F-2P 3265F-8P **and** 1119F **OR** 1121F	**ICD-9**: 070.51, 070.54, 070.70 **and** **CPT**: 99201, 99202, 99203, 99204, 99205, 99212, 99213, 99214, 99215, 99241, 99242, 99243, 99244, 99245
84	Hepatitis C: Ribonucleic Acid (RNA) Testing Before Initiating Treatment	Percentage of patients aged 18 years and older with a diagnosis of chronic hepatitis C who are receiving antiviral treatment for whom quantitative HCV RNA testing was performed within 6 months prior to initiation of treatment	≥ once per reporting period for all patients with a diagnosis of chronic hepatitis C seen during the reporting period	1 of: 3218F 3218F-1P 3218F-8P **and** 4150F **OR** 4151F	**ICD-9**: 070.54 **and** **CPT**: 99201, 99202, 99203, 99204, 99205, 99212, 99213, 99214, 99215, 99241, 99242, 99243, 99244, 99245
85	Hepatitis C: HCV Genotype Testing Prior to Treatment	Percentage of patients aged 18 years and older with a diagnosis of chronic hepatitis C who are receiving antiviral treatment for whom HCV genotype testing was performed prior to initiation of treatment	≥ once per reporting period for all patients with a diagnosis of chronic hepatitis C seen during the reporting period	1 of: 3266F 3266F-8P **and** G8459 **OR** G8458	**ICD-9**: 070.54 **and** **CPT**: 99201, 99202, 99203, 99204, 99205, 99212, 99213, 99214, 99215, 99241, 99242, 99243, 99244, 99245
86	Hepatitis C: Antiviral Treatment Prescribed	Percentage of patients aged 18 years and older with a diagnosis of chronic hepatitis C who were prescribed peginterferon and ribavirin therapy within the 12-month reporting period	≥ once per reporting period for patients with a diagnosis of chronic hepatitis C seen during the reporting period	1 of: 4153F 4153F-1P 4153F-2P 4153F-3P 4153F-8P	**ICD-9**: 070.54 **and** **CPT**: 99201, 99202, 99203, 99204, 99205, 99212, 99213, 99214, 99215, 99241, 99242, 99243, 99244, 99245

CPT only © 2005-2009 American Medical Association. All rights reserved.

#	Title	Description	Reporting Requirements	Numerator Code(s)	Denominator Code(s)
87	Hepatitis C: HCV Ribonucleic Acid (RNA) Testing at Week 12 of Treatment	Percentage of patients aged 18 years and older with a diagnosis of chronic hepatitis C who are receiving antiviral treatment for whom quantitative HCV RNA testing was performed at 12 weeks from the initiation of antiviral treatment	≥ once per reporting period for all patients with a diagnosis of chronic hepatitis C seen during the reporting period	1 of: 3220F 3220F-8P **and** G8461 **OR** 1 of: 3220F-1P 3220F-2P **and** 1 of: G8460 G8461	**ICD-9**: 070.54 **and** **CPT**: 99201, 99202, 99203, 99204, 99205, 99212, 99213, 99214, 99215, 99241, 99242, 99243, 99244, 99245
89	Hepatitis C: Counseling Regarding Risk of Alcohol Consumption	Percentage of patients aged 18 years and older with a diagnosis of hepatitis C who were counseled about the risks of alcohol use at least once within the 12-month reporting period	≥ once per reporting period for patients with a diagnosis of hepatitis C seen during the reporting period	1 of: 4158F 4158F-8P	**ICD-9**: 070.51, 070.54, 070.70 **and** **CPT**: 99201, 99202, 99203, 99204, 99205, 99212, 99213, 99214, 99215, 99241, 99242, 99243, 99244, 99245
90	Hepatitis C: Counseling Regarding Use of Contraception Prior to Antiviral Therapy	Percentage of female patients aged 18 through 44 years and all men aged 18 years and older with a diagnosis of chronic hepatitis C who are receiving antiviral treatment who were counseled regarding contraception prior to the initiation of treatment	≥ once per reporting period for all patients with a diagnosis of chronic hepatitis C seen during the reporting period	1 of: 4159F 4159F-8P **and** G8463 **OR** 4159F-1P **and** 1 of: G8462 G8463	**ICD-9**: 070.54 **and** **CPT**: 99201, 99202, 99203, 99204, 99205, 99212, 99213, 99214, 99215, 99241, 99242, 99243, 99244, 99245
91	Acute Otitis Externa (AOE): Topical Therapy	Percentage of patients aged 2 years and older with a diagnosis of AOE who were prescribed topical preparations	≥ once for each occurrence of AOE during the reporting period. Each unique occurrence is defined as a 30-day period from onset of AOE	1 of: 4130F 4130F-1P 4130F-2P 4130F-8P	**ICD-9**: 380.10, 380.11, 380.12, 380.13, 380.22 **and** **CPT**: 99201, 99202, 99203, 99204, 99205, 99212, 99213, 99214, 99215, 99241, 99242, 99243, 99244, 99245
92	Acute Otitis Externa (AOE): Pain Assessment	Percentage of patient visits for those patients aged 2 years and older with a diagnosis of AOE with assessment for auricular or periauricular pain	each visit for patients with AOE during the reporting period	1 of: 1116F 1116F-1P 1116F-8P	**ICD-9**: 380.10, 380.11, 380.12, 380.13, 380.22 **and** **CPT**: 99201, 99202, 99203, 99204, 99205, 99212, 99213, 99214, 99215, 99241, 99242, 99243, 99244, 99245
93	Acute Otitis Externa (AOE): Systemic Antimicrobial Therapy – Avoidance of Inappropriate Use	Percentage of patients aged 2 years and older with a diagnosis of AOE who were not prescribed systemic antimicrobial therapy	once for each occurrence of AOE during the reporting period	1 of: 4131F 4132F 4132F-1P	**ICD-9**: 380.10, 380.11, 380.12, 380.13, 380.22 **and** **CPT**: 99201, 99202, 99203, 99204, 99205, 99212, 99213, 99214, 99215, 99241, 99242, 99243, 99244, 99245

CPT only © 2005-2009 American Medical Association. All rights reserved.

#	Title	Description	Reporting Requirements	Numerator Code(s)	Denominator Code(s)
94	Otitis Media with Effusion (OME): Diagnostic Evaluation – Assessment of Tympanic Membrane Mobility	Percentage of patient visits for those patients aged 2 months through 12 years with a diagnosis of OME with assessment of tympanic membrane mobility with pneumatic otoscopy or tympanometry	each visit for children with OME during the reporting period	1 of: 2035F 2035F-1P 2035F-2P 2035F-8P	**ICD-9**: 381.10, 381.19, 381.20, 381.29, 381.3, 381.4 **and** **CPT**: 99201, 99202, 99203, 99204, 99205, 99212, 99213, 99214, 99215, 99241, 99242, 99243, 99244, 99245
95	Otitis Media with Effusion (OME): Hearing Testing	Percentage of patients aged 2 months through 12 years with a diagnosis of OME who received tympanostomy tube insertion who had a hearing test performed within 6 months prior to tympanostomy tube insertion	each time a tympanostomy tube insertion procedure is performed during the reporting period for children	1 of: 3230F 3230F-1P 3230F-3P 3230F-8P	**ICD-9**: 381.10, 381.19, 381.20, 381.29, 381.3, 381.4 **and** **CPT**: 69433, 69436
99	Breast Cancer Resection Pathology Reporting: pT Category (Primary Tumor) and pN Category (Regional Lymph Nodes) with Histologic Grade	Percentage of breast cancer resection pathology reports that include the pT category (primary tumor), the pN category (regional lymph nodes), and the histologic grade	each time a breast cancer resection surgical pathology examination is performed during the reporting period for breast cancer patients	1 of: 3250F 3260F 3260F-1P 3260F-8P	**ICD-9**: 174.0, 174.1, 174.2, 174.3, 174.4, 174.5, 174.6, 174.8, 174.9, 175.0, 175.9 **and** **CPT**: 88307, 88309
100	Colorectal Cancer Resection Pathology Reporting: pT Category (Primary Tumor) and pN Category (Regional Lymph Nodes) with Histologic Grade	Percentage of colon and rectum cancer resection pathology reports that include the pT category (primary tumor), the pN category (regional lymph nodes) and the histologic grade	each time a colorectal cancer resection surgical pathology examination is performed during the reporting period for colorectal cancer patients	1 of: 3250F 3260F 3260F-1P 3260F-8P	**ICD-9**: 153.0, 153.1, 153.2, 153.3, 153.4, 153.5, 153.6, 153.7, 153.8, 153.9, 154.0, 154.1, 154.8 **and** **CPT**: 88309

CPT only © 2005-2009 American Medical Association. All rights reserved.

#	Title	Description	Reporting Requirements	Numerator Code(s)	Denominator Code(s)
102	Prostate Cancer: Avoidance of Overuse of Bone Scan for Staging Low-Risk Prostate Cancer Patients	Percentage of patients, regardless of age, with a diagnosis of prostate cancer at low risk of recurrence receiving interstitial prostate brachytherapy, OR external beam radiotherapy to the prostate, OR radical prostatectomy, OR cryotherapy who did not have a bone scan performed at any time since diagnosis of prostate cancer	once per episode of treatment (i.e., interstitial prostate brachytherapy, OR external beam radiotherapy to the prostate, OR radical prostatectomy, OR cryotherapy) for all patients with prostate cancer who receive interstitial prostate brachytherapy, external beam radiotherapy to the prostate, radical prostatectomy, or cryotherapy during the reporting period	1 of: 3269F 3270F **and** 3271F **OR** 1 of: 3269F-1P 3269F-3P **and** 1 of: 3271F 3272F 3273F 3274F	**ICD-9**: 185 **and** **CPT**: 55810, 55812, 55815, 55840, 55842, 55845, 55866, 55873, 77411, 77412, 77413, 77414, 77416, 77418, 77427, 77776, 77777, 77778, 77787
104	Prostate Cancer: Adjuvant Hormonal Therapy for High-Risk Prostate Cancer Patients	Percentage of patients, regardless of age, with a diagnosis of prostate cancer at high risk of recurrence receiving external beam radiotherapy to the prostate who were prescribed adjuvant hormonal therapy (GnRH agonist or antagonist)	once per episode of radiation therapy for all patients with prostate cancer who receive external beam radiotherapy to the prostate during the reporting period	1 of: 4164F 4164F-8P **and** G8465 **OR** 1 of 4164F-1P 4164F-2P **and** 1 of: G8464 G8465	**ICD-9**: 185 **and** **CPT**: 77407, 77408, 77409, 77411, 77412, 77413, 77414, 77416, 77418, 77427
105	Prostate Cancer: Three-dimensional (3D) Radiotherapy	Percentage of patients, regardless of age, with a diagnosis of clinically localized prostate cancer receiving external beam radiotherapy as a primary therapy to the prostate with or without nodal irradiation (no metastases; no salvage therapy). who receive 3D-CRT or IMRT	once per episode of radiation therapy for all patients with prostate cancer who receive external beam radiotherapy to the prostate during the reporting period	1 of: 4165F 4165F-8P **and** 4200F **OR** 4201F	**ICD-9**: 185 **without** **ICD-9**: 197.0, 197.1, 197.2, 197.3, 197.4, 197.5, 197.6, 197.7, 197.8, 198.0, 198.1, 198.2, 198.3, 198.4, 198.5, 198.6, 198.7, 198.81, 198.82, 198.89 **and** **CPT**: 77401, 77402, 77403, 77404, 77406, 77407, 77408, 77409, 77411, 77412, 77413, 77414, 77416, 77418, 77427

CPT only © 2005-2009 American Medical Association. All rights reserved.

#	Title	Description	Reporting Requirements	Numerator Code(s)	Denominator Code(s)
106	Major Depressive Disorder (MDD): Diagnostic Evaluation	Percentage of patients aged 18 years and older with a new diagnosis or recurrent episode of major depressive disorder (MDD) who met the DSM-IV™ criteria during the visit in which the new diagnosis or recurrent episode was identified during the measurement period	≥ once per reporting period for all patients with an active diagnosis of major depressive disorder seen during the reporting period, including episodes of MDD that began prior to the reporting period	1 of: 1040F 1040F-8P	**ICD-9**: 296.20, 296.21, 296.22, 296.23, 296.24, 296.30, 296.31, 296.32, 296.33, 296.34 **and** **CPT**: 90801, 90802, 90804, 90805, 90806, 90807, 90808, 90809, 90810, 90811, 90812, 90813, 90814, 90815, 90845, 90862, 99201, 99202, 99203, 99204, 99205, 99212, 99213, 99214, 99215, 99241, 99242, 99243, 99244, 99245
107	Major Depressive Disorder (MDD): Suicide Risk Assessment	Percentage of patients aged 18 years and older with a new diagnosis or recurrent episode of major depressive disorder (MDD) who had a suicide risk assessment completed at each visit during the measurement period	each visit for a new diagnosis or recurrent episode of MDD, for patients seen individually, during the reporting period	1 of: 3085F 3085F-8P 3094F	**ICD-9**: 296.20, 296.21, 296.22, 296.23, 296.24, 296.30, 296.31, 296.32, 296.33, 296.34 **and** **CPT**: 90801, 90802, 90804, 90805, 90806, 90807, 90808, 90809, 90810, 90811, 90812, 90813, 90814, 90815, 90845, 90862, 99201, 99202, 99203, 99204, 99205, 99212, 99213, 99214, 99215, 99241, 99242, 99243, 99244, 99245
108	Rheumatoid Arthritis (RA): Disease Modifying Anti-Rheumatic Drug (DMARD) Therapy	Percentage of patients aged 18 years and older who were diagnosed with rheumatoid arthritis and were prescribed, dispensed, or administered at least one ambulatory prescription for a disease modifying anti-rheumatic drug (DMARD)	≥ once/ reporting period	1 of: 4187F 4187F-1P 4187F-8P	**ICD-9**: 714.0, 714.1, 714.2, 714.81 **and** **CPT**: 99201, 99202, 99203, 99204, 99205, 99212, 99213, 99214, 99215, 99241, 99242, 99243, 99244, 99245, 99341, 99342, 99343, 99344, 99345, 99347, 99348, 99349, 99350, 99455, 99456
109	Osteoarthritis (OA): Function and Pain Assessment	Percentage of patient visits for patients aged 21 years and older with a diagnosis of osteoarthritis (OA) with assessment for function and pain	each visit occurring during the reporting period for patients with osteoarthritis seen during the reporting period	1 of: 1006F 1006F-8P	**ICD-9**: 715.00, 715.04, 715.09, 715.10, 715.11, 715.12, 715.13, 715.14, 715.15, 715.16, 715.17, 715.18, 715.20, 715.21, 715.22, 715.23, 715.24, 715.25, 715.26, 715.27, 715.28, 715.30, 715.31, 715.32, 715.33, 715.34, 715.35, 715.36, 715.37, 715.38, 715.80, 715.89, 715.90, 715.91, 715.92, 715.93, 715.94, 715.95, 715.96, 715.97, 715.98 **and** **CPT**: 99201, 99202, 99203, 99204, 99205, 99212, 99213, 99214, 99215, 99241, 99242, 99243, 99244, 99245
110	Preventive Care and Screening: Influenza Immunization for Patients ≥ 50 Years Old	Percentage of patients aged 50 years and older who received an influenza immunization during the flu season (September through February)	≥ once per reporting period	1 of: G8482 G8483 G8484	**ICD-9**: Any **and** **CPT**: 99201, 99202, 99203, 99204, 99205, 99212, 99213, 99214, 99215, 99304, 99305, 99306, 99307, 99308, 99309, 99310, 99315, 99316, 99324, 99325, 99326, 99327, 99328, 99334, 99335, 99336, 99337, 99341, 99342, 99343, 99344, 99345, 99347, 99348, 99349, 99350
111	Preventive Care and Screening: Pneumonia Vaccination for Patients 65 Years and Older	Percentage of patients aged 65 years and older who have ever received a pneumococcal vaccine	≥ once per reporting period for patients seen during the reporting period	1 of: 4040F 4040F-1P 4040F-8P	**ICD-9** Any **and** **CPT**: 99201, 99202, 99203, 99204, 99205, 99212, 99213, 99214, 99215, 99218, 99219, 99220, 99241, 99242, 99243, 99244, 99245, 99324, 99325, 99326, 99327, 99328, 99334, 99335, 99336, 99337, 99341, 99342, 99343, 99344, 99345, 99347, 99348, 99349, 99350, 99356, 99357

CPT only © 2005-2009 American Medical Association. All rights reserved.

#	Title	Description	Reporting Requirements	Numerator Code(s)	Denominator Code(s)
112	Preventive Care and Screening: Screening Mammography	Percentage of women aged 40 through 69 years who had a mammogram to screen for breast cancer within 24 months	≥ once per reporting period for female patients seen during the reporting period	1 of: 3014F 3014F-1P 3014F-8P	**ICD-9**: Any **and** **CPT**: 99201, 99202, 99203, 99204, 99205, 99212, 99213, 99214, 99215, 99241, 99242, 99243, 99244, 99245
113	Preventive Care and Screening: Colorectal Cancer Screening	Percentage of patients aged 50 through 80 years who received the appropriate colorectal cancer screening	≥ once per reporting period	1 of: 3017F 3017F-1P 3017F-8P	**ICD-9**: Any **and** **CPT**: 99201, 99202, 99203, 99204, 99205, 99212, 99213, 99214, 99215, 99241, 99242, 99243, 99244, 99245, 99304, 99305, 99306, 99307, 99308, 99309, 99310, 99324, 99325, 99326, 99327, 99328, 99334, 99335, 99336, 99337
114	Preventive Care and Screening: Inquiry Regarding Tobacco Use	Percentage of patients aged 18 years or older who were queried about tobacco use one or more times within 24 months	≥ once per reporting period for all patients seen during the reporting period	1000F **and** 1 of: 1034F 1035F 1036F **OR** 1000F-8P	**ICD-9**: Any **and** **CPT**: 90801, 90802, 90804, 90805, 90806, 90807, 90808, 90809, 90810, 90811, 90812, 90813, 90814, 90815, 90845, 90862, 96150, 96152, 97003, 97004, 99201, 99202, 99203, 99204, 99205, 99212, 99213, 99214, 99215
115	Preventive Care and Screening: Advising Smokers to Quit	Percentage of patients aged 18 years and older and are smokers who received advice to quit smoking	≥ once per reporting period for all patients (whether or not they use tobacco) seen during the reporting period	G8455 **and** 1 of: 4000F 4000F-8P 4001F **OR** 1 of: G8456 G8457	**ICD-9**: Any **and** **CPT**: 99201, 99202, 99203, 99204, 99205, 99212, 99213, 99214, 99215, 99217, 99218, 99219, 99220, 99241, 99242, 99243, 99244, 99245
116	Antibiotic Treatment for Adults with Acute Bronchitis: Avoidance of Inappropriate Use	Percentage of adults aged 18 through 64 years with a diagnosis of acute bronchitis who were not prescribed or dispensed an antibiotic prescription on or within 3 days of the initial date of service	each visit for acute bronchitis during the reporting period	1 of: 4120F 4124F 4124F-1P	**ICD-9**: 466.0 **and** **CPT**: 99201, 99202, 99203, 99204, 99205, 99212, 99213, 99214, 99215, 99217, 99218, 99219, 99220, 99241, 99242, 99243, 99244, 99245
117	Diabetes Mellitus: Dilated Eye Exam in Diabetic Patient	Percentage of patients aged 18 through 75 years with a diagnosis of diabetes mellitus who had a dilated eye exam	≥ once per reporting period for patients with diabetes mellitus seen during the reporting period	1 of: 2022F 2022F-8P 2024F 2024F-8P 2026F 2026F-8P 3072F	**ICD-9**: 250.00, 250.01, 250.02, 250.03, 250.10, 250.11, 250.12, 250.13, 250.20, 250.21, 250.22, 250.23, 250.30, 250.31, 250.32, 250.33, 250.40, 250.41, 250.42, 250.43, 250.50, 250.51, 250.52, 250.53, 250.60, 250.61, 250.62, 250.63, 250.70, 250.71, 250.72, 250.73, 250.80, 250.81, 250.82, 250.83, 250.90, 250.91, 250.92, 250.93, 357.2, 362.01, 362.02, 362.03, 362.04, 362.05, 362.06, 362.07, 366.41, 648.00, 648.01, 648.02, 648.03, 648.04 **and** **CPT**: 92002, 92004, 92012, 92014, 97802, 97803, 97804, 99201, 99202, 99203, 99204, 99205, 99212, 99213, 99214, 99215, 99304, 99305, 99306, 99307, 99308, 99309, 99310, 99324, 99325, 99326, 99327, 99328, 99334, 99335, 99336, 99337, 99341, 99342, 99343, 99344, 99345, 99347, 99348, 99349, 99350, G0270, G0271

CPT only © 2005-2009 American Medical Association. All rights reserved.

#	Title	Description	Reporting Requirements	Numerator Code(s)	Denominator Code(s)
118	Coronary Artery Disease (CAD): Angiotensin-Converting Enzyme (ACE) Inhibitor or Angiotensin Receptor Blocker (ARB) Therapy for Patients with CAD and Diabetes and/or Left Ventricular Systolic Dysfunction (LVSD)	Percentage of patients aged 18 years and older with a diagnosis of coronary artery disease (CAD) who also have diabetes mellitus and/or left ventricular systolic dysfunction (LVSD) who were prescribed ACE Inhibitor or ARB therapy	≥ once per reporting period for all patients with CAD seen during the reporting period	**Option 1:** 1 of: G8468 G8469 G8470 G8471 G8472 **Option 2:** 1 of: G8473 G8474 G8475	**Option 1:** **ICD-9**: 410.00, 410.01, 410.02, 410.10, 410.11, 410.12, 410.20, 410.21, 410.22, 410.30, 410.31, 410.32, 410.40, 410.41, 410.42, 410.50, 410.51, 410.52, 410.60, 410.61, 410.62, 410.70, 410.71, 410.72, 410.80, 410.81, 410.82, 410.90, 410.91, 410.92, 411.0, 411.1, 411.81, 411.89, 412, 413.0, 413.1, 413.9, 414.00, 414.01, 414.02, 414.03, 414.04, 414.05, 414.06, 414.07, 414.8, 414.9, V45.81, V45.82 **and** **CPT**: 99201, 99202, 99203, 99204, 99205, 99212, 99213, 99214, 99215, 99241, 99242, 99243, 99244, 99245, 99304, 99305, 99306, 99307, 99308, 99309, 99310, 99324, 99325, 99326, 99327, 99328, 99334, 99335, 99336, 99337, 99341, 99342, 99343, 99344, 99345, 99347, 99348, 99349, 99350 **Option 2:** **ICD-9**: 410.00, 410.01, 410.02, 410.10, 410.11, 410.12, 410.20, 410.21, 410.22, 410.30, 410.31, 410.32, 410.40, 410.41, 410.42, 410.50, 410.51, 410.52, 410.60, 410.61, 410.62, 410.70, 410.71, 410.72, 410.80, 410.81, 410.82, 410.90, 410.91, 410.92, 411.0, 411.1, 411.81, 411.89, 412, 413.0, 413.1, 413.9, 414.00, 414.01, 414.02, 414.03, 414.04, 414.05, 414.06, 414.07, 414.8, 414.9, V45.81, V45.82 **and** **ICD-9**: 250.00, 250.01, 250.02, 250.03, 250.10, 250.11, 250.12, 250.13, 250.20, 250.21, 250.22, 250.23, 250.30, 250.31, 250.32, 250.33, 250.40, 250.41, 250.42, 250.43, 250.50, 250.51, 250.52, 250.53, 250.60, 250.61, 250.62, 250.63, 250.70, 250.71, 250.72, 250.73, 250.80, 250.81, 250.82, 250.83, 250.90, 250.91, 250.92, 250.93, 648.00, 648.01, 648.02, 648.03, 648.04 **and** **CPT**: 99201, 99202, 99203, 99204, 99205, 99212, 99213, 99214, 99215, 99241, 99242, 99243, 99244, 99245, 99304, 99305, 99306, 99307, 99308, 99309, 99310, 99324, 99325, 99326, 99327, 99328, 99334, 99335, 99336, 99337, 99341, 99342, 99343, 99344, 99345, 99347, 99348, 99349, 99350
119	Diabetes Mellitus: Urine Screening for Microalbumin or Medical Attention for Nephropathy in Diabetic Patients	Percentage of patients aged 18 through 75 years of age with diabetes mellitus who received urine protein screening or medical attention for nephropathy during at least one office visit within 12 months	≥ once per reporting period for all patients with diabetes mellitus seen during the reporting period	1 of: 3060F 3060F-8P 3061F 3061F-8P 3062F 3062F-8P 3066F 4009F	**ICD-9**: 250.00, 250.01, 250.02, 250.03, 250.10, 250.11, 250.12, 250.13, 250.20, 250.21, 250.22, 250.23, 250.30, 250.31, 250.32, 250.33, 250.40, 250.41, 250.42, 250.43, 250.50, 250.51, 250.52, 250.53, 250.60, 250.61, 250.62, 250.63, 250.70, 250.71, 250.72, 250.73, 250.80, 250.81, 250.82, 250.83, 250.90, 250.91, 250.92, 250.93, 357.2, 362.01, 362.02, 362.03, 362.04, 362.05, 362.06, 362.07, 366.41, 648.00, 648.01, 648.02, 648.03, 648.04 **and** **CPT**: 97802, 97803, 97804, 99201, 99202, 99203, 99204, 99205, 99212, 99213, 99214, 99215, 99304, 99305, 99306, 99307, 99308, 99309, 99310, 99324, 99325, 99326, 99327, 99328, 99334, 99335, 99336, 99337, 99341, 99342, 99343, 99344, 99345, 99347, 99348, 99349, 99350, G0270, G0271
121	Chronic Kidney Disease (CKD): Laboratory Testing (Calcium, Phosphorus, Intact Parathyroid Hormone (iPTH) and Lipid Profile)	Percentage of patients aged 18 years and older with a diagnosis of advanced CKD (stage 4 or 5, not receiving Renal Replacement Therapy [RRT]), who had the following laboratory testing ordered at least once during the 12-month reporting period: serum levels of calcium, phosphorus and intact PTH, and lipid profile	≥ once per reporting period for patients with CKD seen during the reporting period.	1 of: 3278F 3278F-1P 3278F-2P 3278F-8P	**ICD-9**: 585.4, 585.5 **and** **CPT**: 99201, 99202, 99203, 99204, 99205, 99212, 99213, 99214, 99215, 99241, 99242, 99243, 99244, 99245

CPT only © 2005-2009 American Medical Association. All rights reserved.

#	Title	Description	Reporting Requirements	Numerator Code(s)	Denominator Code(s)
122	Chronic Kidney Disease (CKD): Blood Pressure Management	Percentage of patient visits for patients aged 18 years and older with a diagnosis of advanced CKD (stage 4 or 5, not receiving Renal Replacement Therapy [RRT]), with a blood pressure < 130/80 mmHg OR blood pressure ≥ 130/80 mmHg with a documented plan of care	each visit for patients with a diagnosis of CKD seen during the reporting period	G8477 **and** 1 of: 0513F 0513F-8P G8478 **OR** G8476 **and** 0513F	**ICD-9**: 585.4, 585.5 **and** **CPT**: 99201, 99202, 99203, 99204, 99205, 99212, 99213, 99214, 99215, 99241, 99242, 99243, 99244, 99245
123	Chronic Kidney Disease (CKD): Plan of Care: Elevated Hemoglobin for Patients Receiving Erythropoiesis-Stimulating Agents (ESA)	Percentage of patient calendar months during the 12-month reporting period in which patients aged 18 years and older with a diagnosis of advanced CKD (stage 4 or 5, not receiving Renal Replacement Therapy [RRT]), receiving ESA therapy, have a hemoglobin < 13 g/dL OR patients whose hemoglobin is ≥ 13 g/dL and have a documented plan of care	each calendar month patients are seen with a diagnosis of advanced CKD (stage 4 or 5) during the reporting period	4171F **and** 1 of: 3280F 3281F 3281F-8P **OR** 3281F-8P **and** 3279F **and** 1 of: 0514F 0514F-8P	**ICD-9**: 585.4, 585.5 **and** **CPT**: 99201, 99202, 99203, 99204, 99205, 99212, 99213, 99214, 99215, 99241, 99242, 99243, 99244, 99245
124	Health Information Technology (HIT): Adoption/Use of Electronic Health Records (EHR)	Documents whether provider has adopted and is using health information technology. To qualify, the provider must have adopted and be using a qualified EHR	each visit occurring during the reporting period for patients seen during the reporting period	1 of: G8447 G8448	**ICD-9**: Any **and** **CPT/HCPCS II**: 90801, 90802, 90804, 90805, 90806, 90807, 90808, 90809, 92002, 92004, 92012, 92014, 92541, 92542, 92543, 92544, 92548, 92552, 92553, 92555, 92557, 92561, 92562, 92563, 92564, 92565, 92567, 92568, 92569, 92571, 92572, 92575, 92576, 92577, 92579, 92582, 92584, 92585, 92586, 92587, 92588, 92601, 92602, 92603, 92604, 92620, 92621, 92625, 92626, 92627, 92640, 95920, 96150, 96151, 96152, 97001, 97002, 97003, 97004, 97750, 97802, 97803, 97804, 98940, 98941, 98942, 99201, 99202, 99203, 99204, 99205, 99211, 99212, 99213, 99214, 99215, 99241, 99242, 99243, 99244, 99245, D7140, D7210, G0101, G0108, G0109, G0270, G0271
126	Diabetes Mellitus: Diabetic Foot and Ankle Care, Peripheral Neuropathy - Neurological Evaluation	Percentage of patients aged 18 years and older with a diagnosis of diabetes mellitus who had a neurological examination of their lower extremities within 12 months	≥ once per reporting period for patients with diabetes mellitus seen during the reporting period	1 of: G8404 G8405 G8406	**ICD-9**: 250.00, 250.01, 250.02, 250.03, 250.10, 250.11, 250.12, 250.13, 250.20, 250.21, 250.22, 250.23, 250.30, 250.31, 250.32, 250.33, 250.40, 250.41, 250.42, 250.43, 250.50, 250.51, 250.52, 250.53, 250.60, 250.61, 250.62, 250.63, 250.70, 250.71, 250.72, 250.73, 250.80, 250.81, 250.82, 250.83, 250.90, 250.91, 250.92, 250.93 **and** **CPT**: 11040, 11041, 11042, 11043, 11044, 11055, 11056, 11057, 11719, 11720, 11721, 11730, 11740, 97001, 97002, 97802, 97803, 99201, 99202, 99203, 99204, 99205, 99212, 99213, 99214, 99215, 99241, 99242, 99243, 99244, 99245, 99251, 99252, 99253, 99254, 99255, 99304, 99305, 99306, 99307, 99308, 99309, 99310, 99324, 99325, 99326, 99327, 99328, 99334, 99335, 99336, 99337, 99341, 99342, 99343, 99344, 99345, 99347, 99348, 99349, 99350

CPT only © 2005-2009 American Medical Association. All rights reserved.

#	Title	Description	Reporting Requirements	Numerator Code(s)	Denominator Code(s)
127	Diabetes Mellitus: Diabetic Foot and Ankle Care, Ulcer Prevention - Evaluation of Footwear	Percentage of patients aged 18 years and older with a diagnosis of diabetes mellitus who were evaluated for proper footwear and sizing	≥ once per reporting period for patients with diabetes mellitus seen during the reporting period	1 of: G8410 G8415 G8416	**ICD-9**: 250.00, 250.01, 250.02, 250.03, 250.10, 250.11, 250.12, 250.13, 250.20, 250.21, 250.22, 250.23, 250.30, 250.31, 250.32, 250.33, 250.40, 250.41, 250.42, 250.43, 250.50, 250.51, 250.52, 250.53, 250.60, 250.61, 250.62, 250.63, 250.70, 250.71, 250.72, 250.73, 250.80, 250.81, 250.82, 250.83, 250.90, 250.91, 250.92, 250.93 **and** **CPT**: 11040, 11041, 11042, 11043, 11044, 11055, 11056, 11057, 11719, 11720, 11721, 11730, 11740, 97001, 97002, 97802, 97803, 99201, 99202, 99203, 99204, 99205, 99212, 99213, 99214, 99215, 99241, 99242, 99243, 99244, 99245, 99251, 99252, 99253, 99254, 99255, 99304, 99305, 99306, 99307, 99308, 99309, 99310, 99324, 99325, 99326, 99327, 99328, 99334, 99335, 99336, 99337, 99341, 99342, 99343, 99344, 99345, 99347, 99348, 99349, 99350
128	Preventive Care and Screening: Body Mass Index (BMI) Screening and Follow-Up	Percentage of patients aged 65 years and older with a calculated Body Mass Index (BMI) within the past six months or during the current visit that is documented in the medical record and if the most recent BMI is outside the parameters, a follow-up plan is documented Parameters: Age ≥ 65 BMI ≥30 or <22 Age 18 – 64 BMI ≥25 or <18.5	≥ once per reporting period for patients seen during the reporting period. The most recent quality code submitted will be used for performance calculation	1 of: G8417 G8418 G8419 G8420 G8421 G8422	**ICD-9**: Any **and** **CPT**: 00100, 00102, 00103, 00104, 00120, 00124, 00126, 00140, 00142, 00144, 00145, 00147, 00148, 00160, 00162, 00164, 00170, 00172, 00174, 00176, 00190, 00192, 00210, 00211, 00212, 00214, 00215, 00216, 00218, 00220, 00222, 00300, 00320, 00322, 00326, 00350, 00352, 00400, 00402, 00404, 00406, 00410, 00450, 00452, 00454, 00470, 00472, 00474, 00500, 00520, 00522, 00524, 00528, 00529, 00530, 00532, 00534, 00537, 00539, 00540, 00541, 00542, 00546, 00548, 00550, 00560, 00561, 00562, 00563, 00566, 00567, 00580, 00600, 00604, 00620, 00622, 00625, 00626, 00630, 00632, 00634, 00635, 00640, 00670, 00700, 00702, 00730, 00740, 00750, 00752, 00754, 00756, 00770, 00790, 00792, 00794, 00796, 00797, 00800, 00802, 00810, 00820, 00830, 00832, 00834, 00836, 00840, 00842, 00844, 00846, 00848, 00851, 00860, 00862, 00864, 00865, 00866, 00868, 00870, 00872, 00873, 00880, 00882, 00902, 00904, 00906, 00908, 00910, 00912, 00914, 00916, 00918, 00920, 00921, 00922, 00924, 00926, 00928, 00930, 00932, 00934, 00936, 00938, 00940, 00942, 00944, 00948, 00950, 00952, 01112, 01120, 01130, 01140, 01150, 01160, 01170, 01173, 01180, 01190, 01200, 01202, 01210, 01212, 01214, 01215, 01220, 01230, 01232, 01234, 01250, 01260, 01270, 01272, 01274, 01320, 01340, 01360, 01380, 01382, 01390, 01392, 01400, 01402, 01404, 01420, 01430, 01432, 01440, 01442, 01444, 01462, 01464, 01470, 01472, 01474, 01480, 01482, 01484, 01486, 01490, 01500, 01502, 01520, 01522, 01610, 01620, 01622, 01630, 01632, 01634, 01636, 01638, 01650, 01652, 01654, 01656, 01670, 01680, 01682, 01710, 01712, 01714, 01716, 01730, 01732, 01740, 01742, 01744, 01756, 01758, 01760, 01770, 01772, 01780, 01782, 01810, 01820, 01829, 01830, 01832, 01840, 01842, 01844, 01850, 01852, 01860, 01916, 01920, 01922, 01924, 01925, 01926, 01930, 01931, 01932, 01933, 01935, 01936, 01951, 01952, 01953, 01958, 01960, 01961, 01962, 01963, 01965, 01966, 01967, 01968, 01969, 01990, 01991, 01992, 01996, 01999, 90801, 90802, 90804, 90805, 90806, 90807, 90808, 90809, 97001, 97003, 97802, 97803, 98960, 99201, 99202, 99203, 99204, 99205, 99211, 99212, 99213, 99214, 99215, 99241, 99242, 99243, 99244, 99245, 99324, 99325, 99326, 99327, 99328, 99334, 99335, 99336, 99337, 99341, 99342, 99343, 99344, 99345, 99347, 99348, 99349, 99350, D7140, D7210, G0101, G0108, G0270

CPT only © 2005-2009 American Medical Association. All rights reserved.

#	Title	Description	Reporting Requirements	Numerator Code(s)	Denominator Code(s)
130	Documentation and Verification of Current Medications in the Medical Record	Percentage of patients aged 18 years and older with a list of current medications with dosages (includes prescription, over-the-counter, herbals, vitamin/mineral/dietary [nutritional] supplements) and verification with the patient or authorized representative is documented by the provider	each visit occurring during the reporting period for patients seen during the reporting period	1 of: G8427 G8428 G8249 G8430 G8507	**ICD-9**: Any **and** **CPT**: 00100, 00102, 00103, 00104, 00120, 00124, 00126, 00140, 00142, 00144, 00145, 00147, 00148, 00160, 00162, 00164, 00170, 00172, 00174, 00176, 00190, 00192, 00210, 00211, 00212, 00214, 00215, 00216, 00218, 00220, 00222, 00300, 00320, 00322, 00326, 00350, 00352, 00400, 00402, 00404, 00406, 00410, 00450, 00452, 00454, 00470, 00472, 00474, 00500, 00520, 00522, 00524, 00528, 00529, 00530, 00532, 00534, 00537, 00539, 00540, 00541, 00542, 00546, 00548, 00550, 00560, 00561, 00562, 00563, 00566, 00567, 00580, 00600, 00604, 00620, 00622, 00625, 00626, 00630, 00632, 00634, 00635, 00640, 00670, 00700, 00702, 00730, 00740, 00750, 00752, 00754, 00756, 00770, 00790, 00792, 00794, 00796, 00797, 00800, 00802, 00810, 00820, 00830, 00832, 00834, 00836, 00840, 00842, 00844, 00846, 00848, 00851, 00860, 00862, 00864, 00865, 00866, 00868, 00870, 00872, 00873, 00880, 00882, 00902, 00904, 00906, 00908, 00910, 00912, 00914, 00916, 00918, 00920, 00921, 00922, 00924, 00926, 00928, 00930, 00932, 00934, 00936, 00938, 00940, 00942, 00944, 00948, 00950, 00952, 01112, 01120, 01130, 01140, 01150, 01160, 01170, 01173, 01180, 01190, 01200, 01202, 01210, 01212, 01214, 01215, 01220, 01230, 01232, 01234, 01250, 01260, 01270, 01272, 01274, 01320, 01340, 01360, 01380, 01382, 01390, 01392, 01400, 01402, 01404, 01420, 01430, 01432, 01440, 01442, 01444, 01462, 01464, 01470, 01472, 01474, 01480, 01482, 01484, 01486, 01490, 01500, 01502, 01520, 01522, 01610, 01620, 01622, 01630, 01632, 01634, 01636, 01638, 01650, 01652, 01654, 01656, 01670, 01680, 01682, 01710, 01712, 01714, 01716, 01730, 01732, 01740, 01742, 01744, 01756, 01758, 01760, 01770, 01772, 01780, 01782, 01810, 01820, 01829, 01830, 01832, 01840, 01842, 01844, 01850, 01852, 01860, 01916, 01920, 01922, 01924, 01925, 01926, 01930, 01931, 01932, 01933, 01935, 01936, 01951, 01952, 01953, 01958, 01960, 01961, 01962, 01963, 01965, 01966, 01967, 01968, 01969, 01990, 01991, 01992, 01996, 01999, 90801, 90802, 92002, 92004, 92012, 92014, 92541, 92542, 92543, 92544, 92545, 92547, 92548, 92557, 92567, 92568, 92569, 92585, 92588, 92626, 96116, 96150, 96152, 97001, 97002, 97003, 97004, 97802, 97803, 98960, 99201, 99202, 99203, 99204, 99205, 99211, 99212, 99213, 99214, 99215, 99241, 99242, 99243, 99244, 99245, G0101, G0108, G0270
131	Pain Assessment Prior to Initiation of Patient Therapy and Follow-up	Percentage of patients aged 18 years and older with documentation of a pain assessment (if pain is present, including location, intensity and description) through discussion with the patient or through use of a standardized tool on each initial evaluation prior to initiation of therapy AND documentation of a follow-up plan	each qualifying visit occurring during the reporting period for patients seen during the reporting period	1 of: G8440 G8441 G8442 G8508 G8509	**ICD-9**: Any **and** **CPT**: 90801, 90802, 96116, 96150, 97001, 97003, 98940, 98941, 98942
134	Screening for Clinical Depression and Follow-Up Plan	Percentage of patients aged 18 years and older screened for clinical depression using a standardized tool	≥ once per reporting period for patients seen during the reporting period	1 of: G8431 G8432 G8433 G8510 G8511	**ICD-9**: Any **and** **CPT**: 90801, 90802, 90804, 90805, 90806, 90807, 90808, 90809, 92557, 92567, 92568, 92625, 97003

 CPT only © 2005-2009 American Medical Association. All rights reserved.

#	Title	Description	Reporting Requirements	Numerator Code(s)	Denominator Code(s)
135	Chronic Kidney Disease (CKD): Influenza Immunization	Percentage of patients aged 18 years and older with a diagnosis of advanced CKD (stage 4 or 5, not receiving Renal Replacement Therapy [RRT]) who received the influenza immunization during the flu season (September through February)	≥ of once per reporting period for advanced CKD patients seen during the reporting period	1 of: 4037F 4037F-1P 4037F-2P 4037F-3P 4037F-8P	**ICD-9**: 585.4, 585.5 and **CPT**: 99201, 99202, 99203, 99204, 99205, 99212, 99213, 99214, 99215, 99241, 99242, 99243, 99244, 99245
136	Melanoma: Follow-Up Aspects of Care	Percentage of patients, regardless of age, with a new diagnosis of melanoma or a history of melanoma who received all of the following aspects of care within 12 months: (1) patient was asked specifically if he/she had any new or changing moles; AND (2) a complete physical skin examination was performed and the morphology, size, and location of new or changing pigmented lesions were noted; AND (3) patient was counseled to perform a monthly self skin examination	≥ of once per reporting period for melanoma patients seen during the reporting period	1 of: 0015F 0015F-3P 0015F-8P	**ICD-9**: 172.0, 172.1, 172.2, 172.3, 172.4, 172.5, 172.6, 172.7, 172.8, 172.9, V10.82 and **CPT**: 99201, 99202, 99203, 99204, 99205, 99212, 99213, 99214, 99215, 99241, 99242, 99243, 99244, 99245
137	Melanoma: Continuity of Care – Recall System	Percentage of patients, regardless of age, with a current diagnosis of melanoma or a history of melanoma who were entered into a recall system with the date for the next complete physical skin examination specified at least once within 12 months	≥ of once per reporting period for melanoma patients seen during the reporting period	1 of: 7010F 7010F-3P 7010F-8P	**ICD-9**: 172.0, 172.1, 172.2, 172.3, 172.4, 172.5, 172.6, 172.7, 172.8, 172.9, V10.82 and **CPT**: 99201, 99202, 99203, 99204, 99205, 99212, 99213, 99214, 99215, 99241, 99242, 99243, 99244, 99245
138	Melanoma: Coordination of Care	Percentage of patient visits, regardless of patient age, with a new occurrence of melanoma who have a treatment plan documented in the chart that was communicated to the physician(s) providing continuing care within one month of diagnosis	each visit occurring during the reporting period for melanoma patients seen during the reporting period	1127F **and** 1 of: 5050F 5050F-2P 5050F-3P 5050F-8P **OR** 1128F	**ICD-9**: 172.0, 172.1, 172.2, 172.3, 172.4, 172.5, 172.6, 172.7, 172.8, 172.9, V10.82 and **CPT**: 99201, 99202, 99203, 99204, 99205, 99212, 99213, 99214, 99215, 99241, 99242, 99243, 99244, 99245
139	Cataracts: Comprehensive Preoperative Assessment for Cataract Surgery with Intraocular Lens (IOL) Placement	Percentage of patients aged 18 years and older with a procedure of cataract surgery with IOL placement who received a comprehensive preoperative assessment of 1) dilated fundus examination; 2) axial length, corneal keratometry measurement, and method of IOL power calculation; and 3) functional or medical indication(s) for surgery prior to the cataract surgery with IOL placement within 12 months prior to cataract surgery	each time a cataract surgery with IOL placement is performed during the reporting period	1 of: 0014F 0014F-8P	**ICD-9**: Any and **CPT**: 66982, 66983, 66984

CPT only © 2005-2009 American Medical Association. All rights reserved.

#	Title	Description	Reporting Requirements	Numerator Code(s)	Denominator Code(s)
140	Age-Related Macular Degeneration (AMD): Counseling on Antioxidant Supplement	Percentage of patients aged 50 years and older with a diagnosis of AMD and/or their caregiver(s) who were counseled within 12 months on the benefits and/or risks of the Age-Related Eye Disease Study (AREDS) formulation for preventing progression of AMD	≥ once per reporting period for AMD patients seen during the reporting period	1 of: 4177F 4177F-3P 4177F-8P	**ICD-9**: 362.50, 362.51, 362.52 and **CPT**: 92002, 92004, 92012, 92014, 99201, 99202, 99203, 99204, 99205, 99212, 99213, 99214, 99215, 99241, 99242, 99243, 99244, 99245, 99307, 99308, 99309, 99310, 99324, 99325, 99326, 99327, 99328, 99334, 99335, 99336, 99337
141	Primary Open-Angle Glaucoma (POAG): Reduction of Intraocular Pressure (IOP) by 15% OR Documentation of a Plan of Care	Percentage of patients aged 18 years and older with a diagnosis of POAG whose glaucoma treatment has not failed (the most recent IOP was reduced by at least 15% from the pre-intervention level) OR if the most recent IOP was not reduced by at least 15% from the pre-intervention level, a plan of care was documented within 12 months	≥ once per reporting period for glaucoma patients seen during the reporting period. It is anticipated that clinicians who provide the primary management of patients with POAG will submit this measure	1 of: 3284F 3284F-8P **OR** 3285F **and** 1 of: 0517F 0517F-3P 0517F-8P	**ICD-9**: 715.00, 715.04, 715.09, 715.10, 715.11, 715.12, 715.13, 715.14, 715.15, 715.16, 715.17, 715.18, 715.20, 715.21, 715.22, 715.23, 715.24, 715.25, 715.26, 715.27, 715.28, 715.30, 715.31, 715.32, 715.33, 715.34, 715.35, 715.36, 715.37, 715.38, 715.80, 715.89, 715.90, 715.91, 715.92, 715.93, 715.94, 715.95, 715.96, 715.97, 715.98 and **CPT**: 99201, 99202, 99203, 99204, 99205, 99212, 99213, 99214, 99215, 99241, 99242, 99243, 99244, 99245
142	Osteoarthritis (OA): Assessment for Use of Anti-Inflammatory or Analgesic Over-the-Counter (OTC) Medications	Percentage of patient visits for patients aged 21 years and older with a diagnosis of OA with an assessment for use of anti-inflammatory or analgesic OTC medications	each visit occurring during the reporting period for OA patients seen during the reporting period	1 of: 1007F 1007F-3P	**ICD-9**: 365.10, 365.11, 365.12, 365.15 and **CPT**: 92002, 92004, 92012, 92014, 99201, 99202, 99203, 99204, 99205, 99212, 99213, 99214, 99215, 99241, 99242, 99243, 99244, 99245, 99307, 99308, 99309, 99310, 99324, 99325, 99326, 99327, 99328, 99334, 99335, 99336, 99337
143	Oncology: Medical and Radiation – Pain Intensity Quantified	Percentage of patient visits, regardless of patient age, with a diagnosis of cancer currently receiving chemotherapy or radiation therapy in which pain intensity is quantified	each visit occurring during the reporting period for patients with a diagnosis of cancer who are seen during the reporting period *(This is a two-part measure which is paired with Measure #144. If pain is present (CPT II code 1125F is submitted), #144 should also be reported.*	1 of: 1125F 1125F-8P 1126F	**ICD-9**: 140.0, 140.1, 140.3, 140.4, 140.5, 140.6, 140.8, 140.9, 141.0, 141.1, 141.2, 141.3, 141.4, 141.5, 141.6, 141.8, 141.9, 142.0, 142.1, 142.2, 142.8, 142.9, 143.0, 143.1, 143.8, 143.9, 144.0, 144.1, 144.8, 144.9, 145.0, 145.1, 145.2, 145.3, 145.4, 145.5, 145.6, 145.8, 145.9, 146.0, 146.1, 146.2, 146.3, 146.4, 146.5, 146.6, 146.7, 146.8, 146.9, 147.0, 147.1, 147.2, 147.3, 147.8, 147.9, 148.0, 148.1, 148.2, 148.3, 148.8, 148.9, 149.0, 149.1, 149.8, 149.9, 150.0, 150.1, 150.2, 150.3, 150.4, 150.5, 150.8, 150.9, 151.0, 151.1, 151.2, 151.3, 151.4, 151.5, 151.6, 151.8, 151.9, 152.0, 152.1, 152.2, 152.3, 152.8, 152.9, 153.0, 153.1, 153.2, 153.3, 153.4, 153.5, 153.6, 153.7, 153.8, 153.9, 154.0, 154.1, 154.2, 154.3, 154.8, 155.0, 155.1, 155.2, 156.0, 156.1, 156.2, 156.8, 156.9, 157.0, 157.1, 157.2, 157.3, 157.4, 157.8, 157.9, 158.0, 158.8, 158.9, 159.0, 159.1, 159.8, 159.9,160.0, 160.1, 160.2, 160.3, 160.4, 160.5, 160.8, 160.9, 161.0, 161.1, 161.2, 161.3, 161.8, 161.9, 162.0, 162.2, 162.3, 162.4, 162.5, 162.8, 162.9, 163.0, 163.1, 163.8, 163.9, 164.0, 164.1, 164.2, 164.3, 164.8, 164.9, 165.0, 165.8, 165.9, 170.0, 170.1, 170.2, 170.3, 170.4, 170.5, 170.6, 170.7, 170.8, 170.9, 171.0, 171.2, 171.3, 171.4, 171.5, 171.6, 171.7, 171.8, 171.9, 172.0, 172.1, 172.2, 172.3, 172.4, 172.5, 172.6, 172.7, 172.8, 172.9, 173.0, 173.1, 173.2, 173.3, 173.4, 173.5, 173.6, 173.7, 173.8, 173.9, 174.0, 174.1, 174.2, 174.3, 174.4, 174.5, 174.6, 174.8, 174.9, 175.0, 175.9, 176.0, 176.1, 176.2, 176.3, 176.4, 176.5, 176.8, 176.9, 179, 180.0, 180.1, 180.8, 180.9, 181, 182.0, 182.1, 182.8, 183.0, 183.2, 183.3, 183.4, 183.5, 183.8, 183.9, 184.0, 184.1, 184.2, 184.3, 184.4, 184.8, 184.9, 185, 186.0, 186.9, 187.1, 187.2, 187.3, 187.4, 187.5, 187.6, 187.7, 187.8, 187.9, 188.0, 188.1, 188.2, 188.3, 188.4, 188.5, 188.6, 188.7, *continued on the next page*

CPT only © 2005-2009 American Medical Association. All rights reserved.

© 2009 MAG Mutual Healthcare Solutions, Inc.

#	Title	Description	Reporting Requirements	Numerator Code(s)	Denominator Code(s)
143	*see previous page*	*see previous page*	*see previous page*	*see previous page*	*continued from previous page* 188.8, 188.9, 189.0, 189.1, 189.2, 189.3, 189.4, 189.8, 189.9, 190.0, 190.1, 190.2, 190.3, 190.4, 190.5, 190.6, 190.7, 190.8, 190.9, 191.0, 191.1, 191.2, 191.3, 191.4, 191.5, 191.6, 191.7, 191.8, 191.9, 192.0, 192.1, 192.2, 192.3, 192.8, 192.9, 193, 194.0, 194.1, 194.3, 194.4, 194.5, 194.6, 194.8, 194.9, 195.0, 195.1, 195.2, 195.3, 195.4, 195.5, 195.8, 196.0, 196.1, 196.2, 196.3, 196.5, 196.6, 196.8, 196.9, 197.0, 197.1, 197.2, 197.3, 197.4, 197.5, 197.6, 197.7, 197.8, 198.0, 198.1, 198.2, 198.3, 198.4, 198.5, 198.6, 198.7, 198.81, 198.82, 198.89, 199.0, 199.1, 199.2, 200.00, 200.01, 200.02, 200.03, 200.04, 200.05, 200.06, 200.07, 200.08, 200.10, 200.11, 200.12, 200.13, 200.14, 200.15, 200.16, 200.17, 200.18, 200.20, 200.21, 200.22, 200.23, 200.24, 200.25, 200.26, 200.27, 200.28, 200.30, 200.31, 200.32, 200.33, 200.34, 200.35, 200.36, 200.37, 200.38, 200.40, 200.41, 200.42, 200.43, 200.44, 200.45, 200.46, 200.47, 200.48; 200.50, 200.51, 200.52, 200.53, 200.54, 200.55, 200.56, 200.57, 200.58, 200.60, 200.61, 200.62, 200.63, 200.64, 200.65, 200.66, 200.67, 200.68, 200.70, 200.71, 200.72, 200.73, 200.74, 200.75, 200.76, 200.77, 200.78, 200.80, 200.81, 200.82, 200.83, 200.84, 200.85, 200.86, 200.87, 200.88, 201.00, 201.01, 201.02, 201.03, 201.04, 201.05, 201.06, 201.07, 201.08, 201.10, 201.11, 201.12, 201.13, 201.14, 201.15, 201.16, 201.17, 201.18, 201.20, 201.21, 201.22, 201.23, 201.24, 201.25, 201.26, 201.27, 201.28, 201.40, 201.41, 201.42, 201.43, 201.44, 201.45, 201.46, 201.47, 201.48, 201.50, 201.51, 201.52, 201.53, 201.54, 201.55, 201.56, 201.57, 201.58, 201.60, 201.61, 201.62, 201.63, 201.64, 201.65, 201.66, 201.67, 201.68, 201.70, 201.71, 201.72, 201.73, 201.74, 201.75, 201.76, 201.77, 201.78, 201.90, 201.91, 201.92, 201.93, 201.94, 201.95, 201.96, 201.97, 201.98, 202.00, 202.01, 202.02, 202.03, 202.04, 202.05, 202.06, 202.07, 202.08, 202.10, 202.11, 202.12, 202.13, 202.14, 202.15, 202.16, 202.17, 202.18, 202.20, 202.21, 202.22, 202.23, 202.24, 202.25, 202.26, 202.27, 202.28, 202.30, 202.31, 202.32, 202.33, 202.34, 202.35, 202.36, 202.37, 202.38, 202.40, 202.41, 202.42, 202.43, 202.44, 202.45, 202.46, 202.47, 202.48, 202.50, 202.51, 202.52, 202.53, 202.54, 202.55, 202.56, 202.57, 202.58, 202.60, 202.61, 202.62, 202.63, 202.64, 202.65, 202.66, 202.67, 202.68, 202.70, 202.71, 202.72, 202.73, 202.74, 202.75, 202.76, 202.77, 202.78, 202.80, 202.81, 202.82, 202.83, 202.84, 202.85, 202.86, 202.87, 202.88, 202.90, 202.91, 202.92, 202.93, 202.94, 202.95, 202.96, 202.97, 202.98, 203.00, 203.01, 203.02, 203.10, 203.11, 203.12, 203.80, 203.81, 203.82, 204.00, 204.01, 204.02, 204.10, 204.11, 204.12, 204.20, 204.21, 204.22, 204.80, 204.81, 204.82, 204.90, 204.91, 204.92, 205.00, 205.01, 205.02, 205.10, 205.11, 205.12, 205.20, 205.21, 205.22, 205.30, 205.31, 205.32, 205.80, 205.81, 205.82, 205.90, 205.91, 205.92, 206.00, 206.01, 206.02, 206.10, 206.11, 206.12, 206.20, 206.21, 206.22, 206.80, 206.81, 206.82, 206.90, 206.91, 206.92, 207.00, 207.01, 207.02, 207.10, 207.11, 207.12, 207.20, 207.21, 207.22, 207.80, 207.81, 207.82, 208.00, 208.01, 208.02, 208.10, 208.11, 208.12, 208.20, 208.21, 208.22, 208.80, 208.81, 208.82, 208.90, 208.91, 208.92, 209.00, 209.01, 209.02, 209.03, 209.10, 209.11, 209.12, 209.13, 209.14, 209.15, 209.16, 209.17, 209.20, 209.21, 209.22, 209.23, 209.24, 209.25, 209.26, 209.27, 209.29, 209.30, 235.0, 235.1, 235.2, 235.3, 235.4, 235.5, 235.6, 235.7, 235.8, 235.9, 236.0, 236.1, 236.2, 236.3, 236.4, 236.5, 236.6, 236.7, 236.90, 236.91, 236.99, 237.0, 237.1, 237.2, 237.3, 237.4, 237.5, 237.6, 237.70, 237.71, 237.72, 237.9, 238.0, 238.1, 238.2, 238.3, 238.4, 238.5, 238.6, 238.71, 238.72, 238.73, 238.74, 238.75, 238.76, 238.77, 238.8, 238.9, 239.0, 239.1, 239.2, 239.3, 239.4, 239.5, 239.6, 239.7, 239.8, 239.9 and **CPT**: 77427, 77431, 77432, 77435, 77470 *continued on the next page*

CPT only © 2005-2009 American Medical Association. All rights reserved.

#	Title	Description	Reporting Requirements	Numerator Code(s)	Denominator Code(s)
143	*see previous page*	*see previous page*	*see previous page*	*see previous page*	*continued from previous page* **OR** **CPT**: 99201, 99202, 99203, 99204, 99205, 99212, 99213, 99214, 99215 and **CPT**: 51720, 96401, 96402, 96405, 96406, 96409, 96411, 96413, 96415, 96416, 96417, 96420, 96422, 96423, 96425, 96440, 96445, 96450, 96521, 96522, 96523, 96542, 96549
144	Oncology: Medical and Radiation – Plan of Care for Pain	Percentage of patient visits, regardless of patient age, with a diagnosis of cancer currently receiving chemotherapy or radiation therapy who report having pain with a documented plan of care to address pain	each visit occurring during the reporting period for patients with a diagnosis of cancer and in which pain is present who are seen during the reporting period *(This is a two-part measure which is paired with Measure #143. This measure should be reported if CPT II code 1125F is submitted for Measure #143.)*	1 of: 0521F 0521F-8P	**ICD-9**: See measure #143 and **CPT**: See measure #143

CPT only © 2005-2009 American Medical Association. All rights reserved.

#	Title	Description	Reporting Requirements	Numerator Code(s)	Denominator Code(s)
145	Radiology: Exposure Time Reported for Procedures Using Fluoroscopy	Percentage of final reports for procedures using fluoroscopy that include documentation of radiation exposure or exposure time	each time fluoroscopy is performed in a hospital or outpatient setting during the reporting period	1 of: 6045F 6045F-8P	**ICD-9**: Any and **CPT/HCPCS**: 0062T, 0075T, 0080T, 24516, 25606, 25651, 26608, 26650, 26676, 26706, 26727, 27235, 27244, 27245, 27506, 27509, 27756, 27759, 28406, 28436, 28456, 28476, 36597, 36598, 37182, 37183, 37184, 37187, 37188, 37210, 43260, 43261, 43262, 43263, 43264, 43265, 43267, 43268, 43269, 43271, 43272, 43752, 44500, 49440, 49441, 49442, 49446, 49450, 49451, 49452, 49460, 49465, 50382, 50384, 50385, 50386, 50387, 50389, 50590, 61623, 62263, 62264, 62280, 62281, 62282, 62318, 62319, 63610, 64510, 64520, 64530, 64561, 64605, 64610, 64620, 64622, 64626, 64680, 64681, 70010, 70015, 70170, 70332, 70370, 70371, 70373, 70390, 71023, 71034, 71040, 71060, 71090, 72240, 72255, 72265, 72270, 72275, 72285, 72291, 72295, 73040, 73085, 73115, 73525, 73542, 73580, 73615, 74190, 74210, 74220, 74230, 74235, 74240, 74241, 74245, 74246, 74247, 74249, 74250, 74251, 74260, 74270, 74280, 74283, 74290, 74291, 74300, 74305, 74320, 74327, 74328, 74329, 74330, 74340, 74355, 74360, 74363, 74400, 74410, 74415, 74420, 74425, 74430, 74440, 74445, 74450, 74455, 74470, 74475, 74480, 74485, 74740, 74742, 75600, 75605, 75625, 75630, 75650, 75658, 75660, 75662, 75665, 75671, 75676, 75680, 75685, 75705, 75710, 75716, 75722, 75724, 75726, 75731, 75733, 75736, 75741, 75743, 75746, 75756, 75790, 75801, 75803, 75805, 75807, 75809, 75810, 75820, 75822, 75825, 75827, 75831, 75833, 75840, 75842, 75860, 75870, 75872, 75880, 75885, 75887, 75889, 75891, 75893, 75894, 75896, 75898, 75900, 75901, 75902, 75940, 75952, 75953, 75954, 75956, 75957, 75958, 75959, 75960, 75961, 75962, 75966, 75970, 75978, 75980, 75982, 75984, 75992, 75994, 75995, 76000, 76001, 76080, 76100, 76101, 76102, 76120, 76150, 76496, 77001, 77002, 77003, 77031, 77053, 77054, 77071, 92611, 93555, 93556, G0106, G0120, G0259, G0260, G0275, G0278, G0365
146	Radiology: Inappropriate Use of "Probably Benign" Assessment Category in Mammography Screening	Percentage of final reports for screening mammograms that are classified as "probably benign"	each time a screening mammogram is performed during the reporting period	1 of: 3040F 3041F 3042F 3043F 3044F 3045F 3050F	**ICD-9**: V76.11, V76.12 and **CPT/HCPCS**: 77057, G0202
147	Nuclear Medicine: Correlation with Existing Imaging Studies for All Patients Undergoing Bone Scintigraphy	Percentage of final reports for all patients, regardless of age, undergoing bone scintigraphy that include physician documentation of correlation with existing relevant imaging studies (eg, x-ray, MRI, CT, etc.) that were performed	each time bone scintigraphy is performed during the reporting period	1 of: 3570F 3570F-3P 3570F-8P	**ICD-9**: Any and **CPT**: 78300, 78305, 78306, 78315, 78320

CPT only © 2005-2009 American Medical Association. All rights reserved.

#	Title	Description	Reporting Requirements	Numerator Code(s)	Denominator Code(s)
148	Back Pain: Initial Visit	The percentage of patients aged 18 through 79 years with a diagnosis of back pain or undergoing back surgery who had back pain and function assessed during the initial visit to the clinician for the episode of back pain	30 consecutive patients meeting patient sample criteria for the measures group **OR** 80% of all patients meeting patient sample criteria for the measures group for the entire reporting period	1 of: 0526F 1130F 1130F-8P	**ICD-9**: 721.3 721.41, 721.42, 721.90, 722.0, 722.10, 722.11, 722.2, 722.30, 722.31, 722.32, 722.39, 722.4, 722.51, 722.52, 722.6, 722.70, 722.71, 722.72, 722.73, 722.80, 722.81, 722.82, 722.83, 722.90, 722.91, 722.92, 722.93, 723.0, 724.00, 724.01, 724.02, 724.09, 724.2, 724.3, 724.4, 724.5, 724.6, 724.70, 724.71, 724.79, 738.4, 738.5, 739.3, 739.4, 756.12, 846.0, 846.1, 846.2, 846.3, 846.8, 846.9, 847.2 and **CPT**: 98940, 98941, 98942, 99201, 99202, 99203, 99204, 99205, 99212, 99213, 99214, 99215, 99241, 99242, 99243, 99244, 99245 **OR** **CPT**: 22210, 22214, 22220, 22222, 22224, 22226, 22532, 22533, 22534, 22548, 22554, 22556, 22558, 22585, 22590, 22595, 22600, 22612, 22614, 22630, 22632, 22818, 22819, 22830, 22840, 22841, 22842, 22843, 22844, 22845, 22846, 22847, 22848, 22849, 63001, 63003, 63005, 63011, 63012, 63015, 63016, 63017, 63020, 63030, 63035, 63040, 63042, 63043, 63044, 63045, 63046, 63047, 63048, 63055, 63056, 63057, 63064, 63066, 63075, 63076, 63077, 63078, 63081, 63082, 63085, 63086, 63087, 63088, 63090, 63091, 63101, 63102, 63103 , 63170, 63172, 63173, 63180, 63182, 63185, 63190, 63191, 63194, 63195, 63196, 63197, 63198, 63199, 63200
149	Back Pain: Physical Exam	Percentage of patients aged 18 through 79 years with a diagnosis of back pain or undergoing back surgery who received a physical examination at the initial visit to the clinician for the episode of back pain	30 consecutive patients meeting patient sample criteria for the measures group **OR** 80% of all patients meeting patient sample criteria for the measures group for the entire reporting period	1 of: 0526F 2040F 2040F-8P	**ICD-9**: 721.3, 721.41, 721.42, 721.90, 722.0, 722.10, 722.11, 722.2, 722.30, 722.31, 722.32, 722.39, 722.4, 722.51, 722.52, 722.6, 722.70, 722.71, 722.72, 722.73, 722.80, 722.81, 722.82, 722.83, 722.90, 722.91, 722.92, 722.93, 723.0, 724.00, 724.01, 724.02, 724.09, 724.2, 724.3, 724.4, 724.5, 724.6, 724.70, 724.71, 724.79, 738.4, 738.5, 739.3, 739.4, 756.12, 846.0, 846.1, 846.2, 846.3, 846.8, 846.9, 847.2 and **CPT**: 98940, 98941, 98942, 99201, 99202, 99203, 99204, 99205, 99212, 99213, 99214, 99215, 99241, 99242, 99243, 99244, 99245 **OR** **CPT**: 22210, 22214, 22220, 22222, 22224, 22226, 22532, 22533, 22534, 22548, 22554, 22556, 22558, 22585, 22590, 22595, 22600, 22612, 22614, 22630, 22632, 22818, 22819, 22830, 22840, 22841, 22842, 22843, 22844, 22845, 22846, 22847, 22848, 22849, 63001, 63003, 63005, 63011, 63012, 63015, 63016, 63017, 63020, 63030, 63035, 63040, 63042, 63043, 63044, 63045, 63046, 63047, 63048, 63055, 63056, 63057, 63064, 63066, 63075, 63076, 63077, 63078, 63081, 63082, 63085, 63086, 63087, 63088, 63090, 63091, 63101, 63102, 63103 , 63170, 63172, 63173, 63180, 63182, 63185, 63190, 63191, 63194, 63195, 63196, 63197, 63198, 63199, 63200

CPT only © 2005-2009 American Medical Association. All rights reserved.

#	Title	Description	Reporting Requirements	Numerator Code(s)	Denominator Code(s)
150	Back Pain: Advice for Normal Activities	The percentage of patients aged 18 through 79 years with a diagnosis of back pain or undergoing back surgery who received advice for normal activities at the initial visit to the clinician for the episode of back pain	30 consecutive patients meeting patient sample criteria for the measures group **OR** 80% of all patients meeting patient sample criteria for the measures group for the entire reporting period	1 of: 0526F 4245F 4245F-8P	**ICD-9**: 721.3, 721.41, 721.42, 721.90, 722.0, 722.10, 722.11, 722.2, 722.30, 722.31, 722.32, 722.39, 722.4, 722.51, 722.52, 722.6, 722.70, 722.71, 722.72, 722.73, 722.80, 722.81, 722.82, 722.83, 722.90, 722.91, 722.92, 722.93, 723.0, 724.00, 724.01, 724.02, 724.09, 724.2, 724.3, 724.4, 724.5, 724.6, 724.70, 724.71, 724.79, 738.4, 738.5, 739.3, 739.4, 756.12, 846.0, 846.1, 846.2, 846.3, 846.8, 846.9, 847.2 and **CPT**: 98940, 98941, 98942, 99201, 99202, 99203, 99204, 99205, 99212, 99213, 99214, 99215, 99241, 99242, 99243, 99244, 99245 **OR** **CPT**: 22210, 22214, 22220, 22222, 22224, 22226, 22532, 22533, 22534, 22548, 22554, 22556, 22558, 22585, 22590, 22595, 22600, 22612, 22614, 22630, 22632, 22818, 22819, 22830, 22840, 22841, 22842, 22843, 22844, 22845, 22846, 22847, 22848, 22849, 63001, 63003, 63005, 63011, 63012, 63015, 63016, 63017, 63020, 63030, 63035, 63040, 63042, 63043, 63044, 63045, 63046, 63047, 63048, 63055, 63056, 63057, 63064, 63066, 63075, 63076, 63077, 63078, 63081, 63082, 63085, 63086, 63087, 63088, 63090, 63091, 63101, 63102, 63103 , 63170, 63172, 63173, 63180, 63182, 63185, 63190, 63191, 63194, 63195, 63196, 63197, 63198, 63199, 63200
151	Back Pain: Advice Against Bed Rest	The percentage of patients aged 18 through 79 years with a diagnosis of back pain or undergoing back surgery who received advice against bed rest lasting four days or longer at the initial visit to the clinician for the episode of back pain	30 consecutive patients meeting patient sample criteria for the measures group **OR** 80% of all patients meeting patient sample criteria for the measures group for the entire reporting period	1 of: 0526F 4248F 4248F-8P	**ICD-9**: 721.3, 721.41, 721.42, 721.90, 722.0, 722.10, 722.11, 722.2, 722.30, 722.31, 722.32, 722.39, 722.4, 722.51, 722.52, 722.6, 722.70, 722.71, 722.72, 722.73, 722.80, 722.81, 722.82, 722.83, 722.90, 722.91, 722.92, 722.93, 723.0, 724.00, 724.01, 724.02, 724.09, 724.2, 724.3, 724.4, 724.5, 724.6, 724.70, 724.71, 724.79, 738.4, 738.5, 739.3, 739.4, 756.12, 846.0, 846.1, 846.2, 846.3, 846.8, 846.9, 847.2 and **CPT**: 98940, 98941, 98942, 99201, 99202, 99203, 99204, 99205, 99212, 99213, 99214, 99215, 99241, 99242, 99243, 99244, 99245 **OR** **CPT**: 22210, 22214, 22220, 22222, 22224, 22226, 22532, 22533, 22534, 22548, 22554, 22556, 22558, 22585, 22590, 22595, 22600, 22612, 22614, 22630, 22632, 22818, 22819, 22830, 22840, 22841, 22842, 22843, 22844, 22845, 22846, 22847, 22848, 22849, 63001, 63003, 63005, 63011, 63012, 63015, 63016, 63017, 63020, 63030, 63035, 63040, 63042, 63043, 63044, 63045, 63046, 63047, 63048, 63055, 63056, 63057, 63064, 63066, 63075, 63076, 63077, 63078, 63081, 63082, 63085, 63086, 63087, 63088, 63090, 63091, 63101, 63102, 63103 , 63170, 63172, 63173, 63180, 63182, 63185, 63190, 63191, 63194, 63195, 63196, 63197, 63198, 63199, 63200
152	Coronary Artery Disease (CAD): Lipid Profile in Patients with CAD	Percentage of patients aged 18 years and older with a diagnosis of CAD who received at least one lipid profile within 12 months	≥ once per reporting period for patients with CAD seen during the reporting period	1 of: 3011F 3011F-8P	**ICD-9**: 410.00, 410.01, 410.02, 410.10, 410.11, 410.12, 410.20, 410.21, 410.22, 410.30, 410.31, 410.32, 410.40, 410.41, 410.42, 410.50, 410.51, 410.52, 410.60, 410.61, 410.62, 410.70, 410.71, 410.72, 410.80, 410.81, 410.82, 410.90, 410.91, 410.92, 411.0, 411.1, 411.81, 411.89, 412, 413.0, 413.1, 413.9, 414.00, 414.01, 414.02, 414.03, 414.04, 414.05, 414.06, 414.07, 414.8, 414.9, V45.81, V45.82 and **CPT**: 99201, 99202, 99203, 99204, 99205, 99212, 99213, 99214, 99215, 99241, 99242, 99243, 99244, 99245, 99304, 99305, 99306, 99307, 99308, 99309, 99310, 99324, 99325, 99326, 99327, 99328, 99334, 99335, 99336, 99337, 99341, 99342, 99343, 99344, 99345, 99347, 99348, 99349, 99350

CPT only © 2005-2009 American Medical Association. All rights reserved.

#	Title	Description	Reporting Requirements	Numerator Code(s)	Denominator Code(s)
153	Chronic Kidney Disease (CKD): Referral for Arteriovenous (AV) Fistula	Percentage of patients aged 18 years and older with the diagnosis of advanced CKD (stage 4 or 5, not receiving Renal Replacement Therapy [RRT]), who were referred for AV fistula at least once during the 12-month reporting period	≥ once per reporting period for patients with a diagnosis of advanced CKD seen during the reporting period.	1 of: 4051F 4051F-1P 4051F-2P 4051F-8P	**ICD-9**: 585.4, 585.5 and **CPT**: 99201, 99202, 99203, 99204, 99205, 99212, 99213, 99214, 99215, 99241, 99242, 99243, 99244, 99245
154	Falls: Risk Assessment	Percentage of patients aged 65 years and older with a history of falls who had a risk assessment for falls completed within 12 months	≥ once per reporting period for patients seen during the reporting period *(This is a two-part measure which is paired with Measure #155. If the falls risk assessment indicates the patient has documentation of two or more falls in the past year or any fall with injury in the past year (CPT II code 1100F is submitted), #155 should also be reported.)*	1100F **and** 1 of: 3288F 3288F-1P 3288F-8P **OR** 3288F-1P **and** 1 of: 1101F 1101F-8P	**ICD-9**: Any and **CPT**: 97001, 97002, 97003, 97004, 99201, 99202, 99203, 99204, 99205, 99212, 99213, 99214, 99215, 99241, 99242, 99243, 99244, 99245, 99304, 99305, 99306, 99307, 99308, 99309, 99310, 99324, 99325, 99326, 99327, 99328, 99334, 99335, 99336, 99337, 99341, 99342, 99343, 99344, 99345, 99347, 99348, 99349, 99350
155	Falls: Plan of Care	Percentage of patients aged 65 years and older with a history of falls who had a plan of care for falls documented within 12 months	≥ once per reporting period for patients seen during the reporting period *This is a two-part measure which is paired with Measure #154.* *This measure should be reported if CPT II code 1100F is submitted for Measure #154.)*	1 of: 0518F 0518F-1P 0518F-8P	**ICD-9**: See measure #155 and **CPT**: See measure #155

CPT only © 2005-2009 American Medical Association. All rights reserved.

#	Title	Description	Reporting Requirements	Numerator Code(s)	Denominator Code(s)
156	Oncology: Radiation Dose Limits to Normal Tissues	Percentage of patients, regardless of age, with a diagnosis of pancreatic or lung cancer receiving 3D conformal radiation therapy with documentation in medical record that radiation dose limits to normal tissues were established prior to the initiation of a course of 3D conformal radiation for a minimum of two tissues	≥ once per reporting period for patients with a diagnosis of cancer receiving 3D conformal radiation therapy seen during the reporting period	1 of: 0520F 0520F-8P	**ICD-9**: 157.0, 157.1, 157.2, 157.3, 157.4, 157.8, 157.9, 162.0, 162.2, 162.3, 162.4, 162.5, 162.8, 162.9 and **CPT**: 77295
157	Thoracic Surgery: Recording of Clinical Stage for Lung Cancer and Esophageal Cancer Resection	Percentage of surgical patients aged 18 years and older undergoing resection for lung or esophageal cancer who had clinical TNM staging provided prior to surgery	each time a major cancer resection of the lung or esophagus is performed	1 of: G8518 G8519 G8520	**ICD-9**: 150.3, 150.4, 150.5, 162.2, 162.3, 162.4, 162.5 and **CPT**: 32440, 32442, 32445, 32480, 32482, 32484, 32486, 32488, 32500, 32503, 32504, 32657, 32663, 43107, 43108, 43112, 43113, 43117, 43118, 43121, 43122, 43123
158	Endarterectomy: Use of Patch During Conventional Endarterectomy	Percentage of patients aged 18 years and older undergoing conventional (non-eversion) endarterectomy who undergo patch closure of the arteriotomy	each time a patient undergoes an endarter-ectomy procedure during the reporting period	1 of: G8524 G8525 G8526	**ICD-9**: Any and **CPT**: 35301
159	HIV/AIDS: CD4+ Cell Count or CD4+ Percentage	Percentage of patients aged 6 months and older with a diagnosis of HIV/AIDS for whom a CD4+ cell count or CD4+ cell percentage was performed at least once every 6 months	twice during the reporting period for patients with HIV/AIDS seen during the reporting period, once during the first half of the year and once in the second half of the year	Registry only (no codes)	**ICD-9**: 042, 079.53, V08 and **CPT**: 99201, 99202, 99203, 99204, 99205, 99212, 99213, 99214, 99215, 99241, 99242, 99243, 99244, 99245
160	HIV/AIDS: Pneumocystis Jiroveci Pneumonia (PCP) Prophylaxis	Percentage of patients aged 6 years and older with a diagnosis of HIV/AIDS and CD4+ cell count <200 cells/mm^3 who were prescribed PCP prophylaxis within 3 months of low CD4+ cell count	≥ once per reporting period for patients with HIV/AIDS seen during the reporting period	Registry only (no codes)	**ICD-9**: 042, 079.53, V08 and **CPT**: 99201, 99202, 99203, 99204, 99205, 99212, 99213, 99214, 99215, 99241, 99242, 99243, 99244, 99245
161	HIV/AIDS: Adolescent and Adult Patients with HIV/AIDS Who Are Prescribed Potent Antiretroviral Therapy	Percentage of patients with a diagnosis of HIV/AIDS aged 13 years and older: who have a history of a nadir CD4+ cell count below 350/mm^3 or who have a history of an AIDS-defining condition, regardless of CD4+ cell count; or who are pregnant, regardless of CD4+ cell count or age, who were prescribed potent antiretroviral therapy	≥ once per reporting period for patients with HIV/AIDS seen during the reporting period	Registry only (no codes)	**ICD-9**: 042, 079.53, V08 and **CPT**: 99201, 99202, 99203, 99204, 99205, 99212, 99213, 99214, 99215, 99241, 99242, 99243, 99244, 99245 **OR, for pregnant patients** **ICD-9**: 042, 079.53, V08 and **ICD-9**: V22.0, V22.1, V22.2, V23.0, V23.1, V23.2, V23.3, V23.41, V23.49, V23.5, V23.7, V23.81, V23.82, V23.83, V23.84, V23.89, V23.9 and **CPT**: 99201, 99202, 99203, 99204, 99205, 99212, 99213, 99214, 99215, 99241, 99242, 99243, 99244, 99245

CPT only © 2005-2009 American Medical Association. All rights reserved.

#	Title	Description	Reporting Requirements	Numerator Code(s)	Denominator Code(s)
162	HIV/AIDS: HIV RNA Control After Six Months of Potent Antiretroviral Therapy	Percentage of patients aged 13 years and older with a diagnosis of HIV/AIDS who are receiving potent antiretroviral therapy, who have a viral load below limits of quantification after at least 6 months of potent antiretroviral therapy or patients whose viral load is not below limits of quantification after at least 6 months of potent antiretroviral therapy and have documentation of a plan of care	≥ once per reporting period for patients with HIV/AIDS who are receiving potent antiretroviral therapy during the reporting period	Registry only (no codes)	**ICD-9**: 042, 079.53, V08 and **CPT**: 99201, 99202, 99203, 99204, 99205, 99212, 99213, 99214, 99215, 99241, 99242, 99243, 99244, 99245
163	Diabetes Mellitus: Foot Exam	The percentage of patients aged 18 through 75 years with diabetes who had a foot examination	≥ once per reporting period for patients with diabetes mellitus seen during the reporting period	1 of: 2028F 2028F-1P 2028F-8P	**ICD-9**: 250.00, 250.01, 250.02, 250.03, 250.10, 250.11, 250.12, 250.13, 250.20, 250.21, 250.22, 250.23, 250.30, 250.31, 250.32, 250.33, 250.40, 250.41, 250.42, 250.43, 250.50, 250.51, 250.52, 250.53, 250.60, 250.61, 250.62, 250.63, 250.70, 250.71, 250.72, 250.73, 250.80, 250.81, 250.82, 250.83, 250.90, 250.91, 250.92, 250.93, 357.2, 362.01, 362.02, 362.03, 362.04, 362.05, 362.06, 362.07, 366.41, 648.00, 648.01, 648.02, 648.03, 648.04 and **CPT/HCPCS**: 97802, 97803, 97804, 99201, 99202, 99203, 99204, 99205, 99212, 99213, 99214, 99215, 99304, 99305, 99306, 99307, 99308, 99309, 99310, 99324, 99325, 99326, 99327, 99328, 99334, 99335, 99336, 99337, 99341, 99342, 99343, 99344, 99345, 99347, 99348, 99349, 99350, G0270, G0271
164	Coronary Artery Bypass Graft (CABG): Prolonged Intubation (Ventilation)	Percentage of patients aged 18 years and older undergoing isolated CABG surgery who require intubation > 24 hours	each time an isolated CABG procedure is performed during the reporting period	Registry only (no codes)	**ICD-9**: Any and **CPT**: 33510, 33511, 33512, 33513, 33514, 33516, 33517, 33518, 33519, 33521, 33522, 33523, 33533, 33534, 33535, 33536
165	Coronary Artery Bypass Graft (CABG): Deep Sternal Wound Infection Rate	Percentage of patients aged 18 years and older undergoing isolated CABG surgery who developed deep sternal wound infection (involving muscle, bone, and/or mediastinum requiring operative intervention) within 30 days postoperatively	each time an isolated CABG procedure is performed during the reporting period	Registry only (no codes)	**ICD-9**: Any and **CPT**: 33510, 33511, 33512, 33513, 33514, 33516, 33517, 33518, 33519, 33521, 33522, 33523, 33533, 33534, 33535, 33536
166	Coronary Artery Bypass Graft (CABG): Stroke/ Cerebrovascular Accident (CVA)	Percentage of patients aged 18 years and older undergoing isolated CABG surgery who had a stroke/CVA	each time an isolated CABG procedure is performed during the reporting period	Registry only (no codes)	**ICD-9**: Any, except V12.54 and **CPT**: 33510, 33511, 33512, 33513, 33514, 33516, 33517, 33518, 33519, 33521, 33522, 33523, 33533, 33534, 33535, 33536
167	Coronary Artery Bypass Graft (CABG): Postoperative Renal Insufficiency	Percentage of patients aged 18 years and older undergoing isolated CABG surgery who develop postoperative renal insufficiency or require dialysis	each time an isolated CABG procedure is performed during the reporting period	Registry only (no codes)	**ICD-9**: Any and **CPT**: 33510, 33511, 33512, 33513, 33514, 33516, 33517, 33518, 33519, 33521, 33522, 33523, 33533, 33534, 33535, 33536

 CPT only © 2005-2009 American Medical Association. All rights reserved.

#	Title	Description	Reporting Requirements	Numerator Code(s)	Denominator Code(s)
168	Coronary Artery Bypass Graft (CABG): Surgical Re-exploration	Percentage of patients aged 18 years and older undergoing isolated CABG surgery who require a return to the operating room (OR) for mediastinal bleeding/tamponade, graft occlusion (due to acute closure, thrombosis, technical or embolic origin), or other cardiac reason	each time an isolated CABG procedure is performed during the reporting period	Registry only (no codes)	**ICD-9**: Any and **CPT**: 33510, 33511, 33512, 33513, 33514, 33516, 33517, 33518, 33519, 33521, 33522, 33523, 33533, 33534, 33535, 33536
169	Coronary Artery Bypass Graft (CABG): Antiplatelet Medications at Discharge	Percentage of patients aged 18 years and older undergoing isolated CABG surgery who have antiplatelet medication at discharge	each time an isolated CABG procedure is performed during the reporting period	Registry only (no codes)	**ICD-9**: Any and **CPT**: 33510, 33511, 33512, 33513, 33514, 33516, 33517, 33518, 33519, 33521, 33522, 33523, 33533, 33534, 33535, 33536
170	Coronary Artery Bypass Graft (CABG): Beta-Blockers Administered at Discharge	Percentage of patients aged 18 years and older undergoing isolated CABG surgery who were discharged on beta-blockers	each time an isolated CABG procedure is performed during the reporting period	Registry only (no codes)	**ICD-9**: Any and **CPT**: 33510, 33511, 33512, 33513, 33514, 33516, 33517, 33518, 33519, 33521, 33522, 33523, 33533, 33534, 33535, 33536
171	Coronary Artery Bypass Graft (CABG): Lipid Management and Counseling	Percentage of patients aged 18 years and older undergoing isolated CABG surgery who have anti-lipid treatment at discharge	each time an isolated CABG procedure is performed during the reporting period	Registry only (no codes)	**ICD-9**: Any and **CPT**: 33510, 33511, 33512, 33513, 33514, 33516, 33517, 33518, 33519, 33521, 33522, 33523, 33533, 33534, 33535, 33536
172	Hemodialysis Vascular Access Decision-Making by Surgeon to Maximize Placement of Autogenous Arterial Venous (AV) Fistula	Percentage of patients aged 18 years and older with a diagnosis of advanced Chronic Kidney Disease (CKD) (stage 4 or 5) or End Stage Renal Disease (ESRD) requiring hemodialysis vascular access documented by surgeon to have received autogenous AV fistula	each time a procedure for hemodialysis access is performed during the reporting period	1 of: G8530 G8531 G8532	**ICD-9**: 585.4, 585.5, 585.6, 996.73 and **CPT**: 36818, 36819, 36820, 36821, 36825, 36830
173	Preventive Care and Screening: Unhealthy Alcohol Use – Screening	Percentage of patients aged 18 years and older who were screened for unhealthy alcohol use using a systematic screening method within 24 months	≥ once per reporting period for patients seen during the reporting period	1 of: 3016F 3016F-1P 3016F-8P	**ICD-9**: Any and **CPT/HCPCS**: 90801, 90802, 90804, 90805, 90806, 90807, 90808, 90809, 90810, 90811, 90812, 90813, 90814, 90815, 90845, 90862, 96150, 96152, 97003, 97004, 97802, 97803, 97804, 98960, 98961, 98962, 99201, 99202, 99203, 99204, 99205, 99212, 99213, 99214, 99215, G0270, G0271
174	Pediatric End Stage Renal Disease (ESRD): Plan of Care for Inadequate Hemodialysis	Percentage of calendar months during the 12-month reporting period in which patients aged 17 years and younger with a diagnosis of ESRD receiving hemodialysis have a single-pool Kt/V ≥ 1.2 or have a single-pool Kt/V < 1.2 with a documented plan of care for inadequate hemodialysis	each calendar month hemodialysis is performed on pediatric ESRD patients seen during the reporting period	Registry only (no codes)	**ICD-9**: 585.6 and **CPT**: 90951, 90952, 90953, 90954, 90955, 90956, 90957, 90958, 90959

CPT only © 2005-2009 American Medical Association. All rights reserved.

#	Title	Description	Reporting Requirements	Numerator Code(s)	Denominator Code(s)
175	Pediatric End Stage Renal Disease (ESRD): Influenza Immunization	Percentage of patients aged 6 months through 17 years with a diagnosis of ESRD and receiving dialysis seen for a visit between November 1 and February 15 who have documented administration of influenza immunization OR patient reported receipt of an influenza immunization from another provider	≥ once for visits occurring between January 1, 2009 and February 15, 2009 for the 2008-2009 influenza season AND a ≥ once for visits occurring between November 1, 2009 and December 31, 2009 for the 2009-2010 influenza season for ESRD patients receiving dialysis seen during the reporting period	1 of: 4274F 4274F-1P 4274F-2P 4274F-3P 4274F-8P	**ICD-9**: 585.6 and **CPT**: 90951, 90952, 90953, 90954, 90955, 90956, 90957, 90958, 90959, 90963, 90964, 90965
176	R heumatoid Arthritis (RA): Tuberculosis Screening	Percentage of patients 18 years and older with a diagnosis of RA who have documentation of a tuberculosis (TB) screening performed and results interpreted within 6 months prior to receiving a first course of therapy using a biologic disease-modifying anti-rheumatic drug (DMARD)	≥ once per reporting period for all RA patients who are being considered or prescribed a first course of biologic disease-modifying anti-rheumatic drug therapy	4195F **and** 1 of: 3455F 3455F-1P 3455F-8P **OR** 4196F	**ICD-9**: 714.0, 714.1, 714.2, 714.81 and **CPT**: 99201, 99202, 99203, 99204, 99205, 99212, 99213, 99214, 99215, 99241, 99242, 99243, 99244, 99245, 99341, 99342, 99343, 99344, 99345, 99347, 99348, 99349, 99350, 99455, 99456
177	Rheumatoid Arthritis (RA): Periodic Assessment of Disease Activity	Percentage of patients 18 years and older with a diagnosis of RA who have an assessment and classification of disease activity within 12 months	≥ once per reporting period for patients with RA seen during the reporting period	1 of: 3470F 3470F-8P 3471F 3472F	**ICD-9**: 714.0, 714.1, 714.2, 714.81 and **CPT**: 99201, 99202, 99203, 99204, 99205, 99212, 99213, 99214, 99215, 99241, 99242, 99243, 99244, 99245, 99341, 99342, 99343, 99344, 99345, 99347, 99348, 99349, 99350, 99455, 99456
178	Rheumatoid Arthritis (RA): Functional Status Assessment	Percentage of patients 18 years and older with a diagnosis of RA for whom a functional status assessment was performed at least once within 12 months	≥ once per reporting period for patients with RA seen during the reporting period	1 of: 1070F 1070F-8P	**ICD-9**: 714.0, 714.1, 714.2, 714.81 and **CPT**: 99201, 99202, 99203, 99204, 99205, 99212, 99213, 99214, 99215, 99241, 99242, 99243, 99244, 99245, 99341, 99342, 99343, 99344, 99345, 99347, 99348, 99349, 99350, 99455, 99456
179	Rheumatoid Arthritis (RA): Assessment and Classification of Disease Prognosis	Percentage of patients 18 years and older with a diagnosis of RA who have an assessment and classification of disease prognosis at least once within 12 months	≥ once per reporting period for patients with RA seen during the reporting period	1 of: 3475F 3475F-8P 3476F	**ICD-9**: 714.0, 714.1, 714.2, 714.81 and **CPT**: 99201, 99202, 99203, 99204, 99205, 99212, 99213, 99214, 99215, 99241, 99242, 99243, 99244, 99245, 99341, 99342, 99343, 99344, 99345, 99347, 99348, 99349, 99350, 99455, 99456

CPT only © 2005-2009 American Medical Association. All rights reserved.

#	Title	Description	Reporting Requirements	Numerator Code(s)	Denominator Code(s)
180	Rheumatoid Arthritis (RA): Glucocorticoid Management	Percentage of patients 18 years and older with a diagnosis of RA who have been assessed for glucocorticoid use and, for those on prolonged doses of prednisone ≥ 10 mg daily (or equivalent) with improvement or no change in disease activity, documentation of glucocorticoid management plan within 12 months	≥ once per reporting period for patients with RA seen during the reporting period.	1 of: 4192F 4193F 4194F-8P **OR** 4194F **and** 1 of: 0540F 0540F-1P 0540F-8P	**ICD-9**: 714.0, 714.1, 714.2, 714.81 and **CPT**: 99201, 99202, 99203, 99204, 99205, 99212, 99213, 99214, 99215, 99241, 99242, 99243, 99244, 99245, 99341, 99342, 99343, 99344, 99345, 99347, 99348, 99349, 99350, 99455, 99456
181	Elder Maltreatment Screen and Follow-Up Plan	Percentage of patients age 65 years and older with documentation of a screen for elder maltreatment AND documented follow-up plan	each initial patient evaluation during the reporting period	1 of: G8534 G8535 G8536 G8537 G8538	**ICD-9**: Any and **CPT/HCPCS**: 90801, 90802, 96116*, 96150, 97003, 97802, 97803*, G0270* * When reporting CPT code 96116, 97803, and G0270, the measure is to be reported each time the code is submitted.
182	Functional Outcome Assessment in Chiropractic Care	Percentage of patients age 18 years and older with documentation of a current functional outcome assessment using a standardized tool AND documentation of a care plan based on identified functional outcome deficiencies	each visit indicating the appropriate numerator code; however, the assessment is required to be current as defined for patients seen during the reporting period	1 of: G8539 G8540 G8541 G8542 G8543	**ICD-9**: Any and **CPT**: 98940, 98941, 98942
183	Hepatitis C: Hepatitis A Vaccination in Patients with HCV	Percentage of patients aged 18 years and older with a diagnosis of hepatitis C who received at least one injection of hepatitis A vaccine, or who have documented immunity to hepatitis A	≥ once per reporting period for patients with a diagnosis of hepatitis C seen during the reporting period *(If reporting Measure #183, Measure #184 must also be reported)*	1 of: 3215F 4148F 4148F-1P 4148F-2P 4148F-8P	**ICD-9**: 070.51, 070.54, 070.70 and **CPT**: 99201, 99202, 99203, 99204, 99205, 99212, 99213, 99214, 99215
184	Hepatitis C: Hepatitis B Vaccination in Patients with HCV	Percentage of patients aged 18 years and older with a diagnosis of hepatitis C who received at least one injection of hepatitis B vaccine, or who have documented immunity to hepatitis B	≥ once per reporting period for patients with a diagnosis of hepatitis C seen during the reporting period *(If reporting Measure #184, Measure #183 must also be reported)*	1 of: 3216F 4149F 4149F-1P 4149F-2P 4149F-8P	**ICD-9**: 070.51, 070.54, 070.70 and **CPT**: 99201, 99202, 99203, 99204, 99205, 99212, 99213, 99214, 99215

CPT only © 2005-2009 American Medical Association. All rights reserved.

#	Title	Description	Reporting Requirements	Numerator Code(s)	Denominator Code(s)
185	Endoscopy & Polyp Surveillance: Colonoscopy Interval for Patients with a History of Adenomatous Polyps – Avoidance of Inappropriate Use	Percentage of patients aged 18 years and older receiving a surveillance colonoscopy and a history of colonic polyp(s) in a previous colonoscopy, who had a follow-up interval of 3 or more years since their last colonoscopy documented in the colonoscopy report	each time a surveillance colonoscopy is performed during the reporting period	1 of: 0529F 0529F-1P 0529F-3P 0529F-8P	**ICD-9**: V12.72 and **CPT/HCPCS**: 44388, 44389, 44392, 44393, 44394, 45355, 45378, 45380, 45381, 45383, 45384, 45385, G0105 **without** **Modifier**: 52, 53, 73, 74
186	Wound Care: Use of Compression System in Patients with Venous Ulcers	Percentage of patients aged 18 years and older with a diagnosis of venous ulcer who were prescribed compression therapy within the 12-month reporting period	≥ once per reporting period for patients with venous ulcer(s) seen during the reporting period	1 of: 4267F 4267F-1P 4267F-2P 4267F-3P 4267F-8P	**ICD-9**: 459.31, 459.33, 459.81 and **ICD-9**: 707.12, 707.13, 707.14, 707.15, 707.19 and **CPT**: 99201, 99202, 99203, 99204, 99205, 99212, 99213, 99214, 99215, 99241, 99242, 99243, 99244, 99245

Copyright attribution and disclaimers

These performance Measures are not clinical guidelines and do not establish a standard of medical care, and have not been tested for all potential applications.

Limited proprietary coding is contained in the Measure specifications for convenience. MAG Mutual Healthcare Solutions, Inc., the AMA, NCQA, ASH, ASCO, NCCN, CAP, APMA, STS, QIO and the Consortium and its members disclaim all liability for use or accuracy of any Current Procedural Terminology (CPT®) or other coding contained in the specifications.

Measures #1, 2, 3, 9, 65, 66, 108, 111, 112, 113, 115, 116, 117, 119, 148, 149, 150, 151 and 163 are © the National Committee for Quality Assurance. All Rights Reserved

Measures #5, 6, 7, 8, 51, 52, 53, 64, 76, 79, 81, 82, 83, 84, 85, 86, 87, 89, 90, 91, 92, 93, 94, 95, 102, 104, 105, 106, 107, 109, 110, 114, 118, 121, 122, 123, 135, 142, 143, 144, 147, 152, 153, 156, 173, 174, 175, 183 and 184 are © 2007-8 American Medical Association. All Rights Reserved

Measures #10, 11, 12, 14, 18, 19, 20, 21, 22, 23, 24, 28, 30, 31, 32, 33, 34, 35, 36, 39, 40, 41, 45, 46, 47, 48, 49, 50, 54, 55, 56, 57, 58, 59, 136, 137, 138, 139, 140, 141, 145, 146, 154, 155, 159, 160, 161 and 162 are © 2004-8 American Medical Association and National Committee for Quality Assurance. All Rights Reserved

Measures #43, 44, 157, 164, 165, 166, 167, 168, 169, 170 and 171 are owned by The Society of Thoracic Surgeons (STS).

Measures #67, 68, 69 and 70 are © 2006-7 American Medical Association and American Society of Hematology. SNOMED CT® © 2004 College of American Pathologists (CAP). All Rights Reserved

Measures #71 and 72 are © 2007 American Medical Association, American Society of Clinical Oncology, and National Comprehensive Cancer Network. All Rights Reserved

Measures #99 and 100 are © 2007 American Medical Association and College of American Pathologists. All Rights Reserved

Measures #124, 128, 130, 131, 134, 181 and 182 were developed by Quality Insights of Pennsylvania as a special project under the Quality Insights' Medicare Quality Improvement Organization (QIO) contract HHSM-500-2005-PA001C with the Centers for Medicare & Medicaid Services. These measures are in the public domain.

Measures #126 and 127 are owned by the American Podiatric Medical Association (APMA).

Measures #176, 177, 178, 179, 180, 185 and 186 are owned by The Society of Thoracic Surgeons (STS).

Measures #158 and 172 are owned by the Society for Vascular Surgery - SVS.

 CPT only © 2005-2009 American Medical Association. All rights reserved.

AAT (alpha-1 antitrypsin) **deficiency** 273.4
AAV (disease) (illness) (infection) - *see* Human immunodeficiency virus (disease) (illness) (infection)
Abactio - *see* Abortion, induced
Abactus venter - *see* Abortion, induced
Abarognosis 781.99
Abasia (-astasia) 307.9
atactica 781.3
choreic 781.3
hysterical 300.11
paroxysmal trepidant 781.3
spastic 781.3
trembling 781.3
trepidans 781.3
Abderhalden-Kaufmann-Lignac syndrome (cystinosis) 270.0
Abdomen, abdominal - *see also* condition
accordion 306.4
acute 789.0 [5th]
angina 557.1
burst 868.00
convulsive equivalent (*see also* Epilepsy) 345.5 [5th]
heart 746.87
muscle deficiency syndrome 756.79
obstipum 756.79
Abdominalgia 789.0 [5th]
periodic 277.31
Abduction contracture, hip or other joint - *see* Contraction, joint
Abercrombie's syndrome (amyloid degeneration) 277.39
Aberrant (congenital) - *see also* Malposition, congenital
adrenal gland 759.1
blood vessel NEC 747.60
arteriovenous NEC 747.60
cerebrovascular 747.81
gastrointestinal 747.61
lower limb 747.64
renal 747.62
spinal 747.82
upper limb 747.63
breast 757.6
endocrine gland NEC 759.2
gastrointestinal vessel (peripheral) 747.61
hepatic duct 751.69
lower limb vessel (peripheral) 747.64
pancreas 751.7
parathyroid gland 759.2
peripheral vascular vessel NEC 747.60
pituitary gland (pharyngeal) 759.2
renal blood vessel 747.62
sebaceous glands, mucous membrane, mouth 750.26
spinal vessel 747.82
spleen 759.0
testis (descent) 752.51
thymus gland 759.2
thyroid gland 759.2
upper limb vessel (peripheral) 747.63
Aberratio
lactis 757.6
testis 752.51
Aberration - *see also* Anomaly
chromosome - *see* Anomaly, chromosome(s)
distantial 368.9
mental (*see also* Disorder, mental, nonpsychotic) 300.9
Abetalipoproteinemia 272.5
Abionarce 780.79
Abiotrophy 799.89
Ablatio
placentae - *see* Placenta, ablatio
retinae (*see also* Detachment, retina) 361.9
Ablation
pituitary (gland) (with hypofunction) 253.7

Ablation – *continued*
placenta - *see* Placenta, ablatio
uterus 621.8
Ablepharia, ablepharon, ablephary 743.62
Ablepsia - *see* Blindness
Ablepsy - *see* Blindness
Ablutomania 300.3
Abnormal, abnormality, abnormalities - *see also* Anomaly
acid-base balance 276.4
fetus or newborn - *see* Distress, fetal
adaptation curve, dark 368.63
alveolar ridge 525.9
amnion 658.9 [5th]
affecting fetus or newborn 762.9
anatomical relationship NEC 759.9
apertures, congenital, diaphragm 756.6
auditory perception NEC 388.40
autosomes NEC 758.5
13 758.1
18 758.2
21 or 22 758.0
D_1 758.1
E_3 758.2
G 758.0
ballistocardiogram 794.39
basal metabolic rate (BMR) 794.7
biosynthesis, testicular androgen 257.2
blood level (of)
cobalt 790.6
copper 790.6
iron 790.6
lead 790.6
lithium 790.6
magnesium 790.6
mineral 790.6
zinc 790.6
blood pressure
elevated (without diagnosis of hypertension) 796.2
low (*see also* Hypotension) 458.9
reading (incidental) (isolated) (nonspecific) 796.3
blood sugar 790.29
bowel sounds 787.5
breathing behavior - *see* Respiration
caloric test 794.19
cervix (acquired) NEC 622.9
congenital 752.40
in pregnancy or childbirth 654.6 [5th]
causing obstructed labor 660.2 [5th]
affecting fetus or newborn 763.1
chemistry, blood NEC 790.6
chest sounds 786.7
chorion 658.9 [5th]
affecting fetus or newborn 762.9
chromosomal NEC 758.89
analysis, nonspecific result 795.2
autosomes (*see also* Abnormal, autosomes NEC) 758.5
fetal, (suspected) affecting management of pregnancy 655.1 [5th]
sex 758.81
clinical findings NEC 796.4
communication - *see* Fistula
configuration of pupils 379.49
coronary
artery 746.85
vein 746.9
cortisol-binding globulin 255.8
course, Eustachian tube 744.24
creatinine clearance 794.4
dentofacial NEC 524.9
functional 524.50
specified type NEC 524.89
development, developmental NEC 759.9
bone 756.9
central nervous system 742.9
direction, teeth 524.30
Dynia (*see also* Defect, coagulation) 286.9
Ebstein 746.2
echocardiogram 793.2
echoencephalogram 794.01

Abnormal, abnormality, abnormalities – *continued*
echogram NEC - *see* Findings, abnormal, structure
electrocardiogram (ECG) (EKG) 794.31
electroencephalogram (EEG) 794.02
electromyogram (EMG) 794.17
ocular 794.14
electro-oculogram (EOG) 794.12
electroretinogram (ERG) 794.11
erythrocytes 289.9
congenital, with perinatal jaundice 282.9 [774.0]
Eustachian valve 746.9
excitability under minor stress 301.9
fat distribution 782.9
feces 787.7
fetal heart rate - *see* Distress, fetal
fetus NEC
affecting management of pregnancy - *see* Pregnancy, management affected by, fetal
causing disproportion 653.7 [5th]
affecting fetus or newborn 763.1
causing obstructed labor 660.1 [5th]
affecting fetus or newborn 763.1
findings without manifest disease - *see* Findings, abnormal
fluid
amniotic 792.3
cerebrospinal 792.0
peritoneal 792.9
pleural 792.9
synovial 792.9
vaginal 792.9
forces of labor NEC 661.9 [5th]
affecting fetus or newborn 763.7
form, teeth 520.2
function studies
auditory 794.15
bladder 794.9
brain 794.00
cardiovascular 794.30
endocrine NEC 794.6
kidney 794.4
liver 794.8
nervous system
central 794.00
peripheral 794.19
oculomotor 794.14
pancreas 794.9
placenta 794.9
pulmonary 794.2
retina 794.11
special senses 794.19
spleen 794.9
thyroid 794.5
vestibular 794.16
gait 781.2
hysterical 300.11
gastrin secretion 251.5
globulin
cortisol-binding 255.8
thyroid-binding 246.8
glucagon secretion 251.4
glucose 790.29
in pregnancy, childbirth, or puerperium 648.8 [5th]
fetus or newborn 775.0
non-fasting 790.29
gravitational (G) forces or states 994.9
hair NEC 704.2
hard tissue formation in pulp 522.3
head movement 781.0
heart
rate
fetus, affecting liveborn infant
before the onset of labor 763.81
during labor 763.82
unspecified as to time of onset 763.83
intrauterine
before the onset of labor 763.81
during labor 763.82

Abnormal, abnormality, abnormalities – *continued*
heart – *continued*
rate – *continued*
intrauterine – *continued*
unspecified as to time of onset 763.83
newborn
before the onset of labor 763.81
during labor 763.82
unspecified as to time of onset 763.83
shadow 793.2
sounds NEC 785.3
hemoglobin (*see also* Disease, hemoglobin) 282.7
trait - *see* Trait, hemoglobin, abnormal
hemorrhage, uterus - *see* Hemorrhage, uterus
histology NEC 795.4
increase in
appetite 783.6
development 783.9
involuntary movement 781.0
jaw closure 524.51
karyotype 795.2
knee jerk 796.1
labor NEC 661.9 [5th]
affecting fetus or newborn 763.7
laboratory findings - *see* Findings, abnormal
length, organ or site, congenital - *see* Distortion
liver function test 790.6
loss of height 781.91
loss of weight 783.21
lung shadow 793.1
mammogram 793.80
calcification 793.89
calculus 793.89
microcalcification 793.81
Mantoux test 795.5
membranes (fetal)
affecting fetus or newborn 762.9
complicating pregnancy 658.8 [5th]
menstruation - *see* Menstruation
metabolism (*see also* condition) 783.9
movement 781.0
disorder NEC 333.90
sleep related, unspecified 780.58
specified NEC 333.99
head 781.0
involuntary 781.0
specified type NEC 333.99
muscle contraction, localized 728.85
myoglobin (Aberdeen) (Annapolis) 289.9
narrowness, eyelid 743.62
optokinetic response 379.57
organs or tissues of pelvis NEC
in pregnancy or childbirth 654.9 [5th]
affecting fetus or newborn 763.89
causing obstructed labor 660.2 [5th]
affecting fetus or newborn 763.1
origin - *see* Malposition, congenital
palmar creases 757.2
Papanicolaou (smear)
anus 796.70
with
atypical squamous cells
cannot exclude high grade squamous intraepithelial lesion (ASC-H) 796.72
of undetermined significance (ASC-US) 796.71
cytologic evidence of malignancy 796.76
high grade squamous intraepithelial lesion (HGSIL) 796.74
low grade squamous intraepithelial lesion (LGSIL) 796.73
glandular 796.70

Abortion – *continued*
- induced – *continued*
  - medical indications - *see* Abortion, legal
  - therapeutic - *see* Abortion, legal
- late - *see* Abortion, spontaneous
- legal (legal indication) (medical indication) (under medical supervision) 635.9 5th
  - with
    - damage to pelvic organ (laceration) (rupture) (tear) 635.2 5th
    - embolism (air) (amniotic fluid) (blood clot) (pulmonary) (pyemic) (septic) (soap) 635.6 5th
    - genital tract and pelvic infection 635.0 5th
    - hemorrhage, delayed or excessive 635.1 5th
    - metabolic disorder 635.4 5th
    - renal failure (acute) 635.3 5th
    - sepsis (genital tract) (pelvic organ) 635.0 5th
      - urinary tract 635.7 5th
    - shock (postoperative) (septic) 635.5 5th
    - specified complication NEC 635.7 5th
    - toxemia 635.3 5th
    - unspecified complication(s) 635.8 5th
    - urinary tract infection 635.7 5th
  - fetus 779.6
- medical indication - *see* Abortion, legal
- mental hygiene problem - *see* Abortion, legal
- missed 632
- operative - *see* Abortion, legal
- psychiatric indication - *see* Abortion, legal
- recurrent - *see* Abortion, spontaneous
- self-induced - *see* Abortion, illegal
- septic - *see* Abortion, by type, with sepsis
- spontaneous 634.9 5th
  - with
    - damage to pelvic organ (laceration) (rupture) (tear) 634.2 5th
    - embolism (air) (amniotic fluid) (blood clot) (pulmonary) (pyemic) (septic) (soap) 634.6 5th
    - genital tract and pelvic infection 634.0 5th
    - hemorrhage, delayed or excessive 634.1 5th
    - metabolic disorder 634.4 5th
    - renal failure 634.3 5th
    - sepsis (genital tract) (pelvic organ) 634.0 5th
      - urinary tract 634.7 5th
    - shock (postoperative) (septic) 634.5 5th
    - specified complication NEC 634.7 5th
    - toxemia 634.3 5th
    - unspecified complication(s) 634.8 5th
    - urinary tract infection 634.7 5th
  - fetus 761.8
  - threatened 640.0 5th
    - affecting fetus or newborn 762.1
- surgical - *see* Abortion, legal
- therapeutic - *see* Abortion, legal
- threatened 640.0 5th
  - affecting fetus or newborn 762.1
- tubal - *see* Pregnancy, tubal
- voluntary - *see* Abortion, legal

Abortus fever 023.9

Aboulomania 301.6

Abrachia 755.20

Abrachiatism 755.20

Abrachiocephalia 759.89

Abrachiocephalus 759.89

Abrami's disease (acquired hemolytic jaundice) 283.9

Abramov-Fiedler myocarditis (acute isolated myocarditis) 422.91

Abrasion - *see also* Injury, superficial, by site
- cornea 918.1
- dental 521.20
  - extending into
    - dentine 521.22
    - pulp 521.23
  - generalized 521.25
  - limited to enamel 521.21
  - localized 521.24
- teeth, tooth (dentifrice) (habitual) (hard tissues) (occupational) (ritual) (traditional) (wedge defect) (*see also* Abrasion, dental) 521.20

Abrikossov's tumor (M9580/0) - *see also* Neoplasm, connective tissue, benign
- malignant (M9580/3) - *see* Neoplasm, connective tissue, malignant

Abrism 988.8

Abruption, placenta - *see* Placenta, abruptio

Abruptio placentae - *see* Placenta, abruptio

Abscess (acute) (chronic) (infectional) (lymphangitic) (metastatic) (multiple) (pyogenic) (septic) (with lymphangitis) (*see also* Cellulitis) 682.9
- abdomen, abdominal
  - cavity 567.22
  - wall 682.2
- abdominopelvic 567.22
- accessory sinus (chronic) (*see also* Sinusitis) 473.9
- adrenal (capsule) (gland) 255.8
- alveolar 522.5
  - with sinus 522.7
- amebic 006.3
  - bladder 006.8
  - brain (with liver or lung abscess) 006.5
  - liver (without mention of brain or lung abscess) 006.3
    - with
      - brain abscess (and lung abscess) 006.5
      - lung abscess 006.4
  - lung (with liver abscess) 006.4
    - with brain abscess 006.5
  - seminal vesicle 006.8
  - specified site NEC 006.8
  - spleen 006.8
- anaerobic 040.0
- ankle 682.6
- anorectal 566
- antecubital space 682.3
- antrum (chronic) (Highmore) (*see also* Sinusitis, maxillary) 473.0
- anus 566
- apical (tooth) 522.5
  - with sinus (alveolar) 522.7
- appendix 540.1
- areola (acute) (chronic) (nonpuerperal) 611.0
  - puerperal, postpartum 675.1 5th
- arm (any part, above wrist) 682.3
- artery (wall) 447.2
- atheromatous 447.2
- auditory canal (external) 380.10
- auricle (ear) (staphylococcal) (streptococcal) 380.10
- axilla, axillary (region) 682.3
  - lymph gland or node 683
- back (any part) 682.2
- Bartholin's gland 616.3
  - with
    - abortion - *see* Abortion, by type, with sepsis
    - ectopic pregnancy (*see also* categories 633.0-633.9) 639.0
    - molar pregnancy (*see also* categories 630-632) 639.0
  - complicating pregnancy or puerperium 646.6 5th

Abscess – *continued*
- Bartholin's gland – *continued*
  - following
    - abortion 639.0
    - ectopic or molar pregnancy 639.0
- bartholinian 616.3
- Bezold's 383.01
- bile, biliary, duct or tract (*see also* Cholecystitis) 576.8
- bilharziasis 120.1
- bladder (wall) 595.89
  - amebic 006.8
- bone (subperiosteal) (*see also* Osteomyelitis) 730.0 5th
  - accessory sinus (chronic) (*see also* Sinusitis) 473.9
  - acute 730.0 5th
  - chronic or old 730.1 5th
  - jaw (lower) (upper) 526.4
  - mastoid - *see* Mastoiditis, acute
  - petrous (*see also* Petrositis) 383.20
  - spinal (tuberculous) (*see also* Tuberculosis) 015.0 5th *[730.88]*
    - nontuberculous 730.08
- bowel 569.5
- brain (any part) 324.0
  - amebic (with liver or lung abscess) 006.5
  - cystic 324.0
  - late effect - *see* category 326
  - otogenic 324.0
  - tuberculous (*see also* Tuberculosis) 013.3 5th
- breast (acute) (chronic) (nonpuerperal) 611.0
  - newborn 771.5
  - puerperal, postpartum 675.1 5th
  - tuberculous (*see also* Tuberculosis) 017.9 5th
- broad ligament (chronic) (*see also* Disease, pelvis, inflammatory) 614.4
  - acute 614.3
- Brodie's (chronic) (localized) (*see also* Osteomyelitis) 730.1 5th
- bronchus 519.19
- buccal cavity 528.3
- bulbourethral gland 597.0
- bursa 727.89
  - pharyngeal 478.29
- buttock 682.5
- canaliculus, breast 611.0
- canthus 372.20
- cartilage 733.99
- cecum 569.5
  - with appendicitis 540.1
- cerebellum, cerebellar 324.0
  - late effect - *see* category 326
- cerebral (embolic) 324.0
  - late effect - *see* category 326
- cervical (neck region) 682.1
  - lymph gland or node 683
  - stump (*see also* Cervicitis) 616.0
- cervix (stump) (uteri) (*see also* Cervicitis) 616.0
- cheek, external 682.0
  - inner 528.3
- chest 510.9
  - with fistula 510.0
  - wall 682.2
- chin 682.0
- choroid 363.00
- ciliary body 364.3
- circumtonsillar 475
- cold (tuberculous) - *see also* Tuberculosis, abscess
  - articular - *see* Tuberculosis, joint
- colon (wall) 569.5
- colostomy or enterostomy 569.61
- conjunctiva 372.00
- connective tissue NEC 682.9
- cornea 370.55
  - with ulcer 370.00
- corpus
  - cavernosum 607.2

Abscess – *continued*
- corpus – *continued*
  - luteum (*see also* Salpingo-oophoritis) 614.2
- Cowper's gland 597.0
- cranium 324.0
- cul-de-sac (Douglas') (posterior) (*see also* Disease, pelvis, inflammatory) 614.4
  - acute 614.3
- dental 522.5
  - with sinus (alveolar) 522.7
- dentoalveolar 522.5
  - with sinus (alveolar) 522.7
- diaphragm, diaphragmatic 567.22
- digit NEC 681.9
- Douglas' cul-de-sac or pouch (*see also* Disease, pelvis, inflammatory) 614.4
  - acute 614.3
- Dubois' 090.5
- ductless gland 259.8
- ear
  - acute 382.00
  - external 380.10
  - inner 386.30
  - middle - *see* Otitis media
- elbow 682.3
- endamebic - *see* Abscess, amebic
- entamebic - *see* Abscess, amebic
- enterostomy 569.61
- epididymis 604.0
- epidural 324.9
  - brain 324.0
  - late effect - *see* category 326
  - spinal cord 324.1
- epiglottis 478.79
- epiploon, epiploic 567.22
- erysipelatous (*see also* Erysipelas) 035
- esophagostomy 530.86
- esophagus 530.19
- ethmoid (bone) (chronic) (sinus) (*see also* Sinusitis, ethmoidal) 473.2
- external auditory canal 380.10
- extradural 324.9
  - brain 324.0
  - late effect - *see* category 326
  - spinal cord 324.1
- extraperitoneal - *see* Abscess, peritoneum
- eye 360.00
- eyelid 373.13
- face (any part, except eye) 682.0
- fallopian tube (*see also* Salpingo-oophoritis) 614.2
- fascia 728.89
- fauces 478.29
- fecal 569.5
- femoral (region) 682.6
- filaria, filarial (*see also* Infestation, filarial) 125.9
- finger (any) (intrathecal) (periosteal) (subcutaneous) (subcuticular) 681.00
- fistulous NEC 682.9
- flank 682.2
- foot (except toe) 682.7
- forearm 682.3
- forehead 682.0
- frontal (sinus) (chronic) (*see also* Sinusitis, frontal) 473.1
- gallbladder (*see also* Cholecystitis, acute) 575.0
- gastric 535.0 5th
- genital organ or tract NEC
  - female 616.9
    - with
      - abortion - *see* Abortion, by type, with sepsis
      - ectopic pregnancy (*see also* categories 633.0-633.9) 639.0
      - molar pregnancy (*see also* categories 630-632) 639.0

- Abscess – *continued*
  - genital organ or tract NEC – *continued*
    - female – *continued*
      - following
        - abortion 639.0
        - ectopic or molar pregnancy 639.0
      - puerperal, postpartum, childbirth 670.8 5th ▲
    - male 608.4
  - genitourinary system, tuberculous (*see also* Tuberculosis) 016.9 5th
  - gingival 523.30
  - gland, glandular (lymph) (acute) NEC 683
  - glottis 478.79
  - gluteal (region) 682.5
  - gonorrheal NEC (*see also* Gonococcus) 098.0
  - groin 682.2
  - gum 523.30
  - hand (except finger or thumb) 682.4
  - head (except face) 682.8
  - heart 429.89
  - heel 682.7
  - helminthic (*see also* Infestation, by specific parasite) 128.9
  - hepatic 572.0
    - amebic (*see also* Abscess, liver, amebic) 006.3
    - duct 576.8
  - hip 682.6
    - tuberculous (active) (*see also* Tuberculosis) 015.1 5th
  - ileocecal 540.1
  - ileostomy (bud) 569.61
  - iliac (region) 682.2
    - fossa 540.1
  - iliopsoas 567.31
    - tuberculous (*see also* Tuberculosis) 015.0 5th *[730.88]*
  - infraclavicular (fossa) 682.3
  - inguinal (region) 682.2
    - lymph gland or node 683
  - intersphincteric (anus) 566
  - intestine, intestinal 569.5
    - rectal 566
  - intra-abdominal (*see also* Abscess, peritoneum) 567.22
    - postoperative 998.59
  - intracranial 324.0
    - late effect - *see* category 326
  - intramammary - *see* Abscess, breast
  - intramastoid (*see also* Mastoiditis, acute) 383.00
  - intraorbital 376.01
  - intraperitoneal 567.22
  - intraspinal 324.1
    - late effect - *see* category 326
  - intratonsillar 475
  - iris 364.3
  - ischiorectal 566
  - jaw (bone) (lower) (upper) 526.4
    - skin 682.0
  - joint (*see also* Arthritis, pyogenic) 711.0 5th
    - vertebral (tuberculous) (*see also* Tuberculosis) 015.0 5th *[730.88]*
      - nontuberculous 724.8
  - kidney 590.2
    - with
      - abortion - *see* Abortion, by type, with urinary tract infection
      - calculus 592.0
      - ectopic pregnancy (*see also* categories 633.0-633.9) 639.8
      - molar pregnancy (*see also* categories 630-632) 639.8
    - complicating pregnancy or puerperium 646.6 5th
      - affecting fetus or newborn 760.1
    - following
      - abortion 639.8
      - ectopic or molar pregnancy 639.8

- Abscess – *continued*
  - knee 682.6
    - joint 711.06
    - tuberculous (active) (*see also* Tuberculosis) 015.2 5th
  - labium (majus) (minus) 616.4
    - complicating pregnancy, childbirth, or puerperium 646.6 5th
  - lacrimal (passages) (sac) (*see also* Dacryocystitis) 375.30
    - caruncle 375.30
    - gland (*see also* Dacryoadenitis) 375.00
  - lacunar 597.0
  - larynx 478.79
  - lateral (alveolar) 522.5
    - with sinus 522.7
  - leg, except foot 682.6
  - lens 360.00
  - lid 373.13
  - lingual 529.0
    - tonsil 475
  - lip 528.5
  - Littre's gland 597.0
  - liver 572.0
    - amebic 006.3
      - with
        - brain abscess (and lung abscess) 006.5
        - lung abscess 006.4
    - due to Entamoeba histolytica 006.3
    - dysenteric (*see also* Abscess, liver, amebic) 006.3
    - pyogenic 572.0
    - tropical (*see also* Abscess, liver, amebic) 006.3
  - loin (region) 682.2
  - lumbar (tuberculous) (*see also* Tuberculosis) 015.0 5th *[730.88]*
    - nontuberculous 682.2
  - lung (miliary) (putrid) 513.0
    - amebic (with liver abscess) 006.4
      - with brain abscess 006.5
  - lymph, lymphatic, gland or node (acute) 683
    - any site, except mesenteric 683
    - mesentery 289.2
  - lymphangitic, acute - *see* Cellulitis
  - malar 526.4
  - mammary gland - *see* Abscess, breast
  - marginal (anus) 566
  - mastoid (process) (*see also* Mastoiditis, acute) 383.00
    - subperiosteal 383.01
  - maxilla, maxillary 526.4
    - molar (tooth) 522.5
      - with sinus 522.7
    - premolar 522.5
    - sinus (chronic) (*see also* Sinusitis, maxillary) 473.0
  - mediastinum 513.1
  - meibomian gland 373.12
  - meninges (*see also* Meningitis) 320.9
  - mesentery, mesenteric 567.22
  - mesosalpinx (*see also* Salpingo-oophoritis) 614.2
  - milk 675.1 5th
  - Monro's (psoriasis) 696.1
  - mons pubis 682.2
  - mouth (floor) 528.3
  - multiple sites NEC 682.9
  - mural 682.2
  - muscle 728.89
    - psoas 567.31
  - myocardium 422.92
  - nabothian (follicle) (*see also* Cervicitis) 616.0
  - nail (chronic) (with lymphangitis) 681.9
    - finger 681.02
    - toe 681.11
  - nasal (fossa) (septum) 478.19
    - sinus (chronic) (*see also* Sinusitis) 473.9
  - nasopharyngeal 478.29
  - nates 682.5

- Abscess – *continued*
  - navel 682.2
    - newborn NEC 771.4
  - neck (region) 682.1
    - lymph gland or node 683
  - nephritic (*see also* Abscess, kidney) 590.2
  - nipple 611.0
    - puerperal, postpartum 675.0 5th
  - nose (septum) 478.19
    - external 682.0
  - omentum 567.22
  - operative wound 998.59
  - orbit, orbital 376.01
  - ossifluent - *see* Abscess, bone
  - ovary, ovarian (corpus luteum) (*see also* Salpingo-oophoritis) 614.2
  - oviduct (*see also* Salpingo-oophoritis) 614.2
  - palate (soft) 528.3
    - hard 526.4
  - palmar (space) 682.4
  - pancreas (duct) 577.0
  - paradontal 523.30
  - parafrenal 607.2
  - parametric, parametrium (chronic) (*see also* Disease, pelvis, inflammatory) 614.4
    - acute 614.3
  - paranephric 590.2
  - parapancreatic 577.0
  - parapharyngeal 478.22
  - pararectal 566
  - parasinus (*see also* Sinusitis) 473.9
  - parauterine (*see also* Disease, pelvis, inflammatory) 614.4
    - acute 614.3
  - paravaginal (*see also* Vaginitis) 616.10
  - parietal region 682.8
  - parodontal 523.30
  - parotid (duct) (gland) 527.3
    - region 528.3
  - parumbilical 682.2
    - newborn 771.4
  - pectoral (region) 682.2
  - pelvirectal 567.22
  - pelvis, pelvic
    - female (chronic) (*see also* Disease, pelvis, inflammatory) 614.4
      - acute 614.3
    - male, peritoneal (cellular tissue) - *see* Abscess, peritoneum
    - tuberculous (*see also* Tuberculosis) 016.9 5th
  - penis 607.2
    - gonococcal (acute) 098.0
      - chronic or duration of 2 months or over 098.2
  - perianal 566
  - periapical 522.5
    - with sinus (alveolar) 522.7
  - periappendiceal 540.1
  - pericardial 420.99
  - pericecal 540.1
  - pericemental 523.30
  - pericholecystic (*see also* Cholecystitis, acute) 575.0
  - pericoronal 523.30
  - peridental 523.30
  - perigastric 535.0 5th
  - perimetric (*see also* Disease, pelvis, inflammatory) 614.4
    - acute 614.3
  - perinephric, perinephritic (*see also* Abscess, kidney) 590.2
  - perineum, perineal (superficial) 682.2
    - deep (with urethral involvement) 597.0
    - urethra 597.0
  - periodontal (parietal) 523.31
    - apical 522.5
  - periosteum, periosteal (*see also* Periostitis) 730.3 5th
    - with osteomyelitis (*see also* Osteomyelitis) 730.2 5th
      - acute or subacute 730.0 5th

- Abscess – *continued*
  - periosteum, periosteal – *continued*
    - with osteomyelitis – *continued*
      - chronic or old 730.1 5th
  - peripleuritic 510.9
    - with fistula 510.0
  - periproctic 566
  - periprostatic 601.2
  - perirectal (staphylococcal) 566
  - perirenal (tissue) (*see also* Abscess, kidney) 590.2
  - perisinuous (nose) (*see also* Sinusitis) 473.9
  - peritoneum, peritoneal (perforated) (ruptured) 567.22
    - with
      - abortion - *see* Abortion, by type, with sepsis
      - appendicitis 540.1
      - ectopic pregnancy (*see also* categories 633.0-633.9) 639.0
      - molar pregnancy (*see also* categories 630-632) 639.0
    - following
      - abortion 639.0
      - ectopic or molar pregnancy 639.0
    - pelvic, female (*see also* Disease, pelvis, inflammatory) 614.4
      - acute 614.3
    - postoperative 998.59
    - puerperal, postpartum, childbirth 670.8 5th ▲
    - tuberculous (*see also* Tuberculosis) 014.0 5th
  - peritonsillar 475
  - perityphlic 540.1
  - periureteral 593.89
  - periurethral 597.0
    - gonococcal (acute) 098.0
      - chronic or duration of 2 months or over 098.2
  - periuterine (*see also* Disease, pelvis, inflammatory) 614.4
    - acute 614.3
  - perivesical 595.89
  - pernicious NEC 682.9
  - petrous bone - *see* Petrositis
  - phagedenic NEC 682.9
    - chancroid 099.0
  - pharynx, pharyngeal (lateral) 478.29
  - phlegmonous NEC 682.9
  - pilonidal 685.0
  - pituitary (gland) 253.8
  - pleura 510.9
    - with fistula 510.0
  - popliteal 682.6
  - postanal 566
  - postcecal 540.1
  - postlaryngeal 478.79
  - postnasal 478.19
  - postpharyngeal 478.24
  - posttonsillar 475
  - posttyphoid 002.0
  - Pott's (*see also* Tuberculosis) 015.0 5th *[730.88]*
  - pouch of Douglas (chronic) (*see also* Disease, pelvis, inflammatory) 614.4
  - premammary - *see* Abscess, breast
  - prepatellar 682.6
  - prostate (*see also* Prostatitis) 601.2
    - gonococcal (acute) 098.12
      - chronic or duration of 2 months or over 098.32
  - psoas 567.31
    - tuberculous (*see also* Tuberculosis) 015.0 5th *[730.88]*
  - pterygopalatine fossa 682.8
  - pubis 682.2
  - puerperal - *see* Puerperal, abscess, by site
  - pulmonary - *see* Abscess, lung
  - pulp, pulpal (dental) 522.0
    - finger 681.01
    - toe 681.10

Abscess – *continued*
- pyemic - *see* septicemia
- pyloric valve 535.0 [5th]
- rectovaginal septum 569.5
- rectovesical 595.89
- rectum 566
- regional NEC 682.9
- renal (*see also* Abscess, kidney) 590.2
- retina 363.00
- retrobulbar 376.01
- retrocecal 567.22
- retrolaryngeal 478.79
- retromammary - *see* Abscess, breast
- retroperineal 682.2
- retroperitoneal 567.38
  - postprocedural 998.59
- retropharyngeal 478.24
  - tuberculous (*see also* Tuberculosis) 012.8 [5th]
- retrorectal 566
- retrouterine (*see also* Disease, pelvis, inflammatory) 614.4
  - acute 614.3
- retrovesical 595.89
- root, tooth 522.5
  - with sinus (alveolar) 522.7
- round ligament (*see also* Disease, pelvis, inflammatory) 614.4
  - acute 614.3
- rupture (spontaneous) NEC 682.9
- sacrum (tuberculous) (*see also* Tuberculosis) 015.0 [5th] *[730.88]*
  - nontuberculous 730.08
- salivary duct or gland 527.3
- scalp (any part) 682.8
- scapular 730.01
- sclera 379.09
- scrofulous (*see also* Tuberculosis) 017.2 [5th]
- scrotum 608.4
- seminal vesicle 608.0
  - amebic 006.8
- septal, dental 522.5
  - with sinus (alveolar) 522.7
- septum (nasal) 478.19
- serous (*see also* Periostitis) 730.3 [5th]
- shoulder 682.3
- side 682.2
- sigmoid 569.5
- sinus (accessory) (chronic) (nasal) (*see also* Sinusitis) 473.9
  - intracranial venous (any) 324.0
    - late effect - *see* category 326
- Skene's duct or gland 597.0
- skin NEC 682.9
  - tuberculous (primary) (*see also* Tuberculosis) 017.0 [5th]
- sloughing NEC 682.9
- specified site NEC 682.8
  - amebic 006.8
- spermatic cord 608.4
- sphenoidal (sinus) (*see also* Sinusitis, sphenoidal) 473.3
- spinal
  - cord (any part) (staphylococcal) 324.1
    - tuberculous (*see also* Tuberculosis) 013.5 [5th]
  - epidural 324.1
- spine (column) (tuberculous) (*see also* Tuberculosis) 015.0 [5th] *[730.88]*
  - nontuberculous 730.08
- spleen 289.59
  - amebic 006.8
- staphylococcal NEC 682.9
- stitch 998.59
- stomach (wall) 535.0 [5th]
- strumous (tuberculous) (*see also* Tuberculosis) 017.2 [5th]
- subarachnoid 324.9
  - brain 324.0
  - cerebral 324.0
  - late effect - *see* category 326
  - spinal cord 324.1
- subareolar - *see also* Abscess, breast
  - puerperal, postpartum 675.1 [5th]

Abscess – *continued*
- subcecal 540.1
- subcutaneous NEC 682.9
- subdiaphragmatic 567.22
- subdorsal 682.2
- subdural 324.9
  - brain 324.0
  - late effect - *see* category 326
  - spinal cord 324.1
- subgaleal 682.8
- subhepatic 567.22
- sublingual 528.3
  - gland 527.3
- submammary - *see* Abscess, breast
- submandibular (region) (space) (triangle) 682.0
  - gland 527.3
- submaxillary (region) 682.0
  - gland 527.3
- submental (pyogenic) 682.0
  - gland 527.3
- subpectoral 682.2
- subperiosteal - *see* Abscess, bone
- subperitoneal 567.22
- subphrenic - *see also* Abscess, peritoneum 567.22
  - postoperative 998.59
- subscapular 682.2
- subungual 681.9
- suburethral 597.0
- sudoriparous 705.89
- suppurative NEC 682.9
- supraclavicular (fossa) 682.3
- suprahepatic 567.22
- suprapelvic (*see also* Disease, pelvis, inflammatory) 614.4
  - acute 614.3
- suprapubic 682.2
- suprarenal (capsule) (gland) 255.8
- sweat gland 705.89
- syphilitic 095.8
- teeth, tooth (root) 522.5
  - with sinus (alveolar) 522.7
  - supporting structures NEC 523.30
- temple 682.0
- temporal region 682.0
- temporosphenoidal 324.0
  - late effect - *see* category 326
- tendon (sheath) 727.89
- testicle - *see* Orchitis
- thecal 728.89
- thigh (acquired) 682.6
- thorax 510.9
  - with fistula 510.0
- throat 478.29
- thumb (intrathecal) (periosteal) (subcutaneous) (subcuticular) 681.00
- thymus (gland) 254.1
- thyroid (gland) 245.0
- toe (any) (intrathecal) (periosteal) (subcutaneous) (subcuticular) 681.10
- tongue (staphylococcal) 529.0
- tonsil(s) (lingual) 475
- tonsillopharyngeal 475
- tooth, teeth (root) 522.5
  - with sinus (alveolar) 522.7
  - supporting structure NEC 523.30
- trachea 478.9
- trunk 682.2
- tubal (*see also* Salpingo-oophoritis) 614.2
- tuberculous - *see* Tuberculosis, abscess
- tubo-ovarian (*see also* Salpingo-oophoritis) 614.2
- tunica vaginalis 608.4
- umbilicus NEC 682.2
  - newborn 771.4
- upper arm 682.3
- upper respiratory 478.9
- urachus 682.2
- urethra (gland) 597.0
- urinary 597.0

Abscess – *continued*
- uterus, uterine (wall) (*see also* Endometritis) 615.9
  - ligament (*see also* Disease, pelvis, inflammatory) 614.4
    - acute 614.3
  - neck (*see also* Cervicitis) 616.0
- uvula 528.3
- vagina (wall) (*see also* Vaginitis) 616.10
- vaginorectal (*see also* Vaginitis) 616.10
- vas deferens 608.4
- vermiform appendix 540.1
- vertebra (column) (tuberculous) (*see also* Tuberculosis) 015.0 [5th] *[730.88]*
  - nontuberculous 730.0 [5th]
- vesical 595.89
- vesicouterine pouch (*see also* Disease, pelvis, inflammatory) 614.4
- vitreous (humor) (pneumococcal) 360.04
- vocal cord 478.5
- von Bezold's 383.01
- vulva 616.4
  - complicating pregnancy, childbirth, or puerperium 646.6 [5th]
- vulvovaginal gland (*see also* Vaginitis) 616.3
- web-space 682.4
- wrist 682.4

Absence (organ or part) (complete or partial)
- acoustic nerve 742.8
- adrenal (gland) (congenital) 759.1
  - acquired V45.79
- albumin (blood) 273.8
- alimentary tract (complete) (congenital) (partial) 751.8
  - lower 751.5
  - upper 750.8
- alpha-fucosidase 271.8
- alveolar process (acquired) 525.8
  - congenital 750.26
- anus, anal (canal) (congenital) 751.2
- aorta (congenital) 747.22
- aortic valve (congenital) 746.89
- appendix, congenital 751.2
- arm (acquired) V49.60
  - above elbow V49.66
  - below elbow V49.65
  - congenital (*see also* Deformity, reduction, upper limb) 755.20
    - lower - *see* Absence, forearm, congenital
    - upper (complete) (partial) (with absence of distal elements, incomplete) 755.24
      - with
        - complete absence of distal elements 755.21
        - forearm (incomplete) 755.23
- artery (congenital) (peripheral) NEC (*see also* Anomaly, peripheral vascular system) 747.60
  - brain 747.81
    - cerebral 747.81
    - coronary 746.85
    - pulmonary 747.3
    - umbilical 747.5
- atrial septum 745.69
- auditory canal (congenital) (external) 744.01
- auricle (ear) (with stenosis or atresia of auditory canal), congenital 744.01
- bile, biliary duct (common) or passage (congenital) 751.61
- bladder (acquired) V45.74
  - congenital 753.8
- bone (congenital) NEC 756.9
  - marrow 284.9
    - acquired (secondary) 284.89
    - congenital 284.09
    - hereditary 284.09
    - idiopathic 284.9
  - skull 756.0
- bowel sounds 787.5

Absence – *continued*
- brain 740.0
  - specified part 742.2
- breast(s) (acquired) V45.71
  - congenital 757.6
- broad ligament (congenital) 752.19
- bronchus (congenital) 748.3
- calvarium, calvaria (skull) 756.0
- canaliculus lacrimalis, congenital 743.65
- carpal(s) (congenital) (complete) (partial) (with absence of distal elements, incomplete) (*see also* Deformity, reduction, upper limb) 755.28
  - with complete absence of distal elements 755.21
- cartilage 756.9
- caudal spine 756.13
- cecum (acquired) (postoperative) (posttraumatic) V45.72
  - congenital 751.2
- cementum 520.4
- cerebellum (congenital) (vermis) 742.2
- cervix (acquired) (uteri) V88.01
  - with remaining uterus V88.03
  - and uterus V88.01
  - congenital 752.49
- chin, congenital 744.89
- cilia (congenital) 743.63
  - acquired 374.89
- circulatory system, part NEC 747.89
- clavicle 755.51
- clitoris (congenital) 752.49
- coccyx, congenital 756.13
- cold sense (*see also* Disturbance, sensation) 782.0
- colon (acquired) (postoperative) V45.72
  - congenital 751.2
- congenital
  - lumen - *see* Atresia
  - organ or site NEC - *see* Agenesis
  - septum - *see* Imperfect, closure
- corpus callosum (congenital) 742.2
- cricoid cartilage 748.3
- diaphragm (congenital) (with hernia) 756.6
  - with obstruction 756.6
- digestive organ(s) or tract, congenital (complete) (partial) 751.8
  - acquired V45.79
  - lower 751.5
  - upper 750.8
- ductus arteriosus 747.89
- duodenum (acquired) (postoperative) V45.72
  - congenital 751.1
- ear, congenital 744.09
  - acquired V45.79
  - auricle 744.01
  - external 744.01
  - inner 744.05
  - lobe, lobule 744.21
  - middle, except ossicles 744.03
    - ossicles 744.04
  - ossicles 744.04
- ejaculatory duct (congenital) 752.89
- endocrine gland NEC (congenital) 759.2
- epididymis (congenital) 752.89
  - acquired V45.77
- epiglottis, congenital 748.3
- epileptic (atonic) (typical) (*see also* Epilepsy) 345.0 [5th]
- erythrocyte 284.9
- erythropoiesis 284.9
  - congenital 284.01
- esophagus (congenital) 750.3
- Eustachian tube (congenital) 744.24
- extremity (acquired)
  - congenital (*see also* Deformity, reduction) 755.4
  - lower V49.70
  - upper V49.60
- extrinsic muscle, eye 743.69
- eye (acquired) V45.78
  - adnexa (congenital) 743.69

- **Absence** – *continued*
  - eye – *continued*
    - congenital 743.00
    - muscle (congenital) 743.69
  - eyelid (fold), congenital 743.62
    - acquired 374.89
  - face
    - bones NEC 756.0
    - specified part NEC 744.89
  - fallopian tube(s) (acquired) V45.77
    - congenital 752.19
  - femur, congenital (complete) (partial) (with absence of distal elements, incomplete) (*see also* Deformity, reduction, lower limb) 755.34
    - with
      - complete absence of distal elements 755.31
      - tibia and fibula (incomplete) 755.33
  - fibrin 790.92
  - fibrinogen (congenital) 286.3
    - acquired 286.6
  - fibula, congenital (complete) (partial) (with absence of distal elements, incomplete) (*see also* Deformity, reduction, lower limb) 755.37
    - with
      - complete absence of distal elements 755.31
      - tibia 755.35
        - with
          - complete absence of distal elements 755.31
          - femur (incomplete) 755.33
            - with complete absence of distal elements 755.31
  - finger (acquired) V49.62
    - congenital (complete) (partial) (*see also* Deformity, reduction, upper limb) 755.29
      - meaning all fingers (complete) (partial) 755.21
      - transverse 755.21
  - fissures of lungs (congenital) 748.5
  - foot (acquired) V49.73
    - congenital (complete) 755.31
  - forearm (acquired) V49.65
    - congenital (complete) (partial) (with absence of distal elements, incomplete) (*see also* Deformity, reduction, upper limb) 755.25
      - with
        - complete absence of distal elements (hand and fingers) 755.21
        - humerus (incomplete) 755.23
  - fovea centralis 743.55
  - fucosidase 271.8
  - gallbladder (acquired) V45.79
    - congenital 751.69
  - gamma globulin (blood) 279.00
  - genital organs
    - acquired V45.77
    - congenital
      - female 752.89
        - external 752.49
        - internal NEC 752.89
      - male 752.89
        - penis 752.69
  - genitourinary organs, congenital NEC 752.89
  - glottis 748.3
  - gonadal, congenital NEC 758.6
  - hair (congenital) 757.4
    - acquired - *see* Alopecia
  - hand (acquired) V49.63
    - congenital (complete) (*see also* Deformity, reduction, upper limb) 755.21
  - heart (congenital) 759.89
    - acquired - *see* Status, organ replacement

- **Absence** – *continued*
  - heat sense (*see also* Disturbance, sensation) 782.0
  - humerus, congenital (complete) (partial) (with absence of distal elements, incomplete) (*see also* Deformity, reduction, upper limb) 755.24
    - with
      - complete absence of distal elements 755.21
      - radius and ulna (incomplete) 755.23
  - hymen (congenital) 752.49
  - ileum (acquired) (postoperative) (posttraumatic) V45.72
    - congenital 751.1
  - immunoglobulin, isolated NEC 279.03
    - IgA 279.01
    - IgG 279.03
    - IgM 279.02
  - incus (acquired) 385.24
    - congenital 744.04
  - internal ear (congenital) 744.05
  - intestine (acquired) (small) V45.72
    - congenital 751.1
      - large 751.2
    - large V45.72
      - congenital 751.2
  - iris (congenital) 743.45
  - jaw - *see* Absence, mandible
  - jejunum (acquired) V45.72
    - congenital 751.1
  - joint, congenital NEC 755.8
  - kidney(s) (acquired) V45.73
    - congenital 753.0
  - labium (congenital) (majus) (minus) 752.49
  - labyrinth, membranous 744.05
  - lacrimal apparatus (congenital) 743.65
  - larynx (congenital) 748.3
  - leg (acquired) V49.70
    - above knee V49.76
    - below knee V49.75
    - congenital (partial) (unilateral) (*see also* Deformity, reduction, lower limb) 755.31
      - lower (complete) (partial) (with absence of distal elements, incomplete) 755.35
        - with
          - complete absence of distal elements (foot and toes) 755.31
          - thigh (incomplete) 755.33
            - with complete absence of distal elements 755.31
      - upper - *see* Absence, femur
  - lens (congenital) 743.35
    - acquired 379.31
  - ligament, broad (congenital) 752.19
  - limb (acquired)
    - congenital (complete) (partial) (*see also* Deformity, reduction) 755.4
      - lower 755.30
        - complete 755.31
        - incomplete 755.32
        - longitudinal - *see* Deficiency, lower limb, longitudinal
        - transverse 755.31
      - upper 755.20
        - complete 755.21
        - incomplete 755.22
        - longitudinal - *see* Deficiency, upper limb, longitudinal
        - transverse 755.21
    - lower NEC V49.70
    - upper NEC V49.60
  - lip 750.26
  - liver (congenital) (lobe) 751.69
  - lumbar (congenital) (vertebra) 756.13
    - isthmus 756.11
    - pars articularis 756.11
  - lumen - *see* Atresia

- **Absence** – *continued*
  - lung (bilateral) (congenital) (fissure) (lobe) (unilateral) 748.5
    - acquired (any part) V45.76
  - mandible (congenital) 524.09
  - maxilla (congenital) 524.09
  - menstruation 626.0
  - metacarpal(s), congenital (complete) (partial) (with absence of distal elements, incomplete) (*see also* Deformity, reduction, upper limb) 755.28
    - with all fingers, complete 755.21
  - metatarsal(s), congenital (complete) (partial) (with absence of distal elements, incomplete) (*see also* Deformity, reduction, lower limb) 755.38
    - with complete absence of distal elements 755.31
  - muscle (congenital) (pectoral) 756.81
    - ocular 743.69
  - musculoskeletal system (congenital) NEC 756.9
  - nail(s) (congenital) 757.5
  - neck, part 744.89
  - nerve 742.8
  - nervous system, part NEC 742.8
  - neutrophil 288.00
  - nipple (congenital) 757.6
    - acquired V45.71
  - nose (congenital) 748.1
    - acquired 738.0
  - nuclear 742.8
  - ocular muscle (congenital) 743.69
  - organ
    - of Corti (congenital) 744.05
    - or site
      - acquired V45.79
      - congenital NEC 759.89
  - osseous meatus (ear) 744.03
  - ovary (acquired) V45.77
    - congenital 752.0
  - oviduct (acquired) V45.77
    - congenital 752.19
  - pancreas (congenital) 751.7
    - acquired (postoperative) (posttraumatic) V45.79
  - parathyroid gland (congenital) 759.2
  - parotid gland(s) (congenital) 750.21
  - patella, congenital 755.64
  - pelvic girdle (congenital) 755.69
  - penis (congenital) 752.69
    - acquired V45.77
  - pericardium (congenital) 746.89
  - perineal body (congenital) 756.81
  - phalange(s), congenital 755.4
    - lower limb (complete) (intercalary) (partial) (terminal) (*see also* Deformity, reduction, lower limb) 755.39
      - meaning all toes (complete) (partial) 755.31
      - transverse 755.31
    - upper limb (complete) (intercalary) (partial) (terminal) (*see also* Deformity, reduction, upper limb) 755.29
      - meaning all digits (complete) (partial) 755.21
      - transverse 755.21
  - pituitary gland (congenital) 759.2
  - postoperative - *see* Absence, by site, acquired
  - prostate (congenital) 752.89
    - acquired V45.77
  - pulmonary
    - artery 747.3
    - trunk 747.3
    - valve (congenital) 746.01
    - vein 747.49
  - punctum lacrimale (congenital) 743.65

- **Absence** – *continued*
  - radius, congenital (complete) (partial) (with absence of distal elements, incomplete) 755.26
    - with
      - complete absence of distal elements 755.21
      - ulna 755.25
        - with
          - complete absence of distal elements 755.21
          - humerus (incomplete) 755.23
  - ray, congenital 755.4
    - lower limb (complete) (partial) (*see also* Deformity, reduction, lower limb) 755.38
      - meaning all rays 755.31
      - transverse 755.31
    - upper limb (complete) (partial) (*see also* Deformity, reduction, upper limb) 755.28
      - meaning all rays 755.21
      - transverse 755.21
  - rectum (congenital) 751.2
    - acquired V45.79
  - red cell 284.9
    - acquired (secondary) 284.81
    - congenital 284.01
    - hereditary 284.01
    - idiopathic 284.9
  - respiratory organ (congenital) NEC 748.9
  - rib (acquired) 738.3
    - congenital 756.3
  - roof of orbit (congenital) 742.0
  - round ligament (congenital) 752.89
  - sacrum, congenital 756.13
  - salivary gland(s) (congenital) 750.21
  - scapula 755.59
  - scrotum, congenital 752.89
  - seminal tract or duct (congenital) 752.89
    - acquired V45.77
  - septum (congenital) - *see also* Imperfect, closure, septum
    - atrial 745.69
      - and ventricular 745.7
    - between aorta and pulmonary artery 745.0
    - ventricular 745.3
      - and atrial 745.7
  - sex chromosomes 758.81
  - shoulder girdle, congenital (complete) (partial) 755.59
  - skin (congenital) 757.39
  - skull bone 756.0
    - with
      - anencephalus 740.0
      - encephalocele 742.0
      - hydrocephalus 742.3
        - with spina bifida (*see also* Spina bifida) 741.0 **5th**
      - microcephalus 742.1
  - spermatic cord (congenital) 752.89
  - spinal cord 742.59
  - spine, congenital 756.13
  - spleen (congenital) 759.0
    - acquired V45.79
  - sternum, congenital 756.3
  - stomach (acquired) (partial) (postoperative) V45.75
    - with postgastric surgery syndrome 564.2
    - congenital 750.7
  - submaxillary gland(s) (congenital) 750.21
  - superior vena cava (congenital) 747.49
  - tarsal(s), congenital (complete) (partial) (with absence of distal elements, incomplete) (*see also* Deformity, reduction, lower limb) 755.38
  - teeth, tooth (congenital) 520.0
    - with abnormal spacing 524.30
    - acquired 525.10
      - with malocclusion 524.30
      - due to
        - caries 525.13

Absence – *continued*
teeth, tooth – *continued*
acquired – *continued*
due to – *continued*
extraction 525.10
periodontal disease 525.12
trauma 525.11
tendon (congenital) 756.81
testis (congenital) 752.89
acquired V45.77
thigh (acquired) 736.89
thumb (acquired) V49.61
congenital 755.29
thymus gland (congenital) 759.2
thyroid (gland) (surgical) 246.8
with hypothyroidism 244.0
cartilage, congenital 748.3
congenital 243
tibia, congenital (complete) (partial) (with absence of distal elements, incomplete) (*see also* Deformity, reduction, lower limb) 755.36
with
complete absence of distal elements 755.31
fibula 755.35
with
complete absence of distal elements 755.31
femur (incomplete) 755.33
with complete absence of distal elements 755.31
toe (acquired) V49.72
congenital (complete) (partial) 755.39
meaning all toes 755.31
transverse 755.31
great V49.71
tongue (congenital) 750.11
tooth, teeth (congenital) 520.0
with abnormal spacing 524.30
acquired 525.10
with malocclusion 524.30
due to
caries 525.13
extraction 525.10
periodontal disease 525.12
trauma 525.11
trachea (cartilage) (congenital) (rings) 748.3
transverse aortic arch (congenital) 747.21
tricuspid valve 746.1
ulna, congenital (complete) (partial) (with absence of distal elements, incomplete) (*see also* Deformity, reduction, upper limb) 755.27
with
complete absence of distal elements 755.21
radius 755.25
with
complete absence of distal elements 755.21
humerus (incomplete) 755.23
umbilical artery (congenital) 747.5
ureter (congenital) 753.4
acquired V45.74
urethra, congenital 753.8
acquired V45.74
urinary system, part NEC, congenital 753.8
acquired V45.74
uterus (acquired) V88.01
with remaining cervical stump V88.02
and cervix V88.01
congenital 752.3
uvula (congenital) 750.26
vagina, congenital 752.49
acquired V45.77
vas deferens (congenital) 752.89
acquired V45.77

Absence – *continued*
vein (congenital) (peripheral) NEC (*see also* Anomaly, peripheral vascular system) 747.60
brain 747.81
great 747.49
portal 747.49
pulmonary 747.49
vena cava (congenital) (inferior) (superior) 747.49
ventral horn cell 742.59
ventricular septum 745.3
vermis of cerebellum 742.2
vertebra, congenital 756.13
vulva, congenital 752.49
Absentia epileptica (*see also* Epilepsy) 345.0 5th
Absinthemia (*see also* Dependence) 304.6 5th
Absinthism (*see also* Dependence) 304.6 5th
Absorbent system disease 459.89
Absorption
alcohol, through placenta or breast milk 760.71
antibiotics, through placenta or breast milk 760.74
anticonvulsants, through placenta or breast milk 760.77
antifungals, through placenta or breast milk 760.74
anti-infective, through placenta or breast milk 760.74
antimetabolics, through placenta or breast milk 760.78
chemical NEC 989.9
specified chemical or substance - *see* Table of Drugs and Chemicals
through placenta or breast milk (fetus or newborn) 760.70
alcohol 760.71
anticonvulsants 760.77
antifungals 760.74
anti-infective agents 760.74
antimetabolics 760.78
cocaine 760.75
"crack" 760.75
diethylstilbestrol [DES] 760.76
hallucinogenic agents 760.73
medicinal agents NEC 760.79
narcotics 760.72
obstetric anesthetic or analgesic drug 763.5
specified agent NEC 760.79
suspected, affecting management of pregnancy 655.5 5th
cocaine, through placenta or breast milk 760.75
drug NEC (*see also* Reaction, drug)
through placenta or breast milk (fetus or newborn) 760.70
alcohol 760.71
anticonvulsants 760.77
antifungals 760.74
anti-infective agents 760.74
antimetabolics 760.78
cocaine 760.75
"crack" 760.75
diethylstilbestrol (DES) 760.76
hallucinogenic agents 760.73
medicinal agents NEC 760.79
narcotics 760.72
obstetric anesthetic or analgesic drug 763.5
specified agent NEC 760.79
suspected, affecting management of pregnancy 655.5 5th
fat, disturbance 579.8
hallucinogenic agents, through placenta or breast milk 760.73
immune sera, through placenta or breast milk 760.79
lactose defect 271.3
medicinal agents NEC, through placenta or breast milk 760.79

Absorption – *continued*
narcotics, through placenta or breast milk 760.72
noxious substance - *see* Absorption, chemical
protein, disturbance 579.8
pus or septic, general - *see* Septicemia
quinine, through placenta or breast milk 760.74
toxic substance - *see* Absorption, chemical
uremic - *see* Uremia
Abstinence symptoms or syndrome
alcohol 291.81
drug 292.0
neonatal 779.5 ●
Abt-Letterer-Siwe syndrome (acute histiocytosis X) (M9722/3) 202.5 5th
Abulia 799.89
Abulomania 301.6
Abuse
adult 995.80
emotional 995.82
multiple forms 995.85
neglect (nutritional) 995.84
physical 995.81
psychological 995.82
sexual 995.83
alcohol (*see also* Alcoholism) 305.0 5th
dependent 303.9 5th
nondependent 305.0 5th
child 995.50
counseling
perpetrator
non-parent V62.83
parent V61.22
victim V61.21
emotional 995.51
multiple forms 995.59
neglect (nutritional) 995.52
physical 995.54
shaken infant syndrome 995.55
psychological 995.51
sexual 995.53
drugs, nondependent 305.9 5th

Note *Use the following fifth-digit subclassification with the following codes: 305.0, 305.2-305.9:*

0 unspecified
1 continuous
2 episodic
3 in remission

amphetamine type 305.7 5th
antidepressants 305.8 5th
anxiolytic 305.4 5th
barbiturates 305.4 5th
caffeine 305.9 5th
cannabis 305.2 5th
cocaine type 305.6 5th
hallucinogens 305.3 5th
hashish 305.2 5th
hypnotic 305.4 5th
inhalant 305.9 5th
LSD 305.3 5th
marijuana 305.2 5th
mixed 305.9 5th
morphine type 305.5 5th
opioid type 305.5 5th
phencyclidine (PCP) 305.9 5th
sedative 305.4 5th
specified NEC 305.9 5th
tranquilizers 305.4 5th
spouse 995.80
tobacco 305.1
Acalcerosis 275.40
Acalcicosis 275.40
Acalculia 784.69
developmental 315.1
Acanthocheilonemiasis 125.4
Acanthocytosis 272.5
Acanthokeratodermia 701.1
Acantholysis 701.8
bullosa 757.39

Acanthoma (benign) (M8070/0) - *see also* Neoplasm, by site, benign
malignant (M8070/3) - *see* Neoplasm, by site, malignant
Acanthosis (acquired) (nigricans) 701.2
adult 701.2
benign (congenital) 757.39
congenital 757.39
glycogenic
esophagus 530.89
juvenile 701.2
tongue 529.8
Acanthrocytosis 272.5
Acapnia 276.3
Acarbia 276.2
Acardia 759.89
Acardiacus amorphus 759.89
Acardiotrophia 429.1
Acardius 759.89
Acariasis 133.9
sarcoptic 133.0
Acaridiasis 133.9
Acarinosis 133.9
Acariosis 133.9
Acarodermatitis 133.9
urticarioides 133.9
Acarophobia 300.29
Acatalasemia 277.89
Acatalasia 277.89
Acatamathesia 784.69
Acataphasia 784.59 ▲
Acathisia 781.0
due to drugs 333.99
Acceleration, accelerated
atrioventricular conduction 426.7
idioventricular rhythm 427.89
Accessory (congenital)
adrenal gland 759.1
anus 751.5
appendix 751.5
atrioventricular conduction 426.7
auditory ossicles 744.04
auricle (ear) 744.1
autosome(s) NEC 758.5
21 or 22 758.0
biliary duct or passage 751.69
bladder 753.8
blood vessels (peripheral) (congenital) NEC (*see also* Anomaly, peripheral vascular system) 747.60
cerebral 747.81
coronary 746.85
bone NEC 756.9
foot 755.67
breast tissue, axilla 757.6
carpal bones 755.56
cecum 751.5
cervix 752.49
chromosome(s) NEC 758.5
13-15 758.1
16-18 758.2
21 or 22 758.0
autosome(s) NEC 758.5
D_1 758.1
E_3 758.2
G 758.0
sex 758.81
coronary artery 746.85
cusp(s), heart valve NEC 746.89
pulmonary 746.09
cystic duct 751.69
digits 755.00
ear (auricle) (lobe) 744.1
endocrine gland NEC 759.2
external os 752.49
eyelid 743.62
eye muscle 743.69
face bone(s) 756.0
fallopian tube (fimbria) (ostium) 752.19
fingers 755.01
foreskin 605
frontonasal process 756.0
gallbladder 751.69

Accessory – *continued*
- genital organ(s)
  - female 752.89
    - external 752.49
    - internal NEC 752.89
  - male NEC 752.89
    - penis 752.69
- genitourinary organs NEC 752.89
- heart 746.89
  - valve NEC 746.89
    - pulmonary 746.09
- hepatic ducts 751.69
- hymen 752.49
- intestine (large) (small) 751.5
- kidney 753.3
- lacrimal canal 743.65
- leaflet, heart valve NEC 746.89
  - pulmonary 746.09
- ligament, broad 752.19
- liver (duct) 751.69
- lobule (ear) 744.1
- lung (lobe) 748.69
- muscle 756.82
- navicular of carpus 755.56
- nervous system, part NEC 742.8
- nipple 757.6
- nose 748.1
- organ or site NEC - *see* Anomaly, specified type NEC
- ovary 752.0
- oviduct 752.19
- pancreas 751.7
- parathyroid gland 759.2
- parotid gland (and duct) 750.22
- pituitary gland 759.2
- placental lobe - *see* Placenta, abnormal
- preauricular appendage 744.1
- prepuce 605
- renal arteries (multiple) 747.62
- rib 756.3
  - cervical 756.2
- roots (teeth) 520.2
- salivary gland 750.22
- sesamoids 755.8
- sinus - *see* condition
- skin tags 757.39
- spleen 759.0
- sternum 756.3
- submaxillary gland 750.22
- tarsal bones 755.67
- teeth, tooth 520.1
  - causing crowding 524.31
- tendon 756.89
- thumb 755.01
- thymus gland 759.2
- thyroid gland 759.2
- toes 755.02
- tongue 750.13
- tragus 744.1
- ureter 753.4
- urethra 753.8
- urinary organ or tract NEC 753.8
- uterus 752.2
- vagina 752.49
- valve, heart NEC 746.89
  - pulmonary 746.09
- vertebra 756.19
- vocal cords 748.3
- vulva 752.49

Accident, accidental - *see also* condition
- birth NEC 767.9
- cardiovascular (*see also* Disease, cardiovascular) 429.2
- cerebral (*see also* Disease, cerebrovascular, acute) 434.91
- cerebrovascular (current) (CVA) (*see also* Disease, cerebrovascular, acute) 434.91
  - aborted 434.91
  - embolic 434.11
  - healed or old V12.54
  - hemorrhagic - *see* Hemorrhage, brain
  - impending 435.9
  - ischemic 434.91

Accident, accidental – *continued*
- cerebrovascular – *continued*
  - late effect - *see* Late effect(s) (of) cerebrovascular disease
  - postoperative 997.02
  - thrombotic 434.01
- coronary (*see also* Infarct, myocardium) 410.9 [5th]
- craniovascular (*see also* Disease, cerebrovascular, acute) 436
- during pregnancy, to mother, affecting fetus or newborn 760.5
- heart, cardiac (*see also* Infarct, myocardium) 410.9 [5th]
- intrauterine 779.89
- vascular - *see* Disease, cerebrovascular, acute

Accommodation
- disorder of 367.51
  - drug-induced 367.89
  - toxic 367.89
- insufficiency of 367.4
- paralysis of 367.51
  - hysterical 300.11
- spasm of 367.53

Accouchement - *see* Delivery

Accreta placenta (without hemorrhage) 667.0 [5th]
- with hemorrhage 666.0 [5th]

Accretio cordis (nonrheumatic) 423.1

Accretions on teeth 523.6

Accumulation secretion, prostate 602.8

Acephalia, acephalism, acephaly 740.0

Acephalic 740.0

Acephalobrachia 759.89

Acephalocardia 759.89

Acephalocardius 759.89

Acephalochiria 759.89

Acephalochirus 759.89

Acephalogaster 759.89

Acephalostomus 759.89

Acephalothorax 759.89

Acephalus 740.0

Acetonemia 790.6
- diabetic 250.1 [5th]
  - due to secondary diabetes 249.1 [5th]

Acetonglycosuria 982.8

Acetonuria 791.6

Achalasia 530.0
- cardia 530.0
- digestive organs congenital NEC 751.8
- esophagus 530.0
- pelvirectal 751.3
- psychogenic 306.4
- pylorus 750.5
- sphincteral NEC 564.89

Achard-Thiers syndrome (adrenogenital) 255.2

Ache(s) - *see* Pain

Acheilia 750.26

Acheiria 755.21

Achillobursitis 726.71

Achillodynia 726.71

Achlorhydria, achlorhydric 536.0
- anemia 280.9
- diarrhea 536.0
- neurogenic 536.0
- postvagotomy 564.2
- psychogenic 306.4
- secondary to vagotomy 564.2

Achloroblepsia 368.52

Achloropsia 368.52

Acholia 575.8

Acholuric jaundice (familial) (splenomegalic) (*see also* Spherocytosis) 282.0
- acquired 283.9

Achondroplasia 756.4

Achrestic anemia 281.8

Achroacytosis, lacrimal gland 375.00
- tuberculous (*see also* Tuberculosis) 017.3 [5th]

Achroma, cutis 709.00

Achromate (congenital) 368.54

Achromatopia 368.54

Achromatopsia (congenital) 368.54

Achromia
- congenital 270.2
- parasitica 111.0
- unguium 703.8

Achylia
- gastrica 536.8
  - neurogenic 536.3
  - psychogenic 306.4
- pancreatica 577.1

Achylosis 536.8

Acid
- burn - *see also* Burn, by site
  - from swallowing acid - *see* Burn, internal organs
- deficiency
  - amide nicotinic 265.2
  - amino 270.9
  - ascorbic 267
  - folic 266.2
  - nicotinic (amide) 265.2
  - pantothenic 266.2
- intoxication 276.2
- peptic disease 536.8
- stomach 536.8
  - psychogenic 306.4

Acidemia 276.2
- arginosuccinic 270.6
- fetal
  - affecting management of pregnancy 656.3 [5th]
  - before onset of labor, in liveborn infant 768.2
  - during labor and delivery, in liveborn infant 768.3
  - intrauterine 656.3 [5th]
  - unspecified as to time of onset, in liveborn infant 768.4
- newborn 775.81
- pipecolic 270.7

Acidity, gastric (high) (low) 536.8
- psychogenic 306.4

Acidocytopenia 288.59

Acidocytosis 288.3

Acidopenia 288.59

Acidosis 276.2
- diabetic 250.1 [5th]
  - due to secondary diabetes 249.1 [5th]
- fetal, affecting management of pregnancy 656.8 [5th]
- fetal, affecting newborn 775.81
- kidney tubular 588.89
- lactic 276.2
- metabolic NEC 276.2
  - with respiratory acidosis 276.4
    - of newborn 775.81
  - late, of newborn 775.7
- newborn 775.81
- renal
  - hyperchloremic 588.89
  - tubular (distal) (proximal) 588.89
- respiratory 276.2
  - complicated by
    - metabolic acidosis 276.4
      - of newborn 775.81
    - metabolic alkalosis 276.4

Aciduria 791.9
- arginosuccinic 270.6
- beta-aminoisobutyric (BAIB) 277.2
- glutaric
  - type I 270.7
  - type II (type IIA, IIB, IIC) 277.85
  - type III 277.86
- glycolic 271.8
- methylmalonic 270.3
  - with glycinemia 270.7
- organic 270.9
- orotic (congenital) (hereditary) (pyrimidine deficiency) 281.4

Acladiosis 111.8
- skin 111.8

Aclasis
- diaphyseal 756.4
- tarsoepiphyseal 756.59

Acleistocardia 745.5

Aclusion 524.4

Acmesthesia 782.0

Acne (pustular) (vulgaris) 706.1
- agminata (*see also* Tuberculosis) 017.0 [5th]
- artificialis 706.1
- atrophica 706.0
- cachecticorum (Hebra) 706.1
- conglobata 706.1
- conjunctiva 706.1
- cystic 706.1
- decalvans 704.09
- erythematosa 695.3
- eyelid 706.1
- frontalis 706.0
- indurata 706.1
- keloid 706.1
- lupoid 706.0
- necrotic, necrotica 706.0
  - miliaris 704.8
- neonatal 706.1
- nodular 706.1
- occupational 706.1
- papulosa 706.1
- rodens 706.0
- rosacea 695.3
- scorbutica 267
- scrofulosorum (Bazin) (*see also* Tuberculosis) 017.0 [5th]
- summer 692.72
- tropical 706.1
- varioliformis 706.0

Acneiform drug eruptions 692.3

Acnitis (primary) (*see also* Tuberculosis) 017.0 [5th]

Acomia 704.00

Acontractile bladder 344.61

Aconuresis (*see also* Incontinence) 788.30

Acosta's disease 993.2

Acousma 780.1

Acoustic - *see* condition

Acousticophobia 300.29

Acquired - *see* condition

Acquired immune deficiency syndrome - *see* Human immunodeficiency virus (disease) (illness) (infection)

Acquired immunodeficiency syndrome - *see* Human immunodeficiency virus (disease) (illness) (infection)

Acragnosis 781.99

Acrania 740.0

Acroagnosis 781.99

Acroasphyxia, chronic 443.89

Acrobrachycephaly 756.0

Acrobystiolith 608.89

Acrobystitis 607.2

Acrocephalopolysyndactyly 755.55

Acrocephalosyndactyly 755.55

Acrocephaly 756.0

Acrochondrohyperplasia 759.82

Acrocyanosis 443.89
- newborn 770.83
  - meaning transient blue hands and feet - omit code

Acrodermatitis 686.8
- atrophicans (chronica) 701.8
- continua (Hallopeau) 696.1
- enteropathica 686.8
- Hallopeau's 696.1
- perstans 696.1
- pustulosa continua 696.1
- recalcitrant pustular 696.1

Acrodynia 985.0

Acrodysplasia 755.55

Acrohyperhidrosis (*see also* Hyperhidrosis) 780.8

Acrokeratosis verruciformis 757.39

Acromastitis 611.0

Acromegaly, acromegalia (skin) 253.0

Acromelalgia 443.82

Acromicria, acromikria 756.59

Accessory – Acromicria, acromikria

- **Acronyx** 703.0
- **Acropachy, thyroid** (*see also* Thyrotoxicosis) 242.9 5th
- **Acropachyderma** 757.39
- **Acroparesthesia** 443.89
  - simple (Schultz's type) 443.89
  - vasomotor (Nothnagel's type) 443.89
- **Acropathy thyroid** (*see also* Thyrotoxicosis) 242.9 5th
- **Acrophobia** 300.29
- **Acroposthitis** 607.2
- **Acroscleriasis** (*see also* Scleroderma) 710.1
- **Acroscleroderma** (*see also* Scleroderma) 710.1
- **Acrosclerosis** (*see also* Scleroderma) 710.1
- **Acrosphacelus** 785.4
- **Acrosphenosyndactylia** 755.55
- **Acrospiroma, eccrine** (M8402/0) - *see* Neoplasm, skin, benign
- **Acrostealgia** 732.9
- **Acrosyndactyly** (*see also* Syndactylism) 755.10
- **Acrotrophodynia** 991.4
- **Actinic** - *see also* condition
  - cheilitis (due to sun) 692.72
    - chronic NEC 692.74
    - due to radiation, except from sun 692.82
  - conjunctivitis 370.24
  - dermatitis (due to sun) (*see also* Dermatitis, actinic) 692.70
    - due to
      - roentgen rays or radioactive substance 692.82
      - ultraviolet radiation, except from sun 692.82
        - sun NEC 692.70
  - elastosis solare 692.74
  - granuloma 692.73
  - keratitis 370.24
  - ophthalmia 370.24
  - reticuloid 692.73
- **Actinobacillosis, general** 027.8
- **Actinobacillus**
  - lignieresii 027.8
  - mallei 024
  - muris 026.1
- **Actinocutitis** NEC (*see also* Dermatitis, actinic) 692.70
- **Actinodermatitis** NEC (*see also* Dermatitis, actinic) 692.70
- **Actinomyces**
  - israelii (infection) - *see* Actinomycosis
  - muris-ratti (infection) 026.1
- **Actinomycosis, actinomycotic** 039.9
  - with
    - pneumonia 039.1
  - abdominal 039.2
  - cervicofacial 039.3
  - cutaneous 039.0
  - pulmonary 039.1
  - specified site NEC 039.8
  - thoracic 039.1
- **Actinoneuritis** 357.89
- **Action, heart**
  - disorder 427.9
    - postoperative 997.1
  - irregular 427.9
    - postoperative 997.1
    - psychogenic 306.2
- **Active** - *see* condition
- **Activity decrease, functional** 780.99
- **Acute** - *see also* condition
  - abdomen NEC 789.0 5th
  - gallbladder (*see also* Cholecystitis, acute) 575.0
- **Acyanoblepsia** 368.53
- **Acyanopsia** 368.53
- **Acystia** 753.8
- **Acystinervia** - *see* Neurogenic, bladder
- **Acystineuria** - *see* Neurogenic, bladder
- **Adactylia, adactyly** (congenital) 755.4
  - lower limb (complete) (intercalary) (partial) (terminal) (*see also* Deformity, reduction, lower limb) 755.39
    - meaning all digits (complete) (partial) 755.31
    - transverse (complete) (partial) 755.31
  - upper limb (complete) (intercalary) (partial) (terminal) (*see also* Deformity, reduction, upper limb) 755.29
    - meaning all digits (complete) (partial) 755.21
    - transverse (complete) (partial) 755.21
- **Adair-Dighton syndrome** (brittle bones and blue sclera, deafness) 756.51
- **Adamantinoblastoma** (M9310/0) - *see* Ameloblastoma
- **Adamantinoma** (M9310/0) - *see* Ameloblastoma
- **Adamantoblastoma** (M9310/0) - *see* Ameloblastoma
- **Adams-Stokes (-Morgagni) disease or syndrome** (syncope with heart block) 426.9
- **Adaptation reaction** (*see also* Reaction, adjustment) 309.9
- **Addiction** - *see also* Dependence
  - absinthe 304.6 5th
  - alcoholic (ethyl) (methyl) (wood) 303.9 5th
    - complicating pregnancy, childbirth, or puerperium 648.4 5th
      - affecting fetus or newborn 760.71
    - suspected damage to fetus affecting management of pregnancy 655.4 5th
  - drug (*see also* Dependence) 304.9 5th
  - ethyl alcohol 303.9 5th
  - heroin 304.0 5th
  - hospital 301.51
  - methyl alcohol 303.9 5th
  - methylated spirit 303.9 5th
  - morphine (-like substances) 304.0 5th
  - nicotine 305.1
  - opium 304.0 5th
  - tobacco 305.1
  - wine 303.9 5th
- **Addison's**
  - anemia (pernicious) 281.0
  - disease (bronze) (primary adrenal insufficiency) 255.41
    - tuberculous (*see also* Tuberculosis) 017.6 5th
  - keloid (morphea) 701.0
  - melanoderma (adrenal cortical hypofunction) 255.41
- **Addison-Biermer anemia** (pernicious) 281.0
- **Addison-Gull disease** - *see* Xanthoma
- **Addisonian crisis or melanosis** (acute adrenocortical insufficiency) 255.41
- **Additional** - *see also* Accessory
  - chromosome(s) 758.5
    - 13-15 758.1
    - 16-18 758.2
    - 21 758.0
    - autosome(s) NEC 758.5
    - sex 758.81
- **Adduction contracture, hip or other joint** - *see* Contraction, joint
- **ADEM** (acute disseminated encephalomyelitis) (postinfectious) 136.9 *[323.61]*
  - infectious 136.9 *[323.61]*
  - noninfectious 323.81
- **Adenasthenia gastrica** 536.0
- **Aden fever** 061
- **Adenitis** (*see also* Lymphadenitis) 289.3
  - acute, unspecified site 683
    - epidemic infectious 075
  - axillary 289.3
    - acute 683
    - chronic or subacute 289.1

Adenitis – *continued*

  - Bartholin's gland 616.89
  - bulbourethral gland (*see also* Urethritis) 597.89
  - cervical 289.3
    - acute 683
    - chronic or subacute 289.1
  - chancroid (Ducrey's bacillus) 099.0
  - chronic (any lymph node, except mesenteric) 289.1
    - mesenteric 289.2
  - Cowper's gland (*see also* Urethritis) 597.89
  - epidemic, acute 075
  - gangrenous 683
  - gonorrheal NEC 098.89
  - groin 289.3
    - acute 683
    - chronic or subacute 289.1
  - infectious 075
  - inguinal (region) 289.3
    - acute 683
    - chronic or subacute 289.1
  - lymph gland or node, except mesenteric 289.3
    - acute 683
    - chronic or subacute 289.1
    - mesenteric (acute) (chronic) (nonspecific) (subacute) 289.2
  - mesenteric (acute) (chronic) (nonspecific) (subacute) 289.2
    - due to Pasteurella multocida (P. septica) 027.2
  - parotid gland (suppurative) 527.2
  - phlegmonous 683
  - salivary duct or gland (any) (recurring) (suppurative) 527.2
  - scrofulous (*see also* Tuberculosis) 017.2 5th
  - septic 289.3
  - Skene's duct or gland (*see also* Urethritis) 597.89
  - strumous, tuberculous (*see also* Tuberculosis) 017.2 5th
  - subacute, unspecified site 289.1
  - sublingual gland (suppurative) 527.2
  - submandibular gland (suppurative) 527.2
  - submaxillary gland (suppurative) 527.2
  - suppurative 683
  - tuberculous - *see* Tuberculosis, lymph gland
  - urethral gland (*see also* Urethritis) 597.89
  - venereal NEC 099.8
  - Wharton's duct (suppurative) 527.2
- **Adenoacanthoma** (M8570/3) - *see* Neoplasm, by site malignant
- **Adenoameloblastoma** (M9300/0) 213.1
  - upper jaw (bone) 213.0
- **Adenocarcinoma** (M8140/3) - *see also* Neoplasm, by site, malignant

Note *The list of adjectival modifiers below is not exhaustive. A description of adenocarcinoma that does not appear in this list should be coded in the same manner as carcinoma with that description. Thus, "mixed acidophil-basophil adenocarcinoma," should be coded in the same manner as "mixed acidophil-basophil carcinoma," which appears in the list under "Carcinoma."*

Except where otherwise indicated, the morphological varieties of adenocarcinoma in the list below should be coded by site as for "Neoplasm, malignant."

  - with
    - apocrine metaplasia (M8573/3)
    - cartilaginous (and osseous) metaplasia (M8571/3)
    - osseous (and cartilaginous) metaplasia (M8571/3)
    - spindle cell metaplasia (M8572/3)
    - squamous metaplasia (M8570/3)

Adenocarcinoma – *continued*

  - acidophil (M8280/3)
    - specified site - *see* Neoplasm, by site, malignant
    - unspecified site 194.3
  - acinar (M8550/3)
  - acinic cell (M8550/3)
  - adrenal cortical (M8370/3) 194.0
  - alveolar (M8251/3)
    - and
      - epidermoid carcinoma, mixed (M8560/3)
      - squamous cell carcinoma, mixed (M8560/3)
  - apocrine (M8401/3)
    - breast - *see* Neoplasm, breast, malignant
    - specified site NEC - *see* Neoplasm, skin, malignant
    - unspecified site 173.9
  - basophil (M8300/3)
    - specified site - *see* Neoplasm, by site, malignant
    - unspecified site 194.3
  - bile duct type (M8160/3)
    - liver 155.1
    - specified site NEC - *see* Neoplasm, by site, malignant
    - unspecified site 155.1
  - bronchiolar (M8250/3) - *see* Neoplasm, lung, malignant
  - ceruminous (M8420/3) 173.2
  - chromophobe (M8270/3)
    - specified site - *see* Neoplasm, by site, malignant
    - unspecified site 194.3
  - clear cell (mesonephroid type) (M8310/3)
  - colloid (M8480/3)
  - cylindroid type (M8200/3)
  - diffuse type (M8145/3)
    - specified site - *see* Neoplasm, by site, malignant
    - unspecified site 151.9
  - duct (infiltrating) (M8500/3)
    - with Paget's disease (M8541/3) - *see* Neoplasm, breast, malignant
    - specified site - *see* Neoplasm, by site, malignant
    - unspecified site 174.9
  - embryonal (M9070/3)
  - endometrioid (M8380/3) - *see* Neoplasm, by site, malignant
  - eosinophil (M8280/3)
    - specified site - *see* Neoplasm, by site, malignant
    - unspecified site 194.3
  - follicular (M8330/3)
    - and papillary (M8340/3) 193
    - moderately differentiated type (M8332/3) 193
    - pure follicle type (M8331/3) 193
    - specified site - *see* Neoplasm, by site, malignant
    - trabecular type (M8332/3) 193
    - unspecified type 193
    - well differentiated type (M8331/3) 193
  - gelatinous (M8480/3)
  - granular cell (M8320/3)
  - Hürthle cell (M8290/3) 193
  - in
    - adenomatous
      - polyp (M8210/3)
      - polyposis coli (M8220/3) 153.9
    - polypoid adenoma (M8210/3)
    - tubular adenoma (M8210/3)
    - villous adenoma (M8261/3)
  - infiltrating duct (M8500/3)
    - with Paget's disease (M8541/3) - *see* Neoplasm, breast, malignant
    - specified site - *see* Neoplasm, by site, malignant
    - unspecified site 174.9

- **Adenocarcinoma** – *continued*
  - inflammatory (M8530/3)
    - specified site - *see* Neoplasm, by site, malignant
    - unspecified site 174.9
  - in situ (M8140/2) - *see* Neoplasm, by site, in situ
  - intestinal type (M8144/3)
    - specified site - *see* Neoplasm, by site, malignant
    - unspecified site 151.9
  - intraductal (noninfiltrating) (M8500/2)
    - papillary (M8503/2)
      - specified site - *see* Neoplasm, by site, in situ
      - unspecified site 233.0
    - specified site - *see* Neoplasm, by site, in situ
    - unspecified site 233.0
  - islet cell (M8150/3)
    - and exocrine, mixed (M8154/3)
      - specified site - *see* Neoplasm, by site, malignant
      - unspecified site 157.9
    - pancreas 157.4
    - specified site NEC - *see* Neoplasm, by site, malignant
    - unspecified site 157.4
  - lobular (M8520/3)
    - specified site - *see* Neoplasm, by site, malignant
    - unspecified site 174.9
  - medullary (M8510/3)
  - mesonephric (M9110/3)
  - mixed cell (M8323/3)
  - mucinous (M8480/3)
  - mucin-producing (M8481/3)
  - mucoid (M8480/3) - *see also* Neoplasm, by site, malignant
    - cell (M8300/3)
      - specified site - *see* Neoplasm, by site, malignant
      - unspecified site 194.3
  - nonencapsulated sclerosing (M8350/3) 193
  - oncocytic (M8290/3)
  - oxyphilic (M8290/3)
  - papillary (M8260/3)
    - and follicular (M8340/3) 193
    - intraductal (noninfiltrating) (M8503/2)
      - specified site - *see* Neoplasm, by site, in situ
      - unspecified site 233.0
    - serous (M8460/3)
      - specified site - *see* Neoplasm, by site, malignant
      - unspecified site 183.0
  - papillocystic (M8450/3)
    - specified site - *see* Neoplasm, by site, malignant
    - unspecified site 183.0
  - pseudomucinous (M8470/3)
    - specified site - *see* Neoplasm, by site, malignant
    - unspecified site 183.0
  - renal cell (M8312/3) 189.0
  - sebaceous (M8410/3)
  - serous (M8441/3) - *see also* Neoplasm, by site, malignant
    - papillary
      - specified site - *see* Neoplasm, by site, malignant
      - unspecified site 183.0
  - signet ring cell (M8490/3)
  - superficial spreading (M8143/3)
  - sweat gland (M8400/3) - *see* Neoplasm, skin, malignant
  - trabecular (M8190/3)
  - tubular (M8211/3)
  - villous (M8262/3)
  - water-clear cell (M8322/3) 194.1
- **Adenofibroma** (M9013/0)
  - clear cell (M8313/0) - *see* Neoplasm, by site, benign
  - endometrioid (M8381/0) 220
    - borderline malignancy (M8381/1) 236.2
    - malignant (M8381/3) 183.0
  - mucinous (M9015/0)
    - specified site - *see* Neoplasm, by site, benign
    - unspecified site 220
  - prostate 600.20
    - with
      - other lower urinary tract symptoms (LUTS) 600.21
      - urinary
        - obstruction 600.21
        - retention 600.21
  - serous (M9014/0)
    - specified site - *see* Neoplasm, by site, benign
    - unspecified site 220
  - specified site - *see* Neoplasm, by site, benign
  - unspecified site 220
- **Adenofibrosis**
  - breast 610.2
  - endometroid 617.0
- **Adenoiditis** 474.01
  - acute 463
  - chronic 474.01
    - with chronic tonsillitis 474.02
- **Adenoids** (congenital) (of nasal fossa) 474.9
  - hypertrophy 474.12
  - vegetations 474.2
- **Adenolipomatosis** (symmetrical) 272.8
- **Adenolymphoma** (M8561/0)
  - specified site - *see* Neoplasm, by site, benign
  - unspecified 210.2
- **Adenoma** (sessile) (M8140/0) - *see also* Neoplasm, by site, benign

Note *Except where otherwise indicated, the morphological varieties of adenoma in the list below should be coded by site as for "Neoplasm, benign."*

  - acidophil (M8280/0)
    - specified site - *see* Neoplasm, by site, benign
    - unspecified site 227.3
  - acinar (cell) (M8550/0)
  - acinic cell (M8550/0)
  - adrenal (cortex) (cortical) (functioning) (M8370/0) 227.0
    - clear cell type (M8373/0) 227.0
    - compact cell type (M8371/0) 227.0
    - glomerulosa cell type (M8374/0) 227.0
    - heavily pigmented variant (M8372/0) 227.0
    - mixed cell type (M8375/0) 227.0
  - alpha cell (M8152/0)
    - pancreas 211.7
    - specified site NEC - *see* Neoplasm, by site, benign
    - unspecified site 211.7
  - alveolar (M8251/0)
  - apocrine (M8401/0)
    - breast 217
    - specified site NEC - *see* Neoplasm, skin, benign
    - unspecified site 216.9
  - basal cell (M8147/0)
  - basophil (M8300/0)
    - specified site - *see* Neoplasm, by site, benign
    - unspecified site 227.3
  - beta cell (M8151/0)
    - pancreas 211.7
    - specified site NEC - *see* Neoplasm, by site, benign
    - unspecified site 211.7
  - bile duct (M8160/0) 211.5
  - black (M8372/0) 227.0
- **Adenoma** – *continued*
  - bronchial (M8140/1) 235.7
    - carcinoid type (M8240/3) - *see* Neoplasm, lung, malignant
    - cylindroid type (M8200/3) - *see* Neoplasm, lung, malignant
  - ceruminous (M8420/0) 216.2
  - chief cell (M8321/0) 227.1
  - chromophobe (M8270/0)
    - specified site - *see* Neoplasm, by site, benign
    - unspecified site 227.3
  - clear cell (M8310/0)
  - colloid (M8334/0)
    - specified site - *see* Neoplasm, by site, benign
    - unspecified site 226
  - cylindroid type, bronchus (M8200/3) - *see* Neoplasm, lung, malignant
  - duct (M8503/0)
  - embryonal (M8191/0)
  - endocrine, multiple (M8360/1)
    - single specified site - *see* Neoplasm, by site, uncertain behavior
    - two or more specified sites 237.4
    - unspecified site 237.4
  - endometrioid (M8380/0) - *see also* Neoplasm, by site, benign
    - borderline malignancy (M8380/1) - *see* Neoplasm, by site, uncertain behavior
  - eosinophil (M8280/0)
    - specified site - *see* Neoplasm, by site, benign
    - unspecified site 227.3
  - fetal (M8333/0)
    - specified site - *see* Neoplasm, by site, benign
    - unspecified site 226
  - follicular (M8330/0)
    - specified site - *see* Neoplasm, by site, benign
    - unspecified site 226
  - hepatocellular (M8170/0) 211.5
  - Hürthle cell (M8290/0) 226
  - intracystic papillary (M8504/0)
  - islet cell (functioning) (M8150/0)
    - pancreas 211.7
    - specified site NEC - *see* Neoplasm, by site, benign
    - unspecified site 211.7
  - liver cell (M8170/0) 211.5
  - macrofollicular (M8334/0)
    - specified site NEC - *see* Neoplasm, by site, benign
    - unspecified site 226
  - malignant, malignum (M8140/3) - *see* Neoplasm, by site, malignant
  - mesonephric (M9110/0)
  - microfollicular (M8333/0)
    - specified site - *see* Neoplasm, by site, benign
    - unspecified site 226
  - mixed cell (M8323/0)
  - monomorphic (M8146/0)
  - mucinous (M8480/0)
  - mucoid cell (M8300/0)
    - specified site - *see* Neoplasm, by site, benign
    - unspecified site 227.3
  - multiple endocrine (M8360/1)
    - single specified site - *see* Neoplasm, by site, uncertain behavior
    - two or more specified sites 237.4
    - unspecified site 237.4
  - nipple (M8506/0) 217
  - oncocytic (M8290/0)
  - oxyphilic (M8290/0)
  - papillary (M8260/0) - *see also* Neoplasm, by site, benign
    - intracystic (M8504/0)
  - papillotubular (M8263/0)
- **Adenoma** – *continued*
  - Pick's tubular (M8640/0)
    - specified site - *see* Neoplasm, by site, benign
    - unspecified site
      - female 220
      - male 222.0
  - pleomorphic (M8940/0)
  - polypoid (M8210/0)
  - prostate (benign) 600.20
    - with
      - other lower urinary tract symptoms (LUTS) 600.21
      - urinary
        - obstruction 600.21
        - retention 600.21
  - rete cell 222.0
  - sebaceous, sebaceum (gland) (senile) (M8410/0) - *see also* Neoplasm, skin, benign
    - disseminata 759.5
  - Sertoli cell (M8640/0)
    - specified site - *see* Neoplasm, by site, benign
    - unspecified site
      - female 220
      - male 222.0
  - skin appendage (M8390/0) - *see* Neoplasm, skin, benign
  - sudoriferous gland (M8400/0) - *see* Neoplasm, skin, benign
  - sweat gland or duct (M8400/0) - *see* Neoplasm, skin, benign
  - testicular (M8640/0)
    - specified site - *see* Neoplasm, by site, benign
    - unspecified site
      - female 220
      - male 222.0
  - thyroid 226
  - trabecular (M8190/0)
  - tubular (M8211/0) - *see also* Neoplasm, by site, benign
    - papillary (M8460/3)
    - Pick's (M8640/0)
      - specified site - *see* Neoplasm, by site, benign
      - unspecified site
        - female 220
        - male 222.0
  - tubulovillous (M8263/0)
  - villoglandular (M8263/0)
  - villous (M8261/1) - *see* Neoplasm, by site, uncertain behavior
  - water-clear cell (M8322/0) 227.1
  - wolffian duct (M9110/0)
- **Adenomatosis** (M8220/0)
  - endocrine (multiple) (M8360/1)
    - single specified site - *see* Neoplasm, by site, uncertain behavior
    - two or more specified sites 237.4
    - unspecified site 237.4
  - erosive of nipple (M8506/0) 217
  - pluriendocrine - *see* Adenomatosis, endocrine
  - pulmonary (M8250/1) 235.7
    - malignant (M8250/3) - *see* Neoplasm, lung, malignant
  - specified site - *see* Neoplasm, by site, benign
  - unspecified site 211.3
- **Adenomatous**
  - cyst, thyroid (gland) - *see* Goiter, nodular
  - goiter (nontoxic) (*see also* Goiter, nodular) 241.9
    - toxic or with hyperthyroidism 242.3 5th
- **Adenomyoma** (M8932/0) - *see also* Neoplasm, by site, benign
  - prostate 600.20
    - with
      - other lower urinary tract symptoms (LUTS) 600.21
      - urinary
        - obstruction 600.21
        - retention 600.21

Adenomyometritis 617.0
Adenomyosis (uterus) (internal) 617.0
Adenopathy (lymph gland) 785.6
- inguinal 785.6
- mediastinal 785.6
- mesentery 785.6
- syphilitic (secondary) 091.4
- tracheobronchial 785.6
  - tuberculous (*see also* Tuberculosis) 012.1 [5th]
    - primary, progressive 010.8 [5th]
- tuberculous (*see also* Tuberculosis, lymph gland) 017.2 [5th]
  - tracheobronchial 012.1 [5th]
    - primary, progressive 010.8 [5th]

Adenopharyngitis 462
Adenophlegmon 683
Adenosalpingitis 614.1
Adenosarcoma (M8960/3) 189.0
Adenosclerosis 289.3
Adenosis
- breast (sclerosing) 610.2
- vagina, congenital 752.49

Adentia (complete) (partial) (*see also* Absence, teeth) 520.0
Adherent
- labium (minus) 624.4
- pericardium (nonrheumatic) 423.1
  - rheumatic 393
- placenta 667.0 [5th]
  - with hemorrhage 666.0 [5th]
- prepuce 605
- scar (skin) NEC 709.2
- tendon in scar 709.2

Adhesion(s), adhesive (postinfectional) (postoperative)
- abdominal (wall) (*see also* Adhesions, peritoneum) 568.0
- amnion to fetus 658.8 [5th]
  - affecting fetus or newborn 762.8
- appendix 543.9
- arachnoiditis - *see* Meningitis
- auditory tube (Eustachian) 381.89
- bands - *see also* Adhesions, peritoneum
  - cervix 622.3
  - uterus 621.5
- bile duct (any) 576.8
- bladder (sphincter) 596.8
- bowel (*see also* Adhesions, peritoneum) 568.0
- cardiac 423.1
  - rheumatic 398.99
- cecum (*see also* Adhesions, peritoneum) 568.0
- cervicovaginal 622.3
  - congenital 752.49
  - postpartal 674.8 [5th]
    - old 622.3
- cervix 622.3
- clitoris 624.4
- colon (*see also* Adhesions, peritoneum) 568.0
- common duct 576.8
- congenital - *see also* Anomaly, specified type NEC
  - fingers (*see also* Syndactylism, fingers) 755.11
  - labium (majus) (minus) 752.49
  - omental, anomalous 751.4
  - ovary 752.0
  - peritoneal 751.4
  - toes (*see also* Syndactylism, toes) 755.13
  - tongue (to gum or roof of mouth) 750.12
- conjunctiva (acquired) (localized) 372.62
  - congenital 743.63
  - extensive 372.63
- cornea - *see* Opacity, cornea
- cystic duct 575.8
- diaphragm (*see also* Adhesions, peritoneum) 568.0
- due to foreign body - *see* Foreign body

Adhesion(s), adhesive – *continued*
- duodenum (*see also* Adhesions, peritoneum) 568.0
  - with obstruction 537.3
- ear, middle - *see* Adhesions, middle ear
- epididymis 608.89
- epidural - *see* Adhesions, meninges
- epiglottis 478.79
- Eustachian tube 381.89
- eyelid 374.46
  - postoperative 997.99
    - surgically created V45.69
- gallbladder (*see also* Disease, gallbladder) 575.8
- globe 360.89
- heart 423.1
  - rheumatic 398.99
- ileocecal (coil) (*see also* Adhesions, peritoneum) 568.0
- ileum (*see also* Adhesions, peritoneum) 568.0
- intestine (postoperative) (*see also* Adhesions, peritoneum) 568.0
  - with obstruction 560.81
    - with hernia - *see also* Hernia, by site, with obstruction
      - gangrenous - *see* Hernia, by site, with gangrene
- intra-abdominal (*see also* Adhesions, peritoneum) 568.0
- iris 364.70
  - to corneal graft 996.79
- joint (*see also* Ankylosis) 718.5 [5th]
- kidney 593.89
- labium (majus) (minus), congenital 752.49
- liver 572.8
- lung 511.0
- mediastinum 519.3
- meninges 349.2
  - cerebral (any) 349.2
    - congenital 742.4
  - congenital 742.8
  - spinal (any) 349.2
    - congenital 742.59
  - tuberculous (cerebral) (spinal) (*see also* Tuberculosis, meninges) 013.0 [5th]
- mesenteric (*see also* Adhesions, peritoneum) 568.0
- middle ear (fibrous) 385.10
  - drum head 385.19
    - to
      - incus 385.11
      - promontorium 385.13
      - stapes 385.12
    - specified NEC 385.19
- nasal (septum) (to turbinates) 478.19
- nerve NEC 355.9
  - spinal 355.9
    - root 724.9
      - cervical NEC 723.4
      - lumbar NEC 724.4
      - lumbosacral 724.4
      - thoracic 724.4
- ocular muscle 378.60
- omentum (*see also* Adhesions, peritoneum) 568.0
- organ or site, congenital NEC - *see* Anomaly, specified type NEC
- ovary 614.6
  - congenital (to cecum, kidney, or omentum) 752.0
- parauterine 614.6
- parovarian 614.6
- pelvic (peritoneal)
  - female (postoperative) (postinfection) 614.6
  - male (postoperative) (postinfection) (*see also* Adhesions, peritoneum) 568.0
  - postpartal (old) 614.6
  - tuberculous (*see also* Tuberculosis) 016.9 [5th]

Adhesion(s), adhesive – *continued*
- penis to scrotum (congenital) 752.69
- periappendiceal (*see also* Adhesions, peritoneum) 568.0
- pericardium (nonrheumatic) 423.1
  - rheumatic 393
  - tuberculous (*see also* Tuberculosis) 017.9 [5th] *[420.0]*
- pericholecystic 575.8
- perigastric (*see also* Adhesions, peritoneum) 568.0
- periovarian 614.6
- periprostatic 602.8
- perirectal (*see also* Adhesions, peritoneum) 568.0
- perirenal 593.89
- peritoneum, peritoneal (fibrous) (postoperative) 568.0
  - with obstruction (intestinal) 560.81
    - with hernia - *see also* Hernia, by site, with obstruction
      - gangrenous - *see* Hernia, by site, with gangrene
  - duodenum 537.3
  - congenital 751.4
  - female (postoperative) (postinfective) 614.6
  - pelvic, female 614.6
  - pelvic, male 568.0
  - postpartal, pelvic 614.6
  - to uterus 614.6
- peritubal 614.6
- periureteral 593.89
- periuterine 621.5
- perivesical 596.8
- perivesicular (seminal vesicle) 608.89
- pleura, pleuritic 511.0
  - tuberculous (*see also* Tuberculosis, pleura) 012.0 [5th]
- pleuropericardial 511.0
- postoperative (gastrointestinal tract) (*see also* Adhesions, peritoneum)
  - pelvic female 614.9
  - pelvic, male 568.0
  - eyelid 997.99
    - surgically created V45.69
  - urethra 598.2
- postpartal, old 624.4
- preputial, prepuce 605
- pulmonary 511.0
- pylorus (*see also* Adhesions, peritoneum) 568.0
- Rosenmüller's fossa 478.29
- sciatic nerve 355.0
- seminal vesicle 608.89
- shoulder (joint) 726.0
- sigmoid flexure (*see also* Adhesions, peritoneum) 568.0
- spermatic cord (acquired) 608.89
  - congenital 752.89
- spinal canal 349.2
  - nerve 355.9
    - root 724.9
      - cervical NEC 723.4
      - lumbar NEC 724.4
      - lumbosacral 724.4
      - thoracic 724.4
- stomach (*see also* Adhesions, peritoneum) 568.0
- subscapular 726.2
- tendonitis 726.90
  - shoulder 726.0
- testicle 608.89
- tongue (congenital) (to gum or roof of mouth) 750.12
  - acquired 529.8
- trachea 519.19
- tubo-ovarian 614.6
- tunica vaginalis 608.89
- ureter 593.89

Adhesion(s), adhesive – *continued*
- uterus 621.5
  - to abdominal wall 614.6
    - in pregnancy or childbirth 654.4 [5th]
      - affecting fetus or newborn 763.89
- vagina (chronic) (postoperative) (postradiation) 623.2
- vaginitis (congenital) 752.49
- vesical 596.8
- vitreous 379.29

Adie (-Holmes) syndrome (tonic pupillary reaction) 379.46
Adiponecrosis neonatorum 778.1
Adiposa dolorosa 272.8
Adiposalgia 272.8
Adiposis
- cerebralis 253.8
- dolorosa 272.8
- tuberosa simplex 272.8

Adiposity 278.02
- heart (*see also* Degeneration, myocardial) 429.1
- localized 278.1

Adiposogenital dystrophy 253.8
Adjustment
- prosthesis or other device - *see* Fitting of
- reaction - *see* Reaction, adjustment

Administration, prophylactic
- antibiotics V07.39
- antitoxin, any V07.2
- antivenin V07.2
- chemotherapeutic agent NEC V07.39
- chemotherapy NEC V07.39
- diphtheria antitoxin V07.2
- fluoride V07.31
- gamma globulin V07.2
- immune sera (gamma globulin) V07.2
- passive immunization agent V07.2
- RhoGAM V07.2

Admission (encounter)
- as organ donor - *see* Donor
- by mistake V68.9
- for
  - adequacy testing (for)
    - hemodialysis V56.31
    - peritoneal dialysis V56.32
  - adjustment (of)
    - artificial
      - arm (complete) (partial) V52.0
      - eye V52.2
      - leg (complete) (partial) V52.1
    - brain neuropacemaker V53.02
    - breast
      - implant V52.4
        - exchange (different material) (different size) V52.4
      - prosthesis V52.4
    - cardiac device V53.39
      - defibrillator, automatic implantable V53.32
      - pacemaker V53.31
        - carotid sinus V53.39
    - catheter
      - non-vascular V58.82
      - vascular V58.81
    - cerebral ventricle (communicating) shunt V53.01
    - colostomy belt V55.3
    - contact lenses V53.1
    - cystostomy device V53.6
    - dental prosthesis V52.3
    - device, unspecified type V53.90
      - abdominal V53.59 ▲
      - cardiac V53.39
        - defibrillator, automatic implantable V53.32
        - pacemaker V53.31
      - carotid sinus V53.39
      - cerebral ventricle (communicating) shunt V53.01
      - gastrointestinal NEC V53.59 ●
      - insulin pump V53.91

- **Admission** - *continued*
  - for - *continued*
    - adjustment (of) - *continued*
      - device, unspecified type - *continued*
        - intestinal V53.50 ●
        - intrauterine contraceptive V25.1
        - nervous system V53.09
        - orthodontic V53.4
        - other device V53.99
        - prosthetic V52.9
          - breast V52.4
          - dental V52.3
          - eye V52.2
          - specified type NEC V52.8
        - special senses V53.09
        - substitution
          - auditory V53.09
          - nervous system V53.09
          - visual V53.09
        - urinary V53.6
      - dialysis catheter
        - extracorporeal V56.1
        - peritoneal V56.2
      - diaphragm (contraceptive) V25.02
      - gastric lap band V53.51 ●
      - gastrointestinal appliance and device NEC V53.59 ●
      - growth rod V54.02
      - hearing aid V53.2
      - ileostomy device V55.2
      - intestinal appliance and ~~or~~ device ~~NEC~~ V53.50 ▲
      - intrauterine contraceptive device V25.1
      - neuropacemaker (brain) (peripheral nerve) (spinal cord) V53.02
      - orthodontic device V53.4
      - orthopedic (device) V53.7
        - brace V53.7
        - cast V53.7
        - shoes V53.7
      - pacemaker
        - brain V53.02
        - cardiac V53.31
        - carotid sinus V53.39
        - peripheral nerve V53.02
        - spinal cord V53.02
      - prosthesis V52.9
        - arm (complete) (partial) V52.0
        - breast V52.4
        - dental V52.3
        - eye V52.2
        - leg (complete) (partial) V52.1
        - specified type NEC V52.8
      - spectacles V53.1
      - wheelchair V53.8
    - adoption referral or proceedings V68.89
    - aftercare (*see also* Aftercare) V58.9
      - cardiac pacemaker V53.31
      - chemotherapy (oral) (intravenous) V58.11 ▲
      - dialysis
        - extracorporeal (renal) V56.0
        - peritoneal V56.8
        - renal V56.0
      - fracture (*see also* Aftercare, fracture) V54.9
      - medical NEC V58.89
      - organ transplant V58.44
      - orthopedic V54.9
        - specified care NEC V54.89
      - pacemaker device
        - brain V53.02
        - cardiac V53.31
        - carotid sinus V53.39
        - nervous system V53.02
        - spinal cord V53.02
      - postoperative NEC V58.49
        - wound closure, planned V58.41
      - postpartum
        - immediately after delivery V24.0
        - routine follow-up V24.2

- **Admission** - *continued*
  - for - *continued*
    - aftercare - *continued*
      - postradiation V58.0
      - radiation therapy V58.0
      - removal of
        - non-vascular catheter V58.82
        - vascular catheter V58.81
      - specified NEC V58.89
      - surgical NEC V58.49
        - wound closure, planned V58.41
      - antineoplastic
        - chemotherapy (oral) (intravenous) V58.11 ▲
        - immunotherapy V58.12
    - artificial insemination V26.1
    - assisted reproductive fertility procedure cycle V26.81
    - attention to artificial opening (of) V55.9
      - artificial vagina V55.7
      - colostomy V55.3
      - cystostomy V55.5
      - enterostomy V55.4
      - gastrostomy V55.1
      - ileostomy V55.2
      - jejunostomy V55.4
      - nephrostomy V55.6
      - specified site NEC V55.8
        - intestinal tract V55.4
        - urinary tract V55.6
      - tracheostomy V55.0
      - ureterostomy V55.6
      - urethrostomy V55.6
    - battery replacement
      - cardiac pacemaker V53.31
    - blood typing V72.86
      - Rh typing V72.86
    - boarding V65.0
    - breast
      - augmentation or reduction V50.1
      - implant exchange (different material) (different size) V52.4
      - reconstruction following mastectomy V51.0
      - removal
        - prophylactic V50.41
        - tissue expander without synchronous insertion of permanent implant V52.4
    - change of
      - cardiac pacemaker (battery) V53.31
      - carotid sinus pacemaker V53.39
      - catheter in artificial opening - *see* Attention to, artificial, opening
      - drains V58.49
      - dressing
        - wound V58.30
          - nonsurgical V58.30
          - surgical V58.31
      - fixation device
        - external V54.89
        - internal V54.01
      - Kirschner wire V54.89
      - neuropacemaker device (brain) (peripheral nerve) (spinal cord) V53.02
      - nonsurgical wound dressing V58.30
      - pacemaker device
        - brain V53.02
        - cardiac V53.31
        - carotid sinus V53.39
        - nervous system V53.02
      - plaster cast V54.89
      - splint, external V54.89
      - Steinmann pin V54.89
      - surgical wound dressing V58.31
      - traction device V54.89
      - wound packing V58.30
        - nonsurgical V58.30
        - surgical V58.31
    - checkup only V70.0

- **Admission** - *continued*
  - for - *continued*
    - chemotherapy, (oral) (intravenous), antineoplastic V58.11 ▲
    - circumcision, ritual or routine (in absence of medical indication) V50.2
    - clinical research investigation (control) (normal comparison) (participant) V70.7
    - closure of artificial opening - *see* Attention to, artificial, opening
    - contraceptive
      - counseling V25.09
        - emergency V25.03
        - postcoital V25.03
      - management V25.9
        - specified type NEC V25.8
    - convalescence following V66.9
      - chemotherapy V66.2
      - psychotherapy V66.3
      - radiotherapy V66.1
      - surgery V66.0
      - treatment (for) V66.5
        - combined V66.6
        - fracture V66.4
        - mental disorder NEC V66.3
        - specified condition NEC V66.5
    - cosmetic surgery NEC V50.1
      - breast reconstruction following mastectomy V51.0
      - following healed injury or operation V51.8
    - counseling (*see also* Counseling) V65.40
      - without complaint or sickness V65.49
      - contraceptive management V25.09
        - emergency V25.03
        - postcoital V25.03
      - dietary V65.3
      - exercise V65.41
      - fertility preservation (prior to cancer therapy) (prior to surgical removal of gonads) V26.42 ●
      - for
        - nonattending third party V65.19
        - pediatric ~~pre-birth visit for expectant mother V65.11~~ ▲
          - pre-adoption visit for adoptive parent(s) V65.11 ●
          - pre-birth visit for expectant parent(s) V65.11 ●
        - victim of abuse
          - child V61.21
          - partner or spouse V61.11
      - genetic V26.33
      - gonorrhea V65.45
      - HIV V65.44
      - human immunodeficiency virus V65.44
      - injury prevention V65.43
      - insulin pump training V65.46
      - natural family planning
        - procreative V26.41
        - to avoid pregnancy V25.04
      - procreative management V26.49
        - using natural family planning V26.41
      - sexually transmitted disease NEC V65.45
        - HIV V65.44
      - specified reason NEC V65.49
      - substance use and abuse V65.42
      - syphilis V65.45
      - victim of abuse
        - child V61.21
        - partner or spouse V61.11
    - desensitization to allergens V07.1

- **Admission** - *continued*
  - for - *continued*
    - dialysis V56.0
      - catheter
        - fitting and adjustment
          - extracorporeal V56.1
          - peritoneal V56.2
        - removal or replacement
          - extracorporeal V56.1
          - peritoneal V56.2
      - extracorporeal (renal) V56.0
      - peritoneal V56.8
      - renal V56.0
    - dietary surveillance and counseling V65.3
    - drug monitoring, therapeutic V58.83
    - ear piercing V50.3
    - elective surgery
      - breast
        - augmentation or reduction V50.1
        - reconstruction following mastectomy V51.0
        - removal, prophylactic V50.41
      - circumcision, ritual or routine (in absence of medical indication) V50.2
      - cosmetic NEC V50.1
        - breast reconstruction following mastectomy V51.0
        - following healed injury or operation V51.8
      - ear piercing V50.3
      - face-lift V50.1
      - hair transplant V50.0
      - plastic
        - breast reconstruction following mastectomy V51.0
        - cosmetic NEC V50.1
        - following healed injury or operation V51.8
      - prophylactic organ removal V50.49
        - breast V50.41
        - ovary V50.42
      - repair of scarred tissue (following healed injury or operation) V51.8
      - specified type NEC V50.8
    - end-of-life care V66.7
    - examination (*see also* Examination) V70.9
      - administrative purpose NEC V70.3
      - adoption V70.3
      - allergy V72.7
      - antibody response V72.61 ●
      - at health care facility V70.0
      - athletic team V70.3
      - camp V70.3
      - cardiovascular, preoperative V72.81
      - clinical research investigation (control) (participant) V70.7
      - dental V72.2
      - developmental testing (child) (infant) V20.2
      - donor (potential) V70.8
      - driver's license V70.3
      - ear V72.19
      - employment V70.5
      - eye V72.0
      - follow-up (routine) - *see* Examination, follow-up
      - for admission to
        - old age home V70.3
        - school V70.3
      - general V70.9
        - specified reason NEC V70.8
      - gynecological V72.31
      - health supervision ~~(child) (infant) V20.2~~ ▲
        - child (over 28 days old) V20.2 ●
        - infant (over 28 days old) V20.2 ●
        - newborn ●
          - 8 to 28 days old V20.32 ●

- **Admission** – *continued*
  - for – *continued*
    - examination – *continued*
      - health supervision – *continued*
        - newborn – *continued*
          - under 8 days old V20.31 ●
      - hearing V72.19
        - following failed hearing screening V72.11
      - immigration V70.3
      - infant, ~~routine V20.2~~ ▲
        - 8 to 28 days old V20.32 ●
        - over 28 days old, routine V20.2 ●
        - under 8 days old V20.31 ●
      - insurance certification V70.3
      - laboratory V72.60 ▲
        - ordered as part of a routine general medical examination V72.62 ●
        - pre-operative V72.63 ●
        - pre-procedural V72.63 ●
        - specified NEC V72.69 ●
      - marriage license V70.3
      - medical (general) (*see also* Examination, medical) V70.9
      - medicolegal reasons V70.4
      - naturalization V70.3
      - pelvic (annual) (periodic) V72.31
      - postpartum checkup V24.2
      - pregnancy (possible) (unconfirmed) V72.40
        - negative result V72.41
        - positive result V72.42
      - preoperative V72.84
        - cardiovascular V72.81
        - respiratory V72.82
        - specified NEC V72.83
      - preprocedural V72.84
        - cardiovascular V72.81
        - general physical V72.83
        - respiratory V72.82
        - specified NEC V72.83
      - prior to chemotherapy V72.83 ●
      - prison V70.3
      - psychiatric (general) V70.2
        - requested by authority V70.1
      - radiological NEC V72.5
      - respiratory, preoperative V72.82
      - school V70.3
      - screening - *see* Screening
      - skin hypersensitivity V72.7
      - specified type NEC V72.85
      - sport competition V70.3
      - vision V72.0
      - well baby and child care V20.2
    - exercise therapy V57.1
    - face-lift, cosmetic reason V50.1
    - fertility preservation (prior to cancer therapy) (prior to surgical removal of gonads) V26.82 ●
    - fitting (of)
      - artificial
        - arm (complete) (partial) V52.0
        - eye V52.2
        - leg (complete) (partial) V52.1
      - biliary drainage tube V58.82
      - brain neuropacemaker V53.02
      - breast V52.4
        - implant V52.4
        - prosthesis V52.4
      - cardiac pacemaker V53.31
      - catheter
        - non-vascular V58.82
        - vascular V58.81
      - cerebral ventricle (communicating) shunt V53.01
      - chest tube V58.82
      - colostomy belt V55.2
      - contact lenses V53.1
      - cystostomy device V53.6
      - dental prosthesis V52.3
      - device, unspecified type V53.90
        - abdominal V53.59 ▲

- **Admission** – *continued*
  - for – *continued*
    - fitting (of) – *continued*
      - device, unspecified type – *continued*
        - cerebral ventricle (communicating) shunt V53.01
        - gastrointestinal NEC V53.59 ●
        - insulin pump V53.91
        - intestinal V53.50 ●
        - intrauterine contraceptive V25.1
        - nervous system V53.09
        - orthodontic V53.4
        - other device V53.99
        - prosthetic V52.9
          - breast V52.4
          - dental V52.3
          - eye V52.2
        - special senses V53.09
        - substitution
          - auditory V53.09
          - nervous system V53.09
          - visual V53.09
      - diaphragm (contraceptive) V25.02
      - gastric lap band V53.51 ●
      - gastrointestinal appliance and device NEC V53.59 ●
      - growth rod V54.02
      - fistula (sinus tract) drainage tube V58.82
      - hearing aid V53.2
      - ileostomy device V55.2
      - intestinal appliance and ~~or~~ device ~~NEC~~ V53.50 ▲
      - intrauterine contraceptive device V25.1
      - neuropacemaker (brain) (peripheral nerve) (spinal cord) V53.02
      - orthodontic device V53.4
      - orthopedic (device) V53.7
        - brace V53.7
        - cast V53.7
        - shoes V53.7
      - pacemaker
        - brain V53.02
        - cardiac V53.31
        - carotid sinus V53.39
        - spinal cord V53.02
      - pleural drainage tube V58.82
      - portacath V58.81
      - prosthesis V52.9
        - arm (complete) (partial) V52.0
        - breast V52.4
        - dental V52.3
        - eye V52.2
        - leg (complete) (partial) V52.1
        - specified type NEC V52.8
      - spectacles V53.1
      - wheelchair V53.8
    - follow-up examination (routine) (following) V67.9
      - cancer chemotherapy V67.2
      - chemotherapy V67.2
      - high-risk medication NEC V67.51
      - injury NEC V67.59
      - psychiatric V67.3
      - psychotherapy V67.3
      - radiotherapy V67.1
      - specified surgery NEC V67.09
      - surgery V67.00
        - vaginal pap smear V67.01
      - treatment (for) V67.9
        - combined V67.6
        - fracture V67.4
        - involving high-risk medication NEC V67.51
        - mental disorder V67.3
        - specified NEC V67.59
    - hair transplant, for cosmetic reason V50.0
    - health advice, education, or instruction V65.4 [5th]

- **Admission** – *continued*
  - for – *continued*
    - hearing conservation and treatment V72.12
    - hormone replacement therapy (postmenopausal) V07.4
    - hospice care V66.7
    - immunizations (childhood) appropriate for age V20.2 ●
    - immunotherapy, antineoplastic V58.12
    - insertion (of)
      - subdermal implantable contraceptive V25.5
    - insulin pump titration V53.91
    - insulin pump training V65.46
    - intrauterine device
      - insertion V25.1
      - management V25.42
    - investigation to determine further disposition V63.8
    - in vitro fertilization cycle V26.81
    - isolation V07.0
    - issue of
      - disability examination certificate V68.01
      - medical certificate NEC V68.09
      - repeat prescription NEC V68.1
        - contraceptive device NEC V25.49
    - kidney dialysis V56.0
    - lengthening of growth rod V54.02
    - mental health evaluation V70.2
      - requested by authority V70.1
    - natural family planning counseling and advice
      - procreative V26.41
      - to avoid pregnancy V25.04
    - nonmedical reason NEC V68.89
    - nursing care evaluation V63.8
    - observation (without need for further medical care) (*see also* Observation) V71.9
      - accident V71.4
      - alleged rape or seduction V71.5
      - criminal assault V71.6
      - following accident V71.4
        - at work V71.3
      - foreign body ingestion V71.89
      - growth and development variations, childhood V21.0
      - inflicted injury NEC V71.6
      - ingestion of deleterious agent or foreign body V71.89
      - injury V71.6
      - malignant neoplasm V71.1
      - mental disorder V71.09
      - newborn - *see* Observation, suspected, condition, newborn
      - rape V71.5
      - specified NEC V71.89
      - suspected
        - abuse V71.81
        - accident V71.4
          - at work V71.3
        - benign neoplasm V71.89
        - cardiovascular V71.7
        - disorder V71.9
        - exposure
          - anthrax V71.82
          - biological agent NEC V71.83
          - SARS V71.83
        - heart V71.7
        - inflicted injury NEC V71.6
        - malignant neoplasm V71.1
        - maternal and fetal problem not found
          - amniotic cavity and membrane V89.01
          - cervical shortening V89.05
          - fetal anomaly V89.03
          - fetal growth V89.04
          - oligohydramnios V89.01
          - other specified NEC V89.09

- **Admission** – *continued*
  - for – *continued*
    - observation – *continued*
      - suspected – *continued*
        - maternal and fetal problem not found – *continued*
          - placenta V89.02
          - polyhydramnios V89.01
        - mental NEC V71.09
        - neglect V71.81
        - specified condition NEC V71.89
        - tuberculosis V71.2
      - tuberculosis V71.2
    - occupational therapy V57.21
    - organ transplant, donor - *see* Donor
    - ovary, ovarian removal, prophylactic V50.42
    - palliative care V66.7
    - Papanicolaou smear
      - cervix V76.2
        - for suspected malignant neoplasm V76.2
          - no disease found V71.1
        - routine, as part of gynecological examination V72.31
        - to confirm findings of recent normal smear following initial abnormal smear V72.32
      - vaginal V76.47
        - following hysterectomy for malignant condition V67.01
    - passage of sounds or bougie in artificial opening - *see* Attention to, artificial, opening
    - paternity testing V70.4
    - peritoneal dialysis V56.32
    - physical therapy NEC V57.1
    - plastic surgery
      - breast reconstruction following mastectomy V51.0
      - cosmetic NEC V50.1
      - following healed injury or operation V51.8
    - postmenopausal hormone replacement therapy V07.4
    - postpartum observation
      - immediately after delivery V24.0
      - routine follow-up V24.2
    - poststerilization (for restoration) V26.0
    - procreative management V26.9
      - assisted reproductive fertility procedure cycle V26.81
      - in vitro fertilization cycle V26.81
      - specified type NEC V26.89
    - prophylactic
      - administration of
        - antibiotics V07.39
        - antitoxin, any V07.2
        - antivenin V07.2
        - chemotherapeutic agent NEC V07.39
        - chemotherapy NEC V07.39
        - diphtheria antitoxin V07.2
        - fluoride V07.31
        - gamma globulin V07.2
        - immune sera (gamma globulin) V07.2
        - RhoGAM V07.2
        - tetanus antitoxin V07.2
      - breathing exercises V57.0
      - chemotherapy NEC V07.39
        - fluoride V07.31
      - measure V07.9
        - specified type NEC V07.8
      - organ removal V50.49
        - breast V50.41
        - ovary V50.42
    - psychiatric examination (general) V70.2
      - requested by authority V70.1
    - radiation management V58.0
    - radiotherapy V58.0

- **Admission** - *continued*
  - for - *continued*
    - reconstruction following mastectomy V51.0
    - reforming of artificial opening - *see* Attention to, artificial, opening
    - rehabilitation V57.9
      - multiple types V57.89
      - occupational V57.21
      - orthoptic V57.4
      - orthotic V57.81
      - physical NEC V57.1
      - specified type NEC V57.89
      - speech(-language) V57.3 ▲
      - vocational V57.22
    - removal of
      - breast tissue expander without synchronous insertion of permanent implant V52.4
      - cardiac pacemaker V53.31
      - cast (plaster) V54.89
      - catheter from artificial opening - *see* Attention to, artificial, opening
      - cerebral ventricle (communicating) shunt V53.01
      - cystostomy catheter V55.5
      - device
        - cerebral ventricle (communicating) shunt V53.01
        - fixation
          - external V54.89
          - internal V54.01
        - intrauterine contraceptive V25.42
        - traction, external V54.89
      - drains V58.49
      - dressing
        - wound V58.30
          - nonsurgical V58.30
          - surgical V58.31
      - fixation device
        - external V54.89
        - internal V54.01
      - intrauterine contraceptive device V25.42
      - Kirschner wire V54.89
      - neuropacemaker (brain) (peripheral nerve) (spinal cord) V53.02
      - nonsurgical wound dressing V58.30
      - orthopedic fixation device
        - external V54.89
        - internal V54.01
      - pacemaker device
        - brain V53.02
        - cardiac V53.31
        - carotid sinus V53.39
        - nervous system V53.02
      - plaster cast V54.89
      - plate (fracture) V54.01
      - rod V54.01
      - screw (fracture) V54.01
      - splint, traction V54.89
      - staples V58.32
      - Steinmann pin V54.89
      - subdermal implantable contraceptive V25.43
      - surgical wound dressing V58.31
      - sutures V58.32
      - traction device, external V54.89
      - ureteral stent V53.6
      - wound packing V58.30
        - nonsurgical V58.30
        - surgical V58.31
    - repair of scarred tissue (following healed injury or operation) V51.8
    - reprogramming of cardiac pacemaker V53.31
    - respirator [ventilator] dependence
      - during
        - mechanical failure V46.14

- **Admission** - *continued*
  - for - *continued*
    - respirator [ventilator] dependence - *continued*
      - during - *continued*
        - power failure V46.12
      - for weaning V46.13
    - restoration of organ continuity (poststerilization) (tuboplasty) (vasoplasty) V26.0
    - Rh typing V72.86
    - routine infant and child vision and hearing testing V20.2 ●
    - sensitivity test - *see also* Test, skin
      - allergy NEC V72.7
      - bacterial disease NEC V74.9
      - Dick V74.8
      - Kveim V82.89
      - Mantoux V74.1
      - mycotic infection NEC V75.4
      - parasitic disease NEC V75.8
      - Schick V74.3
      - Schultz-Charlton V74.8
    - social service (agency) referral or evaluation V63.8
    - speech(-language) therapy V57.3 ▲
    - sterilization V25.2
    - suspected disorder (ruled out) (without need for further care) - *see* Observation
    - terminal care V66.7
    - tests only - *see* Test
    - therapeutic drug monitoring V58.83
    - therapy
      - blood transfusion, without reported diagnosis V58.2
      - breathing exercises V57.0
      - chemotherapy, antineoplastic V58.11
        - prophylactic NEC V07.39
          - fluoride V07.31
      - dialysis (intermittent) (treatment)
        - extracorporeal V56.0
        - peritoneal V56.8
        - renal V56.0
        - specified type NEC V56.8
      - exercise (remedial) NEC V57.1
        - breathing V57.0
      - immunotherapy, antineoplastic V58.12
      - long-term (current) drug use NEC V58.69
        - antibiotics V58.62
        - anticoagulants V58.61
        - anti-inflammatories, non-steroidal (NSAID) V58.64
        - antiplatelets V58.63
        - antithrombotics V58.63
        - aspirin V58.66
        - high-risk medications NEC V58.69
        - insulin V58.67
        - methadone V58.69
        - opiate analgesic V58.69
        - steroids V58.65
      - occupational V57.21
      - orthoptic V57.4
      - physical NEC V57.1
      - radiation V58.0
      - speech(-language) V57.3 ▲
      - vocational V57.22
    - toilet or cleaning
      - of artificial opening - *see* Attention to, artificial, opening
      - of non-vascular catheter V58.82
      - of vascular catheter V58.81
    - tubal ligation V25.2
    - tuboplasty for previous sterilization V26.0
    - ultrasound, routine fetal V28.3
    - vaccination, prophylactic (against)
      - arthropod-borne virus, viral NEC V05.1
        - disease NEC V05.1

- **Admission** - *continued*
  - for - *continued*
    - vaccination, prophylactic (against) - *continued*
      - arthropod-borne virus, viral - *continued*
        - encephalitis V05.0
      - Bacille Calmette Guérin (BCG) V03.2
      - BCG V03.2
      - chickenpox V05.4
      - cholera alone V03.0
        - with typhoid-paratyphoid (cholera + TAB) V06.0
      - common cold V04.7
      - dengue V05.1
      - diphtheria alone V03.5
      - diphtheria-tetanus-pertussis (DTP) (DTaP) V06.1
        - with
          - poliomyelitis (DTP polio) V06.3
          - typhoid-paratyphoid (DTP + TAB) V06.2
      - diphtheria-tetanus [Td] [DT] without pertussis V06.5
      - disease (single) NEC V05.9
        - bacterial NEC V03.9
          - specified type NEC V03.89
        - combinations NEC V06.9
          - specified type NEC V06.8
        - specified type NEC V05.8
        - viral NEC V04.89
      - encephalitis, viral, arthropod-borne V05.0
      - Hemophilus influenzae, type B [Hib] V03.81
      - hepatitis, viral V05.3
      - human papillomavirus (HPV) V04.89
      - immune sera (gamma globulin) V07.2
      - influenza V04.81
        - with
          - Streptococcus pneumoniae [pneumococcus] V06.6
      - Leishmaniasis V05.2
      - measles alone V04.2
      - measles-mumps-rubella (MMR) V06.4
      - mumps alone V04.6
        - with measles and rubella (MMR) V06.4
      - not done because of contraindication V64.09
      - pertussis alone V03.6
      - plague V03.3
      - pneumonia V03.82
      - poliomyelitis V04.0
        - with diphtheria-tetanus-pertussis (DTP polio) V06.3
      - rabies V04.5
      - respiratory syncytial virus (RSV) V04.82
      - rubella alone V04.3
        - with measles and mumps (MMR) V06.4
      - smallpox V04.1
      - specified type NEC V05.8
      - Streptococcus pneumoniae [pneumococcus] V03.82
        - with
          - influenza V06.6
      - tetanus toxoid alone V03.7
        - with diphtheria [Td] [DT] V06.5
          - and pertussis (DTP) (DTaP) V06.1
      - tuberculosis (BCG) V03.2
      - tularemia V03.4

- **Admission** - *continued*
  - for - *continued*
    - vaccination, prophylactic (against) - *continued*
      - typhoid alone V03.1
        - with diphtheria-tetanus-pertussis (TAB + DTP) V06.2
      - typhoid-paratyphoid alone (TAB) V03.1
      - typhus V05.8
      - varicella (chicken pox) V05.4
      - viral encephalitis, arthropod-borne V05.0
      - viral hepatitis V05.3
      - yellow fever V04.4
    - vasectomy V25.2
    - vasoplasty for previous sterilization V26.0
    - vision examination V72.0
    - vocational therapy V57.22
    - waiting period for admission to other facility V63.2
      - undergoing social agency investigation V63.8
    - well baby and child care V20.2
    - x-ray of chest
      - for suspected tuberculosis V71.2
      - routine V72.5
- **Adnexitis** (suppurative) (*see also* Salpingo-oophoritis) 614.2
- **Adolescence** NEC V21.2
- **Adoption**
  - agency referral V68.89
  - examination V70.3
  - held for V68.89
- **Adrenal gland** - *see* condition
- **Adrenalism** 255.9
  - tuberculous (*see also* Tuberculosis) 017.6 [5th]
- **Adrenalitis, adrenitis** 255.8
  - meningococcal hemorrhagic 036.3
- **Adrenarche, precocious** 259.1
- **Adrenocortical syndrome** 255.2
- **Adrenogenital syndrome** (acquired) (congenital) 255.2
  - iatrogenic, fetus or newborn 760.79
- **Adrenoleukodystrophy** 277.86
  - neonatal 277.86
  - x-linked 277.86
- **Adrenomyeloneuropathy** 277.86
- **Adventitious bursa** - *see* Bursitis
- **Adynamia** (episodica) (hereditary) (periodic) 359.3
- **Adynamic**
  - ileus or intestine (*see also* Ileus) 560.1
  - ureter 753.22
- **Aeration lung, imperfect, newborn** 770.5
- **Aerobullosis** 993.3
- **Aerocele** - *see* Embolism, air
- **Aerodermectasia**
  - subcutaneous (traumatic) 958.7
    - surgical 998.81
  - surgical 998.81
- **Aerodontalgia** 993.2
- **Aeroembolism** 993.3
- **Aerogenes capsulatus infection** (*see also* Gangrene, gas) 040.0
- **Aero-otitis media** 993.0
- **Aerophagy, aerophagia** 306.4
  - psychogenic 306.4
- **Aerosinusitis** 993.1
- **Aerotitis** 993.0
- **Affection, affections** - *see also* Disease
  - sacroiliac (joint), old 724.6
  - shoulder region NEC 726.2
- **Afibrinogenemia** 286.3
  - acquired 286.6
  - congenital 286.3
  - postpartum 666.3 [5th]
- **African**
  - sleeping sickness 086.5
  - tick fever 087.1

Admission – African

- **African** – *continued*
  - trypanosomiasis 086.5
    - Gambian 086.3
    - Rhodesian 086.4
- **Aftercare** V58.9
  - amputation stump V54.89
  - artificial openings - *see* Attention to, artificial, opening
  - blood transfusion without reported diagnosis V58.2
  - breathing exercise V57.0
  - cardiac device V53.39
    - defibrillator, automatic implantable V53.32
    - pacemaker V53.31
      - carotid sinus V53.39
  - carotid sinus pacemaker V53.39
  - cerebral ventricle (communicating) shunt V53.01
  - chemotherapy (oral) (intravenous) session (adjunctive) (maintenance) V58.11 ▲
  - defibrillator, automatic implantable cardiac V53.32
  - exercise (remedial) (therapeutic) V57.1
    - breathing V57.0
  - extracorporeal dialysis (intermittent) (treatment) V56.0
  - following surgery NEC V58.49
    - for
      - injury V58.43
      - neoplasm V58.42
      - organ transplant V58.44
      - trauma V58.43
    - joint replacement V54.81
    - of
      - circulatory system V58.73
      - digestive system V58.75
      - genital organs V58.76
      - genitourinary system V58.76
      - musculoskeletal system V58.78
      - nervous sytem V58.72
      - oral cavity V58.75
      - respiratory system V58.74
      - sense organs V58.71
      - skin V58.77
      - subcutaneous tissue V58.77
      - teeth V58.75
      - urinary system V58.76
    - spinal - *see* Aftercare, following surgery, of, specified body system
    - wound closure, planned V58.41
  - fracture V54.9
    - healing V54.89
      - pathologic
        - ankle V54.29
        - arm V54.20
          - lower V54.22
          - upper V54.21
        - finger V54.29
        - foot V54.29
        - hand V54.29
        - hip V54.23
        - leg V54.24
          - lower V54.26
          - upper V54.25
        - pelvis V54.29
        - specified site NEC V54.29
        - toe(s) V54.29
        - vertebrae V54.27
        - wrist V54.29
      - traumatic
        - ankle V54.19
        - arm V54.10
          - lower V54.12
          - upper V54.11
        - finger V54.19
        - foot V54.19
        - hand V54.19
        - hip V54.13
        - leg V54.14
          - lower V54.16
          - upper V54.15
- **Aftercare** – *continued*
  - fracture – *continued*
    - healing – *continued*
      - traumatic – *continued*
        - pelvis V54.19
        - specified site NEC V54.19
        - toe(s) V54.19
        - vertebrae V54.17
        - wrist V54.19
    - removal of
      - external fixation device V54.89
      - internal fixation device V54.01
    - specified care NEC V54.89
  - gait training V57.1
    - for use of artificial limb(s) V57.81
  - internal fixation device V54.09
  - involving
    - dialysis (intermittent) (treatment)
      - extracorporeal V56.0
      - peritoneal V56.8
      - renal V56.0
    - gait training V57.1
      - for use of artificial limb(s) V57.81
    - growth rod
      - adjustment V54.02
      - lengthening V54.02
    - internal fixation device V54.09
    - orthoptic training V57.4
    - orthotic training V57.81
    - radiotherapy session V58.0
    - removal of
      - drains V58.49
      - dressings
        - wound V58.30
          - nonsurgical V58.30
          - surgical V58.31
      - fixation device
        - external V54.89
        - internal V54.01
      - fracture plate V54.01
      - nonsurgical wound dressing V58.30
      - pins V54.01
      - plaster cast V54.89
      - rods V54.01
      - screws V54.01
      - staples V58.32
      - surgical wound dressings V58.31
      - sutures V58.32
      - traction device, external V54.89
      - wound packing V58.30
        - nonsurgical V58.30
        - surgical V58.31
  - neuropacemaker (brain) (peripheral nerve) (spinal cord) V53.02
  - occupational therapy V57.21
  - orthodontic V58.5
  - orthopedic V54.9
    - change of external fixation or traction device V54.89
    - following joint replacement V54.81
    - internal fixation device V54.09
    - removal of fixation device
      - external V54.89
      - internal V54.01
    - specified care NEC V54.89
  - orthoptic training V57.4
  - orthotic training V57.81
  - pacemaker
    - brain V53.02
    - cardiac V53.31
    - carotid sinus V53.39
    - peripheral nerve V53.02
    - spinal cord V53.02
  - peritoneal dialysis (intermittent) (treatment) V56.8
  - physical therapy NEC V57.1
    - breathing exercises V57.0
  - radiotherapy session V58.0
  - rehabilitation procedure V57.9
    - breathing exercises V57.0
    - multiple types V57.89
    - occupational V57.21
    - orthoptic V57.4
    - orthotic V57.81
- **Aftercare** – *continued*
  - rehabilitation procedure – *continued*
    - physical therapy NEC V57.1
    - remedial exercises V57.1
    - specified type NEC V57.89
    - speech(-language) V57.3 ▲
    - therapeutic exercises V57.1
    - vocational V57.22
  - renal dialysis (intermittent) (treatment) V56.0
  - specified type NEC V58.89
    - removal of non-vascular cathether V58.82
    - removal of vascular catheter V58.81
  - speech(-language) therapy V57.3 ▲
  - stump, amputation V54.89
  - vocational rehabilitation V57.22
- **After-cataract** 366.50
  - obscuring vision 366.53
  - specified type, not obscuring vision 366.52
- **Agalactia** 676.4 [5th]
- **Agammaglobulinemia** 279.00
  - with lymphopenia 279.2
  - acquired (primary) (secondary) 279.06
  - Bruton's X-linked 279.04
  - infantile sex-linked (Bruton's) (congenital) 279.04
  - Swiss-type 279.2
- **Aganglionosis** (bowel) (colon) 751.3
- **Age** (old) (*see also* Senile) 797
- **Agenesis** - *see also* Absence, by site, congenital
  - acoustic nerve 742.8
  - adrenal (gland) 759.1
  - alimentary tract (complete) (partial) NEC 751.8
    - lower 751.2
    - upper 750.8
  - anus, anal (canal) 751.2
  - aorta 747.22
  - appendix 751.2
  - arm (complete) (partial) (*see also* Deformity, reduction, upper limb) 755.20
  - artery (peripheral) NEC (*see also* Anomaly, peripheral vascular system) 747.60
    - brain 747.81
    - coronary 746.85
    - pulmonary 747.3
    - umbilical 747.5
  - auditory (canal) (external) 744.01
  - auricle (ear) 744.01
  - bile, biliary duct or passage 751.61
  - bone NEC 756.9
  - brain 740.0
    - specified part 742.2
  - breast 757.6
  - bronchus 748.3
  - canaliculus lacrimalis 743.65
  - carpus NEC (*see also* Deformity, reduction, upper limb) 755.28
  - cartilage 756.9
  - cecum 751.2
  - cerebellum 742.2
  - cervix 752.49
  - chin 744.89
  - cilia 743.63
  - circulatory system, part NEC 747.89
  - clavicle 755.51
  - clitoris 752.49
  - coccyx 756.13
  - colon 751.2
  - corpus callosum 742.2
  - cricoid cartilage 748.3
  - diaphragm (with hernia) 756.6
  - digestive organ(s) or tract (complete) (partial) NEC 751.8
    - lower 751.2
    - upper 750.8
  - ductus arteriosus 747.89
  - duodenum 751.1
  - ear NEC 744.09
    - auricle 744.01
- **Agenesis** – *continued*
  - ear – *continued*
    - lobe 744.21
  - ejaculatory duct 752.89
  - endocrine (gland) NEC 759.2
  - epiglottis 748.3
  - esophagus 750.3
  - Eustachian tube 744.24
  - extrinsic muscle, eye 743.69
  - eye 743.00
    - adnexa 743.69
  - eyelid (fold) 743.62
  - face
    - bones NEC 756.0
    - specified part NEC 744.89
  - fallopian tube 752.19
  - femur NEC (*see also* Absence, femur, congenital) 755.34
  - fibula NEC (*see also* Absence, fibula, congenital) 755.37
  - finger NEC (*see also* Absence, finger, congenital) 755.29
  - foot (complete) (*see also* Deformity, reduction, lower limb) 755.31
  - gallbladder 751.69
  - gastric 750.8
  - genitalia, genital (organ)
    - female 752.89
      - external 752.49
      - internal NEC 752.89
    - male 752.89
      - penis 752.69
  - glottis 748.3
  - gonadal 758.6
  - hair 757.4
  - hand (complete) (*see also* Deformity, reduction, upper limb) 755.21
  - heart 746.89
    - valve NEC 746.89
      - aortic 746.89
      - mitral 746.89
      - pulmonary 746.01
  - hepatic 751.69
  - humerus NEC (*see also* Absence, humerus, congenital) 755.24
  - hymen 752.49
  - ileum 751.1
  - incus 744.04
  - intestine (small) 751.1
    - large 751.2
  - iris (dilator fibers) 743.45
  - jaw 524.09
  - jejunum 751.1
  - kidney(s) (partial) (unilateral) 753.0
  - labium (majus) (minus) 752.49
  - labyrinth, membranous 744.05
  - lacrimal apparatus (congenital) 743.65
  - larynx 748.3
  - leg NEC (*see also* Deformity, reduction, lower limb) 755.30
  - lens 743.35
  - limb (complete) (partial) (*see also* Deformity, reduction) 755.4
    - lower NEC 755.30
    - upper 755.20
  - lip 750.26
  - liver 751.69
  - lung (bilateral) (fissures) (lobe) (unilateral) 748.5
  - mandible 524.09
  - maxilla 524.09
  - metacarpus NEC 755.28
  - metatarsus NEC 755.38
  - muscle (any) 756.81
  - musculoskeletal system NEC 756.9
  - nail(s) 757.5
  - neck, part 744.89
  - nerve 742.8
  - nervous system, part NEC 742.8
  - nipple 757.6
  - nose 748.1
  - nuclear 742.8
  - organ
    - of Corti 744.05

- **Agenesis** – *continued*
  - organ – *continued*
    - or site not listed - *see* Anomaly, specified type NEC
  - osseous meatus (ear) 744.03
  - ovary 752.0
  - oviduct 752.19
  - pancreas 751.7
  - parathyroid (gland) 759.2
  - patella 755.64
  - pelvic girdle (complete) (partial) 755.69
  - penis 752.69
  - pericardium 746.89
  - perineal body 756.81
  - pituitary (gland) 759.2
  - prostate 752.89
  - pulmonary
    - artery 747.3
    - trunk 747.3
    - vein 747.49
  - punctum lacrimale 743.65
  - radioulnar NEC (*see also* Absence, forearm, congenital) 755.25
  - radius NEC (*see also* Absence, radius, congenital) 755.26
  - rectum 751.2
  - renal 753.0
  - respiratory organ NEC 748.9
  - rib 756.3
  - roof of orbit 742.0
  - round ligament 752.89
  - sacrum 756.13
  - salivary gland 750.21
  - scapula 755.59
  - scrotum 752.89
  - seminal duct or tract 752.89
  - septum
    - atrial 745.69
    - between aorta and pulmonary artery 745.0
    - ventricular 745.3
  - shoulder girdle (complete) (partial) 755.59
  - skull (bone) 756.0
    - with
      - anencephalus 740.0
      - encephalocele 742.0
      - hydrocephalus 742.3
        - with spina bifida (*see also* Spina bifida) 741.0 [5th]
      - microcephalus 742.1
  - spermatic cord 752.89
  - spinal cord 742.59
  - spine 756.13
    - lumbar 756.13
      - isthmus 756.11
      - pars articularis 756.11
  - spleen 759.0
  - sternum 756.3
  - stomach 750.7
  - tarsus NEC 755.38
  - tendon 756.81
  - testicular 752.89
  - testis 752.89
  - thymus (gland) 759.2
  - thyroid (gland) 243
    - cartilage 748.3
  - tibia NEC (*see also* Absence, tibia, congenital) 755.36
  - tibiofibular NEC 755.35
  - toe (complete) (partial) (*see also* Absence, toe, congenital) 755.39
  - tongue 750.11
  - trachea (cartilage) 748.3
  - ulna NEC (*see also* Absence, ulna, congenital) 755.27
  - ureter 753.4
  - urethra 753.8
  - urinary tract NEC 753.8
  - uterus 752.3
  - uvula 750.26
  - vagina 752.49
  - vas deferens 752.89

- **Agenesis** – *continued*
  - vein(s) (peripheral) NEC (*see also* Anomaly, peripheral vascular system) 747.60
    - brain 747.81
    - great 747.49
    - portal 747.49
    - pulmonary 747.49
  - vena cava (inferior) (superior) 747.49
  - vermis of cerebellum 742.2
  - vertebra 756.13
    - lumbar 756.13
      - isthmus 756.11
      - pars articularis 756.11
  - vulva 752.49
- **Ageusia** (*see also* Disturbance, sensation) 781.1
- **Aggressiveness** 301.3
- **Aggressive outburst** (*see also* Disturbance, conduct) 312.0 [5th]
  - in children or adolescents 313.9
- **Aging skin** 701.8
- **Agitated** - *see* condition
- **Agitation** 307.9
  - catatonic (*see also* Schizophrenia) 295.2 [5th]
- **Aglossia** (congenital) 750.11
- **Aglycogenosis** 271.0
- **Agnail** (finger) (with lymphangitis) 681.02
- **Agnosia** (body image) (tactile) 784.69
  - verbal 784.69
    - auditory 784.69
      - secondary to organic lesion 784.69
    - developmental 315.8
    - secondary to organic lesion 784.69
  - visual 368.16
    - object 368.16
- **Agoraphobia** 300.22
  - with panic disorder 300.21
- **Agrammatism** 784.69
- **Agranulocytopenia** (*see also* Agranulocytosis) 288.09
- **Agranulocytosis** ~~(angina)~~ (*see also* Neutropenia) 288.09 ▲
  - chronic 288.09
  - cyclical 288.02
  - due to infection 288.04 ●
  - genetic 288.01
  - infantile 288.01
  - periodic 288.02
  - pernicious 288.09
- **Agraphia** (absolute) 784.69
  - with alexia 784.61
  - developmental 315.39
- **Agrypnia** (*see also* Insomnia) 780.52
- **Ague** (*see also* Malaria) 084.6
  - brass-founders' 985.8
  - dumb 084.6
  - tertian 084.1
- **Agyria** 742.2
- **Ahumada-del Castillo syndrome** (nonpuerperal galactorrhea and amenorrhea) 253.1
- **AIDS** 042
- **AIDS-associated retrovirus** (disease) (illness) 042
  - infection - *see* Human immunodeficiency virus, infection
- **AIDS-associated virus** (disease) (illness) 042
  - infection - *see* Human immunodeficiency virus, infection
- **AIDS-like disease** (illness) (syndrome) 042
- **AIDS-related complex** 042
- **AIDS-related conditions** 042
- **AIDS-related virus** (disease) (illness) 042
  - infection - *see* Human immunodeficiency virus, infection
- **AIDS virus** (disease) (illness) 042
  - infection - *see* Human immunodeficiency virus, infection
- **Ailment, heart** - *see* Disease, heart
- **Ailurophobia** 300.29
- **AIN I** [anal intraepithelial neoplasia I] (histologically confirmed) 569.44
- **AIN II** [anal intraepithelial neoplasia II] (histologically confirmed) 569.44
- **AIN III** [anal intraepithelial neoplasia III] 230.6
  - anal canal 230.5
- **Ainhum** (disease) 136.0
- **Air**
  - anterior mediastinum 518.1
  - compressed, disease 993.3
  - embolism (any site) (artery) (cerebral) 958.0
    - with
      - abortion - *see* Abortion, by type, with embolism
      - ectopic pregnancy (*see also* categories 633.0-633.9) 639.6
      - molar pregnancy (*see also* categories 630-632) 639.6
    - due to implanted device - *see* Complications, due to (presence of) any device, implant, or graft classified to 996.0-996.5 NEC
    - following
      - abortion 639.6
      - ectopic or molar pregnancy 639.6
      - infusion, perfusion, or transfusion 999.1
    - in pregnancy, childbirth, or puerperium 673.0 [5th]
    - traumatic 958.0
  - hunger 786.09
    - psychogenic 306.1
  - leak (lung) (pulmonary) (thorax) 512.8
    - iatrogenic 512.1
    - postoperative 512.1
  - rarefied, effects of - *see* Effect, adverse, high altitude
  - sickness 994.6
- **Airplane sickness** 994.6
- **Akathisia, acathisia** 781.0
  - due to drugs 333.99
  - neuroleptic-induced acute 333.99
- **Akinesia algeria** 352.6
- **Akiyami** 100.89
- **Akureyri disease** (epidemic neuromyasthenia) 049.8
- **Alacrima** (congenital) 743.65
- **Alactasia** (hereditary) 271.3
- **Alagille syndrome** 759.89
- **Alalia** 784.3
  - developmental 315.31
    - receptive-expressive 315.32
  - secondary to organic lesion 784.3
- **Alaninemia** 270.8
- **Alastrim** 050.1
- **Albarrán's disease** (colibacilluria) 791.9
- **Albers-Schönberg's disease** (marble bones) 756.52
- **Albert's disease** 726.71
- **Albinism, albino** (choroid) (cutaneous) (eye) (generalized) (isolated) (ocular) (oculocutaneous) (partial) 270.2
- **Albinismus** 270.2
- **Albright (-Martin) (-Bantam) disease** (pseudohypoparathyroidism) 275.49
- **Albright (-McCune) (-Sternberg) syndrome** (osteitis fibrosa disseminata) 756.59
- **Albuminous** - *see* Condition
- **Albuminuria, albuminuric** (acute) (chronic) (subacute) 791.0
  - Bence-Jones 791.0
  - cardiac 785.9
  - complicating pregnancy, childbirth, or puerperium 646.2 [5th]
    - with hypertension - *see* Toxemia, of pregnancy
    - affecting fetus or newborn 760.1
  - cyclic 593.6
  - gestational 646.2 [5th]
  - gravidarum 646.2 [5th]
    - with hypertension - *see* Toxemia, of pregnancy
    - affecting fetus or newborn 760.1
  - heart 785.9

- **Albuminuria, albuminuric** – *continued*
  - idiopathic 593.6
  - orthostatic 593.6
  - postural 593.6
  - pre-eclamptic (mild) 642.4 [5th]
    - affecting fetus or newborn 760.0
    - severe 642.5 [5th]
      - affecting fetus or newborn 760.0
  - recurrent physiologic 593.6
  - scarlatinal 034.1
- **Albumosuria** 791.0
  - Bence-Jones 791.0
  - myelopathic (M9730/3) 203.0 [5th]
- **Alcaptonuria** 270.2
- **Alcohol, alcoholic**
  - abstinence 291.81
  - acute intoxication 305.0 [5th]
    - with dependence 303.0 [5th]
  - addiction (*see also* Alcoholism) 303.9 [5th]
    - maternal
      - with suspected fetal damage affecting management of pregnancy 655.4 [5th]
      - affecting fetus or newborn 760.71
  - amnestic disorder, persisting 291.1
  - anxiety 291.89
  - brain syndrome, chronic 291.2
  - cardiopathy 425.5
  - chronic (*see also* Alcoholism) 303.9 [5th]
  - cirrhosis (liver) 571.2
  - delirium 291.0
    - acute 291.0
    - chronic 291.1
    - tremens 291.0
    - withdrawal 291.0
  - dementia NEC 291.2
  - deterioration 291.2
  - drunkenness (simple) 305.0 [5th]
  - hallucinosis (acute) 291.3
  - induced
    - circadian rhythm sleep disorder 291.82
    - hypersomnia 291.82
    - insomnia 291.82
    - mental disorder 291.9
      - anxiety 291.89
      - mood 291.89
      - sexual 291.89
      - sleep 291.82
      - specified type 291.89
    - parasomnia 291.82
    - persisting
      - amnestic disorder 291.1
      - dementia 291.2
    - psychotic disorder
      - with
        - delusions 291.5
        - hallucinations 291.3
    - sleep disorder 291.82
  - insanity 291.9
  - intoxication (acute) 305.0 [5th]
    - with dependence 303.0 [5th]
    - pathological 291.4
  - jealousy 291.5
  - Korsakoff's, Korsakov's, Korsakow's 291.1
  - liver NEC 571.3
    - acute 571.1
    - chronic 571.2
  - mania (acute) (chronic) 291.9
  - mood 291.89
  - paranoia 291.5
  - paranoid (type) psychosis 291.5
  - pellagra 265.2
  - poisoning, accidental (acute) NEC 980.9
    - specified type of alcohol - *see* Table of Drugs and Chemicals
  - psychosis (*see also* Psychosis, alcoholic) 291.9
    - Korsakoff's, Korsakov's, Korsakow's 291.1
    - polyneuritic 291.1
      - with
        - delusions 291.5
        - hallucinations 291.3
  - related disorder 291.9

Alcohol, alcoholic – *continued*
- withdrawal symptoms, syndrome NEC 291.81
  - delirium 291.0
  - hallucinosis 291.3

Alcoholism 303.9

Note *Use the following fifth-digit subclassification with category 303:*

0 unspecified
1 continuous
2 episodic
3 in remission

- with psychosis (*see also* Psychosis, alcoholic) 291.9
- acute 303.0 [5th]
- chronic 303.9 [5th]
  - with psychosis 291.9
- complicating pregnancy, childbirth, or puerperium 648.4 [5th]
  - affecting fetus or newborn 760.71
- history V11.3
- Korsakoff's, Korsakov's, Korsakow's 291.1
- suspected damage to fetus affecting management of pregnancy 655.4 [5th]

Alder's anomaly or syndrome (leukocyte granulation anomaly) 288.2

Alder-Reilly anomaly (leukocyte granulation) 288.2

Aldosteronism (primary) 255.10
- congenital 255.10
- familial type I 255.11
- glucocorticoid-remediable 255.11
- secondary 255.14

Aldosteronoma (M8370/1) 237.2

Aldrich (-Wiskott) syndrome (eczema-thrombocytopenia) 279.12

Aleppo boil 085.1

Aleukemic - *see* condition

Aleukia
- congenital 288.09
- hemorrhagica 284.9
  - acquired (secondary) 284.89
  - congenital 284.09
  - idiopathic 284.9
- splenica 289.4

Alexia (congenital) (developmental) 315.01
- secondary to organic lesion 784.61

Algoneurodystrophy 733.7

Algophobia 300.29

Alibert-Bazin disease (M9700/3) 202.1 [5th]

Alibert's disease (mycosis fungoides) (M9700/3) 202.1 [5th]

Alice in Wonderland syndrome 293.89

Alienation, mental (*see also* Psychosis) 298.9

Alkalemia 276.3

Alkalosis 276.3
- metabolic 276.3
  - with respiratory acidosis 276.4
- respiratory 276.3

Alkaptonuria 270.2

Allen-Masters syndrome 620.6

Allergic bronchopulmonary aspergillosis 518.6

Allergy, allergic (reaction) 995.3
- air-borne substance (*see also* Fever, hay) 477.9
  - specified allergen NEC 477.8
- alveolitis (extrinsic) 495.9
  - due to
    - Aspergillus clavatus 495.4
    - cryptostroma corticale 495.6
    - organisms (fungal, thermophilic actinomycete, other) growing in ventilation (air conditioning systems) 495.7
  - specified type NEC 495.8
- anaphylactic shock 999.4
  - due to food - *see* Anaphylactic shock, due to, food
- angioneurotic edema 995.1
- animal (cat) (dog) (epidermal) 477.8
  - dander 477.2

Allergy, allergic – *continued*
- animal – *continued*
  - hair 477.2
- arthritis (*see also* Arthritis, allergic) 716.2 [5th]
- asthma - *see* Asthma
- bee sting (anaphylactic shock) 989.5
- biological - *see* Allergy, drug
- bronchial asthma - *see* Asthma
- conjunctivitis (eczematous) 372.14
- dander, animal (cat) (dog) 477.2
- dandruff 477.8
- dermatitis (venenata) - *see* Dermatitis
- diathesis V15.09
- drug, medicinal substance, and biological (any) (correct medicinal substance properly administered) (external) (internal) 995.27
  - wrong substance given or taken NEC 977.9
    - specified drug or substance - *see* Table of Drugs and Chemicals
- dust (house) (stock) 477.8
- eczema - *see* Eczema
- endophthalmitis 360.19
- epidermal (animal) 477.8
- existing dental restorative material 525.66
- feathers 477.8
- food (any) (ingested) 693.1
  - atopic 691.8
  - in contact with skin 692.5
- gastritis 535.4 [5th]
- gastroenteritis 558.3
- gastrointestinal 558.3
- grain 477.0
- grass (pollen) 477.0
  - asthma (*see also* Asthma) 493.0 [5th]
  - hay fever 477.0
- hair, animal (cat) (dog) 477.2
- hay fever (grass) (pollen) (ragweed) (tree) (*see also* Fever, hay) 477.9
- history (of) V15.09
  - to
    - arachnid bite V15.06 ●
    - eggs V15.03
    - food additives V15.05
    - insect bite V15.06
    - latex V15.07
    - milk products V15.02
    - nuts V15.05
      - peanuts V15.01
    - radiographic dye V15.08
    - seafood V15.04
    - specified food NEC V15.05
    - spider bite V15.06
- horse serum - *see* Allergy, serum
- inhalant 477.9
  - dust 477.8
  - pollen 477.0
  - specified allergen other than pollen 477.8
- kapok 477.8
- medicine - *see* Allergy, drug
- migraine 339.00
- milk protein 558.3
- pannus 370.62
- pneumonia 518.3
- pollen (any) (hay fever) 477.0
  - asthma (*see also* Asthma) 493.0 [5th]
- primrose 477.0
- primula 477.0
- purpura 287.0
- ragweed (pollen) (Senecio jacobae) 477.0
  - asthma (*see also* Asthma) 493.0 [5th]
  - hay fever 477.0
- respiratory (*see also* Allergy, inhalant) 477.9
  - due to
    - drug - *see* Allergy, drug
    - food - *see* Allergy, food
- rhinitis (*see also* Fever, hay) 477.9
  - due to food 477.1
- rose 477.0

Allergy, allergic – *continued*
- Senecio jacobae 477.0
- serum (prophylactic) (therapeutic) 999.5
  - anaphylactic shock 999.4
- shock (anaphylactic) (due to adverse effect of correct medicinal substance properly administered) 995.0
  - food - *see* Anaphylactic shock, due to, food
  - from serum or immunization 999.5
    - anaphylactic 999.4
- sinusitis (*see also* Fever, hay) 477.9
- skin reaction 692.9
  - specified substance - *see* Dermatitis, due to
- tree (any) (hay fever) (pollen) 477.0
  - asthma (*see also* Asthma) 493.0 [5th]
- upper respiratory (*see also* Fever, hay) 477.9
- urethritis 597.89
- urticaria 708.0
- vaccine - *see* Allergy, serum

Allescheriosis 117.6

Alligator skin disease (ichthyosis congenita) 757.1
- acquired 701.1

Allocheiria, allochiria (*see also* Disturbance, sensation) 782.0

Almeida's disease (Brazilian blastomycosis) 116.1

Alopecia (atrophicans) (pregnancy) (premature) (senile) 704.00
- adnata 757.4
- areata 704.01
- celsi 704.01
- cicatrisata 704.09
- circumscripta 704.01
- congenital, congenitalis 757.4
- disseminata 704.01
- effluvium (telogen) 704.02
- febrile 704.09
- generalisata 704.09
- hereditaria 704.09
- marginalis 704.01
- mucinosa 704.09
- postinfectional 704.09
- seborrheica 704.09
- specific 091.82
- syphilitic (secondary) 091.82
- telogen effluvium 704.02
- totalis 704.09
- toxica 704.09
- universalis 704.09
- x-ray 704.09

Alpers' disease 330.8

Alpha-lipoproteinemia 272.4

Alpha thalassemia 282.49

Alphos 696.1

Alpine sickness 993.2

Alport's syndrome (hereditary hematurianephropathy-deafness) 759.89

ALPS (autoimmune lymphoproliferative syndrome) 279.41 ●

ALTE (apparent life threatening event) **in newborn and infant** 799.82 ●

Alteration (of)**, altered**
- awareness 780.09
  - transient 780.02
- consciousness 780.09
  - persistent vegetative state 780.03
  - transient 780.02
- mental status 780.97
  - amnesia (retrograde) 780.93
  - memory loss 780.93

Alternaria (infection) 118

Alternating - *see* condition

Altitude, high (effects) - *see* Effect, adverse, high altitude

Aluminosis (of lung) 503

Alvarez syndrome (transient cerebral ischemia) 435.9

Alveolar capillary block syndrome 516.3

Alveolitis
- allergic (extrinsic) 495.9
  - due to organisms (fungal, thermophilic actinomycete, other) growing in ventilation (air conditioning systems) 495.7
  - specified type NEC 495.8
- due to
  - Aspergillus clavatus 495.4
  - Cryptostroma corticale 495.6
- fibrosing (chronic) (cryptogenic) (lung) 516.3
  - idiopathic 516.3
  - rheumatoid 714.81
- jaw 526.5
- sicca dolorosa 526.5

Alveolus, alveolar - *see* condition

Alymphocytosis (pure) 279.2

Alymphoplasia, thymic 279.2

Alzheimer's
- dementia (senile)
  - with behavioral disturbance 331.0 *[294.11]*
  - without behavioral disturbance 331.0 *[294.10]*
- disease or sclerosis 331.0
  - with dementia - *see* Alzheimer's, dementia

Amastia (*see also* Absence, breast) 611.89

Amaurosis (acquired) (congenital) (*see also* Blindness) 369.00
- fugax 362.34
- hysterical 300.11
- Leber's (congenital) 362.76
- tobacco 377.34
- uremic - *see* Uremia

Amaurotic familial idiocy (infantile) (juvenile) (late) 330.1

Ambisexual 752.7

Amblyopia (acquired) (congenital) (partial) 368.00
- color 368.59
  - acquired 368.55
- deprivation 368.02
- ex anopsia 368.00
- hysterical 300.11
- nocturnal 368.60
  - vitamin A deficiency 264.5
- refractive 368.03
- strabismic 368.01
- suppression 368.01
- tobacco 377.34
- toxic NEC 377.34
- uremic - *see* Uremia

Ameba, amebic (histolytica) - *see also* Amebiasis
- abscess 006.3
  - bladder 006.8
  - brain (with liver and lung abscess) 006.5
  - liver 006.3
    - with
      - brain abscess (and lung abscess) 006.5
      - lung abscess 006.4
  - lung (with liver abscess) 006.4
    - with brain abscess 006.5
  - seminal vesicle 006.8
  - spleen 006.8
- carrier (suspected of) V02.2
- meningoencephalitis
  - due to Naegleria (gruberi) 136.29
  - primary 136.29

Amebiasis NEC 006.9
- with
  - brain abscess (with liver or lung abscess) 006.5
  - liver abscess (without mention of brain or lung abscess) 006.3
  - lung abscess (with liver abscess) 006.4
    - with brain abscess 006.5
- acute 006.0
- bladder 006.8
- chronic 006.1

Alcohol, alcoholic – Amebiasis

- **Amebiasis** – *continued*
  - cutaneous 006.6
  - cutis 006.6
  - due to organism other than Entamoeba histolytica 007.8
  - hepatic (*see also* Abscess, liver, amebic) 006.3
  - nondysenteric 006.2
  - seminal vesicle 006.8
  - specified
    - organism NEC 007.8
    - site NEC 006.8
- **Ameboma** 006.8
- **Amelia** 755.4
  - lower limb 755.31
  - upper limb 755.21
- **Ameloblastoma** (M9310/0) 213.1
  - jaw (bone) (lower) 213.1
    - upper 213.0
  - long bones (M9261/3) - *see* Neoplasm, bone, malignant
  - malignant (M9310/3) 170.1
    - jaw (bone) (lower) 170.1
      - upper 170.0
  - mandible 213.1
  - tibial (M9261/3) 170.7
- **Amelogenesis imperfecta** 520.5
  - nonhereditaria (segmentalis) 520.4
- **Amenorrhea** (primary) (secondary) 626.0
  - due to ovarian dysfunction 256.8
  - hyperhormonal 256.8
- **Amentia** (*see also* Retardation, mental) 319
  - Meynert's (nonalcoholic) 294.0
    - alcoholic 291.1
  - nevoid 759.6
- **American**
  - leishmaniasis 085.5
  - mountain tick fever 066.1
  - trypanosomiasis - *see* Trypanosomiasis, American
- **Ametropia** (*see also* Disorder, accommodation) 367.9
- **Amianthosis** 501
- **Amimia** 784.69
- **Amino acid**
  - deficiency 270.9
    - anemia 281.4
  - metabolic disorder (*see also* Disorder, amino acid) 270.9
- **Aminoaciduria** 270.9
  - imidazole 270.5
- **Amnesia** (retrograde) 780.93
  - auditory 784.69
    - developmental 315.31
    - secondary to organic lesion 784.69
  - dissociative 300.12
  - hysterical or dissociative type 300.12
  - psychogenic 300.12
  - transient global 437.7
- **Amnestic** (confabulatory) **syndrome** 294.0
  - alcohol-induced persisting 291.1
  - drug-induced persisting 292.83
  - posttraumatic 294.0
- **Amniocentesis screening** (for) V28.2
  - alphafetoprotein level, raised V28.1
  - chromosomal anomalies V28.0
- **Amnion, amniotic** - *see also* condition
  - nodosum 658.8 5th
- **Amnionitis** (complicating pregnancy) 658.4 5th
  - affecting fetus or newborn 762.7
- **Amoral trends** 301.7
- **Amotio retinae** (*see also* Detachment, retina) 361.9
- **Ampulla**
  - lower esophagus 530.89
  - phrenic 530.89
- **Amputation**
  - any part of fetus, to facilitate delivery 763.89
  - cervix (supravaginal) (uteri) 622.8
    - in pregnancy or childbirth 654.6 5th
      - affecting fetus or newborn 763.89
  - clitoris - *see* Wound, open, clitoris
- **Amputation** – *continued*
  - congenital
    - lower limb 755.31
    - upper limb 755.21
  - neuroma (traumatic) - *see also* Injury, nerve, by site
    - surgical complication (late) 997.61
  - penis - *see* Amputation, traumatic, penis
  - status (without complication) - *see* Absence, by site, acquired
  - stump (surgical) (posttraumatic)
    - abnormal, painful, or with complication (late) 997.60
    - healed or old NEC - *see also* Absence, by site, acquired
      - lower V49.70
      - upper V49.60
  - traumatic (complete) (partial)

Note *"Complicated" includes traumatic amputation with delayed healing, delayed treatment, foreign body, or infection.*

  - arm 887.4
    - at or above elbow 887.2
      - complicated 887.3
    - below elbow 887.0
      - complicated 887.1
    - both (bilateral) (any level(s)) 887.6
      - complicated 887.7
    - complicated 887.5
  - finger(s) (one or both hands) 886.0
    - with thumb(s) 885.0
      - complicated 885.1
    - complicated 886.1
  - foot (except toe(s) only) 896.0
    - and other leg 897.6
      - complicated 897.7
    - both (bilateral) 896.2
      - complicated 896.3
    - complicated 896.1
    - toe(s) only (one or both feet) 895.0
      - complicated 895.1
  - genital organ(s) (external) NEC 878.8
    - complicated 878.9
  - hand (except finger(s) only) 887.0
    - and other arm 887.6
      - complicated 887.7
    - both (bilateral) 887.6
      - complicated 887.7
    - complicated 887.1
    - finger(s) (one or both hands) 886.0
      - with thumb(s) 885.0
        - complicated 885.1
      - complicated 886.1
    - thumb(s) (with fingers of either hand) 885.0
      - complicated 885.1
  - head 874.9
  - late effect - *see* Late, effects (of), amputation
  - leg 897.4
    - and other foot 897.6
      - complicated 897.7
    - at or above knee 897.2
      - complicated 897.3
    - below knee 897.0
      - complicated 897.1
    - both (bilateral) 897.6
      - complicated 897.7
    - complicated 897.5
  - lower limb(s) except toe(s) - *see* Amputation, traumatic, leg
  - nose - *see* Wound, open, nose
  - penis 878.0
    - complicated 878.1
  - sites other than limbs - *see* Wound, open, by site
  - thumb(s) (with finger(s) of either hand) 885.0
    - complicated 885.1
  - toe(s) (one or both feet) 895.0
    - complicated 895.1
- **Amputation** – *continued*
  - upper limb(s) - *see* Amputation traumatic, arm
- **Amputee** (bilateral) (old) - *see also* Absence, by site, acquired V49.70
- **Amusia** 784.69
  - developmental 315.39
  - secondary to organic lesion 784.69
- **Amyelencephalus** 740.0
- **Amyelia** 742.59
- **Amygdalitis** - *see* Tonsillitis
- **Amygdalolith** 474.8
- **Amyloid disease or degeneration** 277.30
  - heart 277.39 *[425.7]*
- **Amyloidosis** (familial) (general) (generalized) (genetic) (primary) 277.30
  - with lung involvement 277.39 *[517.8]*
  - cardiac, hereditary 277.39
  - heart 277.39 *[425.7]*
  - nephropathic 277.39 *[583.81]*
  - neuropathic (Portuguese) (Swiss) 277.39 *[357.4]*
  - pulmonary 277.39 *[517.8]*
  - secondary 277.39
  - systemic, inherited 277.39
- **Amylopectinosis** (brancher enzyme deficiency) 271.0
- **Amylophagia** 307.52
- **Amyoplasia, congenita** 756.89
- **Amyotonia** 728.2
  - congenita 358.8
- **Amyotrophia, amyotrophy, amyotrophic** 728.2
  - congenita 756.89
  - diabetic 250.6 5th *[353.5]*
    - due to secondary diabetes 249.6 5th *[353.5]*
  - lateral sclerosis (syndrome) 335.20
  - neuralgic 353.5
  - sclerosis (lateral) 335.20
  - spinal progressive 335.21
- **Anacidity, gastric** 536.0
  - psychogenic 306.4
- **Anaerosis of newborn** 770.88
- **Analbuminemia** 273.8
- **Analgesia** (*see also* Anesthesia) 782.0
- **Analphalipoproteinemia** 272.5
- **Anaphylactic shock or reaction** (correct substance properly administered) 995.0
  - due to
    - food 995.60
      - additives 995.66
      - crustaceans 995.62
      - eggs 995.68
      - fish 995.65
      - fruits 995.63
      - milk products 995.67
      - nuts (tree) 995.64
      - peanuts 995.61
      - seeds 995.64
      - specified NEC 995.69
      - tree nuts 995.64
      - vegetables 995.63
    - immunization 999.4
    - overdose or wrong substance given or taken 977.9
      - specified drug - *see* Table of Drugs and Chemicals
    - serum 999.4
  - following sting(s) 989.5
  - purpura 287.0
  - serum 999.4
- **Anaphylactoid shock or reaction** - *see* Anaphylactic shock
- **Anaphylaxis** - *see* Anaphylactic shock
- **Anaplasia, cervix** 622.10
- **Anarthria** 784.51 ▲
- **Anarthritic rheumatoid disease** 446.5
- **Anasarca** 782.3
  - cardiac (*see also* Failure, heart) 428.0
  - fetus or newborn 778.0
  - lung 514
- **Anasarca** – *continued*
  - nutritional 262
  - pulmonary 514
  - renal (*see also* Nephrosis) 581.9
- **Anaspadias** 752.62
- **Anastomosis**
  - aneurysmal - *see* Aneurysm
  - arteriovenous, congenital NEC (*see also* Anomaly, arteriovenous) 747.60
    - ruptured, of brain (*see also* Hemorrhage, subarachnoid) 430
  - intestinal 569.89
    - complicated NEC 997.4
      - involving urinary tract 997.5
  - retinal and choroidal vessels 743.58
    - acquired 362.17
- **Anatomical narrow angle** (glaucoma) 365.02
- **Ancylostoma** (infection) (infestation) 126.9
  - americanus 126.1
  - braziliense 126.2
  - caninum 126.8
  - ceylanicum 126.3
  - duodenale 126.0
  - Necator americanus 126.1
- **Ancylostomiasis** (intestinal) 126.9
  - ancylostoma
    - americanus 126.1
    - caninum 126.8
    - ceylanicum 126.3
    - duodenale 126.0
  - braziliense 126.2
  - Necator americanus 126.1
- **Anders' disease or syndrome** (adiposis tuberosa simplex) 272.8
- **Andersen's glycogen storage disease** 271.0
- **Anderson's disease** 272.7
- **Andes disease** 993.2
- **Andrews' disease** (bacterid) 686.8
- **Androblastoma** (M8630/1)
  - benign (M8630/0)
    - specified site - *see* Neoplasm, by site, benign
    - unspecified site
      - female 220
      - male 222.0
  - malignant (M8630/3)
    - specified site - *see* Neoplasm, by site, malignant
    - unspecified site
      - female 183.0
      - male 186.9
  - specified site - *see* Neoplasm, by site, uncertain behavior
  - tubular (M8640/0)
    - with lipid storage (M8641/0)
      - specified site - *see* Neoplasm, by site, benign
      - unspecified site
        - female 220
        - male 222.0
    - specified site - *see* Neoplasm, by site, benign
    - unspecified site
      - female 220
      - male 222.0
  - unspecified site
    - female 236.2
    - male 236.4
- **Android pelvis** 755.69
  - with disproportion (fetopelvic) 653.3 5th
    - affecting fetus or newborn 763.1
    - causing obstructed labor 660.1 5th
      - affecting fetus or newborn 763.1
- **Anectasis, pulmonary** (newborn or fetus) 770.5
- **Anemia** 285.9
  - with
    - disorder of
      - anaerobic glycolysis 282.3
      - pentose phosphate pathway 282.2
    - koilonychia 280.9
  - 6-phosphogluconic dehydrogenase deficiency 282.2
  - achlorhydric 280.9

Anemia – *continued*
- achrestic 281.8
- Addison's (pernicious) 281.0
- Addison-Biermer (pernicious) 281.0
- agranulocytic 288.09
- amino acid deficiency 281.4
- antineoplastic chemotherapy induced 285.3 ●
- aplastic 284.9
  - acquired (secondary) 284.89
  - congenital 284.01
  - constitutional 284.01
  - due to
    - antineoplastic chemotherapy 284.89
    - chronic systemic disease 284.89
    - drugs 284.89
    - infection 284.89
    - radiation 284.89
  - idiopathic 284.9
  - myxedema 244.9
  - of or complicating pregnancy 648.2 5th
  - red cell (acquired) (adult) (with thymoma) 284.81
    - congenital 284.01
    - pure 284.01
  - specified type NEC 284.89
  - toxic (paralytic) 284.89
- aregenerative 284.9
  - congenital 284.01
- asiderotic 280.9
- atypical (primary) 285.9
- autohemolysis of Selwyn and Dacie (type I) 282.2
- autoimmune hemolytic 283.0
- Baghdad Spring 282.2
- Balantidium coli 007.0
- Biermer's (pernicious) 281.0
- blood loss (chronic) 280.0
  - acute 285.1
- bothriocephalus 123.4
- brickmakers' (*see also* Ancylostomiasis) 126.9
- cerebral 437.8
- childhood 282.9
- chlorotic 280.9
- chronica congenita aregenerativa 284.01
- chronic simple 281.9
- combined system disease NEC 281.0 *[336.2]*
  - due to dietary deficiency 281.1 *[336.2]*
- complicating pregnancy or childbirth 648.2 5th
- congenital (following fetal blood loss) 776.5
  - aplastic 284.01
  - due to isoimmunization NEC 773.2
  - Heinz-body 282.7
  - hereditary hemolytic NEC 282.9
  - nonspherocytic
    - type I 282.2
    - type II 282.3
  - pernicious 281.0
  - spherocytic (*see also* Spherocytosis) 282.0
- Cooley's (erythroblastic) 282.49
- crescent - *see* Disease, sickle-cell
- cytogenic 281.0
- Dacie's (nonspherocytic)
  - type I 282.2
  - type II 282.3
- Davidson's (refractory) 284.9
- deficiency 281.9
  - 2, 3 diphosphoglycurate mutase 282.3
  - 2, 3 PG 282.3
  - 6-PGD 282.2
  - 6-phosphogluronic dehydrogenase 282.2
  - amino acid 281.4
  - combined B_{12} and folate 281.3
  - enzyme, drug-induced (hemolytic) 282.2
  - erythrocytic glutathione 282.2
  - folate 281.2
    - dietary 281.2

Anemia – *continued*
- deficiency – *continued*
  - folate – *continued*
    - drug-induced 281.2
  - folic acid 281.2
    - dietary 281.2
    - drug-induced 281.2
  - G-6-PD 282.2
  - GGS-R 282.2
  - glucose-6-phosphate dehydrogenase (G-6-PD) 282.2
  - glucose-phosphate isomerase 282.3
  - glutathione peroxidase 282.2
  - glutathione reductase 282.2
  - glyceraldehyde phosphate dehydrogenase 282.3
  - GPI 282.3
  - G SH 282.2
  - hexokinase 282.3
  - iron (Fe) 280.9
    - specified NEC 280.8
  - nutritional 281.9
    - with
      - poor iron absorption 280.9
      - specified deficiency NEC 281.8
    - due to inadequate dietary iron intake 280.1
    - specified type NEC 281.8
  - of or complicating pregnancy 648.2 5th
  - pentose phosphate pathway 282.2
  - PFK 282.3
  - phosphofructo-aldolase 282.3
  - phosphofructokinase 282.3
  - phosphoglycerate kinase 282.3
  - PK 282.3
  - protein 281.4
  - pyruvate kinase (PK) 282.3
  - TPI 282.3
  - triosephosphate isomerase 282.3
  - vitamin B_{12} NEC 281.1
    - dietary 281.1
    - pernicious 281.0
- Diamond-Blackfan (congenital hypoplastic) 284.01
- dibothriocephalus 123.4
- dimorphic 281.9
- diphasic 281.8
- diphtheritic 032.89
- Diphyllobothrium 123.4
- drepanocytic (*see also* Disease, sickle-cell) 282.60
- due to
  - antineoplastic chemotherapy 285.3 ●
  - blood loss (chronic) 280.0
    - acute 285.1
  - chemotherapy, antineoplastic 285.3 ●
  - defect of Embden-Meyerhof pathway glycolysis 282.3
  - disorder of glutathione metabolism 282.2
  - drug - *see* Anemia, by type (*see also* Table of Drugs and Chemicals)
    - chemotherapy, antineoplastic 285.3 ●
  - fetal blood loss 776.5
  - fish tapeworm (D. latum) infestation 123.4
  - glutathione metabolism disorder 282.2
  - hemorrhage (chronic) 280.0
    - acute 285.1
  - hexose monophosphate (HMP) shunt deficiency 282.2
  - impaired absorption 280.9
  - loss of blood (chronic) 280.0
    - acute 285.1
  - myxedema 244.9
  - Necator americanus 126.1
  - prematurity 776.6
  - selective vitamin B_{12} malabsorption with proteinuria 281.1
- Dyke-Young type (secondary) (symptomatic) 283.9
- dyserythropoietic (congenital) (types I, II, III) 285.8

Anemia – *continued*
- dyshemopoietic (congenital) 285.8
- Egypt (*see also* Ancylostomiasis) 126.9
- elliptocytosis (*see also* Elliptocytosis) 282.1
- enzyme deficiency, drug-induced 282.2
- epidemic (*see also* Ancylostomiasis) 126.9
- EPO resistant 285.21
- erythroblastic
  - familial 282.49
  - fetus or newborn (*see also* Disease, hemolytic) 773.2
    - late 773.5
- erythrocytic glutathione deficiency 282.2
- erythropoietin-resistant (EPO resistant anemia) 285.21
- essential 285.9
- Faber's (achlorhydric anemia) 280.9
- factitious (self-induced bloodletting) 280.0
- familial erythroblastic (microcytic) 282.49
- Fanconi's (congenital pancytopenia) 284.09
- favism 282.2
- fetal 678.0 5th
  - following blood loss, affecting newborn 776.5
- fetus or newborn
  - due to
    - ABO
      - antibodies 773.1
      - incompatibility, maternal/fetal 773.1
      - isoimmunization 773.1
    - Rh
      - antibodies 773.0
      - incompatibility, maternal/fetal 773.0
      - isoimmunization 773.0
  - following fetal blood loss 776.5
- fish tapeworm (D. latum) infestation 123.4
- folate (folic acid) deficiency 281.2
  - dietary 281.2
  - drug-induced 281.2
- folate malabsorption, congenital 281.2
- folic acid deficiency 281.2
  - dietary 281.2
  - drug-induced 281.2
- G-6-PD 282.2
- general 285.9
- glucose-6-phosphate dehydrogenase deficiency 282.2
- glutathione-reductase deficiency 282.2
- goat's milk 281.2
- granulocytic 288.09
- Heinz-body, congenital 282.7
- hemoglobin deficiency 285.9
- hemolytic 283.9
  - acquired 283.9
    - with hemoglobinuria NEC 283.2
    - autoimmune (cold type) (idiopathic) (primary) (secondary) (symptomatic) (warm type) 283.0
    - due to
      - cold reactive antibodies 283.0
      - drug exposure 283.0
      - warm reactive antibodies 283.0
    - fragmentation 283.19
    - idiopathic (chronic) 283.9
    - infectious 283.19
      - autoimmune 283.0
    - non-autoimmune 283.10
    - toxic 283.19
    - traumatic cardiac 283.19
  - acute 283.9
    - due to enzyme deficiency NEC 282.3
    - fetus or newborn (*see also* Disease, hemolytic) 773.2
      - late 773.5
    - Lederer's (acquired infectious hemolytic anemia) 283.19
  - autoimmune (acquired) 283.0

Anemia – *continued*
- hemolytic – *continued*
  - chronic 282.9
    - idiopathic 283.9
  - cold type (secondary) (symptomatic) 283.0
  - congenital (spherocytic) (*see also* Spherocytosis) 282.0
    - nonspherocytic - *see* Anemia, hemolytic, nonspherocytic, congenital
  - drug-induced 283.0
    - enzyme deficiency 282.2
  - due to
    - cardiac conditions 283.19
    - drugs 283.0
    - enzyme deficiency NEC 282.3
      - drug-induced 282.2
    - presence of shunt or other internal prosthetic device 283.19
    - thrombotic thrombocytopenic purpura 446.6
  - elliptocytotic (*see also* Elliptocytosis) 282.1
  - familial 282.9
  - hereditary 282.9
    - due to enzyme deficiency NEC 282.3
    - specified NEC 282.8
  - idiopathic (chronic) 283.9
  - infectious (acquired) 283.19
  - mechanical 283.19
  - microangiopathic 283.19
  - nonautoimmune 283.10
  - nonspherocytic
    - congenital or hereditary NEC 282.3
      - glucose-6-phosphate dehydrogenase deficiency 282.2
      - pyruvate kinase (PK) deficiency 282.3
      - type I 282.2
      - type II 282.3
    - type I 282.2
    - type II 282.3
  - of or complicating pregnancy 648.2 5th
  - resulting from presence of shunt or other internal prosthetic device 283.19
  - secondary 283.19
    - autoimmune 283.0
  - sickle-cell - *see* Disease, sickle-cell
  - Stransky-Regala type (Hb-E) (*see also* Disease, hemoglobin) 282.7
  - symptomatic 283.19
    - autoimmune 283.0
  - toxic (acquired) 283.19
  - uremic (adult) (child) 283.11
  - warm type (secondary) (symptomatic) 283.0
- hemorrhagic (chronic) 280.0
  - acute 285.1
- HEMPAS 285.8
- hereditary erythroblast multinuclearity-positive acidified serum test 285.8
- Herrick's (hemoglobin S disease) 282.61
- hexokinase deficiency 282.3
- high A_2 282.49
- hookworm (*see also* Ancylostomiasis) 126.9
- hypochromic (idiopathic) (microcytic) (normoblastic) 280.9
  - with iron loading 285.0
  - due to blood loss (chronic) 280.0
    - acute 285.1
  - familial sex linked 285.0
  - pyridoxine-responsive 285.0
- hypoplasia, red blood cells 284.81
  - congenital or familial 284.01
- hypoplastic (idiopathic) 284.9
  - congenital 284.01
  - familial 284.01
  - of childhood 284.09

Anemia

Anemia – *continued*
idiopathic 285.9
hemolytic, chronic 283.9
in (due to) (with) ▲
chronic illness NEC 285.29
chronic kidney disease 285.21
end-stage renal disease 285.21
neoplastic disease 285.22
infantile 285.9
infective, infectional 285.9
intertropical (*see also* Ancylostomiasis) 126.9
iron (Fe) deficiency 280.9
due to blood loss (chronic) 280.0
acute 285.1
of or complicating pregnancy 648.2 5th
specified NEC 280.8
Jaksch's (pseudoleukemia infantum) 285.8
Joseph-Diamond-Blackfan (congenital hypoplastic) 284.01
labyrinth 386.50
Lederer's (acquired infectious hemolytic anemia) 283.19
leptocytosis (hereditary) 282.49
leukoerythroblastic 284.2
macrocytic 281.9
nutritional 281.2
of or complicating pregnancy 648.2 5th
tropical 281.2
malabsorption (familial), selective B$_{12}$ with proteinuria 281.1
malarial (*see also* Malaria) 084.6
malignant (progressive) 281.0
malnutrition 281.9
marsh (*see also* Malaria) 084.6
Mediterranean (with hemoglobinopathy) 282.49
megaloblastic 281.9
combined B$_{12}$ and folate deficiency 281.3
nutritional (of infancy) 281.2
of infancy 281.2
of or complicating pregnancy 648.2 5th
refractory 281.3
specified NEC 281.3
megalocytic 281.9
microangiopathic hemolytic 283.19
microcytic (hypochromic) 280.9
due to blood loss (chronic) 280.0
acute 285.1
familial 282.49
hypochromic 280.9
microdrepanocytosis 282.49
miners' (*see also* Ancylostomiasis) 126.9
myelopathic 285.8
myelophthisic (normocytic) 284.2
newborn (*see also* Disease, hemolytic) 773.2
due to isoimmunization (*see also* Disease, hemolytic) 773.2
late, due to isoimmunization 773.5
posthemorrhagic 776.5
nonregenerative 284.9
nonspherocytic hemolytic - *see* Anemia, hemolytic, nonspherocytic
normocytic (infectional) (not due to blood loss) 285.9
due to blood loss (chronic) 280.0
acute 285.1
myelophthisic 284.2
nutritional (deficiency) 281.9
with
poor iron absorption 280.9
specified deficiency NEC 281.8
due to inadequate dietary iron intake 280.1
megaloblastic (of infancy) 281.2
of childhood 282.9
of chronic
disease NEC 285.29
illness NEC 285.29
of or complicating pregnancy 648.2 5th
affecting fetus or newborn 760.8
of prematurity 776.6

Anemia – *continued*
orotic aciduric (congenital) (hereditary) 281.4
osteosclerotic 289.89
ovalocytosis (hereditary) (*see also* Elliptocytosis) 282.1
paludal (*see also* Malaria) 084.6
pentose phosphate pathway deficiency 282.2
pernicious (combined system disease) (congenital) (dorsolateral spinal degeneration) (juvenile) (myelopathy) (neuropathy) (posterior sclerosis) (primary) (progressive) (spleen) 281.0
of or complicating pregnancy 648.2 5th
pleochromic 285.9
of sprue 281.8
portal 285.8
posthemorrhagic (chronic) 280.0
acute 285.1
newborn 776.5
postoperative
due to (acute) blood loss 285.1
chronic blood loss 280.0
other 285.9
postpartum 648.2 5th
pressure 285.9
primary 285.9
profound 285.9
progressive 285.9
malignant 281.0
pernicious 281.0
protein-deficiency 281.4
pseudoleukemica infantum 285.8
puerperal 648.2 5th
pure red cell 284.81
congenital 284.01
pyridoxine-responsive (hypochromic) 285.0
pyruvate kinase (PK) deficiency 282.3
refractoria sideroblastica 238.72
refractory (primary) 238.72
with
excess
blasts-1 (RAEB-1) 238.73
blasts-2 (RAEB-2) 238.72 ▲
hemochromatosis 238.72
ringed sideroblasts (RARS) 238.72
due to
drug 285.0
myelodysplastic syndrome 238.72
toxin 285.0
hereditary 285.0
idiopathic 238.72
megaloblastic 281.3
sideroblastic 238.72
hereditary 285.0
sideropenic 280.9
Rietti-Greppi-Micheli (thalassemia minor) 282.49
scorbutic 281.8
secondary (to) 285.9
blood loss (chronic) 280.0
acute 285.1
hemorrhage 280.0
acute 285.1
inadequate dietary iron intake 280.1
semiplastic 284.9
septic 285.9
sickle-cell (*see also* Disease, sickle-cell) 282.60
sideroachrestic 285.0
sideroblastic (acquired) (any type) (congenital) (drug-induced) (due to disease) (hereditary) (primary) (secondary) (sex-linked hypochromic) (vitamin B$_6$ responsive) 285.0
refractory 238.72
congenital 285.0
drug-induced 285.0
hereditary 285.0
sex-linked hypochromic 285.0

Anemia – *continued*
sideroblastic – *continued*
refractory – *continued*
vitamin B$_6$-responsive 285.0
sideropenic 280.9
due to blood loss (chronic) 280.0
acute 285.1
simple chronic 281.9
specified type NEC 285.8
spherocytic (hereditary) (*see also* Spherocytosis) 282.0
splenic 285.8
familial (Gaucher's) 272.7
splenomegalic 285.8
stomatocytosis 282.8
syphilitic 095.8
target cell (oval) 282.49
thalassemia 282.49
thrombocytopenic (*see also* Thrombocytopenia) 287.5
toxic 284.89
triosephosphate isomerase deficiency 282.3
tropical, macrocytic 281.2
tuberculous (*see also* Tuberculosis) 017.9 5th
Vegan's 281.1
vitamin
B$_6$-responsive 285.0
B$_{12}$ deficiency (dietary) 281.1
pernicious 281.0
von Jaksch's (pseudoleukemia infantum) 285.8
Witts' (achlorhydric anemia) 280.9
Zuelzer (-Ogden) (nutritional megaloblastic anemia) 281.2
Anencephalus, anencephaly 740.0
fetal, affecting management of pregnancy 655.0 5th
Anergasia (*see also* Psychosis, organic) 294.9
senile 290.0
Anesthesia, anesthetic 782.0
complication or reaction NEC 995.22
due to
correct substance properly administered 995.22
overdose or wrong substance given 968.4
specified anesthetic - *see* Table of Drugs and Chemicals
cornea 371.81
death from
correct substance properly administered 995.4
during delivery 668.9 5th
overdose or wrong substance given 968.4
specified anesthetic - *see* Table of Drugs and Chemicals
eye 371.81
functional 300.11
hyperesthetic, thalamic 338.0
hysterical 300.11
local skin lesion 782.0
olfactory 781.1
sexual (psychogenic) 302.72
shock
due to
correct substance properly administered 995.4
overdose or wrong substance given 968.4
specified anesthetic - *see* Table of Drugs and Chemicals
skin 782.0
tactile 782.0
testicular 608.9
thermal 782.0
Anetoderma (maculosum) 701.3
Aneuploidy NEC 758.5
Aneurin deficiency 265.1

Aneurysm (anastomotic) (artery) (cirsoid) (diffuse) (false) (fusiform) (multiple) (ruptured) (saccular) (varicose) 442.9
abdominal (aorta) 441.4
ruptured 441.3
syphilitic 093.0
aorta, aortic (nonsyphilitic) 441.9
abdominal 441.4
dissecting 441.02
ruptured 441.3
syphilitic 093.0
arch 441.2
ruptured 441.1
arteriosclerotic NEC 441.9
ruptured 441.5
ascending 441.2
ruptured 441.1
congenital 747.29
descending 441.9
abdominal 441.4
ruptured 441.3
ruptured 441.5
thoracic 441.2
ruptured 441.1
dissecting 441.00
abdominal 441.02
thoracic 441.01
thoracoabdominal 441.03
due to coarctation (aorta) 747.10
ruptured 441.5
sinus, right 747.29
syphilitic 093.0
thoracoabdominal 441.7
ruptured 441.6
thorax, thoracic (arch) (nonsyphilitic) 441.2
dissecting 441.01
ruptured 441.1
syphilitic 093.0
transverse 441.2
ruptured 441.1
valve (heart) (*see also* Endocarditis, aortic) 424.1
arteriosclerotic NEC 442.9
cerebral 437.3
ruptured (*see also* Hemorrhage, subarachnoid) 430
arteriovenous (congenital) (peripheral) NEC (*see also* Anomaly, arteriovenous) 747.60
acquired NEC 447.0
brain 437.3
ruptured (*see also* Hemorrhage, subarachnoid) 430
coronary 414.11
pulmonary 417.0
brain (cerebral) 747.81
ruptured (*see also* Hemorrhage, subarachnoid) 430
coronary 746.85
pulmonary 747.3
retina 743.58
specified site NEC 747.89
acquired 447.0
traumatic (*see also* Injury, blood vessel, by site) 904.9
basal - *see* Aneurysm, brain
berry (congenital) (ruptured) (*see also* Hemorrhage, subarachnoid) 430
brain 437.3
arteriosclerotic 437.3
ruptured (*see also* Hemorrhage, subarachnoid) 430
arteriovenous 747.81
acquired 437.3
ruptured (*see also* Hemorrhage, subarachnoid) 430
ruptured (*see also* Hemorrhage, subarachnoid) 430
berry (congenital) (ruptured) (*see also* Hemorrhage, subarachnoid) 430
congenital 747.81
ruptured (*see also* Hemorrhage, subarachnoid) 430

- **Aneurysm** - *continued*
  - brain - *continued*
    - meninges 437.3
      - ruptured (*see also* Hemorrhage, subarachnoid) 430
    - miliary (congenital) (ruptured) (*see also* Hemorrhage, subarachnoid) 430
    - mycotic 421.0
      - ruptured (*see also* Hemorrhage, subarachnoid) 430
    - nonruptured 437.3
    - ruptured (*see also* Hemorrhage, subarachnoid) 430
      - syphilitic 094.87
    - syphilitic (hemorrhage) 094.87
    - traumatic - *see* Injury, intracranial
  - cardiac (false) (*see also* Aneurysm, heart) 414.10
  - carotid artery (common) (external) 442.81
    - internal (intracranial portion) 437.3
      - extracranial portion 442.81
      - ruptured into brain (*see also* Hemorrhage, subarachnoid) 430
    - syphilitic 093.89
      - intracranial 094.87
  - cavernous sinus (*see also* Aneurysm, brain) 437.3
    - arteriovenous 747.81
      - ruptured (*see also* Hemorrhage, subarachnoid) 430
    - congenital 747.81
      - ruptured (*see also* Hemorrhage, subarachnoid) 430
  - celiac 442.84
  - central nervous system, syphilitic 094.89
  - cerebral - *see* Aneurysm, brain
  - chest - *see* Aneurysm, thorax
  - circle of Willis (*see also* Aneurysm, brain) 437.3
    - congenital 747.81
      - ruptured (*see also* Hemorrhage, subarachnoid) 430
    - ruptured (*see also* Hemorrhage, subarachnoid) 430
  - common iliac artery 442.2
  - congenital (peripheral) NEC 747.60
    - brain 747.81
      - ruptured (*see also* Hemorrhage, subarachnoid) 430
    - cerebral - *see* Aneurysm, brain, congenital
    - coronary 746.85
    - gastrointestinal 747.61
    - lower limb 747.64
    - pulmonary 747.3
    - renal 747.62
    - retina 743.58
    - specified site NEC 747.89
    - spinal 747.82
    - upper limb 747.63
  - conjunctiva 372.74
  - conus arteriosus (*see also* Aneurysm, heart) 414.10
  - coronary (arteriosclerotic) (artery) (vein) (*see also* Aneurysm, heart) 414.11
    - arteriovenous 746.85
    - congenital 746.85
    - syphilitic 093.89
  - cylindrical 441.9
    - ruptured 441.5
    - syphilitic 093.9
  - dissecting 442.9
    - aorta 441.00
      - abdominal 441.02
      - thoracic 441.01
      - thoracoabdominal 441.03
    - syphilitic 093.9
  - ductus arteriosus 747.0
  - embolic - *see* Embolism, artery
  - endocardial, infective (any valve) 421.0
  - femoral 442.3
  - gastroduodenal 442.84

- **Aneurysm** - *continued*
  - gastroepiploic 442.84
  - heart (chronic or with a stated duration of over 8 weeks) (infectional) (wall) 414.10
    - acute or with a stated duration of 8 weeks or less (*see also* Infarct, myocardium) 410.9 5th
    - congenital 746.89
    - valve - *see* Endocarditis
  - hepatic 442.84
  - iliac (common) 442.2
  - infective (any valve) 421.0
  - innominate (nonsyphilitic) 442.89
    - syphilitic 093.89
  - interauricular septum (*see also* Aneurysm, heart) 414.10
  - interventricular septum (*see also* Aneurysm, heart) 414.10
  - intracranial - *see* Aneurysm, brain
  - intrathoracic (nonsyphilitic) 441.2
    - ruptured 441.1
    - syphilitic 093.0
  - jugular vein 453.89 ▲
  - lower extremity 442.3
  - lung (pulmonary artery) 417.1
  - malignant 093.9
  - mediastinal (nonsyphilitic) 442.89
    - syphilitic 093.89
  - miliary (congenital) (ruptured) (*see also* Hemorrhage, subarachnoid) 430
  - mitral (heart) (valve) 424.0
  - mural (arteriovenous) (heart) (*see also* Aneurysm, heart) 414.10
  - mycotic, any site 421.0
    - without endocarditis - *see* Aneurysm, by site
    - ruptured, brain (*see also* Hemorrhage, subarachnoid) 430
  - myocardium (*see also* Aneurysm, heart) 414.10
  - neck 442.81
  - pancreaticoduodenal 442.84
  - patent ductus arteriosus 747.0
  - peripheral NEC 442.89
    - congenital NEC (*see also* Aneurysm, congenital) 747.60
  - popliteal 442.3
  - pulmonary 417.1
    - arteriovenous 747.3
      - acquired 417.0
    - syphilitic 093.89
    - valve (heart) (*see also* Endocarditis, pulmonary) 424.3
  - racemose 442.9
    - congenital (peripheral) NEC 747.60
  - radial 442.0
  - Rasmussen's (*see also* Tuberculosis) 011.2 5th
  - renal 442.1
  - retinal (acquired) 362.17
    - congenital 743.58
    - diabetic 250.5 5th *[362.01]*
      - due to secondary diabetes 249.5 5th *[362.01]*
  - sinus, aortic (of Valsalva) 747.29
  - specified site NEC 442.89
  - spinal (cord) 442.89
    - congenital 747.82
    - syphilitic (hemorrhage) 094.89
  - spleen, splenic 442.83
  - subclavian 442.82
    - syphilitic 093.89
  - superior mesenteric 442.84
  - syphilitic 093.9
    - aorta 093.0
    - central nervous system 094.89
    - congenital 090.5
    - spine, spinal 094.89
  - thoracoabdominal 441.7
    - ruptured 441.6
  - thorax, thoracic (arch) (nonsyphilitic) 441.2
    - dissecting 441.01

- **Aneurysm** - *continued*
  - thorax, thoracic - *continued*
    - ruptured 441.1
    - syphilitic 093.0
  - traumatic (complication) (early) - *see* Injury, blood vessel, by site
  - tricuspid (heart) (valve) - *see* Endocarditis, tricuspid
  - ulnar 442.0
  - upper extremity 442.0
  - valve, valvular - *see* Endocarditis
  - venous 456.8
    - congenital NEC (*see also* Aneurysm, congenital) 747.60
  - ventricle (arteriovenous) (*see also* Aneurysm, heart) 414.10
  - visceral artery NEC 442.84
- **Angiectasis** 459.89
- **Angiectopia** 459.9
- **Angiitis** 447.6
  - allergic granulomatous 446.4
  - hypersensitivity 446.20
    - Goodpasture's syndrome 446.21
    - specified NEC 446.29
  - necrotizing 446.0
  - Wegener's (necrotizing respiratory granulomatosis) 446.4
- **Angina** (attack) (cardiac) (chest) (effort) (heart) (pectoris) (syndrome) (vasomotor) 413.9
  - abdominal 557.1
  - accelerated 411.1
  - agranulocytic 288.03
  - aphthous 074.0
  - catarrhal 462
  - crescendo 411.1
  - croupous 464.4
  - cruris 443.9
    - due to atherosclerosis NEC (*see also* Arteriosclerosis, extremities) 440.20
  - decubitus 413.0
  - diphtheritic (membranous) 032.0
  - erysipelatous 034.0
  - erythematous 462
  - equivalent 413.9 ●
  - exudative, chronic 476.0
  - faucium 478.29
  - gangrenous 462
    - diphtheritic 032.0
  - infectious 462
  - initial 411.1
  - intestinal 557.1
  - ludovici 528.3
  - Ludwig's 528.3
  - malignant 462
    - diphtheritic 032.0
  - membranous 464.4
    - diphtheritic 032.0
  - mesenteric 557.1
  - monocytic 075
  - nocturnal 413.0
  - phlegmonous 475
    - diphtheritic 032.0
  - preinfarctional 411.1
  - Prinzmetal's 413.1
  - progressive 411.1
  - pseudomembranous 101
  - psychogenic 306.2
  - pultaceous, diphtheritic 032.0
  - scarlatinal 034.1
  - septic 034.0
  - simple 462
  - stable NEC 413.9
  - staphylococcal 462
  - streptococcal 034.0
  - stridulous, diphtheritic 032.3
  - syphilitic 093.9
    - congenital 090.5
  - tonsil 475
  - trachealis 464.4
  - unstable 411.1
  - variant 413.1
  - Vincent's 101

- **Angioblastoma** (M9161/1) - *see* Neoplasm, connective tissue, uncertain behavior
- **Angiocholecystitis** (*see also* Cholecystitis, acute) 575.0
- **Angiocholitis** (*see also* Cholecystitis, acute) 576.1
- **Angiodysgensis spinalis** 336.1
- **Angiodysplasia** (intestinalis) (intestine) 569.84
  - with hemorrhage 569.85
  - duodenum 537.82
    - with hemorrhage 537.83
  - stomach 537.82
    - with hemorrhage 537.83
- **Angioedema** (allergic) (any site) (with urticaria) 995.1
  - hereditary 277.6
- **Angioendothelioma** (M9130/1) - *see also* Neoplasm, by site, uncertain behavior
  - benign (M9130/0) (*see also* Hemangioma, by site) 228.00
  - bone (M9260/3) - *see* Neoplasm, bone, malignant
  - Ewing's (M9260/3) - *see* Neoplasm, bone, malignant
  - nervous system (M9130/0) 228.09
- **Angiofibroma** (M9160/0) - *see also* Neoplasm, by site, benign
  - juvenile (M9160/0) 210.7
    - specified site - *see* Neoplasm, by site, benign
    - unspecified site 210.7
- **Angiohemophilia** (A) (B) 286.4
- **Angioid streaks** (choroid) (retina) 363.43
- **Angiokeratoma** (M9141/0) - *see also* Neoplasm, skin, benign
  - corporis diffusum 272.7
- **Angiokeratosis**
  - diffuse 272.7
- **Angioleiomyoma** (M8894/0) - *see* Neoplasm, connective tissue, benign
- **Angioleucitis** 683
- **Angiolipoma** (M8861/0) (*see also* Lipoma, by site) 214.9
  - infiltrating (M8861/1) - *see* Neoplasm, connective tissue, uncertain behavior
- **Angioma** (M9120/0) (*see also* Hemangioma, by site) 228.00
  - capillary 448.1
  - hemorrhagicum hereditaria 448.0
  - malignant (M9120/3) - *see* Neoplasm, connective tissue, malignant
  - pigmentosum et atrophicum 757.33
  - placenta - *see* Placenta, abnormal
  - plexiform (M9131/0) - *see* Hemangioma, by site
  - senile 448.1
  - serpiginosum 709.1
  - spider 448.1
  - stellate 448.1
- **Angiomatosis** 757.32
  - bacillary 083.8
  - corporis diffusum universale 272.7
  - cutaneocerebral 759.6
  - encephalocutaneous 759.6
  - encephalofacial 759.6
  - encephalotrigeminal 759.6
  - hemorrhagic familial 448.0
  - hereditary familial 448.0
  - heredofamilial 448.0
  - meningo-oculofacial 759.6
  - multiple sites 228.09
  - neuro-oculocutaneous 759.6
  - retina (Hippel's disease) 759.6
  - retinocerebellosa 759.6
  - retinocerebral 759.6
  - systemic 228.09
- **Angiomyolipoma** (M8860/0)
  - specified site - *see* Neoplasm, connective tissue, benign
  - unspecified site 223.0

Aneurysm – Angiomyolipoma

- **Angiomyoliposarcoma** (M8860/3) - *see* Neoplasm, connective tissue, malignant
- **Angiomyoma** (M8894/0) - *see* Neoplasm, connective tissue, benign
- **Angiomyosarcoma** (M8894/3) - *see* Neoplasm, connective tissue, malignant
- **Angioneurosis** 306.2
- **Angioneurotic edema** (allergic) (any site) (with urticaria) 995.1
  - hereditary 277.6
- **Angiopathia, angiopathy** 459.9
  - diabetic (peripheral) 250.7 5th *[443.81]*
    - due to secondary diabetes 249.7 5th *[443.81]*
  - peripheral 443.9
    - diabetic 250.7 5th *[443.81]*
      - due to secondary diabetes 249.7 5th *[443.81]*
    - specified type NEC 443.89
  - retinae syphilitica 093.89
  - retinalis (juvenilis) 362.18
    - background 362.10
    - diabetic 250.5 5th *[362.01]*
      - due to secondary diabetes 249.5 5th *[362.01]*
    - proliferative 362.29
    - tuberculous (*see also* Tuberculosis) 017.3 5th *[362.18]*
- **Angiosarcoma** (M9120/3) - *see* Neoplasm, connective tissue, malignant
- **Angiosclerosis** - *see* Arteriosclerosis
- **Angioscotoma, enlarged** 368.42
- **Angiospasm** 443.9
  - brachial plexus 353.0
  - cerebral 435.9
  - cervical plexus 353.2
  - nerve
    - arm 354.9
      - axillary 353.0
      - median 354.1
      - ulnar 354.2
    - autonomic (*see also* Neuropathy, peripheral, autonomic) 337.9
    - axillary 353.0
    - leg 355.8
      - plantar 355.6
    - lower extremity - *see* Angiospasm, nerve, leg
    - median 354.1
    - peripheral NEC 355.9
    - spinal NEC 355.9
    - sympathetic (*see also* Neuropathy, peripheral, autonomic) 337.9
    - ulnar 354.2
    - upper extremity - *see* Angiospasm, nerve, arm
  - peripheral NEC 443.9
  - traumatic 443.9
    - foot 443.9
    - leg 443.9
  - vessel 443.9
- **Angiospastic disease or edema** 443.9
- **Angle's**
  - class I 524.21
  - class II 524.22
  - class III 524.23
- **Anguillulosis** 127.2
- **Angulation**
  - cecum (*see also* Obstruction, intestine) 560.9
  - coccyx (acquired) 738.6
    - congenital 756.19
  - femur (acquired) 736.39
    - congenital 755.69
  - intestine (large) (small) (*see also* Obstruction, intestine) 560.9
  - sacrum (acquired) 738.5
    - congenital 756.19
  - sigmoid (flexure) (*see also* Obstruction, intestine) 560.9
  - spine (*see also* Curvature, spine) 737.9
- **Angulation** – *continued*
  - tibia (acquired) 736.89
    - congenital 755.69
  - ureter 593.3
  - wrist (acquired) 736.09
    - congenital 755.59
- **Angulus infectiosus** 686.8
- **Anhedonia** 780.99
- **Anhidrosis** (lid) (neurogenic) (thermogenic) 705.0
- **Anhydration** 276.51
  - with
    - hypernatremia 276.0
    - hyponatremia 276.1
- **Anhydremia** 276.52
  - with
    - hypernatremia 276.0
    - hyponatremia 276.1
- **Anidrosis** 705.0
- **Aniridia** (congenital) 743.45
- **Anisakiasis** (infection) (infestation) 127.1
- **Anisakis larva infestation** 127.1
- **Aniseikonia** 367.32
- **Anisocoria** (pupil) 379.41
  - congenital 743.46
- **Anisocytosis** 790.09
- **Anisometropia** (congenital) 367.31
- **Ankle** - *see* condition
- **Ankyloblepharon** (acquired) (eyelid) 374.46
  - filiforme (adnatum) (congenital) 743.62
  - total 743.62
- **Ankylodactly** (*see also* Syndactylism) 755.10
- **Ankyloglossia** 750.0
- **Ankylosis** (fibrous) (osseous) 718.50
  - ankle 718.57
  - any joint, produced by surgical fusion V45.4
  - cricoarytenoid (cartilage) (joint) (larynx) 478.79
  - dental 521.6
  - ear ossicle NEC 385.22
    - malleus 385.21
  - elbow 718.52
  - finger 718.54
  - hip 718.55
  - incostapedial joint (infectional) 385.22
  - joint, produced by surgical fusion NEC V45.4
  - knee 718.56
  - lumbosacral (joint) 724.6
  - malleus 385.21
  - multiple sites 718.59
  - postoperative (status) V45.4
  - sacroiliac (joint) 724.6
  - shoulder 718.51
  - specified site NEC 718.58
  - spine NEC 724.9
  - surgical V45.4
  - teeth, tooth (hard tissues) 521.6
  - temporomandibular joint 524.61
  - wrist 718.53
- **Ankylostoma** - *see* Ancylostoma
- **Ankylostomiasis** (intestinal) - *see* Ancylostomiasis
- **Ankylurethria** (*see also* Stricture, urethra) 598.9
- **Annular** - *see also* condition
  - detachment, cervix 622.8
  - organ or site, congenital NEC - *see* Distortion
  - pancreas (congenital) 751.7
- **Anodontia** (complete) (partial) (vera) 520.0
  - with abnormal spacing 524.30
  - acquired 525.10
    - causing malocclusion 524.30
    - due to
      - caries 525.13
      - extraction 525.10
      - periodontal disease 525.12
      - trauma 525.11
- **Anomaly, anomalous** (congenital) (unspecified type) 759.9
  - abdomen 759.9
  - abdominal wall 756.70
- **Anomaly, anomalous** – *continued*
  - acoustic nerve 742.9
  - adrenal (gland) 759.1
  - Alder (-Reilly) (leukocyte granulation) 288.2
  - alimentary tract 751.9
    - lower 751.5
    - specified type NEC 751.8
    - upper (any part, except tongue) 750.9
      - tongue 750.10
        - specified type NEC 750.19
  - alveolar 524.70
    - ridge (process) 525.8
    - specified NEC 524.79
  - ankle (joint) 755.69
  - anus, anal (canal) 751.5
  - aorta, aortic 747.20
    - arch 747.21
    - coarctation (postductal) (preductal) 747.10
    - cusp or valve NEC 746.9
    - septum 745.0
    - specified type NEC 747.29
  - aorticopulmonary septum 745.0
  - apertures, diaphragm 756.6
  - appendix 751.5
  - aqueduct of Sylvius 742.3
    - with spina bifida (*see also* Spina bifida) 741.0 5th
  - arm 755.50
    - reduction (*see also* Deformity, reduction, upper limb) 755.20
  - arteriovenous (congenital) (peripheral) NEC 747.60
    - brain 747.81
    - cerebral 747.81
    - coronary 746.85
    - gastrointestinal 747.61
      - acquired - *see* Angiodysplasia
    - lower limb 747.64
    - renal 747.62
    - specified site NEC 747.69
    - spinal 747.82
    - upper limb 747.63
  - artery (*see also* Anomaly, peripheral vascular system) NEC 747.60
    - brain 747.81
    - cerebral 747.81
    - coronary 746.85
    - eye 743.9
    - pulmonary 747.3
    - renal 747.62
    - retina 743.9
    - umbilical 747.5
  - arytenoepiglottic folds 748.3
  - atrial
    - bands 746.9
    - folds 746.9
    - septa 745.5
  - atrioventricular
    - canal 745.69
    - common 745.69
    - conduction 426.7
    - excitation 426.7
    - septum 745.4
  - atrium - *see* Anomaly, atrial
  - auditory canal 744.3
    - specified type NEC 744.29
      - with hearing impairment 744.02
  - auricle
    - ear 744.3
      - causing impairment of hearing 744.02
    - heart 746.9
      - septum 745.5
  - autosomes, autosomal NEC 758.5
  - Axenfeld's 743.44
  - back 759.9
  - band
    - atrial 746.9
    - heart 746.9
    - ventricular 746.9
  - Bartholin's duct 750.9
- **Anomaly, anomalous** – *continued*
  - biliary duct or passage 751.60
    - atresia 751.61
  - bladder (neck) (sphincter) (trigone) 753.9
    - specified type NEC 753.8
  - blood vessel 747.9
    - artery - *see* Anomaly, artery
    - peripheral vascular - *see* Anomaly, peripheral vascular system
    - vein - *see* Anomaly, vein
  - bone NEC 756.9
    - ankle 755.69
    - arm 755.50
    - chest 756.3
    - cranium 756.0
    - face 756.0
    - finger 755.50
    - foot 755.67
    - forearm 755.50
    - frontal 756.0
    - head 756.0
    - hip 755.63
    - leg 755.60
    - lumbosacral 756.10
    - nose 748.1
    - pelvic girdle 755.60
    - rachitic 756.4
    - rib 756.3
    - shoulder girdle 755.50
    - skull 756.0
      - with
        - anencephalus 740.0
        - encephalocele 742.0
        - hydrocephalus 742.3
          - with spina bifida (*see also* Spina bifida) 741.0 5th
        - microcephalus 742.1
    - toe 755.66
  - brain 742.9
    - multiple 742.4
    - reduction 742.2
    - specified type NEC 742.4
    - vessel 747.81
  - branchial cleft NEC 744.49
    - cyst 744.42
    - fistula 744.41
    - persistent 744.41
    - sinus (external) (internal) 744.41
  - breast 757.6 ▲
  - broad ligament 752.10
    - specified type NEC 752.19
  - bronchus 748.3
  - bulbar septum 745.0
  - bulbus cordis 745.9
    - persistent (in left ventricle) 745.8
  - bursa 756.9
  - canal of Nuck 752.9
  - canthus 743.9
  - capillary NEC (*see also* Anomaly, peripheral vascular system) 747.60
  - cardiac 746.9
    - septal closure 745.9
      - acquired 429.71
    - valve NEC 746.9
      - pulmonary 746.00
      - specified type NEC 746.89
  - cardiovascular system 746.9
    - complicating pregnancy, childbirth, or puerperium 648.5 5th
  - carpus 755.50
  - cartilage, trachea 748.3
  - cartilaginous 756.9
  - caruncle, lacrimal, lachrymal 743.9
  - cascade stomach 750.7
  - cauda equina 742.59
  - cecum 751.5
  - cerebral - *see also* Anomaly, brain vessels 747.81
  - cerebrovascular system 747.81
  - cervix (uterus) 752.40
    - with doubling of vagina and uterus 752.2
    - in pregnancy or childbirth 654.6 5th
      - affecting fetus or newborn 763.89

Angiomyoliposarcoma – Anomaly, anomalous

Anomaly, anomalous

Anomaly, anomalous

Anomaly, anomalous – *continued*
  specified type NEC – *continued*
    bone(s) – *continued*
      skull 756.0
        with
          anencephalus 740.0
          encephalocele 742.0
          hydrocephalus 742.3
          with spina bifida (*see also* Spina bifida) 741.0 5th
          microcephalus 742.1
    brain 742.4
    breast 757.6
    broad ligament 752.19
    bronchus 748.3
    canal of Nuck 752.89
    cardiac septal closure 745.8
    carpus 755.59
    cartilaginous 756.9
    cecum 751.5
    cervix 752.49
    chest (wall) 756.3
    chin 744.89
    ciliary body 743.46
    circulatory system 747.89
    clavicle 755.51
    clitoris 752.49
    coccyx 756.19
    colon 751.5
    common duct 751.69
    connective tissue 756.89
    cricoid cartilage 748.3
    cystic duct 751.69
    diaphragm 756.6
    digestive organ(s) or tract 751.8
      lower 751.5
      upper 750.8
    duodenum 751.5
    ear 744.29
      auricle 744.29
        causing impairment of hearing 744.02
      causing impairment of hearing 744.09
      inner (causing impairment of hearing) 744.05
      middle, except ossicles 744.03
        ossicles 744.04
    ejaculatory duct 752.89
    endocrine 759.2
    epiglottis 748.3
    esophagus 750.4
    Eustachian tube 744.24
    eye 743.8
      lid 743.63
      muscle 743.69
    face 744.89
      bone(s) 756.0
    fallopian tube 752.19
    fascia 756.89
    femur 755.69
    fibula 755.69
    finger 755.59
    foot 755.67
    fovea centralis 743.55
    gallbladder 751.69
    Gartner's duct 752.89
    gastrointestinal tract 751.8
    genitalia, genital organ(s)
      female 752.89
        external 752.49
        internal NEC 752.89
      male 752.89
        penis 752.69
        scrotal transposition 752.81
    genitourinary tract NEC 752.89
    glottis 748.3
    hair 757.4
    hand 755.59
    heart 746.89
      valve NEC 746.89
        pulmonary 746.09
    hepatic duct 751.69
    hydatid of Morgagni 752.89

Anomaly, anomalous – *continued*
  specified type NEC – *continued*
    hymen 752.49
    integument 757.8
    intestine (large) (small) 751.5
      fixational type 751.4
    iris 743.46
    jejunum 751.5
    joint 755.8
    kidney 753.3
    knee 755.64
    labium (majus) (minus) 752.49
    labyrinth, membranous 744.05
    larynx 748.3
    leg 755.69
    lens 743.39
    limb, except reduction deformity 755.8
      lower 755.69
        reduction deformity (*see also* Deformity, reduction, lower limb) 755.30
      upper 755.59
        reduction deformity (*see also* Deformity, reduction, upper limb) 755.20
    lip 750.26
    liver 751.69
    lung (fissure) (lobe) 748.69
    meatus urinarius 753.8
    metacarpus 755.59
    mouth 750.26
    muscle 756.89
      eye 743.69
    musculoskeletal system, except limbs 756.9
    nail 757.5
    neck 744.89
    nerve 742.8
      acoustic 742.8
      optic 742.8
    nervous system 742.8
    nipple 757.6
    nose 748.1
    organ NEC 759.89
      of Corti 744.05
    osseous meatus (ear) 744.03
    ovary 752.0
    oviduct 752.19
    pancreas 751.7
    parathyroid 759.2
    patella 755.64
    pelvic girdle 755.69
    penis 752.69
    pericardium 746.89
    peripheral vascular system NEC (*see also* Anomaly, peripheral vascular system) 747.60
    pharynx 750.29
    pituitary 759.2
    prostate 752.89
    radius 755.59
    rectum 751.5
    respiratory system 748.8
    rib 756.3
    round ligament 752.89
    sacrum 756.19
    salivary duct or gland 750.26
    scapula 755.59
    sclera 743.47
    scrotum 752.89
      transposition 752.81
    seminal duct or tract 752.89
    shoulder girdle 755.59
    site NEC 759.89
    skin 757.39
    skull (bone(s)) 756.0
      with
        anencephalus 740.0
        encephalocele 742.0
        hydrocephalus 742.3
          with spina bifida (*see also* Spina bifida) 741.0 5th
        microcephalus 742.1
    specified organ or site NEC 759.89

Anomaly, anomalous – *continued*
  specified type NEC – *continued*
    spermatic cord 752.89
    spinal cord 742.59
    spine 756.19
    spleen 759.0
    sternum 756.3
    stomach 750.7
    tarsus 755.67
    tendon 756.89
    testis 752.89
    thorax (wall) 756.3
    thymus 759.2
    thyroid (gland) 759.2
      cartilage 748.3
    tibia 755.69
    toe 755.66
    tongue 750.19
    trachea (cartilage) 748.3
    ulna 755.59
    urachus 753.7
    ureter 753.4
      obstructive 753.29
    urethra 753.8
      obstructive 753.6
    urinary tract 753.8
    uterus 752.3
    uvula 750.26
    vagina 752.49
    vascular NEC (*see also* Anomaly, peripheral vascular system) 747.60
      brain 747.81
    vas deferens 752.89
    vein(s) (peripheral) NEC (*see also* Anomaly, peripheral vascular system) 747.60
      brain 747.81
      great 747.49
      portal 747.49
      pulmonary 747.49
    vena cava (inferior) (superior) 747.49
    vertebra 756.19
    vulva 752.49
  spermatic cord 752.9
  spine, spinal 756.10
    column 756.10
    cord 742.9
      meningocele (*see also* Spina bifida) 741.9 5th
      specified type NEC 742.59
      spina bifida (*see also* Spina bifida) 741.9 5th
      vessel 747.82
    meninges 742.59
    nerve root 742.9
  spleen 759.0
  Sprengel's 755.52
  sternum 756.3
  stomach 750.9
    specified type NEC 750.7
  submaxillary gland 750.9
  superior vena cava 747.40
  talipes - *see* Talipes
  tarsus 755.67
    with complete absence of distal elements 755.31
  teeth, tooth NEC 520.9
    position 524.30
      crowding 524.31
      displacement 524.30
        horizontal 524.33
        vertical 524.34
      distance
        interocclusal
          excessive 524.37
          insufficient 524.36
      excessive spacing 524.32
      rotation 524.35
      specified NEC 524.39
    spacing 524.30
  tendon 756.9
    specified type NEC 756.89

Anomaly, anomalous – *continued*
  termination
    coronary artery 746.85
  testis 752.9
  thebesian valve 746.9
  thigh 755.60
    flexion (*see also* Subluxation, congenital, hip) 754.32
  thorax (wall) 756.3
  throat 750.9
  thumb 755.50
    supernumerary 755.01
  thymus gland 759.2
  thyroid (gland) 759.2
    cartilage 748.3
  tibia 755.60
    saber 090.5
  toe 755.66
    supernumerary 755.02
    webbed (*see also* Syndactylism, toes) 755.13
  tongue 750.10
    specified type NEC 750.19
  trachea, tracheal 748.3
    cartilage 748.3
    rings 748.3
  tragus 744.3
  transverse aortic arch 747.21
  trichromata 368.59
  trichromatopsia 368.59
  tricuspid (leaflet) (valve) 746.9
    atresia 746.1
    Ebstein's 746.2
    specified type NEC 746.89
    stenosis 746.1
  trunk 759.9
  Uhl's (hypoplasia of myocardium, right ventricle) 746.84
  ulna 755.50
  umbilicus 759.9
    artery 747.5
  union, trachea with larynx 748.3
  unspecified site 759.9
  upper extremity 755.50
    vessel 747.63
  urachus 753.7
    specified type NEC 753.7
  ureter 753.9
    obstructive 753.20
    specified type NEC 753.4
      obstructive 753.29
  urethra (valve) 753.9
    obstructive 753.6
    specified type NEC 753.8
  urinary tract or system (any part, except urachus) 753.9
    specified type NEC 753.8
    urachus 753.7
  uterus 752.3
    with only one functioning horn 752.3
    in pregnancy or childbirth 654.0 5th
      affecting fetus or newborn 763.89
      causing obstructed labor 660.2 5th
        affecting fetus or newborn 763.1
  uvula 750.9
  vagina 752.40
  valleculae 748.3
  valve (heart) NEC 746.9
    formation, ureter 753.29
    pulmonary 746.00
    specified type NEC 746.89
  vascular NEC (*see also* Anomaly, peripheral vascular system) 747.60
    ring 747.21
  vas deferens 752.9
  vein(s) (peripheral) NEC (*see also* Anomaly, peripheral vascular system) 747.60
    brain 747.81
    cerebral 747.81
    coronary 746.89
    great 747.40
      specified type NEC 747.49
    portal 747.40

Anomaly, anomalous

Anomaly, anomalous – *continued*
- vein(s) – *continued*
  - pulmonary 747.40
  - retina 743.9
- vena cava (inferior) (superior) 747.40
- venous - *see* Anomaly, vein
- venous return (pulmonary) 747.49
  - partial 747.42
  - total 747.41
- ventricle, ventricular (heart) 746.9
  - bands 746.9
  - folds 746.9
  - septa 745.4
- vertebra 756.10
- vesicourethral orifice 753.9
- vessels NEC (*see also* Anomaly, peripheral vascular system) 747.60
  - optic papilla 743.9
- vitelline duct 751.0
- vitreous humor 743.9
  - specified type NEC 743.51
- vulva 752.40
- wrist (joint) 755.50

Anomia 784.69

Anonychia 757.5
- acquired 703.8

Anophthalmos, anophthalmus (clinical) (congenital) (globe) 743.00
- acquired V45.78

Anopsia (altitudinal) (quadrant) 368.46

Anorchia 752.89

Anorchism, anorchidism 752.89

Anorexia 783.0
- hysterical 300.11
- nervosa 307.1

Anosmia (*see also* Disturbance, sensation) 781.1
- hysterical 300.11
- postinfectional 478.9
- psychogenic 306.7
- traumatic 951.8

Anosognosia 780.99

Anosphrasia 781.1

Anosteoplasia 756.50

Anotia 744.09

Anovulatory cycle 628.0

Anoxemia 799.02
- newborn 770.88

Anoxia 799.02
- altitude 993.2
- cerebral 348.1
  - with
    - abortion - *see* Abortion, by type, with specified complication NEC
    - ectopic pregnancy (*see also* categories 633.0-633.9) 639.8
    - molar pregnancy (*see also* categories 630-632) 639.8
  - complicating
    - delivery (cesarean) (instrumental) 669.4 5th
    - ectopic or molar pregnancy 639.8
    - obstetric anesthesia or sedation 668.2 5th
  - during or resulting from a procedure 997.01
  - following
    - abortion 639.8
    - ectopic or molar pregnancy 639.8
  - newborn (*see also* Distress, fetal, liveborn infant) 770.88
- due to drowning 994.1
- fetal, affecting newborn 770.88
- heart - *see* Insufficiency, coronary
- high altitude 993.2
- intrauterine
  - fetal death (before onset of labor) 768.0
    - during labor 768.1
  - liveborn infant - *see* Distress, fetal, liveborn infant
- myocardial - *see* Insufficiency, coronary
- newborn 768.9
  - mild or moderate 768.6

Anoxia – *continued*
- newborn – *continued*
  - severe 768.5
- pathological 799.02

Anteflexion - *see* Anteversion

Antenatal
- care, normal pregnancy V22.1
  - first V22.0
- sampling
  - chorionic villus V28.89
- screening of mother (for) V28.9
  - based on amniocentesis NEC V28.2
    - chromosomal anomalies V28.0
    - raised alphafetoprotein levels V28.1
  - chromosomal anomalies V28.0
  - fetal growth retardation using ultrasonics V28.4
  - genomic V28.89
  - isoimmunization V28.5
  - malformations using ultrasonics V28.3
  - proteomic V28.89
  - raised alphafetoprotein levels in amniotic fluid V28.1
  - risk
    - pre-term labor V28.82
  - specified condition NEC V28.89
  - Streptococcus B V28.6
- survey
  - fetal anatomic V28.81
- testing
  - nuchal translucency V28.89

Antepartum - *see* condition

Anterior - *see also* condition
- spinal artery compression syndrome 721.1

Antero-occlusion 524.24

Anteversion
- cervix - *see* Anteversion, uterus
- femur (neck), congenital 755.63
- uterus, uterine (cervix) (postinfectional) (postpartal, old) 621.6
  - congenital 752.3
  - in pregnancy or childbirth 654.4 5th
    - affecting fetus or newborn 763.89
    - causing obstructed labor 660.2 5th
      - affecting fetus or newborn 763.1

Anthracosilicosis (occupational) 500

Anthracosis (lung) (occupational) 500
- lingua 529.3

Anthrax 022.9
- with pneumonia 022.1 *[484.5]*
- colitis 022.2
- cutaneous 022.0
- gastrointestinal 022.2
- intestinal 022.2
- pulmonary 022.1
- respiratory 022.1
- septicemia 022.3
- specified manifestation NEC 022.8

Anthropoid pelvis 755.69
- with disproportion (fetopelvic) 653.2 5th
  - affecting fetus or newborn 763.1
  - causing obstructed labor 660.1 5th
    - affecting fetus or newborn 763.1

Anthropophobia 300.29

Antibioma, breast 611.0

Antibodies
- maternal (blood group) (*see also* Incompatibility) 656.2 5th
  - anti-D, cord blood 656.1 5th
    - fetus or newborn 773.0

Antibody deficiency syndrome
- agammaglobulinemic 279.00
- congenital 279.04
- hypogammaglobulinemic 279.00

Anticoagulant, intrinsic, circulating, causing hemorrhagic disorder (*see also* Circulating anticoagulants) 286.5 ▲

Antimongolism syndrome 758.39

Antimonial cholera 985.4

Antisocial personality 301.7

Antithrombinemia (*see also* Circulating anticoagulants) 286.5

Antithromboplastinemia (*see also* Circulating anticoagulants) 286.5

Antithromboplastinogenemia (*see also* Circulating anticoagulants) 286.5

Antitoxin complication or reaction - *see* Complications, vaccination

Anton (-Babinski) syndrome (hemiasomatognosia) 307.9

Antritis (chronic) 473.0
- maxilla 473.0
  - acute 461.0
- stomach 535.4 5th

Antrum, antral - *see* condition

Anuria 788.5
- with
  - abortion - *see* Abortion, by type, with renal failure
  - ectopic pregnancy (*see also* categories 633.0-633.9) 639.3
  - molar pregnancy (*see also* categories 630-632) 639.3
- calculus (impacted) (recurrent) 592.9
  - kidney 592.0
  - ureter 592.1
- congenital 753.3
- due to a procedure 997.5
- following
  - abortion 639.3
  - ectopic or molar pregnancy 639.3
- newborn 753.3
- postrenal 593.4
- puerperal, postpartum, childbirth 669.3 5th
- specified as due to a procedure 997.5
- sulfonamide
  - correct substance properly administered 788.5
  - overdose or wrong substance given or taken 961.0
- traumatic (following crushing) 958.5

Anus, anal - *see also* condition
- high risk human papillomavirus (HPV) DNA test positive 796.75
- low risk human papillomavirus (HPV) DNA test positive 796.79

Anusitis 569.49

Anxiety (neurosis) (reaction) (state) 300.00
- alcohol-induced 291.89
- depression 300.4
- drug-induced 292.89
- due to or associated with physical condition 293.84
- generalized 300.02
- hysteria 300.20
- in
  - acute stress reaction 308.0
  - transient adjustment reaction 309.24
- panic type 300.01
- separation, abnormal 309.21
- syndrome (organic) (transient) 293.84

Aorta, aortic - *see* condition

Aortectasia 441.9

Aortitis (nonsyphilitic) 447.6
- arteriosclerotic 440.0
- calcific 447.6
- Döhle-Heller 093.1
- luetic 093.1rheumatic (*see also* Endocarditis, acute, rheumatic) 391.1
- rheumatoid - *see* Arthritis, rheumatoid
- specific 093.1
- syphilitic 093.1
  - congenital 090.5

Apathetic ~~**thyroid storm** (*see also* Thyrotoxicosis) 242.9~~ 799.25 ▲
- thyroid storm (*see also* Thyrotoxicosis) 242.9 5th ●

Apathy 799.25 ●

Apepsia 536.8
- achlorhydric 536.0
- psychogenic 306.4

Aperistalsis, esophagus 530.0

Apert's syndrome (acrocephalosyndactyly) 755.55

Apert-Gallais syndrome (adrenogenital) 255.2

Apertognathia 524.20

Aphagia 787.20
- psychogenic 307.1

Aphakia (acquired) (bilateral) (postoperative) (unilateral) 379.31
- congenital 743.35

Aphalangia (congenital) 755.4
- lower limb (complete) (intercalary) (partial) (terminal) 755.39
  - meaning all digits (complete) (partial) 755.31
  - transverse 755.31
- upper limb (complete) (intercalary) (partial) (terminal) 755.29
  - meaning all digits (complete) (partial) 755.21
  - transverse 755.21

Aphasia (amnestic) (ataxic) (auditory) (Broca's) (choreatic) (classic) (expressive) (global) (ideational) (ideokinetic) (ideomotor) (jargon) (motor) (nominal) (receptive) (semantic) (sensory) (syntactic) (verbal) (visual) (Wernicke's) 784.3
- developmental 315.31
- syphilis, tertiary 094.89
- uremic - *see* Uremia

Aphemia 784.3
- uremic - *see* Uremia

Aphonia 784.41
- clericorum 784.49
- hysterical 300.11
- organic 784.41
- psychogenic 306.1

Aphthae, aphthous - *see also* condition
- Bednar's 528.2
- cachectic 529.0
- epizootic 078.4
- fever 078.4
- oral 528.2
- stomatitis 528.2
- thrush 112.0
- ulcer (oral) (recurrent) 528.2
  - genital organ(s) NEC
    - female 616.50
    - male 608.89
  - larynx 478.79

Apical - *see* condition

Apical ballooning syndrome 429.83

Aplasia - *see also* Agenesis
- alveolar process (acquired) 525.8
  - congenital 750.26
- aorta (congenital) 747.22
- aortic valve (congenital) 746.89
- axialis extracorticalis (congenital) 330.0
- bone marrow (myeloid) 284.9
  - acquired (secondary) 284.89
  - congenital 284.01
  - idiopathic 284.9
- brain 740.0
  - specified part 742.2
- breast 757.6
- bronchus 748.3
- cementum 520.4
- cerebellar 742.2
- congenital (pure) red cell 284.01
- corpus callosum 742.2
- erythrocyte 284.81
  - congenital 284.01
- extracortical axial 330.0
- eye (congenital) 743.00
- fovea centralis (congenital) 743.55
- germinal (cell) 606.0
- iris 743.45
- labyrinth, membranous 744.05
- limb (congenital) 755.4
  - lower NEC 755.30
  - upper NEC 755.20
- lung (bilateral) (congenital) (unilateral) 748.5
- nervous system NEC 742.8
- nuclear 742.8

Anomaly, anomalous – Aplasia

Aplasia – *continued*
- ovary 752.0
- Pelizaeus-Merzbacher 330.0
- prostate (congenital) 752.89
- red cell (with thymoma) (adult) 284.81
  - acquired (secondary) 284.81
  - congenital 284.01
  - hereditary 284.01
  - of infants 284.01
  - primary 284.01
  - pure 284.01
- round ligament (congenital) 752.89
- salivary gland 750.21
- skin (congenital) 757.39
- spinal cord 742.59
- spleen 759.0
- testis (congenital) 752.89
- thymic, with immunodeficiency 279.2
- thyroid 243
- uterus 752.3
- ventral horn cell 742.59

Apleuria 756.3

Apnea, apneic (spells) 786.03
- newborn, neonatorum 770.81
  - essential 770.81
  - obstructive 770.82
  - primary 770.81
  - sleep 770.81
  - specified NEC 770.82
- psychogenic 306.1
- sleep 780.57
  - with
    - hypersomnia, unspecified 780.53
    - hyposomnia, unspecified 780.51
    - insomnia, unspecified 780.51
    - sleep disturbance 780.57
  - central, in conditions classified elsewhere 327.27
  - obstructive (adult) (pediatric) 327.23
  - organic 327.20
    - other 327.29
  - primary central 327.21

Apneumatosis newborn 770.4

Apodia 755.31

Apophysitis (bone) (*see also* Osteochondrosis) 732.9
- calcaneus 732.5
- juvenile 732.6

Apoplectiform convulsions (*see also* Disease, cerebrovascular, acute) 436

Apoplexia, apoplexy, apoplectic (*see also* Disease, cerebrovascular, acute) 436
- abdominal 569.89
- adrenal 036.3
- attack 436
- basilar (*see also* Disease, cerebrovascular, acute) 436
- brain (*see also* Disease, cerebrovascular, acute) 436
- bulbar (*see also* Disease, cerebrovascular, acute) 436
- capillary (*see also* Disease, cerebrovascular, acute) 436
- cardiac (*see also* Infarct, myocardium) 410.9 [5th]
- cerebral (*see also* Disease, cerebrovascular, acute) 436
- chorea (*see also* Disease, cerebrovascular, acute) 436
- congestive (*see also* Disease, cerebrovascular, acute) 436
  - newborn 767.4
- embolic (*see also* Embolism, brain) 434.1 [5th]
- fetus 767.0
- fit (*see also* Disease, cerebrovascular, acute) 436
- healed or old V12.54
- heart (auricle) (ventricle) (*see also* Infarct, myocardium) 410.9 [5th]
- heat 992.0
- hemiplegia (*see also* Disease, cerebrovascular, acute) 436

Apoplexia, apoplexy, apoplectic – *continued*
- hemorrhagic (stroke) (*see also* Hemorrhage, brain) 432.9
- ingravescent (*see also* Disease, cerebrovascular, acute) 436
- late effect - *see* Late effect(s) (of) cerebrovascular disease
- lung - *see* Embolism, pulmonary
- meninges, hemorrhagic (*see also* Hemorrhage, subarachnoid) 430
- neonatorum 767.0
- newborn 767.0
- pancreatitis 577.0
- placenta 641.2 [5th]
- progressive (*see also* Disease, cerebrovascular, acute) 436
- pulmonary (artery) (vein) - *see* Embolism, pulmonary
- sanguineous (*see also* Disease, cerebrovascular, acute) 436
- seizure (*see also* Disease, cerebrovascular, acute) 436
- serous (*see also* Disease, cerebrovascular, acute) 436
- spleen 289.59
- stroke (*see also* Disease, cerebrovascular, acute) 436
- thrombotic (*see also* Thrombosis, brain) 434.0 [5th]
- uremic - *see* Uremia
- uteroplacental 641.2 [5th]

Appendage
- fallopian tube (cyst of Morgagni) 752.11
- intestine (epiploic) 751.5
- preauricular 744.1
- testicular (organ of Morgagni) 752.89

Appendicitis 541
- with
  - perforation, peritonitis (generalized), or rupture 540.0
    - with peritoneal abscess 540.1
  - peritoneal abscess 540.1
- acute (catarrhal) (fulminating) (gangrenous) (inflammatory) (obstructive) (retrocecal) (suppurative) 540.9
  - with
    - perforation, peritonitis, or rupture 540.0
      - with peritoneal abscess 540.1
    - peritoneal abscess 540.1
- amebic 006.8
- chronic (recurrent) 542
- exacerbation - *see* Appendicitis, acute
- fulminating - *see* Appendicitis, acute
- gangrenous - *see* Appendicitis, acute
- healed (obliterative) 542
- interval 542
- neurogenic 542
- obstructive 542
- pneumococcal 541
- recurrent 542
- relapsing 542
- retrocecal 541
- subacute (adhesive) 542
- subsiding 542
- suppurative - *see* Appendicitis, acute
- tuberculous (*see also* Tuberculosis) 014.8 [5th]

Appendiclausis 543.9

Appendicolithiasis 543.9

Appendicopathia oxyurica 127.4

Appendix, appendicular - *see also* condition
- Morgagni (male) 752.89
  - fallopian tube 752.11

Appetite
- depraved 307.52
- excessive 783.6
  - psychogenic 307.51
- lack or loss (*see also* Anorexia) 783.0
  - nonorganic origin 307.59
- perverted 307.52
  - hysterical 300.11

Apprehension, apprehensiveness (abnormal) (state) 300.00
- specified type NEC 300.09

Approximal wear 521.10

Apraxia (classic) (ideational) (ideokinetic) (ideomotor) (motor) 784.69
- oculomotor, congenital 379.51
- verbal 784.69

Aptyalism 527.7

Aqueous misdirection 365.83

Arabicum elephantiasis (*see also* Infestation, filarial) 125.9

Arachnidism 989.5

Arachnitis - *see* Meningitis

Arachnodactyly 759.82

Arachnoidism 989.5

Arachnoiditis (acute) (adhesive) (basic) (brain) (cerebrospinal) (chiasmal) (chronic) (spinal) (*see also* Meningitis) 322.9
- meningococcal (chronic) 036.0
- syphilitic 094.2
- tuberculous (*see also* Tuberculosis, meninges) 013.0 [5th]

Araneism 989.5

Arboencephalitis, Australian 062.4

Arborization block (heart) 426.6

Arbor virus, arbovirus (infection) NEC 066.9

ARC 042

Arches - *see* condition

Arcuatus uterus 752.3

Arcus (cornea)
- juvenilis 743.43
  - interfering with vision 743.42
- senilis 371.41

Arc-welders' lung 503

Arc-welders' syndrome (photokeratitis) 370.24

Areflexia 796.1

Areola - *see* condition

Argentaffinoma (M8241/1) - *see also* Neoplasm, by site, uncertain behavior
- benign (M8241/0) - *see* Neoplasm, by site, benign
- malignant (M8241/3) - *see* Neoplasm, by site, malignant
- syndrome 259.2

Argentinian hemorrhagic fever 078.7

Arginosuccinicaciduria 270.6

Argonz-Del Castillo syndrome (nonpuerperal galactorrhea and amenorrhea) 253.1

Argyll-Robertson phenomenon, pupil, or syndrome (syphilitic) 094.89
- atypical 379.45
- nonluetic 379.45
- nonsyphilitic 379.45
- reversed 379.45

Argyria, argyriasis NEC 985.8
- conjunctiva 372.55
- cornea 371.16
- from drug or medicinal agent
  - correct substance properly administered 709.09
  - overdose or wrong substance given or taken 961.2

Arhinencephaly 742.2

Arias-Stella phenomenon 621.30

Ariboflavinosis 266.0

Arizona enteritis 008.1

Arm - *see* condition

Armenian disease 277.31

Arnold-Chiari obstruction or syndrome (*see also* Spina bifida) 741.0 [5th]
- type I 348.4
- type II (*see also* Spina bifida) 741.0 [5th]
- type III 742.0
- type IV 742.2

Arousals
- confusional 327.41

Arrest, arrested
- active phase of labor 661.1 [5th]
  - affecting fetus or newborn 763.7

Arrest, arrested – *continued*
- any plane in pelvis
  - complicating delivery 660.1 [5th]
    - affecting fetus or newborn 763.1
- bone marrow (*see also* Anemia, aplastic) 284.9
- cardiac 427.5
  - with
    - abortion - *see* Abortion, by type, with specified complication NEC
    - ectopic pregnancy (*see also* categories 633.0-633.9) 639.8
    - molar pregnancy (*see also* categories 630-632) 639.8
  - complicating
    - anesthesia
      - correct substance properly administered 427.5
      - obstetric 668.1 [5th]
      - overdose or wrong substance given 968.4
        - specified anesthetic - *see* Table of Drugs and Chemicals
    - delivery (cesarean) (instrumental) 669.4 [5th]
    - ectopic or molar pregnancy 639.8
    - surgery (nontherapeutic) (therapeutic) 997.1
  - fetus or newborn 779.85
  - following
    - abortion 639.8
    - ectopic or molar pregnancy 639.8
  - personal history, successfully rescucitated V12.53
  - postoperative (immediate) 997.1
    - long-term effect of cardiac surgery 429.4
- cardiorespiratory (*see also* Arrest, cardiac) 427.5
- deep transverse 660.3 [5th]
  - affecting fetus or newborn 763.1
- development or growth
  - bone 733.91
  - child 783.40
  - fetus 764.9 [5th]
    - affecting management of pregnancy 656.5 [5th]
  - tracheal rings 748.3
- epiphyseal 733.91
- granulopoiesis 288.09
- heart - *see* Arrest, cardiac
- respiratory 799.1
  - newborn 770.87
- sinus 426.6
- transverse (deep) 660.3 [5th]
  - affecting fetus or newborn 763.1

Arrhenoblastoma (M8630/1)
- benign (M8630/0)
  - specified site - *see* Neoplasm, by site, benign
  - unspecified site
    - female 220
    - male 222.0
- malignant (M8630/3)
  - specified site - *see* Neoplasm, by site, malignant
  - unspecified site
    - female 183.0
    - male 186.9
- specified site - *see* Neoplasm, by site, uncertain behavior
- unspecified site
  - female 236.2
  - male 236.4

Arrhinencephaly 742.2
- due to
  - trisomy 13 (13-15) 758.1
  - trisomy 18 (16-18) 758.2

Arrhythmia (auricle) (cardiac) (cordis) (gallop rhythm) (juvenile) (nodal) (reflex) (sinus) (supraventricular) (transitory) (ventricle) 427.9
- bigeminal rhythm 427.89
- block 426.9
- bradycardia 427.89
- contractions, premature 427.60
- coronary sinus 427.89
- ectopic 427.89
- extrasystolic 427.60
- postoperative 997.1
- psychogenic 306.2
- vagal 780.2

Arrillaga-Ayerza syndrome (pulmonary artery sclerosis with pulmonary hypertension) 416.0

Arsenical
- dermatitis 692.4
- keratosis 692.4
- pigmentation 985.1
  - from drug or medicinal agent
    - correct substance properly administered 709.09
    - overdose or wrong substance given or taken 961.1

Arsenism 985.1
- from drug or medicinal agent
  - correct substance properly administered 692.4
  - overdose or wrong substance given or taken 961.1

Arterial - *see* condition

Arteriectasis 447.8

Arteriofibrosis - *see* Arteriosclerosis

Arteriolar sclerosis - *see* Arteriosclerosis

Arteriolith - *see* Arteriosclerosis

Arteriolitis 447.6
- necrotizing, kidney 447.5
- renal - *see* Hypertension, kidney

Arteriolosclerosis - *see* Arteriosclerosis

Arterionephrosclerosis (*see also* Hypertension, kidney) 403.90

Arteriopathy 447.9

Arteriosclerosis, arteriosclerotic (artery) (deformans) (diffuse) (disease) (endarteritis) (general) (obliterans) (obliterative) (occlusive) (senile) (with calcification) 440.9
- with
  - gangrene 440.24
  - psychosis (*see also* Psychosis, arteriosclerotic) 290.40
  - ulceration 440.23
- aorta 440.0
- arteries of extremities - *see* Arteriosclerosis, extremities
- basilar (artery) (*see also* Occlusion, artery, basilar) 433.0 5th
- brain 437.0
- bypass graft
  - coronary artery 414.05
    - autologous artery (gastroepiploic) (internal mammary) 414.04
    - autologous vein 414.02
    - nonautologous biological 414.03
    - of transplanted heart 414.07
  - extremity 440.30
    - autologous vein 440.31
    - nonautologous biological 440.32
- cardiac - *see* Arteriosclerosis, coronary
- cardiopathy - *see* Arteriosclerosis, coronary
- cardiorenal (*see also* Hypertension, cardiorenal) 404.90
- cardiovascular (*see also* Disease, cardiovascular) 429.2
- carotid (artery) (common) (internal) (*see also* Occlusion, artery, carotid) 433.1 5th
- central nervous system 437.0
- cerebral 437.0
  - late effect - *see* Late effect(s) (of) cerebrovascular disease

Arteriosclerosis, arteriosclerotic – *continued*
- cerebrospinal 437.0
- cerebrovascular 437.0
- coronary (artery) 414.00
  - due to lipid rich plaque 414.3
  - graft - *see* Arteriosclerosis, bypass graft
  - native artery 414.01
    - of transplanted heart 414.06
- extremities (native artery) NEC 440.20
  - bypass graft 440.30
    - autologous vein 440.31
    - nonautologous biological 440.32
  - claudication (intermittent) 440.21
    - and
      - gangrene 440.24
      - rest pain 440.22
        - and
          - gangrene 440.24
          - ulceration 440.23
            - and gangrene 440.24
      - ulceration 440.23
        - and gangrene 440.24
  - gangrene 440.24
  - rest pain 440.22
    - and
      - gangrene 440.24
      - ulceration 440.23
        - and gangrene 440.24
  - specified site NEC 440.29
  - ulceration 440.23
    - and gangrene 440.24
- heart (disease) - *see also* Arteriosclerosis, coronary
  - valve 424.99
    - aortic 424.1
    - mitral 424.0
    - pulmonary 424.3
    - tricuspid 424.2
- kidney (*see also* Hypertension, kidney) 403.90
- labyrinth, labyrinthine 388.00
- medial NEC (*see also* Arteriosclerosis, extremities) 440.20
- mesentery (artery) 557.1
- Mönckeberg's (*see also* Arteriosclerosis, extremities) 440.20
- myocarditis 429.0
- nephrosclerosis (*see also* Hypertension, kidney) 403.90
- peripheral (of extremities) - *see* Arteriosclerosis, extremities
- precerebral 433.9 5th
  - specified artery NEC 433.8 5th
- pulmonary (idiopathic) 416.0
- renal (*see also* Hypertension, kidney) 403.90
  - arterioles (*see also* Hypertension, kidney) 403.90
  - artery 440.1
- retinal (vascular) 440.8 *[362.13]*
- specified artery NEC 440.8
  - with gangrene 440.8 *[785.4]*
- spinal (cord) 437.0
- vertebral (artery) (*see also* Occlusion, artery, vertebral) 433.2 5th

Arteriospasm 443.9

Arteriovenous - *see* condition

Arteritis 447.6
- allergic (*see also* Angiitis, hypersensitivity) 446.20
- aorta (nonsyphilitic) 447.6
  - syphilitic 093.1
- aortic arch 446.7
- brachiocephalica 446.7
- brain 437.4
  - syphilitic 094.89
- branchial 446.7
- cerebral 437.4
  - late effect - *see* Late effect(s) (of) cerebrovascular disease
  - sphylitic 094.89

Arteritis – *continued*
- coronary (artery) - *see also* Arteriosclerosis, coronary
  - rheumatic 391.9
    - chronic 398.99
  - syphilitic 093.89
- cranial (left) (right) 446.5
- deformans - *see* Arteriosclerosis
- giant cell 446.5
- necrosing or necrotizing 446.0
- nodosa 446.0
- obliterans - *see also* Arteriosclerosis
  - subclaviocarotica 446.7
- pulmonary 417.8
- retina 362.18
- rheumatic - *see* Fever, rheumatic
- senile - *see* Arteriosclerosis
- suppurative 447.2
- syphilitic (general) 093.89
  - brain 094.89
  - coronary 093.89
  - spinal 094.89
- temporal 446.5
- young female, syndrome 446.7

Artery, arterial - *see* condition

Arthralgia (*see also* Pain, joint) 719.4 5th
- allergic (*see also* Pain, joint) 719.4 5th
- in caisson disease 993.3
- psychogenic 307.89
- rubella 056.71
- Salmonella 003.23
- temporomandibular joint 524.62

Arthritis, arthritic (acute) (chronic) (subacute) 716.9 5th
- meaning Osteoarthritis - *see* Osteoarthrosis

Note *Use the following fifth-digit subclassification with categories 711-712, 715-716:*

0	site unspecified
1	shoulder region
2	upper arm
3	forearm
4	hand
5	pelvic region and thigh
6	lower leg
7	ankle and foot
8	other specified sites
9	multiple sites

- allergic 716.2 5th
- ankylosing (crippling) (spine) 720.0 *[713.2]*
  - sites other than spine 716.9 5th
- atrophic 714.0
  - spine 720.9
- back (*see also* Arthritis, spine) 721.90
- Bechterew's (ankylosing spondylitis) 720.0
- blennorrhagic 098.50 *[711.6]*
- cervical, cervicodorsal (*see also* Spondylosis, cervical) 721.0
- Charcôt's 094.0 *[713.5]*
  - diabetic 250.6 5th *[713.5]*
    - due to secondary diabetes 249.6 5th *[713.5]*
  - syringomyelic 336.0 *[713.5]*
  - tabetic 094.0 *[713.5]*
- chylous (*see also* Filariasis) 125.9 *[711.7]* 5th
- climacteric NEC 716.3 5th
- coccyx 721.8
- cricoarytenoid 478.79
- crystal (-induced) - *see* Arthritis, due to crystals
- deformans (*see also* Osteoarthrosis) 715.9 5th
  - spine 721.90
    - with myelopathy 721.91
- degenerative (*see also* Osteoarthrosis) 715.9 5th
  - idiopathic 715.09
  - polyarticular 715.09

Arthritis, arthritic – *continued*
- degenerative – *continued*
  - spine 721.90
    - with myelopathy 721.91
- dermatoarthritis, lipoid 272.8 *[713.0]*
- due to or associated with
  - acromegaly 253.0 *[713.0]*
  - actinomycosis 039.8 *[711.4]* 5th
  - amyloidosis 277.39 *[713.7]*
  - bacterial disease NEC 040.89 *[711.4]* 5th
  - Behçet's syndrome 136.1 *[711.2]* 5th
  - blastomycosis 116.0 *[711.6]* 5th
  - brucellosis (*see also* Brucellosis) 023.9 *[711.4]* 5th
  - caisson disease 993.3
  - coccidioidomycosis 114.3 *[711.6]* 5th
  - coliform (Escherichia coli) 711.0 5th
  - colitis, ulcerative - (*see also* Colitis, ulcerative) 556.9 *[713.1]*
  - cowpox 051.01 *[711.5]* 5th
  - crystals -(*see also* Gout)
    - dicalcium phosphate 275.49 *[712.1]* 5th
    - pyrophosphate 275.49 *[712.2]* 5th
    - specified NEC 275.49 *[712.8]* 5th
  - dermatoarthritis, lipoid 272.8 *[713.0]*
  - dermatological disorder NEC 709.9 *[713.3]*
  - diabetes 250.6 5th *[713.5]*
    - due to secondary diabetes 249.6 5th *[713.5]*
  - diphtheria 032.89 *[711.4]* 5th
  - dracontiasis 125.7 *[711.7]* 5th
  - dysentery 009.0 *[711.3]* 5th
  - endocrine disorder NEC 259.9 *[713.0]*
  - enteritis NEC 009.1 *[711.3]* 5th
    - infectious (*see also* Enteritis, infectious) 009.0 *[711.3]* 5th
      - specified organism NEC 008.8 *[711.3]* 5th
    - regional (*see also* Enteritis, regional) 555.9 *[713.1]*
    - specified organism NEC 008.8 *[711.3]* 5th
  - epiphyseal slip, nontraumatic (old) 716.8 5th
  - erysipelas 035 *[711.4]* 5th
  - erythema
    - epidemic 026.1
    - multiforme 695.10 *[713.3]*
    - nodosum 695.2 *[713.3]*
  - Escherichia coli 711.0 5th
  - filariasis NEC 125.9 *[711.7]* 5th
  - gastrointestinal condition NEC 569.9 *[713.1]*
  - glanders 024 *[711.4]* 5th
  - Gonococcus 098.50
  - gout 274.00 ▲
  - H. influenzae 711.0 5th
  - helminthiasis NEC 128.9 *[711.7]* 5th
  - hematological disorder NEC 289.9 *[713.2]*
  - hemochromatosis 275.0 *[713.0]*
  - hemoglobinopathy NEC (*see also* Disease, hemoglobin) 282.7 *[713.2]*
  - hemophilia (*see also* Hemophilia) 286.0 *[713.2]*
  - hemophilus influenzae (H. influenzae) 711.0 5th
  - Henoch (-Schönlein) purpura 287.0 *[713.6]*
  - histoplasmosis NEC (*see also* Histoplasmosis) 115.99 *[711.6]* 5th
  - human parvovirus 079.83 *[711.5]* 5th
  - hyperparathyroidism 252.00 *[713.0]*
  - hypersensitivity reaction NEC 995.3 *[713.6]*
  - hypogammaglobulinemia (*see also* Hypogammaglobulinemia) 279.00 *[713.0]*
  - hypothyroidism NEC 244.9 *[713.0]*

- **Arthritis, arthritic** – *continued*
  - due to or associated with – *continued*
    - infection (*see also* Arthritis, infectious) 711.9 5th
    - infectious disease NEC 136.9 *[711.8]* 5th
    - leprosy (*see also* Leprosy) 030.9 *[711.4]* 5th
    - leukemia NEC (M9800/3) 208.9 *[713.2]*
    - lipoid dermatoarthritis 272.8 *[713.0]*
    - Lyme disease 088.81 *[711.8]* 5th
    - Mediterranean fever, familial 277.31 *[713.7]*
    - meningococcal infection 036.82
    - metabolic disorder NEC 277.9 *[713.0]*
    - multiple myelomatosis (M9730/3) 203.0 *[713.2]*
    - mumps 072.79 *[711.5]* 5th
    - mycobacteria 031.8 *[711.4]* 5th
    - mycosis NEC 117.9 *[711.6]* 5th
    - neurological disorder NEC 349.9 *[713.5]*
    - ochronosis 270.2 *[713.0]*
    - O'Nyong Nyong 066.3 *[711.5]* 5th
    - parasitic disease NEC 136.9 *[711.8]* 5th
    - paratyphoid fever (*see also* Fever, paratyphoid) 002.9 *[711.3]* 5th
    - parvovirus B19 079.83 *[711.5]* 5th
    - Pneumococcus 711.0 5th
    - poliomyelitis (*see also* Poliomyelitis) 045.9 5th *[711.5]* 5th
    - Pseudomonas 711.0 5th
    - psoriasis 696.0
    - pyogenic organism (E. coli) (H. influenzae) (Pseudomonas) (Streptococcus) 711.0 5th
    - rat-bite fever 026.1 *[711.4]* 5th
    - regional enteritis (*see also* Enteritis, regional) 555.9 *[713.1]*
    - Reiter's disease 099.3 *[711.1]* 5th
    - respiratory disorder NEC 519.9 *[713.4]*
    - reticulosis, malignant (M9720/3) 202.3 *[713.2]*
    - rubella 056.71
    - salmonellosis 003.23
    - sarcoidosis 135 *[713.7]*
    - serum sickness 999.5 *[713.6]*
    - Staphylococcus 711.0 5th
    - Streptococcus 711.0 5th
    - syphilis (*see also* Syphilis) 094.0 *[711.4]* 5th
    - syringomyelia 336.0 *[713.5]*
    - thalassemia 282.49 *[713.2]*
    - tuberculosis (*see also* Tuberculosis, arthritis) 015.9 5th *[711.4]* 5th
    - typhoid fever 002.0 *[711.3]* 5th
    - ulcerative colitis - (*see also* Colitis, ulcerative) 556.9 *[713.1]*
    - urethritis
      - nongonococcal (*see also* Urethritis, nongonococcal) 099.40 *[711.1]* 5th
      - nonspecific (*see also* Urethritis, nongonococcal) 099.40 *[711.1]* 5th
      - Reiter's 099.3 *[711.1]* 5th
    - viral disease NEC 079.99 *[711.5]* 5th
  - erythema epidemic 026.1
  - gonococcal 098.50
  - gouty ~~(acute)~~ 274.00 ▲
    - acute 274.01 ●
  - hypertrophic (*see also* Osteoarthrosis) 715.9
    - spine 721.90
      - with myelopathy 721.91
  - idiopathic, blennorrheal 099.3
  - in caisson disease 993.3 *[713.8]*
  - infectious or infective (acute) (chronic) (subacute) NEC 711.9 5th
    - nonpyogenic 711.9 5th
    - spine 720.9
  - inflammatory NEC 714.9

- **Arthritis, arthritic** – *continued*
  - juvenile rheumatoid (chronic) (polyarticular) 714.30
    - acute 714.31
    - monoarticular 714.33
    - pauciarticular 714.32
  - lumbar (*see also* Spondylosis, lumbar) 721.3
  - meningococcal 036.82
  - menopausal NEC 716.3 5th
  - migratory - *see* Fever, rheumatic
  - neuropathic (Charcôt's) 094.0 *[713.5]*
    - diabetic 250.6 5th *[713.5]*
      - due to secondary diabetes 249.6 5th *[713.5]*
    - nonsyphilitic NEC 349.9 *[713.5]*
    - syringomyelic 336.0 *[713.5]*
    - tabetic 094.0 *[713.5]*
  - nodosa (*see also* Osteoarthrosis) 715.9 5th
    - spine 721.90
      - with myelopathy 721.91
  - nonpyogenic NEC 716.9 5th
    - spine 721.90
      - with myelopathy 721.91
  - ochronotic 270.2 *[713.0]*
  - palindromic (*see also* Rheumatism, palindromic) 719.3 5th
  - pneumococcal 711.0 5th
  - postdysenteric 009.0 *[711.3]* 5th
  - postrheumatic, chronic (Jaccoud's) 714.4
  - primary progressive 714.0
    - spine 720.9
  - proliferative 714.0
    - spine 720.0
  - psoriatic 696.0
  - purulent 711.0 5th
  - pyogenic or pyemic 711.0 5th
  - rheumatic 714.0
    - acute or subacute - *see* Fever, rheumatic
    - chronic 714.0
    - spine 720.9
  - rheumatoid (nodular) 714.0
    - with
      - splenoadenomegaly and leukopenia 714.1
      - visceral or systemic involvement 714.2
    - aortitis 714.89
    - carditis 714.2
    - heart disease 714.2
    - juvenile (chronic) (polyarticular) 714.30
      - acute 714.31
      - monoarticular 714.33
      - pauciarticular 714.32
    - spine 720.0
  - rubella 056.71
  - sacral, sacroiliac, sacrococcygeal (*see also* Spondylosis, sacral) 721.3
  - scorbutic 267
  - senile or senescent (*see also* Osteoarthrosis) 715.9 5th
    - spine 721.90
      - with myelopathy 721.91
  - septic 711.0 5th
  - serum (nontherapeutic) (therapeutic) 999.5 *[713.6]*
  - specified form NEC 716.8 5th
  - spine 721.90
    - with myelopathy 721.91
    - atrophic 720.9
    - degenerative 721.90
      - with myelopathy 721.91
    - hypertrophic (with deformity) 721.90
      - with myelopathy 721.91
    - infectious or infective NEC 720.9
    - Marie-Strümpell 720.0
    - nonpyogenic 721.90
      - with myelopathy 721.91
    - pyogenic 720.9
    - rheumatoid 720.0
    - traumatic (old) 721.7

- **Arthritis, arthritic** – *continued*
  - spine – *continued*
    - tuberculous (*see also* Tuberculosis) 015.0 5th *[720.81]*
  - staphylococcal 711.0 5th
  - streptococcal 711.0 5th
  - suppurative 711.0 5th
  - syphilitic 094.0 *[713.5]*
    - congenital 090.49 *[713.5]*
  - syphilitica deformans (Charcôt) 094.0 *[713.5]*
  - temporomandibular joint 524.69
  - thoracic (*see also* Spondylosis, thoracic) 721.2
  - toxic of menopause 716.3 5th
  - transient 716.4 5th
  - traumatic (chronic) (old) (post) 716.1 5th
    - current injury - *see* nature of injury
  - tuberculous (*see also* Tuberculosis, arthritis) 015.9 5th *[711.4]* 5th
  - urethritica 099.3 *[711.1]* 5th
  - urica, uratic 274.00 ▲
  - venereal 099.3 *[711.1]* 5th
  - vertebral (*see also* Arthritis, spine) 721.90
  - villous 716.8 5th
  - von Bechterew's 720.0
- **Arthrocele** (*see also* Effusion, joint) 719.0 5th
- **Arthrochondritis** - *see* Arthritis
- **Arthrodesis status** V45.4
- **Arthrodynia** (*see also* Pain, joint) 719.4 5th
  - psychogenic 307.89
- **Arthrodysplasia** 755.9
- **Arthrofibrosis, joint** (*see also* Ankylosis) 718.5 5th
- **Arthrogryposis** 728.3
  - multiplex, congenita 754.89
- **Arthrokatadysis** 715.35
- **Arthrolithiasis** 274.00 ▲
- **Arthro-onychodysplasia** 756.89
- **Arthro-osteo-onychodysplasia** 756.89
- **Arthropathy** (*see also* Arthritis) 716.9 5th

Note *Use the following fifth-digit subclassification with categories 711-712, 716:*

0	site unspecified
1	shoulder region
2	upper arm
3	forearm
4	hand
5	pelvic region and thigh
6	lower leg
7	ankle and foot
8	other specified sites
9	multiple sites

  - Behçet's 136.1 *[711.2]* 5th
  - Charcôt's 094.0 *[713.5]*
    - diabetic 250.6 5th *[713.5]*
      - due to secondary diabetes 249.6 5th *[713.5]*
    - syringomyelic 336.0 *[713.5]*
    - tabetic 094.0 *[713.5]*
  - crystal (-induced) - *see* Arthritis, due to crystals
  - gouty 274.00 ▲
    - acute 274.01 ●
    - chronic (without mention of tophus (tophi)) 274.02 ●
      - with tophus (tophi) 274.03 ●
  - neurogenic, neuropathic (Charcôt's) (tabetic) 094.0 *[713.5]*
    - diabetic 250.6 5th *[713.5]*
      - due to secondary diabetes 249.6 5th *[713.5]*
    - nonsyphilitic NEC 349.9 *[713.5]*
    - syringomyelic 336.0 *[713.5]*
  - postdysenteric NEC 009.0 *[711.3]* 5th
  - postrheumatic, chronic (Jaccoud's) 714.4
  - psoriatic 696.0
  - pulmonary 731.2
  - specified NEC 716.8 5th
  - syringomyelia 336.0 *[713.5]*

- **Arthropathy** – *continued*
  - tabes dorsalis 094.0 *[713.5]*
  - tabetic 094.0 *[713.5]*
  - transient 716.4 5th
  - traumatic 716.1 5th
  - uric acid 274.00 ▲
- **Arthrophyte** (*see also* Loose, body, joint) 718.1 5th
- **Arthrophytis** 719.80
  - ankle 719.87
  - elbow 719.82
  - foot 719.87
  - hand 719.84
  - hip 719.85
  - knee 719.86
  - multiple sites 719.89
  - pelvic region 719.85
  - shoulder (region) 719.81
  - specified site NEC 719.88
  - wrist 719.83
- **Arthropyosis** (*see also* Arthritis, pyogenic) 711.0 5th
- **Arthroscopic surgical procedure converted to open procedure** V64.43
- **Arthrosis** (deformans) (degenerative) (*see also* Osteoarthrosis) 715.9 5th
  - Charcôt's 094.0 *[713.5]*
  - polyarticular 715.09
  - spine (*see also* Spondylosis) 721.90
- **Arthus phenomenon** 995.21
  - due to
    - correct substance properly administered 995.21
    - overdose or wrong substance given or taken 977.9
      - specified drug - *see* Table of Drugs and Chemicals
  - serum 999.5
- **Articular** - *see also* condition
  - disc disorder (reducing or non-reducing) 524.63
  - spondylolisthesis 756.12
- **Articulation**
  - anterior 524.27
  - posterior 524.27
  - reverse 524.27
- **Artificial**
  - device (prosthetic) - *see* Fitting, device
  - insemination V26.1
  - menopause (states) (symptoms) (syndrome) 627.4
  - opening status (functioning) (without complication) V44.9
    - anus (colostomy) V44.3
    - colostomy V44.3
    - cystostomy V44.50
      - appendico-vesicostomy V44.52
      - cutaneous-vesicostomy V44.51
      - specifed type NEC V44.59
    - enterostomy V44.4
    - gastrostomy V44.1
    - ileostomy V44.2
    - intestinal tract NEC V44.4
    - jejunostomy V44.4
    - nephrostomy V44.6
    - specified site NEC V44.8
    - tracheostomy V44.0
    - ureterostomy V44.6
    - urethrostomy V44.6
    - urinary tract NEC V44.6
    - vagina V44.7
    - vagina status V44.7
- **ARV** (disease) (illness) (infection) - *see* Human immunodeficiency virus (disease) (illness) (infection)
- **Arytenoid** - *see* condition
- **Asbestosis** (occupational) 501
- **Asboe-Hansen's disease** (incontinentia pigmenti) 757.33
- **Ascariasis** (intestinal) (lung) 127.0
- **Ascaridiasis** 127.0
- **Ascaridosis** 127.0
- **Ascaris** 127.0
  - lumbricoides (infestation) 127.0

Arthritis, arthritic – Ascaris

Ascaris – *continued*
pneumonia 127.0
Ascending - *see* condition
ASC-H (atypical squamous cells cannot exclude high grade squamous intraepithelial lesion)
anus 796.72
cervix 795.02
vagina 795.12
Aschoff's bodies (*see also* Myocarditis, rheumatic) 398.0
Ascites 789.59
abdominal NEC 789.59
cancerous (M8000/6) 789.51
cardiac 428.0
chylous (nonfilarial) 457.8
filarial (*see also* Infestation, filarial) 125.9
congenital 778.0
due to S. japonicum 120.2
fetal, causing fetopelvic disproportion 653.7 5th
heart 428.0
joint (*see also* Effusion, joint) 719.0
malignant (M8000/6) 789.51
pseudochylous 789.59
syphilitic 095.2
tuberculous (*see also* Tuberculosis) 014.0 5th
Ascorbic acid (vitamin C) **deficiency** (scurvy) 267
ASC-US (atypical squamous cells of undetermined significance)
anus 796.71
cervix 795.01
vagina 795.11
ASCVD (arteriosclerotic cardiovascular disease) 429.2
Aseptic - *see* condition
Asherman's syndrome 621.5
Asialia 527.7
Asiatic cholera (*see also* Cholera) 001.9
Asocial personality or trends 301.7
Asomatognosia 781.8
Aspergillosis 117.3
with pneumonia 117.3 *[484.6]*
allergic bronchopulmonary 518.6
nonsyphilitic NEC 117.3
Aspergillus (flavus) (fumigatus) (infection) (terreus) 117.3
Aspermatogenesis 606.0
Aspermia (testis) 606.0
Asphyxia, asphyxiation (by) 799.01
antenatal - *see* Distress, fetal
bedclothes 994.7
birth (*see also* Asphyxia, newborn) 768.9
bunny bag 994.7
carbon monoxide 986
caul (*see also* Asphyxia, newborn) 768.9
cave-in 994.7
crushing - *see* Injury, internal, intrathoracic organs
constriction 994.7
crushing - *see* Injury, internal, intrathoracic organs
drowning 994.1
fetal, affecting newborn 768.9
food or foreign body (in larynx) 933.1
bronchioles 934.8
bronchus (main) 934.1
lung 934.8
nasopharynx 933.0
nose, nasal passages 932
pharynx 933.0
respiratory tract 934.9
specified part NEC 934.8
throat 933.0
trachea 934.0
gas, fumes, or vapor NEC 987.9
specified - *see* Table of Drugs and Chemicals
gravitational changes 994.7
hanging 994.7
inhalation - *see* Inhalation

Asphyxia, asphyxiation (by) – *continued*
intrauterine
fetal death (before onset of labor) 768.0
during labor 768.1
liveborn infant - *see* Distress, fetal, liveborn infant
local 443.0
mechanical 994.7
during birth (*see also* Distress, fetal) 768.9
mucus 933.1
bronchus (main) 934.1
larynx 933.1
lung 934.8
nasal passages 932
newborn 770.18
pharynx 933.0
respiratory tract 934.9
specified part NEC 934.8
throat 933.0
trachea 934.0
vaginal (fetus or newborn) 770.18
newborn 768.9
with neurologic involvement 768.5
blue 768.6
livida 768.6
mild or moderate 768.6
pallida 768.5
severe 768.5
white 768.5
pathological 799.01
plastic bag 994.7
postnatal (*see also* Asphyxia, newborn) 768.9
mechanical 994.7
pressure 994.7
reticularis 782.61
strangulation 994.7
submersion 994.1
traumatic NEC - *see* Injury, internal, intrathoracic organs
vomiting, vomitus - *see* Asphyxia, food or foreign body
Aspiration
acid pulmonary (syndrome) 997.39
obstetric 668.0 5th
amniotic fluid 770.13
with respiratory symptoms 770.14
bronchitis 507.0
clear amniotic fluid 770.13
with
pneumonia 770.14
pneumonitis 770.14
respiratory symptoms 770.14
contents of birth canal 770.17
with respiratory symptoms 770.18
fetal 770.10
blood 770.15
with
pneumonia 770.16
pneumonitis 770.16
pneumonitis 770.18
food, foreign body, or gasoline (with asphyxiation) - *see* Asphyxia, food or foreign body
meconium 770.11
with
pneumonia 770.12
pneumonitis 770.12
respiratory symptoms 770.12
below vocal cords 770.11
with respiratory symptoms 770.12
mucus 933.1
into
bronchus (main) 934.1
lung 934.8
respiratory tract 934.9
specified part NEC 934.8
trachea 934.0
newborn 770.17
vaginal (fetus or newborn) 770.17
newborn 770.10
with respiratory symptoms 770.18

Aspiration – *continued*
newborn – *continued*
blood 770.15
with
pneumonia 770.16
pneumonitis 770.16
respiratory symptoms 770.16
pneumonia 507.0
fetus or newborn 770.18
meconium 770.12
pneumonitis 507.0
fetus or newborn 770.18
meconium 770.12
obstetric 668.0 5th
postnatal stomach contents 770.85
with
pneumonia 770.86
pneumonitis 770.86
respiratory symptoms 770.86
syndrome of newborn (massive) 770.18
meconium 770.12
vernix caseosa 770.17
Asplenia 759.0
with mesocardia 746.87
Assam fever 085.0
Assimilation, pelvis
with disproportion 653.2 5th
affecting fetus or newborn 763.1
causing obstructed labor 660.1 5th
affecting fetus or newborn 763.1
Assmann's focus (*see also* Tuberculosis) 011.0 5th
Astasia (-abasia) 307.9
hysterical 300.11
Asteatosis 706.8
cutis 706.8
Astereognosis 780.99
Asterixis 781.3
in liver disease 572.8
Asteroid hyalitis 379.22
Asthenia, asthenic 780.79
cardiac (*see also* Failure, heart) 428.9
psychogenic 306.2
cardiovascular (*see also* Failure, heart) 428.9
psychogenic 306.2
heart (*see also* Failure, heart) 428.9
psychogenic 306.2
hysterical 300.11
myocardial (*see also* Failure, heart) 428.9
psychogenic 306.2
nervous 300.5
neurocirculatory 306.2
neurotic 300.5
psychogenic 300.5
psychoneurotic 300.5
psychophysiologic 300.5
reaction, psychoneurotic 300.5
senile 797
Stiller's 780.79
tropical anhidrotic 705.1
Asthenopia 368.13
accommodative 367.4
hysterical (muscular) 300.11
psychogenic 306.7
Asthenospermia 792.2
Asthma, asthmatic (bronchial) (catarrh) (spasmodic) 493.9 5th

Note *The following fifth digit subclassification is for use with codes 493.0-493.2, 493.9:*

0	unspecified
1	with status asthmaticus
2	with (acute) exacerbation

with
chronic obstructive pulmonary disease (COPD) 493.2 5th
hay fever 493.0 5th
rhinitis, allergic 493.0 5th
allergic 493.9 5th
stated cause (external allergen) 493.0 5th
atopic 493.0 5th

Asthma, asthmatic – *continued*
cardiac (*see also* Failure, ventricular, left) 428.1
cardiobronchial (*see also* Failure, ventricular, left) 428.1
cardiorenal (*see also* Hypertension, cardiorenal) 404.90
childhood 493.0 5th
Colliers' 500
cough variant 493.82
croup 493.9 5th
detergent 507.8
due to
detergent 507.8
inhalation of fumes 506.3
internal immunological process 493.0 5th
endogenous (intrinsic) 493.1 5th
eosinophilic 518.3
exercise induced bronchospasm 493.81
exogenous (cosmetics) (dander or dust) (drugs) (dust) (feathers) (food) (hay) (platinum) (pollen) 493.0 5th
extrinsic 493.0 5th
grinders' 502
hay 493.0 5th
heart (*see also* Failure, ventricular, left) 428.1
IgE 493.0 5th
infective 493.1 5th
intrinsic 493.1 5th
Kopp's 254.8
late-onset 493.1 5th
meat-wrappers' 506.9
Millar's (laryngismus stridulus) 478.75
millstone makers' 502
miners' 500
Monday morning 504
New Orleans (epidemic) 493.0 5th
platinum 493.0 5th
pneumoconiotic (occupational) NEC 505
potters' 502
psychogenic 316 *[493.9]* 5th
pulmonary eosinophilic 518.3
red cedar 495.8
Rostan's (*see also* Failure, ventricular, left) 428.1
sandblasters' 502
sequoiosis 495.8
stonemasons' 502
thymic 254.8
tuberculous (*see also* Tuberculosis, pulmonary) 011.9 5th
Wichmann's (laryngismus stridulus) 478.75
wood 495.8
Astigmatism (compound) (congenital) 367.20
irregular 367.22
regular 367.21
Astroblastoma (M9430/3)
nose 748.1
specified site - *see* Neoplasm, by site, malignant
unspecified site 191.9
Astrocytoma (cystic) (M9400/3)
anaplastic type (M9401/3)
specified site - *see* Neoplasm, by site, malignant
unspecified site 191.9
fibrillary (M9420/3)
specified site - *see* Neoplasm, by site, malignant
unspecified site 191.9
fibrous (M9420/3)
specified site - *see* Neoplasm, by site, malignant
unspecified site 191.9
gemistocytic (M9411/3)
specified site - *see* Neoplasm, by site, malignant
unspecified site 191.9

Atresia, atretic – *continued*
- ureteropelvic junction 753.21
- ureterovesical orifice 753.22
- urethra (valvular) 753.6
- urinary tract NEC 753.29
- uterus 752.3
  - acquired 621.8
- vagina (acquired) 623.2
  - congenital 752.49
  - postgonococcal (old) 098.2
  - postinfectional 623.2
  - senile 623.2
- vascular NEC (*see also* Atresia, blood vessel) 747.60
  - cerebral 747.81
- vas deferens 752.89
- vein NEC (*see also* Atresia, blood vessel) 747.60
  - cardiac 746.89
  - great 747.49
  - portal 747.49
  - pulmonary 747.49
- vena cava (inferior) (superior) 747.49
- vesicourethral orifice 753.6
- vulva 752.49
  - acquired 624.8

Atrichia, atrichosis 704.00
- congenital (universal) 757.4

Atrioventricularis commune 745.69

Atrophia - *see also* Atrophy
- alba 709.09
- cutis 701.8
  - idiopathica progressiva 701.8
  - senilis 701.8
- dermatological, diffuse (idiopathic) 701.8
- flava hepatis (acuta) (subacuta) (*see also* Necrosis, liver) 570
- gyrata of choroid and retina (central) 363.54
  - generalized 363.57
- senilis 797
  - dermatological 701.8
- unguium 703.8
  - congenita 757.5

Atrophoderma, atrophodermia 701.9
- diffusum (idiopathic) 701.8
- maculatum 701.3
  - et striatum 701.3
    - due to syphilis 095.8
  - syphilitic 091.3
- neuriticum 701.8
- pigmentosum 757.33
- reticulatum symmetricum faciei 701.8
- senile 701.8
- symmetrical 701.8
- vermiculata 701.8

Atrophy, atrophic
- adrenal (autoimmune) (capsule) (cortex) (gland) 255.41
  - with hypofunction 255.41
- alveolar process or ridge (edentulous) 525.20
  - mandible 525.20
    - minimal 525.21
    - moderate 525.22
    - severe 525.23
  - maxilla 525.20
    - minimal 525.24
    - moderate 525.25
    - severe 525.26
- appendix 543.9
- Aran-Duchenne muscular 335.21
- arm 728.2
- arteriosclerotic - *see* Arteriosclerosis
- arthritis 714.0
  - spine 720.9
- bile duct (any) 576.8
- bladder 596.8
- blanche (of Milian) 701.3
- bone (senile) 733.99
  - due to
    - disuse 733.7
    - infection 733.99
    - tabes dorsalis (neurogenic) 094.0

Atrophy, atrophic – *continued*
- bone – *continued*
  - posttraumatic 733.99
- brain (cortex) (progressive) 331.9
  - with dementia 290.10
  - Alzheimer's 331.0
    - with dementia - *see* Alzheimer's, dementia
  - circumscribed (Pick's) 331.11
    - with dementia
      - with behavioral disturbance 331.11 *[294.11]*
      - without behavioral disturbance 331.11 *[294.10]*
  - congenital 742.4
  - hereditary 331.9
  - senile 331.2
- breast 611.4
  - puerperal, postpartum 676.3 [5th]
- buccal cavity 528.9
- cardiac (brown) (senile) (*see also* Degeneration, myocardial) 429.1
- cartilage (infectional) (joint) 733.99
- cast, plaster of Paris 728.2
- cerebellar - *see* Atrophy, brain
- cerebral - *see* Atrophy, brain
- cervix (endometrium) (mucosa) (myometrium) (senile) (uteri) 622.8
  - menopausal 627.8
- Charcôt-Marie-Tooth 356.1
- choroid 363.40
  - diffuse secondary 363.42
  - hereditary (*see also* Dystrophy, choroid) 363.50
    - gyrate
      - central 363.54
      - diffuse 363.57
      - generalized 363.57
  - senile 363.41
- ciliary body 364.57
- colloid, degenerative 701.3
- conjunctiva (senile) 372.89
- corpus cavernosum 607.89
- cortical (*see also* Atrophy, brain) 331.9
- Cruveilhier's 335.21
- cystic duct 576.8
- dacryosialadenopathy 710.2
- degenerative
  - colloid 701.3
  - senile 701.3
- Déjérine-Thomas 333.0
- diffuse idiopathic, dermatological 701.8
- disuse
  - bone 733.7
  - muscle 728.2
  - pelvic muscles and anal sphincter 618.83
- Duchenne-Aran 335.21
- ear 388.9
- edentulous alveolar ridge 525.20
  - mandible 525.20
    - minimal 525.21
    - moderate 525.22
    - severe 525.23
  - maxilla 525.20
    - minimal 525.24
    - moderate 525.25
    - severe 525.26
- emphysema, lung 492.8
- endometrium (senile) 621.8
  - cervix 622.8
- enteric 569.89
- epididymis 608.3
- eyeball, cause unknown 360.41
- eyelid (senile) 374.50
- facial (skin) 701.9
- facioscapulohumeral (Landouzy-Déjérine) 359.1
- fallopian tube (senile), acquired 620.3
- fatty, thymus (gland) 254.8
- gallbladder 575.8
- gastric 537.89
- gastritis (chronic) 535.1 [5th]
- gastrointestinal 569.89

Atrophy, atrophic – *continued*
- genital organ, male 608.89
- glandular 289.3
- globe (phthisis bulbi) 360.41
- gum (*see also* Recession, gingival) 523.20
- hair 704.2
- heart (brown) (senile) (*see also* Degeneration, myocardial) 429.1
- hemifacial 754.0
  - Romberg 349.89
- hydronephrosis 591
- infantile 261
  - paralysis, acute (*see also* Poliomyelitis, with paralysis) 045.1 [5th]
- intestine 569.89
- iris (generalized) (postinfectional) (sector shaped) 364.59
  - essential 364.51
  - progressive 364.51
  - sphincter 364.54
- kidney (senile) (*see also* Sclerosis, renal) 587
  - with hypertension (*see also* Hypertension, kidney) 403.90
  - congenital 753.0
  - hydronephrotic 591
  - infantile 753.0
- lacrimal apparatus (primary) 375.13
  - secondary 375.14
- Landouzy-Déjérine 359.1
- laryngitis, infection 476.0
- larynx 478.79
- Leber's optic 377.16
- lip 528.5
- liver (acute) (subacute) (*see also* Necrosis, liver) 570
  - chronic (yellow) 571.8
  - yellow (congenital) 570
    - with
      - abortion - *see* Abortion, by type, with specified complication NEC
      - ectopic pregnancy (*see also* categories 633.0-633.9) 639.8
      - molar pregnancy (*see also* categories 630-632) 639.8
    - chronic 571.8
    - complicating pregnancy 646.7 [5th]
    - following
      - abortion 639.8
      - ectopic or molar pregnancy 639.8
    - from injection, inoculation or transfusion (onset within 8 months after administration) - *see* Hepatitis, viral
    - healed 571.5
    - obstetric 646.7 [5th]
    - postabortal 639.8
    - postimmunization - *see* Hepatitis, viral
    - posttransfusion - *see* Hepatitis, viral
    - puerperal, postpartum 674.8 [5th]
- lung (senile) 518.89
  - congenital 748.69
- macular (dermatological) 701.3
  - syphilitic, skin 091.3
    - striated 095.8
- muscle, muscular 728.2
  - disuse 728.2
  - Duchenne-Aran 335.21
  - extremity (lower) (upper) 728.2
  - familial spinal 335.11
  - general 728.2
  - idiopathic 728.2
  - infantile spinal 335.0
  - myelopathic (progressive) 335.10
  - myotonic 359.21
  - neuritic 356.1
  - neuropathic (peroneal) (progressive) 356.1
  - peroneal 356.1
  - primary (idiopathic) 728.2

Atrophy, atrophic – *continued*
- muscle, muscular – *continued*
  - progressive (familial) (hereditary) (pure) 335.21
    - adult (spinal) 335.19
    - infantile (spinal) 335.0
    - juvenile (spinal) 335.11
    - spinal 335.10
      - adult 335.19
      - hereditary or familial 335.11
      - infantile 335.0
  - pseudohypertrophic 359.1
  - spinal (progressive) 335.10
    - adult 335.19
    - Aran-Duchenne 335.21
    - familial 335.11
    - hereditary 335.11
    - infantile 335.0
    - juvenile 335.11
  - syphilitic 095.6
- myocardium (*see also* Degeneration, myocardial) 429.1
- myometrium (senile) 621.8
  - cervix 622.8
- myotatic 728.2
- myotonia 359.21
- nail 703.8
  - congenital 757.5
- nasopharynx 472.2
- nerve - *see also* Disorder, nerve
  - abducens 378.54
  - accessory 352.4
  - acoustic or auditory 388.5
  - cranial 352.9
    - first (olfactory) 352.0
    - second (optic) (*see also* Atrophy, optic nerve) 377.10
    - third (oculomotor) (partial) 378.51
      - total 378.52
    - fourth (trochlear) 378.53
    - fifth (trigeminal) 350.8
    - sixth (abducens) 378.54
    - seventh (facial) 351.8
    - eighth (auditory) 388.5
    - ninth (glossopharyngeal) 352.2
    - tenth (pneumogastric) (vagus) 352.3
    - eleventh (accessory) 352.4
    - twelfth (hypoglossal) 352.5
  - facial 351.8
  - glossopharyngeal 352.2
  - hypoglossal 352.5
  - oculomotor (partial) 378.51
    - total 378.52
  - olfactory 352.0
  - peripheral 355.9
  - pneumogastric 352.3
  - trigeminal 350.8
  - trochlear 378.53
  - vagus (pneumogastric) 352.3
- nervous system, congenital 742.8
- neuritic (*see also* Disorder, nerve) 355.9
- neurogenic NEC 355.9
  - bone
    - tabetic 094.0
- nutritional 261
- old age 797
- olivopontocerebellar 333.0
- optic nerve (ascending) (descending) (infectional) (nonfamilial) (papillomacular bundle) (postretinal) (secondary NEC) (simple) 377.10
  - associated with retinal dystrophy 377.13
  - dominant hereditary 377.16
  - glaucomatous 377.14
  - hereditary (dominant) (Leber's) 377.16
  - Leber's (hereditary) 377.16
  - partial 377.15
  - postinflammatory 377.12
  - primary 377.11
  - syphilitic 094.84
    - congenital 090.49

Atresia, atretic – Atrophy, atrophic

- **Atrophy, atrophic** – *continued*
  - optic nerve – *continued*
    - syphilitic – *continued*
      - tabes dorsalis 094.0
  - orbit 376.45
  - ovary (senile), acquired 620.3
  - oviduct (senile), acquired 620.3
  - palsy, diffuse 335.20
  - pancreas (duct) (senile) 577.8
  - papillary muscle 429.81
  - paralysis 355.9
  - parotid gland 527.0
  - patches skin 701.3
    - senile 701.8
  - penis 607.89
  - pharyngitis 472.1
  - pharynx 478.29
  - pluriglandular 258.8
  - polyarthritis 714.0
  - prostate 602.2
  - pseudohypertrophic 359.1
  - renal (*see also* Sclerosis, renal) 587
  - reticulata 701.8
  - retina (*see also* Degeneration, retina) 362.60
    - hereditary (*see also* Dystrophy, retina) 362.70
  - rhinitis 472.0
  - salivary duct or gland 527.0
  - scar NEC 709.2
  - sclerosis, lobar (of brain) 331.0
    - with dementia
      - with behavioral disturbance 331.0 *[294.11]*
      - without behavioral disturbance 331.0 *[294.10]*
  - scrotum 608.89
  - seminal vesicle 608.89
  - senile 797
    - degenerative, of skin 701.3
  - skin (patches) (senile) 701.8
  - spermatic cord 608.89
  - spinal (cord) 336.8
    - acute 336.8
    - muscular (chronic) 335.10
      - adult 335.19
      - familial 335.11
      - juvenile 335.10
    - paralysis 335.10
      - acute (*see also* Poliomyelitis, with paralysis) 045.1 5th
  - spine (column) 733.99
  - spleen (senile) 289.59
  - spots (skin) 701.3
    - senile 701.8
  - stomach 537.89
  - striate and macular 701.3
    - syphilitic 095.8
  - subcutaneous 701.9
    - due to injection 999.9
  - sublingual gland 527.0
  - submaxillary gland 527.0
  - Sudeck's 733.7
  - suprarenal (autoimmune) (capsule) (gland) 255.41
    - with hypofunction 255.41
  - tarso-orbital fascia, congenital 743.66
  - testis 608.3
  - thenar, partial 354.0
  - throat 478.29
  - thymus (fat) 254.8
  - thyroid (gland) 246.8
    - with
      - cretinism 243
      - myxedema 244.9
    - congenital 243
  - tongue (senile) 529.8
    - papillae 529.4
    - smooth 529.4
  - trachea 519.19
  - tunica vaginalis 608.89
  - turbinate 733.99
  - tympanic membrane (nonflaccid) 384.82
    - flaccid 384.81
  - ulcer (*see also* Ulcer, skin) 707.9
  - upper respiratory tract 478.9
  - uterus, uterine (acquired) (senile) 621.8
    - cervix 622.8
    - due to radiation (intended effect) 621.8
  - vagina (senile) 627.3
  - vascular 459.89
  - vas deferens 608.89
  - vertebra (senile) 733.99
  - vulva (primary) (senile) 624.1
  - Werdnig-Hoffmann 335.0
  - yellow (acute) (congenital) (liver) (subacute) (*see also* Necrosis, liver) 570
    - chronic 571.8
    - resulting from administration of blood, plasma, serum, or other biological substance (within 8 months of administration) - *see* Hepatitis, viral
- **Attack**
  - akinetic (*see also* Epilepsy) 345.0 5th
  - angina - *see* Angina
  - apoplectic (*see also* Disease, cerebrovascular, acute) 436
  - benign shuddering 333.93
  - bilious - *see* Vomiting
  - cataleptic 300.11
  - cerebral (*see also* Disease, cerebrovascular, acute) 436
  - coronary (*see also* Infarct, myocardium) 410.9 5th
  - cyanotic, newborn 770.83
  - epileptic (*see also* Epilepsy) 345.9 5th
  - epileptiform 780.39
  - heart (*see also* Infarct, myocardium) 410.9 5th
  - hemiplegia (*see also* Disease, cerebrovascular, acute) 436
  - hysterical 300.11
  - jacksonian (*see also* Epilepsy) 345.5 5th
  - myocardium, myocardial (*see also* Infarct, myocardium) 410.9 5th
  - myoclonic (*see also* Epilepsy) 345.1 5th
  - panic 300.01
  - paralysis (*see also* Disease, cerebrovascular, acute) 436
  - paroxysmal 780.39
  - psychomotor (*see also* Epilepsy) 345.4 5th
  - salaam (*see also* Epilepsy) 345.6 5th
  - schizophreniform (*see also* Schizophrenia) 295.4 5th
  - sensory and motor 780.39
  - syncope 780.2
  - toxic, cerebral 780.39
  - transient ischemic (TIA) 435.9
  - unconsciousness 780.2
    - hysterical 300.11
  - vasomotor 780.2
  - vasovagal (idiopathic) (paroxysmal) 780.2
- **Attention to**
  - artificial
    - opening (of) V55.9
      - digestive tract NEC V55.4
      - specified site NEC V55.8
      - urinary tract NEC V55.6
    - vagina V55.7
  - colostomy V55.3
  - cystostomy V55.5
  - dressing
    - wound V58.30
      - nonsurgical V58.30
      - surgical V58.31
  - gastrostomy V55.1
  - ileostomy V55.2
  - jejunostomy V55.4
  - nephrostomy V55.6
  - surgical dressings V58.31
  - sutures V58.32
  - tracheostomy V55.0
  - ureterostomy V55.6
  - urethrostomy V55.6
- **Attrition**
  - gum (*see also* Recession, gingival) 523.20
  - teeth (hard tissues) 521.10
    - excessive 521.10
      - extending into
        - dentine 521.12
        - pulp 521.13
      - generalized 521.15
      - limited to enamel 521.11
      - localized 521.14
- **Atypical** - *see also* condition
  - cells
    - endocervical 795.00
    - endometrial 795.00
    - glandular
      - anus 796.70
      - cervical 795.00
      - vaginal 795.10
  - distribution, vessel (congenital) (peripheral) NEC 747.60
  - endometrium 621.9
  - kidney 593.89
- **Atypism, cervix** 622.10
- **Audible tinnitus** (*see also* Tinnitus) 388.30
- **Auditory** - *see* condition
- **Audry's syndrome** (acropachyderma) 757.39
- **Aujeszky's disease** 078.89
- **Aura**
  - jacksonian (see also Epilepsy) 345.5 5th
  - persistent migraine 346.5 5th
    - with cerebral infarction 346.6 5th
    - without cerebral infarction 346.5 5th
- **Aurantiasis, cutis** 278.3
- **Auricle, auricular** - *see* condition
- **Auriculotemporal syndrome** 350.8
- **Australian**
  - Q fever 083.0
  - X disease 062.4
- **Autism, autistic** (child) (infantile) 299.0 5th
- **Autodigestion** 799.89
- **Autoerythrocyte sensitization** 287.2
- **Autographism** 708.3
- **Autoimmune**
  - cold sensitivity 283.0
  - disease NEC 279.49 ▲
  - hemolytic anemia 283.0
  - lymphoproliferative syndrome (ALPS) 279.41 ●
  - thyroiditis 245.2
- **Autoinfection, septic** - *see* Septicemia
- **Autointoxication** 799.89
- **Automatism** 348.89 ▲
  - epileptic (*see also* Epilepsy) 345.4 5th
  - paroxysmal, idiopathic (*see also* Epilepsy) 345.4 5th
- **Autonomic, autonomous**
  - bladder 596.54
    - neurogenic 596.54
      - with cauda equina 344.61
  - dysreflexia 337.3
  - faciocephalalgia (*see also* Neuropathy, peripheral, autonomic) 337.9
  - hysterical seizure 300.11
  - imbalance (*see also* Neuropathy, peripheral, autonomic 337.9
- **Autophony** 388.40
- **Autosensitivity, erythrocyte** 287.2
- **Autotopagnosia** 780.99
- **Autotoxemia** 799.89
- **Autumn - see condition**
- **Avellis' syndrome** 344.89
- **Aviators**
  - disease or sickness (*see also* Effect, adverse, high altitude) 993.2
  - ear 993.0
  - effort syndrome 306.2
- **Avitaminosis** (multiple NEC) (*see also* Deficiency, vitamin) 269.2
  - A 264.9
  - B 266.9
    - with
      - beriberi 265.0
      - pellagra 265.2
  - B_1 265.1
  - B_2 266.0
  - B_6 266.1
  - B_{12} 266.2
  - C (with scurvy) 267
  - D 268.9
    - with
      - osteomalacia 268.2
      - rickets 268.0
  - E 269.1
  - G 266.0
  - H 269.1
  - K 269.0
  - multiple 269.2
  - nicotinic acid 265.2
  - P 269.1
- **Avulsion** (traumatic) 879.8
  - blood vessel - *see* Injury, blood vessel, by site
  - cartilage - *see also* Dislocation, by site
    - knee, current (*see also* Tear, meniscus) 836.2
    - symphyseal (inner), complicating delivery 665.6 5th
  - complicated 879.9
  - diaphragm - *see* Injury, internal, diaphragm
  - ear - *see* Wound, open, ear
  - epiphysis of bone - *see* Fracture, by site
  - external site other than limb - *see* Wound, open, by site
  - eye 871.3
  - fingernail - *see* Wound, open, finger
  - fracture - *see* Fracture, by site
  - genital organs, external - *see* Wound, open, genital organs
  - head (intracranial) NEC - *see also* Injury, intracranial, with open intracranial wound
    - complete 874.9
    - external site NEC 873.8
      - complicated 873.9
  - internal organ or site - *see* Injury, internal, by site
  - joint - *see also* Dislocation, by site
    - capsule - *see* Sprain, by site
  - ligament - *see* Sprain, by site
  - limb - *see also* Amputation, traumatic, by site
    - skin and subcutaneous tissue - *see* Wound, open, by site
  - muscle - *see* Sprain, by site
  - nerve (root) - *see* Injury, nerve, by site
  - scalp - *see* Wound, open, scalp
  - skin and subcutaneous tissue - *see* Wound, open, by site
  - symphyseal cartilage (inner), complicating delivery 665.6 5th
  - tendon - *see also* Sprain, by site
    - with open wound - *see* Wound, open, by site
  - toenail - *see* Wound, open, toe(s)
  - tooth 873.63
    - complicated 873.73
- **Awaiting organ transplant status** V49.83
- **Awareness of heart beat** 785.1
- **Axe grinders' disease** 502
- **Axenfeld's anomaly or syndrome** 743.44
- **Axilla, axillary** - *see also* condition
  - breast 757.6
- **Axonotmesis** - *see* Injury, nerve, by site
- **Ayala's disease** 756.89
- **Ayerza's disease or syndrome** (pulmonary artery sclerosis with pulmonary hypertension) 416.0
- **Azoospermia** 606.0
- **Azorean disease** (of the nervous system) 334.8
- **Azotemia** 790.6
  - meaning uremia (*see also* Uremia) 586
- **Aztec ear** 744.29
- **Azygos lobe, lung** (fissure) 748.69

- **Behavior disorder, disturbance** – *continued*
  - dyssocial, without manifest psychiatric disorder – *continued*
    - child V71.02
  - high-risk- *see* problem
- **Behçet's syndrome** 136.1
- **Behr's disease** 362.50
- **Beigel's disease or morbus** (white piedra) 111.2
- **Bejel** 104.0
- **Bekhterev's disease** (ankylosing spondylitis) 720.0
- **Bekhterev-Strümpell-Marie syndrome** (ankylosing spondylitis) 720.0
- **Belching** (*see also* Eructation) 787.3
- **Bell's**
  - disease (*see also* Psychosis, affective) 296.0 [5th]
  - mania (*see also* Psychosis, affective) 296.0 [5th]
  - palsy, paralysis 351.0
    - infant 767.5
    - newborn 767.5
    - syphilitic 094.89
  - spasm 351.0
- **Bence-Jones albuminuria, albuminosuria, or proteinuria** 791.0
- **Bends** 993.3
- **Benedikt's syndrome** (paralysis) 344.89
- **Benign** - *see also* condition
  - cellular changes, cervix 795.09
  - prostate
    - hyperplasia 600.20
      - with
        - other lower urinary tract symptoms (LUTS) 600.21
        - urinary
          - obstruction 600.21
          - retention 600.21
    - neoplasm 222.2
- **Bennett's**
  - disease (leukemia) 208.9 [5th]
  - fracture (closed) 815.01
    - open 815.11
- **Benson's disease** 379.22
- **Bent**
  - back (hysterical) 300.11
  - nose 738.0
    - congenital 754.0
- **Bereavement** V62.82
  - as adjustment reaction 309.0
- **Berger's paresthesia** (lower limb) 782.0
- **Bergeron's disease** (hysteroepilepsy) 300.11
- **Beriberi** (acute) (atrophic) (chronic) (dry) (subacute) (wet) 265.0
  - with polyneuropathy 265.0 *[357.4]*
  - heart (disease) 265.0 *[425.7]*
  - leprosy 030.1
  - neuritis 265.0 *[357.4]*
- **Berlin's disease or edema** (traumatic) 921.3
- **Berloque dermatitis** 692.72
- **Bernard-Horner syndrome** (*see also* Neuropathy, peripheral, autonomic) 337.9
- **Bernard-Sergent syndrome** (acute adrenocortical insufficiency) 255.41
- **Bernard-Soulier disease or thrombopathy** 287.1
- **Bernhardt's disease or paresthesia** 355.1
- **Bernhardt-Roth disease or syndrome** (parasthesia) 355.1
- **Bernheim's syndrome** (*see also* Failure, heart) 428.0
- **Bertielliasis** 123.8
- **Bertolotti's syndrome** (sacralization of fifth lumbar vertebra) 756.15
- **Berylliosis** (acute) (chronic) (lung) (occupational) 503
- **Besnier's**
  - lupus pernio 135
  - prurigo (atopic dermatitis) (infantile eczema) 691.8
- **Besnier-Boeck disease or sarcoid** 135
- **Besnier-Boeck-Schaumann disease** (sarcoidosis) 135
- **Best's disease** 362.76
- **Bestiality** 302.1
- **Beta-adrenergic hyperdynamic circulatory state** 429.82
- **Beta-aminoisobutyric aciduria** 277.2
- **Beta-mercaptolactate-cysteine disulfiduria** 270.0
- **Beta thalassemia** (major) (minor) (mixed) 282.49
- **Beurmann's disease** (sporotrichosis) 117.1
- **Bezoar** 938
  - intestine 936
  - stomach 935.2
- **Bezold's abscess** (*see also* Mastoiditis) 383.01
- **Bianchi's syndrome** (aphasia-apraxia-alexia) 784.69
- **Bicornuate or bicornis uterus** 752.3
  - in pregnancy or childbirth 654.0 [5th]
    - with obstructed labor 660.2 [5th]
      - affecting fetus or newborn 763.1
    - affecting fetus or newborn 763.89
- **Bicuspid aortic valve** 746.4
- **Biedl-Bardet syndrome** 759.89
- **Bielschowsky's disease** 330.1
- **Bielschowsky-Jansky**
  - amaurotic familial idiocy 330.1
  - disease 330.1
- **Biemond's syndrome** (obesity, polydactyly, and mental retardation) 759.89
- **Biermer's anemia or disease** (pernicious anemia) 281.0
- **Biett's disease** 695.4
- **Bifid** (congenital) - *see also* Imperfect, closure
  - apex, heart 746.89
  - clitoris 752.49
  - epiglottis 748.3
  - kidney 753.3
  - nose 748.1
  - patella 755.64
  - scrotum 752.89
  - toe 755.66
  - tongue 750.13
  - ureter 753.4
  - uterus 752.3
  - uvula 749.02
    - with cleft lip (*see also* Cleft, palate, with cleft lip) 749.20
- **Biforis uterus** (suprasimplex) 752.3
- **Bifurcation** (congenital) - *see also* Imperfect, closure
  - gallbladder 751.69
  - kidney pelvis 753.3
  - renal pelvis 753.3
  - rib 756.3
  - tongue 750.13
  - trachea 748.3
  - ureter 753.4
  - urethra 753.8
  - uvula 749.02
    - with cleft lip (*see also* Cleft, palate, with cleft lip) 749.20
  - vertebra 756.19
- **Bigeminal pulse** 427.89
- **Bigeminy** 427.89
- **Big spleen syndrome** 289.4
- **Bilateral** - *see* condition
- **Bile duct** - *see* condition
- **Bile pigments in urine** 791.4
- **Bilharziasis** (*see also* Schistosomiasis) 120.9
  - chyluria 120.0
  - cutaneous 120.3
  - galacturia 120.0
  - hematochyluria 120.0
  - intestinal 120.1
  - lipemia 120.9
  - lipuria 120.0
  - Oriental 120.2
  - piarhemia 120.9
  - pulmonary 120.2
  - tropical hematuria 120.0
  - vesical 120.0
- **Biliary** - *see* condition
- **Bilious** (attack) - *see also* Vomiting
  - fever, hemoglobinuric 084.8
- **Bilirubinuria** 791.4
- **Biliuria** 791.4
- **Billroth's disease**
  - meningocele (*see also* Spina bifida) 741.9 [5th]
- **Bilobate placenta** - *see* Placenta, abnormal
- **Bilocular**
  - heart 745.7
  - stomach 536.8
- **Bing-Horton syndrome** (histamine cephalgia) 339.00
- **Binswanger's disease or dementia** 290.12
- **Biörck (-Thorson) syndrome** (malignant carcinoid) 259.2
- **Biparta, bipartite** - *see also* Imperfect, closure
  - carpal scaphoid 755.59
  - patella 755.64
  - placenta - *see* Placenta, abnormal
  - vagina 752.49
- **Bird**
  - face 756.0
  - fanciers' lung or disease 495.2
  - flu 488.0 ●
- **Bird's disease** (oxaluria) 271.8
- **Birt-Hogg-Dube syndrome** 759.89
- **Birth**
  - abnormal fetus or newborn 763.9
  - accident, fetus or newborn - *see* Birth, injury
  - complications in mother - *see* Delivery, complicated
  - compression during NEC 767.9
  - defect - *see* Anomaly
  - delayed, fetus 763.9
  - difficult NEC, affecting fetus or newborn 763.9
  - dry, affecting fetus or newborn 761.1
  - forced, NEC, affecting fetus or newborn 763.89
  - forceps, affecting fetus or newborn 763.2
  - hematoma of sternomastoid 767.8
  - immature 765.1 [5th]
    - extremely 765.0 [5th]
  - inattention, after or at 995.52
  - induced, affecting fetus or newborn 763.89
  - infant - *see* Newborn
  - injury NEC 767.9
    - adrenal gland 767.8
    - basal ganglia 767.0
    - brachial plexus (paralysis) 767.6
    - brain (compression) (pressure) 767.0
    - cerebellum 767.0
    - cerebral hemorrhage 767.0
    - conjunctiva 767.8
    - eye 767.8
    - fracture
      - bone, any except clavicle or spine 767.3
      - clavicle 767.2
      - femur 767.3
      - humerus 767.3
      - long bone 767.3
      - radius and ulna 767.3
      - skeleton NEC 767.3
      - skull 767.3
      - spine 767.4
      - tibia and fibula 767.3
    - hematoma 767.8
      - liver (subcapsular) 767.8
      - mastoid 767.8
      - skull 767.19
      - sternomastoid 767.8
      - testes 767.8
      - vulva 767.8
    - intracranial (edema) 767.0
    - laceration
      - brain 767.0
      - by scalpel 767.8
      - peripheral nerve 767.7
    - liver 767.8
- **Birth** – *continued*
  - injury – *continued*
    - meninges
      - brain 767.0
      - spinal cord 767.4
    - nerves (cranial, peripheral) 767.7
      - brachial plexus 767.6
      - facial 767.5
    - paralysis 767.7
      - brachial plexus 767.6
      - Erb (-Duchenne) 767.6
      - facial nerve 767.5
      - Klumpke (-Déjérine) 767.6
      - radial nerve 767.6
      - spinal (cord) (hemorrhage) (laceration) (rupture) 767.4
    - rupture
      - intracranial 767.0
      - liver 767.8
      - spinal cord 767.4
      - spleen 767.8
      - viscera 767.8
    - scalp 767.19
    - scalpel wound 767.8
    - skeleton NEC 767.3
    - specified NEC 767.8
    - spinal cord 767.4
    - spleen 767.8
    - subdural hemorrhage 767.0
    - tentorial, tear 767.0
    - testes 767.8
    - vulva 767.8
  - instrumental, NEC, affecting fetus or newborn 763.2
  - lack of care, after or at 995.52
  - multiple
    - affected by maternal complications of pregnancy 761.5
    - healthy liveborn - *see* Newborn, multiple
  - neglect, after or at 995.52
  - newborn - *see* Newborn
  - palsy or paralysis NEC 767.7
  - precipitate, fetus or newborn 763.6
  - premature (infant) 765.1 [5th]
  - prolonged, affecting fetus or newborn 763.9
  - retarded, fetus or newborn 763.9
  - shock, newborn 779.89
  - strangulation or suffocation
    - due to aspiration of clear amniotic fluid 770.13
      - with respiratory symptoms 770.14
    - mechanical 767.8
  - trauma NEC 767.9
  - triplet
    - affected by maternal complications of pregnancy 761.5
    - healthy liveborn - *see* Newborn, multiple
  - twin
    - affected by maternal complications of pregnancy 761.5
    - healthy liveborn - *see* Newborn, twin
  - ventouse, affecting fetus or newborn 763.3
- **Birthmark** 757.32
- **Bisalbuminemia** 273.8
- **Biskra button** 085.1
- **Bite**(s)
  - with intact skin surface - *see* Contusion
  - animal - *see* Wound, open, by site
    - intact skin surface - *see* Contusion
  - bedbug - *see* Injury, superficial, by site
  - centipede 989.5
  - chigger 133.8
  - fire ant 989.5
  - flea - *see* Injury, superficial, by site
  - human (open wound) - *see also* Wound, open, by site
    - intact skin surface - *see* Contusion
  - insect
    - nonvenomous - *see* Injury, superficial, by site
    - venomous 989.5

Behavior disorder, disturbance – Bite(s)

Bite(s) – *continued*
- mad dog (death from) 071
- open
  - anterior 524.24
  - posterior 524.25
- poisonous 989.5
- red bug 133.8
- reptile 989.5
  - nonvenomous - *see* Wound, open, by site
- snake 989.5
  - nonvenomous - *see* Wound, open, by site
- spider (venomous) 989.5
  - nonvenomous - *see* Injury, superficial, by site
- venomous 989.5

Biting
- cheek or lip 528.9
- nail 307.9

Black
- death 020.9
- eye NEC 921.0
- hairy tongue 529.3
- heel 924.20
- lung disease 500
- palm 923.20

Blackfan-Diamond anemia or syndrome (congenital hypoplastic anemia) 284.01

Blackhead 706.1

Blackout 780.2

Blackwater fever 084.8

Bladder - *see* condition

Blast
- blindness 921.3
- concussion - *see* Blast, injury
- injury 869.0
  - with open wound into cavity 869.1
  - abdomen or thorax - *see* Injury, internal, by site
  - brain (*see also* Concussion, brain) 850.9
    - with skull fracture - *see* Fracture, skull
  - ear (acoustic nerve trauma) 951.5
    - with perforation, tympanic membrane - *see* Wound, open, ear, drum
  - lung (*see also* Injury, internal, lung) 861.20
  - otitic (explosive) 388.11

Blastomycosis, blastomycotic (chronic) (cutaneous) (disseminated) (lung) (pulmonary) (systemic) 116.0
- Brazilian 116.1
- European 117.5
- keloidal 116.2
- North American 116.0
- primary pulmonary 116.0
- South American 116.1

Bleb(s) 709.8
- emphysematous (bullous) (diffuse) (lung) (ruptured) (solitary) 492.0
- filtering, eye (postglaucoma) (status) V45.69
  - with complication 997.99
  - postcataract extraction (complication) 997.99
- lung (ruptured) 492.0
  - congenital 770.5
- subpleural (emphysematous) 492.0

Bleeder (familial) (hereditary) (*see also* Defect, coagulation) 286.9
- nonfamilial 286.9

Bleeding (*see also* Hemorrhage) 459.0
- anal 569.3
- anovulatory 628.0
- atonic, following delivery 666.1 **5th**
- capillary 448.9
- due to subinvolution 621.1
  - puerperal 666.2 **5th**
- ear 388.69
- excessive, associated with menopausal onset 627.0
- familial (*see also* Defect, coagulation) 286.9
- following intercourse 626.7
- gastrointestinal 578.9
- gums 523.8
- hemorrhoids - *see* Hemorrhoids, bleeding
- intermenstrual
  - irregular 626.6
  - regular 626.5
- intraoperative 998.11
- irregular NEC 626.4
- menopausal 627.0
- mouth 528.9
- nipple 611.79
- nose 784.7
- ovulation 626.5
- postclimacteric 627.1
- postcoital 626.7
- postmenopausal 627.1
  - following induced menopause 627.4
- postoperative 998.11
- preclimacteric 627.0
- puberty 626.3
  - excessive, with onset of menstrual periods 626.3
- rectum, rectal 569.3
- tendencies (*see also* Defect, coagulation) 286.9
- throat 784.8
- umbilical stump 772.3
- umbilicus 789.9
- unrelated to menstrual cycle 626.6
- uterus, uterine 626.9
  - climacteric 627.0
  - dysfunctional 626.8
  - functional 626.8
  - unrelated to menstrual cycle 626.6
- vagina, vaginal 623.8
  - functional 626.8
- vicarious 625.8

Blennorrhagia, blennorrhagic - *see* Blennorrhea

Blennorrhea (acute) 098.0
- adultorum 098.40
- alveolaris 523.40
- chronic or duration of 2 months or over 098.2
- gonococcal (neonatorum) 098.40
- inclusion (neonatal) (newborn) 771.6
- neonatorum 098.40

Blepharelosis (*see also* Entropion) 374.00

Blepharitis (eyelid) 373.00
- angularis 373.01
- ciliaris 373.00
  - with ulcer 373.01
- marginal 373.00
  - with ulcer 373.01
- scrofulous (*see also* Tuberculosis) 017.3 **5th** *[373.00]*
- squamous 373.02
- ulcerative 373.01

Blepharochalasis 374.34
- congenital 743.62

Blepharoclonus 333.81

Blepharoconjunctivitis (*see also* Conjunctivitis) 372.20
- angular 372.21
- contact 372.22

Blepharophimosis (eyelid) 374.46
- congenital 743.62

Blepharoplegia 374.89

Blepharoptosis 374.30
- congenital 743.61

Blepharopyorrhea 098.49

Blepharospasm 333.81
- due to drugs 333.85

Blessig's cyst 362.62

Blighted ovum 631

Blind
- bronchus (congenital) 748.3
- eye - *see also* Blindness
  - hypertensive 360.42
  - hypotensive 360.41
- loop syndrome (postoperative) 579.2
- sac, fallopian tube (congenital) 752.19
- spot, enlarged 368.42
- tract or tube (congenital) NEC - *see* Atresia

Blindness (acquired) (congenital) (both eyes) 369.00
- with deafness V49.85
- blast 921.3
  - with nerve injury - *see* Injury, nerve, optic
- Bright's - *see* Uremia
- color (congenital) 368.59
  - acquired 368.55
  - blue 368.53
  - green 368.52
  - red 368.51
  - total 368.54
- concussion 950.9
- cortical 377.75
- day 368.10
  - acquired 368.10
  - congenital 368.10
  - hereditary 368.10
  - specified type NEC 368.10
- due to
  - injury NEC 950.9
  - refractive error - *see* Error, refractive
- eclipse (total) 363.31
- emotional 300.11
- face 368.16
- hysterical 300.11
- legal (both eyes) (USA definition) 369.4
  - with impairment of better (less impaired) eye
    - near-total 369.02
      - with
        - lesser eye impairment 369.02
          - near-total 369.04
          - total 369.03
    - profound 369.05
      - with
        - lesser eye impairment 369.05
          - near-total 369.07
          - profound 369.08
          - total 369.06
    - severe 369.21
      - with
        - lesser eye impairment 369.21
          - blind 369.11
          - near-total 369.13
          - profound 369.14
          - severe 369.22
          - total 369.12
    - total
      - with lesser eye impairment total 369.01
- mind 784.69
- moderate
  - both eyes 369.25
    - with impairment of lesser eye (specified as)
      - blind, not further specified 369.15
      - low vision, not further specified 369.23
      - near-total 369.17
      - profound 369.18
      - severe 369.24
      - total 369.16
  - one eye 369.74
    - with vision of other eye (specified as)
      - near-normal 369.75
      - normal 369.76
- near-total
  - both eyes 369.04
    - with impairment of lesser eye (specified as)
      - blind, not further specified 369.02
      - total 369.03
  - one eye 369.64
    - with vision of other eye (specified as)
      - near-normal 369.65
      - normal 369.66
- night 368.60
  - acquired 368.62
  - congenital (Japanese) 368.61
  - hereditary 368.61
  - specified type NEC 368.69
  - vitamin A deficiency 264.5
- nocturnal - *see* Blindness, night
- one eye 369.60
  - with low vision of other eye 369.10
- profound
  - both eyes 369.08
    - with impairment of lesser eye (specified as)
      - blind, not further specified 369.05
      - near-total 369.07
      - total 369.06
  - one eye 369.67
    - with vision of other eye (specified as)
      - near-normal 369.68
      - normal 369.69
- psychic 784.69
- severe
  - both eyes 369.22
    - with impairment of lesser eye (specified as)
      - blind, not further specified 369.11
      - low vision, not further specified 369.21
      - near-total 369.13
      - profound 369.14
      - total 369.12
  - one eye 369.71
    - with vision of other eye (specified as)
      - near-normal 369.72
      - normal 369.73
- snow 370.24
- sun 363.31
- temporary 368.12
- total
  - both eyes 369.01
  - one eye 369.61
    - with vision of other eye (specified as)
      - near-normal 369.62
      - normal 369.63
- transient 368.12
- traumatic NEC 950.9
- word (developmental) 315.01
  - acquired 784.61
  - secondary to organic lesion 784.61

Blister - *see also* Injury, superficial, by site
- beetle dermatitis 692.89
- due to burn - *see* Burn, by site, second degree
- fever 054.9
- multiple, skin, nontraumatic 709.8

Bloating 787.3

Bloch-Siemens syndrome (incontinentia pigmenti) 757.33

Bloch-Stauffer dyshormonal dermatosis 757.33

Bloch-Sulzberger disease or syndrome (incontinentia pigmenti) (melanoblastosis) 757.33

Block
- alveolar capillary 516.3
- arborization (heart) 426.6
- arrhythmic 426.9
- atrioventricular (AV) (incomplete) (partial) 426.10
  - with
    - 2:1 atrioventricular response block 426.13

- **Block** – *continued*
  - atrioventricular – *continued*
    - with – *continued*
      - atrioventricular dissociation 426.0
    - first degree (incomplete) 426.11
    - second degree (Mobitz type I) 426.13
      - Mobitz (type II) 426.12
    - third degree 426.0
    - complete 426.0
      - congenital 746.86
    - congenital 746.86
    - Mobitz (incomplete)
      - type I (Wenckebach's) 426.13
      - type II 426.12
    - partial 426.13
  - auriculoventricular (*see also* Block, atrioventricular) 426.10
    - complete 426.0
      - congenital 746.86
    - congenital 746.86
  - bifascicular (cardiac) 426.53
  - bundle branch (complete) (false) (incomplete) 426.50
    - bilateral 426.53
    - left (complete) (main stem) 426.3
      - with right bundle branch block 426.53
      - anterior fascicular 426.2
        - with
          - posterior fascicular block 426.3
          - right bundle branch block 426.52
      - hemiblock 426.2
      - incomplete 426.2
        - with right bundle branch block 426.53
      - posterior fascicular 426.2
        - with
          - anterior fascicular block 426.3
          - right bundle branch block 426.51
    - right 426.4
      - with
        - left bundle branch block (incomplete) (main stem) 426.53
        - left fascicular block 426.53
          - anterior 426.52
          - posterior 426.51
    - Wilson's type 426.4
  - cardiac 426.9
  - conduction 426.9
    - complete 426.0
  - Eustachian tube (*see also* Obstruction, Eustachian tube) 381.60
  - fascicular (left anterior) (left posterior) 426.2
  - foramen Magendie (acquired) 331.3
    - congenital 742.3
      - with spina bifida (*see also* Spina bifida) 741.0 [5th]
  - heart 426.9
    - first degree (atrioventricular) 426.11
    - second degree (atrioventricular) 426.13
    - third degree (atrioventricular) 426.0
    - bundle branch (complete) (false) (incomplete) 426.50
      - bilateral 426.53
      - left (*see also* Block, bundle branch, left) 426.3
      - right (*see also* Block, bundle branch, right) 426.4
    - complete (atrioventricular) 426.0
    - congenital 746.86
    - incomplete 426.13
    - intra-atrial 426.6
    - intraventricular NEC 426.6
    - sinoatrial 426.6
    - specified type NEC 426.6
  - hepatic vein 453.0
- **Block** – *continued*
  - intraventricular (diffuse) (myofibrillar) 426.6
    - bundle branch (complete) (false) (incomplete) 426.50
      - bilateral 426.53
      - left (*see also* Block, bundle branch, left) 426.3
      - right (*see also* Block, bundle branch, right) 426.4
  - kidney (*see also* Disease, renal) 593.9
    - postcystoscopic 997.5
  - myocardial (*see also* Block, heart) 426.9
  - nodal 426.10
  - optic nerve 377.49
  - organ or site (congenital) NEC - *see* Atresia
  - parietal 426.6
  - peri-infarction 426.6
  - portal (vein) 452
  - sinoatrial 426.6
  - sinoauricular 426.6
  - spinal cord 336.9
  - trifascicular 426.54
  - tubal 628.2
  - vein NEC 453.9
- **Blocq's disease or syndrome** (astasia-abasia) 307.9
- **Blood**
  - constituents, abnormal NEC 790.6
  - disease 289.9
    - specified NEC 289.89
  - donor V59.01
    - other blood components V59.09
    - stem cells V59.02
    - whole blood V59.01
  - dyscrasia 289.9
    - with
      - abortion - *see* Abortion, by type, with hemorrhage, delayed or excessive
      - ectopic pregnancy (*see also* categories 633.0-633.9) 639.1
      - molar pregnancy (*see also* categories 630-632) 639.1
    - ~~fetus or newborn NEC 776.9~~
    - following
      - abortion 639.1
      - ectopic or molar pregnancy 639.1
    - newborn 776.9 ●
    - puerperal, postpartum 666.3 [5th]
  - flukes NEC (*see also* Infestation, Schistosoma) 120.9
  - in
    - feces (*see also* Melena) 578.1
      - occult 792.1
    - urine (*see also* Hematuria) 599.70
  - mole 631
  - occult 792.1
  - poisoning (*see also* Septicemia) 038.9
  - pressure
    - decreased, due to shock following injury 958.4
    - fluctuating 796.4
    - high (*see also* Hypertension) 401.9
      - incidental reading (isolated) (nonspecific), without diagnosis of hypertension 796.2
    - low (*see also* Hypotension) 458.9
      - incidental reading (isolated) (nonspecific), without diagnosis of hypotension 796.3
  - spitting (*see also* Hemoptysis) 786.3
  - staining cornea 371.12
  - transfusion
    - without reported diagnosis V58.2
    - donor V59.01
      - stem cells V59.02
    - reaction or complication - *see* Complications, transfusion
  - tumor - *see* Hematoma
  - vessel rupture - *see* Hemorrhage
- **Blood** – *continued*
  - vomiting (*see also* Hematemesis) 578.0
- **Blood-forming organ disease** 289.9
- **Bloodgood's disease** 610.1
- **Bloodshot eye** 379.93
- **Bloom (-Machacek) (-Torre) syndrome** 757.39
- **Blotch, palpebral** 372.55
- **Blount's disease** (tibia vara) 732.4
- **Blount-Barber syndrome** (tibia vara) 732.4
- **Blue**
  - baby 746.9
  - bloater 491.20
    - with
      - acute bronchitis 491.22
      - exacerbation (acute) 491.21
  - diaper syndrome 270.0
  - disease 746.9
  - dome cyst 610.0
  - drum syndrome 381.02
  - sclera 743.47
    - with fragility of bone and deafness 756.51
  - toe syndrome 445.02
- **Blueness** (*see also* Cyanosis) 782.5
- **Blurring, visual** 368.8
- **Blushing** (abnormal) (excessive) 782.62
- **BMI** (body mass index)
  - adult
    - 25.0-25.9 V85.21
    - 26.0-26.9 V85.22
    - 27.0-27.9 V85.23
    - 28.0-28.9 V85.24
    - 29.0-29.9 V85.25
    - 30.0-30.9 V85.30
    - 31.0-31.9 V85.31
    - 32.0-32.9 V85.32
    - 33.0-33.9 V85.33
    - 34.0-34.9 V85.34
    - 35.0-35.9 V85.35
    - 36.0-36.9 V85.36
    - 37.0-37.9 V85.37
    - 38.0-38.9 V85.38
    - 39.0-39.9 V85.39
    - 40 and over V85.4
    - between 19-24 V85.1
    - less than 19 V85.0
  - pediatric
    - 5th percentile to less than 85th percentile for age V85.52
    - 85th percentile to less than 95th percentile for age V85.53
    - greater than or equal to 95th percentile for age V85.54
    - less than 5th percentile for age V85.51
- **Boarder, hospital** V65.0
  - infant V65.0
- **Bockhart's impetigo** (superficial folliculitis) 704.8
- **Bodechtel-Guttmann disease** (subacute sclerosing panencephalitis) 046.2
- **Boder-Sedgwick syndrome** (ataxia-telangiectasia) 334.8
- **Body, bodies**
  - Aschoff (*see also* Myocarditis, rheumatic) 398.0
  - asteroid, vitreous 379.22
  - choroid, colloid (degenerative) 362.57
    - hereditary 362.77
  - cytoid (retina) 362.82
  - drusen (retina) (*see also* Drusen) 362.57
    - optic disc 377.21
  - fibrin, pleura 511.0
  - foreign - *see* Foreign body
  - Hassall-Henle 371.41
  - loose
    - joint (*see also* Loose, body, joint) 718.1 [5th]
      - knee 717.6
    - knee 717.6
    - sheath, tendon 727.82
  - Mallory's 034.1
- **Body, bodies** – *continued*
  - mass index (BMI)
    - adult
      - 25.0-25.9 V85.21
      - 26.0-26.9 V85.22
      - 27.0-27.9 V85.23
      - 28.0-28.9 V85.24
      - 29.0-29.9 V85.25
      - 30.0-30.9 V85.30
      - 31.0-31.9 V85.31
      - 32.0-32.9 V85.32
      - 33.0-33.9 V85.33
      - 34.0-34.9 V85.34
      - 35.0-35.9 V85.35
      - 36.0-36.9 V85.36
      - 37.0-37.9 V85.37
      - 38.0-38.9 V85.38
      - 39.0-39.9 V85.39
      - 40 and over V85.4
      - between 19-24 V85.1
      - less than 19 V85.0
    - pediatric
      - 5th percentile to less than 85th percentile for age V85.52
      - 85th percentile to less than 95th percentile for age V85.53
      - greater than or equal to 95th percentile for age V85.54
      - less than 5th percentile for age V85.51
  - Mooser 081.0
  - Negri 071
  - rice (joint) (*see also* Loose, body, joint) 718.1 [5th]
    - knee 717.6
  - rocking 307.3
- **Boeck's**
  - disease (sarcoidosis) 135
  - lupoid (miliary) 135
  - sarcoid 135
- **Boerhaave's syndrome** (spontaneous esophageal rupture) 530.4
- **Boggy**
  - cervix 622.8
  - uterus 621.8
- **Boil** (*see also* Carbuncle) 680.9
  - abdominal wall 680.2
  - Aleppo 085.1
  - ankle 680.6
  - anus 680.5
  - arm (any part, above wrist) 680.3
  - auditory canal, external 680.0
  - axilla 680.3
  - back (any part) 680.2
  - Baghdad 085.1
  - breast 680.2
  - buttock 680.5
  - chest wall 680.2
  - corpus cavernosum 607.2
  - Delhi 085.1
  - ear (any part) 680.0
  - eyelid 373.13
  - face (any part, except eye) 680.0
  - finger (any) 680.4
  - flank 680.2
  - foot (any part) 680.7
  - forearm 680.3
  - Gafsa 085.1
  - genital organ, male 608.4
  - gluteal (region) 680.5
  - groin 680.2
  - hand (any part) 680.4
  - head (any part, except face) 680.8
  - heel 680.7
  - hip 680.6
  - knee 680.6
  - labia 616.4
  - lacrimal (*see also* Dacryocystitis) 375.30
    - gland (*see also* Dacryoadenitis) 375.00
    - passages (duct) (sac) (*see also* Dacryocystitis) 375.30
  - leg, any part, except foot 680.6
  - multiple sites 680.9
  - natal 085.1

Boil – *continued*
- neck 680.1
- nose (external) (septum) 680.0
- orbit, orbital 376.01
- partes posteriores 680.5
- pectoral region 680.2
- penis 607.2
- perineum 680.2
- pinna 680.0
- scalp (any part) 680.8
- scrotum 608.4
- seminal vesicle 608.0
- shoulder 680.3
- skin NEC 680.9
- specified site NEC 680.8
- spermatic cord 608.4
- temple (region) 680.0
- testis 608.4
- thigh 680.6
- thumb 680.4
- toe (any) 680.7
- tropical 085.1
- trunk 680.2
- tunica vaginalis 608.4
- umbilicus 680.2
- upper arm 680.3
- vas deferens 608.4
- vulva 616.4
- wrist 680.4

Bold hives (*see also* Urticaria) 708.9
Bolivian hemorrhagic fever 078.7
Bombé, iris 364.74
Bomford-Rhoads anemia (refractory) 238.72
Bone - *see* condition
Bonnevie-Ullrich syndrome 758.6
Bonnier's syndrome 386.19
Bonvale Dam fever 780.79
Bony block of joint 718.80
- ankle 718.87
- elbow 718.82
- foot 718.87
- hand 718.84
- hip 718.85
- knee 718.86
- multiple sites 718.89
- pelvic region 718.85
- shoulder (region) 718.81
- specified site NEC 718.88
- wrist 718.83

BOOP (bronchiolitis obliterans organized pneumonia) 516.8
Borderline
- intellectual functioning V62.89
- osteopenia 733.90
- pelvis 653.1 [5th]
  - with obstruction during labor 660.1 [5th]
    - affecting fetus or newborn 763.1
- psychosis (*see also* Schizophrenia) 295.5 [5th]
  - of childhood (*see also* Psychosis, childhood) 299.8 [5th]
- schizophrenia (*see also* Schizophrenia) 295.5 [5th]

Borna disease 062.9
Bornholm disease (epidemic pleurodynia) 074.1
Borrelia vincentii (mouth) (pharynx) (tonsils) 101
Bostock's catarrh (*see also* Fever, hay) 477.9
Boston exanthem 048
Botalli, ductus (patent) (persistent) 747.0
Bothriocephalus latus infestation 123.4
Botulism 005.1
- food poisoning 005.1
- infant 040.41
- non-foodborne 040.42
- wound 040.42

Bouba (*see also* Yaws) 102.9
Bouffée délirante 298.3
Bouillaud's disease or syndrome (rheumatic heart disease) 391.9
Bourneville's disease (tuberous sclerosis) 759.5
Boutonneuse fever 082.1
Boutonniere
- deformity (finger) 736.21
- hand (intrinsic) 736.21

Bouveret (-Hoffmann) disease or syndrome (paroxysmal tachycardia) 427.2
Bovine heart - *see* Hypertrophy, cardiac
Bowel - *see* condition
Bowen's
- dermatosis (precancerous) (M8081/2) - *see* Neoplasm, skin, in situ
- disease (M8081/2) - *see* Neoplasm, skin, in situ
- epithelioma (M8081/2) - *see* Neoplasm, skin, in situ
- type
  - epidermoid carcinoma in situ (M8081/2) - *see* Neoplasm, skin, in situ
  - intraepidermal squamous cell carcinoma (M8081/2) - *see* Neoplasm, skin, in situ

Bowing
- femur 736.89
  - congenital 754.42
- fibula 736.89
  - congenital 754.43
- forearm 736.09
  - away from midline (cubitus valgus) 736.01
  - toward midline (cubitus varus) 736.02
- leg(s), long bones, congenital 754.44
- radius 736.09
  - away from midline (cubitus valgus) 736.01
  - toward midline (cubitus varus) 736.02
- tibia 736.89
  - congenital 754.43

Bowleg(s) 736.42
- congenital 754.44
- rachitic 268.1

Boyd's dysentery 004.2
Brachial - *see* condition
Brachman-de Lange syndrome (Amsterdam dwarf, mental retardation, and brachycephaly) 759.89
Brachycardia 427.89
Brachycephaly 756.0
Brachymorphism and ectopia lentis 759.89
Bradley's disease (epidemic vomiting) 078.82
Bradycardia 427.89
- chronic (sinus) 427.81
- newborn 779.81
- nodal 427.89
- postoperative 997.1
- reflex 337.09
- sinoatrial 427.89
  - with paroxysmal tachyarrhythmia or tachycardia 427.81
  - chronic 427.81
- sinus 427.89
  - with paroxysmal tachyarrhythmia or tachycardia 427.81
  - chronic 427.81
  - persistent 427.81
  - severe 427.81
- tachycardia syndrome 427.81
- vagal 427.89

Bradykinesia 781.0 ●
Bradypnea 786.09
Brailsford's disease 732.3
- radial head 732.3
- tarsal scaphoid 732.5

Brailsford-Morquio disease or syndrome (mucopolysaccharidosis IV) 277.5
Brain - *see also* condition
- death 348.89 ▲

Brain – *continued*
- syndrome (acute) (chronic) (nonpsychotic) (organic) (with neurotic reaction) (with behavioral reaction) (*see also* Syndrome, brain) 310.9
  - with
    - presenile brain disease 290.10
    - psychosis, psychotic reaction (*see also* Psychosis, organic) 294.9
  - congenital (*see also* Retardation, mental) 319

Branched-chain amino-acid disease 270.3
Branchial - *see* condition
Brandt's syndrome (acrodermatitis enteropathica) 686.8
Brash (water) 787.1
Brass-founders' ague 985.8
Bravais-Jacksonian epilepsy (*see also* Epilepsy) 345.5 [5th]
Braxton Hicks contractions 644.1 [5th]
Braziers' disease 985.8
Brazilian
- blastomycosis 116.1
- leishmaniasis 085.5

BRBPR (bright red blood per rectum) 569.3
Break
- cardiorenal - *see* Hypertension, cardiorenal
- retina (*see also* Defect, retina) 361.30

Breakbone fever 061
Breakdown
- device, implant, or graft - *see* Complications, mechanical
- nervous (*see also* Disorder, mental, nonpsychotic) 300.9
- perineum 674.2 [5th]

Breast - *see also* condition
- buds 259.1
  - in newborn 779.89
- dense ~~- omit code~~ 793.82 ▲
- nodule 793.89

Breast feeding difficulties 676.8 [5th]
Breath
- foul 784.99
- holder, child 312.81
- holding spells 786.9
- shortness 786.05

Breathing
- asymmetrical 786.09
- bronchial 786.09
- exercises V57.0
- labored 786.09
- mouth 784.99
  - causing malocclusion 524.59
- periodic 786.09
  - high altitude 327.22
- tic 307.20

Breathlessness 786.09
Breda's disease (*see also* Yaws) 102.9
Breech
- delivery, affecting fetus or newborn 763.0
- extraction, affecting fetus or newborn 763.0
- presentation (buttocks) (complete) (frank) 652.2 [5th]
  - with successful version 652.1 [5th]
  - before labor, affecting fetus or newborn 761.7
  - during labor, affecting fetus or newborn 763.0

Breisky's disease (kraurosis vulvae) 624.09
Brennemann's syndrome (acute mesenteric lymphadenitis) 289.2
Brenner's
- tumor (benign) (M9000/0) 220
  - borderline malignancy (M9000/1) 236.2
  - malignant (M9000/3) 183.0
  - proliferating (M9000/1) 236.2

Bretonneau's disease (diphtheritic malignant angina) 032.0
Breus' mole 631
Brevicollis 756.16
Bricklayers' itch 692.89
Brickmakers' anemia 126.9
Bridge
- myocardial 746.85

Bright red blood per rectum (BRBPR) 569.3
Bright's
- blindness - *see* Uremia
- disease (*see also* Nephritis) 583.9
  - arteriosclerotic (*see also* Hypertension, kidney) 403.90

Brill's disease (recrudescent typhus) 081.1
- flea-borne 081.0
- louse-borne 081.1

Brill-Symmers disease (follicular lymphoma) (M9690/3) 202.0 [5th]
Brill-Zinsser disease (recrudescent typhus) 081.1
Brinton's disease (linitis plastica) (M8142/3) 151.9
Brion-Kayser disease (*see also* Fever, paratyphoid) 002.9
Briquet's disorder or syndrome 300.81
Brissaud's
- infantilism (infantile myxedema) 244.9
- motor-verbal tic 307.23

Brissaud-Meige syndrome (infantile myxedema) 244.9
Brittle
- bones (congenital) 756.51
- nails 703.8
  - congenital 757.5

Broad - *see also* condition
- beta disease 272.2
- ligament laceration syndrome 620.6

Brock's syndrome (atelectasis due to enlarged lymph nodes) 518.0
Brocq's disease 691.8
- atopic (diffuse) neurodermatitis 691.8
- lichen simplex chronicus 698.3
- parakeratosis psoriasiformis 696.2
- parapsoriasis 696.2

Brocq-Duhring disease (dermatitis herpetiformis) 694.0
Brodie's
- abscess (localized) (chronic) (*see also* Osteomyelitis) 730.1 [5th]
- disease (joint) (*see also* Osteomyelitis) 730.1 [5th]

Broken
- arches 734
  - congenital 755.67
- back - *see* Fracture, vertebra, by site
- bone - *see* Fracture, by site
- compensation - *see* Disease, heart
- heart syndrome 429.83
- implant or internal device - *see* listing under Complications, mechanical
- neck - *see* Fracture, vertebra, cervical
- nose 802.0
  - open 802.1
- tooth, teeth 873.63
  - complicated 873.73

Bromhidrosis 705.89
Bromidism, bromism
- acute 967.3
  - correct substance properly administered 349.82
  - overdose or wrong substance given or taken 967.3
- chronic (*see also* Dependence) 304.1 [5th]

Bromidrosiphobia 300.23
Bromidrosis 705.89
Bronchi, bronchial - *see* condition
Bronchiectasis (cylindrical) (diffuse) (fusiform) (localized) (moniliform) (postinfectious) (recurrent) (saccular) 494.0
- with acute exacerbation 494.1
- congenital 748.61
- tuberculosis (*see also* Tuberculosis) 011.5 [5th]

Bronchiolectasis - *see* Bronchiectasis

- **Bronchiolitis** (acute) (infectious) (subacute) 466.19
  - with
    - bronchospasm or obstruction 466.19
    - influenza, flu, or grippe 487.1
  - catarrhal (acute) (subacute) 466.19
  - chemical 506.0
    - chronic 506.4
  - chronic (obliterative) 491.8
  - due to external agent - *see* Bronchitis, acute, due to
  - fibrosa obliterans 491.8
  - influenzal 487.1
  - obliterans 491.8
    - with organizing pneumonia (BOOP) 516.8
    - status post lung transplant 996.84
  - obliterative (chronic) (diffuse) (subacute) 491.8
    - due to fumes or vapors 506.4
  - respiratory syncytial virus 466.11
  - vesicular - *see* Pneumonia, broncho-
- **Bronchitis** (diffuse) (hypostatic) (infectious) (inflammatory) (simple) 490
  - with
    - emphysema - *see* Emphysema
    - influenza, flue, or grippe 487.1
    - obstruction airway, chronic 491.20
      - with
        - acute bronchitis 491.22
        - exacerbation (acute) 491.21
    - tracheitis 490
      - acute or subacute 466.0
        - with bronchospasm or obstruction 466.0
      - chronic 491.8
  - acute or subacute 466.0
    - with
      - bronchiectasis 494.1
      - bronchospasm 466.0
      - obstruction 466.0
      - tracheitis 466.0
    - chemical (due to fumes or vapors) 506.0
    - due to
      - fumes or vapors 506.0
      - radiation 508.8
  - allergic (acute) (*see also* Asthma) 493.9 [5th]
  - arachidic 934.1
  - aspiration 507.0
    - due to fumes or vapors 506.0
  - asthmatic (acute) 493.90
    - with
      - acute exacerbation 493.92
      - status asthmaticus 493.91
    - chronic 493.2 [5th]
  - capillary 466.19
    - with bronchospasm or obstruction 466.19
    - chronic 491.8
  - caseous (*see also* Tuberculosis) 011.3 [5th]
  - Castellani's 104.8
  - catarrhal 490
    - acute - *see* Bronchitis, acute
    - chronic 491.0
  - chemical (acute) (subacute) 506.0
    - chronic 506.4
    - due to fumes or vapors (acute) (subactue) 506.0
      - chronic 506.4
  - chronic 491.9
    - with
      - tracheitis (chronic) 491.8
    - asthmatic 493.2 [5th]
    - catarrhal 491.0
    - chemical (due to fumes and vapors) 506.4
    - due to
      - fumes or vapors (chemical) (inhalation) 506.4
      - radiation 508.8
      - tobacco smoking 491.0
    - mucopurulent 491.1

- **Bronchitis** – *continued*
  - chronic – *continued*
    - obstructive 491.20
      - with
        - acute bronchitis 491.22
        - exacerbation (acute) 491.21
    - purulent 491.1
    - simple 491.0
    - specified type NEC 491.8
  - croupous 466.0
    - with bronchospasm or obstruction 466.0
    - due to fumes or vapors 506.0
  - emphysematous 491.20
    - with
      - acute bronchitis 491.22
      - exacerbation (acute) 491.21
  - exudative 466.0
  - fetid (chronic) (recurrent) 491.1
  - fibrinous, acute or subacute 466.0
    - with bronchospasm or obstruction 466.0
  - grippal 487.1
  - influenzal 487.1
  - membranous, acute or subactue 466.0
    - with bronchospasm or obstruction 466.0
  - moulders' 502
  - mucopurulent (chronic) (recurrent) 491.1
    - acute or subacute 466.0
  - obliterans 491.8
  - obstructive (chronic) 491.20
    - with
      - acute bronchitis 491.22
      - exacerbation (acute) 491.21
  - pituitous 491.1
  - plastic (inflammatory) 466.0
  - pneumococcal, acute or subacute 466.0
    - with bronchospasm or obstruction 466.0
  - pseudomembranous 466.0
  - purulent (chronic) (recurrent) 491.1
    - acute or subacute 466.0
      - with bronchospasm or obstruction 466.0
  - putrid 491.1
  - scrofulous (*see also* Tuberculosis) 011.3 [5th]
  - senile 491.9
  - septic, acute or subacute 466.0
    - with bronchospasm or obstruction 466.0
  - smokers' 491.0
  - spirochetal 104.8
  - suffocative, acute or subacute 466.0
  - summer (*see also* Asthma) 493.9 [5th]
  - suppurative (chronic) 491.1
    - acute or subacute 466.0
  - tuberculous (*see also* Tuberculosis) 011.3 [5th]
  - ulcerative 491.8
    - Vincent's 101
  - Vincent's 101
  - viral, acute or subacute 466.0
- **Bronchoalveolitis** 485
- **Bronchoaspergillosis** 117.3
- **Bronchocele**
  - meaning
    - dilatation of bronchus 519.19
    - goiter 240.9
- **Bronchogenic carcinoma** 162.9
- **Bronchohemisporosis** 117.9
- **Broncholithiasis** 518.89
  - tuberculous (*see also* Tuberculosis) 011.3 [5th]
- **Bronchomalacia** 748.3
- **Bronchomoniliasis** 112.89
- **Bronchomycosis** 112.89
- **Bronchonocardiosis** 039.1
- **Bronchopleuropneumonia** - *see* Pneumonia, broncho-
- **Bronchopneumonia** - *see* Pneumonia, broncho-
- **Bronchopneumonitis** - *see* Pneumonia, broncho-

- **Bronchopulmonary** - *see* condition
- **Bronchopulmonitis** - *see* Pneumonia, broncho-
- **Bronchorrhagia** 786.3
  - newborn 770.3
  - tuberculous (*see also* Tuberculosis) 011.3 [5th]
- **Bronchorrhea** (chronic) (purulent) 491.0
  - acute 466.0
- **Bronchospasm** 519.11
  - with
    - asthma - *see* Asthma
    - bronchiolitis, acute 466.19
      - due to respiratory syncytial virus 466.11
    - bronchitis - *see* Bronchitis
    - chronic obstructive pulmonary disease (COPD) 496
    - emphysema - *see* Emphysema
      - due to external agent - *see* Condition, respiratory, acute, due to
  - acute 519.11
  - exercise induced 493.81
- **Bronchospirochetosis** 104.8
- **Bronchostenosis** 519.19
- **Bronchus** - *see* condition
- **Bronze, bronzed**
  - diabetes 275.0
  - disease (Addison's) (skin) 255.41
    - tuberculous (*see also* Tuberculosis) 017.6 [5th]
- **Brooke's disease or tumor** (M8100/0) - *see* Neoplasm, skin, benign
- **Brown's tendon sheath syndrome** 378.61
- **Brown enamel of teeth** (hereditary) 520.5
- **Brown-Séquard's paralysis** (syndrome) 344.89
- **Brow presentation complicating delivery** 652.4 [5th]
- **Brucella, brucellosis** (infection) 023.9
  - abortus 023.1
  - canis 023.3
  - dermatitis, skin 023.9
  - melitensis 023.0
  - mixed 023.8
  - suis 023.2
- **Bruck's disease** 733.99
- **Bruck-de Lange disease or syndrome** (Amsterdam dwart, mental retardation, and brachycephaly) 759.89
- **Brugada syndrome** 746.89
- **Brug's filariasis** 125.1
- **Brugsch's syndrome** (acropachyderma) 757.39
- **Bruhl's disease** (splenic anemia with fever) 285.8
- **Bruise** (skin surface intact) - *see also* Contusion
  - with
    - fracture - Fracture, by site
    - open wound - *see* Wound, open, by site
  - internal organ (abdomen, chest, or pelvis) - *see* Injury, internal, by site
  - umbilical cord 663.6 [5th]
    - affecting fetus or newborn 762.6
- **Bruit** 785.9
  - arterial (abdominal) (carotid) 785.9
  - supraclavicular 785.9
- **Brushburn** - *see* Injury, superficial, by site
- **Bruton's X-linked agammaglobulinemia** 279.04
- **Bruxism** 306.8
  - sleep related 327.53
- **Bubbly lung syndrome** 770.7
- **Bubo** 289.3
  - blennorrhagic 098.89
  - chancroidal 099.0
  - climatic 099.1
  - due to Hemophilus ducreyi 099.0
  - gonococcal 098.89
  - indolent NEC 099.8
  - inguinal NEC 099.8
    - chancroidal 099.0

- **Bubo** – *continued*
  - inguinal – *continued*
    - climatic 099.1
    - due to H. ducreyi 099.0
  - scrofulous (*see also* Tuberculosis) 017.2 [5th]
  - soft chancre 099.0
  - suppurating 683
  - syphilitic 091.0
    - congenital 090.0
  - tropical 099.1
  - venereal NEC 099.8
  - virulent 099.0
- **Bubonic plague** 020.0
- **Bubonocele** - *see* Hernia, inguinal
- **Buccal** - *see* condition
- **Buchanan's disease** (juvenile osteochondrosis of iliac crest) 732.1
- **Buchem's syndrome** (hyperostosis corticalis) 733.3
- **Buchman's disease** (osteochondrosis, juvenile) 732.1
- **Bucket handle fracture** (semilunar cartilage) (*see also* Tear, meniscus) 836.2
- **Budd-Chiari syndrome** (hepatic vein thrombosis) 453.0
- **Budgerigar-fanciers' disease or lung** 495.2
- **Büdinger-Ludloff-Läwen disease** 717.89
- **Buds**
  - breast 259.1
    - in newborn 779.89
- **Buerger's disease** (thromboangiitis obliterans) 443.1
- **Bulbar** - *see* condition
- **Bulbus cordis** 745.9
  - persistent (in left ventricle) 745.8
- **Bulging fontanels** (congenital) 756.0
- **Bulimia** 783.6
  - nervosa 307.51
  - nonorganic origin 307.51
- **Bulky uterus** 621.2
- **Bulla(e)** 709.8
  - lung (emphysematous) (solitary) 492.0
- **Bullet wound** - *see also* Wound, open, by site
  - fracture - *see* Fracture, by site, open
  - internal organ (abdomen, chest, or pelvis) - *see* Injury, internal, by site, with open wound
  - intracranial - *see* Laceration, brain, with open wound
- **Bullis fever** 082.8
- **Bullying** (*see also* Disturbance, conduct) 312.0 [5th]
- **Bundle**
  - branch block (complete) (false) (incomplete) 426.50
    - bilateral 426.53
    - left (*see also* Block, bundle branch, left) 426.3
      - hemiblock 426.2
    - right (*see also* Block, bundle branch, right) 426.4
  - of His - *see* condition
  - of Kent syndrome (anomalous atrioventricular excitation) 426.7
- **Bungpagga** 040.81
- **Bunion** 727.1
- **Bunionette** 727.1
- **Bunyamwera fever** 066.3
- **Buphthalmia, buphthalmos** (congenital) 743.20
  - associated with
    - keratoglobus, congenital 743.22
    - megalocornea 743.22
    - ocular anomalies NEC 743.22
  - isolated 743.21
  - simple 743.21
- **Bürger-Grütz disease or syndrome** (essential familial hyperlipemia) 272.3
- **Buried roots** 525.3
- **Burke's syndrome** 577.8
- **Burkitt's**
  - tumor (M9750/3) 200.2 [5th]

Bronchiolitis – Burkitt's

Burkitt's – *continued*
  type malignant, lymphoma, lymphoblastic, or undifferentiated (M9750/3) 200.2 5th
Burn (acid) (cathode ray) (caustic) (chemical) (electric heating appliance) (electricity) (fire) (flame) (hot liquid or object) (irradiation) (lime) (radiation) (steam) (thermal) (x-ray) 949.0

Note *Use the following fifth-digit subclassification with category 948 to indicate the percent of body surface with third degree burn:*

0	less than 10 percent or unspecified
1	10-19 percent
2	20-29 percent
3	30-39 percent
4	40-49 percent
5	50-59 percent
6	60-69 percent
7	70-79 percent
8	80-89 percent
9	90 percent or more of body surface

  with
    blisters - *see* Burn, by site, second degree
    erythema - *see* Burn, by site, first degree
    skin loss (epidermal) - *see also* Burn, by site, second degree
      full thickness - *see also* Burn, by site, third degree
        with necrosis of underlying tissues - *see* Burn, by site, third degree, deep
  first degree - *see* Burn, by site, first degree
  second degree - *see* Burn, by site, second degree
  third degree - *see also* Burn, by site, third degree
    deep - *see* Burn, by site, third degree, deep
  abdomen, abdominal (muscle) (wall) 942.03
    with
      trunk - *see* Burn, trunk, multiple sites
    first degree 942.13
    second degree 942.23
    third degree 942.33
      deep 942.43
        with loss of body part 942.53
  ankle 945.03
    with
      lower limb(s) - *see* Burn, leg, multiple sites
    first degree 945.13
    second degree 945.23
    third degree 945.33
      deep 945.43
        with loss of body part 945.53
  anus - *see* Burn, trunk, specified site NEC
  arm(s) 943.00
    first degree 943.10
    second degree 943.20
    third degree 943.30
      deep 943.40
        with loss of body part 943.50
    lower - *see* Burn, forearm(s)
    multiple sites, except hand(s) or wrist(s) 943.09
      first degree 943.19
      second degree 943.29
      third degree 943.39
        deep 943.49
          with loss of body part 943.59
    upper 943.03
      first degree 943.13
      second degree 943.23

Burn – *continued*
  arm(s) – *continued*
    upper – *continued*
      third degree 943.33
        deep 943.43
          with loss of body part 943.53
  auditory canal (external) - *see* Burn, ear
  auricle (ear) - *see* Burn, ear
  axilla 943.04
    with
      upper limb(s), except hand(s) or wrist(s) - *see* Burn, arm(s), multiple sites
    first degree 943.14
    second degree 943.24
    third degree 943.34
      deep 943.44
        with loss of body part 943.54
  back 942.04
    with
      trunk - *see* Burn, trunk, multiple sites
    first degree 942.14
    second degree 942.24
    third degree 942.34
      deep 942.44
        with loss of body part 942.54
  biceps
    brachii - *see* Burn, arm(s), upper
    femoris - *see* Burn, thigh
  breast(s) 942.01
    with
      trunk - *see* Burn, trunk, multiple sites
    first degree 942.11
    second degree 942.21
    third degree 942.31
      deep 942.41
        with loss of body part 942.51
  brow - *see* Burn, forehead
  buttock(s) - *see* Burn, back
  canthus (eye) 940.1
    chemical 940.0
  cervix (uteri) 947.4
  cheek (cutaneous) 941.07
    with
      face or head - *see* Burn, head, multiple sites
    first degree 941.17
    second degree 941.27
    third degree 941.37
      deep 941.47
        with loss of body part 941.57
  chest wall (anterior) 942.02
    with
      trunk - *see* Burn, trunk, multiple sites
    first degree 942.12
    second degree 942.22
    third degree 942.32
      deep 942.42
        with loss of body part 942.52
  chin 941.04
    with
      face or head - *see* Burn, head, multiple sites
    first degree 941.14
    second degree 941.24
    third degree 941.34
      deep 941.44
        with loss of body part 941.54
  clitoris - *see* Burn, genitourinary organs, external
  colon 947.3
  conjunctiva (and cornea) 940.4
    chemical
      acid 940.3
      alkaline 940.2
  cornea (and conjunctiva) 940.4
    chemical
      acid 940.3
      alkaline 940.2
  costal region - *see* Burn, chest wall

Burn – *continued*
  due to ingested chemical agent - *see* Burn, internal organs
  ear (auricle) (canal) (drum) (external) 941.01
    with
      face or head - *see* Burn, head, multiple sites
    first degree 941.11
    second degree 941.21
    third degree 941.31
      deep 941.41
        with loss of a body part 941.51
  elbow 943.02
    with
      hand(s) and wrist(s) - *see* Burn, multiple specified sites
      upper limb(s), except hand(s) or wrist(s) - *see also* Burn, arm(s), multiple sites
    first degree 943.12
    second degree 943.22
    third degree 943.32
      deep 943.42
        with loss of body part 943.52
  electricity, electric current - *see* Burn, by site
  entire body - *see* Burn, multiple, specified sites
  epididymis - *see* Burn, genitourinary organs, external
  epigastric region - *see* Burn, abdomen
  epiglottis 947.1
  esophagus 947.2
  extent (percent of body surface)
    less than 10 percent 948.0 5th
    10-19 percent 948.1 5th
    20-29 percent 948.2 5th
    30-39 percent 948.3 5th
    40-49 percent 948.4 5th
    50-59 percent 948.5 5th
    60-69 percent 948.6 5th
    70-79 percent 948.7 5th
    80-89 percent 948.8 5th
    90 percent or more 948.9 5th
  extremity
    lower - *see* Burn, leg
    upper - *see* Burn, arm(s)
  eye(s) (and adnexa) (only) 940.9
    with
      face, head, or neck 941.02
        first degree 941.12
        second degree 941.22
        third degree 941.32
          deep 941.42
            with loss of body part 941.52
      other sites (classifiable to more than one category in 940-945) - *see* Burn, multiple, specified sites
      resulting rupture and destruction of eyeball 940.5
    specified part - *see* Burn, by site
  eyeball - *see also* Burn, eye
    with resulting rupture and destruction of eyeball 940.5
  eyelid(s) 940.1
    chemical 940.0
  face - *see* Burn, head
  finger (nail) (subungual) 944.01
    with
      hand(s) - *see* Burn, hand(s), multiple sites
      other sites - *see* Burn, multiple, specified sites
      thumb 944.04
        first degree 944.14
        second degree 944.24
        third degree 944.34
          deep 944.44
            with loss of body part 944.54
    first degree 944.11

Burn – *continued*
  finger – *continued*
    second degree 944.21
    third degree 944.31
      deep 944.41
        with loss of body part 944.51
    multiple (digits) 944.03
      with thumb - *see* Burn, finger, with thumb
      first degree 944.13
      second degree 944.23
      third degree 944.33
        deep 944.43
          with loss of body part 944.53
  flank - *see* Burn, abdomen
  foot 945.02
    with
      lower limb(s) - *see* Burn, leg, multiple sites
    first degree 945.12
    second degree 945.22
    third degree 945.32
      deep 945.42
        with loss of body part 945.52
  forearm(s) 943.01
    with
      upper limb(s), except hand(s) or wrist(s) - *see* Burn, arm(s), multiple sites
    first degree 943.11
    second degree 943.21
    third degree 943.31
      deep 943.41
        with loss of body part 943.51
  forehead 941.07
    with
      face or head - *see* Burn, head, multiple sites
    first degree 941.17
    second degree 941.27
    third degree 941.37
      deep 941.47
        with loss of body part 941.57
  fourth degree - *see* Burn, by site, third degree, deep
  friction - *see* Injury, superficial, by site
  from swallowing caustic or corrosive substance NEC - *see* Burn, internal organs
  full thickness - *see* Burn, by site, third degree
  gastrointestinal tract 947.3
  genitourinary organs
    external 942.05
      with
        trunk - *see* Burn, trunk, multiple sites
      first degree 942.15
      second degree 942.25
      third degree 942.35
        deep 942.45
          with loss of body part 942.55
    internal 947.8
  globe (eye) - *see* Burn, eyeball
  groin - *see* Burn, abdomen
  gum 947.0
  hand(s) (phalanges) (and wrist) 944.00
    first degree 944.10
    second degree 944.20
    third degree 944.30
      deep 944.40
        with loss of body part 944.50
    back (dorsal surface) 944.06
      first degree 944.16
      second degree 944.26
      third degree 944.36
        deep 944.46
          with loss of body part 944.56
    multiple sites 944.08
      first degree 944.18
      second degree 944.28
      third degree 944.38
        deep 944.48
          with loss of body part 944.58

- **Burn** – *continued*
  - head (and face) 941.00
    - eye(s) only 940.9
      - specified part - *see* Burn, by site
    - first degree 941.10
    - second degree 941.20
    - third degree 941.30
      - deep 941.40
        - with loss of body part 941.50
    - multiple sites 941.09
      - with eyes - *see* Burn, eyes, with face, head, or neck
      - first degree 941.19
      - second degree 941.29
      - third degree 941.39
        - deep 941.49
          - with loss of body part 941.59
  - heel - *see* Burn, foot
  - hip - *see* Burn, trunk, specified site NEC
  - iliac region - *see* Burn, trunk, specified site NEC
  - infected 958.3
  - inhalation (*see also* Burn, internal organs) 947.9
  - internal organs 947.9
    - from caustic or corrosive substance (swallowing) NEC 947.9
    - specified NEC (*see also* Burn, by site) 947.8
  - interscapular region - *see* Burn, back
  - intestine (large) (small) 947.3
  - iris - *see* Burn, eyeball
  - knee 945.05
    - with
      - lower limb(s) - *see* Burn, leg, multiple sites
    - first degree 945.15
    - second degree 945.25
    - third degree 945.35
      - deep 945.45
        - with loss of body part 945.55
  - labium (majus) (minus) - *see* Burn, genitourinary organs, external
  - lacrimal apparatus, duct, gland, or sac 940.1
    - chemical 940.0
  - larynx 947.1
  - late effect - *see* Late, effects (of), burn
  - leg 945.00
    - first degree 945.10
    - second degree 945.20
    - third degree 945.30
      - deep 945.40
        - with loss of body part 945.50
    - lower 945.04
      - with other part(s) of lower limb(s) - *see* Burn, leg, multiple sites
      - first degree 945.14
      - second degree 945.24
      - third degree 945.34
        - deep 945.44
          - with loss of body part 945.54
    - multiple sites 945.09
      - first degree 945.19
      - second degree 945.29
      - third degree 945.39
        - deep 945.49
          - with loss of body part 945.59
    - upper - *see* Burn, thigh
  - lightning - *see* Burn, by site
  - limb(s)
    - lower (including foot or toe(s)) - *see* Burn, leg
    - upper (except wrist and hand) - *see* Burn, arm(s)
  - lip(s) 941.03
    - with
      - face or head - *see* Burn, head, multiple sites
    - first degree 941.13
    - second degree 941.23
    - third degree 941.33
      - deep 941.43
        - with loss of body part 941.53

- **Burn** – *continued*
  - lumbar region - *see* Burn, back
  - lung 947.1
  - malar region - *see* Burn, cheek
  - mastoid region - *see* Burn, scalp
  - membrane, tympanic - *see* Burn, ear
  - midthoracic region - *see* Burn, chest wall
  - mouth 947.0
  - multiple (*see also* Burn, unspecified) 949.0
    - specified sites classifiable to more than one category in 940-945 946.0
      - first degree 946.1
      - second degree 946.2
      - third degree 946.3
        - deep 946.4
          - with loss of body part 946.5
  - muscle, abdominal - *see* Burn, abdomen
  - nasal (septum) - *see* Burn, nose
  - neck 941.08
    - with
      - face or head - *see* Burn, head, multiple sites
    - first degree 941.18
    - second degree 941.28
    - third degree 941.38
      - deep 941.48
        - with loss of body part 941.58
  - nose (septum) 941.05
    - with
      - face or head - *see* Burn, head, multiple sites
    - first degree 941.15
    - second degree 941.25
    - third degree 941.35
      - deep 941.45
        - with loss of body part 941.55
  - occipital region - *see* Burn, scalp
  - orbit region 940.1
    - chemical 940.0
  - oronasopharynx 947.0
  - palate 947.0
  - palm(s) 944.05
    - with
      - hand(s) and wrist(s) - *see* Burn, hand(s), multiple sites
    - first degree 944.15
    - second degree 944.25
    - third degree 944.35
      - deep 944.45
        - with loss of a body part 944.55
  - parietal region - *see* Burn, scalp
  - penis - *see* Burn, genitourinary organs, external
  - perineum - *see* Burn, genitourinary organs, external
  - periocular area 940.1
    - chemical 940.0
  - pharynx 947.0
  - pleura 947.1
  - popliteal space - *see* Burn, knee
  - prepuce - *see* Burn, genitourinary organs, external
  - pubic region - *see* Burn, genitourinary organs, external
  - pudenda - *see* Burn, genitourinary organs, external
  - rectum 947.3
  - sac, lacrimal 940.1
    - chemical 940.0
  - sacral region - *see* Burn, back
  - salivary (ducts) (glands) 947.0
  - scalp 941.06
    - with
      - face or neck - *see* Burn, head, multiple sites
    - first degree 941.16
    - second degree 941.26
    - third degree 941.36
      - deep 941.46
        - with loss of body part 941.56

- **Burn** – *continued*
  - scapular region 943.06
    - with
      - upper limb(s), except hand(s) or wrist(s) - *see* Burn, arm(s), multiple sites
    - first degree 943.16
    - second degree 943.26
    - third degree 943.36
      - deep 943.46
        - with loss of body part 943.56
  - sclera - *see* Burn, eyeball
  - scrotum - *see* Burn, genitourinary organs, external
  - septum, nasal - *see* Burn, nose
  - shoulder(s) 943.05
    - with
      - hand(s) and wrist(s) - *see* Burn, multiple, specified sites
      - upper limb(s), except hand(s) or wrist(s) - *see* Burn, arm(s), multiple sites
    - first degree 943.15
    - second degree 943.25
    - third degree 943.35
      - deep 943.45
        - with loss of body part 943.55
  - skin NEC (*see also* Burn, unspecified) 949.0
  - skull - *see* Burn, head
  - small intestine 947.3
  - sternal region - *see* Burn, chest wall
  - stomach 947.3
  - subconjunctival - *see* Burn, conjunctiva
  - subcutaneous - *see* Burn, by site, third degree
  - submaxillary region - *see* Burn, head
  - submental region - *see* Burn, chin
  - sun - *see* Sunburn
  - supraclavicular fossa - *see* Burn, neck
  - supraorbital - *see* Burn, forehead
  - temple - *see* Burn, scalp
  - temporal region - *see* Burn, scalp
  - testicle - *see* Burn, genitourinary organs, external
  - testis - *see* Burn, genitourinary organs, external
  - thigh 945.06
    - with
      - lower limb(s) - *see* Burn, leg, multiple sites
    - first degree 945.16
    - second degree 945.26
    - third degree 945.36
      - deep 945.46
        - with loss of body part 945.56
  - thorax (external) - *see* Burn, chest wall
  - throat 947.0
  - thumb(s) (nail) (subungual) 944.02
    - with
      - finger(s) - *see* Burn, finger, with other sites, thumb
      - hand(s) and wrist(s) - *see* Burn, hand(s), multiple sites
    - first degree 944.12
    - second degree 944.22
    - third degree 944.32
      - deep 944.42
        - with loss of body part 944.52
  - toe (nail) (subungual) 945.01
    - with
      - lower limb(s) - *see* Burn, leg, multiple sites
    - first degree 945.11
    - second degree 945.21
    - third degree 945.31
      - deep 945.41
        - with loss of body part 945.51
  - tongue 947.0
  - tonsil 947.0
  - trachea 947.1
  - trunk 942.00
    - first degree 942.10
    - second degree 942.20

- **Burn** – *continued*
  - trunk – *continued*
    - third degree 942.30
      - deep 942.40
        - with loss of body part 942.50
    - multiple sites 942.09
      - first degree 942.19
      - second degree 942.29
      - third degree 942.39
        - deep 942.49
          - with loss of body part 942.59
    - specified site NEC 942.09
      - first degree 942.19
      - second degree 942.29
      - third degree 942.39
        - deep 942.49
          - with loss of body part 942.59
  - tunica vaginalis - *see* Burn, genitourinary organs, external
  - tympanic membrane - *see* Burn, ear
  - tympanum - *see* Burn, ear
  - ultraviolet 692.82
  - unspecified site (multiple) 949.0
    - with extent of body surface involved specified
      - less than 10 percent 948.0 [5th]
      - 10-19 percent 948.1 [5th]
      - 20-29 percent 948.2 [5th]
      - 30-39 percent 948.3 [5th]
      - 40-49 percent 948.4 [5th]
      - 50-59 percent 948.5 [5th]
      - 60-69 percent 948.6 [5th]
      - 70-79 percent 948.7 [5th]
      - 80-89 percent 948.8 [5th]
      - 90 percent or more 948.9 [5th]
    - first degree 949.1
    - second degree 949.2
    - third degree 949.3
      - deep 949.4
        - with loss of body part 949.5
  - uterus 947.4
  - uvula 947.0
  - vagina 947.4
  - vulva - *see* Burn, genitourinary organs, external
  - wrist(s) 944.07
    - with
      - hand(s) - *see* Burn, hand(s), multiple sites
    - first degree 944.17
    - second degree 944.27
    - third degree 944.37
      - deep 944.47
        - with loss of body part 944.57
- **Burnett's syndrome** (milk-alkali) 275.42
- **Burnier's syndrome** (hypophyseal dwarfism) 253.3
- **Burning**
  - feet syndrome 266.2
  - sensation (*see also* Disturbance, sensation) 782.0
  - tongue 529.6
- **Burns' disease** (osteochondrosis, lower ulna) 732.3
- **Bursa** - *see also* condition
  - pharynx 478.29
- **Bursitis** NEC 727.3
  - Achilles tendon 726.71
  - adhesive 726.90
    - shoulder 726.0
  - ankle 726.79
  - buttock 726.5
  - calcaneal 726.79
  - collateral ligament
    - fibular 726.63
    - tibial 726.62
  - Duplay's 726.2
  - elbow 726.33
  - finger 726.8
  - foot 726.79
  - gonococcal 098.52
  - hand 726.4
  - hip 726.5
  - infrapatellar 726.69

- **Bursitis** – *continued*
  - ischiogluteal 726.5
  - knee 726.60
  - occupational NEC 727.2
  - olecranon 726.33
  - pes anserinus 726.61
  - pharyngeal 478.29
  - popliteal 727.51
  - prepatellar 726.65
  - radiohumeral 727.3
  - scapulohumeral 726.19
    - adhesive 726.0
  - shoulder 726.10
    - adhesive 726.0
  - subacromial 726.19
    - adhesive 726.0
  - subcoracoid 726.19
  - subdeltoid 726.19
    - adhesive 726.0
  - subpatellar 726.69
  - syphilitic 095.7
  - Thornwaldt's, Tornwaldt's (pharyngeal) 478.29
  - toe 726.79
  - trochanteric area 726.5
  - wrist 726.4
- **Burst stitches or sutures** (complication of surgery) (external) (*see also* Dehiscence) 998.32
  - internal 998.31
- **Buruli ulcer** 031.1
- **Bury's disease** (erythema elevatum diutinum) 695.89
- **Buschke's disease or scleredema** (adultorum) 710.1
- **Busquet's disease** (osteoperiostitis) (*see also* Osteomyelitis) 730.1 5th
- **Busse-Buschke disease** (cryptococcosis) 117.5
- **Buttock** - *see* condition
- **Button**
  - Biskra 085.1
  - Delhi 085.1
  - oriental 085.1
- **Buttonhole hand** (intrinsic) 736.21
- **Bwamba fever** (encephalitis) 066.3
- **Byssinosis** (occupational) 504
- **Bywaters' syndrome** 958.5

C

- **Cacergasia** 300.9
- **Cachexia** 799.4
  - cancerous - *see also* Neoplasm, by site, malignant 799.4
  - cardiac - *see* Disease, heart
  - dehydration 276.51
    - with
      - hypernatremia 276.0
      - hyponatremia 276.1
  - due to malnutrition 799.4
  - exophthalmic 242.0 5th
  - heart - *see* Disease, heart
  - hypophyseal 253.2
  - hypopituitary 253.2
  - lead 984.9
    - specified type of lead - *see* Table of Drugs and Chemicals
  - malaria 084.9
  - malignant - *see also* Neoplasm, by site, malignant 799.4
  - marsh 084.9
  - nervous 300.5
  - old age 797
  - pachydermic - *see* Hypothyroidism
  - paludal 084.9
  - pituitary (postpartum) 253.2
  - renal (*see also* Disease, renal) 593.9
  - saturnine 984.9
    - specified type of lead - *see* Table of Drugs and Chemicals
  - senile 797
- **Cachexia** – *continued*
  - Simmonds' (pituitary cachexia) 253.2
  - splenica 289.59
  - strumipriva (*see also* Hypothyroidism) 244.9
  - tuberculous NEC (*see also* Tuberculosis) 011.9 5th
- **Café au lait spots** 709.09
- **Caffey's disease or syndrome** (infantile cortical hyperostosis) 756.59
- **Caisson disease** 993.3
- **Caked breast** (puerperal, postpartum) 676.2 5th
- **Cake kidney** 753.3
- **Calabar swelling** 125.2
- **Calcaneal spur** 726.73
- **Calcaneoapophysitis** 732.5
- **Calcaneonavicular bar** 755.67
- **Calcareous** - *see* condition
- **Calcicosis** (occupational) 502
- **Calciferol** (vitamin D) **deficiency** 268.9
  - with
    - osteomalacia 268.2
    - rickets (*see also* Rickets) 268.0
- **Calcification**
  - adrenal (capsule) (gland) 255.41
    - tuberculous (*see also* Tuberculosis) 017.6 5th
  - aorta 440.0
  - artery (annular) - *see* Arteriosclerosis
  - auricle (ear) 380.89
  - bladder 596.8
    - due to S. hematobium 120.0
  - brain (cortex) - *see* Calcification, cerebral
  - bronchus 519.19
  - bursa 727.82
  - cardiac (*see also* Degeneration, myocardial) 429.1
  - cartilage (postinfectional) 733.99
  - cerebral (cortex) 348.8<u>9</u> ▲
    - artery 437.0
  - cervix (uteri) 622.8
  - choroid plexus 349.2
  - conjunctiva 372.54
  - corpora cavernosa (penis) 607.89
  - cortex (brain) - *see* Calcification, cerebral
  - dental pulp (nodular) 522.2
  - dentinal papilla 520.4
  - disc, intervertebral 722.90
    - cervical, cervicothoracic 722.91
    - lumbar, lumbosacral 722.93
    - thoracic, thoracolumbar 722.92
  - fallopian tube 620.8
  - falx cerebri - *see* Calcification, cerebral
  - fascia 728.89
  - gallbladder 575.8
  - general 275.40
  - heart (*see also* Degeneration, myocardial) 429.1
    - valve - *see* Endocarditis
  - intervertebral cartilage or disc (postinfectional) 722.90
    - cervical, cervicothoracic 722.91
    - lumbar, lumbosacral 722.93
    - thoracic, thoracolumbar 722.92
  - intracranial - *see* Calcification, cerebral
  - intraspinal ligament 728.89
  - joint 719.80
    - ankle 719.87
    - elbow 719.82
    - foot 719.87
    - hand 719.84
    - hip 719.85
    - knee 719.86
    - multiple sites 719.89
    - pelvic region 719.85
    - shoulder (region) 719.81
    - specified site NEC 719.88
    - wrist 719.83
  - kidney 593.89
    - tuberculous (*see also* Tuberculosis) 016.0 5th
  - larynx (senile) 478.79
  - lens 366.8
- **Calcification** – *continued*
  - ligament 728.89
    - intraspinal 728.89
    - knee (medial collateral) 717.89
  - lung 518.89
    - active 518.89
    - postinfectional 518.89
    - tuberculous (*see also* Tuberculosis, pulmonary) 011.9 5th
  - lymph gland or node (postinfectional) 289.3
    - tuberculous (*see also* Tuberculosis, lymph gland) 017.2 5th
  - mammographic 793.89
  - massive (paraplegic) 728.10
  - medial (*see also* Arteriosclerosis, extremities) 440.20
  - meninges (cerebral) 349.2
  - metastatic 275.40
  - Mönckeberg's - *see* Arteriosclerosis
  - muscle 728.10
    - heterotopic, postoperative 728.13
  - myocardium, myocardial (*see also* Degeneration, myocardial) 429.1
  - ovary 620.8
  - pancreas 577.8
  - penis 607.89
  - periarticular 728.89
  - pericardium (*see also* Pericarditis) 423.8
  - pineal gland 259.8
  - pleura 511.0
    - postinfectional 518.89
    - tuberculous (*see also* Tuberculosis, pleura) 012.0 5th
  - pulp (dental) (nodular) 522.2
  - renal 593.89
  - Rider's bone 733.99
  - sclera 379.16
  - semilunar cartilage 717.89
  - spleen 289.59
  - subcutaneous 709.3
  - suprarenal (capsule) (gland) 255.41
  - tendon (sheath) 727.82
    - with bursitis, synovitis or tenosynovitis 727.82
  - trachea 519.19
  - ureter 593.89
  - uterus 621.8
  - vitreous 379.29
- **Calcified** - *see also* Calcification
  - hematoma NEC 959.9
- **Calcinosis** (generalized) (interstitial) (tumoral) (universalis) 275.49
  - circumscripta 709.3
  - cutis 709.3
  - intervertebralis 275.49 *[722.90]*
  - Raynaud's phenomenonsclerodactyly-telangiectasis (CRST) 710.1
- **Calciphylaxis** (*see also* Calcification, by site) 275.49
- **Calcium**
  - blood
    - high (*see also* Hypercalcemia) 275.42
    - low (*see also* Hypocalcemia) 275.41
  - deposits - *see also* Calcification, by site
    - in bursa 727.82
    - in tendon (sheath) 727.82
      - with bursitis, synovitis or tenosynovitis 727.82
  - salts or soaps in vitreous 379.22
- **Calciuria** 791.9
- **Calculi** - *see* Calculus
- **Calculosis, intrahepatic** - *see* Choledocholithiasis
- **Calculus, calculi, calculous** 592.9
  - ampulla of Vater - *see* Choledocholithiasis
  - anuria (impacted) (recurrent) 592.0
  - appendix 543.9
  - bile duct (any) - *see* Choledocholithiasis
  - biliary - *see* Cholelithiasis
  - bilirubin, multiple - *see* Cholelithiasis
  - bladder (encysted) (impacted) (urinary) 594.1
    - diverticulum 594.0
- **Calculus, calculi, calculous** – *continued*
  - bronchus 518.89
  - calyx (kidney) (renal) 592.0
    - congenital 753.3
  - cholesterol (pure) (solitary) - *see* Cholelithiasis
  - common duct (bile) - *see* Choledocholithiasis
  - conjunctiva 372.54
  - cystic 594.1
    - duct - *see* Cholelithiasis
  - dental 523.6
    - subgingival 523.6
    - supragingival 523.6
  - epididymis 608.89
  - gallbladder - *see also* Cholelithiasis
    - congenital 751.69
  - hepatic (duct) - *see* Choledocholithiasis
  - intestine (impaction) (obstruction) 560.39
  - kidney (impacted) (multiple) (pelvis) (recurrent) (staghorn) 592.0
    - congenital 753.3
  - lacrimal (passages) 375.57
  - liver (impacted) - *see* Choledocholithiasis
  - lung 518.89
  - mammographic 793.89
  - nephritic (impacted) (recurrent) 592.0
  - nose 478.19
  - pancreas (duct) 577.8
  - parotid gland 527.5
  - pelvis, encysted 592.0
  - prostate 602.0
  - pulmonary 518.89
  - renal (impacted) (recurrent) 592.0
    - congenital 753.3
  - salivary (duct) (gland) 527.5
  - seminal vesicle 608.89
  - staghorn 592.0
  - Stensen's duct 527.5
  - sublingual duct or gland 527.5
    - congenital 750.26
  - submaxillary duct, gland, or region 527.5
  - suburethral 594.8
  - tonsil 474.8
  - tooth, teeth 523.6
  - tunica vaginalis 608.89
  - ureter (impacted) (recurrent) 592.1
  - urethra (impacted) 594.2
  - urinary (duct) (impacted) (passage) (tract) 592.9
    - lower tract NEC 594.9
      - specified site 594.8
  - vagina 623.8
  - vesical (impacted) 594.1
  - Wharton's duct 527.5
- **Caliectasis** 593.89
- **California**
  - disease 114.0
  - encephalitis 062.5
- **Caligo cornea** 371.03
- **Callositas, callosity** (infected) 700
- **Callus** (infected) 700
  - bone 726.91
  - excessive, following fracture - *see also* Late, effect (of), fracture
- **Calvé (-Perthes) disease** (osteochondrosis, femoral capital) 732.1
- **Calvities** (*see also* Alopecia) 704.00
- **Cameroon fever** (*see also* Malaria) 084.6
- **Camptocormia** 300.11
- **Camptodactyly** (congenital) 755.59
- **Camurati-Engelmann disease** (diaphyseal sclerosis) 756.59
- **Canal** - *see* condition
- **Canaliculitis** (lacrimal) (acute) 375.31
  - Actinomyces 039.8
  - chronic 375.41
- **Canavan's disease** 330.0

Bursitis – Canavan's disease

Cancer (M8000/3)-*see also* Neoplasm, by site, malignant

Note *The term "cancer" when modified by an adjective or adjectival phrase indicating a morphological type should be coded in the same manner as "carcinoma" with that adjective or phrase. Thus, "squamous-cell cancer" should be coded in the same manner as "squamous-cell carcinoma," which appears in the list under "Carcinoma."*

  bile duct type (M8160/3), liver 155.1
  hepatocellular (M8170/3) 155.0
Cancerous (M8000/3 - *see* Neoplasm, by site, malignant
Cancerphobia 300.29
Cancrum oris 528.1
Candidiasis, candidal 112.9
  with pneumonia 112.4
  balanitis 112.2
  congenital 771.7
  disseminated 112.5
  endocarditis 112.81
  esophagus 112.84
  intertrigo 112.3
  intestine 112.85
  lung 112.4
  meningitis 112.83
  mouth 112.0
  nails 112.3
  neonatal 771.7
  onychia 112.3
  otitis externa 112.82
  otomycosis 112.82
  paronychia 112.3
  perionyxis 112.3
  pneumonia 112.4
  pneumonitis 112.4
  skin 112.3
  specified site NEC 112.89
  systemic 112.5
  urogenital site NEC 112.2
  vagina 112.1
  vulva 112.1
  vulvovaginitis 112.1
Candidiosis - *see* Candidiasis
Candiru infection or infestation 136.8
Canities (premature) 704.3
  congenital 757.4
Canker (mouth) (sore) 528.2
  rash 034.1
Cannabinosis 504
Canton fever 081.9
Cap
  cradle 690.11
Capillariasis 127.5
Capillary - *see* condition
Caplan's syndrome 714.81
Caplan-Colinet syndrome 714.81
Capsule - *see* condition
Capsulitis (joint) 726.90
  adhesive (shoulder)726.0
  hip 726.5
  knee 726.60
  labyrinthine 387.8
  thyroid 245.9
  wrist 726.4
Caput
  crepitus 756.0
  medusae 456.8
  succedaneum 767.19
Carapata disease 087.1
Carate - *see* Pinta
Carboxyhemoglobinemia 986
Carbohydrate-deficient glycoprotein syndrome (CDGS) 271.8
Carbuncle 680.9
  abdominal wall 680.2
  ankle 680.6
  anus 680.5
  arm (any part, above wrist) 680.3
  auditory canal, external 680.0
  axilla 680.3

Carbuncle – *continued*
  back (any part) 680.2
  breast 680.2
  buttock 680.5
  chest wall 680.2
  corpus cavernosum 607.2
  ear (any part) (external) 680.0
  eyelid 373.13
  face (any part, except eye) 680.0
  finger (any) 680.4
  flank 680.2
  foot (any part) 680.7
  forearm 680.3
  genital organ (male) 608.4
  gluteal (region) 680.5
  groin 680.2
  hand (any part) 680.4
  head (any part, except face) 680.8
  heel 680.7
  hip 680.6
  kidney (*see also* Abscess, kidney) 590.2
  knee 680.6
  labia 616.4
  lacrimal
    gland (*see also* Dacryoadenitis) 375.00
    passages (duct) (sac) (*see also* Dacryocystitis) 375.30
  leg, any part except foot 680.6
  lower extremity, any part except foot 680.6
  malignant 022.0
  multiple sites 680.9
  neck 680.1
  nose (external) (septum) 680.0
  orbit, orbital 376.01
  partes posteriores 680.5
  pectoral region 680.2
  penis 607.2
  perineum 680.2
  pinna 680.0
  scalp (any part) 680.8
  scrotum 608.4
  seminal vesicle 608.0
  shoulder 680.3
  skin NEC 680.9
  specified site NEC 680.8
  spermatic cord 608.4
  temple (region) 680.0
  testis 608.4
  thigh 680.6
  thumb 680.4
  toe (any) 680.7
  trunk 680.2
  tunica vaginalis 608.4
  umbilicus 680.2
  upper arm 680.3
  urethra 597.0
  vas deferens 608.4
  vulva 616.4
  wrist 680.4
Carbunculus (*see also* Carbuncle) 680.9
Carcinoid (tumor) (M8240/1) - *see* Tumor, carcinoid
  ~~and struma ovarii (M9091/1) 236.2~~
  ~~argentaffin (M8241/1) - *see* Neoplasm, by site uncertain behavior~~
    ~~malignant (M8241/3) - *see* Neoplasm, by site, malignant~~
  ~~benign (M9091/0) 220~~
  ~~composite (M8244/3) - *see* Neoplasm, by site, malignant~~
  ~~goblet cell (M8243/3) - *see* Neoplasm, by site, malignant~~
    ~~malignant (M8240/3) - *see* Neoplasm, by site, malignant~~
  ~~nonargentaffin (M8242/1) - *see also* Neoplasm, by site, uncertain behavior~~
    ~~malignant (M8242/3) - *see* Neoplasm, by site, malignant~~
  ~~strumal (M9091/1) 236.2~~
  ~~syndrome (intestinal) (metastatic) 259.2~~
  ~~type bronchial adenoma (M8240/3) - *see* Neoplasm, lung, malignant~~
Carcinoidosis 259.2

Carcinoma (M8010/3) - *see also* Neoplasm, by site, malignant

Note *Except where otherwise indicated, the morphological varieties of carcinoma in the list below should be coded by site as for "Neoplasm, malignant."*

  with
    apocrine metaplasia (M8573/3)
    cartilaginous (and osseous) metaplasia (M8571/3)
    osseous (and cartilaginous) metaplasia (M8571/3)
    productive fibrosis (M8141/3)
    spindle cell metaplasia (M8572/3)
    squamous metaplasia (M8570/3)
  acidophil (M8280/3)
    specified site - *see* Neoplasm, by site, malignant
    unspecified site 194.3
  acidophil-basophil, mixed (M8281/3)
    specified site - *see* Neoplasm, by site, malignant
    unspecified site 194.3
  acinar (cell) (M8550/3)
  acinic cell (M8550/3)
  adenocystic (M8200/3)
  adenoid
    cystic (M8200/3)
    squamous cell (M8075/3)
  adenosquamous (M8560/3)
  adnexal (skin) (M8390/3) - *see* Neoplasm, skin, malignant
  adrenal cortical (M8370/3) 194.0
  alveolar (M8251/3)
    cell (M8250/3) - *see* Neoplasm, lung, malignant
  anaplastic type (M8021/3)
  apocrine (M8401/3)
    breast - *see* Neoplasm, breast, malignant
    specified site NEC - *see* Neoplasm, skin, malignant
    unspecified site 173.9
  basal cell (pigmented) (M8090/3) - *see also* Neoplasm, skin, malignant
    fibro-epithelial type (M8093/3) - *see* Neoplasm, skin, malignant
    morphea type (M8092/3) - *see* Neoplasm, skin, malignant
    multicentric (M8091/3) - *see* Neoplasm, skin, malignant
  basaloid (M8123/3)
  basal-squamous cell, mixed (M8094/3) - *see* Neoplasm, skin, malignant
  basophil (M8300/3)
    specified site - *see* Neoplasm, by site, malignant
    unspecified site 194.3
  basophil-acidophil, mixed (M8281/3)
    specified site - *see* Neoplasm, by site, malignant
    unspecified site 194.3
  basosquamous (M8094/3) - *see* Neoplasm, skin, malignant
  bile duct type (M8160/3)
    and hepatocellular, mixed (M8180/3) 155.0
    liver 155.1
    specified site NEC - *see* Neoplasm, by site, malignant
    unspecified site 155.1
  branchial or branchiogenic 146.8
  bronchial or bronchogenic - *see* Neoplasm, lung, malignant
  bronchiolar (terminal) (M8250/3) - *see* Neoplasm, lung, malignant
  bronchiolo-alveolar (M8250/3) - *see* Neoplasm, lung, malignant
  bronchogenic (epidermoid) 162.9
  C cell (M8510/3)
    specified site - *see* Neoplasm, by site, malignant
    unspecified site 193

Carcinoma – *continued*
  ceruminous (M8420/3) 173.2
  chorionic (M9100/3)
    specified site - *see* Neoplasm, by site, malignant
    unspecified site
      female 181
      male 186.9
  chromophobe (M8270/3)
    specified site - *see* Neoplasm, by site, malignant
    unspecified site 194.3
  clear cell (mesonephroid type) (M8310/3)
  cloacogenic (M8124/3)
    specified site - *see* Neoplasm, by site, malignant
    unspecified site 154.8
  colloid (M8480/3)
  cribriform (M8201/3)
  cylindroid type (M8200/3)
  diffuse type (M8145/3)
    specified site - *see* Neoplasm, by site, malignant
    unspecified site 151.9
  duct (cell) (M8500/3)
    with Paget's disease (M8541/3) - *see* Neoplasm, breast, malignant
    infiltrating (M8500/3)
      specified site - *see* Neoplasm, by site, malignant
      unspecified site 174.9
  ductal (M8500/3)
  ductular, infiltrating (M8521/3)
  embryonal (M9070/3)
    and teratoma, mixed (M9081/3)
    combined with choriocarcinoma (M9101/3) - *see* Neoplasm, by site, malignant
    infantile type (M9071/3)
    liver 155.0
    polyembryonal type (M9072/3)
  endometrioid (M8380/3)
  eosinophil (M8280/3)
    specified site - *see* Neoplasm, by site, malignant
    unspecified site 194.3
  epidermoid (M8070/3) - *see also* Carcinoma, squamous cell
    and adenocarcinoma, mixed (M8560/3)
    in situ, Bowen's type (M8081/2) - *see* Neoplasm, skin, in situ
    intradermal - *see* Neoplasm, skin, in situ
  fibroepithelial type basal cell (M8093/3) - *see* Neoplasm, skin, malignant
  follicular (M8330/3)
    and papillary (mixed) (M8340/3) 193
    moderately differentiated type (M8332/3) 193
    pure follicle type (M8331/3) 193
    specified site - *see* Neoplasm, by site, malignant
    trabecular type (M8332/3) 193
    unspecified site 193
    well differentiated type (M8331/3) 193
  gelatinous (M8480/3)
  giant cell (M8031/3)
    and spindle cell (M8030/3)
  granular cell (M8320/3)
  granulosa cell (M8620/3) 183.0
  hepatic cell (M8170/3) 155.0
  hepatocellular (M8170/3) 155.0
    and bile duct, mixed (M8180/3) 155.0
  hepatocholangiolitic (M8180/3) 155.0
  Hürthle cell (thyroid) 193
  hypernephroid (M8311/3)
  in
    adenomatous
      polyp (M8210/3)
      polyposis coli (M8220/3) 153.9
    pleomorphic adenoma (M8940/3)
    polypoid adenoma (M8210/3)
    situ (M8010/3) - *see* Carcinoma, in situ

Cancer – Carcinoma

Carcinoma – *continued*
- in – *continued*
  - tubular adenoma (M8210/3)
  - villous adenoma (M8261/3)
- infiltrating duct (M8500/3)
  - with Paget's disease (M8541/3) - *see* Neoplasm, breast, malignant
  - specified site - *see* Neoplasm, by site, malignant
  - unspecified site 174.9
- inflammatory (M8530/3)
  - specified site - *see* Neoplasm, by site, malignant
  - unspecified site 174.9
- in situ (M8010/2) - *see also* Neoplasm, by site, in situ
  - epidermoid (M8070/2) - *see also* Neoplasm, by site, in situ
    - with questionable stromal invasion (M8076/2)
      - specified site - *see* Neoplasm, by site, in situ
      - unspecified site 233.1
    - Bowen's type (M8081/2) - *see* Neoplasm, skin, in situ
  - intraductal (M8500/2)
    - specified site - *see* Neoplasm, by site, in situ
    - unspecified site 233.0
  - lobular (M8520/2)
    - specified site - *see* Neoplasm, by site, in situ
    - unspecified site 233.0
  - papillary (M8050/2) - *see* Neoplasm, by site, in situ
  - squamous cell (M8070/2) - *see also* Neoplasm, by site, in situ
    - with questionable stromal invasion (M8076/2)
      - specified site - *see* Neoplasm, by site, in situ
      - unspecified site 233.1
  - transitional cell (M8120/2) - *see* Neoplasm, by site, in situ
- intestinal type (M8144/3)
  - specified site - *see* Neoplasm, by site, malignant
  - unspecified site 151.9
- intraductal (noninfiltrating) (M8500/2)
  - papillary (M8503/2)
    - specified site - *see* Neoplasm, by site, in situ
    - unspecified site 233.0
  - specified site - *see* Neoplasm, by site, in situ
  - unspecified site 233.0
- intraepidermal (M8070/2) - *see also* Neoplasm, skin, in situ
  - squamous cell, Bowen's type (M8081/2) - *see* Neoplasm, skin, in situ
- intraepithelial (M8010/2) - *see also* Neoplasm, by site, in situ
  - squamous cell (M8072/2) - *see* Neoplasm, by site, in situ
- intraosseous (M9270/3) 170.1
  - upper jaw (bone) 170.0
- islet cell (M8150/3)
  - and exocrine, mixed (M8154/3)
    - specified site - *see* Neoplasm, by site, malignant
    - unspecified site 157.9
  - pancreas 157.4
  - specified site NEC - *see* Neoplasm, by site, malignant
  - unspecified site 157.4
- juvenile, breast (M8502/3) - *see* Neoplasm, breast, malignant
- Kulchitsky's cell (carcinoid tumor of intestine) 259.2
- large cell (M8012/3)
  - squamous cell, non-keratinizing type (M8072/3)

Carcinoma – *continued*
- Leydig cell (testis) (M8650/3)
  - specified site - *see* Neoplasm, by site, malignant
  - unspecified site 186.9
    - female 183.0
    - male 186.9
- liver cell (M8170/3) 155.0
- lobular (infiltrating) (M8520/3)
  - noninfiltrating (M8520/3)
    - specified site - *see* Neoplasm, by site, in situ
    - unspecified site 233.0
  - specified site - *see* Neoplasm, by site, malignant
  - unspecified site 174.9
- lymphoepithelial (M8082/3)
- medullary (M8510/3)
  - with
    - amyloid stroma (M8511/3)
      - specified site - *see* Neoplasm, by site, malignant
      - unspecified site 193
    - lymphoid stroma (M8512/3)
      - specified site - *see* Neoplasm, by site, malignant
      - unspecified site 174.9
- Merkel cell 209.36 ●
  - buttock 209.36 ●
  - ear 209.31 ●
  - eyelid, including canthus 209.31 ●
  - face 209.31 ●
  - genitals 209.36 ●
  - lip 209.31 ●
  - lower limb 209.34 ●
  - neck 209.32 ●
  - nodal presentation 209.75 ●
  - scalp 209.32 ●
  - secondary (any site) 209.75 ●
  - specified site NEC 209.36 ●
  - trunk 209.35 ●
  - unknown primary site 209.75 ●
  - upper limb 209.33 ●
  - visceral metastatic presentation 209.75 ●
- mesometanephric (M9110/3)
- mesonephric (M9110/3)
- metastatic (M8010/6) - *see* Metastasis, cancer
- metatypical (M8095/3) - *see* Neoplasm, skin, malignant
- morphea type basal cell (M8092/3) - *see* Neoplasm, skin, malignant
- mucinous (M8480/3)
- mucin-producing (M8481/3)
- mucin-secreting (M8481/3)
- mucoepidermoid (M8430/3)
- mucoid (M8480/3)
  - cell (M8300/3)
    - specified site - *see* Neoplasm, by site, malignant
    - unspecified site 194.3
- mucous (M8480/3)
- neuroendocrine
  - high grade (M8240/3) 209.30
  - malignant poorly differentiated (M8240/3) 209.30
- nonencapsulated sclerosing (M8350/3) 193
- noninfiltrating
  - intracystic (M8504/2) - *see* Neoplasm, by site, in situ
  - intraductal (M8500/2)
    - papillary (M8503/2)
      - specified site - *see* Neoplasm, by site, in situ
      - unspecified site 233.0
    - specified site - *see* Neoplasm, by site, in situ
    - unspecified site 233.0
  - lobular (M8520/2)
    - specified site - *see* Neoplasm, by site, in situ
    - unspecified site 233.0

Carcinoma – *continued*
- oat cell (M8042/3)
  - specified site - *see* Neoplasm, by site, malignant
  - unspecified site 162.9
- odontogenic (M9270/3) 170.1
  - upper jaw (bone) 170.0
- onocytic (M8290/3)
- oxyphilic (M8290/3)
- papillary (M8050/3)
  - and follicular (mixed) (M8340/3) 193
  - epidermoid (M8052/3)
  - intraductal (noninfiltrating) (M8503/2)
    - specified site - *see* Neoplasm, by site, in situ
    - unspecified site 233.0
  - serous (M8460/3)
    - specified site - *see* Neoplasm, by site, malignant
    - surface (M8461/3)
      - specified site - *see* Neoplasm, by site, malignant
      - unspecified site 183.0
    - unspecified site 183.0
  - squamous cell (M8052/3)
  - transitional cell (M8130/3)
- papillocystic (M8450/3)
  - specified site - *see* Neoplasm, by site, malignant
  - unspecified site 183.0
- parafollicular cell (M8510/3)
  - specified site - *see* Neoplasm, by site, malignant
  - unspecified site 193
- pleomorphic (M8022/3)
- polygonal cell (M8034/3)
- prickle cell (M8070/3)
- pseudoglandular, squamous cell (M8075/3)
- pseudomucinous (M8470/3)
  - specified site - *see* Neoplasm, by site, malignant
  - unspecified site 183.0
- pseudosarcomatous (M8033/3)
- regaud type (M8082/3) - *see* Neoplasm, nasopharynx, malignant
- renal cell (M8312/3) 189.0
- reserve cell (M8041/3)
- round cell (M8041/3)
- Schmincke (M8082/3) - *see* Neoplasm, nasopharynx, malignant
- Schneiderian (M8121/3)
  - specified site - *see* Neoplasm, by site, malignant
  - unspecified site 160.0
- scirrhous (M8141/3)
- sebaceous (M8410/3) - *see* Neoplasm, skin, malignant
- secondary (M8010/6) - *see* Neoplasm, by site, malignant, secondary
- secretory, breast (M8502/3) - *see* Neoplasm, breast, malignant
- serous (M8441/3)
  - papillary (M8460/3)
    - specified site - *see* Neoplasm, by site, malignant
    - unspecified site 183.0
  - surface, papillary (M8461/3)
    - specified site - *see* Neoplasm, by site, malignant
    - unspecified site 183.0
- Sertoli cell (M8640/3)
  - specified site - *see* Neoplasm, by site, malignant
  - unspecified site 186.9
- signet ring cell (M8490/3)
  - metastatic (M8490/6) - *see* Neoplasm, by site, secondary
- simplex (M8231/3)
- skin appendage (M8390/3) - *see* Neoplasm, skin, malignant
- small cell (M8041/3)
  - fusiform cell type (M8043/3)

Carcinoma – *continued*
- small cell – *continued*
  - squamous cell, nonkeratinizing type (M8073/3)
- solid (M8230/3)
  - with amyloid stroma (M8511/3)
    - specified site - *see* Neoplasm, by site, malignant
    - unspecified site 193
- spheroidal cell (M8035/3)
- spindle cell (M8032/3)
  - and giant cell (M8030/3)
- spinous cell (M8070/3)
- squamous (cell) (M8070/3)
  - adenoid type (M8075/3)
  - and adenocarcinoma, mixed (M8560/3)
  - intraepidermal, Bowen's type - *see* Neoplasm, skin, in situ
  - keratinizing type (large cell) (M8071/3)
  - large cell, nonkeratinizing type (M8072/3)
  - microinvasive (M8076/3)
    - specified site - *see* Neoplasm, by site, malignant
    - unspecified site 180.9
  - nonkeratinizing type (M8072/3)
  - papillary (M8052/3)
  - pseudoglandular (M8075/3)
  - small cell, nonkeratinizing type (M8073/3)
  - spindle cell type (M8074/3)
  - verrucous (M8051/3)
- superficial spreading (M8143/3)
- sweat gland (M8400/3) - *see* Neoplasm, skin, malignant
- theca cell (M8600/3) 183.0
- thymic (M8580/3) 164.0
- trabecular (M8190/3)
- transitional (cell) (M8120/3)
  - papillary (M8130/3)
  - spindle cell type (M8122/3)
- tubular (M8211/3)
- undifferentiated type (M8020/3)
- urothelial (M8120/3)
- ventriculi 151.9
- verrucous (epidermoid) (squamous cell) (M8051/3)
- villous (M8262/3)
- water-clear cell (M8322/3) 194.1
- wolffian duct (M9110/3)

Carcinomaphobia 300.29

Carcinomatosis
- peritonei (M8010/6) 197.6
- specified site NEC (M8010/3) - *see* Neoplasm, by site, malignant
- unspecified site (M8010/6) 199.0

Carcinosarcoma (M8980/3) - *see also* Neoplasm, by site, malignant
- embryonal type (M8981/3) - *see* Neoplasm, by site, malignant

Cardia, cardial - *see* condition

Cardiac - *see also* condition
- death - *see* Disease, heart
- device
  - defibrillator, automatic implantable V45.02
  - in situ NEC V45.00
  - pacemaker
    - cardiac
      - fitting or adjustment V53.31
      - in situ V45.01
    - carotid sinus
      - fitting or adjustment V53.39
      - in situ V45.09
- pacemaker - *see* Cardiac, device, pacemaker
- tamponade 423.3

Cardialgia (*see also* Pain, precordial) 786.51

Cardiectasis - *see* Hypertrophy, cardiac

Cardiochalasia 530.81

Cardiomalacia (*see also* Degeneration, myocardial) 429.1

Cardiomegalia glycogenica diffusa 271.0

- **Cardiomegaly** (*see also* Hypertrophy, cardiac) 429.3
  - congenital 746.89
  - glycogen 271.0
  - hypertensive (*see also* Hypertension, heart) 402.90
  - idiopathic 425.4
- **Cardiomyoliposis** (*see also* Degeneration, myocardial) 429.1
- **Cardiomyopathy** (congestive) (constrictive) (familial) (infiltrative) (obstructive) (restrictive) (sporadic) 425.4
  - alcoholic 425.5
  - amyloid 277.39 *[425.7]*
  - beriberi 265.0 *[425.7]*
  - cobalt-beer 425.5
  - congenital 425.3
  - due to
    - amyloidosis 277.39 *[425.7]*
    - beriberi 265.0 *[425.7]*
    - cardiac glycogenosis 271.0 *[425.7]*
    - Chagas' disease 086.0
    - Friedreich's ataxia 334.0 *[425.8]*
    - hypertension - *see* Hypertension, with, heart involvement
    - mucopolysaccharidosis 277.5 *[425.7]*
    - myotonia atrophica 359.21 *[425.8]*
    - progressive muscular dystrophy 359.1 *[425.8]*
    - sarcoidosis 135 *[425.8]*
  - glycogen storage 271.0 *[425.7]*
  - hypertensive - *see* Hypertension, with, heart involvement
  - hypertrophic
    - nonobstructive 425.4
    - obstructive 425.1
      - congenital 746.84
  - idiopathic (concentric) 425.4
  - in
    - Chagas' disease 086.0
    - sarcoidosis 135 *[425.8]*
  - ischemic 414.8
  - metabolic NEC 277.9 *[425.7]*
    - amyloid 277.39 *[425.7]*
    - thyrotoxic (*see also* Thyrotoxicosis) 242.9 5th *[425.7]*
    - thyrotoxicosis (*see also* Thyrotoxicosis) 242.9 5th *[425.7]*
  - newborn 425.4
    - congenital 425.3
  - takotsubo 429.83
  - nutritional 269.9 *[425.7]*
    - beriberi 265.0 *[425.7]*
  - obscure of Africa 425.2
  - peripartum 674.5 5th
  - postpartum 674.5 5th
  - primary 425.4
  - secondary 425.9
  - stress induced 429.83
  - thyrotoxic (*see also* Thyrotoxicosis) 242.9 5th *[425.7]*
  - toxic NEC 425.9
  - tuberculous (*see also* Tuberculosis) 017.9 5th *[425.8]*
- **Cardionephritis** - *see* Hypertension, cardiorenal
- **Cardionephropathy** - *see* Hypertension, cardiorenal
- **Cardionephrosis** - *see* Hypertension, cardiorenal
- **Cardioneurosis** 306.2
- **Cardiopathia nigra** 416.0
- **Cardiopathy** (*see also* Disease, heart) 429.9
  - hypertensive (*see also* Hypertension, heart) 402.90
  - idiopathic 425.4
  - mucopolysaccharidosis 277.5 *[425.7]*
- **Cardiopericarditis** (*see also* Pericarditis) 423.9
- **Cardiophobia** 300.29
- **Cardioptosis** 746.87
- **Cardiorenal** - *see* condition
- **Cardiorrhexis** (*see also* Infarct, myocardium) 410.9 5th
- **Cardiosclerosis** - *see* Arteriosclerosis, coronary
- **Cardiosis** - *see* Disease, heart
- **Cardiospasm** (esophagus) (reflex) (stomach) 530.0
  - congenital 750.7
- **Cardiostenosis** - *see* Disease, heart
- **Cardiosymphysis** 423.1
- **Cardiothyrotoxicosis** - *see* Hyperthyroidism
- **Cardiovascular** - *see* condition
- **Carditis** (acute) (bacterial) (chronic) (subacute) 429.89
  - Coxsackie 074.20
  - hypertensive (*see also* Hypertension, heart) 402.90
  - meningococcal 036.40
  - rheumatic - *see* Disease, heart, rheumatic
  - rheumatoid 714.2
- **Care** (of)
  - child (routine) V20.1
  - convalescent following V66.9
    - chemotherapy V66.2
    - medical NEC V66.5
    - psychotherapy V66.3
    - radiotherapy V66.1
    - surgery V66.0
    - surgical NEC V66.0
    - treatment (for) V66.5
      - combined V66.6
      - fracture V66.4
      - mental disorder NEC V66.3
      - specified type NEC V66.5
  - end-of-life V66.7
  - family member (handicapped) (sick)
    - creating problem for family V61.49
    - provided away from home for holiday relief V60.5
    - unavailable, due to
      - absence (person rendering care) (sufferer) V60.4
      - inability (any reason) of person rendering care V60.4
  - holiday relief V60.5
  - hospice V66.7
  - lack of (at or after birth) (infant) (child) 995.52
    - adult 995.84
  - lactation of mother V24.1
  - palliative V66.7
  - postpartum
    - immediately after delivery V24.0
    - routine follow-up V24.2
  - prenatal V22.1
    - first pregnancy V22.0
    - high-risk pregnancy V23.9
      - specified problem NEC V23.89
  - terminal V66.7
  - unavailable, due to
    - absence of person rendering care V60.4
    - inability (any reason) of person rendering care V60.4
  - well baby V20.1
- **Caries** (bone) (*see also* Tuberculosis, bone) 015.9 5th *[730.8]* 5th
  - arrested 521.04
  - cementum 521.03
  - cerebrospinal (tuberculous) 015.0 5th *[730.88]*
  - dental (acute) (chronic) (incipient) (infected) 521.00
    - with pulp exposure 521.03
    - extending to
      - dentine 521.02
      - pulp 521.03
    - other specified NEC 521.09
    - pit and fissure 521.06
    - primary
      - pit and fissure origin 521.06
      - root surface 521.08
      - smooth surface origin 521.07
    - root surface 521.08
    - smooth surface 521.07
  - dentin (acute) (chronic) 521.02

- **Caries** – *continued*
  - enamel (acute) (chronic) (incipient) 521.01
  - external meatus 380.89
  - hip (*see also* Tuberculosis) 015.1 5th *[730.85]*
  - initial 521.01
  - knee 015.2 5th *[730.86]*
  - labyrinth 386.8
  - limb NEC 015.7 5th *[730.88]*
  - mastoid (chronic) (process) 383.1
  - middle ear 385.89
  - nose 015.7 5th *[730.88]*
  - orbit 015.7 5th *[730.88]*
  - ossicle 385.24
  - petrous bone 383.20
  - sacrum (tuberculous) 015.0 5th *[730.88]*
  - spine, spinal (column) (tuberculous) 015.0 5th *[730.88]*
  - syphilitic 095.5
    - congenital 090.0 *[730.8]* 5th
  - teeth (internal) 521.00
    - initial 521.01
  - vertebra (column) (tuberculous) 015.0 5th *[730.88]*
- **Carini's syndrome** (ichthyosis congenita) 757.1
- **Carious teeth** 521.00
- **Carneous mole** 631
- **Carnosinemia** 270.5
- **Carotid body or sinus syndrome** 337.01
- **Carotidynia** 337.01
- **Carotinemia** (dietary) 278.3
- **Carotinosis** (cutis) (skin) 278.3
- **Carpal tunnel syndrome** 354.0
- **Carpenter's syndrome** 759.89
- **Carpopedal spasm** (*see also* Tetany) 781.7
- **Carpoptosis** 736.05
- **Carrier** (suspected) **of**
  - amebiasis V02.2
  - bacterial disease (meningococcal, staphylococcal) NEC V02.59
  - cholera V02.0
  - cystic fibrosis gene V83.81
  - defective gene V83.89
  - diphtheria V02.4
  - dysentery (bacillary) V02.3
    - amebic V02.2
  - Endamoeba histolytica V02.2
  - gastrointestinal pathogens NEC V02.3
  - genetic defect V83.89
  - gonorrhea V02.7
  - group B streptococcus V02.51
  - HAA (hepatitis Australian-antigen) V02.61
  - hemophilia A (asymptomatic) V83.01
    - symptomatic V83.02
  - hepatitis V02.60
    - Australian-antigen (HAA) V02.61
    - B V02.61
    - C V02.62
    - specified type NEC V02.69
    - serum V02.61
    - viral V02.60
  - infective organism NEC V02.9
  - malaria V02.9
  - paratyphoid V02.3
  - Salmonella V02.3
    - typhosa V02.1
  - serum hepatitis V02.61
  - Shigella V02.3
  - Staphylococcus NEC V02.59
    - methicillin
      - resistant Staphylococcus aureus V02.54
      - susceptible Staphylococcus aureus V02.53
  - Streptococcus NEC V02.52
    - group B V02.51
  - typhoid V02.1
  - venereal disease NEC V02.8
- **Carrión's disease** (Bartonellosis) 088.0
- **Car sickness** 994.6
- **Carter's**
  - relapsing fever (Asiatic) 087.0
- **Cartilage** - *see* condition
- **Caruncle** (inflamed)
  - abscess, lacrimal (*see also* Dacryocystitis) 375.30
  - conjunctiva 372.00
    - acute 372.00
  - eyelid 373.00
  - labium (majus) (minus) 616.89
  - lacrimal 375.30
  - urethra (benign) 599.3
  - vagina (wall) 616.89
- **Cascade stomach** 537.6
- **Caseation lymphatic gland** (*see also* Tuberculosis) 017.2 5th
- **Caseous**
  - bronchitis - *see* Tuberculosis, pulmonary
  - meningitis 013.0 5th
  - pneumonia - *see* Tuberculosis, pulmonary
- **Cassidy (-Scholte) syndrome** (malignant carcinoid) 259.2
- **Castellani's bronchitis** 104.8
- **Castleman's tumor or lymphoma** (mediastinal lymph node hyperplasia) 785.6
- **Castration, traumatic** 878.2
  - complicated 878.3
- **Casts in urine** 791.7
- **Cat's ear** 744.29
- **Catalepsy** 300.11
  - catatonic (acute) (*see also* Schizophrenia) 295.2 5th
  - hysterical 300.11
  - schizophrenic (*see also* Schizophrenia) 295.2 5th
- **Cataphasia** 307.0
- **Cataplexy** (idiopathic) *see also* Narcolepsy
- **Cataract** (anterior cortical) (anterior polar) (black) (capsular) (central) (cortical) (hypermature) (immature) (incipient) (mature) 366.9
  - anterior
    - and posterior axial embryonal 743.33
    - pyramidal 743.31
    - subcapsular polar
      - infantile, juvenile, or presenile 366.01
      - senile 366.13
  - associated with
    - calcinosis 275.40 *[366.42]*
    - craniofacial dysostosis 756.0 *[366.44]*
    - galactosemia 271.1 *[366.44]*
    - hypoparathyroidism 252.1 *[366.42]*
    - myotonic disorders 359.21 *[366.43]*
    - neovascularization 366.33
  - blue dot 743.39
  - cerulean 743.39
  - complicated NEC 366.30
  - congenital 743.30
    - capsular or subcapsular 743.31
    - cortical 743.32
    - nuclear 743.33
    - specified type NEC 743.39
    - total or subtotal 743.34
    - zonular 743.32
  - coronary (congenital) 743.39
    - acquired 366.12
  - cupuliform 366.14
  - diabetic 250.5 5th *[366.41]*
    - due to secondary diabetes 249.5 5th *[366.41]*
  - drug-induced 366.45
  - due to
    - chalcosis 360.24 *[366.34]*
    - chronic choroiditis (*see also* Choroiditis) 363.20 *[366.32]*
    - degenerative myopia 360.21 *[366.34]*
    - glaucoma (*see also* Glaucoma) 365.9 *[366.31]*
    - infection, intraocular NEC 366.32
    - inflammatory ocular disorder NEC 366.32
    - iridocyclitis, chronic 364.10 *[366.33]*

Cataract – *continued*
- due to – *continued*
  - pigmentary retinal dystrophy 362.74 *[366.34]*
  - radiation 366.46
- electric 366.46
- glassblowers' 366.46
- heat ray 366.46
- heterochromic 366.33
- in eye disease NEC 366.30
- infantile (*see also* Cataract, juvenile) 366.00
- intumescent 366.12
- irradiational 366.46
- juvenile 366.00
  - anterior subcapsular polar 366.01
  - combined forms 366.09
  - cortical 366.03
  - lamellar 366.03
  - nuclear 366.04
  - posterior subcapsular polar 366.02
  - specified NEC 366.09
  - zonular 366.03
- lamellar 743.32
  - infantile juvenile, or presenile 366.03
- morgagnian 366.18
- myotonic 359.21 *[366.43]*
- myxedema 244.9 *[366.44]*
- nuclear 366.16
- posterior, polar (capsular) 743.31
  - infantile, juvenile, or presenile 366.02
  - senile 366.14
- presenile (*see also* Cataract, juvenile) 366.00
- punctate
  - acquired 366.12
  - congenital 743.39
- secondary (membrane) 366.50
  - obscuring vision 366.53
  - specified type, not obscuring vision 366.52
- senile 366.10
  - anterior subcapsular polar 366.13
  - combined forms 366.19
  - cortical 366.15
  - hypermature 366.18
  - immature 366.12
  - incipient 366.12
  - mature 366.17
  - nuclear 366.16
  - posterior subcapsular polar 366.14
  - specified NEC 366.19
  - total or subtotal 366.17
- snowflake 250.5 [5th] *[366.41]*
  - due to secondary diabetes 249.5 [5th] *[366.41]*
- specified NEC 366.8
- subtotal (senile) 366.17
  - congenital 743.34
- sunflower 360.24 *[366.34]*
- tetanic NEC 252.1 *[366.42]*
- total (mature) (senile) 366.17
  - congenital 743.34
  - localized 366.21
  - traumatic 366.22
- toxic 366.45
- traumatic 366.20
  - partially resolved 366.23
  - total 366.22
- zonular (perinuclear) 743.32
  - infantile, juvenile, or presenile 366.03

Cataracta 366.10
- brunescens 366.16
- cerulea 743.39
- complicata 366.30
- congenita 743.30
- coralliformis 743.39
- coronaria (congenital) 743.39
  - acquired 366.12
- diabetic 250.5 [5th] *[366.41]*
  - due to secondary diabetes 249.5 [5th] *[366.41]*
- floriformis 360.24 *[366.34]*

Cataracta – *continued*
- membranacea
  - accreta 366.50
  - congenita 743.39
- nigra 366.16

Catarrh, catarrhal (inflammation) (*see also* condition) 460
- acute 460
- asthma, asthmatic (*see also* Asthma) 493.9 [5th]
- Bostock's (*see also* Fever, hay) 477.9
- bowel - *see* Enteritis
- bronchial 490
  - acute 466.0
  - chronic 491.0
  - subacute 466.0
- cervix, cervical (canal) (uteri) - *see* Cervicitis
- chest (*see also* Bronchitis) 490
- chronic 472.0
- congestion 472.0
- conjunctivitis 372.03
- due to syphilis 095.9
  - congenital 090.0
- enteric - *see* Enteritis
- epidemic 487.1
- Eustachian 381.50
- eye (acute) (vernal) 372.03
- fauces (*see also* Pharyngitis) 462
- febrile 460
- fibrinous acute 466.0
- gastroenteric - *see* Enteritis
- gastrointestinal - *see* Enteritis
- gingivitis 523.00
- hay (*see also* Fever, hay) 477.9
- infectious 460
- intestinal - *see* Enteritis
- larynx (*see also* Laryngitis, chronic) 476.0
- liver 070.1
  - with hepatic coma 070.0
- lung (*see also* Bronchitis) 490
  - acute 466.0
  - chronic 491.0
- middle ear (chronic) - *see* Otitis media, chronic
- mouth 528.00
- nasal (chronic) (*see also* Rhinitis) 472.0
  - acute 460
- nasobronchial 472.2
- nasopharyngeal (chronic) 472.2
  - acute 460
- nose - *see* Catarrh, nasal
- ophthalmia 372.03
- pneumococcal, acute 466.0
- pulmonary (*see also* Bronchitis) 490
  - acute 466.0
  - chronic 491.0
- spring (eye) 372.13
- suffocating (*see also* Asthma) 493.9 [5th]
- summer (hay) (*see also* Fever, hay) 477.9
- throat 472.1
- tracheitis 464.10
  - with obstruction 464.11
- tubotympanal 381.4
  - acute (*see also* Otitis media, acute, nonsuppurative) 381.00
  - chronic 381.10
- vasomotor (*see also* Fever, hay) 477.9
- vesical (bladder) - *see* Cystitis

Catarrhus aestivus (*see also* Fever, hay) 477.9

Catastrophe, cerebral (*see also* Disease, cerebrovascular, acute) 436

Catatonia, catatonic (acute) 781.99
- with
  - affective psychosis - *see* Psychosis, affective
- agitation 295.2 [5th]
- dementia (praecox) 295.2 [5th]
- due to or associated with physical condition 293.89
- excitation 295.2 [5th]
- excited type 295.2 [5th]
- in conditions classified elsewhere 293.89
- schizophrenia 295.2 [5th]

Catatonia, catatonic – *continued*
- stupor 295.2 [5th]

Cat-scratch - *see also* Injury, superficial
- disease or fever 078.3

Cauda equina - *see also* condition
- syndrome 344.60

Cauliflower ear 738.7

Caul over face 768.9

Causalgia 355.9
- lower limb 355.71
- upper limb 354.4

Cause
- external, general effects NEC 994.9
- not stated 799.9
- unknown 799.9

Caustic burn - *see also* Burn, by site
- from swallowing caustic or corrosive substance - *see* Burn, internal organs

Cavare's disease (familial periodic paralysis) 359.3

Cave-in, injury
- crushing (severe) (*see also* Crush, by site) 869.1
- suffocation 994.7

Cavernitis (penis) 607.2
- lymph vessel - *see* Lymphangioma

Cavernositis 607.2

Cavernous - *see* condition

Cavitation of lung (*see also* Tuberculosis) 011.2 [5th]
- nontuberculous 518.89
- primary, progressive 010.8 [5th]

Cavity
- lung - *see* Cavitation of lung
- optic papilla 743.57
- pulmonary - *see* Cavitation of lung
- teeth 521.00
- vitreous (humor) 379.21

Cavovarus foot, congenital 754.59

Cavus foot (congenital) 754.71
- acquired 736.73

Cazenave's
- disease (pemphigus) NEC 694.4
- lupus (erythematosus) 695.4

CDGS (carbohydrate-deficient glycoprotein syndrome) 271.8

Cecitis - *see* Appendicitis

Cecocele - *see* Hernia

Cecum - *see* condition

Celiac
- artery compression syndrome 447.4
- disease 579.0
- infantilism 579.0

Cell, cellular - *see also* condition
- anterior chamber (eye) (positive aqueous ray) 364.04

Cellulitis (diffuse) (with lymphangitis) (*see also* Abscess) 682.9
- abdominal wall 682.2
- anaerobic (*see also* Gas gangrene) 040.0
- ankle 682.6
- anus 566
- areola 611.0
- arm (any part, above wrist) 682.3
- auditory canal (external) 380.10
- axilla 682.3
- back (any part) 682.2
- breast 611.0
  - postpartum 675.1 [5th]
- broad ligament (*see also* Disease, pelvis, inflammatory) 614.4
  - acute 614.3
- buttock 682.5
- cervical (neck region) 682.1
- cervix (uteri) (*see also* Cervicitis) 616.0
- cheek, external 682.0
  - internal 528.3
- chest wall 682.2
- chronic NEC 682.9
- colostomy 569.61
- corpus cavernosum 607.2
- digit 681.9

Cellulitis – *continued*
- Douglas' cul-de-sac or pouch (chronic) (*see also* Disease, pelvis, inflammatory) 614.4
  - acute 614.3
- drainage site (following operation) 998.59
- ear, external 380.10
- enterostomy 569.61
- erysipelar (*see also* Erysipelas) 035
- esophagostomy 530.86
- eyelid 373.13
- face (any part, except eye) 682.0
- finger (intrathecal) (periosteal) (subcutaneous) (subcuticular) 681.00
- flank 682.2
- foot (except toe) 682.7
- forearm 682.3
- gangrenous (*see also* Gangrene) 785.4
- genital organ NEC
  - female - *see* Abscess, genital organ, female
  - male 608.4
- glottis 478.71
- gluteal (region) 682.5
- gonococcal NEC 098.0
- groin 682.2
- hand (except finger or thumb) 682.4
- head (except face) NEC 682.8
- heel 682.7
- hip 682.6
- jaw (region) 682.0
- knee 682.6
- labium (majus) (minus) (*see also* Vulvitis) 616.10
- larynx 478.71
- leg, except foot 682.6
- lip 528.5
- mammary gland 611.0
- mouth (floor) 528.3
- multiple sites NEC 682.9
- nasopharynx 478.21
- navel 682.2
  - newborn NEC 771.4
- neck (region) 682.1
- nipple 611.0
- nose 478.19
  - external 682.0
- orbit, orbital 376.01
- palate (soft) 528.3
- pectoral (region) 682.2
- pelvis, pelvic
  - with
    - abortion - *see* Abortion, by type, with sepsis
    - ectopic pregnancy (*see also* categories 633.0-633.9) 639.0
    - molar pregnancy (*see also* categories 630-632) 639.0
  - female (*see also* Disease, pelvis, inflammatory) 614.4
    - acute 614.3
  - following
    - abortion 639.0
    - ectopic or molar pregnancy 639.0
  - male 567.21
  - puerperal, postpartum, childbirth 670.8 [5th] ▲
- penis 607.2
- perineal, perineum 682.2
- perirectal 566
- peritonsillar 475
- periurethral 597.0
- periuterine (*see also* Disease, pelvis, inflammatory) 614.4
  - acute 614.3
- pharynx 478.21
- phlegmonous NEC 682.9
- rectum 566
- retromammary 611.0
- retroperitoneal (*see also* Peritonitis) 567.38

- **Cellulitis** – *continued*
  - round ligament (*see also* Disease, pelvis, inflammatory) 614.4
    - acute 614.3
  - scalp (any part) 682.8
    - dissecting 704.8
  - scrotum 608.4
  - seminal vesicle 608.0
  - septic NEC 682.9
  - shoulder 682.3
  - specified sites NEC 682.8
  - spermatic cord 608.4
  - submandibular (region) (space) (triangle) 682.0
    - gland 527.3
  - submaxillary 528.3
    - gland 527.3
  - submental (pyogenic) 682.0
    - gland 527.3
  - suppurative NEC 682.9
  - testis 608.4
  - thigh 682.6
  - thumb (intrathecal) (periosteal) (subcutaneous) (subcuticular) 681.00
  - toe (intrathecal) (periosteal) (subcutaneous) (subcuticular) 681.10
  - tonsil 475
  - trunk 682.2
  - tuberculous (primary) (*see also* Tuberculosis) 017.0 5th
  - tunica vaginalis 608.4
  - umbilical 682.2
    - newborn NEC 771.4
  - vaccinal 999.39
  - vagina - *see* Vaginitis
  - vas deferens 608.4
  - vocal cords 478.5
  - vulva (*see also* Vulvitis) 616.10
  - wrist 682.4
- **Cementoblastoma, benign** (M9273/0) 213.1
  - upper jaw (bone) 213.0
- **Cementoma** (M9273/0) 213.1
  - gigantiform (M9276/0) 213.1
    - upper jaw (bone) 213.0
  - upper jaw (bone) 213.0
- **Cementoperiostitis** 523.40
  - acute 523.33
  - apical 523.40
- **Cephalgia, cephalagia** (*see also* Headache) 784.0
  - histamine 339.00
  - nonorganic origin 307.81
  - other trigeminal autonomic (TACS) 339.09
  - psychogenic 307.81
  - tension 307.81
- **Cephalhematocele, cephalematocele**
  - due to birth injury 767.19
  - fetus or newborn 767.19
  - traumatic (*see also* Contusion, head) 920
- **Cephalhematoma, cephalematoma** (calcified)
  - due to birth injury 767.19
  - fetus or newborn 767.19
  - traumatic (*see also* Contusion, head) 920
- **Cephalic** - *see* condition
- **Cephalitis** - *see* Encephalitis
- **Cephalocele** 742.0
- **Cephaloma** - *see* Neoplasm, by site, malignant
- **Cephalomenia** 625.8
- **Cephalopelvic** - *see* condition
- **Cercomoniasis** 007.3
- **Cerebellitis** - *see* Encephalitis
- **Cerebellum** (cerebellar) - *see* condition
- **Cerebral** - *see* condition
- **Cerebritis** - *see* Encephalitis
- **Cerebrohepatorenal syndrome** 759.89
- **Cerebromacular degeneration** 330.1
- **Cerebromalacia** (*see also* Softening, brain) 434.9 5th
- **Cerebrosidosis** 272.7
- **Cerebrospasticity** - *see* Palsy, cerebral
- **Cerebrospinal** - *see* condition
- **Cerebrum** - *see* condition
- **Ceroid storage disease** 272.7
- **Cerumen** (accumulation) (impacted) 380.4
- **Cervical** - *see also* condition
  - auricle 744.43
  - high risk human papillomavirus (HPV) DNA test positive 795.05
  - intraepithelial glandular neoplasia 233.1
  - low risk human papillomavirus (HPV) DNA test positive 795.09
  - rib 756.2
  - shortening - *see* Short, cervical
- **Cervicalgia** 723.1
- **Cervicitis** (acute) (chronic) (nonvenereal) (subacute) (with erosion or ectropion) 616.0
  - with
    - abortion - *see* Abortion, by type, with sepsis
    - ectopic pregnancy (*see also* categories 633.0-633.9) 639.0
    - molar pregnancy (*see also* categories 630-632) 639.0
    - ulceration 616.0
  - chlamydial 099.53
  - complicating pregnancy or puerperium 646.6 5th
    - affecting fetus or newborn 760.8
  - following
    - abortion 639.0
    - ectopic or molar pregnancy 639.0
  - gonococcal (acute) 098.15
    - chronic or duration of 2 months or more 098.35
  - senile (atrophic) 616.0
  - syphilitic 095.8
  - trichomonal 131.09
  - tuberculous (*see also* Tuberculosis) 016.7 5th
- **Cervicoaural fistula** 744.49
- **Cervicocolpitis** (emphysematosa) (*see also* Cervicitis) 616.0
- **Cervix** - *see* condition
- **Cesarean delivery, operation or section** NEC 669.7 5th
  - affecting fetus or newborn 763.4
  - post mortem, affecting fetus or newborn 761.6
  - previous, affecting management of pregnancy 654.2 5th
- **Céstan's syndrome** 344.89
- **Céstan-Chenais paralysis** 344.89
- **Céstan-Raymond syndrome** 433.8 5th
- **Cestode infestation NEC** 123.9
  - specified type NEC 123.8
- **Cestodiasis** 123.9
- **CGF** (congenital generalized fibromatosis) 759.89
- **Chabert's disease** 022.9
- **Chacaleh** 266.2
- **Chafing** 709.8
- **Chagas' disease** (*see also* Trypanosomiasis, American) 086.2
  - with heart involvement 086.0
- **Chagres fever** 084.0
- **Chalasia** (cardiac sphincter) 530.81
- **Chalazion** 373.2
- **Chalazoderma** 757.39
- **Chalcosis** 360.24
  - cornea 371.15
  - crystalline lens 360.24 [366.34
  - retina 360.24
- **Chalicosis** (occupational) (pulmonum) 502
- **Chancre** (any genital site) (hard) (indurated) (infecting) (primary) (recurrent) 091.0
  - congenital 090.0
  - conjunctiva 091.2
  - Ducrey's 099.0
  - extragenital 091.2
  - eyelid 091.2
  - Hunterian 091.0
  - lip (syphilis) 091.2
  - mixed 099.8
- **Chancre** – *continued*
  - nipple 091.2
  - Nisbet's 099.0
  - of
    - carate 103.0
    - pinta 103.0
  - yaws 102.0
  - palate, soft 091.2
  - phagedenic 099.0
  - Ricord's 091.0
  - Rollet's (syphilitic) 091.0
  - seronegative 091.0
  - seropositive 091.0
  - simple 099.0
  - soft 099.0
    - bubo 099.0
  - urethra 091.0
  - yaws 102.0
- **Chancriform syndrome** 114.1
- **Chancroid** 099.0
  - anus 099.0
  - penis (Ducrey's bacillus) 099.0
  - perineum 099.0
  - rectum 099.0
  - scrotum 099.0
  - urethra 099.0
  - vulva 099.0
- **Chandipura fever** 066.8
- **Chandler's disease** (osteochondritis dissecans, hip) 732.7
- **Change**(s) (of) - *see also* Removal of
  - arteriosclerotic - *see* Arteriosclerosis
  - battery
    - cardiac pacemaker V53.31
  - bone 733.90
    - diabetic 250.8 5th *[731.8]*
      - due to secondary diabetes 249.8 5th *[731.8]*
    - in disease, unknown cause 733.90
  - bowel habits 787.99
  - cardiorenal (vascular) (*see also* Hypertension, cardiorenal) 404.90
  - cardiovascular - *see* Disease, cardiovascular
  - circulatory 459.9
  - cognitive or personality change of other type, nonpsychotic 310.1
  - color, teeth, tooth
    - during formation 520.8
    - extrinsic 523.6
    - intrinsic posteruptive 521.7
  - contraceptive device V25.42
  - cornea, corneal
    - degenerative NEC 371.40
    - membrane NEC 371.30
    - senile 371.41
  - coronary (*see also* Ischemia, heart) 414.9
  - degenerative
    - chamber angle (anterior) (iris) 364.56
    - ciliary body 364.57
    - spine or vertebra (*see also* Spondylosis) 721.90
  - dental pulp, regressive 522.2
  - drains V58.49
  - dressing
    - wound V58.30
      - nonsurgical V58.30
      - surgical V58.31
  - fixation device V54.89
    - external V54.89
    - internal V54.01
  - heart - *see also* Disease, heart
  - hip joint 718.95
  - hyperplastic larynx 478.79
  - hypertrophic
    - nasal sinus (*see also* Sinusitis) 473.9
    - turbinate, nasal 478.0
    - upper respiratory tract 478.9
  - inflammatory - *see* Inflammation
  - joint (*see also* Derangement, joint) 718.90
    - sacroiliac 724.6
  - Kirschner wire V54.89
  - knee 717.9
  - macular, congenital 743.55
- **Change**(s) (of) – *continued*
  - malignant (M----/3) - *see also* Neoplasm, by site, malignant

Note *For malignant change occurring in a neoplasm, use the appropriate M code with behavior digit/3 e.g., malignant change in uterine fibroidM8890/3. For malignant change occurring in a nonneoplastic condition (e.g., gastric ulcer) use the M code M8000/3.*

  - mental (status) NEC 780.97
    - due to or associated with physical condition - *see* Syndrome, brain
  - myocardium, myocardial - *see* Degeneration, myocardial
  - of life (*see also* Menopause) 627.2
  - pacemaker battery (cardiac) V53.31
  - peripheral nerve 355.9
  - personality (nonpsychotic) NEC 310.1
  - plaster cast V54.89
  - refractive, transient 367.81
  - regressive, dental pulp 522.2
  - retina 362.9
    - myopic (degenerative) (malignant) 360.21
    - vascular appearance 362.13
  - sacroiliac joint 724.6
  - scleral 379.19
    - degenerative 379.16
  - senile (*see also* Senility) 797
  - sensory (*see also* Disturbance, sensation) 782.0
  - skin texture 782.8
  - spinal cord 336.9
  - splint, external V54.89
  - subdermal implantable contraceptive V25.5
  - suture V58.32
  - traction device V54.89
  - trophic 355.9
    - arm NEC 354.9
    - leg NEC 355.8
    - lower extremity NEC 355.8
    - upper extremity NEC 354.9
  - vascular 459.9
  - vasomotor 443.9
  - voice 784.49
    - psychogenic 306.1
  - wound packing V58.30
    - nonsurgical V58.30
    - surgical V58.31
- **Changing sleep-work schedule, affecting sleep** 327.36
- **Changuinola fever** 066.0
- **Chapping skin** 709.8
- **Character**
  - depressive 301.12
- **Charcôt's**
  - arthropathy 094.0 *[713.5]*
  - cirrhosis - *see* Cirrhosis, biliary
  - disease 094.0
    - spinal cord 094.0
  - fever (biliary) (hepatic) (intermittent) - *see* Choledocholithiasis
  - joint (disease) 094.0 *[713.5]*
    - diabetic 250.6 5th *[713.5]*
      - due to secondary diabetes 249.6 5th *[713.5]*
    - syringomyelic 336.0 *[713.5]*
  - syndrome (intermittent claudication) 443.9
    - due to atherosclerosis 440.21
- **Charcôt-Marie-Tooth disease, paralysis, or syndrome** 356.1
- **CHARGE association** (syndrome) 759.89
- **Charleyhorse** (quadriceps) 843.8
  - muscle, except quadriceps - *see* Sprain, by site
- **Charlouis' disease** (*see also* Yaws) 102.9
- **Chauffeur's fracture** - *see* Fracture, ulna, lower end
- **Cheadle (-Möller) (-Barlow) disease or syndrome** (infantile scurvy) 267

Cellulitis – Cheadle (-Möller) (-Barlow) disease or syndrome

Checking (of)
- contraceptive device (intrauterine) V25.42
- device
  - fixation V54.89
    - external V54.89
    - internal V54.09
  - traction V54.89
- Kirschner wire V54.89
- plaster cast V54.89
- splint, external V54.89

Checkup
- following treatment - *see* Examination
- health V70.0
- infant (over 28 days old) (not sick) V20.2 ▲
- newborn, routine
  - 8 to 28 days old V20.32 ●
  - ~~initial V20.2~~
  - over 28 days old, routine V20.2 ●
  - ~~subsequent V20.2~~
  - under 8 days old V20.31 ●
  - weight V20.32 ●
- pregnancy (normal) V22.1
  - first V22.0
  - high-risk pregnancy V23.9
    - specified problem NEC V23.89

Chédiak-Higashi (-Steinbrinck) anomaly, disease, or syndrome (congenital gigantism of peroxidase granules) 288.2

Cheek - *see also* condition
- biting 528.9

Cheese itch 133.8

Cheese washers' lung 495.8

Cheilitis 528.5
- actinic (due to sun) 692.72
  - chronic NEC 692.74
    - due to radiation, except from sun 692.82
  - due to radiation, except from sun 692.82
- acute 528.5
- angular 528.5
- catarrhal 528.5
- chronic 528.5
- exfoliative 528.5
- gangrenous 528.5
- glandularis apostematosa 528.5
- granulomatosa 351.8
- infectional 528.5
- membranous 528.5
- Miescher's 351.8
- suppurative 528.5
- ulcerative 528.5
- vesicular 528.5

Cheilodynia 528.5

Cheilopalatoschisis (*see also* Cleft, palate, with cleft lip) 749.20

Cheilophagia 528.9

Cheiloschisis (*see also* Cleft, lip) 749.10

Cheilosis 528.5
- with pellagra 265.2
- angular 528.5
- due to
  - dietary deficiency 266.0
  - vitamin deficiency 266.0

Cheiromegaly 729.89

Cheiropompholyx 705.81

Cheloid (*see also* Keloid) 701.4

Chemical burn - *see also* Burn, by site
- from swallowing chemical - *see* Burn, internal organs

Chemodectoma (M8693/1) - *see* Paraganglioma, nonchromaffin

Chemoprophylaxis NEC V07.39

Chemosis, conjunctiva 372.73

Chemotherapy
- convalescence V66.2
- encounter (for) (oral) (intravenous) V58.11 ▲
- maintenance (oral) (intravenous) V58.11 ▲
- prophylactic NEC V07.39
  - fluoride V07.31

Cherubism 526.89

Chest - *see* condition

Cheyne-Stokes respiration (periodic) 786.04

Chiari's
- disease or syndrome (hepatic vein thrombosis) 453.0
- malformation
  - type I 348.4
  - type II (*see also* Spina bifida) 741.0 [5th]
  - type III 742.0
  - type IV 742.2
- network 746.89

Chiari-Frommel syndrome 676.6 [5th]

Chicago disease (North American blastomycosis) 116.0

Chickenpox (*see also* Varicella) 052.9
- exposure to V01.71
- vaccination and inoculation (prophylactic) V05.4

Chiclero ulcer 085.4

Chiggers 133.8

Chignon 111.2
- fetus or newborn (from vacuum extraction) 767.19

Chigoe disease 134.1

Chikungunya fever 066.3

Chilaiditi's syndrome (subphrenic displacement, colon) 751.4

Chilblains 991.5
- lupus 991.5

Child
- behavior causing concern V61.20
  - adopted child V61.24 ●
  - biological child V61.23 ●
  - foster child V61.25 ●

Childbed fever 670.8 [5th] ▲

Childbirth - *see also* Delivery
- puerperal complications - *see* Puerperal

Childhood, period of rapid growth V21.0

Chill(s) 780.64
- with fever 780.60
- without fever 780.64
- congestive 780.99
  - in malarial regions 084.6
- septic - *see* Septicemia
- urethral 599.84

Chilomastigiasis 007.8

Chin - *see* condition

Chinese dysentery 004.9

Chiropractic dislocation (*see also* Lesion, nonallopathic, by site) 739.9

Chitral fever 066.0

Chlamydia, chlamydial - *see* condition

Chloasma 709.09
- cachecticorum 709.09
- eyelid 374.52
  - congenital 757.33
  - hyperthyroid 242.0 [5th]
- gravidarum 646.8 [5th]
- idiopathic 709.09
- skin 709.09
- symptomatic 709.09

Chloroma (M9930/3) 205.3 [5th]

Chlorosis 280.9
- Egyptian (*see also* Ancylostomiasis) 126.9
- miners' (*see also* Ancylostomiasis) 126.9

Chlorotic anemia 280.9

Chocolate cyst (ovary) 617.1

Choked
- disk or disc - *see* Papilledema
- on food, phlegm, or vomitus NEC (*see also* Asphyxia, food) 933.1
- phlegm 933.1
- while vomiting NEC (*see also* Asphyxia, food) 933.1

Chokes (resulting from bends) 993.3

Choking sensation 784.99

Cholangiectasis (*see also* Disease, gallbladder) 575.8

Cholangiocarcinoma (M8160/3)
- and hepatocellular carcinoma, combined (M8180/3) 155.0
- liver 155.1

Cholangiocarcinoma – *continued*
- specified site NEC - *see* Neoplasm, by site, malignant
- unspecified site 155.1

Cholangiohepatitis 575.8
- due to fluke infestation 121.1

Cholangiohepatoma (M8180/3) 155.0

Cholangiolitis (acute) (chronic) (extrahepatic) (gangrenous) 576.1
- intrahepatic 575.8
- paratyphoidal (*see also* Fever, paratyphoid) 002.9
- typhoidal 002.0

Cholangioma (M8160/0) 211.5
- malignant - *see* Cholangiocarcinoma

Cholangitis (acute) (ascending) (catarrhal) (chronic) (infective) (malignant) (primary) (recurrent) (sclerosing) (secondary) (stenosing) (suppurative) 576.1
- chronic nonsuppurative destructive 571.6
- nonsuppurative destructive (chronic) 571.6

Cholecystdocholithiasis - *see* Choledocholithiasis

Cholecystitis 575.10
- with
  - calculus, stones in
    - bile duct (common) (hepatic) - *see* Choledocholithiasis
    - gallbladder - *see* Cholelithiasis
- acute 575.0
- acute and chronic 575.12
- chronic 575.11
- emphysematous (acute) (*see also* Cholecystitis, acute) 575.0
- gangrenous (*see also* Cholecystitis, acute) 575.0
- paratyphoidal, current (*see also* Fever, paratyphoid) 002.9
- suppurative (*see also* Cholecystitis, acute) 575.0
- typhoidal 002.0

Choledochitis (suppurative) 576.1

Choledocholith - *see* Choledocholithiasis

Choledocholithiasis 574.5 [5th]

Note *Use the following fifth-digit subclassification with category 574:*

0	without mention of obstruction
1	with obstruction

- with
  - cholecystitis 574.4 [5th]
    - acute 574.3 [5th]
    - chronic 574.4 [5th]
  - cholelithiasis 574.9 [5th]
    - with
      - cholecystitis 574.7 [5th]
        - acute 574.6 [5th]
          - and chronic 574.8 [5th]
        - chronic 574.7 [5th]

Cholelithiasis (impacted) (multiple) 574.2 [5th]

Note *Use the following fifth-digit subclassification with category 574:*

0	without mention of obstruction
1	with obstruction

- with
  - cholecystitis 574.1 [5th]
    - acute 574.0 [5th]
    - chronic 574.1 [5th]
  - choledocholithiasis 574.9 [5th]
    - with
      - cholecystitis 574.7 [5th]
        - acute 574.6 [5th]
          - and chronic 574.8 [5th]
        - chronic cholecystitis 574.7 [5th]

Cholemia (*see also* Jaundice) 782.4
- familial 277.4
- Gilbert's (familial nonhemolytic) 277.4

Cholemic gallstone - *see* Cholelithiasis

Choleperitoneum, choleperitonitis (*see also* Disease, gallbladder) 567.81

Cholera (algid) (Asiatic) (asphyctic) (epidemic) (gravis) (Indian) (malignant) (morbus) (pestilential) (spasmodic) 001.9
- antimonial 985.4
- carrier (suspected) of V02.0
- classical 001.0
- contact V01.0
- due to
  - Vibrio
    - cholerae (Inaba, Ogawa, Hikojima serotypes) 001.0
      - El Tor 001.1
- El Tor 001.1
- exposure to V01.0
- vaccination, prophylactic (against) V03.0

Cholerine (*see also* Cholera) 001.9

Cholestasis 576.8
- due to total parenteral nutrition (TPN) 573.8

Cholesteatoma (ear) 385.30
- attic (primary) 385.31
- diffuse 385.35
- external ear (canal) 380.21
- marginal (middle ear) 385.32
  - with involvement of mastoid cavity 385.33
  - secondary (with middle ear involvement) 385.33
- mastoid cavity 385.30
- middle ear (secondary) 385.32
  - with involvement of mastoid cavity 385.33
- postmastoidectomy cavity (recurrent) 383.32
- primary 385.31
- recurrent, postmastoidectomy cavity 383.32
- secondary (middle ear) 385.32
  - with involvement of mastoid cavity 385.33

Cholesteatosis (middle ear) (*see also* Cholesteatoma) 385.30
- diffuse 385.35

Cholesteremia 272.0

Cholesterin
- granuloma, middle ear 385.82
- in vitreous 379.22

Cholesterol
- deposit
  - retina 362.82
  - vitreous 379.22
- elevated (high) 272.0
  - with elevated (high) triglycerides 272.2
- imbibition of gallbladder (*see also* Disease, gallbladder) 575.6

Cholesterolemia 272.0
- essential 272.0
- familial 272.0
- hereditary 272.0

Cholesterosis, cholesterolosis (gallbladder) 575.6
- with
  - cholecystitis - *see* Cholecystitis
  - cholelithiasis - *see* Cholelithiasis
- middle ear (*see also* Cholesteatoma) 385.30

Cholocolic fistula (*see also* Fistula, gallbladder) 575.5

Choluria 791.4

Chondritis (purulent) 733.99
- auricle 380.03
- costal 733.6
  - Tietze's 733.6
- patella, posttraumatic 717.7
- pinna 380.03
- posttraumatica patellae 717.7
- tuberculous (active) (*see also* Tuberculosis) 015.9 [5th]
  - intervertebral 015.0 [5th] *[730.88]*

Chondroangiopathia calcarea seu punctate 756.59

- **Chondroblastoma** (M9230/0) - *see also* Neoplasm, bone, benign
  - malignant (M9230/3) - *see* Neoplasm, bone, malignant
- **Chondrocalcinosis** (articular) (crystal deposition) (dihydrate) (*see also* Arthritis, due to, crystals) 275.49 *[712.3]* [5th]
  - due to
    - calcium pyrophosphate 275.49 *[712.2]* [5th]
    - dicalcium phosphate crystals 275.49 *[712.1]* [5th]
    - pyrophosphate crystals 275.49 *[712.2]* [5th]
- **Chondrodermatitis nodularis helicis** 380.00
- **Chondrodysplasia** 756.4
  - angiomatose 756.4
  - calcificans congenita 756.59
  - epiphysialis punctata 756.59
  - hereditary deforming 756.4
  - rhizomelic punctata 277.86
- **Chondrodystrophia** (fetalis) 756.4
  - calcarea 756.4
  - calcificans congenita 756.59
  - fetalis hypoplastica 756.59
  - hypoplastica calcinosa 756.59
  - punctata 756.59
  - tarda 277.5
- **Chondrodystrophy** (familial) (hypoplastic) 756.4
  - myotonic (congenital) 359.23
- **Chondroectodermal dysplasia** 756.55
- **Chondrolysis** 733.99
- **Chondroma** (M9220/0) - *see also* Neoplasm cartilage, benign
  - juxtacortical (M9221/0) - *see* Neoplasm, bone, benign
  - periosteal (M9221/0) - *see* Neoplasm, bone, benign
- **Chondromalacia** 733.92
  - epiglottis (congenital) 748.3
  - generalized 733.92
  - knee 717.7
  - larynx (congenital) 748.3
  - localized, except patella 733.92
  - patella, patellae 717.7
  - systemic 733.92
  - tibial plateau 733.92
  - trachea (congenital) 748.3
- **Chondromatosis** (M9220/1) - *see* Neoplasm, cartilage, uncertain behavior
- **Chondromyxosarcoma** (M9220/3) - *see* Neoplasm, cartilage, malignant
- **Chondro-osteodysplasia** (Morquio-Brailsford type) 277.5
- **Chondro-osteodystrophy** 277.5
- **Chondro-osteoma** (M9210/0) - *see* Neoplasm, bone, benign
- **Chondropathia tuberosa** 733.6
- **Chondrosarcoma** (M9220/3) - *see also* Neoplasm, cartilage, malignant
  - juxtacortical (M9221/3) - *see* Neoplasm, bone, malignant
  - mesenchymal (M9240/3) - *see* Neoplasm, connective tissue, malignant
- **Chordae tendineae rupture** (chronic) 429.5
- **Chordee** (nonvenereal) 607.89
  - congenital 752.63
  - gonococcal 098.2
- **Chorditis** (fibrinous) (nodosa) (tuberosa) 478.5
- **Chordoma** (M9370/3) - *see* Neoplasm, by site, malignant
- **Chorea** (gravis) (minor) (spasmodic) 333.5
  - with
    - heart involvement - *see* Chorea with rheumatic heart disease
    - rheumatic heart disease (chronic, inactive, or quiescent) (conditions classifiable to 393-398) - *see* rheumatic heart condition involved
      - active or acute (conditions classifiable to 391) 392.0
  - acute - *see* Chorea, Sydenham's
  - apoplectic (*see also* Disease, cerebrovascular, acute) 436
  - chronic 333.4
  - electric 049.8
  - gravidarum - *see* Eclampsia, pregnancy
  - habit 307.22
  - hereditary 333.4
  - Huntington's 333.4
  - posthemiplegic 344.89
  - pregnancy - *see* Eclampsia, pregnancy
  - progressive 333.4
    - chronic 333.4
    - hereditary 333.4
  - rheumatic (chronic) 392.9
    - with heart disease or involvement - *see* Chorea, with rheumatic heart disease
  - senile 333.5
  - Sydenham's 392.9
    - with heart involvement - *see* Chorea, with rheumatic heart disease
    - nonrheumatic 333.5
  - variabilis 307.23
- **Choreoathetosis** (paroxysmal) 333.5
- **Chorioadenoma** (destruens) (M9100/1) 236.1
- **Chorioamnionitis** 658.4 [5th]
  - affecting fetus or newborn 762.7
- **Chorioangioma** (M9120/0) 219.8
- **Choriocarcinoma** (M9100/3)
  - combined with
    - embryonal carcinoma (M9101/3) - *see* Neoplasm, by site, malignant
    - teratoma (M9101/3) - *see* Neoplasm, by site, malignant
  - specified site - *see* Neoplasm, by site, malignant
  - unspecified site
    - female 181
    - male 186.9
- **Chorioencephalitis, lymphocytic** (acute) (serous) 049.0
- **Chorioepithelioma** (M9100/3) - *see* Choriocarcinoma
- **Choriomeningitis** (acute) (benign) (lymphocytic) (serous) 049.0
- **Chorionepithelioma** (M9100/3) - *see* Choriocarcinoma
- **Chorionitis** (*see also* Scleroderma) 710.1
- **Chorioretinitis** 363.20
  - disseminated 363.10
    - generalized 363.13
    - in
      - neurosyphilis 094.83
      - secondary syphilis 091.51
    - peripheral 363.12
    - posterior pole 363.11
    - tuberculous (*see also* Tuberculosis) 017.3 [5th] *[363.13]*
  - due to
    - histoplasmosis (*see also* Histoplasmosis) 115.92
    - toxoplasmosis (acquired) 130.2
      - congenital (active) 771.2
  - focal 363.00
    - juxtapapillary 363.01
    - peripheral 363.04
    - posterior pole NEC 363.03
  - juxtapapillaris, juxtapapillary 363.01
  - progressive myopia (degeneration) 360.21
  - syphilitic (secondary) 091.51
    - congenital (early) 090.0 *[363.13]*
      - late 090.5 *[363.13]*
    - late 095.8 *[363.13]*

Chorioretinitis – *continued*

  - tuberculous (*see also* Tuberculosis) 017.3 [5th] *[363.13]*
- **Choristoma** - *see* Neoplasm, by site, benign
- **Choroid** - *see* condition
- **Choroideremia, choroidermia** (initial stage) (late stage) (partial or total atrophy) 363.55
- **Choroiditis** (*see also* Chorioretinitis) 363.20
  - leprous 030.9 *[363.13]*
  - senile guttate 363.41
  - sympathetic 360.11
  - syphilitic (secondary) 091.51
    - congenital (early) 090.0 *[363.13]*
      - late 090.5 *[363.13]*
    - late 095.8 *[363.13]*
  - Tay's 363.41
  - tuberculous (*see also* Tuberculosis) 017.3 [5th] *[363.13]*
- **Choroidopathy** NEC 363.9
  - degenerative (*see also* Degeneration, choroid) 363.40
  - hereditary (*see also* Dystrophy, choroid) 363.50
  - specified type NEC 363.8
- **Choroidoretinitis** - *see* Chorioretinitis
- **Choroidosis, central serous** 362.41
- **Choroidretinopathy, serous** 362.41
- **Christian's syndrome** (chronic histiocytosis X) 277.89
- **Christian-Weber disease** (nodular nonsuppurative panniculitis) 729.30
- **Christmas disease** 286.1
- **Chromaffinoma** (M8700/0) - *see also* Neoplasm, by site, benign
  - malignant (M8700/3) - *see* Neoplasm, by site, malignant
- **Chromatopsia** 368.59
- **Chromhidrosis, chromidrosis** 705.89
- **Chromoblastomycosis** 117.2
- **Chromomycosis** 117.2
- **Chromophytosis** 111.0
- **Chromotrichomycosis** 111.8
- **Chronic** - *see* condition
- **Churg-Strauss syndrome** 446.4
- **Chyle cyst, mesentery** 457.8
- **Chylocele** (nonfilarial) 457.8
  - filarial (*see also* Infestation, filarial) 125.9
  - tunica vaginalis (nonfilarial) 608.84
    - filarial (*see also* Infestation, filarial) 125.9
- **Chylomicronemia** (fasting) (with hyperprebetalipoproteinemia) 272.3
- **Chylopericardium** (acute) 420.90
- **Chylothorax** (nonfilarial) 457.8
  - filarial (*see also* Infestation, filarial) 125.9
- **Chylous**
  - ascites 457.8
  - cyst of peritoneum 457.8
  - hydrocele 603.9
  - hydrothorax (nonfilarial) 457.8
    - filarial (*see also* Infestation, filarial) 125.9
- **Chyluria** 791.1
  - bilharziasis 120.0
  - due to
    - Brugia (malayi) 125.1
    - Wuchereria (bancrofti) 125.0
      - malayi 125.1
  - filarial (*see also* Infestation, filarial) 125.9
  - filariasis (*see also* Infestation, filarial) 125.9
  - nonfilarial 791.1
- **Cicatricial** (deformity) - *see* Cicatrix
- **Cicatrix** (adherent) (contracted) (painful) (vicious) 709.2
  - adenoid 474.8
  - alveolar process 525.8
  - anus 569.49
  - auricle 380.89
  - bile duct (*see also* Disease, biliary) 576.8
  - bladder 596.8
  - bone 733.99
  - brain 348.89 ▲

Cicatrix – *continued*

  - cervix (postoperative) (postpartal) 622.3
    - in pregnancy or childbirth 654.6 [5th]
      - causing obstructed labor 660.2 [5th]
  - chorioretinal 363.30
    - disseminated 363.35
    - macular 363.32
    - peripheral 363.34
    - posterior pole NEC 363.33
  - choroid - *see* Cicatrix, chorioretinal
  - common duct (*see also* Disease, biliary) 576.8
  - congenital 757.39
  - conjunctiva 372.64
  - cornea 371.00
    - tuberculous (*see also* Tuberculosis) 017.3 [5th] *[371.05]*
  - duodenum (bulb) 537.3
  - esophagus 530.3
  - eyelid 374.46
    - with
      - ectropion - *see* Ectropion
      - entropion - *see* Entropion
  - hypopharynx 478.29
  - knee, semilunar cartilage 717.5
  - lacrimal
    - canaliculi 375.53
    - duct
      - acquired 375.56
      - neonatal 375.55
    - punctum 375.52
    - sac 375.54
  - larynx 478.79
  - limbus (cystoid) 372.64
  - lung 518.89
  - macular 363.32
    - disseminated 363.35
    - peripheral 363.34
  - middle ear 385.89
  - mouth 528.9
  - muscle 728.89
  - nasolacrimal duct
    - acquired 375.56
    - neonatal 375.55
  - nasopharynx 478.29
  - palate (soft) 528.9
  - penis 607.89
  - prostate 602.8
  - rectum 569.49
  - retina 363.30
    - disseminated 363.35
    - macular 363.32
    - peripheral 363.34
    - posterior pole NEC 363.33
  - semilunar cartilage - *see* Derangement, meniscus
  - seminal vesicle 608.89
  - skin 709.2
    - infected 686.8
    - postinfectional 709.2
    - tuberculous (*see also* Tuberculosis) 017.0 [5th]
  - specified site NEC 709.2
  - throat 478.29
  - tongue 529.8
  - tonsil (and adenoid) 474.8
  - trachea 478.9
  - tuberculous NEC (*see also* Tuberculosis) 011.9 [5th]
  - ureter 593.89
  - urethra 599.84
  - uterus 621.8
  - vagina 623.4
    - in pregnancy or childbirth 654.7 [5th]
      - causing obstructed labor 660.2 [5th]
  - vocal cord 478.5
  - wrist, constricting (annular) 709.2
- **CIDP** (chronic inflammatory demyelinating polyneuropathy) 357.81
- **CIN I** [cervical intraepithelial neoplasia I] 622.11
- **CIN II** [cervical intraepithelial neoplasia II] 622.12

Chondroblastoma – CIN II

- **CIN III** [cervical intraepithelial neoplasia III] 233.1
- **Cinchonism**
  - correct substance properly administered 386.9
  - overdose or wrong substance given or taken 961.4
- **Circine herpes** 110.5
- **Circle of Willis** - *see* condition
- **Circular** - *see also* condition
  - hymen 752.49
- **Circulating, intrinsic anticoagulants causing hemorrhagic disorder** 286.5 ▲
  - following childbirth 666.3 5th
  - postpartum 666.3 5th
- **Circulation**
  - collateral (venous), any site 459.89
  - defective 459.9
    - congenital 747.9
    - lower extremity 459.89
  - embryonic 747.9
  - failure 799.89
    - fetus or newborn 779.89
    - peripheral 785.59
  - fetal, persistent 747.83
  - heart, incomplete 747.9
- **Circulatory system** - *see* condition
- **Circulus senilis** 371.41
- **Circumcision**
  - in absence of medical indication V50.2
  - ritual V50.2
  - routine V50.2
- **Circumscribed** - *see* condition
- **Circumvallata placenta** - *see* Placenta, abnormal
- **Cirrhosis, cirrhotic** 571.5
  - with alcoholism 571.2
  - alcoholic (liver) 571.2
  - atrophic (of liver) - *see* Cirrhosis, portal
  - Baumgarten-Cruveilhier 571.5
  - biliary (cholangiolitic) (cholangitic) (cholestatic) (extrahepatic) (hypertrophic) (intrahepatic) (nonobstructive) (obstructive) (pericholangiolitic) (posthepatic) (primary) (secondary) (xanthomatous) 571.6
    - due to
      - clonorchiasis 121.1
      - flukes 121.3
  - brain 331.9
  - capsular - *see* Cirrhosis, portal
  - cardiac 571.5
    - alcoholic 571.2
  - central (liver) - *see* Cirrhosis, liver
  - Charcôt's 571.6
  - cholangiolitic - *see* Cirrhosis, biliary
  - cholangitic - *see* Cirrhosis, biliary
  - cholestatic - *see* Cirrhosis, biliary
  - clitoris (hypertrophic) 624.2
  - coarsely nodular 571.5
  - congestive (liver) - *see* Cirrhosis, cardiac
  - Cruveilhier-Baumgarten 571.5
  - cryptogenic (of liver) 571.5
    - alcoholic 571.2
  - dietary (*see also* Cirrhosis, portal) 571.5
  - due to
    - bronzed diabetes 275.0
    - congestive hepatomegaly - *see* Cirrhosis, cardiac
    - cystic fibrosis 277.00
    - hemochromatosis 275.0
    - hepatolenticular degeneration 275.1
    - passive congestion (chronic) - *see* Cirrhosis, cardiac
    - Wilson's disease 275.1
    - xanthomatosis 272.2
  - extrahepatic (obstructive) - *see* Cirrhosis, biliary
  - fatty 571.8
    - alcoholic 571.0
  - florid 571.2
  - Glisson's - *see* Cirrhosis, portal

Cirrhosis, cirrhotic – *continued*

  - Hanot's (hypertrophic) - *see* Cirrhosis, biliary
  - hepatic - *see* Cirrhosis, liver
  - hepatolienal - *see* Cirrhosis, liver
  - hobnail - *see* Cirrhosis, portal
  - hypertrophic - *see also* Cirrhosis, liver
    - biliary - *see* Cirrhosis, biliary
    - Hanot's - *see* Cirrhosis, biliary
  - infectious NEC - *see* Cirrhosis, portal
  - insular - *see* Cirrhosis, portal
  - intrahepatic (obstructive) (primary) (secondary) - *see* Cirrhosis, biliary
  - juvenile (*see also* Cirrhosis, portal) 571.5
  - kidney (*see also* Sclerosis, renal) 587
  - Laennec's (of liver) 571.2
    - nonalcoholic 571.5
  - liver (chronic) (hepatolienal) (hypertrophic) (nodular) (splenomegalic) (unilobar) 571.5
    - with alcoholism 571.2
    - alcoholic 571.2
    - congenital (due to failure of obliteration of umbilical vein) 777.8
    - cryptogenic 571.5
      - alcoholic 571.2
    - fatty 571.8
      - alcoholic 571.0
    - macronodular 571.5
      - alcoholic 571.2
    - micronodular 571.5
      - alcoholic 571.2
    - nodular, diffuse 571.5
      - alcoholic 571.2
    - pigmentary 275.0
    - portal 571.5
      - alcoholic 571.2
    - postnecrotic 571.5
      - alcoholic 571.2
    - syphilitic 095.3
  - lung (chronic) (*see also* Fibrosis, lung) 515
  - macronodular (of liver) 571.5
    - alcoholic 571.2
  - malarial 084.9
  - metabolic NEC 571.5
  - micronodular (of liver) 571.5
    - alcoholic 571.2
  - monolobular - *see* Cirrhosis, portal
  - multilobular - *see* Cirrhosis, portal
  - nephritis (*see also* Sclerosis, renal) 587
  - nodular - *see* Cirrhosis, liver
  - nutritional (fatty) 571.5
  - obstructive (biliary) (extrahepatic) (intrahepatic) - *see* Cirrhosis, biliary
  - ovarian 620.8
  - paludal 084.9
  - pancreas (duct) 577.8
  - pericholangiolitic - *see* Cirrhosis, biliary
  - periportal - *see* Cirrhosis, portal
  - pigment, pigmentary (of liver) 275.0
  - portal (of liver) 571.5
    - alcoholic 571.2
  - posthepatitic (*see also* Cirrhosis, postnecrotic) 571.5
  - postnecrotic (of liver) 571.5
    - alcoholic 571.2
  - primary (intrahepatic) - *see* Cirrhosis, biliary
  - pulmonary (*see also* Fibrosis, lung) 515
  - renal (*see also* Sclerosis, renal) 587
  - septal (*see also* Cirrhosis, postnecrotic) 571.5
  - spleen 289.51
  - splenomegalic (of liver) - *see* Cirrhosis, liver
  - stasis (liver) - *see* Cirrhosis, liver
  - stomach 535.4 5th
  - Todd's (*see also* Cirrhosis, biliary) 571.6
  - toxic (nodular) - *see* Cirrhosis, postnecrotic
  - trabecular - *see* Cirrhosis, postnecrotic
  - unilobar - *see* Cirrhosis, liver
  - vascular (of liver) - *see* Cirrhosis, liver

Cirrhosis, cirrhotic – *continued*

  - xanthomatous (biliary) (*see also* Cirrhosis, biliary) 571.6
    - due to xanthomatosis (familial) (metabolic) (primary) 272.2
- **Cistern, subarachnoid** 793.0
- **Citrullinemia** 270.6
- **Citrullinuria** 270.6
- **Ciuffini-Pancoast tumor** (M8010/3) (carcinoma, pulmonary apex) 162.3
- **Civatte's disease or poikiloderma** 709.09
- **CJD** (Creutzfeldt-Jakob disease) 046.19
  - variant (vCJD) 046.11
- **Clam diggers' itch** 120.3
- **Clap** - *see* Gonorrhea
- **Clark's paralysis** 343.9
- **Clarke-Hadfield syndrome** (pancreatic infantilism) 577.8
- **Clastothrix** 704.2
- **Claude's syndrome** 352.6
- **Claude Bernard-Horner syndrome** (*see also* Neuropathy, peripheral, autonomic) 337.9
- **Claudication, intermittent** 443.9
  - cerebral (artery) (*see also* Ischemia, cerebral, transient) 435.9
  - due to atherosclerosis 440.21
  - spinal cord (arteriosclerotic) 435.1
    - syphilitic 094.89
  - spinalis 435.1
  - venous (axillary) 453.89 ▲
- **Claudicatio venosa intermittens** 453.89 ▲
- **Claustrophobia** 300.29
- **Clavus** (infected) 700
- **Clawfoot** (congenital) 754.71
  - acquired 736.74
- **Clawhand** (acquired) 736.06
  - congenital 755.59
- **Clawtoe** (congenital) 754.71
  - acquired 735.5
- **Clay eating** 307.52
- **Clay shovelers' fracture** - *see* Fracture, vertebra, cervical
- **Cleansing of artificial opening** (*see also* Attention to artificial opening) V55.9
- **Cleft** (congenital) - *see also* Imperfect, closure
  - alveolar process 525.8
  - branchial (persistent) 744.41
    - cyst 744.42
  - clitoris 752.49
  - cricoid cartilage, posterior 748.3
  - facial (*see also* Cleft, lip) 749.10
  - lip 749.10
    - with cleft palate 749.20
      - bilateral (lip and palate) 749.24
        - with unilateral lip or palate 749.25
        - complete 749.23
        - incomplete 749.24
      - unilateral (lip and palate) 749.22
        - with bilateral lip or palate 749.25
        - complete 749.21
        - incomplete 749.22
    - bilateral 749.14
      - with cleft palate, unilateral 749.25
      - complete 749.13
      - incomplete 749.14
    - unilateral 749.12
      - with cleft palate, bilateral 749.25
      - complete 749.11
      - incomplete 749.12
  - nose 748.1
  - palate 749.00
    - with cleft lip 749.20
      - bilateral (lip and palate) 749.24
        - with unilateral lip or palate 749.25
        - complete 749.23
        - incomplete 749.24
      - unilateral (lip and palate) 749.22
        - with bilateral lip or palate 749.25
        - complete 749.21
        - incomplete 749.22

Cleft – *continued*

  - palate – *continued*
    - bilateral 749.04
      - with cleft lip, unilateral 749.25
      - complete 749.03
      - incomplete 749.04
    - unilateral 749.02
      - with cleft lip, bilateral 749.25
      - complete 749.01
      - incomplete 749.02
  - penis 752.69
  - posterior, cricoid cartilage 748.3
  - scrotum 752.89
  - sternum (congenital) 756.3
  - thyroid cartilage (congenital) 748.3
  - tongue 750.13
  - uvula 749.02
    - with cleft lip (*see also* Cleft, lip, with cleft palate) 749.20
  - water 366.12
- **Cleft hand** (congenital) 755.58
- **Cleidocranial dysostosis** 755.59
- **Cleidotomy, fetal** 763.89
- **Cleptomania** 312.32
- **Clérambault's syndrome** 297.8
  - erotomania 302.89
- **Clergyman's sore throat** 784.49
- **Click, clicking**
  - systolic syndrome 785.2
- **Clifford's syndrome** (postmaturity) 766.22
- **Climacteric** (*see also* Menopause) 627.2
  - arthritis NEC (*see also* Arthritis, climacteric) 716.3 5th
  - depression (*see also* Psychosis, affective) 296.2 5th
  - disease 627.2
    - recurrent episode 296.3 5th
    - single episode 296.2 5th
  - female (symptoms) 627.2
  - male (symptoms) (syndrome) 608.89
  - melancholia (*see also* Psychosis, affective) 296.2 5th
    - recurrent episode 296.3 5th
    - single episode 296.2 5th
  - paranoid state 297.2
  - paraphrenia 297.2
  - polyarthritis NEC 716.39
    - male 608.89
  - symptoms (female) 627.2
- **Clinical research investigation** (control) (participant) V70.7
- **Clinodactyly** 755.59
- **Clitoris** - *see* condition
- **Cloaca, persistent** 751.5
- **Clonorchiasis** 121.1
- **Clonorchiosis** 121.1
- **Clonorchis infection, liver** 121.1
- **Clonus** 781.0
- **Closed bite** 524.20
- **Closed surgical procedure converted to open procedure**
  - arthroscopic V64.43
  - laparoscopic V64.41
  - thoracoscopic V64.42
- **Closure**
  - artificial opening (*see also* Attention to artificial opening) V55.9
  - congenital, nose 748.0
  - cranial sutures, premature 756.0
  - defective or imperfect NEC - *see* Imperfect, closure
  - fistula, delayed - *see* Fistula
  - fontanelle, delayed 756.0
  - foramen ovale, imperfect 745.5
  - hymen 623.3
  - interauricular septum, defective 745.5
  - interventricular septum, defective 745.4
  - lacrimal duct 375.56
    - congenital 743.65
    - neonatal 375.55
  - nose (congenital) 748.0
    - acquired 738.0
  - vagina 623.2
  - valve - *see* Endocarditis

- **Closure** – *continued*
  - vulva 624.8
- **Clot** (blood)
  - artery (obstruction) (occlusion) (*see also* Embolism) 444.9
  - atrial appendage 429.89
  - bladder 596.7
  - brain (extradural or intradural) (*see also* Thrombosis, brain) 434.0 [5th]
    - late effect - *see* Late effect(s) (of) cerebrovascular disease
  - circulation 444.9
  - heart (*see also* Infarct, myocardium) 410.9 [5th]
    - without myocardial infarction 429.89
  - vein (*see also* Thrombosis) 453.9
- **Clotting defect** NEC (*see also* Defect, coagulation) 286.9
- **Clouded state** 780.09
  - epileptic (*see also* Epilepsy) 345.9 [5th]
  - paroxysmal (idiopathic) (*see also* Epilepsy) 345.9 [5th]
- **Clouding**
  - corneal graft 996.51
- **Cloudy**
  - antrum, antra 473.0
  - dialysis effluent 792.5
- **Clouston's** (hidrotic) **ectodermal dysplasia** 757.31
- **Clubbing of fingers** 781.5
- **Clubfinger** 736.29
  - acquired 736.29
  - congenital 754.89
- **Clubfoot** (congenital) 754.70
  - acquired 736.71
  - equinovarus 754.51
  - paralytic 736.71
- **Club hand** (congenital) 754.89
  - acquired 736.07
- **Clubnail** (acquired) 703.8
  - congenital 757.5
- **Clump kidney** 753.3
- **Clumsiness** 781.3
  - syndrome 315.4
- **Cluttering** 307.0
- **Clutton's joints** 090.5
- **Coagulation, intravascular** (diffuse) (disseminated) (*see also* Fibrinolysis) 286.6
  - newborn 776.2
- **Coagulopathy** (*see also* Defect, coagulation) 286.9
  - consumption 286.6
  - intravascular (disseminated) NEC 286.6
    - newborn 776.2
- **Coalition**
  - calcaneoscaphoid 755.67
  - calcaneus 755.67
  - tarsal 755.67
- **Coal miners'**
  - elbow 727.2
  - lung 500
- **Coal workers' lung or pneumoconiosis** 500
- **Coarctation**
  - aorta (postductal) (preductal) 747.10
  - pulmonary artery 747.3
- **Coated tongue** 529.3
- **Coats' disease** 362.12
- **Cocainism** (*see also* Dependence) 304.2 [5th]
- **Coccidioidal granuloma** 114.3
- **Coccidioidomycosis** 114.9
  - with pneumonia 114.0
  - cutaneous (primary) 114.1
  - disseminated 114.3
  - extrapulmonary (primary) 114.1
  - lung 114.5
    - acute 114.0
    - chronic 114.4
    - primary 114.0
  - meninges 114.2
  - primary (pulmonary) 114.0
    - acute 114.0
  - prostate 114.3
- **Coccidioidomycosis** – *continued*
  - pulmonary 114.5
    - acute 114.0
    - chronic 114.4
    - primary 114.0
  - specified site NEC 114.3
- **Coccidioidosis** 114.9
  - lung 114.5
    - acute 114.0
    - chronic 114.4
    - primary 114.0
  - meninges 114.2
- **Coccidiosis** (colitis) (diarrhea) (dysentery) 007.2
- **Cocciuria** 791.9
- **Coccus in urine** 791.9
- **Coccydynia** 724.79
- **Coccygodynia** 724.79
- **Coccyx** - *see* condition
- **Cochin-China**
  - diarrhea 579.1
    - anguilluliasis 127.2
  - ulcer 085.1
- **Cock's peculiar tumor** 706.2
- **Cockayne's disease or syndrome** (microcephaly and dwarfism) 759.89
- **Cockayne-Weber syndrome** (epidermolysis bullosa) 757.39
- **Cocked-up toe** 735.2
- **Codman's tumor** (benign chondroblastoma) (M9230/0) - *see* Neoplasm, bone, benign
- **Coenurosis** 123.8
- **Coffee workers' lung** 495.8
- **Cogan's syndrome** 370.52
  - congenital oculomotor apraxia 379.51
  - nonsyphilitic interstitial keratitis 370.52
- **Coiling, umbilical cord** - *see* Complications, umbilical cord
- **Coitus, painful** (female) 625.0
  - male 608.89
  - psychogenic 302.76
- **Cold** 460
  - with influenza, flu, or grippe 487.1
  - abscess - *see also* Tuberculosis, abscess
    - articular - *see* Tuberculosis, joint
  - agglutinin
    - disease (chronic) or syndrome 283.0
    - hemoglobinuria 283.0
      - paroxysmal (cold) (nocturnal) 283.2
  - allergic (*see also* Fever, hay) 477.9
  - bronchus or chest - *see* Bronchitis
    - with grippe or influenza 487.1
  - common (head) 460
    - vaccination, prophylactic (against) V04.7
  - deep 464.10
  - effects of 991.9
    - specified effect NEC 991.8
  - excessive 991.9
    - specified effect NEC 991.8
  - exhaustion from 991.8
  - exposure to 991.9
    - specified effect NEC 991.8
  - grippy 487.1
  - head 460
  - injury syndrome (newborn) 778.2
  - intolerance 780.99
  - on lung - *see* Bronchitis
  - rose 477.0
  - sensitivity, autoimmune 283.0
  - virus 460
- **Coldsore** (*see also* Herpes, simplex) 054.9
- **Colibacillosis** 041.4
  - generalized 038.42
- **Colibacilluria** 791.9
- **Colic** (recurrent) 789.7 ▲
  - abdomen 789.7 ▲
    - psychogenic 307.89
  - appendicular 543.9
  - appendix 543.9
  - bile duct - *see* Choledocholithiasis
  - biliary - *see* Cholelithiasis
- **Colic** – *continued*
  - bilious - *see* Cholelithiasis
  - common duct - *see* Choledocholithiasis
  - Devonshire NEC 984.9
    - specified type of lead - *see* Table of Drugs and Chemicals
  - flatulent 787.3
  - gallbladder or gallstone - *see* Cholelithiasis
  - gastric 536.8
  - hepatic (duct) - *see* Choledocholithiasis
  - hysterical 300.11
  - in ●
    - adult 789.0 [5th] ●
    - child over 12 months old 789.0 [5th] ●
    - infant 789.7 ●
  - infantile 789.7 ▲
  - intestinal 789.7 ▲
  - kidney 788.0
  - lead NEC 984.9
    - specified type of lead - *see* Table of Drugs and Chemicals
  - liver (duct) - *see* Choledocholithiasis
  - mucous 564.9
    - psychogenic 316 *[564.9]*
  - nephritic 788.0
  - Painter's NEC 984.9
  - pancreas 577.8
  - psychogenic 306.4
  - renal 788.0
  - saturnine NEC 984.9
    - specified type of lead - *see* Table of Drugs and Chemicals
  - spasmodic 789.7 ▲
  - ureter 788.0
  - urethral 599.84
    - due to calculus 594.2
  - uterus 625.8
    - menstrual 625.3
  - vermicular 543.9
  - virus 460
  - worm NEC 128.9
- **Colicystitis** (*see also* Cystitis) 595.9
- **Colitis** (acute) (catarrhal) (croupous) (cystica superficialis) (exudative) (hemorrhagic) (noninfectious) (phlegmonous) (presumed noninfectious) 558.9
  - adaptive 564.9
  - allergic 558.3
  - amebic (*see also* Amebiasis) 006.9
    - nondysenteric 006.2
  - anthrax 022.2
  - bacillary (*see also* Infection, Shigella) 004.9
  - balantidial 007.0
  - chronic 558.9
    - ulcerative (*see also* Colitis, ulcerative) 556.9
  - coccidial 007.2
  - dietetic 558.9
  - due to radiation 558.1
  - eosinophilic 558.42 ▲
  - functional 558.9
  - gangrenous 009.0
  - giardial 007.1
  - granulomatous 555.1
  - gravis (*see also* Colitis, ulcerative) 556.9
  - infectious (*see also* Enteritis, due to, specific organism) 009.0
    - presumed 009.1
  - ischemic 557.9
    - acute 557.0
    - chronic 557.1
    - due to mesenteric artery insufficiency 557.1
  - membranous 564.9
    - psychogenic 316 *[564.9]*
  - mucous 564.9
    - psychogenic 316 *[564.9]*
  - necrotic 009.0
  - polyposa (*see also* Colitis, ulcerative) 556.9
  - protozoal NEC 007.9
  - pseudomembranous 008.45
  - pseudomucinous 564.9
- **Colitis** – *continued*
  - regional 555.1
  - segmental 555.1
  - septic (*see also* Enteritis, due to, specific organism) 009.0
  - spastic 564.9
    - psychogenic 316 *[564.9]*
  - Staphylococcus 008.41
    - food 005.0
  - thromboulcerative 557.0
  - toxic 558.2
  - transmural 555.1
  - trichomonal 007.3
  - tuberculous (ulcerative) 014.8 [5th]
  - ulcerative (chronic) (idiopathic) (nonspecific) 556.9
    - entero- 556.0
    - fulminant 557.0
    - ileo- 556.1
    - left-sided 556.5
    - procto- 556.2
    - proctosigmoid 556.3
    - psychogenic 316 *[556]* [4th]
    - specified NEC 556.8
    - universal 556.6
- **Collagen disease** NEC 710.9
  - nonvascular 710.9
  - vascular (allergic) (*see also* Angiitis, hypersensitivity) 446.20
- **Collagenosis** (*see also* Collagen disease) 710.9
  - cardiovascular 425.4
  - mediastinal 519.3
- **Collapse** 780.2
  - adrenal 255.8
  - cardiorenal (*see also* Hypertension, cardiorenal) 404.90
  - cardiorespiratory 785.51
    - fetus or newborn 779.85
  - cardiovascular (*see also* Disease, heart) 785.51
    - fetus or newborn 779.85
  - circulatory (peripheral) 785.59
    - with
      - abortion - *see* Abortion, by type, with shock
      - ectopic pregnancy (*see also* categories 633.0-633.9) 639.5
      - molar pregnancy (*see also* categories 630-632) 639.5
    - during or after labor and delivery 669.1 [5th]
    - fetus or newborn 779.85
    - following
      - abortion 639.5
      - ectopic or molar pregnancy 639.5
  - during or after labor and delivery 669.1 [5th]
    - fetus or newborn 779.89
  - external ear canal 380.50
    - secondary to
      - inflammation 380.53
      - surgery 380.52
      - trauma 380.51
  - general 780.2
  - heart - *see* Disease, heart
  - heat 992.1
  - hysterical 300.11
  - labyrinth, membranous (congenital) 744.05
  - lung (massive) (*see also* Atelectasis) 518.0
    - pressure, during labor 668.0 [5th]
  - myocardial - *see* Disease, heart
  - nervous (*see also* Disorder, mental, nonpsychotic) 300.9
  - neurocirculatory 306.2
  - nose 738.0
  - postoperative (cardiovascular) 998.0
  - pulmonary (*see also* Atelectasis) 518.0
    - fetus or newborn 770.5
      - partial 770.5
      - primary 770.4
  - thorax 512.8
    - iatrogenic 512.1
    - postoperative 512.1

Closure – Collapse

- **Collapse** – *continued*
  - trachea 519.19
  - valvular - *see* Endocarditis
  - vascular (peripheral) 785.59
    - with
      - abortion - *see* Abortion, by type, with shock
      - ectopic pregnancy (*see also* categories 633.0-633.9) 639.5
      - molar pregnancy (*see also* categories 630-632) 639.5
    - cerebral (*see also* Disease, cerebrovascular, acute) 436
    - during or after labor and delivery 669.1 [5th]
    - fetus or newborn 779.89
    - following
      - abortion 639.5
      - ectopic or molar pregnancy 639.5
  - vasomotor 785.59
  - vertebra 733.13
- **Collateral** - *see also* condition
  - circulation (venous) 459.89
  - dilation, veins 459.89
- **Colles' fracture** (closed) (reversed) (separation) 813.41
  - open 813.51
- **Collet's syndrome** 352.6
- **Collet-Sicard syndrome** 352.6
- **Colliculitis urethralis** (*see also* Urethritis) 597.89
- **Colliers'**
  - asthma 500
  - lung 500
  - phthisis (*see also* Tuberculosis) 011.4 [5th]
- **Collodion baby** (ichthyosis congenita) 757.1
- **Colloid milium** 709.3
- **Coloboma** NEC 743.49
  - choroid 743.59
  - fundus 743.52
  - iris 743.46
  - lens 743.36
  - lids 743.62
  - optic disc (congenital) 743.57
    - acquired 377.23
  - retina 743.56
  - sclera 743.47
- **Coloenteritis** - *see* Enteritis
- **Colon** - *see* condition
- **Colonization**
  - MRSA (methicillin resistant Staphylococcus aureus) V02.54
  - MSSA (methicillin susceptible Staphylococcus aureus) V02.53
- **Coloptosis** 569.89
- **Color**
  - amblyopia NEC 368.59
    - acquired 368.55
  - blindness NEC (congenital) 368.59
    - acquired 368.55
- **Colostomy**
  - attention to V55.3
  - fitting or adjustment V55.3
  - malfunctioning 569.62
  - status V44.3
- **Colpitis** (*see also* Vaginitis) 616.10
- **Colpocele** 618.6
- **Colpocystitis** (*see also* Vaginitis) 616.10
- **Colporrhexis** 665.4 [5th]
- **Colpospasm** 625.1
- **Column, spinal, vertebral** - *see* condition
- **Coma** 780.01
  - apoplectic (*see also* Disease, cerebrovascular, acute) 436
  - diabetic (with ketoacidosis) 250.3 [5th]
    - due to secondary diabetes 249.3 [5th]
    - hyperosmolar 250.2 [5th]
      - due to secondary diabetes 249.2 [5th]
  - eclamptic (*see also* Eclampsia) 780.39
  - epileptic 345.3
  - hepatic 572.2
  - hyperglycemic 250.2
    - due to secondary diabetes 249.2 [5th]
- **Coma** – *continued*
  - hyperosmolar (diabetic) (nonketotic) 250.2 [5th]
    - due to secondary diabetes 249.2 [5th]
  - hypoglycemic 251.0
    - diabetic 250.3 [5th]
      - due to secondary diabetes 249.3 [5th]
  - insulin 250.3 [5th]
    - due to secondary diabetes 249.3 [5th]
    - hyperosmolar 250.2 [5th]
      - due to secondary diabetes 249.2 [5th]
    - nondiabetic 251.0
    - organic hyperinsulinism 251.0
  - Kussmaul's (diabetic) 250.3 [5th]
    - due to secondary diabetes 249.3 [5th]
  - liver 572.2
  - newborn 779.2
  - prediabetic 250.2 [5th]
    - due to secondary diabetes 249.2 [5th]
  - uremic - *see* Uremia
- **Combat fatigue** (*see also* Reaction, stress, acute) 308.9
- **Combined** - *see* condition
- **Comedo** 706.1
- **Comedocarcinoma** (M8501/3) - *see also* Neoplasm, breast, malignant
  - noninfiltrating (M8501/2)
    - specified site - *see* Neoplasm, by site, in situ
    - unspecified site 233.0
- **Comedomastitis** 610.4
- **Comedones** 706.1
  - lanugo 757.4
- **Comma bacillus, carrier** (suspected) **of** V02.3
- **Comminuted fracture** - *see* Fracture, by site
- **Common**
  - aortopulmonary trunk 745.0
  - atrioventricular canal (defect) 745.69
  - atrium 745.69
  - cold (head) 460
    - vaccination, prophylactic (against) V04.7
  - truncus (arteriosus) 745.0
  - ventricle 745.3
- **Commotio** (current)
  - cerebri (*see also* Concussion, brain) 850.9
    - with skull fracture - *see* Fracture, skull, by site
  - retinae 921.3
  - spinalis - *see* Injury, spinal, by site
- **Commotion** (current)
  - brain (without skull fracture) (*see also* Concussion, brain) 850.9
    - with skull fracture - *see* Fracture, skull, by site
  - spinal cord - *see* Injury, spinal, by site
- **Communication**
  - abnormal - *see also* Fistula
    - between
      - base of aorta and pulmonary artery 745.0
      - left ventricle and right atrium 745.4
      - pericardial sac and pleural sac 748.8
      - pulmonary artery and pulmonary vein 747.3
    - congenital, between uterus and anterior abdominal wall 752.3
      - bladder 752.3
      - intestine 752.3
      - rectum 752.3
  - left ventricular-right atrial 745.4
  - pulmonary artery-pulmonary vein 747.3
- **Compartment syndrome** - *see* Syndrome, compartment
- **Compensation**
  - broken - *see* Failure, heart
  - failure - *see* Failure, heart
  - neurosis, psychoneurosis 300.11
- **Complaint** - *see also* Disease
  - bowel, functional 564.9
    - psychogenic 306.4
  - intestine, functional 564.9
    - psychogenic 306.4
- **Complaint** – *continued*
  - kidney (*see also* Disease, renal) 593.9
  - liver 573.9
  - miners' 500
- **Complete** - *see* condition
- **Complex**
  - cardiorenal (*see also* Hypertension, cardiorenal) 404.90
  - castration 300.9
  - Costen's 524.60
  - ego-dystonic homosexuality 302.0
  - Eisenmenger's (ventricular septal defect) 745.4
  - homosexual, ego-dystonic 302.0
  - hypersexual 302.89
  - inferiority 301.9
  - jumped process
    - spine - *see* Dislocation, vertebra
  - primary, tuberculosis (*see also* Tuberculosis) 010.0 [5th]
  - regional pain syndrome 355.9
    - type I 337.20
      - lower limb 337.22
      - specified site NEC 337.29
      - upper limb 337.21
    - type II
      - lower limb 355.71
      - upper limb 354.4
  - Taussig-Bing (transposition, aorta and overriding pulmonary artery) 745.11
- **Complications**
  - abortion NEC - *see* categories 634-639
  - accidental puncture or laceration during a procedure 998.2
  - amniocentesis, fetal 679.1 [5th]
  - amputation stump (late) (surgical) 997.60
    - traumatic - *see* Amputation, traumatic
  - anastomosis (and bypass) - *see also* Complications, due to (presence of) any device, implant, or graft classified to 996.0-996.5 NEC
    - hemorrhage NEC 998.11
    - intestinal (internal) NEC 997.4
      - involving urinary tract 997.5
    - mechanical - *see* Complications, mechanical, graft
    - urinary tract (involving intestinal tract) 997.5
  - anesthesia, anesthetic NEC (*see also* Anesthesia, complication) 995.22
    - in labor and delivery 668.9 [5th]
      - affecting fetus or newborn 763.5
      - cardiac 668.1 [5th]
      - central nervous system 668.2 [5th]
      - pulmonary 668.0 [5th]
      - specified type NEC 668.8 [5th]
  - aortocoronary (bypass) graft 996.03
    - atherosclerosis - *see* Arteriosclerosis, coronary
      - embolism 996.72
      - occlusion NEC 996.72
      - thrombus 996.72
  - arthroplasty (*see also* Complications, prosthetic joint) 996.49
  - artificial opening
    - cecostomy 569.60
    - colostomy 569.60
    - cystostomy 997.5
    - enterostomy 569.60
    - esophagostomy 530.87
      - infection 530.86
      - mechanical 530.87
    - gastrostomy 536.40
    - ileostomy 569.60
    - jejunostomy 569.60
    - nephrostomy 997.5
    - tracheostomy 519.00
    - ureterostomy 997.5
    - urethrostomy 997.5
  - bariatric surgery 997.4
  - bile duct implant (prosthetic) NEC 996.79
    - infection or inflammation 996.69
    - mechanical 996.59
- **Complications** – *continued*
  - bleeding (intraoperative) (postoperative) 998.11
  - blood vessel graft 996.1
    - aortocoronary 996.03
      - atherosclerosis - *see* Arteriosclerosis, coronary
      - embolism 996.72
      - occlusion NEC 996.72
      - thrombus 996.72
    - atherosclerosis - *see* Arteriosclerosis, extremities
    - embolism 996.74
    - occlusion NEC 996.74
    - thrombus 996.74
  - bone growth stimulator NEC 996.78
    - infection or inflammation 996.67
  - bone marrow transplant 996.85
  - breast implant (prosthetic) NEC 996.79
    - infection or inflammation 996.69
    - mechanical 996.54
  - bypass - *see also* Complications, anastomosis
    - aortocoronary 996.03
      - atherosclerosis - *see* Arteriosclerosis, coronary
      - embolism 996.72
      - occlusion NEC 996.72
      - thrombus 996.72
    - carotid artery 996.1
      - atherosclerosis - *see* Arteriosclerosis, coronary
      - embolism 996.74
      - occlusion NEC 996.74
      - thrombus 996.74
  - cardiac (*see also* Disease, heart) 429.9
    - device, implant, or graft NEC 996.72
      - infection or inflammation 996.61
      - long-term effect 429.4
      - mechanical (*see also* Complications, mechanical, by type) 996.00
      - valve prosthesis 996.71
        - infection or inflammation 996.61
    - postoperative NEC 997.1
      - long-term effect 429.4
  - cardiorenal (*see also* Hypertension, cardiorenal) 404.90
  - carotid artery bypass graft 996.1
    - atherosclerosis - *see* Arteriosclerosis, coronary
    - embolism 996.74
    - occlusion NEC 996.74
    - thrombus 996.74
  - cataract fragments in eye 998.82
  - catheter device NEC - *see also* Complications, due to (presence of) any device, implant, or graft classified to 996.0-996.5 NEC
    - mechanical - *see* Complications, mechanical, catheter
  - cecostomy 569.60
  - cesarean section wound 674.3 [5th]
  - chemotherapy (antineoplastic) 995.29
  - chin implant (prosthetic) NEC 996.79
    - infection or inflammation 996.69
    - mechanical 996.59
  - colostomy (enterostomy) 569.60
    - specified type NEC 569.69
  - contraceptive device, intrauterine NEC 996.76
    - infection 996.65
    - inflammation 996.65
    - mechanical 996.32
  - cord (umbilical) - *see* Complications, umbilical cord
  - cornea
    - due to
      - contact lens 371.82
  - coronary (artery) bypass (graft) NEC 996.03
    - atherosclerosis - *see* Arteriosclerosis, coronary
    - embolism 996.72

Complications – *continued*
- coronary (artery) bypass (graft) – *continued*
  - infection or inflammation 996.61
  - mechanical 996.03
  - occlusion NEC 996.72
  - specified type NEC 996.72
  - thrombus 996.72
- cystostomy 997.5
- delivery 669.9 [5th]
  - procedure (instrumental) (manual) (surgical) 669.4 [5th]
  - specified type NEC 669.8 [5th]
- dialysis (hemodialysis) (peritoneal) (renal) NEC 999.9
  - catheter NEC - *see also* Complications, due to (presence of) any device, implant, or graft classified to 996.0-996.5 NEC
    - infection or inflammation 996.62
      - peritoneal 996.68
    - mechanical 996.1
      - peritoneal 996.56
- drug NEC 995.29
- due to (presence of) any device, implant, or graft classified to 996.0-996.5 NEC 996.70
  - with infection or inflammation - *see* Complications, infection or inflammation, due to (presence of) any device, implant, or graft classified to 996.0-996.5 NEC
  - arterial NEC 996.74
    - coronary NEC 996.03
      - atherosclerosis - *see* Arteriosclerosis, coronary
      - embolism 996.72
      - occlusion NEC 996.72
      - specified type NEC 996.72
      - thrombus 996.72
    - renal dialysis 996.73
  - arteriovenous fistula or shunt NEC 996.74
  - bone growth stimulator 996.78
  - breast NEC 996.79
  - cardiac NEC 996.72
    - defibrillator 996.72
    - pacemaker 996.72
    - valve prosthesis 996.71
  - catheter NEC 996.79
    - spinal 996.75
    - urinary, indwelling 996.76
    - vascular NEC 996.74
      - renal dialysis 996.73
    - ventricular shunt 996.75
  - coronary (artery) bypass (graft) NEC 996.03
    - atherosclerosis - *see* Arteriosclerosis, coronary
    - embolism 996.72
    - occlusion NEC 996.72
    - thrombus 996.72
  - electrodes
    - brain 996.75
    - heart 996.72
  - esophagostomy 530.87
  - gastrointestinal NEC 996.79
  - genitourinary NEC 996.76
  - heart valve prosthesis NEC 996.71
  - infusion pump 996.74
  - insulin pump 996.57
  - internal
    - joint prosthesis 996.77
    - orthopedic NEC 996.78
    - specified type NEC 996.79
  - intrauterine contraceptive device NEC 996.76
  - joint prosthesis, internal NEC 996.77
  - mechanical - *see* Complications, mechanical
  - nervous system NEC 996.75
  - ocular lens NEC 996.79
  - orbital NEC 996.79

Complications – *continued*
- due to (presence of) any device, implant, or graft classified to 996.0-996.5 NEC 996.70 – *continued*
  - orthopedic NEC 996.78
    - joint, internal 996.77
  - renal dialysis 996.73
  - specified type NEC 996.79
  - urinary catheter, indwelling 996.76
  - vascular NEC 996.74
  - ventricular shunt 996.75
- during dialysis NEC 999.9
- ectopic or molar pregnancy NEC 639.9
- electroshock therapy NEC 999.9
- enterostomy 569.60
  - specified type NEC 569.69
- esophagostomy 530.87
  - infection 530.86
  - mechanical 530.87
- external (fixation) device with internal component(s) NEC 996.78
  - infection or inflammation 996.67
  - mechanical 996.49
- extracorporeal circulation NEC 999.9
- eye implant (prosthetic) NEC 996.79
  - infection or inflammation 996.69
  - mechanical
    - ocular lens 996.53
    - orbital globe 996.59
- fetal, from amniocentesis 679.1 [5th]
- gastrointestinal, postoperative NEC (*see also* Complications, surgical procedures) 997.4
- gastrostomy 536.40
  - specified type NEC 536.49
- genitourinary device, implant or graft NEC 996.76
  - infection or inflammation 996.65
    - urinary catheter, indwelling 996.64
  - mechanical (*see also* Complications, mechanical, by type) 996.30
    - specified NEC 996.39
- graft (bypass) (patch) - *see also* Complications, due to (presence of) any device, implant, or graft classified to 996.0-996.5 NEC
  - bone marrow 996.85
  - corneal NEC 996.79
    - infection or inflammation 996.69
    - rejection or reaction 996.51
  - mechanical - *see* Complications, mechanical, graft
  - organ (immune or nonimmune cause) (partial) (total) 996.80
    - bone marrow 996.85
    - heart 996.83
    - intestines 996.87
    - kidney 996.81
    - liver 996.82
    - lung 996.84
    - pancreas 996.86
    - specified NEC 996.89
  - skin NEC 996.79
    - infection or inflammation 996.69
    - rejection 996.52
      - artificial 996.55
      - decellularized allodermis 996.55
- heart - *see also* Disease, heart transplant (immune or nonimmune cause) 996.83
- hematoma (intraoperative) (postoperative) 998.12
- hemorrhage (intraoperative) (postoperative) 998.11
- hyperalimentation therapy NEC 999.9
- immunization (procedure) - *see* Complications, vaccination
- implant - *see also* Complications, due to (presence of) any device, implant, or graft classified to 996.0-996.5 NEC
  - dental placement, hemorrhagic 525.71
  - mechanical, - *see* Complications, mechanical, implant

Complications – *continued*
- infection and inflammation
  - due to (presence of) any device, implant or graft classified to 996.0-996.5 NEC 996.60
    - arterial NEC 996.62
      - coronary 996.61
      - renal dialysis 996.62
    - arteriovenous fistula or shunt 996.62
    - artificial heart 996.61
    - bone growth stimulator 996.67
    - breast 996.69
    - cardiac 996.61
    - catheter NEC 996.69
      - central venous 999.31
      - Hickman 999.31
      - peripherally inserted central (PICC) 999.31
      - peritoneal 996.68
      - portacath (port-a-cath) 999.31
      - spinal 996.63
      - triple lumen 999.31
      - umbilical venous 999.31
      - urinary, indwelling 996.64
      - vascular (arterial) (dialysis) (peripheral venous) NEC 996.62
      - ventricular shunt 996.63
    - central venous catheter 999.31
    - coronary artery bypass 996.61
    - electrodes
      - brain 996.63
      - heart 996.61
    - gastrointestinal NEC 996.69
    - genitourinary NEC 996.65
      - indwelling urinary catheter 996.64
    - heart assist device 996.61
    - heart valve 996.61
    - Hickman catheter 999.31
    - infusion pump 996.62
    - insulin pump 996.69
    - intrauterine contraceptive device 996.65
    - joint prosthesis, internal 996.66
    - ocular lens 996.69
    - orbital (implant) 996.69
    - orthopedic NEC 996.67
      - joint, internal 996.66
    - peripherally inserted central catheter (PICC) 999.31
    - portacath (port-a-cath) 999.31
    - specified type NEC 996.69
    - triple lumen catheter 999.31
    - umbilical venous catheter 999.31
    - urinary catheter, indwelling 996.64
    - ventricular shunt 996.63
- infusion (procedure) 999.88
  - blood - *see* Complications, transfusion
  - infection NEC 999.39
  - sepsis NEC 999.39
- inhalation therapy NEC 999.9
- injection (procedure) 999.9
  - drug reaction (*see also* Reaction, drug) 995.27
  - infection NEC 999.39
  - sepsis NEC 999.39
  - serum (prophylactic) (therapeutic) - *see* Complications, vaccination
  - vaccine (any) - *see* Complications, vaccination
- inoculation (any) - *see* Complications, vaccination
- insulin pump 996.57
- internal device (catheter) (electronic) (fixation) (prosthetic) - *see also* Complications, due to (presence of) any device, implant, or graft classified to 996.0-996.5 NEC
  - mechanical - *see* Complications, mechanical
- intestinal pouch, specified NEC 569.79 ●

Complications – *continued*
- intestinal transplant (immune or nonimmune cause) 996.87
- intraoperative bleeding or hemorrhage 998.11
- intrauterine contraceptive device (*see also* Complications, contraceptive device) 996.76
  - with fetal damage affecting management of pregnancy 655.8 [5th]
  - infection or inflammation 996.65
- in utero procedure
  - fetal 679.1 [5th]
  - maternal 679.0 [5th]
- jejunostomy 569.60
- kidney transplant (immune or nonimmune cause) 996.81
- labor 669.9 [5th]
  - specified condition NEC 669.8 [5th]
- liver transplant (immune or nonimmune cause) 996.82
- lumbar puncture 349.0
- mechanical
  - anastomosis - *see* Complications, mechanical, graft
  - artificial heart 996.09
  - bypass - *see* Complications, mechanical, graft
  - catheter NEC 996.59
    - cardiac 996.09
    - cystostomy 996.39
    - dialysis (hemodialysis) 996.1
      - peritoneal 996.56
    - during a procedure 998.2
    - urethral, indwelling 996.31
  - colostomy 569.62
  - device NEC 996.59
    - balloon (counterpulsation), intra-aortic 996.1
    - cardiac 996.00
      - automatic implantable defibrillator 996.04
      - long-term effect 429.4
      - specified NEC 996.09
    - contraceptive, intrauterine 996.32
    - counterpulsation, intra-aortic 996.1
    - fixation, external, with internal components 996.49
    - fixation, internal (nail, rod, plate) 996.40
    - genitourinary 996.30
      - specified NEC 996.39
    - insulin pump 996.57
    - nervous system 996.2
    - orthopedic, internal 996.40
      - prosthetic joint (*see also* Complications, mechanical, device, orthopedic, prosthetic, joint) 996.47
    - prosthetic NEC 996.59
      - joint ~~(*see also* Complications, prosthetic joint)~~ 996.47 ▲
        - articular bearing surface wear 996.46
        - aseptic loosening 996.41
        - breakage 996.43
        - dislocation 996.42
        - failure 996.47 ▲
        - fracture 996.43
          - around prosthetic 996.44
          - peri-prosthetic 996.44
        - instability 996.42
        - loosening 996.41
        - peri-prosthetic osteolysis 996.45
        - subluxation 996.42
        - wear 996.46
    - umbrella, vena cava 996.1
    - vascular 996.1
  - dorsal column stimulator 996.2
  - electrode NEC 996.59
    - brain 996.2

Complications

- **Complications** - *continued*
  - mechanical - *continued*
    - electrode - *continued*
      - cardiac 996.01
      - spinal column 996.2
    - enterostomy 569.62
    - esophagostomy 530.87
    - fistula, arteriovenous, surgically created 996.1
    - gastrostomy 536.42
    - graft NEC 996.52
      - aortic (bifurcation) 996.1
      - aortocoronary bypass 996.03
      - blood vessel NEC 996.1
      - bone 996.49
      - cardiac 996.00
      - carotid artery bypass 996.1
      - cartilage 996.49
      - corneal 996.51
      - coronary bypass 996.03
      - decellularized allodermis 996.55
      - genitourinary 996.30
        - specified NEC 996.39
      - muscle 996.49
      - nervous system 996.2
      - organ (immune or nonimmune cause) 996.80
        - heart 996.83
        - intestines 996.87
        - kidney 996.81
        - liver 996.82
        - lung 996.84
        - pancreas 996.86
        - specified NEC 996.89
      - orthopedic, internal 996.49
      - peripheral nerve 996.2
      - prosthetic NEC 996.59
      - skin 996.52
        - artificial 996.55
      - specified NEC 996.59
      - tendon 996.49
      - tissue NEC 996.52
      - tooth 996.59
      - ureter, without mention of resection 996.39
      - vascular 996.1
    - heart valve prosthesis 996.02
      - long-term effect 429.4
    - implant NEC 996.59
      - cardiac 996.00
        - automatic implantable defibrillator 996.04
        - long-term effect 429.4
        - specified NEC 996.09
      - electrode NEC 996.59
        - brain 996.2
        - cardiac 996.01
        - spinal column 996.2
      - genitourinary 996.30
      - nervous system 996.2
      - orthopedic, internal 996.49
      - prosthetic NEC 996.59
        - in
          - bile duct 996.59
          - breast 996.54
          - chin 996.59
          - eye
            - ocular lens 996.53
            - orbital globe 996.59
      - vascular 996.1
    - insulin pump 996.57
    - nonabsorbable surgical material 996.59
    - pacemaker NEC 996.59
      - brain 996.2
      - cardiac 996.01
      - nerve (phrenic) 996.2
    - patch - *see* Complications, mechanical, graft
    - prosthesis NEC 996.59
      - bile duct 996.59
      - breast 996.54
      - chin 996.59
      - ocular lens 996.53
      - reconstruction, vas deferens 996.39
    - reimplant NEC 996.59
      - extremity (*see also* Complications, reattached, extremity) 996.90
      - organ (*see also* Complications, transplant, organ, by site) 996.80
    - repair - *see* Complications, mechanical, graft
    - respirator [ventilator] V46.14
    - shunt NEC 996.59
      - arteriovenous, surgically created 996.1
      - ventricular (communicating) 996.2
    - stent NEC 996.59
    - tracheostomy 519.02
    - vas deferens reconstruction 996.39
    - ventilator [respirator] V46.14
  - medical care NEC 999.9
    - cardiac NEC 997.1
    - gastrointestinal NEC 997.4
    - nervous system NEC 997.00
    - peripheral vascular NEC 997.2
    - respiratory NEC 997.39
    - urinary NEC 997.5
    - vascular
      - mesenteric artery 997.71
      - other vessels 997.79
      - peripheral vessels 997.2
      - renal artery 997.72
  - nephrostomy 997.5
  - nervous system
    - device, implant, or graft NEC 349.1
      - mechanical 996.2
    - postoperative NEC 997.00
  - obstetric 669.9 [5th]
    - procedure (instrumental) (manual) (surgical) 669.4 [5th]
    - specified NEC 669.8 [5th]
    - surgical wound 674.3 [5th]
  - ocular lens implant NEC 996.79
    - infection or inflammation 996.69
    - mechanical 996.53
  - organ transplant - *see* Complications, transplant, organ, by site
  - orthopedic device, implant, or graft
    - internal (fixation) (nail) (plate) (rod) NEC 996.78
      - infection or inflammation 996.67
      - joint prosthesis 996.77
        - infection or inflammation 996.66
      - mechanical 996.40
  - pacemaker (cardiac) 996.72
    - infection or inflammation 996.61
    - mechanical 996.01
  - pancreas transplant (immune or nonimmune cause) 996.86
  - perfusion NEC 999.9
  - perineal repair (obstetrical) 674.3 [5th]
    - disruption 674.2 [5th]
  - pessary (uterus) (vagina) - *see* Complications, contraceptive device
  - phototherapy 990
  - postcystoscopic 997.5
  - postmastoidectomy NEC 383.30
  - postoperative - *see* Complications, surgical procedures
  - pregnancy NEC 646.9 [5th]
    - affecting fetus or newborn 761.9
  - prosthetic device, internal - *see also* Complications, due to (presence of) any device, implant or graft classified to 996.0-996.5 NEC
    - mechanical NEC (*see also* Complications, mechanical) 996.59
  - puerperium NEC (*see also* Puerperal) 674.9 [5th]
  - puncture, spinal 349.0
  - pyelogram 997.5
  - radiation 990
  - radiotherapy 990
  - reattached
    - body part, except extremity 996.99
    - extremity (infection) (rejection) 996.90
      - arm(s) 996.94
      - digit(s) (hand) 996.93
        - foot 996.95
      - finger(s) 996.93
      - foot 996.95
      - forearm 996.91
      - hand 996.92
      - leg 996.96
      - lower NEC 996.96
      - toe(s) 996.95
      - upper NEC 996.94
  - reimplant NEC - *see also* Complications, due to (presence of) any device, implant, or graft classified to 996.0-996.5 NEC
    - bone marrow 996.85
    - extremity (*see also* Complications, reattached, extremity) 996.90
      - due to infection 996.90
    - mechanical - *see* Complications, mechanical, reimplant
    - organ (immune or nonimmune cause) (partial) (total) (*see also* Complications, transplant, organ, by site) 996.80
  - renal allograft 996.81
  - renal dialysis - *see* Complications, dialysis
  - respirator [ventilator], mechanical V46.14
  - respiratory 519.9
    - device, implant or graft NEC 996.79
      - infection or inflammation 996.69
      - mechanical 996.59
    - distress syndrome, adult, following trauma or surgery 518.5
    - insufficiency, acute, postoperative 518.5
    - postoperative NEC 997.39
    - therapy NEC 999.9
  - sedation during labor and delivery 668.9 [5th]
    - affecting fetus or newborn 763.5
    - cardiac 668.1 [5th]
    - central nervous system 668.2 [5th]
    - pulmonary 668.0 [5th]
    - specified type NEC 668.8 [5th]
  - seroma (intraoperative) (postoperative) (noninfected) 998.13
    - infected 998.51
  - shunt - *see also* Complications, due to (presence of) any device, implant, or graft classified to 996.0-996.5 NEC
    - mechanical - *see* Complications, mechanical, shunt
  - specified body system NEC
    - device, implant, or graft - *see* Complications, due to (presence of) any device, implant, or graft classified to 996.0-996.5 NEC
    - postoperative NEC 997.99
  - spinal puncture or tap 349.0
  - stoma, external
    - gastrointestinal tract
      - colostomy 569.60
      - enterostomy 569.60
      - esophagostomy 530.87
        - infection 530.86
        - mechanical 530.87
      - gastrostomy 536.40
    - urinary tract 997.5
  - stomach banding 997.4
  - stomach stapling 997.4
  - surgical procedures 998.9
    - accidental puncture or laceration 998.2
    - amputation stump (late) 997.60
    - anastomosis - *see* Complications, anastomosis
    - burst stitches or sutures (external) (*see also* Dehiscence) 998.32
      - internal 998.31
- **Complications** - *continued*
  - surgical procedures - *continued*
    - cardiac 997.1
      - long-term effect following cardiac surgery 429.4
      - catheter device - *see* Complications, catheter device
    - cataract fragments in eye 998.82
    - cecostomy malfunction 569.62
    - colostomy malfunction 569.62
    - cystostomy malfunction 997.5
    - dehiscence (of incision) (external) (*see also* Dehiscence) 998.32
      - internal 998.31
    - dialysis NEC (*see also* Complications, dialysis) 999.9
    - disruption (*see also* Dehiscence)
      - anastomosis (internal) - *see* Complications, mechanical, graft
      - internal suture (line) 998.31
      - wound (external) 998.32
        - internal 998.31
    - dumping syndrome (postgastrectomy) 564.2
    - elephantiasis or lymphedema 997.99
      - postmastectomy 457.0
    - emphysema (surgical) 998.81
    - enterostomy malfunction 569.62
    - esophagostomy malfunction 530.87
    - evisceration 998.32
    - fistula (persistent postoperative) 998.6
    - foreign body inadvertently left in wound (sponge) (suture) (swab) 998.4
    - from nonabsorbable surgical material (Dacron) (mesh) (permanent suture) (reinforcing) (Teflon) - *see* Complications due to (presence of) any device, implant, or graft classified to 996.0-996.5 NEC
    - gastrointestinal NEC 997.4
    - gastrostomy malfunction 536.42
    - hematoma 998.12
    - hemorrhage 998.11
    - ileostomy malfunction 569.62
    - internal prosthetic device NEC (*see also* Complications, internal device) 996.70
      - hemolytic anemia 283.19
      - infection or inflammation 996.60
      - malfunction - *see* Complications, mechanical
      - mechanical complication - *see* Complications, mechanical
      - thrombus 996.70
    - jejunostomy malfunction 569.62
    - nervous system NEC 997.00
    - obstruction, internal anastomosis - *see* Complications, mechanical, graft
    - other body system NEC 997.99
    - peripheral vascular NEC 997.2
    - postcardiotomy syndrome 429.4
    - postcholecystectomy syndrome 576.0
    - postcommissurotomy syndrome 429.4
    - postgastrectomy dumping syndrome 564.2
    - postmastectomy lymphedema syndrome 457.0
    - postmastoidectomy 383.30
      - cholesteatoma, recurrent 383.32
      - cyst, mucosal 383.31
      - granulation 383.33
      - inflammation, chronic 383.33
    - postvagotomy syndrome 564.2
    - postvalvulotomy syndrome 429.4
    - reattached extremity (infection) (rejection) (*see also* Complications, reattached, extremity) 996.90
    - respiratory NEC 997.39
    - seroma 998.13

- **Concussion** – *continued*
  - blast – *continued*
    - ear (acoustic nerve trauma) 951.5
      - with perforation, tympanic membrane - *see* Wound, open, ear drum
    - thorax - *see* Injury, internal, intrathoracic organs NEC
  - brain or cerebral (without skull fracture) 850.9
    - with
      - loss of consciousness 850.5
        - brief (less than one hour)
          - 30 minutes or less 850.11
          - 31-59 minutes 850.12
        - moderate (1-24 hours) 850.2
        - prolonged (more than 24 hours) (with complete recovery) (with return to pre-existing conscious level) 850.3
          - without return to pre-existing conscious level 850.4
      - mental confusion or disorientation (without loss of consciousness) 850.0
        - with loss of consciousness - *see* Concussion, brain, with, loss of consciousness
      - skull fracture - *see* Fracture, skull, by site
    - without loss of consciousness 850.0
  - cauda equina 952.4
  - cerebral - *see* Concussion, brain
  - conus medullaris (spine) 952.4
  - hydraulic - *see* Concussion, blast
  - internal organs - *see* Injury, internal, by site
  - labyrinth - *see* Injury, intracranial
  - ocular 921.3
  - osseous labyrinth - *see* Injury, intracranial
  - spinal (cord) - *see also* Injury, spinal, by site
    - due to
      - broken
        - back - *see* Fracture, vertebra, by site, with spinal cord injury
        - neck - *see* Fracture, vertebra, cervical, with spinal cord injury
      - fracture, fracture dislocation, or compression fracture of spine or vertebra - *see* Fracture, vertebra, by site, with spinal cord injury
  - syndrome 310.2
  - underwater blast - *see* Concussion, blast
- **Condition** - *see also* Disease
  - fetal hematologic 678.0 [5th]
  - psychiatric 298.9
  - respiratory NEC 519.9
    - acute or subacute NEC 519.9
      - due to
        - external agent 508.9
          - specified type NEC 508.8
        - fumes or vapors (chemical) (inhalation) 506.3
        - radiation 508.0
    - chronic NEC 519.9
      - due to
        - external agent 508.9
          - specified type NEC 508.8
        - fumes or vapors (chemical) (inhalation) 506.4
        - radiation 508.1
    - due to
      - external agent 508.9
        - specified type NEC 508.8
      - fumes or vapors (chemical) inhalation 506.9
- **Conduct disturbance** (*see also* Disturbance, conduct) 312.9
  - adjustment reaction 309.3
  - hyperkinetic 314.2
- **Condyloma** NEC 078.11
  - acuminatum 078.11
  - gonorrheal 098.0
  - latum 091.3
  - syphilitic 091.3
    - congenital 090.0
  - venereal, syphilitic 091.3
- **Confinement** - *see* Delivery
- **Conflagration** - *see also* Burn, by site
  - asphyxia (by inhalation of smoke, gases, fumes, or vapors) 987.9
    - specified agent - *see* Table of Drugs and Chemicals
- **Conflict**
  - family V61.9
    - specified circumstance NEC V61.8
  - interpersonal NEC V62.81
  - marital V61.10
    - involving
      - divorce V61.03
      - estrangement V61.09
  - parent (guardian)-child V61.20 ▲
    - adopted child V61.24 ●
    - biological child V61.23 ●
    - foster child V61.25 ●
  - partner V61.10
- **Confluent** - *see* condition
- **Confusion, confused** (mental) (state) (*see also* State, confusional) 298.9
  - acute 293.0
  - epileptic 293.0
  - postoperative 293.9
  - psychogenic 298.2
  - reactive (from emotional stress, psychological trauma) 298.2
  - subacute 293.1
- **Confusional arousals** 327.41
- **Congelation** 991.9
- **Congenital** - *see also* condition
  - aortic septum 747.29
  - generalized fibromatosis (CGF) 759.89
  - intrinsic factor deficiency 281.0
  - malformation - *see* Anomaly
- **Congestion, congestive**
  - asphyxia, newborn 768.9
  - bladder 596.8
  - bowel 569.89
  - brain (*see also* Disease, cerebrovascular NEC) 437.8
    - malarial 084.9
  - breast 611.79
  - bronchi 519.19
  - bronchial tube 519.19
  - catarrhal 472.0
  - cerebral - *see* Congestion, brain
  - cerebrospinal - *see* Congestion, brain
  - chest 786.9
  - chill 780.99
    - malarial (*see also* Malaria) 084.6
  - circulatory NEC 459.9
  - conjunctiva 372.71
  - due to disturbance of circulation 459.9
  - duodenum 537.3
  - enteritis - *see* Enteritis
  - eye 372.71
  - fibrosis syndrome (pelvic) 625.5
  - gastroenteritis - *see* Enteritis
  - general 799.89
  - glottis 476.0
  - heart (*see also* Failure, heart) 428.0
  - hepatic 573.0
  - hypostatic (lung) 514
  - intestine 569.89
  - intracranial - *see* Congestion, brain
  - kidney 593.89
  - labyrinth 386.50
  - larynx 476.0
  - liver 573.0

- **Congestion, congestive** – *continued*
  - lung 786.9
    - active or acute (*see also* Pneumonia) 486
      - congenital 770.0
    - chronic 514
    - hypostatic 514
    - idiopathic, acute 518.5
    - passive 514
  - malaria, malarial (brain) (fever) (*see also* Malaria) 084.6
  - medulla - *see* Congestion, brain
  - nasal 478.19
  - nose 478.19
  - orbit, orbital 376.33
    - inflammatory (chronic) 376.10
      - acute 376.00
  - ovary 620.8
  - pancreas 577.8
  - pelvic, female 625.5
  - pleural 511.0
  - prostate (active) 602.1
  - pulmonary - *see* Congestion, lung
  - renal 593.89
  - retina 362.89
  - seminal vesicle 608.89
  - spinal cord 336.1
  - spleen 289.51
    - chronic 289.51
  - stomach 537.89
  - trachea 464.11
  - urethra 599.84
  - uterus 625.5
    - with subinvolution 621.1
  - viscera 799.89
- **Congestive** - *see* Congestion
- **Conical**
  - cervix 622.6
  - cornea 371.60
  - teeth 520.2
- **Conjoined twins** 759.4
  - causing disproportion (fetopelvic) 678.1 [5th]
  - fetal 678.1 [5th]
- **Conjugal maladjustment** V61.10
  - involving
    - divorce V61.03
    - estrangement V61.09
- **Conjunctiva** - *see* condition
- **Conjunctivitis** (exposure) (infectious) (nondiphtheritic) (pneumococcal) (pustular) (staphylococcal) (streptococcal) NEC 372.30
  - actinic 370.24
  - acute 372.00
    - atopic 372.05
    - chemical 372.06 ●
    - contagious 372.03
    - follicular 372.02
    - hemorrhagic (viral) 077.4
    - toxic 372.06 ●
  - adenoviral (acute) 077.3
  - allergic (chronic) 372.14
    - with hay fever 372.05
  - anaphylactic 372.05
  - angular 372.03
  - Apollo (viral) 077.4
  - atopic 372.05
  - blennorrhagic (neonatorum) 098.40
  - catarrhal 372.03
  - chemical 372.06 ▲
    - allergic 372.05
    - meaning corrosion - *See* Burn, conjunctiva
  - chlamydial 077.98
    - due to
      - Chlamydia trachomatis - *see* Trachoma
      - paratrachoma 077.0
  - chronic 372.10
    - allergic 372.14
    - follicular 372.12
    - simple 372.11
    - specified type NEC 372.14
- **Conjunctivitis** – *continued*
  - chronic – *continued*
    - vernal 372.13
  - diphtheritic 032.81
  - due to
    - dust 372.05
    - enterovirus type 70 077.4
    - erythema multiforme 695.10 *[372.33]*
    - filariasis (*see also* Filariasis) 125.9 *[372.15]*
    - mucocutaneous
      - disease NEC 372.33
      - leishmaniasis 085.5 *[372.15]*
    - Reiter's disease 099.3 *[372.33]*
    - syphilis 095.8 *[372.10]*
    - toxoplasmosis (acquired) 130.1
      - congenital (active) 771.2
    - trachoma - *see* Trachoma
  - dust 372.05
  - eczematous 370.31
  - epidemic 077.1
    - hemorrhagic 077.4
  - follicular (acute) 372.02
    - adenoviral (acute) 077.3
    - chronic 372.12
  - glare 370.24
  - gonococcal (neonatorum) 098.40
  - granular (trachomatous) 076.1
    - late effect 139.1
  - hemorrhagic (acute) (epidemic) 077.4
  - herpetic (simplex) 054.43
    - zoster 053.21
  - inclusion 077.0
  - infantile 771.6
  - influenzal 372.03
  - Koch-Weeks 372.03
  - light 372.05
  - medicamentosa 372.05
  - membranous 372.04
  - meningococcic 036.89
  - Morax-Axenfeld 372.02
  - mucopurulent NEC 372.03
  - neonatal 771.6
    - gonococcal 098.40
  - Newcastle's 077.8
  - nodosa 360.14
  - of Beal 077.3
  - parasitic 372.15
    - filariasis (*see also* Filariasis) 125.9 *[372.15]*
    - mucocutaneous leishmaniasis 085.5 *[372.15]*
  - Parinaud's 372.02
  - petrificans 372.39
  - phlyctenular 370.31
  - pseudomembranous 372.04
    - diphtheritic 032.81
  - purulent 372.03
  - Reiter's 099.3 *[372.33]*
  - rosacea 695.3 *[372.31]*
  - serous 372.01
    - viral 077.99
  - simple chronic 372.11
  - specified NEC 372.39
  - sunlamp 372.04
  - swimming pool 077.0
  - toxic 372.06 ●
  - trachomatous (follicular) 076.1
    - acute 076.0
    - late effect 139.1
  - traumatic NEC 372.39
  - tuberculous (*see also* Tuberculosis) 017.3 [5th] *[370.31]*
  - tularemic 021.3
  - tularensis 021.3
  - vernal 372.13
    - limbar 372.13 *[370.32]*
  - viral 077.99
    - acute hemorrhagic 077.4
    - specified NEC 077.8
- **Conjunctoblepharitis** - *see* Conjunctivitis
- **Conjunctivochalasis** 372.81
- **Conn (-Louis) syndrome** (primary aldosteronism) 255.12

Connective tissue - *see* condition
Conradi (-Hünermann) syndrome or disease (chondrodysplasia calcificans congenita) 756.59
Consanguinity V19.7
Consecutive - *see* condition
Consolidated lung (base) - *see* Pneumonia, lobar
Constipation 564.00
 atonic 564.09
 drug induced
  correct substance properly administered 564.09
  overdose or wrong substance given or taken 977.9
   specified drug - *see* Table of Drugs and Chemicals
 neurogenic 564.09
 other specified NEC 564.09
 outlet dysfunction 564.02
 psychogenic 306.4
 simple 564.00
 slow transit 564.01
 spastic 564.09
Constitutional - *see also* condition
 arterial hypotension (*see also* Hypotension) 458.9
 obesity 278.00
  morbid 278.01
 psychopathic state 301.9
 short stature in childhood 783.43
 state, developmental V21.9
  specified development NEC V21.8
 substandard 301.6
Constitutionally substandard 301.6
Constriction
 anomalous, meningeal bands or folds 742.8
 aortic arch (congenital) 747.10
 asphyxiation or suffocation by 994.7
 bronchus 519.19
 canal, ear (*see also* Stricture, ear canal, acquired) 380.50
 duodenum 537.3
 gallbladder (*see also* Obstruction, gallbladder) 575.2
  congenital 751.69
 intestine (*see also* Obstruction, intestine) 560.9
 larynx 478.74
  congenital 748.3
 meningeal bands or folds, anomalous 742.8
 organ or site, congenital NEC - *see* Atresia
 prepuce (congenital) 605
 pylorus 537.0
  adult hypertrophic 537.0
  congenital or infantile 750.5
  newborn 750.5
 ring (uterus) 661.4 [5th]
  affecting fetus or newborn 763.7
 spastic - *see also* Spasm
  ureter 593.3
  urethra - *see* Stricture, urethra
 stomach 537.89
 ureter 593.3
 urethra - *see* Stricture, urethra
 visual field (functional) (peripheral) 368.45
Constrictive - *see* condition
Consultation V65.9
 medical - *see also* Counseling, medical
 specified reason NEC V65.8
 without complaint or sickness V65.9
  feared complaint unfounded V65.5
  specified reason NEC V65.8
Consumption - *see* Tuberculosis
Contact
 with
  AIDS virus V01.79
  anthrax V01.81
  asbestos V15.84 ●
  cholera V01.0

Contact – *continued*
 with – *continued*
  communicable disease V01.9
   specified type NEC V01.89
   viral NEC V01.79
  Escherichia coli (E. coli) V01.83
  German measles V01.4
  gonorrhea V01.6
  HIV V01.79
  human immunodeficiency virus V01.79
  lead V15.86 ●
  meningococcus V01.84
  parasitic disease NEC V01.89
  poliomyelitis V01.2
  potentially hazardous body fluids V15.85 ●
  rabies V01.5
  rubella V01.4
  SARS-associated coronavirus V01.82
  smallpox V01.3
  syphilis V01.6
  tuberculosis V01.1
  varicella V01.71
  venereal disease V01.6
  viral disease NEC V01.79
 dermatitis - *see* Dermatitis
Contamination, food (*see also* Poisoning, food) 005.9
Contraception, contraceptive
 advice NEC V25.09
  family planning V25.09
  fitting of diaphragm V25.02
  prescribing or use of
   oral contraceptive agent V25.01
   specified agent NEC V25.02
 counseling NEC V25.09
  emergency V25.03
  family planning V25.09
  fitting of diaphragm V25.02
  prescribing or use of
   oral contraceptive agent V25.01
    emergency V25.03
    postcoital V25.03
   specified agent NEC V25.02
 device (in situ) V45.59
  causing menorrhagia 996.76
  checking V25.42
  complications 996.32
  insertion V25.1
  intrauterine V45.51
  reinsertion V25.42
  removal V25.42
  subdermal V45.52
 fitting of diaphragm V25.02
 insertion
  intrauterine contraceptive device V25.1
  subdermal implantable V25.5
 maintenance V25.40
  examination V25.40
   intrauterine device V25.42
   oral contraceptive V25.41
   specified method NEC V25.49
   subdermal implantable V25.43
  intrauterine device V25.42
  oral contraceptive V25.41
  specified method NEC V25.49
  subdermal implantable V25.43
 management NEC V25.49
 prescription
  oral contraceptive agent V25.01
   emergency V25.03
   postcoital V25.03
   repeat V25.41
  specified agent NEC V25.02
   repeat V25.49
 sterilization V25.2
 surveillance V25.40
  intrauterine device V25.42
  oral contraceptive agent V25.41
  specified method NEC V25.49
  subdermal implantable V25.43

Contraction, contracture, contracted
 Achilles tendon (*see also* Short, tendon, Achilles) 727.81
 anus 564.89
 axilla 729.90
 bile duct (*see also* Disease, biliary) 576.8
 bladder 596.8
  neck or sphincter 596.0
 bowel (*see also* Obstruction, intestine) 560.9
 Braxton Hicks 644.1 [5th]
 breast implant, capsular 611.83
 bronchus 519.19
 burn (old) - *see* Cicatrix
 capsular, of breast implant 611.83
 cecum (*see also* Obstruction, intestine) 560.9
 cervix (*see also* Stricture, cervix) 622.4
  congenital 752.49
 cicatricial - *see* Cicatrix
 colon (*see also* Obstruction, intestine) 560.9
 conjunctiva trachomatous, active 076.1
  late effect 139.1
 Dupuytren's 728.6
 eyelid 374.41
 eye socket (after enucleation) 372.64
 face 729.90
 fascia (lata) (postural) 728.89
  Dupuytren's 728.6
  palmar 728.6
  plantar 728.71
 finger NEC 736.29
  congenital 755.59
  joint (*see also* Contraction, joint) 718.44
 flaccid, paralytic
  joint (*see also* Contraction, joint) 718.4 [5th]
  muscle 728.85
   ocular 378.50
 gallbladder (*see also* Obstruction, gallbladder) 575.2
 hamstring 728.89
  tendon 727.81
 heart valve - *see* Endocarditis
 Hicks' 644.1 [5th]
 hip (*see also* Contraction, joint) 718.4 [5th]
 hourglass
  bladder 596.8
   congenital 753.8
  gallbladder (*see also* Obstruction, gallbladder) 575.2
   congenital 751.69
  stomach 536.8
   congenital 750.7
   psychogenic 306.4
  uterus 661.4 [5th]
   affecting fetus or newborn 763.7
 hysterical 300.11
 infantile (*see also* Epilepsy) 345.6 [5th]
 internal os (*see also* Stricture, cervix) 622.4
 intestine (*see also* Obstruction, intestine) 560.9
 joint (abduction) (acquired) (adduction) (flexion) (rotation) 718.40
  ankle 718.47
  congenital NEC 755.8
   generalized or multiple 754.89
    lower limb joints 754.89
   hip (*see also* Subluxation, congenital, hip) 754.32
   lower limb (including pelvic girdle) not involving hip 754.89
   upper limb (including shoulder girdle) 755.59
  elbow 718.42
  foot 718.47
  hand 718.44
  hip 718.45
  hysterical 300.11
  knee 718.46
  multiple sites 718.49

Contraction, contracture, contracted – *continued*
 joint – *continued*
  pelvic region 718.45
  shoulder (region) 718.41
  specified site NEC 718.48
  wrist 718.43
 kidney (granular) (secondary) (*see also* Sclerosis, renal) 587
  congenital 753.3
  hydronephritic 591
  pyelonephritic (*see also* Pyelitis, chronic) 590.00
  tuberculous (*see also* Tuberculosis) 016.0 [5th]
 ligament 728.89
  congenital 756.89
 liver - *see* Cirrhosis, liver
 muscle (postinfectional) (postural) NEC 728.85
  congenital 756.89
   sternocleidomastoid 754.1
  extraocular 378.60
  eye (extrinsic) (*see also* Strabismus) 378.9
   paralytic (*see also* Strabismus, paralytic) 378.50
  flaccid 728.85
  hysterical 300.11
  ischemic (Volkmann's) 958.6
  paralytic 728.85
  posttraumatic 958.6
  psychogenic 306.0
   specified as conversion reaction 300.11
 myotonic 728.85
 neck (*see also* Torticollis) 723.5
  congenital 754.1
  psychogenic 306.0
 ocular muscle (*see also* Strabismus) 378.9
  paralytic (*see also* Strabismus, paralytic) 378.50
 organ or site, congenital NEC - *see* Atresia
 outlet (pelvis) - *see* Contraction, pelvis
 palmar fascia 728.6
 paralytic
  joint (*see also* Contraction, joint) 718.4 [5th]
  muscle 728.85
   ocular (*see also* Strabismus, paralytic) 378.50
 pelvis (acquired) (general) 738.6
  affecting fetus or newborn 763.1
  complicating delivery 653.1 [5th]
   causing obstructed labor 660.1 [5th]
   generally contracted 653.1 [5th]
    causing obstructed labor 660.1 [5th]
   inlet 653.2 [5th]
    causing obstructed labor 660.1 [5th]
   midpelvic 653.8 [5th]
    causing obstructed labor 660.1 [5th]
   midplane 653.8 [5th]
    causing obstructed labor 660.1 [5th]
   outlet 653.3 [5th]
    causing obstructed labor 660.1 [5th]
 plantar fascia 728.71
 premature
  atrial 427.61
  auricular 427.61
  auriculoventricular 427.61
  heart (junctional) (nodal) 427.60
  supraventricular 427.61
  ventricular 427.69
 prostate 602.8
 pylorus (*see also* Pylorospasm) 537.81
 rectosigmoid (*see also* Obstruction, intestine) 560.9
 rectum, rectal (sphincter) 564.89
  psychogenic 306.4

Contraction, contracture, contracted – *continued*
- ring (Bandl's) 661.4 [5th]
  - affecting fetus or newborn 763.7
- scar - *see* Cicatrix
- sigmoid (*see also* Obstruction, intestine) 560.9
- socket, eye 372.64
- spine (*see also* Curvature, spine) 737.9
- stomach 536.8
  - hourglass 536.8
    - congenital 750.7
    - psychogenic 306.4
  - psychogenic 306.4
- tendon (sheath) (*see also* Short, tendon) 727.81
- toe 735.8
- ureterovesical orifice (postinfectional) 593.3
- urethra 599.84
- uterus 621.8
  - abnormal 661.9 [5th]
    - affecting fetus or newborn 763.7
  - clonic, hourglass or tetanic 661.4 [5th]
    - affecting fetus or newborn 763.7
  - dyscoordinate 661.4 [5th]
    - affecting fetus or newborn 763.7
  - hourglass 661.4 [5th]
    - affecting fetus or newborn 763.7
  - hypotonic NEC 661.2 [5th]
    - affecting fetus or newborn 763.7
  - incoordinate 661.4 [5th]
    - affecting fetus or newborn 763.7
  - inefficient or poor 661.2 [5th]
    - affecting fetus or newborn 763.7
  - irregular 661.2 [5th]
    - affecting fetus or newborn 763.7
  - tetanic 661.4 [5th]
    - affecting fetus or newborn 763.7
- vagina (outlet) 623.2
- vesical 596.8
  - neck or urethral orifice 596.0
- visual field, generalized 368.45
- Volkmann's (ischemic) 958.6

Contusion (skin surface intact) 924.9
- with
  - crush injury - *see* Crush
  - dislocation - *see* Dislocation, by site
  - fracture - *see* Fracture, by site
  - internal injury - *see also* Injury, internal, by site
    - heart - *see* Contusion, cardiac
    - kidney - *see* Contusion, kidney
    - liver - *see* Contusion, liver
    - lung - *see* Contusion, lung
    - spleen - *see* Contusion, spleen
  - intracranial injury - *see* Injury, intracranial
  - nerve injury - *see* Injury, nerve
  - open wound - *see* Wound, open, by site
- abdomen, abdominal (muscle) (wall) 922.2
  - organ(s) NEC 868.00
- adnexa, eye NEC 921.9
- ankle 924.21
  - with other parts of foot 924.20
- arm 923.9
  - lower (with elbow) 923.10
  - upper 923.03
    - with shoulder or axillary region 923.09
- auditory canal (external) (meatus) (and other part(s) of neck, scalp, or face, except eye) 920
- auricle, ear (and other part(s) of neck, scalp, or face except eye) 920
- axilla 923.02
  - with shoulder or upper arm 923.09
- back 922.31
- bone NEC 924.9

Contusion – *continued*
- brain (cerebral) (membrane) (with hemorrhage) 851.8 [5th]

Note *Use the following fifth-digit subclassification with categories 851-854:*

0	unspecified state of consciousness
1	with no loss of consciousness
2	with brief [less than one hour] loss of consciousness
3	with moderate [1-24 hours] loss of consciousness
4	with prolonged [more than 24 hours] loss of consciousness and return to pre-existing conscious level
5	with prolonged [more than 24 hours] loss of consciousness, without return to pre-existing conscious level Use fifth-digit 5 to designate when a patient is unconscious and dies before regaining consciousness, regardless of the duration of the loss of consciousness
6	with loss of consciousness of unspecified duration
9	with concussion, unspecified

  - with
    - open intracranial wound 851.9 [5th]
    - skull fracture - *see* Fracture, skull, by site
  - cerebellum 851.4 [5th]
    - with open intracranial wound 851.5 [5th]
  - cortex 851.0 [5th]
    - with open intracranial wound 851.1 [5th]
  - occipital lobe 851.4 [5th]
    - with open intracranial wound 851.5 [5th]
  - stem 851.4 [5th]
    - with open intracranial wound 851.5 [5th]
- breast 922.0
- brow (and other part(s) of neck, scalp, or face, except eye) 920
- buttock 922.32
- canthus 921.1
- cardiac 861.01
  - with open wound into thorax 861.11
- cauda equina (spine) 952.4
- cerebellum - *see* Contusion, brain, cerebellum
- cerebral - *see* Contusion, brain
- cheek(s) (and other part(s) of neck, scalp, or face, except eye) 920
- chest (wall) 922.1
- chin (and other part(s) of neck, scalp, or face, except eye) 920
- clitoris 922.4
- conjunctiva 921.1
- conus medullaris (spine) 952.4
- cornea 921.3
- corpus cavernosum 922.4
- cortex (brain) (cerebral) - *see* Contusion, brain, cortex
- costal region 922.1
- ear (and other part(s) of neck, scalp, or face except eye) 920
- elbow 923.11
  - with forearm 923.10
- epididymis 922.4
- epigastric region 922.2
- eye NEC 921.9
- eyeball 921.3
- eyelid(s) (and periocular area) 921.1
- face (and neck, or scalp, any part, except eye) 920
- femoral triangle 922.2
- fetus or newborn 772.6
- finger(s) (nail) (subungual) 923.3
- flank 922.2
- foot (with ankle) (excluding toe(s)) 924.20

Contusion – *continued*
- forearm (and elbow) 923.10
- forehead (and other part(s) of neck, scalp, or face, except eye) 920
- genital organs, external 922.4
- globe (eye) 921.3
- groin 922.2
- gum(s) (and other part(s) of neck, scalp, or face, except eye) 920
- hand(s) (except fingers alone) 923.20
- head (any part, except eye) (and face) (and neck) 920
- heart - *see* Contusion, cardiac
- heel 924.20
- hip 924.01
  - with thigh 924.00
- iliac region 922.2
- inguinal region 922.2
- internal organs (abdomen, chest, or pelvis) NEC - *see* Injury, internal, by site
- interscapular region 922.33
- iris (eye) 921.3
- kidney 866.01
  - with open wound into cavity 866.11
- knee 924.11
  - with lower leg 924.10
- labium (majus) (minus) 922.4
- lacrimal apparatus, gland, or sac 921.1
- larynx (and other part(s) of neck, scalp, or face, except eye) 920
- late effect - *see* Late, effects (of), contusion
- leg 924.5
  - lower (with knee) 924.10
- lens 921.3
- lingual (and other part(s) of neck, scalp, or face, except eye) 920
- lip(s) (and other part(s) of neck, scalp, or face, except eye) 920
- liver 864.01
  - with
    - laceration - *see* Laceration, liver
    - open wound into cavity 864.11
- lower extremity 924.5
  - multiple sites 924.4
- lumbar region 922.31
- lung 861.21
  - with open wound into thorax 861.31
- malar region (and other part(s) of neck, scalp, or face, except eye) 920
- mandibular joint (and other part(s) of neck, scalp, or face, except eye) 920
- mastoid region (and other part(s) of neck, scalp, or face, except eye) 920
- membrane, brain - *see* Contusion, brain
- midthoracic region 922.1
- mouth (and other part(s) of neck, scalp, or face, except eye) 920
- multiple sites (not classifiable to same three-digit category) 924.8
  - lower limb 924.4
  - trunk 922.8
  - upper limb 923.8
- muscle NEC 924.9
- myocardium - *see* Contusion, cardiac
- nasal (septum) (and other part(s) of neck, scalp, or face, except eye) 920
- neck (and scalp, or face, any part, except eye) 920
- nerve - *see* Injury, nerve, by site
- nose (and other part(s) of neck, scalp, or face, except eye) 920
- occipital region (scalp) (and neck or face, except eye) 920
  - lobe - *see* Contusion, brain, occipital lobe
- orbit (region) (tissues) 921.2
- palate (soft) (and other part(s) of neck, scalp, or face, except eye) 920
- parietal region (scalp) (and neck, or face, except eye) 920
  - lobe - *see* Contusion, brain
- penis 922.4
- pericardium - *see* Contusion, cardiac

Contusion – *continued*
- perineum 922.4
- periocular area 921.1
- pharynx (and other part(s) of neck, scalp, or face, except eye) 920
- popliteal space (*see also* Contusion, knee) 924.11
- prepuce 922.4
- pubic region 922.4
- pudenda 922.4
- pulmonary - *see* Contusion, lung
- quadriceps femoralis 924.00
- rib cage 922.1
- sacral region 922.32
- salivary ducts or glands (and other part(s) of neck, scalp, or face, except eye) 920
- scalp (and neck, or face any part, except eye) 920
- scapular region 923.01
  - with shoulder or upper arm 923.09
- sclera (eye) 921.3
- scrotum 922.4
- shoulder 923.00
  - with upper arm or axillar regions 923.09
- skin NEC 924.9
- skull 920
- spermatic cord 922.4
- spinal cord - *see also* Injury, spinal, by site
  - cauda equina 952.4
  - conus medullaris 952.4
- spleen 865.01
  - with open wound into cavity 865.11
- sternal region 922.1
- stomach - *see* Injury, internal, stomach
- subconjunctival 921.1
- subcutaneous NEC 924.9
- submaxillary region (and other part(s) of neck, scalp, or face, except eye) 920
- submental region (and other part(s) of neck, scalp, or face, except eye) 920
- subperiosteal NEC 924.9
- supraclavicular fossa (and other part(s) of neck, scalp, or face, except eye) 920
- supraorbital (and other part(s) of neck, scalp, or face, except eye) 920
- temple (region) (and other part(s) of neck, scalp, or face, except eye) 920
- testis 922.4
- thigh (and hip) 924.00
- thorax 922.1
  - organ - *see* Injury, internal, intrathoracic
- throat (and other part(s) of neck, scalp, or face, except eye) 920
- thumb(s) (nail) (subungual) 923.3
- toe(s) (nail) (subungual) 924.3
- tongue (and other part(s) of neck, scalp, or face, except eye) 920
- trunk 922.9
  - multiple sites 922.8
  - specified site - *see* Contusion, by site
- tunica vaginalis 922.4
- tympanum (membrane) (and other part(s) of neck, scalp, or face, except eye) 920
- upper extremity 923.9
  - multiple sites 923.8
- uvula (and other part(s) of neck, scalp, or face, except eye) 920
- vagina 922.4
- vocal cord(s) (and other part(s) of neck, scalp, or face, except eye) 920
- vulva 922.4
- wrist 923.21
  - with hand(s), except finger(s) alone 923.20

Conus (any type) (congenital) 743.57
- acquired 371.60
- medullaris syndrome 336.8

Convalescence (following) V66.9
- chemotherapy V66.2
- medical NEC V66.5

Convalescence (following) – *continued*
- psychotherapy V66.3
- radiotherapy V66.1
- surgery NEC V66.0
- treatment (for) NEC V66.5
  - combined V66.6
  - fracture V66.4
  - mental disorder NEC V66.3
  - specified disorder NEC V66.5

Conversion
- hysteria, hysterical, any type 300.11
- closed surgical procedure to open procedure
  - arthroscopic V64.43
  - laparoscopic V64.41
  - thoracoscopic V64.42
- neurosis, any 300.11
- reaction, any 300.11

Converter, tuberculosis (test reaction) 795.5

Convulsions (idiopathic) 780.39
- apoplectiform (*see also* Disease, cerebrovascular, acute) 436
- brain 780.39
- cerebral 780.39
- cerebrospinal 780.39
- due to trauma NEC - *see* Injury, intracranial
- eclamptic (*see also* Eclampsia) 780.39
- epileptic (*see also* Epilepsy) 345.9 5th
- epileptiform (*see also* Seizure, epileptiform) 780.39
- epileptoid (*see also* Seizure, epileptiform) 780.39
- ether
  - anesthetic
    - correct substance properly administered 780.39
    - overdose or wrong substance given 968.2
  - other specified type - *see* Table of Drugs and Chemicals
- febrile (simple) 780.31
  - complex 780.32
- generalized 780.39
- hysterical 300.11
- infantile 780.39
  - epilepsy - *see* Epilepsy
- internal 780.39
- jacksonian (*see also* Epilepsy) 345.5 5th
- myoclonic 333.2
- newborn 779.0
- paretic 094.1
- pregnancy (nephritic) (uremic) - *see* Eclampsia, pregnancy
- psychomotor (*see also* Epilepsy) 345.4 5th
- puerperal, postpartum - *see* Eclampsia, pregnancy
- recurrent 780.39
  - epileptic - *see* Epilepsy
- reflex 781.0
- repetitive 780.39
  - epileptic - *see* Epilepsy
- salaam (*see also* Epilepsy) 345.6 5th
- scarlatinal 034.1
- spasmodic 780.39
- tetanus, tetanic (*see also* Tetanus) 037
- thymic 254.8
- uncinate 780.39
- uremic 586

Convulsive - *see also* Convulsions
- disorder or state 780.39
  - epileptic - *see* Epilepsy
- equivalent, abdominal (*see also* Epilepsy) 345.5 5th

Cooke-Apert-Gallais syndrome (adrenogenital) 255.2

Cooley's anemia (erythroblastic) 282.49

Coolie itch 126.9

Cooper's
- disease 610.1
- hernia - *see* Hernia, Cooper's

Coordination disturbance 781.3

Copper wire arteries, retina 362.13

Copra itch 133.8

Coprolith 560.39

Coprophilia 302.89

Coproporphyria, hereditary 277.1

Coprostasis 560.39
- with hernia - *see also* Hernia, by site, with obstruction
  - gangrenous - *see* Hernia, by site, with gangrene

Cor
- biloculare 745.7
- bovinum - *see* Hypertrophy, cardiac
- bovis - *see also* Hypertrophy, cardiac
- pulmonale (chronic) 416.9
  - acute 415.0
- triatriatum, triatrium 746.82
- triloculare 745.8
  - biatriatum 745.3
  - biventriculare 745.69

Corbus' disease 607.1

Cord - *see also* condition
- around neck (tightly) (with compression)
  - affecting fetus or newborn 762.5
  - complicating delivery 663.1 5th
    - without compression 663.3 5th
      - affecting fetus or newborn 762.6
- bladder NEC 344.61
  - tabetic 094.0
- prolapse
  - affecting fetus or newborn 762.4
  - complicating delivery 663.0 5th

Cord's angiopathy (*see also* Tuberculosis) 017.3 5th *[362.18]*

Cordis ectopia 746.87

Corditis (spermatic) 608.4

Corectopia 743.46

Cori type glycogen storage disease - see Disease, glycogen storage

Cork-handlers' disease or lung 495.3

Corkscrew esophagus 530.5

Corlett's pyosis (impetigo) 684

Corn (infected) 700

Cornea - *see also* condition
- donor V59.5
- guttata (dystrophy) 371.57
- plana 743.41

Cornelia de Lange's syndrome (Amsterdam dwarf, mental retardation, and brachycephaly) 759.89

Cornual gestation or pregnancy - *see* Pregnancy, cornual

Cornu cutaneum 702.8

Coronary (artery) - *see also* condition
- arising from aorta or pulmonary trunk 746.85

Corpora - *see also* condition
- amylacea (prostate) 602.8
- cavernosa - *see* condition

Corpulence (*see also* Obesity)

Corpus - *see* condition

Corrigan's disease - *see* Insufficiency, aortic

Corrosive burn - *see* Burn, by site

Corsican fever (*see also* Malaria) 084.6

Cortical - *see also* condition
- blindness 377.75
- necrosis, kidney (bilateral) 583.6

Corticoadrenal - *see* condition

Corticosexual syndrome 255.2

Coryza (acute) 460
- with grippe or influenza 487.1
- syphilitic 095.8
  - congenital (chronic) 090.0

Costen's syndrome or complex 524.60

Costiveness (*see also* Constipation) 564.00

Costochondritis 733.6

Cotard's syndrome (paranoia) 297.1

Cot death 798.0

Cotia virus 059.8

Cotungo's disease 724.3

Cough 786.2
- with hemorrhage (*see also* Hemoptysis) 786.3
- affected 786.2
- bronchial 786.2
  - with grippe or influenza 487.1

Cough – *continued*
- chronic 786.2
- epidemic 786.2
- functional 306.1
- hemorrhagic 786.3
- hysterical 300.11
- laryngeal, spasmodic 786.2
- nervous 786.2
- psychogenic 306.1
- smokers' 491.0
- tea tasters' 112.89

Counseling NEC V65.40
- without complaint or sickness V65.49
- abuse victim NEC V62.89
  - child V61.21
  - partner V61.11
  - spouse V61.11
- child abuse, maltreatment, or neglect V61.21
- contraceptive NEC V25.09
  - device (intrauterine) V25.02
  - maintenance V25.40
    - intrauterine contraceptive device V25.42
    - oral contraceptive (pill) V25.41
    - specified type NEC V25.49
    - subdermal implantable V25.43
  - management NEC V25.9
  - oral contraceptive (pill) V25.01
    - emergency V25.03
    - postcoital V25.03
  - prescription NEC V25.02
    - oral contraceptive (pill) V25.01
      - emergency V25.03
      - postcoital V25.03
      - repeat prescription V25.41
    - repeat prescription V25.40
  - subdermal implantable V25.43
  - surveillance NEC V25.40
- dietary V65.3
- exercise V65.41
- expectant parent(s) ~~mother, pediatric pre-birth visit V65.11~~ ▲
  - pediatric pre-adoption visit V65.11 ●
  - pediatric pre-birth visit V65.11 ●
- explanation of
  - investigation finding NEC V65.49
  - medication NEC V65.49
- family planning V25.09
  - natural
    - procreative V26.41
    - to avoid pregnancy V25.04
- for nonattending third party V65.19
- genetic V26.33
- gonorrhea V65.45
- health (advice) (education) (instruction) NEC V65.49
- HIV V65.44
- human immunodeficiency virus V65.44
- injury prevention V65.43
- insulin pump training V65.46
- marital V61.10
- medical (for) V65.9
  - boarding school resident V60.6
  - condition not demonstrated V65.5
  - feared complaint and no disease found V65.5
  - institutional resident V60.6
  - on behalf of another V65.19
  - person living alone V60.3
- natural family planning
  - procreative V26.41
  - to avoid pregnancy V25.04
- parent (guardian)-child conflict V61.20 ▲
  - adopted child V61.24 ●
  - biological child V61.23 ●
  - foster child V61.25 ●
  - specified problem NEC V61.29
- partner abuse
  - perpetrator V61.12
  - victim V61.11

Counseling – *continued*
- pediatric ~~pre-birth visit for expectant mother V65.11~~ ▲
  - pre-adoption visit for adoptive parent(s) V65.11 ●
  - pre-birth visit for expectant parents V65.11 ●
- perpetrator of
  - child abuse V62.83
    - parental V61.22
  - partner abuse V61.12
  - spouse abuse V61.12
- procreative V65.49
- sex NEC V65.49
  - transmitted disease NEC V65.45
    - HIV V65.44
- specified reason NEC V65.49
- spousal abuse
  - perpetrator V61.12
  - victim V61.11
- substance use and abuse V65.42
- syphilis V65.45
- victim (of)
  - abuse NEC V62.89
  - child abuse V61.21
  - partner abuse V61.11
  - spousal abuse V61.11

Coupled rhythm 427.89

Couvelaire uterus (complicating delivery) - *see* Placenta, separation

Cowper's gland - *see* condition

Cowperitis (*see also* Urethritis) 597.89
- gonorrheal (acute) 098.0
  - chronic or duration of 2 months or over 098.2

Cowpox (abortive) 051.01
- due to vaccination 999.0
- eyelid 051.01 *[373.5]*
  - postvaccination 999.0 *[373.5]*

Coxa
- plana 732.1
- valga (acquired) 736.31
  - congenital 755.61
  - late effect of rickets 268.1
- vara (acquired) 736.32
  - congenital 755.62
  - late effect of rickets 268.1

Coxae malum senilis 715.25

Coxalgia (nontuberculous) 719.45
- tuberculous (*see also* Tuberculosis) 015.1 5th *[730.85]*

Coxalgic pelvis 736.30

Coxitis 716.65

Coxsackie (infection) (virus) 079.2
- central nervous system NEC 048
- endocarditis 074.22
- enteritis 008.67
- meningitis (aseptic) 047.0
- myocarditis 074.23
- pericarditis 074.21
- pharyngitis 074.0
- pleurodynia 074.1
- specific disease NEC 074.8

Crabs, meaning pubic lice 132.2

Crack baby 760.75

Cracked
- nipple 611.2
  - puerperal, postpartum 676.1 5th
- tooth 521.81

Cradle cap 690.11

Craft neurosis 300.89

Craigiasis 007.8

Cramp(s) 729.82
- abdominal 789.0 5th
- bathing 994.1
- colic 789.7 ▲
  - infantile 789.7 ●
  - psychogenic 306.4
- due to immersion 994.1
- extremity (lower) (upper) NEC 729.82
- fireman 992.2
- heat 992.2
- hysterical 300.11
- immersion 994.1

Convalescence – Cramp(s)

Cramp(s) – Cuban itch

- **Cubitus**
  - valgus (acquired) 736.01
    - congenital 755.59
    - late effect of rickets 268.1
  - varus (acquired) 736.02
    - congenital 755.59
    - late effect of rickets 268.1
- **Cultural deprivation** V62.4
- **Cupping of optic disc** 377.14
- **Curling's ulcer** - *see* Ulcer, duodenum
- **Curling esophagus** 530.5
- **Curschmann (-Batten) (-Steinert) disease or syndrome** 359.21
- **Curvature**
  - organ or site, congenital NEC - *see* Distortion
  - penis (lateral) 752.69
  - Pott's (spinal) (*see also* Tuberculosis) 015.0 5th *[737.43]*
  - radius, idiopathic, progressive (congenital) 755.54
  - spine (acquired) (angular) (idiopathic) (incorrect) (postural) 737.9
    - congenital 754.2
    - due to or associated with
      - Charcôt-Marie-Tooth disease 356.1 *[737.40]*
      - mucopolysaccharidosis 277.5 *[737.40]*
      - neurofibromatosis 237.71 *[737.40]*
      - osteitis
        - deformans 731.0 *[737.40]*
        - fibrosa cystica 252.01 *[737.40]*
      - osteoporosis (*see also* Osteoporosis) 733.00 *[737.40]*
      - poliomyelitis (*see also* Poliomyelitis) 138 *[737.40]*
      - tuberculosis (Pott's curvature) (*see also* Tuberculosis) 015.0 5th *[737.43]*
    - kyphoscoliotic (*see also* Kyphoscoliosis) 737.30
    - kyphotic (*see also* Kyphosis) 737.10
    - late effect of rickets 268.1 *[737.40]*
    - Pott's 015.0 5th *[737.40]*
    - scoliotic (*see also* Scoliosis) 737.30
    - specified NEC 737.8
    - tuberculous 015.0 5th *[737.40]*
- **Cushing's**
  - basophilism, disease, or syndrome (iatrogenic) (idiopathic) (pituitary basophilism) (pituitary dependent) 255.0
  - ulcer - *see* Ulcer, peptic
- **Cushingoid due to steroid therapy**
  - correct substance properly administered 255.0
  - overdose or wrong substance given or taken 962.0
- **Cut** (external) - *see* Wound, open, by site
- **Cutaneous** - *see also* condition
  - hemorrhage 782.7
  - horn (cheek) (eyelid) (mouth) 702.8
  - larva migrans 126.9
- **Cutis** - *see also* condition
  - hyperelastic 756.83
    - acquired 701.8
  - laxa 756.83
    - senilis 701.8
  - marmorata 782.61
  - osteosis 709.3
  - pendula 756.83
    - acquired 701.8
  - rhomboidalis nuchae 701.8
  - verticis gyrata 757.39
    - acquired 701.8
- **Cyanopathy, newborn** 770.83
- **Cyanosis** 782.5
  - autotoxic 289.7
  - common atrioventricular canal 745.69
  - congenital 770.83
  - conjunctiva 372.71
  - due to
    - endocardial cushion defect 745.60

- **Cyanosis** – *continued*
  - due to – *continued*
    - nonclosure, foramen botalli 745.5
    - patent foramen botalli 745.5
    - persistent foramen ovale 745.5
  - enterogenous 289.7
  - fetus or newborn 770.83
  - ostium primum defect 745.61
  - paroxysmal digital 443.0
  - retina, retinal 362.10
- **Cycle**
  - anovulatory 628.0
  - menstrual, irregular 626.4
- **Cyclencephaly** 759.89
- **Cyclical vomiting** 536.2
  - associated with migraine 346.2 5th
  - psychogenic 306.4
- **Cyclitic membrane** 364.74
- **Cyclitis** (*see also* Iridocyclitis) 364.3
  - acute 364.00
    - primary 364.01
    - recurrent 364.02
  - chronic 364.10
    - in
      - sarcoidosis 135 *[364.11]*
      - tuberculosis (*see also* Tuberculosis) 017.3 5th *[364.11]*
  - Fuchs' heterochromic 364.21
  - granulomatous 364.10
  - lens induced 364.23
  - nongranulomatous 364.00
  - posterior 363.21
  - primary 364.01
  - recurrent 364.02
  - secondary (noninfectious) 364.04
    - infectious 364.03
  - subacute 364.00
    - primary 364.01
    - recurrent 364.02
- **Cyclokeratitis** - *see* Keratitis
- **Cyclophoria** 378.44
- **Cyclopia, cyclops** 759.89
- **Cycloplegia** 367.51
- **Cyclospasm** 367.53
- **Cyclosporiasis** 007.5
- **Cyclothymia** 301.13
- **Cyclothymic personality** 301.13
- **Cyclotropia** 378.33
- **Cyesis** - *see* Pregnancy
- **Cylindroma** (M8200/3) - *see also* Neoplasm, by site, malignant
  - eccrine dermal (M8200/0) - *see* Neoplasm, skin, benign
  - skin (M8200/0) - *see* Neoplasm, skin, benign
- **Cylindruria** 791.7
- **Cyllosoma** 759.89
- **Cynanche**
  - diphtheritic 032.3
  - tonsillaris 475
- **Cynorexia** 783.6
- **Cyphosis** - *see* Kyphosis
- **Cyprus fever** (*see also* Brucellosis) 023.9
- **Cyriax's syndrome** (slipping rib) 733.99

- **Cyst** (mucus) (retention) (serous) (simple)

Note *In general, cysts are not neoplastic and are classified to the appropriate category for disease of the specified anatomical site. This generalization does not apply to certain types of cysts which are neoplastic in nature, for example, dermoid, nor does it apply to cysts of certain structures, for example, branchial cleft, which are classified as developmental anomalies.*

The following listing includes some of the most frequently reported sites of cysts as well as qualifiers which indicate the type of cyst. The latter qualifiers usually are not repeated under the anatomical sites. Since the code assignment for a given site may vary depending upon the type of cyst, the coder should refer to the listings under the specified type of cyst before consideration is given to the site.

  - accessory, fallopian tube 752.11
  - adenoid (infected) 474.8
  - adrenal gland 255.8
    - congenital 759.1
  - air, lung 518.89
  - allantoic 753.7
  - alveolar process (jaw bone) 526.2
  - amnion, amniotic 658.8 5th
  - anterior chamber (eye) 364.60
    - exudative 364.62
    - implantation (surgical) (traumatic) 364.61
    - parasitic 360.13
  - anterior nasopalatine 526.1
  - antrum 478.19
  - anus 569.49
  - apical (periodontal) (tooth) 522.8
  - appendix 543.9
  - arachnoid, brain 348.0
  - arytenoid 478.79
  - auricle 706.2
  - Baker's (knee) 727.51
    - tuberculous (*see also* Tuberculosis) 015.2 5th
  - Bartholin's gland or duct 616.2
  - bile duct (*see also* Disease, biliary) 576.8
  - bladder (multiple) (trigone) 596.8
  - Blessig's 362.62
  - blood, endocardial (*see also* Endocarditis) 424.90
  - blue dome 610.0
  - bone (local) 733.20
    - aneurysmal 733.22
    - jaw 526.2
      - developmental (odontogenic) 526.0
      - fissural 526.1
      - latent 526.89
    - solitary 733.21
    - unicameral 733.21
  - brain 348.0
    - congenital 742.4
    - hydatid (*see also* Echinococcus) 122.9
    - third ventricle (colloid) 742.4
  - branchial (cleft) 744.42
  - branchiogenic 744.42
  - breast (benign) (blue dome) (pedunculated) (solitary) (traumatic) 610.0
    - involution 610.4
    - sebaceous 610.8
  - broad ligament (benign) 620.8
    - embryonic 752.11
  - bronchogenic (mediastinal) (sequestration) 518.89
    - congenital 748.4
  - buccal 528.4
  - bulbourethral gland (Cowper's) 599.89
  - bursa, bursal 727.49
    - pharyngeal 478.26

- **Cyst** – *continued*
  - calcifying odontogenic (M9301/0) 213.1
    - upper jaw (bone) 213.0
  - canal of Nuck (acquired) (serous) 629.1
    - congenital 752.41
  - canthus 372.75
  - carcinomatous (M8010/3) - *see* Neoplasm, by site, malignant
  - cartilage (joint) - *see* Derangement, joint
  - cauda equina 336.8
  - cavum septi pellucidi NEC 348.0
  - celomic (pericardium) 746.89
  - cerebellopontine (angle) - *see* Cyst, brain
  - cerebellum - *see* Cyst, brain
  - cerebral - *see* Cyst, brain
  - cervical lateral 744.42
  - cervix 622.8
    - embryonal 752.41
    - nabothian (gland) 616.0
  - chamber, anterior (eye) 364.60
    - exudative 364.62
    - implantation (surgical) (traumatic) 364.61
    - parasitic 360.13
  - chiasmal, optic NEC (*see also* Lesion, chiasmal) 377.54
  - chocolate (ovary) 617.1
  - choledochal (congenital) 751.69
    - acquired 576.8
  - choledochus 751.69
  - chorion 658.8 5th
  - choroid plexus 348.0
  - chyle, mesentery 457.8
  - ciliary body 364.60
    - exudative 364.64
    - implantation 364.61
    - primary 364.63
  - clitoris 624.8
  - coccyx (*see also* Cyst, bone) 733.20
  - colloid
    - third ventricle (brain) 742.4
    - thyroid gland - *see* Goiter
  - colon 569.89
  - common (bile) duct (*see also* Disease, biliary) 576.8
  - congenital NEC 759.89
    - adrenal glands 759.1
    - epiglottis 748.3
    - esophagus 750.4
    - fallopian tube 752.11
    - kidney 753.10
      - multiple 753.19
      - single 753.11
    - larynx 748.3
    - liver 751.62
    - lung 748.4
    - mediastinum 748.8
    - ovary 752.0
    - oviduct 752.11
    - pancreas 751.7
    - periurethral (tissue) 753.8
    - prepuce NEC 752.69
      - penis 752.69
    - sublingual 750.26
    - submaxillary gland 750.26
    - thymus (gland) 759.2
    - tongue 750.19
    - ureterovesical orifice 753.4
    - vulva 752.41
  - conjunctiva 372.75
  - cornea 371.23
  - corpora quadrigemina 348.0
  - corpus
    - albicans (ovary) 620.2
    - luteum (ruptured) 620.1
  - Cowper's gland (benign) (infected) 599.89
  - cranial meninges 348.0
  - craniobuccal pouch 253.8
  - craniopharyngeal pouch 253.8
  - cystic duct (*see also* Disease, gallbladder) 575.8
  - Cysticercus (any site) 123.1

Cubitus – Cyst

Cyst

Cyst – *continued*
  rectum (epithelium) (mucous) 569.49
  renal - *see* Cyst, kidney
  residual (radicular) 522.8
  retention (ovary) 620.2
  retina 361.19
    macular 362.54
    parasitic 360.13
    primary 361.13
    secondary 361.14
  retroperitoneal 568.89
  sacrococcygeal (dermoid) 685.1
    with abscess 685.0
  salivary gland or duct 527.6
    mucous extravasation or retention 527.6
  Sampson's 617.1
  sclera 379.19
  scrotum (sebaceous) 706.2
    sweat glands 706.2
  sebaceous (duct) (gland) 706.2
    breast 610.8
    eyelid 374.84
    genital organ NEC
      female 629.89
      male 608.89
    scrotum 706.2
  semilunar cartilage (knee) (multiple) 717.5
  seminal vesicle 608.89
  serous (ovary) 620.2
  sinus (antral) (ethmoidal) (frontal) (maxillary) (nasal) (sphenoidal) 478.19
  Skene's gland 599.89
  skin (epidermal) (epidermoid, inclusion) (epithelial) (inclusion) (retention) (sebaceous) 706.2
    breast 610.8
    eyelid 374.84
    genital organ NEC
      female 629.89
      male 608.89
    neoplastic 216.3
    scrotum 706.2
    sweat gland or duct 705.89
  solitary
    bone 733.21
    kidney 593.2
  spermatic cord 608.89
  sphenoid sinus 478.19
  spinal meninges 349.2
  spine (*see also* Cyst, bone) 733.20
  spleen NEC 289.59
    congenital 759.0
    hydatid (*see also* Echinococcus) 122.9
  spring water (pericardium) 746.89
  subarachnoid 348.0
    intrasellar 793.0
  subdural (cerebral) 348.0
    spinal cord 349.2
  sublingual gland 527.6
    mucous extravasation or retention 527.6
  submaxillary gland 527.6
    mucous extravasation or retention 527.6
  suburethral 599.89
  suprarenal gland 255.8
  suprasellar - *see* Cyst, brain
  sweat gland or duct 705.89
  sympathetic nervous system 337.9
  synovial 727.40
    popliteal space 727.51
  Tarlov's 355.9
  tarsal 373.2
  tendon (sheath) 727.42
  testis 608.89
  theca-lutein (ovary) 620.2
  Thornwaldt's, Tornwaldt's 478.26
  thymus (gland) 254.8
  thyroglossal (duct) (infected) (persistent) 759.2

Cyst – *continued*
  thyroid (gland) 246.2
    adenomatous - *see* Goiter, nodular
    colloid (*see also* Goiter) 240.9
  thyrolingual duct (infected) (persistent) 759.2
  tongue (mucous) 529.8
  tonsil 474.8
  tooth (dental root) 522.8
  tubo-ovarian 620.8
    inflammatory 614.1
  tunica vaginalis 608.89
  turbinate (nose) (*see also* Cyst, bone) 733.20
  Tyson's gland (benign) (infected) 607.89
  umbilicus 759.89
  urachus 753.7
  ureter 593.89
  ureterovesical orifice 593.89
    congenital 753.4
  urethra 599.84
  urethral gland (Cowper's) 599.89
  uterine
    ligament 620.8
      embryonic 752.11
    tube 620.8
  uterus (body) (corpus) (recurrent) 621.8
    embryonal 752.3
  utricle (ear) 386.8
    prostatic 599.89
  utriculus masculinus 599.89
  vagina, vaginal (squamous cell) (wall) 623.8
    embryonal 752.41
    implantation 623.8
    inclusion 623.8
  vallecula, vallecular 478.79
  ventricle, neuroepithelial 348.0
  verumontanum 599.89
  vesical (orifice) 596.8
  vitreous humor 379.29
  vulva (sweat glands) 624.8
    congenital 752.41
    implantation 624.8
    inclusion 624.8
    sebaceous gland 624.8
  vulvovaginal gland 624.8
  wolffian 752.89
Cystadenocarcinoma (M8440/3) - *see also* Neoplasm, by site, malignant
  bile duct type (M8161/3) 155.1
  endometrioid (M8380/3) - *see* Neoplasm, by site, malignant
  mucinous (M8470/3)
    papillary (M8471/3)
      specified site - *see* Neoplasm, by site, malignant
      unspecified site 183.0
    specified site - *see* Neoplasm, by site, malignant
    unspecified site 183.0
  papillary (M8450/3)
    mucinous (M8471/3)
      specified site - *see* Neoplasm, by site, malignant
      unspecified site 183.0
    pseudomucinous (M8471/3)
      specified site - *see* Neoplasm, by site, malignant
      unspecified site 183.0
    serous (M8460/3)
      specified site - *see* Neoplasm, by site, malignant
      unspecified site 183.0
    specified site - *see* Neoplasm, by site, malignant
    unspecified 183.0
  pseudomucinous (M8470/3)
    papillary (M8471/3)
      specified site - *see* Neoplasm, by site, malignant
      unspecified site 183.0
    specified site - *see* Neoplasm, by site, malignant

Cystadenocarcinoma – *continued*
  pseudomucinous – *continued*
    unspecified site 183.0
  serous (M8441/3)
    papillary (M8460/3)
      specified site - *see* Neoplasm, by site, malignant
      unspecified site 183.0
    specified site - *see* Neoplasm, by site, malignant
    unspecified site 183.0
Cystadenofibroma (M9013/0)
  clear cell (M8313/0) - *see* Neoplasm, by site, benign
  endometrioid (M8381/0) 220
    borderline malignancy (M8381/1) 236.2
    malignant (M8381/3) 183.0
  mucinous (M9015/0)
    specified site - *see* Neoplasm, by site, benign
    unspecified site 220
  serous (M9014/0)
    specified site - *see* Neoplasm, by site, benign
    unspecified site 220
  specified site - *see* Neoplasm, by site, benign
  unspecified site 220
Cystadenoma (M8440/0) - *see also* Neoplasm, by site, benign
  bile duct (M8161/0) 211.5
  endometrioid (M8380/0) - *see also* Neoplasm, by site, benign
    borderline malignancy (M8380/1) - *see* Neoplasm, by site, uncertain behavior
  malignant (M8440/3) - *see* Neoplasm, by site, malignant
  mucinous (M8470/0)
    borderline malignancy (M8470/1)
      specified site - *see* Neoplasm, uncertain behavior
      unspecified site 236.2
    papillary (M8471/0)
      borderline malignancy (M8471/1)
        specified site - *see* Neoplasm, by site, uncertain behavior
        unspecified site 236.2
      specified site - *see* Neoplasm, by site, benign
      unspecified site 220
    specified site - *see* Neoplasm, by site, benign
    unspecified site 220
  papillary (M8450/0)
    borderline malignancy (M8450/1)
      specified site - *see* Neoplasm, by site, uncertain behavior
      unspecified site 236.2
    lymphomatosum (M8561/0) 210.2
    mucinous (M8471/0)
      borderline malignancy (M8471/1)
        specified site - *see* Neoplasm, by site, uncertain behavior
        unspecified site 236.2
      specified site - *see* Neoplasm, by site, benign
      unspecified site 220
    pseudomucinous (M8471/0)
      borderline malignancy (M8471/1)
        specified site - *see* Neoplasm, by site uncertain behavior
        unspecified site 236.2
      specified site - *see* Neoplasm, by site, benign
      unspecified site 220
    serous (M8460/0)
      borderline malignancy (M8460/1)
        specified site - *see* Neoplasm, by site, uncertain behavior
        unspecified site 236.2
      specified site - *see* Neoplasm, by site, benign

Cystadenoma – *continued*
  papillary – *continued*
    serous – *continued*
      unspecified site 220
    specified site - *see* Neoplasm, by site, benign
    unspecified site 220
  pseudomucinous (M8470/0)
    borderline malignancy (M8470/1)
      specified site - *see* Neoplasm, by site uncertain behavior
      unspecified site 236.2
    papillary (M8471/0)
      borderline malignancy (M8471/1)
        specified site - *see* Neoplasm, by site uncertain behavior
        unspecified site 236.2
      specified site - *see* Neoplasm, by site, benign
      unspecified site 220
    specified site - *see* Neoplasm, by site, benign
    unspecified site 220
  serous (M8441/0)
    borderline malignancy (M8441/1)
      specified site - *see* Neoplasm, by site, uncertain behavior
      unspecified site 236.2
    papillary (M8460/0)
      borderline malignancy (M8460/1)
        specified site - *see* Neoplasm, by site, uncertain behavior
        unspecified site 236.2
      specified site - *see* Neoplasm, by site, benign
      unspecified site 220
    specified site - *see* Neoplasm, by site, benign
    unspecified site 220
  thyroid 226
Cystathioninemia 270.4
Cystathioninuria 270.4
Cystic - *see also* condition
  breast, chronic 610.1
  corpora lutea 620.1
  degeneration, congenital
    brain 742.4
    kidney (*see also* Cystic, disease, kidney) 753.10
  disease
    breast, chronic 610.1
    kidney, congenital 753.10
      medullary 753.16
      multiple 753.19
      polycystic - *see* Polycystic, kidney
      single 753.11
      specified NEC 753.19
    liver, congenital 751.62
    lung 518.89
      congenital 748.4
    pancreas, congenital 751.7
    semilunar cartilage 717.5
  duct - *see* condition
  eyeball, congenital 743.03
  fibrosis (pancreas) 277.00
    with
      manifestations
        gastrointestinal 277.03
        pulmonary 277.02
        specified NEC 277.09
      meconium ileus 277.01
      pulmonary exacerbation 277.02
  hygroma (M9173/0) 228.1
  kidney, congenital 753.10
    medullary 753.16
    multiple 753.19
    polycystic - *see* Polycystic, kidney
    single 753.11
    specified NEC 753.19
  liver, congenital 751.62
  lung 518.89
    congenital 748.4
  mass - *see* Cyst
  mastitis, chronic 610.1

Cystic – *continued*
- ovary 620.2
- pancreas, congenital 751.7

Cysticerciasis 123.1
Cysticercosis (mammary) (subretinal) 123.1
Cysticercus 123.1
- cellulosae infestation 123.1

Cystinosis (malignant) 270.0
Cystinuria 270.0
Cystitis (bacillary) (colli) (diffuse) (exudative) (hemorrhagic) (purulent) (recurrent) (septic) (suppurative) (ulcerative) 595.9
- with
  - abortion - *see* Abortion, by type, with urinary tract infection
  - ectopic pregnancy (*see also* categories 633.0-633.9) 639.8
  - fibrosis 595.1
  - leukoplakia 595.1
  - malakoplakia 595.1
  - metaplasia 595.1
  - molar pregnancy (*see also* categories 630-632) 639.8
- actinomycotic 039.8 *[595.4]*
- acute 595.0
  - of trigone 595.3
- allergic 595.89
- amebic 006.8 *[595.4]*
- bilharzial 120.9 *[595.4]*
- blennorrhagic (acute) 098.11
  - chronic or duration of 2 months or more 098.31
- bullous 595.89
- calculous 594.1
- chlamydial 099.53
- chronic 595.2
  - interstitial 595.1
  - of trigone 595.3
- complicating pregnancy, childbirth, or puerperium 646.6 5th
  - affecting fetus or newborn 760.1
- cystic(a) 595.81
- diphtheritic 032.84
- echinococcal
  - glanulosus 122.3 *[595.4]*
  - multilocularis 122.6 *[595.4]*
- emphysematous 595.89
- encysted 595.81
- follicular 595.3
- following
  - abortion 639.8
  - ectopic or molar pregnancy 639.8
- gangrenous 595.89
- glandularis 595.89
- gonococcal (acute) 098.11
  - chronic or duration of 2 months or more 098.31
- incrusted 595.89
- interstitial 595.1
- irradiation 595.82
- irritation 595.89
- malignant 595.89
- monilial 112.2
- of trigone 595.3
- panmural 595.1
- polyposa 595.89
- prostatic 601.3
- radiation 595.82
- Reiter's (abacterial) 099.3
- specified NEC 595.89
- subacute 595.2
- submucous 595.1
- syphilitic 095.8
- trichomoniasis 131.09
- tuberculous (*see also* Tuberculosis) 016.1 5th
- ulcerative 595.1

Cystocele
- female (without uterine prolapse) 618.01
  - with uterine prolapse 618.4
    - complete 618.3
    - incomplete 618.2
  - lateral 618.02

Cystocele – *continued*
- female – *continued*
  - midline 618.01
  - paravaginal 618.02
- in pregnancy or childbirth 654.4 5th
  - affecting fetus or newborn 763.89
  - causing obstructed labor 660.2 5th
    - affecting fetus or newborn 763.1
- male 596.8

Cystoid
- cicatrix limbus 372.64
- degeneration macula 362.53

Cystolithiasis 594.1
Cystoma (M8440/0) - *see also* Neoplasm, by site, benign
- endometrial, ovary 617.1
- mucinous (M8470/0)
  - specified site - *see* Neoplasm, by site, benign
  - unspecified site 220
- serous (M8441/0)
  - specified site - *see* Neoplasm, by site, benign
  - unspecified site 220
- simple (ovary) 620.2

Cystoplegia 596.53
Cystoptosis 596.8
Cystopyelitis (*see also* Pyelitis) 590.80
Cystorrhagia 596.8
Cystosarcoma phyllodes (M9020/1) 238.3
- benign (M9020/0) 217
- malignant (M9020/3) - *see* Neoplasm, breast, malignant

Cystostomy status V44.50
- with complication 997.5
- appendico-vesicostomy V44.52
- cutaneous-vesicostomy V44.51
- specifed type NEC V44.59

Cystourethritis (*see also* Urethritis) 597.89
Cystourethrocele (*see also* Cystocele)
- female (without uterine prolapse) 618.09
  - with uterine prolapse 618.4
    - complete 618.3
    - incomplete 618.2
- male 596.8

Cytomegalic inclusion disease 078.5
- congenital 771.1

Cytomycosis, reticuloendothelial (*see also* Histoplasmosis, American) 115.00
Cytopenia 289.9
- refractory
  - with
    - multilineage dysplasia (RCMD) 238.72
      - and ringed sideroblasts (RCMD-RS) 238.72

D

Daae (-Finsen) disease (epidemic pleurodynia) 074.1
Dabney's grip 074.1
Da Costa's syndrome (neurocirculatory asthenia) 306.2
Dacryoadenitis, dacryadenitis 375.00
- acute 375.01
- chronic 375.02

Dacryocystitis 375.30
- acute 375.32
- chronic 375.42
- neonatal 771.6
- phlegmonous 375.33
- syphilitic 095.8
  - congenital 090.0
- trachomatous, active 076.1
  - late effect 139.1
- tuberculous (*see also* Tuberculosis) 017.3 5th

Dacryocystoblenorrhea 375.42
Dacryocystocele 375.43
Dacryolith, dacryolithiasis 375.57
Dacryoma 375.43
Dacryopericystitis (acute) (subacute) 375.32
- chronic 375.42

Dacryops 375.11
Dacryosialadenopathy, atrophic 710.2
Dacryostenosis 375.56
- congenital 743.65

Dactylitis
- bone (*see also* Osteomyelitis) 730.2 5th
- sickle-cell 282.62
  - Hb-C 282.64
  - Hb-SS 282.62
  - specified NEC 282.69
- syphilitic 095.5
- tuberculous (*see also* Tuberculosis) 015.5 5th

Dactylolysis spontanea 136.0
Dactylosymphysis (*see also* Syndactylism) 755.10
Damage
- arteriosclerotic - *see* Arteriosclerosis
- brain 348.9
  - anoxic, hypoxic 348.1
    - during or resulting from a procedure 997.01
    - ischemic, in newborn 768.7<u>0</u> ▲
      - mild 768.71 ●
      - moderate 768.72 ●
      - severe 768.73 ●
  - child NEC 343.9
  - due to birth injury 767.0
  - minimal (child) (*see also* Hyperkinesia) 314.9
  - newborn 767.0
- cardiac - *see also* Disease, heart
- cardiorenal (vascular) (*see also* Hypertension, cardiorenal) 404.90
- central nervous system - *see* Damage, brain
- cerebral NEC - *see* Damage, brain
- coccyx, complicating delivery 665.6 5th
- coronary (*see also* Ischemia, heart) 414.9
- eye, birth injury 767.8
- heart - *see also* Disease, heart
  - valve - *see* Endocarditis
- hypothalamus NEC 348.9
- liver 571.9
  - alcoholic 571.3
- medication 995.20
- myocardium (*see also* Degeneration, myocardial) 429.1
- pelvic
  - joint or ligament, during delivery 665.6 5th
  - organ NEC
    - with
      - abortion - *see* Abortion, by type, with damage to pelvic organs
      - ectopic pregnancy (*see also* categories 633.0-633.9) 639.2
      - molar pregnancy (*see also* categories 630-632) 639.2
    - during delivery 665.5 5th
    - following
      - abortion 639.2
      - ectopic or molar pregnancy 639.2
- renal (*see also* Disease, renal) 593.9
- skin, solar 692.79
  - acute 692.72
  - chronic 692.74
- subendocardium, subendocardial (*see also* Degeneration, myocardial) 429.1
- vascular 459.9

Dameshek's syndrome (erythroblastic anemia) 282.49
Dana-Putnam syndrome (subacute combined sclerosis with pernicious anemia) 281.0 *[336.2]*
Danbolt (-Closs) syndrome (acrodermatitis enteropathica) 686.8
Dandruff 690.18
Dandy fever 061
Dandy-Walker deformity or syndrome (atresia, foramen of Magendie) 742.3
- with spina bifida (*see also* Spina bifida) 741.0 5th

Dangle foot 736.79
Danielssen's disease (anesthetic leprosy) 030.1
Danlos' syndrome 756.83
Darier's disease (congenital) (keratosis follicularis) 757.39
- due to vitamin A deficiency 264.8
- meaning erythema annulare centrifugum 695.0

Darier-Roussy sarcoid 135
Dark area on retina 239.81 ●
Darling's
- disease (*see also* Histoplasmosis, American) 115.00
- histoplasmosis (*see also* Histoplasmosis, American) 115.00

Dartre 054.9
Darwin's tubercle 744.29
Davidson's anemia (refractory) 284.9
Davies' disease 425.0
Davies-Colley syndrome (slipping rib) 733.99
Dawson's encephalitis 046.2
Day blindness (*see also* Blindness, day) 368.60
Dead
- fetus
  - retained (in utero) 656.4 5th
    - early pregnancy (death before 22 completed weeks gestation) 632
    - late (death after 22 completed weeks gestation) 656.4 5th
  - syndrome 641.3 5th
- labyrinth 386.50
- ovum, retained 631

Deaf and dumb NEC 389.7
Deaf mutism (acquired) (congenital) NEC 389.7
- endemic 243
- hysterical 300.11
- syphilitic, congenital 090.0

Deafness (acquired) (complete) (congenital) (hereditary) (middle ear) (partial) 389.9
- with
  - blindness V49.85
  - blue sclera and fragility of bone 756.51
- auditory fatigue 389.9
- aviation 993.0
  - nerve injury 951.5
- boilermakers' 951.5
- central 389.14
  - with conductive hearing loss 389.20
    - bilateral 389.22
    - unilateral 389.21
- conductive (air) 389.00
  - with sensorineural hearing loss 389.20
    - bilateral 389.22
    - unilateral 389.21
  - bilateral 389.06
  - combined types 389.08
  - external ear 389.01
  - inner ear 389.04
  - middle ear 389.03
  - multiple types 389.08
  - tympanic membrane 389.02
  - unilateral 389.05
- emotional (complete) 300.11
- functional (complete) 300.11
- high frequency 389.8
- hysterical (complete) 300.11
- injury 951.5
- low frequency 389.8
- mental 784.69
- mixed conductive and sensorineural 389.20
  - bilateral 389.22
  - unilateral 389.21

- **Deafness** – *continued*
  - nerve
    - with conductive hearing loss 389.20
      - bilateral 389.22
      - unilateral 389.21
    - bilateral 389.12
    - unilateral 389.13
  - neural
    - with conductive hearing loss 389.20
      - bilateral 389.22
      - unilateral 389.21
    - bilateral 389.12
    - unilateral 389.13
  - noise-induced 388.12
    - nerve injury 951.5
  - nonspeaking 389.7
  - perceptive 389.10
    - with conductive hearing loss 389.20
      - bilateral 389.22
      - unilateral 389.21
    - central 389.14
    - neural
      - bilateral 389.12
      - unilateral 389.13
    - sensorineural 389.10
      - asymmetrical 389.16
      - bilateral 389.18
      - unilateral 389.15
    - sensory
      - bilateral 389.11
      - unilateral 389.17
  - psychogenic (complete) 306.7
  - sensorineural (*see also* Deafness, perceptive) 389.10
    - asymmetrical 389.16
    - bilateral 389.18
    - unilateral 389.15
  - sensory
    - with conductive hearing loss 389.20
      - bilateral 389.22
      - unilateral 389.21
    - bilateral 389.11
    - unilateral 389.17
  - specified type NEC 389.8
  - sudden NEC 388.2
  - syphilitic 094.89
  - transient ischemic 388.02
  - transmission - *see* Deafness, conductive
  - traumatic 951.5
  - word (secondary to organic lesion) 784.69
    - developmental 315.31
- **Death**
  - after delivery (cause not stated) (sudden) 674.9 [5th]
  - anesthetic
    - due to
      - correct substance properly administered 995.4
      - overdose or wrong substance given 968.4
        - specified anesthetic - *see* Table of Drugs and Chemicals
    - during delivery 668.9 [5th]
  - brain 348.82 ▲
  - cardiac (sudden) (SCD) - code to underlying condition
    - family history of V17.41
    - personal history of, successfully resuscitated V12.53
  - cause unknown 798.2
  - cot (infant) 798.0
  - crib (infant) 798.0
  - fetus, fetal (cause not stated) (intrauterine) 779.9
    - early, with retention (before 22 completed weeks gestation) 632
    - from asphyxia or anoxia (before labor) 768.0
      - during labor 768.1
    - late, affecting management of pregnancy (after 22 completed weeks gestation) 656.4 [5th]
  - from pregnancy NEC 646.9 [5th]
  - instantaneous 798.1
- **Death** – *continued*
  - intrauterine (*see also* Death, fetus) 779.9
    - complicating pregnancy 656.4 [5th]
  - maternal, affecting fetus or newborn 761.6
  - neonatal NEC 779.9
  - sudden (cause unknown) 798.1
    - cardiac (SCD)
      - family history of V17.41
      - personal history of, successfully resuscitated V12.53
    - during delivery 669.9 [5th]
      - under anesthesia NEC 668.9
    - infant, syndrome (SIDS) 798.0
    - puerperal, during puerperium 674.9 [5th]
  - unattended (cause unknown) 798.9
  - under anesthesia NEC
    - due to
      - correct substance properly administered 995.4
      - overdose or wrong substance given 968.4
        - specified anesthetic - *see* Table of Drugs and Chemicals
    - during delivery 668.9 [5th]
  - violent 798.1
- **de Beurmann-Gougerot disease** (sporotrichosis) 117.1
- **Debility** (general) (infantile) (postinfectional) 799.3
  - with nutritional difficulty 269.9
  - congenital or neonatal NEC 779.9
  - nervous 300.5
  - old age 797
  - senile 797
- **Débove's disease** (splenomegaly) 789.2
- **Decalcification**
  - bone (*see also* Osteoporosis) 733.00
  - teeth 521.89
- **Decapitation** 874.9
  - fetal (to facilitate delivery) 763.89
- **Decapsulation, kidney** 593.89
- **Decay**
  - dental 521.00
  - senile 797
  - tooth, teeth 521.00
- **Decensus, uterus** - *see* Prolapse, uterus
- **Deciduitis** (acute)
  - with
    - abortion - *see* Abortion, by type, with sepsis
    - ectopic pregnancy (*see also* categories 633.0-633.9) 639.0
    - molar pregnancy (*see also* categories 630-632) 639.0
  - affecting fetus or newborn 760.8
  - following
    - abortion 639.0
    - ectopic or molar pregnancy 639.0
  - in pregnancy 646.6 [5th]
  - puerperal, postpartum 670.1 [5th] ▲
- **Deciduoma malignum** (M9100/3) 181
- **Deciduous tooth** (retained) 520.6
- **Decline** (general) (*see also* Debility) 799.3
- **Decompensation**
  - cardiac (acute) (chronic) (*see also* Disease, heart) 429.9
    - failure - *see* Failure, heart
  - cardiorenal (*see also* Hypertension, cardiorenal) 404.90
  - cardiovascular (*see also* Disease, cardiovascular) 429.2
  - heart (*see also* Disease, heart) 429.9
    - failure - *see* Failure, heart
  - hepatic 572.2
  - myocardial (acute) (chronic) (*see also* Disease, heart) 429.9
    - failure - *see* Failure, heart
  - respiratory 519.9
- **Decompression sickness** 993.3
- **Decrease, decreased**
  - blood
    - platelets (*see also* Thrombocytopenia) 287.5
- **Decrease, decreased** – *continued*
  - blood – *continued*
    - pressure 796.3
      - due to shock following
        - injury 958.4
        - operation 998.0
    - white cell count 288.50
      - specified NEC 288.59
  - cardiac reserve - *see* Disease, heart
  - estrogen 256.39
    - postablative 256.2
  - fetal movements 655.7 [5th]
  - fragility of erythrocytes 289.89
  - function
    - adrenal (cortex) 255.41
      - medulla 255.5
    - ovary in hypopituitarism 253.4
    - parenchyma of pancreas 577.8
    - pituitary (gland) (lobe) (anterior) 253.2
      - posterior (lobe) 253.8
  - functional activity 780.99
  - glucose 790.29
  - haptoglobin (serum) NEC 273.8
  - leukocytes 288.50
  - libido 799.81
  - lymphocytes 288.51
  - platelets (*see also* Thrombocytopenia) 287.5
  - pulse pressure 785.9
  - respiration due to shock following injury 958.4
  - sexual desire 799.81
  - tear secretion NEC 375.15
  - tolerance
    - fat 579.8
    - salt and water 276.9
  - vision NEC 369.9
  - white blood cell count 288.50
- **Decubital gangrene** (*see also* Ulcer, pressure) 707.00 *[785.4]*
- **Decubiti** (*see also* Ulcer, pressure) 707.00
- **Decubitus** (ulcer) (*see also* Ulcer, pressure) 707.00
  - with gangrene 707.00 *[785.4]*
  - ankle 707.06
  - back
    - lower 707.03
    - upper 707.02
  - buttock 707.05
  - coccyx 707.03 ●
  - elbow 707.01
  - head 707.09
  - heel 707.07
  - hip 707.04
  - other site 707.09
  - sacrum 707.03
  - shoulder blades 707.02
- **Deepening acetabulum** 718.85
- **Defect, defective** 759.9
  - 3-beta-hydroxysteroid dehydrogenase 255.2
  - 11-hydroxylase 255.2
  - 21-hydroxylase 255.2
  - abdominal wall, congenital 756.70
  - aorticopulmonary septum 745.0
  - aortic septal 745.0
  - atrial septal (ostium secundum type) 745.5
    - acquired 429.71
    - ostium primum type 745.61
    - sinus venosus 745.8
  - atrioventricular
    - canal 745.69
    - septum 745.4
      - acquired 429.71
  - atrium secundum 745.5
    - acquired 429.71
  - auricular septal 745.5
    - acquired 429.71
  - bilirubin excretion 277.4
  - biosynthesis, testicular androgen 257.2
  - bridge 525.60
  - bulbar septum 745.0
- **Defect, defective** – *continued*
  - butanol-insoluble iodide 246.1
  - chromosome - *see* Anomaly, chromosome
  - circulation (acquired) 459.9
    - congenital 747.9
    - newborn 747.9
  - clotting NEC (*see also* Defect, coagulation) 286.9
  - coagulation (factor) (*see also* Deficiency, coagulation factor) 286.9
    - with
      - abortion - *see* Abortion, by type, with hemorrhage
      - ectopic pregnancy (*see also* categories 634-638) 639.1
      - molar pregnancy (*see also* categories 630-632) 639.1
    - acquired (any) 286.7
    - antepartum or intrapartum 641.3 [5th]
      - affecting fetus or newborn 762.1
    - causing hemorrhage of pregnancy or delivery 641.3 [5th]
    - complicating pregnancy, childbirth, or puerperium 649.3 [5th]
    - due to
      - liver disease 286.7
      - vitamin K deficiency 286.7
    - newborn, transient 776.3
    - postpartum 666.3 [5th]
    - specified type NEC 286.9
  - conduction (heart) 426.9
    - bone (*see also* Deafness, conductive) 389.00
  - congenital, organ or site NEC - *see also* Anomaly
    - circulation 747.9
    - Descemet's membrane 743.9
      - specified type NEC 743.49
    - diaphragm 756.6
    - ectodermal 757.9
    - esophagus 750.9
    - pulmonic cusps - *see* Anomaly, heart valve
    - respiratory system 748.9
      - specified type NEC 748.8
  - crown 525.60
  - cushion endocardial 745.60
  - dental restoration 525.60
  - dentin (hereditary) 520.5
  - Descemet's membrane (congenital) 743.9
    - acquired 371.30
    - specific type NEC 743.49
  - deutan 368.52
  - developmental - *see also* Anomaly, by site
    - cauda equina 742.59
    - left ventricle 746.9
      - with atresia or hypoplasia of aortic orifice or valve, with hypoplasia of ascending aorta 746.7
      - in hypoplastic left heart syndrome 746.7
    - testis 752.9
    - vessel 747.9
  - diaphragm
    - with elevation, eventration, or hernia - *see* Hernia, diaphragm
    - congenital 756.6
      - with elevation, eventration, or hernia 756.6
      - gross (with elevation, eventration, or hernia) 756.6
  - ectodermal, congenital 757.9
  - Eisenmenger's (ventricular septal defect) 745.4
  - endocardial cushion 745.60
    - specified type NEC 745.69
  - esophagus, congenital 750.9
  - extensor retinaculum 728.9
  - fibrin polymerization (*see also* Defect, coagulation) 286.3
  - filling
    - biliary tract 793.3
    - bladder 793.5

Defect, defective – *continued*
- filling – *continued*
  - dental 525.60
  - gallbladder 793.3
  - kidney 793.5
  - stomach 793.4
  - ureter 793.5
- fossa ovalis 745.5
- gene, carrier (suspected) of V83.89
- Gerbode 745.4
- glaucomatous, without elevated tension 365.89
- Hageman (factor) (*see also* Defect, coagulation) 286.3
- hearing (*see also* Deafness) 389.9
- high grade 317
- homogentisic acid 270.2
- interatrial septal 745.5
  - acquired 429.71
- interauricular septal 745.5
  - acquired 429.71
- interventricular septal 745.4
  - with pulmonary stenosis or atresia, dextraposition of aorta, and hypertrophy of right ventricle 745.2
  - acquired 429.71
  - in tetralogy of Fallot 745.2
- iodide trapping 246.1
- iodotyrosine dehalogenase 246.1
- kynureninase 270.2
- learning, specific 315.2
- major osseous 731.3
- mental (*see also* Retardation, mental) 319
- osseous, major 731.3
- osteochondral NEC 738.8
- ostium
  - primum 745.61
  - secundum 745.5
- pericardium 746.89
- peroxidase-binding 246.1
- placental blood supply - *see* Placenta, insufficiency
- platelet (qualitative) 287.1
  - constitutional 286.4
- postural, spine 737.9
- protan 368.51
- pulmonic cusps, congenital 746.00
- renal pelvis 753.9
  - obstructive 753.29
  - specified type NEC 753.3
- respiratory system, congenital 748.9
  - specified type NEC 748.8
- retina, retinal 361.30
  - with detachment (*see also* Detachment, retina, with retinal defect) 361.00
  - multiple 361.33
    - with detachment 361.02
  - nerve fiber bundle 362.85
  - single 361.30
    - with detachment 361.01
- septal (closure) (heart) NEC 745.9
  - acquired 429.71
  - atrial 745.5
  - specified type NEC 745.8
- speech NEC 784.5<u>9</u> ▲
  - developmental 315.39
  - late effect of cerebrovascular disease - *see* Late effect(s) (of) cerebrovascular disease, speech and language deficit ●
  - secondary to organic lesion 784.5<u>9</u> ▲
- Taussig-Bing (transposition, aorta and overriding pulmonary artery) 745.11
- teeth, wedge 521.20
- thyroid hormone synthesis 246.1
- tritan 368.53
- ureter 753.9
  - obstructive 753.29
- vascular (acquired) (local) 459.9
  - congenital (peripheral) NEC 747.60
    - gastrointestinal 747.61

Defect, defective – *continued*
- vascular – *continued*
  - congenital – *continued*
    - lower limb 747.64
    - renal 747.62
    - specified NEC 747.69
    - spinal 747.82
    - upper limb 747.63
- ventricular septal 745.4
  - with pulmonary stenosis or atresia, dextraposition of aorta, and hypertrophy of right ventricle 745.2
  - acquired 429.71
  - atrioventricular canal type 745.69
  - between infundibulum and anterior portion 745.4
  - in tetralogy of Fallot 745.2
  - isolated anterior 745.4
- vision NEC 369.9
- visual field 368.40
  - arcuate 368.43
  - heteronymous, bilateral 368.47
  - homonymous, bilateral 368.46
  - localized NEC 368.44
  - nasal step 368.44
  - peripheral 368.44
  - sector 368.43
- voice <u>and resonance</u> 784.40 ▲
- wedge, teeth (abrasion) 521.20

Defeminization syndrome 255.2

Deferentitis 608.4
- gonorrheal (acute) 098.14
  - chronic or duration of 2 months or over 098.34

Defibrination syndrome (*see also* Fibrinolysis) 286.6

Deficiency, deficient
- 3-beta-hydroxysteroid dehydrogenase 255.2
- 6-phosphogluconic dehydrogenase (anemia) 282.2
- 11-beta-hydroxylase 255.2
- 17-alpha-hydroxylase 255.2
- 18-hydroxysteroid dehydrogenase 255.2
- 20-alpha-hydroxylase 255.2
- 21-hydroxylase 255.2
- AAT (alpha-1 antitrypsin) 273.4
- abdominal muscle syndrome 756.79
- accelerator globulin (Ac G) (blood) (*see also* Defect, coagulation) 286.3
- AC globulin (congenital) (*see also* Defect, coagulation) 286.3
  - acquired 286.7
- activating factor (blood) (*see also* Defect, coagulation) 286.3
- adenohypophyseal 253.2
- adenosine deaminase 277.2
- aldolase (hereditary) 271.2
- alpha-1-antitrypsin 273.4
- alpha-1-trypsin inhibitor 273.4
- alpha-fucosidase 271.8
- alpha-lipoprotein 272.5
- alpha-mannosidase 271.8
- amino acid 270.9
- anemia - *see* Anemia, deficiency
- aneurin 265.1
  - with beriberi 265.0
- antibody NEC 279.00
- antidiuretic hormone 253.5
- antihemophilic
  - factor (A) 286.0
    - B 286.1
    - C 286.2
  - globulin (AHG) NEC 286.0
- antithrombin III 289.81
- antitrypsin 273.4
- argininosuccinate synthetase or lyase 270.6
- ascorbic acid (with scurvy) 267
- autoprothrombin
  - I (*see also* Defect, coagulation) 286.3
  - II 286.1
  - C (*see also* Defect, coagulation) 286.3

Deficiency, deficient – *continued*
- bile salt 579.8
- biotin 266.2
- biotinidase 277.6
- bradykinase-1 277.6
- brancher enzyme (amylopectinosis) 271.0
- calciferol 268.9
  - with
    - osteomalacia 268.2
    - rickets (*see also* Rickets) 268.0
- calcium 275.40
  - dietary 269.3
- calorie, severe 261
- carbamyl phosphate synthetase 270.6
- cardiac (*see also* Insufficiency, myocardial) 428.0
- carnitine 277.81
  - due to
    - hemodialysis 277.83
    - inborn errors of metabolism 277.82
    - valproic acid therapy 277.83
  - iatrogenic 277.83
  - palmitoyltransferase (CPT1, CPT2) 277.85
  - palmityl transferase (CPT1, CPT2) 277.85
  - primary 277.81
  - secondary 277.84
- carotene 264.9
- Carr factor (*see also* Defect, coagulation) 286.9
- central nervous system 349.9
- ceruloplasmin 275.1
- cevitamic acid (with scurvy) 267
- choline 266.2
- Christmas factor 286.1
- chromium 269.3
- citrin 269.1
- clotting (blood) (*see also* Defect, coagulation) 286.9
- coagulation factor NEC 286.9
  - with
    - abortion - *see* Abortion, by type, with hemorrhage
    - ectopic pregnancy (*see also* categories 634-638) 639.1
    - molar pregnancy (*see also* categories 630-632) 639.1
  - acquired (any) 286.7
  - antepartum or intrapartum 641.3 [5th]
    - affecting fetus or newborn 762.1
  - complicating pregnancy, childbirth, or puerperium 649.3 [5th]
  - due to
    - liver disease 286.7
    - vitamin K deficiency 286.7
  - newborn, transient 776.3
  - postpartum 666.3 [5th]
  - specified type NEC 286.3
- color vision (congenital) 368.59
  - acquired 368.55
- combined glucocorticoid and mineralocorticoid 255.41
- combined, two or more coagulation factors (*see also* Defect, coagulation) 286.9
- complement factor NEC 279.8
- contact factor (*see also* Defect, coagulation) 286.3
- copper NEC 275.1
- corticoadrenal 255.41
- craniofacial axis 756.0
- cyanocobalamin (vitamin B_{12}) 266.2
- debrancher enzyme (limit dextrinosis) 271.0
- desmolase 255.2
- diet 269.9
- dihydrofolate reductase 281.2
- dihydropteridine reductase 270.1
- disaccharidase (intestinal) 271.3
- disease NEC 269.9
- ear(s) V48.8
- edema 262
- endocrine 259.9

Deficiency, deficient – *continued*
- enzymes, circulating NEC (*see also* Deficiency, by specific enzyme) 277.6
- ergosterol 268.9
  - with
    - osteomalacia 268.2
    - rickets (*see also* Rickets) 268.0
- erythrocytic glutathione (anemia) 282.2
- eyelid(s) V48.8
- factor (*see also* Defect, coagulation) 286.9
  - I (congenital) (fibrinogen) 286.3
    - antepartum or intrapartum 641.3 [5th]
      - affecting fetus or newborn 762.1
    - newborn, transient 776.3
    - postpartum 666.3 [5th]
  - II (congenital) (prothrombin) 286.3
  - V (congenital) (labile) 286.3
  - VII (congenital) (stable) 286.3
  - VIII (congenital) (functional) 286.0
    - with
      - functional defect 286.0
      - vascular defect 286.4
  - IX (Christmas) (congenital) (functional) 286.1
  - X (congenital) (Stuart-Prower) 286.3
  - XI (congenital) (plasma thromboplastin antecedent) 286.2
  - XII (congenital) (Hageman) 286.3
  - XIII (congenital) (fibrin stabilizing) 286.3
  - hageman 286.3
  - multiple (congenital) 286.9
    - acquired 286.7
- fibrinase (*see also* Defect, coagulation) 286.3
- fibrinogen (congenital) (*see also* Defect, coagulation) 286.3
  - acquired 286.6
- fibrin-stabilizing factor (congenital) (*see also* Defect, coagulation) 286.3
  - acquired 286.7
- finger - *see* Absence, finger
- fletcher factor (*see also* Defect, coagulation) 286.9
- fluorine 269.3
- folate, anemia 281.2
- folic acid (vitamin B_c) 266.2
  - anemia 281.2
- follicle-stimulating hormone (FSH) 253.4
- fructokinase 271.2
- fructose-1, 6-diphosphate 271.2
- fructose-1-phosphate aldolase 271.2
- FSH (follicle-stimulating hormone) 253.4
- fucosidase 271.8
- galactokinase 271.1
- galactose-1-phosphate uridyl transferase 271.1
- gamma globulin in blood 279.00
- glass factor (*see also* Defect, coagulation) 286.3
- glucocorticoid 255.41
- glucose-6-phosphatase 271.0
- glucose-6-phosphate dehydrogenase anemia 282.2
- glucuronyl transferase 277.4
- glutathione-reductase (anemia) 282.2
- glycogen synthetase 271.0
- growth hormone 253.3
- Hageman factor (congenital) (*see also* Defect, coagulation) 286.3
- head V48.0
- hemoglobin (*see also* Anemia) 285.9
- hepatophosphorylase 271.0
- hexose monophosphate (HMP) shunt 282.2
- HGH (human growth hormone) 253.3
- HG-PRT 277.2
- homogentisic acid oxidase 270.2

Deficiency, deficient – *continued*
- hormone - *see also* Deficiency, by specific hormone
  - anterior pituitary (isolated) (partial) NEC 253.4
    - growth (human) 253.3
  - follicle-stimulating 253.4
  - growth (human) (isolated) 253.3
  - human growth 253.3
  - interstitial cell-stimulating 253.4
  - luteinizing 253.4
  - melanocyte-stimulating 253.4
  - testicular 257.2
- human growth hormone 253.3
- humoral 279.00
  - with
    - hyper-IgM 279.05
      - autosomal recessive 279.05
      - X-linked 279.05
    - increased IgM 279.05
  - congenital hypogammaglobulinemia 279.04
    - non-sex-linked 279.06
  - selective immunoglobulin NEC 279.03
    - IgA 279.01
    - IgG 279.03
    - IgM 279.02
      - increased 279.05
  - specified NEC 279.09
- hydroxylase 255.2
- hypoxanthine-guanine phosphoribosyltransferase (HG-PRT) 277.2
- ICSH (interstitial cell-stimulating hormone) 253.4
- immunity NEC 279.3
  - cell-mediated 279.10
    - with
      - hyperimmunoglobulinemia 279.2
      - thrombocytopenia and eczema 279.12
    - specified NEC 279.19
  - combined (severe) 279.2
    - syndrome 279.2
  - common variable 279.06
  - humoral NEC 279.00
  - IgA (secretory) 279.01
  - IgG 279.03
  - IgM 279.02
- immunoglobulin, selective NEC 279.03
  - IgA 279.01
  - IgG 279.03
  - IgM 279.02
- inositol (B complex) 266.2
- interferon 279.49 ▲
- internal organ V47.0
- interstitial cell-stimulating hormone (ICSH) 253.4
- intrinsic factor (Castle's) (congenital) 281.0
- intrinsic (urethral) sphincter (ISD) 599.82
- invertase 271.3
- iodine 269.3
- iron, anemia 280.9
- labile factor (congenital) (*see also* Defect, coagulation) 286.3
  - acquired 286.7
- lacrimal fluid (acquired) 375.15
  - congenital 743.64
- lactase 271.3
- laki-Lorand factor (*see also* Defect, coagulation) 286.3
- lecithin-cholesterol acyltranferase 272.5
- LH (luteinizing hormone) 253.4
- limb V49.0
  - lower V49.0
    - congenital (*see also* Deficiency, lower limb, congenital) 755.30
  - upper V49.0
    - congenital (*see also* Deficiency, upper limb, congenital) 755.20

Deficiency, deficient – *continued*
- lipocaic 577.8
- lipoid (high-density) 272.5
- lipoprotein (familial) (high-density) 272.5
- liver phosphorylase 271.0
- long chain 3-hydroxyacyl CoA dehydrogenase (LCHAD) 277.85
- long chain/very long chain acyl CoA dehydrogenase (LCAD, VLCAD) 277.85
- lower limb V49.0
  - congenital 755.30
    - with complete absence of distal elements 755.31
    - longitudinal (complete) (partial) (with distal deficiencies, incomplete) 755.32
      - with complete absence of distal elements 755.31
      - combined femoral, tibial, fibular (incomplete) 755.33
      - femoral 755.34
      - fibular 755.37
      - metatarsal(s) 755.38
      - phalange(s) 755.39
        - meaning all digits 755.31
      - tarsal(s) 755.38
      - tibia 755.36
      - tibiofibular 755.35
    - transverse 755.31
- luteinizing hormone (LH) 253.4
- lysosomal alpha-1, 4 glucosidase 271.0
- magnesium 275.2
- mannosidase 271.8
- medium chain acyl CoA dehydrogenase (MCAD) 277.85
- melanocyte-stimulating hormone (MSH) 253.4
- menadione (vitamin K) 269.0
  - newborn 776.0
- mental (familial) (hereditary) (*see also* Retardation, mental) 319
- methylenetetrahydrofolate reductase (MTHFR) 270.4
- mineral NEC 269.3
- mineralocorticoid 255.42
- molybdenum 269.3
- moral 301.7
- multiple, syndrome 260
- myocardial (*see also* Insufficiency, myocardial) 428.0
- myophosphorylase 271.0
- NADH (DPNH) -methemoglobin-reductase (congenital) 289.7
- NADH diaphorase or reductase (congenital) 289.7
- neck V48.1
- niacin (amide) (-tryptophan) 265.2
- nicotinamide 265.2
- nicotinic acid (amide) 265.2
- nose V48.8
- number of teeth (*see also* Anodontia) 520.0
- nutrition, nutritional 269.9
  - specified NEC 269.8
- ornithine transcarbamylase 270.6
- ovarian 256.39
- oxygen (*see also* Anoxia) 799.02
- pantothenic acid 266.2
- parathyroid (gland) 252.1
- phenylalanine hydroxylase 270.1
- phosphoenolpyruvate carboxykinase 271.8
- phosphofructokinase 271.2
- phosphoglucomutase 271.0
- phosphohexosisomerase 271.0
- phosphomannomutase 271.8
- phosphomannose isomerase 271.8
- phosphomannosyl mutase 271.8
- phosphorylase kinase, liver 271.0
- pituitary (anterior) 253.2
  - posterior 253.5
- placenta - *see* Placenta, insufficiency
- plasma
  - cell 279.00

Deficiency, deficient – *continued*
- plasma – *continued*
  - protein (paraproteinemia) (pyroglobulinemia) 273.8
    - gamma globulin 279.00
  - thromboplastin
    - antecedent (PTA) 286.2
    - component (PTC) 286.1
- platelet NEC 287.1
  - constitutional 286.4
- polyglandular 258.9
- potassium (K) 276.8
- proaccelerin (congenital) (*see also* Defect, congenital) 286.3
  - acquired 286.7
- proconvertin factor (congenital) (*see also* Defect, coagulation) 286.3
  - acquired 286.7
- prolactin 253.4
- protein 260
  - anemia 281.4
  - C 289.81
  - plasma - *see* Deficiency, plasma, protein
  - S 289.81
- prothrombin (congenital) (*see also* Defect, coagulation) 286.3
  - acquired 286.7
- Prower factor (*see also* Defect, coagulation) 286.3
- PRT 277.2
- pseudocholinesterase 289.89
- psychobiological 301.6
- PTA 286.2
- PTC 286.1
- purine nucleoside phosphorylase 277.2
- pyracin (alpha) (beta) 266.1
- pyridoxal 266.1
- pyridoxamine 266.1
- pyridoxine (derivatives) 266.1
- pyruvate carboxylase 271.8
- pyruvate dehydrogenase 271.8
- pyruvate kinase (PK) 282.3
- riboflavin (vitamin B_2) 266.0
- saccadic eye movements 379.57
- salivation 527.7
- salt 276.1
- secretion
  - ovary 256.39
  - salivary gland (any) 527.7
  - urine 788.5
- selenium 269.3
- serum
  - antitrypsin, familial 273.4
  - protein (congenital) 273.8
- short chain acyl CoA dehydrogenase (SCAD) 277.85
- short stature homeobox gene (SHOX)
  - with
    - dyschondrosteosis 756.89
    - short stature (idiopathic) 783.43
    - Turner's syndrome 758.6
- smooth pursuit movements (eye) 379.58
- sodium (Na) 276.1
- SPCA (*see also* Defect, coagulation) 286.3
- specified NEC 269.8
- stable factor (congenital) (*see also* Defect, coagulation) 286.3
  - acquired 286.7
- Stuart (-Prower) factor (*see also* Defect, coagulation) 286.3
- sucrase 271.3
- sucrase-isomaltase 271.3
- sulfite oxidase 270.0
- syndrome, multiple 260
- thiamine, thiaminic (chloride) 265.1
- thrombokinase (*see also* Defect, coagulation) 286.3
  - newborn 776.0
- thrombopoieten 287.39
- thymolymphatic 279.2
- thyroid (gland) 244.9
- tocopherol 269.1
- toe - *see* Absence, toe

Deficiency, deficient – *continued*
- tooth bud (*see also* Anodontia) 520.0
- trunk V48.1
- UDPG-glycogen transferase 271.0
- upper limb V49.0
  - congenital 755.20
    - with complete absence of distal elements 755.21
    - longitudinal (complete) (partial) (with distal deficiencies, incomplete) 755.22
      - carpal(s) 755.28
      - combined humeral, radial, ulnar (incomplete) 755.23
      - humeral 755.24
      - metacarpal(s) 755.28
      - phalange(s) 755.29
        - meaning all digits 755.21
      - radial 755.26
      - radioulnar 755.25
      - ulnar 755.27
    - transverse (complete) (partial) 755.21
- vascular 459.9
- vasopressin 253.5
- viosterol (*see also* Deficiency, calciferol) 268.9
- vitamin (multiple) NEC 269.2
  - A 264.9
    - with
      - Bitôt's spot 264.1
        - corneal 264.2
          - with corneal ulceration 264.3
      - keratomalacia 264.4
      - keratosis, follicular 264.8
      - night blindness 264.5
      - scar of cornea, xerophthalmic 264.6
      - specified manifestation NEC 264.8
        - ocular 264.7
    - xeroderma 264.8
    - xerophthalmia 264.7
    - xerosis
      - conjunctival 264.0
        - with Bitôt's spot 264.1
      - corneal 264.2
        - with corneal ulceration 264.3
  - B (complex) NEC 266.9
    - with
      - beriberi 265.0
      - pellagra 265.2
    - specified type NEC 266.2
  - B_1 NEC 265.1
    - beriberi 265.0
  - B_2 266.0
  - B_6 266.1
  - B_{12} 266.2
  - B_C (folic acid) 266.2
  - C (ascorbic acid) (with scurvy) 267
  - D (calciferol) (ergosterol) 268.9
    - with
      - osteomalacia 268.2
      - rickets (*see also* Rickets) 268.0
  - E 269.1
  - folic acid 266.2
  - G 266.0
  - H 266.2
  - K 269.0
    - of newborn 776.0
  - nicotinic acid 265.2
  - P 269.1
  - PP 265.2
  - specified NEC 269.1
- zinc 269.3

Deficient - *see also* Deficiency
- blink reflex 374.45
- craniofacial axis 756.0
- number of teeth (*see also* Anodontia) 520.0
- secretion of urine 788.5

Deficit
- cognitive 294.9

Deficit – *continued*
- neurologic NEC 781.99
  - due to
    - cerebrovascular lesion (*see also* Disease, cerebrovascular, acute) 436
      - late effect - *see* Late effect(s) (of) cerebrovascular disease
    - transient ischemic attack 435.9
  - ischemic
    - reversible (RIND) 434.91
      - history of (personal) V12.54
      - prolonged (PRIND) 434.91
        - history of (personal) V12.54
- oxygen 799.02

Deflection
- radius 736.09
- septum (acquired) (nasal) (nose) 470
- spine - *see* Curvature, spine
- turbinate (nose) 470

Defluvium
- capillorum (*see also* Alopecia) 704.00
- ciliorum 374.55
- unguium 703.8

Deformity 738.9
- abdomen, congenital 759.9
- abdominal wall
  - acquired 738.8
  - congenital 756.70
    - muscle deficiency syndrome 756.79
- acquired (unspecified site) 738.9
  - specified site NEC 738.8
- adrenal gland (congenital) 759.1
- alimentary tract, congenital 751.9
  - lower 751.5
  - specified type NEC 751.8
  - upper (any part, except tongue) 750.9
    - specified type NEC 750.8
    - tongue 750.10
      - specified type NEC 750.19
- ankle (joint) (acquired) 736.70
  - abduction 718.47
  - congenital 755.69
  - contraction 718.47
  - specified NEC 736.79
- anus (congenital) 751.5
  - acquired 569.49
- aorta (congenital) 747.20
  - acquired 447.8
  - arch 747.21
    - acquired 447.8
  - coarctation 747.10
- aortic
  - arch 747.21
    - acquired 447.8
  - cusp or valve (congenital) 746.9
    - acquired (*see also* Endocarditis, aortic) 424.1
  - ring 747.21
- appendix 751.5
- arm (acquired) 736.89
  - congenital 755.50
- arteriovenous (congenital) (peripheral) NEC 747.60
  - gastrointestinal 747.61
  - lower limb 747.64
  - renal 747.62
  - specified NEC 747.69
  - spinal 747.82
  - upper limb 747.63
- artery (congenital) (peripheral) NEC (*see also* Deformity, vascular) 747.60
  - acquired 447.8
  - cerebral 747.81
  - coronary (congenital) 746.85
    - acquired (*see also* Ischemia, heart) 414.9
  - retinal 743.9
  - umbilical 747.5
- atrial septal (congenital) (heart) 745.5
- auditory canal (congenital) (external) (*see also* Deformity, ear) 744.3
  - acquired 380.50

Deformity – *continued*
- auricle
  - ear (congenital) (*see also* Deformity, ear) 744.3
    - acquired 380.32
  - heart (congenital) 746.9
- back (acquired) - *see* Deformity, spine
- Bartholin's duct (congenital) 750.9
- bile duct (congenital) 751.60
  - acquired 576.8
    - with calculus, choledocholithiasis, or stones - *see* Choledocholithiasis
- biliary duct or passage (congenital) 751.60
  - acquired 576.8
    - with calculus, choledocholithiasis, or stones - *see* Choledocholithiasis
- bladder (neck) (sphincter) (trigone) (acquired) 596.8
  - congenital 753.9
- bone (acquired) NEC 738.9
  - congenital 756.9
  - turbinate 738.0
- boutonniere (finger) 736.21
- brain (congenital) 742.9
  - acquired 348.89 ▲
  - multiple 742.4
  - reduction 742.2
  - vessel (congenital) 747.81
- breast (acquired) 611.89
  - congenital 757.6 ▲
  - reconstructed 612.0
- bronchus (congenital) 748.3
  - acquired 519.19
- bursa, congenital 756.9
- canal of Nuck 752.9
- canthus (congenital) 743.9
  - acquired 374.89
- capillary (acquired) 448.9
  - congenital NEC (*see also* Deformity, vascular) 747.60
- cardiac - *see* Deformity, heart
- cardiovascular system (congenital) 746.9
- caruncle, lacrimal (congenital) 743.9
  - acquired 375.69
- cascade, stomach 537.6
- cecum (congenital) 751.5
  - acquired 569.89
- cerebral (congenital) 742.9
  - acquired 348.89 ▲
- cervix (acquired) (uterus) 622.8
  - congenital 752.40
- cheek (acquired) 738.19
  - congenital 744.9
- chest (wall) (acquired) 738.3
  - congenital 754.89
  - late effect of rickets 268.1
- chin (acquired) 738.19
  - congenital 744.9
- choroid (congenital) 743.9
  - acquired 363.8
  - plexus (congenital) 742.9
    - acquired 349.2
- cicatricial - *see* Cicatrix
- cilia (congenital) 743.9
  - acquired 374.89
- circulatory system (congenital) 747.9
- clavicle (acquired) 738.8
  - congenital 755.51
- clitoris (congenital) 752.40
  - acquired 624.8
- clubfoot - *see* Clubfoot
- coccyx (acquired) 738.6
  - congenital 756.10
- colon (congenital) 751.5
  - acquired 569.89
- concha (ear) (congenital) (*see also* Deformity, ear) 744.3
  - acquired 380.32
- congenital, organ or site not listed (*see also* Anomaly) 759.9
- cornea (congenital) 743.9
  - acquired 371.70

Deformity – *continued*
- coronary artery (congenital) 746.85
  - acquired (*see also* Ischemia, heart) 414.9
- cranium (acquired) 738.19
  - congenital (*see also* Deformity, skull, congenital) 756.0
- cricoid cartilage (congenital) 748.3
  - acquired 478.79
- cystic duct (congenital) 751.60
  - acquired 575.8
- Dandy-Walker 742.3
  - with spina bifida (*see also* Spina bifida) 741.0 [5th]
- diaphragm (congenital) 756.6
  - acquired 738.8
- digestive organ(s) or system (congenital) NEC 751.9
  - specified type NEC 751.8
- ductus arteriosus 747.0
- duodenal bulb 537.89
- duodenum (congenital) 751.5
  - acquired 537.89
- dura (congenital) 742.9
  - brain 742.4
    - acquired 349.2
  - spinal 742.59
    - acquired 349.2
- ear (congenital) 744.3
  - acquired 380.32
  - auricle 744.3
    - causing impairment of hearing 744.02
  - causing impairment of hearing 744.00
  - external 744.3
    - causing impairment of hearing 744.02
  - internal 744.05
  - lobule 744.3
  - middle 744.03
    - ossicles 744.04
  - ossicles 744.04
- ectodermal (congenital) NEC 757.9
  - specified type NEC 757.8
- ejaculatory duct (congenital) 752.9
  - acquired 608.89
- elbow (joint) (acquired) 736.00
  - congenital 755.50
  - contraction 718.42
- endocrine gland NEC 759.2
- epididymis (congenital) 752.9
  - acquired 608.89
  - torsion 608.24
- epiglottis (congenital) 748.3
  - acquired 478.79
- esophagus (congenital) 750.9
  - acquired 530.89
- Eustachian tube (congenital) NEC 744.3
  - specified type NEC 744.24
- extremity (acquired) 736.9
  - congenital, except reduction deformity 755.9
    - lower 755.60
    - upper 755.50
  - reduction - *see* Deformity, reduction
- eye (congenital) 743.9
  - acquired 379.8
  - muscle 743.9
- eyebrow (congenital) 744.89
- eyelid (congenital) 743.9
  - acquired 374.89
  - specified type NEC 743.62
- face (acquired) 738.19
  - congenital (any part) 744.9
    - due to intrauterine malposition and pressure 754.0
- fallopian tube (congenital) 752.10
  - acquired 620.8
- femur (acquired) 736.89
  - congenital 755.60
- fetal
  - with fetopelvic disproportion 653.7 [5th]
    - affecting fetus or newborn 763.1
  - causing obstructed labor 660.1 [5th]
    - affecting fetus or newborn 763.1

Deformity – *continued*
- fetal – *continued*
  - known or suspected, affecting management of pregnancy 655.9 [5th]
- finger (acquired) 736.20
  - boutonniere type 736.21
  - congenital 755.50
  - flexion contracture 718.44
  - swan neck 736.22
- flexion (joint) (acquired) 736.9
  - congenital NEC 755.9
  - hip or thigh (acquired) 736.39
    - congenital (*see also* Subluxation, congenital, hip) 754.32
- foot (acquired) 736.70
  - cavovarus 736.75
    - congenital 754.59
  - congenital NEC 754.70
    - specified type NEC 754.79
  - valgus (acquired) 736.79
    - congenital 754.60
      - specified type NEC 754.69
  - varus (acquired) 736.79
    - congenital 754.50
      - specified type NEC 754.59
- forearm (acquired) 736.00
  - congenital 755.50
- forehead (acquired) 738.19
  - congenital (*see also* Deformity, skull, congenital) 756.0
- frontal bone (acquired) 738.19
  - congenital (*see also* Deformity, skull, congenital) 756.0
- gallbladder (congenital) 751.60
  - acquired 575.8
- gastrointestinal tract (congenital) NEC 751.9
  - acquired 569.89
  - specified type NEC 751.8
- genitalia, genital organ(s) or system NEC
  - congenital 752.9
  - female (congenital) 752.9
    - acquired 629.89
    - external 752.40
    - internal 752.9
  - male (congenital) 752.9
    - acquired 608.89
- globe (eye) (congenital) 743.9
  - acquired 360.89
- gum (congenital) 750.9
  - acquired 523.9
- gunstock 736.02
- hand (acquired) 736.00
  - claw 736.06
  - congenital 755.50
  - minus (and plus) (intrinsic) 736.09
  - pill roller (intrinsic) 736.09
  - plus (and minus) (intrinsic) 736.09
  - swan neck (intrinsic) 736.09
- head (acquired) 738.10
  - congenital (*see also* Deformity, skull, congenital) 756.0
  - specified NEC 738.19
- heart (congenital) 746.9
  - auricle (congenital) 746.9
  - septum 745.9
    - auricular 745.5
    - specified type NEC 745.8
    - ventricular 745.4
  - valve (congenital) NEC 746.9
    - acquired - *see* Endocarditis
    - pulmonary (congenital) 746.00
    - specified type NEC 746.89
  - ventricle (congenital) 746.9
- heel (acquired) 736.76
  - congenital 755.67
- hepatic duct (congenital) 751.60
  - acquired 576.8
    - with calculus, choledocholithiasis, or stones - *see* Choledocholithiasis
- hip (joint) (acquired) 736.30
  - congenital NEC 755.63

Deficit – Deformity

- **Deformity** – *continued*
  - hip – *continued*
    - flexion 718.45
      - congenital (*see also* Subluxation, congenital, hip) 754.32
  - hourglass - *see* Contraction, hourglass
  - humerus (acquired) 736.89
    - congenital 755.50
  - hymen (congenital) 752.40
  - hypophyseal (congenital) 759.2
  - ileocecal (coil) (valve) (congenital) 751.5
    - acquired 569.89
  - ileum (intestine) (congenital) 751.5
    - acquired 569.89
  - ilium (acquired) 738.6
    - congenital 755.60
  - integument (congenital) 757.9
  - intervertebral cartilage or disc (acquired) - *see also* Displacement, intervertebral disc
    - congenital 756.10
  - intestine (large) (small) (congenital) 751.5
    - acquired 569.89
  - iris (acquired) 364.75
    - congenital 743.9
    - prolapse 364.89
  - ischium (acquired) 738.6
    - congenital 755.60
  - jaw (acquired) (congenital) NEC 524.9
    - due to intrauterine malposition and pressure 754.0
  - joint (acquired) NEC 738.8
    - congenital 755.9
    - contraction (abduction) (adduction) (extension) (flexion) - *see* Contraction, joint
  - kidney(s) (calyx) (pelvis) (congenital) 753.9
    - acquired 593.89
    - vessel 747.62
      - acquired 459.9
  - Klippel-Feil (brevicollis) 756.16
  - knee (acquired) NEC 736.6
    - congenital 755.64
  - labium (majus) (minus) (congenital) 752.40
    - acquired 624.8
  - lacrimal apparatus or duct (congenital) 743.9
    - acquired 375.69
  - larynx (muscle) (congenital) 748.3
    - acquired 478.79
    - web (glottic) (subglottic) 748.2
  - leg (lower) (upper) (acquired) NEC 736.89
    - congenital 755.60
      - reduction - *see* Deformity, reduction, lower limb
  - lens (congenital) 743.9
    - acquired 379.39
  - lid (fold) (congenital) 743.9
    - acquired 374.89
  - ligament (acquired) 728.9
    - congenital 756.9
  - limb (acquired) 736.9
    - congenital, except reduction deformity 755.9
      - lower 755.60
        - reduction (*see also* Deformity, reduction, lower limb) 755.30
      - upper 755.50
        - reduction (*see also* Deformity, reduction, lower limb) 755.20
    - specified NEC 736.89
  - lip (congenital) NEC 750.9
    - acquired 528.5
    - specified type NEC 750.26
  - liver (congenital) 751.60
    - acquired 573.8
    - duct (congenital) 751.60
      - acquired 576.8
        - with calculus, choledocholithiasis, or stones - *see* Choledocholithiasis
  - lower extremity - *see* Deformity, leg
  - lumbosacral (joint) (region) (congenital) 756.10
    - acquired 738.5
  - lung (congenital) 748.60
    - acquired 518.89
    - specified type NEC 748.69
  - lymphatic system, congenital 759.9
  - Madelung's (radius) 755.54
  - maxilla (acquired) (congenital) 524.9
  - meninges or membrane (congenital) 742.9
    - brain 742.4
      - acquired 349.2
    - spinal (cord) 742.59
      - acquired 349.2
  - mesentery (congenital) 751.9
    - acquired 568.89
  - metacarpus (acquired) 736.00
    - congenital 755.50
  - metatarsus (acquired) 736.70
    - congenital 754.70
  - middle ear, except ossicles (congenital) 744.03
    - ossicles 744.04
  - mitral (leaflets) (valve) (congenital) 746.9
    - acquired - *see* Endocarditis, mitral
    - Ebstein's 746.89
    - parachute 746.5
    - specified type NEC 746.89
    - stenosis, congenital 746.5
  - mouth (acquired) 528.9
    - congenital NEC 750.9
      - specified type NEC 750.26
  - multiple, congenital NEC 759.7
    - specified type NEC 759.89
  - muscle (acquired) 728.9
    - congenital 756.9
      - specified type NEC 756.89
      - sternocleidomastoid (due to intrauterine malposition and pressure) 754.1
  - musculoskeletal system, congenital NEC 756.9
    - specified type NEC 756.9
  - nail (acquired) 703.9
    - congenital 757.9
  - nasal - *see* Deformity, nose
  - neck (acquired) NEC 738.2
    - congenital (any part) 744.9
      - sternocleidomastoid 754.1
  - nervous system (congenital) 742.9
  - nipple (congenital) 757.<u>6</u> ▲
    - acquired 611.89
  - nose, nasal (cartilage) (acquired) 738.0
    - bone (turbinate) 738.0
    - congenital 748.1
      - bent 754.0
      - squashed 754.0
    - saddle 738.0
      - syphilitic 090.5
    - septum 470
      - congenital 748.1
    - sinus (wall) (congenital) 748.1
      - acquired 738.0
    - syphilitic (congenital) 090.5
      - late 095.8
  - ocular muscle (congenital) 743.9
    - acquired 378.60
  - opticociliary vessels (congenital) 743.9
  - orbit (congenital) (eye) 743.9
    - acquired NEC 376.40
      - associated with craniofacial deformities 376.44
      - due to
        - bone disease 376.43
        - surgery 376.47
        - trauma 376.47
  - organ of Corti (congenital) 744.05
  - ovary (congenital) 752.0
    - acquired 620.8
  - oviduct (congenital) 752.10
    - acquired 620.8
  - palate (congenital) 750.9
    - acquired 526.89
    - cleft (congenital) (*see also* Cleft, palate) 749.00
    - hard, acquired 526.89
    - soft, acquired 528.9
  - pancreas (congenital) 751.7
    - acquired 577.8
  - parachute, mitral valve 746.5
  - parathyroid (gland) 759.2
  - parotid (gland) (congenital) 750.9
    - acquired 527.8
  - patella (acquired) 736.6
    - congenital 755.64
  - pelvis, pelvic (acquired) (bony) 738.6
    - with disproportion (fetopelvic) 653.0 [5th]
      - affecting fetus or newborn 763.1
      - causing obstructed labor 660.1 [5th]
        - affecting fetus or newborn 763.1
    - congenital 755.60
    - rachitic (late effect) 268.1
  - penis (glans) (congenital) 752.9
    - acquired 607.89
  - pericardium (congenital) 746.9
    - acquired - *see* Pericarditis
  - pharynx (congenital) 750.9
    - acquired 478.29
  - Pierre Robin (congenital) 756.0
  - pinna (acquired) 380.32
    - congenital 744.3
  - pituitary (congenital) 759.2
  - pleural folds (congenital) 748.8
  - portal vein (congenital) 747.40
  - posture - *see* Curvature, spine
  - prepuce (congenital) 752.9
    - acquired 607.89
  - prostate (congenital) 752.9
    - acquired 602.8
  - pulmonary valve - *see* Endocarditis, pulmonary
  - pupil (congenital) 743.9
    - acquired 364.75
  - pylorus (congenital) 750.9
    - acquired 537.89
  - rachitic (acquired), healed or old 268.1
  - radius (acquired) 736.00
    - congenital 755.50
      - reduction - *see* Deformity, reduction, upper limb
  - rectovaginal septum (congenital) 752.40
    - acquired 623.8
  - rectum (congenital) 751.5
    - acquired 569.49
  - reduction (extremity) (limb) 755.4
    - brain 742.2
    - lower limb 755.30
      - with complete absence of distal elements 755.31
      - longitudinal (complete) (partial) (with distal deficiencies, incomplete) 755.32
        - with complete absence of distal elements 755.31
        - combined femoral, tibial, fibular (incomplete) 755.33
        - femoral 755.34
        - fibular 755.37
        - metatarsal(s) 755.38
        - phalange(s) 755.39
          - meaning all digits 755.31
        - tarsal(s) 755.38
        - tibia 755.36
        - tibiofibular 755.35
      - transverse 755.31
    - upper limb 755.20
      - with complete absence of distal elements 755.21
      - longitudinal (complete) (partial) (with distal deficiencies, incomplete) 755.22
        - with complete absence of distal elements 755.21
        - carpal(s) 755.28
        - combined humeral, radial, ulnar (incomplete) 755.23
        - humeral 755.24
        - metacarpal(s) 755.28
        - phalange(s) 755.29
          - meaning all digits 755.21
        - radial 755.26
        - radioulnar 755.25
        - ulnar 755.27
      - transverse (complete) (partial) 755.21
  - renal - *see* Deformity, kidney
  - respiratory system (congenital) 748.9
    - specified type NEC 748.8
  - rib (acquired) 738.3
    - congenital 756.3
      - cervical 756.2
  - rotation (joint) (acquired) 736.9
    - congenital 755.9
    - hip or thigh 736.39
      - congenital (*see also* Subluxation, congenital, hip) 754.32
  - sacroiliac joint (congenital) 755.69
    - acquired 738.5
  - sacrum (acquired) 738.5
    - congenital 756.10
  - saddle
    - back 737.8
    - nose 738.0
      - syphilitic 090.5
  - salivary gland or duct (congenital) 750.9
    - acquired 527.8
  - scapula (acquired) 736.89
    - congenital 755.50
  - scrotum (congenital) 752.9
    - acquired 608.89
  - sebaceous gland, acquired 706.8
  - seminal tract or duct (congenital) 752.9
    - acquired 608.89
  - septum (nasal) (acquired) 470
    - congenital 748.1
  - shoulder (joint) (acquired) 736.89
    - congenital 755.50
      - specified type NEC 755.59
    - contraction 718.41
  - sigmoid (flexure) (congenital) 751.5
    - acquired 569.89
  - sinus of Valsalva 747.29
  - skin (congenital) 757.9
    - acquired NEC 709.8
  - skull (acquired) 738.19
    - congenital 756.0
      - with
        - anencephalus 740.0
        - encephalocele 742.0
        - hydrocephalus 742.3
          - with spina bifida (*see also* Spina bifida) 741.0 [5th]
        - microcephalus 742.1
      - due to intrauterine malposition and pressure 754.0
  - soft parts, organs or tissues (of pelvis)
    - in pregnancy or childbirth NEC 654.9 [5th]
      - affecting fetus or newborn 763.89
      - causing obstructed labor 660.2 [5th]
        - affecting fetus or newborn 763.1
  - spermatic cord (congenital) 752.9
    - acquired 608.89
      - torsion 608.22
        - extravaginal 608.21

Deformity

Deformity – *continued*
spermatic cord – *continued*
acquired – *continued*
torsion – *continued*
intravaginal 608.22
spinal
column - *see* Deformity, spine
cord (congenital) 742.9
acquired 336.8
vessel (congenital) 747.82
nerve root (congenital) 742.9
acquired 724.9
spine (acquired) NEC 738.5
congenital 756.10
due to intrauterine malposition and pressure 754.2
kyphoscoliotic (*see also* Kyphoscoliosis) 737.30
kyphotic (*see also* Kyphosis) 737.10
lordotic (*see also* Lordosis) 737.20
rachitic 268.1
scoliotic (*see also* Scoliosis) 737.30
spleen
acquired 289.59
congenital 759.0
Sprengel's (congenital) 755.52
sternum (acquired) 738.3
congenital 756.3
stomach (congenital) 750.9
acquired 537.89
submaxillary gland (congenital) 750.9
acquired 527.8
swan neck (acquired)
finger 736.22
hand 736.09
talipes - *see* Talipes
teeth, tooth NEC 520.9
testis (congenital) 752.9
acquired 608.89
torsion 608.20
thigh (acquired) 736.89
congenital 755.60
thorax (acquired) (wall) 738.3
congenital 754.89
late effect of rickets 268.1
thumb (acquired) 736.20
congenital 755.50
thymus (tissue) (congenital) 759.2
thyroid (gland) (congenital) 759.2
cartilage 748.3
acquired 478.79
tibia (acquired) 736.89
congenital 755.60
saber 090.5
toe (acquired) 735.9
congenital 755.66
specified NEC 735.8
tongue (congenital) 750.10
acquired 529.8
tooth, teeth NEC 520.9
trachea (rings) (congenital) 748.3
acquired 519.19
transverse aortic arch (congenital) 747.21
tricuspid (leaflets) (valve) (congenital) 746.9
acquired - *see* Endocarditis, tricuspid
atresia or stenosis 746.1
specified type NEC 746.89
trunk (acquired) 738.3
congenital 759.9
ulna (acquired) 736.00
congenital 755.50
upper extremity - *see* Deformity, arm
urachus (congenital) 753.7
ureter (opening) (congenital) 753.9
acquired 593.89
urethra (valve) (congenital) 753.9
acquired 599.84
urinary tract or system (congenital) 753.9
urachus 753.7
uterus (congenital) 752.3
acquired 621.8
uvula (congenital) 750.9
acquired 528.9

Deformity – *continued*
vagina (congenital) 752.40
acquired 623.8
valve, valvular (heart) (congenital) 746.9
acquired - *see* Endocarditis
pulmonary 746.00
specified type NEC 746.89
vascular (congenital) (peripheral) NEC 747.60
acquired 459.9
gastrointestinal 747.61
lower limb 747.64
renal 747.62
specified site NEC 747.69
spinal 747.82
upper limb 747.63
vas deferens (congenital) 752.9
acquired 608.89
vein (congenital) NEC (*see also* Deformity, vascular) 747.60
brain 747.81
coronary 746.9
great 747.40
vena cava (inferior) (superior) (congenital) 747.40
vertebra - *see* Deformity, spine
vesicourethral orifice (acquired) 596.8
congenital NEC 753.9
specified type NEC 753.8
vessels of optic papilla (congenital) 743.9
visual field (contraction) 368.45
vitreous humor (congenital) 743.9
acquired 379.29
vulva (congenital) 752.40
acquired 624.8
wrist (joint) (acquired) 736.00
congenital 755.50
contraction 718.43
valgus 736.03
congenital 755.59
varus 736.04
congenital 755.59

Degeneration, degenerative
adrenal (capsule) (gland) 255.8
with hypofunction 255.41
fatty 255.8
hyaline 255.8
infectional 255.8
lardaceous 277.39
amyloid (any site) (general) 277.39
anterior cornua, spinal cord 336.8
anterior labral 840.8
aorta, aortic 440.0
fatty 447.8
valve (heart) (*see also* Endocarditis, aortic) 424.1
arteriovascular - *see* Arteriosclerosis
artery, arterial (atheromatous) (calcareous) - *see also* Arteriosclerosis
amyloid 277.39
lardaceous 277.39
medial NEC (*see also* Arteriosclerosis, extremities) 440.20
articular cartilage NEC (*see also* Disorder, cartilage, articular) 718.0 5th
elbow 718.02
knee 717.5
patella 717.7
shoulder 718.01
spine (*see also* Spondylosis) 721.90
atheromatous - *see* Arteriosclerosis
bacony (any site) 277.39
basal nuclei or ganglia NEC 333.0
bone 733.90
brachial plexus 353.0
brain (cortical) (progressive) 331.9
arteriosclerotic 437.0
childhood 330.9
specified type NEC 330.8
congenital 742.4
cystic 348.0
congenital 742.4
familial NEC 331.89

Degeneration, degenerative – *continued*
brain – *continued*
grey matter 330.8
heredofamilial NEC 331.89
in
alcoholism 303.9 5th *[331.7]*
beriberi 265.0 *[331.7]*
cerebrovascular disease 437.9 *[331.7]*
congenital hydrocephalus 742.3 *[331.7]*
with spina bifida (*see also* Spina bifida) 741.0 5th *[331.7]*
Babry's disease 272.7 *[330.2]*
Gaucher's disease 272.7 *[330.2]*
Hunter's disease or syndrome 277.5 *[330.3]*
lipidosis
cerebral 330.1
generalized 272.7 *[330.2]*
mucopolysaccharidosis 277.5 *[330.3]*
myxedema (*see also* Myxedema) 244.9 *[331.7]*
neoplastic disease NEC (M8000/1) 239.9 *[331.7]*
Niemann-Pick disease 272.7 *[330.2]*
sphingolipidosis 272.7 *[330.2]*
vitamin B_{12} deficiency 266.2 *[331.7]*
motor centers 331.89
senile 331.2
specified type NEC 331.89
breast - *see* Disease, breast
Bruch's membrane 363.40
bundle of His 426.50
left 426.3
right 426.4
calcareous NEC 275.49
capillaries 448.9
amyloid 277.39
fatty 448.9
lardaceous 277.39
cardiac (brown) (calcareous) (fatty) (fibrous) (hyaline) (mural) (muscular) (pigmentary) (senile) (with arteriosclerosis) (*see also* Degeneration, myocardial) 429.1
valve, valvular - *see* Endocarditis
cardiorenal (*see also* Hypertension, cardiorenal) 404.90
cardiovascular (*see also* Disease, cardiovascular) 429.2
renal (*see also* Hypertension, cardiorenal) 404.90
cartilage (joint) - *see* Derangement, joint
cerebellar NEC 334.9
primary (hereditary) (sporadic) 334.2
cerebral - *see* Degeneration, brain
cerebromacular 330.1
cerebrovascular 437.1
due to hypertension 437.2
late effect - *see* Late effect(s) (of) cerebrovascular disease
cervical plexus 353.2
cervix 622.8
due to radiation (intended effect) 622.8
adverse effect or misadventure 622.8
changes, spine or vertebra (*see also* Spondylosis) 721.90
chitinous 277.39
chorioretinal 363.40
congenital 743.53
hereditary 363.50
choroid (colloid) (drusen) 363.40
hereditary 363.50
senile 363.41
diffuse secondary 363.42
cochlear 386.8
collateral ligament (knee) (medial) 717.82
lateral 717.81

Degeneration, degenerative – *continued*
combined (spinal cord) (subacute) 266.2 *[336.2]*
with anemia (pernicious) 281.0 *[336.2]*
due to dietary deficiency 281.1 *[336.2]*
due to vitamin B_{12} deficiency anemia (dietary) 281.1 *[336.2]*
conjunctiva 372.50
amyloid 277.39 *[372.50]*
cornea 371.40
calcerous 371.44
familial (hereditary) (*see also* Dystrophy, cornea) 371.50
macular 371.55
reticular 371.54
hyaline (of old scars) 371.41
marginal (Terrien's) 371.48
mosaic (shagreen) 371.41
nodular 371.46
peripheral 371.48
senile 371.41
cortical (cerebellar) (parenchymatous) 334.2
alcoholic 303.9 5th *[334.4]*
diffuse, due to arteriopathy 437.0
corticostriatal-spinal 334.8
cretinoid 243
cruciate ligament (knee) (posterior) 717.84
anterior 717.83
cutis 709.3
amyloid 277.39
dental pulp 522.2
disc disease - *see* Degeneration, intervertebral disc
dorsolateral (spinal cord) - *see* Degeneration, combined
endocardial 424.90
extrapyramidal NEC 333.90
eye NEC 360.40
macular (*see also* Degeneration, macula) 362.50
congenital 362.75
hereditary 362.76
fatty (diffuse) (general) 272.8
liver 571.8
alcoholic 571.0
localized site - *see* Degeneration, by site, fatty
placenta - *see* Placenta, abnormal
globe (eye) NEC 360.40
macular - *see* Degeneration, macula
grey matter 330.8
heart (brown) (calcareous) (fatty) (fibrous) (hyaline) (mural) (muscular) (pigmentary) (senile) (with arteriosclerosis) (*see also* Degeneration, myocardial) 429.1
amyloid 277.39 *[425.7]*
atheromatous - *see* Arteriosclerosis, coronary
gouty 274.82
hypertensive (*see also* Hypertension, heart) 402.90
ischemic 414.9
valve, valvular - *see* Endocarditis
hepatolenticular (Wilson's) 275.1
hepatorenal 572.4
heredofamilial
brain NEC 331.89
spinal cord NEC 336.8
hyaline (diffuse) (generalized) 728.9
localized - *see also* Degeneration, by site
cornea 371.41
keratitis 371.41
hypertensive vascular - *see* Hypertension
infrapatellar fat pad 729.31
internal semilunar cartilage 717.3
intervertebral disc 722.6
with myelopathy 722.70
cervical, cervicothoracic 722.4
with myelopathy 722.71

Degeneration, degenerative – Dehiscence

- **Dehydration** (cachexia) 276.51
  - with
    - hypernatremia 276.0
    - hyponatremia 276.1
  - newborn 775.5
- **Deiters' nucleus syndrome** 386.19
- **Déjérine's disease** 356.0
- **Déjérine-Klumpke paralysis** 767.6
- **Déjérine-Roussy syndrome** 338.0
- **Déjérine-Sottas disease or neuropathy** (hypertrophic) 356.0
- **Déjérine-Thomas atrophy or syndrome** 333.0
- **de Lange's syndrome** (Amsterdam dwarf, mental retardation, and brachycephaly) 759.89
- **Delay, delayed**
  - adaptation, cones or rods 368.63
  - any plane in pelvis
    - affecting fetus or newborn 763.1 5th
    - complicating delivery 660.1 5th
  - birth or delivery NEC 662.1
    - affecting fetus or newborn 763.9
    - second twin, triplet, or multiple mate 662.3 5th
  - closure - *see also* Fistula
    - cranial suture 756.0
    - fontanel 756.0
  - coagulation NEC 790.92
  - conduction (cardiac) (ventricular) 426.9
  - delivery NEC 662.1 5th
    - second twin, triplet, etc. 662.3 5th
      - affecting fetus or newborn 763.89
  - development
    - in childhood 783.40
      - physiological 783.40
    - intellectual NEC 315.9
    - learning NEC 315.2
    - reading 315.00
    - sexual 259.0
    - speech 315.39
      - and language due to hearing loss 315.34
      - associated with hyperkinesis 314.1
    - spelling 315.09
  - gastric emptying 536.8
  - menarche 256.39
    - due to pituitary hypofunction 253.4
  - menstruation (cause unknown) 626.8
  - milestone in childhood 783.42
  - motility - *see* Hypomotility
  - passage of meconium (newborn) 777.1
  - primary respiration 768.9
  - puberty 259.0
  - separation of umbilical cord 779.83
  - sexual maturation, female 259.0
  - vaccination V64.00
- **Del Castillo's syndrome** (germinal aplasia) 606.0
- **Deleage's disease** 359.89
- **Deletion syndrome**
  - 5p 758.31
  - 22q11.2 758.32
  - autosomal NEC 758.39
  - constitutional 5q deletion 758.39
- **Delhi** (boil) (button) (sore) 085.1
- **Delinquency** (juvenile) 312.9
  - group (*see also* Disturbance, conduct) 312.2 5th
  - neurotic 312.4
- **Delirium, delirious** 780.09
  - acute (psychotic) 293.0
  - alcoholic 291.0
    - acute 291.0
    - chronic 291.1
  - alcoholicum 291.0
  - chronic (*see also* Psychosis) 293.89
    - due to or associated with physical condition - *see* Psychosis, organic
  - drug-induced 292.81
  - due to conditions classified elsewhere 293.0
  - eclamptic (*see also* Eclampsia) 780.39

- **Delirium, delirious** – *continued*
  - exhaustion (*see also* Reaction, stress, acute) 308.9
  - hysterical 300.11
  - in
    - presenile dementia 290.11
    - senile dementia 290.3
  - induced by drug 292.81
  - manic, maniacal (acute) (*see also* Psychosis, affective) 296.0 5th
    - recurrent episode 296.1 5th
    - single episode 296.0 5th
  - puerperal 293.9
  - senile 290.3
  - subacute (psychotic) 293.1
  - thyroid (*see also* Thyrotoxicosis) 242.9 5th
  - traumatic - *see also* Injury, intracranial
    - with
      - lesion, spinal cord - *see* Injury, spinal, by site
      - shock, spinal - *see* Injury, spinal, by site
  - tremens (impending) 291.0
  - uremic - *see* Uremia
  - withdrawal
    - alcoholic (acute) 291.0
      - chronic 291.1
    - drug 292.0
- **Delivery**

Note *Use the following fifth-digit subclassification with categories 640-649, 651-676:*

0	unspecified as to episode of care
1	delivered, with or without mention of antepartum condition
2	delivered, with mention of postpartum complication
3	antepartum condition or complication
4	postpartum condition or complication

  - breech (assisted) (buttocks) (complete) (frank) (spontaneous) 652.2 5th
    - affecting fetus or newborn 763.0
    - extraction NEC 669.6 5th
  - cesarean (for) 669.7 5th
    - abnormal
      - cervix 654.6 5th
      - pelvic organs or tissues 654.9 5th
      - pelvis (bony) (major) NEC 653.0 5th
      - presentation or position 652.9 5th
        - in multiple gestation 652.6 5th
      - size, fetus 653.5 5th
      - soft parts (of pelvis) 654.9 5th
      - uterus, congenital 654.0 5th
      - vagina 654.7 5th
      - vulva 654.8 5th
    - abruptio placentae 641.2 5th
    - acromion presentation 652.8 5th
    - affecting fetus or newborn 763.4
    - anteversion, cervix or uterus 654.4 5th
    - atony, uterus 661.2 5th
      - with hemorrhage 666.1 5th
    - bicornis or bicornuate uterus 654.0 5th
    - breech presentation (buttocks) (complete) (frank) 652.2 5th
    - brow presentation 652.4 5th
    - cephalopelvic disproportion (normally formed fetus) 653.4 5th
    - chin presentation 652.4 5th
    - cicatrix of cervix 654.6 5th
    - contracted pelvis (general) 653.1 5th
      - inlet 653.2 5th
      - outlet 653.3 5th
    - cord presentation or prolapse 663.0 5th
    - cystocele 654.4 5th
    - deformity (acquired) (congenital)
      - pelvic organs or tissues NEC 654.9 5th
      - pelvis (bony) NEC 653.0 5th
    - displacement, uterus NEC 654.4 5th
    - disproportion NEC 653.9 5th

- **Delivery** – *continued*
  - cesarean (for) – *continued*
    - distress
      - fetal 656.8 5th
      - maternal 669.0 5th
    - eclampsia 642.6 5th
    - face presentation 652.4 5th
    - failed
      - forceps 660.7 5th
      - trial of labor NEC 660.6 5th
      - vacuum extraction 660.7 5th
      - ventouse 660.7 5th
    - fetal deformity 653.7 5th
    - fetal-maternal hemorrhage 656.0 5th
    - fetus, fetal
      - distress 656.8 5th
      - prematurity 656.8 5th
    - fibroid (tumor) (uterus) 654.1 5th
    - footling 652.8 5th
      - with successful version 652.1 5th
    - hemorrhage (antepartum) (intrapartum) NEC 641.9 5th
    - hydrocephalic fetus 653.6 5th
    - incarceration of uterus 654.3 5th
    - incoordinate uterine action 661.4 5th
    - inertia, uterus 661.2 5th
      - primary 661.0 5th
      - secondary 661.1 5th
    - lateroversion, uterus or cervix 654.4 5th
    - mal lie 652.9 5th
    - malposition
      - fetus 652.9 5th
        - in multiple gestation 652.6 5th
      - pelvic organs or tissues NEC 654.9 5th
      - uterus NEC or cervix 654.4 5th
    - malpresentation NEC 652.9 5th
      - in multiple gestation 652.6 5th
    - maternal
      - diabetes mellitus (conditions classifiable to 249 and 250) 648.0 5th
      - heart disease NEC 648.6 5th
    - meconium in liquor 656.8 5th
      - staining only 792.3
    - oblique presentation 652.3 5th
    - oversize fetus 653.5 5th
    - pelvic tumor NEC 654.9 5th
    - placental insufficiency 656.5 5th
    - placenta previa 641.0 5th
      - with hemorrhage 641.1 5th
    - poor dilation, cervix 661.0 5th
    - pre-eclampsia 642.4 5th
      - severe 642.5 5th
    - previous
      - cesarean delivery, section 654.2 5th
      - surgery (to)
        - cervix 654.6 5th
        - gynecological NEC 654.9 5th
        - rectum 654.8 5th
        - uterus NEC 654.9 5th
          - previous cesarean delivery, section 654.2 5th
        - vagina 654.7 5th
    - prolapse
      - arm or hand 652.7 5th
      - uterus 654.4 5th
    - prolonged labor 662.1 5th
    - rectocele 654.4 5th
    - retroversion, uterus or cervix 654.3 5th
    - rigid
      - cervix 654.6 5th
      - pelvic floor 654.4 5th
      - perineum 654.8 5th
      - vagina 654.7 5th
      - vulva 654.8 5th
    - sacculation, pregnant uterus 654.4 5th
    - scar(s)
      - cervix 654.6 5th
      - cesarean delivery, section 654.2 5th
      - uterus NEC 654.9 5th
        - due to previous cesarean delivery, section 654.2 5th
    - Shirodkar suture in situ 654.5 5th

- **Delivery** – *continued*
  - cesarean (for) – *continued*
    - shoulder presentation 652.8 5th
    - stenosis or stricture, cervix 654.6 5th
    - transverse presentation or lie 652.3 5th
    - tumor, pelvic organs or tissues NEC 654.4 5th
    - umbilical cord presentation or prolapse 663.0 5th
  - completely normal case - *see* category 650
  - complicated (by) NEC 669.9 5th
    - abdominal tumor, fetal 653.7 5th
      - causing obstructed labor 660.1 5th
    - abnormal, abnormality of
      - cervix 654.6 5th
        - causing obstructed labor 660.2 5th
      - forces of labor 661.9 5th
      - formation of uterus 654.0 5th
      - pelvic organs or tissues 654.9 5th
        - causing obstructed labor 660.2 5th
      - pelvis (bony) (major) NEC 653.0 5th
        - causing obstructed labor 660.1 5th
      - presentation or position NEC 652.9 5th
        - causing obstructed labor 660.0 5th
      - size, fetus 653.5 5th
        - causing obstructed labor 660.1 5th
      - soft parts (of pelvis) 654.9 5th
        - causing obstructed labor 660.2 5th
      - uterine contractions NEC 661.9 5th
      - uterus (formation) 654.0 5th
        - causing obstructed labor 660.2 5th
      - vagina 654.7 5th
        - causing obstructed labor 660.2 5th
    - abnormally formed uterus (any type) (congenital) 654.0 5th
      - causing obstructed labor 660.2 5th
    - acromion presentation 652.8 5th
      - causing obstructed labor 660.0 5th
    - adherent placenta 667.0 5th
      - with hemorrhage 666.0 5th
    - adhesions, uterus (to abdominal wall) 654.4 5th
    - advanced maternal age NEC 659.6 5th
      - multigravida 659.6 5th
      - primigravida 659.5 5th
    - air embolism 673.0 5th
    - amnionitis 658.4 5th
    - amniotic fluid embolism 673.1 5th
    - anesthetic death 668.9 5th
    - annular detachment, cervix 665.3 5th
    - antepartum hemorrhage - *see* Delivery, complicated, hemorrhage
    - anteversion, cervix or uterus 654.4 5th
      - causing obstructed labor 660.2 5th
    - apoplexy 674.0 5th
      - placenta 641.2 5th
    - arrested active phase 661.1 5th
    - asymmetrical pelvis bone 653.0 5th
      - causing obstructed labor 660.1 5th
    - atony, uterus with hemorrhage (hypotonic) (inertia) 666.1 5th
      - hypertonic 661.4 5th
    - Bandl's ring 661.4 5th
    - Battledore placenta - *see* Placenta, abnormal
    - bicornis or bicornuate uterus 654.0 5th
      - causing obstructed labor 660.2 5th
    - birth injury to mother NEC 665.9 5th
    - bleeding (*see also* Delivery, complicated, hemorrhage) 641.9 5th
    - breech presentation (assisted) (buttocks) (complete) (frank) (spontaneous) 652.2 5th
      - with successful version 652.1 5th

- **Delivery** – *continued*
  - complicated (by) – *continued*
    - brow presentation 652.4 5th
    - cephalopelvic disproportion (normally formed fetus) 653.4 5th
      - causing obstructed labor 660.1 5th
    - cerebral hemorrhage 674.0 5th
    - cervical dystocia 661.2 5th
    - chin presentation 652.4 5th
      - causing obstructed labor 660.0 5th
    - cicatrix
      - cervix 654.6 5th
        - causing obstructed labor 660.2 5th
      - vagina 654.7 5th
        - causing obstructed labor 660.2 5th
    - coagulation defect 649.3 5th
    - colporrhexis 665.4 5th
      - with perineal laceration 664.0 5th
    - compound presentation 652.8 5th
      - causing obstructed labor 660.0 5th
    - compression of cord (umbilical) 663.2 5th
      - around neck 663.1 5th
      - cord prolapsed 663.0 5th
    - contraction, contracted pelvis 653.1 5th
      - causing obstructed labor 660.1 5th
      - general 653.1 5th
        - causing obstructed labor 660.1 5th
      - inlet 653.2 5th
        - causing obstructed labor 660.1 5th
      - midpelvic 653.8 5th
        - causing obstructed labor 660.1 5th
      - midplane 653.8 5th
        - causing obstructed labor 660.1 5th
      - outlet 653.3 5th
        - causing obstructed labor 660.1 5th
    - contraction ring 661.4 5th
    - cord (umbilical) 663.9 5th
      - around neck, tightly or with compression 663.1 5th
        - without compression 663.3 5th
      - bruising 663.6 5th
      - complication NEC 663.9 5th
        - specified type NEC 663.8 5th
      - compression NEC 663.2 5th
      - entanglement NEC 663.3 5th
        - with compression 663.2 5th
      - forelying 663.0 5th
      - hematoma 663.6 5th
      - marginal attachment 663.8 5th
      - presentation 663.0 5th
      - prolapse (complete) (occult) (partial) 663.0 5th
      - short 663.4 5th
      - specified complication NEC 663.8 5th
      - thrombosis (vessels) 663.6 5th
      - vascular lesion 663.6 5th
      - velamentous insertion 663.8 5th
    - Couvelaire uterus 641.2 5th
    - cretin pelvis (dwarf type) (male type) 653.1 5th
      - causing obstructed labor 660.1 5th
    - crossbirth 652.3 5th
      - with successful version 652.1 5th
      - causing obstructed labor 660.0 5th
    - cyst (Gartner's duct) 654.7 5th
    - cystocele 654.4 5th
      - causing obstructed labor 660.2 5th
    - death of fetus (near term) 656.4 5th
      - early (before 22 completed weeks gestation) 632
    - deformity (acquired) (congenital)
      - fetus 653.7 5th
        - causing obstructed labor 660.1 5th

- **Delivery** – *continued*
  - complicated (by) – *continued*
    - deformity – *continued*
      - pelvic organs or tissues NEC 654.9 5th
        - causing obstructed labor 660.2 5th
      - pelvis (bony) NEC 653.0 5th
        - causing obstructed labor 660.1 5th
    - delay, delayed
      - delivery in multiple pregnancy 662.3 5th
        - due to locked mates 660.5 5th
      - following rupture of membranes (spontaneous) 658.2 5th
        - artificial 658.3 5th
    - depressed fetal heart tones 659.7 5th
    - diastasis recti 665.8 5th
    - dilatation
      - bladder 654.4 5th
        - causing obstructed labor 660.2 5th
      - cervix, incomplete, poor or slow 661.0 5th
    - diseased placenta 656.7 5th
    - displacement uterus NEC 654.4 5th
      - causing obstructed labor 660.2 5th
    - disproportion NEC 653.9 5th
      - causing obstructed labor 660.1 5th
    - disruptio uteri - *see* Delivery, complicated, rupture, uterus
    - distress
      - fetal 656.8 5th
      - maternal 669.0 5th
    - double uterus (congenital) 654.0 5th
      - causing obstructed labor 660.2 5th
    - dropsy amnion 657 5th
    - dysfunction, uterus 661.9 5th
      - hypertonic 661.4 5th
      - hypotonic 661.2 5th
        - primary 661.0 5th
        - secondary 661.1 5th
      - incoordinate 661.4 5th
    - dystocia
      - cervical 661.2 5th
      - fetal - *see* Delivery, complicated, abnormal, presentation
      - maternal - *see* Delivery, complicated, prolonged labor
      - pelvic - *see* Delivery, complicated, contraction pelvis
      - positional 652.8 5th
      - shoulder girdle 660.4 5th
    - eclampsia 642.6 5th
    - ectopic kidney 654.4 5th
      - causing obstructed labor 660.2 5th
    - edema, cervix 654.6 5th
      - causing obstructed labor 660.2 5th
    - effusion, amniotic fluid 658.1 5th
    - elderly multigravida 659.6 5th
    - elderly primigravida 659.5 5th
    - embolism (pulmonary) 673.2 5th
      - air 673.0 5th
      - amniotic fluid 673.1 5th
      - blood-clot 673.2 5th
      - cerebral 674.0 5th
      - fat 673.8 5th
      - pyemic 673.3 5th
      - septic 673.3 5th
    - entanglement, umbilical cord 663.3 5th
      - with compression 663.2 5th
      - around neck (with compression) 663.1 5th
    - eversion, cervix or uterus 665.2 5th
    - excessive
      - fetal growth 653.5 5th
        - causing obstructed labor 660.1 5th
      - size of fetus 653.5 5th
        - causing obstructed labor 660.1 5th
    - face presentation 652.4 5th
      - causing obstructed labor 660.0 5th

- **Delivery** – *continued*
  - complicated (by) – *continued*
    - face presentation – *continued*
      - to pubes 660.3 5th
    - failure, fetal head to enter pelvic brim 652.5 5th
      - causing obstructed labor 660.0 5th
    - female genital mutilation 660.8 5th
    - fetal
      - acid-base balance 656.8 5th
      - death (near term) NEC 656.4 5th
        - early (before 22 completed weeks gestation) 632
      - deformity 653.7 5th
        - causing obstructed labor 660.1 5th
      - distress 656.8 5th
      - heart rate or rhythm 659.7 5th
      - reduction of multiple fetuses reduced to single fetus 651.7 5th
    - fetopelvic disproportion 653.4 5th
      - causing obstructed labor 660.1 5th
    - fever during labor 659.2 5th
    - fibroid (tumor) (uterus) 654.1 5th
      - causing obstructed labor 660.2 5th
    - fibromyomata 654.1 5th
      - causing obstructed labor 660.2 5th
    - forelying umbilical cord 663.0 5th
    - fracture of coccyx 665.6 5th
    - hematoma 664.5 5th
      - broad ligament 665.7 5th
      - ischial spine 665.7 5th
      - pelvic 665.7 5th
      - perineum 664.5 5th
      - soft tissues 665.7 5th
      - subdural 674.0 5th
      - umbilical cord 663.6 5th
      - vagina 665.7 5th
      - vulva or perineum 664.5 5th
    - hemorrhage (uterine) (antepartum) (intrapartum) (pregnancy) 641.9 5th
      - accidental 641.2 5th
      - associated with
        - afibrinogenemia 641.3 5th
        - coagulation defect 641.3 5th
          - hyperfibrinolysis 641.3 5th
          - hypofibrinogenemia 641.3 5th
      - cerebral 674.0 5th
      - due to
        - low-lying placenta 641.1 5th
        - placenta previa 641.1 5th
        - premature separation of placenta (normally implanted) 641.2 5th
        - retained placenta 666.0 5th
        - trauma 641.8 5th
        - uterine leiomyoma 641.8 5th
      - marginal sinus rupture 641.2 5th
      - placenta NEC 641.9 5th
      - postpartum (atonic) (immediate) (within 24 hours) 666.1 5th
        - with retained or trapped placenta 666.0 5th
        - delayed 666.2 5th
        - secondary 666.2 5th
        - third stage 666.0 5th
    - hourglass contraction, uterus 661.4 5th
    - hydramnios 657 5th
    - hydrocephalic fetus 653.6 5th
      - causing obstructed labor 660.1 5th
    - hydrops fetalis 653.7 5th
      - causing obstructed labor 660.1 5th
    - hypertension - *see* Hypertension, complicating pregnancy
    - hypertonic uterine dysfunction 661.4 5th
    - hypotonic uterine dysfunction 661.2 5th
    - impacted shoulders 660.4 5th
    - incarceration, uterus 654.3 5th
      - causing obstructed labor 660.2 5th

- **Delivery** – *continued*
  - complicated (by) – *continued*
    - incomplete dilation (cervix) 661.0 5th
    - incoordinate uterus 661.4 5th
    - indication NEC 659.9 5th
      - specified type NEC 659.8 5th
    - inertia, uterus 661.2 5th
      - hypertonic 661.4 5th
      - hypotonic 661.2 5th
      - primary 661.0 5th
      - secondary 661.1 5th
    - infantile
      - genitalia 654.4 5th
        - causing obstructed labor 660.2 5th
      - uterus (os) 654.4 5th
        - causing obstructed labor 660.2 5th
    - injury (to mother) NEC 665.9 5th
    - intrauterine fetal death (near term) NEC 656.4 5th
      - early (before 22 completed weeks gestation) 632
    - inversion, uterus 665.2 5th
    - kidney, ectopic 654.4 5th
      - causing obstructed labor 660.2 5th
    - knot (true), umbilical cord 663.2 5th
    - labor, premature (before 37 completed weeks gestation) 644.2 5th
    - laceration 664.9 5th
      - anus (sphincter) (healed) (old) 654.8 5th
        - with mucosa 664.3 5th
        - not associated with third-degree perineal laceration 664.6 5th
      - bladder (urinary) 665.5 5th
      - bowel 665.5 5th
      - central 664.4 5th
      - cervix (uteri) 665.3 5th
      - fourchette 664.0 5th
      - hymen 664.0 5th
      - labia (majora) (minora) 664.0 5th
      - pelvic
        - floor 664.1 5th
        - organ NEC 665.5 5th
      - perineum, perineal 664.4 5th
        - first degree 664.0 5th
        - second degree 664.1 5th
        - third degree 664.2 5th
        - fourth degree 664.3 5th
        - central 664.4 5th
        - extensive NEC 664.4 5th
        - muscles 664.1 5th
        - skin 664.0 5th
        - slight 664.0 5th
      - peritoneum 665.5 5th
      - periurethral tissue 664.8 5th
      - rectovaginal (septum) (without perineal laceration) 665.4 5th
        - with perineum 664.2 5th
          - with anal or rectal mucosa 664.3 5th
      - skin (perineum) 664.0 5th
      - specified site or type NEC 664.8 5th
      - sphincter ani (healed) (old) 654.8 5th
        - with mucosa 664.3 5th
        - not associated with third-degree perineal laceration 664.6 5th
      - urethra 665.5 5th
      - uterus 665.1 5th
        - before labor 665.0 5th
      - vagina, vaginal (deep) (high) (sulcus) (wall) (without perineal laceration) 665.4 5th
        - with perineum 664.0 5th
        - muscles, with perineum 664.1 5th
      - vulva 664.0 5th
    - lateroversion, uterus or cervix 654.4 5th
      - causing obstructed labor 660.2 5th
    - locked mates 660.5 5th

- **Delivery** – *continued*
  - complicated (by) – *continued*
    - low implantation of placenta - *see* Delivery, complicated, placenta, previa
    - mal lie 652.9 5th
    - malposition
      - fetus NEC 652.9 5th
        - causing obstructed labor 660.0 5th
      - pelvic organs or tissues NEC 654.9 5th
        - causing obstructed labor 660.2 5th
      - placenta 641.1 5th
        - without hemorrhage 641.0 5th
      - uterus NEC or cervix 654.4 5th
        - causing obstructed labor 660.2 5th
    - malpresentation 652.9 5th
      - causing obstructed labor 660.0 5th
    - marginal sinus (bleeding) (rupture) 641.2 5th
    - maternal hypotension syndrome 669.2 5th
    - meconium in liquor 656.8 5th
    - membranes, retained - *see* Delivery, complicated, placenta, retained
    - mentum presentation 652.4 5th
      - causing obstructed labor 660.0 5th
    - metrorrhagia (myopathia) - *see* Delivery, complicated, hemorrhage
    - metrorrhexis - *see* Delivery, complicated, rupture, uterus
    - multiparity (grand) 659.4 5th
    - myelomeningocele, fetus 653.7 5th
      - causing obstructed labor 660.1 5th
    - Nägele's pelvis 653.0 5th
      - causing obstructed labor 660.1 5th
    - nonengagement, fetal head 652.5 5th
      - causing obstructed labor 660.0 5th
    - oblique presentation 652.3 5th
      - causing obstructed labor 660.0 5th
    - obstetric
      - shock 669.1 5th
      - trauma NEC 665.9 5th
    - obstructed labor 660.9 5th
      - due to
        - abnormality of pelvic organs or tissues (conditions classifiable to 654.0-654.9) 660.2 5th
        - deep transverse arrest 660.3 5th
        - impacted shoulders 660.4 5th
        - locked twins 660.5 5th
        - malposition and malpresentation of fetus (conditions classifiable to 652.0-652.9) 660.0 5th
        - persistent occipitoposterior 660.3 5th
        - shoulder dystocia 660.4 5th
    - occult prolapse of umbilical cord 663.0 5th
    - oversize fetus 653.5 5th
      - causing obstructed labor 660.1 5th
    - pathological retraction ring, uterus 661.4 5th
    - pelvic
      - arrest (deep) (high) (of fetal head) (transverse) 660.3 5th
      - deformity (bone) - *see also* Deformity, pelvis, with disproportion
        - soft tissue 654.9 5th
          - causing obstructed labor 660.2 5th
      - tumor NEC 654.9 5th
        - causing obstructed labor 660.2 5th
    - penetration, pregnant uterus by instrument 665.1 5th
    - perforation - *see* Delivery, complicated, laceration
    - persistent
      - hymen 654.8 5th
        - causing obstructed labor 660.2 5th
      - occipitoposterior 660.3 5th
    - placenta, placental
      - ablatio 641.2 5th
      - abnormality 656.7 5th
        - with hemorrhage 641.2 5th
      - abruptio 641.2 5th
      - accreta 667.0 5th
        - with hemorrhage 666.0 5th
      - adherent (without hemorrhage) 667.0 5th
        - with hemorrhage 666.0 5th
      - apoplexy 641.2 5th
      - battledore- *see* Placenta, abnormal
      - detachment (premature) 641.2 5th
      - disease 656.7 5th
      - hemorrhage NEC 641.9 5th
      - increta (without hemorrhage) 667.0 5th
        - with hemorrhage 666.0 5th
      - low (implantation) 641.1 5th
        - without hemorrhage 641.0 5th
      - malformation 656.7 5th
        - with hemorrhage 641.2 5th
      - malposition 641.1 5th
        - without hemorrhage 641.0 5th
      - marginal sinus rupture 641.2 5th
      - percreta 667.0 5th
        - with hemorrhage 666.0 5th
      - premature separation 641.2 5th
      - previa (central) (lateral) (marginal) (partial) 641.1 5th
        - without hemorrhage 641.0 5th
      - retained (with hemorrhage) 666.0 5th
        - without hemorrhage 667.0 5th
      - rupture of marginal sinus 641.2 5th
      - separation (premature) 641.2 5th
      - trapped 666.0 5th
        - without hemorrhage 667.0 5th
      - vicious insertion 641.1 5th
    - polyhydramnios 657 5th
    - polyp, cervix 654.6 5th
      - causing obstructed labor 660.2 5th
    - precipitate labor 661.3 5th
    - premature
      - labor (before 37 completed weeks gestation) 644.2 5th
      - rupture, membranes 658.1 5th
        - delayed delivery following 658.2 5th
    - presenting umbilical cord 663.0 5th
    - previous
      - cesarean delivery, section 654.2 5th
      - surgery
        - cervix 654.6 5th
          - causing obstructed labor 660.2 5th
        - gynecological NEC 654.9 5th
          - causing obstructed labor 660.2 5th
        - perineum 654.8 5th
        - rectum 654.8 5th
        - uterus NEC 654.9 5th
          - due to previous cesarean delivery, section 654.2 5th
        - vagina 654.7 5th
          - causing obstructed labor 660.2 5th
        - vulva 654.8 5th
    - primary uterine inertia 661.0 5th
    - primipara, elderly or old 659.5 5th
    - prolapse
      - arm or hand 652.7 5th
        - causing obstructed labor 660.0 5th

- **Delivery** – *continued*
  - complicated (by) – *continued*
    - prolapse – *continued*
      - cord (umbilical) 663.0 5th
      - fetal extremity 652.8 5th
      - foot or leg 652.8 5th
        - causing obstructed labor 660.0 5th
      - umbilical cord (complete) (occult) (partial) 663.0 5th
      - uterus 654.4 5th
        - causing obstructed labor 660.2 5th
    - prolonged labor 662.1 5th
      - first stage 662.0 5th
      - second stage 662.2 5th
      - active phase 661.2 5th
      - due to
        - cervical dystocia 661.2 5th
        - contraction ring 661.4 5th
        - tetanic uterus 661.4 5th
        - uterine inertia 661.2 5th
          - primary 661.0 5th
          - secondary 661.1 5th
      - latent phase 661.0 5th
    - pyrexia during labor 659.2 5th
    - rachitic pelvis 653.2 5th
      - causing obstructed labor 660.1 5th
    - rectocele 654.4 5th
      - causing obstructed labor 660.2 5th
    - retained membranes or portions of placenta 666.2 5th
      - without hemorrhage 667.1 5th
    - retarded (prolonged) birth 662.1 5th
    - retention secundines (with hemorrhage) 666.2 5th
      - without hemorrhage 667.1 5th
    - retroversion, uterus or cervix 654.3 5th
      - causing obstructed labor 660.2 5th
    - rigid
      - cervix 654.6 5th
        - causing obstructed labor 660.2 5th
      - pelvic floor 654.4 5th
        - causing obstructed labor 660.2 5th
      - perineum or vulva 654.8 5th
        - causing obstructed labor 660.2 5th
      - vagina 654.7 5th
        - causing obstructed labor 660.2 5th
    - Robert's pelvis 653.0 5th
      - causing obstructed labor 660.1 5th
    - rupture - *see also* Delivery, complicated, laceration
      - bladder (urinary) 665.5 5th
      - cervix 665.3 5th
      - marginal sinus 641.2 5th
      - membranes, premature 658.1 5th
      - pelvic organ NEC 665.5 5th
      - perineum (without mention of other laceration) - *see* Delivery, complicated, laceration, perineum
      - peritoneum 665.5 5th
      - urethra 665.5 5th
      - uterus (during labor) 665.1 5th
        - before labor 665.0 5th
    - sacculation, pregnant uterus 654.4 5th
    - sacral teratomas, fetal 653.7 5th
      - causing obstructed labor 660.1 5th
    - scar(s)
      - cervix 654.6 5th
        - causing obstructed labor 660.2 5th
      - cesarean delivery, section 654.2 5th
        - causing obstructed labor 660.2 5th
      - perineum 654.8 5th
        - causing obstructed labor 660.2 5th

- **Delivery** – *continued*
  - complicated (by) – *continued*
    - scar(s) – *continued*
      - uterus NEC 654.9 5th
        - causing obstructed labor 660.2 5th
        - due to previous cesarean delivery, section 654.2 5th
      - vagina 654.7 5th
        - causing obstructed labor 660.2 5th
      - vulva 654.8 5th
        - causing obstructed labor 660.2 5th
    - scoliotic pelvis 653.0 5th
      - causing obstructed labor 660.1 5th
    - secondary uterine inertia 661.1 5th
    - secundines, retained - *see* Delivery, complicated, placenta, retained
    - separation
      - placenta (premature) 641.2 5th
      - pubic bone 665.6 5th
      - symphysis pubis 665.6 5th
    - septate vagina 654.7 5th
      - causing obstructed labor 660.2 5th
    - shock (birth) (obstetric) (puerperal) 669.1 5th
    - short cord syndrome 663.4 5th
    - shoulder
      - girdle dystocia 660.4 5th
      - presentation 652.8 5th
        - causing obstructed labor 660.0 5th
    - Siamese twins 678.1 5th
      - ~~causing obstructed labor 660.1~~
    - slow slope active phase 661.2 5th
    - spasm
      - cervix 661.4 5th
      - uterus 661.4 5th
    - spondylolisthesis, pelvis 653.3 5th
      - causing obstructed labor 660.1 5th
    - spondylolysis (lumbosacral) 653.3 5th
      - causing obstructed labor 660.1 5th
    - spondylosis 653.0 5th
      - causing obstructed labor 660.1 5th
    - stenosis or stricture
      - cervix 654.6 5th
        - causing obstructed labor 660.2 5th
      - vagina 654.7 5th
        - causing obstructed labor 660.2 5th
    - sudden death, unknown cause 669.9 5th
    - tear (pelvic organ) (*see also* Delivery, complicated, laceration) 664.9 5th
      - anal sphincter (healed) (old) 654.8 5th
        - not associated with third-degree perineal laceration 664.6 5th
    - teratomas, sacral, fetal 653.7 5th
      - causing obstructed labor 660.1 5th
    - tetanic uterus 661.4 5th
    - tipping pelvis 653.0 5th
      - causing obstructed labor 660.1 5th
    - transverse
      - arrest (deep) 660.3 5th
      - presentation or lie 652.3 5th
        - with successful version 652.1 5th
        - causing obstructed labor 660.0 5th
    - trauma (obstetrical) NEC 665.9 5th
    - tumor
      - abdominal, fetal 653.7 5th
        - causing obstructed labor 660.1 5th
      - pelvic organs or tissues NEC 654.9 5th
        - causing obstructed labor 660.2 5th

- **Delivery** – *continued*
  - complicated (by) – *continued*
    - umbilical cord (*see also* Delivery, complicated, cord) 663.9 5th
      - around neck tightly, or with compression 663.1 5th
      - entanglement NEC 663.3 5th
        - with compression 663.2 5th
      - prolapse (complete) (occult) (partial) 663.0 5th
    - unstable lie 652.0 5th
      - causing obstructed labor 660.0 5th
    - uterine
      - inertia (*see also* Delivery, complicated, inertia, uterus) 661.2 5th
      - spasm 661.4 5th
    - vasa previa 663.5 5th
    - velamentous insertion of cord 663.8 5th
    - young maternal age 659.8 5th
  - delayed NEC 662.1 5th
    - following rupture of membranes (spontaneous) 658.2 5th
      - artificial 658.3 5th
    - second twin, triplet, etc. 662.3 5th
  - difficult NEC 669.9 5th
    - previous, affecting management of pregnancy or childbirth V23.49
    - specified type NEC 669.8 5th
  - early onset (spontaneous) 644.2 5th
  - footling 652.8 5th
    - with successful version 652.1 5th
  - forceps NEC 669.5 5th
    - affecting fetus or newborn 763.2
  - missed (at or near term) 656.4 5th
  - multiple gestation NEC 651.9 5th
    - with fetal loss and retention of one or more fetus(es) 651.6 5th
    - following (elective) fetal reduction 651.7 5th
    - specified type NEC 651.8 5th
      - with fetal loss and retention of one or more fetus(es) 651.6 5th
      - following (elective) fetal reduction 651.7 5th
  - nonviable infant 656.4 5th
  - normal - *see* category 650
  - precipitate 661.3 5th
    - affecting fetus or newborn 763.6
  - premature NEC (before 37 completed weeks gestation) 644.2 5th
    - previous, affecting management of pregnancy V23.41
  - quadruplet NEC 651.2 5th
    - with fetal loss and retention of one or more fetus(es) 651.5 5th
    - following (elective) fetal reduction 651.7 5th
  - quintuplet NEC 651.8 5th
    - with fetal loss and retention of one or more fetus(es) 651.6 5th
    - following (elective) fetal reduction 651.7 5th
  - sextuplet NEC 651.8 5th
    - with fetal loss and retention of one or more fetus(es) 651.6 5th
    - following (elective) fetal reduction 651.7 5th
  - specified complication NEC 669.8 5th
  - stillbirth (near term) NEC 656.4 5th
    - early (before 22 completed weeks gestation) 632
  - term pregnancy (live birth) NEC - *see* category 650
    - stillbirth NEC 656.4 5th
  - threatened premature 644.2 5th
  - triplets NEC 651.1 5th
    - with fetal loss and retention of one or more fetus(es) 651.4 5th
    - delayed delivery (one or more mates) 662.3 5th
    - following (elective) fetal reduction 651.7 5th
    - locked mates 660.5 5th

- **Delivery** – *continued*
  - twins NEC 651.0 5th
    - with fetal loss and retention of one fetus 651.3 5th
    - delayed delivery (one or more mates) 662.3 5th
    - following (elective) fetal reduction 651.7 5th
    - locked mates 660.5 5th
  - uncomplicated - *see* category 650
  - vacuum extractor NEC 669.5 5th
    - affecting fetus or newborn 763.3
  - ventouse NEC 669.5 5th
    - affecting fetus or newborn 763.3
- **Dellen, cornea** 371.41
- **Delusions** (paranoid) 297.9
  - grandiose 297.1
  - parasitosis 300.29
  - systematized 297.1
- **Dementia** 294.8
  - alcohol-induced persisting (*see also* Psychosis, alcoholic) 291.2
  - Alzheimer's - *see* Alzheimer's, dementia
  - arteriosclerotic (simple type) (uncomplicated) 290.40
    - with
      - acute confusional state 290.41
      - delirium 290.41
      - delusions 290.42
      - depressed mood 290.43
    - depressed type 290.43
    - paranoid type 290.42
  - Binswanger's 290.12
  - catatonic (acute) (*see also* Schizophrenia) 295.2 5th
  - congenital (*see also* Retardation, mental) 319
  - degenerative 290.9
    - presenile-onset - *see* Dementia, presenile
    - senile-onset - *see* Dementia, senile
  - developmental (*see also* Schizophrenia) 295.9 5th
  - dialysis 294.8
    - transient 293.9
  - drug-induced persisting (*see also* Psychosis, drug) 292.82
  - due to or associated with condition(s) classified elsewhere
    - Alzheimer's
      - with behavioral disturbance 331.0 *[294.11]*
      - without behavioral disturbance 331.0 *[294.10]*
    - cerebral lipidoses
      - with behavioral disturbance 330.1 *[294.11]*
      - without behavioral disturbance 330.1 *[294.10]*
    - epilepsy
      - with behavioral disturbance 345.9 5th *[294.11]*
      - without behavioral disturbance 345.9 5th *[294.10]*
    - hepatolenticular degeneration
      - with behavioral disturbance 275.1 *[294.11]*
      - without behavioral disturbance 275.1 *[294.10]*
    - HIV
      - with behavioral disturbance 042 *[294.11]*
      - without behavioral disturbance 042 *[294.10]*
    - Huntington's chorea
      - with behavioral disturbance 333.4 *[294.11]*
      - without behavioral disturbance 333.4 *[294.10]*
    - Jakob-Creutzfeldt disease (CJD)
      - with behavioral disturbance 046.19 *[294.11]*
      - without behavioral disturbance 046.19 *[294.10]*

- **Dementia** – *continued*
  - due to or associated with condition(s) classified elsewhere – *continued*
    - Jakob-Creutzfeldt disease (CJD) – *continued*
      - variant (vCJD) 046.11
        - with dementia
          - with behavioral disturbance 046.11 *[294.11]*
          - without behavioral disturbance 046.11 *[294.10]*
    - Lewy bodies
      - with behavioral disturbance 331.82 *[294.11]*
      - without behavioral disturbance 331.82 *[294.10]*
    - multiple sclerosis
      - with behavioral disturbance 340 *[294.11]*
      - without behavioral disturbance 340 *[294.10]*
    - neurosyphilis
      - with behavioral disturbance 094.9 *[294.11]*
      - without behavioral disturbance 094.9 *[294.10]*
    - Parkinsonism
      - with behavioral disturbance 331.82 *[294.11]*
      - without behavioral disturbance 331.82 *[294.10]*
    - Pelizaeus-Merzbacher disease
      - with behavioral disturbance 333.0 *[294.11]*
      - without behavioral disturbance 333.0 *[294.10]*
    - Pick's disease
      - with behavioral disturbance 331.11 *[294.11]*
      - without behavioral disturbance 331.11 *[294.10]*
    - polyarteritis nodosa
      - with behavioral disturbance 446.0 *[294.11]*
      - without behavioral disturbance 446.0 *[294.10]*
    - syphilis
      - with behavioral disturbance 094.1 *[294.11]*
      - without behavioral disturbance 094.1 *[294.10]*
    - Wilson's disease
      - with behavioral disturbance 275.1 *[294.11]*
      - without behavioral disturbance 275.1 *[294.10]*
  - frontal 331.19
    - with behavioral disturbance 331.19 *[294.11]*
    - without behavioral disturbance 331.19 *[294.10]*
  - frontotemporal 331.19
    - with behavioral disturbance 331.19 *[294.11]*
    - without behavioral disturbance 331.19 *[294.10]*
  - hebephrenic (acute) 295.1 5th
  - Heller's (infantile psychosis) (*see also* Psychosis, childhood) 299.1 5th
  - idiopathic 290.9
    - presenile-onset - *see* Dementia, presenile
    - senile-onset - *see* Dementia, senile
  - in
    - arteriosclerotic brain disease 290.40
    - senility 290.0
  - induced by drug 292.82
  - infantile, infantilia (*see also* Psychosis, childhood) 299.0 5th
  - Lewy body 331.82
    - with behavioral disturbance 331.82 *[294.11]*

- **Dementia** – *continued*
  - Lewy body – *continued*
    - without behavioral disturbance 331.82 *[294.10]*
  - multi-infarct (cerebrovascular) (*see also* Dementia, arteriosclerotic) 290.40
  - old age 290.0
  - paralytica, paralytic 094.1
    - juvenilis 090.40
    - syphilitic 094.1
      - congenital 090.40
    - tabetic form 094.1
  - paranoid (*see also* Schizophrenia) 295.3 5th
  - paraphrenic (*see also* Schizophrenia) 295.3 5th
  - paretic 094.1
  - praecox (*see also* Schizophrenia) 295.9 5th
  - presenile 290.10
    - with
      - acute confusional state 290.11
      - delirium 290.11
      - delusional features 290.12
      - depressive features 290.13
    - depressed type 290.13
    - paranoid type 290.12
    - simple type 290.10
    - uncomplicated 290.10
  - primary (acute) (*see also* Schizophrenia) 295.0 5th
  - progressive, syphilitic 094.1
  - puerperal - *see* Psychosis, puerperal
  - schizophrenic (*see also* Schizophrenia) 295.9 5th
  - senile 290.0
    - with
      - acute confusional state 290.3
      - delirium 290.3
      - delusional features 290.20
      - depressive features 290.21
    - depressed type 290.21
    - exhaustion 290.0
    - paranoid type 290.20
  - simple type (acute) (*see also* Schizophrenia) 295.0 5th
  - simplex (acute) (*see also* Schizophrenia) 295.0 5th
  - syphilitic 094.1
  - uremic - *see* Uremia
  - vascular 290.40
    - with
      - delirium 290.41
      - delusions 290.42
      - depressed mood 290.43
- **Demerol dependence** (*see also* Dependence) 304.0 5th
- **Demineralization, ankle** (*see also* Osteoporosis) 733.00
- **Demodex folliculorum** (infestation) 133.8
- **Demoralization** 799.25 ●
- **de Morgan's spots** (senile angiomas) 448.1
- **Demyelinating**
  - polyneuritis, chronic inflammatory 357.81
- **Demyelination, demyelinization**
  - central nervous system 341.9
    - specified NEC 341.8
  - corpus callosum (central) 341.8
  - global 340
- **Dengue** (fever) 061
  - sandfly 061
  - vaccination, prophylactic (against) V05.1
  - virus hemorrhagic fever 065.4
- **Dens**
  - evaginatus 520.2
  - in dente 520.2
  - invaginatus 520.2
- **Dense**
  - breast(s) - omit code
- **Density**
  - increased, bone (disseminated) (generalized) (spotted) 733.99
  - lung (nodular) 518.89
- **Dental** - *see also* condition
  - examination only V72.2

Dentia praecox 520.6
Denticles (in pulp) 522.2
Dentigerous cyst 526.0
Dentin
- irregular (in pulp) 522.3
- opalescent 520.5
- secondary (in pulp) 522.3
- sensitive 521.89

Dentinogenesis imperfecta 520.5
Dentinoma (M9271/0) 213.1
- upper jaw (bone) 213.0

Dentition 520.7
- abnormal 520.6
- anomaly 520.6
- delayed 520.6
- difficult 520.7
- disorder of 520.6
- precocious 520.6
- retarded 520.6

Denture sore (mouth) 528.9
Dependence

Note *Use the following fifth-digit subclassification with category 304:*

- **0** unspecified
- **1** continuous
- **2** episodic
- **3** in remission

- with
  - withdrawal symptoms
    - alcohol 291.81
    - drug 292.0
- 14-hydroxy-dihydromorphinone 304.0 5th
- absinthe 304.6 5th
- acemorphan 304.0 5th
- acetanilid(e) 304.6 5th
- acetophenetidin 304.6 5th
- acetorphine 304.0 5th
- acetyldihydrocodeine 304.0 5th
- acetyldihydrocodeinone 304.0 5th
- Adalin 304.1 5th
- afghanistan black 304.3 5th
- agrypnal 304.1 5th
- alcohol, alcoholic (ethyl) (methyl) (wood) 303.9 5th
  - maternal, with suspected fetal damage affecting management of pregnancy 655.4 5th
- allobarbitone 304.1 5th
- allonal 304.1 5th
- allylisopropylacetylurea 304.1 5th
- alphaprodine (hydrochloride) 304.0 5th
- Alurate 304.1 5th
- Alvodine 304.0 5th
- amethocaine 304.6 5th
- amidone 304.0 5th
- amidopyrine 304.6 5th
- aminopyrine 304.6 5th
- amobarbital 304.1 5th
- amphetamine(s) (type) (drugs classifiable to 969.7) 304.4 5th
- amylene hydrate 304.6 5th
- amylobarbitone 304.1 5th
- amylocaine 304.6 5th
- Amytal (sodium) 304.1 5th
- analgesic (drug) NEC 304.6 5th
  - synthetic with morphine-like effect 304.0 5th
- anesthetic (agent) (drug) (gas) (general) (local) NEC 304.6 5th
- Angel dust 304.6 5th
- anileridine 304.0 5th
- antipyrine 304.6 5th
- anxiolytic 304.1 5th
- aprobarbital 304.1 5th
- aprobarbitone 304.1 5th
- atropine 304.6 5th
- Avertin (bromide) 304.6 5th
- barbenyl 304.1 5th
- barbital(s) 304.1 5th
- barbitone 304.1 5th
- barbiturate(s) (compounds) (drugs classifiable to 967.0) 304.1 5th

Dependence – *continued*
- barbituric acid (and compounds) 304.1 5th
- benzedrine 304.4 5th
- benzylmorphine 304.0 5th
- Beta-chlor 304.1 5th
- bhang 304.3 5th
- blue velvet 304.0 5th
- Brevital 304.1 5th
- bromal (hydrate) 304.1 5th
- bromide(s) NEC 304.1 5th
- bromine compounds NEC 304.1 5th
- bromisovalum 304.1 5th
- bromoform 304.1 5th
- Bromo-seltzer 304.1 5th
- bromural 304.1 5th
- butabarbital (sodium) 304.1 5th
- butabarpal 304.1 5th
- butallylonal 304.1 5th
- butethal 304.1 5th
- buthalitone (sodium) 304.1 5th
- Butisol 304.1 5th
- butobarbitone 304.1 5th
- butyl chloral (hydrate) 304.1 5th
- caffeine 304.4 5th
- cannabis (indica) (sativa) (resin) (derivatives) (type) 304.3 5th
- carbamazepine 304.6 5th
- Carbrital 304.1 5th
- carbromal 304.1 5th
- carisoprodol 304.6 5th
- Catha (edulis) 304.4 5th
- chloral (betaine) (hydrate) 304.1 5th
- chloralamide 304.1 5th
- chloralformamide 304.1 5th
- chloralose 304.1 5th
- chlordiazepoxide 304.1 5th
- Chloretone 304.1 5th
- chlorobutanol 304.1 5th
- chlorodyne 304.1 5th
- chloroform 304.6 5th
- Cliradon 304.0 5th
- coca (leaf) and derivatives 304.2 5th
- cocaine 304.2 5th
  - hydrochloride 304.2 5th
  - salt (any) 304.2 5th
- codeine 304.0 5th
- combination of drugs (excluding morphine or opioid type drug) NEC 304.8 5th
  - morphine or opioid type drug with any other drug 304.7 5th
- croton-chloral 304.1 5th
- cyclobarbital 304.1 5th
- cyclobarbitone 304.1 5th
- dagga 304.3 5th
- Delvinal 304.1 5th
- Demerol 304.0 5th
- desocodeine 304.0 5th
- desomorphine 304.0 5th
- desoxyephedrine 304.4 5th
- DET 304.5 5th
- dexamphetamine 304.4 5th
- dexedrine 304.4 5th
- dextromethorphan 304.0 5th
- dextromoramide 304.0 5th
- dextronorpseudoephedrine 304.4 5th
- dextrorphan 304.0 5th
- diacetylmorphine 304.0 5th
- Dial 304.1 5th
- diallylbarbituric acid 304.1 5th
- diamorphine 304.0 5th
- diazepam 304.1 5th
- dibucaine 304.6 5th
- dichloroethane 304.6 5th
- diethyl barbituric acid 304.1 5th
- diethylsulfone-diethylmethane 304.1 5th
- difencloxazine 304.0 5th
- dihydrocodeine 304.0 5th
- dihydrocodeinone 304.0 5th
- dihydrohydroxycodeinone 304.0 5th
- dihydroisocodeine 304.0 5th
- dihydromorphine 304.0 5th
- dihydromorphinone 304.0 5th
- dihydroxcodeinone 304.0 5th

Dependence – *continued*
- Dilaudid 304.0 5th
- dimenhydrinate 304.6 5th
- dimethylmeperidine 304.0 5th
- dimethyltriptamine 304.5 5th
- Dionin 304.0 5th
- diphenoxylate 304.6 5th
- dipipanone 304.0 5th
- d-lysergic acid diethylamide 304.5 5th
- DMT 304.5 5th
- Dolophine 304.0 5th
- DOM 304.2 5th
- doriden 304.1 5th
- dormiral 304.1 5th
- Dormison 304.1 5th
- Dromoran 304.0 5th
- drug NEC 304.9 5th
  - analgesic NEC 304.6 5th
  - combination (excluding morphine or opioid type drug) NEC 304.8 5th
    - morphine or opioid type drug with any other drug 304.7 5th
  - complicating pregnancy, childbirth, or puerperium 648.3 5th
    - affecting fetus or newborn 779.5
  - hallucinogenic 304.5 5th
  - hypnotic NEC 304.1 5th
  - narcotic NEC 304.9 5th
  - psychostimulant NEC 304.4 5th
  - sedative 304.1 5th
  - soporific NEC 304.1 5th
  - specified type NEC 304.6 5th
  - suspected damage to fetus affecting management of pregnancy 655.5 5th
  - synthetic, with morphine-like effect 304.0 5th
  - tranquilizing 304.1 5th
- duboisine 304.6 5th
- ectylurea 304.1 5th
- Endocaine 304.6 5th
- Equanil 304.1 5th
- Eskabarb 304.1 5th
- ethchlorvynol 304.1 5th
- ether (ethyl) (liquid) (vapor) (vinyl) 304.6 5th
- ethidene 304.6 5th
- ethinamate 304.1 5th
- ethoheptazine 304.6 5th
- ethyl
  - alcohol 303.9 5th
  - bromide 304.6 5th
  - carbamate 304.6 5th
  - chloride 304.6 5th
  - morphine 304.0 5th
- ethylene (gas) 304.6 5th
  - dichloride 304.6 5th
- ethylidene chloride 304.6 5th
- etilfen 304.1 5th
- etorphine 304.0 5th
- etoval 304.1 5th
- eucodal 304.0 5th
- euneryl 304.1 5th
- Evipal 304.1 5th
- Evipan 304.1 5th
- fentanyl 304.0 5th
- ganja 304.3 5th
- gardenal 304.1 5th
- gardenpanyl 304.1 5th
- gelsemine 304.6 5th
- Gelsemium 304.6 5th
- Gemonil 304.1 5th
- glucochloral 304.1 5th
- glue (airplane) (sniffing) 304.6 5th
- glutethimide 304.1 5th
- hallucinogenics 304.5 5th
- hashish 304.3 5th
- headache powder NEC 304.6 5th
- Heavenly Blue 304.5 5th
- hedonal 304.1 5th
- hemp 304.3 5th
- heptabarbital 304.1 5th
- Heptalgin 304.0 5th
- heptobarbitone 304.1 5th

Dependence – *continued*
- heroin 304.0 5th
  - salt (any) 304.0 5th
- hexethal (sodium) 304.1 5th
- hexobarbital 304.1 5th
- Hycodan 304.0 5th
- hydrocodone 304.0 5th
- hydromorphinol 304.0 5th
- hydromorphinone 304.0 5th
- hydromorphone 304.0 5th
- hydroxycodeine 304.0 5th
- hypnotic NEC 304.1 5th
- Indian hemp 304.3 5th
- inhalant 304.6 5th
- intranarcon 304.1 5th
- Kemithal 304.1 5th
- ketobemidone 304.0 5th
- khat 304.4 5th
- kif 304.3 5th
- Lactuca (virosa) extract 304.1 5th
- lactucarium 304.1 5th
- laudanum 304.0 5th
- Lebanese red 304.3 5th
- Leritine 304.0 5th
- lettuce opium 304.1 5th
- Levanil 304.1 5th
- Levo-Dromoran 304.0 5th
- levo-iso-methadone 304.0 5th
- levorphanol 304.0 5th
- Librium 304.1 5th
- Lomotil 304.6 5th
- Lotusate 304.1 5th
- LSD (-25) (and derivatives) 304.5 5th
- Luminal 304.1 5th
- lysergic acid 304.5 5th
  - amide 304.5 5th
- maconha 304.3 5th
- magic mushroom 304.5 5th
- marihuana 304.3 5th
- MDA (methylene dioxyamphetamine) 304.4 5th
- Mebaral 304.1 5th
- Medinal 304.1 5th
- Medomin 304.1 5th
- megahallucinogenics 304.5 5th
- meperidine 304.0 5th
- mephobarbital 304.1 5th
- meprobamate 304.1 5th
- mescaline 304.5 5th
- methadone 304.0 5th
- methamphetamine(s) 304.4 5th
- methaqualone 304.1 5th
- metharbital 304.1 5th
- methitural 304.1 5th
- methobarbitone 304.1 5th
- methohexital 304.1 5th
- methopholine 304.6 5th
- methyl
  - alcohol 303.9 5th
  - bromide 304.6 5th
  - morphine 304.0 5th
  - sulfonal 304.1 5th
- methylated spirit 303.9 5th
- methylbutinol 304.6 5th
- methyldihydromorphinone 304.0 5th
- methylene
  - chloride 304.6 5th
  - dichloride 304.6 5th
  - dioxyamphetamine (MDA) 304.4 5th
- methylparafynol 304.1 5th
- methylphenidate 304.4 5th
- methyprylone 304.1 5th
- metopon 304.0 5th
- Miltown 304.1 5th
- morning glory seeds 304.5 5th
- morphinan(s) 304.0 5th
- morphine (sulfate) (sulfite) (type) (drugs classifiable to 965.00-965.09) 304.0 5th
- morphine or opioid type drug (drugs classifiable to 965.00-965.09) with any other drug 304.7 5th
- morphinol(s) 304.0 5th
- morphinon 304.0 5th

Dependence – *continued*
- morpholinylethylmorphine 304.0 5th
- mylomide 304.1 5th
- myristicin 304.5 5th
- narcotic (drug) NEC 304.9 5th
- nealbarbital 304.1 5th
- nealbarbitone 304.1 5th
- Nembutal 304.1 5th
- Neonal 304.1 5th
- Neraval 304.1 5th
- Neravan 304.1 5th
- neurobarb 304.1 5th
- nicotine 305.1
- Nisentil 304.0 5th
- nitrous oxide 304.6 5th
- Noctec 304.1 5th
- Noludar 304.1 5th
- nonbarbiturate sedatives and tranquilizers with similar effect 304.1 5th
- noptil 304.1 5th
- normorphine 304.0 5th
- noscapine 304.0 5th
- Novocaine 304.6 5th
- Numorphan 304.0 5th
- nunol 304.1 5th
- Nupercaine 304.6 5th
- Oblivon 304.1 5th
- on
  - aspirator V46.0
  - hemodialysis V45.11
  - hyperbaric chamber V46.8
  - iron lung V46.11
  - machine (enabling) V46.9
    - specified type NEC V46.8
  - peritoneal dialysis V45.11
  - Possum (patient-operated-selector-mechanism) V46.8
  - renal dialysis machine V45.11
  - respirator [ventilator] V46.11
    - encounter
      - during
        - power failure V46.12
        - mechanical failure V46.14
      - for weaning V46.13
  - supplemental oxygen V46.2
  - wheelchair V46.3
- opiate 304.0 5th
- opioids 304.0 5th
- opioid type drug 304.0 5th
  - with any other drug 304.7 5th
- opium (alkaloids) (derivatives) (tincture) 304.0 5th
- ortal 304.1 5th
- Oxazepam 304.1 5th
- oxycodone 304.0 5th
- oxymorphone 304.0 5th
- Palfium 304.0 5th
- Panadol 304.6 5th
- pantopium 304.0 5th
- pantopon 304.0 5th
- papaverine 304.0 5th
- paracetamol 304.6 5th
- paracodin 304.0 5th
- paraldehyde 304.1 5th
- paregoric 304.0 5th
- Parzone 304.0 5th
- PCP (phencyclidine) 304.6 5th
- Pearly Gates 304.5 5th
- pentazocine 304.0 5th
- pentobarbital 304.1 5th
- pentobarbitone (sodium) 304.1 5th
- Pentothal 304.1 5th
- Percaine 304.6 5th
- Percodan 304.0 5th
- Perichlor 304.1 5th
- Pernocton 304.1 5th
- Pernoston 304.1 5th
- peronine 304.0 5th
- pethidine (hydrochloride) 304.0 5th
- petrichloral 304.1 5th
- peyote 304.5 5th
- Phanodorn 304.1 5th
- phenacetin 304.6 5th
- phenadoxone 304.0 5th

Dependence – *continued*
- phenaglycodol 304.1 5th
- phenazocine 304.0 5th
- phencyclidine 304.6 5th
- phenmetrazine 304.4 5th
- phenobal 304.1 5th
- phenobarbital 304.1 5th
- phenobarbitone 304.1 5th
- phenomorphan 304.0 5th
- phenonyl 304.1 5th
- phenoperidine 304.0 5th
- pholcodine 304.0 5th
- piminodine 304.0 5th
- Pipadone 304.0 5th
- Pitkin's solution 304.6 5th
- Placidyl 304.1 5th
- polysubstance 304.8 5th
- Pontocaine 304.6 5th
- pot 304.3 5th
- potassium bromide 304.1 5th
- Preludin 304.4 5th
- Prinadol 304.0 5th
- probarbital 304.1 5th
- procaine 304.6 5th
- propanal 304.1 5th
- propoxyphene 304.6 5th
- psilocibin 304.5 5th
- psilocin 304.5 5th
- psilocybin 304.5 5th
- psilocyline 304.5 5th
- psilocyn 304.5 5th
- psychedelic agents 304.5 5th
- psychostimulant NEC 304.4 5th
- psychotomimetic agents 304.5 5th
- pyrahexyl 304.3 5th
- Pyramidon 304.6 5th
- quinalbarbitone 304.1 5th
- racemoramide 304.0 5th
- racemorphan 304.0 5th
- Rela 304.6 5th
- scopolamine 304.6 5th
- secobarbital 304.1 5th
- seconal 304.1 5th
- sedative NEC 304.1 5th
  - nonbarbiturate with barbiturate effect 304.1 5th
- Sedormid 304.1 5th
- sernyl 304.1 5th
- sodium bromide 304.1 5th
- Soma 304.6 5th
- Somnal 304.1 5th
- Somnos 304.1 5th
- Soneryl 304.1 5th
- soporific (drug) NEC 304.1 5th
- specified drug NEC 304.6 5th
- speed 304.4 5th
- spinocaine 304.6 5th
- stovaine 304.6 5th
- STP 304.5 5th
- stramonium 304.6 5th
- Sulfonal 304.1 5th
- sulfonethylmethane 304.1 5th
- sulfonmethane 304.1 5th
- Surital 304.1 5th
- synthetic drug with morphine-like effect 304.0 5th
- talbutal 304.1 5th
- tetracaine 304.6 5th
- tetrahydrocannabinol 304.3 5th
- tetronal 304.1 5th
- THC 304.3 5th
- thebacon 304.0 5th
- thebaine 304.0 5th
- thiamil 304.1 5th
- thiamylal 304.1 5th
- thiopental 304.1 5th
- tobacco 305.1
- toluene, toluol 304.6 5th
- tranquilizer NEC 304.1 5th
  - nonbarbiturate with barbiturate effect 304.1 5th
- tribromacetaldehyde 304.6 5th
- tribromethanol 304.6 5th
- tribromomethane 304.6 5th

Dependence – *continued*
- trichloroethanol 304.6 5th
- trichoroethyl phosphate 304.1 5th
- triclofos 304.1 5th
- Trional 304.1 5th
- Tuinal 304.1 5th
- Turkish green 304.3 5th
- urethan(e) 304.6 5th
- Valium 304.1 5th
- Valmid 304.1 5th
- veganin 304.0 5th
- veramon 304.1 5th
- Veronal 304.1 5th
- versidyne 304.6 5th
- vinbarbital 304.1 5th
- vinbarbitone 304.1 5th
- vinyl bitone 304.1 5th
- vitamin B_6 266.1
- wine 303.9 5th
- Zactane 304.6 5th

Dependency
- passive 301.6
- reactions 301.6

Depersonalization (episode, in neurotic state) (neurotic) (syndrome) 300.6

Depletion
- carbohydrates 271.9
- complement factor 279.8
- extracellular fluid 276.52
- plasma 276.52
- potassium 276.8
  - nephropathy 588.89
- salt or sodium 276.1
  - causing heat exhaustion or prostration 992.4
  - nephropathy 593.9
- volume 276.50
  - extracellular fluid 276.52
  - plasma 276.52

Deployment (military) ●
- personal history of V62.22 ●
- returned from V62.22 ●
- status V62.21 ●

Deposit
- argentous, cornea 371.16
- bone, in Boeck's sarcoid 135
- calcareous, calcium - *see* Calcification
- cholesterol
  - retina 362.82
  - skin 709.3
  - vitreous (humor) 379.22
- conjunctival 372.56
- cornea, corneal NEC 371.10
  - argentous 371.16
  - in
    - cystinosis 270.0 *[371.15]*
    - mucopolysaccharidosis 277.5 *[371.15]*
- crystalline, vitreous (humor) 379.22
- hemosiderin, in old scars of cornea 371.11
- metallic, in lens 366.45
- skin 709.3
- teeth, tooth (betel) (black) (green) (materia alba) (orange) (soft) (tobacco) 523.6
- urate, in kidney (*see also* Disease, renal) 593.9

Depraved appetite 307.52

Depression 311
- acute (*see also* Psychosis, affective) 296.2 5th
  - recurrent episode 296.3 5th
  - single episode 296.2 5th
- agitated (*see also* Psychosis, affective) 296.2 5th
  - recurrent episode 296.3 5th
  - single episode 296.2 5th
- anaclitic 309.21
- anxiety 300.4
- arches 734
  - congenital 754.61
- autogenous (*see also* Psychosis, affective) 296.2 5th
  - recurrent episode 296.3 5th

Depression – *continued*
- autogenous – *continued*
  - single episode 296.2 5th
- basal metabolic rate (BMR) 794.7
- bone marrow 289.9
- central nervous system 799.1
  - newborn 779.2
- cerebral 331.9
  - newborn 779.2
- cerebrovascular 437.8
  - newborn 779.2
- chest wall 738.3
- endogenous (*see also* Psychosis, affective) 296.2 5th
  - recurrent episode 296.3 5th
  - single episode 296.2 5th
- functional activity 780.99
- hysterical 300.11
- involutional, climacteric, or menopausal (*see also* Psychosis, affective) 296.2 5th
  - recurrent episode 296.3 5th
  - single episode 296.2 5th
- manic (*see also* Psychosis, affective) 296.80
- medullary 348.89 ▲
  - newborn 779.2
- mental 300.4
- metatarsal heads - *see* Depression, arches
- metatarsus - *see* Depression, arches
- monopolar (*see also* Psychosis, affective) 296.2 5th
  - recurrent episode 296.3 5th
  - single episode 296.2 5th
- nervous 300.4
- neurotic 300.4
- nose 738.0
- postpartum 648.4 5th
- psychogenic 300.4
  - reactive 298.0
- psychoneurotic 300.4
- psychotic (*see also* Psychosis, affective) 296.2 5th
  - reactive 298.0
  - recurrent episode 296.3 5th
  - single episode 296.2 5th
- reactive 300.4
  - neurotic 300.4
  - psychogenic 298.0
  - psychoneurotic 300.4
  - psychotic 298.0
- recurrent 296.3 5th
- respiratory center 348.89 ▲
  - newborn 770.89
- scapula 736.89
- senile 290.21
- situational (acute) (brief) 309.0
  - prolonged 309.1
- skull 754.0
- sternum 738.3
- visual field 368.40

Depressive reaction - *see also* Reaction, depressive
- acute (transient) 309.0
  - with anxiety 309.28
- prolonged 309.1
- situational (acute) 309.0
  - prolonged 309.1

Deprivation
- cultural V62.4
- emotional V62.89
  - affecting
    - adult 995.82
    - infant or child 995.51
- food 994.2
  - specific substance NEC 269.8
- protein (familial) (kwashiorkor) 260
- sleep V69.4
- social V62.4
  - affecting
    - adult 995.82
    - infant or child 995.51
- symptoms, syndrome
  - alcohol 291.81
  - drug 292.0

Dependence – Deprivation

- **Deprivation** – *continued*
  - vitamins (*see also* Deficiency, vitamin) 269.2
  - water 994.3
- **de Quervain's**
  - disease (tendon sheath) 727.04
  - syndrome 259.51
  - thyroiditis (subacute granulomatous thyroiditis) 245.1
- **Derangement**
  - ankle (internal) 718.97
    - current injury (*see also* Dislocation, ankle) 837.0
    - recurrent 718.37
  - cartilage (articular) NEC (*see also* Disorder, cartilage, articular) 718.0 [5th]
    - knee 717.9
      - recurrent 718.36
    - recurrent 718.3 [5th]
  - collateral ligament (knee) (medial) (tibial) 717.82
    - current injury 844.1
      - lateral (fibular) 844.0
    - lateral (fibular) 717.81
      - current injury 844.0
  - cruciate ligament (knee) (posterior) 717.84
    - anterior 717.83
      - current injury 844.2
    - current injury 844.2
  - elbow (internal) 718.92
    - current injury (*see also* Dislocation, elbow) 832.00
    - recurrent 718.32
  - gastrointestinal 536.9
  - heart - *see* Disease, heart
  - hip (joint) (internal) (old) 718.95
    - current injury (*see also* Dislocation, hip) 835.00
    - recurrent 718.35
  - intervertebral disc - *see* Displacement, intervertebral disc
  - joint (internal) 718.90
    - ankle 718.97
    - current injury - *see also* Dislocation, by site
      - knee, meniscus or cartilage (*see also* Tear, meniscus) 836.2
    - elbow 718.92
    - foot 718.97
    - hand 718.94
    - hip 718.95
    - knee 717.9
    - multiple sites 718.99
    - pelvic region 718.95
    - recurrent 718.30
      - ankle 718.37
      - elbow 718.32
      - foot 718.37
      - hand 718.34
      - hip 718.35
      - knee 718.36
      - multiple sites 718.39
      - pelvic region 718.35
      - shoulder (region) 718.31
      - specified site NEC 718.38
      - temporomandibular (old) 524.69
      - wrist 718.33
    - shoulder (region) 718.91
    - specified site NEC 718.98
    - spine NEC 724.9
    - temporomandibular 524.69
    - wrist 718.93
  - knee (cartilage) (internal) 717.9
    - current injury (*see also* Tear, meniscus) 836.2
    - ligament 717.89
      - capsular 717.85
      - collateral - *see* Derangement, collateral ligament
      - cruciate - *see* Derangement, cruciate ligament
      - specified NEC 717.85

- **Derangement** – *continued*
  - knee – *continued*
    - recurrent 718.36
  - low back NEC 724.9
  - meniscus NEC (knee) 717.5
    - current injury (*see also* Tear, meniscus) 836.2
    - lateral 717.40
      - anterior horn 717.42
      - posterior horn 717.43
      - specified NEC 717.49
    - medial 717.3
      - anterior horn 717.1
      - posterior horn 717.2
    - recurrent 718.3 [5th]
    - site other than knee - *see* Disorder, cartilage, articular
  - mental (*see also* Psychosis) 298.9
  - rotator cuff (recurrent) (tear) 726.10
    - current 840.4
  - sacroiliac (old) 724.6
    - current - *see* Dislocation, sacroiliac
  - semilunar cartilage (knee) 717.5
    - current injury 836.2
      - lateral 836.1
      - medial 836.0
    - recurrent 718.3 [5th]
  - shoulder (internal) 718.91
    - current injury (*see also* Dislocation, shoulder) 831.00
    - recurrent 718.31
  - spine (recurrent) NEC 724.9
    - current - *see* Dislocation, spine
  - temporomandibular (internal) (joint) (old) 524.69
    - current - *see* Dislocation, jaw
- **Dercum's disease or syndrome** (adiposis dolorosa) 272.8
- **Derealization** (neurotic) 300.6
- **Dermal** - *see* condition
- **Dermaphytid** - *see* Dermatophytosis
- **Dermatergosis** - *see* Dermatitis
- **Dermatitis** (allergic) (contact) (occupational) (venenata) 692.9
  - ab igne 692.82
  - acneiform 692.9
  - actinic (due to sun) 692.70
    - acute 692.72
    - chronic NEC 692.74
    - other than from sun NEC 692.82
  - ambustionis
    - due to
      - burn or scald - *see* Burn, by site
      - sunburn (*see also* Sunburn) 692.71
  - amebic 006.6
  - ammonia 691.0
  - anaphylactoid NEC 692.9
  - arsenical 692.4
  - artefacta 698.4
    - psychogenic 316 *[698.4]*
  - asthmatic 691.8
  - atopic (allergic) (intrinsic) 691.8
    - psychogenic 316 *[691.8]*
  - atrophicans 701.8
    - diffusa 701.8
    - maculosa 701.3
  - autoimmune progesterone 279.49 ●
  - berlock, berloque 692.72
  - blastomycetic 116.0
  - blister beetle 692.89
  - Brucella NEC 023.9
  - bullosa 694.9
    - striata pratensis 692.6
  - bullous 694.9
    - mucosynechial, atrophic 694.60
      - with ocular involvement 694.61
    - seasonal 694.8
  - calorica
    - due to
      - burn or scald - *see* Burn, by site
      - cold 692.89
      - sunburn (*see also* Sunburn) 692.71
  - caterpillar 692.89
  - cercarial 120.3

- **Dermatitis** – *continued*
  - combustionis
    - due to
      - burn or scald - *see* Burn, by site
      - sunburn (*see also* Sunburn) 692.71
  - congelationis 991.5
  - contusiformis 695.2
  - diabetic 250.8 [5th]
  - diaper 691.0
  - diphtheritica 032.85
  - due to
    - acetone 692.2
    - acids 692.4
    - adhesive plaster 692.4
    - alcohol (skin contact) (substances classifiable to 980.0-980.9) 692.4
      - taken internally 693.8
    - alkalis 692.4
    - allergy NEC 692.9
    - ammonia (household) (liquid) 692.4
    - animal
      - dander (cat) (dog) 692.84
      - hair (cat) (dog) 692.84
    - arnica 692.3
    - arsenic 692.4
      - taken internally 693.8
    - blister beetle 692.89
    - cantharides 692.3
    - carbon disulphide 692.2
    - caterpillar 692.89
    - caustics 692.4
    - cereal (ingested) 693.1
      - contact with skin 692.5
    - chemical(s) NEC 692.4
      - internal 693.8
      - irritant NEC 692.4
      - taken internally 693.8
    - chlorocompounds 692.2
    - coffee (ingested) 693.1
      - contact with skin 692.5
    - cold weather 692.89
    - cosmetics 692.81
    - cyclohexanes 692.2
    - dander, animal (cat) (dog) 692.84
    - deodorant 692.81
    - detergents 692.0
    - dichromate 692.4
    - drugs and medicinals (correct substance properly administered) (internal use) 693.0
      - external (in contact with skin) 692.3
        - wrong substance given or taken 976.9
          - specified substance - *see* Table of Drugs and Chemicals
      - wrong substance given or taken 977.9
        - specified substance - *see* Table of Drugs and Chemicals
    - dyes 692.89
      - hair 692.89
    - epidermophytosis - *see* Dermatophytosis
    - esters 692.2
    - external irritant NEC 692.9
      - specified agent NEC 692.89
    - eye shadow 692.81
    - fish (ingested) 693.1
      - contact with skin 692.5
    - flour (ingested) 693.1
      - contact with skin 692.5
    - food (ingested) 693.1
      - in contact with skin 692.5
    - fruit (ingested) 693.1
      - contact with skin 692.5
    - fungicides 692.3
    - furs 692.84
    - glycols 692.2
    - greases NEC 692.1
    - hair, animal (cat) (dog) 692.84
    - hair dyes 692.89

- **Dermatitis** – *continued*
  - due to – *continued*
    - hot
      - objects and materials - *see* Burn, by site
      - weather or places 692.89
    - hydrocarbons 692.2
    - infrared rays, except from sun 692.82
      - solar NEC (*see also* Dermatitis, due to, sun) 692.70
    - ingested substance 693.9
      - drugs and medicinals (*see also* Dermatitis, due to, drugs and medicinals) 693.0
      - food 693.1
      - specified substance NEC 693.8
    - ingestion or injection of
      - chemical 693.8
      - drug (correct substance properly administered) 693.0
        - wrong substance given or taken 977.9
          - specified substance - *see* Table of Drugs and Chemicals
    - insecticides 692.4
    - internal agent 693.9
      - drugs and medicinals (*see also* Dermatitis, due to, drugs and medicinals) 693.0
      - food (ingested) 693.1
        - in contact with skin 692.5
      - specified agent NEC 693.8
    - iodine 692.3
    - iodoform 692.3
    - irradiation 692.82
    - jewelry 692.83
    - keratolytics 692.3
    - ketones 692.2
    - lacquer tree (Rhus verniciflua) 692.6
    - light (sun) NEC (*see also* Dermatitis, due to, sun) 692.70
      - other 692.82
    - low temperature 692.89
    - mascara 692.81
    - meat (ingested) 693.1
      - contact with skin 692.5
    - mercury, mercurials 692.3
    - metals 692.83
    - milk (ingested) 693.1
      - contact with skin 692.5
    - Neomycin 692.3
    - nylon 692.4
    - oils NEC 692.1
    - paint solvent 692.2
    - pediculocides 692.3
    - petroleum products (substances classifiable to 981) 692.4
    - phenol 692.3
    - photosensitiveness, photosensitivity (sun) 692.72
      - other light 692.82
    - plants NEC 692.6
    - plasters, medicated (any) 692.3
    - plastic 692.4
    - poison
      - ivy (Rhus toxicodendron) 692.6
      - oak (Rhus diversiloba) 692.6
      - plant or vine 692.6
      - sumac (Rhus venenata) 692.6
      - vine (Rhus radicans) 692.6
    - preservatives 692.89
    - primrose (primula) 692.6
    - primula 692.6
    - radiation 692.82
      - sun NEC (*see also* Dermatitis, due to, sun) 692.70
      - tanning bed 692.82
    - radioactive substance 692.82
    - radium 692.82
    - ragweed (Senecio jacobae) 692.6
    - Rhus (diversiloba) (radicans) (toxicodendron) (venenata) (verniciflua) 692.6

- **Dermatitis** – *continued*
  - due to – *continued*
    - rubber 692.4
    - scabicides 692.3
    - Senecio jacobae 692.6
    - solar radiation - *see* Dermatitis, due to, sun
    - solvents (any) (substances classifiable to (982.0-982.8) 692.2
      - chlorocompound group 692.2
      - cyclohexane group 692.2
      - ester group 692.2
      - glycol group 692.2
      - hydrocarbon group 692.2
      - ketone group 692.2
      - paint 692.2
    - specified agent NEC 692.89
    - sun 692.70
      - acute 692.72
      - chronic NEC 692.74
      - specified NEC 692.79
    - sunburn (*see also* Sunburn) 692.71
    - sunshine NEC (*see also* Dermatitis, due to, sun) 692.70
    - tanning bed 692.82
    - tetrachlorethylene 692.2
    - toluene 692.2
    - topical medications 692.3
    - turpentine 692.2
    - ultraviolet rays, except from sun 692.82
      - sun NEC (*see also* Dermatitis, due to, sun) 692.70
    - vaccine or vaccination (correct substance properly administered) 693.0
      - wrong substance given or taken
        - bacterial vaccine 978.8
          - specified - *see* Table of Drugs and Chemicals
        - other vaccines NEC 979.9
          - specified - *see* Table of Drugs and Chemicals
    - varicose veins (*see also* Varicose, vein, inflamed or infected) 454.1
    - x-rays 692.82
  - dyshydrotic 705.81
  - dysmenorrheica 625.8
  - eczematoid NEC 692.9
    - infectious 690.8
  - eczematous NEC 692.9
  - epidemica 695.89
  - erysipelatosa 695.81
  - escharotica - *see* Burn, by site
  - exfoliativa, exfoliative 695.89
    - generalized 695.89
    - infantum 695.81
    - neonatorum 695.81
  - eyelid 373.31
    - allergic 373.32
    - contact 373.32
    - eczematous 373.31
    - herpes (zoster) 053.20
      - simplex 054.41
    - infective 373.5
      - due to
        - actinomycosis 039.3 *[373.5]*
        - herpes
          - simplex 054.41
          - zoster 053.20
        - impetigo 684 *[373.5]*
        - leprosy (*see also* Leprosy) 030.0 *[373.4]*
        - lupus vulgaris (tuberculous) (*see also* Tuberculosis) 017.0 [5th] *[373.4]*
        - mycotic dermatitis (*see also* Dermatomycosis) 111.9 *[373.5]*
        - vaccinia 051.02 *[373.5]*
          - postvaccination 999.0 *[373.5]*
      - yaws (*see also* Yaws) 102.9 *[373.4]*
  - facta, factitia 698.4
    - psychogenic 316 *[698.4]*

- **Dermatitis** – *continued*
  - ficta 698.4
    - psychogenic 316 *[698.4]*
  - flexural 691.8
  - follicularis 704.8
  - friction 709.8
  - fungus 111.9
    - specified type NEC 111.8
  - gangrenosa, gangrenous (infantum) (*see also* Gangrene) 785.4
  - gestationis 646.8 [5th]
  - gonococcal 098.89
  - gouty 274.89
  - harvest mite 133.8
  - heat 692.89
  - herpetiformis (bullous) (erythematous) (pustular) (vesicular) 694.0
    - juvenile 694.2
    - senile 694.5
  - hiemalis 692.89
  - hypostatic, hypostatica 454.1
    - with ulcer 454.2
  - impetiginous 684
  - infantile (acute) (chronic) (intertriginous) (intrinsic) (seborrheic) 690.12
  - infectiosa eczematoides 690.8
  - infectious (staphylococcal) (streptococcal) 686.9
    - eczematoid 690.8
  - infective eczematoid 690.8
  - Jacquet's (diaper dermatitis) 691.0
  - leptus 133.8
  - lichenified NEC 692.9
  - lichenoid, chronic 701.0
  - lichenoides purpurica pigmentosa 709.1
  - meadow 692.6
  - medicamentosa (correct substance properly administered) (internal use) (*see also* Dermatitis, due to, drugs or medicinals) 693.0
    - due to contact with skin 692.3
  - mite 133.8
  - multiformis 694.0
    - juvenile 694.2
    - senile 694.5
  - napkin 691.0
  - neuro 698.3
  - neurotica 694.0
  - nummular NEC 692.9
  - osteatosis, osteatotic 706.8
  - papillaris capillitii 706.1
  - pellagrous 265.2
  - perioral 695.3
  - perstans 696.1
  - photosensitivity (sun) 692.72
    - other light 692.82
  - pigmented purpuric lichenoid 709.1
  - polymorpha dolorosa 694.0
  - primary irritant 692.9
  - pruriginosa 694.0
  - pruritic NEC 692.9
  - psoriasiform nodularis 696.2
  - psychogenic 316
  - purulent 686.00
  - pustular contagious 051.2
  - pyococcal 686.00
  - pyocyaneus 686.09
  - pyogenica 686.00
  - radiation 692.82
  - repens 696.1
  - Ritter's (exfoliativa) 695.81
  - Schamberg's (progressive pigmentary dermatosis) 709.09
  - schistosome 120.3
  - seasonal bullous 694.8
  - seborrheic 690.10
    - infantile 690.12
  - sensitization NEC 692.9
  - septic (*see also* Septicemia) 686.00
    - gonococcal 098.89
  - solar, solare NEC (*see also* Dermatitis, due to, sun) 692.70

- **Dermatitis** – *continued*
  - stasis 454.1
    - due to
      - postphlebitic syndrome 459.12
        - with ulcer 459.13
      - varicose veins - *see* Varicose
    - ulcerated or with ulcer (varicose) 454.2
  - sunburn (*see also* Sunburn) 692.71
  - suppurative 686.00
  - traumatic NEC 709.8
  - trophoneurotica 694.0
  - ultraviolet, except from sun 692.82
    - due to sun NEC (*see also* Dermatitis, due to, sun) 692.70
  - varicose 454.1
    - with ulcer 454.2
  - vegetans 686.8
  - verrucosa 117.2
  - xerotic 706.8
- **Dermatoarthritis, lipoid** 272.8 *[713.0]*
- **Dermatochalasia, dermatochalasis** 374.87
- **Dermatofibroma** (lenticulare) (M8832/0) - *see also* Neoplasm, skin, benign
  - protuberans (M8832/1) - *see* Neoplasm, skin, uncertain behavior
- **Dermatofibrosarcoma** (protuberans) (M8832/3) - *see* Neoplasm, skin, malignant
- **Dermatographia** 708.3
- **Dermatolysis** (congenital) (exfoliativa) 757.39
  - acquired 701.8
  - eyelids 374.34
  - palpebrarum 374.34
  - senile 701.8
- **Dermatomegaly NEC** 701.8
- **Dermatomucomyositis** 710.3
- **Dermatomycosis** 111.9
  - furfuracea 111.0
  - specified type NEC 111.8
- **Dermatomyositis** (acute) (chronic) 710.3
- **Dermatoneuritis of children** 985.0
- **Dermatophiliasis** 134.1
- **Dermatophytide** - *see* Dermatophytosis
- **Dermatophytosis** (Epidermophyton) (infection) (microsporum) (tinea) (Trichophyton) 110.9
  - beard 110.0
  - body 110.5
  - deep seated 110.6
  - fingernails 110.1
  - foot 110.4
  - groin 110.3
  - hand 110.2
  - nail 110.1
  - perianal (area) 110.3
  - scalp 110.0
  - scrotal 110.8
  - specified site NEC 110.8
  - toenails 110.1
  - vulva 110.8
- **Dermatopolyneuritis** 985.0
- **Dermatorrhexis** 756.83
  - acquired 701.8
- **Dermatosclerosis** (*see also* Scleroderma) 710.1
  - localized 701.0
- **Dermatosis** 709.9
  - Andrews' 686.8
  - atopic 691.8
  - Bowen's (M8081/2) - *see* Neoplasm, skin, in situ
  - bullous 694.9
    - specified type NEC 694.8
  - erythematosquamous 690.8
  - exfoliativa 695.89
  - factitial 698.4
  - gonococcal 098.89
  - herpetiformis 694.0
    - juvenile 694.2
    - senile 694.5
  - hysterical 300.11
  - linear IgA 694.8
  - menstrual NEC 709.8

- **Dermatosis** – *continued*
  - neutrophilic, acute febrile 695.89
  - occupational (*see also* Dermatitis) 692.9
  - papulosa nigra 709.8
  - pigmentary NEC 709.00
    - progressive 709.09
    - Schamberg's 709.09
    - Siemens-Bloch 757.33
  - progressive pigmentary 709.09
  - psychogenic 316
  - pustular subcorneal 694.1
  - Schamberg's (progressive pigmentary) 709.09
  - senile NEC 709.3
  - specified NEC 702.8
  - Unna's (seborrheic dermatitis) 690.10
- **Dermographia** 708.3
- **Dermographism** 708.3
- **Dermoid** (cyst) (M9084/0) - *see also* Neoplasm, by site, benign
  - with malignant transformation (M9084/3) 183.0
- **Dermopathy**
  - infiltrative, with thyrotoxicosis 242.0 [5th]
  - nephrogenic fibrosing 701.8
  - senile NEC 709.3
- **Dermophytosis** - *see* Dermatophytosis
- **Descemet's membrane** - *see* condition
- **Descemetocele** 371.72
- **Descending** - *see* condition
- **Descensus uteri** (complete) (incomplete) (partial) (without vaginal wall prolapse) 618.1
  - with mention of vaginal wall prolapse - *see* Prolapse, uterovaginal
- **Desensitization to allergens** V07.1
- **Desert**
  - rheumatism 114.0
  - sore (*see also* Ulcer, skin) 707.9
- **Desertion** (child) (newborn) 995.52
  - adult 995.84
- **Desmoid** (extra-abdominal) (tumor) (M8821/1) - *see also* Neoplasm, connective tissue, uncertain behavior
  - abdominal (M8822/1) - *see* Neoplasm, connective tissue, uncertain behavior
- **Despondency** 300.4
- **Desquamative dermatitis NEC** 695.89
- **Destruction**
  - articular facet (*see also* Derangement, joint) 718.9 [5th]
    - vertebra 724.9
  - bone 733.90
    - syphilitic 095.5
  - joint (*see also* Derangement, joint) 718.9 [5th]
    - sacroiliac 724.6
  - kidney 593.89
  - live fetus to facilitate birth NEC 763.89
  - ossicles (ear) 385.24
  - rectal sphincter 569.49
  - septum (nasal) 478.19
  - tuberculous NEC (*see also* Tuberculosis) 011.9 [5th]
  - tympanic membrane 384.82
  - tympanum 385.89
  - vertebral disc - *see* Degeneration, intervertebral disc
- **Destructiveness** (*see also* Disturbance, conduct) 312.9
  - adjustment reaction 309.3
- **Detachment**
  - cartilage - *see also* Sprain, by site
    - knee - *see* Tear, meniscus
  - cervix, annular 622.8
    - complicating delivery 665.3 [5th]
  - choroid (old) (postinfectional) (simple) (spontaneous) 363.70
    - hemorrhagic 363.72
    - serous 363.71
  - knee, medial meniscus (old) 717.3
    - current injury 836.0
  - ligament - *see* Sprain, by site

Dermatitis – Detachment

- **Detachment** – *continued*
  - placenta (premature) - *see* Placenta, separation
  - retina (recent) 361.9
    - with retinal defect (rhegmatogenous) 361.00
      - giant tear 361.03
      - multiple 361.02
      - partial
        - with
          - giant tear 361.03
          - multiple defects 361.02
          - retinal dialysis (juvenile) 361.04
          - single defect 361.01
      - retinal dialysis (juvenile) 361.04
      - single 361.01
      - subtotal 361.05
      - total 361.05
    - delimited (old) (partial) 361.06
    - old
      - delimited 361.06
      - partial 361.06
      - total or subtotal 361.07
    - pigment epithelium (RPE) (serous) 362.42
      - exudative 362.42
      - hemorrhagic 362.43
    - rhegmatogenous (*see also* Detachment, retina, with retinal defect) 361.00
    - serous (without retinal defect) 361.2
    - specified type NEC 361.89
    - traction (with vitreoretinal organization) 361.81
  - vitreous humor 379.21
- **Detergent asthma** 507.8
- **Deterioration**
  - epileptic
    - with behavioral disturbance 345.9 5th *[294.11]*
    - without behavioral disturbance 345.9 5th *[294.10]*
  - heart, cardiac (*see also* Degeneration, myocardial) 429.1
  - mental (*see also* Psychosis) 298.9
  - myocardium, myocardial (*see also* Degeneration, myocardial) 429.1
  - senile (simple) 797
    - transplanted organ - *see* Complications, transplant, organ, by site
- **de Toni-Fanconi syndrome** (cystinosis) 270.0
- **Deuteranomaly** 368.52
- **Deuteranopia** (anomalous trichromat) (complete) (incomplete) 368.52
- **Deutschländer's disease** - *see* Fracture, foot
- **Development**
  - abnormal, bone 756.9
  - arrested 783.40
    - bone 733.91
    - child 783.40
    - due to malnutrition (protein-calorie) 263.2
    - fetus or newborn 764.9 5th
    - tracheal rings (congenital) 748.3
  - defective, congenital - *see also* Anomaly
    - cauda equina 742.59
    - left ventricle 746.9
      - with atresia or hypoplasia of aortic orifice or valve with hypoplasia of ascending aorta 746.7
      - in hypoplastic left heart syndrome 746.7
  - delayed (*see also* Delay, development) 783.40
    - arithmetical skills 315.1
    - language (skills) 315.31
      - and speech due to hearing loss 315.34
      - expressive 315.31
      - mixed receptive-expressive 315.32
    - learning skill, specified NEC 315.2

- **Development** – *continued*
  - delayed – *continued*
    - mixed skills 315.5
    - motor coordination 315.4
    - reading 315.00
    - specified
      - learning skill NEC 315.2
      - type NEC, except learning 315.8
    - speech 315.39
      - and language due to hearing loss 315.34
      - associated with hyperkinesia 314.1
      - phonological 315.39
    - spelling 315.09
    - written expression 315.2
  - imperfect, congenital - *see also* Anomaly
    - heart 746.9
    - lungs 748.60
  - improper (fetus or newborn) 764.9 5th
  - incomplete (fetus or newborn) 764.9 5th
    - affecting management of pregnancy 656.5 5th
    - bronchial tree 748.3
    - organ or site not listed - *see* Hypoplasia
    - respiratory system 748.9
  - sexual, precocious NEC 259.1
  - tardy, mental (*see also* Retardation, mental) 319
- **Developmental** - *see* condition
- **Devergie's disease** (pityriasis rubra pilaris) 696.4
- **Deviation**
  - conjugate (eye) 378.87
    - palsy 378.81
    - spasm, spastic 378.82
  - esophagus 530.89
  - eye, skew 378.87
  - mandible, opening and closing 524.53
  - midline (jaw) (teeth) 524.29
    - specified site NEC - *see* Malposition
  - organ or site, congenital NEC - *see* Malposition, congenital
  - occlusal plane 524.76
  - septum (acquired) (nasal) 470
    - congenital 754.0
  - sexual 302.9
    - bestiality 302.1
    - coprophilia 302.89
    - ego-dystonic
      - homosexuality 302.0
      - lesbianism 302.0
    - erotomania 302.89
      - Clérambault's 297.8
    - exhibitionism (sexual) 302.4
    - fetishism 302.81
      - transvestic 302.3
    - frotteurism 302.89
    - homosexuality, ego-dystonic 302.0
      - pedophilic 302.2
    - lesbianism, ego-dystonic 302.0
    - masochism 302.83
    - narcissism 302.89
    - necrophilia 302.89
    - nymphomania 302.89
    - pederosis 302.2
    - pedophilia 302.2
    - sadism 302.84
    - sadomasochism 302.84
    - satyriasis 302.89
    - specified type NEC 302.89
    - transvestic fetishism 302.3
    - transvestism 302.3
    - voyeurism 302.82
    - zoophilia (erotica) 302.1
  - teeth, midline 524.29
  - trachea 519.19
  - ureter (congenital) 753.4
- **Devic's disease** 341.0
- **Device**
  - cerebral ventricle (communicating) in situ V45.2
  - contraceptive - *see* Contraceptive, device
  - drainage, cerebrospinal fluid V45.2

- **Devil's**
  - grip 074.1
  - pinches (purpura simplex) 287.2
- **Devitalized tooth** 522.9
- **Devonshire colic** 984.9
  - specified type of lead - *see* Table of Drugs and Chemicals
- **Dextraposition, aorta** 747.21
  - with ventricular septal defect, pulmonary stenosis or atresia, and hypertrophy of right ventricle 745.2
  - in tetralogy of Fallot 745.2
- **Dextratransposition, aorta** 745.11
- **Dextrinosis, limit** (debrancher enzyme deficiency) 271.0
- **Dextrocardia** (corrected) (false) (isolated) (secondary) (true) 746.87
  - with
    - complete transposition of viscera 759.3
    - situs inversus 759.3
- **Dextroversion, kidney (left)** 753.3
- **Dhobie itch** 110.3
- **Diabetes, diabetic** (brittle) (congenital) (familial) (mellitus) ~~(poorly controlled)~~ (severe) (slight) (without complication) 250.0 5th ▲

Note *Use the following fifth-digit subclassification with category 250:*

0 type II or unspecified type, not stated as uncontrolled

Fifth-digit 0 is for use for type II patients, even if the patient requires insulin

1 type I [juvenile type], not stated as uncontrolled

2 type II or unspecified type, uncontrolled

Fifth-digit 2 is for use for type II patients, even if the patient requires insulin

3 type I [juvenile type], uncontrolled

- with
  - coma (with ketoacidosis) 250.3 5th
    - due to secondary diabetes 249.3 5th
    - hyperosmolar (nonketotic) 250.2 5th
      - due to secondary diabetes 249.2 5th
  - complication NEC 250.9 5th
    - due to secondary diabetes 249.9 5th
    - specified NEC 250.8 5th
      - due to secondary diabetes 249.8 5th
  - gangrene 250.7 5th *[785.4]*
    - due to secondary diabetes 249.7 5th *[785.4]*
  - hyperglycemia - code to Diabetes, by type, with 5th digit for not stated as uncontrolled
  - hyperosmolarity 250.2 5th
    - due to secondary diabetes 249.2 5th
  - ketosis, ketoacidosis 250.1 5th
    - due to secondary diabetes 249.1 5th
  - osteomyelitis 250.8 5th *[731.8]*
    - due to secondary diabetes 249.8 5th *[731.8]*
  - specified manifestations NEC 250.8 5th
    - due to secondary diabetes 249.8 5th
- acetonemia 250.1 5th
  - due to secondary diabetes 249.1 5th
- acidosis 250.1 5th
  - due to secondary diabetes 249.1 5th
- amyotrophy 250.6 5th *[353.5]*
  - due to secondary diabetes 249.6 5th *[353.5]*
- angiopathy, peripheral 250.7 5th *[443.81]*
  - due to secondary diabetes 249.7 5th *[443.81]*
- asymptomatic 790.29

- **Diabetes, diabetic** – *continued*
  - autonomic neuropathy (peripheral) 250.6 5th *[337.1]*
    - due to secondary diabetes 249.6 5th *[337.1]*
  - bone change 250.8 5th *[731.8]*
    - due to secondary diabetes 249.8 5th *[731.8]*
  - bronze, bronzed 275.0
  - cataract 250.5 5th *[366.41]*
    - due to secondary diabetes 249.5 5th *[366.41]*
  - chemical induced - *see* Diabetes, secondary
    - complicating pregnancy, childbirth, or puerperium 648.0 5th
  - coma (with ketoacidosis) 250.3 5th
    - due to secondary diabetes 249.3 5th
    - hyperglycemic 250.3 5th
      - due to secondary diabetes 249.3 5th
    - hyperosmolar (nonketotic) 250.2 5th
      - due to secondary diabetes 249.2 5th
    - hypoglycemic 250.3 5th
      - due to secondary diabetes 249.3 5th
    - insulin 250.3 5th
      - due to secondary diabetes 249.3 5th
  - complicating pregnancy, childbirth, or puerperium (maternal) (conditions classifiable to 249 and 250) 648.0 5th
    - affecting fetus or newborn 775.0
  - complication NEC 250.9 5th
    - due to secondary diabetes 249.9 5th
    - specified NEC 250.8 5th
      - due to secondary diabetes 249.8 5th
  - dorsal sclerosis 250.6 5th *[340]*
    - due to secondary diabetes 249.6 5th *[340]*
  - drug-induced - *see also* Diabetes, secondary
    - overdose or wrong substance given or taken - *see* Table of Drugs and Chemicals
  - due to
    - cystic fibrosis - *see* Diabetes, secondary
    - infection - *see* Diabetes, secondary
  - dwarfism-obesity syndrome 258.1
  - gangrene 250.7 5th *[785.4]*
    - due to secondary diabetes 249.7 5th *[785.4]*
  - gastroparesis 250.6 5th *[536.3]*
    - due to secondary diabetes 249.6 5th *[536.3]*
  - gestational 648.8 5th
    - complicating pregnancy, childbirth, or puerperium 648.8 5th
  - glaucoma 250.5 5th *[365.44]*
    - due to secondary diabetes 249.5 5th *[365.44]*
  - glomerulosclerosis (intercapillary) 250.4 5th *[581.81]*
    - due to secondary diabetes 249.4 5th *[581.81]*
  - glycogenosis, secondary 250.8 5th *[259.8]*
    - due to secondary diabetes 249.8 5th *[259.8]*
  - hemochromatosis 275.0
  - hyperosmolar coma 250.2 5th
    - due to secondary diabetes 249.2 5th
  - hyperosmolarity 250.2 5th
    - due to secondary diabetes 249.2 5th
  - hypertension-nephrosis syndrome 250.4 5th *[581.81]*
    - due to secondary diabetes 249.4 5th *[581.81]*
  - hypoglycemia 250.8 5th
    - due to secondary diabetes 249.8 5th
  - hypoglycemic shock 250.8 5th
    - due to secondary diabetes 249.8 5th
  - inadequately controlled - code to Diabetes, by type, with 5th digit for not stated as uncontrolled
  - insipidus 253.5
    - nephrogenic 588.1

- **Diabetes, diabetic** – *continued*
  - insipidus – *continued*
    - pituitary 253.5
    - vasopressin-resistant 588.1
  - intercapillary glomerulosclerosis 250.4 5th *[581.81]*
    - due to secondary diabetes 249.4 5th *[581.81]*
  - iritis 250.5 5th *[364.42]*
    - due to secondary diabetes 249.5 5th *[364.42]*
  - ketosis, ketoacidosis 250.1 5th
    - due to secondary diabetes 249.1 5th
  - Kimmelstiel (-Wilson) disease or syndrome (intercapillary glomerulosclerosis) 250.4 5th *[581.81]*
    - due to secondary diabetes 249.4 5th *[581.81]*
  - Lancereaux's (diabetes mellitus with marked emaciation) 250.8 5th *[261]*
    - due to secondary diabetes 249.8 5th *[261]*
  - latent (chemical) - *see* Diabetes, secondary
    - complicating pregnancy, childbirth, or puerperium 648.0 5th
  - lipoidosis 250.8 5th *[272.7]*
    - due to secondary diabetes 249.8 5th *[272.7]*
  - macular edema 250.5 5th *[362.07]*
    - due to secondary diabetes 249.5 5th *[362.07]*
  - maternal
    - with manifest disease in the infant 775.1
    - affecting fetus or newborn 775.0
  - microaneurysms, retinal 250.5 5th *[362.01]*
    - due to secondary diabetes 249.5 5th *[362.01]*
  - mononeuropathy 250.6 5th *[355.9]*
    - due to secondary diabetes 249.6 5th *[355.9]*
  - neonatal, transient 775.1
  - nephropathy 250.4 5th *[583.81]*
    - due to secondary diabetes 249.4 5th *[583.81]* ▲
  - nephrosis (syndrome) 250.4 5th *[581.81]*
    - due to secondary diabetes 249.4 5th *[581.81]*
  - neuralgia 250.6 5th *[357.2]*
    - due to secondary diabetes 249.6 5th *[357.2]*
  - neuritis 250.6 5th *[357.2]*
    - due to secondary diabetes 249.6 5th *[357.2]*
  - neurogenic arthropathy 250.6 5th *[713.5]*
    - due to secondary diabetes 249.6 5th *[713.5]*
  - neuropathy 250.6 5th *[357.2]*
    - autonomic (peripheral) 250.6 5th *[337.1]* ●
      - due to secondary diabetes 249.6 5th *[337.1]* ●
    - due to secondary diabetes 249.6 5th *[357.2]*
  - nonclinical 790.29
  - osteomyelitis 250.8 5th *[731.8]*
    - due to secondary diabetes 249.8 5th *[731.8]*
  - out of control - code to Diabetes, by type, with 5th digit for uncontrolled
  - peripheral autonomic neuropathy 250.6 5th *[337.1]*
    - due to secondary diabetes 249.6 5th *[337.1]*
  - phosphate 275.3
  - polyneuropathy 250.6 5th *[357.2]*
    - due to secondary diabetes 249.6 5th *[357.2]*
  - poorly controlled - code to Diabetes, by type, with 5th digit for not stated as uncontrolled
  - renal (true) 271.4

- **Diabetes, diabetic** – *continued*
  - retinal
    - edema 250.5 5th *[362.07]*
      - due to secondary diabetes 249.5 5th *[362.07]*
    - hemorrhage 250.5 5th *[362.01]*
      - due to secondary diabetes 249.5 5th *[362.01]*
    - microaneurysms 250.5 5th *[362.01]*
      - due to secondary diabetes 249.5 5th *[362.01]*
  - retinitis 250.5 5th *[362.01]*
    - due to secondary diabetes 249.5 5th *[362.01]*
  - retinopathy 250.5 5th *[362.01]*
    - background 250.5 5th *[362.01]*
      - due to secondary diabetes 249.5 5th *[362.01]*
    - due to secondary diabetes 249.5 5th *[362.01]*
    - nonproliferative 250.5 5th *[362.03]*
      - due to secondary diabetes 249.5 5th *[362.03]*
      - mild 250.5 5th *[362.04]*
        - due to secondary diabetes 249.5 5th *[362.04]*
      - moderate 250.5 5th *[362.05]*
        - due to secondary diabetes 249.5 5th *[362.05]*
      - severe 250.5 5th *[362.06]*
        - due to secondary diabetes 249.5 5th *[362.06]*
    - proliferative 250.5 5th *[362.02]*
      - due to secondary diabetes 249.5 5th *[362.02]*
  - secondary (chemical-induced) (due to chronic condition) (due to infection) (drug-induced) 249.0 5th
    - with
      - coma (with ketoacidosis) 249.3 5th
        - hyperosmolar (nonketotic) 249.2 5th
      - complication NEC 249.9 5th
        - specified NEC 249.8 5th
      - gangrene 249.7 5th *[785.4]*
      - hyperosmolarity 249.2 5th
      - ketosis, ketoacidosis 249.1 5th
      - osteomyelitis 249.8 5th *[731.8]*
      - specified manifestations NEC 249.8 5th
    - acetonemia 249.1 5th
    - acidosis 249.1 5th
    - amyotrophy 249.6 5th *[353.5]*
    - angiopathy, peripheral 249.7 5th *[443.81]*
    - autonomic neuropathy (peripheral) 249.6 5th *[337.1]*
    - bone change 249.8 5th *[731.8]*
    - cataract 249.5 5th *[366.41]*
    - coma (with ketoacidosis) 249.3 5th
      - hyperglycemic 249.3 5th
      - hyperosmolar (nonketotic) 249.2 5th
      - hypoglycemic 249.3 5th
      - insulin 249.3 5th
    - complicating pregnancy, childbirth, or puerperium (maternal) 648.0 5th
      - affecting fetus or newborn 775.0
      - complication NEC 249.9 5th
      - specified NEC 249.8 5th
    - dorsal sclerosis 249.6 5th *[340]*
    - due to overdose or wrong substance given or taken - *see* Table of Drugs and Chemicals
    - gangrene 249.7 5th *[785.4]*
    - gastroparesis 249.6 5th *[536.3]*
    - glaucoma 249.5 5th *[365.44]*
    - glomerulosclerosis (intercapillary) 249.4 5th *[581.81]*
    - glycogenosis, secondary 249.8 5th *[259.8]*
    - hyperosmolar coma 249.2 5th
    - hyperosmolarity 249.2 5th

- **Diabetes, diabetic** – *continued*
  - secondary – *continued*
    - hypertension-nephrosis syndrome 249.4 5th *[581.81]*
    - hypoglycemia 249.8 5th
    - hypoglycemic shock 249.8 5th
    - intercapillary glomerulosclerosis 249.4 5th *[581.81]*
    - iritis 249.5 5th *[364.42]*
    - ketosis, ketoacidosis 249.1 5th
    - Kimmelstiel (-Wilson) disease or syndrome (intercapillary glomerulosclerosis) 249.4 5th *[581.81]*
    - Lancereaux's (diabetes mellitus with marked emaciation) 249.8 5th *[261]*
    - lipoidosis 249.8 5th *[272.7]*
    - macular edema 249.5 5th *[362.07]*
    - maternal
      - with manifest disease in the infant 775.1
      - affecting fetus or newborn 775.0
    - microaneurysms, retinal 249.5 5th *[362.01]*
    - mononeuropathy 249.6 5th *[355.9]*
    - nephropathy 249.4 5th *[583.81]* ▲
    - nephrosis (syndrome) 249.4 5th *[581.81]*
    - neuralgia 249.6 5th *[357.2]*
    - neuritis 249.6 5th *[357.2]*
    - neurogenic arthropathy 249.6 5th *[713.5]*
    - neuropathy 249.6 5th *[357.2]*
      - autonomic (peripheral) 249.6 5th *[337.1]* ●
    - osteomyelitis 249.8 5th *[731.8]*
    - peripheral autonomic neuropathy 249.6 5th *[337.1]*
    - polyneuropathy 249.6 5th *[357.2]*
    - retinal
      - edema 249.5 5th *[362.07]*
      - hemorrhage 249.5 5th *[362.01]*
      - microaneurysms 249.5 5th *[362.01]*
    - retinitis 249.5 5th *[362.01]*
    - retinopathy 249.5 5th *[362.01]*
      - background 249.5 5th *[362.01]*
      - nonproliferative 249.5 5th *[362.03]*
        - mild 249.5 5th *[362.04]*
        - moderate 249.5 5th *[362.05]*
        - severe 249.5 5th *[362.06]*
      - proliferative 249.5 5th *[362.02]*
    - ulcer (skin) 249.8 5th *[707.9]*
      - lower extremity 249.8 5th *[707.10]*
        - ankle 249.8 5th *[707.13]*
        - calf 249.8 5th *[707.12]*
        - foot 249.8 5th *[707.15]*
        - heel 249.8 5th *[707.14]*
        - knee 249.8 5th *[707.19]*
        - specified site NEC 249.8 5th *[707.19]*
        - thigh 249.8 5th *[707.11]*
        - toes 249.8 5th *[707.15]*
      - specified site NEC 249.8 5th *[707.8]*
    - xanthoma 249.8 5th *[272.2]*
  - steroid induced - *see also* Diabetes, secondary
    - overdose or wrong substance given or taken 962.0
  - stress 790.29
  - subclinical 790.29
  - subliminal 790.29
  - sugar 250.0 5th
  - ulcer (skin) 250.8 5th *[707.9]*
    - due to secondary diabetes 249.8 5th *[707.9]*
    - lower extremity 250.8 5th *[707.10]*
      - ankle 250.8 5th *[707.13]*
        - due to secondary diabetes 249.8 5th *[707.13]*
      - calf 250.8 5th *[707.12]*
        - due to secondary diabetes 249.8 5th *[707.12]*

- **Diabetes, diabetic** – *continued*
  - ulcer – *continued*
    - lower extremity – *continued*
      - due to secondary diabetes 249.8 5th *[707.10]*
      - foot 250.8 5th *[707.15]*
        - due to secondary diabetes 249.8 5th *[707.15]*
      - heel 250.8 5th *[707.14]*
        - due to secondary diabetes 249.8 5th *[707.14]*
      - knee 250.8 5th *[707.19]*
        - due to secondary diabetes 249.8 5th *[707.19]*
      - specified site NEC 250.8 5th *[707.19]*
        - due to secondary diabetes 249.8 5th *[707.19]*
      - thigh 250.8 5th *[707.11]*
        - due to secondary diabetes 249.8 5th *[707.11]*
      - toes 250.8 5th *[707.15]*
        - due to secondary diabetes 249.8 5th *[707.15]*
    - specified site NEC 250.8 5th *[707.8]*
      - due to secondary diabetes 249.8 5th *[707.8]*
  - xanthoma 250.8 5th *[272.2]*
    - due to secondary diabetes 249.8 5th *[272.2]*
- **Diacyclothrombopathia** 287.1
- **Diagnosis deferred** 799.9
- **Dialysis** (intermittent) (treatment)
  - anterior retinal (juvenile) (with detachment) 361.04
  - extracorporeal V56.0
  - hemodialysis V56.0
    - status only V45.11
  - peritoneal V56.8
    - status only V45.11
  - renal V56.0
    - status only V45.11
  - specified type NEC V56.8
- **Diamond-Blackfan anemia or syndrome** (congenital hypoplastic anemia) 284.01
- **Diamond-Gardener syndrome** (autoerythrocyte sensitization) 287.2
- **Diaper rash** 691.0
- **Diaphoresis** (excessive) **NEC** (*see also* Hyperhidrosis) 780.8
- **Diaphragm** - *see* condition
- **Diaphragmalgia** 786.52
- **Diaphragmitis** 519.4
- **Diaphyseal aclasis** 756.4
- **Diaphysitis** 733.99
- **Diarrhea, diarrheal** (acute) (autumn) (bilious) (bloody) (catarrhal) (choleraic) (chronic) (gravis) (green) (infantile) (lienteric) (noninfectious) (presumed noninfectious) (putrefactive) (secondary) (sporadic) (summer) (symptomatic) (thermic) 787.91
  - achlorhydric 536.0
  - allergic 558.3
  - amebic (*see also* Amebiasis) 006.9
    - with abscess - *see* Abscess, amebic
    - acute 006.0
    - chronic 006.1
    - nondysenteric 006.2
  - bacillary - *see* Dysentery, bacillary
  - bacterial NEC 008.5
  - balantidial 007.0
  - bile salt-induced 579.8
  - cachectic NEC 787.91
  - chilomastix 007.8
  - choleriformis 001.1
  - coccidial 007.2
  - Cochin-China 579.1
    - anguilluliasis 127.2
    - psilosis 579.1
  - Dientamoeba 007.8
  - dietetic 787.91

Diabetes, diabetic – Diarrhea, diarrheal

- **Diarrhea, diarrheal** – *continued*
  - due to
    - achylia gastrica 536.8
    - Aerobacter aerogenes 008.2
    - Bacillus coli - *see* Enteritis, E. coli
    - bacteria NEC 008.5
    - bile salts 579.8
    - Capillaria
      - hepatica 128.8
      - philippinensis 127.5
    - Clostridium perfringens (C) (F) 008.46
    - Enterobacter aerogenes 008.2
    - enterococci 008.49
    - Escherichia coli - *see* Enteritis, E. coli
    - Giardia lamblia 007.1
    - Heterophyes heterophyes 121.6
    - irritating foods 787.91
    - Metagonimus yokogawai 121.5
    - Necator americanus 126.1
    - Paracolobactrum arizonae 008.1
    - Paracolon bacillus NEC 008.47
      - Arizona 008.1
    - Proteus (bacillus) (mirabilis) (Morganii) 008.3
    - Pseudomonas aeruginosa 008.42
    - S. japonicum 120.2
    - specified organism NEC 008.8
      - bacterial 008.49
      - viral NEC 008.69
    - Staphylococcus 008.41
    - Streptococcus 008.49
      - anaerobic 008.46
    - Strongyloides stercoralis 127.2
    - Trichuris trichiuria 127.3
    - virus NEC (*see also* Enteritis, viral) 008.69
  - dysenteric 009.2
    - due to specified organism NEC 008.8
  - dyspeptic 787.91
  - endemic 009.3
    - due to specified organism NEC 008.8
  - epidemic 009.2
    - due to specified organism NEC 008.8
  - fermentative 787.91
  - flagellate 007.9
  - Flexner's (ulcerative) 004.1
  - functional 564.5
    - following gastrointestinal surgery 564.4
    - psychogenic 306.4
  - giardial 007.1
  - Giardia lamblia 007.1
  - hill 579.1
  - hyperperistalsis (nervous) 306.4
  - infectious 009.2
    - due to specified organism NEC 008.8
    - presumed 009.3
  - inflammatory 787.91
    - due to specified organism NEC 008.8
  - malarial (*see also* Malaria) 084.6
  - mite 133.8
  - mycotic 117.9
  - nervous 306.4
  - neurogenic 564.5
  - parenteral NEC 009.2
  - postgastrectomy 564.4
  - postvagotomy 564.4
  - prostaglandin induced 579.8
  - protozoal NEC 007.9
  - psychogenic 306.4
  - septic 009.2
    - due to specified organism NEC 008.8
  - specified organism NEC 008.8
    - bacterial 008.49
    - viral NEC 008.69
  - Staphylococcus 008.41
  - Streptococcus 008.49
    - anaerobic 008.46
  - toxic 558.2
  - travelers' 009.2
    - due to specified organism NEC 008.8
  - trichomonal 007.3
  - tropical 579.1
  - tuberculous 014.8 [5th]
- **Diarrhea, diarrheal** – *continued*
  - ulcerative (chronic) (*see also* Colitis, ulcerative) 556.9
  - viral (*see also* Enteritis, viral) 008.8
  - zymotic NEC 009.2
- **Diastasis**
  - cranial bones 733.99
    - congenital 756.0
  - joint (traumatic) - *see* Dislocation, by site
  - muscle 728.84
    - congenital 756.89
  - recti (abdomen) 728.84
    - complicating delivery 665.8 [5th]
    - congenital 756.79
- **Diastema, teeth, tooth** 524.30
- **Diastematomyelia** 742.51
- **Diataxia, cerebral, infantile** 343.0
- **Diathesis**
  - allergic V15.09
  - bleeding (familial) 287.9
  - cystine (familial) 270.0
  - gouty 274.9
  - hemorrhagic (familial) 287.9
    - newborn NEC 776.0
  - oxalic 271.8
  - scrofulous (*see also* Tuberculosis) 017.2 [5th]
  - spasmophilic (*see also* Tetany) 781.7
  - ulcer 536.9
  - uric acid 274.9
- **Diaz's disease or osteochondrosis** 732.5
- **Dibothriocephaliasis** 123.4
  - larval 123.5
- **Dibothriocephalus** (infection) (infestation) (latus) 123.4
  - larval 123.5
- **Dicephalus** 759.4
- **Dichotomy, teeth** 520.2
- **Dichromat, dichromata** (congenital) 368.59
- **Dichromatopsia** (congenital) 368.59
- **Dichuchwa** 104.0
- **Dicroceliasis** 121.8
- **Didelphys, didelphic** (*see also* Double uterus) 752.2
- **Didymitis** (*see also* Epididymitis) 604.90
- **Died** - *see also* Death
  - without
    - medical attention (cause unknown) 798.9
    - sign of disease 798.2
- **Dientamoeba diarrhea** 007.8
- **Dietary**
  - inadequacy or deficiency 269.9
  - surveillance and counseling V65.3
- **Dietl's crisis** 593.4
- **Dieulafoy lesion** (hemorrhagic)
  - of
    - duodenum 537.84
    - esophagus 530.82
    - intestine 569.86
    - stomach 537.84
- **Difficult**
  - birth, affecting fetus or newborn 763.9
  - delivery NEC 669.9 [5th]
- **Difficulty**
  - feeding 783.3
    - adult 783.3
    - breast 676.8 [5th]
    - child 783.3
    - elderly 783.3
    - infant 783.3
    - newborn 779.3<u>1</u> ▲
    - nonorganic (infant) NEC 307.59
  - mechanical, gastroduodenal stoma 537.89
  - reading 315.00
  - specific, spelling 315.09
  - swallowing (*see also* Dysphagia) 787.20
  - walking 719.7
- **Diffuse** - *see* condition
- **Diffused ganglion** 727.42
- **Di George's syndrome** (thymic hypoplasia) 279.11
- **Digestive** - *see* condition
- **Di Guglielmo's disease or syndrome** (M9841/3) 207.0 [5th]
- **Diktyoma** (M9051/3) - *see* Neoplasm, by site, malignant
- **Dilaceration, tooth** 520.4
- **Dilatation**
  - anus 564.89
    - venule - *see* Hemorrhoids
  - aorta (focal) (general) (*see also* Aneurysm, aorta) 441.9
    - congenital 747.29
    - infectional 093.0
    - ruptured 441.5
    - syphilitic 093.0
  - appendix (cystic) 543.9
  - artery 447.8
  - bile duct (common) (cystic) (congenital) 751.69
    - acquired 576.8
  - bladder (sphincter) 596.8
    - congenital 753.8
    - in pregnancy or childbirth 654.4 [5th]
      - causing obstructed labor 660.2 [5th]
        - affecting fetus or newborn 763.1
  - blood vessel 459.89
  - bronchus, bronchi 494.0
    - with acute exacerbation 494.1
  - calyx (due to obstruction) 593.89
  - capillaries 448.9
  - cardiac (acute) (chronic) (*see also* Hypertrophy, cardiac) 429.3
    - congenital 746.89
      - valve NEC 746.89
        - pulmonary 746.09
    - hypertensive (*see also* Hypertension, heart) 402.90
  - cavum septi pellucidi 742.4
  - cecum 564.89
    - psychogenic 306.4
  - cervix (uteri) - *see also* Incompetency, cervix
    - incomplete, poor, slow
      - affecting fetus or newborn 763.7
      - complicating delivery 661.0 [5th]
        - affecting fetus or newborn 763.7
  - colon 564.7
    - congenital 751.3
    - due to mechanical obstruction 560.89
    - psychogenic 306.4
  - common bile duct (congenital) 751.69
    - acquired 576.8
      - with calculus, choledocholithiasis, or stones - *see* Choledocholithiasis
  - cystic duct 751.69
    - acquired (any bile duct) 575.8
  - duct, mammary 610.4
  - duodenum 564.89
  - esophagus 530.89
    - congenital 750.4
    - due to
      - achalasia 530.0
      - cardiospasm 530.0
  - Eustachian tube, congenital 744.24
  - fontanel 756.0
  - gallbladder 575.8
    - congenital 751.69
  - gastric 536.8
    - acute 536.1
    - psychogenic 306.4
  - heart (acute) (chronic) (*see also* Hypertrophy, cardiac) 429.3
    - congenital 746.89
    - hypertensive (*see also* Hypertension, heart) 402.90
    - valve - *see also* Endocarditis
      - congenital 746.89
  - ileum 564.89
    - psychogenic 306.4
  - inguinal rings - *see* Hernia, inguinal
  - jejunum 564.89
    - psychogenic 306.4
  - kidney (calyx) (collecting structures) (cystic) (parenchyma) (pelvis) 593.89
  - lacrimal passages 375.69
- **Dilatation** – *continued*
  - lymphatic vessel 457.1
  - mammary duct 610.4
  - Meckel's diverticulum (congenital) 751.0
  - meningeal vessels, congenital 742.8
  - myocardium (acute) (chronic) (*see also* Hypertrophy, cardiac) 429.3
  - organ or site, congenital NEC - *see* Distortion
  - pancreatic duct 577.8
  - pelvis, kidney 593.89
  - pericardium - *see* Pericarditis
  - pharynx 478.29
  - prostate 602.8
  - pulmonary
    - artery (idiopathic) 417.8
      - congenital 747.3
    - valve, congenital 746.09
  - pupil 379.43
  - rectum 564.89
  - renal 593.89
  - saccule vestibularis, congenital 744.05
  - salivary gland (duct) 527.8
  - sphincter ani 564.89
  - stomach 536.8
    - acute 536.1
    - psychogenic 306.4
  - submaxillary duct 527.8
  - trachea, congenital 748.3
  - ureter (idiopathic) 593.89
    - congenital 753.20
    - due to obstruction 593.5
  - urethra (acquired) 599.84
  - vasomotor 443.9
  - vein 459.89
  - ventricular, ventricle (acute) (chronic) (*see also* Hypertrophy, cardiac) 429.3
    - cerebral, congenital 742.4
    - hypertensive (*see also* Hypertension, heart) 402.90
  - venule 459.89
    - anus - *see* Hemorrhoids
  - vesical orifice 596.8
- **Dilated, dilation** - *see* Dilatation
- **Diminished**
  - hearing (acuity) (*see also* Deafness) 389.9
  - pulse pressure 785.9
  - vision NEC 369.9
  - vital capacity 794.2
- **Diminuta taenia** 123.6
- **Diminution, sense or sensation** (cold) (heat) (tactile) (vibratory) (*see also* Disturbance, sensation) 782.0
- **Dimitri-Sturge-Weber disease** (encephalocutaneous angiomatosis) 759.6
- **Dimple**
  - parasacral 685.1
    - with abscess 685.0
  - pilonidal 685.1
    - with abscess 685.0
  - postanal 685.1
    - with abscess 685.0
- **Dioctophyma renale** (infection) (infestation) 128.8
- **Dipetalonemiasis** 125.4
- **Diphallus** 752.69
- **Diphtheria, diphtheritic** (gangrenous) (hemorrhagic) 032.9
  - carrier (suspected) of V02.4
  - cutaneous 032.85
  - cystitis 032.84
  - faucial 032.0
  - infection of wound 032.85
  - inoculation (anti) (not sick) V03.5
  - laryngeal 032.3
  - myocarditis 032.82
  - nasal anterior 032.2
  - nasopharyngeal 032.1
  - neurological complication 032.89
  - peritonitis 032.83
  - specified site NEC 032.89
- **Diphyllobothriasis** (intestine) 123.4
  - larval 123.5

- **Diplacusis** 388.41
- **Diplegia** (upper limbs) 344.2
  - brain or cerebral 437.8
  - congenital 343.0
  - facial 351.0
    - congenital 352.6
  - infantile or congenital (cerebral) (spastic) (spinal) 343.0
  - lower limbs 344.1
  - syphilitic, congenital 090.49
- **Diplococcus, diplococcal** - *see* condition
- **Diplomyelia** 742.59
- **Diplopia** 368.2
  - refractive 368.15
- **Dipsomania** (*see also* Alcoholism) 303.9 [5th]
  - with psychosis (*see also* Psychosis, alcoholic) 291.9
- **Dipylidiasis** 123.8
  - intestine 123.8
- **Direction, teeth, abnormal** 524.30
- **Dirt-eating child** 307.52
- **Disability**
  - heart - *see* Disease, heart
  - learning NEC 315.2
  - special spelling 315.09
- **Disarticulation** (*see also* Derangement, joint) 718.9
  - meaning
    - amputation
      - status - *see* Absence, by site
      - traumatic - *see* Amputation, traumatic
    - dislocation, traumatic or congenital - *see* Dislocation
- **Disaster, cerebrovascular** (*see also* Disease, cerebrovascular, acute) 436
- **Discharge**
  - anal NEC 787.99
  - breast (female) (male) 611.79
  - conjunctiva 372.89
  - continued locomotor idiopathic (*see also* Epilepsy) 345.5 [5th]
  - diencephalic autonomic idiopathic (*see also* Epilepsy) 345.5 [5th]
  - ear 388.60
    - blood 388.69
    - cerebrospinal fluid 388.61
  - excessive urine 788.42
  - eye 379.93
  - nasal 478.19
  - nipple 611.79
  - patterned motor idiopathic (*see also* Epilepsy) 345.5 [5th]
  - penile 788.7
  - postnasal - *see* Sinusitis
  - sinus, from mediastinum 510.0
  - umbilicus 789.9
  - urethral 788.7
    - bloody 599.84
  - vaginal 623.5
- **Discitis** 722.90
  - cervical, cervicothoracic 722.91
  - lumbar, lumbosacral 722.93
  - thoracic, thoracolumbar 722.92
- **Discogenic syndrome** - *see* Displacement, intervertebral disc
- **Discoid**
  - kidney 753.3
  - meniscus, congenital 717.5
  - semilunar cartilage 717.5
- **Discoloration**
  - mouth 528.9
  - nails 703.8
  - teeth 521.7
    - due to
      - drugs 521.7
      - metals (copper) (silver) 521.7
      - pulpal bleeding 521.7
    - during formation 520.8
    - extrinsic 523.6
    - intrinsic posteruptive 521.7
- **Discomfort**
  - chest 786.59
  - visual 368.13
- **Discomycosis** - *see* Actinomycosis
- **Discontinuity, ossicles, ossicular chain** 385.23
- **Discrepancy**
  - centric occlusion
    - maximum intercuspation 524.55
    - of teeth 524.55
  - leg length (acquired) 736.81
    - congenital 755.30
  - uterine size-date 649.6 [5th]
- **Discrimination**
  - political V62.4
  - racial V62.4
  - religious V62.4
  - sex V62.4
- **Disease, diseased** - *see also* Syndrome
  - Abrami's (acquired hemolytic jaundice) 283.9
  - absorbent system 459.89
  - accumulation - *see* Thesaurismosis
  - acid-peptic 536.8
  - Acosta's 993.2
  - Adams-Stokes (-Morgagni) (syncope with heart block) 426.9
  - Addison's (bronze) (primary adrenal insufficiency) 255.41
    - anemia (pernicious) 281.0
    - tuberculous (*see also* Tuberculosis) 017.6 [5th]
  - Addison-Gull - *see* Xanthoma
  - adenoids (and tonsils) (chronic) 474.9
  - adrenal (gland) (capsule) (cortex) 255.9
    - hyperfunction 255.3
    - hypofunction 255.41
    - specified type NEC 255.8
  - ainhum (dactylolysis spontanea) 136.0
  - akamushi (scrub typhus) 081.2
  - Akureyri (epidemic neuromyasthenia) 049.8
  - Albarrán's (colibacilluria) 791.9
  - Albers-Schönberg's (marble bones) 756.52
  - Albert's 726.71
  - Albright (-Martin) (-Bantam) 275.49
  - Alibert's (mycosis fungoides) (M9700/3) 202.1 [5th]
  - Alibert-Bazin (M9700/3) 202.1 [5th]
  - alimentary canal 569.9
  - alligator skin (ichthyosis congenita) 757.1
    - acquired 701.1
  - Almeida's (Brazilian blastomycosis) 116.1
  - Alpers' 330.8
  - alpine 993.2
  - altitude 993.2
  - alveoli, teeth 525.9
  - Alzheimer's - *see* Alzheimer's
  - amyloid (any site) 277.30
  - anarthritic rheumatoid 446.5
  - Anders' (adiposis tuberosa simplex) 272.8
  - Andersen's (glycogenosis IV) 271.0
  - Anderson's (angiokeratoma corporis diffusum) 272.7
  - Andes 993.2
  - Andrews' (bacterid) 686.8
  - angiopastic, angiospasmodic 443.9
    - cerebral 435.9
      - with transient neurologic deficit 435.9
    - vein 459.89
  - anterior
    - chamber 364.9
    - horn cell 335.9
      - specified type NEC 335.8
  - antral (chronic) 473.0
    - acute 461.0
  - anus NEC 569.49
  - aorta (nonsyphilitic) 447.9
    - syphilitic NEC 093.89
  - aortic (heart) (valve) (*see also* Endocarditis, aortic) 424.1
  - apollo 077.4
  - aponeurosis 726.90
  - appendix 543.9
  - aqueous (chamber) 364.9
  - arc-welders' lung 503

Disease, diseased – *continued*

- Armenian 277.31
- Arnold-Chiari (*see also* Spina bifida) 741.0 [5th]
- arterial 447.9
  - occlusive (*see also* Occlusion, by site) 444.22
    - with embolus or thrombus - *see* Occlusion, by site
    - due to stricture or stenosis 447.1
  - specified type NEC 447.8
- arteriocardiorenal (*see also* Hypertension, cardiorenal) 404.90
- arteriolar (generalized) (obliterative) 447.90
  - specified type NEC 447.8
- arteriorenal - *see* Hypertension, kidney
- arteriosclerotic - *see also* Arteriosclerosis
  - cardiovascular 429.2
  - coronary - *see* Arteriosclerosis, coronary
  - heart - *see* Arteriosclerosis, coronary
  - vascular - *see* Arteriosclerosis
- artery 447.9
  - cerebral 437.9
  - coronary - *see* Arteriosclerosis, coronary
  - specified type NEC 447.8
- arthropod-borne NEC 088.9
  - specified type NEC 088.89
- Asboe-Hansen's (incontinentia pigmenti) 757.33
- atticoantral, chronic (with posterior or superior marginal perforation of ear drum) 382.2
- auditory canal, ear 380.9
- Aujeszky's 078.89
- auricle, ear NEC 380.30
- Australian X 062.4
- autoimmune NEC 279.49 ▲
  - hemolytic (cold type) (warm type) 283.0
  - parathyroid 252.1
  - thyroid 245.2
- aviators' (*see also* Effect, adverse, high altitude) 993.2
- ax(e)-grinders' 502
- Ayala's 756.89
- Ayerza's (pulmonary artery sclerosis with pulmonary hypertension) 416.0
- Azorean (of the nervous system) 334.8
- Babington's (familial hemorrhagic telangiectasia) 448.0
- back bone NEC 733.90
- bacterial NEC 040.89
  - zoonotic NEC 027.9
    - specified type NEC 027.8
- Baehr-Schiffrin (thrombotic thrombocytopenic purpura) 446.6
- Baelz's (cheilitis glandularis apostematosa) 528.5
- Baerensprung's (eczema marginatum) 110.3
- Balfour's (chloroma) 205.3 [5th]
- balloon (*see also* Effect, adverse, high altitude) 993.2
- Baló's 341.1
- Bamberger (-Marie) (hypertrophic pulmonary osteoarthropathy) 731.2
- Bang's (Brucella abortus) 023.1
- Bannister's 995.1
- Banti's (with cirrhosis) (with portal hypertension) - *see* Cirrhosis, liver
- Barcoo (*see also* Ulcer, skin) 707.9
- barium lung 503
- Barlow (-Möller) (infantile scurvy) 267
- barometer makers' 985.0
- Barraquer (-Simons) (progressive lipodystrophy) 272.6
- basal ganglia 333.90
  - degenerative NEC 333.0
  - specified NEC 333.89
- Basedow's (exophthalmic goiter) 242.0 [5th]

Disease, diseased – *continued*

- basement membrane NEC 583.89
  - with
    - pulmonary hemorrhage (Goodpasture's syndrome) 446.21 *[583.81]*
- Bateman's 078.0
  - purpura (senile) 287.2
- Batten's 330.1 *[362.71]*
- Batten-Mayou (retina) 330.1 *[362.71]*
- Batten-Steinert 359.21
- Battey 031.0
- Baumgarten-Cruveilhier (cirrhosis of liver) 571.5
- bauxite-workers' 503
- Bayle's (dementia paralytica) 094.1
- Bazin's (primary) (*see also* Tuberculosis) 017.1 [5th]
- Beard's (neurasthenia) 300.5
- Beau's (*see also* Degeneration, myocardial) 429.1
- Bechterew's (ankylosing spondylitis) 720.0
- Becker's
  - idiopathic mural endomyocardial disease 425.2
  - myotonia congenita, recessive form 359.22
- Begbie's (exophthalmic goiter) 242.0 [5th]
- Behr's 362.50
- Beigel's (white piedra) 111.2
- Bekhterev's (ankylosing spondylitis) 720.0
- Bell's (*see also* Psychosis, affective) 296.0 [5th]
- Bennett's (leukemia) 208.9 [5th]
- Benson's 379.22
- Bergeron's (hysteroepilepsy) 300.11
- Berlin's 921.3
- Bernard-Soulier (thrombopathy) 287.1
- Bernhardt (-Roth) 355.1
- beryllium 503
- Besnier-Boeck (-Schaumann) (sarcoidosis) 135
- Best's 362.76
- Beurmann's (sporotrichosis) 117.1
- Bielschowsky (-Jansky) 330.1
- Biermer's (pernicious anemia) 281.0
- Biett's (discoid lupus erythematosus) 695.4
- bile duct (*see also* Disease, biliary) 576.9
- biliary (duct) (tract) 576.9
  - with calculus, choledocholithiasis, or stones - *see* Choledocholithiasis
- Billroth's (meningocele) (*see also* Spina bifida) 741.9 [5th]
- Binswanger's 290.12
- Bird's (oxaluria) 271.8
- bird fanciers' 495.2
- black lung 500
- bladder 596.9
  - specified NEC 596.8
- bleeder's 286.0
- Bloch-Sulzberger (incontinentia pigmenti) 757.33
- Blocq's (astasia-abasia) 307.9
- blood (-forming organs) 289.9
  - specified NEC 289.89
  - vessel 459.9
- Bloodgood's 610.1
- Blount's (tibia vara) 732.4
- blue 746.9
- Bodechtel-Guttmann (subacute sclerosing panencephalitis) 046.2
- Boeck's (sarcoidosis) 135
- bone 733.90
  - fibrocystic NEC 733.29
    - jaw 526.2
  - marrow 289.9
  - Paget's (osteitis deformans) 731.0
  - specified type NEC 733.99
  - von Recklinghausen's (osteitis fibrosa cystica) 252.01
- Bonfils' - *see* Disease, Hodgkin's
- Borna 062.9
- Bornholm (epidemic pleurodynia) 074.1
- Bostock's (*see also* Fever, hay) 477.9

- **Disease, diseased** – *continued*
  - Bouchard's (myopathic dilatation of the stomach) 536.1
  - Bouillaud's (rheumatic heart disease) 391.9
  - Bourneville (-Brissaud) (tuberous sclerosis) 759.5
  - Bouveret (-Hoffmann) (paroxysmal tachycardia) 427.2
  - bowel 569.9
    - functional 564.9
      - psychogenic 306.4
  - Bowen's (M8081/2) - *see* Neoplasm, skin, in situ
  - Bozzolo's (multiple myeloma) (M9730/3) 203.0 [5th]
  - Bradley's (epidemic vomiting) 078.82
  - Brailsford's 732.3
    - radius, head 732.3
    - tarsal, scaphoid 732.5
  - Brailsford-Morquio (mucopolysaccharidosis IV) 277.5
  - brain 348.9
    - Alzheimer's 331.0
      - with dementia - *see* Alzheimer's, dementia
    - arterial, artery 437.9
    - arteriosclerotic 437.0
    - congenital 742.9
    - degenerative - *see* Degeneration, brain
    - inflammatory - *see also* Encephalitis
      - late effect - *see* category 326
    - organic 348.9
      - arteriosclerotic 437.0
    - parasitic NEC 123.9
    - Pick's 331.11
      - with dementia
        - with behavioral disturbance 331.11 *[294.11]*
        - without behavioral disturbance 331.11 *[294.10]*
    - senile 331.2
  - braziers' 985.8
  - breast 611.9
    - cystic (chronic) 610.1
    - fibrocystic 610.1
    - inflammatory 611.0
    - Paget's (M8540/3) 174.0
    - puerperal, postpartum NEC 676.3 [5th]
    - specified NEC 611.89
  - Breda's (*see also* Yaws) 102.9
  - Breisky's (kraurosis vulvae) 624.09
  - Bretonneau's (diphtheritic malignant angina) 032.0
  - Bright's (*see also* Nephritis) 583.9
    - arteriosclerotic (*see also* Hypertension, kidney) 403.90
  - Brill's (recrudescent typhus) 081.1
    - flea-borne 081.0
    - louse-borne 081.1
  - Brill-Symmers (follicular lymphoma) (M9690/3) 202.0 [5th]
  - Brill-Zinsser (recrudescent typhus) 081.1
  - Brinton's (leather bottle stomach) (M8142/3) 151.9
  - Brion-Kayser (*see also* Fever, paratyphoid) 002.9
  - broad
    - beta 272.2
    - ligament, noninflammatory 620.9
      - specified NEC 620.8
  - Brocq's 691.8
    - meaning
      - atopic (diffuse) neurodermatitis 691.8
      - dermatitis herpetiformis 694.0
      - lichen simplex chronicus 698.3
      - parapsoriasis 696.2
      - prurigo 698.2
  - Brocq-Duhring (dermatitis herpetiformis) 694.0
  - Brodie's (joint) (*see also* Osteomyelitis) 730.1 [5th]
  - bronchi 519.19

- **Disease, diseased** – *continued*
  - bronchopulmonary 519.19
  - bronze (Addison's) 255.41
    - tuberculous (*see also* Tuberculosis) 017.6 [5th]
  - Brown-Séquard 344.89
  - Bruck's 733.99
  - Bruck-de Lange (Amsterdam dwarf, mental retardation, and brachycephaly) 759.89
  - Bruhl's (splenic anemia with fever) 285.8
  - Bruton's (X-linked agammaglobulinemia) 279.04
  - buccal cavity 528.9
  - Buchanan's (juvenile osteochondrosis, iliac crest) 732.1
  - Buchman's (osteochondrosis juvenile) 732.1
  - Budgerigar-Fanciers' 495.2
  - Budinger-Ludloff-Läwen 717.89
  - Büerger's (thromboangiitis obliterans) 443.1
  - Bürger-Grütz (essential familial hyperlipemia) 272.3
  - Burns' (lower ulna) 732.3
  - bursa 727.9
  - Bury's (erythema elevatum diutinum) 695.89
  - Buschke's 710.1
  - Busquet's (*see also* Osteomyelitis) 730.1 [5th]
  - Busse-Buschke (cryptococcosis) 117.5
  - C_2 (*see also* Alcoholism) 303.9 [5th]
  - caffey's (infantile cortical hyperostosis) 756.59
  - caisson 993.3
  - calculous 592.9
  - California 114.0
  - Calvé (-Perthes) (osteochondrosis, femoral capital) 732.1
  - Camurati-Engelmann (diaphyseal sclerosis) 756.59
  - Canavan's 330.0
  - capillaries 448.9
  - Carapata 087.1
  - cardiac - *see* Disease, heart
  - cardiopulmonary, chronic 416.9
  - cardiorenal (arteriosclerotic) (hepatic) (hypertensive) (vascular) (*see also* Hypertension, cardiorenal) 404.90
  - cardiovascular (arteriosclerotic) 429.2
    - congenital 746.9
    - hypertensive (*see also* Hypertension, heart) 402.90
      - benign 402.10
      - malignant 402.00
    - renal (*see also* Hypertension, cardiorenal) 404.90
    - syphilitic (asymptomatic) 093.9
  - carotid gland 259.8
  - Carrión's (Bartonellosis) 088.0
  - cartilage NEC 733.90
    - specified NEC 733.99
  - Castellani's 104.8
  - cat-scratch 078.3
  - Cavare's (familial periodic paralysis) 359.3
  - Cazenave's (pemphigus) 694.4
  - cecum 569.9
  - celiac (adult) 579.0
    - infantile 579.0
  - cellular tissue NEC 709.9
  - central core 359.0
  - cerebellar, cerebellum - *see* Disease, brain
  - cerebral (*see also* Disease, brain) 348.9
    - arterial, artery 437.9
    - degenerative - *see* Degeneration, brain
  - cerebrospinal 349.9
  - cerebrovascular NEC 437.9
    - acute 436
      - embolic - *see* Embolism, brain
      - late effect - *see* Late effect(s) (of) cerebrovascular disease
      - puerperal, postpartum, childbirth 674.0 [5th]
      - thrombotic - *see* Thrombosis, brain

- **Disease, diseased** – *continued*
  - cerebrovascular – *continued*
    - arteriosclerotic 437.0
    - embolic - *see* Embolism, brain
    - ischemic, generalized NEC 437.1
    - late effect - *see* Late effect(s) (of) cerebrovascular disease
    - occlusive 437.1
    - puerperal, postpartum, childbirth 674.0 [5th]
    - specified type NEC 437.8
    - thrombotic - *see* Thrombosis, brain
  - ceroid storage 272.7
  - cervix (uteri)
    - inflammatory 616.0
    - noninflammatory 622.9
      - specified NEC 622.8
  - Chabert's 022.9
  - Chagas' (*see also* Trypanosomiasis, American) 086.2
  - Chandler's (osteochondritis dissecans, hip) 732.7
  - Charcôt's (joint) 094.0 *[713.5]*
    - spinal cord 094.0
  - Charcôt-Marie-Tooth 356.1
  - Charlouis' (*see also* Yaws) 102.9
  - Cheadle (-Möller) (-Barlow) (infantile scurvy) 267
  - Chédiak-Steinbrinck (-Higashi) (congenital gigantism of peroxidase granules) 288.2
  - cheek, inner 528.9
  - chest 519.9
  - Chiari's (hepatic vein thrombosis) 453.0
  - Chicago (North American blastomycosis) 116.0
  - chignon (white piedra) 111.2
  - chigoe, chigo (jigger) 134.1
  - childhood granulomatous 288.1
  - Chinese liver fluke 121.1
  - chlamydial NEC 078.88
  - cholecystic (*see also* Disease, gallbladder) 575.9
  - choroid 363.9
    - degenerative (*see also* Degeneration, choroid) 363.40
    - hereditary (*see also* Dystrophy, choroid) 363.50
    - specified type NEC 363.8
  - Christian's (chronic histiocytosis X) 277.89
  - Christian-Weber (nodular nonsuppurative panniculitis) 729.30
  - Christmas 286.1
  - ciliary body 364.9
    - specified NEC 364.89
  - circulatory (system) NEC 459.9
    - chronic, maternal, affecting fetus or newborn 760.3
    - specified NEC 459.89
    - syphilitic 093.9
      - congenital 090.5
  - Civatte's (poikiloderma) 709.09
  - climacteric 627.2
    - male 608.89
  - coagulation factor deficiency (congenital) (*see also* Defect, coagulation) 286.9
  - Coats' 362.12
  - coccidioidal pulmonary 114.5
    - acute 114.0
    - chronic 114.4
    - primary 114.0
    - residual 114.4
  - Cockayne's (microcephaly and dwarfism) 759.89
  - Cogan's 370.52
  - cold
    - agglutinin 283.0
      - or hemoglobinuria 283.0
        - paroxysmal (cold) (nocturnal) 283.2
    - hemagglutinin (chronic) 283.0
  - collagen NEC 710.9
    - nonvascular 710.9
    - specified NEC 710.8

- **Disease, diseased** – *continued*
  - collagen – *continued*
    - vascular (allergic) (*see also* Angiitis, hypersensitivity) 446.20
  - colon 569.9
    - functional 564.9
      - congenital 751.3
    - ischemic 557.0
  - combined system (of spinal cord) 266.2 *[336.2]*
    - with anemia (pernicious) 281.0 *[336.2]*
  - compressed air 993.3
  - Concato's (pericardial polyserositis) 423.2
    - peritoneal 568.82
    - pleural - *see* Pleurisy
  - congenital NEC 799.89
  - conjunctiva 372.9
    - chlamydial 077.98
      - specified NEC 077.8
    - specified type NEC 372.89
    - viral 077.99
      - specified NEC 077.8
  - connective tissue, diffuse (*see also* Disease, collagen) 710.9
  - Conor and Bruch's (boutonneuse fever) 082.1
  - Conradi (-Hünermann) 756.59
  - Cooley's (erythroblastic anemia) 282.49
  - Cooper's 610.1
  - Corbus' 607.1
  - cork-handlers' 495.3
  - cornea (*see also* Keratopathy) 371.9
  - coronary (*see also* Ischemia, heart) 414.9
    - congenital 746.85
    - ostial, syphilitic 093.20
      - aortic 093.22
      - mitral 093.21
      - pulmonary 093.24
      - tricuspid 093.23
  - Corrigan's - *see* Insufficiency, aortic
  - Cotugno's 724.3
  - Coxsackie (virus) NEC 074.8
  - cranial nerve NEC 352.9
  - Creutzfeldt-Jakob (CJD) 046.19
    - with dementia
      - with behavioral disturbance 046.19 *[294.11]*
      - without behavioral disturbance 046.19 *[294.10]*
    - familial 046.19
    - iatrogenic 046.19
    - specified NEC 046.19
    - sporadic 046.19
    - variant (vCJD) 046.11
      - with dementia
        - with behavioral disturbance 046.11 *[294.11]*
        - without behavioral disturbance 046.11 *[294.10]*
  - Crigler-Najjar (congenital hyperbilirubinemia) 277.4
  - Crocq's (acrocyanosis) 443.89
  - Crohn's (intestine) (*see also* Enteritis, regional) 555.9
  - Crouzon's (craniofacial dysostosis) 756.0
  - Cruchet's (encephalitis lethargica) 049.8
  - Cruveilhier's 335.21
  - Cruz-Chagas (*see also* Trypanosomiasis, American) 086.2
  - crystal deposition (*see also* Arthritis, due to, crystals) 712.9 [5th]
  - Csillag's (lichen sclerosus et atrophicus) 701.0
  - Curschmann's 359.21
  - Cushing's (pituitary basophilism) 255.0
  - cystic
    - breast (chronic) 610.1
    - kidney, congenital (*see also* Cystic, disease, kidney) 753.10
    - liver, congenital 751.62
    - lung 518.89
      - congenital 748.4

Disease, diseased – *continued*
  cystic – *continued*
    pancreas 577.2
      congenital 751.7
    renal, congenital (*see also* Cystic, disease, kidney) 753.10
    semilunar cartilage 717.5
  cysticercus 123.1
  cystine storage (with renal sclerosis) 270.0
  cytomegalic inclusion (generalized) 078.5
    with
      pneumonia 078.5 *[484.1]*
    congenital 771.1
  Daae (-Finsen) (epidemic pleurodynia) 074.1
  dancing 297.8
  Danielssen's (anesthetic leprosy) 030.1
  Darier's (congenital) (keratosis follicularis) 757.39
    erythema annulare centrifugum 695.0
    vitamin A deficiency 264.8
  Darling's (histoplasmosis) (*see also* Histoplasmosis, American) 115.00
  davies' 425.0
  de Beurmann-Gougerot (sporotrichosis) 117.1
  Débove's (splenomegaly) 789.2
  deer fly (*see also* Tularemia) 021.9
  deficiency 269.9
  degenerative - *see also* Degeneration
    disc - *see* Degeneration, intervertebral disc
  degos' 447.8
  Déjérine (-Sottas) 356.0
  Déleage's 359.89
  demyelinating, demyelinizating (brain stem) (central nervous system) 341.9
    multiple sclerosis 340
    specified NEC 341.8
  de Quervain's (tendon sheath) 727.04
    thyroid (subacute granulomatous thyroiditis) 245.1
  Dercum's (adiposis dolorosa) 272.8
  Deutschländer's - *see* Fracture, foot
  Devergie's (pityriasis rubra pilaris) 696.4
  Devic's 341.0
  diaphorase deficiency 289.7
  diaphragm 519.4
  diarrheal, infectious 009.2
  diatomaceous earth 502
  Diaz's (osteochondrosis astragalus) 732.5
  digestive system 569.9
  Di Guglielmo's (erythemic myelosis) (M9841/3) 207.0 5th
  Dimitri-Sturge-Weber (encephalocutaneous angiomatosis) 759.6
  disc, degenerative - *see* Degeneration, intervertebral disc
  discogenic (*see also* Disease, intervertebral disc) 722.90
  diverticular - *see* Diverticula
  Down's (mongolism) 758.0
  Dubini's (electric chorea) 049.8
  Dubois' (thymus gland) 090.5
  Duchenne's 094.0
    locomotor ataxia 094.0
    muscular dystrophy 359.1
    paralysis 335.22
    pseudohypertrophy, muscles 359.1
  Duchenne-Griesinger 359.1
  ductless glands 259.9
  Duhring's (dermatitis herpetiformis) 694.0
  Dukes (-Filatov) 057.8
  duodenum NEC 537.9
    specified NEC 537.89
  Duplay's 726.2
  Dupré's (meningism) 781.6
  Dupuytren's (muscle contracture) 728.6
  Durand-Nicolas-Favre (climatic bubo) 099.1
  Duroziez's (congenital mitral stenosis) 746.5

Disease, diseased – *continued*
  Dutton's (trypanosomiasis) 086.9
  Eales' 362.18
  ear (chronic) (inner) NEC 388.9
    middle 385.9
      adhesive (*see also* Adhesions, middle ear) 385.10
      specified NEC 385.89
  Eberth's (typhoid fever) 002.0
  Ebstein's
    heart 746.2
    meaning diabetes 250.4 5th *[581.81]*
      due to secondary diabetes 249.4 5th *[581.81]*
  Echinococcus (*see also* Echinococcus) 122.9
  ECHO virus NEC 078.89
  Economo's (encephalitis lethargica) 049.8
  Eddowes' (brittle bones and blue sclera) 756.51
  Edsall's 992.2
  Eichstedt's (pityriasis versicolor) 111.0
  Ellis-van Creveld (chondroectodermal dysplasia) 756.55
  endocardium - *see* Endocarditis
  endocrine glands or system NEC 259.9
    specified NEC 259.8
  endomyocardial, idiopathic mural 425.2
  Engel-von Recklinghausen (osteitis fibrosa cystica) 252.01
  Engelmann's (diaphyseal sclerosis) 756.59
  English (rickets) 268.0
  Engman's (infectious eczematoid dermatitis) 690.8
  enteroviral, enterovirus NEC 078.89
    central nervous system NEC 048
  epidemic NEC 136.9
  epididymis 608.9
  epigastric, functional 536.9
    psychogenic 306.4
  Erb (-Landouzy) 359.1
  Erb-Goldflam 358.00
  Erdheim-Chester (ECD) 277.89 ●
  Erichsen's (railway spine) 300.16
  esophagus 530.9
    functional 530.5
    psychogenic 306.4
  Eulenburg's (congenital paramyotonia) 359.29
  Eustachian tube 381.9
  Evans' (thrombocytopenic purpura) 287.32
  external auditory canal 380.9
  extrapyramidal NEC 333.90
  eye 379.90
    anterior chamber 364.9
    inflammatory NEC 364.3
    muscle 378.9
  eyeball 360.9
  eyelid 374.9
  eyeworm of Africa 125.2
  Fabry's (angiokeratoma corporis diffusum) 272.7
  facial nerve (seventh) 351.9
    newborn 767.5
  Fahr-Volhard (malignant nephrosclerosis) 403.00
  fallopian tube, noninflammatory 620.9
    specified NEC 620.8
  familial periodic 277.31
    paralysis 359.3
  Fanconi's (congenital pancytopenia) 284.09
  Farber's (disseminated lipogranulomatosis) 272.8
  fascia 728.9
    inflammatory 728.9
  Fauchard's (periodontitis) 523.40
  Favre-Durand-Nicolas (climatic bubo) 099.1
  Favre-Racouchot (elastoidosis cutanea nodularis) 701.8
  Fede's 529.0
  Feer's 985.0

Disease, diseased – *continued*
  Felix's (juvenile osteochondrosis, hip) 732.1
  Fenwick's (gastric atrophy) 537.89
  Fernels' (aortic aneurysm) 441.9
  fibrocaseous, of lung (*see also* Tuberculosis, pulmonary) 011.9 5th
  fibrocystic - *see also* Fibrocystic, disease
    newborn 277.01
  Fiedler's (leptospiral jaundice) 100.0
  fifth 057.0
  Filatoff's (infectious mononucleosis) 075
  Filatov's (infectious mononucleosis) 075
  file-cutters' 984.9
    specified type of lead - *see* Table of Drugs and Chemicals
  filterable virus NEC 078.89
  fish skin 757.1
    acquired 701.1
  Flajani (-Basedow) (exophthalmic goiter) 242.0 5th
  Flatau-Schilder 341.1
  flax-dressers' 504
  Fleischner's 732.3
  flint 502
  fluke - *see* Infestation, fluke
  Følling's (phenylketonuria) 270.1
  foot and mouth 078.4
  foot process 581.3
  Forbes' (glycogenosis III) 271.0
  Fordyce's (ectopic sebaceous glands) (mouth) 750.26
  Fordyce-Fox (apocrine miliaria) 705.82
  Fothergill's
    meaning scarlatina anginosa 034.1
    neuralgia (*see also* Neuralgia, trigeminal) 350.1
  Fournier's 608.83
  fourth 057.8
  Fox (-Fordyce) (apocrine miliaria) 705.82
  Francis' (*see also* Tularemia) 021.9
  Franklin's (heavy chain) 273.2
  Frei's (climatic bubo) 099.1
  Freiberg's (flattening metatarsal) 732.5
  Friedländer's (endarteritis obliterans) - *see* Arteriosclerosis
  Friedreich's
    combined systemic or ataxia 334.0
    facial hemihypertrophy 756.0
    myoclonia 333.2
  Fröhlich's (adiposogenital dystrophy) 253.8
  Frommel's 676.6 5th
  frontal sinus (chronic) 473.1
    acute 461.1
  Fuller's earth 502
  fungus, fungous NEC 117.9
  Gaisböck's (polycythemia hypertonica) 289.0
  gallbladder 575.9
    congenital 751.60
  Gamna's (siderotic splenomegaly) 289.51
  Gamstorp's (adynamia episodica hereditaria) 359.3
  Gandy-Nanta (siderotic splenomegaly) 289.51
  Gannister (occupational) 502
  Garré's (*see also* Osteomyelitis) 730.1 5th
  gastric (*see also* Disease, stomach) 537.9
  gastroesophageal reflux (GERD) 530.81
  gastrointestinal (tract) 569.9
    amyloid 277.39
    functional 536.9
      psychogenic 306.4
  Gaucher's (adult) (cerebroside lipidosis) (infantile) 272.7
  Gayet's (superior hemorrhagic polioencephalitis) 265.1
  Gee (-Herter) (-Heubner) (-Thaysen) (nontropical sprue) 579.0
  generalized neoplastic (M8000/6) 199.0
  genital organs NEC
    female 629.9
      specified NEC 629.89

Disease, diseased – *continued*
  genital organs NEC – *continued*
    male 608.9
  Gerhardt's (erythromelalgia) 443.82
  Gerlier's (epidemic vertigo) 078.81
  Gibert's (pityriasis rosea) 696.3
  Gibney's (perispondylitis) 720.9
  Gierke's (glycogenosis I) 271.0
  Gilbert's (familial nonhemolytic jaundice) 277.4
  Gilchrist's (North American blastomycosis) 116.0
  Gilford (-Hutchinson) (progeria) 259.8
  Gilles de la Tourette's (motor-verbal tic) 307.23
  Giovannini's 117.9
  gland (lymph) 289.9
  Glanzmann's (hereditary hemorrhagic thrombasthenia) 287.1
  glassblowers' 527.1
  Glénard's (enteroptosis) 569.89
  Glisson's (*see also* Rickets) 268.0
  glomerular
    membranous, idiopathic 581.1
    minimal change 581.3
  glycogen storage (Andersen's) (Cori types 1-7) (Forbes') (McArdle-Schmid-Pearson) (Pompe's) (types I-VII) 271.0
    cardiac 271.0 *[425.7]*
    generalized 271.0
    glucose-6-phosphatase deficiency 271.0
    heart 271.0 *[425.7]*
    hepatorenal 271.0
    liver and kidneys 271.0
    myocardium 271.0 *[425.7]*
    von Gierke's (glycogenosis I) 271.0
  Goldflam-Erb 358.00
  Goldscheider's (epidermolysis bullosa) 757.39
  Goldstein's (familial hemorrhagic telangiectasia) 448.0
  gonococcal NEC 098.0
  Goodall's (epidemic vomiting) 078.82
  Gordon's (exudative enteropathy) 579.8
  Gougerot's (trisymptomatic) 709.1
  Gougerot-Carteaud (confluent reticulate papillomatosis) 701.8
  Gougerot-Hailey-Hailey (benign familial chronic pemphigus) 757.39
  graft-versus-host 279.50
    acute 279.51
      on chronic 279.53
    chronic 279.52
  grain-handlers' 495.8
  Grancher's (splenopneumonia) - *see* Pneumonia
  granulomatous (childhood) (chronic) 288.1
  graphite lung 503
  Graves' (exophthalmic goiter) 242.0 5th
  Greenfield's 330.0
  green monkey 078.89
  Griesinger's (*see also* Ancylostomiasis) 126.9
  grinders' 502
  Grisel's 723.5
  Gruby's (tinea tonsurans) 110.0
  Guertin's (electric chorea) 049.8
  Guillain-Barré 357.0
  Guinon's (motor-verbal tic) 307.23
  Gull's (thyroid atrophy with myxedema) 244.8
  Gull and Sutton's - *see* Hypertension, kidney
  gum NEC 523.9
  Günther's (congenital erythropoietic porphyria) 277.1
  gynecological 629.9
    specified NEC 629.89
  H 270.0
  Haas' 732.3

- **Disease, diseased** – *continued*
  - Habermann's (acute parapsoriasis varioliformis) 696.2
  - Haff 985.1
  - Hageman (congenital factor XII deficiency) (*see also* Defect, congenital) 286.3
  - Haglund's (osteochondrosis os tibiale externum) 732.5
  - Hagner's (hypertrophic pulmonary osteoarthropathy) 731.2
  - Hailey-Hailey (benign familial chronic pemphigus) 757.39
  - hair (follicles) NEC 704.9
    - specified type NEC 704.8
  - Hallervorden-Spatz 333.0
  - Hallopeau's (lichen sclerosus et atrophicus) 701.0
  - Hamman's (spontaneous mediastinal emphysema) 518.1
  - hand, foot, and mouth 074.3
  - Hand-Schüller-Christian (chronic histiocytosis X) 277.89
  - Hanot's - *see* Cirrhosis, biliary
  - Hansen's (leprosy) 030.9
    - benign form 030.1
    - malignant form 030.0
  - Harada's 363.22
  - Harley's (intermittent hemoglobinuria) 283.2
  - Hart's (pellagra-cerebellar ataxia-renal aminoaciduria) 270.0
  - Hartnup (pellagra-cerebellar ataxia-renal aminoaciduria) 270.0
  - Hashimoto's (struma lymphomatosa) 245.2
  - Hb - *see* Disease, hemoglobin
  - heart (organic) 429.9
    - with
      - acute pulmonary edema (*see also* Failure, ventricular, left) 428.1
        - hypertensive 402.91
          - with renal failure 404.92
          - benign 402.11
            - with renal failure 404.12
          - malignant 402.01
            - with renal failure 404.02
        - kidney disease - *see* Hypertension, cardiorenal
        - rheumatic fever (conditions classifiable to 390)
          - active 391.9
            - with chorea 392.0
          - inactive or quiescent (with chorea) 398.90
    - amyloid 277.39 *[425.7]*
    - aortic (valve) (*see also* Endocarditis, aortic) 424.1
    - arteriosclerotic or sclerotic (minimal) (senile) - *see* Arteriosclerosis, coronary
    - artery, arterial - *see* Arteriosclerosis, coronary
    - atherosclerotic - *see* Arteriosclerosis, coronary
    - beer drinkers' 425.5
    - beriberi 265.0 *[425.7]*
    - black 416.0
    - congenital NEC 746.9
      - cyanotic 746.9
      - maternal, affecting fetus or newborn 760.3
      - specified type NEC 746.89
    - congestive (*see also* Failure, heart) 428.0
    - coronary 414.9
    - cryptogenic 429.9
    - due to
      - amyloidosis 277.39 *[425.7]*
      - beriberi 265.0 *[425.7]*
      - cardiac glycogenosis 271.0 *[425.7]*
      - Friedreich's ataxia 334.0 *[425.8]*
      - gout 274.82

- **Disease, diseased** – *continued*
  - heart – *continued*
    - due to – *continued*
      - mucopolysaccharidosis 277.5 *[425.7]*
      - myotonia atrophica 359.21 *[425.8]*
      - progressive muscular dystrophy 359.1 *[425.8]*
      - sarcoidosis 135 *[425.8]*
    - fetal 746.9
      - inflammatory 746.89
    - fibroid (*see also* Myocarditis) 429.0
    - functional 427.9
      - postoperative 997.1
      - psychogenic 306.2
    - glycogen storage 271.0 *[425.7]*
    - gonococcal NEC 098.85
    - gouty 274.82
    - hypertensive (*see also* Hypertension, heart) 402.90
      - benign 402.10
      - malignant 402.00
    - hyperthyroid (*see also* Hyperthyroidism) 242.9 [5th] *[425.7]*
    - incompletely diagnosed - *see* Disease, heart
    - ischemic (chronic) (*see also* Ischemia, heart) 414.9
      - acute (*see also* Infarct, myocardium) 410.9 [5th]
        - without myocardial infarction 411.89
          - with coronary (artery) occlusion 411.81
      - asymptomatic 412
      - diagnosed on ECG or other special investigation but currently presenting no symptoms 412
    - kyphoscoliotic 416.1
    - mitral (*see also* Endocarditis, mitral) 394.9
    - muscular (*see also* Degeneration, myocardial) 429.1
    - postpartum 674.8 [5th]
    - psychogenic (functional) 306.2
    - pulmonary (chronic) 416.9
      - acute 415.0
      - specified NEC 416.8
    - rheumatic (chronic) (inactive) (old) (quiescent) (with chorea) 398.90
      - active or acute 391.9
        - with chorea (active) (rheumatic) (Sydenham's) 392.0
        - specified type NEC 391.8
      - maternal, affecting fetus or newborn 760.3
    - rheumatoid - *see* Arthritis, rheumatoid
    - sclerotic - *see* Arteriosclerosis, coronary
    - senile (*see also* Myocarditis) 429.0
    - specified type NEC 429.89
    - syphilitic 093.89
      - aortic 093.1
        - aneurysm 093.0
      - asymptomatic 093.89
      - congenital 090.5
    - thyroid (gland) (*see also* Hyperthyroidism) 242.9 [5th] *[425.7]*
    - thyrotoxic (*see also* Thyrotoxicosis) 242.9 [5th] *[425.7]*
    - tuberculous (*see also* Tuberculosis) 017.9 [5th] *[425.8]*
    - valve, valvular (obstructive) (regurgitant) - *see also* Endocarditis
      - congenital NEC (*see also* Anomaly, heart, valve) 746.9
        - pulmonary 746.00
        - specified type NEC 746.89
    - vascular - *see* Disease, cardiovascular
  - heavy-chain (gamma G) 273.2
  - Heberden's 715.04

- **Disease, diseased** – *continued*
  - Hebra's
    - dermatitis exfoliativa 695.89
    - erythema multiforme exudativum 695.19
    - pityriasis
      - maculata et circinata 696.3
      - rubra 695.89
        - pilaris 696.4
    - prurigo 698.2
  - Heerfordt's (uveoparotitis) 135
  - Heidenhain's 290.10
    - with dementia 290.10
  - Heilmeyer-Schöner (M9842/3) 207.1 [5th]
  - Heine-Medin (*see also* Poliomyelitis) 045.9 [5th]
  - Heller's (*see also* Psychosis, childhood) 299.1 [5th]
  - Heller-Döhle (syphilitic aortitis) 093.1
  - hematopoietic organs 289.9
  - hemoglobin (Hb) 282.7
    - with thalassemia 282.49
    - abnormal (mixed) NEC 282.7
      - with thalassemia 282.49
    - AS genotype 282.5
    - Bart's 282.49
    - C (Hb-C) 282.7
      - with other abnormal hemoglobin NEC 282.7
      - elliptocytosis 282.7
      - Hb-S (without crisis) 282.63
        - with
          - crisis 282.64
          - vaso-occlusive pain 282.64
      - sickle-cell (without crisis) 282.63
        - with
          - crisis 282.64
          - vaso-occlusive pain 282.64
      - thalassemia 282.49
    - constant spring 282.7
    - D (Hb-D) 282.7
      - with other abnormal hemoglobin NEC 282.7
      - Hb-S (without crisis) 282.68
        - with crisis 282.69
      - sickle-cell (without crisis) 282.68
        - with crisis 282.69
      - thalassemia 282.49
    - E (Hb-E) 282.7
      - with other abnormal hemoglobin NEC 282.7
      - Hb-S (without crisis) 282.68
        - with crisis 282.69
      - sickle-cell (without crisis) 282.68
        - with crisis 282.69
      - thalassemia 282.49
    - elliptocytosis 282.7
    - F (Hb-F) 282.7
    - G (Hb-G) 282.7
    - H (Hb-H) 282.49
    - hereditary persistence, fetal (HPFH) ("Swiss variety") 282.7
    - high fetal gene 282.7
    - I thalassemia 282.49
    - M 289.7
    - S - *see also* Disease, sickle-cell, Hb-S
      - thalassemia (without crisis) 282.41
        - with
          - crisis 282.42
          - vaso-occlusive pain 282.42
    - spherocytosis 282.7
    - unstable, hemolytic 282.7
    - Zurich (Hb-Zurich) 282.7
  - hemolytic (fetus) (newborn) 773.2
    - autoimmune (cold type) (warm type) 283.0
    - due to or with
      - incompatibility
        - ABO (blood group) 773.1
        - blood (group) (Duffy) (Kell) (Kidd) (Lewis) (M) (S) NEC 773.2
        - Rh (blood group) (factor) 773.0
      - Rh negative mother 773.0

- **Disease, diseased** – *continued*
  - hemolytic – *continued*
    - unstable hemoglobin 282.7
  - hemorrhagic 287.9
    - newborn 776.0
  - Henoch (-Schönlein) (purpura nervosa) 287.0
  - hepatic - *see* Disease, liver
  - hepatolenticular 275.1
  - heredodegenerative NEC
    - brain 331.89
    - spinal cord 336.8
  - Hers' (glycogenosis VI) 271.0
  - Herter (-Gee) (-Heubner) (nontropical sprue) 579.0
  - Herxheimer's (diffuse idiopathic cutaneous atrophy) 701.8
  - Heubner's 094.89
  - Heubner-Herter (nontropical sprue) 579.0
  - high fetal gene or hemoglobin thalassemia 282.49
  - Hildenbrand's (typhus) 081.9
  - hip (joint) NEC 719.95
    - congenital 755.63
    - suppurative 711.05
    - tuberculous (*see also* Tuberculosis) 015.1 [5th] *[730.85]*
  - Hippel's (retinocerebral angiomatosis) 759.6
  - Hirschfeld's (acute diabetes mellitus) (*see also* Diabetes) 250.0 [5th]
    - due to secondary diabetes 249.0 [5th]
  - Hirschsprung's (congenital megacolon) 751.3
  - His (-Werner) (trench fever) 083.1
  - HIV 042
  - Hodgkin's (M9650/3) 201.9 [5th]

Note *Use the following fifth-digit subclassification with category 201:*

0	unspecified site
1	lymph nodes of head, face, and neck
2	intrathoracic lymph nodes
3	intra-abdominal lymph nodes
4	lymph nodes of axilla and upper limb
5	lymph nodes of inguinal region and lower limb
6	intrapelvic lymph nodes
7	spleen
8	lymph nodes of multiple sites

  - Hodgkin's – (continued)
    - lymphocytic
      - depletion (M9653/3) 201.7 [5th]
        - diffuse fibrosis (M9654/3) 201.7 [5th]
        - reticular type (M9655/3) 201.7 [5th]
      - predominance (M9651/3) 201.4 [5th]
    - lymphocytic-histiocytic predominance (M9651/3) 201.4 [5th]
    - mixed cellularity (M9652/3) 201.6 [5th]
    - nodular sclerosis (M9656/3) 201.5 [5th]
      - cellular phase (M9657/3) 201.5 [5th]
  - Hodgson's 441.9
    - ruptured 441.5
  - Hoffa (-Kastert) (liposynovitis prepatellaris) 272.8
  - Holla (*see also* Spherocytosis) 282.0
  - homozygous-Hb-S 282.61
  - hoof and mouth 078.4
  - hookworm (*see also* Ancylostomiasis) 126.9
  - Horton's (temporal arteritis) 446.5
  - host-versus-graft (immune or nonimmune cause) 279.50
  - HPFH (hereditary persistence of fetal hemoglobin) ("Swiss variety") 282.7
  - Huchard's (continued arterial hypertension) 401.9
  - Huguier's (uterine fibroma) 218.9
  - human immunodeficiency (virus) 042
  - hunger 251.1

Disease, diseased

- **Disease, diseased** – *continued*
  - lung – *continued*
    - fibroid (chronic) (*see also* Fibrosis, lung) 515
    - fluke 121.2
      - oriental 121.2
    - in
      - amyloidosis 277.39 *[517.8]*
      - polymyositis 710.4 *[517.8]*
      - sarcoidosis 135 *[517.8]*
      - Sjögren's syndrome 710.2 *[517.8]*
      - syphilis 095.1
      - systemic lupus erythematosus 710.0 *[517.8]*
      - systemic sclerosis 710.1 *[517.2]*
    - interstitial (chronic) 515
      - acute 136.3
    - nonspecific, chronic 496
    - obstructive (chronic) (COPD) 496
      - with
        - acute
          - bronchitis 491.22
          - exacerbation NEC 491.21
        - alveolitis, allergic (*see also* Alveolitis, allergic) 495.9
        - asthma (chronic) (obstructive) 493.2 5th
        - bronchiectasis 494.0
          - with acute exacerbation 494.1
        - bronchitis (chronic) 491.20
          - with
            - acute bronchitis 491.22
            - exacerbation (acute) 491.21
        - decompensated 491.21
          - with exacerbation 491.21
        - emphysema NEC 492.8
      - diffuse (with fibrosis) 496
    - polycystic 518.89
      - asthma (chronic) (obstructive) 493.2 5th
      - congenital 748.4
    - purulent (cavitary) 513.0
    - restrictive 518.89
    - rheumatoid 714.81
      - diffuse interstitial 714.81
    - specified NEC 518.89
  - Lutembacher's (atrial septal defect with mitral stenosis) 745.5
  - Lutz-Miescher (elastosis perforans serpiginosa) 701.1
  - Lutz-Splendore-de Almeida (Brazilian blastomycosis) 116.1
  - Lyell's (toxic epidermal necrolysis) 695.15
    - due to drug
      - correct substance properly administered 695.15
      - overdose or wrong substance given or taken 977.9
        - specific drug - *see* Table of Drugs and Chemicals
  - Lyme 088.81
  - lymphatic (gland) (system) 289.9
    - channel (noninfective) 457.9
    - vessel (noninfective) 457.9
      - specified NEC 457.8
  - lymphoproliferative (chronic) (M9970/1) 238.79
  - Machado-Joseph 334.8
  - Madelung's (lipomatosis) 272.8
  - Madura (actinomycotic) 039.9
    - mycotic 117.4
  - Magitot's 526.4
  - Majocchi's (purpura annularis telangiectodes) 709.1
  - malarial (*see also* Malaria) 084.6
  - Malassez's (cystic) 608.89
  - Malibu 919.8
    - infected 919.9
  - malignant (M8000/3) - *see also* Neoplasm, by site, malignant
    - previous, affecting management of pregnancy V23.89

- **Disease, diseased** – *continued*
  - Manson's 120.1
  - maple bark 495.6
  - maple syrup (urine) 270.3
  - Marburg (virus) 078.89
  - Marchiafava (-Bignami) 341.8
  - Marfan's 090.49
    - congenital syphilis 090.49
    - meaning Marfan's syndrome 759.82
  - Marie-Bamberger (hypertrophic pulmonary osteoarthropathy) (secondary) 731.2
    - primary or idiopathic (acropachyderma) 757.39
    - pulmonary (hypertrophic osteoarthropathy) 731.2
  - Marie-Strümpell (ankylosing spondylitis) 720.0
  - Marion's (bladder neck obstruction) 596.0
  - Marsh's (exophthalmic goiter) 242.0 5th
  - Martin's 715.27
  - mast cell 757.33
    - systemic (M9741/3) 202.6 5th
  - mastoid (*see also* Mastoiditis) 383.9
    - process 385.9
  - maternal, unrelated to pregnancy NEC, affecting fetus or newborn 760.9
  - Mathieu's (leptospiral jaundice) 100.0
  - Mauclaire's 732.3
  - Mauriac's (erythema nodosum syphiliticum) 091.3
  - Maxcy's 081.0
  - McArdle (-Schmid-Pearson) (glycogenosis V) 271.0
  - mediastinum NEC 519.3
  - Medin's (*see also* Poliomyelitis) 045.9 5th
  - Mediterranean (with hemoglobinopathy) 282.49
  - medullary center (idiopathic) (respiratory) 348.89 ▲
  - Meige's (chronic hereditary edema) 757.0
  - Meleda 757.39
  - Ménétrier's (hypertrophic gastritis) 535.2 5th
  - Ménière's (active) 386.00
    - cochlear 386.02
    - cochleovestibular 386.01
    - inactive 386.04
    - in remission 386.04
    - vestibular 386.03
  - meningeal - *see* Meningitis
  - mental (*see also* Psychosis) 298.9
  - Merzbacher-Pelizaeus 330.0
  - mesenchymal 710.9
  - mesenteric embolic 557.0
  - metabolic NEC 277.9
  - metal polishers' 502
  - metastatic - *see* Metastasis
  - Mibelli's 757.39
  - microdrepanocytic 282.49
  - microvascular - code to condition
  - Miescher's 709.3
  - Mikulicz's (dryness of mouth, absent or decreased lacrimation) 527.1
  - Milkman (-Looser) (osteomalacia with pseudofractures) 268.2
  - Miller's (osteomalacia) 268.2
  - Mills' 335.29
  - Milroy's (chronic hereditary edema) 757.0
  - Minamata 985.0
  - Minor's 336.1
  - Minot's (hemorrhagic disease, newborn) 776.0
  - Minot-von Willebrand-Jürgens (angiohemophilia) 286.4
  - Mitchell's (erythromelalgia) 443.82
  - mitral - *see* Endocarditis, mitral
  - Mljet (mal de Meleda) 757.39
  - Möbius, Moebius' 346.2 5th
  - Möeller's 267
  - Möller (-Barlow) (infantile scurvy) 267
  - Mönckeberg's (*see also* Arteriosclerosis, extremities) 440.20

- **Disease, diseased** – *continued*
  - Mondor's (thrombophlebitis of breast) 451.89
  - Monge's 993.2
  - Morel-Kraepelin (*see also* Schizophrenia) 295.9 5th
  - Morgagni's (syndrome) (hyperostosis frontalis interna) 733.3
  - Morgagni-Adams-Stokes (syncope with heart block) 426.9
  - Morquio (-Brailsford) (-Ullrich) (mucopolysaccharidosis IV) 277.5
  - Morton's (with metatarsalgia) 355.6
  - Morvan's 336.0
  - motor neuron (bulbar) (mixed type) 335.20
  - Mouchet's (juvenile osteochondrosis, foot) 732.5
  - mouth 528.9
  - Moyamoya 437.5
  - Mucha's (acute parapsoriasis varioliformis) 696.2
  - mu-chain 273.2
  - mucolipidosis (I) (II) (III) 272.7
  - Münchmeyer's (exostosis luxurians) 728.11
  - Murri's (intermittent hemoglobinuria) 283.2
  - muscle 359.9
    - inflammatory 728.9
    - ocular 378.9
  - musculoskeletal system 729.90
  - mushroom workers' 495.5
  - Mya's (congenital dilation, colon) 751.3
  - mycotic 117.9
  - myeloproliferative (chronic) (M9960/1) 238.79
  - myocardium, myocardial (*see also* Degeneration, myocardial) 429.1
    - hypertensive (*see also* Hypertension, heart) 402.90
    - primary (idiopathic) 425.4
  - myoneural 358.9
  - Naegeli's 287.1
  - nail 703.9
    - specified type NEC 703.8
  - nairobi sheep 066.1
  - nasal 478.19
    - cavity NEC 478.19
    - sinus (chronic) - *see* Sinusitis
  - navel (newborn) NEC 779.89
    - delayed separation of umbilical cord 779.83
  - nemaline body 359.0
  - neoplastic, generalized (M8000/6) 199.0
  - nerve - *see* Disorder, nerve
  - nervous system (central) 349.9
    - autonomic, peripheral (*see also* Neuropathy, peripheral, autonomic) 337.9
    - congenital 742.9
    - inflammatory - *see* Encephalitis
    - parasympathetic (*see also* Neuropathy, peripheral, autonomic) 337.9
    - peripheral NEC 355.9
    - prion NEC 046.79
    - specified NEC 349.89
    - sympathetic (*see also* Neuropathy, peripheral, autonomic) 337.9
    - vegetative (*see also* Neuropathy, peripheral, autonomic) 337.9
  - Nettleship's (urticaria pigmentosa) 757.33
  - Neumann's (pemphigus vegetans) 694.4
  - neurologic (central) NEC (*see also* Disease, nervous system) 349.9
    - peripheral NEC 355.9
  - neuromuscular system NEC 358.9
  - Newcastle 077.8
  - Nicolas (-Durand) -Favre (climatic bubo) 099.1
  - Niemann-Pick (lipid histiocytosis) 272.7
  - nipple 611.9
    - paget's (M8540/3) 174.0
  - Nishimoto (-Takeuchi) 437.5

- **Disease, diseased** – *continued*
  - nonarthropod-borne NEC 078.89
    - central nervous system NEC 049.9
    - enterovirus NEC 078.89
  - nonautoimmune hemolytic NEC 283.10
  - Nonne-Milroy-Meige (chronic hereditary edema) 757.0
  - Norrie's (congenital progressive oculoacousticocerebral degeneration) 743.8
  - nose 478.19
  - nucleus pulposus - *see* Disease, intervertebral disc
  - nutritional 269.9
    - maternal, affecting fetus or newborn 760.4
  - oasthouse, urine 270.2
  - obliterative vascular 447.1
  - Odelberg's (juvenile osteochondrosis) 732.1
  - Oguchi's (retina) 368.61
  - Ohara's (*see also* Tularemia) 021.9
  - Ollier's (chondrodysplasia) 756.4
  - Opitz's (congestive splenomegaly) 289.51
  - Oppenheim's 358.8
  - Oppenheim-Urbach (necrobiosis lipoidica diabeticorum) 250.8 5th *[709.3]*
    - due to secondary diabetes 249.8 5th *[709.3]*
  - optic nerve NEC 377.49
  - orbit 376.9
    - specified NEC 376.89
  - Oriental liver fluke 121.1
  - Oriental lung fluke 121.2
  - Ormond's 593.4
  - Osgood's tibia (tubercle) 732.4
  - Osgood-Schlatter 732.4
  - Osler (-Vaquez) (polycythemia vera) (M9950/1) 238.4
  - Osler-Rendu (familial hemorrhagic telangiectasia) 448.0
  - osteofibrocystic 252.01
  - Otto's 715.35
  - outer ear 380.9
  - ovary (noninflammatory) NEC 620.9
    - cystic 620.2
    - polycystic 256.4
    - specified NEC 620.8
  - Owren's (congenital) (*see also* Defect, coagulation) 286.3
  - Paas' 756.59
  - Paget's (osteitis deformans) 731.0
    - with infiltrating duct carcinoma of the breast (M8541/3) - *see* Neoplasm, breast, malignant
    - bone 731.0
      - osteosarcoma in (M9184/3) - *see* Neoplasm, bone, malignant
    - breast (M8540/3) 174.0
    - extramammary (M8542/3) - *see also* Neoplasm, skin, malignant
      - anus 154.3
        - skin 173.5
    - malignant (M8540/3)
      - breast 174.0
      - specified site NEC (M8542/3) - *see* Neoplasm, skin, malignant
      - unspecified site 174.0
    - mammary (M8540/3) 174.0
    - nipple (M8540/3) 174.0
  - palate (soft) 528.9
  - Paltauf-Sternberg 201.9 5th
  - pancreas 577.9
    - cystic 577.2
      - congenital 751.7
    - fibrocystic 277.00
  - Panner's 732.3
    - capitellum humeri 732.3
    - head of humerus 732.3
    - tarsal navicular (bone) (osteochondrosis) 732.5
  - panvalvular - *see* Endocarditis, mitral
  - parametrium 629.9

Disease, diseased – *continued*
- parasitic NEC 136.9
  - cerebral NEC 123.9
  - intestinal NEC 129
  - mouth 112.0
  - skin NEC 134.9
  - specified type - *see* Infestation
  - tongue 112.0
- parathyroid (gland) 252.9
  - specified NEC 252.8
- Parkinson's 332.0
- parodontal 523.9
- Parrot's (syphilitic osteochondritis) 090.0
- Parry's (exophthalmic goiter) 242.0 5th
- Parson's (exophthalmic goiter) 242.0 5th
- Pavy's 593.6
- Paxton's (white piedra) 111.2
- Payr's (splenic flexure syndrome) 569.89
- pearl-workers' (chronic osteomyelitis) (*see also* Osteomyelitis) 730.1 5th
- Pel-Ebstein - *see* Disease, Hodgkin's
- Pelizaeus-Merzbacher 330.0
  - with dementia
    - with behavioral disturbance 330.0 *[294.11]*
    - without behavioral disturbance 330.0 *[294.10]*
- Pellegrini-Stieda (calcification, knee joint) 726.62
- pelvis, pelvic
  - female NEC 629.9
    - specified NEC 629.89
  - gonococcal (acute) 098.19
    - chronic or duration of 2 months or over 098.39
  - infection (*see also* Disease, pelvis, inflammatory) 614.9
  - inflammatory (female) (PID) 614.9
    - with
      - abortion - *see* Abortion, by type, with sepsis
      - ectopic pregnancy (*see also* categories 633.0-633.9) 639.0
      - molar pregnancy (*see also* categories 630-632) 639.0
    - acute 614.3
    - chronic 614.4
    - complicating pregnancy 646.6 5th
      - affecting fetus or newborn 760.8
    - following
      - abortion 639.0
      - ectopic or molar pregnancy 639.0
    - peritonitis (acute) 614.5
      - chronic NEC 614.7
    - puerperal, postpartum, childbirth 670.8 5th ▲
    - specified NEC 614.8
  - organ, female NEC 629.9
    - specified NEC 629.89
  - peritoneum, female NEC 629.9
    - specified NEC 629.89
- penis 607.9
  - inflammatory 607.2
- peptic NEC 536.9
  - acid 536.8
- periapical tissues NEC 522.9
- pericardium 423.9
  - specified type NEC 423.8
- perineum
  - female
    - inflammatory 616.9
      - specified NEC 616.89
    - noninflammatory 624.9
      - specified NEC 624.8
  - male (inflammatory) 682.2
- periodic (familial) (Reimann's) NEC 277.31
  - paralysis 359.3
- periodontal NEC 523.9
  - specified NEC 523.8
- periosteum 733.90

Disease, diseased – *continued*
- peripheral
  - arterial 443.9
  - autonomic nervous system (*see also* Neuropathy, autonomic) 337.9
  - nerve NEC (*see also* Neuropathy) 356.9
    - multiple - *see* Polyneuropathy
  - vascular 443.9
    - specified type NEC 443.89
- peritoneum 568.9
  - pelvic, female 629.9
    - specified NEC 629.89
- Perrin-Ferraton (snapping hip) 719.65
- persistent mucosal (middle ear) (with posterior or superior marginal perforation of ear drum) 382.2
- Perthes' (capital femoral osteochondrosis) 732.1
- Petit's (*see also* Hernia, lumbar) 553.8
- Peutz-Jeghers 759.6
- Peyronie's 607.85
- Pfeiffer's (infectious mononucleosis) 075
- pharynx 478.20
- Phocas' 610.1
- photochromogenic (acid-fast bacilli) (pulmonary) 031.0
  - nonpulmonary 031.9
- Pick's
  - brain 331.11
    - with dementia
      - with behavioral disturbance 331.11 *[294.11]*
      - without behavioral disturbance 331.11 *[294.10]*
  - cerebral atrophy 331.11
    - with dementia
      - with behavioral disturbance 331.11 *[294.11]*
      - without behavioral disturbance 331.11 *[294.10]*
  - lipid histiocytosis 272.7
  - liver (pericardial pseudocirrhosis of liver) 423.2
  - pericardium (pericardial pseudocirrhosis of liver) 423.2
  - polyserositis (pericardial pseudocirrhosis of liver) 423.2
- Pierson's (osteochondrosis) 732.1
- pigeon fanciers' or breeders' 495.2
- pineal gland 259.8
- pink 985.0
- Pinkus' (lichen nitidus) 697.1
- pinworm 127.4
- pituitary (gland) 253.9
  - hyperfunction 253.1
  - hypofunction 253.2
- pituitary snuff-takers' 495.8
- placenta
  - affecting fetus or newborn 762.2
  - complicating pregnancy or childbirth 656.7 5th
- pleura (cavity) (*see also* Pleurisy) 511.0
- Plummer's (toxic nodular goiter) 242.3 5th
- pneumatic
  - drill 994.9
  - hammer 994.9
- policeman's 729.2
- Pollitzer's (hidradenitis suppurativa) 705.83
- polycystic (congenital) 759.89
  - kidney or renal 753.12
    - adult type (APKD) 753.13
    - autosomal dominant 753.13
    - autosomal recessive 753.14
    - childhood type (CPKD) 753.14
    - infantile type 753.14
  - liver or hepatic 751.62
  - lung or pulmonary 518.89
    - congenital 748.4
  - ovary, ovaries 256.4
  - spleen 759.0
- Pompe's (glycogenosis II) 271.0
- Poncet's (tuberculous rheumatism) (*see also* Tuberculosis) 015.9 5th

Disease, diseased – *continued*
- Posada-Wernicke 114.9
- Potain's (pulmonary edema) 514
- Pott's (*see also* Tuberculosis) 015.0 5th *[730.88]*
  - osteomyelitis 015.0 5th *[730.88]*
  - paraplegia 015.0 5th *[730.88]*
  - spinal curvature 015.0 5th *[737.43]*
  - spondylitis 015.0 5th *[720.81]*
- Potter's 753.0
- Poulet's 714.2
- pregnancy NEC (*see also* Pregnancy) 646.9 5th
- Preiser's (osteoporosis) 733.09
- Pringle's (tuberous sclerosis) 759.5
- Profichet's 729.90
- prostate 602.9
  - specified type NEC 602.8
- protozoal NEC 136.8
  - intestine, intestinal NEC 007.9
- pseudo-Hurler's (mucolipidosis III) 272.7
- psychiatric (*see also* Psychosis) 298.9
- psychotic (*see also* Psychosis) 298.9
- Puente's (simple glandular cheilitis) 528.5
- puerperal NEC (*see also* Puerperal) 674.9 5th
- pulmonary - *see also* Disease, lung
  - amyloid 277.39 *[517.8]*
  - artery 417.9
  - circulation, circulatory 417.9
    - specified NEC 417.8
  - diffuse obstructive (chronic) 496
    - with
      - acute bronchitis 491.22
      - asthma (chronic) (obstructive) 493.2 5th
      - exacerbation NEC (acute) 491.21
  - heart (chronic) 416.9
    - specified NEC 416.8
  - hypertensive (vascular) 416.0
    - cardiovascular 416.0
  - obstructive diffuse (chronic) 496
    - with
      - acute bronchitis 491.22
      - asthma (chronic) (obstructive) 493.2 5th
      - bronchitis (chronic) 491.20
        - with
          - exacerbation (acute) 491.21
        - acute 491.22
      - exacerbation NEC (acute) 491.21
    - decompensated 491.21
      - with exacerbation 491.21
  - valve (*see also* Endocarditis, pulmonary) 424.3
- pulp (dental) NEC 522.9
- pulseless 446.7
- Putnam's (subacute combined sclerosis with pernicious anemia) 281.0 *[336.2]*
- Pyle (-Cohn) (craniometaphyseal dysplasia) 756.89
- pyramidal tract 333.90
- Quervain's
  - tendon sheath 727.04
  - thyroid (subacute granulomatous thyroiditis) 245.1
- Quincke's - *see* Edema, angioneurotic
- Quinquaud (acne decalvans) 704.09
- rag sorters' 022.1
- Raynaud's (paroxysmal digital cyanosis) 443.0
- reactive airway - *see* Asthma
- Recklinghausen's (M9540/1) 237.71
  - bone (osteitis fibrosa cystica) 252.01
- Recklinghausen-Applebaum (hemochromatosis) 275.0
- Reclus' (cystic) 610.1
- rectum NEC 569.49
- Refsum's (heredopathia atactica polyneuritiformis) 356.3
- Reichmann's (gastrosuccorrhea) 536.8
- Reimann's (periodic) 277.31

Disease, diseased – *continued*
- Reiter's 099.3
- renal (functional) (pelvis) (*see also* Disease, kidney) 593.9
  - with
    - edema (*see also* Nephrosis) 581.9
    - exudative nephritis 583.89
    - lesion of interstitial nephritis 583.89
    - stated generalized cause - *see* Nephritis
  - acute 593.9
  - basement membrane NEC 583.89
    - with pulmonary hemorrhage (Goodpasture's syndrome) 446.21 *[583.81]*
  - chronic (*see also* Disease, kidney, chronic) 585.9
  - complicating pregnancy or puerperium NEC 646.2 5th
    - with hypertension - *see* Toxemia, of pregnancy
    - affecting fetus or newborn 760.1
  - cystic, congenital (*see also* Cystic, disease, kidney) 753.10
  - diabetic 250.4 5th *[583.81]*
    - due to secondary diabetes 249.4 5th *[583.81]*
  - due to
    - amyloidosis 277.39 *[583.81]*
    - diabetes mellitus 250.4 5th *[583.81]*
      - due to secondary diabetes 249.4 5th *[583.81]*
    - systemic lupus erythematosis 710.0 *[583.81]*
  - end-stage 585.6
  - exudative 583.89
  - fibrocystic (congenital) 753.19
  - gonococcal 098.19 *[583.81]*
  - gouty 274.10
  - hypertensive (*see also* Hypertension, kidney) 403.90
  - immune complex NEC 583.89
  - interstitial (diffuse) (focal) 583.89
  - lupus 710.0 *[583.81]*
  - maternal, affecting fetus or newborn 760.1
    - hypertensive 760.0
  - phosphate-losing (tubular) 588.0
  - polycystic (congenital) 753.12
    - adult type (APKD) 753.13
    - autosomal dominant 753.13
    - autosomal recessive 753.14
    - childhood type (CPKD) 753.14
    - infantile type 753.14
  - specified lesion or cause NEC (*see also* Glomerulonephritis) 583.89
  - subacute 581.9
  - syphilitic 095.4
  - tuberculous (*see also* Tuberculosis) 016.0 5th *[583.81]*
  - tubular (*see also* Nephrosis, tubular) 584.5
- Rendu-Osler-Weber (familial hemorrhagic telangiectasia) 448.0
- renovascular (arteriosclerotic) (*see also* Hypertension, kidney) 403.90
- respiratory (tract) 519.9
  - acute or subacute (upper) NEC 465.9
    - due to fumes or vapors 506.3
    - multiple sites NEC 465.8
    - noninfectious 478.9
    - streptococcal 034.0
  - chronic 519.9
    - arising in the perinatal period 770.7
    - due to fumes or vapors 506.4
  - due to
    - aspiration of liquids or solids 508.9
    - external agents NEC 508.9
      - specified NEC 508.8
    - fumes or vapors 506.9
      - acute or subacute NEC 506.3
      - chronic 506.4
  - fetus or newborn NEC 770.9
  - obstructive 496

Disease, diseased – *continued*
Urbach-Oppenheim (necrobiosis lipoidica diabeticorum) 250.8 5th *[709.3]*
due to secondary diabetes 249.8 5th *[709.3]*
Urbach-Wiethe (lipoid proteinosis) 272.8
ureter 593.9
urethra 599.9
specified type NEC 599.84
urinary (tract) 599.9
bladder 596.9
specified NEC 596.8
maternal, affecting fetus or newborn 760.1
Usher-Senear (pemphigus erythematosus) 694.4
uterus (organic) 621.9
infective (*see also* Endometritis) 615.9
inflammatory (*see also* Endometritis) 615.9
noninflammatory 621.9
specified type NEC 621.8
uveal tract
anterior 364.9
posterior 363.9
vagabonds' 132.1
vagina, vaginal
inflammatory 616.10
noninflammatory 623.9
specified NEC 623.8
Valsuani's (progressive pernicious anemia, puerperal) 648.2 5th
complicating pregnancy or puerperium 648.2 5th
valve, valvular - *see also* Endocarditis
congenital NEC (*see also* Anomaly, heart, valve) 746.9
pulmonary 746.00
specified type NEC 746.89
van Bogaert-Nijssen (-Peiffer) 330.0
van Creveld-von Gierke (glycogenosis I) 271.0
van den Bergh's (enterogenous cyanosis) 289.7
van Neck's (juvenile osteochondrosis) 732.1
Vaquez (-Osler) (polycythemia vera) (M9950/1) 238.4
vascular 459.9
arteriosclerotic - *see* Arteriosclerosis
hypertensive - *see* Hypertension
obliterative 447.1
peripheral 443.9
occlusive 459.9
peripheral (occlusive) 443.9
in (due to) (with) diabetes mellitus 250.7 5th *[443.81]* ▲
in (due to) (with) secondary diabetes 249.7 5th *[443.81]* ▲
specified type NEC 443.89
vas deferens 608.9
vasomotor 443.9
vasospastic 443.9
vein 459.9
venereal 099.9
chlamydial NEC 099.50
anus 099.52
bladder 099.53
cervix 099.53
epididymis 099.54
genitourinary NEC 099.55
lower 099.53
specified NEC 099.54
pelvic inflammatory disease 099.54
perihepatic 099.56
peritoneum 099.56
pharynx 099.51
rectum 099.52
specified site NEC 099.59
testis 099.54
vagina 099.53
vulva 099.53

Disease, diseased – *continued*
venereal – *continued*
complicating pregnancy, childbirth, or puerperium 647.2 5th
fifth 099.1
sixth 099.1
specified nature or type NEC 099.8
chlamydial - *see* Disease, venereal, chlamydial
Verneuil's (syphilitic bursitis) 095.7
Verse's (calcinosis intervertebralis) 275.49 *[722.90]*
vertebra, vertebral NEC 733.90
disc - *see* Disease, Intervertebral disc
vibration NEC 994.9
Vidal's (lichen simplex chronicus) 698.3
Vincent's (trench mouth) 101
Virchow's 733.99
virus (filterable) NEC 078.89
arbovirus NEC 066.9
arthropod-borne NEC 066.9
central nervous system NEC 049.9
specified type NEC 049.8
complicating pregnancy, childbirth, or puerperium 647.6 5th
contact (with) V01.79
varicella V01.71
exposure to V01.79
varicella V01.71
Marburg 078.89
maternal
with fetal damage affecting management of pregnancy 655.3 5th
nonarthropod-borne NEC 078.89
central nervous system NEC 049.9
specified NEC 049.8
vaccination, prophylactic (against) V04.89
vitreous 379.29
vocal cords NEC 478.5
Vogt's (Cecile) 333.71
Vogt-Spielmeyer 330.1
Volhard-Fahr (malignant nephrosclerosis) 403.00
Volkmann's
acquired 958.6
von Bechterew's (ankylosing spondylitis) 720.0
von Economo's (encephalitis lethargica) 049.8
von Eulenburg's (congenital paramyotonia) 359.29
von Gierke's (glycogenosis I) 271.0
von Graefe's 378.72
von Hippel's (retinocerebral angiomatosis) 759.6
von Hippel-Lindau (angiomatosis retinocerebellosa) 759.6
von Jaksch's (pseudoleukemia infantum) 285.8
von Recklinghausen's (M9540/1) 237.71
bone (osteitis fibrosa cystica) 252.01
von Recklinghausen-Applebaum (hemochromatosis) 275.0
von Willebrand (-Jürgens) (angiohemophilia) 286.4
von Zambusch's (lichen sclerosus et atrophicus) 701.0
Voorhoeve's (dyschondroplasia) 756.4
Vrolik's (osteogenesis imperfecta) 756.51
vulva
inflammatory 616.10
noninflammatory 624.9
specified NEC 624.8
Wagner's (colloid milium) 709.3
Waldenström's (osteochondrosis capital femoral) 732.1
Wallgren's (obstruction of splenic vein with collateral circulation) 459.89
Wardrop's (with lymphangitis) 681.9
finger 681.02
toe 681.11
Wassilieff's (leptospiral jaundice) 100.0

Disease, diseased – *continued*
wasting NEC 799.4
due to malnutrition 261
paralysis 335.21
Waterhouse-Friderichsen 036.3
waxy (any site) 277.39
Weber-Christian (nodular nonsuppurative panniculitis) 729.30
Wegner's (syphilitic osteochondritis) 090.0
Weil's (leptospiral jaundice) 100.0
of lung 100.0
Weir Mitchell's (erythromelalgia) 443.82
Werdnig-Hoffmann 335.0
Werlhof's (*see also* Purpura, thrombocytopenic) 287.39
Wermer's 258.01
Werner's (progeria adultorum) 259.8
Werner-His (trench fever) 083.1
Werner-Schultz (agranulocytosis) 288.09
Wernicke's (superior hemorrhagic polioencephalitis) 265.1
Wernicke-Posadas 114.9
Whipple's (intestinal lipodystrophy) 040.2
whipworm 127.3
white
blood cell 288.9
specified NEC 288.8
spot 701.0
White's (congenital) (keratosis follicularis) 757.39
Whitmore's (melioidosis) 025
Widal-Abrami (acquired hemolytic jaundice) 283.9
Wilkie's 557.1
Wilkinson-Sneddon (subcorneal pustular dermatosis) 694.1
Willis' (diabetes mellitus) (*see also* Diabetes) 250.0 5th
due to secondary diabetes 249.0 5th
Wilson's (hepatolenticular degeneration) 275.1
Wilson-Brocq (dermatitis exfoliativa) 695.89
winter vomiting 078.82
Wise's 696.2
Wohlfart-Kugelberg-Welander 335.11
Woillez's (acute idiopathic pulmonary congestion) 518.5
Wolman's (primary familial xanthomatosis) 272.7
wool-sorters' 022.1
Zagari's (xerostomia) 527.7
Zahorsky's (exanthem subitum) 058.10
Ziehen-Oppenheim 333.6
zoonotic, bacterial NEC 027.9
specified type NEC 027.8
Disfigurement (due to scar) 709.2
head V48.6
limb V49.4
neck V48.7
trunk V48.7
Disgerminoma - *see* Dysgerminoma
Disinsertion, retina 361.04
Disintegration, complete, of the body 799.89
traumatic 869.1
Disk kidney 753.3
Dislocatable hip, congenital (*see also* Dislocation, hip, congenital) 754.30

Dislocation (articulation) (closed) (displacement) (simple) (subluxation) 839.8

Note *"Closed" includes simple, complete, partial, uncomplicated, and unspecified dislocation.*

"Open" includes dislocation specified as infected or compound and dislocation with foreign body.

"Chronic," "habitual," "old," or "recurrent" dislocations should be coded as indicated under the entry "Dislocation, recurrent"; and "pathological" as indicated under the entry "Dislocation, pathological."

For late effect of dislocation see Late, effect, dislocation.

with fracture - *see* Fracture, by site
acromioclavicular (joint) (closed) 831.04
open 831.14
anatomical site (closed)
specified NEC 839.69
open 839.79
unspecified or ill-defined 839.8
open 839.9
ankle (scaphoid bone) (closed) 837.0
open 837.1
arm (closed) 839.8
open 839.9
astragalus (closed) 837.0
open 837.1
atlanto-axial (closed) 839.01
open 839.11
atlas (closed) 839.01
open 839.11
axis (closed) 839.02
open 839.12
back (closed) 839.8
open 839.9
Bell-Daly 723.8
breast bone (closed) 839.61
open 839.71
capsule, joint - *see* Dislocation, by site
carpal (bone) - *see* Dislocation, wrist
carpometacarpal (joint) (closed) 833.04
open 833.14
cartilage (joint) - *see also* Dislocation, by site
knee - *see* Tear, meniscus
cervical, cervicodorsal, or cervicothoracic (spine) (vertebra) - *see* Dislocation, vertebra, cervical
chiropractic (*see also* Lesion, nonallopathic) 739.9
chondrocostal - *see* Dislocation, costochondral
chronic - *see* Dislocation, recurrent
clavicle (closed) 831.04
open 831.14
coccyx (closed) 839.41
open 839.51
collar bone (closed) 831.04
open 831.14
compound (open) NEC 839.9
congenital NEC 755.8
hip (*see also* Dislocation, hip, congenital) 754.30
lens 743.37
rib 756.3
sacroiliac 755.69
spine NEC 756.19
vertebra 756.19
coracoid (closed) 831.09
open 831.19
costal cartilage (closed) 839.69
open 839.79
costochondral (closed) 839.69
open 839.79
cricoarytenoid articulation (closed) 839.69
open 839.79

Disease, diseased – Dislocation

Dislocation – *continued*
- cricothyroid (cartilage) articulation (closed) 839.69
  - open 839.79
- dorsal vertebrae (closed) 839.21
  - open 839.31
- ear ossicle 385.23
- elbow (closed) 832.00
  - anterior (closed) 832.01
    - open 832.11
  - congenital 754.89
  - divergent (closed) 832.09
    - open 832.19
  - lateral (closed) 832.04
    - open 832.14
  - medial (closed) 832.03
    - open 832.13
  - open 832.10
  - posterior (closed) 832.02
    - open 832.12
  - recurrent 718.32
  - specified type NEC 832.09
    - open 832.19
- eye 360.81
  - lateral 376.36
- eyeball 360.81
  - lateral 376.36
- femur
  - distal end (closed) 836.50
    - anterior 836.52
      - open 836.62
    - lateral 836.54 ▲
      - open 836.64 ▲
    - medial 836.53 ▲
      - open 836.63 ▲
    - open 836.60
    - posterior 836.51
      - open 836.61
  - proximal end (closed) 835.00
    - anterior (pubic) 835.03
      - open 835.13
    - obturator 835.02
      - open 835.12
    - open 835.10
    - posterior 835.01
      - open 835.11
- fibula
  - distal end (closed) 837.0
    - open 837.1
  - proximal end (closed) 836.59
    - open 836.69
- finger(s) (phalanx) (thumb) (closed) 834.00
  - interphalangeal (joint) 834.02
    - open 834.12
  - metacarpal (bone), distal end 834.01
    - open 834.11
  - metacarpophalangeal (joint) 834.01
    - open 834.11
  - open 834.10
  - recurrent 718.34
- foot (closed) 838.00
  - open 838.10
  - recurrent 718.37
- forearm (closed) 839.8
  - open 839.9
- fracture - *see* Fracture, by site
- glenoid (closed) 831.09
  - open 831.19
- habitual - *see* Dislocation, recurrent
- hand (closed) 839.8
  - open 839.9
- hip (closed) 835.00
  - anterior 835.03
    - obturator 835.02
      - open 835.12
    - open 835.13
  - congenital (unilateral) 754.30
    - with subluxation of other hip 754.35
    - bilateral 754.31
  - developmental 718.75
  - open 835.10

Dislocation – *continued*
- hip (closed) – *continued*
  - posterior 835.01
    - open 835.11
  - recurrent 718.35
- humerus (closed) 831.00
  - distal end (*see also* Dislocation, elbow) 832.00
  - open 831.10
  - proximal end (closed) 831.00
    - anterior (subclavicular) (subcoracoid) (subglenoid) (closed) 831.01
      - open 831.11
    - inferior (closed) 831.03
      - open 831.13
    - open 831.10
    - posterior (closed) 831.02
      - open 831.12
- implant - *see* Complications, mechanical
- incus 385.23
- infracoracoid (closed) 831.01
  - open 831.11
- innominate (pubic junction) (sacral junction) (closed) 839.69
  - acetabulum (*see also* Dislocation, hip) 835.00
  - open 839.79
- interphalangeal (joint)
  - finger or hand (closed) 834.02
    - open 834.12
  - foot or toe (closed) 838.06
    - open 838.16
- jaw (cartilage) (meniscus) (closed) 830.0
  - open 830.1
  - recurrent 524.69
- joint NEC (closed) 839.8
  - developmental 718.7 5th
  - open 839.9
  - pathological - *see* Dislocation, pathological
  - recurrent - *see* Dislocation, recurrent
- knee (closed) 836.50
  - anterior 836.51
    - open 836.61
  - congenital (with genu recurvatum) 754.41
  - habitual 718.36
  - lateral 836.54
    - open 836.64
  - medial 836.53
    - open 836.63
  - old 718.36
  - open 836.60
  - posterior 836.52
    - open 836.62
  - recurrent 718.36
  - rotatory 836.59
    - open 836.69
- lacrimal gland 375.16
- leg (closed) 839.8
  - open 839.9
- lens (crystalline) (complete) (partial) 379.32
  - anterior 379.33
  - congenital 743.37
  - ocular implant 996.53
  - posterior 379.34
  - traumatic 921.3
- ligament - *see* Dislocation, by site
- lumbar (vertebrae) (closed) 839.20
  - open 839.30
- lumbosacral (vertebrae) (closed) 839.20
  - congenital 756.19
  - open 839.30
- mandible (closed) 830.0
  - open 830.1
- maxilla (inferior) (closed) 830.0
  - open 830.1
- meniscus (knee) - *see also* Tear, meniscus
  - other sites - *see* Dislocation, by site
- metacarpal (bone)
  - distal end (closed) 834.01
    - open 834.11

Dislocation – *continued*
- metacarpal (bone) – *continued*
  - proximal end (closed) 833.05
    - open 833.15
- metacarpophalangeal (joint) (closed) 834.01
  - open 834.11
- metatarsal (bone) (closed) 838.04
  - open 838.14
- metatarsophalangeal (joint) (closed) 838.05
  - open 838.15
- midcarpal (joint) (closed) 833.03
  - open 833.13
- midtarsal (joint) (closed) 838.02
  - open 838.12
- Monteggia's - *see* Dislocation, hip
- multiple locations (except fingers only or toes only) (closed) 839.8
  - open 839.9
- navicular (bone) foot (closed) 837.0
  - open 837.1
- neck (*see also* Dislocation, vertebra, cervical) 839.00
- Nélaton's - *see* Dislocation, ankle
- nontraumatic (joint) - *see* Dislocation, pathological
- nose (closed) 839.69
  - open 839.79
- not recurrent, not current injury - *see* Dislocation, pathological
- occiput from atlas (closed) 839.01
  - open 839.11
- old - *see* Dislocation, recurrent
- open (compound) NEC 839.9
- ossicle, ear 385.23
- paralytic (flaccid) (spastic) - *see* Dislocation, pathological
- patella (closed) 836.3
  - congenital 755.64
  - open 836.4
- pathological NEC 718.20
  - ankle 718.27
  - elbow 718.22
  - foot 718.27
  - hand 718.24
  - hip 718.25
  - knee 718.26
  - lumbosacral joint 724.6
  - multiple sites 718.29
  - pelvic region 718.25
  - sacroiliac 724.6
  - shoulder (region) 718.21
  - specified site NEC 718.28
  - spine 724.8
    - sacroiliac 724.6
  - wrist 718.23
- pelvis (closed) 839.69
  - acetabulum (*see also* Dislocation, hip) 835.00
  - open 839.79
- phalanx
  - foot or toe (closed) 838.09
    - open 838.19
  - hand or finger (*see also* Dislocation, finger) 834.00
- postpoliomyelitic - *see* Dislocation, pathological
- prosthesis, internal - *see* Complications, mechanical
- radiocarpal (joint) (closed) 833.02
  - open 833.12
- radioulnar (joint)
  - distal end (closed) 833.01
    - open 833.11
  - proximal end (*see also* Dislocation, elbow) 832.00
- radius
  - distal end (closed) 833.00
    - open 833.10
  - proximal end (closed) 832.01
    - open 832.11

Dislocation – *continued*
- recurrent (*see also* Derangement, joint, recurrent) 718.3 5th
  - elbow 718.32
  - hip 718.35
  - joint NEC 718.38
  - knee 718.36
  - lumbosacral (joint) 724.6
  - patella 718.36
  - sacroiliac 724.6
  - shoulder 718.31
  - temporomandibular 524.69
- rib (cartilage) (closed) 839.69
  - congenital 756.3
  - open 839.79
- sacrococcygeal (closed) 839.42
  - open 839.52
- sacroiliac (joint) (ligament) (closed) 839.42
  - congenital 755.69
  - open 839.52
  - recurrent 724.6
- sacrum (closed) 839.42
  - open 839.52
- scaphoid (bone)
  - ankle or foot (closed) 837.0
    - open 837.1
  - wrist (closed) (*see also* Dislocation, wrist) 833.00
    - open 833.10
- scapula (closed) 831.09
  - open 831.19
- semilunar cartilage, knee - *see* Tear, meniscus
- septal cartilage (nose) (closed) 839.69
  - open 839.79
- septum (nasal) (old) 470
- sesamoid bone - *see* Dislocation, by site
- shoulder (blade) (ligament) (closed) 831.00
  - anterior (subclavicular) (subcoracoid) (subglenoid) (closed) 831.01
    - open 831.11
  - chronic 718.31
  - inferior 831.03
    - open 831.13
  - open 831.10
  - posterior (closed) 831.02
    - open 831.12
  - recurrent 718.31
- skull - *see* Injury, intracranial
- Smith's - *see* Dislocation, foot
- spine (articular process) (*see also* Dislocation, vertebra) (closed) 839.40
  - atlanto-axial (closed) 839.01
    - open 839.11
    - recurrent 723.8
  - cervical, cervicodorsal, cervicothoracic (closed) (*see also* Dislocation, vertebrae, cervical) 839.00
    - open 839.10
    - recurrent 723.8
  - coccyx 839.41
    - open 839.51
  - congenital 756.19
  - due to birth trauma 767.4
  - open 839.50
  - recurrent 724.9
  - sacroiliac 839.42
    - recurrent 724.6
  - sacrum (sacrococcygeal) (sacroiliac) 839.42
    - open 839.52
- spontaneous - *see* Dislocation, pathological
- sternoclavicular (joint) (closed) 839.61
  - open 839.71
- sternum (closed) 839.61
  - open 839.71
- subastragalar - *see* Dislocation, foot
- subglenoid (closed) 831.01
  - open 831.11

Dislocation

Dislocation – *continued*
- symphysis
  - jaw (closed) 830.0
    - open 830.1
  - mandibular (closed) 830.0
    - open 830.1
  - pubis (closed) 839.69
    - open 839.79
- tarsal (bone) (joint) 838.01
  - open 838.11
- tarsometatarsal (joint) 838.03
  - open 838.13
- temporomandibular (joint) (closed) 830.0
  - open 830.1
  - recurrent 524.69
- thigh
  - distal end (*see also* Dislocation, femur, distal end) 836.50
  - proximal end (*see also* Dislocation, hip) 835.00
- thoracic (vertebrae) (closed) 839.21
  - open 839.31
- thumb(s) (*see also* Dislocation, finger) 834.00
- thyroid cartilage (closed) 839.69
  - open 839.79
- tibia
  - distal end (closed) 837.0
    - open 837.1
  - proximal end (closed) 836.50
    - anterior 836.51
      - open 836.61
    - lateral 836.54
      - open 836.64
    - medial 836.53
      - open 836.63
    - open 836.60
    - posterior 836.52
      - open 836.62
    - rotatory 836.59
      - open 836.69
- tibiofibular
  - distal (closed) 837.0
    - open 837.1
  - superior (closed) 836.59
    - open 836.69
- toe(s) (closed) 838.09
  - open 838.19
- trachea (closed) 839.69
  - open 839.79
- ulna
  - distal end (closed) 833.09
    - open 833.19
  - proximal end - *see* Dislocation, elbow
- vertebra (articular process) (body) (closed) (traumatic) 839.40
  - cervical, cervicodorsal or cervicothoracic (closed) 839.00
    - first (atlas) 839.01
      - open 839.11
    - second (axis) 839.02
      - open 839.12
    - third 839.03
      - open 839.13
    - fourth 839.04
      - open 839.14
    - fifth 839.05
      - open 839.15
    - sixth 839.06
      - open 839.16
    - seventh 839.07
      - open 839.17
    - congenital 756.19
    - multiple sites 839.08
      - open 839.18
    - open 839.10
  - congenital 756.19
  - dorsal 839.21
    - open 839.31
    - recurrent 724.9
  - lumbar, lumbosacral 839.20
    - open 839.30
  - non-traumatic - *see* Displacement, intervertebral disc

Dislocation – *continued*
- vertebra – *continued*
  - open NEC 839.50
  - recurrent 724.9
  - specified region NEC 839.49
    - open 839.59
  - thoracic 839.21
    - open 839.31
- wrist (carpal bone) (scaphoid) (semilunar) (closed) 833.00
  - carpometacarpal (joint) 833.04
    - open 833.14
  - metacarpal bone, proximal end 833.05
    - open 833.15
  - midcarpal (joint) 833.03
    - open 833.13
  - open 833.10
  - radiocarpal (joint) 833.02
    - open 833.12
  - radioulnar (joint) 833.01
    - open 833.11
  - recurrent 718.33
  - specified site NEC 833.09
    - open 833.19
- xiphoid cartilage (closed) 839.61
  - open 839.71

Dislodgement
- artificial skin graft 996.55
- decellularized allodermis graft 996.55

Disobedience, hostile (covert) (overt) (*see also* Disturbance, conduct) 312.0 5th

Disorder - *see also* Disease
- academic underachievement, childhood and adolescence 313.83
- accommodation 367.51
  - drug-induced 367.89
  - toxic 367.89
- adjustment (*see also* Reaction, adjustment) 309.9
  - with
    - anxiety 309.24
    - anxiety and depressed mood 309.28
    - depressed mood 309.0
    - disturbance of conduct 309.3
    - disturbance of emotions and conduct 309.4
- adrenal (capsule) (cortex) (gland) 255.9
  - specified type NEC 255.8
- adrenogenital 255.2
- affective (*see also* Psychosis, affective) 296.90
  - atypical 296.81
- aggressive, unsocialized (*see also* Disturbance, conduct) 312.0 5th
- alcohol, alcoholic (*see also* Alcohol) 291.9
- allergic - *see* Allergy
- amino acid (metabolic) (*see also* Disturbance, metabolism, amino acid) 270.9
  - albinism 270.2
  - alkaptonuria 270.2
  - argininosuccinicaciduria 270.6
  - beta-amino-isobutyricaciduria 277.2
  - cystathioninuria 270.4
  - cystinosis 270.0
  - cystinuria 270.0
  - glycinuria 270.0
  - homocystinuria 270.4
  - imidazole 270.5
  - maple syrup (urine) disease 270.3
  - neonatal, transitory 775.89
  - oasthouse urine disease 270.2
  - ochronosis 270.2
  - phenylketonuria 270.1
  - phenylpyruvic oligophrenia 270.1
  - purine NEC 277.2
  - pyrimidine NEC 277.2
  - renal transport NEC 270.0
  - specified type NEC 270.8
  - transport NEC 270.0
    - renal 270.0
  - xanthinuria 277.2

Disorder – *continued*
- amnestic (*see also* Amnestic syndrome) 294.8
  - alcohol-induced peristing 291.1
  - drug-induced persisting 292.83
  - in conditions classified elsewhere 294.0
- anaerobic glycolysis with anemia 282.3
- anxiety (*see also* Anxiety) 300.00
  - due to or associated with physical condition 293.84
- arteriole 447.9
  - specified type NEC 447.8
- artery 447.9
  - specified type NEC 447.8
- articulation - *see* Disorder, joint
- Asperger's 299.8 5th
- attachment of infancy or early childhood 313.89
- attention deficit 314.00
  - with hyperactivity 314.01
  - predominantly
    - combined hyperactive/inattentive 314.01
    - hyperactive/impulsive 314.01
    - inattentive 314.00
  - residual type 314.8
- auditory processing disorder 388.45
  - acquired 388.45
  - developmental 315.32
- autistic 299.0 5th
- autoimmune NEC 279.49 ▲
  - hemolytic (cold type) (warm type) 283.0
  - parathyroid 252.1
  - thyroid 245.2
- avoidant, childhood or adolescence 313.21
- balance
  - acid-base 276.9
    - mixed (with hypercapnia) 276.4
  - electrolyte 276.9
  - fluid 276.9
- behavior NEC (*see also* Disturbance, conduct) 312.9
  - disruptive 312.9
- bilirubin excretion 277.4
- bipolar (affective) (alternating) 296.80

Note *Use the following fifth-digit subclassification with categories 296.0-296.6:*

0	unspecified
1	mild
2	moderate
3	severe, without mention of psychotic behavior
4	severe, specified as with psychotic behavior
5	in partial or unspecified remission
6	in full remission

  - atypical 296.7
  - specified type NEC 296.89
  - type I 296.7
    - most recent episode (or current)
      - depressed 296.5 5th
      - hypomanic 296.4 5th
      - manic 296.4 5th
      - mixed 296.6 5th
      - unspecified 296.7
    - single manic episode 296.0 5th
  - type II (recurrent major depressive episodes with hypomania) 296.89
- bladder 596.9
  - functional NEC 596.59
  - specified NEC 596.8
- bleeding 286.9
- bone NEC 733.90
  - specified NEC 733.99
- brachial plexus 353.0
- branched-chain amino-acid degradation 270.3
- breast 611.9
  - puerperal, postpartum 676.3 5th

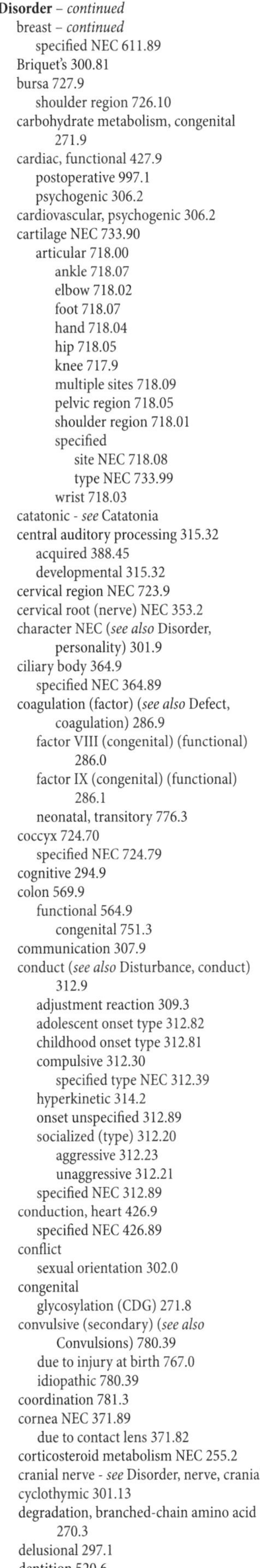

Disorder – *continued*
- breast – *continued*
  - specified NEC 611.89
- Briquet's 300.81
- bursa 727.9
  - shoulder region 726.10
- carbohydrate metabolism, congenital 271.9
- cardiac, functional 427.9
  - postoperative 997.1
  - psychogenic 306.2
- cardiovascular, psychogenic 306.2
- cartilage NEC 733.90
  - articular 718.00
    - ankle 718.07
    - elbow 718.02
    - foot 718.07
    - hand 718.04
    - hip 718.05
    - knee 717.9
    - multiple sites 718.09
    - pelvic region 718.05
    - shoulder region 718.01
    - specified
      - site NEC 718.08
      - type NEC 733.99
    - wrist 718.03
- catatonic - *see* Catatonia
- central auditory processing 315.32
  - acquired 388.45
  - developmental 315.32
- cervical region NEC 723.9
- cervical root (nerve) NEC 353.2
- character NEC (*see also* Disorder, personality) 301.9
- ciliary body 364.9
  - specified NEC 364.89
- coagulation (factor) (*see also* Defect, coagulation) 286.9
  - factor VIII (congenital) (functional) 286.0
  - factor IX (congenital) (functional) 286.1
  - neonatal, transitory 776.3
- coccyx 724.70
  - specified NEC 724.79
- cognitive 294.9
- colon 569.9
  - functional 564.9
    - congenital 751.3
- communication 307.9
- conduct (*see also* Disturbance, conduct) 312.9
  - adjustment reaction 309.3
  - adolescent onset type 312.82
  - childhood onset type 312.81
  - compulsive 312.30
    - specified type NEC 312.39
  - hyperkinetic 314.2
  - onset unspecified 312.89
  - socialized (type) 312.20
    - aggressive 312.23
    - unaggressive 312.21
  - specified NEC 312.89
- conduction, heart 426.9
  - specified NEC 426.89
- conflict
  - sexual orientation 302.0
- congenital
  - glycosylation (CDG) 271.8
- convulsive (secondary) (*see also* Convulsions) 780.39
  - due to injury at birth 767.0
  - idiopathic 780.39
- coordination 781.3
- cornea NEC 371.89
  - due to contact lens 371.82
- corticosteroid metabolism NEC 255.2
- cranial nerve - *see* Disorder, nerve, cranial
- cyclothymic 301.13
- degradation, branched-chain amino acid 270.3
- delusional 297.1
- dentition 520.6

Dislocation – Disorder

Disorder – *continued*
- depersonalization 300.6
- depressive NEC 311
  - atypical 296.82
  - major (*see also* Psychosis, affective) 296.2 [5th]
    - recurrent episode 296.3 [5th]
    - single episode 296.2 [5th]
- development, specific 315.9
  - associated with hyperkinesia 314.1
  - coordination 315.4
  - language 315.31
    - and speech due to hearing loss 315.34
  - learning 315.2
    - arithmetical 315.1
    - reading 315.00
  - mixed 315.5
  - motor coordination 315.4
  - specified type NEC 315.8
  - speech 315.39
    - and language due to hearing loss 315.34
- diaphragm 519.4
- digestive 536.9
  - fetus or newborn 777.9
    - specified NEC 777.8
  - psychogenic 306.4
- disintegrative,childhood 299.1 [5th]
- dissociative 300.15
  - identity 300.14
  - nocturnal 307.47
- drug-related 292.9
- dysmorphic body 300.7
- dysthymic 300.4
- ear 388.9
  - degenerative NEC 388.00
  - external 380.9
    - specified 380.89
  - pinna 380.30
  - specified type NEC 388.8
  - vascular NEC 388.00
- eating NEC 307.50
- electrolyte NEC 276.9
  - with
    - abortion - *see* Abortion, by type, with metabolic disorder
    - ectopic pregnancy (*see also* categories 633.0-633.9) 639.4
    - molar pregnancy (*see also* categories 630-632) 639.4
  - acidosis 276.2
    - metabolic 276.2
    - respiratory 276.2
  - alkalosis 276.3
    - metabolic 276.3
    - respiratory 276.3
  - following
    - abortion 639.4
    - ectopic or molar pregnancy 639.4
  - neonatal, transitory NEC 775.5
- emancipation as adjustment reaction 309.22
- emotional (*see also* Disorder, mental, nonpsychotic) V40.9
- endocrine 259.9
  - specified type NEC 259.8
- esophagus 530.9
  - functional 530.5
  - psychogenic 306.4
- explosive
  - intermittent 312.34
  - isolated 312.35
- expressive language 315.31
- eye 379.90
  - globe - *see* Disorder, globe
  - ill-defined NEC 379.99
  - limited duction NEC 378.63
  - specified NEC 379.8
- eyelid 374.9
  - degenerative 374.50
  - sensory 374.44
  - specified type NEC 374.89
  - vascular 374.85

Disorder – *continued*
- factitious (with combined psychological and physical signs and symptoms) (with predominantly physical signs and symptoms) 300.19
  - with predominantly psychological signs and symptoms 300.16
- factor, coagulation (*see also* Defect, coagulation) 286.9
  - VIII (congenital) (functional) 286.0
  - IX (congenital) (functional) 286.1
- fascia 728.9
- fatty acid oxidation 277.85
- feeding - *see* Feeding
- female sexual arousal 302.72
- fluid NEC 276.9
- gastric (functional) 536.9
  - motility 536.8
  - psychogenic 306.4
  - secretion 536.8
- gastrointestinal (functional) NEC 536.9
  - newborn (neonatal) 777.9
    - specified NEC 777.8
  - psychogenic 306.4
- gender (child) 302.6
  - adult 302.85
- gender identity (childhood) 302.6
  - adolescents 302.85
  - adults (-life) 302.85
- genitourinary system, psychogenic 306.50
- globe 360.9
  - degenerative 360.20
    - specified NEC 360.29
  - specified type NEC 360.89
- hearing - *see also* Deafness
  - conductive type (air) (*see also* Deafness, conductive) 389.00
  - mixed conductive and sensorineural 389.20
    - bilateral 389.22
    - unilateral 389.21
  - nerve
    - bilateral 389.12
    - unilateral 389.13
  - perceptive (*see also* Deafness, perceptive) 389.10
  - sensorineural type NEC (*see also* Deafness, sensorineural) 389.10
- heart action 427.9
  - postoperative 997.1
- hematological, transient neonatal 776.9
  - specified type NEC 776.8
- hematopoietic organs 289.9
- hemorrhagic NEC 287.9
  - due to intrinsic circulating anticoagulants 286.5
  - specified type NEC 287.8
- hemostasis (*see also* Defect, coagulation) 286.9
- homosexual conflict 302.0
- hypomanic (chronic) 301.11
- identity
  - childhood and adolescence 313.82
    - gender 302.6
- immune mechanism (immunity) 279.9
  - single complement (C_1-C_9) 279.8
  - specified type NEC 279.8
- impulse control (*see also* Disturbance, conduct, compulsive) 312.30
- infant sialic acid storage 271.8
- integument, fetus or newborn 778.9
  - specified type NEC 778.8
- interactional psychotic (childhood) (*see also* Psychosis, childhood) 299.1 [5th]
- intermittent explosive 312.34
- intervertebral disc 722.90
  - cervical, cervicothoracic 722.91
  - lumbar, lumbosacral 722.93
  - thoracic, thoracolumbar 722.92
- intestinal 569.9
  - functional NEC 564.9
    - congenital 751.3
    - postoperative 564.4
  - psychogenic 306.4

Disorder – *continued*
- introverted, of childhood and adolescence 313.22
- involuntary emotional expression (IEED) 310.8
- iris 364.9
  - specified NEC 364.89
- iron, metabolism 275.0
- isolated explosive 312.35
- joint NEC 719.90
  - ankle 719.97
  - elbow 719.92
  - foot 719.97
  - hand 719.94
  - hip 719.95
  - knee 719.96
  - multiple sites 719.99
  - pelvic region 719.95
  - psychogenic 306.0
  - shoulder (region) 719.91
  - specified site NEC 719.98
  - temporomandibular 524.60
    - sounds on opening or closing 524.64
    - specified NEC 524.69
  - wrist 719.93
- kidney 593.9
  - functional 588.9
    - specified NEC 588.89
- labyrinth, labyrinthine 386.9
  - specified type NEC 386.8
- lactation 676.9 [5th]
- language (developmental) (expressive) 315.31
  - mixed receptive-expressive 315.32
- learning 315.9
- ligament 728.9
- ligamentous attachments, peripheral - *see also* Enthesopathy
  - spine 720.1
- limb NEC 729.90
  - psychogenic 306.0
- lipid
  - metabolism, congenital 272.9
  - storage 272.7
- lipoprotein deficiency (familial) 272.5
- low back NEC 724.9
  - psychogenic 306.0
- lumbosacral
  - plexus 353.1
  - root (nerve) NEC 353.4
- lymphoproliferative (chronic) NEC (M9970/1) 238.79
  - post-transplant (PTLD) 238.77
- major depressive (*see also* Psychosis, affective) 296.2 [5th]
  - recurrent episode 296.3 [5th]
  - single episode 296.2 [5th]
- male erectile 607.84
  - nonorganic origin 302.72
- manic (*see also* Psychosis, affective) 296.0 [5th]
  - atypical 296.81
- mathematics 315.1
- meniscus NEC (*see also* Disorder, cartilage, articular) 718.0 [5th]
- menopausal 627.9
  - specified NEC 627.8
- menstrual 626.9
  - psychogenic 306.52
  - specified NEC 626.8
- mental (nonpsychotic) 300.9
  - affecting management of pregnancy, childbirth, or puerperium 648.4 [5th]
  - drug-induced 292.9
    - hallucinogen persisting perception 292.89
    - specified type NEC 292.89
  - due to or associated with
    - alcoholism 291.9
    - drug consumption NEC 292.9
      - specified type NEC 292.89
    - physical condition NEC 293.9

Disorder – *continued*
- mental – *continued*
  - induced by drug 292.9
    - specified type NEC 292.89
  - neurotic (*see also* Neurosis) 300.9
  - of infancy, childhood or adolescence 313.9
  - persistent
    - other
      - due to conditions classified elsewhere 294.8
    - unspecified
      - due to conditions classified elsewhere 294.9
  - presenile 310.1
    - psychotic NEC 290.10
  - previous, affecting management of pregnancy V23.89
  - psychoneurotic (*see also* Neurosis) 300.9
  - psychotic (*see also* Psychosis) 298.9
    - brief 298.8
    - senile 290.20
  - specific, following organic brain damage 310.9
    - cognitive or personality change of other type 310.1
    - frontal lobe syndrome 310.0
    - postconcussional syndrome 310.2
    - specified type NEC 310.8
  - transient
    - in conditions classified elsewhere 293.9
- metabolism NEC 277.9
  - with
    - abortion - *see* Abortion, by type, with metabolic disorder
    - ectopic pregnancy (*see also* categories 633.0-633.9) 639.4
    - molar pregnancy (*see also* categories 630-632) 639.4
  - alkaptonuria 270.2
  - amino acid (*see also* Disorder, amino acid) 270.9
    - specified type NEC 270.8
  - ammonia 270.6
  - arginine 270.6
  - argininosuccinic acid 270.6
  - basal 794.7
  - bilirubin 277.4
  - calcium 275.40
  - carbohydrate 271.9
    - specified type NEC 271.8
  - cholesterol 272.9
  - citrulline 270.6
  - copper 275.1
  - corticosteroid 255.2
  - cystine storage 270.0
  - cystinuria 270.0
  - fat 272.9
  - fatty acid oxidation 277.85
  - following
    - abortion 639.4
    - ectopic or molar pregnancy 639.4
  - fructosemia 271.2
  - fructosuria 271.2
  - fucosidosis 271.8
  - galactose-1-phosphate uridyl transferase 271.1
  - glutamine 270.7
  - glycine 270.7
  - glycogen storage NEC 271.0
    - hepatorenal 271.0
  - hemochromatosis 275.0
  - in labor and delivery 669.0 [5th]
  - iron 275.0
  - lactose 271.3
  - lipid 272.9
    - specified type NEC 272.8
    - storage 272.7
  - lipoprotein - *see also* Hyperlipemia
    - deficiency (familial) 272.5
  - lysine 270.7
  - magnesium 275.2

Disorder

- **Disorder** – *continued*
  - metabolism – *continued*
    - mannosidosis 271.8
    - mineral 275.9
      - specified type NEC 275.8
    - mitochondrial 277.87
    - mucopolysaccharide 277.5
    - nitrogen 270.9
    - ornithine 270.6
    - oxalosis 271.8
    - pentosuria 271.8
    - phenylketonuria 270.1
    - phosphate 275.3
    - phosphorus 275.3
    - plasma protein 273.9
      - specified type NEC 273.8
    - porphyrin 277.1
    - purine 277.2
    - pyrimidine 277.2
    - serine 270.7
    - sodium 276.9
    - specified type NEC 277.89
    - steroid 255.2
    - threonine 270.7
    - urea cycle 270.6
    - xylose 271.8
  - micturition NEC 788.69
    - psychogenic 306.53
  - misery and unhappiness, of childhood and adolescence 313.1
  - mitochondrial metabolism 277.87
  - mitral valve 424.0
  - mood- (*see also* Disorder, bipolar) 296.90
    - episodic 296.90
      - specified NEC 296.99
    - in conditions classified elsewhere 293.83
  - motor tic 307.20
    - chronic 307.22
    - transient (childhood) 307.21
  - movement NEC 333.90
    - hysterical 300.11
    - medication-induced 333.90
    - periodic limb 327.51
    - sleep related, unspecified 780.58
      - other organic 327.59
    - specified type NEC 333.99
    - stereotypic 307.3
  - mucopolysaccharide 277.5
  - muscle 728.9
    - psychogenic 306.0
    - specified type NEC 728.3
  - muscular attachments, peripheral - *see also* Enthesopathy
    - spine 720.1
  - musculoskeletal system NEC 729.90
    - psychogenic 306.0
  - myeloproliferative (chronic) NEC (M9960/1) 238.79
  - myoneural 358.9
    - due to lead 358.2
    - specified type NEC 358.8
    - toxic 358.2
  - myotonic 359.29
  - neck region NEC 723.9
  - nerve 349.9
    - abducens NEC 378.54
    - accessory 352.4
    - acoustic 388.5
    - auditory 388.5
    - auriculotemporal 350.8
    - axillary 353.0
    - cerebral - *see* Disorder, nerve, cranial
    - cranial 352.9
      - first 352.0
      - second 377.49
      - third
        - partial 378.51
        - total 378.52
      - fourth 378.53
      - fifth 350.9
      - sixth 378.54
      - seventh NEC 351.9
      - eighth 388.5

- **Disorder** – *continued*
  - nerve – *continued*
    - cranial – *continued*
      - ninth 352.2
      - tenth 352.3
      - eleventh 352.4
      - twelfth 352.5
      - multiple 352.6
    - entrapment - *see* Neuropathy, entrapment
    - facial 351.9
      - specified NEC 351.8
    - femoral 355.2
    - glossopharyngeal NEC 352.2
    - hypoglossal 352.5
    - iliohypogastric 355.79
    - ilioinguinal 355.79
    - intercostal 353.8
    - lateral
      - cutaneous of thigh 355.1
      - popliteal 355.3
    - lower limb NEC 355.8
    - medial, popliteal 355.4
    - median NEC 354.1
    - obturator 355.79
    - oculomotor
      - partial 378.51
      - total 378.52
    - olfactory 352.0
    - optic 377.49
      - hypoplasia 377.43
      - ischemic 377.41
      - nutritional 377.33
      - toxic 377.34
    - peroneal 355.3
    - phrenic 354.8
    - plantar 355.6
    - pneumogastric 352.3
    - posterior tibial 355.5
    - radial 354.3
    - recurrent laryngeal 352.3
    - root 353.9
      - specified NEC 353.8
    - saphenous 355.79
    - sciatic NEC 355.0
    - specified NEC 355.9
      - lower limb 355.79
      - upper limb 354.8
    - spinal 355.9
    - sympathetic NEC 337.9
    - trigeminal 350.9
      - specified NEC 350.8
    - trochlear 378.53
    - ulnar 354.2
    - upper limb NEC 354.9
    - vagus 352.3
  - nervous system NEC 349.9
    - autonomic (peripheral) (*see also* Neuropathy, peripheral, autonomic) 337.9
    - cranial 352.9
    - parasympathetic (*see also* Neuropathy, peripheral, autonomic) 337.9
    - specified type NEC 349.89
    - sympathetic (*see also* Neuropathy, peripheral, autonomic) 337.9
    - vegetative (*see also* Neuropathy, peripheral, autonomic) 337.9
  - neurohypophysis NEC 253.6
  - neurological NEC 781.99
    - peripheral NEC 355.9
  - neuromuscular NEC 358.9
    - hereditary NEC 359.1
    - specified NEC 358.8
    - toxic 358.2
  - neurotic 300.9
    - specified type NEC 300.89
  - neutrophil, polymorphonuclear (functional) 288.1
  - nightmare 307.47
  - night terror 307.46
  - obsessive-compulsive 300.3
  - oppositional defiant, childhood and adolescence 313.81

- **Disorder** – *continued*
  - optic
    - chiasm 377.54
      - associated with
        - inflammatory disorders 377.54
        - neoplasm NEC 377.52
          - pituitary 377.51
        - pituitary disorders 377.51
        - vascular disorders 377.53
    - nerve 377.49
    - radiations 377.63
    - tracts 377.63
  - orbit 376.9
    - specified NEC 376.89
  - orgasmic
    - female 302.73
    - male 302.74
  - overanxious, of childhood and adolescence 313.0
  - oxidation, fatty acid 277.85
  - pancreas, internal secretion (other than diabetes mellitus) 251.9
    - specified type NEC 251.8
  - panic 300.01
    - with agoraphobia 300.21
  - papillary muscle NEC 429.81
  - paranoid 297.9
    - induced 297.3
    - shared 297.3
  - parathyroid 252.9
    - specified type NEC 252.8
  - paroxysmal, mixed 780.39
  - pentose phosphate pathway with anemia 282.2
  - periodic limb movement 327.51
  - peroxisomal 277.86
  - personality 301.9
    - affective 301.10
    - aggressive 301.3
    - amoral 301.7
    - anancastic, anankastic 301.4
    - antisocial 301.7
    - asocial 301.7
    - asthenic 301.6
    - avoidant 301.82
    - borderline 301.83
    - compulsive 301.4
    - cyclothymic 301.13
    - dependent-passive 301.6
    - dyssocial 301.7
    - emotional instability 301.59
    - epileptoid 301.3
    - explosive 301.3
    - following organic brain damage 310.1
    - histrionic 301.50
    - hyperthymic 301.11
    - hypomanic (chronic) 301.11
    - hypothymic 301.12
    - hysterical 301.50
    - immature 301.89
    - inadequate 301.6
    - introverted 301.21
    - labile 301.59
    - moral deficiency 301.7
    - narcissistic 301.81
    - obsessional 301.4
    - obsessive-compulsive 301.4
    - overconscientious 301.4
    - paranoid 301.0
    - passive (-dependent) 301.6
    - passive-aggressive 301.84
    - pathological NEC 301.9
    - pseudosocial 301.7
    - psychopathic 301.9
    - schizoid 301.20
      - introverted 301.21
      - schizotypal 301.22
    - schizotypal 301.22
    - seductive 301.59
    - type A 301.4
    - unstable 301.59
  - pervasive developmental 299.9 [5th]
    - childhood-onset 299.8 [5th]
    - specified NEC 299.8 [5th]

- **Disorder** – *continued*
  - phonological 315.39
  - pigmentation, choroid (congenital) 743.53
  - pinna 380.30
    - specified type NEC 380.39
  - pituitary, thalamic 253.9
    - anterior NEC 253.4
    - iatrogenic 253.7
    - postablative 253.7
    - specified NEC 253.8
  - pityriasis-like NEC 696.8
  - platelets (blood) 287.1
  - polymorphonuclear neutrophils (functional) 288.1
  - porphyrin metabolism 277.1
  - postmenopausal 627.9
    - specified type NEC 627.8
  - post-transplant lymphoproliferative (PTLD) 238.77
  - post-traumatic stress (PTSD) 309.81
  - posttraumatic stress 309.81
    - acute 309.81
    - brief 309.81
    - chronic 309.81
  - premenstrual dysphoric (PMDD) 625.4
  - psoriatic-like NEC 696.8
  - psychic, with diseases classified elsewhere 316
  - psychogenic NEC (*see also* condition) 300.9
    - allergic NEC
      - respiratory 306.1
    - anxiety 300.00
      - atypical 300.00
      - generalized 300.02
    - appetite 307.59
    - articulation, joint 306.0
    - asthenic 300.5
    - blood 306.8
    - cardiovascular (system) 306.2
    - compulsive 300.3
    - cutaneous 306.3
    - depressive 300.4
    - digestive (system) 306.4
    - dysmenorrheic 306.52
    - dyspneic 306.1
    - eczematous 306.3
    - endocrine (system) 306.6
    - eye 306.7
    - feeding 307.59
    - functional NEC 306.9
    - gastric 306.4
    - gastrointestinal (system) 306.4
    - genitourinary (system) 306.50
    - heart (function) (rhythm) 306.2
    - hemic 306.8
    - hyperventilatory 306.1
    - hypochondriacal 300.7
    - hysterical 300.10
    - intestinal 306.4
    - joint 306.0
    - learning 315.2
    - limb 306.0
    - lymphatic (system) 306.8
    - menstrual 306.52
    - micturition 306.53
    - monoplegic NEC 306.0
    - motor 307.9
    - muscle 306.0
    - musculoskeletal 306.0
    - neurocirculatory 306.2
    - obsessive 300.3
    - occupational 300.89
    - organ or part of body NEC 306.9
    - organs of special sense 306.7
    - paralytic NEC 306.0
    - phobic 300.20
    - physical NEC 306.9
    - pruritic 306.3
    - rectal 306.4
    - respiratory (system) 306.1
    - rheumatic 306.0
    - sexual (function) 302.70
      - specified type NEC 302.79

- **Disorder** – *continued*
  - psychogenic – *continued*
    - sexual orientation conflict 302.0
    - skin (allergic) (eczematous) (pruritic) 306.3
    - sleep 307.40
      - initiation or maintenance 307.41
        - persistent 307.42
        - transient 307.41
      - movement 780.58
      - specified type NEC 307.49
      - sleep terror 307.46
    - specified part of body NEC 306.8
    - stomach 306.4
  - psychomotor NEC 307.9
    - hysterical 300.11
  - psychoneurotic (*see also* Neurosis) 300.9
    - mixed NEC 300.89
  - psychophysiologic (*see also* Disorder, psychosomatic) 306.9
  - psychosexual identity (childhood) 302.6
    - adult-life 302.85
  - psychosomatic NEC 306.9
    - allergic NEC
      - respiratory 306.1
    - articulation, joint 306.0
    - cardiovascular (system) 306.2
    - cutaneous 306.3
    - digestive (system) 306.4
    - dysmenorrheic 306.52
    - dyspneic 306.1
    - endocrine (system) 306.6
    - eye 306.7
    - gastric 306.4
    - gastrointestinal (system) 306.4
    - genitourinary (system) 306.50
    - heart (functional) (rhythm) 306.2
    - hyperventilatory 306.1
    - intestinal 306.4
    - joint 306.0
    - limb 306.0
    - lymphatic (system) 306.8
    - menstrual 306.52
    - micturition 306.53
    - monoplegic NEC 306.0
    - muscle 306.0
    - musculoskeletal 306.0
    - neurocirculatory 306.2
    - organs of special sense 306.7
    - paralytic NEC 306.0
    - pruritic 306.3
    - rectal 306.4
    - respiratory (system) 306.1
    - rheumatic 306.0
    - sexual (function) 302.70
      - specified type NEC 302.79
    - skin 306.3
    - specified part of body NEC 306.8
    - stomach 306.4
  - psychotic (*see also* Psychosis) 298.9
    - brief 298.8
  - purine metabolism NEC 277.2
  - pyrimidine metabolism NEC 277.2
  - reactive attachment of infancy or early childhood 313.89
  - reading, developmental 315.00
  - reflex 796.1
  - REM sleep behavior 327.42
  - renal function, impaired 588.9
    - specified type NEC 588.89
  - renal transport NEC 588.89
  - respiration, respiratory NEC 519.9
    - due to
      - aspiration of liquids or solids 508.9
      - inhalation of fumes or vapors 506.9
    - psychogenic 306.1
  - retina 362.9
    - specified type NEC 362.89
  - rumination 307.53
  - sacroiliac joint NEC 724.6
  - sacrum 724.6
  - schizo-affective (*see also* Schizophrenia) 295.7 [5th]
  - schizoid, childhood or adolescence 313.22

- **Disorder** – *continued*
  - schizophreniform 295.4 [5th]
  - schizotypal personality 301.22
  - secretion, thyrocalcitonin 246.0
  - seizure 345.9 [5th]
    - recurrent 345.9 [5th]
      - epileptic - *see* Epilepsy
  - semantic pragmatic 315.39
    - with autism 299.0 [5th]
  - sense of smell 781.1
    - psychogenic 306.7
  - separation anxiety 309.21
  - sexual (*see also* Deviation, sexual) 302.9
    - aversion 302.79
    - desire, hypoactive 302.71
    - function, psychogenic 302.70
  - shyness, of childhood and adolescence 313.21
  - single complement (C_1-C_9) 279.8
  - skin NEC 709.9
    - fetus or newborn 778.9
      - specified type 778.8
    - psychogenic (allergic) (eczematous) (pruritic) 306.3
    - specified type NEC 709.8
    - vascular 709.1
  - sleep 780.50
    - with apnea - *see* Apnea, sleep
    - alcohol induced 291.82
    - arousal 307.46
      - confusional 327.41
    - circadian rhythm 327.30
      - advanced sleep phase type 327.32
      - alcohol induced 291.82
      - delayed sleep phase type 327.31
      - drug induced 292.85
      - free running type 327.34
      - in conditions classified elsewhere 327.37
      - irregular sleep-wake type 327.33
      - jet lag type 327.35
      - other 327.39
      - shift work type 327.36
    - drug induced 292.85
    - initiation or maintenance (*see also* Insomnia) 780.52
      - nonorganic origin (transient) 307.41
        - persistent 307.42
    - nonorganic origin 307.40
      - specified type NEC 307.49
    - organic specified type NEC 327.8
    - periodic limb movement 327.51
    - specified NEC 780.59
    - wake
      - cycle - *see* Disorder, sleep, circadian rhythm
      - schedule - *see* Disorder, sleep, circadian rhythm
  - social, of childhood and adolescence 313.22
  - soft tissue 729.90
    - specified type NEC 729.99
  - somatization 300.81
  - somatoform (atypical) (undifferentiated) 300.82
    - severe 300.81
    - specified type NEC 300.89
  - speech NEC 784.59 ▲
    - nonorganic origin 307.9
  - spine NEC 724.9
    - ligamentous or muscular attachments, peripheral 720.1
  - steroid metabolism NEC 255.2
  - stomach (functional) (*see also* Disorder, gastric) 536.9
    - psychogenic 306.4
  - storage, iron 275.0
  - stress (*see also* Reaction, stress, acute) 308.3
    - posttraumatic
      - acute 309.81
      - brief 309.81
      - chronic (motor or vocal) 309.81

- **Disorder** – *continued*
  - substitution 300.11
  - suspected - *see* Observation
  - synovium 727.9
  - temperature regulation, fetus or newborn 778.4
  - temporomandibular joint NEC 524.60
    - sounds on opening or closing 524.64
    - specified NEC 524.69
  - tendon 727.9
    - shoulder region 726.10
  - thoracic root (nerve) NEC 353.3
  - thyrocalcitonin secretion 246.0
  - thyroid (gland) NEC 246.9
    - specified type NEC 246.8
  - tic 307.20
    - chronic (motor or vocal) 307.22
    - motor-verbal 307.23
    - organic origin 333.1
    - transient (of childhood) 307.21
  - tooth NEC 525.9
    - development NEC 520.9
      - specified type NEC 520.8
    - eruption 520.6
    - specified type NEC 525.8
  - Tourette's 307.23
  - transport, carbohydrate 271.9
    - specified type NEC 271.8
  - tubular, phosphate-losing 588.0
  - tympanic membrane 384.9
  - unaggressive, unsocialized (*see also* Disturbance, conduct) 312.1 [5th]
  - undersocialized, unsocialized (*see also* Disturbance, conduct)
    - aggressive (type) 312.0 [5th]
    - unaggressive (type) 312.1 [5th]
  - vision, visual NEC 368.9
    - binocular NEC 368.30
    - cortex 377.73
      - associated with
        - inflammatory disorders 377.73
        - neoplasms 377.71
        - vascular disorders 377.72
    - pathway NEC 377.63
      - associated with
        - inflammatory disorders 377.63
        - neoplasms 377.61
        - vascular disorders 377.62
  - vocal tic
    - chronic 307.22
  - wakefulness (*see also* Hypersomnia) 780.54
    - nonorganic origin (transient) 307.43
      - persistent 307.44
  - written expression 315.2
- **Disorganized globe** 360.29
- **Displacement, displaced**

Note *For acquired displacement of bones, cartilage, joints, tendons, due to injury, see also Dislocation.*

Displacements at ages under one year should be considered congenital, provided there is no indication the condition was acquired after birth.

  - acquired traumatic of bone, cartilage, joint, tendon NEC (without fracture) (*see also* Dislocation) 839.8
    - with fracture - *see* Fracture, by site
  - adrenal gland (congenital) 759.1
  - alveolus and teeth, vertical 524.75
  - appendix, retrocecal (congenital) 751.5
  - auricle (congenital) 744.29
  - bladder (acquired) 596.8
    - congenital 753.8
  - brachial plexus (congenital) 742.8
  - brain stem, caudal 742.4
  - canaliculus lacrimalis 743.65
  - cardia, through esophageal hiatus 750.6
  - cerebellum, caudal 742.4
  - cervix - *see* Displacement, uterus
  - colon (congenital) 751.4

- **Displacement, displaced** – *continued*
  - device, implant, or graft - *see* Complications, mechanical
  - epithelium
    - columnar of cervix 622.10
    - cuboidal, beyond limits of external os (uterus) 752.49
  - esophageal mucosa into cardia of stomach, congenital 750.4
  - esophagus (acquired) 530.89
    - congenital 750.4
  - eyeball (acquired) (old) 376.36
    - congenital 743.8
    - current injury 871.3
    - lateral 376.36
  - fallopian tube (acquired) 620.4
    - congenital 752.19
    - opening (congenital) 752.19
  - gallbladder (congenital) 751.69
  - gastric mucosa 750.7
    - into
      - duodenum 750.7
      - esophagus 750.7
      - Meckel's diverticulum, congenital 750.7
  - globe (acquired) (lateral) (old) 376.36
    - current injury 871.3
  - graft
    - artificial skin graft 996.55
    - decellularized allodermis graft 996.55
  - heart (congenital) 746.87
    - acquired 429.89
  - hymen (congenital) (upward) 752.49
  - internal prosthesis NEC - *see* Complications, mechanical
  - intervertebral disc (with neuritis, radiculitis, sciatica, or other pain) 722.2
    - with myelopathy 722.70
    - cervical, cervicodorsal, cervicothoracic 722.0
      - with myelopathy 722.71
      - due to major trauma - *see* Dislocation, vertebra, cervical
    - due to trauma - *see* Dislocation, vertebra
    - lumbar, lumbosacral 722.10
      - with myelopathy 722.73
      - due to major trauma - *see* Dislocation, vertebra, lumbar
    - thoracic, thoracolumbar 722.11
      - with myelopathy 722.72
      - due to major trauma - *see* Dislocation, vertebra, thoracic
  - intrauterine device 996.32
  - kidney (acquired) 593.0
    - congenital 753.3
  - lacrimal apparatus or duct (congenital) 743.65
  - macula (congenital) 743.55
  - Meckel's diverticulum (congenital) 751.0
  - nail (congenital) 757.5
    - acquired 703.8
  - opening of Wharton's duct in mouth 750.26
  - organ or site, congenital NEC - *see* Malposition, congenital
  - ovary (acquired) 620.4
    - congenital 752.0
    - free in peritoneal cavity (congenital) 752.0
    - into hernial sac 620.4
  - oviduct (acquired) 620.4
    - congenital 752.19
  - parathyroid (gland) 252.8
  - parotid gland (congenital) 750.26
  - punctum lacrimale (congenital) 743.65
  - sacroiliac (congenital) (joint) 755.69
    - current injury - *see* Dislocation, sacroiliac
    - old 724.6
  - spine (congenital) 756.19

Distortion (congenital) – *continued*
tibia 755.69
toe(s) 755.66
tongue 750.19
trachea (cartilage) 748.3
ulna 755.59
ureter 753.4
causing obstruction 753.20
urethra 753.8
causing obstruction 753.6
uterus 752.3
vagina 752.49
vein (peripheral) NEC (*see also* Distortion, peripheral vascular system) 747.60
great 747.49
portal 747.49
pulmonary 747.49
vena cava (inferior) (superior) 747.49
vertebra 756.19
visual NEC 368.15
shape or size 368.14
vulva 752.49
wrist (bones) (joint) 755.59
Distress
abdomen 789.0 5th
colon 564.9
emotional V40.9
epigastric 789.0 5th
fetal (syndrome) 768.4
affecting management of pregnancy or childbirth 656.8 5th
liveborn infant 768.4
first noted
before onset of labor 768.2
during labor and delivery 768.3
stillborn infant (death before onset of labor) 768.0
death during labor 768.1
gastrointestinal (functional) 536.9
psychogenic 306.4
intestinal (functional) NEC 564.9
psychogenic 306.4
intrauterine -*see* Distress, fetal
leg 729.5
maternal 669.0 5th
mental V40.9
respiratory 786.09
acute (adult) 518.82
adult syndrome (following shock, surgery, or trauma) 518.5
specified NEC 518.82
fetus or newborn 770.89
syndrome (idiopathic) (newborn) 769
stomach 536.9
psychogenic 306.4
Distribution vessel, atypical NEC 747.60
coronary artery 746.85
spinal 747.82
Districhiasis 704.2
Disturbance - *see also* Disease
absorption NEC 579.9
calcium 269.3
carbohydrate 579.8
fat 579.8
protein 579.8
specified type NEC 579.8
vitamin (*see also* Deficiency, vitamin) 269.2
acid-base equilibrium 276.9
activity and attention, simple, with hyperkinesis 314.01
amino acid (metabolic) (*see also* Disorder, amino acid) 270.9
imidazole 270.5
maple syrup (urine) disease 270.3
transport 270.0
assimilation, food 579.9
attention, simple 314.00
with hyperactivity 314.01
auditory, nerve, except deafness 388.5
behavior (*see also* Disturbance, conduct) 312.9

Disturbance – *continued*
blood clotting (hypoproteinemia) (mechanism) (*see also* Defect, coagulation) 286.9
central nervous system NEC 349.9
cerebral nerve NEC 352.9
circulatory 459.9
conduct 312.9
adjustment reaction 309.3
adolescent onset type 312.82
childhood onset type 312.81

Note *Use the following fifth-digit subclassification with categories 312.0-312.2:*

0	unspecified
1	mild
2	moderate
3	severe

compulsive 312.30
intermittent explosive disorder 312.34
isolated explosive disorder 312.35
kleptomania 312.32
pathological gambling 312.31
pyromania 312.33
hyperkinetic 314.2
intermittent explosive 312.34
isolated explosive 312.35
mixed with emotions 312.4
socialized (type) 312.20
aggressive 312.23
unaggressive 312.21
specified type NEC 312.89
undersocialized, unsocialized
aggressive (type) 312.0 5th
unaggressive (type) 312.1 5th
coordination 781.3
cranial nerve NEC 352.9
deep sensibility - *see* Disturbance, sensation
digestive 536.9
psychogenic 306.4
electrolyte - *see* Imbalance, electrolyte
emotions specific to childhood or adolescence 313.9
with
academic underachievement 313.83
anxiety and fearfulness 313.0
elective mutism 313.23
identity disorder 313.82
jealousy 313.3
misery and unhappiness 313.1
oppositional defiant disorder 313.81
overanxiousness 313.0
sensitivity 313.21
shyness 313.21
social withdrawal 313.22
withdrawal reaction 313.22
involving relationship problems 313.3
mixed 313.89
specified type NEC 313.89
endocrine (gland) 259.9
neonatal, transitory 775.9
specified NEC 775.89
equilibrium 780.4
feeding (elderly) (infant) 783.3
newborn 779.31 ▲
nonorganic origin NEC 307.59
psychogenic NEC 307.59
fructose metabolism 271.2
gait 781.2
hysterical 300.11
gastric (functional) 536.9
motility 536.8
psychogenic 306.4
secretion 536.8
gastrointestinal (functional) 536.9
psychogenic 306.4
habit, child 307.9
hearing, except deafness 388.40

Disturbance – *continued*
heart, functional (conditions classifiable to 426, 427, 428)
due to presence of (cardiac) prosthesis 429.4
postoperative (immediate) 997.1
long-term effect of cardiac surgery 429.4
psychogenic 306.2
hormone 259.9
innervation uterus, sympathetic, parasympathetic 621.8
keratinization NEC
gingiva 523.10
lip 528.5
oral (mucosa) (soft tissue) 528.79
residual ridge mucosa
excessive 528.72
minimal 528.71
tongue 528.79
labyrinth, labyrinthine (vestibule) 386.9
learning, specific NEC 315.2
memory (*see also* Amnesia) 780.93
mild, following organic brain damage 310.8
mental (*see also* Disorder, mental) 300.9
associated with diseases classified elsewhere 316
metabolism (acquired) (congenital) (*see also* Disorder, metabolism) 277.9
with
abortion - *see* Abortion, by type, with metabolic disorder
ectopic pregnancy (*see also* categories 633.0-633.9) 639.4
molar pregnancy (*see also* categories 630-632) 639.4
amino acid (*see also* Disorder, amino acid) 270.9
aromatic NEC 270.2
branched-chain 270.3
specified type NEC 270.8
straight-chain NEC 270.7
sulfur-bearing 270.4
transport 270.0
ammonia 270.6
arginine 270.6
argininosuccinic acid 270.6
carbohydrate NEC 271.9
cholesterol 272.9
citrulline 270.6
cystathionine 270.4
fat 272.9
following
abortion 639.4
ectopic or molar pregnancy 639.4
general 277.9
carbohydrate 271.9
iron 275.0
phosphate 275.3
sodium 276.9
glutamine 270.7
glycine 270.7
histidine 270.5
homocystine 270.4
in labor or delivery 669.0 5th
iron 275.0
isoleucine 270.3
leucine 270.3
lipoid 272.9
specified type NEC 272.8
lysine 270.7
methionine 270.4
neonatal, transitory 775.9
specified type NEC 775.89
nitrogen 788.99
ornithine 270.6
phosphate 275.3
phosphatides 272.7
serine 270.7
sodium NEC 276.9
threonine 270.7
tryptophan 270.2
tyrosine 270.2

Disturbance – *continued*
metabolism – *continued*
urea cycle 270.6
valine 270.3
motor 796.1
nervous functional 799.21 ▲
neuromuscular mechanism (eye) due to syphilis 094.84
nutritional 269.9
nail 703.8
ocular motion 378.87
psychogenic 306.7
oculogyric 378.87
psychogenic 306.7
oculomotor NEC 378.87
psychogenic 306.7
olfactory nerve 781.1
optic nerve NEC 377.49
oral epithelium, including tongue 528.79
residual ridge mucosa
excessive 528.72
minimal 528.71
personality (pattern) (trait) (*see also* Disorder, personality) 301.9
following organic brain damage 310.1
polyglandular 258.9
psychomotor 307.9
pupillary 379.49
reflex 796.1
rhythm, heart 427.9
postoperative (immediate) 997.1
long-term effect of cardiac surgery 429.4
psychogenic 306.2
salivary secretion 527.7
sensation (cold) (heat) (localization) (tactile discrimination localization) (texture) (vibratory) NEC 782.0
hysterical 300.11
skin 782.0
smell 781.1
taste 781.1
sensory (*see also* Disturbance, sensation) 782.0
innervation 782.0
situational (transient) (*see also* Reaction, adjustment) 309.9
acute 308.3
sleep 780.50
with apnea - *see* Apnea, sleep
initiation or maintenance (*see also* Insomnia) 780.52
nonorganic origin 307.41
nonorganic origin 307.40
specified type NEC 307.49
specified NEC 780.59
nonorganic origin 307.49
wakefulness (*see also* Hypersomnia) 780.54
nonorganic origin 307.43
sociopathic 301.7
speech NEC 784.59 ▲
developmental 315.39
associated with hyperkinesis 314.1
secondary to organic lesion 784.59 ▲
stomach (functional) (*see also* Disturbance, gastric) 536.9
sympathetic (nerve) (*see also* Neuropathy, peripheral, autonomic) 337.9
temperature sense 782.0
hysterical 300.11
tooth
eruption 520.6
formation 520.4
structure, hereditary NEC 520.5
touch (*see also* Disturbance, sensation) 782.0
vascular 459.9
arteriosclerotic - *see* Arteriosclerosis
vasomotor 443.9
vasospastic 443.9
vestibular labyrinth 386.9
vision, visual NEC 368.9
psychophysical 368.16

- **Dropsy, dropsical** – *continued*
  - cardiac (*see also* Failure, heart) 428.0
  - cardiorenal (*see also* Hypertension, cardiorenal) 404.90
  - chest 511.9
  - fetus or newborn 778.0
    - due to isoimmunization 773.3
  - gangrenous (*see also* Gangrene) 785.4
  - heart (*see also* Failure, heart) 428.0
  - hepatic - *see* Cirrhosis, liver
  - infantile - *see* Hydrops, fetalis
  - kidney (*see also* Nephrosis) 581.9
  - liver - *see* Cirrhosis, liver
  - lung 514
  - malarial (*see also* Malaria) 084.9
  - neonatorum - *see* Hydrops, fetalis
  - nephritic 581.9
  - newborn - *see* Hydrops, fetalis
  - nutritional 269.9
  - ovary 620.8
  - pericardium (*see also* Pericarditis) 423.9
  - renal (*see also* Nephrosis) 581.9
  - uremic - *see* Uremia
- **Drowned, drowning** (near) 994.1
  - lung 518.5
- **Drowsiness** 780.09
- **Drug** - *see also* condition
  - addiction (*see also* Dependence) 304.9 [5th]
  - adverse effect NEC, correct substance properly administered 995.20
  - allergy 995.27
  - dependence (*see also* Dependence) 304.9 [5th]
  - habit (*see also* Dependence) 304.9 [5th]
  - hypersensitivity 995.27
  - induced
    - circadian rhythm sleep disorder 292.85
    - hypersomnia 292.85
    - insomnia 292.85
    - mental disorder 292.9
      - anxiety 292.89
      - mood 292.84
      - sexual 292.89
      - sleep 292.85
      - specified type 292.89
    - parasomnia 292.85
    - persisting
      - amnestic disorder 292.83
      - dementia 292.82
    - psychotic disorder
      - with
        - delusions 292.11
        - hallucinations 292.12
    - sleep disorder 292.85
  - intoxication 292.89
  - overdose - *see* Table of Drugs and Chemicals
  - poisoning - *see* Table of Drugs and Chemicals
  - therapy (maintenance) status NEC
    - chemotherapy, antineoplastic V58.11
    - immunotherapy, antineoplastic V58.12
    - long-term (current) use V58.69
      - antibiotics V58.62
      - anticoagulants V58.61
      - anti-inflammatories, non-steroidal (NSAID) V58.64
      - antiplatelets V58.63
      - antithrombotics V58.63
      - aspirin V58.66
      - high-risk medications NEC V58.69
      - insulin V58.67
      - methadone V58.69
      - opiate analgesic V58.69
      - steroids V58.65
  - wrong substance given or taken in error - *see* Table of Drugs and Chemicals
- **Drunkenness** (*see also* Abuse, drugs, nondependent) 305.0 [5th]
  - acute in alcoholism (*see also* Alcoholism) 303.0 [5th]
  - chronic (*see also* Alcoholism) 303.9 [5th]
  - pathologic 291.4
- **Drunkenness** – *continued*
  - simple (acute) 305.0 [5th]
    - in alcoholism 303.0 [5th]
  - sleep 307.47
- **Drusen**
  - optic disc or papilla 377.21
  - retina (colloid) (hyaloid degeneration) 362.57
    - hereditary 362.77
- **Drusenfieber** 075
- **Dry, dryness** - *see also* condition
  - eye 375.15
    - syndrome 375.15
  - larynx 478.79
  - mouth 527.7
  - nose 478.19
  - skin syndrome 701.1
  - socket (teeth) 526.5
  - throat 478.29
- **DSAP** (disseminated superficial actinic porokeratosis) 692.75
- **Duane's retraction syndrome** 378.71
- **Duane-Stilling-Türk syndrome** (ocular retraction syndrome) 378.71
- **Dubin-Johnson disease or syndrome** 277.4
- **Dubini's disease** (electric chorea) 049.8
- **Dubois' abscess or disease** 090.5
- **Duchenne's**
  - disease 094.0
    - locomotor ataxia 094.0
    - muscular dystrophy 359.1
    - pseudohypertrophy, muscles 359.1
  - paralysis 335.22
  - syndrome 335.22
- **Duchenne-Aran myelopathic, muscular atrophy** (nonprogressive) (progressive) 335.21
- **Duchenne-Griesinger disease** 359.1
- **Ducrey's**
  - bacillus 099.0
  - chancre 099.0
  - disease (chancroid) 099.0
- **Duct, ductus** - *see* condition
- **Duengero** 061
- **Duhring's disease** (dermatitis herpetiformis) 694.0
- **Dukes (-Filatov) disease** 057.8
- **Dullness**
  - cardiac (decreased) (increased) 785.3
- **Dumb ague** (*see also* Malaria) 084.6
- **Dumbness** (*see also* Aphasia) 784.3
- **Dumdum fever** 085.0
- **Dumping syndrome** (postgastrectomy) 564.2
  - nonsurgical 536.8
- **Duodenitis** (nonspecific) (peptic) 535.60
  - with hemorrhage 535.61
  - due to
    - strongyloides stercoralis 127.2
- **Duodenocholangitis** 575.8
- **Duodenum, duodenal** - *see* condition
- **Duplay's disease, periarthritis, or syndrome** 726.2
- **Duplex** - *see also* Accessory
  - kidney 753.3
  - placenta - *see* Placenta, abnormal
  - uterus 752.2
- **Duplication** - *see also* Accessory
  - anus 751.5
  - aortic arch 747.21
  - appendix 751.5
  - biliary duct (any) 751.69
  - bladder 753.8
  - cecum 751.5
    - and appendix 751.5
  - clitoris 752.49
  - cystic duct 751.69
  - digestive organs 751.8
  - duodenum 751.5
  - esophagus 750.4
  - fallopian tube 752.19
  - frontonasal process 756.0
  - gallbladder 751.69
  - ileum 751.5
  - intestine (large) (small) 751.5
- **Duplication** – *continued*
  - jejunum 751.5
  - kidney 753.3
  - liver 751.69
  - nose 748.1
  - pancreas 751.7
  - penis 752.69
  - respiratory organs NEC 748.9
  - salivary duct 750.22
  - spinal cord (incomplete) 742.51
  - stomach 750.7
  - ureter 753.4
  - vagina 752.49
  - vas deferens 752.89
  - vocal cords 748.3
- **Dupré's disease or syndrome** (meningism) 781.6
- **Dupuytren's**
  - contraction 728.6
  - disease (muscle contracture) 728.6
  - fracture (closed) 824.4
    - ankle (closed) 824.4
      - open 824.5
    - fibula (closed) 824.4
      - open 824.5
    - open 824.5
    - radius (closed) 813.42
      - open 813.52
  - muscle contracture 728.6
- **Durand-Nicolas-Favre disease** (climatic bubo) 099.1
- **Durotomy, incidental** (inadvertent) (*see also* Tear, dural) 349.31
- **Duroziez's disease** (congenital mitral stenosis) 746.5
- **Dust**
  - conjunctivitis 372.05
  - reticulation (occupational) 504
- **Dutton's**
  - disease (trypanosomiasis) 086.9
  - relapsing fever (West African) 087.1
- **Dwarf, dwarfism** 259.4
  - with infantilism (hypophyseal) 253.3
  - achondroplastic 756.4
  - Amsterdam 759.89
  - bird-headed 759.89
  - congenital 259.4
  - constitutional 259.4
  - hypophyseal 253.3
  - infantile 259.4
  - Levi type 253.3
  - Lorain-Levi (pituitary) 253.3
  - Lorain type (pituitary) 253.3
  - metatropic 756.4
  - nephrotic-glycosuric, with hypophosphatemic rickets 270.0
  - nutritional 263.2
  - ovarian 758.6
  - pancreatic 577.8
  - pituitary 253.3
  - polydystrophic 277.5
  - primordial 253.3
  - psychosocial 259.4
  - renal 588.0
    - with hypertension - *see* Hypertension, kidney
  - Russell's (uterine dwarfism and craniofacial dysostosis) 759.89
- **Dyke-Young anemia or syndrome** (acquired macrocytic hemolytic anemia) (secondary) (symptomatic) 283.9
- **Dynia abnormality** (*see also* Defect, coagulation) 286.9
- **Dysacousis** 388.40
- **Dysadrenocortism** 255.9
  - hyperfunction 255.3
  - hypofunction 255.41
- **Dysarthria** 784.51 ▲
  - due to late effect of cerebrovascular disease (*see also* Late effect(s) (of) cerebrovascular disease) 438.13 ●
- **Dysautonomia** (*see also* Neuropathy, peripheral, autonomic) 337.9
  - familial 742.8
- **Dysbarism** 993.3
- **Dysbasia** 719.7
  - angiosclerotica intermittens 443.9
    - due to atherosclerosis 440.21
  - hysterical 300.11
  - lordotica (progressiva) 333.6
  - nonorganic origin 307.9
  - psychogenic 307.9
- **Dysbetalipoproteinemia** (familial) 272.2
- **Dyscalculia** 315.1
- **Dyschezia** (*see also* Constipation) 564.00
- **Dyschondroplasia** (with hemangiomata) 756.4
  - Voorhoeve's 756.4
- **Dyschondrosteosis** 756.59
- **Dyschromia** 709.00
- **Dyscollagenosis** 710.9
- **Dyscoria** 743.41
- **Dyscraniopyophalangy** 759.89
- **Dyscrasia**
  - blood 289.9
    - with antepartum hemorrhage 641.3 [5th]
    - ~~fetus or newborn NEC 776.9~~
    - hemorrhage, subungual 287.8
    - puerperal, postpartum 666.3 [5th]
  - ovary 256.8
  - plasma cell 273.9
  - pluriglandular 258.9
  - polyglandular 258.9
- **Dysdiadochokinesia** 781.3
- **Dysectasia, vesical neck** 596.8
- **Dysendocrinism** 259.9
- **Dysentery, dysenteric** (bilious) (catarrhal) (diarrhea) (epidemic) (gangrenous) (hemorrhagic) (infectious) (sporadic) (tropical) (ulcerative) 009.0
  - abscess, liver (*see also* Abscess, amebic) 006.3
  - amebic (*see also* Amebiasis) 006.9
    - with abscess - *see* Abscess, amebic
    - acute 006.0
    - carrier (suspected) of V02.2
    - chronic 006.1
  - arthritis (*see also* Arthritis, due to, dysentery) 009.0 *[711.3]* [5th]
    - bacillary 004.9 *[711.3]* [5th]
  - asylum 004.9
  - bacillary 004.9
    - arthritis 004.9 *[711.3]* [5th]
    - boyd 004.2
    - flexner 004.1
    - schmitz (-Stutzer) 004.0
    - shiga 004.0
    - shigella 004.9
      - group A 004.0
      - group B 004.1
      - group C 004.2
      - group D 004.3
      - specified type NEC 004.8
    - sonne 004.3
    - specified type NEC 004.8
  - bacterium 004.9
  - balantidial 007.0
  - balantidium coli 007.0
  - Boyd's 004.2
  - Chilomastix 007.8
  - Chinese 004.9
  - choleriform 001.1
  - coccidial 007.2
  - Dientamoeba fragilis 007.8
  - due to specified organism NEC - *see* Enteritis, due to, by organism
  - Embadomonas 007.8
  - Endolimax nana - *see* Dysentery, amebic
  - Entamoba, entamebic - *see* Dysentery, amebic
  - Flexner's 004.1
  - Flexner-Boyd 004.2
  - giardial 007.1
  - Giardia lamblia 007.1
  - Hiss-Russell 004.1
  - lamblia 007.1
  - leishmanial 085.0
  - malarial (*see also* Malaria) 084.6

- **Dysentery, dysenteric** – *continued*
  - metazoal 127.9
  - Monilia 112.89
  - protozoal NEC 007.9
  - Russell's 004.8
  - salmonella 003.0
  - schistosomal 120.1
  - Schmitz (-Stutzer) 004.0
  - Shiga 004.0
  - Shigella NEC (*see also* Dysentery, bacillary) 004.9
    - boydii 004.2
    - dysenteriae 004.0
      - schmitz 004.0
      - shiga 004.0
    - flexneri 004.1
    - group A 004.0
    - group B 004.1
    - group C 004.2
    - group D 004.3
    - Schmitz 004.0
    - Shiga 004.0
    - Sonnei 004.3
  - Sonne 004.3
  - strongyloidiasis 127.2
  - trichomonal 007.3
  - tuberculous (*see also* Tuberculosis) 014.8 [5th]
  - viral (*see also* Enteritis, viral) 008.8
- **Dysequilibrium** 780.4
- **Dysesthesia** 782.0
  - hysterical 300.11
- **Dysfibrinogenemia (congenital)** (*see also* **Defect, coagulation**) 286.3
- **Dysfunction**
  - adrenal (cortical) 255.9
    - hyperfunction 255.3
    - hypofunction 255.41
  - associated with sleep stages or arousal from sleep 780.56
    - nonorganic origin 307.47
  - bladder NEC 596.59
  - bleeding, uterus 626.8
  - brain, minimal (*see also* Hyperkinesia) 314.9
  - cerebral 348.30
  - colon 564.9
    - psychogenic 306.4
  - colostomy or enterostomy 569.62
  - cystic duct 575.8
  - diastolic 429.9
    - with heart failure - *see* Failure, heart
    - due to
      - cardiomyopathy - *see* Cardiomyopathy
      - hypertension - *see* Hypertension, heart
  - endocrine NEC 259.9
  - endometrium 621.8
  - enteric stoma 569.62
  - enterostomy 569.62
  - erectile 607.84
    - nonorganic origin 302.72
  - esophagostomy 530.87
  - Eustachian tube 381.81
  - gallbladder 575.8
  - gastrointestinal 536.9
  - gland, glandular NEC 259.9
  - heart 427.9
    - postoperative (immediate) 997.1
      - long-term effect of cardiac surgery 429.4
  - hemoglobin 289.89
  - hepatic 573.9
  - hepatocellular NEC 573.9
  - hypophysis 253.9
    - hyperfunction 253.1
    - hypofunction 253.2
    - posterior lobe 253.6
      - hypofunction 253.5
  - kidney (*see also* Disease, renal) 593.9
  - labyrinthine 386.50
    - specified NEC 386.58
- **Dysfunction** – *continued*
  - liver 573.9
    - constitutional 277.4
  - minimal brain (child) (*see also* Hyperkinesia) 314.9
  - ovary, ovarian 256.9
    - hyperfunction 256.1
      - estrogen 256.0
    - hypofunction 256.39
      - postablative 256.2
    - postablative 256.2
    - specified NEC 256.8
  - papillary muscle 429.81
    - with myocardial infarction 410.8 [5th]
  - parathyroid 252.8
    - hyperfunction 252.00
    - hypofunction 252.1
  - pineal gland 259.8
  - pituitary (gland) 253.9
    - hyperfunction 253.1
    - hypofunction 253.2
    - posterior 253.6
      - hypofunction 253.5
  - placental - *see* Placenta, insufficiency
  - platelets (blood) 287.1
  - polyglandular 258.9
    - specified NEC 258.8
  - psychosexual 302.70
    - with
      - dyspareunia (functional) (psychogenic) 302.76
      - frigidity 302.72
      - impotence 302.72
      - inhibition
        - orgasm
          - female 302.73
          - male 302.74
        - sexual
          - desire 302.71
          - excitement 302.72
      - premature ejaculation 302.75
      - sexual aversion 302.79
      - specified disorder NEC 302.79
      - vaginismus 306.51
  - pylorus 537.9
  - rectum 564.9
    - psychogenic 306.4
  - segmental (*see also* Dysfunction, somatic) 739.9
  - senile 797
  - sexual 302.70
  - sinoatrial node 427.81
  - somatic 739.9
    - abdomen 739.9
    - acromioclavicular 739.7
    - cervical 739.1
    - cervicothoracic 739.1
    - costochondral 739.8
    - costovertebral 739.8
    - extremities
      - lower 739.6
      - upper 739.7
    - head 739.0
    - hip 739.5
    - lumbar, lumbosacral 739.3
    - occipitocervical 739.0
    - pelvic 739.5
    - pubic 739.5
    - rib cage 739.8
    - sacral 739.4
    - sacrococcygeal 739.4
    - sacroiliac 739.4
    - specified site NEC 739.9
    - sternochondral 739.8
    - sternoclavicular 739.7
    - temporomandibular 739.0
    - thoracic, thoracolumbar 739.2
  - stomach 536.9
    - psychogenic 306.4
  - suprarenal 255.9
    - hyperfunction 255.3
    - hypofunction 255.41
  - systolic 429.9
    - with heart failure - *see* Failure, heart
- **Dysfunction** – *continued*
  - symbolic NEC 784.60
    - specified type NEC 784.69
  - temporomandibular (joint) (joint-pain-syndrome) NEC 524.60
    - sounds on opening or closing 524.64
    - specified NEC 524.69
  - testicular 257.9
    - hyperfunction 257.0
    - hypofunction 257.2
    - specified type NEC 257.8
  - thymus 254.9
  - thyroid 246.9
    - complicating pregnancy, childbirth, or puerperium 648.1 [5th]
    - hyperfunction - *see* Hyperthyroidism
    - hypofunction - *see* Hypothyroidism
  - uterus, complicating delivery 661.9 [5th]
    - affecting fetus or newborn 763.7
    - hypertonic 661.4 [5th]
    - hypotonic 661.2 [5th]
      - primary 661.0 [5th]
      - secondary 661.1 [5th]
  - velopharyngeal (acquired) 528.9
    - congenital 750.29
  - ventricular 429.9
    - with congestive heart failure (*see also* Failure, heart) 428.0
    - due to
      - cardiomyopathy - *see* Cardiomyopathy
      - hypertension - *see* Hypertension, heart
    - left, reversible following sudden emotional stress 429.83
  - vesicourethral NEC 596.59
  - vestibular 386.50
    - specified type NEC 386.58
- **Dysgammaglobulinemia** 279.06
- **Dysgenesis**
  - gonadal (due to chromosomal anomaly) 758.6
    - pure 752.7
  - kidney(s) 753.0
  - ovarian 758.6
  - renal 753.0
  - reticular 279.2
  - seminiferous tubules 758.6
  - tidal platelet 287.31
- **Dysgerminoma** (M9060/3)
  - specified site - *see* Neoplasm, by site, malignant
  - unspecified site
    - female 183.0
    - male 186.9
- **Dysgeusia** 781.1
- **Dysgraphia** 781.3
- **Dyshidrosis** 705.81
- **Dysidrosis** 705.81
- **Dysinsulinism** 251.8
- **Dyskaryotic cervical smear** 795.09
- **Dyskeratosis** (*see also* Keratosis) 701.1
  - bullosa hereditaria 757.39
  - cervix 622.10
  - congenital 757.39
  - follicularis 757.39
    - vitamin A deficiency 264.8
  - gingiva 523.8
  - oral soft tissue NEC 528.79
  - tongue 528.79
  - uterus NEC 621.8
- **Dyskinesia** 781.3
  - biliary 575.8
  - esophagus 530.5
  - hysterical 300.11
  - intestinal 564.89
  - neuroleptic-induced tardive 333.85
  - nonorganic origin 307.9
  - orofacial 333.82
    - due to drugs 333.85
  - psychogenic 307.9
  - subacute, due to drugs 333.85
  - tardive (oral) 333.85
- **Dyslalia** 784.59 ▲
  - developmental 315.39
- **Dyslexia** 784.61
  - developmental 315.02
  - secondary to organic lesion 784.61
- **Dyslipidemia** 272.4
- **Dysmaturity** (*see also* Immaturity) 765.1 [5th]
  - lung 770.4
  - pulmonary 770.4
- **Dysmenorrhea** (essential) (exfoliative) (functional) (intrinsic) (membranous) (primary) (secondary) 625.3
  - psychogenic 306.52
- **Dysmetabolic syndrome X** 277.7
- **Dysmetria** 781.3
- **Dysmorodystrophia mesodermalis congenita** 759.82
- **Dysnomia** 784.3
- **Dysorexia** 783.0
  - hysterical 300.11
- **Dysostosis**
  - cleidocranial, cleidocranialis 755.59
  - craniofacial 756.0
  - Fairbank's (idiopathic familial generalized osteophytosis) 756.50
  - mandibularis 756.0
  - mandibulofacial, incomplete 756.0
  - multiplex 277.5
  - orodigitofacial 759.89
- **Dyspareunia** (female) 625.0
  - male 608.89
  - psychogenic 302.76
- **Dyspepsia** (allergic) (congenital) (fermentative) (flatulent) (functional) (gastric) (gastrointestinal) (neurogenic) (occupational) (reflex) 536.8
  - acid 536.8
  - atonic 536.3
    - psychogenic 306.4
  - diarrhea 787.91
    - psychogenic 306.4
  - intestinal 564.89
    - psychogenic 306.4
  - nervous 306.4
  - neurotic 306.4
  - psychogenic 306.4
- **Dysphagia** 787.20
  - cervical 787.29
  - functional 300.11
  - hysterical 300.11
  - nervous 300.11
  - neurogenic 787.29
  - oral phase 787.21
  - oropharyngeal phase 787.22
  - pharyngeal phase 787.23
  - pharyngoesophageal phase 787.24
  - psychogenic 306.4
  - sideropenic 280.8
  - spastica 530.5
  - specified NEC 787.29
- **Dysphagocytosis, congenital** 288.1
- **Dysphasia** 784.59 ▲
- **Dysphonia** 784.42 ▲
  - clericorum 784.49
  - functional 300.11
  - hysterical 300.11
  - psychogenic 306.1
  - spastica 478.79
- **Dyspigmentation** - *see also* Pigmentation
  - eyelid (acquired) 374.52
- **Dyspituitarism** 253.9
  - hyperfunction 253.1
  - hypofunction 253.2
  - posterior lobe 253.6
- **Dysplasia** - *see also* Anomaly
  - anus 569.44
    - intraepithelial neoplasia I [AIN I] (histologically confirmed) 569.44
    - intraepithelial neoplasia II [AIN II] (histologically confirmed) 569.44

Dysentery, dysenteric – Dysplasia

- **Dysplasia** – *continued*
  - anus – *continued*
    - intraepithelial neoplasia III [AIN III] 230.6
      - anal canal 230.5
    - mild (histologically confirmed) 569.44
    - moderate (histologically confirmed) 569.44
    - severe 230.6
      - anal canal 230.5
  - artery
    - fibromuscular NEC 447.8
      - carotid 447.8
      - renal 447.3
  - bladder 596.8
  - bone (fibrous) NEC 733.29
    - diaphyseal, progressive 756.59
    - jaw 526.89
    - monostotic 733.29
    - polyostotic 756.54
    - solitary 733.29
  - brain 742.9
  - bronchopulmonary, fetus or newborn 770.7
  - cervix (uteri) 622.10
    - cervical intraepithelial neoplasia I [CIN I] 622.11
    - cervical intraepithelial neoplasia II [CIN II] 622.12
    - cervical intraepithelial neoplasia III [CIN III] 233.1
    - CIN I 622.11
    - CIN II 622.12
    - CIN III 233.1
    - mild 622.11
    - moderate 622.12
    - severe 233.1
  - chondroectodermal 756.55
  - chondromatose 756.4
  - colon 211.3
  - craniocarpotarsal 759.89
  - craniometaphyseal 756.89
  - dentinal 520.5
  - diaphyseal, progressive 756.59
  - ectodermal (anhidrotic) (Bason) (Clouston's) (congenital) (Feinmesser) (hereditary) (hidrotic) (Marshall) (Robinson's) 757.31
  - epiphysealis 756.9
    - multiplex 756.56
    - punctata 756.59
  - epiphysis 756.9
    - multiple 756.56
  - epithelial
    - epiglottis 478.79
    - uterine cervix 622.10
  - erythroid NEC 289.89
  - eye (*see also* Microphthalmos) 743.10
  - familial metaphyseal 756.89
  - fibromuscular, artery NEC 447.8
    - carotid 447.8
    - renal 447.3
  - fibrous
    - bone NEC 733.29
    - diaphyseal, progressive 756.59
    - jaw 526.89
    - monostotic 733.29
    - polyostotic 756.54
    - solitary 733.29
  - high grade, focal - *see* Neoplasm, by site, benign
  - hip (congenital) 755.63
    - with dislocation (*see also* Dislocation, hip, congenital) 754.30
  - hypohidrotic ectodermal 757.31
  - joint 755.8
  - kidney 753.15
  - leg 755.69
  - linguofacialis 759.89
  - lung 748.5
  - macular 743.55
  - mammary (benign) (gland) 610.9
    - cystic 610.1
    - specified type NEC 610.8
- **Dysplasia** – *continued*
  - metaphyseal 756.9
    - familial 756.89
  - monostotic fibrous 733.29
  - muscle 756.89
  - myeloid NEC 289.89
  - nervous system (general) 742.9
  - neuroectodermal 759.6
  - oculoauriculovertebral 756.0
  - oculodentodigital 759.89
  - olfactogenital 253.4
  - osteo-onycho-arthro (hereditary) 756.89
  - periosteum 733.99
  - polyostotic fibrous 756.54
  - progressive diaphyseal 756.59
  - prostate 602.3
    - intraepithelial neoplasia I [PIN I] 602.3
    - intraepithelial neoplasia II [PIN II] 602.3
    - intraepithelial neoplasia III [PIN III] 233.4
  - renal 753.15
  - renofacialis 753.0
  - retinal NEC 743.56
  - retrolental (*see also* Retinopathy of prematurity) 362.21
  - skin 709.8
  - spinal cord 742.9
  - thymic, with immunodeficiency 279.2
  - vagina 623.0
    - mild 623.0
    - moderate 623.0
    - severe 233.31
  - vocal cord 478.5
  - vulva 624.8
    - intraepithelial neoplasia I [VIN I] 624.01
    - intraepithelial neoplasia II [VIN II] 624.02
    - intraepithelial neoplasia III [VIN III] 233.32
    - mild 624.01
    - moderate 624.02
    - severe 233.32
    - VIN I 624.01
    - VIN II 624.02
    - VIN III 233.32
- **Dyspnea** (nocturnal) (paroxysmal) 786.09
  - asthmatic (bronchial) (*see also* Asthma) 493.9 5th
    - with bronchitis (*see also* Asthma) 493.9
      - chronic 493.2 5th
    - cardiac (*see also* Failure, ventricular, left) 428.1
  - cardiac (*see also* Failure, ventricular, left) 428.1
  - functional 300.11
  - hyperventilation 786.01
  - hysterical 300.11
  - Monday morning 504
  - newborn 770.89
  - psychogenic 306.1
  - uremic - *see* Uremia
- **Dyspraxia** 781.3
  - syndrome 315.4
- **Dysproteinemia** 273.8
  - transient with copper deficiency 281.4
- **Dysprothrombinemia** (constitutional) (*see also* Defect, coagulation) 286.3
- **Dysreflexia, autonomic** 337.3
- **Dysrhythmia**
  - cardiac 427.9
    - postoperative (immediate) 997.1
      - long-term effect of cardiac surgery 429.4
    - specified type NEC 427.89
  - cerebral or cortical 348.30
- **Dyssecretosis, mucoserous** 710.2
- **Dyssocial reaction, without manifest psychiatric disorder**
  - adolescent V71.02
  - adult V71.01
  - child V71.02
- **Dyssomnia** NEC 780.56
  - nonorganic origin 307.47
- **Dyssplenism** 289.4
- **Dyssynergia**
  - biliary (*see also* Disease, biliary) 576.8
  - cerebellaris myoclonica 334.2
  - detrusor sphincter (bladder) 596.55
  - ventricular 429.89
- **Dystasia, hereditary areflexic** 334.3
- **Dysthymia** 300.4
- **Dysthymic disorder** 300.4
- **Dysthyroidism** 246.9
- **Dystocia** 660.9
  - affecting fetus or newborn 763.1
  - cervical 661.2 5th
    - affecting fetus or newborn 763.7
  - contraction ring 661.4 5th
    - affecting fetus or newborn 763.7
  - fetal 660.9 5th
    - abnormal size 653.5 5th
    - affecting fetus or newborn 763.1
    - deformity 653.7 5th
  - maternal 660.9 5th
    - affecting fetus or newborn 763.1
  - positional 660.0 5th
    - affecting fetus or newborn 763.1
  - shoulder (girdle) 660.4 5th
    - affecting fetus or newborn 763.1
  - uterine NEC 661.4 5th
    - affecting fetus or newborn 763.7
- **Dystonia**
  - acute
    - due to drugs 333.72
    - neuroleptic-induced acute 333.72
  - deformans progressiva 333.6
  - lenticularis 333.6
  - musculorum deformans 333.6
  - torsion (idiopathic) 333.6
    - acquired 333.79
    - fragments (of) 333.89
    - genetic 333.6
    - symptomatic 333.79
- **Dystonic**
  - movements 781.0
- **Dystopia kidney** 753.3
- **Dystrophy, dystrophia** 783.9
  - adiposogenital 253.8
  - asphyxiating thoracic 756.4
  - Becker's type 359.22
  - brevicollis 756.16
  - Bruch's membrane 362.77
  - cervical (sympathetic) NEC 337.09
  - chondro-osseus with punctate epiphyseal dysplasia 756.59
  - choroid (hereditary) 363.50
    - central (areolar) (partial) 363.53
      - total (gyrate) 363.54
    - circinate 363.53
    - circumpapillary (partial) 363.51
      - total 363.52
    - diffuse
      - partial 363.56
      - total 363.57
    - generalized
      - partial 363.56
      - total 363.57
    - gyrate
      - central 363.54
      - generalized 363.57
    - helicoid 363.52
    - peripapillary - *see* Dystrophy, choroid, circumpapillary
    - serpiginous 363.54
  - cornea (hereditary) 371.50
    - anterior NEC 371.52
    - Cogan's 371.52
    - combined 371.57
    - crystalline 371.56
    - endothelial (Fuchs') 371.57
    - epithelial 371.50
      - juvenile 371.51
      - microscopic cystic 371.52
    - granular 371.53
    - lattice 371.54
- **Dystrophy, dystrophia** – *continued*
  - cornea – *continued*
    - macular 371.55
    - marginal (Terrien's) 371.48
    - meesman's 371.51
    - microscopic cystic (epithelial) 371.52
    - nodular, Salzmann's 371.46
    - polymorphous 371.58
    - posterior NEC 371.58
    - ring-like 371.52
    - Salzmann's nodular 371.46
    - stromal NEC 371.56
  - dermatochondrocorneal 371.50
  - Duchenne's 359.1
  - due to malnutrition 263.9
  - Erb's 359.1
  - familial
    - hyperplastic periosteal 756.59
    - osseous 277.5
  - foveal 362.77
  - Fuchs', cornea 371.57
  - Gowers' muscular 359.1
  - hair 704.2
  - hereditary, progressive muscular 359.1
  - hypogenital, with diabetic tendency 759.81
  - Landouzy-Déjérine 359.1
  - Leyden-Möbius 359.1
  - mesodermalis congenita 759.82
  - muscular 359.1
    - congenital (hereditary) 359.0
      - myotonic 359.22
    - distal 359.1
    - Duchenne's 359.1
    - Erb's 359.1
    - fascioscapulohumeral 359.1
    - Gowers' 359.1
    - hereditary (progressive) 359.1
    - Landouzy-Déjérine 359.1
    - limb-girdle 359.1
    - myotonic 359.21
    - progressive (hereditary) 359.1
      - Charcôt-Marie-Tooth 356.1
    - pseudohypertrophic (infantile) 359.1
  - myocardium, myocardial (*see also* Degeneration, myocardial) 429.1
  - myotonic 359.21
  - myotonica 359.21
  - nail 703.8
    - congenital 757.5
  - neurovascular (traumatic) (*see also* Neuropathy, peripheral, autonomic) 337.9
  - nutritional 263.9
  - ocular 359.1
  - oculocerebrorenal 270.8
  - oculopharyngeal 359.1
  - ovarian 620.8
  - papillary (and pigmentary) 701.1
  - pelvicrural atrophic 359.1
  - pigmentary (*see also* Acanthosis) 701.2
  - pituitary (gland) 253.8
  - polyglandular 258.8
  - posttraumatic sympathetic - *see* Dystrophy, symphatic
  - progressive ophthalmoplegic 359.1
  - reflex neuromuscular - *see* Dystrophy, sympathetic
  - retina, retinal (hereditary) 362.70
    - albipunctate 362.74
    - Bruch's membrane 362.77
    - cone, progressive 362.75
    - hyaline 362.77
    - in
      - Bassen-Kornzweig syndrome 272.5 *[362.72]*
      - cerebroretinal lipidosis 330.1 *[362.71]*
      - Refsum's disease 356.3 *[362.72]*
      - systemic lipidosis 272.7 *[362.71]*
    - juvenile (Stargardt's) 362.75
    - pigmentary 362.74
    - pigment epithelium 362.76
    - progressive cone (-rod) 362.75

Edema, edematous – *continued*
- intracranial 348.5
  - due to injury at birth 767.8
- iris 364.89
- joint (*see also* Effusion, joint) 719.0 [5th]
- larynx (*see also* Edema, glottis) 478.6
- legs 782.3
  - due to venous obstruction 459.2
  - hereditary 757.0
- localized 782.3
  - due to venous obstruction 459.2
    - lower extremity 459.2
- lower extremities - *see* Edema, legs
- lung 514
  - acute 518.4
    - with heart disease or failure (*see also* Failure, ventricular, left) 428.1
      - congestive 428.0
    - chemical (due to fumes or vapors) 506.1
    - due to
      - external agent(s) NEC 508.9
        - specified NEC 508.8
      - fumes and vapors (chemical) (inhalation) 506.1
      - radiation 508.0
  - chemical (acute) 506.1
    - chronic 506.4
  - chronic 514
    - chemical (due to fumes or vapors) 506.4
    - due to
      - external agent(s) NEC 508.9
        - specified NEC 508.8
      - fumes or vapors (chemical) (inhalation) 506.4
      - radiation 508.1
  - due to
    - external agent 508.9
      - specified NEC 508.8
    - high altitude 993.2
    - near drowning 994.1
  - postoperative 518.4
  - terminal 514
- lymphatic 457.1
  - due to mastectomy operation 457.0
- macula 362.83
  - cystoid 362.53
  - diabetic 250.5 [5th] *[362.07]*
    - due to secondary diabetes 249.5 [5th] *[362.07]*
- malignant (*see also* Gangrene, gas) 040.0
- Milroy's 757.0
- nasopharynx 478.25
- neonatorum 778.5
- nutritional (newborn) 262
  - with dyspigmentation, skin and hair 260
- optic disc or nerve - *see* Papilledema
- orbit 376.33
  - circulatory 459.89
- palate (soft) (hard) 528.9
- pancreas 577.8
- penis 607.83
- periodic 995.1
  - hereditary 277.6
- pharynx 478.25
- pitting 782.3
- pulmonary - *see* Edema, lung
- Quincke's 995.1
  - hereditary 277.6
- renal (*see also* Nephrosis) 581.9
- retina (localized) (macular) (peripheral) 362.83
  - cystoid 362.53
  - diabetic 250.5 [5th] *[362.07]*
    - due to secondary diabetes 249.5 [5th] *[362.07]*
- salt 276.0
- scrotum 608.86
- seminal vesicle 608.86
- spermatic cord 608.86
- spinal cord 336.1

Edema, edematous – *continued*
- stasis (*see also* Hypertension, venous) 459.30
- starvation 262
- subconjunctival 372.73
- subglottic (*see also* Edema, glottis) 478.6
- supraglottic (*see also* Edema, glottis) 478.6
- testis 608.86
- toxic NEC 782.3
- traumatic NEC 782.3
- tunica vaginalis 608.86
- vas deferens 608.86
- vocal cord - *see* Edema, glottis
- vulva (acute) 624.8

Edentia (complete) (partial) (*see also* Absence, tooth) 520.0
- acquired (*see also* Edentulism) 525.40
  - due to
    - caries 525.13
    - extraction 525.10
    - periodontal disease 525.12
    - specified NEC 525.19
    - trauma 525.11
- causing malocclusion 524.30
- congenital (deficiency of tooth buds) 520.0

Edentulism 525.40
- complete 525.40
  - class I 525.41
  - class II 525.42
  - class III 525.43
  - class IV 525.44
- partial 525.50
  - class I 525.51
  - class II 525.52
  - class III 525.53
  - class IV 525.54

Edsall's disease 992.2

Educational handicap V62.3

Edwards' syndrome 758.2

Effect, adverse NEC
- abnormal gravitational (G) forces or states 994.9
- air pressure - *see* Effect, adverse, atmospheric pressure
- altitude (high) - *see* Effect, adverse, high altitude
- anesthetic
  - in labor and delivery NEC 668.9 [5th]
    - affecting fetus or newborn 763.5
- antitoxin - *see* Complications, vaccination
- atmospheric pressure 993.9
  - due to explosion 993.4
  - high 993.3
  - low - *see* Effect, adverse, high altitude
  - specified effect NEC 993.8
- biological, correct substance properly administered (*see also* Effect, adverse, drug) 995.20
- blood (derivatives) (serum) (transfusion) - *see* Complications, transfusion
- chemical substance NEC 989.9
  - specified - *see* Table of Drugs and Chemicals
- cobalt, radioactive (*see also* Effect, adverse, radioactive substance) 990
- cold (temperature) (weather) 991.9
  - chilblains 991.5
  - frostbite - *see* Frostbite
  - specified effect NEC 991.8
- drugs and medicinals 995.20
  - correct substance properly administered 995.20
  - overdose or wrong substance given or taken 977.9
    - specified drug - *see* Table of Drugs and Chemicals
- electric current (shock) 994.8
  - burn - *see* Burn, by site
- electricity (electrocution) (shock) 994.8
  - burn - *see* Burn, by site
- exertion (excessive) 994.5
- exposure 994.9
  - exhaustion 994.4
- external cause NEC 994.9

Effect, adverse NEC – *continued*
- fallout (radioactive) NEC 990
- fluoroscopy NEC 990
- foodstuffs
  - allergic reaction (*see also* Allergy, food) 693.1
  - anaphylactic shock due to food NEC 995.60
  - noxious 988.9
    - specified type NEC (*see also* Poisoning, by name of noxious foodstuff) 988.8
- gases, fumes, or vapors - *see* Table of Drugs and Chemicals
- glue (airplane) sniffing 304.6 [5th]
- heat - *see* Heat
- high altitude NEC 993.2
  - anoxia 993.2
  - on
    - ears 993.0
    - sinuses 993.1
  - polycythemia 289.0
- hot weather - *see* Heat
- hunger 994.2
- immersion, foot 991.4
- immunization - *see* Complications, vaccination
- immunological agents - *see* Complications, vaccination
- implantation (removable) of isotope or radium NEC 990
- infrared (radiation) (rays) NEC 990
  - burn - *see* Burn, by site
  - dermatitis or eczema 692.82
- infusion - *see* Complications, infusion
- ingestion or injection of isotope (therapeutic) NEC 990
- irradiation NEC (*see also* Effect, adverse, radiation) 990
- isotope (radioactive) NEC 990
- lack of care (child) (infant) (newborn) 995.52
  - adult 995.84
- lightning 994.0
  - burn - *see* Burn, by site
- Lirugin - *see* Complications, vaccination
- mesothorium NEC 990
- motion 994.6
- noise, inner ear 388.10
- medicinal substance, correct, properly administered (*see also* Effect, adverse, drugs) 995.20
- other drug, medicinal and biological substance 995.29
- overheated places - *see* Heat
- polonium NEC 990
- psychosocial, of work environment V62.1
- radiation (diagnostic) (fallout) (infrared) (natural source) (therapeutic) (tracer) (ultraviolet) (x-ray) NEC 990
  - with pulmonary manifestations
    - acute 508.0
    - chronic 508.1
  - dermatitis or eczema 692.82
    - due to sun NEC (*see also* Dermatitis, due to, sun) 692.70
  - fibrosis of lungs 508.1
  - maternal with suspected damage to fetus affecting management of pregnancy 655.6 [5th]
  - pneumonitis 508.0
- radioactive substance NEC 990
  - dermatitis or eczema 692.82
- radioactivity NEC 990
- radiotherapy NEC 990
  - dermatitis or eczema 692.82
- radium NEC 990
- reduced temperature 991.9
  - frostbite - *see* Frostbite
  - immersion, foot (hand) 991.4
  - specified effect NEC 991.8
- roentgenography NEC 990

Effect, adverse NEC – *continued*
- roentgenoscopy NEC 990
- roentgen rays NEC 990
- serum (prophylactic) (therapeutic) NEC 999.5
- specified NEC 995.89
  - external cause NEC 994.9
- strangulation 994.7
- submersion 994.1
- teletherapy NEC 990
- thirst 994.3
- transfusion - *see* Complications, transfusion
- ultraviolet (radiation) (rays) NEC 990
  - burn - *see also* Burn, by site
    - from sun (*see also* Sunburn) 692.71
  - dermatitis or eczema 692.82
    - due to sun NEC (*see also* Dermatitis, due to, sun) 692.70
- uranium NEC 990
- vaccine (any) - *see* Complications, vaccination
- weightlessness 994.9
- whole blood - *see also* Complications, transfusion
  - overdose or wrong substance given (*see also* Table of Drugs and Chemicals) 964.7
- working environment V62.1
  - x-rays NEC 990
    - dermatitis or eczema 692.82

Effect, remote
- of cancer-*see* condition

Effects, late - *see* Late, effect (of)

Effluvium, telogen 704.02

Effort
- intolerance 306.2
- syndrome (aviators) (psychogenic) 306.2

Effusion
- amniotic fluid (*see also* Rupture, membranes, premature) 658.1 [5th]
- brain (serous) 348.5
- bronchial (*see also* Bronchitis) 490
- cerebral 348.5
- cerebrospinal (*see also* Meningitis) 322.9
  - vessel 348.5
- chest - *see* Effusion, pleura
- intracranial 348.5
- joint 719.00
  - ankle 719.07
  - elbow 719.02
  - foot 719.07
  - hand 719.04
  - hip 719.05
  - knee 719.06
  - multiple sites 719.09
  - pelvic region 719.05
  - shoulder (region) 719.01
  - specified site NEC 719.08
  - wrist 719.03
- meninges (*see also* Meningitis) 322.9
- pericardium, pericardial (*see also* Pericarditis) 423.9
  - acute 420.90
- peritoneal (chronic) 568.82
- pleura, pleurisy, pleuritic, pleuropericardial 511.9
  - bacterial, nontuberculous 511.1
  - fetus or newborn 511.9
  - malignant 511.81
  - nontuberculous 511.9
    - bacterial 511.1
  - pneumococcal 511.1
  - staphylococcal 511.1
  - streptococcal 511.1
  - traumatic 862.29
    - with open wound 862.39
  - tuberculous (*see also* Tuberculosis, pleura) 012.0 [5th]
    - primary progressive 010.1 [5th]
- pulmonary - *see* Effusion, pleura
- spinal (*see also* Meningitis) 322.9
- thorax, thoracic - *see* Effusion, pleura

Egg (oocyte) (ovum)
  donor V59.70
    over age 35 V59.73
      anonymous recipient V59.73
      designated recipient V59.74
    under age 35 V59.71
      anonymous recipient V59.71
      designated recipient V59.72
Eggshell nails 703.8
  congenital 757.5
Ego-dystonic
  homosexuality 302.0
  lesbianism 302.0
  sexual orientation 302.0
Egyptian splenomegaly 120.1
Ehlers-Danlos syndrome 756.83
Ehrlichiosis 082.40
  chaffeensis 082.41
  specified type NEC 082.49
Eichstedt's disease (pityriasis versicolor) 111.0
EIN (endometrial intraepithelial neoplasia) 621.35 ●
Eisenmenger's complex or syndrome (ventricular septal defect) 745.4
Ejaculation, semen
  painful 608.89
    psychogenic 306.59
  premature 302.75
  retrograde 608.87
Ekbom syndrome (restless legs) 333.94
Ekman's syndrome (brittle bones and blue sclera) 756.51
Elastic skin 756.83
  acquired 701.8
Elastofibroma (M8820/0) - *see* Neoplasm, connective tissue, benign
Elastoidosis
  cutanea nodularis 701.8
  cutis cystica et comedonica 701.8
Elastoma 757.39
  juvenile 757.39
  Miescher's (elastosis perforans serpiginosa) 701.1
Elastomyofibrosis 425.3
Elastosis 701.8
  atrophicans 701.8
  perforans serpiginosa 701.1
  reactive perforating 701.1
  senilis 701.8
  solar (actinic) 692.74
Elbow - *see* condition
Electric
  current, electricity, effects (concussion) (fatal) (nonfatal) (shock) 994.8
    burn - *see* Burn, by site
  feet (foot) syndrome 266.2
  shock from electroshock gun (taser) 994.8
Electrocution 994.8
Electrolyte imbalance 276.9
  with
    abortion - *see* Abortion, by type, with metabolic disorder
    ectopic pregnancy (*see also* categories 633.0-633.9) 639.4
    hyperemesis gravidarum (before 22 completed weeks gestation) 643.1 [5th]
    molar pregnancy (*see also* categories 630-632) 639.4
  following
    abortion 639.4
    ectopic or molar pregnancy 639.4
Elephant man syndrome 237.71
Elephantiasis (nonfilarial) 457.1
  arabicum (*see also* Infestation, filarial) 125.9
  congenita hereditaria 757.0
  congenital (any site) 757.0
  due to
    Brugia (malayi) 125.1
    mastectomy operation 457.0
    Wuchereria (bancrofti) 125.0
      malayi 125.1

Elephantiasis – *continued*
  eyelid 374.83
  filarial (*see also* Infestation, filarial) 125.9
  filariensis (*see also* Infestation, filarial) 125.9
  gingival 523.8
  glandular 457.1
  graecorum 030.9
  lymphangiectatic 457.1
  lymphatic vessel 457.1
    due to mastectomy operation 457.0
  neuromatosa 237.71
  postmastectomy 457.0
  scrotum 457.1
  streptococcal 457.1
  surgical 997.99
    postmastectomy 457.0
  telangiectodes 457.1
  vulva (nonfilarial) 624.8
Elevated - *see* Elevation
  findings on laboratory examination - *see* Findings, abnormal, without diagnosis (examination) (laboratory test) ●
  GFR (glomerular filtration rate) - *see* Findings, abnormal, without diagnosis (examination) (laboratory test) ●
Elevation
  17-ketosteroids 791.9
  acid phosphatase 790.5
  alkaline phosphatase 790.5
  amylase 790.5
  antibody titers 795.79
  basal metabolic rate (BMR) 794.7
  blood pressure (*see also* Hypertension) 401.9
    reading (incidental) (isolated) (nonspecific), no diagnosis of hypertension 796.2
  blood sugar 790.29
  body temperature (of unknown origin) (*see also* Pyrexia) 780.60
  C-reactive protein (CRP) 790.95
  cancer antigen 125 [CA 125] 795.82
  carcinoembryonic antigen [CEA] 795.81
  cholesterol 272.0
    with high triglycerides 272.2
  conjugate, eye 378.81
  CRP (C-reactive protein) 790.95
  diaphragm, congenital 756.6
  GFR (glomerular filtration rate) - *see* Findings, abnormal, without diagnosis (examination) (laboratory test) ●
  glucose
    fasting 790.21
    tolerance test 790.22
  immunoglobulin level 795.79
  indolacetic acid 791.9
  lactic acid dehydrogenase (LDH) level 790.4
  leukocytes 288.60
  lipase 790.5
  lipoprotein a level 272.8
  liver function test (LFT) 790.6
    alkaline phosphatase 790.5
    aminotransferase 790.4
    bilirubin 782.4
    hepatic enzyme NEC 790.5
    lactate dehydrogenase 790.4
  lymphocytes 288.61
  prostate specific antigen (PSA) 790.93
  renin 790.99
    in hypertension (*see also* Hypertension, renovascular) 405.91
  Rh titer 999.7
  scapula, congenital 755.52
  sedimentation rate 790.1
  SGOT 790.4
  SGPT 790.4
  transaminase 790.4
  triglycerides 272.1
    with high cholesterol 272.2

Elevation – *continued*
  vanillylmandelic acid 791.9
  venous pressure 459.89
  VMA 791.9
  white blood cell count 288.60
    specified NEC 288.69
Elliptocytosis (congenital) (hereditary) 282.1
  Hb-C (disease) 282.7
  hemoglobin disease 282.7
  sickle-cell (disease) 282.60
    trait 282.5
Ellis-van Creveld disease or syndrome (chondroectodermal dysplasia) 756.55
Ellison-Zollinger syndrome (gastric hypersecretion with pancreatic islet cell tumor) 251.5
Elongation, elongated (congenital) - *see also* Distortion
  bone 756.9
  cervix (uteri) 752.49
    acquired 622.6
    hypertrophic 622.6
  colon 751.5
  common bile duct 751.69
  cystic duct 751.69
  frenulum, penis 752.69
  labia minora, acquired 624.8
  ligamentum patellae 756.89
  petiolus (epiglottidis) 748.3
  styloid bone (process) 733.99
  tooth, teeth 520.2
  uvula 750.26
    acquired 528.9
Elschnig bodies or pearls 366.51
El Tor cholera 001.1
Emaciation (due to malnutrition) 261
Emancipation disorder 309.22
Embadomoniasis 007.8
Embarrassment heart, cardiac - *see* Disease, heart
Embedded tooth, teeth 520.6
  root only 525.3
Embolic - *see* condition
Embolism 444.9
  with
    abortion - *see* Abortion, by type, with embolism
    ectopic pregnancy (*see also* categories 633.0-633.9) 639.6
    molar pregnancy (*see also* categories 630-632) 639.6
  air (any site) 958.0
    with
      abortion - *see* Abortion, by type, with embolism
      ectopic pregnancy (*see also* categories 633.0-633.9) 639.6
      molar pregnancy (*see also* categories 630-632) 639.6
    due to implanted device - *see* Complications, due to (presence of) any device, implant, or graft classified to 996.0-996.5 NEC
    following
      abortion 639.6
      ectopic or molar pregnancy 639.6
      infusion, perfusion, or transfusion 999.1
    in pregnancy, childbirth, or puerperium 673.0 [5th]
    traumatic 958.0
  amniotic fluid (pulmonary) 673.1 [5th]
    with
      abortion - *see* Abortion, by type, with embolism
      ectopic pregnancy (*see also* categories 633.0-633.9) 639.6
      molar pregnancy (*see also* categories 630-632) 639.6
    following
      abortion 639.6
      ectopic or molar pregnancy 639.6
  aorta, aortic 444.1
    abdominal 444.0

Embolism – *continued*
  aorta, aortic – *continued*
    bifurcation 444.0
    saddle 444.0
    thoracic 444.1
  artery 444.9
    auditory, internal 433.8 [5th]
    basilar (*see also* Occlusion, artery, basilar) 433.0 [5th]
    bladder 444.89
    carotid (common) (internal) (*see also* Occlusion, artery, carotid) 433.1 [5th]
    cerebellar (anterior inferior) (posterior inferior) (superior) 433.8 [5th]
    cerebral (*see also* Embolism, brain) 434.1 [5th]
    choroidal (anterior) 433.8 [5th]
    communicating posterior 433.8 [5th]
    coronary (*see also* Infarct, myocardium) 410.9 [5th]
      without myocardial infarction 411.81
    extremity 444.22
      lower 444.22
      upper 444.21
    hypophyseal 433.8 [5th]
    mesenteric (with gangrene) 557.0
    ophthalmic (*see also* Occlusion, retina) 362.30
    peripheral 444.22
    pontine 433.8 [5th]
    precerebral NEC - *see* Occlusion, artery, precerebral
    pulmonary - *see* Embolism, pulmonary
    pyemic 449
      pulmonary 415.12
    renal 593.81
    retinal (*see also* Occlusion, retina) 362.30
    septic 449
      pulmonary 415.12
    specified site NEC 444.89
    vertebral (*see also* Occlusion, artery, vertebral) 433.2 [5th]
  auditory, internal 433.8 [5th]
  basilar (artery) (*see also* Occlusion, artery, basilar) 433.0 [5th]
  birth, mother - *see* Embolism, obstetrical
  blood-clot
    with
      abortion - *see* Abortion, by type, with embolism
      ectopic pregnancy (*see also* categories 633.0-633.9) 639.6
      molar pregnancy (*see also* categories 630-632) 639.6
    following
      abortion 639.6
      ectopic or molar pregnancy 639.6
    in pregnancy, childbirth, or puerperium 673.2 [5th]
  brain 434.1 [5th]
    with
      abortion - *see* Abortion, by type, with embolism
      ectopic pregnancy (*see also* categories 633.0-633.9) 639.6
      molar pregnancy (*see also* categories 630-632) 639.6
    following
      abortion 639.6
      ectopic or molar pregnancy 639.6
    late effect - *see* Late effect(s) (of) cerebrovascular disease
    puerperal, postpartum, childbirth 674.0 [5th]
  capillary 448.9
  cardiac (*see also* Infarct, myocardium) 410.9 [5th]
  carotid (artery) (common) (internal) (*see also* Occlusion, artery, carotid) 433.1 [5th]

Embolism – *continued*
cavernous sinus (venous) - *see* Embolism, intracranial venous sinus
cerebral (*see also* Embolism, brain) 434.1 5th
cholesterol - *see* Atheroembolism
choroidal (anterior) (artery) 433.8 5th
coronary (artery or vein) (systemic) (*see also* Infarct, myocardium) 410.9 5th
without myocardial infarction 411.81
due to (presence of) any device, implant, or graft classifiable to 996.0-996.5 - *see* Complications, due to (presence of) any device, implant, or graft classified to 996.0-996.5 NEC
encephalomalacia (*see also* Embolism, brain) 434.1 5th
extremities 444.22
lower 444.22
upper 444.21
eye 362.30
fat (cerebral) (pulmonary) (systemic) 958.1
with
abortion - *see* Abortion, by type, with embolism
ectopic pregnancy (*see also* categories 633.0-633.9) 639.6
molar pregnancy (*see also* categories 630-632) 639.6
complicating delivery or puerperium 673.8 5th
following
abortion 639.6
ectopic or molar pregnancy 639.6
in pregnancy, childbirth, or the puerperium 673.8 5th
femoral (artery) 444.22
vein 453.6 ▲
deep 453.41
following
abortion 639.6
ectopic or molar pregnancy 639.6
infusion, perfusion, or transfusion
air 999.1
thrombus 999.2
heart (fatty) (*see also* Infarct, myocardium) 410.9 5th
hepatic (vein) 453.0
iliac (artery) 444.81
iliofemoral 444.81
in pregnancy, childbirth, or puerperium (pulmonary) - *see* Embolism, obstetrical
intestine (artery) (vein) (with gangrene) 557.0
intracranial (*see also* Embolism, brain) 434.1 5th
venous sinus (any) 325
late effect - *see* category 326
nonpyogenic 437.6
in pregnancy or puerperium 671.5 5th
kidney (artery) 593.81
lateral sinus (venous) - *see* Embolism, intracranial venous sinus
longitudinal sinus (venous) - *see* Embolism, intracranial venous sinus
lower extremity 444.22
lung (massive) - *see* Embolism, pulmonary
meninges (*see also* Embolism, brain) 434.1 5th
mesenteric (artery) (with gangrene) 557.0
multiple NEC 444.9
obstetrical (pulmonary) 673.2 5th
air 673.0 5th
amniotic fluid (pulmonary) 673.1 5th
blood-clot 673.2 5th
cardiac 674.8 5th
fat 673.8 5th
heart 674.8 5th
pyemic 673.3 5th
septic 673.3 5th

Embolism – *continued*
obstetrical – *continued*
specified NEC 674.8 5th
ophthalmic (*see also* Occlusion, retina) 362.30
paradoxical NEC 444.9
penis 607.82
peripheral arteries NEC 444.22
lower 444.22
upper 444.21
pituitary 253.8
popliteal (artery) 444.22
portal (vein) 452
postoperative NEC 997.2
cerebral 997.02
mesenteric artery 997.71
other vessels 997.79
peripheral vascular 997.2
pulmonary 415.11
septic 415.11
renal artery 997.72
precerebral artery (*see also* Occlusion, artery, precerebral) 433.9 5th
puerperal - *see* Embolism, obstetrical
pulmonary (acute) (artery) (vein) 415.19 ▲
with
abortion - *see* Abortion, by type, with embolism
ectopic pregnancy (*see also* categories 633.0-633.9) 639.6
molar pregnancy (*see also* categories 630-632) 639.6
chronic 416.2 ●
following
abortion 639.6
ectopic or molar pregnancy 639.6
healed or old V12.51 ●
iatrogenic 415.11
in pregnancy, childbirth, or puerperium - *see* Embolism, obstetrical
personal history of V12.51 ●
postoperative 415.11
septic 415.12
pyemic (multiple) (*see also* Septicemia) 415.12
with
abortion - *see* Abortion, by type, with embolism
ectopic pregnancy (*see also* categories 633.0-633.9) 639.6
molar pregnancy (*see also* categories 630-632) 639.6
Aerobacter aerogenes 415.12
enteric gram-negative bacilli 415.12
Enterobacter aerogenes 415.12
Escherichia coli 415.12
following
abortion 639.6
ectopic or molar pregnancy 639.6
Hemophilus influenzae 415.12
pneumococcal 415.12
Proteus vulgaris 415.12
Pseudomonas (aeruginosa) 415.12
puerperal, postpartum, childbirth (any organism) 673.3 5th
Serratia 415.12
specified organism NEC 415.12
staphylococcal 415.12
aureus 415.12
specified organism NEC 415.12
streptococcal 415.12
renal (artery) 593.81
vein 453.3
retina, retinal (*see also* Occlusion, retina) 362.30
saddle (aorta) 444.0
septic 415.12
arterial 449
septicemic - *see* Embolism, pyemic
sinus - *see* Embolism, intracranial venous sinus

Embolism – *continued*
soap
with
abortion - *see* Abortion, by type, with embolism
ectopic pregnancy (*see also* categories 633.0-633.9) 639.6
molar pregnancy (*see also* categories 630-632) 639.6
following
abortion 639.6
ectopic or molar pregnancy 639.6
spinal cord (nonpyogenic) 336.1
in pregnancy or puerperium 671.5 5th
pyogenic origin 324.1
late effect - *see* category 326
spleen, splenic (artery) 444.89
thrombus (thromboembolism) following infusion, perfusion, or transfusion 999.2
upper extremity 444.21
vein 453.9
with inflammation or phlebitis - *see* Thrombophlebitis
antecubital ●
acute 453.81 ●
chronic 453.71 ●
axillary ●
acute 453.84 ●
chronic 453.74 ●
basilic ●
acute 453.81 ●
chronic 453.71 ●
brachial ●
acute 453.82 ●
chronic 453.72 ●
brachiocephalic (innominate) ●
acute 453.87 ●
chronic 453.77 ●
cephalic ●
acute 453.81 ●
chronic 453.71 ●
cerebral (*see also* Embolism, brain) 434.1 5th
coronary (*see also* Infarct, myocardium) 410.9 5th
without myocardial infarction 411.81
hepatic 453.0
internal jugular ●
acute 453.86 ●
chronic 453.76 ●
lower extremity (superficial) 453.6 ▲
deep 453.40
acute 453.40 ●
calf 453.42 ●
distal (lower leg) 453.42 ●
femoral 453.41 ●
iliac 453.41 ●
lower leg 453.42 ●
peroneal 453.42 ●
popliteal 453.41 ●
proximal (upper leg) 453.41 ●
thigh 453.41 ●
tibial 453.42 ●
~~calf 453.42~~
chronic 453.50 ●
calf 453.52 ●
distal (lower leg) 453.52 ●
femoral 453.51 ●
iliac 453.51 ●
lower leg 453.52 ●
peroneal 453.52 ●
popliteal 453.51 ●
proximal (upper leg) 453.51 ●
thigh 453.51 ●
tibial 453.52 ●
~~distal (lower leg) 453.42~~
~~femoral 453.41~~
~~iliac 453.41~~
~~lower leg 453.42~~
~~peroneal 453.42~~

Embolism – *continued*
vein – *continued*
lower extremity – *continued*
deep – *continued*
~~popliteal 453.41~~
~~proximal (upper leg) 453.41~~
~~thigh 453.41~~
~~tibial 453.42~~
saphenous (greater) (lesser) 453.6 ●
superficial 453.6 ●
mesenteric (with gangrene) 557.0
portal 452
pulmonary - *see* Embolism, pulmonary
radial ●
acute 453.82 ●
chronic 453.72 ●
renal 453.3
saphenous (greater) (lesser) 453.6 ●
specified NEC (acute) 453.89 ▲
with inflammation or phlebitis - *see* Thrombophlebitis
chronic 453.79 ●
subclavian ●
acute 453.85 ●
chronic 453.75 ●
superior vena cava ●
acute 453.87 ●
chronic 453.77 ●
thoracic ●
acute 453.87 ●
chronic 453.77 ●
ulnar ●
acute 453.82 ●
chronic 453.72 ●
upper extremity 453.83 ●
acute 453.83 ●
deep 453.82 ●
superficial 453.81 ●
chronic 453.73 ●
deep 453.72 ●
superficial 453.71 ●
vena cava ~~(inferior) (superior) 453.2~~
inferior 453.2 ●
superior ●
acute 453.87 ●
chronic 453.77 ●
vessels of brain (*see also* Embolism, brain) 434.1 5th
Embolization - *see* Embolism
Embolus - *see* Embolism
Embryoma (M9080/1) - *see also* Neoplasm, by site, uncertain behavior
benign (M9080/0) - *see* Neoplasm, by site, benign
kidney (M8960/3) 189.0
liver (M8970/3) 155.0
malignant (M9080/3) - *see also* Neoplasm, by site, malignant
kidney (M8960/3) 189.0
liver (M8970/3) 155.0
testis (M9070/3) 186.9
undescended 186.0
testis (M9070/3) 186.9
undescended 186.0
Embryonic
circulation 747.9
heart 747.9
vas deferens 752.89
Embryopathia NEC 759.9
Embryotomy, fetal 763.89
Embryotoxon 743.43
interfering with vision 743.42
Emesis - *see also* Vomiting
bilious 787.04 ●
gravidarum - *see* Hyperemesis, gravidarum
Emissions, nocturnal (semen) 608.89
Emotional
crisis - *see* Crisis, emotional
disorder (*see also* Disorder, mental) 300.9
instability (excessive) 301.3
lability 799.24 ●
overlay - *see* Reaction, adjustment

4th Fourth Digit Required 5th Fifth Digit Required | *[code]* Manifestation Code | ● New Line ▲ Revised Line text New Text ~~text~~ Deleted text

Emotional - *continued*
- upset 300.9

Emotionality, pathological 301.3
Emotogenic disease (*see also* Disorder, psychogenic) 306.9
Emphysema (atrophic) (centriacinar) (centrilobular) (chronic) (diffuse) (essential) (hypertrophic) (interlobular) (lung) (obstructive) (panlobular) (paracicatricial) (paracinar) (postural) (pulmonary) (senile) (subpleural) (traction) (unilateral) (unilobular) (vesicular) 492.8
- with bronchitis
  - chronic 491.20
    - with
      - acute bronchitis 491.22
      - exacerbation (acute) 491.21
- bullous (giant) 492.0
- cellular tissue 958.7
  - surgical 998.81
- compensatory 518.2
- congenital 770.2
- conjunctiva 372.89
- connective tissue 958.7
  - surgical 998.81
- due to fumes or vapors 506.4
- eye 376.89
- eyelid 374.85
  - surgical 998.81
  - traumatic 958.7
- fetus or newborn (interstitial) (mediastinal) (unilobular) 770.2
- heart 416.9
- interstitial 518.1
  - congenital 770.2
  - fetus or newborn 770.2
- laminated tissue 958.7
  - surgical 998.81
- mediastinal 518.1
  - fetus or newborn 770.2
- newborn (interstitial) (mediastinal) (unilobular) 770.2
- obstructive diffuse with fibrosis 492.8
- orbit 376.89
- subcutaneous 958.7
  - due to trauma 958.7
  - nontraumatic 518.1
  - surgical 998.81
- surgical 998.81
- thymus (gland) (congenital) 254.8
- traumatic 958.7
- tuberculous (*see also* Tuberculosis, pulmonary) 011.9 [5th]

Employment examination (certification) V70.5
Empty sella (turcica) **syndrome** 253.8
Empyema (chest) (diaphragmatic) (double) (encapsulated) (general) (interlobar) (lung) (medial) (necessitatis) (perforating chest wall) (pleura) (pneumococcal) (residual) (sacculated) (streptococcal) (supradiaphragmatic) 510.9
- with fistula 510.0
- accessory sinus (chronic) (*see also* Sinusitis) 473.9
- acute 510.9
  - with fistula 510.0
- antrum (chronic) (*see also* Sinusitis, maxillary) 473.0
- brain (any part) (*see also* Abscess, brain) 324.0
- ethmoidal (sinus) (chronic) (*see also* Sinusitis, ethmoidal) 473.2
- extradural (*see also* Abscess, extradural) 324.9
- frontal (sinus) (chronic) (*see also* Sinusitis, frontal) 473.1
- gallbladder (*see also* Cholecystitis, acute) 575.0
- mastoid (process) (acute) (*see also* Mastoiditis, acute) 383.00

Empyema - *continued*
- maxilla, maxillary 526.4
  - sinus (chronic) (*see also* Sinusitis, maxillary) 473.0
- nasal sinus (chronic) (*see also* Sinusitis) 473.9
- sinus (accessory) (nasal) (*see also* Sinusitis) 473.9
- sphenoidal (chronic) (sinus) (*see also* Sinusitis, sphenoidal) 473.3
- subarachnoid (*see also* Abscess, extradural) 324.9
- subdural (*see also* Abscess, extradural) 324.9
- tuberculous (*see also* Tuberculosis, pleura) 012.0 [5th]
- ureter (*see also* Ureteritis) 593.89
- ventricular (*see also* Abscess, brain) 324.0

Enameloma 520.2
Encephalitis (bacterial) (chronic) (hemorrhagic) (idiopathic) (nonepidemic) (spurious) (subacute) 323.9
- acute - *see also* Encephalitis, viral
  - disseminated (postinfectious) NEC 136.9 *[323.61]*
    - postimmunization or postvaccination 323.51
  - inclusional 049.8
  - inclusion body 049.8
  - necrotizing 049.8
- arboviral, arbovirus NEC 064
- arthropod-borne (*see also* Encephalitis, viral, arthropod-borne) 064
- Australian X 062.4
- Bwamba fever 066.3
- California (virus) 062.5
- Central European 063.2
- Czechoslovakian 063.2
- Dawson's (inclusion body) 046.2
- diffuse sclerosing 046.2
- due to
  - actinomycosis 039.8 *[323.41]*
  - cat-scratch disease 078.3 *[323.01]*
  - human herpesvirus 6 058.21
  - human herpesvirus 7 058.29
  - human herpesvirus NEC 058.29
  - infection classified elsewhere 136.9 *[323.41]*
  - infectious mononucleosis 075 *[323.01]*
  - malaria (*see also* Malaria) 084.6 *[323.2]*
  - negishi virus 064
  - ornithosis 073.7 *[323.01]*
  - prophylactic inoculation against smallpox 323.51
  - rickettsiosis (*see also* Rickettsiosis) 083.9 *[323.1]*
  - rubella 056.01
  - toxoplasmosis (acquired) 130.0
    - congenital (active) 771.2 *[323.41]*
  - typhus (fever) (*see also* Typhus) 081.9 *[323.1]*
  - vaccination (smallpox) 323.51
- Eastern equine 062.2
- endemic 049.8
- epidemic 049.8
- equine (acute) (infectious) (viral) 062.9
  - eastern 062.2
  - venezuelan 066.2
  - western 062.1
- Far Eastern 063.0
- following vaccination or other immunization procedure 323.51
- herpes 054.3
- human herpesvirus 6 058.21
- human herpesvirus 7 058.29
- human herpesvirus NEC 058.29
- ilheus (virus) 062.8
- inclusion body 046.2
- infectious (acute) (virus) NEC 049.8
- influenzal 487.8 *[323.41]*
  - lethargic 049.8
- Japanese (B type) 062.0
- La Crosse 062.5

Encephalitis - *continued*
- Langat 063.8
- late effect - *see* Late, effect, encephalitis
- lead 984.9 *[323.71]*
- lethargic (acute) (infectious) (influenzal) 049.8
- lethargica 049.8
- louping ill 063.1
- lupus 710.0 *[323.81]*
- lymphatica 049.0
- Mengo 049.8
- meningococcal 036.1
- mumps 072.2
- Murray Valley 062.4
- myoclonic 049.8
- Negishi virus 064
- otitic NEC 382.4 *[323.41]*
- parasitic NEC 123.9 *[323.41]*
- periaxialis (concentrica) (diffusa) 341.1
- postchickenpox 052.0
- postexanthematous NEC 057.9 *[323.62]*
- postimmunization 323.51
- postinfectious NEC 136.9 *[323.62]*
- postmeasles 055.0
- posttraumatic 323.81
- postvaccinal (smallpox) 323.51
- postvaricella 052.0
- postviral NEC 079.99 *[323.62]*
  - postexanthematous 057.9 *[323.62]*
    - specified NEC 057.8 *[323.62]*
- Powassan 063.8
- progressive subcortical (Binswanger's) 290.12
- Rasmussen 323.81
- Rio Bravo 049.8
- rubella 056.01
- Russian
  - autumnal 062.0
  - spring-summer type (taiga) 063.0
- saturnine 984.9 *[323.71]*
- Semliki Forest 062.8
- serous 048
- slow-acting virus NEC 046.8
- specified cause NEC 323.81
- St. Louis type 062.3
- subacute sclerosing 046.2
- subcorticalis chronica 290.12
- summer 062.0
- suppurative 324.0
- syphilitic 094.81
  - congenital 090.41
- tick-borne 063.9
- torula, torular 117.5 *[323.41]*
- toxic NEC 989.9 *[323.71]*
- toxoplasmic (acquired) 130.0
  - congenital (active) 771.2 *[323.41]*
- trichinosis 124 *[323.41]*
- Trypanosomiasis (*see also* Trypanosomiasis) 086.9 *[323.2]*
- tuberculous (*see also* Tuberculosis) 013.6 [5th]
- type B (Japanese) 062.0
- type C 062.3
- van Bogaert's 046.2
- Venezuelan 066.2
- Vienna type 049.8
- viral, virus 049.9
  - arthropod-borne NEC 064
    - mosquito-borne 062.9
      - Australian X disease 062.4
      - California virus 062.5
      - Eastern equine 062.2
      - Ilheus virus 062.8
      - Japanese (B type) 062.0
      - Murray Valley 062.4
      - specified type NEC 062.8
      - St. Louis 062.3
      - type B 062.0
      - type C 062.3
      - Western equine 062.1
    - tick-borne 063.9
      - biundulant 063.2
      - Central European 063.2
      - Czechoslovakian 063.2

Encephalitis - *continued*
- viral, virus - *continued*
  - arthropod-borne - *continued*
    - tick-borne - *continued*
      - diphasic meningoencephalitis 063.2
      - Far Eastern 063.0
      - Langat 063.8
      - louping ill 063.1
      - Powassan 063.8
      - Russian spring-summer (taiga) 063.0
      - specified type NEC 063.8
    - vector unknown 064
  - slow acting NEC 046.8
  - specified type NEC 049.8
  - vaccination, prophylactic (against) V05.0
- von Economo's 049.8
- Western equine 062.1
- West Nile type 066.41

Encephalocele 742.0
- orbit 376.81

Encephalocystocele 742.0
Encephalomalacia (brain) (cerebellar) (cerebral) (cerebrospinal) (*see also* Softening, brain) 434.9 [5th]
- due to
  - hemorrhage (*see also* Hemorrhage, brain) 431
  - recurrent spasm of artery 435.9
- embolic (cerebral) (*see also* Embolism, brain) 434.1 [5th]
- subcorticalis chronicus arteriosclerotica 290.12
- thrombotic (*see also* Thrombosis, brain) 434.0 [5th]

Encephalomeningitis - *see* Meningoencephalitis
Encephalomeningocele 742.0
Encephalomeningomyelitis - *see* Meningoencephalitis
Encephalomeningopathy (*see also* Meningoencephalitis) 349.9
Encephalomyelitis (chronic) (granulomatous) (myalgic, benign) (*see also* Encephalitis) 323.9
- abortive disseminated 049.8
- acute disseminated (ADEM) (postinfectious) 136.9 *[323.61]*
  - infectious 136.9 *[323.61]*
  - noninfectious 323.81
  - postimmunization 323.51
- due to
  - cat-scratch disease 078.3 *[323.01]*
  - infectious mononucleosis 075 *[323.01]*
  - ornithosis 073.7 *[323.01]*
  - vaccination (any) 323.51
- equine (acute) (infectious) 062.9
  - eastern 062.2
  - venezuelan 066.2
  - western 062.1
- funicularis infectiosa 049.8
- late effect - *see* Late, effect, encephalitis
- Munch-Peterson's 049.8
- postchickenpox 052.0
- postimmunization 323.51
- postmeasles 055.0
- postvaccinal (smallpox) 323.51
- rubella 056.01
- specified cause NEC 323.81
- syphilitic 094.81
- West Nile 066.41

Encephalomyelocele 742.0
Encephalomyelomeningitis - *see* Meningoencephalitis
Encephalomyeloneuropathy 349.9
Encephalomyelopathy 349.9
- subacute necrotizing (infantile) 330.8

Encephalomyeloradiculitis (acute) 357.0
Encephalomyeloradiculoneuritis (acute) 357.0
Encephalomyeloradiculopathy 349.9
Encephalomyocarditis 074.23

Emotional – Encephalomyocarditis

Encephalopathia hyperbilirubinemica, newborn – Endocarditis

Encephalopathia hyperbilirubinemica, newborn 774.7
- due to isoimmunization (conditions classifiable to 773.0-773.2) 773.4

Encephalopathy (acute) 348.30
- alcoholic 291.2
- anoxic - *see* Damage, brain, anoxic
- arteriosclerotic 437.0
  - late effect - *see* Late effect(s) (of) cerebrovascular disease
- bilirubin, newborn 774.7
  - due to isoimmunization 773.4
- congenital 742.9
- demyelinating (callosal) 341.8
- due to
  - birth injury (intracranial) 767.8
  - dialysis 294.8
    - transient 293.9
  - drugs - (*see also* Table of Drugs and Chemicals) 348.39
  - hyperinsulinism - *see* Hyperinsulinism
  - influenza (virus) 487.8
  - lack of vitamin (*see also* Deficiency, vitamin) 269.2
  - nicotinic acid deficiency 291.2
  - serum (nontherapeutic) (therapeutic) 999.5
  - syphilis 094.81
  - trauma (postconcussional) 310.2
    - current (*see also* Concussion, brain) 850.9
      - with skull fracture - *see* Fracture, skull, by site, with intracranial injury
  - vaccination 323.51
- hepatic 572.2
- hyperbilirubinemic, newborn 774.7
  - due to isoimmunization (conditions classifiable to 773.0-773.2) 773.4
- hypertensive 437.2
- hypoglycemic 251.2
- hypoxic - *see also* Damage, brain, anoxic
  - ischemic (HIE) 768.70 ▲
    - mild 768.71 ●
    - moderate 768.72 ●
    - severe 768.73 ●
- infantile cystic necrotizing (congenital) 341.8
- lead 984.9 *[323.71]*
- leukopolio 330.0
- metabolic (*see also* Delirium) 348.31
  - toxic 349.82
- necrotizing
  - hemorrhagic (acute) 323.61
  - subacute 330.8
- other specified type NEC 348.39
- pellagrous 265.2
- portal-systemic 572.2
- postcontusional 310.2
- posttraumatic 310.2
- saturnine 984.9 *[323.71]*
- septic 348.31
- spongioform, subacute (viral) 046.19
- subacute
  - necrotizing 330.8
  - spongioform 046.19
  - viral, spongioform 046.19
- subcortical progressive (Schilder) 341.1
  - chronic (Binswanger's) 290.12
- toxic 349.82
  - metabolic 349.82
- traumatic (postconcussional) 310.2
  - current (*see also* Concussion, brain) 850.9
    - with skull fracture - *see* Fracture, skull, by site, with intracranial injury
- vitamin B deficiency NEC 266.9
- Wernicke's (superior hemorrhagic polioencephalitis) 265.1

Encephalorrhagia (*see also* Hemorrhage, brain) 432.9
- healed or old V12.54

Encephalorrhagia – *continued*
- late effect - *see* Late effect(s) (of) cerebrovascular disease

Encephalosis, posttraumatic 310.2

Enchondroma (M9220/0) - *see also* Neoplasm, bone, benign
- multiple, congenital 756.4

Enchondromatosis (cartilaginous) (congenital) (multiple) 756.4

Enchondroses, multiple (cartilaginous) (congenital) 756.4

Encopresis (*see also* Incontinence, feces) 787.6
- nonorganic origin 307.7

Encounter for - *see also* Admission for
- administrative purpose only V68.9
  - referral of patient without examination or treatment V68.81
  - specified purpose NEC V68.89
- chemotherapy, (oral) (intravenous), antineoplastic V58.11 ▲
- dialysis
  - extracorporeal (renal) V56.0
  - peritoneal V56.8
- disability examination V68.01
- end-of-life care V66.7
- hospice care V66.7
- immunizations (childhood) appropriate for age V20.2 ●
- immunotherapy, antineoplastic V58.12
- screening mammogram NEC V76.12
  - for high-risk patient V76.11
- palliative care V66.7
- paternity testing V70.4
- radiotherapy V58.0
- respirator [ventilator] dependence
  - during
    - mechanical failure V46.14
    - power failure V46.12
  - for weaning V46.13
- routine infant and child vision and hearing testing V20.2 ●
- school examination V70.3 ●
  - following surgery V67.09 ●
- terminal care V66.7
- weaning from respirator [ventilator] V46.13

Encystment - *see* Cyst

End of life
- artificial heart valve 996.02
- pacemaker lead or battery V53.31
- joint prosthesis (*see also* Complications, mechanical, devices NEC, prosthetic NEC, joint) 996.47

End-of-life care V66.7

Endamebiasis - *see* Amebiasis

Endamoeba - *see* Amebiasis

Endarteritis (bacterial, subacute) (infective) (septic) 447.6
- brain, cerebral or cerebrospinal 437.4
  - late effect - *see* Late effect(s) (of) cerebrovascular disease
- coronary (artery) - *see* Arteriosclerosis, coronary
- deformans - *see* Arteriosclerosis
- embolic (*see also* Embolism) 444.9
- obliterans - *see also* Arteriosclerosis
  - pulmonary 417.8
- pulmonary 417.8
- retina 362.18
- senile - *see* Arteriosclerosis
- syphilitic 093.89
  - brain or cerebral 094.89
  - congenital 090.5
  - spinal 094.89
- tuberculous (*see also* Tuberculosis) 017.9 [5th]

Endemic - *see* condition

Endocarditis (chronic) (indeterminate) (interstitial) (marantic) (nonbacterial thrombotic) (residual) (sclerotic) (sclerous) (senile) (valvular) 424.90
- with
  - rheumatic fever (conditions classifiable to 390)
    - active - *see* Endocarditis, acute, rheumatic
    - inactive or quiescent (with chorea) 397.9
- acute or subacute 421.9
  - rheumatic (aortic) (mitral) (pulmonary) (tricuspid) 391.1
    - with chorea (acute) (rheumatic) (Sydenham's) 392.0
- aortic (heart) (nonrheumatic) (valve) 424.1
  - with
    - mitral (valve) disease 396.9
      - active or acute 391.1
        - with chorea (acute) (rheumatic) (Sydenham's) 392.0
      - bacterial 421.0
    - rheumatic fever (conditions classifiable to 390)
      - active - *see* Endocarditis, acute, rheumatic
      - inactive or quiescent (with chorea) 395.9
        - with mitral disease 396.9
  - acute or subacute 421.9
  - arteriosclerotic 424.1
  - congenital 746.89
  - hypertensive 424.1
  - rheumatic (chronic) (inactive) 395.9
    - with mitral (valve) disease 396.9
      - active or acute 391.1
        - with chorea (acute) (rheumatic) (Sydenham's) 392.0
    - active or acute 391.1
      - with chorea (acute) (rheumatic) (Sydenham's) 392.0
  - specified cause, except rheumatic 424.1
  - syphilitic 093.22
- arteriosclerotic or due to arteriosclerosis 424.99
- atypical verrucous (Libman-Sacks) 710.0 *[424.91]*
- bacterial (acute) (any valve) (chronic) (subacute) 421.0
- blastomycotic 116.0 *[421.1]*
- candidal 112.81
- congenital 425.3
- constrictive 421.0
- Coxsackie 074.22
- due to
  - blastomycosis 116.0 *[421.1]*
  - candidiasis 112.81
  - coxsackie (virus) 074.22
  - disseminated lupus erythematosus 710.0 *[424.91]*
  - histoplasmosis (*see also* Histoplasmosis) 115.94
  - hypertension (benign) 424.99
  - moniliasis 112.81
  - prosthetic cardiac valve 996.61
  - Q fever 083.0 *[421.1]*
  - serratia marcescens 421.0
  - typhoid (fever) 002.0 *[421.1]*
- fetal 425.3
- gonococcal 098.84
- hypertensive 424.99
- infectious or infective (acute) (any valve) (chronic) (subacute) 421.0
- lenta (acute) (any valve) (chronic) (subacute) 421.0
- Libman-Sacks 710.0 *[424.91]*
- Loeffler's (parietal fibroplastic) 421.0
- malignant (acute) (any valve) (chronic) (subacute) 421.0
- meningococcal 036.42

Endocarditis – *continued*
- mitral (chronic) (double) (fibroid) (heart) (inactive) (valve) (with chorea) 394.9
  - with
    - aortic (valve) disease 396.9
      - active or acute 391.1
        - with chorea (acute) (rheumatic) (Sydenham's) 392.0
    - rheumatic fever (conditions classifiable to 390)
      - active - *see* Endocarditis, acute, rheumatic
      - inactive or quiescent (with chorea) 394.9
        - with aortic valve disease 396.9
  - active or acute 391.1
    - with chorea (acute) (rheumatic) (Sydenham's) 392.0
    - bacterial 421.0
  - arteriosclerotic 424.0
  - congenital 746.89
  - hypertensive 424.0
  - nonrheumatic 424.0
    - acute or subacute 421.9
  - syphilitic 093.21
- monilial 112.81
- mycotic (acute) (any valve) (chronic) (subacute) 421.0
- pneumococcic (acute) (any valve) (chronic) (subacute) 421.0
- pulmonary (chronic) (heart) (valve) 424.3
  - with
    - rheumatic fever (conditions classifiable to 390)
      - active - *see* Endocarditis, acute, rheumatic
      - inactive or quiescent (with chorea) 397.1
  - acute or subacute 421.9
    - rheumatic 391.1
      - with chorea (acute) (rheumatic) (Sydenham's) 392.0
  - arteriosclerotic or due to arteriosclerosis 424.3
  - congenital 746.09
  - hypertensive or due to hypertension (benign) 424.3
  - rheumatic (chronic) (inactive) (with chorea) 397.1
    - active or acute 391.1
      - with chorea (acute) (rheumatic) (Sydenham's) 392.0
  - syphilitic 093.24
- purulent (acute) (any valve) (chronic) (subacute) 421.0
- rheumatic (chronic) (inactive) (with chorea) 397.9
  - active or acute (aortic) (mitral) (pulmonary) (tricuspid) 391.1
    - with chorea (acute) (rheumatic) (Sydenham's) 392.0
- septic (acute) (any valve) (chronic) (subacute) 421.0
- specified cause, except rheumatic 424.99
- streptococcal (acute) (any valve) (chronic) (subacute) 421.0
- subacute - *see* Endocarditis, acute
- suppurative (any valve) (acute) (chronic) (subacute) 421.0
- syphilitic NEC 093.20
- toxic (*see also* Endocarditis, acute) 421.9
- tricuspid (chronic) (heart) (inactive) (rheumatic) (valve) (with chorea) 397.0
  - with
    - rheumatic fever (conditions classifiable to 390)
      - active - *see* Endocarditis, acute, rheumatic
      - inactive or quiescent (with chorea) 397.0

- **Endocarditis** – *continued*
  - tricuspid – *continued*
    - active or acute 391.1
      - with chorea (acute) (rheumatic) (Sydenham's) 392.0
    - arteriosclerotic 424.2
    - congenital 746.89
    - hypertensive 424.2
    - nonrheumatic 424.2
      - acute or subacute 421.9
    - specified cause, except rheumatic 424.2
    - syphilitic 093.23
  - tuberculous (*see also* Tuberculosis) 017.9 5th *[424.91]*
  - typhoid 002.0 *[421.1]*
  - ulcerative (acute) (any valve) (chronic) (subacute) 421.0
  - vegetative (acute) (any valve) (chronic) (subacute) 421.0
  - verrucous (acute) (any valve) (chronic) (subacute) NEC 710.0 *[424.91]*
    - nonbacterial 710.0 *[424.91]*
    - nonrheumatic 710.0 *[424.91]*
- **Endocardium, endocardial** - *see also* condition
  - cushion defect 745.60
    - specified type NEC 745.69
- **Endocervicitis** (*see also* Cervicitis) 616.0
  - due to
    - intrauterine (contraceptive) device 996.65
  - gonorrheal (acute) 098.15
    - chronic or duration of 2 months or over 098.35
- **Endocervicitis** – *continued*
  - hyperplastic 616.0
  - syphilitic 095.8
  - trichomonal 131.09
  - tuberculous (*see also* Tuberculosis) 016.7 5th
- **Endocrine** - *see* condition
- **Endocrinopathy, pluriglandular** 258.9
- **Endodontitis** 522.0
- **Endomastoiditis** (*see also* Mastoiditis) 383.9
- **Endometrioma** 617.9
- **Endometriosis** 617.9
  - appendix 617.5
  - bladder 617.8
  - bowel 617.5
  - broad ligament 617.3
  - cervix 617.0
  - colon 617.5
  - cul-de-sac (Douglas') 617.3
  - exocervix 617.0
  - fallopian tube 617.2
  - female genital organ NEC 617.8
  - gallbladder 617.8
  - in scar of skin 617.6
  - internal 617.0
  - intestine 617.5
  - lung 617.8
  - myometrium 617.0
  - ovary 617.1
  - parametrium 617.3
  - pelvic peritoneum 617.3
  - peritoneal (pelvic) 617.3
  - rectovaginal septum 617.4
  - rectum 617.5
  - round ligament 617.3
  - skin 617.6
  - specified site NEC 617.8
  - stromal (M8931/1) 236.0
  - umbilicus 617.8
  - uterus 617.0
    - internal 617.0
  - vagina 617.4
  - vulva 617.8
- **Endometritis** (nonspecific) (purulent) (septic) (suppurative) 615.9
  - with
    - abortion - *see* Abortion, by type, with sepsis
    - ectopic pregnancy (*see also* categories 633.0-633.9) 639.0
- **Endometritis** – *continued*
  - with – *continued*
    - molar pregnancy (*see also* categories 630-632) 639.0
  - acute 615.0
  - blennorrhagic 098.16
    - acute 098.16
    - chronic or duration of 2 months or over 098.36
  - cervix, cervical (*see also* Cervicitis) 616.0
    - hyperplastic 616.0
  - chronic 615.1
  - complicating pregnancy 670.1 5th ▲
    - affecting fetus or newborn 760.8
    - septic 670.2 5th ●
  - decidual 615.9
  - following
    - abortion 639.0
    - ectopic or molar pregnancy 639.0
  - gonorrheal (acute) 098.16
    - chronic or duration of 2 months or over 098.36
  - hyperplastic (*see also* Hyperplasia, endometrium) 621.30
    - cervix 616.0
  - polypoid - *see* Endometritis, hyperplastic
  - puerperal, postpartum, childbirth 670.1 5th ▲
    - septic 670.2 5th ●
  - senile (atrophic) 615.9
  - subacute 615.0
  - tuberculous (*see also* Tuberculosis) 016.7 5th
- **Endometrium** - *see* condition
- **Endomyocardiopathy, South African** 425.2
- **Endomyocarditis** - *see* Endocarditis
- **Endomyofibrosis** 425.0
- **Endomyometritis** (*see also* Endometritis) 615.9
- **Endopericarditis** - *see* Endocarditis
- **Endoperineuritis** - *see* Disorder, nerve
- **Endophlebitis** (*see also* Phlebitis) 451.9
  - leg 451.2
    - deep (vessels) 451.19
    - superficial (vessels) 451.0
  - portal (vein) 572.1
  - retina 362.18
  - specified site NEC 451.89
  - syphilitic 093.89
- **Endophthalmia** (*see also* Endophthalmitis) 360.00
  - gonorrheal 098.42
- **Endophthalmitis** (globe) (infective) (metastatic) (purulent) (subacute) 360.00
  - acute 360.01
  - bleb associated 379.63
  - chronic 360.03
  - parasitic 360.13
  - phacoanaphylactic 360.19
  - specified type NEC 360.19
  - sympathetic 360.11
- **Endosalpingioma** (M9111/1) 236.2
- **Endosalpingiosis** 629.89
- **Endosteitis** - *see* Osteomyelitis
- **Endothelioma, bone** (M9260/3) - *see* Neoplasm, bone, malignant
- **Endotheliosis** 287.8
  - hemorrhagic infectional 287.8
- **Endotoxemia** - code to condition
- **Endotoxic shock** 785.52
- **Endotrachelitis** (*see also* Cervicitis) 616.0
- **Enema rash** 692.89
- **Engel-von Recklinghausen disease or syndrome** (osteitis fibrosa cystica) 252.01
- **Engelmann's disease** (diaphyseal sclerosis) 756.59
- **English disease** (*see also* Rickets) 268.0
- **Engman's disease** (infectious eczematoid dermatitis) 690.8
- **Engorgement**
  - breast 611.79
    - newborn 778.7
- **Engorgement** – *continued*
  - breast – *continued*
    - puerperal, postpartum 676.2 5th
  - liver 573.9
  - lung 514
  - pulmonary 514
  - retina, venous 362.37
  - stomach 536.8
  - venous, retina 362.37
- **Enlargement, enlarged** - *see also* Hypertrophy
  - abdomen 789.3 5th
  - adenoids 474.12
    - and tonsils 474.10
  - alveolar process or ridge 525.8
  - apertures of diaphragm (congenital) 756.6
  - blind spot, visual field 368.42
  - gingival 523.8
  - heart, cardiac (*see also* Hypertrophy, cardiac) 429.3
  - lacrimal gland, chronic 375.03
  - liver (*see also* Hypertrophy, liver) 789.1
  - lymph gland or node 785.6
  - orbit 376.46
  - organ or site, congenital NEC - *see* Anomaly, specified type NEC
  - parathyroid (gland) 252.01
  - pituitary fossa 793.0
  - prostate (simple) (soft) 600.00
    - with
      - other lower urinary tract symptoms (LUTS) 600.01
      - urinary
        - obstruction 600.01
        - retention 600.01
  - sella turcica 793.0
  - spleen (*see also* Splenomegaly) 789.2
    - congenital 759.0
  - thymus (congenital) (gland) 254.0
  - thyroid (gland) (*see also* Goiter) 240.9
  - tongue 529.8
  - tonsils 474.11
    - and adenoids 474.10
  - uterus 621.2
- **Enophthalmos** 376.50
  - due to
    - atrophy of orbital tissue 376.51
    - surgery 376.52
    - trauma 376.52
- **Enostosis** 526.89
- **Entamebiasis** - *see* Amebiasis
- **Entamebic** - *see* Amebiasis
- **Entanglement, umbilical cord**(s) 663.3 5th
  - with compression 663.2 5th
  - affecting fetus or newborn 762.5
  - around neck with compression 663.1 5th
  - twins in monoamniotic sac 663.2 5th
- **Enteralgia** 789.0
- **Enteric** - *see* condition
- **Enteritis** (acute) (catarrhal) (choleraic) (chronic) (congestive) (diarrheal) (exudative) (follicular) (hemorrhagic) (infantile) (lienteric) (noninfectious) (perforative) (phlegmonous) (presumed noninfectious) (pseudomembranous) 558.9
  - adaptive 564.9
  - aertrycke infection 003.0
  - allergic 558.3
  - amebic (*see also* Amebiasis) 006.9
    - with abscess - *see* Abscess, amebic
    - acute 006.0
      - with abscess - *see* Abscess, amebic
      - nondysenteric 006.2
    - chronic 006.1
      - with abscess - *see* Abscess, amebic
      - nondysenteric 006.2
    - nondysenteric 006.2
  - anaerobic (cocci) (gram-negative) (gram-positive) (mixed) NEC 008.46
  - bacillary NEC 004.9
  - bacterial NEC 008.5
    - specified NEC 008.49
- **Enteritis** – *continued*
  - Bacteroides (fragilis) (melaninogeniscus) (oralis) 008.46
  - Butyrivibrio (fibriosolvens) 008.46
  - Campylobacter 008.43
  - Candida 112.85
  - Chilomastix 007.8
  - choleriformis 001.1
  - chronic 558.9
    - ulcerative (*see also* Colitis, ulcerative) 556.9
  - cicatrizing (chronic) 555.0
  - Clostridium
    - botulinum 005.1
    - difficile 008.45
    - haemolyticum 008.46
    - novyi 008.46
    - perfringens (C) (F) 008.46
    - specified type NEC 008.46
  - coccidial 007.2
  - dietetic 558.9
  - due to
    - achylia gastrica 536.8
    - adenovirus 008.62
    - Aerobacter aerogenes 008.2
    - anaerobes (*see also* Enteritis, anaerobic) 008.46
    - Arizona (bacillus) 008.1
    - astrovirus 008.66
    - Bacillus coli - *see* Enteritis, E. coli
    - bacteria NEC 008.5
      - specified NEC 008.49
    - Bacteroides (*see also* Enteritis, Bacteroides) 008.46
    - Butyrivibrio (fibriosolvens) 008.46
    - calicivirus 008.65 ▲
    - Camplyobacter 008.43
    - Clostridium - *see* Enteritis, Clostridium
    - Cockle agent 008.64
    - Coxsackie (virus) 008.67
    - Ditchling agent 008.64
    - ECHO virus 008.67
    - Enterobacter aerogenes 008.2
    - enterococci 008.49
    - enterovirus NEC 008.67
    - Escherichia coli - *see* Enteritis, E. coli
    - Eubacterium 008.46
    - Fusobacterium (nucleatum) 008.46
    - gram-negative bacteria NEC 008.47
      - anaerobic NEC 008.46
    - Hawaii agent 008.63
    - irritating foods 558.9
    - Klebsiella aerogenes 008.47
    - Marin County agent 008.66
    - Montgomery County agent 008.63
    - norovirus 008.63 ●
    - Norwalk-like agent 008.63
    - Norwalk virus 008.63
    - Otofuke agent 008.63
    - Paracolobactrum arizonae 008.1
    - paracolon bacillus NEC 008.47
      - arizona 008.1
    - Paramatta agent 008.64
    - Peptococcus 008.46
    - Peptostreptococcus 008.46
    - Proprionibacterium 008.46
    - Proteus (bacillus) (mirabilis) (morganii) 008.3
    - Pseudomonas aeruginosa 008.42
    - Rotavirus 008.61
    - Sapporo agent 008.63
    - small round virus (SRV) NEC 008.64
      - featureless NEC 008.63
      - structured NEC 008.63
    - Snow Mountain (SM) agent 008.63
    - specified
      - bacteria NEC 008.49
      - organism, nonbacterial NEC 008.8
      - virus NEC 008.69
    - Staphylococcus 008.41
    - Streptococcus 008.49
      - anaerobic 008.46
    - Taunton agent 008.63
    - Torovirus 008.69

Endocarditis – Enteritis

4th Fourth Digit Required | 5th Fifth Digit Required | *[code]* Manifestation Code | ● New Line | ▲ Revised Line | text New Text | ~~text~~ Deleted text

Enteritis – *continued*
  due to – *continued*
    Treponema 008.46
    Veillonella 008.46
    virus 008.8
      specified type NEC 008.69
    Wollan (W) agent 008.64
    Yersinia enterocolitica 008.44
  dysentery - *see* Dysentery
  E. coli 008.00
    enterohemorrhagic 008.04
    enteroinvasive 008.03
    enteropathogenic 008.01
    enterotoxigenic 008.02
    specified type NEC 008.09
  El Tor 001.1
  embadomonial 007.8
  eosinophilic 558.41
  epidemic 009.0
  Eubacterium 008.46
  fermentative 558.9
  fulminant 557.0
  Fusobacterium (nucleatum) 008.46
  gangrenous (*see also* Enteritis, due to, by organism) 009.0
  giardial 007.1
  gram-negative bacteria NEC 008.47
    anaerobic NEC 008.46
  infectious NEC (*see also* Enteritis, due to, by organism) 009.0
    presumed 009.1
  influenzal 487.8
  ischemic 557.9
    acute 557.0
    chronic 557.1
    due to mesenteric artery insufficiency 557.1
  membranous 564.9
  mucous 564.9
  myxomembranous 564.9
  necrotic (*see also* Enteritis, due to, by organism) 009.0
  necroticans 005.2
  necrotizing of fetus or newborn (*see also* Enterocolitis, necrotizing, newborn) 777.50
  neurogenic 564.9
  newborn 777.8
    necrotizing (*see also* Enterocolitis, necrotizing, newborn) 777.50
  parasitic NEC 129
  paratyphoid (fever) (*see also* Fever, paratyphoid) 002.9
  Peptococcus 008.46
  Peptostreptococcus 008.46
  Proprionibacterium 008.46
  protozoal NEC 007.9
  radiation 558.1
  regional (of) 555.9
    intestine
      large (bowel, colon, or rectum) 555.1
        with small intestine 555.2
      small (duodenum, ileum, or jejunum) 555.0
        with large intestine 555.2
  Salmonella infection 003.0
  salmonellosis 003.0
  segmental (*see also* Enteritis, regional) 555.9
  septic (*see also* Enteritis, due to, by organism) 009.0
  Shigella 004.9
  simple 558.9
  spasmodic 564.9
  spastic 564.9
  staphylococcal 008.41
    due to food 005.0
  streptococcal 008.49
    anaerobic 008.46
  toxic 558.2
  Treponema (denticola) (macrodentium) 008.46
  trichomonal 007.3

Enteritis – *continued*
  tuberculous (*see also* Tuberculosis) 014.8 5th
  typhosa 002.0
  ulcerative (chronic) (*see also* Colitis, ulcerative) 556.9
  Veillonella 008.46
  viral 008.8
    adenovirus 008.62
    enterovirus 008.67
    specified virus NEC 008.69
  Yersinia enterocolitica 008.44
  zymotic 009.0
Enteroarticular syndrome 099.3
Enterobiasis 127.4
Enterobius vermicularis 127.4
Enterocele (*see also* Hernia) 553.9
  pelvis, pelvic (acquired) (congenital) 618.6
  vagina, vaginal (acquired) (congenital) 618.6
Enterocolitis - *see also* Enteritis
  fetus or newborn (*see also* Enterocolitis, necrotizing, newborn) 777.8
    necrotizing 777.50
  fulminant 557.0
  granulomatous 555.2
  hemorrhagic (acute) 557.0
    chronic 557.1
  necrotizing (acute) (membranous) 557.0
    newborn 777.50
      with
        perforation 777.53
        pneumatosis without perforation 777.52
        pneumatosis and perforation 777.53
      without pneumatosis, without perforation 777.51 ●
      stage I 777.51
      stage II 777.52
      stage III 777.53
  primary necrotizing (*see also* Enterocolitis, necrotizing, newborn) 777.50
  pseudomembranous 008.45
    newborn 008.45 ●
  radiation 558.1
    newborn (*see also* Enterocolitis, necrotizing, newborn) 777.50
  ulcerative 556.0
Enterocystoma 751.5
Enterogastritis - *see* Enteritis
Enterogenous cyanosis 289.7
Enterolith, enterolithiasis (impaction) 560.39
  with hernia - *see also* Hernia, by site, with obstruction
    gangrenous - *see* Hernia, by site, with gangrene
Enteropathy 569.9
  exudative (of Gordon) 579.8
  gluten 579.0
  hemorrhagic, terminal 557.0
  protein-losing 579.8
Enteroperitonitis (*see also* Peritonitis) 567.9
Enteroptosis 569.89
Enterorrhagia 578.9
Enterospasm 564.9
  psychogenic 306.4
Enterostenosis (*see also* Obstruction, intestine) 560.9
Enterostomy status V44.4
  with complication 569.60
Enthesopathy 726.90
  ankle and tarsus 726.70
  elbow region 726.30
    specified NEC 726.39
  hip 726.5
  knee 726.60
  peripheral NEC 726.8
  shoulder region 726.10
    adhesive 726.0
  spinal 720.1
  wrist and carpus 726.4
Entrance, air into vein - *see* Embolism, air

Entrapment, nerve - *see* Neuropathy, entrapment
Entropion (eyelid) 374.00
  cicatricial 374.04
  congenital 743.62
  late effect of trachoma (healed) 139.1
  mechanical 374.02
  paralytic 374.02
  senile 374.01
  spastic 374.03
Enucleation of eye (current) (traumatic) 871.3
Enuresis 788.30
  habit disturbance 307.6
  nocturnal 788.36
    psychogenic 307.6
  nonorganic origin 307.6
  psychogenic 307.6
Enzymopathy 277.9
Eosinopenia 288.59
Eosinophilia 288.3
  allergic 288.3
  hereditary 288.3
  idiopathic 288.3
  infiltrative 518.3
  Loeffler's 518.3
  myalgia syndrome 710.5
  pulmonary (tropical) 518.3
  secondary 288.3
  tropical 518.3
Eosinophilic - *see also* condition
  fasciitis 728.89
  granuloma (bone) 277.89
  infiltration lung 518.3
Ependymitis (acute) (cerebral) (chronic) (granular) (*see also* Meningitis) 322.9
Ependymoblastoma (M9392/3)
  specified site - *see* Neoplasm, by site, malignant
  unspecified site 191.9
Ependymoma (epithelial) (malignant) (M9391/3)
  anaplastic type (M9392/3)
    specified site - *see* Neoplasm, by site, malignant
    unspecified site 191.9
  benign (M9391/0)
    specified site - *see* Neoplasm, by site, benign
    unspecified site 225.0
  myxopapillary (M9394/1) 237.5
  papillary (M9393/1) 237.5
  specified site - *see* Neoplasm, by site, malignant
  unspecified site 191.9
Ependymopathy 349.2
  spinal cord 349.2
Ephelides, ephelis 709.09
Ephemeral fever (*see also* Pyrexia) 780.60
Epiblepharon (congenital) 743.62
Epicanthus, epicanthic fold (congenital) (eyelid) 743.63
Epicondylitis (elbow) (lateral) 726.32
  medial 726.31
Epicystitis (*see also* Cystitis) 595.9
Epidemic - *see* condition
Epidermidalization, cervix - *see* condition
Epidermidization, cervix - *see* condition
Epidermis, epidermal - *see* condition
Epidermization, cervix - *see* condition
Epidermodysplasia verruciformis 078.19
Epidermoid
  cholesteatoma - *see* Cholesteatoma
  inclusion (*see also* Cyst, skin) 706.2
Epidermolysis
  acuta (combustiformis) (toxica) 695.15
  bullosa 757.39
  necroticans combustiformis 695.15
    due to drug
      correct substance properly administered 695.15

Epidermolysis – *continued*
  necroticans combustiformis – *continued*
    due to drug – *continued*
      overdose or wrong substance given or taken 977.9
        specified drug - *see* Table of Drugs and Chemicals
Epidermophytid - *see* Dermatophytosis
Epidermophytosis (infected) - *see* Dermatophytosis
Epidermosis, ear (middle) (*see also* Cholesteatoma) 385.30
Epididymis - *see* condition
Epididymitis (nonvenereal) 604.90
  with abscess 604.0
  acute 604.99
  blennorrhagic (acute) 098.0
    chronic or duration of 2 months or over 098.2
  caseous (*see also* Tuberculosis) 016.4 5th
  chlamydial 099.54
  diphtheritic 032.89 *[604.91]*
  filarial 125.9 *[604.91]*
  gonococcal (acute) 098.0
    chronic or duration of 2 months or over 098.2
  recurrent 604.99
  residual 604.99
  syphilitic 095.8 *[604.91]*
  tuberculous (*see also* Tuberculosis) 016.4 5th
Epididymo-orchitis (*see also* Epididymitis) 604.90
  with abscess 604.0
  chlamydial 099.54
  gonococcal (acute) 098.13
    chronic or duration of 2 months or over 098.33
Epidural - *see* condition
Epigastritis (*see also* Gastritis) 535.5 5th
Epigastrium, epigastric - *see* condition
Epigastrocele (*see also* Hernia, epigastric) 553.29
Epiglottiditis (acute) 464.30
  with obstruction 464.31
  chronic 476.1
  viral 464.30
    with obstruction 464.31
Epiglottis - *see* condition
Epiglottitis (acute) 464.30
  with obstruction 464.31
  chronic 476.1
  viral 464.30
    with obstruction 464.31
Epignathus 759.4
Epilepsia
  partialis continua (*see also* Epilepsy) 345.7 5th
  procursiva (*see also* Epilepsy) 345.8 5th
Epilepsy, epileptic (idiopathic) 345.9 5th

Note *Use the following fifth-digit subclassifications with categories 345.0, 345.1, 345.4-345.9*

0 without mention of intractable epilepsy
1 with intractable epilepsy
  pharmacoresistant (pharmacologically resistant) ●
  poorly controlled ●
  refractory (medically) ●
  treatment resistant ●

  abdominal 345.5 5th
  absence (attack) 345.0 5th
  akinetic 345.0 5th
    psychomotor 345.4 5th
  automatism 345.4 5th
  autonomic diencephalic 345.5 5th
  brain 345.9 5th
  Bravais-Jacksonian 345.5 5th
  cerebral 345.9 5th
  climacteric 345.9 5th
  clonic 345.1 5th

- **Epilepsy, epileptic** – *continued*
  - clouded state 345.9 [5th]
  - coma 345.3
  - communicating 345.4 [5th]
  - complicating pregnancy, childbirth, or the puerperium 649.4 [5th]
  - congenital 345.9 [5th]
  - convulsions 345.9 [5th]
  - cortical (focal) (motor) 345.5 [5th]
  - cursive (running) 345.8 [5th]
  - cysticercosis 123.1
  - deterioration
    - with behavioral disturbance 345.9 [5th] *[294.11]*
    - without behavioral disturbance 345.9 [5th] *[294.10]*
  - due to syphilis 094.89
  - equivalent 345.5 [5th]
  - fit 345.9 [5th]
  - focal (motor) 345.5 [5th]
  - gelastic 345.8 [5th]
  - generalized 345.9 [5th]
    - convulsive 345.1 [5th]
    - flexion 345.1 [5th]
    - nonconvulsive 345.0 [5th]
  - grand mal (idiopathic) 345.1 [5th]
  - Jacksonian (motor) (sensory) 345.5 [5th]
  - Kojevnikoff's, Kojevnikov's, Kojewnikoff's 345.7 [5th]
  - laryngeal 786.2
  - limbic system 345.4 [5th]
  - localization related (focal) (partial) and epileptic syndromes
    - with
      - complex partial seizures 345.4 [5th]
      - simple partial seizures 345.5 [5th]
  - major (motor) 345.1 [5th]
  - minor 345.0 [5th]
  - mixed (type) 345.9 [5th]
  - motor partial 345.5 [5th]
  - musicogenic 345.1 [5th]
  - myoclonus, myoclonic 345.1 [5th]
    - progressive (familial) 345.1 [5th] ▲
  - nonconvulsive, generalized 345.0 [5th]
  - parasitic NEC 123.9
  - partial (focalized) 345.5 [5th]
    - with
      - impairment of consciousness 345.4 [5th]
      - memory and ideational disturbances 345.4 [5th]
    - without impairment of consciousness 345.5 [5th]
    - abdominal type 345.5 [5th]
    - motor type 345.5 [5th]
    - psychomotor type 345.4 [5th]
    - psychosensory type 345.4 [5th]
    - secondarily generalized 345.4 [5th]
    - sensory type 345.5 [5th]
    - somatomotor type 345.5 [5th]
    - somatosensory type 345.5 [5th]
    - temporal lobe type 345.4 [5th]
    - visceral type 345.5 [5th]
    - visual type 345.5 [5th]
  - peripheral 345.9 [5th]
  - petit mal 345.0 [5th]
  - photokinetic 345.8 [5th]
  - progressive myoclonic (familial) 345.1 [5th] ▲
  - psychic equivalent 345.5 [5th]
  - psychomotor 345.4 [5th]
  - psychosensory 345.4 [5th]
  - reflex 345.1 [5th]
  - seizure 345.9 [5th]
  - senile 345.9 [5th]
  - sensory-induced 345.5 [5th]
  - sleep (*see also* Narcolepsy) 347.00
  - somatomotor type 345.5 [5th]
  - somatosensory 345.5 [5th]
  - specified type NEC 345.8 [5th]
  - status (grand mal) 345.3
    - focal motor 345.7 [5th]
    - petit mal 345.2
    - psychomotor 345.7 [5th]
    - temporal lobe 345.7 [5th]
  - symptomatic 345.9 [5th]
  - temporal lobe 345.4 [5th]
  - tonic (-clonic) 345.1 [5th]
  - traumatic (injury unspecified) 907.0
    - injury specified - *see* Late, effect (of) specified injury
  - twilight 293.0
  - uncinate (gyrus) 345.4 [5th]
  - Unverricht (-Lundborg) (familial myoclonic) 345.1 [5th] ▲
  - visceral 345.5 [5th]
  - visual 345.5 [5th]
- **Epileptiform**
  - convulsions 780.39
  - seizure 780.39
- **Epiloia** 759.5
- **Epimenorrhea** 626.2
- **Epipharyngitis** (*see also* Nasopharyngitis) 460
- **Epiphora** 375.20
  - due to
    - excess lacrimation 375.21
    - insufficient drainage 375.22
- **Epiphyseal arrest** 733.91
  - femoral head 732.2
- **Epiphyseolysis, epiphysiolysis** (*see also* Osteochondrosis) 732.9
- **Epiphysitis** (*see also* Osteochondrosis) 732.9
  - juvenile 732.6
  - marginal (Scheuermann's) 732.0
  - os calcis 732.5
  - syphilitic (congenital) 090.0
  - vertebral (Scheuermann's) 732.0
- **Epiplocele** (*see also* Hernia) 553.9
- **Epiploitis** (*see also* Peritonitis) 567.9
- **Epiplosarcomphalocele** (*see also* Hernia, umbilicus) 553.1
- **Episcleritis** 379.00
  - gouty 274.89 *[379.09]*
  - nodular 379.02
  - periodica fugax 379.01
    - angioneurotic - *see* Edema, angioneurotic
  - specified NEC 379.09
  - staphylococcal 379.00
  - suppurative 379.00
  - syphilitic 095.0
  - tuberculous (*see also* Tuberculosis) 017.3 [5th] *[379.09]*
- **Episode**
  - brain (*see also* Disease, cerebrovascular, acute) 436
  - cerebral (*see also* Disease, cerebrovascular, acute) 436
  - depersonalization (in neurotic state) 300.6
  - hyporesponsive 780.09
  - psychotic (*see also* Psychosis) 298.9
    - organic, transient 293.9
  - schizophrenic (acute) NEC (*see also* Schizophrenia) 295.4 [5th]
- **Epispadias**
  - female 753.8
  - male 752.62
- **Episplenitis** 289.59
- **Epistaxis** (multiple) 784.7
  - hereditary 448.0
  - vicarious menstruation 625.8
- **Epithelioma** (malignant) (M8011/3) - *see also* Neoplasm, by site, malignant
  - adenoides cysticum (M8100/0) - *see* Neoplasm, skin, benign
  - basal cell (M8090/3) - *see* Neoplasm, skin, malignant
  - benign (M8011/0) - *see* Neoplasm, by site, benign
  - Bowen's (M8081/2) - *see* Neoplasm, skin, in situ
  - calcifying (benign) (Malherbe's) (M8110/0) - *see* Neoplasm, skin, benign
  - external site - *see* Neoplasm, skin, malignant
  - intraepidermal, Jadassohn (M8096/0) - *see* Neoplasm, skin, benign
  - squamous cell (M8070/3) - *see* Neoplasm, by site, malignant
- **Epitheliopathy**
  - pigment, retina 363.15
  - posterior multifocal placoid (acute) 363.15
- **Epithelium, epithelial** - *see* condition
- **Epituberculosis** (allergic) (with atelectasis) (*see also* Tuberculosis) 010.8 [5th]
- **Eponychia** 757.5
- **Epstein's**
  - nephrosis or syndrome (*see also* Nephrosis) 581.9
  - pearl (mouth) 528.4
- **Epstein-Barr infection** (viral) 075
  - chronic 780.79 *[139.8]*
- **Epulis** (giant cell) (gingiva) 523.8
- **Equinia** 024
- **Equinovarus** (congenital) 754.51
  - acquired 736.71
- **Equivalent**
  - angina 413.9 ●
  - convulsive (abdominal) (*see also* Epilepsy) 345.5 [5th]
  - epileptic (psychic) (*see also* Epilepsy) 345.5 [5th]
- **Erb's**
  - disease 359.1
  - palsy, paralysis (birth) (brachial) (newborn) 767.6
    - spinal (spastic) syphilitic 094.89
  - pseudohypertrophic muscular dystrophy 359.1
- **Erb (-Duchenne) paralysis** (birth injury) (newborn) 767.6
- **Erb-Goldflam disease or syndrome** 358.00
- **Erdheim-Chester disease** (ECD) 277.89 ●
- **Erdheim's syndrome** (acromegalic macrospondylitis) 253.0
- **Erection, painful** (persistent) 607.3
- **Ergosterol deficiency** (vitamin D) 268.9
  - with
    - osteomalacia 268.2
    - rickets (*see also* Rickets) 268.0
- **Ergotism** (ergotized grain) 988.2
  - from ergot used as drug (migraine therapy)
    - correct substance properly administered 349.82
    - overdose or wrong substance given or taken 975.0
- **Erichsen's disease** (railway spine) 300.16
- **Erlacher-Blount syndrome** (tibia vara) 732.4
- **Erosio interdigitalis blastomycetica** 112.3
- **Erosion**
  - arteriosclerotic plaque - *see* Arteriosclerosis, by site
  - artery NEC 447.2
    - without rupture 447.8
  - bone 733.99
  - bronchus 519.19
  - cartilage (joint) 733.99
  - cervix (uteri) (acquired) (chronic) (congenital) 622.0
    - with mention of cervicitis 616.0
  - cornea (recurrent) (*see also* Keratitis) 371.42
    - traumatic 918.1
  - dental (idiopathic) (occupational) 521.30
    - extending into
      - dentine 521.32
      - pulp 521.33
    - generalized 521.35
    - limited to enamel 521.31
    - localized 521.34
  - duodenum, postpyloric - *see* Ulcer, duodenum
  - esophagus 530.89
  - gastric 535.4 [5th]
  - intestine 569.89
  - lymphatic vessel 457.8
  - pylorus, pyloric (ulcer) 535.4 [5th]
  - sclera 379.16
  - spine, aneurysmal 094.89
  - spleen 289.59
  - stomach 535.4 [5th]
  - teeth (idiopathic) (occupational) (*see also* Erosion, dental) 521.30
    - due to
      - medicine 521.30
      - persistent vomiting 521.30
  - urethra 599.84
  - uterus 621.8
  - vertebra 733.99
- **Erotomania** 302.89
  - Clerambault's 297.8
- **Error**
  - in diet 269.9
  - refractive 367.9
    - astigmatism (*see also* Astigmatism) 367.20
    - drug-induced 367.89
    - hypermetropia 367.0
    - hyperopia 367.0
    - myopia 367.1
    - presbyopia 367.4
    - toxic 367.89
- **Eructation** 787.3
  - nervous 306.4
  - psychogenic 306.4
- **Eruption**
  - creeping 126.9
  - drug - *see* Dermatitis, due to, drug
  - Hutchinson, summer 692.72
  - Kaposi's varicelliform 054.0
  - napkin (psoriasiform) 691.0
  - polymorphous
    - light (sun) 692.72
      - other source 692.82
  - psoriasiform, napkin 691.0
  - recalcitrant pustular 694.8
  - ringed 695.89
  - skin (*see also* Dermatitis) 782.1
    - creeping (meaning hookworm) 126.9
    - due to
      - chemical(s) NEC 692.4
        - internal use 693.8
      - drug - *see* Dermatitis, due to, drug
      - prophylactic inoculation or vaccination against disease - *see* Dermatitis, due to, vaccine
      - smallpox vaccination NEC - *see* Dermatitis, due to, vaccine
    - erysipeloid 027.1
    - feigned 698.4
    - hutchinson, summer 692.72
    - kaposi's, varicelliform 054.0
      - vaccinia 999.0
    - lichenoid, axilla 698.3
    - polymorphous, due to light 692.72
    - toxic NEC 695.0
    - vesicular 709.8
  - teeth, tooth
    - accelerated 520.6
    - delayed 520.6
    - difficult 520.6
    - disturbance of 520.6
    - in abnormal sequence 520.6
    - incomplete 520.6
    - late 520.6
    - natal 520.6
    - neonatal 520.6
    - obstructed 520.6
    - partial 520.6
    - persistent primary 520.6
    - premature 520.6
    - prenatal 520.6
  - vesicular 709.8
- **Erysipelas** (gangrenous) (infantile) (newborn) (phlegmonous) (suppurative) 035
  - external ear 035 *[380.13]*

- **Erysipelas** – *continued*
  - puerperal, postpartum, childbirth 670.8 5th ▲
- **Erysipelatoid** (Rosenbach's) 027.1
- **Erysipeloid** (Rosenbach's) 027.1
- **Erythema, erythematous** (generalized) 695.9
  - ab igne - *see* Burn, by site, first degree
  - annulare (centrifugum) (rheumaticum) 695.0
  - arthriticum epidemicum 026.1
  - brucellum (*see also* Brucellosis) 023.9
  - bullosum 695.19
  - caloricum - *see* Burn, by site, first degree
  - chronicum migrans 088.81
  - circinatum 695.19
  - diaper 691.0
  - due to
    - chemical (contact) NEC 692.4
      - internal 693.8
    - drug (internal use) 693.0
      - contact 692.3
  - elevatum diutinum 695.89
  - endemic 265.2
  - epidemic, arthritic 026.1
  - figuratum perstans 695.0
  - gluteal 691.0
  - gyratum (perstans) (repens) 695.19
  - heat - *see* Burn, by site, first degree
  - ichthyosiforme congenitum 757.1
  - induratum (primary) (scrofulosorum) (*see also* Tuberculosis) 017.1 5th
    - nontuberculous 695.2
  - infantum febrile 057.8
  - infectional NEC 695.9
  - infectiosum 057.0
  - inflammation NEC 695.9
  - intertrigo 695.89
  - iris 695.10
  - lupus (discoid) (localized) (*see also* Lupus, erythematosus) 695.4
  - marginatum 695.0
    - rheumaticum - *see* Fever, rheumatic
  - medicamentosum - *see* Dermatitis, due to, drug
  - migrans 529.1
    - chronicum 088.81
  - multiforme 695.10
    - bullosum 695.19
    - conjunctiva 695.19
    - exudativum (Hebra) 695.19
    - major 695.12
    - minor 695.11
    - pemphigoides 694.5
  - napkin 691.0
  - neonatorum 778.8
  - nodosum 695.2
    - tuberculous (*see also* Tuberculosis) 017.1 5th
  - nummular, nummulare 695.19
  - palmar 695.0
  - palmaris hereditarium 695.0
  - pernio 991.5
  - perstans solare 692.72
  - rash, newborn 778.8
  - scarlatiniform (exfoliative) (recurrent) 695.0
  - simplex marginatum 057.8
  - solare - (*see also* Sunburn) 692.71
  - streptogenes 696.5
  - toxic, toxicum NEC 695.0
    - newborn 778.8
  - tuberculous (primary) (*see also* Tuberculosis) 017.0 5th
  - venenatum 695.0
- **Erythematosus** - *see* condition
- **Erythematous** - *see* condition
- **Erythermalgia** (primary) 443.82
- **Erythralgia** 443.82
- **Erythrasma** 039.0
- **Erythredema** 985.0
  - polyneuritica 985.0
  - polyneuropathy 985.0
- **Erythremia** (acute) (M9841/3) 207.0 5th
  - chronic (M9842/3) 207.1 5th
  - secondary 289.0
- **Erythroblastopenia** (acquired) 284.89
  - congenital 284.01
- **Erythroblastophthisis** 284.01
- **Erythroblastosis** (fetalis) (newborn) 773.2
  - due to
    - ABO
      - antibodies 773.1
      - incompatibility, maternal/fetal 773.1
      - isoimmunization 773.1
    - Rh
      - antibodies 773.0
      - incompatibility, maternal/fetal 773.0
      - isoimmunization 773.0
- **Erythrocyanosis** (crurum) 443.89
- **Erythrocythemia** - *see* Erythremia
- **Erythrocytopenia** 285.9
- **Erythrocytosis** (megalosplenic)
  - familial 289.6
  - oval, hereditary (*see also* Elliptocytosis) 282.1
  - secondary 289.0
  - stress 289.0
- **Erythroderma** (*see also* Erythema) 695.9
  - desquamativa (in infants) 695.89
  - exfoliative 695.89
  - ichthyosiform, congenital 757.1
  - infantum 695.89
  - maculopapular 696.2
  - neonatorum 778.8
  - psoriaticum 696.1
  - secondary 695.9
- **Erythrodysesthesia, palmar plantar** (PPE) 693.0
- **Erythrogenesis imperfecta** 284.09
- **Erythroleukemia** (M9840/3) 207.0 5th
- **Erythromelalgia** 443.82
- **Erythromelia** 701.8
- **Erythropenia** 285.9
- **Erythrophagocytosis** 289.9
- **Erythrophobia** 300.23
- **Erythroplakia**
  - oral mucosa 528.79
  - tongue 528.79
- **Erythroplasia** (Queyrat) (M8080/2)
  - specified site - *see* Neoplasm, skin, in situ
  - unspecified site 233.5
- **Erythropoiesis, idiopathic ineffective** 285.0
- **Escaped beats, heart** 427.60
  - postoperative 997.1
- **Esoenteritis** - *see* Enteritis
- **Esophagalgia** 530.89
- **Esophagectasis** 530.89
  - due to cardiospasm 530.0
- **Esophagismus** 530.5
- **Esophagitis** (alkaline) (chemical) (chronic) (infectional) (necrotic) (peptic) (postoperative) (regurgitant) 530.10
  - acute 530.12
  - candidal 112.84
  - eosinophilic 530.13
  - reflux 530.11
  - specified NEC 530.19
  - tuberculous (*see also* Tuberculosis) 017.8 5th
  - ulcerative 530.19
- **Esophagocele** 530.6
- **Esophagodynia** 530.89
- **Esophagomalacia** 530.89
- **Esophagoptosis** 530.89
- **Esophagospasm** 530.5
- **Esophagostenosis** 530.3
- **Esophagostomiasis** 127.7
- **Esophagostomy**
  - complication 530.87
    - infection 530.86
    - malfunctioning 530.87
    - mechanical 530.87
- **Esophagotracheal** - *see* condition
- **Esophagus** - *see* condition
- **Esophoria** 378.41
  - convergence, excess 378.84
  - divergence, insufficiency 378.85
- **Esotropia** (nonaccommodative) 378.00
  - accommodative 378.35
  - alternating 378.05
    - with
      - A pattern 378.06
      - specified noncomitancy NEC 378.08
      - V pattern 378.07
      - X pattern 378.08
      - Y pattern 378.08
    - intermittent 378.22
  - intermittent 378.20
    - alternating 378.22
    - monocular 378.21
  - monocular 378.01
    - with
      - A pattern 378.02
      - specified noncomitancy NEC 378.04
      - V pattern 378.03
      - X pattern 378.04
      - Y pattern 378.04
    - intermittent 378.21
- **Espundia** 085.5
- **Essential** - *see* condition
- **Esterapenia** 289.89
- **Esthesioneuroblastoma** (M9522/3) 160.0
- **Esthesioneurocytoma** (M9521/3) 160.0
- **Esthesioneuroepithelioma** (M9523/3) 160.0
- **Esthiomene** 099.1
- **Estivo-autumnal**
  - fever 084.0
  - malaria 084.0
- **Estrangement** V61.09
- **Estriasis** 134.0
- **Ethanolaminuria** 270.8
- **Ethanolism** (*see also* Alcoholism) 303.9 5th
- **Ether dependence, dependency** (*see also* Dependence) 304.6 5th
- **Etherism** (*see also* Dependence) 304.6 5th
- **Ethmoid, ethmoidal** - *see* condition
- **Ethmoiditis** (chronic) (nonpurulent) (purulent) (*see also* Sinusitis, ethmoidal) 473.2
  - influenzal 487.1
  - Woakes' 471.1
- **Ethylism** (*see also* Alcoholism) 303.9
- **Eulenburg's disease** (congenital paramyotonia) 359.29
- **Eunuchism** 257.2
- **Eunuchoidism** 257.2
  - hypogonadotropic 257.2
- **European blastomycosis** 117.5
- **Eustachian** - *see* condition
- **Euthyroid sick syndrome** 790.94
- **Euthyroidism** 244.9
- **Evaluation**
  - fetal lung maturity 659.8 5th
  - for suspected condition (*see also* Observation) V71.9
    - abuse V71.81
    - exposure
      - anthrax V71.82
      - biologic agent NEC V71.83
      - SARS V71.83
    - neglect V71.81
    - newborn - *see* Observation, suspected, condition, newborn
    - specified condition NEC V71.89
  - mental health V70.2
    - requested by authority V70.1
  - nursing care V63.8
  - social service V63.8
- **Evans' syndrome** (thrombocytopenic purpura) 287.32
- **Event, apparent life threatening, in newborn and infant** (ALTE) 799.82 ●
- **Eventration**
  - colon into chest - *see* Hernia, diaphragm
  - diaphragm (congenital) 756.6
- **Eversion**
  - bladder 596.8
  - cervix (uteri) 622.0
    - with mention of cervicitis 616.0
  - foot NEC 736.79
    - congenital 755.67
  - lacrimal punctum 375.51
  - punctum lacrimale (postinfectional) (senile) 375.51
  - ureter (meatus) 593.89
  - urethra (meatus) 599.84
  - uterus 618.1
    - complicating delivery 665.2 5th
      - affecting fetus or newborn 763.89
    - puerperal, postpartum 674.8 5th
- **Evidence**
  - of malignancy
    - cytologic
      - without histologic confirmation
        - anus 796.76
        - cervix 795.06
        - vagina 795.16
- **Evisceration**
  - birth injury 767.8
  - bowel (congenital) - *see* Hernia, ventral
  - congenital (*see also* Hernia, ventral) 553.29
  - operative wound 998.32
  - traumatic NEC 869.1
    - eye 871.3
- **Evulsion** - *see* Avulsion
- **Ewing's**
  - angioendothelioma (M9260/3) - *see* Neoplasm, bone, malignant
  - sarcoma (M9260/3) - *see* Neoplasm, bone, malignant
  - tumor (M9260/3) - *see* Neoplasm, bone, malignant
- **Exaggerated lumbosacral angle** (with impinging spine) 756.12
- **Examination** (general) (routine) (of) (for) V70.9
  - allergy V72.7
  - annual V70.0
  - cardiovascular preoperative V72.81
  - cervical Papanicolaou smear V76.2
    - as a part of routine gynecological examination V72.31
    - to confirm findings of recent normal smear following initial abnormal smear V72.32
  - child care (routine) V20.2
  - clinical research investigation (normal control patient) (participant) V70.7
  - dental V72.2
  - developmental testing (child) (infant) V20.2
  - donor (potential) V70.8
  - ear V72.19
  - eye V72.0
  - following
    - accident (motor vehicle) V71.4
    - alleged rape or seduction (victim or culprit) V71.5
    - inflicted injury (victim or culprit) NEC V71.6
    - rape or seduction, alleged (victim or culprit) V71.5
    - treatment (for) V67.9
      - combined V67.6
      - fracture V67.4
      - involving high-risk medication NEC V67.51
      - mental disorder V67.3
      - specified condition NEC V67.59
  - follow-up (routine) (following) V67.9
    - cancer chemotherapy V67.2
    - chemotherapy V67.2
    - disease NEC V67.59
    - high-risk medication NEC V67.51
    - injury NEC V67.59
    - population survey V70.6
    - postpartum V24.2
    - psychiatric V67.3

- **Examination** – *continued*
  - follow-up – *continued*
    - psychotherapy V67.3
    - radiotherapy V67.1
    - specified surgery NEC V67.09
    - surgery V67.00
      - vaginal pap smear V67.01
  - gynecological V72.31
    - for contraceptive maintenance V25.40
      - intrauterine device V25.42
      - pill V25.41
      - specified method NEC V25.49
  - health (of)
    - armed forces personnel V70.5
    - checkup V70.0
    - child, routine V20.2
    - defined subpopulation NEC V70.5
    - inhabitants of institutions V70.5
    - occupational V70.5
    - pre-employment screening V70.5
    - preschool children V70.5
      - for admission to school V70.3
    - prisoners V70.5
      - for entrance into prison V70.3
    - prostitutes V70.5
    - refugees V70.5
    - school children V70.5
    - students V70.5
  - hearing V72.19
    - following failed hearing screening V72.11
  - infant ~~V20.2~~ ▲
    - 8 to 28 days old V20.32 ●
    - over 28 days old, routine V20.2 ●
    - under 8 days old V20.31 ●
  - laboratory V72.60 ▲
    - ordered as part of a routine general medical examination V72.62 ●
    - pre-operative V72.63 ●
    - pre-procedural V72.63 ●
    - specified NEC V72.69 ●
  - lactating mother V24.1
  - medical (for) (of) V70.9
    - administrative purpose NEC V70.3
    - admission to
      - old age home V70.3
      - prison V70.3
      - school V70.3
    - adoption V70.3
    - armed forces personnel V70.5
    - at health care facility V70.0
    - camp V70.3
    - child, routine V20.2
    - clinical research (control) (normal comparison) (participant) V70.7
    - defined subpopulation NEC V70.5
    - donor (potential) V70.8
    - driving license V70.3
    - general V70.9
      - routine V70.0
      - specified reason NEC V70.8
    - immigration V70.3
    - inhabitants of institutions V70.5
    - insurance certification V70.3
    - marriage V70.3
    - medicolegal reasons V70.4
    - naturalization V70.3
    - occupational V70.5
    - population survey V70.6
    - pre-employment V70.5
    - preschool children V70.5
      - for admission to school V70.3
    - prison V70.3
    - prisoners V70.5
      - for entrance into prison V70.3
    - prostitutes V70.5
    - refugees V70.5
    - school children V70.5
    - specified reason NEC V70.8
    - sport competition V70.3
    - students V70.5
  - medicolegal reason V70.4
  - pelvic (annual) (periodic) V72.31
  - periodic (annual) (routine) V70.0

- **Examination** – *continued*
  - postpartum
    - immediately after delivery V24.0
    - routine follow-up V24.2
  - pregnancy (unconfirmed) (possible) V72.40
    - negative result V72.41
    - positive result V72.42
  - prenatal V22.1
    - first pregnancy V22.0
    - high-risk pregnancy V23.9
      - specified problem NEC V23.89
  - preoperative V72.84
    - cardiovascular V72.81
    - respiratory V72.82
    - specified NEC V72.83
  - preprocedural V72.84
    - cardiovascular V72.81
    - general physical V72.83
    - respiratory V72.82
    - specified NEC V72.83
  - prior to chemotherapy V72.83 ●
  - psychiatric V70.2
    - follow-up not needing further care V67.3
    - requested by authority V70.1
  - radiological NEC V72.5
  - respiratory preoperative V72.82
  - screening - *see* Screening
  - sensitization V72.7
  - skin V72.7
    - hypersensitivity V72.7
  - special V72.9
  - specified type or reason NEC V72.85
    - preoperative V72.83
      - specified NEC V72.83
  - teeth V72.2
  - vaginal Papanicolaou smear V76.47
    - following hysterectomy for malignant condition V67.01
  - victim or culprit following
    - alleged rape or seduction V71.5
    - inflicted injury NEC V71.6
  - vision V72.0
  - well baby V20.2
- **Exanthem, exanthema** (*see also* Rash) 782.1
  - Boston 048
  - epidemic, with meningitis 048
  - lichenoid psoriasiform 696.2
  - subitum 058.10
    - due to
      - human herpesvirus 6 058.11
      - human herpesvirus 7 058.12
  - viral, virus NEC 057.9
    - specified type NEC 057.8
- **Excess, excessive, excessively**
  - alcohol level in blood 790.3
  - carbohydrate tissue, localized 278.1
  - carotene (dietary) 278.3
  - cold 991.9
    - specified effect NEC 991.8
  - convergence 378.84
  - crying 780.95
    - of
      - adolescent 780.95
      - adult 780.95
      - baby 780.92
      - child 780.95
      - infant (baby) 780.92
      - newborn 780.92
  - development, breast 611.1
  - diaphoresis (*see also* Hyperhidrosis) 780.8
  - distance, interarch 524.28
  - divergence 378.85
  - drinking (alcohol) NEC (*see also* Abuse, drugs, nondependent) 305.0 [5th]
    - continual (*see also* Alcoholism) 303.9 [5th]
    - habitual (*see also* Alcoholism) 303.9 [5th]
  - eating 783.6
  - eyelid fold (congenital) 743.62
  - fat 278.02
    - in heart (*see also* Degeneration, myocardial) 429.1

- **Excess, excessive, excessively** – *continued*
  - fat – *continued*
    - tissue, localized 278.1
  - foreskin 605
  - gas 787.3
  - gastrin 251.5
  - glucagon 251.4
  - heat (*see also* Heat) 992.9
  - horizontal
    - overjet 524.26
    - overlap 524.26
  - interarch distance 524.28
  - intermaxillary vertical dimension 524.37
  - interocclusal distance of teeth 524.37
  - large
    - colon 564.7
      - congenital 751.3
    - fetus or infant 766.0
      - with obstructed labor 660.1 [5th]
      - affecting management of pregnancy 656.6 [5th]
      - causing disproportion 653.5 [5th]
    - newborn (weight of 4500 grams or more) 766.0
    - organ or site, congenital NEC - *see* Anomaly, specified type NEC
  - lid fold (congenital) 743.62
  - long
    - colon 751.5
    - organ or site, congenital NEC - *see* Anomaly, specified type NEC
    - umbilical cord (entangled)
      - affecting fetus or newborn 762.5
      - in pregnancy or childbirth 663.3 [5th]
        - with compression 663.2 [5th]
  - menstruation 626.2
  - number of teeth 520.1
    - causing crowding 524.31
  - nutrients (dietary) NEC 783.6
  - potassium (K) 276.7
  - salivation (*see also* Ptyalism) 527.7
  - secretion - *see also* Hypersecretion
    - milk 676.6 [5th]
    - sputum 786.4
    - sweat (*see also* Hyperhidrosis) 780.8
  - short
    - organ or site, congenital NEC - *see* Anomaly, specified type NEC
    - umbilical cord
      - affecting fetus or newborn 762.6
      - in pregnancy or childbirth 663.4 [5th]
  - skin NEC 701.9
    - eyelid 743.62
      - acquired 374.30
  - sodium (Na) 276.0
  - spacing of teeth 524.32
  - sputum 786.4
  - sweating (*see also* Hyperhidrosis) 780.8
  - tearing (ducts) (eye) (*see also* Epiphora) 375.20
  - thirst 783.5
    - due to deprivation of water 994.3
  - tissue in reconstructed breast 612.0
  - tuberosity 524.07
  - vitamin
    - A (dietary) 278.2
      - administered as drug (chronic) (prolonged excessive intake) 278.2
        - reaction to sudden overdose 963.5
    - D (dietary) 278.4
      - administered as drug (chronic) (prolonged excessive intake) 278.4
        - reaction to sudden overdose 963.5
  - weight 278.02
    - gain 783.1
      - of pregnancy 646.1 [5th]
    - loss 783.21
- **Excitability, abnormal, under minor stress** 309.29

- **Excitation**
  - catatonic (*see also* Schizophrenia) 295.2 [5th]
  - psychogenic 298.1
  - reactive (from emotional stress, psychological trauma) 298.1
- **Excitement**
  - manic (*see also* Psychosis, affective) 296.0 [5th]
    - recurrent episode 296.1 [5th]
    - single episode 296.0 [5th]
  - mental, reactive (from emotional stress, psychological trauma) 298.1
  - state, reactive (from emotional stress, psychological trauma) 298.1
- **Excluded pupils** 364.76
- **Excoriation** (traumatic) (*see also* Injury, superficial, by site) 919.8
  - neurotic 698.4
- **Excyclophoria** 378.44
- **Excyclotropia** 378.33
- **Exencephalus, exencephaly** 742.0
- **Exercise**
  - breathing V57.0
  - remedial NEC V57.1
  - therapeutic NEC V57.1
- **Exfoliation**
  - skin
    - due to erythematous condition 695.50
      - involving (percent of body surface)
        - less than 10 percent 695.50
        - 10-19 percent 695.51
        - 20-29 percent 695.52
        - 30-39 percent 695.53
        - 40-49 percent 695.54
        - 50-59 percent 695.55
        - 60-69 percent 695.56
        - 70-79 percent 695.57
        - 80-89 percent 695.58
        - 90 percent or more 695.59
  - teeth
    - due to systemic causes 525.0
- **Exfoliative** - *see also* condition
  - dermatitis 695.89
- **Exhaustion, exhaustive** (physical NEC) 780.79
  - battle (*see also* Reaction, stress, acute) 308.9
  - cardiac (*see also* Failure, heart) 428.9
  - delirium (*see also* Reaction, stress, acute) 308.9
  - due to
    - cold 991.8
    - excessive exertion 994.5
    - exposure 994.4
    - overexertion 994.5
  - fetus or newborn 779.89
  - heart (*see also* Failure, heart) 428.9
  - heat 992.5
    - due to
      - salt depletion 992.4
      - water depletion 992.3
  - manic (*see also* Psychosis, affective) 296.0 [5th]
    - recurrent episode 296.1 [5th]
    - single episode 296.0 [5th]
  - maternal, complicating delivery 669.8 [5th]
    - affecting fetus or newborn 763.89
  - mental 300.5
  - myocardium, myocardial (*see also* Failure, heart) 428.9
  - nervous 300.5
  - old age 797
  - postinfectional NEC 780.79
  - psychogenic 300.5
  - psychosis (*see also* Reaction, stress, acute) 308.9
  - senile 797
    - dementia 290.0
- **Exhibitionism (sexual)** 302.4
- **Exomphalos** 756.72 ▲
- **Exophoria** 378.42
  - convergence, insufficiency 378.83
  - divergence, excess 378.85

Examination – Exophoria

- **Exophthalmic**
  - cachexia 242.0 [5th]
  - goiter 242.0 [5th]
  - ophthalmoplegia 242.0 [5th] *[376.22]*
- **Exophthalmos** 376.30
  - congenital 743.66
  - constant 376.31
  - endocrine NEC 259.9 *[376.22]*
  - hyperthyroidism 242.0 [5th] *[376.21]*
  - intermittent NEC 376.34
  - malignant 242.0 [5th] *[376.21]*
  - pulsating 376.35
    - endocrine NEC 259.9 *[376.22]*
  - thyrotoxic 242.0 [5th] *[376.21]*
- **Exostosis** 726.91
  - cartilaginous (M9210/0) - *see* Neoplasm, bone, benign
  - congenital 756.4
  - ear canal, external 380.81
  - gonococcal 098.89
  - hip 726.5
  - intracranial 733.3
  - jaw (bone) 526.81
  - luxurians 728.11
  - multiple (cancellous) (congenital) (hereditary) 756.4
  - nasal bones 726.91
  - orbit, orbital 376.42
  - osteocartilaginous (M9210/0) - *see* Neoplasm, bone, benign
  - spine 721.8
    - with spondylosis - *see* Spondylosis
  - syphilitic 095.5
  - wrist 726.4
- **Exotropia** 378.10
  - alternating 378.15
    - with
      - A pattern 378.16
      - specified noncomitancy NEC 378.18
      - V pattern 378.17
      - X pattern 378.18
      - Y pattern 378.18
    - intermittent 378.24
  - intermittent 378.20
    - alternating 378.24
    - monocular 378.23
  - monocular 378.11
    - with
      - A pattern 378.12
      - specified noncomitancy NEC 378.14
      - V pattern 378.13
      - X pattern 378.14
      - Y pattern 378.14
    - intermittent 378.23
- **Explanation of**
  - investigation finding V65.4 [5th]
  - medication V65.4 [5th]
- **Exposure** (suspected) 994.9 ▲
  - algae bloom V87.32 ●
  - cold 991.9
    - specified effect NEC 991.8
  - effects of 994.9
  - exhaustion due to 994.4
  - to
    - AIDS virus V01.79
    - anthrax V01.81
    - aromatic
      - amines V87.11
      - dyes V87.19
    - arsenic V87.01
    - asbestos V15.84
    - benzene V87.12
    - body fluids (hazardous) V15.85
    - cholera V01.0
    - chromium compounds V87.09
    - communicable disease V01.9
      - specified type NEC V01.89
    - dyes V87.2
      - aromatic V87.19
    - Escherichia coli (E. coli) V01.83
    - German measles V01.4
    - gonorrhea V01.6

- **Exposure** (suspected) – *continued*
  - to – *continued*
    - hazardous
      - aromatic compounds NEC V87.19
      - body fluids V15.85
      - chemicals NEC V87.2
      - metals V87.09
      - substances V87.39
    - HIV V01.79
    - human immunodeficiency virus V01.79
    - lead V15.86
    - meningococcus V01.84
    - mold V87.31
    - nickel dust V87.09
    - parasitic disease V01.89
    - poliomyelitis V01.2
    - polycyclic aromatic hydrocarbons V87.19
    - potentially hazardous body fluids V15.85
    - SARS-associated coronavirus V01.82
    - rabies V01.5
    - rubella V01.4
    - smallpox V01.3
    - syphilis V01.6
    - tuberculosis V01.1
    - varicella V01.71
    - venereal disease V01.6
    - viral disease NEC V01.79
      - varicella V01.71
- **Exsanguination, fetal** 772.0
- **Exstrophy**
  - abdominal content 751.8
  - bladder (urinary) 753.5
- **Extensive** - *see* condition
- **Extra** - *see also* Accessory
  - rib 756.3
    - cervical 756.2
- **Extraction**
  - with hook 763.89
  - breech NEC 669.6 [5th]
    - affecting fetus or newborn 763.0
  - cataract postsurgical V45.61
  - manual NEC 669.8 [5th]
    - affecting fetus or newborn 763.89
- **Extrasystole** 427.60
  - atrial 427.61
  - postoperative 997.1
  - ventricular 427.69
- **Extrauterine gestation or pregnancy** - *see* Pregnancy, ectopic
- **Extravasation**
  - blood 459.0
    - lower extremity 459.0
  - chemotherapy, vesicant 999.81 ▲
  - chyle into mesentery 457.8
  - pelvicalyceal 593.4
  - pyelosinus 593.4
  - urine 788.8
    - from ureter 788.8
  - vesicant
    - agent NEC 999.82 ▲
    - chemotherapy 999.81 ▲
- **Extremity** - *see* condition
- **Extrophy** - *see* Exstrophy
- **Extroversion**
  - bladder 753.5
  - uterus 618.1
    - complicating delivery 665.2 [5th]
      - affecting fetus or newborn 763.89
    - postpartal (old) 618.1
- **Extruded tooth** 524.34
- **Extrusion**
  - alveolus and teeth 524.75
  - breast implant (prosthetic) 996.54
  - device, implant, or graft - *see* Complications, mechanical
  - eye implant (ball) (globe) 996.59
  - intervertebral disc - *see* Displacement, intervertebral disc
  - lacrimal gland 375.43
  - mesh (reinforcing) 996.59
  - ocular lens implant 996.53

- **Extrusion** – *continued*
  - prosthetic device NEC - *see* Complications, mechanical
  - vitreous 379.26
- **Exudate, pleura** - *see* Effusion, pleura
- **Exudates, retina** 362.82
- **Exudative** - *see* condition
- **Eye, eyeball, eyelid** - *see* condition
- **Eyestrain** 368.13
- **Eyeworm disease of Africa** 125.2

F

- **Faber's anemia or syndrome** (achlorhydric anemia) 280.9
- **Fabry's disease** (angiokeratoma corporis diffusum) 272.7
- **Face, facial** - *see* condition
- **Facet of cornea** 371.44
- **Faciocephalalgia, autonomic** (*see also* Neuropathy, peripheral, autonomic) 337.9
- **Facioscapulohumeral myopathy** 359.1
- **Factitious disorder, illness** - *see* Illness, factitious
- **Factor**
  - deficiency - *see* Deficiency, factor
  - psychic, associated with diseases classified elsewhere 316
  - risk-*see* problem
- **Fahr-Volhard disease** (malignant nephrosclerosis) 403.00
- **Failure, failed**
  - adenohypophyseal 253.2
  - attempted abortion (legal) (*see also* Abortion, failed) 638.9
  - bone marrow (anemia) 284.9
    - acquired (secondary) 284.89
    - congenital 284.09
    - idiopathic 284.9
  - cardiac (*see also* Failure, heart) 428.9
    - newborn 779.89
  - cardiorenal (chronic) 428.9
    - hypertensive (*see also* Hypertension, cardiorenal) 404.93
  - cardiorespiratory 799.1
    - specified during or due to a procedure 997.1
      - long-term effect of cardiac surgery 429.4
  - cardiovascular (chronic) 428.9
  - cerebrovascular 437.8
  - cervical dilatation in labor 661.0 [5th]
    - affecting fetus or newborn 763.7
  - circulation, circulatory 799.89
    - fetus or newborn 779.89
    - peripheral 785.50
  - compensation - *see* Disease, heart
  - congestive (*see also* Failure, heart) 428.0
  - conscious sedation, during procedure 995.24 ●
  - coronary (*see also* Insufficiency, coronary) 411.89
  - dental implant 525.79
    - due to
      - infection 525.71
      - lack of attached gingiva 525.72
      - occlusal trauma (caused by poor prosthetic design) 525.72
      - parafunctional habits 525.72
      - periodontal infection (peri-implantitis) 525.72
      - poor oral hygiene 525.72
      - unintentional loading 525.71
    - endosseous NEC 525.79
    - mechanical 525.73
    - osseointegration 525.71
      - due to
        - complications of systemic disease 525.71
        - poor bone quality 525.71
        - premature loading 525.71

- **Failure, failed** – *continued*
  - dental implant – *continued*
    - osseointegration – *continued*
      - ~~following intentional prosthetic loading 525.72~~
      - iatrogenic 525.71
      - prior to intentional prosthetic loading 525.71
    - post-osseointegration
      - biological 525.72
        - iatrogenic 525.72
      - due to complications of systemic disease 525.72
      - mechanical 525.73
    - pre-integration 525.71
    - pre-osseointegration 525.71
  - dental prosthesis causing loss of dental implant 525.73
  - dental restoration
    - marginal integrity 525.61
    - periodontal anatomical integrity 525.65
  - descent of head (at term) 652.5 [5th]
    - affecting fetus or newborn 763.1
    - in labor 660.0 [5th]
      - affecting fetus or newborn 763.1
  - device, implant, or graft - *see* Complications, mechanical
  - engagement of head NEC 652.5 [5th]
    - in labor 660.0
  - extrarenal 788.99
  - fetal head to enter pelvic brim 652.5 [5th]
    - affecting fetus or newborn 763.1
    - in labor 660.0 [5th]
      - affecting fetus or newborn 763.1
  - forceps NEC 660.7 [5th]
    - affecting fetus or newborn 763.1
  - fusion (joint) (spinal) 996.49
  - growth in childhood 783.43
  - heart (acute) (sudden) 428.9
    - with
      - abortion - *see* Abortion, by type, with specified complication NEC
      - acute pulmonary edema (*see also* Failure, ventricular, left) 428.1
        - with congestion (*see also* Failure, heart) 428.0
      - decompensation (*see also* Failure, heart) 428.0
      - dilation - *see* Disease, heart
      - ectopic pregnancy (*see also* categories 633.0-633.9) 639.8
      - molar pregnancy (*see also* categories 630-632) 639.8
    - arteriosclerotic 440.9
    - combined left-right sided 428.0
    - combined systolic and diastolic 428.40
      - acute 428.41
      - acute on chronic 428.43
      - chronic 428.42
    - compensated (*see also* Failure, heart) 428.0
    - complicating
      - abortion - *see* Abortion, by type, with specified complication NEC
      - delivery (cesarean) (instrumental) 669.4 [5th]
      - ectopic pregnancy (*see also* categories 633.0-633.9) 639.8
      - molar pregnancy (*see also* categories 630-632) 639.8
      - obstetric anesthesia or sedation 668.1 [5th]
      - surgery 997.1
    - congestive (compensated) (decompensated) (*see also* Failure, heart) 428.0
      - with rheumatic fever (conditions classifiable to 390)
        - active 391.8

- **Failure, failed** – *continued*
  - heart – *continued*
    - congestive – *continued*
      - with rheumatic fever – *continued*
        - inactive or quiescent (with chorea) 398.91
      - fetus or newborn 779.89
      - hypertensive (*see also* Hypertension, heart) 402.91
        - with renal disease (*see also* Hypertension, cardiorenal) 404.91
          - with renal failure 404.93
        - benign 402.11
        - malignant 402.01
      - rheumatic (chronic) (inactive) (with chorea) 398.91
        - active or acute 391.8
          - with chorea (Sydenham's) 392.0
    - decompensated (*see also* Failure, heart) 428.0
    - degenerative (*see also* Degeneration, myocardial) 429.1
    - diastolic 428.30
      - acute 428.31
      - acute on chronic 428.33
      - chronic 428.32
    - due to presence of (cardiac) prosthesis 429.4
    - fetus or newborn 779.89
    - following
      - abortion 639.8
      - cardiac surgery 429.4
      - ectopic or molar pregnancy 639.8
    - high output NEC 428.9
    - hypertensive (*see also* Hypertension, heart) 402.91
      - with renal disease (*see also* Hypertension, cardiorenal) 404.91
        - with renal failure 404.93
      - benign 402.11
      - malignant 402.01
    - left (ventricular) (*see also* Failure, ventricular, left) 428.1
      - with right-sided failure (*see also* Failure, heart) 428.0
    - low output (syndrome) NEC 428.9
    - organic - *see* Disease, heart
    - postoperative (immediate) 997.1
      - long term effect of cardiac surgery 429.4
    - rheumatic (chronic) (congestive) (inactive) 398.91
    - right (secondary to left heart failure, conditions classifiable to 428.1) (ventricular) (*see also* Failure, heart) 428.0
    - senile 797
    - specified during or due to a procedure 997.1
      - long-term effect of cardiac surgery 429.4
    - systolic 428.20
      - acute 428.21
      - acute on chronic 428.23
      - chronic 428.22
    - thyrotoxic (*see also* Thyrotoxicosis) 242.9 [5th] *[425.7]*
    - valvular - *see* Endocarditis
  - hepatic 572.8
    - acute 570
    - due to a procedure 997.4
  - hepatorenal 572.4
  - hypertensive heart (*see also* Hypertension, heart) 402.91
    - benign 402.11
    - malignant 402.01
  - induction (of labor) 659.1 [5th]
    - abortion (legal) (*see also* Abortion, failed) 638.9
    - affecting fetus or newborn 763.89
    - by oxytocic drugs 659.1 [5th]

- **Failure, failed** – *continued*
  - induction – *continued*
    - instrumental 659.0 [5th]
    - mechanical 659.0 [5th]
    - medical 659.1 [5th]
    - surgical 659.0 [5th]
  - initial alveolar expansion, newborn 770.4
  - involution, thymus (gland) 254.8
  - kidney - *see* Failure, renal
  - lactation 676.4 [5th]
  - Leydig's cell, adult 257.2
  - liver 572.8
    - acute 570
  - medullary 799.89
  - mitral - *see* Endocarditis, mitral
  - moderate sedation, during procedure 995.24 ●
  - myocardium, myocardial (*see also* Failure, heart) 428.9
    - chronic (*see also* Failure, heart) 428.0
    - congestive (*see also* Failure, heart) 428.0
  - ovarian (primary) 256.39
    - iatrogenic 256.2
    - postablative 256.2
    - postirradiation 256.2
    - postsurgical 256.2
  - ovulation 628.0
  - prerenal 788.99
  - renal (kidney) 586 ▲
    - with
      - abortion - *see* Abortion, by type, with renal failure
      - ectopic pregnancy (*see also* categories 633.0-633.9) 639.3
      - edema (*see also* Nephrosis) 581.9
      - hypertension (*see also* Hypertension, kidney) 403.91
      - hypertensive heart disease (conditions classifiable to 402) 404.92
        - with heart failure 404.93
        - benign 404.12
          - with heart failure 404.13
        - malignant 404.02
          - with heart failure 404.03
      - molar pregnancy (*see also* categories 630-632) 639.3
      - tubular necrosis (acute) 584.5
    - acute 584.9
      - with lesion of
        - necrosis
          - cortical (renal) 584.6
          - medullary (renal) (papillary) 584.7
          - tubular 584.5
        - specified pathology NEC 584.8
    - chronic 585.9
      - hypertensive or with hypertension (*see also* Hypertension, kidney) 403.91
    - due to a procedure 997.5
    - following
      - abortion 639.3
      - crushing 958.5
      - ectopic or molar pregnancy 639.3
      - labor and delivery (acute) 669.3
    - hypertensive (*see also* Hypertension, kidney) 403.91
    - puerperal, postpartum 669.3
  - respiration, respiratory 518.81
    - acute 518.81
    - acute and chronic 518.84
    - center 348.89 ▲
      - newborn 770.84
    - chronic 518.83
    - due to trauma, surgery or shock 518.5
    - newborn 770.84
  - rotation
    - cecum 751.4
    - colon 751.4
    - intestine 751.4
    - kidney 753.3

- **Failure, failed** – *continued*
  - sedation, during procedure ●
    - conscious 995.24 ●
    - moderate 995.24 ●
  - segmentation - *see also* Fusion
    - fingers (*see also* Syndactylism, fingers) 755.11
    - toes (*see also* Syndactylism, toes) 755.13
  - seminiferous tubule, adult 257.2
  - senile (general) 797
    - with psychosis 290.20
  - testis, primary (seminal) 257.2
  - to progress 661.2 [5th]
  - to thrive
    - adult 783.7
    - child 783.41
    - newborn 779.34 ●
  - transplant 996.80
    - bone marrow 996.85
    - organ (immune or nonimmune cause) 996.80
      - bone marrow 996.85
      - heart 996.83
      - intestines 996.87
      - kidney 996.81
      - liver 996.82
      - lung 996.84
      - pancreas 996.86
      - specified NEC 996.89
    - skin 996.52
      - artificial 996.55
      - decellularized allodermis 996.55
      - temporary allograft or pigskin graft - omit code
  - trial of labor NEC 660.6 [5th]
    - affecting fetus or newborn 763.1
  - tubal ligation 998.89
  - urinary 586
  - vacuum extraction
    - abortion - *see* Abortion, failed
    - delivery NEC 660.7 [5th]
      - affecting fetus or newborn 763.1
  - vasectomy 998.89
  - ventouse NEC 660.7 [5th]
    - affecting fetus or newborn 763.1
  - ventricular (*see also* Failure, heart) 428.9
    - left 428.1
      - with rheumatic fever (conditions classifiable to 390)
        - active 391.8
          - with chorea 392.0
        - inactive or quiescent (with chorea) 398.91
      - hypertensive (*see also* Hypertension, heart) 402.91
        - benign 402.11
        - malignant 402.01
      - rheumatic (chronic) (inactive) (with chorea) 398.91
        - active or acute 391.8
          - with chorea 392.0
    - right (*see also* Failure, heart) 428.0
  - vital centers, fetus or newborn 779.89
  - weight gain in childhood 783.41
- **Fainting** (fit) (spell) 780.2
- **Falciform hymen** 752.49
- **Fall, maternal, affecting fetus or newborn** 760.5
- **Fallen arches** 734
- **Falling, any organ or part** - *see* Prolapse
- **Fallopian**
  - insufflation
    - fertility testing V26.21
    - following sterilization reversal V26.22
  - tube - *see* condition
- **Fallot's**
  - pentalogy 745.2
  - tetrad or tetralogy 745.2
  - triad or trilogy 746.09
- **Fallout, radioactive** (adverse effect) NEC 990
- **False** - *see also* condition
  - bundle branch block 426.50

- **False** – *continued*
  - bursa 727.89
  - croup 478.75
  - joint 733.82
  - labor (pains) 644.1 [5th]
  - opening, urinary, male 752.69
  - passage, urethra (prostatic) 599.4
  - positive
    - serological test for syphilis 795.6
    - Wassermann reaction 795.6
  - pregnancy 300.11
- **Family, familial** - *see also* condition
  - affected by
    - family member
      - currently on deployment (military) V61.01
      - returned from deployment (military) (current or past conflict) V61.02
  - disruption (*see also* Disruption, family) V61.09
  - estrangement V61.09
  - hemophagocytic
    - lymphohistiocytosis 288.4
    - reticulosis 288.4
  - Li-Fraumeni (syndrome) V84.01
  - planning advice V25.09
    - natural
      - procreative V26.41
      - to avoid pregnancy V25.04
  - problem V61.9
    - specified circumstance NEC V61.8
  - retinoblastoma (syndrome) 190.5
- **Famine** 994.2
  - edema 262
- **Fanconi's anemia** (congenital pancytopenia) 284.09
- **Fanconi (-de Toni) (-Debré) syndrome** (cystinosis) 270.0
- **Farber (-Uzman) syndrome or disease** (disseminated lipogranulomatosis) 272.8
- **Farcin** 024
- **Farcy** 024
- **Farmers'**
  - lung 495.0
  - skin 692.74
- **Farsightedness** 367.0
- **Fascia** - *see* condition
- **Fasciculation** 781.0
- **Fasciculitis optica** 377.32
- **Fasciitis** 729.4
  - eosinophilic 728.89
  - necrotizing 728.86
  - nodular 728.79
  - perirenal 593.4
  - plantar 728.71
  - pseudosarcomatous 728.79
  - traumatic (old) NEC 728.79
    - current - *see* Sprain, by site
- **Fasciola hepatica infestation** 121.3
- **Fascioliasis** 121.3
- **Fasciolopsiasis** (small intestine) 121.4
- **Fasciolopsis** (small intestine) 121.4
- **Fast pulse** 785.0
- **Fat**
  - embolism (cerebral) (pulmonary) (systemic) 958.1
    - with
      - abortion - *see* Abortion, by type, with embolism
      - ectopic pregnancy (*see also* categories 633.0-633.9) 639.6
      - molar pregnancy (*see also* categories 630-632) 639.6
    - complicating delivery or puerperium 673.8 [5th]
    - following
      - abortion 639.6
      - ectopic or molar pregnancy 639.6
    - in pregnancy, childbirth, or the puerperium 673.8 [5th]

- **Fever** - *continued*
  - hemorrhagic - *continued*
    - tick-borne NEC 065.3
  - hepatic (*see also* Cholecystitis) 575.8
    - intermittent (Charcôt's) - *see* Choledocholithiasis
  - herpetic (*see also* Herpes) 054.9
  - hyalomma tick 065.0
  - icterohemorrhagic 100.0
  - inanition 780.60
    - newborn 778.4
  - in conditions classified elsewhere 780.61
  - infective NEC 136.9
  - intermittent (bilious) (*see also* Malaria) 084.6
    - hepatic (Charcôt) - *see* Choledocholithiasis
    - of unknown origin (*see also* Pyrexia) 780.60
    - pernicious 084.0
  - iodide
    - correct substance properly administered 780.60
    - overdose or wrong substance given or taken 975.5
  - Japanese river 081.2
  - jungle yellow 060.0
  - Junin virus, hemorrhagic 078.7
  - Katayama 120.2
  - Kedani 081.2
  - Kenya 082.1
  - Korean hemorrhagic 078.6
  - Lassa 078.89
  - Lone Star 082.8
  - lung - *see* Pneumonia
  - Machupo virus, hemorrhagic 078.7
  - malaria, malarial (*see also* Malaria) 084.6
  - Malta (*see also* Brucellosis) 023.9
  - Marseilles 082.1
  - marsh (*see also* Malaria) 084.6
  - Mayaro (viral) 066.3
  - Mediterranean (*see also* Brucellosis) 023.9
    - familial 277.31
    - tick 082.1
  - meningeal - *see* Meningitis
  - metal fumes NEC 985.8
  - Meuse 083.1
  - Mexican - *see* Typhus, Mexican
  - Mianeh 087.1
  - miasmatic (*see also* Malaria) 084.6
  - miliary 078.2
  - milk, female 672 5th
  - mill 504
  - mite-borne hemorrhagic 065.8
  - Monday 504
  - mosquito-borne NEC 066.3
    - hemorrhagic NEC 065.4
  - mountain 066.1
    - meaning
      - Rocky Mountain spotted 082.0
      - undulant fever (*see also* Brucellosis) 023.9
    - tick (American) 066.1
  - Mucambo (viral) 066.3
  - mud 100.89
  - Neapolitan (*see also* Brucellosis) 023.9
  - neutropenic 288.00
  - newborn (environmentally-induced) 778.4
  - nine-mile 083.0
  - nonexanthematous tick 066.1
  - North Asian tick-borne typhus 082.2
  - Omsk hemorrhagic 065.1
  - O'nyong nyong (viral) 066.3
  - Oropouche (viral) 066.3
  - Oroya 088.0
  - paludal (*see also* Malaria) 084.6
  - Panama 084.0
  - pappataci 066.0
  - paratyphoid 002.9
    - A 002.1
    - B (Schottmüller's) 002.2
    - C (Hirschfeld) 002.3
  - parrot 073.9
  - periodic 277.31
  - pernicious, acute 084.0
  - persistent (of unknown origin) (*see also* Pyrexia) 780.60
  - petechial 036.0
  - pharyngoconjunctival 077.2
    - adenoviral type 3 077.2
  - Philippine hemorrhagic 065.4
  - phlebotomus 066.0
  - Piry 066.8
  - Pixuna (viral) 066.3
  - Plasmodium ovale 084.3
  - pleural (*see also* Pleurisy) 511.0
  - pneumonic - *see* Pneumonia
  - polymer fume 987.8
  - postimmunization 780.63
  - postoperative 780.62
    - due to infection 998.59
  - postvaccination 780.63
  - pretibial 100.89
  - puerperal, postpartum 672 5th
  - putrid - *see* Septicemia
  - pyemic - *see* Septicemia
  - Q 083.0
    - with pneumonia 083.0 *[484.8]*
  - quadrilateral 083.0
  - quartan (malaria) 084.2
  - Queensland (coastal) 083.0
    - seven-day 100.89
  - Quintan (A) 083.1
  - quotidian 084.0
  - rabbit (*see also* Tularemia) 021.9
  - rat-bite 026.9
    - due to
      - Spirillum minor or minus 026.0
      - Spirochaeta morsus muris 026.0
      - Streptobacillus moniliformis 026.1
  - recurrent - *see* Fever, relapsing
  - relapsing 087.9
    - Carter's (Asiatic) 087.0
    - Dutton's (West African) 087.1
    - Koch's 087.9
    - louse-borne (epidemic) 087.0
    - Novy's (American) 087.1
    - Obermeyer's (European) 087.0
    - spirillum NEC 087.9
    - tick-borne (endemic) 087.1
  - remittent (bilious) (congestive) (gastric) (*see also* Malaria) 084.6
  - rheumatic (active) (acute) (chronic) (subacute) 390
    - with heart involvement 391.9
      - carditis 391.9
      - endocarditis (aortic) (mitral) (pulmonary) (tricuspid) 391.1
      - multiple sites 391.8
      - myocarditis 391.2
      - pancarditis, acute 391.8
      - pericarditis 391.0
      - specified type NEC 391.8
      - valvulitis 391.1
    - inactive or quiescent with
      - cardiac hypertrophy 398.99
      - carditis 398.90
      - endocarditis 397.9
        - aortic (valve) 395.9
          - with mitral (valve) disease 396.9
        - mitral (valve) 394.9
          - with aortic (valve) disease 396.9
        - pulmonary (valve) 397.1
        - tricuspid (valve) 397.0
      - heart conditions (classifiable to 429.3, 429.6, 429.9) 398.99
        - failure (congestive) (conditions classifiable to 428.0, 428.9) 398.91
      - left ventricular failure (conditions classifiable to 428.1) 398.91

- **Fever** - *continued*
  - rheumatic - *continued*
    - inactive or quiescent with - *continued*
      - myocardial degeneration (conditions classifiable to 429.1) 398.0
      - myocarditis (conditions classifiable to 429.0) 398.0
      - pancarditis 398.99
      - pericarditis 393
  - Rift Valley (viral) 066.3
  - Rocky Mountain spotted 082.0
  - rose 477.0
  - Ross river (viral) 066.3
  - Russian hemorrhagic 078.6
  - sandfly 066.0
  - San Joaquin (valley) 114.0
  - Sao Paulo 082.0
  - scarlet 034.1
  - septic - *see* Septicemia
  - seven-day 061
    - Japan 100.89
    - Queensland 100.89
  - shin bone 083.1
  - Singapore hemorrhagic 065.4
  - solar 061
  - sore 054.9
  - South African tick-bite 087.1
  - Southeast Asia hemorrhagic 065.4
  - spinal - *see* Meningitis
  - spirillary 026.0
  - splenic (*see also* Anthrax) 022.9
  - spotted (Rocky Mountain) 082.0
    - American 082.0
    - Brazilian 082.0
    - Colombian 082.0
    - meaning
      - cerebrospinal meningitis 036.0
      - typhus 082.9
  - spring 309.23
  - steroid
    - correct substance properly administered 780.60
    - overdose or wrong substance given or taken 962.0
  - streptobacillary 026.1
  - subtertian 084.0
  - Sumatran mite 081.2
  - sun 061
  - swamp 100.89
  - sweating 078.2
  - swine 003.8
  - sylvatic yellow 060.0
  - Tahyna 062.5
  - tertian - *see* Malaria, tertian
  - Thailand hemorrhagic 065.4
  - thermic 992.0
  - three day 066.0
    - with Coxsackie exanthem 074.8
  - tick
    - American mountain 066.1
    - Colorado 066.1
    - Kemerovo 066.1
    - Mediterranean 082.1
    - mountain 066.1
    - nonexanthematous 066.1
    - Quaranfil 066.1
  - tick-bite NEC 066.1
  - tick-borne NEC 066.1
    - hemorrhagic NEC 065.3
  - transitory of newborn 778.4
  - trench 083.1
  - tsutsugamushi 081.2
  - typhogastric 002.0
  - typhoid (abortive) (ambulant) (any site) (hemorrhagic) (infection) (intermittent) (malignant) (rheumatic) 002.0
  - typhomalarial (*see also* Malaria) 084.6
  - typhus - *see* Typhus
  - undulant (*see also* Brucellosis) 023.9
  - unknown origin (*see also* Pyrexia) 780.60
  - uremic - *see* Uremia
  - uveoparotid 135

- **Fever** - *continued*
  - valley (Coccidioidomycosis) 114.0
  - Venezuelan equine 066.2
  - Volhynian 083.1
  - Wesselsbron (viral) 066.3
  - West
    - African 084.8
    - Nile (viral) 066.40
      - with
        - cranial nerve disorders 066.42
        - encephalitis 066.41
        - optic neuritis 066.42
        - other complications 066.49
        - other neurologic manifestations 066.42
        - polyradiculitis 066.42
  - Whitmore's 025
  - Wolhynian 083.1
  - worm 128.9
  - Yaroslav hemorrhagic 078.6
  - yellow 060.9
    - jungle 060.0
    - sylvatic 060.0
    - urban 060.1
    - vaccination, prophylactic (against) V04.4
  - Zika (viral) 066.3
- **Fibrillation**
  - atrial (established) (paroxysmal) 427.31
  - auricular (atrial) (established) 427.31
  - cardiac (ventricular) 427.41
  - coronary (*see also* Infarct, myocardium) 410.9 5th
  - heart (ventricular) 427.41
  - muscular 728.9
  - postoperative 997.1
  - ventricular 427.41
- **Fibrin**
  - ball or bodies, pleural (sac) 511.0
  - chamber, anterior (eye) (gelatinous exudate) 364.04
- **Fibrinogenolysis** (hemorrhagic) - *see* Fibrinolysis
- **Fibrinogenopenia** (congenital) (hereditary) (*see also* Defect, coagulation) 286.3
  - acquired 286.6
- **Fibrinolysis** (acquired) (hemorrhagic) (pathologic) 286.6
  - with
    - abortion - *see* Abortion, by type, with hemorrhage, delayed or excessive
    - ectopic pregnancy (*see also* categories 633.0-633.9) 639.1
    - molar pregnancy (*see also* categories 630-632) 639.1
  - antepartum or intrapartum 641.3 5th
    - affecting fetus or newborn 762.1
  - following
    - abortion 639.1
    - ectopic or molar pregnancy 639.1
  - newborn, transient 776.2
  - postpartum 666.3 5th
- **Fibrinopenia** (hereditary) (*see also* Defect, coagulation) 286.3
  - acquired 286.6
- **Fibrinopurulent** - *see* condition
- **Fibrinous** - *see* condition
- **Fibroadenoma** (M9010/0)
  - cellular intracanalicular (M9020/0) 217
  - giant (intracanalicular) (M9020/0) 217
  - intracanalicular (M9011/0)
    - cellular (M9020/0) 217
    - giant (M9020/0) 217
    - specified site - *see* Neoplasm, by site, benign
    - unspecified site 217
  - juvenile (M9030/0) 217
  - pericanicular (M9012/0)
    - specified site - *see* Neoplasm, by site, benign
    - unspecified site 217
  - phyllodes (M9020/0) 217

- **Fibroadenoma** – *continued*
  - prostate 600.20
    - with
      - other lower urinary tract symptoms (LUTS) 600.21
      - urinary
        - obstruction 600.21
        - retention 600.21
  - specified site - *see* Neoplasm, by site, benign
  - unspecified site 217
- **Fibroadenosis, breast** (chronic) (cystic) (diffuse) (periodic) (segmental) 610.2
- **Fibroangioma** (M9160/0) - *see also* Neoplasm, by site, benign
  - juvenile (M9160/0)
    - specified site - *see* Neoplasm, by site, benign
    - unspecified site 210.7
- **Fibrocellulitis progressiva ossificans** 728.11
- **Fibrochondrosarcoma** (M9220/3) - *see* Neoplasm, cartilage, malignant
- **Fibrocystic**
  - disease 277.00
    - bone NEC 733.29
    - breast 610.1
    - jaw 526.2
    - kidney (congenital) 753.19
    - liver 751.62
    - lung 518.89
      - congenital 748.4
    - pancreas 277.00
  - kidney (congenital) 753.19
- **Fibrodysplasia ossificans multiplex** (progressiva) 728.11
- **Fibroelastosis** (cordis) (endocardial) (endomyocardial) 425.3
- **Fibroid** (tumor) (M8890/0) - *see also* Neoplasm, connective tissue, benign
  - disease, lung (chronic) (*see also* Fibrosis, lung) 515
  - heart (disease) (*see also* Myocarditis) 429.0
  - induration, lung (chronic) (*see also* Fibrosis, lung) 515
  - in pregnancy or childbirth 654.1 [5th]
    - affecting fetus or newborn 763.89
    - causing obstructed labor 660.2 [5th]
      - affecting fetus or newborn 763.1
  - liver - *see* Cirrhosis, liver
  - lung (*see also* Fibrosis, lung) 515
  - pneumonia (chronic) (*see also* Fibrosis, lung) 515
  - uterus (M8890/0) (*see also* Leiomyoma, uterus) 218.9
- **Fibrolipoma** (M8851/0) (*see also* Lipoma, by site) 214.9
- **Fibroliposarcoma** (M8850/3) - *see* Neoplasm, connective tissue, malignant
- **Fibroma** (M8810/0) - *see also* Neoplasm, connective tissue, benign
  - ameloblastic (M9330/0) 213.1
    - upper jaw (bone) 213.0
  - bone (nonossifying) 733.99
    - ossifying (M9262/0) - *see* Neoplasm, bone, benign
  - cementifying (M9274/0) - *see* Neoplasm, bone, benign
  - chondromyxoid (M9241/0) - *see* Neoplasm, bone, benign
  - desmoplastic (M8823/1) - *see* Neoplasm, connective tissue, uncertain behavior
  - facial (M8813/0) - *see* Neoplasm, connective tissue, benign
  - invasive (M8821/1) - *see* Neoplasm, connective tissue, uncertain behavior
  - molle (M8851/0) (*see also* Lipoma, by site) 214.9
  - myxoid (M8811/0) - *see* Neoplasm, connective tissue, benign
- **Fibroma** – *continued*
  - nasopharynx, nasopharyngeal (juvenile) (M9160/0) 210.7
  - nonosteogenic (nonossifying) - *see* Dysplasia, fibrous
  - odontogenic (M9321/0) 213.1
    - upper jaw (bone) 213.0
  - ossifying (M9262/0) - *see* Neoplasm, bone, benign
  - periosteal (M8812/0) - *see* Neoplasm, bone, benign
  - prostate 600.20
    - with
      - other lower urinary tract symptoms (LUTS) 600.21
      - urinary
        - obstruction 600.21
        - retention 600.21
  - soft (M8851/0) (*see also* Lipoma, by site) 214.9
- **Fibromatosis** 728.79
  - abdominal (M8822/1) - *see* Neoplasm, connective tissue, uncertain behavior
  - aggressive (M8821/1) - *see* Neoplasm, connective tissue, uncertain behavior
  - congenital generalized (CGF) 759.89
  - Dupuytren's 728.6
  - gingival 523.8
  - plantar fascia 728.71
  - proliferative 728.79
  - pseudosarcomatous (proliferative) (subcutaneous) 728.79
  - subcutaneous pseudosarcomatous (proliferative) 728.79
- **Fibromyalgia** 729.1
- **Fibromyoma** (M8890/0) - *see also* Neoplasm, connective tissue, benign
  - uterus (corpus) (*see also* Leiomyoma, uterus) 218.9
    - in pregnancy or childbirth 654.1 [5th]
      - affecting fetus or newborn 763.89
      - causing obstructed labor 660.2 [5th]
        - affecting fetus or newborn 763.1
- **Fibromyositis** (*see also* Myositis) 729.1
  - scapulohumeral 726.2
- **Fibromyxolipoma** (M8852/0) (*see also* Lipoma, by site) 214.9
- **Fibromyxoma** (M8811/0) - *see* Neoplasm, connective tissue, benign
- **Fibromyxosarcoma** (M8811/3) - *see* Neoplasm, connective tissue, malignant
- **Fibro-odontoma, ameloblastic** (M9290/0) 213.1
  - upper jaw (bone) 213.0
- **Fibro-osteoma** (M9262/0) - *see* Neoplasm, bone, benign
- **Fibroplasia, retrolental** (*see also* Retinopathy of prematurity) 362.21
- **Fibropurulent** - *see* condition
- **Fibrosarcoma** (M8810/3) - *see also* Neoplasm, connective tissue, malignant
  - ameloblastic (M9330/3) 170.1
    - upper jaw (bone) 170.0
  - congenital (M8814/3) - *see* Neoplasm, connective tissue, malignant
  - fascial (M8813/3) - *see* Neoplasm, connective tissue, malignant
  - infantile (M8814/3) - *see* Neoplasm, connective tissue, malignant
  - odontogenic (M9330/3) 170.1
    - upper jaw (bone) 170.0
  - periosteal (M8812/3) - *see* Neoplasm, bone, malignant
- **Fibrosclerosis**
  - breast 610.3
  - corpora cavernosa (penis) 607.89
  - familial multifocal NEC 710.8
  - multifocal (idiopathic) NEC 710.8
  - penis (corpora cavernosa) 607.89
- **Fibrosis, fibrotic**
  - adrenal (gland) 255.8
  - alveolar (diffuse) 516.3
  - amnion 658.8 [5th]
  - anal papillae 569.49
  - anus 569.49
  - appendix, appendiceal, noninflammatory 543.9
  - arteriocapillary - *see* Arteriosclerosis
  - bauxite (of lung) 503
  - biliary 576.8
    - due to Clonorchis sinensis 121.1
  - bladder 596.8
    - interstitial 595.1
    - localized submucosal 595.1
    - panmural 595.1
  - bone, diffuse 756.59
  - breast 610.3
  - capillary - *see also* Arteriosclerosis
    - lung (chronic) (*see also* Fibrosis, lung) 515
  - cardiac (*see also* Myocarditis) 429.0
  - cervix 622.8
  - chorion 658.8 [5th]
  - corpus cavernosum 607.89
  - cystic (of pancreas) 277.00
    - with
      - manifestations
        - gastrointestinal 277.03
        - pulmonary 277.02
        - specified NEC 277.09
      - meconium ileus 277.01
      - pulmonary exacerbation 277.02
  - due to (presence of) any device, implant, or graft - *see* Complications, due to (presence of) any device, implant, or graft classified to 996.0-996.5 NEC
  - ejaculatory duct 608.89
  - endocardium (*see also* Endocarditis) 424.90
  - endomyocardial (African) 425.0
  - epididymis 608.89
  - eye muscle 378.62
  - graphite (of lung) 503
  - heart (*see also* Myocarditis) 429.0
  - hepatic - *see also* Cirrhosis, liver
    - due to Clonorchis sinensis 121.1
  - hepatolienal - *see* Cirrhosis, liver
  - hepatosplenic - *see* Cirrhosis, liver
  - infrapatellar fat pad 729.31
  - interstitial pulmonary, newborn 770.7
  - intrascrotal 608.89
  - kidney (*see also* Sclerosis, renal) 587
  - liver - *see* Cirrhosis, liver
  - lung (atrophic) (capillary) (chronic) (confluent) (massive) (perialveolar) (peribronchial) 515
    - with
      - anthracosilicosis (occupational) 500
      - anthracosis (occupational) 500
      - asbestosis (occupational) 501
      - bagassosis (occupational) 495.1
      - bauxite 503
      - berylliosis (occupational) 503
      - byssinosis (occupational) 504
      - calcicosis (occupational) 502
      - chalicosis (occupational) 502
      - dust reticulation (occupational) 504
      - farmers' lung 495.0
      - gannister disease (occupational) 502
      - graphite 503
      - pneumonoconiosis (occupational) 505
      - pneumosiderosis (occupational) 503
      - siderosis (occupational) 503
      - silicosis (occupational) 502
      - tuberculosis (*see also* Tuberculosis) 011.4 [5th]
    - diffuse (idiopathic) (interstitial) 516.3
    - due to
      - bauxite 503
- **Fibrosis, fibrotic** – *continued*
  - lung – *continued*
    - due to – *continued*
      - fumes or vapors (chemical) (inhalation) 506.4
      - graphite 503
    - following radiation 508.1
    - postinflammatory 515
    - silicotic (massive) (occupational) 502
    - tuberculous (*see also* Tuberculosis) 011.4 [5th]
  - lymphatic gland 289.3
  - median bar 600.90
    - with
      - other lower urinary tract symptoms (LUTS) 600.91
      - urinary
        - obstruction 600.91
        - retention 600.91
  - mediastinum (idiopathic) 519.3
  - meninges 349.2
  - muscle NEC 728.2
    - iatrogenic (from injection) 999.9
  - myocardium, myocardial (*see also* Myocarditis) 429.0
  - oral submucous 528.8
  - ovary 620.8
  - oviduct 620.8
  - pancreas 577.8
    - cystic 277.00
      - with
        - manifestations
          - gastrointestinal 277.03
          - pulmonary 277.02
          - specified NEC 277.09
        - meconium ileus 277.01
        - pulmonary exacerbation 277.02
  - penis 607.89
  - periappendiceal 543.9
  - periarticular (*see also* Ankylosis) 718.5 [5th]
  - pericardium 423.1
  - perineum, in pregnancy or childbirth 654.8 [5th]
    - affecting fetus or newborn 763.89
    - causing obstructed labor 660.2 [5th]
      - affecting fetus or newborn 763.1
  - perineural NEC 355.9
    - foot 355.6
  - periureteral 593.89
  - placenta - *see* Placenta, abnormal
  - pleura 511.0
  - popliteal fat pad 729.31
  - preretinal 362.56
  - prostate (chronic) 600.90
    - with
      - other lower urinary tract symptoms (LUTS) 600.91
      - urinary
        - obstruction 600.91
        - retention 600.91
  - pulmonary (chronic) (*see also* Fibrosis, lung) 515
    - alveolar capillary block 516.3
    - interstitial
      - diffuse (idiopathic) 516.3
      - newborn 770.7
  - radiation - *see* Effect, adverse, radiation
  - rectal sphincter 569.49
  - retroperitoneal, idiopathic 593.4
  - sclerosing mesenteric (idiopathic) 567.82
  - scrotum 608.89
  - seminal vesicle 608.89
  - senile 797
  - skin NEC 709.2
  - spermatic cord 608.89
  - spleen 289.59
    - bilharzial (*see also* Schistosomiasis) 120.9
  - subepidermal nodular (M8832/0) - *see* Neoplasm, skin, benign
  - submucous NEC 709.2
    - oral 528.8
    - tongue 528.8
  - syncytium - *see* Placenta, abnormal

Fibroadenoma – Fibrosis, fibrotic

- **Fibrosis, fibrotic** – *continued*
  - testis 608.89
    - chronic, due to syphilis 095.8
  - thymus (gland) 254.8
  - tunica vaginalis 608.89
  - ureter 593.89
  - urethra 599.84
  - uterus (nonneoplastic) 621.8
    - bilharzial (*see also* Schistosomiasis) 120.9
    - neoplastic (*see also* Leiomyoma, uterus) 218.9
  - vagina 623.8
  - valve, heart (*see also* Endocarditis) 424.90
  - vas deferens 608.89
  - vein 459.89
    - lower extremities 459.89
  - vesical 595.1
- **Fibrositis** (periarticular) (rheumatoid) 729.0
  - humeroscapular region 726.2
  - nodular, chronic
    - Jaccoud's 714.4
    - rheumatoid 714.4
  - ossificans 728.11
  - scapulohumeral 726.2
- **Fibrothorax** 511.0
- **Fibrotic** - *see* Fibrosis
- **Fibrous** - *see* condition
- **Fibroxanthoma** (M8831/0) - *see also* Neoplasm, connective tissue, benign
  - atypical (M8831/1) - *see* Neoplasm, connective tissue, uncertain behavior
  - malignant (M8831/3) - *see* Neoplasm, connective tissue, malignant
- **Fibroxanthosarcoma** (M8831/3) - *see* Neoplasm, connective tissue, malignant
- **Fiedler's**
  - disease (leptospiral jaundice) 100.0
  - myocarditis or syndrome (acute isolated myocarditis) 422.91
- **Fiessinger-Leroy (-Reiter) syndrome** 099.3
- **Fiessinger-Rendu syndrome** (erythema muliforme exudativum) 695.19
- **Fifth disease** (eruptive) 057.0
  - venereal 099.1
- **Filaria, filarial** - *see* Infestation, filarial
- **Filariasis** (*see also* Infestation, filarial) 125.9
  - bancroftian 125.0
  - brug's 125.1
  - due to
    - bancrofti 125.0
    - Brugia (Wuchereria) (malayi) 125.1
    - loa loa 125.2
    - malayi 125.1
    - organism NEC 125.6
    - Wuchereria (bancrofti) 125.0
      - malayi 125.1
  - Malayan 125.1
  - ozzardi 125.5
  - specified type NEC 125.6
- **Filatoff's, Filatov's, Filatow's disease** (infectious mononucleosis) 075
- **File-cutters' disease** 984.9
  - specified type of lead - *see* Table of Drugs and Chemicals
- **Filling defect**
  - biliary tract 793.3
  - bladder 793.5
  - duodenum 793.4
  - gallbladder 793.3
  - gastrointestinal tract 793.4
  - intestine 793.4
  - kidney 793.5
  - stomach 793.4
  - ureter 793.5
- **Filtering bleb, eye** (postglaucoma) (status) V45.69
  - with complication or rupture 997.99
  - postcataract extraction (complication) 997.99
- **Fimbrial cyst** (congenital) 752.11
- **Fimbriated hymen** 752.49
- **Financial problem affecting care** V60.2
- **Findings, (abnormal), without diagnosis** (examination) (laboratory test) 796.4 ▲
  - 17-ketosteroids, elevated 791.9
  - acetonuria 791.6
  - acid phosphatase 790.5
  - albumin-globulin ratio 790.99
  - albuminuria 791.0
  - alcohol in blood 790.3
  - alkaline phosphatase 790.5
  - amniotic fluid 792.3
  - amylase 790.5
  - antenatal screening 796.5
  - anisocytosis 790.09
  - anthrax, positive 795.31
  - antibody titers, elevated 795.79
  - anticardiolipin antibody 795.79
  - antigen-antibody reaction 795.79
  - antiphospholipid antibody 795.79
  - bacteriuria 791.9
  - ballistocardiogram 794.39
  - bicarbonate 276.9
  - bile in urine 791.4
  - bilirubin 277.4
  - bleeding time (prolonged) 790.92
  - blood culture, positive 790.7
  - blood gas level (arterial) 790.91
  - blood sugar level 790.29
    - high 790.29
      - fasting glucose 790.21
      - glucose tolerance test 790.22
    - low 251.2
  - C-reactive protein (CRP) 790.95
  - calcium 275.40
  - cancer antigen 125 [CA 125] 795.82
  - carbonate 276.9
  - carcinoembryonic antigen [CEA] 795.81
  - casts, urine 791.7
  - catecholamines 791.9
  - cells, urine 791.7
  - cerebrospinal fluid (color) (content) (pressure) 792.0
  - cervical
    - high risk human papillomavirus (HPV) DNA test positive 795.05
    - low risk human papillomavirus (HPV) DNA test positive 795.09
  - chloride 276.9
  - cholesterol 272.9
    - high 272.0
      - with high triglycerides 272.2
  - chromosome analysis 795.2
  - chyluria 791.1
  - circulation time 794.39
  - cloudy dialysis effluent 792.5
  - cloudy urine 791.9
  - coagulation study 790.92
  - cobalt, blood 790.6
  - color of urine (unusual) NEC 791.9
  - copper, blood 790.6
  - creatinine clearance 794.4
  - crystals, urine 791.9
  - culture, positive NEC 795.39
    - blood 790.7
    - HIV V08
    - human immunodeficiency virus V08
    - nose 795.39
      - Staphylococcus - *see* Carrier (suspected) of, Staphylococcus
    - skin lesion NEC 795.39
    - spinal fluid 792.0
    - sputum 795.39
    - stool 792.1
    - throat 795.39
    - urine 791.9
    - viral
      - human immunodeficiency V08
    - wound 795.39
  - cytology specified site NEC 796.9 ●
  - echocardiogram 793.2
  - echoencephalogram 794.01
  - echogram NEC - *see* Findings, abnormal, structure
  - electrocardiogram (ECG) (EKG) 794.31
  - electroencephalogram (EEG) 794.02
  - electrolyte level, urinary 791.9
  - electromyogram (EMG) 794.17
    - ocular 794.14
  - electro-oculogram (EOG) 794.12
  - electroretinogram (ERG) 794.11
  - enzymes, serum NEC 790.5
  - fibrinogen titer coagulation study 790.92
  - filling defect - *see* Filling defect
  - function study NEC 794.9
    - auditory 794.15
    - bladder 794.9
    - brain 794.00
    - cardiac 794.30
    - endocrine NEC 794.6
      - thyroid 794.5
    - kidney 794.4
    - liver 794.8
    - nervous system
      - central 794.00
      - peripheral 794.19
    - oculomotor 794.14
    - pancreas 794.9
    - placenta 794.9
    - pulmonary 794.2
    - retina 794.11
    - special senses 794.19
    - spleen 794.9
    - vestibular 794.16
  - gallbladder, nonvisualization 793.3
  - glucose 790.29
    - elevated
      - fasting 790.21
      - tolerance test 790.22
  - glycosuria 791.5
  - heart
    - shadow 793.2
    - sounds 785.3
  - hematinuria 791.2
  - hematocrit
    - drop (precipitous) 790.01
    - elevated 282.7
    - low 285.9
  - hematologic NEC 790.99
  - hematuria 599.70
  - hemoglobin
    - drop 790.01 ●
    - elevated 282.7
    - low 285.9
  - hemoglobinuria 791.2
  - histological NEC 795.4
  - hormones 259.9
  - immunoglobulins, elevated 795.79
  - indolacetic acid, elevated 791.9
  - iron 790.6
  - karyotype 795.2
  - ketonuria 791.6
  - lactic acid dehydrogenase (LDH) 790.4
  - lead 790.6
  - lipase 790.5
  - lipids NEC 272.9
  - lithium, blood 790.6
  - liver function test 790.6
  - lung field (coin lesion) (shadow) 793.1
  - magnesium, blood 790.6
  - mammogram 793.80
    - calcification 793.89
    - calculus 793.89
    - dense breasts 793.82 ●
    - inconclusive 793.82 ●
      - due to dense breasts 793.82 ●
    - microcalcification 793.81
  - mediastinal shift 793.2
  - melanin, urine 791.9
  - microbiologic NEC 795.39
  - mineral, blood NEC 790.6
  - myoglobinuria 791.3
  - nasal swab, anthrax 795.31
  - neonatal screening 796.6
  - nitrogen derivatives, blood 790.6
  - nonvisualization of gallbladder 793.3
  - nose culture, positive 795.39
  - odor of urine (unusual) NEC 791.9
  - oxygen saturation 790.91
  - Papanicolaou (smear) 796.9
    - anus 796.70
      - with
        - atypical squamous cells
          - cannot exclude high grade squamous intraepithelial lesion (ASC-H) 796.72
          - of undetermined significance (ASC-US) 796.71
        - cytologic evidence of malignancy 796.76
        - high grade squamous intraepithelial lesion (HGSIL) 796.74
        - low grade squamous intraepithelial lesion (LGSIL) 796.73
      - glandular 796.70
      - specified finding NEC 796.79
    - cervix 795.00
      - with
        - atypical squamous cells
          - cannot exclude high grade squamous intraepithelial lesion (ASC-H) 795.02
          - of undetermined significance (ASC-US) 795.01
        - cytologic evidence of malignancy 795.06
        - high grade squamous intraepithelial lesion (HGSIL) 795.04
        - low grade squamous intraepithelial lesion (LGSIL) 795.03
      - dyskaryotic 795.09
      - nonspecific finding NEC 795.09
    - other site 796.9
    - vagina 795.10
      - with
        - atypical squamous cells
          - cannot exclude high grade squamous intraepithelial lesion (ASC-H) 795.12
          - of undetermined significance (ASC-US) 795.11
        - cytologic evidence of malignancy 795.16
        - high grade squamous intraepithelial lesion (HGSIL) 795.14
        - low grade squamous intraepithelial lesion (LGSIL) 795.13
      - glandular 795.10
      - specified NEC 795.19
  - peritoneal fluid 792.9
  - phonocardiogram 794.39
  - phosphorus 275.3
  - pleural fluid 792.9
  - pneumoencephalogram 793.0
  - PO_2-oxygen ratio 790.91
  - poikilocytosis 790.09
  - potassium
    - deficiency 276.8
    - excess 276.7
  - PPD 795.5
  - prostate specific antigen (PSA) 790.93
  - protein, serum NEC 790.99
  - proteinuria 791.0
  - prothrombin time (prolonged) (partial) (PT) (PTT) 790.92
  - pyuria 791.9

Findings, (abnormal), without diagnosis – Fistula

- **Fistula** – *continued*
  - common duct (bile duct) 576.4
  - congenital, NEC - *see* Anomaly, specified type NEC
  - cornea, causing hypotony 360.32
  - coronary, arteriovenous 414.19
    - congenital 746.85
  - costal region 510.0
  - cul-de-sac, Douglas' 619.8
  - cutaneous 686.9
  - cystic duct (*see also* Fistula, gallbladder) 575.5
    - congenital 751.69
  - dental 522.7
  - diaphragm 510.0
    - bronchovisceral 510.0
    - pleuroperitoneal 510.0
    - pulmonoperitoneal 510.0
  - duodenum 537.4
  - ear (canal) (external) 380.89
  - enterocolic 569.81
  - enterocutaneous 569.81
  - enteroenteric 569.81
  - entero-uterine 619.1
    - congenital 752.3
  - enterovaginal 619.1
    - congenital 752.49
  - enterovesical 596.1
  - epididymis 608.89
    - tuberculous (*see also* Tuberculosis) 016.4 5th
  - esophagobronchial 530.89
    - congenital 750.3
  - esophagocutaneous 530.89
  - esophagopleurocutaneous 530.89
  - esophagotracheal 530.84
    - congenital 750.3
  - esophagus 530.89
    - congenital 750.4
  - ethmoid (*see also* Sinusitis, ethmoidal) 473.2
  - eyeball (cornea) (sclera) 360.32
  - eyelid 373.11
  - fallopian tube (external) 619.2
  - fecal 569.81
    - congenital 751.5
  - from periapical lesion 522.7
  - frontal sinus (*see also* Sinusitis, frontal) 473.1
  - gallbladder 575.5
    - with calculus, cholelithiasis, stones (*see also* Cholelithiasis) 574.2 5th
    - congenital 751.69
  - gastric 537.4
  - gastrocolic 537.4
    - congenital 750.7
    - tuberculous (*see also* Tuberculosis) 014.8 5th
  - gastroenterocolic 537.4
  - gastroesophageal 537.4
  - gastrojejunal 537.4
  - gastrojejunocolic 537.4
  - genital
    - organs
      - female 619.9
        - specified site NEC 619.8
      - male 608.89
    - tract-skin (female) 619.2
  - hepatopleural 510.0
  - hepatopulmonary 510.0
  - horseshoe 565.1
  - ileorectal 569.81
  - ileosigmoidal 569.81
  - ileostomy 569.69
  - ileovesical 596.1
  - ileum 569.81
  - in ano 565.1
    - tuberculous (*see also* Tuberculosis) 014.8 5th
  - inner ear (*see also* Fistula, labyrinth) 386.40
  - intestine 569.81
  - intestinocolonic (abdominal) 569.81
  - intestinoureteral 593.82

- **Fistula** – *continued*
  - intestinouterine 619.1
  - intestinovaginal 619.1
    - congenital 752.49
  - intestinovesical 596.1
  - involving female genital tract 619.9
    - digestive-genital 619.1
    - genital tract-skin 619.2
    - specified site NEC 619.8
    - urinary-genital 619.0
  - ischiorectal (fossa) 566
  - jejunostomy 569.69
  - jejunum 569.81
  - joint 719.80
    - ankle 719.87
    - elbow 719.82
    - foot 719.87
    - hand 719.84
    - hip 719.85
    - knee 719.86
    - multiple sites 719.89
    - pelvic region 719.85
    - shoulder (region) 719.81
    - specified site NEC 719.88
    - tuberculous - *see* Tuberculosis, joint
    - wrist 719.83
  - kidney 593.89
  - labium (majus) (minus) 619.8
  - labyrinth, labyrinthine NEC 386.40
    - combined sites 386.48
    - multiple sites 386.48
    - oval window 386.42
    - round window 386.41
    - semicircular canal 386.43
  - lacrimal, lachrymal (duct) (gland) (sac) 375.61
  - lacrimonasal duct 375.61
  - laryngotracheal 748.3
  - larynx 478.79
  - lip 528.5
    - congenital 750.25
  - lumbar, tuberculous (*see also* Tuberculosis) 015.0 5th *[730.8]* 5th
  - lung 510.0
  - lymphatic (node) (vessel) 457.8
  - mamillary 611.0
  - mammary (gland) 611.0
    - puerperal, postpartum 675.1 5th
  - mastoid (process) (region) 383.1
  - maxillary (*see also* Sinusitis, maxillary) 473.0
  - mediastinal 510.0
  - mediastinobronchial 510.0
  - mediastinocutaneous 510.0
  - middle ear 385.89
  - mouth 528.3
  - nasal 478.19
    - sinus (*see also* Sinusitis) 473.9
  - nasopharynx 478.29
  - nipple - *see* Fistula, breast
  - nose 478.19
  - oral (cutaneous) 528.3
    - maxillary (*see also* Sinusitis, maxillary) 473.0
    - nasal (with cleft palate) (*see also* Cleft, palate) 749.00
  - orbit, orbital 376.10
  - oro-antral (*see also* Sinusitis, maxillary) 473.0
  - oval window (internal ear) 386.42
  - oviduct (external) 619.2
  - palate (hard) 526.89
    - soft 528.9
  - pancreatic 577.8
  - pancreaticoduodenal 577.8
  - parotid (gland) 527.4
    - region 528.3
  - pelvoabdominointestinal 569.81
  - penis 607.89
  - perianal 565.1
  - pericardium (pleura) (sac) (*see also* Pericarditis) 423.8
  - pericecal 569.81
  - perineal - *see* Fistula, perineum

- **Fistula** – *continued*
  - perineorectal 569.81
  - perineosigmoidal 569.81
  - perineo-urethroscrotal 608.89
  - perineum, perineal (with urethral involvement) NEC 599.1
    - tuberculous (*see also* Tuberculosis) 017.9 5th
    - ureter 593.82
  - perirectal 565.1
    - tuberculous (*see also* Tuberculosis) 014.8 5th
  - peritoneum (*see also* Peritonitis) 567.22
  - periurethral 599.1
  - pharyngo-esophageal 478.29
  - pharynx 478.29
    - branchial cleft (congenital) 744.41
  - pilonidal (infected) (rectum) 685.1
    - with abscess 685.0
  - pleura, pleural, pleurocutaneous, pleuroperitoneal 510.0
    - stomach 510.0
    - tuberculous (*see also* Tuberculosis) 012.0 5th
  - pleuropericardial 423.8
  - postauricular 383.81
  - postoperative, persistent 998.6
  - preauricular (congenital) 744.46
  - prostate 602.8
  - pulmonary 510.0
    - arteriovenous 417.0
      - congenital 747.3
    - tuberculous (*see also* Tuberculosis, pulmonary) 011.9 5th
  - pulmonoperitoneal 510.0
  - rectolabial 619.1
  - rectosigmoid (intercommunicating) 569.81
  - rectoureteral 593.82
  - rectourethral 599.1
    - congenital 753.8
  - rectouterine 619.1
    - congenital 752.3
  - rectovaginal 619.1
    - congenital 752.49
    - old, postpartal 619.1
    - tuberculous (*see also* Tuberculosis) 014.8 5th
  - rectovesical 596.1
    - congenital 753.8
  - rectovesicovaginal 619.1
  - rectovulvar 619.1
    - congenital 752.49
  - rectum (to skin) 565.1
    - tuberculous (*see also* Tuberculosis) 014.8 5th
  - renal 593.89
  - retroauricular 383.81
  - round window (internal ear) 386.41
  - salivary duct or gland 527.4
    - congenital 750.24
  - sclera 360.32
  - scrotum (urinary) 608.89
    - tuberculous (*see also* Tuberculosis) 016.5 5th
  - semicircular canals (internal ear) 386.43
  - sigmoid 569.81
    - vesicoabdominal 596.1
  - sigmoidovaginal 619.1
    - congenital 752.49
  - skin 686.9
    - ureter 593.82
    - vagina 619.2
  - sphenoidal sinus (*see also* Sinusitis, sphenoidal) 473.3
  - splenocolic 289.59
  - stercoral 569.81
  - stomach 537.4
  - sublingual gland 527.4
    - congenital 750.24
  - submaxillary
    - gland 527.4
      - congenital 750.24
    - region 528.3

- **Fistula** – *continued*
  - thoracic 510.0
    - duct 457.8
  - thoracicoabdominal 510.0
  - thoracicogastric 510.0
  - thoracicointestinal 510.0
  - thoracoabdominal 510.0
  - thoracogastric 510.0
  - thorax 510.0
  - thyroglossal duct 759.2
  - thyroid 246.8
  - trachea (congenital) (external) (internal) 748.3
  - tracheoesophageal 530.84
    - congenital 750.3
    - following tracheostomy 519.09
  - traumatic
    - arteriovenous (*see also* Injury, blood vessel, by site) 904.9
      - brain - *see* Injury, intracranial
  - tuberculous - *see* Tuberculosis, by site
  - typhoid 002.0
  - umbilical 759.89
  - umbilico-urinary 753.8
  - urachal, urachus 753.7
  - ureter (persistent) 593.82
  - ureteroabdominal 593.82
  - ureterocervical 593.82
  - ureterorectal 593.82
  - ureterosigmoido-abdominal 593.82
  - ureterovaginal 619.0
  - ureterovesical 596.2
  - urethra 599.1
    - congenital 753.8
    - tuberculous (*see also* Tuberculosis) 016.3 5th
  - urethroperineal 599.1
  - urethroperineovesical 596.2
  - urethrorectal 599.1
    - congenital 753.8
  - urethroscrotal 608.89
  - urethrovaginal 619.0
  - urethrovesical 596.2
  - urethrovesicovaginal 619.0
  - urinary (persistent) (recurrent) 599.1
  - uteroabdominal (anterior wall) 619.2
    - congenital 752.3
  - uteroenteric 619.1
  - uterofecal 619.1
  - uterointestinal 619.1
    - congenital 752.3
  - uterorectal 619.1
    - congenital 752.3
  - uteroureteric 619.0
  - uterovaginal 619.8
  - uterovesical 619.0
    - congenital 752.3
  - uterus 619.8
  - vagina (wall) 619.8
    - postpartal, old 619.8
  - vaginocutaneous (postpartal) 619.2
  - vaginoileal (acquired) 619.1
  - vaginoperineal 619.2
  - vesical NEC 596.2
  - vesicoabdominal 596.2
  - vesicocervicovaginal 619.0
  - vesicocolic 596.1
  - vesicocutaneous 596.2
  - vesicoenteric 596.1
  - vesicointestinal 596.1
  - vesicometrorectal 619.1
  - vesicoperineal 596.2
  - vesicorectal 596.1
    - congenital 753.8
  - vesicosigmoidal 596.1
  - vesicosigmoidovaginal 619.1
  - vesicoureteral 596.2
  - vesicoureterovaginal 619.0
  - vesicourethral 596.2
  - vesicourethrorectal 596.1
  - vesicouterine 619.0
    - congenital 752.3
  - vesicovaginal 619.0

- **Fistula** – *continued*
  - vulvorectal 619.1
    - congenital 752.49
- **Fit** 780.39
  - apoplectic (*see also* Disease, cerebrovascular, acute) 436
    - late effect - *see* Late effect(s) (of) cerebrovascular disease
  - epileptic (*see also* Epilepsy) 345.9 [5th]
  - fainting 780.2
  - hysterical 300.11
  - newborn 779.0
- **Fitting** (of)
  - artificial
    - arm (complete) (partial) V52.0
    - breast V52.4
      - implant exchange (different material) (different size) V52.4
    - eye(s) V52.2
    - leg(s) (complete) (partial) V52.1
  - brain neuropacemaker V53.02
  - cardiac pacemaker V53.31
  - carotid sinus pacemaker V53.39
  - cerebral ventricle (communicating) shunt V53.01
  - colostomy belt V55.3
  - contact lenses V53.1
  - cystostomy device V53.6
  - defibrillator, automatic implantable cardiac V53.32
  - dentures V52.3
  - device, unspecified type V53.90
    - abdominal V53.59 ▲
    - cardiac
      - defibrillator, automatic implantable V53.32
      - pacemaker V53.31
      - specified NEC V53.39
    - cerebral ventricle (communicating) shunt V53.01
    - gastrointestinal NEC V53.59 ●
    - insulin pump V53.91
    - intestinal V53.50 ●
    - intrauterine contraceptive V25.1
    - nervous system V53.09
    - orthodontic V53.4
    - orthoptic V53.1
    - other device V53.99
    - prosthetic V52.9
      - breast V52.4
      - dental V52.3
      - eye V52.2
      - specified type NEC V52.8
    - special senses V53.09
    - substitution
      - auditory V53.09
      - nervous system V53.09
      - visual V53.09
    - urinary V53.6
  - diaphragm (contraceptive) V25.02
  - gastric lap band V53.51 ●
  - gastrointestinal appliance and device NEC V53.59 ●
  - glasses (reading) V53.1
  - growth rod V54.02
  - hearing aid V53.2
  - ileostomy device V55.2
  - intestinal appliance and ~~or~~ device ~~NEC~~ V53.50 ▲
  - intrauterine contraceptive device V25.1
  - neuropacemaker (brain) (peripheral nerve) (spinal cord) V53.02
  - orthodontic device V53.4
  - orthopedic (device) V53.7
    - brace V53.7
    - cast V53.7
    - corset V53.7
    - shoes V53.7
  - pacemaker (cardiac) V53.31
    - brain V53.02
    - carotid sinus V53.39
    - peripheral nerve V53.02
    - spinal cord V53.02
- **Fitting** (of) – *continued*
  - prosthesis V52.9
    - arm (complete) (partial) V52.0
    - breast V52.4
      - implant exchange (different material) (different size) V52.4
    - dental V52.3
    - eye V52.2
    - leg (complete) (partial) V52.1
    - specified type NEC V52.8
  - spectacles V53.1
  - wheelchair V53.8
- **Fitz's syndrome** (acute hemorrhagic pancreatitis) 577.0
- **Fitz-Hugh and Curtis syndrome** 098.86
  - due to
    - Chlamydia trachomatis 099.56
    - Neisseria gonorrhoeae (gonococcal peritonitis) 098.86
- **Fixation**
  - joint - *see* Ankylosis
  - larynx 478.79
  - pupil 364.76
  - stapes 385.22
    - deafness (*see also* Deafness, conductive) 389.04
  - uterus (acquired) - *see* Malposition, uterus
  - vocal cord 478.5
- **Flaccid** - *see also* condition
  - foot 736.79
  - forearm 736.09
  - palate, congenital 750.26
- **Flail**
  - chest 807.4
    - newborn 767.3
  - joint (paralytic) 718.80
    - ankle 718.87
    - elbow 718.82
    - foot 718.87
    - hand 718.84
    - hip 718.85
    - knee 718.86
    - multiple sites 718.89
    - pelvic region 718.85
    - shoulder (region) 718.81
    - specified site NEC 718.88
    - wrist 718.83
- **Flajani (-Basedow) syndrome or disease** (exophthalmic goiter) 242.0 [5th]
- **Flap, liver** 572.8
- **Flare, anterior chamber** (aqueous) (eye) 364.04
- **Flashback phenomena** (drug) (hallucinogenic) 292.89
- **Flat**
  - chamber (anterior) (eye) 360.34
  - chest, congenital 754.89
  - electroencephalogram (EEG) 348.89 ▲
  - foot (acquired) (fixed type) (painful) (postural) (spastic) 734
    - congenital 754.61
      - rocker bottom 754.61
      - vertical talus 754.61
    - rachitic 268.1
    - rocker bottom (congenital) 754.61
    - vertical talus, congenital 754.61
  - organ or site, congenital NEC - *see* Anomaly, specified type NEC
  - pelvis 738.6
    - with disproportion (fetopelvic) 653.2 [5th]
      - affecting fetus or newborn 763.1
      - causing obstructed labor 660.1 [5th]
        - affecting fetus or newborn 763.1
    - congenital 755.69
- **Flatau-Schilder disease** 341.1
- **Flattening**
  - head, femur 736.39
  - hip 736.39
  - lip (congenital) 744.89
  - nose (congenital) 754.0
    - acquired 738.0
- **Flatulence** 787.3
- **Flatus** 787.3
  - vaginalis 629.89
- **Flax dressers' disease** 504
- **Flea bite** - *see* Injury, superficial, by site
- **Fleischer (-Kayser) ring** (corneal pigmentation) 275.1 *[371.14]*
- **Fleischner's disease** 732.3
- **Fleshy mole** 631
- **Flexibilitas cerea** (*see also* Catalepsy) 300.11
- **Flexion**
  - cervix - *see* Flexion, uterus
  - contracture, joint (*see also* Contraction, joint) 718.4 [5th]
  - deformity, joint (*see also* Contraction, joint) 736.9
    - hip, congenital (*see also* Subluxation, congenital, hip) 754.32
  - uterus (*see also* Malposition, uterus) 621.6
- **Flexner's**
  - bacillus 004.1
  - diarrhea (ulcerative) 004.1
  - dysentery 004.1
- **Flexner-Boyd dysentery** 004.2
- **Flexure** - *see* condition
- **Floater, vitreous** 379.24
- **Floating**
  - cartilage (joint) (*see also* Disorder, cartilage, articular) 718.0 [5th]
    - knee 717.6
  - gallbladder (congenital) 751.69
  - kidney 593.0
    - congenital 753.3
  - liver (congenital) 751.69
  - rib 756.3
  - spleen 289.59
- **Flooding** 626.2
- **Floor** - *see* condition
- **Floppy**
  - infant NEC 781.99
  - iris syndrome 364.81
  - valve syndrome (mitral) 424.0
- **Flu** - *see also* Influenza
  - bird 488.0 ●
  - gastric NEC 008.8
  - swine 488.1 ●
- **Fluctuating blood pressure** 796.4
- **Fluid**
  - abdomen 789.59
  - chest (*see also* Pleurisy, with effusion) 511.9
  - heart (*see also* Failure, heart) 428.0
  - joint (*see also* Effusion, joint) 719.0 [5th]
  - loss (acute) 276.50
    - with
      - hypernatremia 276.0
      - hyponatremia 276.1
  - lung - *see also* Edema, lung
    - encysted 511.89
  - peritoneal cavity 789.59
    - malignant 789.51
  - pleural cavity (*see also* Pleurisy, with effusion) 511.9
  - retention 276.6
- **Flukes** NEC (*see also* Infestation, fluke) 121.9
  - blood NEC (*see also* Infestation, Schistosoma) 120.9
  - liver 121.3
- **Fluor** (albus) (vaginalis) 623.5
  - trichomonal (Trichomonas vaginalis) 131.00
- **Fluorosis** (dental) (chronic) 520.3
- **Flushing** 782.62
  - menopausal 627.2
- **Flush syndrome** 259.2
- **Flutter**
  - atrial or auricular 427.32
  - heart (ventricular) 427.42
    - atrial 427.32
  - impure 427.32
  - postoperative 997.1
  - ventricular 427.42
- **Flux** (bloody) (serosanguineous) 009.0
- **Focal** - *see* condition
- **Fochier's abscess** - *see* Abscess, by site
- **Focus, Assmann's** (*see also* Tuberculosis) 011.0 [5th]
- **Fogo selvagem** 694.4
- **Foix-Alajouanine syndrome** 336.1
- **Folds, anomalous** - *see also* Anomaly, specified type NEC
  - Bowman's membrane 371.31
  - Descemet's membrane 371.32
  - epicanthic 743.63
  - heart 746.89
  - posterior segment of eye, congenital 743.54
- **Folie a deux** 297.3
- **Follicle**
  - cervix (nabothian) (ruptured) 616.0
  - graafian, ruptured, with hemorrhage 620.0
  - nabothian 616.0
- **Folliclis** (primary) (*see also* Tuberculosis) 017.0 [5th]
- **Follicular** - *see also* condition
  - cyst (atretic) 620.0
- **Folliculitis** 704.8
  - abscedens et suffodiens 704.8
  - decalvans 704.09
  - gonorrheal (acute) 098.0
    - chronic or duration of 2 months or more 098.2
  - keloid, keloidalis 706.1
  - pustular 704.8
  - ulerythematosa reticulata 701.8
- **Folliculosis, conjunctival** 372.02
- **Følling's disease** (phenylketonuria) 270.1
- **Follow-up** (examination) (routine) (following) V67.9
  - cancer chemotherapy V67.2
  - chemotherapy V67.2
  - fracture V67.4
  - high-risk medication V67.51
  - injury NEC V67.59
  - postpartum
    - immediately after delivery V24.0
    - routine V24.2
  - psychiatric V67.3
  - psychotherapy V67.3
  - radiotherapy V67.1
  - specified condition NEC V67.59
  - specified surgery NEC V67.09
  - surgery V67.00
    - vaginal pap smear V67.01
  - treatment V67.9
    - combined NEC V67.6
    - fracture V67.4
    - involving high-risk medication NEC V67.51
    - mental disorder V67.3
    - specified NEC V67.59
- **Fong's syndrome** (hereditary osteoonychodysplasia) 756.89
- **Food**
  - allergy 693.1
  - anaphylactic shock - *see* Anaphylactic shock, due to food
  - asphyxia (from aspiration or inhalation) (*see also* Asphyxia, food) 933.1
  - choked on (*see also* Asphyxia, food) 933.1
  - deprivation 994.2
    - specified kind of food NEC 269.8
  - intoxication (*see also* Poisoning, food) 005.9
  - lack of 994.2
  - poisoning (*see also* Poisoning, food) 005.9
  - refusal or rejection NEC 307.59
  - strangulation or suffocation (*see also* Asphyxia, food) 933.1
  - toxemia (*see also* Poisoning, food) 005.9
- **Foot** - *see also* condition
  - and mouth disease 078.4
  - process disease 581.3
- **Foramen ovale** (nonclosure) (patent) (persistent) 745.5
- **Forbes'** (glycogen storage) **disease** 271.0
- **Forbes-Albright syndrome** (nonpuerperal amenorrhea and lactation associated with pituitary tumor) 253.1

Forced birth or delivery NEC 669.8 [5th]
- affecting fetus or newborn NEC 763.89

Forceps
- delivery NEC 669.5 [5th]
  - affecting fetus or newborn 763.2

Fordyce's disease (ectopic sebaceous glands) (mouth) 750.26

Fordyce-Fox disease (apocrine miliaria) 705.82

Forearm - *see* condition

Foreign body

Note *For foreign body with open wound or other injury, see Wound, open, or the type of injury specified.*

  - accidentally left during a procedure 998.4
  - anterior chamber (eye) 871.6
    - magnetic 871.5
      - retained or old 360.51
    - retained or old 360.61
- ciliary body (eye) 871.6
  - magnetic 871.5
    - retained or old 360.52
  - retained or old 360.62
- entering through orifice (current) (old)
  - accessory sinus 932
  - air passage (upper) 933.0
    - lower 934.8
  - alimentary canal 938
  - alveolar process 935.0
  - antrum (Highmore) 932
  - anus 937
  - appendix 936
  - asphyxia due to (*see also* Asphyxia, food) 933.1
  - auditory canal 931
  - auricle 931
  - bladder 939.0
  - bronchioles 934.8
  - bronchus (main) 934.1
  - buccal cavity 935.0
  - canthus (inner) 930.1
  - cecum 936
  - cervix (canal) uterine 939.1
  - coil, ileocecal 936
  - colon 936
  - conjunctiva 930.1
  - conjunctival sac 930.1
  - cornea 930.0
  - digestive organ or tract NEC 938
  - duodenum 936
  - ear (external) 931
  - esophagus 935.1
  - eye (external) 930.9
    - combined sites 930.8
    - intraocular - *see* Foreign body, by site
    - specified site NEC 930.8
  - eyeball 930.8
    - intraocular - *see* Foreign body, intraocular
  - eyelid 930.1
    - retained or old 374.86
  - frontal sinus 932
  - gastrointestinal tract 938
  - genitourinary tract 939.9
  - globe 930.8
    - penetrating 871.6
      - magnetic 871.5
        - retained or old 360.50
      - retained or old 360.60
  - gum 935.0
  - Highmore's antrum 932
  - hypopharynx 933.0
  - ileocecal coil 936
  - ileum 936
  - inspiration (of) 933.1
  - intestine (large) (small) 936
  - lacrimal apparatus, duct, gland, or sac 930.2
  - larynx 933.1
  - lung 934.8
  - maxillary sinus 932

Foreign body – *continued*
- entering through orifice – *continued*
  - mouth 935.0
  - nasal sinus 932
  - nasopharynx 933.0
  - nose (passage) 932
  - nostril 932
  - oral cavity 935.0
  - palate 935.0
  - penis 939.3
  - pharynx 933.0
  - pyriform sinus 933.0
  - rectosigmoid 937
    - junction 937
  - rectum 937
  - respiratory tract 934.9
    - specified part NEC 934.8
  - sclera 930.1
  - sinus 932
    - accessory 932
    - frontal 932
    - maxillary 932
    - nasal 932
    - pyriform 933.0
  - small intestine 936
  - stomach (hairball) 935.2
  - suffocation by (*see also* Asphyxia, food) 933.1
  - swallowed 938
    - tongue 933.0
  - tear ducts or glands 930.2
  - throat 933.0
  - tongue 935.0
    - swallowed 933.0
  - tonsil, tonsillar 933.0
    - fossa 933.0
  - trachea 934.0
  - ureter 939.0
  - urethra 939.0
  - uterus (any part) 939.1
  - vagina 939.2
  - vulva 939.2
  - wind pipe 934.0
- feeling of, in throat 784.99
- granuloma (old) 728.82
  - bone 733.99
  - in operative wound (inadvertently left) 998.4
    - due to surgical material intentionally left - *see* Complications, due to (presence of) any device, implant, or graft classified to 996.0-996.5 NEC
  - muscle 728.82
  - skin 709.4
  - soft tissue NEC 709.4
  - subcutaneous tissue 709.4
- in
  - bone (residual) 733.99
  - open wound - *see* Wound, open, by site complicated
  - soft tissue (residual) 729.6
- inadvertently left in operation wound (causing adhesions, obstruction, or perforation) 998.4
- ingestion, ingested NEC 938
- inhalation or inspiration (*see also* Asphyxia, food) 933.1
- internal organ, not entering through an orifice - *see* Injury, internal, by site, with open wound
- intraocular (nonmagnetic) 871.6
  - combined sites 871.6
    - magnetic 871.5
      - retained or old 360.59
    - retained or old 360.69
  - magnetic 871.5
    - retained or old 360.50
  - retained or old 360.60
  - specified site NEC 871.6
    - magnetic 871.5
      - retained or old 360.59
    - retained or old 360.69

Foreign body – *continued*
- iris (nonmagnetic) 871.6
  - magnetic 871.5
    - retained or old 360.52
  - retained or old 360.62
- lens (nonmagnetic) 871.6
  - magnetic 871.5
    - retained or old 360.53
  - retained or old 360.63
- lid, eye 930.1
- ocular muscle 870.4
  - retained or old 376.6
- old or residual
  - bone 733.99
  - eyelid 374.86
  - middle ear 385.83
  - muscle 729.6
    - ocular 376.6
  - retrobulbar 376.6
  - skin 729.6
    - with granuloma 709.4
  - soft tissue 729.6
    - with granuloma 709.4
  - subcutaneous tissue 729.6
    - with granuloma 709.4
- operation wound, left accidentally 998.4
- orbit 870.4
  - retained or old 376.6
- posterior wall, eye 871.6
  - magnetic 871.5
    - retained or old 360.55
  - retained or old 360.65
- respiratory tree 934.9
  - specified site NEC 934.8
- retained (old) (nonmagnetic) (in)
  - anterior chamber (eye) 360.61
    - magnetic 360.51
  - ciliary body 360.62
    - magnetic 360.52
  - eyelid 374.86
  - globe 360.60
    - magnetic 360.50
  - intraocular 360.60
    - magnetic 360.50
    - specified site NEC 360.69
      - magnetic 360.59
  - iris 360.62
    - magnetic 360.52
  - lens 360.63
    - magnetic 360.53
  - muscle 729.6
  - orbit 376.6
  - posterior wall of globe 360.65
    - magnetic 360.55
  - retina 360.65
    - magnetic 360.55
  - retrobulbar 376.6
  - skin 729.6
    - with granuloma 709.4
  - soft tissue 729.6
    - with granuloma 709.4
  - subcutaneous tissue 729.6
    - with granuloma 709.4
  - vitreous 360.64
    - magnetic 360.54
- retina 871.6
  - magnetic 871.5
    - retained or old 360.55
  - retained or old 360.65
- superficial, without major open wound (*see also* Injury, superficial, by site) 919.6
- swallowed NEC 938
- throat, feeling of 784.99
- vitreous (humor) 871.6
  - magnetic 871.5
    - retained or old 360.54
  - retained or old 360.64

Forking, aqueduct of Sylvius 742.3
- with spina bifida (*see also* Spina bifida) 741.0 [5th]

Formation
- bone in scar tissue (skin) 709.3
- connective tissue in vitreous 379.25

Formation – *continued*
- Elschnig pearls (postcataract extraction) 366.51
- hyaline in cornea 371.49
- sequestrum in bone (due to infection) (*see also* Osteomyelitis) 730.1 [5th]
- valve
  - colon, congenital 751.5
  - ureter (congenital) 753.29

Formication 782.0

Fort Bragg fever 100.89

Fossa - *see also* condition
- pyriform - *see* condition

Foster care (status) V60.81 ●

Foster-Kennedy syndrome 377.04

Fothergill's
- disease, meaning scarlatina anginosa 034.1
- neuralgia (*see also* Neuralgia, trigeminal) 350.1

Foul breath 784.99

Found dead (cause unknown) 798.9

Foundling V20.0

Fournier's disease (idiopathic gangrene) 608.83

Fourth
- cranial nerve - *see* condition
- disease 057.8
- molar 520.1

Foville's syndrome 344.89

Fox's
- disease (apocrine miliaria) 705.82
- impetigo (contagiosa) 684

Fox-Fordyce disease (apocrine miliaria) 705.82

Fracture (abduction) (adduction) (avulsion) (compression) (crush) (dislocation) (oblique) (separation) (closed) 829.0

Note *For fracture of any of the following sites with fracture of other bones – see Fracture, multiple.*

"Closed" includes the following descriptions of fractures, with or without delayed healing, unless they are specified as open or compound:

comminuted
depressed
elevated
fissured
greenstick
impacted
linear
simple
slipped epiphysis
spiral
unspecified

"Open" includes the following descriptions of fractures, with or without delayed healing:

compound
infected
missile
puncture
with foreign body

For late effect of fracture, see Late, effect, fracture, by site.

- with
  - internal injuries in same region (conditions classifiable to 860-869) - *see also* Injury, internal, by site
    - pelvic region - *see* Fracture, pelvis
- acetabulum (with visceral injury) (closed) 808.0
  - open 808.1
- acromion (process) (closed) 811.01
  - open 811.11
- alveolus (closed) 802.8
  - open 802.9
- ankle (malleolus) (closed) 824.8
  - bimalleolar (Dupuytren's) (Pott's) 824.4
    - open 824.5

Forced birth or delivery – Fracture

- **Fracture** – *continued*
  - ankle – *continued*
    - bone 825.21
      - open 825.31
    - lateral malleolus only (fibular) 824.2
      - open 824.3
    - medial malleolus only (tibial) 824.0
      - open 824.1
    - open 824.9
    - pathologic 733.16
    - talus 825.21
      - open 825.31
    - trimalleolar 824.6
      - open 824.7
  - antrum - *see* Fracture, skull, base
  - arm (closed) 818.0
    - and leg(s) (any bones) 828.0
      - open 828.1
    - both (any bones) (with rib(s)) (with sternum) 819.0
      - open 819.1
    - lower 813.80
      - open 813.90
    - open 818.1
    - upper - *see* Fracture, humerus
  - astragalus (closed) 825.21
    - open 825.31
  - atlas - *see* Fracture, vertebra, cervical, first
  - axis - *see* Fracture, vertebra, cervical, second
  - back - *see* Fracture, vertebra, by site
  - Barton's - *see* Fracture, radius, lower end
  - basal (skull) - *see* Fracture, skull, base
  - Bennett's (closed) 815.01
    - open 815.11
  - bimalleolar (closed) 824.4
    - open 824.5
  - bone (closed) NEC 829.0
    - birth injury NEC 767.3
    - open 829.1
    - pathological NEC (*see also* Fracture, pathologic) 733.10
    - stress NEC (*see also* Fracture, stress) 733.95
  - boot top - *see* Fracture, fibula
  - boxers' - *see* Fracture, metacarpal bone(s)
  - breast bone - *see* Fracture, sternum
  - bucket handle (semilunar cartilage) - *see* Tear, meniscus
  - buckle - *see* Fracture, torus ●
  - burst - *see* Fracture, traumatic, by site
  - bursting - *see* Fracture, phalanx, hand, distal
  - calcaneus (closed) 825.0
    - open 825.1
  - capitate (bone) (closed) 814.07
    - open 814.17
  - capitellum (humerus) (closed) 812.49
    - open 812.59
  - carpal bone(s) (wrist NEC) (closed) 814.00
    - open 814.10
    - specified site NEC 814.09
      - open 814.19
  - cartilage, knee (semilunar) - *see* Tear, meniscus
  - cervical - *see* Fracture, vertebra, cervical
  - chauffeur's - *see* Fracture, ulna, lower end
  - chisel - *see* Fracture, radius, upper end
  - chronic - *see* Fracture, pathologic ●
  - clavicle (interligamentous part) (closed) 810.00
    - acromial end 810.03
      - open 810.13
    - due to birth trauma 767.2
    - open 810.10
    - shaft (middle third) 810.02
      - open 810.12
    - sternal end 810.01
      - open 810.11
  - clayshovelers' - *see* Fracture, vertebra, cervical
  - coccyx - *see also* Fracture, vertebra, coccyx
    - complicating delivery 665.6 [5th]

- **Fracture** – *continued*
  - collar bone - *see* Fracture, clavicle
  - Colles' (reversed) (closed) 813.41
    - open 813.51
  - comminuted - *see* Fracture, by site
  - compression - *see also* Fracture, by site
    - nontraumatic - *see* Fracture, pathologic
  - congenital 756.9
  - coracoid process (closed) 811.02
    - open 811.12
  - coronoid process (ulna) (closed) 813.02
    - mandible (closed) 802.23
      - open 802.33
    - open 813.12
  - corpus cavernosum penis 959.13
  - costochondral junction - *see* Fracture, rib
  - costosternal junction - *see* Fracture, rib
  - cranium - *see* Fracture, skull, by site
  - cricoid cartilage (closed) 807.5
    - open 807.6
  - cuboid (ankle) (closed) 825.23
    - open 825.33
  - cuneiform
    - foot (closed) 825.24
      - open 825.34
    - wrist (closed) 814.03
      - open 814.13
  - dental implant 525.73
  - dental restorative material
    - with loss of material 525.64
    - without loss of material 525.63
  - due to
    - birth injury - *see* Birth injury, fracture
    - gunshot - *see* Fracture, by site, open
    - neoplasm - *see* Fracture, pathologic
    - osteoporosis - *see* Fracture, pathologic
  - Dupuytren's (ankle) (fibula) (closed) 824.4
    - open 824.5
    - radius 813.42
      - open 813.52
  - Duverney's - *see* Fracture, ilium
  - elbow - *see also* Fracture, humerus, lower end
    - olecranon (process) (closed) 813.01
      - open 813.11
    - supracondylar (closed) 812.41
      - open 812.51
  - ethmoid (bone) (sinus) - *see* Fracture, skull, base
  - face bone(s) (closed) NEC 802.8
    - with
      - other bone(s) - *see* Fracture, multiple, skull
      - skull - *see also* Fracture, skull
        - involving other bones - *see* Fracture, multiple, skull
    - open 802.9
  - fatigue - *see* Fracture, march
  - femur, femoral (closed) 821.00
    - cervicotrochanteric 820.03
      - open 820.13
    - condyles, epicondyles 821.21
      - open 821.31
    - distal end - *see* Fracture, femur, lower end
    - epiphysis (separation)
      - capital 820.01
        - open 820.11
      - head 820.01
        - open 820.11
      - lower 821.22
        - open 821.32
      - trochanteric 820.01
        - open 820.11
      - upper 820.01
        - open 820.11
    - head 820.09
      - open 820.19
    - lower end or extremity (distal end) (closed) 821.20
      - condyles, epicondyles 821.21
        - open 821.31
      - epiphysis (separation) 821.22
        - open 821.32

- **Fracture** – *continued*
  - femur, femoral – *continued*
    - lower end or extremity – *continued*
      - multiple sites 821.29
        - open 821.39
      - open 821.30
      - specified site NEC 821.29
        - open 821.39
      - supracondylar 821.23
        - open 821.33
      - T-shaped 821.21
        - open 821.31
    - neck (closed) 820.8
      - base (cervicotrochanteric) 820.03
        - open 820.13
      - extracapsular 820.20
        - open 820.30
      - intertrochanteric (section) 820.21
        - open 820.31
      - intracapsular 820.00
        - open 820.10
      - intratrochanteric 820.21
        - open 820.31
      - midcervical 820.02
        - open 820.12
      - open 820.9
      - pathologic 733.14
        - specified part NEC 733.15
      - specified site NEC 820.09
        - open 820.19
      - transcervical 820.02
        - open 820.12
      - transtrochanteric 820.20
        - open 820.30
    - open 821.10
    - pathologic 733.14
      - specified part NEC 733.15
    - peritrochanteric (section) 820.20
      - open 820.30
    - shaft (lower third) (middle third) (upper third) 821.01
      - open 821.11
    - subcapital 820.09
      - open 820.19
    - subtrochanteric (region) (section) 820.22
      - open 820.32
    - supracondylar 821.23
      - open 821.33
    - transepiphyseal 820.01
      - open 820.11
    - trochanter (greater) (lesser) (*see also* Fracture, femur, neck, by site) 820.20
      - open 820.30
    - T-shaped, into knee joint 821.21
      - open 821.31
    - upper end 820.8
      - open 820.9
  - fibula (closed) 823.81
    - with tibia 823.82
      - open 823.92
    - distal end 824.8
      - open 824.9
    - epiphysis
      - lower 824.8
        - open 824.9
      - upper - *see* Fracture, fibula, upper end
    - head - *see* Fracture, fibula, upper end
    - involving ankle 824.2
      - open 824.3
    - lower end or extremity 824.8
      - open 824.9
    - malleolus (external) (lateral) 824.2
      - open 824.3
    - open NEC 823.91
    - pathologic 733.16
    - proximal end - *see* Fracture, fibula, upper end
    - shaft 823.21
      - with tibia 823.22
        - open 823.32
      - open 823.31

- **Fracture** – *continued*
  - fibula (closed) – *continued*
    - stress 733.93
    - torus 823.41
      - with tibia 823.42
    - upper end or extremity (epiphysis) (head) (proximal end) (styloid) 823.01
      - with tibia 823.02
        - open 823.12
      - open 823.11
  - finger(s), of one hand (closed) (*see also* Fracture, phalanx, hand) 816.00
    - with
      - metacarpal bone(s), of same hand 817.0
        - open 817.1
      - thumb of same hand 816.03
        - open 816.13
    - open 816.10
  - foot, except toe(s) alone (closed) 825.20
    - open 825.30
  - forearm (closed) NEC 813.80
    - lower end (distal end) (lower epiphysis) 813.40
      - open 813.50
    - open 813.90
    - shaft 813.20
      - open 813.30
    - upper end (proximal end) (upper epiphysis) 813.00
      - open 813.10
  - fossa, anterior, middle, or posterior - *see* Fracture, skull, base
  - frontal (bone) - *see also* Fracture, skull, vault
    - sinus - *see* Fracture, skull, base
  - Galeazzi's - *see* Fracture, radius, lower end
  - glenoid (cavity) (fossa) (scapula) (closed) 811.03
    - open 811.13
  - Gosselin's - *see* Fracture, ankle
  - greenstick - *see* Fracture, by site
  - grenade-throwers' - *see* Fracture, humerus, shaft
  - gutter - *see* Fracture, skull, vault
  - hamate (closed) 814.08
    - open 814.18
  - hand, one (closed) 815.00
    - carpals 814.00
      - open 814.10
      - specified site NEC 814.09
        - open 814.19
    - metacarpals 815.00
      - open 815.10
    - multiple, bones of one hand 817.0
      - open 817.1
    - open 815.10
    - phalanges (*see also* Fracture, phalanx, hand) 816.00
      - open 816.10
  - healing
    - aftercare (*see also* Aftercare, fracture) V54.89
    - change of cast V54.89
    - complications - *see* condition
    - convalescence V66.4
    - removal of
      - cast V54.89
      - fixation device
        - external V54.89
        - internal V54.01
  - heel bone (closed) 825.0
    - open 825.1
  - Hill-Sachs 812.09
  - hip (closed) (*see also* Fracture, femur, neck) 820.8
    - open 820.9
    - pathologic 733.14
  - humerus (closed) 812.20
    - anatomical neck 812.02
      - open 812.12

- **Fracture** - *continued*
  - humerus (closed) - *continued*
    - articular process (*see also* Fracture humerus, condyle(s)) 812.44
      - open 812.54
    - capitellum 812.49
      - open 812.59
    - condyle(s) 812.44
      - lateral (external) 812.42
        - open 812.52
      - medial (internal epicondyle) 812.43
        - open 812.53
      - open 812.54
    - distal end - *see* Fracture, humerus, lower end
    - epiphysis
      - lower (*see also* Fracture, humerus, condyle(s)) 812.44
        - open 812.54
      - upper 812.09
        - open 812.19
    - external condyle 812.42
      - open 812.52
    - great tuberosity 812.03
      - open 812.13
    - head 812.09
      - open 812.19
    - internal epicondyle 812.43
      - open 812.53
    - lesser tuberosity 812.09
      - open 812.19
    - lower end or extremity (distal end) (*see also* Fracture, humerus, by site) 812.40
      - multiple sites NEC 812.49
        - open 812.59
      - open 812.50
      - specified site NEC 812.49
        - open 812.59
    - neck 812.01
      - open 812.11
    - open 812.30
    - pathologic 733.11
    - proximal end - *see* Fracture, humerus, upper end
    - shaft 812.21
      - open 812.31
    - supracondylar 812.41
      - open 812.51
    - surgical neck 812.01
      - open 812.11
    - trochlea 812.49
      - open 812.59
    - T-shaped 812.44
      - open 812.54
    - tuberosity - *see* Fracture, humerus, upper end
    - upper end or extremity (proximal end) (*see also* Fracture, humerus, by site) 812.00
      - open 812.10
      - specified site NEC 812.09
        - open 812.19
  - hyoid bone (closed) 807.5
    - open 807.6
  - hyperextension - *see* Fracture, radius, lower end
  - ilium (with visceral injury) (closed) 808.41
    - open 808.51
  - impaction, impacted - *see* Fracture, by site
  - incus - *see* Fracture, skull, base
  - innominate bone (with visceral injury) (closed) 808.49
    - open 808.59
  - instep, of one foot (closed) 825.20
    - with toe(s) of same foot 827.0
      - open 827.1
    - open 825.30
  - insufficiency - *see* Fracture, pathologic, by site
  - internal
    - ear - *see* Fracture, skull, base

- **Fracture** - *continued*
  - internal - *continued*
    - semilunar cartilage, knee - *see* Tear, meniscus, medial
  - intertrochanteric - *see* Fracture, femur, neck, intertrochanteric
  - ischium (with visceral injury) (closed) 808.42
    - open 808.52
  - jaw (bone) (lower) (closed) (*see also* Fracture, mandible) 802.20
    - angle 802.25
      - open 802.35
    - open 802.30
    - upper - *see* Fracture, maxilla
  - knee
    - cap (closed) 822.0
      - open 822.1
    - cartilage (semilunar) - *see* Tear, meniscus
  - labyrinth (osseous) - *see* Fracture, skull, base
  - larynx (closed) 807.5
    - open 807.6
  - late effect - *see* Late, effects (of), fracture
  - Le Fort's - *see* Fracture, maxilla
  - leg (closed) 827.0
    - with rib(s) or sternum 828.0
      - open 828.1
    - both (any bones) 828.0
      - open 828.1
    - lower - *see* Fracture, tibia
    - open 827.1
    - upper - *see* Fracture, femur
  - limb
    - lower (multiple) (closed) NEC 827.0
      - open 827.1
    - upper (multiple) (closed) NEC 818.0
      - open 818.1
  - long bones, due to birth trauma - *see* Birth injury, fracture
  - lumbar - *see* Fracture, vertebra, lumbar
  - lunate bone (closed) 814.02
    - open 814.12
  - malar bone (closed) 802.4
    - open 802.5
  - Malgaigne's (closed) 808.43
    - open 808.53
  - malleolus (closed) 824.8
    - bimalleolar 824.4
      - open 824.5
    - lateral 824.2
      - and medial - *see also* Fracture, malleolus, bimalleolar
        - with lip of tibia - *see* Fracture, malleolus, trimalleolar
      - open 824.3
    - medial (closed) 824.0
      - and lateral - *see also* Fracture, malleolus, bimalleolar
        - with lip of tibia - *see* Fracture, malleolus, trimalleolar
      - open 824.1
    - open 824.9
    - trimalleolar (closed) 824.6
      - open 824.7
  - malleus - *see* Fracture, skull, base
  - malunion 733.81
  - mandible (closed) 802.20
    - angle 802.25
      - open 802.35
    - body 802.28
      - alveolar border 802.27
        - open 802.37
      - open 802.38
      - symphysis 802.26
        - open 802.36
    - condylar process 802.21
      - open 802.31
    - coronoid process 802.23
      - open 802.33
    - multiple sites 802.29
      - open 802.39
    - open 802.30

- **Fracture** - *continued*
  - mandible (closed) - *continued*
    - ramus NEC 802.24
      - open 802.34
    - subcondylar 802.22
      - open 802.32
  - manubrium - *see* Fracture, sternum
  - march 733.95
    - fibula 733.93
    - metatarsals 733.94
    - tibia 733.93
  - maxilla, maxillary (superior) (upper jaw) (closed) 802.4
    - inferior - *see* Fracture, mandible
    - open 802.5
  - meniscus, knee - *see* Tear, meniscus
  - metacarpus, metacarpal (bone(s)), of one hand (closed) 815.00
    - with phalanx, phalanges, hand (finger(s)) (thumb) of same hand 817.0
      - open 817.1
    - base 815.02
      - first metacarpal 815.01
        - open 815.11
      - open 815.12
      - thumb 815.01
        - open 815.11
    - multiple sites 815.09
      - open 815.19
    - neck 815.04
      - open 815.14
    - open 815.10
    - shaft 815.03
      - open 815.13
  - metatarsus, metatarsal (bone(s)), of one foot (closed) 825.25
    - with tarsal bone(s) 825.29
      - open 825.39
    - open 825.35
  - monteggia's (closed) 813.03
    - open 813.13
  - Moore's - *see* Fracture, radius, lower end
  - multangular bone (closed)
    - larger 814.05
      - open 814.15
    - smaller 814.06
      - open 814.16
  - multiple (closed) 829.0

Note *Multiple fractures of sites classifiable to the same three-or four-digit category are coded to that category, except for sites classifiable to 810-818 or 820-827 in different limbs.*

Multiple fractures of sites classifiable to different fourth-digit subdivisions within the same three-digit category should be dealt with according to coding rules.

Multiple fractures of sites classifiable to different three-digit categories (identifiable from the listing under "Fracture"), and of sites classifiable to 810-818 or 820-827 in different limbs should be coded according to the following list, which should be referred to in the following priority order: skull or face bones, pelvis or vertebral column, legs, arms.

- arm (multiple bones in same arm except in hand alone) (sites classifiable to 810-817 with sites classifiable to a different three-digit category in 810-817 in same arm) (closed) 818.0
  - open 818.1
- arms, both or arm(s) with rib(s) or sternum (sites classifiable to 810-818 with sites classifiable to same range of categories in other limb or to 807) (closed) 819.0
  - open 819.1

- **Fracture** - *continued*
  - multiple (closed) - *continued*
    - bones of trunk NEC (closed) 809.0
      - open 809.1
    - hand, metacarpal bone(s) with phalanx or phalanges of same hand (sites classifiable to 815 with sites classifiable to 816 in same hand) (closed) 817.0
      - open 817.1
    - leg (multiple bones in same leg) (sites classifiable to 820-826 with sites classifiable to a different three-digit category in that range in same leg) (closed) 827.0
      - open 827.1
    - legs, both or leg(s) with arm(s), rib(s), or sternum (sites classifiable to 820-827 with sites classifiable to same range of categories in other leg or to 807 or 810-819) (closed) 828.0
      - open 828.1
    - open 829.1
    - pelvis with other bones except skull or face bones (sites classifiable to 808 with sites classifiable to 805-807 or 810-829) (closed) 809.0
      - open 809.1
    - skull, specified or unspecified bones, or face bone(s) with any other bone(s) (sites classifiable to 800-803 with sites classifiable to 805-829) (closed) 804.0 5th

Note *Use the following fifth-digit subclassification with categories 800, 801, 803, and 804:*

0	unspecified state of consciousness
1	with no loss of consciousness
2	with brief [less than one hour] loss of consciousness
3	with moderate [1-24 hours] loss of consciousness
4	with prolonged [more than 24 hours] loss of consciousness and return to pre-existing conscious level
5	with prolonged [more than 24 hours] loss of consciousness, without return to pre-existing conscious level
	Use fifth-digit 5 to designate when a patient is unconscious and dies before regaining consciousness, regardless of the duration of the loss of consciousness
6	with loss of consciousness of unspecified duration
9	with concussion, unspecified

- with
  - contusion, cerebral 804.1 5th
  - epidural hemorrhage 804.2 5th
  - extradural hemorrhage 804.2 5th
  - hemorrhage (intracranial) NEC 804.3 5th
  - intracranial injury NEC 804.4 5th
  - laceration, cerebral 804.1 5th
  - subarachnoid hemorrhage 804.2 5th
  - subdural hemorrhage 804.2 5th
- open 804.5 5th
  - with
    - contusion, cerebral 804.6 5th
    - epidural hemorrhage 804.7 5th
    - extradural hemorrhage 804.7 5th
    - hemorrhage (intracranial) NEC 804.8 5th
    - intracranial injury NEC 804.9 5th
    - laceration, cerebral 804.6 5th

Fracture

Fracture – *continued*
- multiple (closed) – *continued*
  - skull, specified or unspecified bones, or face bone(s) with any other bone(s) – *continued*
    - open – *continued*
      - with – *continued*
        - subarachnoid hemorrhage 804.7 5th
        - subdural hemorrhage 804.7 5th
  - vertebral column with other bones, except skull or face bones (sites classifiable to 805 or 806 with sites classifiable to 807-808 or 810-829) (closed) 809.0
    - open 809.1
- nasal (bone(s)) (closed) 802.0
  - open 802.1
  - sinus - *see* Fracture, skull, base
- navicular
  - carpal (wrist) (closed) 814.01
    - open 814.11
  - tarsal (ankle) (closed) 825.22
    - open 825.32
- neck - *see* Fracture, vertebra, cervical
- neural arch - *see* Fracture, vertebra, by site
- nonunion 733.82
- nose, nasal, (bone) (septum) (closed) 802.0
  - open 802.1
- occiput - *see* Fracture, skull, base
- odontoid process - *see* Fracture, vertebra, cervical
- olecranon (process) (ulna) (closed) 813.01
  - open 813.11
- open 829.1
- orbit, orbital (bone) (region) (closed) 802.8
  - floor (blow-out) 802.6
    - open 802.7
  - open 802.9
  - roof - *see* Fracture, skull, base
  - specified part NEC 802.8
    - open 802.9
- os
  - calcis (closed) 825.0
    - open 825.1
  - magnum (closed) 814.07
    - open 814.17
  - pubis (with visceral injury) (closed) 808.2
    - open 808.3
  - triquetrum (closed) 814.03
    - open 814.13
- osseous
  - auditory meatus - *see* Fracture, skull, base
  - labyrinth - *see* Fracture, skull, base
- ossicles, auditory (incus) (malleus) (stapes) - *see* Fracture, skull, base
- osteoporotic - *see* Fracture, pathologic
- palate (closed) 802.8
  - open 802.9
- paratrooper - *see* Fracture, tibia, lower end
- parietal bone - *see* Fracture, skull, vault
- parry - *see* Fracture, Monteggia's
- patella (closed) 822.0
  - open 822.1
- pathologic (cause unknown) 733.10
  - ankle 733.16
  - femur (neck) 733.14
    - specified NEC 733.15
  - fibula 733.16
  - hip 733.14
  - humerus 733.11
  - radius (distal) 733.12
  - specified site NEC 733.19
  - tibia 733.16
  - ulna 733.12
  - vertebrae (collapse) 733.13
  - wrist 733.12
- pedicle (of vertebral arch) - *see* Fracture, vertebra, by site
- pelvis, pelvic (bone(s)) (with visceral injury) (closed) 808.8
  - multiple (with disruption of pelvic circle) 808.43
    - open 808.53
  - open 808.9
  - rim (closed) 808.49
    - open 808.59
- peritrochanteric (closed) 820.20
  - open 820.30
- phalanx, phalanges, of one
  - foot (closed) 826.0
    - with bone(s) of same lower limb 827.0
      - open 827.1
    - open 826.1
  - hand (closed) 816.00
    - with metacarpal bone(s) of same hand 817.0
      - open 817.1
    - distal 816.02
      - open 816.12
    - middle 816.01
      - open 816.11
    - multiple sites NEC 816.03
      - open 816.13
    - open 816.10
    - proximal 816.01
      - open 816.11
- pisiform (closed) 814.04
  - open 814.14
- pond - *see* Fracture, skull, vault
- Pott's (closed) 824.4
  - open 824.5
- prosthetic device, internal - *see* Complications, mechanical
- pubis (with visceral injury) (closed) 808.2
  - open 808.3
- Quervain's (closed) 814.01
  - open 814.11
- radius (alone) (closed) 813.81
  - with ulna NEC 813.83
    - open 813.93
  - distal end - *see* Fracture, radius, lower end
  - epiphysis
    - lower - *see* Fracture, radius, lower end
    - upper - *see* Fracture, radius, upper end
  - head - *see* Fracture, radius, upper end
  - lower end or extremity (distal end) (lower epiphysis) 813.42
    - with ulna (lower end) 813.44
      - open 813.54
    - open 813.52
    - torus 813.45
      - with ulna 813.47 ●
  - neck - *see* Fracture, radius, upper end
  - open NEC 813.91
  - pathologic 733.12
  - proximal end - *see* Fracture, radius, upper end
  - shaft (closed) 813.21
    - with ulna (shaft) 813.23
      - open 813.33
    - open 813.31
  - upper end 813.07
    - with ulna (upper end) 813.08
      - open 813.18
    - epiphysis 813.05
      - open 813.15
    - head 813.05
      - open 813.15
    - multiple sites 813.07
      - open 813.17
    - neck 813.06
      - open 813.16
    - open 813.17
    - specified site NEC 813.07
      - open 813.17
- ramus
  - inferior or superior (with visceral injury) (closed) 808.2
    - open 808.3
  - ischium - *see* Fracture, ischium
  - mandible 802.24
    - open 802.34
- rib(s) (closed) 807.0 5th

Note *Use the following fifth-digit subclassification with categories 807.0-807.1:*

0	rib(s), unspecified
1	one rib
2	two ribs
3	three ribs
4	four ribs
5	five ribs
6	six ribs
7	seven ribs
8	eight or more ribs
9	multiple ribs, unspecified

  - with flail chest (open) 807.4
  - open 807.1 5th
- root, tooth 873.63
  - complicated 873.73
- sacrum - *see* Fracture, vertebra, sacrum
- scaphoid
  - ankle (closed) 825.22
    - open 825.32
  - wrist (closed) 814.01
    - open 814.11
- scapula (closed) 811.00
  - acromial, acromion (process) 811.01
    - open 811.11
  - body 811.09
    - open 811.19
  - coracoid process 811.02
    - open 811.12
  - glenoid (cavity) (fossa) 811.03
    - open 811.13
  - neck 811.03
    - open 811.13
  - open 811.10
- semilunar
  - bone, wrist (closed) 814.02
    - open 814.12
  - cartilage (interior) (knee) - *see* Tear, meniscus
- sesamoid bone - *see* Fracture, by site
- shepherd's (closed) 825.21
  - open 825.31
- shoulder - *see also* Fracture, humerus, upper end
  - blade - *see* Fracture, scapula
- silverfork - *see* Fracture, radius, lower end
- sinus (ethmoid) (frontal) (maxillary) (nasal) (sphenoidal) - *see* Fracture, skull, base
- Skillern's - *see* Fracture, radius, shaft
- skull (multiple NEC) (with face bones) (closed) 803.0 5th

Note *Use the following fifth-digit subclassification with categories 800, 801, 803, and 804:*

0	unspecified state of consciousness
1	with no loss of consciousness
2	with brief [less than one hour] loss of consciousness
3	with moderate [1-24 hours] loss of consciousness
4	with prolonged [more than 24 hours] loss of consciousness and return to pre-existing conscious level
5	with prolonged [more than 24 hours] loss of consciousness, without return to pre-existing conscious level
	Use fifth-digit 5 to designate when a patient is unconscious and dies before regaining consciousness, regardless of the duration of the loss of consciousness
6	with loss of consciousness of unspecified duration
9	with concussion, unspecified

  - with
    - contusion, cerebral 803.1 5th
    - epidural hemorrhage 803.2 5th
    - extradural hemorrhage 803.2 5th
    - hemorrhage (intracranial) NEC 803.3 5th
    - intracranial injury NEC 803.4 5th
    - laceration, cerebral 803.1 5th
    - other bones - *see* Fracture, multiple, skull
    - subarachnoid hemorrhage 803.2 5th
    - subdural hemorrhage 803.2 5th
  - base (antrum) (ethmoid bone) (fossa) (internal ear) (nasal sinus) (occiput) (sphenoid) (temporal bone) (closed) 801.0 5th
    - with
      - contusion, cerebral 801.1 5th
      - epidural hemorrhage 801.2 5th
      - extradural hemorrhage 801.2 5th
      - hemorrhage (intracranial) NEC 801.3 5th
      - intracranial injury NEC 801.4 5th
      - laceration, cerebral 801.1 5th
      - subarachnoid hemorrhage 801.2 5th
      - subdural hemorrhage 801.2 5th
    - open 801.5 5th
      - with
        - contusion, cerebral 801.6 5th
        - epidural hemorrhage 801.7 5th
        - extradural hemorrhage 801.7 5th
        - hemorrhage (intracranial) NEC 801.8 5th
        - intracranial injury NEC 801.9 5th
        - laceration, cerebral 801.6 5th
        - subarachnoid hemorrhage 801.7 5th
        - subdural hemorrhage 801.7 5th
  - birth injury 767.3
  - face bones - *see* Fracture, face bones
  - open 803.5 5th
    - with
      - contusion, cerebral 803.6 5th
      - epidural hemorrhage 803.7 5th
      - extradural hemorrhage 803.7 5th
      - hemorrhage (intracranial) NEC 803.8 5th
      - intracranial injury NEC 803.9 5th
      - laceration, cerebral 803.6 5th

Fracture

- **Fracture** - *continued*
  - skull (closed) - *continued*
    - open - *continued*
      - with - *continued*
        - subarachnoid hemorrhage 803.7 5th
        - subdural hemorrhage 803.7 5th
    - vault (frontal bone) (parietal bone) (vertex) (closed) 800.0 5th
      - with
        - contusion, cerebral 800.1 5th
        - epidural hemorrhage 800.2 5th
        - extradural hemorrhage 800.2 5th
        - hemorrhage (intracranial) NEC 800.3 5th
        - intracranial injury NEC 800.4 5th
        - laceration, cerebral 800.1 5th
        - subarachnoid hemorrhage 800.2 5th
        - subdural hemorrhage 800.2 5th
      - open 800.5 5th
        - with
          - contusion, cerebral 800.6 5th
          - epidural hemorrhage 800.7 5th
          - extradural hemorrhage 800.7 5th
          - hemorrhage (intracranial) NEC 800.8 5th
          - intracranial injury NEC 800.9 5th
          - laceration, cerebral 800.6 5th
          - subarachnoid hemorrhage 800.7 5th
          - subdural hemorrhage 800.7 5th
  - Smith's 813.41
    - open 813.51
  - sphenoid (bone) (sinus) - *see* Fracture, skull, base
  - spine - *see also* Fracture, vertebra, by site
    - due to birth trauma 767.4
  - spinous process - *see* Fracture, vertebra, by site
  - spontaneous - *see* Fracture, pathologic
  - sprinters' - *see* Fracture, ilium
  - stapes - *see* Fracture, skull, base
  - stave - *see also* Fracture, metacarpus, metacarpal bone(s)
    - spine - *see* Fracture, tibia, upper end
  - sternum (closed) 807.2
    - with flail chest (open) 807.4
    - open 807.3
  - Stieda's - *see* Fracture, femur, lower end
  - stress 733.95
    - fibula 733.93
    - metatarsals 733.94
    - specified site NEC 733.95
    - tibia 733.93
  - styloid process
    - metacarpal (closed) 815.02
      - open 815.12
    - radius - *see* Fracture, radius, lower end
    - temporal bone - *see* Fracture, skull, base
    - ulna - *see* Fracture, ulna, lower end
  - supracondylar, elbow 812.41
    - open 812.51
  - symphysis pubis (with visceral injury) (closed) 808.2
    - open 808.3
  - talus (ankle bone) (closed) 825.21
    - open 825.31
  - tarsus, tarsal bone(s) (with metatarsus) of one foot (closed) NEC 825.29
    - open 825.39
  - temporal bone (styloid) - *see* Fracture, skull, base
  - tendon - *see* Sprain, by site
  - thigh - *see* Fracture, femur, shaft
  - thumb (and finger(s)) of one hand (closed) (*see also* Fracture, phalanx, hand) 816.00
    - with metacarpal bone(s) of same hand 817.0
      - open 817.1
    - metacarpal(s) - *see* Fracture, metacarpus
    - open 816.10
  - thyroid cartilage (closed) 807.5
    - open 807.6
  - tibia (closed) 823.80
    - with fibula 823.82
      - open 823.92
    - condyles - *see* Fracture, tibia, upper end
    - distal end 824.8
      - open 824.9
    - epiphysis
      - lower 824.8
        - open 824.9
      - upper - *see* Fracture, tibia, upper end
    - head (involving knee joint) - *see* Fracture, tibia, upper end
    - intercondyloid eminence - *see* Fracture, tibia, upper end
    - involving ankle 824.0
      - open 824.1
    - lower end or extremity (anterior lip) (posterior lip) 824.8
      - open 824.9
    - malleolus (internal) (medial) 824.0
      - open 824.1
    - open NEC 823.90
    - pathologic 733.16
    - proximal end - *see* Fracture, tibia, upper end
    - shaft 823.20
      - with fibula 823.22
        - open 823.32
      - open 823.30
    - spine - *see* Fracture, tibia, upper end
    - stress 733.93
    - torus 823.40
      - with fibula 823.42
    - tuberosity - *see* Fracture, tibia, upper end
    - upper end or extremity (condyle) (epiphysis) (head) (spine) (proximal end) (tuberosity) 823.00
      - with fibula 823.02
        - open 823.12
      - open 823.10
  - toe(s), of one foot (closed) 826.0
    - with bone(s) of same lower limb 827.0
      - open 827.1
    - open 826.1
  - tooth (root) 873.63
    - complicated 873.73
  - torus
    - fibula 823.41
      - with tibia 823.42
    - humerus 812.49 ●
    - radius <u>(alone)</u> 813.45 ▲
      - with ulna 813.47 ●
    - tibia 823.40
      - with fibula 823.42
    - ulna (alone) 813.46 ●
      - with radius 813.47 ●
  - trachea (closed) 807.5
    - open 807.6
  - transverse process - *see* Fracture, vertebra, by site
  - trapezium (closed) 814.05
    - open 814.15
  - trapezoid bone (closed) 814.06
    - open 814.16
  - trimalleolar (closed) 824.6
    - open 824.7
  - triquetral (bone) (closed) 814.03
    - open 814.13
  - trochanter (greater) (lesser) (closed) (*see also* Fracture, femur, neck, by site) 820.20
    - open 820.30
  - trunk (bones) (closed) 809.0
    - open 809.1
  - tuberosity (external) - *see* Fracture, by site
  - ulna (alone) (closed) 813.82
    - with radius NEC 813.83
      - open 813.93
    - coronoid process (closed) 813.02
      - open 813.12
    - distal end - *see* Fracture, ulna, lower end
    - epiphysis
      - lower - *see* Fracture, ulna, lower end
      - upper - *see* Fracture, ulna, upper, end
    - head - *see* Fracture, ulna, lower end
    - lower end (distal end) (head) (lower epiphysis) (styloid process) 813.43
      - with radius (lower end) 813.44
        - open 813.54
      - open 813.53
    - olecranon process (closed) 813.01
      - open 813.11
    - open NEC 813.92
    - pathologic 733.12
    - proximal end - *see* Fracture, ulna, upper end
    - shaft 813.22
      - with radius (shaft) 813.23
        - open 813.33
      - open 813.32
    - styloid process - *see* Fracture, ulna, lower end
    - torus 813.46 ●
      - with radius 813.47 ●
    - transverse - *see* Fracture, ulna, by site
    - upper end (epiphysis) 813.04
      - with radius (upper end) 813.08
        - open 813.18
      - multiple sites 813.04
        - open 813.14
      - open 813.14
      - specified site NEC 813.04
        - open 813.14
  - unciform (closed) 814.08
    - open 814.18
  - vertebra, vertebral (back) (body) (column) (neural arch) (pedicle) (spine) (spinous process) (transverse process) (closed) 805.8
    - with
      - hematomyelia - *see* Fracture, vertebra, by site, with spinal cord injury
      - injury to
        - cauda equina - *see* Fracture, vertebra, sacrum, with spinal cord injury
        - nerve - *see* Fracture, vertebra, by site, with spinal cord injury
      - paralysis - *see* Fracture, vertebra, by site, with spinal cord injury
      - paraplegia - *see* Fracture, vertebra, by site, with spinal cord injury
      - quadriplegia - *see* Fracture, vertebra, by site, with spinal cord injury
      - spinal concussion - *see* Fracture, vertebra, by site, with spinal cord injury
      - spinal cord injury (closed) NEC 806.8

Fracture - *continued*
vertebra, vertebral (closed) - *continued*

Note *Use the following fifth-digit subclassification with categories 806.0-806.3:*

C_1-C_4 or unspecified level and D_1-D_6 (T_1-T_6) or unspecified level with:

0 unspecified spinal cord injury
1 complete lesion of cord
2 anterior cord syndrome
3 central cord syndrome
4 specified injury NEC

C_5-C_7 level and D_7-D_{12} level with:

5 unspecified spinal cord injury
6 complete lesion of cord
7 anterior cord syndrome
8 central cord syndrome
9 specified injury NEC

- with (continued)
  - spinal cord injury (closed) NEC 806.8 (continued)
    - cervical 806.0 5th
      - open 806.1 5th
    - chronic 733.13
    - dorsal, dorsolumbar 806.2 5th
      - open 806.3 5th
      - open 806.9
    - thoracic, thoracolumbar 806.2 5th
      - open 806.3 5th
- atlanto-axial - *see* Fracture, vertebra, cervical
- cervical (hangman) (teardrop) (closed) 805.00
  - with spinal cord injury - *see* Fracture, vertebra, with spinal cord injury, cervical
  - first (atlas) 805.01
    - open 805.11
  - second (axis) 805.02
    - open 805.12
  - third 805.03
    - open 805.13
  - fourth 805.04
    - open 805.14
  - fifth 805.05
    - open 805.15
  - sixth 805.06
    - open 805.16
  - seventh 805.07
    - open 805.17
  - multiple sites 805.08
    - open 805.18
  - open 805.10
- coccyx (closed) 805.6
  - with spinal cord injury (closed) 806.60
    - cauda equina injury 806.62
      - complete lesion 806.61
        - open 806.71
      - open 806.72
    - open 806.70
    - specified type NEC 806.69
      - open 806.79
  - open 805.7
- collapsed 733.13
- compression, not due to trauma 733.13
- dorsal (closed) 805.2
  - with spinal cord injury - *see* Fracture, vertebra, with spinal cord injury, dorsal
  - open 805.3
- dorsolumbar (closed) 805.2
  - with spinal cord injury - *see* Fracture, vertebra, with spinal cord injury, dorsal
  - open 805.3
- due to osteoporosis 733.13
- fetus or newborn 767.4
- lumbar (closed) 805.4
  - with spinal cord injury (closed) 806.4
    - open 806.5
  - open 805.5

Fracture

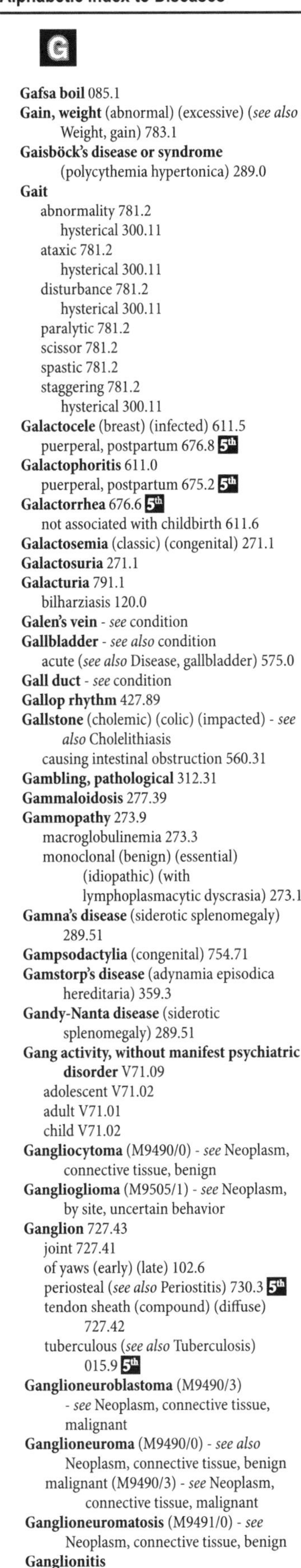

G

Gafsa boil 085.1
Gain, weight (abnormal) (excessive) (*see also* Weight, gain) 783.1
Gaisböck's disease or syndrome (polycythemia hypertonica) 289.0
Gait
- abnormality 781.2
  - hysterical 300.11
- ataxic 781.2
  - hysterical 300.11
- disturbance 781.2
  - hysterical 300.11
- paralytic 781.2
- scissor 781.2
- spastic 781.2
- staggering 781.2
  - hysterical 300.11

Galactocele (breast) (infected) 611.5
- puerperal, postpartum 676.8 5th

Galactophoritis 611.0
- puerperal, postpartum 675.2 5th

Galactorrhea 676.6 5th
- not associated with childbirth 611.6

Galactosemia (classic) (congenital) 271.1
Galactosuria 271.1
Galacturia 791.1
- bilharziasis 120.0

Galen's vein - *see* condition
Gallbladder - *see also* condition
- acute (*see also* Disease, gallbladder) 575.0

Gall duct - *see* condition
Gallop rhythm 427.89
Gallstone (cholemic) (colic) (impacted) - *see also* Cholelithiasis
- causing intestinal obstruction 560.31

Gambling, pathological 312.31
Gammaloidosis 277.39
Gammopathy 273.9
- macroglobulinemia 273.3
- monoclonal (benign) (essential) (idiopathic) (with lymphoplasmacytic dyscrasia) 273.1

Gamna's disease (siderotic splenomegaly) 289.51
Gampsodactylia (congenital) 754.71
Gamstorp's disease (adynamia episodica hereditaria) 359.3
Gandy-Nanta disease (siderotic splenomegaly) 289.51
Gang activity, without manifest psychiatric disorder V71.09
- adolescent V71.02
- adult V71.01
- child V71.02

Gangliocytoma (M9490/0) - *see* Neoplasm, connective tissue, benign
Ganglioglioma (M9505/1) - *see* Neoplasm, by site, uncertain behavior
Ganglion 727.43
- joint 727.41
- of yaws (early) (late) 102.6
- periosteal (*see also* Periostitis) 730.3 5th
- tendon sheath (compound) (diffuse) 727.42
- tuberculous (*see also* Tuberculosis) 015.9 5th

Ganglioneuroblastoma (M9490/3) - *see* Neoplasm, connective tissue, malignant
Ganglioneuroma (M9490/0) - *see also* Neoplasm, connective tissue, benign
- malignant (M9490/3) - *see* Neoplasm, connective tissue, malignant

Ganglioneuromatosis (M9491/0) - *see* Neoplasm, connective tissue, benign
Ganglionitis
- fifth nerve (*see also* Neuralgia, trigeminal) 350.1
- gasserian 350.1
- geniculate 351.1
  - herpetic 053.11

Ganglionitis – *continued*
- geniculate – *continued*
  - newborn 767.5
- herpes zoster 053.11
- herpetic geniculate (Hunt's syndrome) 053.11

Gangliosidosis 330.1
Gangosa 102.5
Gangrene, gangrenous (anemia) (artery) (cellulitis) (dermatitis) (dry) (infective) (moist) (pemphigus) (septic) (skin) (stasis) (ulcer) 785.4
- with
  - arteriosclerosis (native artery) 440.24
    - bypass graft 440.30
      - autologous vein 440.31
      - nonautologous biological 440.32
  - diabetes (mellitus) 250.7 5th *[785.4]*
    - due to secondary diabetes 249.7 5th *[785.4]*
- abdomen (wall) 785.4
- adenitis 683
- alveolar 526.5
- angina 462
  - diphtheritic 032.0
- anus 569.49
- appendices epiploicae - *see* Gangrene, mesentery
- appendix - *see* Appendicitis, acute
- arteriosclerotic - *see* Arteriosclerosis, with, gangrene
- auricle 785.4
- Bacillus welchii (*see also* Gangrene, gas) 040.0
- bile duct (*see also* Cholangitis) 576.8
- bladder 595.89
- bowel - *see* Gangrene, intestine
- cecum - *see* Gangrene, intestine
- Clostridium perfringens or welchii (*see also* Gangrene, gas) 040.0
- colon - *see* Gangrene, intestine
- connective tissue 785.4
- cornea 371.40
- corpora cavernosa (infective) 607.2
  - noninfective 607.89
- cutaneous, spreading 785.4
- decubital (*see also* Ulcer, pressure) 707.00 *[785.4]*
- diabetic (any site) 250.7 5th *[785.4]*
  - due to secondary diabetes 249.7 5th *[785.4]*
- dropsical 785.4
- emphysematous (*see also* Gangrene, gas) 040.0
- epidemic (ergotized grain) 988.2
- epididymis (infectional) (*see also* Epididymitis) 604.99
- erysipelas (*see also* Erysipelas) 035
- extremity (lower) (upper) 785.4
- gallbladder or duct (*see also* Cholecystitis, acute) 575.0
- gas (bacillus) 040.0
  - with
    - abortion - *see* Abortion, by type, with sepsis
    - ectopic pregnancy (*see also* categories 633.0-633.9) 639.0
    - molar pregnancy (*see also* categories 630-632) 639.0
  - following
    - abortion 639.0
    - ectopic or molar pregnancy 639.0
  - puerperal, postpartum, childbirth 670.8 5th ▲
- glossitis 529.0
- gum 523.8
- hernia - *see* Hernia, by site, with gangrene
- hospital noma 528.1
- intestine, intestinal (acute) (hemorrhagic) (massive) 557.0
  - with
    - hernia - *see* Hernia, by site, with gangrene

Gangrene, gangrenous – *continued*
- intestine, intestinal – *continued*
  - with – *continued*
    - mesenteric embolism or infarction 557.0
    - obstruction (*see also* Obstruction, intestine) 560.9
- laryngitis 464.00
  - with obstruction 464.01
- liver 573.8
- lung 513.0
  - spirochetal 104.8
- lymphangitis 457.2
- Meleney's (cutaneous) 686.09
- mesentery 557.0
  - with
    - embolism or infarction 557.0
    - intestinal obstruction (*see also* Obstruction, intestine) 560.9
- mouth 528.1
- noma 528.1
- orchitis 604.90
- ovary (*see also* Salpingo-oophoritis) 614.2
- pancreas 577.0
- penis (infectional) 607.2
  - noninfective 607.89
- perineum 785.4
- pharynx 462
  - septic 034.0
- pneumonia 513.0
- Pott's 440.24
- presenile 443.1
- pulmonary 513.0
- pulp, tooth 522.1
- quinsy 475
- Raynaud's (symmetric gangrene) 443.0 *[785.4]*
- rectum 569.49
- retropharyngeal 478.24
- rupture - *see* Hernia, by site, with gangrene
- scrotum 608.4
  - noninfective 608.83
- senile 440.24
- sore throat 462
- spermatic cord 608.4
  - noninfective 608.89
- spine 785.4
- spirochetal NEC 104.8
- spreading cutaneous 785.4
- stomach 537.89
- stomatitis 528.1
- symmetrical 443.0 *[785.4]*
- testis (infectional) (*see also* Orchitis) 604.99
  - noninfective 608.89
- throat 462
  - diphtheritic 032.0
- thyroid (gland) 246.8
- tonsillitis (acute) 463
- tooth (pulp) 522.1
- tuberculous NEC (*see also* Tuberculosis) 011.9 5th
- tunica vaginalis 608.4
  - noninfective 608.89
- umbilicus 785.4
- uterus (*see also* Endometritis) 615.9
- uvulitis 528.3
- vas deferens 608.4
  - noninfective 608.89
- vulva (*see also* Vulvitis) 616.10

Gannister disease (occupational) 502
- with tuberculosis - *see* Tuberculosis, pulmonary

Ganser's syndrome, hysterical 300.16
Gardner-Diamond syndrome (autoerythrocyte sensitization) 287.2
Gargoylism 277.5
Garré's
- disease (*see also* Osteomyelitis) 730.1 5th
- osteitis (sclerosing) (*see also* Osteomyelitis) 730.1 5th
- osteomyelitis (*see also* Osteomyelitis) 730.1 5th

Garrod's pads, knuckle 728.79
Gartner's duct
- cyst 752.41
- persistent 752.41

Gas 787.3
- asphyxia, asphyxiation, inhalation, poisoning, suffocation NEC 987.9
  - specified gas - *see* Table of Drugs and Chemicals
- bacillus gangrene or infection - *see* Gas, gangrene
- cyst, mesentery 568.89
- excessive 787.3
- gangrene 040.0
  - with
    - abortion - *see* Abortion, by type, with sepsis
    - ectopic pregnancy (*see also* categories 633.0-633.9) 639.0
    - molar pregnancy (*see also* categories 630-632) 639.0
  - following
    - abortion 639.0
    - ectopic or molar pregnancy 639.0
  - puerperal, postpartum, childbirth 670.8 5th ▲
- on stomach 787.3
- pains 787.3

Gastradenitis 535.0 5th
Gastralgia 536.8
- psychogenic 307.89

Gastrectasis, gastrectasia 536.1
- psychogenic 306.4

Gastric - *see* condition
Gastrinoma (M8153/1)
- malignant (M8153/3)
  - pancreas 157.4
  - specified site NEC - *see* Neoplasm, by site, malignant
  - unspecified site 157.4
- specified site - *see* Neoplasm, by site, uncertain behavior
- unspecified site 235.5

Gastritis 535.5 5th

Note *Use the following fifth-digit subclassification for category 535:*

0 without mention of hemorrhage
1 with hemorrhage

- acute 535.0 5th
- alcoholic 535.3 5th
- allergic 535.4 5th
- antral 535.4 5th
- atrophic 535.1 5th
- atrophic-hyperplastic 535.1 5th
- bile-induced 535.4 5th
- catarrhal 535.0 5th
- chronic (atrophic) 535.1 5th
- cirrhotic 535.4 5th
- corrosive (acute) 535.4 5th
- dietetic 535.4 5th
- due to diet deficiency 269.9 *[535.4]* 5th
- eosinophilic 535.7 5th
- erosive 535.4 5th
- follicular 535.4 5th
  - chronic 535.1 5th
- giant hypertrophic 535.2 5th
- glandular 535.4 5th
  - chronic 535.1 5th
- hypertrophic (mucosa) 535.2 5th
  - chronic giant 211.1
- irritant 535.4 5th
- nervous 306.4
- phlegmonous 535.0 5th
- psychogenic 306.4
- sclerotic 535.4 5th
- spastic 536.8
- subacute 535.0 5th
- superficial 535.4 5th
- suppurative 535.0 5th
- toxic 535.4 5th
- tuberculous (*see also* Tuberculosis) 017.9 5th

Gastrocarcinoma (M8010/3) 151.9

Gafsa boil – Gastrocarcinoma

- **Gastrocolic** - *see* condition
- **Gastrocolitis** - *see* Enteritis
- **Gastrodisciasis** 121.8
- **Gastroduodenitis** (*see also* Gastritis) 535.5 5th
  - catarrhal 535.0 5th
  - infectional 535.0 5th
  - virus, viral 008.8
    - specified type NEC 008.69
- **Gastrodynia** 536.8
- **Gastroenteritis** (acute) (catarrhal) (congestive) (hemorrhagic) (noninfectious) (*see also* Enteritis) 558.9
  - aertrycke infection 003.0
  - allergic 558.3
  - chronic 558.9
    - ulcerative (*see also* Colitis, ulcerative) 556.9
  - dietetic 558.9
  - due to
    - antineoplastic chemotherapy 558.9
    - food poisoning (*see also* Poisoning, food) 005.9
    - radiation 558.1
  - eosinophilic 558.41
  - epidemic 009.0
  - functional 558.9
  - infectious (*see also* Enteritis, due to, by organism) 009.0
    - presumed 009.1
  - salmonella 003.0
  - septic (*see also* Enteritis, due to, by organism) 009.0
  - toxic 558.2
  - tuberculous (*see also* Tuberculosis) 014.8 5th
  - ulcerative (*see also* Colitis, ulcerative) 556.9
  - viral NEC 008.8
    - specified type NEC 008.69
  - zymotic 009.0
- **Gastroenterocolitis** - *see* Enteritis
- **Gastroenteropathy, protein-losing** 579.8
- **Gastroenteroptosis** 569.89
- **Gastroesophageal laceration-hemorrhage syndrome** 530.7
- **Gastroesophagitis** 530.19
- **Gastrohepatitis** (*see also* Gastritis) 535.5 5th
- **Gastrointestinal** - *see* condition
- **Gastrojejunal** - *see* condition
- **Gastrojejunitis** (*see also* Gastritis) 535.5 5th
- **Gastrojejunocolic** - *see* condition
- **Gastroliths** 537.89
- **Gastromalacia** 537.89
- **Gastroparalysis** 536.3
  - diabetic 250.6 5th *[536.3]*
    - due to secondary diabetes 249.6 5th *[536.3]*
- **Gastroparesis** 536.3
  - diabetic 250.6 5th *[536.3]*
    - due to secondary diabetes 249.6 5th *[536.3]*
- **Gastropathy** 537.9
  - congestive portal 537.89
  - erythematous 535.5 5th
  - exudative 579.8
  - portal hypertensive 537.89
- **Gastroptosis** 537.5
- **Gastrorrhagia** 578.0
- **Gastrorrhea** 536.8
  - psychogenic 306.4
- **Gastroschisis** (congenital) 756.73 ▲
  - acquired 569.89
- **Gastrospasm** (neurogenic) (reflex) 536.8
  - neurotic 306.4
  - psychogenic 306.4
- **Gastrostaxis** 578.0
- **Gastrostenosis** 537.89
- **Gastrostomy**
  - attention to V55.1
  - complication 536.40
    - specified type 536.49
  - infection 536.41
- **Gastrostomy** – *continued*
  - malfunctioning 536.42
  - status V44.1
- **Gastrosuccorrhea** (continuous) (intermittent) 536.8
  - neurotic 306.4
  - psychogenic 306.4
- **Gaucher's**
  - disease (adult) (cerebroside lipidosis) (infantile) 272.7
  - hepatomegaly 272.7
  - splenomegaly (cerebroside lipidosis) 272.7
- **GAVE** (gastric antral vascular ectasia) 537.82
  - with hemorrhage 537.83
  - without hemorrhage 537.82
- **Gayet's disease** (superior hemorrhagic polioencephalitis) 265.1
- **Gayet-Wernicke's syndrome** (superior hemorrhagic polioencephalitis) 265.1
- **Gee (-Herter) (-Heubner) (-Thaysen) disease or syndrome** (nontropical sprue) 579.0
- **Gélineau's syndrome** (*see also* Narcolepsy) 347.00
- **Gemination, teeth** 520.2
- **Gemistocytoma** (M9411/3)
  - specified site - *see* Neoplasm, by site, malignant
  - unspecified site 191.9
- **Genetic**
  - susceptibility to
    - MEN (multiple endocrine neoplasia) V84.81
    - neoplasia
      - multiple endocrine [MEN] V84.81
    - neoplasm
      - malignant, of
        - breast V84.01
        - endometrium V84.04
        - other V84.09
        - ovary V84.02
        - prostate V84.03
    - specified disease NEC V84.89
- **General, generalized** - *see* condition
- **Genital** - *see* condition
  - warts 078.11
- **Genito-anorectal syndrome** 099.1
- **Genitourinary system** - *see* condition
- **Genu**
  - congenital 755.64
  - extrorsum (acquired) 736.42
    - congenital 755.64
    - late effects of rickets 268.1
  - introrsum (acquired) 736.41
    - congenital 755.64
    - late effects of rickets 268.1
  - rachitic (old) 268.1
  - recurvatum (acquired) 736.5
    - congenital 754.40
      - with dislocation of knee 754.41
    - late effects of rickets 268.1
  - valgum (acquired) (knock-knee) 736.41
    - congenital 755.64
    - late effects of rickets 268.1
  - varum (acquired) (bowleg) 736.42
    - congenital 755.64
    - late effect of rickets 268.1
- **Geographic tongue** 529.1
- **Geophagia** 307.52
- **Geotrichosis** 117.9
  - intestine 117.9
  - lung 117.9
  - mouth 117.9
- **Gephyrophobia** 300.29
- **Gerbode defect** 745.4
- **GERD** (gastroesophageal reflux disease) 530.81
- **Gerhardt's**
  - disease (erythromelalgia) 443.82
  - syndrome (vocal cord paralysis) 478.30
- **Gerlier's disease** (epidemic vertigo) 078.81
- **German measles** 056.9
  - exposure to V01.4
- **Germinoblastoma** (diffuse) (M9614/3) 202.8 5th
  - follicular (M9692/3) 202.0 5th
- **Germinoma** (M9064/3) - *see* Neoplasm, by site, malignant
- **Gerontoxon** 371.41
- **Gerstmann's syndrome** (finger agnosia) 784.69
- **Gerstmann-Sträussler-Scheinker syndrome** (GSS) 046.71
- **Gestation** (period) - *see also* Pregnancy
  - ectopic NEC (*see also* Pregnancy, ectopic) 633.90
    - with intrauterine pregnancy 633.91
- **Gestational proteinuria** 646.2 5th
  - with hypertension - *see* Toxemia, of pregnancy
- **Ghon tubercle primary infection** (*see also* Tuberculosis) 010.0 5th
- **Ghost**
  - teeth 520.4
  - vessels, cornea 370.64
- **Ghoul hand** 102.3
- **Gianotti Crosti syndrome** 057.8
  - due to known virus- *see* Infection, virus
  - due to unknown virus 057.8
- **Giant**
  - cell
    - epulis 523.8
    - peripheral (gingiva) 523.8
    - tumor, tendon sheath 727.02
  - colon (congenital) 751.3
  - esophagus (congenital) 750.4
  - kidney 753.3
  - urticaria 995.1
    - hereditary 277.6
- **Giardia lamblia infestation** 007.1
- **Giardiasis** 007.1
- **Gibert's disease** (pityriasis rosea) 696.3
- **Gibraltar fever** - *see* Brucellosis
- **Giddiness** 780.4
  - hysterical 300.11
  - psychogenic 306.9
- **Gierke's disease** (glycogenosis I) 271.0
- **Gigantism** (cerebral) (hypophyseal) (pituitary) 253.0
- **Gilbert's disease or cholemia** (familial nonhemolytic jaundice) 277.4
- **Gilchrist's disease** (North American blastomycosis) 116.0
- **Gilford (-Hutchinson) disease or syndrome** (progeria) 259.8
- **Gilles de la Tourette's disease** (motor-verbal tic) 307.23
- **Gillespie's syndrome** (dysplasia oculodentodigitalis) 759.89
- **Gingivitis** 523.10
  - acute 523.00
    - necrotizing 101
    - non-plaque induced 523.01
    - plaque induced 523.00
  - catarrhal 523.00
  - chronic 523.10
    - non-plaque induced 523.11
  - desquamative 523.10
  - expulsiva 523.40
  - hyperplastic 523.10
  - marginal, simple 523.10
  - necrotizing, acute 101
  - non-plaque induced 523.11
  - pellagrous 265.2
  - plaque induced 523.10
  - ulcerative 523.10
    - acute necrotizing 101
  - Vincent's 101
- **Gingivoglossitis** 529.0
- **Gingivopericementitis** 523.40
- **Gingivosis** 523.10
- **Gingivostomatitis** 523.10
  - herpetic 054.2
- **Giovannini's disease** 117.9
- **GISA** (glycopeptide intermediate staphylococcus aureus) V09.8 5th
- **Gland, glandular** - *see* condition
- **Glanders** 024
- **Glanzmann (-Naegeli) disease or thrombasthenia** 287.1
- **Glassblowers' disease** 527.1
- **Glaucoma** (capsular) (inflammatory) (noninflammatory) (primary) 365.9
  - with increased episcleral venous pressure 365.82
  - absolute 360.42
  - acute 365.22
    - narrow angle 365.22
    - secondary 365.60
  - angle closure 365.20
    - acute 365.22
    - chronic 365.23
    - intermittent 365.21
    - interval 365.21
    - residual stage 365.24
    - subacute 365.21
  - borderline 365.00
  - chronic 365.11
    - noncongestive 365.11
    - open angle 365.11
    - simple 365.11
  - closed angle - *see* Glaucoma, angle closure
  - congenital 743.20
    - associated with other eye anomalies 743.22
    - simple 743.21
  - congestive - *see* Glaucoma, narrow angle
  - corticosteroid-induced (glaucomatous stage) 365.31
    - residual stage 365.32
  - hemorrhagic 365.60
  - hypersecretion 365.81
  - in or with
    - aniridia 365.42
    - Axenfeld's anomaly 365.41
    - congenital syndromes NEC 759.89 *[365.44]*
    - disorder of lens NEC 365.59
    - inflammation, ocular 365.62 ●
    - iris
      - anomalies NEC 365.42
      - atrophy, essential 365.42
      - bombé 365.61
    - microcornea 365.43
    - neurofibromatosis 237.71 *[365.44]*
    - ocular
      - cysts NEC 365.64
      - disorders NEC 365.60
      - trauma 365.65
      - tumors NEC 365.64
    - pupillary block or seclusion 365.61
    - Rieger's anomaly or syndrome 365.41
    - seclusion of pupil 365.61
    - Sturge-Weber (-Dimitri) syndrome 759.6 *[365.44]*
    - systemic syndrome NEC 365.44
    - tumor of globe 365.64
    - vascular disorders NEC 365.63
  - infantile 365.14
    - congenital 743.20
      - associated with other eye anomalies 743.22
      - simple 743.21
  - juvenile 365.14
  - low tension 365.12
  - malignant 365.83
  - narrow angle (primary) 365.20
    - acute 365.22
    - chronic 365.23
    - intermittent 365.21
    - interval 365.21
    - residual stage 365.24
    - subacute 365.21
  - newborn 743.20
    - associated with other eye anomalies 743.22
    - simple 743.21
  - noncongestive (chronic) 365.11
  - nonobstructive (chronic) 365.11
  - obstructive 365.60
    - due to lens changes 365.59

Glaucoma – *continued*
open angle 365.10
with
borderline intraocular pressure 365.01
cupping of optic discs 365.01
primary 365.11
residual stage 365.15
phacolytic 365.51
pigmentary 365.13
postinfectious 365.60
pseudoexfoliation 365.52
secondary NEC 365.60
simple (chronic) 365.11
simplex 365.11
steroid responders 365.03
suspect 365.00
syphilitic 095.8
traumatic NEC 365.65
newborn 767.8
wide angle (*see also* Glaucoma, open angle) 365.10
Glaucomatous flecks (subcapsular) 366.31
Glazed tongue 529.4
Gleet 098.2
Glénard's disease or syndrome (enteroptosis) 569.89
Glinski-Simmonds syndrome (pituitary cachexia) 253.2
Glioblastoma (multiforme) (M9440/3)
with sarcomatous component (M9442/3)
specified site - *see* Neoplasm, by site, malignant
unspecified site 191.9
giant cell (M9441/3)
specified site - *see* Neoplasm, by site, malignant
unspecified site 191.9
specified site - *see* Neoplasm, by site, malignant
unspecified site 191.9
Glioma (malignant) (M9380/3)
astrocytic (M9400/3)
specified site - *see* Neoplasm, by site, malignant
unspecified site 191.9
mixed (M9382/3)
specified site - *see* Neoplasm, by site, malignant
unspecified site 191.9
nose 748.1
specified site NEC - *see* Neoplasm, by site, malignant
subependymal (M9383/1) 237.5
unspecified site 191.9
Gliomatosis cerebri (M9381/3) 191.0
Glioneuroma (M9505/1) - *see* Neoplasm, by site, uncertain behavior
Gliosarcoma (M9380/3)
specified site - *see* Neoplasm, by site, malignant
unspecified site 191.9
Gliosis (cerebral) 349.89
spinal 336.0
Glisson's
cirrhosis - *see* Cirrhosis, portal
disease (*see also* Rickets) 268.0
Glissonitis 573.3
Globinuria 791.2
Globus 306.4
hystericus 300.11
Glomangioma (M8712/0) (*see also* Hemangioma) 228.00
Glomangiosarcoma (M8710/3) - *see* Neoplasm, connective tissue, malignant
Glomerular nephritis (*see also* Nephritis) 583.9
Glomerulitis (*see also* Nephritis) 583.9
Glomerulonephritis (*see also* Nephritis) 583.9
with
edema (*see also* Nephrosis) 581.9

Glomerulonephritis – *continued*
with – *continued*
lesion of
exudative nephritis 583.89
interstitial nephritis (diffuse) (focal) 583.89
necrotizing glomerulitis 583.4
acute 580.4
chronic 582.4
renal necrosis 583.9
cortical 583.6
medullary 583.7
specified pathology NEC 583.89
acute 580.89
chronic 582.89
necrosis, renal 583.9
cortical 583.6
medullary (papillary) 583.7
specified pathology or lesion NEC 583.89
acute 580.9
with
exudative nephritis 580.89
interstitial nephritis (diffuse) (focal) 580.89
necrotizing glomerulitis 580.4
extracapillary with epithelial crescents 580.4
poststreptococcal 580.0
proliferative (diffuse) 580.0
rapidly progressive 580.4
specified pathology NEC 580.89
arteriolar (*see also* Hypertension, kidney) 403.90
arteriosclerotic (*see also* Hypertension, kidney) 403.90
ascending (*see also* Pyelitis) 590.80
basement membrane NEC 583.89
with
pulmonary hemorrhage (Goodpasture's syndrome) 446.21 *[583.81]*
chronic 582.9
with
exudative nephritis 582.89
interstitial nephritis (diffuse) (focal) 582.89
necrotizing glomerulitis 582.4
specified pathology or lesion NEC 582.89
endothelial 582.2
extracapillary with epithelial crescents 582.4
hypocomplementemic persistent 582.2
lobular 582.2
membranoproliferative 582.2
membranous 582.1
and proliferative (mixed) 582.2
sclerosing 582.1
mesangiocapillary 582.2
mixed membranous and proliferative 582.2
proliferative (diffuse) 582.0
rapidly progressive 582.4
sclerosing 582.1
cirrhotic - *see* Sclerosis, renal
desquamative - *see* Nephrosis
due to or associated with
amyloidosis 277.39 *[583.81]*
with nephrotic syndrome 277.39 *[581.81]*
chronic 277.39 *[582.81]*
diabetes mellitus 250.4 [5th] *[583.81]*
with nephrotic syndrome 250.4 [5th] *[581.81]*
due to secondary diabetes 249.4 [5th] *[581.81]*
due to secondary diabetes 249.4 [5th] *[581.81]*
diphtheria 032.89 *[580.81]*
gonococcal infection (acute) 098.19 *[583.81]*
chronic or duration of 2 months or over 098.39 *[583.81]*

Glomerulonephritis – *continued*
due to or associated with – *continued*
infectious hepatitis 070.9 *[580.81]*
malaria (with nephrotic syndrome) 084.9 *[581.81]*
mumps 072.79 *[580.81]*
polyarteritis (nodosa) (with nephrotic syndrome) 446.0 *[581.81]*
specified pathology NEC 583.89
acute 580.89
chronic 582.89
streptotrichosis 039.8 *[583.81]*
subacute bacterial endocarditis 421.0 *[580.81]*
syphilis (late) 095.4
congenital 090.5 *[583.81]*
early 091.69 *[583.81]*
systemic lupus erythematosus 710.0 *[583.81]*
with nephrotic syndrome 710.0 *[581.81]*
chronic 710.0 *[582.81]*
tuberculosis (*see also* Tuberculosis) 016.0 [5th] *[583.81]*
typhoid fever 002.0 *[580.81]*
extracapillary with epithelial crescents 583.4
acute 580.4
chronic 582.4
exudative 583.89
acute 580.89
chronic 582.89
focal (*see also* Nephritis) 583.9
embolic 580.4
granular 582.89
granulomatous 582.89
hydremic (*see also* Nephrosis) 581.9
hypocomplementemic persistent 583.2
with nephrotic syndrome 581.2
chronic 582.2
immune complex NEC 583.89
infective (*see also* Pyelitis) 590.80
interstitial (diffuse) (focal) 583.89
with nephrotic syndrome 581.89
acute 580.89
chronic 582.89
latent or quiescent 582.9
lobular 583.2
with nephrotic syndrome 581.2
chronic 582.2
membranoproliferative 583.2
with nephrotic syndrome 581.2
chronic 582.2
membranous 583.1
with nephrotic syndrome 581.1
and proliferative (mixed) 583.2
with nephrotic syndrome 581.2
chronic 582.2
chronic 582.1
sclerosing 582.1
with nephrotic syndrome 581.1
mesangiocapillary 583.2
with nephrotic syndrome 581.2
chronic 582.2
minimal change 581.3
mixed membranous and proliferative 583.2
with nephrotic syndrome 581.2
chronic 582.2
necrotizing 583.4
acute 580.4
chronic 582.4
nephrotic (*see also* Nephrosis) 581.9
old - *see* Glomerulonephritis, chronic
parenchymatous 581.89
poststreptococcal 580.0
proliferative (diffuse) 583.0
with nephrotic syndrome 581.0
acute 580.0
chronic 582.0
purulent (*see also* Pyelitis) 590.80
quiescent - *see* Nephritis, chronic
rapidly progressive 583.4
acute 580.4

Glomerulonephritis – *continued*
rapidly progressive – *continued*
chronic 582.4
sclerosing membranous (chronic) 582.1
with nephrotic syndrome 581.1
septic (*see also* Pyelitis) 590.80
specified pathology or lesion NEC 583.89
with nephrotic syndrome 581.89
acute 580.89
chronic 582.89
suppurative (acute) (disseminated) (*see also* Pyelitis) 590.80
toxic - *see* Nephritis, acute
tubal, tubular - *see* Nephrosis, tubular
type II (Ellis) - *see* Nephrosis
vascular - *see* Hypertension, kidney
Glomerulosclerosis (*see also* Sclerosis, renal) 587
focal 582.1
with nephrotic syndrome 581.1
intercapillary (nodular) (with diabetes) 250.4 [5th] *[581.81]*
due to secondary diabetes 249.4 [5th] *[581.81]*
Glossagra 529.6
Glossalgia 529.6
Glossitis 529.0
areata exfoliativa 529.1
atrophic 529.4
benign migratory 529.1
gangrenous 529.0
Hunter's 529.4
median rhomboid 529.2
Moeller's 529.4
pellagrous 265.2
Glossocele 529.8
Glossodynia 529.6
exfoliativa 529.4
Glossoncus 529.8
Glossophytia 529.3
Glossoplegia 529.8
Glossoptosis 529.8
Glossopyrosis 529.6
Glossotrichia 529.3
Glossy skin 701.9
Glottis - *see* condition
Glottitis - *see* Glossitis
Glucagonoma (M8152/0)
malignant (M8152/3)
pancreas 157.4
specified site NEC - *see* Neoplasm, by site, malignant
unspecified site 157.4
pancreas 211.7
specified site NEC - *see* Neoplasm, by site, benign
unspecified site 211.7
Glucoglycinuria 270.7
Glue ear syndrome 381.20
Glue sniffing (airplane glue) (*see also* Dependence) 304.6 [5th]
Glycinemia (with methylmalonic acidemia) 270.7
Glycinuria (renal) (with ketosis) 270.0
Glycogen
infiltration (*see also* Disease, glycogen storage) 271.0
storage disease (*see also* Disease, glycogen storage) 271.0
Glycogenosis (*see also* Disease, glycogen storage) 271.0
cardiac 271.0 *[425.7]*
Cori, types I-VII 271.0
diabetic, secondary 250.8 [5th] *[259.8]*
due to secondary diabetes 249.8 [5th] *[259.8]*
diffuse (with hepatic cirrhosis) 271.0
generalized 271.0
glucose-6-phosphatase deficiency 271.0
hepatophosphorylase deficiency 271.0
hepatorenal 271.0
myophosphorylase deficiency 271.0
Glycopenia 251.2

Glaucoma – Glycopenia

Glycopeptide
- intermediate staphylococcus aureus (GISA) V09.8 [5th]
- resistant
  - enterococcus V09.8 [5th]
  - staphylococcus aureus (GRSA) V09.8 [5th]

Glycoprolinuria 270.8
Glycosuria 791.5
- renal 271.4

Gnathostoma (spinigerum) (infection) (infestation) 128.1
- wandering swellings from 128.1

Gnathostomiasis 128.1
Goiter (adolescent) (colloid) (diffuse) (dipping) (due to iodine deficiency) (endemic) (euthyroid) (heart) (hyperplastic) (internal) (intrathoracic) (juvenile) (mixed type) (nonendemic) (parenchymatous) (plunging) (sporadic) (subclavicular) (substernal) 240.9
- with
  - hyperthyroidism (recurrent) (*see also* Goiter, toxic) 242.0 [5th]
  - thyrotoxicosis (*see also* Goiter, toxic) 242.0 [5th]
- adenomatous (*see also* Goiter, nodular) 241.9
- cancerous (M8000/3) 193
- complicating pregnancy, childbirth, or puerperium 648.1 [5th]
- congenital 246.1
- cystic (*see also* Goiter, nodular) 241.9
- due to enzyme defect in synthesis of thyroid hormone (butane-insoluble iodine) (coupling) (deiodinase) (iodide trapping or organification) (iodotyrosine dehalogenase) (peroxidase) 246.1
- dyshormonogenic 246.1
- exophthalmic (*see also* Goiter, toxic) 242.0 [5th]
- familial (with deaf-mutism) 243
- fibrous 245.3
- lingual 759.2
- lymphadenoid 245.2
- malignant (M8000/3) 193
- multinodular (nontoxic) 241.1
  - toxic or with hyperthyroidism (*see also* Goiter, toxic) 242.2 [5th]
- nodular (nontoxic) 241.9
  - with
    - hyperthyroidism (*see also* Goiter, toxic) 242.3 [5th]
    - thyrotoxicosis (*see also* Goiter, toxic) 242.3 [5th]
  - endemic 241.9
  - exophthalmic (diffuse) (*see also* Goiter, toxic) 242.0 [5th]
  - multinodular (nontoxic) 241.1
  - sporadic 241.9
  - toxic (*see also* Goiter, toxic) 242.3 [5th]
  - uninodular (nontoxic) 241.0
- nontoxic (nodular) 241.9
  - multinodular 241.1
  - uninodular 241.0
- pulsating (*see also* Goiter, toxic) 242.0 [5th]
- simple 240.0
- toxic 242.0 [5th]

Note *Use the following fifth-digit subclassification with category 242:*

0 without mention of thyrotoxic crisis or storm

1 with mention of thyrotoxic crisis or storm

  - adenomatous 242.3 [5th]
    - multinodular 242.2 [5th]
    - uninodular 242.1 [5th]
  - multinodular 242.2 [5th]
  - nodular 242.3 [5th]
    - multinodular 242.2 [5th]
    - uninodular 242.1 [5th]

Goiter – *continued*
- toxic – *continued*
  - uninodular 242.1 [5th]
- uninodular (nontoxic) 241.0 [5th]
  - toxic or with hyperthyroidism (*see also* Goiter, toxic) 242.1 [5th]

Goldberg (-Maxwell) (-Morris) syndrome (testicular feminization) 259.51
Goldblatt's
- hypertension 440.1
- kidney 440.1

Goldenhar's syndrome (oculoauriculovertebral dysplasia) 756.0
Goldflam-Erb disease or syndrome 358.00
Goldscheider's disease (epidermolysis bullosa) 757.39
Goldstein's disease (familial hemorrhagic telangiectasia) 448.0
Golfer's elbow 726.32
Goltz-Gorlin syndrome (dermal hypoplasia) 757.39
Gonadoblastoma (M9073/1)
- specified site - *see* Neoplasm, by site uncertain behavior
- unspecified site
  - female 236.2
  - male 236.4

Gonecystitis (*see also* Vesiculitis) 608.0
Gongylonemiasis 125.6
- mouth 125.6

Goniosynechiae 364.73
Gonococcemia 098.89
Gonococcus, gonococcal (disease) (infection) (*see also* condition) 098.0
- anus 098.7
- bursa 098.52
- chronic NEC 098.2
- complicating pregnancy, childbirth, or puerperium 647.1 [5th]
  - affecting fetus or newborn 760.2
- conjunctiva, conjunctivitis (neonatorum) 098.40
- dermatosis 098.89
- endocardium 098.84
- epididymo-orchitis 098.13
  - chronic or duration of 2 months or over 098.33
- eye (newborn) 098.40
- fallopian tube (chronic) 098.37
  - acute 098.17
- genitourinary (acute) (organ) (system) (tract) (*see also* Gonorrhea) 098.0
  - lower 098.0
    - chronic 098.2
  - upper 098.10
    - chronic 098.30
- heart NEC 098.85
- joint 098.50
- keratoderma 098.81
- keratosis (blennorrhagica) 098.81
- lymphatic (gland) (node) 098.89
- meninges 098.82
- orchitis (acute) 098.13
  - chronic or duration of 2 months or over 098.33
- pelvis (acute) 098.19
  - chronic or duration of 2 months or over 098.39
- pericarditis 098.83
- peritonitis 098.86
- pharyngitis 098.6
- pharynx 098.6
- proctitis 098.7
- pyosalpinx (chronic) 098.37
  - acute 098.17
- rectum 098.7
- septicemia 098.89
- skin 098.89
- specified site NEC 098.89
- synovitis 098.51
- tendon sheath 098.51
- throat 098.6

Gonococcus, gonococcal – *continued*
- urethra (acute) 098.0
  - chronic or duration of 2 months or over 098.2
- vulva (acute) 098.0
  - chronic or duration of 2 months or over 098.2

Gonocytoma (M9073/1)
- specified site - *see* Neoplasm, by site, uncertain behavior
- unspecified site
  - female 236.2
  - male 236.4

Gonorrhea 098.0
- acute 098.0
- Bartholin's gland (acute) 098.0
  - chronic or duration of 2 months or over 098.2
- bladder (acute) 098.11
  - chronic or duration of 2 months or over 098.31
- carrier (suspected of) V02.7
- cervix (acute) 098.15
  - chronic or duration of 2 months or over 098.35
- chronic 098.2
- complicating pregnancy, childbirth, or puerperium 647.1
  - affecting fetus or newborn 760.2
- conjunctiva, conjunctivitis (neonatorum) 098.40
- contact V01.6
- Cowper's gland (acute) 098.0
  - chronic or duration of 2 months or over 098.2
- duration of 2 months or over 098.2
- exposure to V01.6
- fallopian tube (chronic) 098.37
  - acute 098.17
- genitourinary (acute) (organ) (system) (tract) 098.0
  - chronic 098.2
  - duration of 2 months or over 098.2
- kidney (acute) 098.19
  - chronic or duration of 2 months or over 098.39
- ovary (acute) 098.19
  - chronic or duration of 2 months or over 098.39
- pelvis (acute) 098.19
  - chronic or duration of 2 months or over 098.39
- penis (acute) 098.0
  - chronic or duration of 2 months or over 098.2
- prostate (acute) 098.12
  - chronic or duration of 2 months or over 098.32
- seminal vesicle (acute) 098.14
  - chronic or duration of 2 months or over 098.34
- specified site NEC - *see* Gonococcus
- spermatic cord (acute) 098.14
  - chronic or duration of 2 months or over 098.34
- urethra (acute) 098.0
  - chronic or duration of 2 months or over 098.2
- vagina (acute) 098.0
  - chronic or duration of 2 months or over 098.2
- vas deferens (acute) 098.14
  - chronic or duration of 2 months or over 098.34
- vulva (acute) 098.0
  - chronic or duration of 2 months or over 098.2

Goodpasture's syndrome (pneumorenal) 446.21
Good's syndrome 279.06
Gopalan's syndrome (burning feet) 266.2
Gordon's disease (exudative enteropathy) 579.8
Gorlin-Chaudhry-Moss syndrome 759.89
Gougerot's syndrome (trisymptomatic) 709.1
Gougerot-Blum syndrome (pigmented purpuric lichenoid dermatitis) 709.1
Gougerot-Carteaud disease or syndrome (confluent reticulate papillomatosis) 701.8
Gougerot-Hailey-Hailey disease (benign familial chronic pemphigus) 757.39
Gougerot (-Houwer)-Sjögren syndrome (keratoconjunctivitis sicca) 710.2
Gouley's syndrome (constrictive pericarditis) 423.2
Goundou 102.6
Gout, gouty 274.9
- with ~~specified manifestations NEC 274.89~~
  - specified manifestations NEC 274.89 ●
  - tophi (tophus) 274.03 ●
- acute 274.01 ●
- arthritis ~~(acute)~~ 274.00 ▲
  - acute 274.01 ●
- arthropathy 274.00 ▲
  - acute 274.01 ●
  - chronic (without mention of tophus (tophi)) 274.02 ●
    - with tophus (tophi) 274.03 ●
- attack 274.01 ●
- chronic 274.02 ●
  - tophaceous 274.03 ●
- degeneration, heart 274.82
- diathesis 274.9
- eczema 274.89
- episcleritis 274.89 *[379.09]*
- external ear (tophus) 274.81
- flare 274.01 ●
- glomerulonephritis 274.10
- iritis 274.89 *[364.11]*
- joint 274.00 ▲
- kidney 274.10
- lead 984.9
  - specified type of lead - *see* Table of Drugs and Chemicals
- nephritis 274.10
- neuritis 274.89 *[357.4]*
- phlebitis 274.89 *[451.9]*
- rheumatic 714.0
- saturnine 984.9
  - specified type of lead - *see* Table of Drugs and Chemicals
- spondylitis 274.00 ▲
- synovitis 274.00 ▲
- syphilitic 095.8
- tophi 274.03 ▲
  - ear 274.81
  - heart 274.82
  - specified site NEC 274.82

Gowers'
- muscular dystrophy 359.1
- syndrome (vasovagal attack) 780.2

Gowers-Paton-Kennedy syndrome 377.04
Gradenigo's syndrome 383.02
Graft-versus-host disease 279.50
- ~~bone marrow 996.85~~
- due to organ transplant NEC - *see* Complications, transplant, organ

Graham Steell's murmur (pulmonic regurgitation) (*see also* Endocarditis, pulmonary) 424.3
Grain-handlers' disease or lung 495.8
Grain mite (itch) 133.8
Grand
- mal (idiopathic) (*see also* Epilepsy) 345.1 [5th]
  - hysteria of Charcôt 300.11
  - nonrecurrent or isolated 780.39
- multipara
  - affecting management of labor and delivery 659.4 [5th]
  - status only (not pregnant) V61.5

Granite workers' lung 502
Granular - *see also* condition
- inflammation, pharynx 472.1
- kidney (contracting) (*see also* Sclerosis, renal) 587

Granular – *continued*
- liver - *see* Cirrhosis, liver
- nephritis - *see* Nephritis

Granulation tissue, abnormal - *see also* Granuloma
- abnormal or excessive 701.5
- postmastoidectomy cavity 383.33
- postoperative 701.5
- skin 701.5

Granulocytopenia, granulocytopenic (primary) 288.00
- malignant 288.09

Granuloma NEC 686.1
- abdomen (wall) 568.89
  - skin (pyogenicum) 686.1
    - from residual foreign body 709.4
- annulare 695.89
- anus 569.49
- apical 522.6
- appendix 543.9
- aural 380.23
- beryllium (skin) 709.4
  - lung 503
- bone (*see also* Osteomyelitis) 730.1 5th
  - eosinophilic 277.89
  - from residual foreign body 733.99
- canaliculus lacrimalis 375.81
- cerebral 348.89 ▲
- cholesterin, middle ear 385.82
- coccidioidal (progressive) 114.3
  - lung 114.4
  - meninges 114.2
  - primary (lung) 114.0
- colon 569.89
- conjunctiva 372.61
- dental 522.6
- ear, middle (cholesterin) 385.82
  - with otitis media - *see* Otitis media
- eosinophilic 277.89
  - bone 277.89
  - lung 277.89
  - oral mucosa 528.9
- exuberant 701.5
- eyelid 374.89
- facial
  - lethal midline 446.3
  - malignant 446.3
- faciale 701.8
- fissuratum (gum) 523.8
- foot NEC 686.1
- foreign body (in soft tissue) NEC 728.82
  - bone 733.99
  - in operative wound 998.4
  - muscle 728.82
  - skin 709.4
  - subcutaneous tissue 709.4
- fungoides 202.1 5th
- gangraenescens 446.3
- giant cell (central) (jaw) (reparative) 526.3
  - gingiva 523.8
  - peripheral (gingiva) 523.8
- gland (lymph) 289.3
- Hodgkin's (M9661/3) 201.1 5th
- ileum 569.89
- infectious NEC 136.9
- inguinale (Donovan) 099.2
  - venereal 099.2
- intestine 569.89
- iridocyclitis 364.10
- jaw (bone) 526.3
  - reparative giant cell 526.3
- kidney (*see also* Infection, kidney) 590.9
- lacrimal sac 375.81
- larynx 478.79
- lethal midline 446.3
- lipid 277.89
- lipoid 277.89
- liver 572.8
- lung (infectious) (*see also* Fibrosis, lung) 515
  - coccidioidal 114.4
  - eosinophilic 277.89
- lymph gland 289.3
- Majocchi's 110.6

Granuloma – *continued*
- malignant, face 446.3
- mandible 526.3
- mediastinum 519.3
- midline 446.3
- monilial 112.3
- muscle 728.82
  - from residual foreign body 728.82
- nasal sinus (*see also* Sinusitis) 473.9
- operation wound 998.59
  - foreign body 998.4
  - stitch (external) 998.89
    - internal wound 998.89
  - talc 998.7
- oral mucosa, eosinophilic or pyogenic 528.9
- orbit, orbital 376.11
- paracoccidioidal 116.1
- penis, venereal 099.2
- periapical 522.6
- peritoneum 568.89
  - due to ova of helminths NEC (*see also* Helminthiasis) 128.9
- postmastoidectomy cavity 383.33
- postoperative - *see* Granuloma, operation wound
- prostate 601.8
- pudendi (ulcerating) 099.2
- pudendorum (ulcerative) 099.2
- pulp, internal (tooth) 521.49
- pyogenic, pyogenicum (skin) 686.1
  - maxillary alveolar ridge 522.6
  - oral mucosa 528.9
- rectum 569.49
- reticulohistiocytic 277.89
- rubrum nasi 705.89
- sarcoid 135
- Schistosoma 120.9
- septic (skin) 686.1
- silica (skin) 709.4
- sinus (accessory) (infectional) (nasal) (*see also* Sinusitis) 473.9
- skin (pyogenicum) 686.1
  - from foreign body or material 709.4
- sperm 608.89
- spine
  - syphilitic (epidural) 094.89
  - tuberculous (*see also* Tuberculosis) 015.0 5th *[730.88]*
- stitch (postoperative) 998.89
  - internal wound 998.89
- suppurative (skin) 686.1
- suture (postoperative) 998.89
  - internal wound 998.89
- swimming pool 031.1
- talc 728.82
  - in operation wound 998.7
- telangiectaticum (skin) 686.1
- tracheostomy 519.09
- trichophyticum 110.6
- tropicum 102.4
- umbilicus 686.1
  - newborn 771.4
- urethra 599.84
- uveitis 364.10
- vagina 099.2
- venereum 099.2
- vocal cords 478.5
- Wegener's (necrotizing respiratory granulomatosis) 446.4

Granulomatosis NEC 686.1
- disciformis chronica et progressiva 709.3
- infantiseptica 771.2
- lipoid 277.89
- lipophagic, intestinal 040.2
- miliary 027.0
- necrotizing, respiratory 446.4
- progressive, septic 288.1
- Wegener's (necrotizing respiratory) 446.4

Granulomatous tissue - *see* Granuloma

Granulosis rubra nasi 705.89

Graphite fibrosis (of lung) 503

Graphospasm 300.89
- organic 333.84

Grating scapula 733.99

Gravel (urinary) (*see also* Calculus) 592.9

Graves' disease (exophthalmic goiter) (*see also* Goiter, toxic) 242.0 5th

Gravis - *see* condition

Grawitz's tumor (hypernephroma) (M8312/3) 189.0

Grayness, hair (premature) 704.3
- congenital 757.4

Gray or grey syndrome (chloramphenicol) (newborn) 779.4

Greenfield's disease 330.0

Green sickness 280.9

Greenstick fracture - *see* Fracture, by site

Greig's syndrome (hypertelorism) 756.0

Grief 309.0

Griesinger's disease (*see also* Ancylostomiasis) 126.9

Grinders'
- asthma 502
- lung 502
- phthisis (*see also* Tuberculosis) 011.4 5th

Grinding, teeth 306.8

Grip
- Dabney's 074.1
- devil's 074.1

Grippe, grippal - *see also* Influenza
- Balkan 083.0
- intestinal 487.8
- summer 074.8

Grippy cold 487.1

Grisel's disease 723.5

Groin - *see* condition

Grooved
- nails (transverse) 703.8
- tongue 529.5
  - congenital 750.13

Ground itch 126.9

Growing pains, children 781.99

Growth (fungoid) (neoplastic) (new) (M8000/1) - *see also* Neoplasm, by site, unspecified nature
- adenoid (vegetative) 474.12
  - benign (M8000/0) - *see* Neoplasm, by site, benign
- fetal, poor 764.9 5th
  - affecting management of pregnancy 656.5 5th
- malignant (M8000/3) - *see* Neoplasm, by site, malignant
- rapid, childhood V21.0
- secondary (M8000/6) - *see* Neoplasm, by site, malignant, secondary

GRSA (glycopeptide resistant staphylococcus aureus) V09.8 5th

Gruber's hernia - *see* Hernia, Gruber's

Gruby's disease (tinea tonsurans) 110.0

GSS (Gerstmann-Sträussler-Scheinker syndrome) 046.71

G-trisomy 758.0

Guama fever 066.3

Gubler (-Millard) paralysis or syndrome 344.89

Guérin-Stern syndrome (arthrogryposis multiplex congenita) 754.89

Guertin's disease (electric chorea) 049.8

Guillain-Barré disease or syndrome 357.0

Guinea worms (infection) (infestation) 125.7

Guinon's disease (motor-verbal tic) 307.23

Gull's disease (thyroid atrophy with myxedema) 244.8

Gull and Sutton's disease - *see* Hypertension, kidney

Gum - *see* condition

Gumboil 522.7

Gumma (syphilitic) 095.9
- artery 093.89
  - cerebral or spinal 094.89
- bone 095.5
  - of yaws (late) 102.6
- brain 094.89
- cauda equina 094.89
- central nervous system NEC 094.9
- ciliary body 095.8 *[364.11]*

Gumma – *continued*
- congenital 090.5
  - testis 090.5
- eyelid 095.8 *[373.5]*
- heart 093.89
- intracranial 094.89
- iris 095.8 *[364.11]*
- kidney 095.4
- larynx 095.8
- leptomeninges 094.2
- liver 095.3
- meninges 094.2
- myocardium 093.82
- nasopharynx 095.8
- neurosyphilitic 094.9
- nose 095.8
- orbit 095.8
- palate (soft) 095.8
- penis 095.8
- pericardium 093.81
- pharynx 095.8
- pituitary 095.8
- scrofulous (*see also* Tuberculosis) 017.0 5th
- skin 095.8
- specified site NEC 095.8
- spinal cord 094.89
- tongue 095.8
- tonsil 095.8
- trachea 095.8
- tuberculous (*see also* Tuberculosis) 017.0 5th
- ulcerative due to yaws 102.4
- ureter 095.8
- yaws 102.4
  - bone 102.6

Gunn's syndrome (jaw-winking syndrome) 742.8

Gunshot wound - *see also* Wound, open, by site
- fracture - *see* Fracture, by site, open
- internal organs (abdomen, chest, or pelvis) - *see* Injury, internal, by site, with open wound
- intracranial - *see* Laceration, brain, with open intracranial wound

Günther's disease or syndrome (congenital erythropoietic porphyria) 277.1

Gustatory hallucination 780.1

Gynandrism 752.7

Gynandroblastoma (M8632/1)
- specified site - *see* Neoplasm, by site, uncertain behavior
- unspecified site
  - female 236.2
  - male 236.4

Gynandromorphism 752.7

Gynatresia (congenital) 752.49

Gynecoid pelvis, male 738.6

Gynecological examination V72.31
- for contraceptive maintenance V25.40

Gynecomastia 611.1

Gynephobia 300.29

Gyrate scalp 757.39

H

Haas' disease (osteochondrosis head of humerus) 732.3

Habermann's disease (acute parapsoriasis varioliformis) 696.2

Habit, habituation
- chorea 307.22
  - disturbance, child 307.9
- drug (*see also* Dependence) 304.9 5th
- laxative (*see also* Abuse, drugs, nondependent) 305.9 5th
- spasm 307.20
  - chronic 307.22
  - transient (of childhood) 307.21
- tic 307.20
  - chronic 307.22
  - transient (of childhood) 307.21

- **Helminthiasis** – *continued*
  - mixed types (intestinal) (types classifiable to more than one of the categories 120.0-127.7) 127.8
  - Necator americanus 126.1
  - specified type NEC 128.8
  - Trichinella 124
- **Heloma** 700
- **Hemangioblastoma** (M9161/1) - *see also* Neoplasm, connective tissue, uncertain behavior
  - malignant (M9161/3) - *see* Neoplasm, connective tissue, malignant
- **Hemangioblastomatosis, cerebelloretinal** 759.6
- **Hemangioendothelioma** (M9130/1) - *see also* Neoplasm, by site, uncertain behavior
  - benign (M9130/0) 228.00
  - bone (diffuse) (M9130/3) - *see* Neoplasm, bone, malignant
  - malignant (M9130/3) - *see* Neoplasm, connective tissue, malignant
  - nervous system (M9130/0) 228.09
- **Hemangioendotheliosarcoma** (M9130/3) - *see* Neoplasm, connective tissue, malignant
- **Hemangiofibroma** (M9160/0) - *see* Neoplasm, by site, benign
- **Hemangiolipoma** (M8861/0) - *see* Lipoma
- **Hemangioma** (M9120/0) 228.00
  - arteriovenous (M9123/0) - *see* Hemangioma, by site
  - brain 228.02
  - capillary (M9131/0) - *see* Hemangioma, by site
  - cavernous (M9121/0) - *see* Hemangioma, by site
  - central nervous system NEC 228.09
  - choroid 228.09
  - heart 228.09
  - infantile (M9131/0) - *see* Hemangioma, by site
  - intra-abdominal structures 228.04
  - intracranial structures 228.02
  - intramuscular (M9132/0) - *see* Hemangioma, by site
  - iris 228.09
  - juvenile (M9131/0) - *see* Hemangioma, by site
  - malignant (M9120/3) - *see* Neoplasm, connective tissue, malignant
  - meninges 228.09
    - brain 228.02
    - spinal cord 228.09
  - peritoneum 228.04
  - placenta - *see* Placenta, abnormal
  - plexiform (M9131/0) - *see* Hemangioma, by site
  - racemose (M9123/0) - *see* Hemangioma, by site
  - retina 228.03
  - retroperitoneal tissue 228.04
  - sclerosing (M8832/0) - *see* Neoplasm, skin, benign
  - simplex (M9131/0) - *see* Hemangioma, by site
  - skin and subcutaneous tissue 228.01
  - specified site NEC 228.09
  - spinal cord 228.09
  - venous (M9122/0) - *see* Hemangioma, by site
  - verrucous keratotic (M9142/0) - *see* Hemangioma, by site
- **Hemangiomatosis** (systemic) 757.32
  - involving single site - *see* Hemangioma
- **Hemangiopericytoma** (M9150/1) - *see also* Neoplasm, connective tissue, uncertain behavior
  - benign (M9150/0) - *see* Neoplasm, connective tissue, benign
  - malignant (M9150/3) - *see* Neoplasm, connective tissue, malignant
- **Hemangiosarcoma** (M9120/3) - *see* Neoplasm, connective tissue, malignant
- **Hemarthrosis** (nontraumatic) 719.10
  - ankle 719.17
  - elbow 719.12
  - foot 719.17
  - hand 719.14
  - hip 719.15
  - knee 719.16
  - multiple sites 719.19
  - pelvic region 719.15
  - shoulder (region) 719.11
  - specified site NEC 719.18
  - traumatic - *see* Sprain, by site
  - wrist 719.13
- **Hematemesis** 578.0
  - with ulcer - *see* Ulcer, by site, with hemorrhage
  - due to S. japonicum 120.2
  - Goldstein's (familial hemorrhagic telangiectasia) 448.0
  - newborn 772.4
    - due to swallowed maternal blood 777.3
- **Hematidrosis** 705.89
- **Hematinuria** (*see also* Hemoglobinuria) 791.2
  - malarial 084.8
  - paroxysmal 283.2
- **Hematite miners' lung** 503
- **Hematobilia** 576.8
- **Hematocele** (congenital) (diffuse) (idiopathic) 608.83
  - broad ligament 620.7
  - canal of Nuck 629.0
  - cord, male 608.83
  - fallopian tube 620.8
  - female NEC 629.0
  - ischiorectal 569.89
  - male NEC 608.83
  - ovary 629.0
  - pelvis, pelvic
    - female 629.0
      - with ectopic pregnancy (*see also* Pregnancy, ectopic) 633.90
        - with intrauterine pregnancy 633.91
    - male 608.83
  - periuterine 629.0
  - retrouterine 629.0
  - scrotum 608.83
  - spermatic cord (diffuse) 608.83
  - testis 608.84
  - traumatic - *see* Injury, internal, pelvis
  - tunica vaginalis 608.83
  - uterine ligament 629.0
  - uterus 621.4
  - vagina 623.6
  - vulva 624.5
- **Hematocephalus** 742.4
- **Hematochezia** (*see also* Melena) 578.1
- **Hematochyluria** (*see also* Infestation, filarial) 125.9
- **Hematocolpos** 626.8
- **Hematocornea** 371.12
- **Hematogenous** - *see* condition
- **Hematoma** (skin surface intact) (traumatic) - *see also* Contusion

Note *Hematomas are coded according to origin and the nature and site of the hematoma or the accompanying injury. Hematomas of unspecified origin are coded as injuries of the sites involved, except:*

(a) hematomas of genital organs which are coded as diseases of the organ involved unless they complicate pregnancy or delivery

(b) hematomas of the eye which are coded as diseases of the eye.

For late effect of hematoma classifiable to 920-924 see Late, effect, contusion.

  - with
    - crush injury - *see* Crush
    - fracture - *see* Fracture, by site
    - injury of internal organs - *see also* Injury, internal, by site
      - kidney - *see* Hematoma, kidney, traumatic
      - liver - *see* Hematoma, liver, traumatic
      - spleen - *see* Hematoma, spleen
    - nerve injury - *see* Injury, nerve
    - open wound - *see* Wound, open, by site
    - skin surface intact - *see* Contusion
  - abdomen (wall) - *see* Contusion, abdomen
  - amnion 658.8 [5th]
  - aorta, dissecting 441.00
    - abdominal 441.02
    - thoracic 441.01
    - thoracoabdominal 441.03
  - arterial (complicating trauma) 904.9
    - specified site - *see* Injury, blood vessel, by site
  - auricle (ear) 380.31
  - birth injury 767.8
    - skull 767.19
  - brain (traumatic) 853.0 [5th]

Note *Use the following fifth-digit subclassification with categories 851-854:*

0	unspecified state of consciousness
1	with no loss of consciousness
2	with brief [less than one hour] loss of consciousness
3	with moderate [1-24 hours] loss of consciousness
4	with prolonged [more than 24 hours] loss of consciousness and return to pre-existing conscious level
5	with prolonged [more than 24 hours] loss of consciousness, without return to pre-existing conscious level *Use fifth-digit 5 to designate when a patient is unconscious and dies before regaining consciousness, regardless of the duration of the loss of consciousness*
6	with loss of consciousness of unspecified duration
9	with concussion, unspecified

    - with
      - cerebral
        - contusion - *see* Contusion, brain
        - laceration - *see* Laceration, brain
      - open intracranial wound 853.1 [5th]
      - skull fracture - *see* Fracture, skull, by site
    - extradural or epidural 852.4 [5th]
      - with open intracranial wound 852.5 [5th]
      - fetus or newborn 767.0
      - nontraumatic 432.0
    - fetus or newborn NEC 767.0

- **Hematoma** – *continued*
  - brain – *continued*
    - nontraumatic (*see also* Hemorrhage, brain) 431
      - epidural or extradural 432.0
      - newborn NEC 772.8
      - subarachnoid, arachnoid, or meningeal (*see also* Hemorrhage, subarachnoid) 430
      - subdural (*see also* Hemorrhage, subdural) 432.1
    - subarachnoid, arachnoid, or meningeal 852.0 [5th]
      - with open intracranial wound 852.1 [5th]
      - fetus or newborn 772.2
      - nontraumatic (*see also* Hemorrhage, subarachnoid) 430
    - subdural 852.2 [5th]
      - with open intracranial wound 852.3 [5th]
      - fetus or newborn (localized) 767.0
      - nontraumatic (*see also* Hemorrhage, subdural) 432.1
  - breast (nontraumatic) 611.89
  - broad ligament (nontraumatic) 620.7
    - complicating delivery 665.7 [5th]
    - traumatic - *see* Injury, internal, broad ligament
  - calcified NEC 959.9
  - capitis 920
    - due to birth injury 767.19
    - newborn 767.19
  - cerebral - *see* Hematoma, brain
  - cesarean section wound 674.3 [5th]
  - chorion - *see* Placenta, abnormal
  - complicating delivery (perineum) (vulva) 664.5 [5th]
    - pelvic 665.7 [5th]
    - vagina 665.7 [5th]
  - corpus
    - cavernosum (nontraumatic) 607.82
    - luteum (nontraumatic) (ruptured) 620.1
  - dura (mater) - *see* Hematoma, brain, subdural
  - epididymis (nontraumatic) 608.83
  - epidural (traumatic) - *see also* Hematoma, brain, extradural
    - spinal - *see* Injury, spinal, by site
  - episiotomy 674.3 [5th]
  - external ear 380.31
  - extradural - *see also* Hematoma, brain, extradural
    - fetus or newborn 767.0
    - nontraumatic 432.0
      - fetus or newborn 767.0
  - fallopian tube 620.8
  - genital organ (nontraumatic)
    - female NEC 629.89
    - male NEC 608.83
    - traumatic (external site) 922.4
      - internal - *see* Injury, internal, genital organ
  - graafian follicle (ruptured) 620.0
  - internal organs (abdomen, chest, or pelvis) - *see also* Injury, internal, by site
    - kidney - *see* Hematoma, kidney, traumatic
    - liver - *see* Hematoma, liver, traumatic
    - spleen - *see* Hematoma, spleen
  - intracranial - *see* Hematoma, brain
  - kidney, cystic 593.81
    - traumatic 866.01
      - with open wound into cavity 866.11
  - labia (nontraumatic) 624.5
  - lingual (and other parts of neck, scalp, or face, except eye) 920
  - liver (subcapsular) 573.8
    - birth injury 767.8
    - fetus or newborn 767.8

Helminthiasis – Hematoma

Hematoma – *continued*
  liver – *continued*
    traumatic NEC 864.01
      with
        laceration - *see* Laceration, liver
        open wound into cavity 864.11
  mediastinum - *see* Injury, internal, mediastinum
  meninges, meningeal (brain) - *see also* Hematoma, brain, subarachnoid
    spinal - *see* Injury, spinal, by site
  mesosalpinx (nontraumatic) 620.8
    traumatic - *see* Injury, internal, pelvis
  muscle (traumatic) - *see* Contusion, by site
    nontraumatic 729.92
  nasal (septum) (and other part(s) of neck, scalp, or face, except eye) 920
  obstetrical surgical wound 674.3 [5th]
  orbit, orbital (nontraumatic) 376.32
    traumatic 921.2
  ovary (corpus luteum) (nontraumatic) 620.1
    traumatic - *see* Injury, internal, ovary
  pelvis (female) (nontraumatic) 629.89
    complicating delivery 665.7 [5th]
    male 608.83
    traumatic - *see also* Injury, internal, pelvis
      specified organ NEC (*see also* Injury, internal, pelvis) 867.6
  penis (nontraumatic) 607.82
  pericranial (and neck, or face any part, except eye) 920
    due to injury at birth 767.19
  perineal wound (obstetrical) 674.3 [5th]
    complicating delivery 664.5 [5th]
  perirenal, cystic 593.81
  pinna 380.31
  placenta - *see* Placenta, abnormal
  postoperative 998.12
  retroperitoneal (nontraumatic) 568.81
    traumatic - *see* Injury, internal, retroperitoneum
  retropubic, male 568.81
  scalp (and neck, or face any part, except eye) 920
    fetus or newborn 767.19
  scrotum (nontraumatic) 608.83
    traumatic 922.4
  seminal vesicle (nontraumatic) 608.83
    traumatic - *see* Injury, internal, seminal, vesicle
  soft tissue 729.92
  spermatic cord - *see also* Injury, internal, spermatic cord
    nontraumatic 608.83
  spinal (cord) (meninges) - *see also* Injury, spinal, by site
    fetus or newborn 767.4
    nontraumatic 336.1
  spleen 865.01
    with
      laceration - *see* Laceration, spleen
      open wound into cavity 865.11
  sternocleidomastoid, birth injury 767.8
  sternomastoid, birth injury 767.8
  subarachnoid - *see also* Hematoma, brain, subarachnoid
    fetus or newborn 772.2
    nontraumatic (*see also* Hemorrhage, subarachnoid) 430
      newborn 772.2
  subdural - *see also* Hematoma, brain, subdural
    fetus or newborn (localized) 767.0
    nontraumatic (*see also* Hemorrhage, subdural) 432.1
  subperiosteal (syndrome) 267
    traumatic - *see* Hematoma, by site
  superficial, fetus or newborn 772.6
  syncytium - *see* Placenta, abnormal
  testis (nontraumatic) 608.83
    birth injury 767.8
    traumatic 922.4

Hematoma – *continued*
  tunica vaginalis (nontraumatic) 608.83
  umbilical cord 663.6 [5th]
    affecting fetus or newborn 762.6
  uterine ligament (nontraumatic) 620.7
    traumatic - *see* Injury, internal, pelvis
  uterus 621.4
    traumatic - *see* Injury, internal, pelvis
  vagina (nontraumatic) (ruptured) 623.6
    complicating delivery 665.7 [5th]
    traumatic 922.4
  vas deferens (nontraumatic) 608.83
    traumatic - *see* Injury, internal, vas deferens
  vitreous 379.23
  vocal cord 920
  vulva (nontraumatic) 624.5
    complicating delivery 664.5 [5th]
    fetus or newborn 767.8
    traumatic 922.4
Hematometra 621.4
Hematomyelia 336.1
  with fracture of vertebra (*see also* Fracture, vertebra, by site, with spinal cord injury) 806.8
  fetus or newborn 767.4
Hematomyelitis 323.9
  late effect - *see* category 326
Hematoperitoneum (*see also* Hemoperitoneum) 568.81
Hematopneumothorax (*see also* Hemothorax) 511.89
Hematopoiesis, cyclic 288.02
Hematoporphyria (acquired) (congenital) 277.1
Hematoporphyrinuria (acquired) (congenital) 277.1
Hematorachis, hematorrhachis 336.1
  fetus or newborn 767.4
Hematosalpinx 620.8
  with
    ectopic pregnancy (*see also* categories 633.0-633.9) 639.2
    molar pregnancy (*see also* categories 630-632) 639.2
  infectional (*see also* Salpingo-oophoritis) 614.2
Hematospermia 608.82
Hematothorax (*see also* Hemothorax) 511.89
Hematotympanum 381.03
Hematuria (benign) (essential) (idiopathic) 599.70
  due to S. hematobium 120.0
  endemic 120.0
  gross 599.71
  intermittent 599.70
  malarial 084.8
  microscopic 599.72
  paroxysmal 599.70
  sulfonamide
    correct substance properly administered 599.70
    overdose or wrong substance given or taken 961.0
  tropical (bilharziasis) 120.0
  tuberculous (*see also* Tuberculosis) 016.9 [5th]
Hematuric bilious fever 084.8
Hemeralopia 368.10
Hemiabiotrophy 799.89
Hemi-akinesia 781.8
Hemianalgesia (*see also* Disturbance, sensation) 782.0
Hemianencephaly 740.0
Hemianesthesia (*see also* Disturbance, sensation) 782.0
Hemianopia, hemianopsia (altitudinal) (homonymous) 368.46
  binasal 368.47
  bitemporal 368.47
  heteronymous 368.47
  syphilitic 095.8
Hemiasomatognosia 307.9
Hemiathetosis 781.0

Hemiatrophy 799.89
  cerebellar 334.8
  face 349.89
    progressive 349.89
  fascia 728.9
  leg 728.2
  tongue 529.8
Hemiballism (us) 333.5
Hemiblock (cardiac) (heart) (left) 426.2
Hemicardia 746.89
Hemicephalus, hemicephaly 740.0
Hemichorea 333.5
Hemicrania 346.9 [5th]
  congenital malformation 740.0
  continua 339.41
  paroxysmal 339.03
    chronic 339.04
    episodic 339.03
Hemidystrophy - *see* Hemiatrophy
Hemiectromelia 755.4
Hemihypalgesia (*see also* Disturbance, sensation) 782.0
Hemihypertrophy (congenital) 759.89
  cranial 756.0
Hemihypesthesia (*see also* Disturbance, sensation) 782.0
Hemi-inattention 781.8
Hemimelia 755.4
  lower limb 755.30
    paraxial (complete) (incomplete) (intercalary) (terminal) 755.32
      fibula 755.37
      tibia 755.36
    transverse (complete) (partial) 755.31
  upper limb 755.20
    paraxial (complete) (incomplete) (intercalary) (terminal) 755.22
      radial 755.26
      ulnar 755.27
    transverse (complete) (partial) 755.21
Hemiparalysis (*see also* Hemiplegia) 342.9 [5th]
Hemiparesis (*see also* Hemiplegia) 342.9 [5th]
Hemiparesthesia (*see also* Disturbance, sensation) 782.0
Hemiplegia 342.9 [5th]
  acute (*see also* Disease, cerebrovascular, acute) 436
  alternans facialis 344.89
  apoplectic (*see also* Disease, cerebrovascular, acute) 436
    late effect or residual
      affecting
        dominant side 438.21
        nondominant side 438.22
        unspecified side 438.20
  arteriosclerotic 437.0
    late effect or residual
      affecting
        dominant side 438.21
        nondominant side 438.22
        unspecified side 438.20
  ascending (spinal) NEC 344.89
  attack (*see also* Disease, cerebrovascular, acute) 436
  brain, cerebral (current episode) 437.8
    congenital 343.1
  cerebral - *see* Hemiplegia, brain
  congenital (cerebral) (spastic) (spinal) 343.1
  conversion neurosis (hysterical) 300.11
  cortical - *see* Hemiplegia, brain
  due to
    arteriosclerosis 437.0
      late effect or residual
        affecting
          dominant side 438.21
          nondominant side 438.22
          unspecified side 438.20

Hemiplegia – *continued*
  due to – *continued*
    cerebrovascular lesion (*see also* Disease, cerebrovascular, acute) 436
      late effect
        affecting
          dominant side 438.21
          nondominant side 438.22
          unspecified side 438.20
  embolic (current) (*see also* Embolism, brain) 434.1 [5th]
    late effect
      affecting
        dominant side 438.21
        nondominant side 438.22
        unspecified side 438.20
  flaccid 342.0 [5th]
  hypertensive (current episode) 437.8
  infantile (postnatal) 343.4
  late effect
    birth injury, intracranial or spinal 343.4
    cerebrovascular lesion - *see* Late effect(s) (of) cerebrovascular disease
    viral encephalitis 139.0
  middle alternating NEC 344.89
  newborn NEC 767.0
  seizure (current episode) (*see also* Disease, cerebrovascular, acute) 436
  spastic 342.1 [5th]
    congenital or infantile 343.1
  specified NEC 342.8
  thrombotic (current) (*see also* Thrombosis, brain) 434.0 [5th]
    late effect - *see* Late effect(s) (of) cerebrovascular disease
Hemisection, spinal cord - *see* Fracture, vertebra, by site, with spinal cord injury
Hemispasm 781.0
  facial 781.0
Hemispatial neglect 781.8
Hemisporosis 117.9
Hemitremor 781.0
Hemivertebra 756.14
Hemobilia 576.8
Hemocholecyst 575.8
Hemochromatosis (acquired) (diabetic) (hereditary) (liver) (myocardium) (primary idiopathic) (secondary) 275.0
  with refractory anemia 238.72
Hemodialysis V56.0
Hemoglobin - *see also* condition
  abnormal (disease) - *see* Disease, hemoglobin
  AS genotype 282.5
  fetal, hereditary persistence 282.7
  high-oxygen-affinity 289.0
  low NEC 285.9
  S (Hb-S), heterozygous 282.5
Hemoglobinemia 283.2
  due to blood transfusion NEC 999.89
    bone marrow 996.85
  paroxysmal 283.2
Hemoglobinopathy (mixed) (*see also* Disease, hemoglobin) 282.7
  with thalassemia 282.49
  sickle-cell 282.60
    with thalassemia (without crisis) 282.41
      with
        crisis 282.42
        vaso-occlusive pain 282.42
Hemoglobinuria, hemoglobinuric 791.2
  with anemia, hemolytic, acquired (chronic) NEC 283.2
  cold (agglutinin) (paroxysmal) (with Raynaud's syndrome) 283.2
  due to
    exertion 283.2
    hemolysis (from external causes) NEC 283.2

Hematoma – Hemoglobinuria, hemoglobinuric

- **Hemoglobinuria, hemoglobinuric** – *continued*
  - exercise 283.2
  - fever (malaria) 084.8
  - infantile 791.2
  - intermittent 283.2
  - malarial 084.8
  - march 283.2
  - nocturnal (paroxysmal) 283.2
  - paroxysmal (cold) (nocturnal) 283.2
- **Hemolymphangioma** (M9175/0) 228.1
- **Hemolysis**
  - fetal - *see* Jaundice, fetus or newborn
  - intravascular (disseminated) NEC 286.6
    - with
      - abortion - *see* Abortion, by type, with hemorrhage, delayed or excessive
      - ectopic pregnancy (*see also* categories 633.0-633.9) 639.1
      - hemorrhage of pregnancy 641.3 [5th]
        - affecting fetus or newborn 762.1
      - molar pregnancy (*see also* categories 630-632) 639.1
    - acute 283.2
    - following
      - abortion 639.1
      - ectopic or molar pregnancy 639.1
  - neonatal - *see* Jaundice, fetus or newborn
  - transfusion NEC 999.89
    - bone marrow 996.85
- **Hemolytic** - *see also* condition
  - anemia - *see* Anemia, hemolytic
  - uremic syndrome 283.11
- **Hemometra** 621.4
- **Hemopericardium** (with effusion) 423.0
  - newborn 772.8
  - traumatic (*see also* Hemothorax, traumatic) 860.2
    - with open wound into thorax 860.3
- **Hemoperitoneum** 568.81
  - infectional (*see also* Peritonitis) 567.29
  - traumatic - *see* Injury, internal, peritoneum
- **Hemophagocytic syndrome** 288.4
  - infection-associated 288.4
- **Hemophilia** (familial) (hereditary) 286.0
  - A 286.0
    - carrier (asymptomatic) V83.01
      - symptomatic V83.02
  - acquired 286.5
  - B (Leyden) 286.1
  - C 286.2
  - calcipriva (*see also* Fibrinolysis) 286.7
  - classical 286.0
  - nonfamilial 286.7
  - secondary 286.5
  - vascular 286.4
- **Hemophilus influenzae** NEC 041.5
  - arachnoiditis (basic) (brain) (spinal) 320.0
    - late effect - *see* category 326
  - bronchopneumonia 482.2
  - cerebral ventriculitis 320.0
    - late effect - *see* category 326
  - cerebrospinal inflammation 320.0
    - late effect - *see* category 326
  - infection NEC 041.5
  - leptomeningitis 320.0
    - late effect - *see* category 326
  - meningitis (cerebral) (cerebrospinal) (spinal) 320.0
    - late effect - *see* category 326
  - meningomyelitis 320.0
    - late effect - *see* category 326
  - pachymeningitis (adhesive) (fibrous) (hemorrhagic) (hypertrophic) (spinal) 320.0
    - late effect - *see* category 326
  - pneumonia (broncho-) 482.2
- **Hemophthalmos** 360.43
- **Hemopneumothorax** (*see also* Hemothorax) 511.89
  - traumatic 860.4
    - with open wound into thorax 860.5
- **Hemoptysis** 786.3
  - due to Paragonimus (westermani) 121.2
  - newborn 770.3
  - tuberculous (*see also* Tuberculosis, pulmonary) 011.9 [5th]
- **Hemorrhage, hemorrhagic** (nontraumatic) 459.0
  - abdomen 459.0
  - accidental (antepartum) 641.2 [5th]
    - affecting fetus or newborn 762.1
  - adenoid 474.8
  - adrenal (capsule) (gland) (medulla) 255.41
    - newborn 772.5
  - after labor - *see* Hemorrhage, postpartum
  - alveolar
    - lung, newborn 770.3
    - process 525.8
  - alveolus 525.8
  - amputation stump (surgical) 998.11
    - secondary, delayed 997.69
  - anemia (chronic) 280.0
    - acute 285.1
  - antepartum - *see* Hemorrhage, pregnancy
  - anus (sphincter) 569.3
  - apoplexy (stroke) 432.9
  - arachnoid - *see* Hemorrhage, subarachnoid
  - artery NEC 459.0
    - brain (*see also* Hemorrhage, brain) 431
    - middle meningeal - *see* Hemorrhage, subarachnoid
  - basilar (ganglion) (*see also* Hemorrhage, brain) 431
  - bladder 596.8
  - blood dyscrasia 289.9
  - bowel 578.9
    - newborn 772.4
  - brain (miliary) (nontraumatic) 431
    - with
      - birth injury 767.0
    - arachnoid - *see* Hemorrhage, subarachnoid
    - due to
      - birth injury 767.0
      - rupture of aneurysm (congenital) (*see also* Hemorrhage, subarachnoid) 430
        - mycotic 431
      - syphilis 094.89
    - epidural or extradural - *see* Hemorrhage, extradural
    - fetus or newborn (anoxic) (hypoxic) (due to birth trauma) (nontraumatic) 767.0
      - intraventricular 772.10
        - grade I 772.11
        - grade II 772.12
        - grade III 772.13
        - grade IV 772.14
    - iatrogenic 997.02
    - postoperative 997.02
    - puerperal, postpartum, childbirth 674.0 [5th]
    - stem 431
    - subarachnoid, arachnoid, or meningeal - *see* Hemorrhage, subarachnoid
    - subdural - *see* Hemorrhage, subdural

- **Hemorrhage, hemorrhagic** – *continued*
  - brain – *continued*
    - traumatic NEC 853.0 [5th]

Note *Use the following fifth-digit subclassification with categories 851-854:*

0	unspecified state of consciousness
1	with no loss of consciousness
2	with brief [less than one hour] loss of consciousness
3	with moderate [1-24 hours] loss of consciousness
4	with prolonged [more than 24 hours] loss of consciousness and return to pre-existing conscious level
5	with prolonged [more than 24 hours] loss of consciousness, without return to pre-existing conscious level
	Use fifth-digit 5 to designate when a patient is unconscious and dies before regaining consciousness, regardless of the duration of the loss of consciousness
6	with loss of consciousness of unspecified duration
9	with concussion, unspecified

  - with
    - cerebral
      - contusion - *see* Contusion, brain
      - laceration - *see* Laceration, brain
    - open intracranial wound 853.1 [5th]
    - skull fracture - *see* Fracture, skull, by site
  - extradural or epidural 852.4 [5th]
    - with open intracranial wound 852.5 [5th]
  - subarachnoid 852.0 [5th]
    - with open intracranial wound 852.1 [5th]
  - subdural 852.2 [5th]
    - with open intracranial wound 852.3 [5th]
- breast 611.79
- bronchial tube - *see* Hemorrhage, lung
- bronchopulmonary - *see* Hemorrhage, lung
- bronchus (cause unknown) (*see also* Hemorrhage, lung) 786.3
- bulbar (*see also* Hemorrhage, brain) 431
- bursa 727.89
- capillary 448.9
  - primary 287.8
- capsular - *see* Hemorrhage, brain
- cardiovascular 429.89
- cecum 578.9
- cephalic (*see also* Hemorrhage, brain) 431
- cerebellar (*see also* Hemorrhage, brain) 431
- cerebellum (*see also* Hemorrhage, brain) 431
- cerebral (*see also* Hemorrhage, brain) 431
  - fetus or newborn (anoxic) (traumatic) 767.0
- cerebromeningeal (*see also* Hemorrhage, brain) 431
- cerebrospinal (*see also* Hemorrhage, brain) 431
- cerebrovascular accident - *see* Hemorrhage, brain
- cerebrum (*see also* Hemorrhage, brain) 431
- cervix (stump) (uteri) 622.8
- cesarean section wound 674.3
- chamber, anterior (eye) 364.41
- childbirth - *see* Hemorrhage, complicating, delivery
- choroid 363.61
  - expulsive 363.62
- ciliary body 364.41

- **Hemorrhage, hemorrhagic** – *continued*
  - cochlea 386.8
  - colon - *see* Hemorrhage, intestine
  - complicating
    - delivery 641.9 [5th]
      - affecting fetus or newborn 762.1
      - associated with
        - afibrinogenemia 641.3 [5th]
          - affecting fetus or newborn 763.89
        - coagulation defect 641.3 [5th]
          - affecting fetus or newborn 763.89
        - hyperfibrinolysis 641.3 [5th]
          - affecting fetus or newborn 763.89
        - hypofibrinogenemia 641.3 [5th]
          - affecting fetus or newborn 763.89
      - due to
        - low-lying placenta 641.1 [5th]
          - affecting fetus or newborn 762.0
        - placenta previa 641.1 [5th]
          - affecting fetus or newborn 762.0
        - premature separation of placenta 641.2 [5th]
          - affecting fetus or newborn 762.1
        - retained
          - placenta 666.0 [5th]
          - secundines 666.2 [5th]
        - trauma 641.8 [5th]
          - affecting fetus or newborn 763.89
        - uterine leiomyoma 641.8 [5th]
          - affecting fetus or newborn 763.89
  - complication(s)
    - of dental implant placement 525.71
    - surgical procedure 998.11
  - concealed NEC 459.0
  - congenital 772.9
  - conjunctiva 372.72
    - newborn 772.8
  - cord, newborn 772.0
    - slipped ligature 772.3
    - stump 772.3
  - corpus luteum (ruptured) 620.1
  - cortical (*see also* Hemorrhage, brain) 431
  - cranial 432.9
  - cutaneous 782.7
    - newborn 772.6
  - cyst, pancreas 577.2
  - cystitis - *see* Cystitis
  - delayed
    - with
      - abortion - *see* Abortion, by type, with hemorrhage, delayed or excessive
      - ectopic pregnancy (*see also* categories 633.0-633.9) 639.1
      - molar pregnancy (*see also* categories 630-632) 639.1
    - following
      - abortion 639.1
      - ectopic or molar pregnancy 639.1
    - postpartum 666.2 [5th]
  - diathesis (familial) 287.9
    - newborn 776.0
  - disease 287.9
    - newborn 776.0
    - specified type NEC 287.8
  - disorder 287.9
    - due to intrinsic circulating anticoagulants 286.5
    - specified type NEC 287.8

Hemoglobinuria, hemoglobinuric – Hemorrhage, hemorrhagic

- **Hemorrhage, hemorrhagic** – *continued*
  - pregnancy – *continued*
    - due to – *continued*
      - placenta previa 641.1 [5th]
        - affecting fetus or newborn 762.0
      - premature separation of placenta (normally implanted) 641.2 [5th]
        - affecting fetus or newborn 762.1
      - threatened abortion 640.0 [5th]
        - affecting fetus or newborn 762.1
      - trauma 641.8 [5th]
        - affecting fetus or newborn 762.1
    - early (before 22 completed weeks gestation) 640.9 [5th]
      - affecting fetus or newborn 762.1
    - previous, affecting management of pregnancy or childbirth V23.49
    - unavoidable - *see* Hemorrhage, pregnancy, due to placenta previa
  - prepartum (mother) - *see* Hemorrhage, pregnancy
  - preretinal, cause unspecified 362.81
  - prostate 602.1
  - puerperal (*see also* Hemorrhage, postpartum) 666.1 [5th]
  - pulmonary - *see also* Hemorrhage, lung
    - newborn (massive) 770.3
    - renal syndrome 446.21
  - purpura (primary) (*see also* Purpura, thrombocytopenic) 287.39
  - rectum (sphincter) 569.3
  - recurring, following initial hemorrhage at time of injury 958.2
  - renal 593.81
    - pulmonary syndrome 446.21
  - respiratory tract (*see also* Hemorrhage, lung) 786.3
  - retina, retinal (deep) (superficial) (vessels) 362.81
    - diabetic 250.5 [5th] *[362.01]*
      - due to secondary diabetes 249.5 [5th] *[362.01]*
    - due to birth injury 772.8
  - retrobulbar 376.89
  - retroperitoneal 459.0
  - retroplacental (*see also* Placenta, separation) 641.2 [5th]
  - scalp 459.0
    - due to injury at birth 767.19
  - scrotum 608.83
  - secondary (nontraumatic) 459.0
    - following initial hemorrhage at time of injury 958.2
  - seminal vesicle 608.83
  - skin 782.7
    - newborn 772.6
  - spermatic cord 608.83
  - spinal (cord) 336.1
    - aneurysm (ruptured) 336.1
      - syphilitic 094.89
    - due to birth injury 767.4
    - fetus or newborn 767.4
  - spleen 289.59
  - spontaneous NEC 459.0
    - petechial 782.7
  - stomach 578.9
    - newborn 772.4
    - ulcer - *see* Ulcer, stomach, with hemorrhage
  - subaponeurotic, newborn 767.11
    - massive (birth injury) 767.11
  - subarachnoid (nontraumatic) 430
    - fetus or newborn (anoxic) (traumatic) 772.2
    - puerperal, postpartum, childbirth 674.0 [5th]
    - traumatic - *see* Hemorrhage, brain, traumatic, subarachnoid
  - subconjunctival 372.72
    - due to birth injury 772.8
    - newborn 772.8
- **Hemorrhage, hemorrhagic** – *continued*
  - subcortical (*see also* Hemorrhage, brain) 431
  - subcutaneous 782.7
  - subdiaphragmatic 459.0
  - subdural (nontraumatic) 432.1
    - due to birth injury 767.0
    - fetus or newborn (anoxic) (hypoxic) (due to birth trauma) 767.0
    - puerperal, postpartum, childbirth 674.0 [5th]
    - spinal 336.1
    - traumatic - *see* Hemorrhage, brain, traumatic, subdural
  - subgaleal 767.11
  - subhyaloid 362.81
  - subperiosteal 733.99
  - subretinal 362.81
  - subtentorial (*see also* Hemorrhage, subdural) 432.1
  - subungual 703.8
    - due to blood dyscrasia 287.8
  - suprarenal (capsule) (gland) 255.41
    - fetus or newborn 772.5
  - tentorium (traumatic) - *see also* Hemorrhage, brain, traumatic
    - fetus or newborn 767.0
    - nontraumatic - *see* Hemorrhage, subdural
  - testis 608.83
  - thigh 459.0
  - third stage 666.0 [5th]
  - thorax - *see* Hemorrhage, lung
  - throat 784.8
  - thrombocythemia 238.71
  - thymus (gland) 254.8
  - thyroid (gland) 246.3
    - cyst 246.3
  - tongue 529.8
  - tonsil 474.8
    - postoperative 998.11
  - tooth socket (postextraction) 998.11
  - trachea - *see* Hemorrhage, lung
  - traumatic - *see also* nature of injury
    - brain - *see* Hemorrhage, brain, traumatic
    - recurring or secondary (following initial hemorrhage at time of injury) 958.2
  - tuberculous NEC (*see also* Tuberculosis, pulmonary) 011.9 [5th]
  - tunica vaginalis 608.83
  - ulcer - *see* Ulcer, by site, with hemorrhage
  - umbilicus, umbilical cord 772.0
    - after birth, newborn 772.3
    - complicating delivery 663.8 [5th]
      - affecting fetus or newborn 772.0
    - slipped ligature 772.3
    - stump 772.3
  - unavoidable (due to placenta previa) 641.1 [5th]
    - affecting fetus or newborn 762.0
  - upper extremity 459.0
  - urethra (idiopathic) 599.84
  - uterus, uterine (abnormal) 626.9
    - climacteric 627.0
    - complicating delivery - *see* Hemorrhage, complicating, delivery
    - due to
      - intrauterine contraceptive device 996.76
        - perforating uterus 996.32
    - functional or dysfunctional 626.8
    - in pregnancy - *see* Hemorrhage, pregnancy
    - intermenstrual 626.6
      - irregular 626.6
      - regular 626.5
    - postmenopausal 627.1
    - postpartum (*see also* Hemorrhage, postpartum) 666.1 [5th]
    - prepubertal 626.8
    - pubertal 626.3
- **Hemorrhage, hemorrhagic** – *continued*
  - uterus, uterine – *continued*
    - puerperal (immediate) 666.1 [5th]
  - vagina 623.8
  - vasa previa 663.5 [5th]
    - affecting fetus or newborn 772.0
  - vas deferens 608.83
  - ventricular (*see also* Hemorrhage, brain) 431
  - vesical 596.8
  - viscera 459.0
    - newborn 772.8
  - vitreous (humor) (intraocular) 379.23
  - vocal cord 478.5
  - vulva 624.8
- **Hemorrhoids** (anus) (rectum) (without complication) 455.6
  - bleeding, prolapsed, strangulated, or ulcerated NEC 455.8
    - external 455.5
    - internal 455.2
  - complicated NEC 455.8
  - complicating pregnancy and puerperium 671.8 [5th]
  - external 455.3
    - with complication NEC 455.5
    - bleeding, prolapsed, strangulated, or ulcerated 455.5
    - thrombosed 455.4
  - internal 455.0
    - with complication NEC 455.2
    - bleeding, prolapsed, strangulated, or ulcerated 455.2
    - thrombosed 455.1
  - residual skin tag 455.9
  - sentinel pile 455.9
  - thrombosed NEC 455.7
    - external 455.4
    - internal 455.1
- **Hemosalpinx** 620.8
- **Hemosiderosis** 275.0
  - dietary 275.0
  - pulmonary (idiopathic) 275.0 *[516.1]*
  - transfusion NEC 999.89
    - bone marrow 996.85
- **Hemospermia** 608.82
- **Hemothorax** 511.89
  - bacterial, nontuberculous 511.1
  - newborn 772.8
  - nontuberculous 511.89
    - bacterial 511.1
  - pneumococcal 511.1
  - postoperative 998.11
  - staphylococcal 511.1
  - streptococcal 511.1
  - traumatic 860.2
    - with
      - open wound into thorax 860.3
      - pneumothorax 860.4
        - with open wound into thorax 860.5
  - tuberculous (*see also* Tuberculosis, pleura) 012.0 [5th]
- **Hemotympanum** 385.89
- **Hench-Rosenberg syndrome** (palindromic arthritis) (*see also* Rheumatism, palindromic) 719.3 [5th]
- **Henle's warts** 371.41
- **Henoch (-Schönlein)**
  - disease or syndrome (allergic purpura) 287.0
  - purpura (allergic) 287.0
- **Henpue, henpuye** 102.6
- **Heparin-induced thrombocytopenia** (HIT) 289.84
- **Heparitinuria** 277.5
- **Hepar lobatum** 095.3
- **Hepatalgia** 573.8
- **Hepatic** - *see also* condition
  - flexure syndrome 569.89
- **Hepatitis** 573.3
  - acute (*see also* Necrosis, liver) 570
    - alcoholic 571.1
- **Hepatitis** – *continued*
  - acute – *continued*
    - infective 070.1
      - with hepatic coma 070.0
  - alcoholic 571.1
  - amebic - *see* Abscess, liver, amebic
  - anicteric (acute) - *see* Hepatitis, viral
  - antigen-associated (HAA) - *see* Hepatitis, viral, type B
  - Australian antigen (positive) - *see* Hepatitis, viral, type B
  - autoimmune 571.42
  - catarrhal (acute) 070.1
    - with hepatic coma 070.0
    - chronic 571.40
    - newborn 070.1
      - with hepatic coma 070.0
  - chemical 573.3
  - cholangiolitic 573.8
  - cholestatic 573.8
  - chronic 571.40
    - active 571.49
      - viral - *see* Hepatitis, viral
    - aggressive 571.49
    - persistent 571.41
    - viral - *see* Hepatitis, viral
  - cytomegalic inclusion virus 078.5 *[573.1]*
  - diffuse 573.3
  - "dirty needle" - *see* Hepatitis, viral
  - drug-induced 573.3
  - due to
    - Coxsackie 074.8 *[573.1]*
    - cytomegalic inclusion virus 078.5 *[573.1]*
    - infectious mononucleosis 075 *[573.1]*
    - malaria 084.9 *[573.2]*
    - mumps 072.71
    - secondary syphilis 091.62
    - toxoplasmosis (acquired) 130.5
      - congenital (active) 771.2
  - epidemic - *see* Hepatitis, viral, type A
  - fetus or newborn 774.4
  - fibrous (chronic) 571.49
    - acute 570
  - from injection, inoculation, or transfusion (blood) (other substance) (plasma) (serum) (onset within 8 months after administration) - *see* Hepatitis, viral
  - fulminant (viral) (*see also* Hepatitis, viral) 070.9
    - with hepatic coma 070.6
    - type A 070.1
      - with hepatic coma 070.0
    - type B - *see* Hepatitis, viral, type B
  - giant cell (neonatal) 774.4
  - hemorrhagic 573.8
  - history of
    - B V12.09
    - C V12.09
  - homologous serum - *see* Hepatitis, viral
  - hypertrophic (chronic) 571.49
    - acute 570
  - infectious, infective (acute) (chronic) (subacute) 070.1
    - with hepatic coma 070.0
  - inoculation - *see* Hepatitis, viral
  - interstitial (chronic) 571.49
    - acute 570
  - lupoid 571.49
  - malarial 084.9 *[573.2]*
  - malignant (*see also* Necrosis, liver) 570
  - neonatal (toxic) 774.4
  - newborn 774.4
  - parenchymatous (acute) (*see also* Necrosis, liver) 570
  - peliosis 573.3
  - persistent, chronic 571.41
  - plasma cell 571.49
  - postimmunization - *see* Hepatitis, viral
  - postnecrotic 571.49
  - posttransfusion - *see* Hepatitis, viral
  - recurrent 571.49
  - septic 573.3

- **Hepatitis** – *continued*
  - serum - *see* Hepatitis, viral
    - carrier (suspected of) V02.61
  - subacute (*see also* Necrosis, liver) 570
  - suppurative (diffuse) 572.0
  - syphilitic (late) 095.3
    - congenital (early) 090.0 *[573.2]*
      - late 090.5 *[573.2]*
    - secondary 091.62
  - toxic (noninfectious) 573.3
    - fetus or newborn 774.4
  - tuberculous (*see also* Tuberculosis) 017.9 5th
  - viral (acute) (anicteric) (cholangiolitic) (cholestatic) (chronic) (subacute) 070.9
    - with hepatic coma 070.6
    - AU-SH type virus - *see* Hepatitis, viral, type B
    - australian antigen - *see* Hepatitis, viral, type B
    - B-antigen - *see* Hepatitis, viral, type B
    - Coxsackie 074.8 *[573.1]*
    - cytomegalic inclusion 078.5 *[573.1]*
    - IH (virus) - *see* Hepatitis, viral, type A
    - infectious hepatitis virus - *see* Hepatitis, viral, type A
    - serum hepatitis virus - *see* Hepatitis, viral, type B
    - SH - *see* Hepatitis, viral, type B
    - specified type NEC 070.59
      - with hepatic coma 070.49
    - type A 070.1
      - with hepatic coma 070.0
    - type B (acute) 070.30
      - with
        - hepatic coma 070.20
      - carrier status V02.61
      - chronic 070.32
        - with
          - hepatic coma 070.22
            - with hepatitis delta 070.23
          - hepatitis delta 070.33
            - with hepatic coma 070.23
          - with hepatitis delta 070.21
        - hepatitis delta 070.31
          - with hepatic coma 070.21
    - type C
      - acute 070.51
        - with hepatic coma 070.41
      - carrier status V02.62
      - chronic 070.54
        - with hepatic coma 070.44
      - in remission 070.54
      - unspecified 070.70
        - with hepatic coma 070.71
    - type delta (with hepatitis B carrier state) 070.52
      - with
        - active hepatitis B disease - *see* Hepatitis, viral, type B
        - hepatic coma 070.42
    - type E 070.53
      - with hepatic coma 070.43
    - vaccination and inoculation (prophylactic) V05.3
  - Waldenström's (lupoid hepatitis) 571.49
- **Hepatization, lung** (acute) - *see also* Pneumonia, lobar
  - chronic (*see also* Fibrosis, lung) 515
- **Hepatoblastoma** (M8970/3) 155.0
- **Hepatocarcinoma** (M8170/3) 155.0
- **Hepatocholangiocarcinoma** (M8180/3) 155.0
- **Hepatocholangioma, benign** (M8180/0) 211.5
- **Hepatocholangitis** 573.8
- **Hepatocystitis** (*see also* Cholecystitis) 575.10
- **Hepatodystrophy** 570
- **Hepatolenticular degeneration** 275.1
- **Hepatolithiasis - see Choledocholithiasis**
- **Hepatoma** (malignant) (M8170/3) 155.0
  - benign (M8170/0) 211.5
  - congenital (M8970/3) 155.0
- **Hepatoma** – *continued*
  - embryonal (M8970/3) 155.0
- **Hepatomegalia glycogenica diffusa** 271.0
- **Hepatomegaly** (*see also* Hypertrophy, liver) 789.1
  - congenital 751.69
    - syphilitic 090.0
  - due to Clonorchis sinensis 121.1
  - Gaucher's 272.7
  - syphilitic (congenital) 090.0
- **Hepatoptosis** 573.8
- **Hepatorrhexis** 573.8
- **Hepatosis, toxic** 573.8
- **Hepatosplenomegaly** 571.8
  - due to S. japonicum 120.2
  - hyperlipemic (Bürger-Grutz type) 272.3
- **Herald patch** 696.3
- **Hereditary** - *see* condition
- **Heredodegeneration** 330.9
  - macular 362.70
- **Heredopathia atactica polyneuritiformis** 356.3
- **Heredosyphilis** (*see also* Syphilis, congenital) 090.9
- **Hermaphroditism** (true) 752.7
  - with specified chromosomal anomaly - *see* Anomaly, chromosomes, sex
- **Hernia, hernial** (acquired) (recurrent) 553.9
  - with
    - gangrene (obstructed) NEC 551.9
    - obstruction NEC 552.9
      - and gangrene 551.9
  - abdomen (wall) - *see* Hernia, ventral
  - abdominal, specified site NEC 553.8
    - with
      - gangrene (obstructed) 551.8
      - obstruction 552.8
        - and gangrene 551.8
  - appendix 553.8
    - with
      - gangrene (obstructed) 551.8
      - obstruction 552.8
        - and gangrene 551.8
  - bilateral (inguinal) - *see* Hernia, inguinal
  - bladder (sphincter)
    - congenital (female) (male) 756.71
    - female (*see also* Cystocele, female) 618.01
    - male 596.8
  - brain 348.4
    - congenital 742.0
  - broad ligament 553.8
  - cartilage, vertebral - *see* Displacement, intervertebral disc
  - cerebral 348.4
    - congenital 742.0
    - endaural 742.0
  - ciliary body 364.89
    - traumatic 871.1
  - colic 553.9
    - with
      - gangrene (obstructed) 551.9
      - obstruction 552.9
        - and gangrene 551.9
  - colon 553.9
    - with
      - gangrene (obstructed) 551.9
      - obstruction 552.9
        - and gangrene 551.9
  - colostomy (stoma) 569.69
  - Cooper's (retroperitoneal) 553.8
    - with
      - gangrene (obstructed) 551.8
      - obstruction 552.8
        - and gangrene 551.8
  - crural - *see* Hernia, femoral
  - diaphragm, diaphragmatic 553.3
    - with
      - gangrene (obstructed) 551.3
      - obstruction 552.3
        - and gangrene 551.3
    - congenital 756.6
    - due to gross defect of diaphragm 756.6
- **Hernia, hernial** – *continued*
  - diaphragm, diaphragmatic – *continued*
    - traumatic 862.0
      - with open wound into cavity 862.1
  - direct (inguinal) - *see* Hernia, inguinal
  - disc, intervertebral - *see* Displacement, intervertebral disc
  - diverticulum, intestine 553.9
    - with
      - gangrene (obstructed) 551.9
      - obstruction 552.9
        - and gangrene 551.9
  - double (inguinal) - *see* Hernia, inguinal
  - due to adhesion with obstruction 560.81
  - duodenojejunal 553.8
    - with
      - gangrene (obstructed) 551.8
      - obstruction 552.8
        - and gangrene 551.8
  - en glissade - *see* Hernia, inguinal
  - enterostomy (stoma) 569.69
  - epigastric 553.29
    - with
      - gangrene (obstruction) 551.29
      - obstruction 552.29
        - and gangrene 551.29
    - recurrent 553.21
      - with
        - gangrene (obstructed) 551.21
        - obstruction 552.21
          - and gangrene 551.21
  - esophageal hiatus (sliding) 553.3
    - with
      - gangrene (obstructed) 551.3
      - obstruction 552.3
        - and gangrene 551.3
    - congenital 750.6
  - external (inguinal) - *see* Hernia, inguinal
  - fallopian tube 620.4
  - fascia 728.89
  - fat 729.30
    - eyelid 374.34
    - orbital 374.34
    - pad 729.30
      - eye, eyelid 374.34
      - knee 729.31
      - orbit 374.34
      - popliteal (space) 729.31
      - specified site NEC 729.39
  - femoral (unilateral) 553.00
    - with
      - gangrene (obstructed) 551.00
      - obstruction 552.00
        - with gangrene 551.00
    - bilateral 553.02
      - gangrenous (obstructed) 551.02
      - obstructed 552.02
        - with gangrene 551.02
      - recurrent 553.03
        - gangrenous (obstructed) 551.03
        - obstructed 552.03
          - with gangrene 551.03
    - recurrent (unilateral) 553.01
      - bilateral 553.03
        - gangrenous (obstructed) 551.03
        - obstructed 552.03
          - with gangrene 551.03
      - gangrenous (obstructed) 551.01
      - obstructed 552.01
        - with gangrene 551.01
  - foramen
    - Bochdalek 553.3
      - with
        - gangrene (obstructed) 551.3
        - obstruction 552.3
          - and gangrene 551.3
      - congenital 756.6
    - magnum 348.4
    - Morgagni, Morgagnian 553.3
      - with
        - gangrene 551.3
        - obstruction 552.3
          - and gangrene 551.3
      - congenital 756.6
- **Hernia, hernial** – *continued*
  - funicular (umbilical) 553.1
    - with
      - gangrene (obstructed) 551.1
      - obstruction 552.1
        - and gangrene 551.1
    - spermatic cord - *see* Hernia, inguinal
  - gangrenous - *see* Hernia, by site, with gangrene
  - gastrointestinal tract 553.9
    - with
      - gangrene (obstructed) 551.9
      - obstruction 552.9
        - and gangrene 551.9
  - gluteal - *see* Hernia, femoral
  - Gruber's (internal mesogastric) 553.8
    - with
      - gangrene (obstructed) 551.8
      - obstruction 552.8
        - and gangrene 551.8
  - Hesselbach's 553.8
    - with
      - gangrene (obstructed) 551.8
      - obstruction 552.8
        - and gangrene 551.8
  - hiatal (esophageal) (sliding) 553.3
    - with
      - gangrene (obstructed) 551.3
      - obstruction 552.3
        - and gangrene 551.3
    - congenital 750.6
  - incarcerated (*see also* Hernia, by site, with obstruction) 552.9
    - gangrenous (*see also* Hernia, by site, with gangrene) 551.9
  - incisional 553.21
    - with
      - gangrene (obstructed) 551.21
      - obstruction 552.21
        - and gangrene 551.21
    - lumbar - *see* Hernia, lumbar
      - recurrent 553.21
      - with
        - gangrene (obstructed) 551.21
        - obstruction 552.21
          - and gangrene 551.21
  - indirect (inguinal) - *see* Hernia, inguinal
  - infantile - *see* Hernia, inguinal
  - infrapatellar fat pad 729.31
  - inguinal (direct) (double) (encysted) (external) (funicular) (indirect) (infantile) (internal) (interstitial) (oblique) (scrotal) (sliding) 550.9 5th

Note *Use the following fifth-digit subclassification with category 550:*

0	unilateral or unspecified (not specified as recurrent)
1	unilateral or unspecified, recurrent
2	bilateral (not specified as recurrent)
3	bilateral, recurrent

-
    - with
      - gangrene (obstructed) 550.0 5th
      - obstruction 550.1 5th
        - and gangrene 550.0 5th
  - internal 553.8
    - with
      - gangrene (obstructed) 551.8
      - obstruction 552.8
        - and gangrene 551.8
    - inguinal - *see* Hernia, inguinal
  - interstitial 553.9
    - with
      - gangrene (obstructed) 551.9
      - obstruction 552.9
        - and gangrene 551.9
    - inguinal - *see* Hernia, inguinal
  - intervertebral cartilage or disc - *see* Displacement, intervertebral disc
  - intestine, intestinal 553.9
    - with
      - gangrene (obstructed) 551.9

- **Hernia, hernial** – *continued*
  - intestine, intestinal – *continued*
    - with – *continued*
      - obstruction 552.9
        - and gangrene 551.9
  - intra-abdominal 553.9
    - with
      - gangrene (obstructed) 551.9
      - obstruction 552.9
        - and gangrene 551.9
  - intraparietal 553.9
    - with
      - gangrene (obstructed) 551.9
      - obstruction 552.9
        - and gangrene 551.9
  - iris 364.89
    - traumatic 871.1
  - irreducible (*see also* Hernia, by site, with obstruction) 552.9
    - gangrenous (with obstruction) (*see also* Hernia, by site, with gangrene) 551.9
  - ischiatic 553.8
    - with
      - gangrene (obstructed) 551.8
      - obstruction 552.8
        - and gangrene 551.8
  - ischiorectal 553.8
    - with
      - gangrene (obstructed) 551.8
      - obstruction 552.8
        - and gangrene 551.8
  - lens 379.32
    - traumatic 871.1
  - linea
    - alba - *see* Hernia, epigastric
    - semilunaris - *see* Hernia, spigelian
  - Littre's (diverticular) 553.9
    - with
      - gangrene (obstructed) 551.9
      - obstruction 552.9
        - and gangrene 551.9
  - lumbar 553.8
    - with
      - gangrene (obstructed) 551.8
      - obstruction 552.8
        - and gangrene 551.8
    - intervertebral disc 722.10
  - lung (subcutaneous) 518.89
    - congenital 748.69
  - mediastinum 519.3
  - mesenteric (internal) 553.8
    - with
      - gangrene (obstructed) 551.8
      - obstruction 552.8
        - and gangrene 551.8
  - mesocolon 553.8
    - with
      - gangrene (obstructed) 551.8
      - obstruction 552.8
        - and gangrene 551.8
  - muscle (sheath) 728.89
  - nucleus pulposus - *see* Displacement, intervertebral disc
  - oblique (inguinal) - *see* Hernia, inguinal
  - obstructive (*see also* Hernia, by site, with obstruction) 552.9
    - gangrenous (with obstruction) (*see also* Hernia, by site, with gangrene) 551.9
  - obturator 553.8
    - with
      - gangrene (obstructed) 551.8
      - obstruction 552.8
        - and gangrene 551.8
  - omental 553.8
    - with
      - gangrene (obstructed) 551.8
      - obstruction 552.8
        - and gangrene 551.8
  - orbital fat (pad) 374.34
  - ovary 620.4
  - oviduct 620.4
  - paracolostomy (stoma) 569.69

- **Hernia, hernial** – *continued*
  - paraduodenal 553.8
    - with
      - gangrene (obstructed) 551.8
      - obstruction 552.8
        - and gangrene 551.8
  - paraesophageal 553.3
    - with
      - gangrene (obstructed) 551.3
      - obstruction 552.3
        - and gangrene 551.3
    - congenital 750.6
  - parahiatal 553.3
    - with
      - gangrene (obstructed) 551.3
      - obstruction 552.3
        - and gangrene 551.3
  - paraumbilical 553.1
    - with
      - gangrene (obstructed) 551.1
      - obstruction 552.1
        - and gangrene 551.1
  - parietal 553.9
    - with
      - gangrene (obstructed) 551.9
      - obstruction 552.9
        - and gangrene 551.9
  - perineal 553.8
    - with
      - gangrene (obstructed) 551.8
      - obstruction 552.8
        - and gangrene 551.8
  - peritoneal sac, lesser 553.8
    - with
      - gangrene (obstructed) 551.8
      - obstruction 552.8
        - and gangrene 551.8
  - popliteal fat pad 729.31
  - postoperative 553.21
    - with
      - gangrene (obstructed) 551.21
      - obstruction 552.21
        - and gangrene 551.21
  - pregnant uterus 654.4 [5th]
  - prevesical 596.8
  - properitoneal 553.8
    - with
      - gangrene (obstructed) 551.8
      - obstruction 552.8
        - and gangrene 551.8
  - pudendal 553.8
    - with
      - gangrene (obstructed) 551.8
      - obstruction 552.8
        - and gangrene 551.8
  - rectovaginal 618.6
  - retroperitoneal 553.8
    - with
      - gangrene (obstructed) 551.8
      - obstruction 552.8
        - and gangrene 551.8
  - Richter's (parietal) 553.9
    - with
      - gangrene (obstructed) 551.9
      - obstruction 552.9
        - and gangrene 551.9
  - Rieux's, Riex's (retrocecal) 553.8
    - with
      - gangrene (obstructed) 551.8
      - obstruction 552.8
        - and gangrene 551.8
  - sciatic 553.8
    - with
      - gangrene (obstructed) 551.8
      - obstruction 552.8
        - and gangrene 551.8
  - scrotum, scrotal - *see* Hernia, inguinal
  - sliding (inguinal) - *see also* Hernia, inguinal
    - hiatus - *see* Hernia, hiatal
  - spigelian 553.29
    - with
      - gangrene (obstructed) 551.29

- **Hernia, hernial** – *continued*
  - spigelian – *continued*
    - with – *continued*
      - obstruction 552.29
        - and gangrene 551.29
  - spinal (*see also* Spina bifida) 741.9 [5th]
    - with hydrocephalus 741.0 [5th]
  - strangulated (*see also* Hernia, by site, with obstruction) 552.9
    - gangrenous (with obstruction) (*see also* Hernia, by site, with gangrene) 551.9
  - supraumbilicus (linea alba) - *see* Hernia, epigastric
  - tendon 727.9
  - testis (nontraumatic) 550.9 [5th]
    - meaning
      - scrotal hernia 550.9 [5th]
      - symptomatic late syphilis 095.8
  - Treitz's (fossa) 553.8
    - with
      - gangrene (obstructed) 551.8
      - obstruction 552.8
        - and gangrene 551.8
  - tunica
    - albuginea 608.89
    - vaginalis 752.89
  - umbilicus, umbilical 553.1
    - with
      - gangrene (obstructed) 551.1
      - obstruction 552.1
        - and gangrene 551.1
  - ureter 593.89
    - with obstruction 593.4
  - uterus 621.8
    - pregnant 654.4 [5th]
  - vaginal (posterior) 618.6
  - velpeau's (femoral) (*see also* Hernia, femoral) 553.00
  - ventral 553.20
    - with
      - gangrene (obstructed) 551.20
      - obstruction 552.20
        - and gangrene 551.20
    - incisional 553.21
    - recurrent 553.21
      - with
        - gangrene (obstructed) 551.21
        - obstruction 552.21
          - and gangrene 551.21
  - vesical
    - congenital (female) (male) 756.71
    - female (*see also* Cystocele, female) 618.01
    - male 596.8
  - vitreous (into anterior chamber) 379.21
    - traumatic 871.1
- **Herniation** - *see also* Hernia
  - brain (stem) 348.4
  - cerebral 348.4
  - gastric mucosa (into duodenal bulb) 537.89
  - mediastinum 519.3
  - nucleus pulposus - *see* Displacement, intervertebral disc
- **Herpangina** 074.0
- **Herpes, herpetic** 054.9
  - auricularis (zoster) 053.71
    - simplex 054.73
  - blepharitis (zoster) 053.20
    - simplex 054.41
  - circinate 110.5
  - circinatus 110.5
    - bullous 694.5
  - conjunctiva (simplex) 054.43
    - zoster 053.21
  - cornea (simplex) 054.43
    - disciform (simplex) 054.43
    - zoster 053.21
  - encephalitis 054.3
  - eye (zoster) 053.29
    - simplex 054.40
  - eyelid (zoster) 053.20
    - simplex 054.41

- **Herpes, herpetic** – *continued*
  - febrilis 054.9
  - fever 054.9
  - geniculate ganglionitis 053.11
  - genital, genitalis 054.10
    - specified site NEC 054.19
  - gestationis 646.8 [5th]
  - gingivostomatitis 054.2
  - iridocyclitis (simplex) 054.44
    - zoster 053.22
  - iris (any site) 695.10
  - iritis (simplex) 054.44
  - keratitis (simplex) 054.43
    - dendritic 054.42
    - disciform 054.43
    - interstitial 054.43
    - zoster 053.21
  - keratoconjunctivitis (simplex) 054.43
    - zoster 053.21
  - labialis 054.9
    - meningococcal 036.89
  - lip 054.9
  - meningitis (simplex) 054.72
    - zoster 053.0
  - ophthalmicus (zoster) 053.20
    - simplex 054.40
  - otitis externa (zoster) 053.71
    - simplex 054.73
  - penis 054.13
  - perianal 054.10
  - pharyngitis 054.79
  - progenitalis 054.10
  - scrotum 054.19
  - septicemia 054.5
  - simplex 054.9
    - complicated 054.8
      - ophthalmic 054.40
        - specified NEC 054.49
      - specified NEC 054.79
    - congenital 771.2
    - external ear 054.73
    - keratitis 054.43
      - dendritic 054.42
    - meningitis 054.72
    - myelitis 054.74
    - neuritis 054.79
    - specified complication NEC 054.79
      - ophthalmic 054.49
    - visceral 054.71
  - stomatitis 054.2
  - tonsurans 110.0
    - maculosus (of Hebra) 696.3
  - visceral 054.71
  - vulva 054.12
  - vulvovaginitis 054.11
  - whitlow 054.6
  - zoster 053.9
    - auricularis 053.71
    - complicated 053.8
      - specified NEC 053.79
    - conjunctiva 053.21
    - cornea 053.21
    - ear 053.71
    - eye 053.29
    - geniculate 053.11
    - keratitis 053.21
      - interstitial 053.21
    - myelitis 053.14
    - neuritis 053.10
    - ophthalmicus(a) 053.20
    - oticus 053.71
    - otitis externa 053.71
    - specified complication NEC 053.79
    - specified site NEC 053.9
  - zosteriform, intermediate type 053.9
- **Herrick's**
  - anemia (hemoglobin S disease) 282.61
  - syndrome (hemoglobin S disease) 282.61
- **Hers' disease** (glycogenosis VI) 271.0
- **Herter's infantilism** (nontropical sprue) 579.0
- **Herter** (-Gee) **disease or syndrome** (nontropical sprue) 579.0

Hernia, hernial – Herter disease or syndrome

- **Herxheimer's disease** (diffuse idiopathic cutaneous atrophy) 701.8
- **Herxheimer's reaction** 995.0
- **Hesitancy, urinary** 788.64
- **Hesselbach's hernia** - *see* Hernia, Hesselbach's
- **Heterochromia** (congenital) 743.46
  - acquired 364.53
  - cataract 366.33
  - cyclitis 364.21
  - hair 704.3
  - iritis 364.21
  - retained metallic foreign body 360.62
    - magnetic 360.52
  - uveitis 364.21
- **Heterophoria** 378.40
  - alternating 378.45
  - vertical 378.43
- **Heterophyes, small intestine** 121.6
- **Heterophyiasis** 121.6
- **Heteropsia** 368.8
- **Heterotopia, heterotopic** - *see also* Malposition, congenital
  - cerebralis 742.4
  - pancreas, pancreatic 751.7
  - spinalis 742.59
- **Heterotropia** 378.30
  - intermittent 378.20
    - vertical 378.31
  - vertical (constant) (intermittent) 378.31
- **Heubner's disease** 094.89
- **Heubner-Herter disease or syndrome** (nontropical sprue) 579.0
- **Hexadactylism** 755.00
- **Heyd's syndrome** (hepatorenal) 572.4
- **HGSIL** (high grade squamous intraepithelial lesion) (cytologic finding) (Pap smear finding)
  - anus 796.74
  - cervix 795.04
    - biopsy finding - code to CIN II or CIN III
  - vagina 795.14
- **Hibernoma** (M8880/0) - *see* Lipoma
- **Hiccough** 786.8
  - epidemic 078.89
  - psychogenic 306.1
- **Hiccup** (*see also* Hiccough) 786.8
- **Hicks (-Braxton) contractures** 644.1 [5th]
- **Hidden penis** 752.65
- **Hidradenitis** (axillaris) (suppurative) 705.83
- **Hidradenoma** (nodular) (M8400/0) - *see also* Neoplasm, skin, benign
  - clear cell (M8402/0) - *see* Neoplasm, skin, benign
  - papillary (M8405/0) - *see* Neoplasm, skin, benign
- **Hidrocystoma** (M8404/0) - *see* Neoplasm, skin, benign
- **HIE** (hypoxic-ischemic encephalopathy) 768.7<u>0</u> ▲
  - mild 768.71 ●
  - moderate 768.72 ●
  - severe 768.73 ●
- **High**
  - A_2 anemia 282.49
  - altitude effects 993.2
    - anoxia 993.2
    - on
      - ears 993.0
      - sinuses 993.1
    - polycythemia 289.0
  - arch
    - foot 755.67
    - palate 750.26
  - artery (arterial) tension (*see also* Hypertension) 401.9
    - without diagnosis of hypertension 796.2
  - basal metabolic rate (BMR) 794.7
- **High** – *continued*
  - blood pressure (*see also* Hypertension) 401.9
    - incidental reading (isolated) (nonspecific), no diagnosis of hypertension 796.2
  - cholesterol 272.0
    - with high triglycerides 272.2
  - compliance bladder 596.4
  - diaphragm (congenital) 756.6
  - frequency deafness (congenital) (regional) 389.8
  - head at term 652.5 [5th]
    - affecting fetus or newborn 763.1
  - output failure (cardiac) (*see also* Failure, heart) 428.9
  - oxygen-affinity hemoglobin 289.0
  - palate 750.26
  - risk
    - behavior - *see* problem
    - family situation V61.9
      - specified circumstance NEC V61.8
    - human papillomavirus (HPV) DNA test positive
      - anal 796.75
      - cervical 795.05
      - vaginal 795.15
    - individual NEC V62.89
    - infant NEC V20.1
    - patient taking drugs (prescribed) V67.51
      - nonprescribed (*see also* Abuse, drugs, nondependent) 305.9 [5th]
    - pregnancy V23.9
      - inadequate prenatal care V23.7
      - specified problem NEC V23.89
  - temperature (of unknown origin) (*see also* Pyrexia) 780.60
  - thoracic rib 756.3
  - triglycerides 272.1
    - with high cholesterol 272.2
- **Hildenbrand's disease** (typhus) 081.9
- **Hilger's syndrome** 337.09
- **Hill diarrhea** 579.1
- **Hilliard's lupus** (*see also* Tuberculosis) 017.0 [5th]
- **Hilum** - *see* condition
- **Hip** - *see* condition
- **Hippel's disease** (retinocerebral angiomatosis) 759.6
- **Hippus** 379.49
- **Hirschfeld's disease** (acute diabetes mellitus) (*see also* Diabetes) 250.0 [5th]
  - due to secondary diabetes 249.0 [5th]
- **Hirschsprung's disease or megacolon** (congenital) 751.3
- **Hirsuties** (*see also* Hypertrichosis) 704.1
- **Hirsutism** (*see also* Hypertrichosis) 704.1
- **Hirudiniasis** (external) (internal) 134.2
- **His-Werner disease** (trench fever) 083.1
- **Hiss-Russell dysentery** 004.1
- **Histamine cephalgia** 339.00 [5th]
- **Histidinemia** 270.5
- **Histidinuria** 270.5
- **Histiocytic syndromes** 288.4
- **Histiocytoma** (M8832/0) - *see also* Neoplasm, skin, benign
  - fibrous (M8830/0) - *see also* Neoplasm, skin, benign
    - atypical (M8830/1) - *see* Neoplasm, connective tissue, uncertain behavior
    - malignant (M8830/3) - *see* Neoplasm, connective tissue, malignant
- **Histiocytosis** (acute) (chronic) (subacute) 277.89
  - acute differentiated progressive (M9722/3) 202.5 [5th]
  - cholesterol 277.89
  - essential 277.89
  - lipid, lipoid (essential) 272.7
  - lipochrome (familial) 288.1
  - malignant (M9720/3) 202.3 [5th]
- **Histiocytosis** – *continued*
  - non-Langerhans cell 277.89 ●
  - polyostotic sclerosing 277.89 ●
  - X (chronic) 277.89
    - acute (progressive) (M9722/3) 202.5 [5th]
- **Histoplasmosis** 115.90
  - with
    - endocarditis 115.94
    - meningitis 115.91
- **Histoplasmosis** – *continued*
  - with – *continued*
    - pericarditis 115.93
    - pneumonia 115.95
    - retinitis 115.92
    - specified manifestation NEC 115.99
  - African (due to Histoplasma duboisii) 115.10
    - with
      - endocarditis 115.14
      - meningitis 115.11
      - pericarditis 115.13
      - pneumonia 115.15
      - retinitis 115.12
      - specified manifestation NEC 115.19
  - American (due to Histoplasma capsulatum) 115.00
    - with
      - endocarditis 115.04
      - meningitis 115.01
      - pericarditis 115.03
      - pneumonia 115.05
      - retinitis 115.02
      - specified manifestation NEC 115.09
  - Darling's - *see* Histoplasmosis, American
  - large form (*see also* Histoplasmosis, African) 115.10
  - lung 115.05
  - small form (*see also* Histoplasmosis, American) 115.00
- **History** (personal) **of**
  - abuse
    - emotional V15.42
    - neglect V15.42
    - physical V15.41
    - sexual V15.41
  - affective psychosis V11.1
  - alcoholism V11.3
    - specified as drinking problem (*see also* Abuse, drugs, nondependent) 305.0 [5th]
  - allergy to
    - analgesic agent NEC V14.6
    - anesthetic NEC V14.4
    - antibiotic agent NEC V14.1
      - penicillin V14.0
    - anti-infective agent NEC V14.3
    - arachnid bite V15.06 ●
    - diathesis V15.09
    - drug V14.9
      - specified type NEC V14.8
    - eggs V15.03
    - food additives V15.05
    - insect bite V15.06
    - latex V15.07
    - medicinal agents V14.9
      - specified type NEC V14.8
    - milk products V15.02
    - narcotic agent NEC V14.5
    - nuts V15.05
      - peanuts V15.01
    - penicillin V14.0
    - radiographic dye V15.08
    - seafood V15.04
    - serum V14.7
    - specified food NEC V15.05
    - specified nonmedicinal agents NEC V15.09
    - spider bite V15.06
    - sulfa V14.2
    - sulfonamides V14.2
    - therapeutic agent NEC V15.09
    - vaccine V14.7
  - anemia V12.3
- **History** (personal) **of** – *continued*
  - arthritis V13.4
  - arrest, sudden cardiac V12.53
  - attack, transient ischemic (TIA) V12.54
  - benign neoplasm of brain V12.41
  - blood disease V12.3
  - calculi, urinary V13.01
  - cardiovascular disease V12.50
    - myocardial infarction 412
  - chemotherapy, antineoplastic V87.41
  - child abuse V15.41
  - cigarette smoking V15.82
  - circulatory system disease V12.50
    - myocardial infarction 412
  - congenital malformation V13.69
  - contraception V15.7
  - death, sudden, successfully resuscitated V12.53
  - deficit
    - prolonged reversible ischemic neurologic (PRIND) V12.54
    - reversible ischemic neurologic (RIND) V12.54
  - diathesis, allergic V15.09
  - digestive system disease V12.70
    - peptic ulcer V12.71
    - polyps, colonic V12.72
    - specified NEC V12.79
  - disease (of) V13.9
    - blood V12.3
    - blood-forming organs V12.3
    - cardiovascular system V12.50
    - circulatory system V12.50
      - specified NEC V12.59
    - digestive system V12.70
      - peptic ulcer V12.71
      - polyps, colonic V12.72
      - specified NEC V12.79
    - infectious V12.00
      - malaria V12.03
      - methicillin resistant Staphylococcus aureus (MRSA) V12.04
      - MRSA (methicillin resistant Staphylococcus aureus) V12.04
      - poliomyelitis V12.02
      - specified NEC V12.09
      - tuberculosis V12.01
    - parasitic V12.00
      - specified NEC V12.09
    - respiratory system V12.60
      - pneumonia V12.61
      - specified NEC V12.69
    - skin V13.3
    - specified site NEC V13.8
    - subcutaneous tissue V13.3
    - trophoblastic V13.1
      - affecting management of pregnancy V23.1
  - disorder (of) V13.9
    - endocrine V12.2
    - genital system V13.29
    - hematological V12.3
    - immunity V12.2
    - mental V11.9
      - affective type V11.1
      - manic-depressive V11.1
      - neurosis V11.2
      - schizophrenia V11.0
      - specified type NEC V11.8
    - metabolic V12.2
    - musculoskeletal NEC V13.59
    - nervous system V12.40
      - specified type NEC V12.49
    - obstetric V13.29
      - affecting management of current pregnancy V23.49
        - pre-term labor V23.41
      - pre-term labor V13.21
    - sense organs V12.40
      - specified type NEC V12.49
    - specified site NEC V13.8
    - urinary system V13.00
      - calculi V13.01

- **History** (personal) **of** – *continued*
  - disorder (of) – *continued*
    - urinary system – *continued*
      - infection V13.02
      - nephrotic syndrome V13.03
      - specified NEC V13.09
  - drug use
    - nonprescribed (*see also* Abuse, drugs, nondependent) 305.9 [5th]
    - patent (*see also* Abuse, drugs, nondependent) 305.9 [5th]
  - dysplasia
    - cervical (conditions classifiable to 622.10-622.12) V13.22
  - extracorporeal membrane oxygenation (ECMO) V15.87
  - effect NEC of external cause V15.89
  - embolism (pulmonary) V12.51
  - emotional abuse V15.42
  - encephalitis V12.42
  - endocrine disorder V12.2
  - estrogen therapy V87.43 ●
  - failed ●
    - conscious sedation V15.80 ●
    - moderate sedation V15.80 ●
  - falling V15.88
  - family
    - allergy V19.6
    - anemia V18.2
    - arteriosclerosis V17.49
    - arthritis V17.7
    - asthma V17.5
    - blindness V19.0
    - blood disorder NEC V18.3
    - cardiovascular disease V17.49
    - carrier, genetic disease V18.9
    - cerebrovascular disease V17.1
    - chronic respiratory condition NEC V17.6
    - colonic polyps V18.51
    - congenital anomalies V19.5
    - consanguinity V19.7
    - coronary artery disease V17.3
    - cystic fibrosis V18.19
    - deafness V19.2
    - diabetes mellitus V18.0
    - digestive disorders V18.59
    - disease or disorder (of)
      - allergic V19.6
      - blood NEC V18.3
      - cardiovascular NEC V17.49
      - cerebrovascular V17.1
      - colonic polyps V18.51
      - coronary artery V17.3
      - death, sudden cardiac (SCD) V17.41
      - digestive V18.59
      - ear NEC V19.3
      - endocrine V18.19
        - multiple neoplasia [MEN] syndrome V18.11
      - eye NEC V19.1
      - genitourinary NEC V18.7
      - hypertensive V17.49
      - infectious V18.8
      - ischemic heart V17.3
      - kidney V18.69
        - polycystic V18.61
      - mental V17.0
      - metabolic V18.19
      - musculoskeletal NEC V17.89
        - osteoporosis V17.81
      - neurological NEC V17.2
      - parasitic V18.8
      - psychiatric condition V17.0
      - skin condition V19.4
    - ear disorder NEC V19.3
    - endocrine disease V18.19
      - multiple neoplasia [MEN] syndrome V18.11
    - epilepsy V17.2
    - eye disorder NEC V19.1
    - genetic disease carrier V18.9
    - genitourinary disease NEC V18.7

- **History** (personal) **of** – *continued*
  - family – *continued*
    - glomerulonephritis V18.69
    - gout V18.19
    - hay fever V17.6
    - hearing loss V19.2
    - hematopoietic neoplasia V16.7
    - Hodgkin's disease V16.7
    - Huntington's chorea V17.2
    - hydrocephalus V19.5
    - hypertension V17.49
    - infarction, myocardial V17.3
    - infectious disease V18.8
    - ischemic heart disease V17.3
    - kidney disease V18.69
      - polycystic V18.61
    - leukemia V16.6
    - lymphatic malignant neoplasia NEC V16.7
    - malignant neoplasm (of) NEC V16.9
      - anorectal V16.0
      - anus V16.0
      - appendix V16.0
      - bladder V16.52
      - bone V16.8
      - brain V16.8
      - breast V16.3
        - male V16.8
      - bronchus V16.1
      - cecum V16.0
      - cervix V16.49
      - colon V16.0
      - duodenum V16.0
      - esophagus V16.0
      - eye V16.8
      - gallbladder V16.0
      - gastrointestinal tract V16.0
      - genital organs V16.40
      - hemopoietic NEC V16.7
      - ileum V16.0
      - ilium V16.8
      - intestine V16.0
      - intrathoracic organs NEC V16.2
      - kidney V16.51
      - larynx V16.2
      - liver V16.0
      - lung V16.1
      - lymphatic NEC V16.7
      - ovary V16.41
      - oviduct V16.41
      - pancreas V16.0
      - penis V16.49
      - prostate V16.42
      - rectum V16.0
      - respiratory organs NEC V16.2
      - skin V16.8
      - specified site NEC V16.8
      - stomach V16.0
      - testis V16.43
      - trachea V16.1
      - ureter V16.59
      - urethra V16.59
      - urinary organs V16.59
      - uterus V16.49
      - vagina V16.49
      - vulva V16.49
    - MEN (multiple endocrine neoplasia syndrome) V18.11
    - mental retardation V18.4
    - metabolic disease NEC V18.19
    - mongolism V19.5
    - ~~monoclonal drug therapy V87.42~~
    - multiple
      - endocrine neoplasia [MEN] syndrome V18.11
      - myeloma V16.7
    - musculoskeletal disease NEC V17.89
      - osteoporosis V17.81
    - myocardial infarction V17.3
    - nephritis V18.69
    - nephrosis V18.69
    - osteoporosis V17.81
    - parasitic disease V18.8
    - polycystic kidney disease V18.61

- **History** (personal) **of** – *continued*
  - family – *continued*
    - psychiatric disorder V17.0
    - psychosis V17.0
    - retardation, mental V18.4
    - retinitis pigmentosa V19.1
    - schizophrenia V17.0
    - skin conditions V19.4
    - specified condition NEC V19.8
    - stroke (cerebrovascular) V17.1
    - sudden cardiac death (SCD) V17.41
    - visual loss V19.0
  - fracture, healed
    - pathologic V13.51
    - stress V13.52
    - traumatic V15.51
  - genital system disorder V13.29
    - pre-term labor V13.21
  - health hazard V15.9
    - falling V15.88
    - specified cause NEC V15.89
  - hepatitis
    - B V12.09
    - C V12.09
  - Hodgkin's disease V10.72
  - hypospadias V13.61
  - immunity disorder V12.2
  - immunosuppression therapy V87.46 ●
  - infarction, cerebral, without residual deficits V12.54
  - infection
    - central nervous system V12.42
    - urinary (tract) V13.02
  - infectious disease V12.00
    - malaria V12.03
    - methicillin resistant Staphylococcus aureus (MRSA) V12.04
    - MRSA (methicillin resistant Staphylococcus aureus) V12.04
    - poliomyelitis V12.02
    - specified NEC V12.09
    - tuberculosis V12.01
  - injury NEC V15.59
    - traumatic brain V15.52 ●
  - insufficient prenatal care V23.7
  - in utero procedure
    - during pregnancy V15.21
    - while a fetus V15.22
  - irradiation V15.3
  - leukemia V10.60
    - lymphoid V10.61
    - monocytic V10.63
    - myeloid V10.62
    - specified type NEC V10.69
  - little or no prenatal care V23.7
  - low birth weight (*see also* Status, low birth weight) V21.30
  - lymphosarcoma V10.71
  - malaria V12.03
  - malignant carcinoid tumor V10.91 ●
  - malignant neoplasm (of) V10.90 ▲
    - accessory sinus V10.22
    - adrenal V10.88
    - anus V10.06
    - bile duct V10.09
    - bladder V10.51
    - bone V10.81
    - brain V10.85
    - breast V10.3
    - bronchus V10.11
    - cervix uteri V10.41
    - colon V10.05
    - connective tissue NEC V10.89
    - corpus uteri V10.42
    - digestive system V10.00
      - specified part NEC V10.09
    - duodenum V10.09
    - endocrine gland NEC V10.88
    - epididymis V10.48
    - esophagus V10.03
    - eye V10.84
    - fallopian tube V10.44
    - female genital organ V10.40
      - specified site NEC V10.44

- **History** (personal) **of** – *continued*
  - malignant neoplasm (of) – *continued*
    - gallbladder V10.09
    - gastrointestinal tract V10.00
    - gum V10.02
    - hematopoietic NEC V10.79
    - hypopharynx V10.02
    - ileum V10.09
    - intrathoracic organs NEC V10.20
    - jejunum V10.09
    - kidney V10.52
    - large intestine V10.05
    - larynx V10.21
    - lip V10.02
    - liver V10.07
    - lung V10.11
    - lymphatic NEC V10.79
    - lymph glands or nodes NEC V10.79
    - male genital organ V10.45
      - specified site NEC V10.49
    - mediastinum V10.29
    - melanoma (of skin) V10.82
    - middle ear V10.22
    - mouth V10.02
      - specified part NEC V10.02
    - nasal cavities V10.22
    - nasopharynx V10.02
    - nervous system NEC V10.86
    - nose V10.22
    - oropharynx V10.02
    - ovary V10.43
    - pancreas V10.09
    - parathyroid V10.88
    - penis V10.49
    - pharynx V10.02
    - pineal V10.88
    - pituitary V10.88
    - placenta V10.44
    - pleura V10.29
    - prostate V10.46
    - rectosigmoid junction V10.06
    - rectum V10.06
    - renal pelvis V10.53
    - respiratory organs NEC V10.20
    - salivary gland V10.02
    - skin V10.83
      - melanoma V10.82
    - small intestine NEC V10.09
    - soft tissue NEC V10.89
    - specified site NEC V10.89
    - stomach V10.04
    - testis V10.47
    - thymus V10.29
    - thyroid V10.87
    - tongue V10.01
    - trachea V10.12
    - ureter V10.59
    - urethra V10.59
    - urinary organ V10.50
    - uterine adnexa V10.44
    - uterus V10.42
    - vagina V10.44
    - vulva V10.44
  - malignant neuroendocrine tumor V10.91 ●
  - manic-depressive psychosis V11.1
  - meningitis V12.42
  - mental disorder V11.9
    - affective type V11.1
    - manic-depressive V11.1
    - neurosis V11.2
    - schizophrenia V11.0
    - specified type NEC V11.8
  - Merkel cell carcinoma V10.91 ●
  - metabolic disorder V12.2
  - methicillin resistant Staphylococcus aureus (MRSA) V12.04
  - MRSA (methicillin resistant Staphylococcus aureus) V12.04
  - musculoskeletal disorder NEC V13.59
  - myocardial infarction 412
  - neglect (emotional) V15.42
  - nephrotic syndrome V13.03

History of – Hydralazine lupus or syndrome

History (personal) **of** – *continued*
- nervous system disorder V12.40
  - specified type NEC V12.49
- neurosis V11.2
- noncompliance with medical treatment V15.81
- nutritional deficiency V12.1
- obstetric disorder V13.29
  - affecting management of current pregnancy V23.49
    - pre-term labor V23.41
  - pre-term labor V13.21
- parasitic disease V12.00
  - specified NEC V12.09
- perinatal problems V13.7
  - low birth weight (*see also* Status, low birth weight) V21.30
- physical abuse V15.41
- poisoning V15.6
- poliomyelitis V12.02
- polyps, colonic V12.72
- poor obstetric V13.29
  - affecting management of current pregnancy V23.49
    - pre-term labor V23.41
  - pre-term labor V13.21
- prolonged reversible ischemic neurologic deficit (PRIND) V12.54
- psychiatric disorder V11.9
  - affective type V11.1
  - manic-depressive V11.1
  - neurosis V11.2
  - schizophrenia V11.0
  - specified type NEC V11.8
- psychological trauma V15.49
  - emotional abuse V15.42
  - neglect V15.42
  - physical abuse V15.41
  - rape V15.41
- psychoneurosis V11.2
- radiation therapy V15.3
- rape V15.41
- respiratory system disease V12.60
  - pneumonia V12.61
  - specified NEC V12.69
- reticulosarcoma V10.71
- return from military deployment V62.22
- reversible ischemic neurologic deficit (RIND) V12.54
- schizophrenia V11.0
- skin disease V13.3
- smoking (tobacco) V15.82
- steroid therapy V87.45 ●
  - inhaled V87.44 ●
  - systemic V87.45 ●
- stroke without residual deficits V12.54
- subcutaneous tissue disease V13.3
- sudden
  - cardiac
    - arrest V12.53
    - death (successfully resuscitated) V12.53
- surgery to
  - great vessels V15.1
  - heart V15.1
  - in utero
    - during pregnancy V15.21
    - while a fetus V15.22
  - organs NEC V15.29
- syndrome, nephrotic V13.03
- therapy
  - antineoplastic drug V87.41
  - drug NEC V87.49
  - estrogen V87.43 ●
  - monoclonal drug V87.42
  - immunosuppression V87.46 ●
  - steroid V87.45 ●
    - inhaled V87.44 ●
    - systemic V87.45 ●
- thrombophlebitis V12.52
- thrombosis V12.51
- tobacco use V15.82

History (personal) **of** – *continued*
- trophoblastic disease V13.1
  - affecting management of pregnancy V23.1
- tuberculosis V12.01
- ulcer, peptic V12.71
- urinary system disorder V13.00
  - calculi V13.01
  - infection V13.02
  - nephrotic syndrome V13.03
  - specified NEC V13.09

HIT (heparin-induced thrombocytopenia) 289.84

HIV infection (disease) (illness) - *see* Human immunodeficiency virus (disease) (illness) (infection)

Hives (bold) (*see also* Urticaria) 708.9

Hoarseness 784.42 ▲

Hobnail liver - *see* Cirrhosis, portal

Hobo, hoboism V60.0

Hodgkin's
- disease (M9650/3) 201.9 [5th]
  - lymphocytic
    - depletion (M9653/3) 201.7 [5th]
      - diffuse fibrosis (M9654/3) 201.7 [5th]
      - reticular type (M9655/3) 201.7 [5th]
    - predominance (M9651/3) 201.4 [5th]
  - lymphocytic-histiocytic predominance (M9651/3) 201.4 [5th]
  - mixed cellularity (M9652/3) 201.6 [5th]
  - nodular sclerosis (M9656/3) 201.5 [5th]
    - cellular phase (M9657/3) 201.5 [5th]
- granuloma (M9661/3) 201.1 [5th]
- lymphogranulomatosis (M9650/3) 201.9 [5th]
- lymphoma (M9650/3) 201.9 [5th]
- lymphosarcoma (M9650/3) 201.9 [5th]
- paragranuloma (M9660/3) 201.0 [5th]
- sarcoma (M9662/3) 201.2 [5th]

Hodgson's disease (aneurysmal dilatation of aorta) 441.9
- ruptured 441.5

Hodi-potsy 111.0

Hoffa (-Kastert) disease or syndrome (liposynovitis prepatellaris) 272.8

Hoffmann's syndrome 244.9 *[359.5]*

Hoffmann-Bouveret syndrome (paroxysmal tachycardia) 427.2

Hole
- macula 362.54
- optic disc, crater-like 377.22
- retina (macula) 362.54
  - round 361.31
    - with detachment 361.01

Holla disease (*see also* Spherocytosis) 282.0

Holländer-Simons syndrome (progressive lipodystrophy) 272.6

Hollow foot (congenital) 754.71
- acquired 736.73

Holmes' syndrome (visual disorientation) 368.16

Holoprosencephaly 742.2
- due to
  - trisomy 13 758.1
  - trisomy 18 758.2

Holthouse's hernia - *see* Hernia, inguinal

Homesickness 309.89

Homocystinemia 270.4

Homocystinuria 270.4

Homologous serum jaundice (prophylactic) (therapeutic) - *see* Hepatitis, viral

Homosexuality - omit code
- ego-dystonic 302.0
- pedophilic 302.2
- problems with 302.0

Homozygous Hb-S disease 282.61

Honeycomb lung 518.89
- congenital 748.4

Hong Kong ear 117.3

HOOD (hereditary osteo-onychodysplasia) 756.89

Hooded
- clitoris 752.49
- penis 752.69

Hookworm (anemia) (disease) (infestation) - *see* Ancylostomiasis

Hoppe-Goldflam syndrome 358.00

Hordeolum (external) (eyelid) 373.11
- internal 373.12

Horn
- cutaneous 702.8
  - cheek 702.8
  - eyelid 702.8
  - penis 702.8
- iliac 756.89
- nail 703.8
  - congenital 757.5
- papillary 700

Horner's
- syndrome (*see also* Neuropathy, peripheral, autonomic) 337.9
  - traumatic 954.0
- teeth 520.4

Horseshoe kidney (congenital) 753.3

Horton's
- disease (temporal arteritis) 446.5
- headache or neuralgia 339.00

Hospice care V66.7

Hospitalism (in children) NEC 309.83

Hourglass contraction, contracture
- bladder 596.8
- gallbladder 575.2
  - congenital 751.69
- stomach 536.8
  - congenital 750.7
  - psychogenic 306.4
- uterus 661.4 [5th]
  - affecting fetus or newborn 763.7

Household circumstance affecting care V60.9
- specified type NEC V60.89 ▲

Housemaid's knee 727.2

Housing circumstance affecting care V60.9
- specified type NEC V60.89 ▲

HTLV-I infection 079.51

HTLV-II infection 079.52

HTLV-III (disease) (illness) (infection) - *see* Human immunodeficiency virus (disease) (illness) (infection)

HTLV-III/LAV (disease) (illness) (infection) - *see* Human immunodeficiency virus (disease) (illness) (infection)

Huchard's disease (continued arterial hypertension) 401.9

Hudson-Stähli lines 371.11

Huguier's disease (uterine fibroma) 218.9

Hum, venous - omit code

Human bite (open wound) - (*see also* Wound, open, by site)
- intact skin surface - *see* Contusion

Human immunodeficiency virus (disease) (illness) 042
- infection V08
  - with symptoms, symptomatic 042

Human immunodeficiency virus-2 infection 079.53

Human immunovirus - *see* Human immunodeficiency virus (disease) (illness) (infection)

Human papillomavirus 079.4
- high risk, DNA test positive
  - anal 796.75
  - cervical 795.05
  - vaginal 795.15
- low risk, DNA test positive
  - anal 796.79
  - cervical 795.09
  - vaginal 795.19

Human parvovirus 079.83

Human T-cell lymphotrophic virus I infection 079.51

Human T-cell lymphotrophic virus II infection 079.52

Human T-cell lymphotropic virus-III (disease) (illness) (infection) - *see* Human immunodeficiency virus (disease) (illness) (infection)

Humpback (acquired) 737.9
- congenital 756.19

Hunchback (acquired) 737.9
- congenital 756.19

Hunger 994.2
- air, psychogenic 306.1
- disease 251.1

Hungry bone syndrome 275.5

Hunner's ulcer (*see also* Cystitis) 595.1

Hunt's
- neuralgia 053.11
- syndrome (herpetic geniculate ganglionitis) 053.11
  - dyssynergia cerebellaris myoclonica 334.2

Hunter's glossitis 529.4

Hunter (-Hurler) syndrome (mucopolysaccharidosis II) 277.5

Hunterian chancre 091.0

Huntington's
- chorea 333.4
- disease 333.4

Huppert's disease (multiple myeloma) (M9730/3) 203.0 [5th]

Hurler (-Hunter) disease or syndrome (mucopolysaccharidosis II) 277.5

Hürthle cell
- adenocarcinoma (M8290/3) 193
- adenoma (M8290/0) 226
- carcinoma (M8290/3) 193
- tumor (M8290/0) 226

Hutchinson's
- disease meaning
  - angioma serpiginosum 709.1
  - cheiropompholyx 705.81
  - prurigo estivalis 692.72
  - summer eruption, or summer prurigo 692.72
- incisors 090.5
- melanotic freckle (M8742/2) - *see also* Neoplasm, skin, in situ
  - malignant melanoma in (M8742/3) - *see* Melanoma
- teeth or incisors (congenital syphilis) 090.5

Hutchinson-Boeck disease or syndrome (sarcoidosis) 135

Hutchinson-Gilford disease or syndrome (progeria) 259.8

Hyaline
- degeneration (diffuse) (generalized) 728.9
  - localized - *see* Degeneration, by site
- membrane (disease) (lung) (newborn) 769

Hyalinosis cutis et mucosae 272.8

Hyalin plaque, sclera, senile 379.16

Hyalitis (asteroid) 379.22
- syphilitic 095.8

Hydatid
- cyst or tumor - *see also* Echinococcus
  - fallopian tube 752.11
- mole - *see* Hydatidiform mole
- Morgagni (congenital) 752.89
  - fallopian tube 752.11

Hydatidiform mole (benign) (complicating pregnancy) (delivered) (undelivered) 630
- invasive (M9100/1) 236.1
- malignant (M9100/1) 236.1
- previous, affecting management of pregnancy V23.1

Hydatidosis - *see* Echinococcus

Hyde's disease (prurigo nodularis) 698.3

Hydradenitis 705.83

Hydradenoma (M8400/0) - *see* Hidradenoma

Hydralazine lupus or syndrome
- correct substance properly administered 695.4
- overdose or wrong substance given or taken 972.6

Hydramnios 657 5th
- affecting fetus or newborn 761.3

Hydrancephaly 742.3
- with spina bifida (*see also* Spina bifida) 741.0 5th

Hydranencephaly 742.3
- with spina bifida (*see also* Spina bifida) 741.0 5th

Hydrargyrism NEC 985.0

Hydrarthrosis (*see also* Effusion, joint) 719.0
- gonococcal 098.50
- intermittent (*see also* Rheumatism, palindromic) 719.3 5th
- of yaws (early) (late) 102.6
- syphilitic 095.8
  - congenital 090.5

Hydremia 285.9

Hydrencephalocele (congenital) 742.0

Hydrencephalomeningocele (congenital) 742.0

Hydroa 694.0
- aestivale 692.72
- gestationis 646.8 5th
- herpetiformis 694.0
- pruriginosa 694.0
- vacciniforme 692.72

Hydroadenitis 705.83

Hydrocalycosis (*see also* Hydronephrosis) 591
- congenital 753.29

Hydrocalyx (*see also* Hydronephrosis) 591

Hydrocele (calcified) (chylous) (idiopathic) (infantile) (inguinal canal) (recurrent) (senile) (spermatic cord) (testis) (tunica vaginalis) 603.9
- canal of Nuck (female) 629.1
  - male 603.9
- congenital 778.6
- encysted 603.0
  - congenital 778.6
- female NEC 629.89
- infected 603.1
- round ligament 629.89
- specified type NEC 603.8
  - congenital 778.6
- spinalis (*see also* Spina bifida) 741.9 5th
- vulva 624.8

Hydrocephalic fetus
- affecting management or pregnancy 655.0 5th
- causing disproportion 653.6 5th
  - with obstructed labor 660.1 5th
    - affecting fetus or newborn 763.1

Hydrocephalus (acquired) (external) (internal) (malignant) (noncommunicating) (obstructive) (recurrent) 331.4
- aqueduct of Sylvius stricture 742.3
  - with spina bifida (*see also* Spina bifida) 741.0 5th
- chronic 742.3
  - with spina bifida (*see also* Spina bifida) 741.0 5th
- communicating 331.3
- congenital (external) (internal) 742.3
  - with spina bifida (*see also* Spina bifida) 741.0 5th
- due to
  - stricture of aqueduct of Sylvius 742.3
    - with spina bifida (*see also* Spina bifida) 741.0 5th
  - toxoplasmosis (congenital) 771.2
- fetal affecting management of pregnancy 655.0 5th
- foramen Magendie block (acquired) 331.3
  - congenital 742.3
    - with spina bifida (*see also* Spina bifida) 741.0 5th
- newborn 742.3
  - with spina bifida (*see also* Spina bifida) 741.0 5th
- normal pressure 331.5
  - idiopathic (INPH) 331.5
  - secondary 331.3
- otitic 348.2
- syphilitic, congenital 090.49
- tuberculous (*see also* Tuberculosis) 013.8 5th

Hydrocolpos (congenital) 623.8

Hydrocystoma (M8404/0) - *see* Neoplasm, skin, benign

Hydroencephalocele (congenital) 742.0

Hydroencephalomeningocele (congenital) 742.0

Hydrohematopneumothorax (*see also* Hemothorax) 511.89

Hydromeningitis - *see* Meningitis

Hydromeningocele (spinal) (*see also* Spina bifida) 741.9 5th
- cranial 742.0

Hydrometra 621.8

Hydrometrocolpos 623.8

Hydromicrocephaly 742.1

Hydromphalus (congenital) (since birth) 757.39

Hydromyelia 742.53

Hydromyelocele (*see also* Spina bifida) 741.9 5th

Hydronephrosis 591
- atrophic 591
- congenital 753.29
- due to S. hematobium 120.0
- early 591
- functionless (infected) 591
- infected 591
- intermittent 591
- primary 591
- secondary 591
- tuberculous (*see also* Tuberculosis) 016.0 5th

Hydropericarditis (*see also* Pericarditis) 423.9

Hydropericardium (*see also* Pericarditis) 423.9

Hydroperitoneum 789.59

Hydrophobia 071

Hydrophthalmos (*see also* Buphthalmia) 743.20

Hydropneumohemothorax (*see also* Hemothorax) 511.89

Hydropneumopericarditis (*see also* Pericarditis) 423.9

Hydropneumopericardium (*see also* Pericarditis) 423.9

Hydropneumothorax 511.89
- nontuberculous 511.89
  - bacterial 511.1
- pneumococcal 511.1
- staphylococcal 511.1
- streptococcal 511.1
- traumatic 860.0
  - with open wound into thorax 860.1
- tuberculous (*see also* Tuberculosis, pleura) 012.0 5th

Hydrops 782.3
- abdominis 789.59
- amnii (complicating pregnancy) (*see also* Hydramnios) 657 5th
- articulorum intermittens (*see also* Rheumatism, palindromic) 719.3 5th
- cardiac (*see also* Failure, heart) 428.0
- congenital - *see* Hydrops, fetalis
- endolymphatic (*see also* Disease, Ménière's) 386.00
- fetal(is) or newborn 778.0
  - due to isoimmunization 773.3
  - not due to isoimmunization 778.0
- gallbladder 575.3
- idiopathic (fetus or newborn) 778.0
- joint (*see also* Effusion, joint) 719.0 5th
- labyrinth (*see also* Disease, Ménière's) 386.00
- meningeal NEC 331.4
- nutritional 262
- pericardium - *see* Pericarditis
- pleura (*see also* Hydrothorax) 511.89
- renal (*see also* Nephrosis) 581.9
- spermatic cord (*see also* Hydrocele) 603.9

Hydropyonephrosis (*see also* Pyelitis) 590.80
- chronic 590.00

Hydrorachis 742.53

Hydrorrhea (nasal) 478.19
- gravidarum 658.1 5th
- pregnancy 658.1 5th

Hydrosadenitis 705.83

Hydrosalpinx (fallopian tube) (follicularis) 614.1

Hydrothorax (double) (pleural) 511.89
- chylous (nonfilarial) 457.8
  - filaria (*see also* Infestation, filarial) 125.9
- nontuberculous 511.89
  - bacterial 511.1
- pneumococcal 511.1
- staphylococcal 511.1
- streptococcal 511.1
- traumatic 862.29
  - with open wound into thorax 862.39
- tuberculous (*see also* Tuberculosis, pleura) 012.0 5th

Hydroureter 593.5
- congenital 753.22

Hydroureteronephrosis (*see also* Hydronephrosis) 591

Hydrourethra 599.84

Hydroxykynureninuria 270.2

Hydroxyprolinemia 270.8

Hydroxyprolinuria 270.8

Hygroma (congenital) (cystic) (M9173/0) 228.1
- prepatellar 727.3
- subdural - *see* Hematoma, subdural

Hymen - *see* condition

Hymenolepiasis (diminuta) (infection) (infestation) (nana) 123.6

Hymenolepsis (diminuta) (infection) (infestation) (nana) 123.6

Hypalgesia (*see also* Disturbance, sensation) 782.0

Hyperabduction syndrome 447.8

Hyperacidity, gastric 536.8
- psychogenic 306.4

Hyperactive, hyperactivity 314.01
- basal cell, uterine cervix 622.10
- bladder 596.51
- bowel (syndrome) 564.9
  - sounds 787.5
- cervix epithelial (basal) 622.10
- child 314.01
- colon 564.9
- gastrointestinal 536.8
  - psychogenic 306.4
- intestine 564.9
- labyrinth (unilateral) 386.51
  - with loss of labyrinthine reactivity 386.58
  - bilateral 386.52
- nasal mucous membrane 478.19
- stomach 536.8
- thyroid (gland) (*see also* Thyrotoxicosis) 242.9 5th

Hyperacusis 388.42

Hyperadrenalism (cortical) 255.3
- medullary 255.6

Hyperadrenocorticism 255.3
- congenital 255.2
- iatrogenic
  - correct substance properly administered 255.3
  - overdose or wrong substance given or taken 962.0

Hyperaffectivity 301.11

Hyperaldosteronism (atypical) (hyperplastic) (normoaldosteronal) (normotensive) (primary) 255.10
- secondary 255.14

Hyperalgesia (*see also* Disturbance, sensation) 782.0

Hyperalimentation 783.6
- carotene 278.3
- specified NEC 278.8
- vitamin A 278.2
- vitamin D 278.4

Hyperaminoaciduria 270.9
- arginine 270.6
- citrulline 270.6
- cystine 270.0
- glycine 270.0
- lysine 270.7
- ornithine 270.6
- renal (types I, II, III) 270.0

Hyperammonemia (congenital) 270.6

Hyperamnesia 780.99

Hyperamylasemia 790.5

Hyperaphia 782.0

Hyperazotemia 791.9

Hyperbetalipoproteinemia (acquired) (essential) (familial) (hereditary) (primary) (secondary) 272.0
- with prebetalipoproteinemia 272.2

Hyperbilirubinemia 782.4
- congenital 277.4
- constitutional 277.4
- neonatal (transient) (*see also* Jaundice, fetus or newborn) 774.6
  - of prematurity 774.2

Hyperbilirubinemica encephalopathia, newborn 774.7
- due to isoimmunization 773.4

Hypercalcemia, hypercalcemic (idiopathic) 275.42
- nephropathy 588.89

Hypercalcinuria 275.40

Hypercapnia 786.09
- with mixed acid-based disorder 276.4
- fetal, affecting newborn 770.89

Hypercarotinemia 278.3

Hypercementosis 521.5

Hyperchloremia 276.9

Hyperchlorhydria 536.8
- neurotic 306.4
- psychogenic 306.4

Hypercholesterinemia - *see* Hypercholesterolemia

Hypercholesterolemia 272.0
- with hyperglyceridemia, endogenous 272.2
- essential 272.0
- familial 272.0
- hereditary 272.0
- primary 272.0
- pure 272.0

Hypercholesterolosis 272.0

Hyperchylia gastrica 536.8
- psychogenic 306.4

Hyperchylomicronemia (familial) (with hyperbetalipoproteinemia) 272.3

Hypercoagulation syndrome (primary) 289.81
- secondary 289.82

Hypercorticosteronism
- correct substance properly administered 255.3
- overdose or wrong substance given or taken 962.0

Hypercortisonism
- correct substance properly administered 255.3
- overdose or wrong substance given or taken 962.0

Hyperdynamic beta-adrenergic state or syndrome (circulatory) 429.82

Hyperekplexia 759.89

Hyperelectrolytemia 276.9

Hyperemesis 536.2
- arising during pregnancy - *see* Hyperemesis, gravidarum
- gravidarum (mild) (before 22 completed weeks gestation) 643.0 5th
  - with
    - carbohydrate depletion 643.1 5th
    - dehydration 643.1 5th

- **Hyperemesis** – *continued*
  - gravidarum – *continued*
    - with – *continued*
      - electrolyte imbalance 643.1 [5th]
      - metabolic disturbance 643.1 [5th]
    - affecting fetus or newborn 761.8
    - severe (with metabolic disturbance) 643.1 [5th]
  - psychogenic 306.4
- **Hyperemia** (acute) 780.99
  - anal mucosa 569.49
  - bladder 596.7
  - cerebral 437.8
  - conjunctiva 372.71
  - ear, internal, acute 386.30
  - enteric 564.89
  - eye 372.71
  - eyelid (active) (passive) 374.82
  - intestine 564.89
  - iris 364.41
  - kidney 593.81
  - labyrinth 386.30
  - liver (active) (passive) 573.8
  - lung 514
  - ovary 620.8
  - passive 780.99
  - pulmonary 514
  - renal 593.81
  - retina 362.89
  - spleen 289.59
  - stomach 537.89
- **Hyperesthesia** (body surface) (*see also* Disturbance, sensation) 782.0
  - larynx (reflex) 478.79
    - hysterical 300.11
  - pharynx (reflex) 478.29
- **Hyperestrinism** 256.0
- **Hyperestrogenism** 256.0
- **Hyperestrogenosis** 256.0
- **Hyperexplexia** 759.89
- **Hyperextension, joint** 718.80
  - ankle 718.87
  - elbow 718.82
  - foot 718.87
  - hand 718.84
  - hip 718.85
  - knee 718.86
  - multiple sites 718.89
  - pelvic region 718.85
  - shoulder (region) 718.81
  - specified site NEC 718.88
  - wrist 718.83
- **Hyperfibrinolysis** - *see* Fibrinolysis
- **Hyperfolliculinism** 256.0
- **Hyperfructosemia** 271.2
- **Hyperfunction**
  - adrenal (cortex) 255.3
    - androgenic, acquired benign 255.3
    - medulla 255.6
    - virilism 255.2
  - corticoadrenal NEC 255.3
  - labyrinth - *see* Hyperactive, labyrinth
  - medulloadrenal 255.6
  - ovary 256.1
    - estrogen 256.0
  - pancreas 577.8
  - parathyroid (gland) 252.00
  - pituitary (anterior) (gland) (lobe) 253.1
  - testicular 257.0
- **Hypergammaglobulinemia** 289.89
  - monoclonal, benign (BMH) 273.1
  - polyclonal 273.0
  - Waldenström's 273.0
- **Hyperglobulinemia** 273.8
- **Hyperglycemia** 790.29
  - maternal
    - affecting fetus or newborn 775.0
    - manifest diabetes in infant 775.1
  - postpancreatectomy (complete) (partial) 251.3
- **Hyperglyceridemia** 272.1
  - endogenous 272.1
  - essential 272.1
  - familial 272.1
- **Hyperglyceridemia** – *continued*
  - hereditary 272.1
  - mixed 272.3
  - pure 272.1
- **Hyperglycinemia** 270.7
- **Hypergonadism**
  - ovarian 256.1
  - testicular (infantile) (primary) 257.0
- **Hyperheparinemia** (*see also* Circulating anticoagulants) 286.5
- **Hyperhidrosis, hyperidrosis** 705.21
  - axilla 705.21
  - face 705.21
  - focal (localized) 705.21
    - primary 705.21
      - axilla 705.21
      - face 705.21
      - palms 705.21
      - soles 705.21
    - secondary 705.22
      - axilla 705.22
      - face 705.22
      - palms 705.22
      - soles 705.22
  - generalized 780.8
  - palms 705.21
  - psychogenic 306.3
  - secondary 780.8
  - soles 705.21
- **Hyperhistidinemia** 270.5
- **Hyperinsulinism** (ectopic) (functional) (organic) NEC 251.1
  - iatrogenic 251.0
  - reactive 251.2
  - spontaneous 251.2
  - therapeutic misadventure (from administration of insulin) 962.3
- **Hyperiodemia** 276.9
- **Hyperirritability** (cerebral), **in newborn** 779.1
- **Hyperkalemia** 276.7
- **Hyperkeratosis** (*see also* Keratosis) 701.1
  - cervix 622.2
  - congenital 757.39
  - cornea 371.89
  - due to yaws (early) (late) (palmar or plantar) 102.3
  - eccentrica 757.39
  - figurata centrifuga atrophica 757.39
  - follicularis 757.39
    - in cutem penetrans 701.1
  - limbic (cornea) 371.89
  - palmoplantaris climacterica 701.1
  - pinta (carate) 103.1
  - senile (with pruritus) 702.0
  - tongue 528.79
  - universalis congenita 757.1
  - vagina 623.1
  - vocal cord 478.5
  - vulva 624.09
- **Hyperkinesia, hyperkinetic** (disease) (reaction) (syndrome) 314.9
  - with
    - attention deficit - *see* Disorder, attention deficit
    - conduct disorder 314.2
    - developmental delay 314.1
    - simple disturbance of activity and attention 314.01
    - specified manifestation NEC 314.8
  - heart (disease) 429.82
  - of childhood or adolescence NEC 314.9
- **Hyperlacrimation** (*see also* Epiphora) 375.20
- **Hyperlipemia** (*see also* Hyperlipidemia) 272.4
- **Hyperlipidemia** 272.4
  - carbohydrate-induced 272.1
  - combined 272.2 ▲
  - endogenous 272.1
  - exogenous 272.3
  - fat-induced 272.3
  - group
    - A 272.0
    - B 272.1
- **Hyperlipidemia** – *continued*
  - group – *continued*
    - C 272.2
    - D 272.3
  - mixed 272.2
  - specified type NEC 272.4
- **Hyperlipidosis** 272.7
  - hereditary 272.7
- **Hyperlipoproteinemia** (acquired) (essential) (familial) (hereditary) (primary) (secondary) 272.4
  - Fredrickson type
    - I 272.3
    - IIA 272.0
    - IIB 272.2
    - III 272.2
    - IV 272.1
    - V 272.3
  - low-density-lipoid-type (LDL) 272.0
  - very-low-density-lipoid-type [VLDL] 272.1
- **Hyperlucent lung, unilateral** 492.8
- **Hyperluteinization** 256.1
- **Hyperlysinemia** 270.7
- **Hypermagnesemia** 275.2
  - neonatal 775.5
- **Hypermaturity** (fetus or newborn)
  - post-term infant 766.21
  - prolonged gestation infant 766.22
- **Hypermenorrhea** 626.2
- **Hypermetabolism** 794.7
- **Hypermethioninemia** 270.4
- **Hypermetropia** (congenital) 367.0
- **Hypermobility**
  - cecum 564.9
  - coccyx 724.71
  - colon 564.9
    - psychogenic 306.4
  - ileum 564.89
  - joint (acquired) 718.80
    - ankle 718.87
    - elbow 718.82
    - foot 718.87
    - hand 718.84
    - hip 718.85
    - knee 718.86
    - multiple sites 718.89
    - pelvic region 718.85
    - shoulder (region) 718.81
    - specified site NEC 718.88
    - wrist 718.83
  - kidney, congenital 753.3
  - meniscus (knee) 717.5
  - scapula 718.81
  - stomach 536.8
    - psychogenic 306.4
  - syndrome 728.5
  - testis, congenital 752.52
  - urethral 599.81
- **Hypermotility**
  - gastrointestinal 536.8
  - intestine 564.9
    - psychogenic 306.4
  - stomach 536.8
- **Hypernasality** 784.43 ▲
- **Hypernatremia** 276.0
  - with water depletion 276.0
- **Hypernephroma** (M8312/3) 189.0
- **Hyperopia** 367.0
- **Hyperorexia** 783.6
- **Hyperornithinemia** 270.6
- **Hyperosmia** (*see also* Disturbance, sensation) 781.1
- **Hyperosmolality** 276.0
- **Hyperosteogenesis** 733.99
- **Hyperostosis** 733.99
  - calvarial 733.3
  - cortical 733.3
    - infantile 756.59
  - frontal, internal of skull 733.3
  - interna frontalis 733.3
  - monomelic 733.99
  - skull 733.3
    - congenital 756.0
- **Hyperostosis** – *continued*
  - vertebral 721.8
    - with spondylosis - *see* Spondylosis ankylosing 721.6
- **Hyperovarianism** 256.1
- **Hyperovarism, hyperovaria** 256.1
- **Hyperoxaluria** (primary) 271.8
- **Hyperoxia** 987.8
- **Hyperparathyroidism** 252.00
  - ectopic 259.3
  - other 252.08
  - primary 252.01
  - secondary(of renal origin) 588.81
    - non-renal 252.02
  - tertiary 252.08
- **Hyperpathia** (*see also* Disturbance, sensation) 782.0
  - psychogenic 307.80
- **Hyperperistalsis** 787.4
  - psychogenic 306.4
- **Hyperpermeability, capillary** 448.9
- **Hyperphagia** 783.6
- **Hyperphenylalaninemia** 270.1
- **Hyperphoria** 378.40
  - alternating 378.45
- **Hyperphosphatemia** 275.3
- **Hyperpiesia** (*see also* Hypertension) 401.9
- **Hyperpiesis** (*see also* Hypertension) 401.9
- **Hyperpigmentation** - *see* Pigmentation
- **Hyperpinealism** 259.8
- **Hyperpipecolatemia** 270.7
- **Hyperpituitarism** 253.1
- **Hyperplasia, hyperplastic**
  - adenoids (lymphoid tissue) 474.12
    - and tonsils 474.10
  - adrenal (capsule) (cortex) (gland) 255.8
    - with
      - sexual precocity (male) 255.2
      - virilism, adrenal 255.2
      - virilization (female) 255.2
    - congenital 255.2
    - due to excess ACTH (ectopic) (pituitary) 255.0
    - medulla 255.8
  - alpha cells (pancreatic)
    - with
      - gastrin excess 251.5
      - glucagon excess 251.4
  - appendix (lymphoid) 543.0
  - artery, fibromuscular NEC 447.8
    - carotid 447.8
    - renal 447.3
  - bone 733.99
    - marrow 289.9
  - breast (*see also* Hypertrophy, breast) 611.1
    - ductal 610.8 ●
      - atypical 610.8 ●
  - carotid artery 447.8
  - cementation, cementum (teeth) (tooth) 521.5
  - cervical gland 785.6
  - cervix (uteri) 622.10
    - basal cell 622.10
    - congenital 752.49
    - endometrium 622.10
    - polypoid 622.10
  - chin 524.05
  - clitoris, congenital 752.49
  - dentin 521.5
  - endocervicitis 616.0
  - endometrium, endometrial (adenomatous) (atypical) (cystic) (glandular) (polypoid) (uterus) 621.30
    - with atypia 621.33
    - without atypia
      - complex 621.32
      - simple 621.31
    - benign 621.34 ●
    - cervix 622.10
  - epithelial 709.8
    - focal, oral, including tongue 528.79
    - mouth (focal) 528.79
    - nipple 611.89

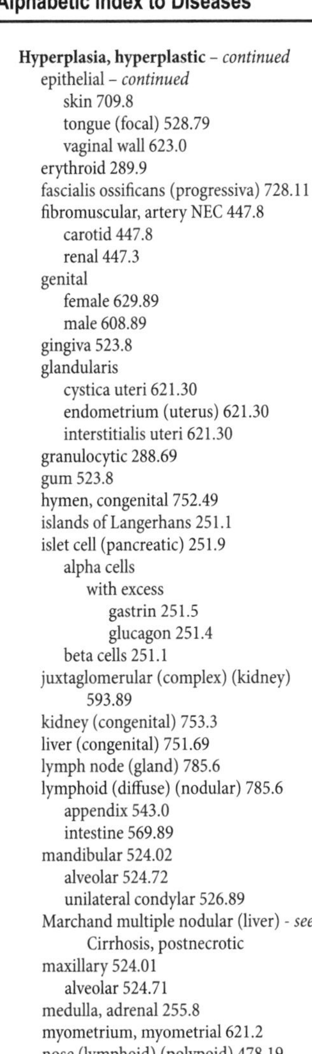

- **Hyperplasia, hyperplastic** – *continued*
  - epithelial – *continued*
    - skin 709.8
    - tongue (focal) 528.79
    - vaginal wall 623.0
  - erythroid 289.9
  - fascialis ossificans (progressiva) 728.11
  - fibromuscular, artery NEC 447.8
    - carotid 447.8
    - renal 447.3
  - genital
    - female 629.89
    - male 608.89
  - gingiva 523.8
  - glandularis
    - cystica uteri 621.30
    - endometrium (uterus) 621.30
    - interstitialis uteri 621.30
  - granulocytic 288.69
  - gum 523.8
  - hymen, congenital 752.49
  - islands of Langerhans 251.1
  - islet cell (pancreatic) 251.9
    - alpha cells
      - with excess
        - gastrin 251.5
        - glucagon 251.4
    - beta cells 251.1
  - juxtaglomerular (complex) (kidney) 593.89
  - kidney (congenital) 753.3
  - liver (congenital) 751.69
  - lymph node (gland) 785.6
  - lymphoid (diffuse) (nodular) 785.6
    - appendix 543.0
    - intestine 569.89
  - mandibular 524.02
    - alveolar 524.72
    - unilateral condylar 526.89
  - Marchand multiple nodular (liver) - *see* Cirrhosis, postnecrotic
  - maxillary 524.01
    - alveolar 524.71
  - medulla, adrenal 255.8
  - myometrium, myometrial 621.2
  - nose (lymphoid) (polypoid) 478.19
  - oral soft tissue (inflammatory) (irritative) (mucosa) NEC 528.9
    - gingiva 523.8
    - tongue 529.8

- **Hyperplasia, hyperplastic** – *continued*
  - organ or site, congenital NEC - *see* Anomaly, specified type NEC
  - ovary 620.8
  - palate, papillary 528.9
  - pancreatic islet cells 251.9
    - alpha
      - with excess
        - gastrin 251.5
        - glucagon 251.4
    - beta 251.1
  - parathyroid (gland) 252.01
  - persistent, vitreous (primary) 743.51
  - pharynx (lymphoid) 478.29
  - prostate 600.90
    - with
      - other lower urinary tract symptoms (LUTS) 600.91
      - urinary
        - obstruction 600.91
        - retention 600.91
    - adenofibromatous 600.20
      - with
        - other lower urinary tract symptoms (LUTS) 600.21
        - urinary
          - obstruction 600.21
          - retention 600.21
    - nodular 600.10
      - with
        - urinary
          - obstruction 600.11
          - retention 600.11
  - renal artery (fibromuscular) 447.3
  - reticuloendothelial (cell) 289.9
  - salivary gland (any) 527.1
  - Schimmelbusch's 610.1
  - suprarenal (capsule) (gland) 255.8
  - thymus (gland) (persistent) 254.0
  - thyroid (*see also* Goiter) 240.9
    - primary 242.0 [5th]
    - secondary 242.2 [5th]
  - tonsil (lymphoid tissue) 474.11
    - and adenoids 474.10
  - urethrovaginal 599.89
  - uterus, uterine (myometrium) 621.2
    - endometrium (*see also* Hyperplasia, endometrium) 621.30
  - vitreous (humor), primary persistent 743.51
  - vulva 624.3
  - zygoma 738.11

- **Hyperpnea** 786.01
- **Hyperpotassemia** 276.7
- **Hyperprebetalipoproteinemia** 272.1
  - with chylomicronemia 272.3
  - familial 272.1
- **Hyperprolactinemia** 253.1
- **Hyperprolinemia** 270.8
- **Hyperproteinemia** 273.8
- **Hyperprothrombinemia** 289.89
- **Hyperpselaphesia** 782.0
- **Hyperpyrexia** 780.60
  - heat (effects of) 992.0
  - malarial (*see also* Malaria) 084.6
  - malignant, due to anesthetic 995.86
  - rheumatic - *see* Fever, rheumatic
  - unknown origin (*see also* Pyrexia) 780.60
- **Hyperreactor, vascular** 780.2
- **Hyperreflexia** 796.1
  - bladder, autonomic 596.54
    - with cauda equina 344.61
  - detrusor 344.61
- **Hypersalivation** (*see also* Ptyalism) 527.7
- **Hypersarcosinemia** 270.8
- **Hypersecretion**
  - ACTH 255.3
  - androgens (ovarian) 256.1
  - calcitonin 246.0
  - corticoadrenal 255.3
  - cortisol 255.0
  - estrogen 256.0
  - gastric 536.8
    - psychogenic 306.4
  - gastrin 251.5
  - glucagon 251.4
  - hormone
    - ACTH 255.3
    - anterior pituitary 253.1
    - growth NEC 253.0
    - ovarian androgen 256.1
    - testicular 257.0
    - thyroid stimulating 242.8 [5th]
  - insulin - *see* Hyperinsulinism
  - lacrimal glands (*see also* Epiphora) 375.20
  - medulloadrenal 255.6
  - milk 676.6 [5th]
  - ovarian androgens 256.1
  - pituitary (anterior) 253.1
  - salivary gland (any) 527.7
  - testicular hormones 257.0
  - thyrocalcitonin 246.0
  - upper respiratory 478.9

- **Hypersegmentation, hereditary** 288.2
  - eosinophils 288.2
  - neutrophil nuclei 288.2
- **Hypersensitive, hypersensitiveness, hypersensitivity** - *see also* Allergy
  - angiitis 446.20
    - specified NEC 446.29
  - carotid sinus 337.01
  - colon 564.9
    - psychogenic 306.4
  - DNA (deoxyribonucleic acid) NEC 287.2
  - drug (*see also* Allergy, drug) 995.27
  - esophagus 530.89
  - insect bites - *see* Injury, superficial, by site
  - labyrinth 386.58
  - pain (*see also* Disturbance, sensation) 782.0
  - pneumonitis NEC 495.9
  - reaction (*see also* Allergy) 995.3
    - upper respiratory tract NEC 478.8
  - stomach (allergic) (nonallergic) 536.8
    - psychogenic 306.4
- **Hypersomatotropism** (classic) 253.0
- **Hypersomnia, unspecified** 780.54
  - with sleep apnea, unspecified 780.53
  - alcohol induced 291.82
  - drug induced 292.85
  - due to
    - medical condition classified elsewhere 327.14
    - mental disorder 327.15
  - idiopathic
    - with long sleep time 327.11
    - without long sleep time 327.12
  - menstrual related 327.13
  - nonorganic origin 307.43
    - persistent (primary) 307.44
    - transient 307.43
  - organic 327.10
    - other 327.19
  - primary 307.44
  - recurrent 327.13
- **Hypersplenia** 289.4
- **Hypersplenism** 289.4
- **Hypersteatosis** 706.3
- **Hyperstimulation, ovarian** 256.1
- **Hypersuprarenalism** 255.3
- **Hypersusceptibility - see Allergy**
- **Hyper-TBG-nemia** 246.8
- **Hypertelorism** 756.0
  - orbit, orbital 376.41

Hypertension, hypertensive	Malignant	Benign	Unspecified
Hypertension, hypertensive (arterial) (arteriolar) (crisis) (degeneration) (disease) (essential) (fluctuating) (idiopathic) (intermittent) (labile) (low renin) (orthostatic) (paroxysmal) (primary) (systemic) (uncontrolled) (vascular)	401.0	401.1	401.9
with			
chronic kidney disease			
stage I through stage IV, or unspecified	403.00	403.10	403.90
stage V or end stage renal disease	403.01	403.11	403.91
heart involvement (conditions classifiable to 429.0-429.3, 429.8, 429.9 due to hypertension) (*see also* Hypertension, heart)	402.00	402.10	402.90
with kidney involvement - *see* Hypertension, cardiorenal			
renal (kidney) involvement (only conditions classifiable to 585~~, 586, 587~~) (excludes conditions classifiable to 584) (*see also* Hypertension, kidney) ▲	403.00	403.10	403.90
with heart involvement - *see* Hypertension, cardiorenal failure (and sclerosis) (*see also* Hypertension, kidney)	403.01	403.11	403.91
sclerosis without failure (*see also* Hypertension, kidney)	403.00	403.10	403.90
accelerated (*see also* Hypertension, by type, malignant)	401.0	–	–
antepartum - *see* Hypertension, complicating pregnancy, childbirth, or the puerperium			
cardiorenal (disease)	404.00	404.10	404.90
with			
chronic kidney disease			
stage I through stage IV, or unspecified	404.00	404.10	404.90
and heart failure	404.01	404.11	404.91
stage V or end stage renal disease	404.02	404.12	404.92
and heart failure	404.03	404.13	404.93
heart failure	404.01	404.11	404.91
and chronic kidney disease	404.01	404.11	404.91
stage I through stage IV or unspecified	404.01	404.11	404.91
stage V or end stage renal disease	404.03	404.13	404.93
cardiovascular disease (arteriosclerotic) (sclerotic)	402.00	402.10	402.90
with			
heart failure	402.01	402.11	402.91
renal involvement (conditions classifiable to 403) (*see also* Hypertension, cardiorenal)	404.00	404.10	404.90
cardiovascular renal (disease) (sclerosis) (*see also* Hypertension, cardiorenal)	404.00	404.10	404.9
cerebrovascular disease NEC	437.2	437.2	437.2
complicating pregnancy, childbirth, or the puerperium	642.2 5th	642.0 5th	642.9 5th
with			
albuminuria (and edema) (mild)	–	–	642.4 5th
severe	–	–	642.5 5th
chronic kidney disease	642.2 5th	642.2 5th	642.2 5th
and heart disease	642.2 5th	642.2 5th	642.2 5th
edema (mild)	–	–	642.4 5th
severe	–	–	642.5 5th
heart disease	642.2 5th	642.2 5th	642.2 5th
and chronic kidney disease	642.2 5th	642.2 5th	642.2 5th
renal disease	642.2 5th	642.2 5th	642.2 5th
and heart disease	642.2 5th	642.2 5th	642.2 5th
chronic	642.2 5th	642.0 5th	642.0 5th
with pre-eclampsia or eclampsia	642.7 5th	642.7 5th	642.7 5th
fetus or newborn	760.0	760.0	760.0
essential	–	642.0 5th	642.0 5th
with pre-eclampsia or eclampsia	–	642.7	642.7 5th
fetus or newborn	760.0	760.0	760.0
fetus or newborn	760.0	760.0	760.0
gestational	–	–	642.3 5th
pre-existing	642.2 5th	642.0 5th	642.0 5th
with pre-eclampsia or eclampsia	642.7 5th	642.7 5th	642.7 5th
fetus or newborn	760.0	760.0	760.0
secondary to renal disease	642.1 5th	642.1 5th	642.1 5th
with pre-eclampsia or eclampsia	642.7 5th	642.7 5th	642.7 5th
fetus or newborn	760.0	760.0	760.0
transient	–	–	642.3 5th
due to			
aldosteronism, primary	405.09	405.19	405.99
brain tumor	405.09	405.19	405.99
bulbar poliomyelitis	405.09	405.19	405.99
calculus			
kidney	405.09	405.19	405.99
ureter	405.09	405.19	405.99
coarctation, aorta	405.09	405.19	405.99

Hypertension, hypertensive	Malignant	Benign	Unspecified
due to – *continued*			
Cushing's disease	405.09	405.19	405.99
glomerulosclerosis (*see also* Hypertension, kidney)	403.00	403.10	403.90
periarteritis nodosa	405.09	405.19	405.99
pheochromocytoma	405.09	405.19	405.99
polycystic kidney(s)	405.09	405.19	405.99
polycythemia	405.09	405.19	405.99
porphyria	405.09	405.19	405.99
pyelonephritis	405.09	405.19	405.99
renal (artery)			
aneurysm	405.01	405.11	405.91
anomaly	405.01	405.11	405.91
embolism	405.01	405.11	405.91
fibromuscular hyperplasia	405.01	405.11	405.91
occlusion	405.01	405.11	405.91
stenosis	405.01	405.11	405.91
thrombosis	405.01	405.11	405.91
encephalopathy	437.2	437.2	437.2
gestational (transient) NEC	–	–	642.3 5th
Goldblatt's	440.1	440.1	440.1
heart (disease) (conditions classifiable to 429.0-429.3, 429.8, 429.9 due to hypertension)	402.00	402.10	402.90
with			
heart failure	402.01	402.11	402.91
hypertensive kidney disease (conditions classifiable to 403) (*see also* Hypertension, cardiorenal)	404.00	404.10	404.90
renal sclerosis (*see also* Hypertension, cardiorenal)	404.00	404.10	404.90
intracranial, benign	–	348.2	–
intraocular	–	–	365.04
kidney	403.00	403.10	403.90
with			
chronic kidney disease			
stage I through stage IV, or unspecified	403.00	403.10	403.90
stage V or end stage renal disease	403.01	403.11	403.91
heart involvement (conditions classifiable to 429.0-429.3, 429.8, 429.9 due to hypertension) (*see also* Hypertension, cardiorenal)	404.00	404.10	404.90
hypertensive heart (disease) (conditions classifiable to 402) (*see also* Hypertension, cardiorenal)	404.00	404.10	404.90
lesser circulation	–	–	416.0
necrotizing	401.0	–	–
ocular	–	–	365.04
pancreatic duct - code to underlying condition			
with			
chronic pancreatitis	–	–	577.1
portal (due to chronic liver disease)	–	–	572.3
postoperative			997.91
psychogenic	–	–	306.2
puerperal, postpartum *see* Hypertension, complicating pregnancy, childbirth, or the puerperium			
pulmonary (artery)	–	–	416.8
with cor pulmonale (chronic)	–	–	416.8
acute	–	–	415.0
idiopathic	–	–	416.0
primary	–	–	416.0
of newborn	–	–	747.83
secondary	–	–	416.8
renal (disease) (*see also* Hypertension, kidney)	403.00	403.10	403.90
renovascular NEC	405.01	405.11	405.91
secondary NEC	405.09	405.19	405.99
due to			
aldosteronism, primary	405.09	405.19	405.99
brain tumor	405.09	405.19	405.99
bulbar poliomyelitis	405.09	405.19	405.99
calculus			
kidney	405.09	405.19	405.99
ureter	405.09	405.19	405.99
coarctation, aorta	405.09	405.19	405.99
Cushing's disease	405.09	405.19	405.99
glomerulosclerosis (*see also* Hypertension, kidney)	403.00	403.10	403.90
periarteritis nodosa	405.09	405.19	405.99
pheochromocytoma	405.09	405.19	405.99
polycystic kidney(s)	405.09	405.19	405.99
polycythemia	405.09	405.19	405.99
porphyria	405.09	405.19	405.99
pyelonephritis	405.09	405.19	405.99
renal (artery)			
aneurysm	405.01	405.11	405.91

Hypertension, hypertensive	Malignant	Benign	Unspecified
secondary – *continued*			
due to – *continued*			
renal (artery) – *continued*			
anomaly	405.01	405.11	405.91
embolism	405.01	405.11	405.91
fibromuscular hyperplasia	405.01	405.11	405.91
occlusion	405.01	405.11	405.91
stenosis	405.01	405.11	405.91
thrombosis	405.01	405.11	405.91
transient	–	–	796.2
of pregnancy	–	–	642.3 5th

Hypertension, hypertensive	Malignant	Benign	Unspecified
venous, chronic (asymptomatic) (idiopathic)	–	–	459.30
with			
complication, NEC	–	–	459.39
inflammation	–	–	459.32
with ulcer	–	–	459.33
ulcer	–	–	459.31
with inflammation	–	–	459.33
due to			
deep vein thrombosis (*see also* Syndrome, postphlebitic)	–	–	459.10

Hyperthecosis, ovary 256.8
Hyperthermia (of unknown origin) (*see also* Pyrexia) 780.60
- malignant (due to anesthesia) 995.86
- newborn 778.4

Hyperthymergasia (*see also* Psychosis, affective) 296.0 5th
- reactive (from emotional stress, psychological trauma) 298.1
- recurrent episode 296.1 5th
- single episode 296.0 5th

Hyperthymism 254.8
Hyperthyroid (recurrent) - *see* Hyperthyroidism
Hyperthyroidism (latent) (preadult) (recurrent) (without goiter) 242.9 5th

Note *Use the following fifth-digit subclassification with category 242:*

0 without mention of thyrotoxic crisis or storm

1 with mention of thyrotoxic crisis or storm

- with
  - goiter (diffuse) 242.0 5th
    - adenomatous 242.3 5th
      - multinodular 242.2 5th
      - uninodular 242.1 5th
    - nodular 242.3 5th
      - multinodular 242.2 5th
      - uninodular 242.1 5th
  - thyroid nodule 242.1 5th
- complicating pregnancy, childbirth, or puerperium 648.1 5th
- neonatal (transient) 775.3

Hypertonia - *see* Hypertonicity
Hypertonicity
- bladder 596.51
- fetus or newborn 779.89
- gastrointestinal (tract) 536.8
- infancy 779.89
  - due to electrolyte imbalance 779.89
- muscle 728.85
- stomach 536.8
  - psychogenic 306.4
- uterus, uterine (contractions) 661.4 5th
  - affecting fetus or newborn 763.7

Hypertony - *see* Hypertonicity
Hypertransaminemia 790.4
Hypertrichosis 704.1
- congenital 757.4
- eyelid 374.54
- lanuginosa 757.4
  - acquired 704.1

Hypertriglyceridemia, essential 272.1
Hypertrophy, hypertrophic
- adenoids (infectional) 474.12
  - and tonsils (faucial) (infective) (lingual) (lymphoid) 474.10
- adrenal 255.8
- alveolar process or ridge 525.8
- anal papillae 569.49
- apocrine gland 705.82
- artery NEC 447.8
  - carotid 447.8
  - congenital (peripheral) NEC 747.60
    - gastrointestinal 747.61
    - lower limb 747.64
    - renal 747.62
    - specified NEC 747.69
    - spinal 747.82
    - upper limb 747.63
  - renal 447.3
- arthritis (chronic) (*see also* Osteoarthrosis) 715.9 5th
  - spine (*see also* Spondylosis) 721.90
- arytenoid 478.79
- asymmetrical (heart) 429.9
- auricular - *see* Hypertrophy, cardiac
- Bartholin's gland 624.8
- bile duct 576.8
- bladder (sphincter) (trigone) 596.8
- blind spot, visual field 368.42
- bone 733.99

Hypertrophy, hypertrophic – *continued*
- brain 348.89 ▲
- breast 611.1
  - cystic 610.1
  - fetus or newborn 778.7
  - fibrocystic 610.1
  - massive pubertal 611.1
  - puerperal, postpartum 676.3 5th
  - senile (parenchymatous) 611.1
- cardiac (chronic) (idiopathic) 429.3
  - with
    - rheumatic fever (conditions classifiable to 390)
      - active 391.8
        - with chorea 392.0
      - inactive or quiescent (with chorea) 398.99
  - congenital NEC 746.89
  - fatty (*see also* Degeneration, myocardial) 429.1
  - hypertensive (*see also* Hypertension, heart) 402.90
  - rheumatic (with chorea) 398.99
    - active or acute 391.8
      - with chorea 392.0
  - valve (*see also* Endocarditis) 424.90
    - congenital NEC 746.89
- cartilage 733.99
- cecum 569.89
- cervix (uteri) 622.6
  - congenital 752.49
  - elongation 622.6
- clitoris (cirrhotic) 624.2
  - congenital 752.49
- colon 569.89
  - congenital 751.3
- conjunctiva, lymphoid 372.73
- cornea 371.89
- corpora cavernosa 607.89
- duodenum 537.89
- endometrium (uterus) (*see also* Hyperplasia, endometrium) 621.30
  - cervix 622.6
- epididymis 608.89
- esophageal hiatus (congenital) 756.6
  - with hernia - *see* Hernia, diaphragm
- eyelid 374.30
- falx, skull 733.99
- fat pad 729.30
  - infrapatellar 729.31
  - knee 729.31
  - orbital 374.34
  - popliteal 729.31
  - prepatellar 729.31
  - retropatellar 729.31
  - specified site NEC 729.39
- foot (congenital) 755.67
- frenum, frenulum (tongue) 529.8
  - linguae 529.8
  - lip 528.5
- gallbladder or cystic duct 575.8
- gastric mucosa 535.2 5th
- gingiva 523.8
- gland, glandular (general) NEC 785.6
- gum (mucous membrane) 523.8
- heart (idiopathic) - *see also* Hypertrophy, cardiac
  - valve - *see also* Endocarditis
    - congenital NEC 746.89
- hemifacial 754.0
- hepatic - *see* Hypertrophy, liver
- hiatus (esophageal) 756.6
- hilus gland 785.6
- hymen, congenital 752.49
- ileum 569.89
- infrapatellar fat pad 729.31
- intestine 569.89
- jejunum 569.89
- kidney (compensatory) 593.1
  - congenital 753.3
- labial frenulum 528.5
- labium (majus) (minus) 624.3
- lacrimal gland, chronic 375.03

Hypertrophy, hypertrophic – *continued*
- ligament 728.9
  - spinal 724.8
- linguae frenulum 529.8
- lingual tonsil (infectional) 474.11
- lip (frenum) 528.5
  - congenital 744.81
- liver 789.1
  - acute 573.8
  - cirrhotic - *see* Cirrhosis, liver
  - congenital 751.69
  - fatty - *see* Fatty, liver
- lymph gland 785.6
  - tuberculous - *see* Tuberculosis, lymph gland
- mammary gland - *see* Hypertrophy, breast
- maxillary frenulum 528.5
- Meckel's diverticulum (congenital) 751.0
- medial meniscus, acquired 717.3
- median bar 600.90
  - with
    - other lower urinary tract symptoms (LUTS) 600.91
    - urinary
      - obstruction 600.91
      - retention 600.91
- mediastinum 519.3
- meibomian gland 373.2
- meniscus, knee, congenital 755.64
- metatarsal head 733.99
- metatarsus 733.99
- mouth 528.9
- mucous membrane
  - alveolar process 523.8
  - nose 478.19
  - turbinate (nasal) 478.0
- muscle 728.9
- muscular coat, artery NEC 447.8
  - carotid 447.8
  - renal 447.3
- myocardium (*see also* Hypertrophy, cardiac) 429.3
  - idiopathic 425.4
- myometrium 621.2
- nail 703.8
  - congenital 757.5
- nasal 478.19
  - alae 478.19
  - bone 738.0
  - cartilage 478.19
  - mucous membrane (septum) 478.19
  - sinus (*see also* Sinusitis) 473.9
  - turbinate 478.0
- nasopharynx, lymphoid (infectional) (tissue) (wall) 478.29
- neck, uterus 622.6
- nipple 611.1
- normal aperture diaphragm (congenital) 756.6
- nose (*see also* Hypertrophy, nasal) 478.19
- orbit 376.46
- organ or site, congenital NEC - *see* Anomaly, specified type NEC
- osteoarthropathy (pulmonary) 731.2
- ovary 620.8
- palate (hard) 526.89
  - soft 528.9
- pancreas (congenital) 751.7
- papillae
  - anal 569.49
  - tongue 529.3
- parathyroid (gland) 252.01
- parotid gland 527.1
- penis 607.89
- phallus 607.89
  - female (clitoris) 624.2
- pharyngeal tonsil 474.12
- pharyngitis 472.1
- pharynx 478.29
  - lymphoid (infectional) (tissue) (wall) 478.29
- pituitary (fossa) (gland) 253.8
- popliteal fat pad 729.31

Hypertrophy, hypertrophic – *continued*
- preauricular (lymph) gland (Hampstead) 785.6
- prepuce (congenital) 605
  - female 624.2
- prostate (asymptomatic) (early) (recurrent) 600.90
  - with
    - other lower urinary tract symptoms (LUTS) 600.91
    - urinary
      - obstruction 600.91
      - retention 600.91
  - adenofibromatous 600.20
    - with
      - other lower urinary tract symptoms (LUTS) 600.21
      - urinary
        - obstruction 600.21
        - retention 600.21
  - benign 600.00
    - with
      - other lower urinary tract symptoms (LUTS) 600.01
      - urinary
        - obstruction 600.01
        - retention 600.01
  - congenital 752.89
- pseudoedematous hypodermal 757.0
- pseudomuscular 359.1
- pylorus (muscle) (sphincter) 537.0
  - congenital 750.5
  - infantile 750.5
- rectal sphincter 569.49
- rectum 569.49
- renal 593.1
- rhinitis (turbinate) 472.0
- salivary duct or gland 527.1
  - congenital 750.26
- scaphoid (tarsal) 733.99
- scar 701.4
- scrotum 608.89
- sella turcica 253.8
- seminal vesicle 608.89
- sigmoid 569.89
- skin condition NEC 701.9
- spermatic cord 608.89
- spinal ligament 724.8
- spleen - *see* Splenomegaly
- spondylitis (spine) (*see also* Spondylosis) 721.90
- stomach 537.89
- subaortic stenosis (idiopathic) 425.1
- sublingual gland 527.1
  - congenital 750.26
- submaxillary gland 527.1
- suprarenal (gland) 255.8
- tendon 727.9
- testis 608.89
  - congenital 752.89
- thymic, thymus (congenital) (gland) 254.0
- thyroid (gland) (*see also* Goiter) 240.9
  - primary 242.0 5th
  - secondary 242.2 5th
- toe (congenital) 755.65
  - acquired 735.8
- tongue 529.8
  - congenital 750.15
  - frenum 529.8
  - papillae (foliate) 529.3
- tonsil (faucial) (infective) (lingual) (lymphoid) 474.11
  - with
    - adenoiditis 474.01
    - tonsillitis 474.00
      - and adenoiditis 474.02
  - and adenoids 474.10
- tunica vaginalis 608.89
- turbinate (mucous membrane) 478.0
- ureter 593.89
- urethra 599.84
- uterus 621.2
  - puerperal, postpartum 674.8 5th
- uvula 528.9

- **Hypertrophy, hypertrophic** – *continued*
  - vagina 623.8
  - vas deferens 608.89
  - vein 459.89
  - ventricle, ventricular (heart) (left) (right) - *see also* Hypertrophy, cardiac
    - congenital 746.89
    - due to hypertension (left) (right) (*see also* Hypertension, heart) 402.90
      - benign 402.10
      - malignant 402.00
    - right with ventricular septal defect, pulmonary stenosis or atresia, and dextraposition of aorta 745.2
  - verumontanum 599.89
  - vesical 596.8
  - vocal cord 478.5
  - vulva 624.3
    - stasis (nonfilarial) 624.3
- **Hypertropia** (intermittent) (periodic) 378.31
- **Hypertyrosinemia** 270.2
- **Hyperuricemia** 790.6
- **Hypervalinemia** 270.3
- **Hyperventilation** (tetany) 786.01
  - hysterical 300.11
  - psychogenic 306.1
  - syndrome 306.1
- **Hyperviscidosis** 277.00
- **Hyperviscosity** (of serum) (syndrome) NEC 273.3
  - polycythemic 289.0
  - sclerocythemic 282.8
- **Hypervitaminosis** (dietary) NEC 278.8
  - A (dietary) 278.2
  - D (dietary) 278.4
  - from excessive administration or use of vitamin preparations (chronic) 278.8
    - reaction to sudden overdose 963.5
    - vitamin A 278.2
      - reaction to sudden overdose 963.5
    - vitamin D 278.4
      - reaction to sudden overdose 963.5
    - vitamin K
      - correct substance properly administered 278.8
      - overdose or wrong substance given or taken 964.3
- **Hypervolemia** 276.6
- **Hypesthesia** (*see also* Disturbance, sensation) 782.0
  - cornea 371.81
- **Hyphema** (anterior chamber) (ciliary body) (iris) 364.41
  - traumatic 921.3
- **Hyphemia** - *see* Hyphema
- **Hypoacidity, gastric** 536.8
  - psychogenic 306.4
- **Hypoactive labyrinth** (function) - *see* Hypofunction, labyrinth
- **Hypoadrenalism** 255.41
  - tuberculous (*see also* Tuberculosis) 017.6 5th
- **Hypoadrenocorticism** 255.41
  - pituitary 253.4
- **Hypoalbuminemia** 273.8
- **Hypoaldosteronism** 255.42
- **Hypoalphalipoproteinemia** 272.5
- **Hypobarism** 993.2
- **Hypobaropathy** 993.2
- **Hypobetalipoproteinemia** (familial) 272.5
- **Hypocalcemia** 275.41
  - cow's milk 775.4
  - dietary 269.3
  - neonatal 775.4
  - phosphate-loading 775.4
- **Hypocalcification, teeth** 520.4
- **Hypochloremia** 276.9
- **Hypochlorhydria** 536.8
  - neurotic 306.4
  - psychogenic 306.4
- **Hypocholesteremia** 272.5
- **Hypochondria** (reaction) 300.7
- **Hypochondriac** 300.7
- **Hypochondriasis** 300.7
- **Hypochromasia blood cells** 280.9
- **Hypochromic anemia** 280.9
  - due to blood loss (chronic) 280.0
    - acute 285.1
  - microcytic 280.9
- **Hypocoagulability** (*see also* Defect, coagulation) 286.9
- **Hypocomplementemia** 279.8
- **Hypocythemia** (progressive) 284.9
- **Hypodontia** (*see also* Anodontia) 520.0
- **Hypoeosinophilia** 288.59
- **Hypoesthesia** (*see also* Disturbance, sensation) 782.0
  - cornea 371.81
  - tactile 782.0
- **Hypoestrinism** 256.39
- **Hypoestrogenism** 256.39
- **Hypoferremia** 280.9
  - due to blood loss (chronic) 280.0
- **Hypofertility**
  - female 628.9
  - male 606.1
- **Hypofibrinogenemia** 286.3
  - acquired 286.6
  - congenital 286.3
- **Hypofunction**
  - adrenal (gland) 255.41
    - cortex 255.41
    - medulla 255.5
    - specified NEC 255.5
  - cerebral 331.9
  - corticoadrenal NEC 255.41
  - intestinal 564.89
  - labyrinth (unilateral) 386.53
    - with loss of labyrinthine reactivity 386.55
    - bilateral 386.54
      - with loss of labyrinthine reactivity 386.56
  - Leydig cell 257.2
  - ovary 256.39
    - postablative 256.2
  - pituitary (anterior) (gland) (lobe) 253.2
    - posterior 253.5
  - testicular 257.2
    - iatrogenic 257.1
    - postablative 257.1
    - postirradiation 257.1
    - postsurgical 257.1
- **Hypogammaglobulinemia** 279.00
  - acquired primary 279.06
  - non-sex-linked, congenital 279.06
  - sporadic 279.06
  - transient of infancy 279.09
- **Hypogenitalism** (congenital) (female) (male) 752.89
  - penis 752.69
- **Hypoglycemia** (spontaneous) 251.2
  - coma 251.0
    - diabetic 250.3 5th
      - due to secondary diabetes 249.3 5th
  - diabetic 250.8 5th
    - due to secondary diabetes 249.8 5th
  - due to insulin 251.0
    - therapeutic misadventure 962.3
  - familial (idiopathic) 251.2
  - following gastrointestinal surgery 579.3
  - infantile (idiopathic) 251.2
  - in infant of diabetic mother 775.0
  - leucine-induced 270.3
  - neonatal 775.6
  - reactive 251.2
  - specified NEC 251.1
- **Hypoglycemic shock** 251.0
  - diabetic 250.8 5th
    - due to secondary diabetes 249.8 5th
  - due to insulin 251.0
  - functional (syndrome) 251.1
- **Hypogonadism**
  - female 256.39
  - gonadotrophic (isolated) 253.4
- **Hypogonadism** – *continued*
  - hypogonadotropic (isolated) (with anosmia) 253.4
  - isolated 253.4
  - male 257.2
    - hereditary familial (Reifenstein's syndrome) 259.52
  - ovarian (primary) 256.39
  - pituitary (secondary) 253.4
  - testicular (primary) (secondary) 257.2
- **Hypohidrosis** 705.0
- **Hypohidrotic ectodermal dysplasia** 757.31
- **Hypoidrosis** 705.0
- **Hypoinsulinemia, postsurgical** 251.3
  - postpancreatectomy (complete) (partial) 251.3
- **Hypokalemia** 276.8
- **Hypokinesia** 780.99
- **Hypoleukia splenica** 289.4
- **Hypoleukocytosis** 288.50
- **Hypolipidemia** 272.5
- **Hypolipoproteinemia** 272.5
- **Hypomagnesemia** 275.2
  - neonatal 775.4
- **Hypomania, hypomanic reaction** (*see also* Psychosis, affective) 296.0 5th
  - recurrent episode 296.1 5th
  - single episode 296.0 5th
- **Hypomastia** (congenital) 611.82
- **Hypomenorrhea** 626.1
- **Hypometabolism** 783.9
- **Hypomotility**
  - gastrointestinal tract 536.8
    - psychogenic 306.4
  - intestine 564.89
    - psychogenic 306.4
  - stomach 536.8
    - psychogenic 306.4
- **Hyponasality** 784.4<u>4</u> ▲
- **Hyponatremia** 276.1
- **Hypo-ovarianism** 256.39
- **Hypo-ovarism** 256.39
- **Hypoparathyroidism** (idiopathic) (surgically induced) 252.1
  - neonatal 775.4
- **Hypopharyngitis** 462
- **Hypophoria** 378.40
- **Hypophosphatasia** 275.3
- **Hypophosphatemia** (acquired) (congenital) (familial) 275.3
  - renal 275.3
- **Hypophyseal, hypophysis** - *see also* condition
  - dwarfism 253.3
  - gigantism 253.0
  - syndrome 253.8
- **Hypophyseothalamic syndrome** 253.8
- **Hypopiesis** - *see* Hypotension
- **Hypopigmentation** 709.00
  - eyelid 374.53
- **Hypopinealism** 259.8
- **Hypopituitarism** (juvenile) (syndrome) 253.2
  - due to
    - hormone therapy 253.7
    - hypophysectomy 253.7
    - radiotherapy 253.7
  - postablative 253.7
  - postpartum hemorrhage 253.2
- **Hypoplasia, hypoplasis** 759.89
  - adrenal (gland) 759.1
  - alimentary tract 751.8
    - lower 751.2
    - upper 750.8
  - anus, anal (canal) 751.2
  - aorta 747.22
  - aortic
    - arch (tubular) 747.10
    - orifice or valve with hypoplasia of ascending aorta and defective development of left ventricle (with mitral valve atresia) 746.7
  - appendix 751.2
  - areola 757.6
- **Hypoplasia, hypoplasis** – *continued*
  - arm (*see also* Absence, arm, congenital) 755.20
  - artery (congenital) (peripheral) 747.60
    - brain 747.81
    - cerebral 747.81
    - coronary 746.85
    - gastrointestinal 747.61
    - lower limb 747.64
    - pulmonary 747.3
    - renal 747.62
    - retinal 743.58
    - specified NEC 747.69
    - spinal 747.82
    - umbilical 747.5
    - upper limb 747.63
  - auditory canal 744.29
    - causing impairment of hearing 744.02
  - biliary duct (common) or passage 751.61
  - bladder 753.8
  - bone NEC 756.9
    - face 756.0
    - malar 756.0
    - mandible 524.04
      - alveolar 524.74
    - marrow 284.9
      - acquired (secondary) 284.89
      - congenital 284.09
      - idiopathic 284.9
    - maxilla 524.03
      - alveolar 524.73
    - skull (*see also* Hypoplasia, skull) 756.0
  - brain 742.1
    - gyri 742.2
    - specified part 742.2
  - breast (areola) 611.82
  - bronchus (tree) 748.3
  - cardiac 746.89
    - valve - *see* Hypoplasia, heart, valve
    - vein 746.89
  - carpus (*see also* Absence, carpal, congenital) 755.28
  - cartilaginous 756.9
  - cecum 751.2
  - cementum 520.4
    - hereditary 520.5
  - cephalic 742.1
  - cerebellum 742.2
  - cervix (uteri) 752.49
  - chin 524.06
  - clavicle 755.51
  - coccyx 756.19
  - colon 751.2
  - corpus callosum 742.2
  - cricoid cartilage 748.3
  - dermal, focal (Goltz) 757.39
  - digestive organ(s) or tract NEC 751.8
    - lower 751.2
    - upper 750.8
  - ear 744.29
    - auricle 744.23
    - lobe 744.29
    - middle, except ossicles 744.03
      - ossicles 744.04
    - ossicles 744.04
  - enamel of teeth (neonatal) (postnatal) (prenatal) 520.4
    - hereditary 520.5
  - endocrine (gland) NEC 759.2
  - endometrium 621.8
  - epididymis 752.89
  - epiglottis 748.3
  - erythroid, congenital 284.01
  - erythropoietic, chronic acquired 284.81
  - esophagus 750.3
  - Eustachian tube 744.24
  - eye (*see also* Microphthalmos) 743.10
    - lid 743.62
  - face 744.89
    - bone(s) 756.0
  - fallopian tube 752.19
  - femur (*see also* Absence, femur, congenital) 755.34

Hypoplasia, hypoplasis – *continued*
  fibula (*see also* Absence, fibula, congenital) 755.37
  finger (*see also* Absence, finger, congenital) 755.29
  focal dermal 757.39
  foot 755.31
  gallbladder 751.69
  genitalia, genital organ(s)
    female 752.89
      external 752.49
      internal NEC 752.89
    in adiposogenital dystrophy 253.8
    male 752.89
      penis 752.69
  glottis 748.3
  hair 757.4
  hand 755.21
  heart 746.89
    left (complex) (syndrome) 746.7
    valve NEC 746.89
      pulmonary 746.01
  humerus (*see also* Absence, humerus, congenital) 755.24
  hymen 752.49
  intestine (small) 751.1
    large 751.2
  iris 743.46
  jaw 524.09
  kidney(s) 753.0
  labium (majus) (minus) 752.49
  labyrinth, membranous 744.05
  lacrimal duct (apparatus) 743.65
  larynx 748.3
  leg (*see also* Absence, limb, congenital, lower) 755.30
  limb 755.4
    lower (*see also* Absence, limb, congenital, lower) 755.30
    upper (*see also* Absence, limb, congenital, upper) 755.20
  liver 751.69
  lung (lobe) 748.5
  mammary (areolar) 611.82
  mandibular 524.04
    alveolar 524.74
    unilateral condylar 526.89
  maxillary 524.03
    alveolar 524.73
  medullary 284.9
  megakaryocytic 287.30
  metacarpus (*see also* Absence, metacarpal, congenital) 755.28
  metatarsus (*see also* Absence, metatarsal, congenital) 755.38
  muscle 756.89
    eye 743.69
  myocardium (congenital) (Uhl's anomaly) 746.84
  nail(s) 757.5
  nasolacrimal duct 743.65
  nervous system NEC 742.8
  neural 742.8
  nose, nasal 748.1
  ophthalmic (*see also* Microphthalmos) 743.10
  optic nerve 377.43
  organ
    of Corti 744.05
    or site NEC - *see* Anomaly, by site
  osseous meatus (ear) 744.03
  ovary 752.0
  oviduct 752.19
  pancreas 751.7
  parathyroid (gland) 759.2
  parotid gland 750.26
  patella 755.64
  pelvis, pelvic girdle 755.69
  penis 752.69
  peripheral vascular system (congenital) NEC 747.60
    gastrointestinal 747.61
    lower limb 747.64
    renal 747.62

Hypoplasia, hypoplasis – *continued*
  peripheral vascular system – *continued*
    specified NEC 747.69
    spinal 747.82
    upper limb 747.63
  pituitary (gland) 759.2
  pulmonary 748.5
    arteriovenous 747.3
    artery 747.3
    valve 746.01
  punctum lacrimale 743.65
  radioulnar (*see also* Absence, radius, congenital, with ulna) 755.25
  radius (*see also* Absence, radius, congenital) 755.26
  rectum 751.2
  respiratory system NEC 748.9
  rib 756.3
  sacrum 756.19
  scapula 755.59
  shoulder girdle 755.59
  skin 757.39
  skull (bone) 756.0
    with
      anencephalus 740.0
      encephalocele 742.0
      hydrocephalus 742.3
        with spina bifida (*see also* Spina bifida) 741.0 **5th**
      microcephalus 742.1
  spinal (cord) (ventral horn cell) 742.59
    vessel 747.82
  spine 756.19
  spleen 759.0
  sternum 756.3
  tarsus (*see also* Absence, tarsal, congenital) 755.38
  testis, testicle 752.89
  thymus (gland) 279.11
  thyroid (gland) 243
    cartilage 748.3
  tibiofibular (*see also* Absence, tibia, congenital, with fibula) 755.35
  toe (*see also* Absence, toe, congenital) 755.39
  tongue 750.16
  trachea (cartilage) (rings) 748.3
  Turner's (tooth) 520.4
  ulna (*see also* Absence, ulna, congenital) 755.27
  umbilical artery 747.5
  ureter 753.29
  uterus 752.3
  vagina 752.49
  vascular (peripheral) NEC (*see also* Hypoplasia, peripheral vascular system) 747.60
    brain 747.81
  vein(s) (peripheral) NEC (*see also* Hypoplasia, peripheral vascular system) 747.60
    brain 747.81
    cardiac 746.89
    great 747.49
    portal 747.49
    pulmonary 747.49
  vena cava (inferior) (superior) 747.49
  vertebra 756.19
  vulva 752.49
  zonule (ciliary) 743.39
  zygoma 738.12
Hypopotassemia 276.8
Hypoproaccelerinemia (*see also* Defect, coagulation) 286.3
Hypoproconvertinemia (congenital) (*see also* Defect, coagulation) 286.3
Hypoproteinemia (essential) (hypermetabolic) (idiopathic) 273.8
Hypoproteinosis 260
Hypoprothrombinemia (congenital) (hereditary) (idiopathic) (*see also* Defect, coagulation) 286.3
  acquired 286.7
  newborn 776.3

Hypopselaphesia 782.0
Hypopyon (anterior chamber) (eye) 364.05
  iritis 364.05
  ulcer (cornea) 370.04
Hypopyrexia 780.99
Hyporeflex 796.1
Hyporeninemia, extreme 790.99
  in primary aldosteronism 255.10
Hyporesponsive episode 780.09
Hyposecretion
  ACTH 253.4
  ovary 256.39
    postablative 256.2
  salivary gland (any) 527.7
Hyposegmentation of neutrophils, hereditary 288.2
Hyposiderinemia 280.9
Hyposmolality 276.1
  syndrome 276.1
Hyposomatotropism 253.3
Hyposomnia, unspecified (*see also* Insomnia) 780.52
  with sleep apnea, unspecified 780.51
Hypospadias (male) 752.61
  female 753.8
Hypospermatogenesis 606.1
Hyposphagma 372.72
Hyposplenism 289.59
Hypostasis, pulmonary 514
Hypostatic - *see* condition
Hyposthenuria 593.89
Hyposuprarenalism 255.41
Hypo-TBG-nemia 246.8
Hypotension (arterial) (constitutional) 458.9
  chronic 458.1
  iatrogenic 458.29
  maternal, syndrome (following labor and delivery) 669.2 **5th**
  of hemodialysis 458.21
  orthostatic (chronic) 458.0
    dysautonomic-dyskinetic syndrome 333.0
  permanent idiopathic 458.1
  postoperative 458.29
  postural 458.0
  specified type NEC 458.8
  transient 796.3
Hypothermia (accidental) 991.6
  anesthetic 995.89
  associated with low environmental temperature 991.6
  newborn NEC 778.3
  not associated with low environmental temperature 780.65
Hypothymergasia (*see also* Psychosis, affective) 296.2 **5th**
  recurrent episode 296.3 **5th**
  single episode 296.2 **5th**
Hypothyroidism (acquired) 244.9
  complicating pregnancy, childbirth, or puerperium 648.1 **5th**
  congenital 243
  due to
    ablation 244.1
      radioactive iodine 244.1
      surgical 244.0
    iodine (administration) (ingestion) 244.2
      radioactive 244.1
    irradiation therapy 244.1
    p-aminosalicylic acid (PAS) 244.3
    phenylbutazone 244.3
    resorcinol 244.3
    specified cause NEC 244.8
    surgery 244.0
  goitrous (sporadic) 246.1
  iatrogenic NEC 244.3
  iodine 244.2
  pituitary 244.8
  postablative NEC 244.1
  postsurgical 244.0
  primary 244.9
  secondary NEC 244.8
  specified cause NEC 244.8

Hypothyroidism – *continued*
  sporadic goitrous 246.1
Hypotonia, hypotonicity, hypotony 781.3
  benign congenital 358.8
  bladder 596.4
  congenital 779.89
    benign 358.8
  eye 360.30
    due to
      fistula 360.32
      ocular disorder NEC 360.33
    following loss of aqueous or vitreous 360.33
    primary 360.31
  infantile muscular (benign) 359.0
  muscle 728.9
  uterus, uterine (contractions) - *see* Inertia, uterus
Hypotrichosis 704.09
  congenital 757.4
  lid (congenital) 757.4
    acquired 374.55
  postinfectional NEC 704.09
Hypotropia 378.32
Hypoventilation 786.09
  congenital central alveolar syndrome 327.25
  idiopathic sleep related nonobstructive alveolar 327.24
  sleep related, in conditions classifiable elsewhere 327.26
Hypovitaminosis (*see also* Deficiency, vitamin) 269.2
Hypovolemia 276.52
  surgical shock 998.0
  traumatic (shock) 958.4
Hypoxemia (*see also* Anoxia) 799.02
  sleep related, in conditions classifiable elsewhere 327.26
Hypoxia (*see also* Anoxia) 799.02
  cerebral 348.1
    during or resulting from a procedure 997.01
    newborn 770.88
      mild or moderate 768.6
      severe 768.5
  fetal, affecting newborn 770.88
  intrauterine - *see* Distress, fetal
  myocardial (*see also* Insufficiency, coronary) 411.89
    arteriosclerotic - *see* Arteriosclerosis, coronary
  newborn 770.88
  sleep related 327.24
Hypoxic-ischemic encephalopathy (HIE) 768.70 ▲
  mild 768.71 ●
  moderate 768.72 ●
  severe 768.73 ●
Hypsarrhythmia (*see also* Epilepsy) 345.6 **5th**
Hysteralgia, pregnant uterus 646.8 **5th**
Hysteria, hysterical 300.10
  anxiety 300.20
  Charcôt's gland 300.11
  conversion (any manifestation) 300.11
  dissociative type NEC 300.15
  psychosis, acute 298.1
Hysteroepilepsy 300.11
Hysterotomy, affecting fetus or newborn 763.89

I

Iatrogenic syndrome of excess cortisol 255.0
IBM (inclusion body myositis) 359.71 ●
Iceland disease (epidemic neuromyasthenia) 049.8
Ichthyosis (congenita) 757.1
  acquired 701.1
  fetalis gravior 757.1
  follicularis 757.1

Hypoplasia, hypoplasis – Ichthyosis

- **Ichthyosis** – *continued*
  - hystrix 757.39
  - lamellar 757.1
  - lingual 528.6
  - palmaris and plantaris 757.39
  - simplex 757.1
  - vera 757.1
  - vulgaris 757.1
- **Ichthyotoxism** 988.0
  - bacterial (*see also* Poisoning, food) 005.9
- **Icteroanemia, hemolytic** (acquired) 283.9
  - congenital (*see also* Spherocytosis) 282.0
- **Icterus** (*see also* Jaundice) 782.4
  - catarrhal - *see* Icterus, infectious
  - conjunctiva 782.4
    - newborn 774.6
  - epidemic - *see* Icterus, infectious
  - febrilis - *see* Icterus, infectious
  - fetus or newborn - *see* Jaundice, fetus or newborn
  - gravis (*see also* Necrosis, liver) 570
    - complicating pregnancy 646.7 [5th]
      - affecting fetus or newborn 760.8
    - fetus or newborn NEC 773.0
    - obstetrical 646.7 [5th]
      - affecting fetus or newborn 760.8
  - hematogenous (acquired) 283.9
  - hemolytic (acquired) 283.9
    - congenital (*see also* Spherocytosis) 282.0
  - hemorrhagic (acute) 100.0
    - leptospiral 100.0
    - newborn 776.0
    - spirochetal 100.0
  - infectious 070.1
    - with hepatic coma 070.0
    - leptospiral 100.0
    - spirochetal 100.0
  - intermittens juvenilis 277.4
  - malignant (*see also* Necrosis, liver) 570
  - neonatorum (*see also* Jaundice, fetus or newborn) 774.6
  - pernicious (*see also* Necrosis, liver) 570
  - spirochetal 100.0
- **Ictus solaris, solis** 992.0
- **Identity disorder** 313.82
  - dissociative 300.14
  - gender role (child) 302.6
    - adult 302.85
  - psychosexual (child) 302.6
    - adult 302.85
- **Idioglossia** 307.9
- **Idiopathic** - *see* condition
- **Idiosyncrasy** (*see also* Allergy) 995.3
  - drug, medicinal substance, and biological - *see* Allergy, drug
- **Idiot, idiocy** (congenital) 318.2
  - amaurotic (Bielschowsky) (-Jansky) (family) (infantile (late)) (juvenile (late)) (Vogt-Spielmeyer) 330.1
  - microcephalic 742.1
  - Mongolian 758.0
  - oxycephalic 756.0
- **Id reaction** (due to bacteria) 692.89
- **Ideation**
  - suicidal V62.84
- **IEED** (involuntary emotional expression disorder) 310.8
- **IFIS** (intraoperative floppy iris syndrome) 364.81
- **IgE asthma** 493.0 [5th]
- **Ileitis** (chronic) (*see also* Enteritis) 558.9
  - infectious 009.0
  - noninfectious 558.9
  - regional (ulcerative) 555.0
    - with large intestine 555.2
  - segmental 555.0
    - with large intestine 555.2
  - terminal (ulcerative) 555.0
    - with large intestine 555.2
- **Ileocolitis** (*see also* Enteritis) 558.9
  - infectious 009.0
  - regional 555.2
  - ulcerative 556.1
- **Ileostomy status** V44.2
  - with complication 569.60
- **Ileotyphus** 002.0
- **Ileum** - *see* condition
- **Ileus** (adynamic) (bowel) (colon) (inhibitory) (intestine) (neurogenic) (paralytic) 560.1
  - arteriomesenteric duodenal 537.2
  - due to gallstone (in intestine) 560.31
  - duodenal, chronic 537.2
  - following gastrointestinal surgery 997.4
  - gallstone 560.31
  - mechanical (*see also* Obstruction, intestine) 560.9
  - meconium 777.1
    - due to cystic fibrosis 277.01
  - myxedema 564.89
  - postoperative 997.4
  - transitory, newborn 777.4
- **Iliac** - *see* condition
- **Iliotibial band friction syndrome** 728.89
- **Ill, louping** 063.1
- **Illegitimacy** V61.6
- **Illness** - *see also* Disease
  - factitious 300.19
    - with
      - combined psychological and physical signs and symptoms 300.19
      - physical symptoms 300.19
      - predominantly
        - physical signs and symptoms 300.19
        - psychological symptoms 300.16
    - chronic (with physical symptoms) 301.51
  - heart - *see* Disease, heart
  - manic-depressive (*see also* Psychosis, affective) 296.80
  - mental (*see also* Disorder, mental) 300.9
- **Imbalance** 781.2
  - autonomic (*see also* Neuropathy, peripheral, autonomic) 337.9
  - electrolyte 276.9
    - with
      - abortion - *see* Abortion, by type, with metabolic disorder
      - ectopic pregnancy (*see also* categories 633.0-633.9) 639.4
      - hyperemesis gravidarum (before 22 completed weeks gestation) 643.1 [5th]
      - molar pregnancy (*see also* categories 630-632) 639.4
    - following
      - abortion 639.4
      - ectopic or molar pregnancy 639.4
    - neonatal, transitory NEC 775.5
  - endocrine 259.9
  - eye muscle NEC 378.9
    - heterophoria - *see* Heterophoria
  - glomerulotubular NEC 593.89
  - hormone 259.9
  - hysterical (*see also* Hysteria) 300.10
  - labyrinth NEC 386.50
  - posture 729.90
  - sympathetic (*see also* Neuropathy, peripheral, autonomic) 337.9
- **Imbecile, imbecility** 318.0
  - moral 301.7
  - old age 290.9
  - senile 290.9
  - specified IQ - *see* IQ
  - unspecified IQ 318.0
- **Imbedding, intrauterine device** 996.32
- **Imbibition, cholesterol** (gallbladder) 575.6
- **Imerslund (-Gräsbeck) syndrome** (anemia due to familial selective vitamin B_{12} malabsorption) 281.1
- **Iminoacidopathy** 270.8
- **Iminoglycinuria, familial** 270.8
- **Immature** - *see also* Immaturity
  - personality 301.89
- **Immaturity** 765.1 [5th]
  - extreme 765.0 [5th]
  - fetus or infant light-for-dates - *see* Light-for-dates
  - lung, fetus or newborn 770.4
  - organ or site NEC - *see* Hypoplasia
  - pulmonary, fetus or newborn 770.4
  - reaction 301.89
  - sexual (female) (male) 259.0
- **Immersion** 994.1
  - foot 991.4
  - hand 991.4
- **Immobile, immobility**
  - complete
    - due to severe physical disability or frality 780.72
  - intestine 564.89
  - joint - *see* Ankylosis
  - syndrome (paraplegic) 728.3
- **Immunization**
  - ABO
    - affecting management of pregnancy 656.2 [5th]
      - fetus or newborn 773.1
  - complication - *see* Complications, vaccination
  - Rh factor
    - affecting management of pregnancy 656.1 [5th]
      - fetus or newborn 773.0
    - from transfusion 999.7
- **Immunodeficiency** 279.3
  - with
    - adenosine-deaminase deficiency 279.2
    - defect, predominant
      - B-cell 279.00
      - T-cell 279.10
    - hyperimmunoglobulinemia 279.2
    - lymphopenia, hereditary 279.2
    - thrombocytopenia and eczema 279.12
    - thymic
      - aplasia 279.2
      - dysplasia 279.2
  - autosomal recessive, Swiss-type 279.2
  - common variable 279.06
  - severe combined (SCID) 279.2
  - to Rh factor
    - affecting management of pregnancy 656.1 [5th]
      - fetus or newborn 773.0
  - X-linked, with increased IgM 279.05
- **Immunotherapy, prophylactic** V07.2
  - antineoplastic V58.12
- **Impaction, impacted**
  - bowel, colon, rectum 560.30
    - with hernia - *see also* Hernia, by site, with, obstruction
      - gangrenous - *see* Hernia, by site, with gangrene
    - by
      - calculus 560.39
      - gallstone 560.31
    - fecal 560.39
    - specified type NEC 560.39
  - calculus - *see* Calculus
  - cerumen (ear) (external) 380.4
  - cuspid 520.6
  - dental 520.6
  - fecal, feces 560.39
    - with hernia - *see also* Hernia, by site, with obstruction
      - gangrenous - *see* Hernia, by site, with gangrene
  - fracture - *see* Fracture, by site
  - gallbladder - *see* Cholelithiasis
  - gallstone(s) - *see* Cholelithiasis
    - in intestine (any part) 560.31
  - intestine(s) 560.30
    - with hernia - *see also* Hernia, by site, with obstruction
      - gangrenous - *see* Hernia, by site, with gangrene
    - by
      - calculus 560.39
- **Impaction, impacted** – *continued*
  - intestine(s) – *continued*
    - by – *continued*
      - gallstone 560.31
    - fecal 560.39
    - specified type NEC 560.39
  - intrauterine device (IUD) 996.32
  - molar 520.6
  - shoulder 660.4 [5th]
    - affecting fetus or newborn 763.1
  - tooth, teeth 520.6
  - turbinate 733.99
- **Impaired, impairment** (function)
  - arm V49.1
    - movement, involving
      - musculoskeletal system V49.1
      - nervous system V49.2
  - auditory discrimination 388.43
  - back V48.3
  - body (entire) V49.89
  - combined visual hearing V49.85
  - cognitive, mild, so stated 331.83
  - dual sensory V49.85
  - glucose
    - fasting 790.21
    - tolerance test (oral) 790.22
  - hearing (*see also* Deafness) 389.9
    - combined with visual impairment V49.85
  - heart - *see* Disease, heart
  - kidney (*see also* Disease, renal) 593.9
    - disorder resulting from 588.9
      - specified NEC 588.89
  - leg V49.1
    - movement, involving
      - musculoskeletal system V49.1
      - nervous system V49.2
  - limb V49.1
    - movement, involving
      - musculoskeletal system V49.1
      - nervous system V49.2
  - liver 573.8
  - mastication 524.9
  - mild cognitive, so stated 331.83
  - mobility
    - ear ossicles NEC 385.22
    - incostapedial joint 385.22
    - malleus 385.21
  - myocardium, myocardial (*see also* Insufficiency, myocardial) 428.0
  - neuromusculoskeletal NEC V49.89
    - back V48.3
    - head V48.2
    - limb V49.2
    - neck V48.3
    - spine V48.3
    - trunk V48.3
  - rectal sphincter 787.99
  - renal (*see also* Disease, renal) 593.9
    - disorder resulting from 588.9
      - specified NEC 588.89
  - spine V48.3
  - vision NEC 369.9
    - both eyes NEC 369.3
    - combined with hearing impairment V49.85
    - moderate 369.74
      - both eyes 369.25
        - with impairment of lesser eye (specified as)
          - blind, not further specified 369.15
          - low vision, not further specified 369.23
          - near-total 369.17
          - profound 369.18
          - severe 369.24
          - total 369.16
      - one eye 369.74
        - with vision of other eye (specified as)
          - near-normal 369.75
          - normal 369.76

Impaired, impairment (function) – *continued*
- vision – *continued*
  - near-total 369.64
    - both eyes 369.04
      - with impairment of lesser eye (specified as)
        - blind, not further specified 369.02
        - total 369.03
    - one eye 369.64
      - with vision of other eye (specified as)
        - near-normal 369.65
        - normal 369.66
  - one eye 369.60
    - with low vision of other eye 369.10
  - profound 369.67
    - both eyes 369.08
      - with impairment of lesser eye (specified as)
        - blind, not further specified 369.05
        - near-total 369.07
        - total 369.06
    - one eye 369.67
      - with vision of other eye (specified as)
        - near-normal 369.68
        - normal 369.69
  - severe 369.71
    - both eyes 369.22
      - with impairment of lesser eye (specified as)
        - blind, not further specified 369.11
        - low vision, not further specified 369.21
        - near-total 369.13
        - profound 369.14
        - total 369.12
    - one eye 369.71
      - with vision of other eye (specified as)
        - near-normal 369.72
        - normal 369.73
  - total
    - both eyes 369.01
    - one eye 369.61
      - with vision of other eye (specified as)
        - near-normal 369.62
        - normal 369.63

Impaludism - *see* Malaria

Impediment, speech NEC 784.59 ▲
- psychogenic 307.9
- secondary to organic lesion 784.59 ▲

Impending
- cerebrovascular accident or attack 435.9
- coronary syndrome 411.1
- delirium tremens 291.0
- myocardial infarction 411.1

Imperception, auditory (acquired) (congenital) 389.9

Imperfect
- aeration, lung (newborn) 770.5
- closure (congenital)
  - alimentary tract NEC 751.8
    - lower 751.5
    - upper 750.8
  - atrioventricular ostium 745.69
  - atrium (secundum) 745.5
    - primum 745.61
  - branchial cleft or sinus 744.41
  - choroid 743.59
  - cricoid cartilage 748.3
  - cusps, heart valve NEC 746.89
    - pulmonary 746.09
  - ductus
    - arteriosus 747.0
    - Botalli 747.0
  - ear drum 744.29
    - causing impairment of hearing 744.03

Imperfect – *continued*
- closure (congenital) – *continued*
  - endocardial cushion 745.60
  - epiglottis 748.3
  - esophagus with communication to bronchus or trachea 750.3
  - Eustachian valve 746.89
  - eyelid 743.62
  - face, facial (*see also* Cleft, lip) 749.10
  - foramen
    - Botalli 745.5
    - ovale 745.5
  - genitalia, genital organ(s) or system
    - female 752.89
      - external 752.49
      - internal NEC 752.89
      - uterus 752.3
    - male 752.89
      - penis 752.69
  - glottis 748.3
  - heart valve (cusps) NEC 746.89
  - interatrial ostium or septum 745.5
  - interauricular ostium or septum 745.5
  - interventricular ostium or septum 745.4
  - iris 743.46
  - kidney 753.3
  - larynx 748.3
  - lens 743.36
  - lip (*see also* Cleft, lip) 749.10
  - nasal septum or sinus 748.1
  - nose 748.1
  - omphalomesenteric duct 751.0
  - optic nerve entry 743.57
  - organ or site NEC - *see* Anomaly, specified type, by site
  - ostium
    - interatrial 745.5
    - interauricular 745.5
    - interventricular 745.4
  - palate (*see also* Cleft, palate) 749.00
  - preauricular sinus 744.46
  - retina 743.56
  - roof of orbit 742.0
  - sclera 743.47
  - septum
    - aortic 745.0
    - aorticopulmonary 745.0
    - atrial (secundum) 745.5
      - primum 745.61
    - between aorta and pulmonary artery 745.0
    - heart 745.9
    - interatrial (secundum) 745.5
      - primum 745.61
    - interauricular (secundum) 745.5
      - primum 745.61
    - interventricular 745.4
      - with pulmonary stenosis or atresia, dextraposition of aorta, and hypertrophy of right ventricle 745.2
      - in tetralogy of Fallot 745.2
    - nasal 748.1
    - ventricular 745.4
      - with pulmonary stenosis or atresia, dextraposition of aorta, and hypertrophy of right ventricle 745.2
      - in tetralogy of Fallot 745.2
  - skull 756.0
    - with
      - anencephalus 740.0
      - encephalocele 742.0
      - hydrocephalus 742.3
        - with spina bifida (*see also* Spina bifida) 741.0 5th
      - microcephalus 742.1
  - spine (with meningocele) (*see also* Spina bifida) 741.90
  - thyroid cartilage 748.3
  - trachea 748.3

Imperfect – *continued*
- closure (congenital) – *continued*
  - tympanic membrane 744.29
    - causing impairment of hearing 744.03
  - uterus (with communication to bladder, intestine, or rectum) 752.3
  - uvula 749.02
    - with cleft lip (*see also* Cleft, palate, with cleft lip) 749.20
  - vitelline duct 751.0
- development - *see* Anomaly, by site
- erection 607.84
- fusion - *see* Imperfect, closure
- inflation lung (newborn) 770.5
- intestinal canal 751.5
- poise 729.90
- rotation - *see* Malrotation
- septum, ventricular 745.4

Imperfectly descended testis 752.51

Imperforate (congenital) - *see also* Atresia
- anus 751.2
- bile duct 751.61
- cervix (uteri) 752.49
- esophagus 750.3
- hymen 752.42
- intestine (small) 751.1
  - large 751.2
- jejunum 751.1
- pharynx 750.29
- rectum 751.2
- salivary duct 750.23
- urethra 753.6
- urinary meatus 753.6
- vagina 752.49

Impervious (congenital) - *see also* Atresia
- anus 751.2
- bile duct 751.61
- esophagus 750.3
- intestine (small) 751.1
  - large 751.5
- rectum 751.2
- urethra 753.6

Impetiginization of other dermatoses 684

Impetigo (any organism) (any site) (bullous) (circinate) (contagiosa) (neonatorum) (simplex) 684
- Bockhart's (superficial folliculitis) 704.8
- external ear 684 *[380.13]*
- eyelid 684 *[373.5]*
- Fox's (contagiosa) 684
- furfuracea 696.5
- herpetiformis 694.3
  - nonobstetrical 694.3
- staphylococcal infection 684
- ulcerative 686.8
- vulgaris 684

Impingement, soft tissue between teeth 524.89
- anterior 524.81
- posterior 524.82

Implant, endometrial 617.9

Implantation
- anomalous - *see also* Anomaly, specified type, by site
  - ureter 753.4
- cyst
  - external area or site (skin) NEC 709.8
  - iris 364.61
  - vagina 623.8
  - vulva 624.8
- dermoid (cyst)
  - external area or site (skin) NEC 709.8
  - iris 364.61
  - vagina 623.8
  - vulva 624.8
- placenta, low or marginal - *see* Placenta previa

Impotence (sexual) 607.84
- organic origin NEC 607.84
- psychogenic 302.72

Impoverished blood 285.9

Impression, basilar 756.0

Imprisonment V62.5

Improper
- development, infant 764.9 5th

Improperly tied umbilical cord (causing hemorrhage) 772.3

Impulses, obsessional 300.3

Impulsive ~~neurosis 300.3~~ 799.23 ▲
- neurosis 300.3 ●

Impulsiveness 799.23 ●

Inaction, kidney (*see also* Disease, renal) 593.9

Inactive - *see* condition

Inadequate, inadequacy
- aesthetics of dental restoration 525.67
- biologic 301.6
- cardiac and renal - *see* Hypertension, cardiorenal
- constitutional 301.6
- development
  - child 783.40
  - fetus 764.9 5th
    - affecting management of pregnancy 656.5 5th
  - genitalia
    - after puberty NEC 259.0
    - congenital - *see* Hypoplasia, genitalia
  - lungs 748.5
  - organ or site NEC - *see* Hypoplasia, by site
- dietary 269.9
- distance, interarch 524.28
- education V62.3
- environment
  - economic problem V60.2
  - household condition NEC V60.1
  - poverty V60.2
  - unemployment V62.0
- functional 301.6
- household care, due to
  - family member
    - handicapped or ill V60.4
    - temporarily away from home V60.4
      - on vacation V60.5
  - technical defects in home V60.1
  - temporary absence from home of person rendering care V60.4
- housing (heating) (space) V60.1
- interarch distance 524.28
- material resources V60.2
- mental (*see also* Retardation, mental) 319
- nervous system 799.29 ▲
- personality 301.6
- prenatal care in current pregnancy V23.7
- pulmonary
  - function 786.09
    - newborn 770.89
  - ventilation, newborn 770.89
- respiration 786.09
  - newborn 770.89
- sample
  - cytology
    - anal 796.78
    - cervical 795.08
    - vaginal 795.18
- social 301.6

Inanition 263.9
- with edema 262
- due to
  - deprivation of food 994.2
  - malnutrition 263.9
- fever 780.60

Inappropriate secretion
- ACTH 255.0
- antidiuretic hormone (ADH) (excessive) 253.6
  - deficiency 253.5
- ectopic hormone NEC 259.3
- pituitary (posterior) 253.6

Inattention after or at birth 995.52

Inborn errors of metabolism - *see* Disorder, metabolism

4th Fourth Digit Required 5th Fifth Digit Required | *[code]* Manifestation Code | ● New Line ▲ Revised Line text New Text ~~text~~ Deleted text

- **Incarceration, incarcerated**
  - bubonocele - *see also* Hernia, inguinal, with obstruction
    - gangrenous - *see* Hernia, inguinal, with gangrene
  - colon (by hernia) - *see also* Hernia, by site with obstruction
    - gangrenous - *see* Hernia, by site, with gangrene
  - enterocele 552.9
    - gangrenous 551.9
  - epigastrocele 552.29
    - gangrenous 551.29
  - epiplocele 552.9
    - gangrenous 551.9
  - exomphalos 552.1
    - gangrenous 551.1
  - fallopian tube 620.8
  - hernia - *see also* Hernia, by site, with obstruction
    - gangrenous - *see* Hernia, by site, with gangrene
  - iris, in wound 871.1
  - lens, in wound 871.1
  - merocele (*see also* Hernia, femoral, with obstruction) 552.00
  - omentum (by hernia) - *see also* Hernia, by site, with obstruction
    - gangrenous - *see* Hernia, by site, with gangrene
  - omphalocele 756.72 ▲
  - rupture (meaning hernia) (*see also* Hernia, by site, with obstruction) 552.9
    - gangrenous (*see also* Hernia, by site, with gangrene) 551.9
  - sarcoepiplocele 552.9
    - gangrenous 551.9
  - sarcoepiplomphalocele 552.1
    - with gangrene 551.1
  - uterus 621.8
    - gravid 654.3 [5th]
      - causing obstructed labor 660.2 [5th]
        - affecting fetus or newborn 763.1
- **Incident, cerebrovascular** (*see also* Disease, cerebrovascular, acute) 436
- **Incineration** (entire body) (from fire, conflagration, electricity, or lightning) - *see* Burn, multiple, specified sites
- **Incised wound**
  - external - *see* Wound, open, by site
  - internal organs (abdomen, chest, or pelvis) - *see* Injury, internal, by site, with open wound
- **Incision, incisional**
  - hernia - *see* Hernia, incisional
  - surgical, complication - *see* Complications, surgical procedures
  - traumatic
    - external - *see* Wound, open, by site
    - internal organs (abdomen, chest, or pelvis) - *see* Injury, internal, by site, with open wound
- **Inclusion**
  - azurophilic leukocytic 288.2
  - blennorrhea (neonatal) (newborn) 771.6
  - cyst - *see* Cyst, skin
  - gallbladder in liver (congenital) 751.69
- **Incompatibility**
  - ABO
    - affecting management of pregnancy 656.2 [5th]
    - fetus or newborn 773.1
    - infusion or transfusion reaction 999.6
  - blood (group) (Duffy) (E) (K(ell)) (Kidd) (Lewis) (M) (N) (P) (S) NEC 999.89 ▲
    - affecting management of pregnancy 656.2 [5th]
    - fetus or newborn 773.2
    - infusion or transfusion reaction 999.89 ▲
  - contour of existing restoration of tooth with oral health 525.65

- **Incompatibility** – *continued*
  - marital V61.10
    - involving
      - divorce V61.03
      - estrangement V61.09
  - Rh (blood group) (factor)
    - affecting management of pregnancy 656.1 [5th]
    - fetus or newborn 773.0
    - infusion or transfusion reaction 999.7
  - Rhesus - *see* Incompatibility, Rh
- **Incompetency, incompetence, incompetent**
  - annular
    - aortic (valve) (*see also* Insufficiency, aortic) 424.1
    - mitral (valve) - (*see also* Insufficiency, mitral) 424.0
    - pulmonary valve (heart) (*see also* Endocarditis, pulmonary) 424.3
  - aortic (valve) (*see also* Insufficiency, aortic) 424.1
    - syphilitic 093.22
  - cardiac (orifice) 530.0
    - valve - *see* Endocarditis
  - cervix, cervical (os) 622.5
    - in pregnancy 654.5 [5th]
      - affecting fetus or newborn 761.0
  - chronotropic 426.89
    - with
      - autonomic dysfunction 337.9
      - ischemic heart disease 414.9
      - left ventricular dysfunction 429.89 ▲
      - sinus node dysfunction 427.81
  - esophagogastric (junction) (sphincter) 530.0
  - heart valve, congenital 746.89
  - mitral (valve) - *see* Insufficiency, mitral
  - papillary muscle (heart) 429.81
  - pelvic fundus
    - pubocervical tissue 618.81
    - rectovaginal tissue 618.82
  - pulmonary valve (heart) (*see also* Endocarditis, pulmonary) 424.3
    - congenital 746.09
  - tricuspid (annular) (rheumatic) (valve) (*see also* Endocarditis, tricuspid) 397.0
  - valvular - *see* Endocarditis
  - vein, venous (saphenous) (varicose) (*see also* Varicose, vein) 454.9
  - velopharyngeal (closure)
    - acquired 528.9
    - congenital 750.29
- **Incomplete** - *see also* condition
  - bladder emptying 788.21
  - expansion lungs (newborn) 770.5
  - gestation (liveborn) - *see* Immaturity
  - rotation - *see* Malrotation
- **Inconclusive** ●
  - image test due to excess body fat 793.91 ●
  - mammogram, mammography 793.82 ●
    - due to dense breasts 793.82 ●
- **Incontinence** 788.30
  - without sensory awareness 788.34
  - anal sphincter 787.6
  - continuous leakage 788.37
  - feces 787.6
    - due to hysteria 300.11
    - nonorganic origin 307.7
  - hysterical 300.11
  - mixed (male) (female) (urge and stress) 788.33
  - overflow 788.38
  - paradoxical 788.39
  - rectal 787.6
  - specified NEC 788.39
  - stress (female) 625.6
    - male NEC 788.32
  - urethral sphincter 599.84
  - urge 788.31
    - and stress (male) (female) 788.33
  - urine 788.30
    - active 788.30

- **Incontinence** – *continued*
  - urine – *continued*
    - due to
      - cognitive impairment 788.91
      - immobility 788.91
      - severe physical disability 788.91
    - functional 788.91
    - male 788.30
      - stress 788.32
        - and urge 788.33
    - neurogenic 788.39
    - nonorganic origin 307.6
    - stress (female) 625.6
      - male NEC 788.32
    - urge 788.31
      - and stress 788.33
- **Incontinentia pigmenti** 757.33
- **Incoordinate**
  - uterus (action) (contractions) 661.4 [5th]
    - affecting fetus or newborn 763.7
- **Incoordination**
  - esophageal-pharyngeal (newborn) 787.24
  - muscular 781.3
  - papillary muscle 429.81
- **Increase, increased**
  - abnormal, in development 783.9
  - androgens (ovarian) 256.1
  - anticoagulants (antithrombin) (anti-VIIIa) (anti-IXa) (anti-Xa) (anti-XIa) 286.5
    - postpartum 666.3 [5th]
  - cold sense (*see also* Disturbance, sensation) 782.0
  - estrogen 256.0
  - function
    - adrenal (cortex) 255.3
      - medulla 255.6
    - pituitary (anterior) (gland) (lobe) 253.1
      - posterior 253.6
  - heat sense (*see also* Disturbance, sensation) 782.0
  - intracranial pressure 781.99
    - injury at birth 767.8
  - light reflex of retina 362.13
  - permeability, capillary 448.9
  - pressure
    - intracranial 781.99
      - injury at birth 767.8
    - intraocular 365.00
  - pulsations 785.9
  - pulse pressure 785.9
  - sphericity, lens 743.36
  - splenic activity 289.4
  - venous pressure 459.89
    - portal 572.3
- **Incrustation, cornea, lead, or zinc** 930.0
- **Incyclophoria** 378.44
- **Incyclotropia** 378.33
- **Indeterminate sex** 752.7
- **India rubber skin** 756.83
- **Indicanuria** 270.2
- **Indigestion** (bilious) (functional) 536.8
  - acid 536.8
  - catarrhal 536.8
  - due to decomposed food NEC 005.9
  - fat 579.8
  - nervous 306.4
  - psychogenic 306.4
- **Indirect** - *see* condition
- **Indolent bubo NEC** 099.8
- **Induced**
  - abortion - *see* Abortion, induced
  - birth, affecting fetus or newborn 763.89
  - delivery - *see* Delivery
  - labor - *see* Delivery
- **Induration, indurated**
  - brain 348.89 ▲
  - breast (fibrous) 611.79
    - puerperal, postpartum 676.3 [5th]
  - broad ligament 620.8
  - chancre 091.0
    - anus 091.1
    - congenital 090.0

- **Induration, indurated** – *continued*
  - chancre – *continued*
    - extragenital NEC 091.2
  - corpora cavernosa (penis) (plastic) 607.89
  - liver (chronic) 573.8
    - acute 573.8
  - lung (black) (brown) (chronic) (fibroid) (*see also* Fibrosis, lung) 515
    - essential brown 275.0 *[516.1]*
  - penile 607.89
  - phlebitic - *see* Phlebitis
  - skin 782.8
  - stomach 537.89
- **Induratio penis plastica** 607.89
- **Industrial** - *see* condition
- **Inebriety** (*see also* Abuse, drugs, nondependent) 305.0 [5th]
- **Inefficiency**
  - kidney (*see also* Disease, renal) 593.9
  - thyroid (acquired) (gland) 244.9
- **Inelasticity, skin** 782.8
- **Inequality, leg** (acquired) (length) 736.81
  - congenital 755.30
- **Inertia**
  - bladder 596.4
    - neurogenic 596.54
      - with cauda equina syndrome 344.61
  - stomach 536.8
    - psychogenic 306.4
  - uterus, uterine 661.2 [5th]
    - affecting fetus or newborn 763.7
    - primary 661.0 [5th]
    - secondary 661.1 [5th]
  - vesical 596.4
    - neurogenic 596.54
      - with cauda equina 344.61
- **Infant** - *see also* condition
  - excessive crying of 780.92
  - fussy (baby) 780.91
  - held for adoption V68.89
  - newborn - *see* Newborn
  - post-term (gestation period over 40 completed weeks to 42 completed weeks) 766.21
  - prolonged gestation of (period over 42 completed weeks) 766.22
  - syndrome of diabetic mother 775.0
- **"Infant Hercules" syndrome** 255.2
- **Infantile** - *see also* condition
  - genitalia, genitals 259.0
    - in pregnancy or childbirth NEC 654.4 [5th]
      - affecting fetus or newborn 763.89
      - causing obstructed labor 660.2 [5th]
        - affecting fetus or newborn 763.1
  - heart 746.9
  - kidney 753.3
  - lack of care 995.52
  - macula degeneration 362.75
  - melanodontia 521.05
  - os, uterus (*see also* Infantile, genitalia) 259.0
  - pelvis 738.6
    - with disproportion (fetopelvic) 653.1 [5th]
      - affecting fetus or newborn 763.1
      - causing obstructed labor 660.1 [5th]
        - affecting fetus or newborn 763.1
  - penis 259.0
  - testis 257.2
  - uterus (*see also* Infantile, genitalia) 259.0
  - vulva 752.49
- **Infantilism** 259.9
  - with dwarfism (hypophyseal) 253.3
  - Brissaud's (infantile myxedema) 244.9
  - celiac 579.0
  - Herter's (nontropical sprue) 579.0
  - hypophyseal 253.3
  - hypothalamic (with obesity) 253.8
  - idiopathic 259.9
  - intestinal 579.0
  - pancreatic 577.8
  - pituitary 253.3
  - renal 588.0

Incarceration, incarcerated – Infantilism

Infantilism – *continued*
sexual (with obesity) 259.0
Infants, healthy liveborn - *see* Newborn
Infarct, infarction
adrenal (capsule) (gland) 255.41
amnion 658.8 [5th]
anterior (with contiguous portion of intraventricular septum) NEC (*see also* Infarct, myocardium) 410.1 [5th]
appendices epiploicae 557.0
bowel 557.0
brain (stem) 434.91
embolic (*see also* Embolism, brain) 434.11
healed or old without residuals V12.54
iatrogenic 997.02
lacunar 434.91
late effect - *see* Late effect(s) (of) cerebrovascular disease
postoperative 997.02
puerperal, postpartum, childbirth 674.0 [5th]
thrombotic (*see also* Thrombosis, brain) 434.01
breast 611.89
Brewer's (kidney) 593.81
cardiac (*see also* Infarct, myocardium) 410.9 [5th]
cerebellar (*see also* Infarct, brain) 434.91
embolic (*see also* Embolism, brain) 434.11
cerebral (*see also* Infarct, brain) 434.91
aborted 434.91
embolic (*see also* Embolism, brain) 434.11
thrombotic (*see also* Infarct, brain) 434.01
chorion 658.8 [5th]
colon (acute) (agnogenic) (embolic) (hemorrhagic) (nonocclusive) (nonthrombotic) (occlusive) (segmental) (thrombotic) (with gangrene) 557.0
coronary artery (*see also* Infarct, myocardium) 410.9 [5th]
cortical 434.91
embolic (*see also* Embolism) 444.9
fallopian tube 620.8
gallbladder 575.8
heart (*see also* Infarct, myocardium) 410.9 [5th]
hepatic 573.4
hypophysis (anterior lobe) 253.8
impending (myocardium) 411.1
intestine (acute) (agnogenic) (embolic) (hemorrhagic) (nonocclusive) (nonthrombotic) (occlusive) (thrombotic) (with gangrene) 557.0
kidney 593.81
lacunar 434.91
liver 573.4
lung (embolic) (thrombotic) 415.19
with
abortion - *see* Abortion, by type, with, embolism
ectopic pregnancy (*see also* categories 633.0-633.9) 639.6
molar pregnancy (*see also* categories 630-632) 639.6
following
abortion 639.6
ectopic or molar pregnancy 639.6
iatrogenic 415.11
in pregnancy, childbirth, or puerperium - *see* Embolism, obstetrical
postoperative 415.11
septic 415.12
lymph node or vessel 457.8
medullary (brain) - *see* Infarct, brain
meibomian gland (eyelid) 374.85
mesentery, mesenteric (embolic) (thrombotic) (with gangrene) 557.0
midbrain - *see* Infarct, brain

Infarct, infarction – *continued*
myocardium, myocardial (acute or with a stated duration of 8 weeks or less) (with hypertension) 410.9 [5th]

Note *Use the following fifth-digit subclassification with category 410:*

0	episode unspecified
1	initial episode
2	subsequent episode without recurrence

with symptoms after 8 weeks from date of infarction 414.8 [5th]
anterior (wall) (with contiguous portion of intraventricular septum) NEC 410.1 [5th]
anteroapical (with contiguous portion of intraventricular septum) 410.1 [5th]
anterolateral (wall) 410.0 [5th]
anteroseptal (with contiguous portion of intraventricular septum) 410.1 [5th]
apical-lateral 410.5 [5th]
atrial 410.8 [5th]
basal-lateral 410.5 [5th]
chronic (with symptoms after 8 weeks from date of infarction) 414.8
diagnosed on ECG, but presenting no symptoms 412
diaphragmatic wall (with contiguous portion of intraventricular septum) 410.4
healed or old, currently presenting no symptoms 412
high lateral 410.5 [5th]
impending 411.1
inferior (wall) (with contiguous portion of intraventricular septum) 410.4 [5th]
inferolateral (wall) 410.2 [5th]
inferoposterior wall 410.3 [5th]
intraoperative 997.1
lateral wall 410.5 [5th]
non-Q wave 410.7 [5th]
non-ST elevation (NSTEMI) 410.7 [5th]
nontransmural 410.7 [5th]
papillary muscle 410.8 [5th]
past (diagnosed on ECG or other special investigation, but currently presenting no symptoms) 412
with symptoms NEC 414.8
posterior (strictly) (true) (wall) 410.6 [5th]
posterobasal 410.6 [5th]
posteroinferior 410.3 [5th]
posterolateral 410.5 [5th]
postprocedural 997.1
previous, currently presenting no symptoms 412
Q wave (*see also* Infarct, myocardium, by site) 410.9 [5th]
septal 410.8 [5th]
specified site NEC 410.8 [5th]
ST elevation (STEMI) 410.9 [5th]
anterior (wall) 410.1 [5th]
anterolateral (wall) 410.0 [5th]
inferior (wall) 410.4 [5th]
inferolateral (wall) 410.2 [5th]
inferoposterior wall 410.3 [5th]
lateral wall 410.5 [5th]
posterior (strictly) (true) (wall) 410.6 [5th]
specified site NEC 410.8 [5th]
subendocardial 410.7 [5th]
syphilitic 093.82
non-ST elevation myocardial infarction (NSTEMI) 410.7 [5th]
nontransmural 410.7 [5th]
omentum 557.0
ovary 620.8
pancreas 577.8

Infarct, infarction – *continued*
papillary muscle (*see also* Infarct, myocardium) 410.8 [5th]
parathyroid gland 252.8
pituitary (gland) 253.8
placenta (complicating pregnancy) 656.7 [5th]
affecting fetus or newborn 762.2
pontine - *see* Infarct, brain
posterior NEC (*see also* Infarct, myocardium) 410.6 [5th]
prostate 602.8
pulmonary (artery) (hemorrhagic) (vein) 415.19
with
abortion - *see* Abortion, by type, with embolism
ectopic pregnancy (*see also* categories 633.0-633.9) 639.6
molar pregnancy (*see also* categories 630-632) 639.6
following
abortion 639.6
ectopic or molar pregnancy 639.6
iatrogenic 415.11
in pregnancy, childbirth, or puerperium - *see* Embolism, obstetrical
postoperative 415.11
septic 415.12
renal 593.81
embolic or thrombotic 593.81
retina, retinal 362.84
with occlusion - *see* Occlusion, retina
spinal (acute) (cord) (embolic) (nonembolic) 336.1
spleen 289.59
embolic or thrombotic 444.89
subchorionic - *see* Infarct, placenta
subendocardial (*see also* Infarct, myocardium) 410.7 [5th]
suprarenal (capsule) (gland) 255.41
syncytium - *see* Infarct, placenta
testis 608.83
thrombotic (*see also* Thrombosis) 453.9
artery, arterial - *see* Embolism
thyroid (gland) 246.3
ventricle (heart) (*see also* Infarct, myocardium) 410.9 [5th]
Infecting - *see* condition
Infection, infected, infective (opportunistic) 136.9
with lymphangitis - *see* Lymphangitis
abortion - *see* Abortion, by type, with, sepsis
abscess (skin) - *see* Abscess, by site
Absidia 117.7
acanthamoeba 136.21
Acanthocheilonema (perstans) 125.4
streptocerca 125.6
accessory sinus (chronic) (*see also* Sinusitis) 473.9
Achorion - *see* Dermatophytosis
Acremonium falciforme 117.4
acromioclavicular (joint) 711.91
actinobacillus
lignieresii 027.8
mallei 024
muris 026.1
actinomadura - *see* Actinomycosis
Actinomyces (israelii) - *see also* Actinomycosis
muris-ratti 026.1
Actinomycetales (actinomadura) (Actinomyces) (Nocardia) (Streptomyces) - *see* Actinomycosis
actinomycotic NEC (*see also* Actinomycosis) 039.9
adenoid (chronic) 474.01
acute 463
and tonsil (chronic) 474.02
acute or subacute 463

Infection, infected, infective – *continued*
adenovirus NEC 079.0
in diseases classified elsewhere - *see* category 079
unspecified nature or site 079.0
Aerobacter aerogenes NEC 041.85
enteritis 008.2
aerogenes capsulatus (*see also* Gangrene, gas) 040.0
aertrycke (*see also* Infection, Salmonella) 003.9
ajellomyces dermatitidis 116.0
alimentary canal NEC (*see also* Enteritis, due to, by organism) 009.0
Allescheria boydii 117.6
Alternaria 118
alveolus, alveolar (process) (pulpal origin) 522.4
ameba, amebic (histolytica) (*see also* Amebiasis) 006.9
acute 006.0
chronic 006.1
free-living 136.29
hartmanni 007.8
specified
site NEC 006.8
type NEC 007.8
amniotic fluid or cavity 658.4 [5th]
affecting fetus or newborn 762.7
anaerobes (cocci) (gram-negative) (gram-positive) (mixed) NEC 041.84
anal canal 569.49
Ancylostoma braziliense 126.2
angiostrongylus cantonensis 128.8
anisakiasis 127.1
Anisakis larva 127.1
anthrax (*see also* Anthrax) 022.9
antrum (chronic) (*see also* Sinusitis, maxillary) 473.0
anus (papillae) (sphincter) 569.49
arbor virus NEC 066.9
arbovirus NEC 066.9
argentophil-rod 027.0
Ascaris lumbricoides 127.0
ascomycetes 117.4
Aspergillus (flavus) (fumigatus) (terreus) 117.3
atypical
acid-fast (bacilli) (*see also* Mycobacterium, atypical) 031.9
mycobacteria (*see also* Mycobacterium, atypical) 031.9
auditory meatus (circumscribed) (diffuse) (external) (*see also* Otitis, externa) 380.10
auricle (ear) (*see also* Otitis, externa) 380.10
axillary gland 683
Babesiasis 088.82
Babesiosis 088.82
Bacillus NEC 041.89
abortus 023.1
anthracis (*see also* Anthrax) 022.9
cereus (food poisoning) 005.89
coli - *see* Infection, Escherichia coli
coliform NEC 041.85
Ducrey's (any location) 099.0
Flexner's 004.1
Friedländer's NEC 041.3
fusiformis 101
gas (gangrene) (*see also* Gangrene, gas) 040.0
mallei 024
melitensis 023.0
paratyphoid, paratyphosus 002.9
A 002.1
B 002.2
C 002.3
Schmorl's 040.3
Shiga 004.0
suipestifer (*see also* Infection, Salmonella) 003.9
swimming pool 031.1
typhosa 002.0

Infection, infected, infective – *continued*
- Bacillus – *continued*
  - welchii (*see also* Gangrene, gas) 040.0
  - Whitmore's 025
- bacterial NEC 041.9
  - specified NEC 041.89
    - anaerobic NEC 041.84
    - gram-negative NEC 041.85
      - anaerobic NEC 041.84
- Bacterium
  - paratyphosum 002.9
    - A 002.1
    - B 002.2
    - C 002.3
  - typhosum 002.9
- Bacteroides (fragilis) (melaninogenicus) (oralis) NEC 041.82
- balantidium coli 007.0
- Bartholin's gland 616.89
- Basidiobolus 117.7
- Bedsonia 079.98
  - specified NEC 079.88
- bile duct 576.1
- bladder (*see also* Cystitis) 595.9
- Blastomyces, blastomycotic 116.0
  - brasiliensis 116.1
  - dermatitidis 116.0
  - European 117.5
  - loboi 116.2
  - North American 116.0
  - South American 116.1
- bleb
  - postprocedural 379.60
    - stage 1 379.61
    - stage 2 379.62
    - stage 3 379.63
- blood stream - *see also* Septicemia
  - catheter-related (CRBSI) 999.31
- bone 730.9 [5th]
  - specified - *see* Osteomyelitis
- Bordetella 033.9
  - bronchiseptica 033.8
  - parapertussis 033.1
  - pertussis 033.0
- Borrelia
  - bergdorfi 088.81
  - vincentii (mouth) (pharynx) (tonsil) 101
- bovine stomatitis 059.11
- brain (*see also* Encephalitis) 323.9
  - late effect - *see* category 326
  - membranes - (*see also* Meningitis) 322.9
  - septic 324.0
    - late effect - *see* category 326
    - meninges (*see also* Meningitis) 320.9
- branchial cyst 744.42
- breast 611.0
  - puerperal, postpartum 675.2 [5th]
    - with nipple 675.9 [5th]
      - specified type NEC 675.8 [5th]
    - nonpurulent 675.2 [5th]
    - purulent 675.1 [5th]
- bronchus (*see also* Bronchitis) 490
  - fungus NEC 117.9
- Brucella 023.9
  - abortus 023.1
  - canis 023.3
  - melitensis 023.0
  - mixed 023.8
  - suis 023.2
- Brugia (Wuchereria) malayi 125.1
- bursa - *see* Bursitis
- buttocks (skin) 686.9
- Candida (albicans) (tropicalis) (*see also* Candidiasis) 112.9
  - congenital 771.7
- Candiru 136.8
- Capillaria
  - hepatica 128.8
  - philippinensis 127.5
- cartilage 733.99
- cat liver fluke 121.0

Infection, infected, infective – *continued*
- catheter-related bloodstream (CRBSI) 999.31
- cellulitis - *see* Cellulitis, by site
- Cephalosporum falciforme 117.4
- Cercomonas hominis (intestinal) 007.3
- cerebrospinal (*see also* Meningitis) 322.9
  - late effect - *see* category 326
- cervical gland 683
- cervix (*see also* Cervicitis) 616.0
- cesarean section wound 674.3 [5th]
- Chilomastix (intestinal) 007.8
- Chlamydia 079.98
  - specified NEC 079.88
- Cholera (*see also* Cholera) 001.9
- chorionic plate 658.8 [5th]
- Cladosporium
  - bantianum 117.8
  - carrionii 117.2
  - mansoni 111.1
  - trichoides 117.8
  - wernecki 111.1
- Clonorchis (sinensis) (liver) 121.1
- Clostridium (haemolyticum) (novyi) NEC 041.84
  - botulinum 005.1
  - histolyticum (*see also* Gangrene, gas) 040.0
  - oedematiens (*see also* Gangrene, gas) 040.0
  - perfringens 041.83
    - due to food 005.2
  - septicum (*see also* Gangrene, gas) 040.0
  - sordellii (*see also* Gangrene, gas) 040.0
  - welchii (*see also* Gangrene, gas) 040.0
    - due to food 005.2
- Coccidioides (immitis) (*see also* Coccidioidomycosis) 114.9
- coccus NEC 041.89
- colon (*see also* Enteritis, due to, by organism) 009.0
  - bacillus - *see* Infection, Escherichia coli
- colostomy or enterostomy 569.61
- common duct 576.1
- complicating pregnancy, childbirth, or puerperium NEC 647.9 [5th]
  - affecting fetus or newborn 760.2
- Condiobolus 117.7
- congenital NEC 771.89
  - Candida albicans 771.7
  - chronic 771.2
  - Cytomegalovirus 771.1
  - hepatitis, viral 771.2
  - herpes simplex 771.2
  - listeriosis 771.2
  - malaria 771.2
  - poliomyelitis 771.2
  - rubella 771.0
  - toxoplasmosis 771.2
  - tuberculosis 771.2
  - urinary (tract) 771.82
  - vaccinia 771.2
- coronavirus 079.89
  - SARS-associated 079.82
- corpus luteum (*see also* Salpingo-oophoritis) 614.2
- Corynebacterium diphtheriae - *see* Diphtheria
- cotia virus 059.8
- Coxsackie (*see also* Coxsackie) 079.2
  - endocardium 074.22
  - heart NEC 074.20
  - in diseases classified elsewhere - *see* category 079
  - meninges 047.0
  - myocardium 074.23
  - pericardium 074.21
  - pharynx 074.0
  - specified disease NEC 074.8
  - unspecified nature or site 079.2
- Cryptococcus neoformans 117.5
- Cryptosporidia 007.4
- Cunninghamella 117.7
- cyst - *see* Cyst

Infection, infected, infective – *continued*
- Cysticercus cellulosae 123.1
- cytomegalovirus 078.5
  - congenital 771.1
- dental (pulpal origin) 522.4
- deuteromycetes 117.4
- Dicrocoelium dendriticum 121.8
- Dipetalonema (perstans) 125.4
  - streptocerca 125.6
- diphtherial - *see* Diphtheria
- Diphyllobothrium (adult) (latum) (pacificum) 123.4
  - larval 123.5
- Diplogonoporus (grandis) 123.8
- Dipylidium (caninum) 123.8
- Dirofilaria 125.6
- dog tapeworm 123.8
- Dracunculus medinensis 125.7
- Dreschlera 118
  - hawaiiensis 117.8
- Ducrey's bacillus (any site) 099.0
- due to or resulting from
  - central venous catheter 999.31
  - device, implant, or graft (any) (presence of) - *see* Complications, infection and inflammation, due to (presence of) any device, implant, or graft classified to 996.0-996.5 NEC
  - injection, inoculation, infusion, transfusion, or vaccination (prophylactic) (therapeutic) 999.39
  - injury NEC - *see* Wound, open, by site, complicated
  - surgery 998.59
- duodenum 535.6 [5th]
- ear - *see also* Otitis
  - external (*see also* Otitis, externa) 380.10
  - inner (*see also* Labyrinthitis) 386.30
  - middle - *see* Otitis, media
- Eaton's agent NEC 041.81
- Eberthella typhosa 002.0
- Ebola 078.89
- echinococcosis 122.9
- Echinococcus (*see also* Echinococcus) 122.9
- Echinostoma 121.8
- ECHO virus 079.1
  - in diseases classified elsewhere - *see* category 079
  - unspecified nature or site 079.1
- Ehrlichiosis 082.40
  - chaffeensis 082.41
  - specified type NEC 082.49
- Endamoeba - *see* Infection, ameba
- endocardium (*see also* Endocarditis) 421.0
- endocervix (*see also* Cervicitis) 616.0
- Entamoeba - *see* Infection, ameba
- enteric (*see also* Enteritis, due to, by organism) 009.0
- Enterobacter aerogenes NEC 041.85
- Enterobacter sakazakii 041.85
- Enterobius vermicularis 127.4
- enterococcus NEC 041.04
- enterovirus NEC 079.89
  - central nervous system NEC 048
  - enteritis 008.67
  - meningitis 047.9
- Entomophthora 117.7
- Epidermophyton - *see* Dermatophytosis
- epidermophytosis - *see* Dermatophytosis
- episiotomy 674.3 [5th]
- Epstein-Barr virus 075
  - chronic 780.79 *[139.8]*
- erysipeloid 027.1
- Erysipelothrix (insidiosa) (rhusiopathiae) 027.1
- erythema infectiosum 057.0
- Escherichia coli NEC 041.4
  - enteritis - *see* Enteritis, E. coli
  - generalized 038.42
  - intestinal - *see* Enteritis, E. coli

Infection, infected, infective – *continued*
- esophagostomy 530.86
- ethmoidal (chronic) (sinus) (*see also* Sinusitis, ethmoidal) 473.2
- Eubacterium 041.84
- Eustachian tube (ear) 381.50
  - acute 381.51
  - chronic 381.52
- exanthema subitum (*see also* Exanthem subitum) 058.10
- external auditory canal (meatus) (*see also* Otitis, externa) 380.10
- eye NEC 360.00
- eyelid 373.9
  - specified NEC 373.8
- fallopian tube (*see also* Salpingo-oophoritis) 614.2
- fascia 728.89
- Fasciola
  - gigantica 121.3
  - hepatica 121.3
- Fasciolopsis (buski) 121.4
- fetus (intra-amniotic) - *see* Infection, congenital
- filarial - *see* Infestation, filarial
- finger (skin) 686.9
  - abscess (with lymphangitis) 681.00
    - pulp 681.01
  - cellulitis (with lymphangitis) 681.00
  - distal closed space (with lymphangitis) 681.00
  - nail 681.02
    - fungus 110.1
- fish tapeworm 123.4
  - larval 123.5
- flagellate, intestinal 007.9
- fluke - *see* Infestation, fluke
- focal
  - teeth (pulpal origin) 522.4
  - tonsils 474.00
    - and adenoids 474.02
- Fonsecaea
  - compactum 117.2
  - pedrosoi 117.2
- food (*see also* Poisoning, food) 005.9
- foot (skin) 686.9
  - fungus 110.4
- Francisella tularensis (*see also* Tularemia) 021.9
- frontal sinus (chronic) (*see also* Sinusitis, frontal) 473.1
- fungus NEC 117.9
  - beard 110.0
  - body 110.5
  - dermatiacious NEC 117.8
  - foot 110.4
  - groin 110.3
  - hand 110.2
  - nail 110.1
  - pathogenic to compromised host only 118
  - perianal (area) 110.3
  - scalp 110.0
  - scrotum 110.8
  - skin 111.9
    - foot 110.4
    - hand 110.2
  - toenails 110.1
  - trachea 117.9
- Fusarium 118
- Fusobacterium 041.84
- gallbladder (*see also* Cholecystitis, acute) 575.0
- Gardnerella vaginalis 041.89
- gas bacillus (*see also* Gas, gangrene) 040.0
- gastric (*see also* Gastritis) 535.5 [5th]
- Gastrodiscoides hominis 121.8
- gastroenteric (*see also* Enteritis, due to, by organism) 009.0
- gastrointestinal (*see also* Enteritis, due to, by organism) 009.0
- gastrostomy 536.41
- generalized NEC (*see also* Septicemia) 038.9

Infection, infected, infective – *continued*
- Petriellidium boydii 117.6
- pharynx 478.29
  - Coxsackie virus 074.0
  - phlegmonous 462
  - posterior, lymphoid 474.00
- Phialophora
  - gougerotii 117.8
  - jeanselmei 117.8
  - verrucosa 117.2
- Piedraia hortai 111.3
- pinna, acute 380.11
- pinta 103.9
  - intermediate 103.1
  - late 103.2
  - mixed 103.3
  - primary 103.0
- pinworm 127.4
- pityrosporum furfur 111.0
- pleuropneumonia-like organisms NEC (PPLO) 041.81
- pneumococcal NEC 041.2
  - generalized (purulent) 038.2
- Pneumococcus NEC 041.2
- postoperative wound 998.59
- posttraumatic NEC 958.3
- postvaccinal 999.39
- poxvirus 059.9
  - specified NEC 059.8
- prepuce NEC 607.1
- Proprionibacterium 041.84
- prostate (capsule) (*see also* Prostatitis) 601.9
- Proteus (mirabilis) (morganii) (vulgaris) NEC 041.6
  - enteritis 008.3
- protozoal NEC 136.8
  - intestinal NEC 007.9
- Pseudomonas NEC 041.7
  - mallei 024
  - pneumonia 482.1
  - pseudomallei 025
- psittacosis 073.9
- puerperal, postpartum (major) 670.0 [5th] ▲
  - minor 646.6 [5th]
- pulmonary - *see* Infection, lung
- purulent - *see* Abscess
- putrid, generalized - *see* Septicemia
- pyemic - *see* Septicemia
- Pyrenochaeta romeroi 117.4
- Q fever 083.0
- rabies 071
- rectum (sphincter) 569.49
- renal (*see also* Infection, kidney) 590.9
  - pelvis and ureter 590.3
- resistant to drugs - *see* Resistance (to), drugs by microorganisms
- respiratory 519.8
  - chronic 519.8
  - influenzal (acute) (upper) 487.1
  - lung 518.89
  - rhinovirus 460
  - syncytial virus 079.6
  - upper (acute) (infectious) NEC 465.9
    - with flu, grippe, or influenza 487.1
    - influenzal 487.1
    - multiple sites NEC 465.8
    - streptococcal 034.0
    - viral NEC 465.9
- respiratory syncytial virus (RSV) 079.6
- resulting from presence of shunt or other internal prosthetic device - *see* Complications, infection and inflammation, due to (presence of) any device, implant, or graft classified to 996.0-996.5 NEC
- retroperitoneal 567.39
- retrovirus 079.50
  - human immunodeficiency virus type 2 [HIV 2] 079.53
  - human T-cell lymphotrophic virus type I [HTLV-I] 079.51

Infection, infected, infective – *continued*
- retrovirus – *continued*
  - human T-cell lymphotrophic virus type II [HTLV-II] 079.52
  - specified NEC 079.59
- Rhinocladium 117.1
- Rhinosporidium (seeberi) 117.0
- rhinovirus
  - in diseases classified elsewhere - *see* category 079
  - unspecified nature or site 079.3
- Rhizopus 117.7
- rickettsial 083.9
- rickettsialpox 083.2
- rubella (*see also* Rubella) 056.9
  - congenital 771.0
- Saccharomyces (*see also* Candidiasis) 112.9
- Saksenaea 117.7
- salivary duct or gland (any) 527.2
- Salmonella (aertrycke) (callinarum) (choleraesuis) (enteritidis) (suipestifer) (typhimurium) 003.9
  - with
    - arthritis 003.23
    - gastroenteritis 003.0
    - localized infection 003.20
      - specified type NEC 003.29
    - meningitis 003.21
    - osteomyelitis 003.24
    - pneumonia 003.22
    - septicemia 003.1
    - specified manifestation NEC 003.8
  - due to food (poisoning) (any serotype) (*see also* Poisoning, food, due to, Salmonella)
  - hirschfeldii 002.3
  - localized 003.20
    - specified type NEC 003.29
  - paratyphi 002.9
    - A 002.1
    - B 002.2
    - C 002.3
  - schottmuelleri 002.2
  - specified type NEC 003.8
  - typhi 002.0
  - typhosa 002.0
- saprophytic 136.8
- Sarcocystis, lindemanni 136.5
- SARS-associated coronavirus 079.82
- scabies 133.0
- Schistosoma - *see* Infestation, Schistosoma
- Schmorl's bacillus 040.3
- scratch or other superficial injury - *see* Injury, superficial, by site
- scrotum (acute) NEC 608.4
- sealpox 059.12
- secondary, burn or open wound (dislocation) (fracture) 958.3
- seminal vesicle (*see also* Vesiculitis) 608.0
- septic
  - generalized - *see* Septicemia
  - localized, skin (*see also* Abscess) 682.9
- septicemic - *see* Septicemia
- seroma 998.51
- Serratia (marcescens) 041.85
  - generalized 038.44
- sheep liver fluke 121.3
- Shigella 004.9
  - boydii 004.2
  - dysenteriae 004.0
  - Flexneri 004.1
  - group
    - A 004.0
    - B 004.1
    - C 004.2
    - D 004.3
  - Schmitz (-Stutzer) 004.0
  - Schmitzii 004.0
  - Shiga 004.0
  - Sonnei 004.3
  - specified type NEC 004.8
- Sin Nombre virus 079.81

Infection, infected, infective – *continued*
- sinus (*see also* Sinusitis) 473.9
  - pilonidal 685.1
    - with abscess 685.0
  - skin NEC 686.9
- Skene's duct or gland (*see also* Urethritis) 597.89
- skin (local) (staphylococcal) (streptococcal) NEC 686.9
  - abscess - *see* Abscess, by site
  - cellulitis - *see* Cellulitis, by site
  - due to fungus 111.9
    - specified type NEC 111.8
  - mycotic 111.9
    - specified type NEC 111.8
  - ulcer (*see also* Ulcer, skin) 707.9
- slow virus 046.9
  - specified condition NEC 046.8
- Sparganum (mansoni) (proliferum) 123.5
- spermatic cord NEC 608.4
- sphenoidal (chronic) (sinus) (*see also* Sinusitis, sphenoidal) 473.3
- Spherophorus necrophorus 040.3
- spinal cord NEC (*see also* Encephalitis) 323.9
  - abscess 324.1
    - late effect - *see* category 326
  - late effect - *see* category 326
  - meninges - *see* Meningitis
  - streptococcal 320.2
- Spirillum
  - minus or minor 026.0
  - morsus muris 026.0
  - obermeieri 087.0
- spirochetal NEC 104.9
  - lung 104.8
  - specified nature or site NEC 104.8
- spleen 289.59
- Sporothrix schenckii 117.1
- Sporotrichum (schenckii) 117.1
- Sporozoa 136.8
- staphylococcal NEC 041.10
  - aureus 041.11
    - methicillin
      - resistant (MRSA) 041.12
      - susceptible MSSA) 041.11
  - food poisoning 005.0
  - generalized (purulent) 038.10
    - aureus 038.11
      - methicillin
        - resistant 038.12
        - susceptible 038.11
    - specified organism NEC 038.19
  - pneumonia 482.40
    - aureus 482.41
      - methicillin
        - resistant (MRSA) 482.42
        - susceptible (MSSA) 482.41
    - MRSA (methicillin resistant staphylococcus aureus) 482.42
    - MSSA (methicillin susceptible staphylococcus aureus) 482.41
    - specified type NEC 482.49
  - septicemia 038.10
    - aureus 038.11
      - methicillin
        - resistant (MRSA) 038.12
        - susceptible (MSSA) 038.11
    - MRSA (methicillin resistant staphylococcus aureus) 038.12
    - MSSA (methicillin susceptible staphylococcus aureus) 038.11
    - specified organism NEC 038.19
  - specified NEC 041.19
- steatoma 706.2
- Stellantchasmus falcatus 121.6
- Streptobacillus moniliformis 026.1
- streptococcal NEC 041.00
  - generalized (purulent) 038.0

Infection, infected, infective – *continued*
- streptococcal – *continued*
  - group
    - A 041.01
    - B 041.02
    - C 041.03
    - D [enterococcus] 041.04
    - G 041.05
  - pneumonia - *see* Pneumonia, streptococcal
  - septicemia 038.0
  - sore throat 034.0
  - specified NEC 041.09
- Streptomyces - *see* Actinomycosis
- streptotrichosis - *see* Actinomycosis
- Strongyloides (stercoralis) 127.2
- stump (amputation) (posttraumatic) (surgical) 997.62
  - traumatic - *see* Amputation, traumatic, by site, complicated
- subcutaneous tissue, local NEC 686.9
- submaxillary region 528.9
- suipestifer (*see also* Infection, Salmonella) 003.9
- swimming pool bacillus 031.1
- syphilitic - *see* Syphilis
- systemic - *see* Septicemia
- Taenia - *see* Infestation, Taenia
- Taeniarhynchus saginatus 123.2
- tanapox 059.21
- tapeworm - *see* Infestation, tapeworm
- tendon (sheath) 727.89
- Ternidens diminutus 127.7
- testis (*see also* Orchitis) 604.90
- thigh (skin) 686.9
- threadworm 127.4
- throat 478.29
  - pneumococcal 462
  - staphylococcal 462
  - streptococcal 034.0
  - viral NEC (*see also* Pharyngitis) 462
- thumb (skin) 686.9
  - abscess (with lymphangitis) 681.00
    - pulp 681.01
  - cellulitis (with lymphangitis) 681.00
  - nail 681.02
- thyroglossal duct 529.8
- toe (skin) 686.9
  - abscess (with lymphangitis) 681.10
  - cellulitis (with lymphangitis) 681.10
  - nail 681.11
    - fungus 110.1
- tongue NEC 529.0
  - parasitic 112.0
- tonsil (faucial) (lingual) (pharyngeal) 474.00
  - acute or subacute 463
  - and adenoid 474.02
  - tag 474.00
- tooth, teeth 522.4
  - periapical (pulpal origin) 522.4
  - peridental 523.30
  - periodontal 523.31
  - pulp 522.0
  - socket 526.5
- TORCH - *see* Infection, congenital NEC
  - without active infection 760.2
- Torula histolytica 117.5
- Toxocara (cani) (cati) (felis) 128.0
- Toxoplasma gondii (*see also* Toxoplasmosis) 130.9
- trachea, chronic 491.8
  - fungus 117.9
- traumatic NEC 958.3
- trematode NEC 121.9
- trench fever 083.1
- Treponema
  - denticola 041.84
  - macrodenticum 041.84
  - pallidum (*see also* Syphilis) 097.9
- Trichinella (spiralis) 124
- Trichomonas 131.9
  - bladder 131.09
  - cervix 131.09

Infection, infected, infective – *continued*
- Trichomonas – *continued*
  - hominis 007.3
  - intestine 007.3
  - prostate 131.03
  - specified site NEC 131.8
  - urethra 131.02
  - urogenitalis 131.00
  - vagina 131.01
  - vulva 131.01
- Trichophyton, trichophytid - *see* Dermatophytosis
- Trichosporon (beigelii) cutaneum 111.2
- Trichostrongylus 127.6
- Trichuris (trichiuria) 127.3
- Trombicula (irritans) 133.8
- Trypanosoma (*see also* Trypanosomiasis) 086.9
  - cruzi 086.2
- tubal (*see also* Salpingo-oophoritis) 614.2
- tuberculous NEC (*see also* Tuberculosis) 011.9 [5th]
- tubo-ovarian (*see also* Salpingo-oophoritis) 614.2
- tunica vaginalis 608.4
- tympanic membrane - *see* Myringitis
- typhoid (abortive) (ambulant) (bacillus) 002.0
- typhus 081.9
  - flea-borne (endemic) 081.0
  - louse-borne (epidemic) 080
  - mite-borne 081.2
  - recrudescent 081.1
  - tick-borne 082.9
    - African 082.1
    - North Asian 082.2
- umbilicus (septic) 686.9
  - newborn NEC 771.4
- ureter 593.89
- urethra (*see also* Urethritis) 597.80
- urinary (tract) NEC 599.0
  - with
    - abortion - *see* Abortion, by type, with urinary tract infection
    - ectopic pregnancy (*see also* categories 633.0-633.9) 639.8
    - molar pregnancy (*see also* categories 630-632) 639.8
  - candidal 112.2
  - complicating pregnancy, childbirth, or puerperium 646.6 [5th]
    - affecting fetus or newborn 760.1
  - asymptomatic 646.5 [5th]
    - affecting fetus or newborn 760.1
  - diplococcal (acute) 098.0
    - chronic 098.2
  - due to Trichomonas (vaginalis) 131.00
  - following
    - abortion 639.8
    - ectopic or molar pregnancy 639.8
  - gonococcal (acute) 098.0
    - chronic or duration of 2 months or over 098.2
  - newborn 771.82
  - trichomonal 131.00
  - tuberculous (*see also* Tuberculosis) 016.3 [5th]
- uterus, uterine (*see also* Endometritis) 615.9
- utriculus masculinus NEC 597.89
- vaccination 999.39
- vagina (granulation tissue) (wall) (*see also* Vaginitis) 616.10
- varicella 052.9
- varicose veins - *see* Varicose, veins
- variola 050.9
  - major 050.0
  - minor 050.1
- vas deferens NEC 608.4
- Veillonella 041.84
- verumontanum 597.89
- vesical (*see also* Cystitis) 595.9

Infection, infected, infective – *continued*
- Vibrio
  - cholerae 001.0
    - El Tor 001.1
  - parahaemolyticus (food poisoning) 005.4
  - vulnificus 041.85
- Vincent's (gums) (mouth) (tonsil) 101
- virus, viral 079.99
  - adenovirus
    - in diseases classified elsewhere - *see* category 079
    - unspecified nature or site 079.0
  - central nervous system NEC 049.9
    - enterovirus 048
      - meningitis 047.9
        - specified type NEC 047.8
    - slow virus 046.9
      - specified condition NEC 046.8
  - chest 519.8
  - conjunctivitis 077.99
    - specified type NEC 077.89
  - coronavirus 079.89
    - SARS-associated 079.82
  - Coxsackie (*see also* Infection, Coxsackie) 079.2
  - Ebola 065.8
  - ECHO
    - in diseases classified elsewhere - *see* category 079
    - unspecified nature or site 079.1
  - encephalitis 049.9
    - arthropod-borne NEC 064
    - tick-borne 063.9
      - specified type NEC 063.8
  - enteritis NEC (*see also* Enteritis, viral) 008.8
  - exanthem NEC 057.9
  - Hantavirus 079.81
  - human papilloma 079.4
  - in diseases classified elsewhere - *see* category 079
  - intestine (*see also* Enteritis, viral) 008.8
  - Lung - *see* Pneumonia, viral
  - respiratory syncytial (RSV) 079.6
  - Retrovirus 079.50
  - rhinovirus
    - in diseases classified elsewhere - *see* category 079
    - unspecified nature or site 079.3
  - salivary gland disease 078.5
  - slow 046.9
    - specified condition NEC 046.8
  - specified type NEC 079.89
    - in diseases classified elsewhere - *see* category 079
  - unspecified nature or site 079.99
  - warts 078.10
    - specified NEC 078.19
  - yaba monkey tumor 059.22
- vulva (*see also* Vulvitis) 616.10
- whipworm 127.3
- Whitmore's bacillus 025
- wound (local) (posttraumatic) NEC 958.3
  - with
    - dislocation - *see* Dislocation, by site, open
    - fracture - *see* Fracture, by site, open
    - open wound - *see* Wound, open, by site, complicated
  - postoperative 998.59
  - surgical 998.59
- Wuchereria 125.0
  - bancrofti 125.0
  - malayi 125.1
- yaba monkey tumor virus 059.22
- yatapoxvirus 059.20
- yaws - *see* Yaws
- yeast (*see also* Candidiasis) 112.9
- yellow fever (*see also* Fever, yellow) 060.9
- Yersinia pestis (*see also* Plague) 020.9
- Zeis' gland 373.12
- zoonotic bacterial NEC 027.9
- Zopfia senegalensis 117.4

Infective, infectious - *see* condition

Inferiority complex 301.9
- constitutional psychopathic 301.9

Infertility
- female 628.9
  - age related 628.8
  - associated with
    - adhesions, peritubal 614.6 *[628.2]*
    - anomaly
      - cervical mucus 628.4
      - congenital
        - cervix 628.4
        - fallopian tube 628.2
        - uterus 628.3
        - vagina 628.4
    - anovulation 628.0
    - dysmucorrhea 628.4
    - endometritis, tuberculous (*see also* Tuberculosis) 016.7 [5th] *[628.3]*
    - Stein-Leventhal syndrome 256.4 *[628.0]*
  - due to
    - adiposogenital dystrophy 253.8 *[628.1]*
    - anterior pituitary disorder NEC 253.4 *[628.1]*
      - hyperfunction 253.1 *[628.1]*
    - cervical anomaly 628.4
    - fallopian tube anomaly 628.2
    - ovarian failure 256.39 *[628.0]*
    - Stein-Leventhal syndrome 256.4 *[628.0]*
    - uterine anomaly 628.3
    - vaginal anomaly 628.4
  - nonimplantation 628.3
  - origin
    - cervical 628.4
    - pituitary-hypothalamus NEC 253.8 *[628.1]*
      - anterior pituitary NEC 253.4 *[628.1]*
        - hyperfunction NEC 253.1 *[628.1]*
      - dwarfism 253.3 *[628.1]*
      - panhypopituitarism 253.2 *[628.1]*
    - specified NEC 628.8
    - tubal (block) (occlusion) (stenosis) 628.2
      - adhesions 614.6 *[628.2]*
    - uterine 628.3
    - vaginal 628.4
  - previous, requiring supervision of pregnancy V23.0
- male 606.9
  - absolute 606.0
  - due to
    - azoospermia 606.0
    - drug therapy 606.8
    - extratesticular cause NEC 606.8
    - germinal cell
      - aplasia 606.0
      - desquamation 606.1
    - hypospermatogenesis 606.1
    - infection 606.8
    - obstruction, afferent ducts 606.8
    - oligospermia 606.1
    - radiation 606.8
    - spermatogenic arrest (complete) 606.0
      - incomplete 606.1
    - systemic disease 606.8

Infestation 134.9
- Acanthocheilonema (perstans) 125.4
  - streptocerca 125.6
- Acariasis 133.9
  - demodex folliculorum 133.8
  - sarcoptes scabiei 133.0
  - trombiculae 133.8
- Agamofilaria streptocerca 125.6
- Ancylostoma, Ankylostoma 126.9
  - americanum 126.1
  - braziliense 126.2

Infestation – *continued*
- Ancylostoma, Ankylostoma – *continued*
  - canium 126.8
  - ceylanicum 126.3
  - duodenale 126.0
  - new world 126.1
  - old world 126.0
- Angiostrongylus cantonensis 128.8
- anisakiasis 127.1
- Anisakis larva 127.1
- arthropod NEC 134.1
- Ascaris lumbricoides 127.0
- Bacillus fusiformis 101
- Balantidium coli 007.0
- beef tapeworm 123.2
- Bothriocephalus (latus) 123.4
  - larval 123.5
- broad tapeworm 123.4
  - larval 123.5
- Brugia malayi 125.1
- Candiru 136.8
- Capillaria
  - hepatica 128.8
  - philippinensis 127.5
- cat liver fluke 121.0
- Cercomonas hominis (intestinal) 007.3
- cestodes 123.9
  - specified type NEC 123.8
- chigger 133.8
- chigoe 134.1
- Chilomastix 007.8
- Clonorchis (sinensis) (liver) 121.1
- coccidia 007.2
- complicating pregnancy, childbirth, or puerperium 647.9 [5th]
  - affecting fetus or newborn 760.8
- Cysticercus cellulosae 123.1
- Demodex folliculorum 133.8
- Dermatobia (hominis) 134.0
- Dibothriocephalus (latus) 123.4
  - larval 123.5
- Dicrocoelium dendriticum 121.8
- Diphyllobothrium (adult) (intestinal) (latum) (pacificum) 123.4
  - larval 123.5
- Diplogonoporus (grandis) 123.8
- Dipylidium (caninum) 123.8
- Distoma hepaticum 121.3
- dog tapeworm 123.8
- Dracunculus medinensis 125.7
- dragon worm 125.7
- dwarf tapeworm 123.6
- Echinococcus (*see also* Echinococcus) 122.9
- Echinostoma ilocanum 121.8
- Embadomonas 007.8
- Endamoeba (histolytica) - *see* Infection, ameba
- Entamoeba (histolytica) - *see* Infection, ameba
- Enterobius vermicularis 127.4
- Epidermophyton - *see* Dermatophytosis
- eyeworm 125.2
- Fasciola
  - gigantica 121.3
  - hepatica 121.3
- Fasciolopsis (buski) (small intestine) 121.4
- filarial 125.9
  - due to
    - acanthocheilonema (perstans) 125.4
      - streptocerca 125.6
    - Brugia (Wuchereria) malayi 125.1
    - Dracunculus medinensis 125.7
    - guinea worms 125.7
    - Mansonella (ozzardi) 125.5
    - Onchocerca volvulus 125.3
      - eye 125.3 *[360.13]*
      - eyelid 125.3 *[373.6]*
    - Wuchereria (bancrofti) 125.0
      - malayi 125.1
  - specified type NEC 125.6
- fish tapeworm 123.4
  - larval 123.5

Infestation – *continued*
- fluke 121.9
  - blood NEC (*see also* Schistosomiasis) 120.9
  - cat liver 121.0
  - intestinal (giant) 121.4
  - liver (sheep) 121.3
    - cat 121.0
    - Chinese 121.1
    - clonorchiasis 121.1
    - fascioliasis 121.3
    - oriental 121.1
  - lung (oriental) 121.2
  - sheep liver 121.3
- fly larva 134.0
- Gasterophilus (intestinalis) 134.0
- Gastrodiscoides hominis 121.8
- Giardia lamblia 007.1
- Gnathostoma (spinigerum) 128.1
- Gongylonema 125.6
- guinea worm 125.7
- helminth NEC 128.9
  - intestinal 127.9
    - mixed (types classifiable to more than one category in 120.0-127.7) 127.8
    - specified type NEC 127.7
  - specified type NEC 128.8
- Heterophyes heterophyes (small intestine) 121.6
- hookworm (*see also* Infestation, ancylostoma) 126.9
- Hymenolepis (diminuta) (nana) 123.6
- intestinal NEC 129
- leeches (aquatic) (land) 134.2
- Leishmania - *see* Leishmaniasis
- lice (*see also* infestation, pediculus) 132.9
- Linguatulidae, linguatula (pentastoma) (serrata) 134.1
- Loa loa 125.2
  - eyelid 125.2 *[373.6]*
- louse (*see also* Infestation, pediculus) 132.9
  - body 132.1
  - head 132.0
  - pubic 132.2
- maggots 134.0
- Mansonella (ozzardi) 125.5
- medina 125.7
- Metagonimus yokogawai (small intestine) 121.5
- Microfilaria streptocerca 125.3
  - eye 125.3 *[360.13]*
  - eyelid 125.3 *[373.6]*
- Microsporon furfur 111.0
- microsporum - *see* Dermatophytosis
- mites 133.9
  - scabic 133.0
  - specified type NEC 133.8
- monilia (albicans) (*see also* Candidiasis) 112.9
  - vagina 112.1
  - vulva 112.1
- mouth 112.0
- Necator americanus 126.1
- nematode (intestinal) 127.9
  - Ancylostoma (*see also* Ancylostoma) 126.9
  - Ascaris lumbricoides 127.0
  - conjunctiva NEC 128.9
  - Dioctophyma 128.8
  - Enterobius vermicularis 127.4
  - Gnathostoma spinigerum 128.1
  - Oesophagostomum (apiostomum) 127.7
  - Physaloptera 127.4
  - specified type NEC 127.7
  - Strongyloides stercoralis 127.2
  - Ternidens diminutus 127.7
  - Trichinella spiralis 124
  - Trichostrongylus 127.6
  - Trichuris (trichiuria) 127.3
- Oesophagostomum (apiostomum) 127.7
- Oestrus ovis 134.0

Infestation – *continued*
- Onchocerca (volvulus) 125.3
  - eye 125.3 *[360.13]*
  - eyelid 125.3 *[373.6]*
- Opisthorchis (felineus) (tenuicollis) (viverrini) 121.0
- Oxyuris vermicularis 127.4
- Paragonimus (westermani) 121.2
- parasite, parasitic NEC 136.9
  - eyelid 134.9 *[373.6]*
  - intestinal 129
  - mouth 112.0
  - orbit 376.13
  - skin 134.9
  - tongue 112.0
- pediculus 132.9
  - capitis (humanus) (any site) 132.0
  - corporis (humanus) (any site) 132.1
  - eyelid 132.0 *[373.6]*
  - mixed (classifiable to more than one category in 132.0-132.2) 132.3
  - pubis (any site) 132.2
- phthirus (pubis) (any site) 132.2
  - with any infestation classifiable to 132.0 and 132.1 132.3
- pinworm 127.4
- pork tapeworm (adult) 123.0
- protozoal NEC 136.8
- pubic louse 132.2
- rat tapeworm 123.6
- red bug 133.8
- roundworm (large) NEC 127.0
- sand flea 134.1
- saprophytic NEC 136.8
- Sarcoptes scabiei 133.0
- scabies 133.0
- Schistosoma 120.9
  - bovis 120.8
  - cercariae 120.3
  - hematobium 120.0
  - intercalatum 120.8
  - japonicum 120.2
  - mansoni 120.1
  - mattheii 120.8
  - specified
    - site - *see* Schistosomiasis
    - type NEC 120.8
  - spindale 120.8
- screw worms 134.0
- skin NEC 134.9
- Sparganum (mansoni) (proliferum) 123.5
  - larval 123.5
- specified type NEC 134.8
- Spirometra larvae 123.5
- Sporozoa NEC 136.8
- Stellantchasmus falcatus 121.6
- Strongyloides 127.2
- Strongylus (gibsoni) 127.7
- Taenia 123.3
  - diminuta 123.6
  - Echinococcus (*see also* Echinococcus) 122.9
  - mediocanellata 123.2
  - nana 123.6
  - saginata (mediocanellata) 123.2
  - solium (intestinal form) 123.0
    - larval form 123.1
- Taeniarhynchus saginatus 123.2
- tapeworm 123.9
  - beef 123.2
  - broad 123.4
    - larval 123.5
  - dog 123.8
  - dwarf 123.6
  - fish 123.4
    - larval 123.5
  - pork 123.0
  - rat 123.6
- Ternidens diminutus 127.7
- Tetranychus molestissimus 133.8
- threadworm 127.4
- tongue 112.0
- Toxocara (cani) (cati) (felis) 128.0
- trematode(s) NEC 121.9

Infestation – *continued*
- Trichina spiralis 124
- Trichinella spiralis 124
- Trichocephalus 127.3
- Trichomonas 131.9
  - bladder 131.09
  - cervix 131.09
  - intestine 007.3
  - prostate 131.03
  - specified site NEC 131.8
  - urethra (female) (male) 131.02
  - urogenital 131.00
  - vagina 131.01
  - vulva 131.01
- Trichophyton - *see* Dermatophytosis
- Trichostrongylus instabilis 127.6
- Trichuris (trichiuria) 127.3
- Trombicula (irritans) 133.8
- Trypanosoma - *see* Trypanosomiasis
- Tunga penetrans 134.1
- Uncinaria americana 126.1
- whipworm 127.3
- worms NEC 128.9
  - intestinal 127.9
- Wuchereria 125.0
  - bancrofti 125.0
  - malayi 125.1

Infiltrate, infiltration
- with an iron compound 275.0
- amyloid (any site) (generalized) 277.39
- calcareous (muscle) NEC 275.49
  - localized - *see* Degeneration, by site
- calcium salt (muscle) 275.49
- chemotherapy, vesicant 999.81 ▲
- corneal (*see also* Edema, cornea) 371.20
- eyelid 373.9
- fatty (diffuse) (generalized) 272.8
  - localized - *see* Degeneration, by site, fatty
- glycogen, glycogenic (*see also* Disease, glycogen storage) 271.0
- heart, cardiac
  - fatty (*see also* Degeneration, myocardial) 429.1
  - glycogenic 271.0 *[425.7]*
- inflammatory in vitreous 379.29
- kidney (*see also* Disease, renal) 593.9
- leukemic (M9800/3) - *see* Leukemia
- liver 573.8
  - fatty - *see* Fatty, liver
  - glycogen (*see also* Disease, glycogen storage) 271.0
- lung (*see also* Infiltrate, pulmonary) 518.3
  - eosinophilic 518.3
  - x-ray finding only 793.1
- lymphatic (*see also* Leukemia, lymphatic) 204.9 5th
  - gland, pigmentary 289.3
- muscle, fatty 728.9
- myelogenous (*see also* Leukemia, myeloid) 205.9 5th
- myocardium, myocardial
  - fatty (*see also* Degeneration, myocardial) 429.1
  - glycogenic 271.0 *[425.7]*
- pulmonary 518.3
  - with
    - eosinophilia 518.3
    - pneumonia - *see* Pneumonia, by type
    - x-ray finding only 793.1
  - Ranke's primary (*see also* Tuberculosis) 010.0 5th
- skin, lymphocytic (benign) 709.8
- thymus (gland) (fatty) 254.8
- urine 788.8
- vitreous humor 379.29

Infirmity 799.89
- senile 797

Inflammation, inflamed, inflammatory (with exudation)
- abducens (nerve) 378.54
- accessory sinus (chronic) (*see also* Sinusitis) 473.9

Inflammation, inflamed, inflammatory – *continued*
- adrenal (gland) 255.8
- alimentary canal - *see* Enteritis
- alveoli (teeth) 526.5
  - scorbutic 267
- amnion - *see* Amnionitis
- anal canal 569.49
- antrum (chronic) (*see also* Sinusitis, maxillary) 473.0
- anus 569.49
- appendix (*see also* Appendicitis) 541
- arachnoid - *see* Meningitis
- areola 611.0
  - puerperal, postpartum 675.0 5th
- areolar tissue NEC 686.9
- artery - *see* Arteritis
- auditory meatus (external) (*see also* Otitis, externa) 380.10
- Bartholin's gland 616.89
- bile duct or passage 576.1
- bladder (*see also* Cystitis) 595.9
- bleb
  - postprocedural 379.60
    - stage 1 379.61
    - stage 2 379.62
    - stage 3 379.63
- bone - *see* Osteomyelitis
- bowel (*see also* Enteritis) 558.9
- brain (*see also* Encephalitis) 323.9
  - late effect - *see* category 326
  - membrane - *see* Meningitis
- breast 611.0
  - puerperal, postpartum 675.2 5th
- broad ligament (*see also* Disease, pelvis, inflammatory) 614.4
  - acute 614.3
- bronchus - *see* Bronchitis
- bursa - *see* Bursitis
- capsule
  - liver 573.3
  - spleen 289.59
- catarrhal (*see also* Catarrh) 460
  - vagina 616.10
- cecum (*see also* Appendicitis) 541
- cerebral (*see also* Encephalitis) 323.9
  - late effect - *see* category 326
  - membrane - *see* Meningitis
- cerebrospinal (*see also* Meningitis) 322.9
  - late effect - *see* category 326
  - meningococcal 036.0
  - tuberculous (*see also* Tuberculosis) 013.6 5th
- cervix (uteri) (*see also* Cervicitis) 616.0
- chest 519.9
- choroid NEC (*see also* Choroiditis) 363.20
- cicatrix (tissue) - *see* Cicatrix
- colon (*see also* Enteritis) 558.9
  - granulomatous 555.1
  - newborn 558.9
- connective tissue (diffuse) NEC 728.9
- cornea (*see also* Keratitis) 370.9
  - with ulcer (*see also* Ulcer, cornea) 370.00
- corpora cavernosa (penis) 607.2
- cranial nerve - *see* Disorder, nerve, cranial
- diarrhea - *see* Diarrhea
- disc (intervertebral) (space) 722.90
  - cervical, cervicothoracic 722.91
  - lumbar, lumbosacral 722.93
  - thoracic, thoracolumbar 722.92
- Douglas' cul-de-sac or pouch (chronic) (*see also* Disease, pelvis, inflammatory) 614.4
  - acute 614.3
- due to (presence of) any device, implant, or graft classifiable to 996.0-996.5 - *see* Complications, infection and inflammation, due to (presence of) any device, implant, or graft classified to 996.0-996.5 NEC
- duodenum 535.6 5th
- dura mater - *see* Meningitis

Infestation – Inflammation, inflamed, inflammatory

- **Inflammation, inflamed, inflammatory** – *continued*
  - ear - *see also* Otitis
    - external (*see also* Otitis, externa) 380.10
    - inner (*see also* Labyrinthitis) 386.30
    - middle - *see* Otitis media
  - esophagus 530.10
  - ethmoidal (chronic) (sinus) (*see also* Sinusitis, ethmoidal) 473.2
  - Eustachian tube (catarrhal) 381.50
    - acute 381.51
    - chronic 381.52
  - extrarectal 569.49
  - eye 379.99
  - eyelid 373.9
    - specified NEC 373.8
  - fallopian tube (*see also* Salpingo-oophoritis) 614.2
  - fascia 728.9
  - fetal membranes (acute) 658.4 5th
    - affecting fetus or newborn 762.7
  - follicular, pharynx 472.1
  - frontal (chronic) (sinus) (*see also* Sinusitis, frontal) 473.1
  - gallbladder (*see also* Cholecystitis, acute) 575.0
  - gall duct (*see also* Cholecystitis) 575.10
  - gastrointestinal (*see also* Enteritis) 558.9
  - genital organ (diffuse) (internal)
    - female 614.9
      - with
        - abortion - *see* Abortion, by type, with sepsis
        - ectopic pregnancy (*see also* categories 633.0-633.9) 639.0
        - molar pregnancy (*see also* categories 630-632) 639.0
      - complicating pregnancy, childbirth, or puerperium 646.6 5th
        - affecting fetus or newborn 760.8
      - following
        - abortion 639.0
        - ectopic or molar pregnancy 639.0
    - male 608.4
  - gland (lymph) (*see also* Lymphadenitis) 289.3
  - glottis (*see also* Laryngitis) 464.00
    - with obstruction 464.01
  - granular, pharynx 472.1
  - gum 523.10
  - heart (*see also* Carditis) 429.89
  - hepatic duct 576.8
  - hernial sac - *see* Hernia, by site
  - ileum (*see also* Enteritis) 558.9
    - terminal or regional 555.0
      - with large intestine 555.2
  - intervertebral disc 722.90
    - cervical, cervicothoracic 722.91
    - lumbar, lumbosacral 722.93
    - thoracic, thoracolumbar 722.92
  - intestine (*see also* Enteritis) 558.9
  - jaw (acute) (bone) (chronic) (lower) (suppurative) (upper) 526.4
  - jejunum - *see* Enteritis
  - joint NEC (*see also* Arthritis) 716.9 5th
    - sacroiliac 720.2
  - kidney (*see also* Nephritis) 583.9
  - knee (joint) 716.66
    - tuberculous (active) (*see also* Tuberculosis) 015.2 5th
  - labium (majus) (minus) (*see also* Vulvitis) 616.10
  - lacrimal
    - gland (*see also* Dacryoadenitis) 375.00
    - passages (duct) (sac) (*see also* Dacryocystitis) 375.30
  - larynx (*see also* Laryngitis) 464.00
    - with obstruction 464.01
    - diphtheritic 032.3
  - leg NEC 686.9
  - lip 528.5
  - liver (capsule) (*see also* Hepatitis) 573.3
    - acute 570
    - chronic 571.40
    - suppurative 572.0
  - lung (acute) (*see also* Pneumonia) 486
    - chronic (interstitial) 518.89
  - lymphatic vessel (*see also* Lymphangitis) 457.2
  - lymph node or gland (*see also* Lymphadenitis) 289.3
  - mammary gland 611.0
    - puerperal, postpartum 675.2 5th
  - maxilla, maxillary 526.4
    - sinus (chronic) (*see also* Sinusitis, maxillary) 473.0
  - membranes of brain or spinal cord - *see* Meningitis
  - meninges - *see* Meningitis
  - mouth 528.00
  - muscle 728.9
  - myocardium (*see also* Myocarditis) 429.0
  - nasal sinus (chronic) (*see also* Sinusitis) 473.9
  - nasopharynx - *see* Nasopharyngitis
  - navel 686.9
    - newborn NEC 771.4
  - nerve NEC 729.2
  - nipple 611.0
    - puerperal, postpartum 675.0 5th
  - nose 478.19
    - suppurative 472.0
  - oculomotor nerve 378.51
  - optic nerve 377.30
  - orbit (chronic) 376.10
    - acute 376.00
    - chronic 376.10
  - ovary (*see also* Salpingo-oophoritis) 614.2
  - oviduct (*see also* Salpingo-oophoritis) 614.2
  - pancreas - *see* Pancreatitis
  - parametrium (chronic) (*see also* Disease, pelvis, inflammatory) 614.4
    - acute 614.3
  - parotid region 686.9
    - gland 527.2
  - pelvis, female (*see also* Disease, pelvis, inflammatory) 614.9
  - penis (corpora cavernosa) 607.2
  - perianal 569.49
  - pericardium (*see also* Pericarditis) 423.9
  - perineum (female) (male) 686.9
  - perirectal 569.49
  - peritoneum (*see also* Peritonitis) 567.9
  - periuterine (*see also* Disease, pelvis, inflammatory) 614.9
  - perivesical (*see also* Cystitis) 595.9
  - petrous bone (*see also* Petrositis) 383.20
  - pharynx (*see also* Pharyngitis) 462
    - follicular 472.1
    - granular 472.1
  - pia mater - *see* Meningitis
  - pleura - *see* Pleurisy
  - postmastoidectomy cavity 383.30
    - chronic 383.33
  - pouch, internal ileoanal 569.71 ●
  - prostate (*see also* Prostatitis) 601.9
  - rectosigmoid - *see* Rectosigmoiditis
  - rectum (*see also* Proctitis) 569.49
  - respiratory, upper (*see also* Infection, respiratory, upper) 465.9
    - chronic, due to external agent - *see* Condition, respiratory, chronic, due to, external agent
    - due to
      - fumes or vapors (chemical) (inhalation) 506.2
      - radiation 508.1
  - retina (*see also* Retinitis) 363.20
  - retrocecal (*see also* Appendicitis) 541
  - retroperitoneal (*see also* Peritonitis) 567.9
  - salivary duct or gland (any) (suppurative) 527.2
  - scorbutic, alveoli, teeth 267
  - scrotum 608.4
  - sigmoid - *see* Enteritis
  - sinus (*see also* Sinusitis) 473.9
  - Skene's duct or gland (*see also* Urethritis) 597.89
  - skin 686.9
  - spermatic cord 608.4
  - sphenoidal (sinus) (*see also* Sinusitis, sphenoidal) 473.3
  - spinal
    - cord (*see also* Encephalitis) 323.9
      - late effect - *see* category 326
    - membrane - *see* Meningitis
    - nerve - *see* Disorder, nerve
  - spine (*see also* Spondylitis) 720.9
  - spleen (capsule) 289.59
  - stomach - *see* Gastritis
  - stricture, rectum 569.49
  - subcutaneous tissue NEC 686.9
  - suprarenal (gland) 255.8
  - synovial (fringe) (membrane) - *see* Bursitis
  - tendon (sheath) NEC 726.90
  - testis (*see also* Orchitis) 604.90
  - thigh 686.9
  - throat (*see also* Sore throat) 462
  - thymus (gland) 254.8
  - thyroid (gland) (*see also* Thyroiditis) 245.9
  - tongue 529.0
  - tonsil - *see* Tonsillitis
  - trachea - *see* Tracheitis
  - trochlear nerve 378.53
  - tubal (*see also* Salpingo-oophoritis) 614.2
  - tuberculous NEC (*see also* Tuberculosis) 011.9 5th
  - tubo-ovarian (*see also* Salpingo-oophoritis) 614.2
  - tunica vaginalis 608.4
  - tympanic membrane - *see* Myringitis
  - umbilicus, umbilical 686.9
    - newborn NEC 771.4
  - uterine ligament (*see also* Disease, pelvis, inflammatory) 614.4
    - acute 614.3
  - uterus (catarrhal) (*see also* Endometritis) 615.9
  - uveal tract (anterior) (*see also* Iridocyclitis) 364.3
    - posterior - *see* Chorioretinitis
    - sympathetic 360.11
  - vagina (*see also* Vaginitis) 616.10
  - vas deferens 608.4
  - vein (*see also* Phlebitis) 451.9
    - thrombotic 451.9
      - cerebral (*see also* Thrombosis, brain) 434.0 5th
      - leg 451.2
        - deep (vessels) NEC 451.19
        - superficial (vessels) 451.0
      - lower extremity 451.2
        - deep (vessels) NEC 451.19
        - superficial (vessels) 451.0
  - vesicant
    - agent NEC 998.82
    - chemotherapy 998.81
  - vocal cord 478.5
  - vulva (*see also* Vulvitis) 616.10
- **Inflation, lung imperfect** (newborn) 770.5
- **Influenza, influenzal** 487.1
  - with
    - bronchitis 487.1
    - bronchopneumonia 487.0
    - cold (any type) 487.1
    - digestive manifestations 487.8
    - hemoptysis 487.1
    - involvement of
      - gastrointestinal tract 487.8
      - nervous system 487.8
    - laryngitis 487.1
    - manifestations NEC 487.8
      - respiratory 487.1
        - pneumonia 487.0
    - pharyngitis 487.1
    - pneumonia (any form classifiable to 480-483, 485-486) 487.0
    - respiratory manifestations NEC 487.1
    - sinusitis 487.1
    - sore throat 487.1
    - tonsillitis 487.1
    - tracheitis 487.1
    - upper respiratory infection (acute) 487.1
  - abdominal 487.8
  - A/H5N1 488.0 ●
  - Asian 487.1
  - avian 488.0 ●
  - bronchial 487.1
  - bronchopneumonia 487.0
  - catarrhal 487.1
  - due to identified ~~avian influenza virus 488~~ ▲
    - avian influenza virus 488.0 ●
    - novel H1N1 influenza virus 488.1 ●
  - epidemic 487.1
  - gastric 487.8
  - intestinal 487.8
  - laryngitis 487.1
  - maternal affecting fetus or newborn 760.2
    - manifest influenza in infant 771.2
  - novel (2009) H1N1 488.1 ●
  - novel A/H1N1 488.1 ●
  - pharyngitis 487.1
  - pneumonia (any form) 487.0
  - respiratory (upper) 487.1
  - specified NEC 487.1 ●
  - stomach 487.8
  - vaccination, prophylactic (against) V04.81
- **Influenza-like disease** 487.1
- **Infraction, Freiberg's** (metatarsal head) 732.5
- **Infraeruption, teeth** 524.34
- **Infusion complication, misadventure, or reaction** - *see* Complication, infusion
- **Ingestion**
  - chemical - *see* Table of Drugs and Chemicals
  - drug or medicinal substance
    - overdose or wrong substance given or taken 977.9
      - specified drug - *see* Table of Drugs and Chemicals
  - foreign body NEC (*see also* Foreign body) 938
- **Ingrowing**
  - hair 704.8
  - nail (finger) (toe) (infected) 703.0
- **Inguinal** - *see also* condition
  - testis 752.51
- **Inhalation**
  - carbon monoxide 986
  - flame
    - mouth 947.0
    - lung 947.1
  - food or foreign body (*see also* Asphyxia, food or foreign body) 933.1
  - gas, fumes, or vapor (noxious) 987.9
    - specified agent - *see* Table of Drugs and Chemicals
  - liquid or vomitus (*see also* Asphyxia, food or foreign body) 933.1
    - lower respiratory tract NEC 934.9
  - meconium (fetus or newborn) 770.11
    - with respiratory symptoms 770.12
  - mucus (*see also* Asphyxia, mucus) 933.1
  - oil (causing suffocation) (*see also* Asphyxia, food or foreign body) 933.1
  - pneumonia - *see* Pneumonia, aspiration
  - smoke 987.9
  - steam 987.9

- **Inhalation** – *continued*
  - stomach contents or secretions (*see also* Asphyxia, food or foreign body) 933.1
    - in labor and delivery 668.0 [5th]
- **Inhibition, inhibited**
  - academic as adjustment reaction 309.23
  - orgasm
    - female 302.73
    - male 302.74
  - sexual
    - desire 302.71
    - excitement 302.72
  - work as adjustment reaction 309.23
- **Inhibitor, systemic lupus erythematosus (presence of)** 286.5
- **Iniencephalus, iniencephaly** 740.2
- **Injected eye** 372.74
- **Injury** 959.9

Note *For abrasion, insect bite (nonvenomous), blister, or scratch, see Injury, superficial.*

For laceration, traumatic rupture, tear, or penetrating wound of internal organs, such as heart, lung, liver, kidney, pelvic organs, whether or not accompanied by open wound in the same region, see Injury, internal.

For nerve injury, see Injury, nerve.

For late effect of injuries classifiable to 850-854, 860-869, 900-919, 950-959, see Late, effect, injury, by type.

- abdomen, abdominal (viscera) - *see also* Injury, internal, abdomen
  - muscle or wall 959.12
- acoustic, resulting in deafness 951.5
- adenoid 959.09
- adrenal (gland) - *see* Injury, internal, adrenal
- alveolar (process) 959.09
- ankle (and foot) (and knee) (and leg, except thigh) 959.7
- anterior chamber, eye 921.3
- anus 959.19
- aorta (thoracic) 901.0
  - abdominal 902.0
- appendix - *see* Injury, internal, appendix
- arm, upper (and shoulder) 959.2
- artery (complicating trauma) (*see also* Injury, blood vessel, by site) 904.9
  - cerebral or meningeal (*see also* Hemorrhage, brain, traumatic, subarachnoid) 852.0 [5th]
- auditory canal (external) (meatus) 959.09
- auricle, auris, ear 959.09
- axilla 959.2
- back 959.19
- bile duct - *see* Injury, internal, bile duct
- birth - *see also* Birth, injury
  - canal NEC, complicating delivery 665.9 [5th]
- bladder (sphincter) - *see* Injury, internal, bladder
- blast (air) (hydraulic) (immersion) (underwater) NEC 869.0
  - with open wound into cavity NEC 869.1
  - abdomen or thorax - *see* Injury, internal, by site
  - brain - *see* Concussion, brain
  - ear (acoustic nerve trauma) 951.5
    - with perforation of tympanic membrane - *see* Wound, open, ear, drum
- blood vessel NEC 904.9
  - abdomen 902.9
    - multiple 902.87
    - specified NEC 902.89
  - aorta (thoracic) 901.0
    - abdominal 902.0
  - arm NEC 903.9

Injury – *continued*
- blood vessel – *continued*
  - axillary 903.00
    - artery 903.1
    - vein 903.02
  - azygos vein 901.89
  - basilic vein 903.1
  - brachial (artery) (vein) 903.1
  - bronchial 901.89
  - carotid artery 900.00
    - common 900.01
    - external 900.02
    - internal 900.03
  - celiac artery 902.20
    - specified branch NEC 902.24
  - cephalic vein (arm) 903.1
  - colica dextra 902.26
  - cystic
    - artery 902.24
    - vein 902.39
  - deep plantar 904.6
  - digital (artery) (vein) 903.5
  - due to accidental puncture or laceration during procedure 998.2
  - extremity
    - lower 904.8
      - multiple 904.7
      - specified NEC 904.7
    - upper 903.9
      - multiple 903.8
      - specified NEC 903.8
  - femoral
    - artery (superficial) 904.1
      - above profunda origin 904.0
      - common 904.0
    - vein 904.2
  - gastric
    - artery 902.21
    - vein 902.39
  - head 900.9
    - intracranial - *see* Injury, intracranial
    - multiple 900.82
    - specified NEC 900.89
  - hemiazygos vein 901.89
  - hepatic
    - artery 902.22
    - vein 902.11
  - hypogastric 902.59
    - artery 902.51
    - vein 902.52
  - ileocolic
    - artery 902.26
    - vein 902.31
  - iliac 902.50
    - artery 902.53
    - specified branch NEC 902.59
    - vein 902.54
  - innominate
    - artery 901.1
    - vein 901.3
  - intercostal (artery) (vein) 901.81
  - jugular vein (external) 900.81
    - internal 900.1
  - leg NEC 904.8
  - mammary (artery) (vein) 901.82
  - mesenteric
    - artery 902.20
      - inferior 902.27
      - specified branch NEC 902.29
      - superior (trunk) 902.25
        - branches, primary 902.26
    - vein 902.39
      - inferior 902.32
      - superior (and primary subdivisions) 902.31
  - neck 900.9
    - multiple 900.82
    - specified NEC 900.89
  - ovarian 902.89
    - artery 902.81
    - vein 902.82
  - palmar artery 903.4

Injury – *continued*
- blood vessel – *continued*
  - pelvis 902.9
    - multiple 902.87
    - specified NEC 902.89
  - plantar (deep) (artery) (vein) 904.6
  - popliteal 904.40
    - artery 904.41
    - vein 904.42
  - portal 902.33
  - pulmonary 901.40
    - artery 901.41
    - vein 901.42
  - radial (artery) (vein) 903.2
  - renal 902.40
    - artery 902.41
    - specified NEC 902.49
    - vein 902.42
  - saphenous
    - artery 904.7
    - vein (greater) (lesser) 904.3
  - splenic
    - artery 902.23
    - vein 902.34
  - subclavian
    - artery 901.1
    - vein 901.3
  - suprarenal 902.49
  - thoracic 901.9
    - multiple 901.83
    - specified NEC 901.89
  - tibial 904.50
    - artery 904.50
      - anterior 904.51
      - posterior 904.53
    - vein 904.50
      - anterior 904.52
      - posterior 904.54
  - ulnar (artery) (vein) 903.3
  - uterine 902.59
    - artery 902.55
    - vein 902.56
  - vena cava
    - inferior 902.10
      - specified branches NEC 902.19
    - superior 901.2
- brachial plexus 953.4
  - newborn 767.6
- brain (traumatic) NEC (*see also* Injury, intracranial) 854.0 [5th] ▲
  - due to fracture of skull - *see* Fracture, skull, by site ●
- breast 959.19
- broad ligament - *see* Injury, internal, broad ligament
- bronchus, bronchi - *see* Injury, internal, bronchus
- brow 959.09
- buttock 959.19
- canthus, eye 921.1
- cathode ray 990
- cauda equina 952.4
  - with fracture, vertebra - *see* Fracture, vertebra, sacrum
- cavernous sinus (*see also* Injury, intracranial) 854.0 [5th]
- cecum - *see* Injury, internal, cecum
- celiac ganglion or plexus 954.1
- cerebellum (*see also* Injury, intracranial) 854.0 [5th]
- cervix (uteri) - *see* Injury, internal, cervix
- cheek 959.09
- chest - *see* Injury, internal, chest
  - wall 959.11
- childbirth - *see also* Birth, injury
  - maternal NEC 665.9 [5th]
- chin 959.09
- choroid (eye) 921.3
- clitoris 959.14
- coccyx 959.19
  - complicating delivery 665.6 [5th]
- colon - *see* Injury, internal, colon
- common duct - *see* Injury, internal, common duct

Injury – *continued*
- conjunctiva 921.1
  - superficial 918.2
- cord
  - spermatic - *see* Injury, internal, spermatic cord
  - spinal - *see* Injury, spinal, by site
- cornea 921.3
  - abrasion 918.1
  - due to contact lens 371.82
  - penetrating - *see* Injury, eyeball, penetrating
  - superficial 918.1
    - due to contact lens 371.82
- cortex (cerebral) (*see also* Injury, intracranial) 854.0 [5th]
  - visual 950.3
- costal region 959.11
- costochondral 959.11
- cranial
  - bones - *see* Fracture, skull, by site
  - cavity (*see also* Injury, intracranial) 854.0 [5th]
  - nerve - *see* Injury, nerve, cranial
- crushing - *see* Crush
- cutaneous sensory nerve
  - lower limb 956.4
  - upper limb 955.5
- deep tissue - *see* Contusion, by site
  - meaning pressure ulcer 707.25
- delivery - *see also* Birth, injury
  - maternal NEC 665.9 [5th]
- Descemet's membrane - *see* Injury, eyeball, penetrating
- diaphragm - *see* Injury, internal, diaphragm
- diffuse axonal - *see* Injury, intracranial
- duodenum - *see* Injury, internal, duodenum
- ear (auricle) (canal) (drum) (external) 959.09
- elbow (and forearm) (and wrist) 959.3
- epididymis 959.14
- epigastric region 959.12
- epiglottis 959.09
- epiphyseal, current - *see* Fracture, by site
- esophagus - *see* Injury, internal, esophagus
- Eustachian tube 959.09
- extremity (lower) (upper) NEC 959.8
- eye 921.9
  - penetrating eyeball - *see* Injury, eyeball, penetrating
  - superficial 918.9
- eyeball 921.3
  - penetrating 871.7
    - with
      - partial loss (of intraocular tissue) 871.2
      - prolapse or exposure (of intraocular tissue) 871.1
    - without prolapse 871.0
    - foreign body (nonmagnetic) 871.6
      - magnetic 871.5
  - superficial 918.9
- eyebrow 959.09
- eyelid(s) 921.1
  - laceration - *see* Laceration, eyelid
  - superficial 918.0
- face (and neck) 959.09
- fallopian tube - *see* Injury, internal, fallopian tube
- fingers(s) (nail) 959.5
- flank 959.19
- foot (and ankle) (and knee) (and leg, except thigh) 959.7
- forceps NEC 767.9
  - scalp 767.19
- forearm (and elbow) (and wrist) 959.3
- forehead 959.09
- gallbladder - *see* Injury, internal, gallbladder
- gasserian ganglion 951.2
- gastrointestinal tract - *see* Injury, internal, gastrointestinal tract

Inhalation – Injury

Injury – *continued*
- genital organ(s)
  - with
    - abortion - *see* Abortion, by type, with, damage to pelvic organs
    - ectopic pregnancy (*see also* categories 633.0-633.9) 639.2
    - molar pregnancy (*see also* categories 630-632) 639.2
  - external 959.14
    - fracture of corpus cavernosum penis 959.13
  - following
    - abortion 639.2
    - ectopic or molar pregnancy 639.2
  - internal - *see* Injury, internal, genital organs
  - obstetrical trauma NEC 665.9 [5th]
    - affecting fetus or newborn 763.89
- gland
  - lacrimal 921.1
    - laceration 870.8
  - parathyroid 959.09
  - salivary 959.09
  - thyroid 959.09
- globe (eye) (*see also* Injury, eyeball) 921.3
- grease gun - *see* Wound, open, by site, complicated
- groin 959.19
- gum 959.09
- hand(s) (except fingers) 959.4
- head NEC 959.01
  - with
    - loss of consciousness 850.5
    - skull fracture - *see* Fracture, skull, by site
- heart - *see* Injury, internal, heart
- heel 959.7
- hip (and thigh) 959.6
- hymen 959.14
- hyperextension (cervical) (vertebra) 847.0
- ileum - *see* Injury, internal, ileum
- iliac region 959.19
- infrared rays NEC 990
- instrumental (during surgery) 998.2
  - birth injury - *see* Birth, injury
  - nonsurgical (*see also* Injury, by site) 959.9
  - obstetrical 665.9 [5th]
    - affecting fetus or newborn 763.89
    - bladder 665.5 [5th]
    - cervix 665.3 [5th]
    - high vaginal 665.4 [5th]
    - perineal NEC 664.9 [5th]
    - urethra 665.5 [5th]
    - uterus 665.5 [5th]
- internal 869.0

Note *For injury of internal organ(s) by foreign body entering through a natural orifice (e.g., inhaled, ingested, or swallowed)see Foreign body, entering through orifice.*

For internal injury of any of the following sites with internal injury of any other of the sitessee Injury, internal, multiple.

  - with
    - fracture
      - pelvis - *see* Fracture, pelvis
      - specified site, except pelvis - *see* Injury, internal, by site
    - open wound into cavity 869.1
  - abdomen, abdominal (viscera) NEC 868.00
    - with
      - fracture, pelvis - *see* Fracture, pelvis
      - open wound into cavity 868.10
    - specified site NEC 868.09
      - with open wound into cavity 868.19

Injury – *continued*
- internal – *continued*
  - adrenal (gland) 868.01
    - with open wound into cavity 868.11
  - aorta (thoracic) 901.0
    - abdominal 902.0
  - appendix 863.85
    - with open wound into cavity 863.95
  - bile duct 868.02
    - with open wound into cavity 868.12
  - bladder (sphincter) 867.0
    - with
      - abortion - *see* Abortion, by type, with, damage to pelvic organs
      - ectopic pregnancy (*see also* categories 633.0-633.9) 639.2
      - molar pregnancy (*see also* categories 630-632) 639.2
      - open wound into cavity 867.1
    - following
      - abortion 639.2
      - ectopic or molar pregnancy 639.2
    - obstetrical trauma 665.5 [5th]
      - affecting fetus or newborn 763.89
  - blood vessel - *see* Injury, blood vessel, by site
  - broad ligament 867.6
    - with open wound into cavity 867.7
  - bronchus, bronchi 862.21
    - with open wound into cavity 862.31
  - cecum 863.89
    - with open wound into cavity 863.99
  - cervix (uteri) 867.4
    - with
      - abortion - *see* Abortion, by type, with damage to pelvic organs
      - ectopic pregnancy (*see also* categories 633.0-633.9) 639.2
      - molar pregnancy (*see also* categories 630-632) 639.2
      - open wound into cavity 867.5
    - following
      - abortion 639.2
      - ectopic or molar pregnancy 639.2
    - obstetrical trauma 665.3
      - affecting fetus or newborn 763.89
  - chest (*see also* Injury, internal, intrathoracic organs) 862.8
    - with open wound into cavity 862.9
  - colon 863.40
    - with
      - open wound into cavity 863.50
      - rectum 863.46
        - with open wound into cavity 863.56
    - ascending (right) 863.41
      - with open wound into cavity 863.51
    - descending (left) 863.43
      - with open wound into cavity 863.53
    - multiple sites 863.46
      - with open wound into cavity 863.56
    - sigmoid 863.44
      - with open wound into cavity 863.54
    - specified site NEC 863.49
      - with open wound into cavity 863.59
    - transverse 863.42
      - with open wound into cavity 863.52
  - common duct 868.02
    - with open wound into cavity 868.12

Injury – *continued*
- internal – *continued*
  - complicating delivery 665.9 [5th]
    - affecting fetus or newborn 763.89
  - diaphragm 862.0
    - with open wound into cavity 862.1
  - duodenum 863.21
    - with open wound into cavity 863.31
  - esophagus (intrathoracic) 862.22
    - with open wound into cavity 862.32
    - cervical region 874.4
      - complicated 874.5
  - fallopian tube 867.6
    - with open wound into cavity 867.7
  - gallbladder 868.02
    - with open wound into cavity 868.12
  - gastrointestinal tract NEC 863.80
    - with open wound into cavity 863.90
  - genital organ NEC 867.6
    - with open wound into cavity 867.7
  - heart 861.00
    - with open wound into thorax 861.10
  - ileum 863.29
    - with open wound into cavity 863.39
  - intestine NEC 863.89
    - with open wound into cavity 863.99
    - large NEC 863.40
      - with open wound into cavity 863.50
    - small NEC 863.20
      - with open wound into cavity 863.30
  - intra-abdominal (organ) 868.00
    - with open wound into cavity 868.10
    - multiple sites 868.09
      - with open wound into cavity 868.19
    - specified site NEC 868.09
      - with open wound into cavity 868.19
  - intrathoracic organs (multiple) 862.8
    - with open wound into cavity 862.9
    - diaphragm (only) - *see* Injury, internal, diaphragm
    - heart (only) - *see* Injury, internal, heart
    - lung (only) - *see* Injury, internal, lung
    - specified site NEC 862.29
      - with open wound into cavity 862.39
  - intrauterine (*see also* Injury, internal, uterus) 867.4
    - with open wound into cavity 867.5
  - jejunum 863.29
    - with open wound into cavity 863.39
  - kidney (subcapsular) 866.00
    - with
      - disruption of parenchyma (complete) 866.03
        - with open wound into cavity 866.13
      - hematoma (without rupture of capsule) 866.01
        - with open wound into cavity 866.11
      - laceration 866.02
        - with open wound into cavity 866.12
      - open wound into cavity 866.10
  - liver 864.00
    - with
      - contusion 864.01
        - with open wound into cavity 864.11
      - hematoma 864.01
        - with open wound into cavity 864.11
      - laceration 864.05
        - with open wound into cavity 864.15

Injury – *continued*
- internal – *continued*
  - liver – *continued*
    - with – *continued*
      - laceration – *continued*
        - major (disruption of hepatic parenchyma) 864.04
          - with open wound into cavity 864.14
        - minor (capsule only) 864.02
          - with open wound into cavity 864.12
        - moderate (involving parenchyma) 864.03
          - with open wound into cavity 864.13
        - multiple 864.04
        - stellate 864.04
          - with open wound into cavity 864.14
      - open wound into cavity 864.10
  - lung 861.20
    - with open wound into thorax 861.30
    - hemopneumothorax - *see* Hemopneumothorax, traumatic
    - hemothorax - *see* Hemothorax, traumatic
    - pneumohemothorax - *see* Pneumohemothorax, traumatic
    - pneumothorax - *see* Pneumothorax, traumatic
    - transfusion related, acute (TRALI) 518.7
  - mediastinum 862.29
    - with open wound into cavity 862.39
  - mesentery 863.89
    - with open wound into cavity 863.99
  - mesosalpinx 867.6
    - with open wound into cavity 867.7
  - multiple 869.0

Note *Multiple internal injuries of sites classifiable to the same three-or four-digit category should be classified to that category.*

Multiple injuries classifiable to different fourth-digit subdivisions of 861.- (heart and lung injuries) should be dealt with according to coding rules.

    - internal 869.0
      - with open wound into cavity 869.1
    - intra-abdominal organ (sites classifiable to 863-868)
      - with
        - intrathoracic organ(s) (sites classifiable to 861-862) 869.0
          - with open wound into cavity 869.1
        - other intra-abdominal organ(s) (sites classifiable to 863-868, except where classifiable to the same three-digit category) 868.09
          - with open wound into cavity 868.19
    - intrathoracic organ (sites classifiable to 861-862)
      - with
        - intra-abdominal organ(s) (sites classifiable to 863-868) 869.0
          - with open wound into cavity 869.1

- **Injury** – *continued*
  - internal – *continued*
    - multiple – *continued*
      - intrathoracic organ – *continued*
        - other intrathoracic organs(s) (sites classifiable to 861-862, except where classifiable to the same three-digit category) 862.8
          - with open wound into cavity 862.9
    - myocardium - *see* Injury, internal, heart
    - ovary 867.6
      - with open wound into cavity 867.7
    - pancreas (multiple sites) 863.84
      - with open wound into cavity 863.94
      - body 863.82
        - with open wound into cavity 863.92
      - head 863.81
        - with open wound into cavity 863.91
      - tail 863.83
        - with open wound into cavity 863.93
    - pelvis, pelvic (organs) (viscera) 867.8
      - with
        - fracture, pelvis - *see* Fracture, pelvis
        - open wound into cavity 867.9
      - specified site NEC 867.6
        - with open wound into cavity 867.7
    - peritoneum 868.03
      - with open wound into cavity 868.13
    - pleura 862.29
      - with open wound into cavity 862.39
    - prostate 867.6
      - with open wound into cavity 867.7
    - rectum 863.45
      - with
        - colon 863.46
          - with open wound into cavity 863.56
        - open wound into cavity 863.55
    - retroperitoneum 868.04
      - with open wound into cavity 868.14
    - round ligament 867.6
      - with open wound into cavity 867.7
    - seminal vesicle 867.6
      - with open wound into cavity 867.7
    - spermatic cord 867.6
      - with open wound into cavity 867.7
      - scrotal - *see* Wound, open, spermatic cord
    - spleen 865.00
      - with
        - disruption of parenchyma (massive) 865.04
          - with open wound into cavity 865.14
        - hematoma (without rupture of capsule) 865.01
          - with open wound into cavity 865.11
        - open wound into cavity 865.10
        - tear, capsular 865.02
          - with open wound into cavity 865.12
          - extending into parenchyma 865.03
            - with open wound into cavity 865.13
    - stomach 863.0
      - with open wound into cavity 863.1
    - suprarenal gland (multiple) 868.01
      - with open wound into cavity 868.11
    - thorax, thoracic (cavity) (organs) (multiple) (*see also* Injury, internal, intrathoracic organs) 862.8
      - with open wound into cavity 862.9

- **Injury** – *continued*
  - internal – *continued*
    - thymus (gland) 862.29
      - with open wound into cavity 862.39
    - trachea (intrathoracic) 862.29
      - with open wound into cavity 862.39
      - cervical region (*see also* Wound, open, trachea) 874.02
    - ureter 867.2
      - with open wound into cavity 867.3
    - urethra (sphincter) 867.0
      - with
        - abortion - *see* Abortion, by type, with, damage to pelvic organs
        - ectopic pregnancy (*see also* categories 633.0-633.9) 639.2
        - molar pregnancy (*see also* categories 630-632) 639.2
        - open wound into cavity 867.1
      - following
        - abortion 639.2
        - ectopic or molar pregnancy 639.2
      - obstetrical trauma 665.5 [5th]
        - affecting fetus or newborn 763.89
    - uterus 867.4
      - with
        - abortion - *see* Abortion, by type, with, damage to pelvic organs
        - ectopic pregnancy (*see also* categories 633.0-633.9) 639.2
        - molar pregnancy (*see also* categories 630-632) 639.2
        - open wound into cavity 867.5
      - following
        - abortion 639.2
        - ectopic or molar pregnancy 639.2
      - obstetrical trauma NEC 665.5 [5th]
        - affecting fetus or newborn 763.89
    - vas deferens 867.6
      - with open wound into cavity 867.7
    - vesical (sphincter) 867.0
      - with open wound into cavity 867.1
    - viscera (abdominal) (*see also* Injury, internal, multiple) 868.00
      - with
        - fracture, pelvis - *see* Fracture, pelvis
        - open wound into cavity 868.10
      - thoracic NEC (*see also* Injury, internal, intrathoracic organs) 862.8
        - with open wound into cavity 862.9
  - interscapular region 959.19
  - intervertebral disc 959.19
  - intestine - *see* Injury, internal, intestine
  - intra-abdominal (organs) NEC - *see* Injury, internal, intra-abdominal

- **Injury** – *continued*
  - intracranial (traumatic) 854.0 [5th] ▲

Note *Use the following fifth-digit subclassification with categories 851-854:*

0 unspecified state of consciousness
1 with no loss of consciousness
2 with brief [less than one hour] loss of consciousness
3 with moderate [1-24 hours] loss of consciousness
4 with prolonged [more than 24 hours] loss of consciousness and return to pre-existing conscious level
5 with prolonged [more than 24 hours] loss of consciousness, without return to pre-existing conscious level

Use fifth-digit 5 to designate when a patient is unconscious and dies before regaining consciousness, regardless of the duration of the loss of consciousness

6 with loss of consciousness of unspecified duration
9 with concussion, unspecified

- with
  - open intracranial wound 854.1 [5th]
  - skull fracture - *see* Fracture, skull, by site
- contusion 851.8 [5th]
  - with open intracranial wound 851.9 [5th]
  - brain stem 851.4 [5th]
    - with open intracranial wound 851.5 [5th]
  - cerebellum 851.4 [5th]
    - with open intracranial wound 851.5 [5th]
  - cortex (cerebral) 851.0 [5th]
    - with open intracranial wound 851.2 [5th]
  - hematoma - *see* Injury, intracranial, hemorrhage
  - hemorrhage 853.0 [5th]
    - with
      - laceration - *see* Injury, intracranial, laceration
      - open intracranial wound 853.1 [5th]
    - extradural 852.4 [5th]
      - with open intracranial wound 852.5 [5th]
    - subarachnoid 852.0 [5th]
      - with open intracranial wound 852.1 [5th]
    - subdural 852.2 [5th]
      - with open intracranial wound 852.3 [5th]
  - laceration 851.8 [5th]
    - with open intracranial wound 851.9 [5th]
    - brain stem 851.6 [5th]
      - with open intracranial wound 851.7 [5th]
    - cerebellum 851.6 [5th]
      - with open intracranial wound 851.7 [5th]
    - cortex (cerebral) 851.2 [5th]
      - with open intracranial wound 851.3 [5th]

- intraocular - *see* Injury, eyeball, penetrating
- intrathoracic organs (multiple) - *see* Injury, internal, intrathoracic organs
- intrauterine - *see* Injury, internal, intrauterine
- iris 921.3
  - penetrating - *see* Injury, eyeball, penetrating
- jaw 959.09
- jejunum - *see* Injury, internal, jejunum

- **Injury** – *continued*
  - joint NEC 959.9
    - old or residual 718.80
      - ankle 718.87
      - elbow 718.82
      - foot 718.87
      - hand 718.84
      - hip 718.85
      - knee 718.86
      - multiple sites 718.89
      - pelvic region 718.85
      - shoulder (region) 718.81
      - specified site NEC 718.88
      - wrist 718.83
  - kidney - *see* Injury, internal, kidney
    - acute (nontraumatic) 584.9
  - knee (and ankle) (and foot) (and leg, except thigh) 959.7
  - labium (majus) (minus) 959.14
  - labyrinth, ear 959.09
  - lacrimal apparatus, gland, or sac 921.1
    - laceration 870.8
  - larynx 959.09
  - late effect - *see* Late, effects (of), injury
  - leg, except thigh (and ankle) (and foot) (and knee) 959.7
    - upper or thigh 959.6
  - lens, eye 921.3
    - penetrating - *see* Injury, eyeball, penetrating
  - lid, eye - *see* Injury, eyelid
  - lip 959.09
  - liver - *see* Injury, internal, liver
  - lobe, parietal - *see* Injury, intracranial
  - lumbar (region) 959.19
    - plexus 953.5
  - lumbosacral (region) 959.19
    - plexus 953.5
  - lung - *see* Injury, internal, lung
  - malar region 959.09
  - mastoid region 959.09
  - maternal, during pregnancy, affecting fetus or newborn 760.5
  - maxilla 959.09
  - mediastinum - *see* Injury, internal, mediastinum
  - membrane
    - brain (*see also* Injury, intracranial) 854.0 [5th]
    - tympanic 959.09
  - meningeal artery - *see* Hemorrhage, brain, traumatic, subarachnoid
  - meninges (cerebral) - *see* Injury, intracranial
  - mesenteric
    - artery - *see* Injury, blood vessel, mesenteric, artery
    - plexus, inferior 954.1
    - vein - *see* Injury, blood vessel, mesenteric, vein
  - mesentery - *see* Injury, internal, mesentery
  - mesosalpinx - *see* Injury, internal, mesosalpinx
  - middle ear 959.09
  - midthoracic region 959.11
  - mouth 959.09
  - multiple (sites not classifiable to the same four-digit category in 959.0-959.7) 959.8
    - internal 869.0
      - with open wound into cavity 869.1
  - musculocutaneous nerve 955.4
  - nail
    - finger 959.5
    - toe 959.7
  - nasal (septum) (sinus) 959.09
  - nasopharynx 959.09
  - neck (and face) 959.09
  - nerve 957.9
    - abducens 951.3
    - abducent 951.3
    - accessory 951.6
    - acoustic 951.5
    - ankle and foot 956.9

Injury

Injury – *continued*
- nerve – *continued*
  - anterior crural, femoral 956.1
  - arm (*see also* Injury, nerve, upper limb) 955.9
  - auditory 951.5
  - axillary 955.0
  - brachial plexus 953.4
  - cervical sympathetic 954.0
  - cranial 951.9
    - first or olfactory 951.8
    - second or optic 950.0
    - third or oculomotor 951.0
    - fourth or trochlear 951.1
    - fifth or trigeminal 951.2
    - sixth or abducens 951.3
    - seventh or facial 951.4
    - eighth, acoustic, or auditory 951.5
    - ninth or glossopharyngeal 951.8
    - tenth, pneumogastric, or vagus 951.8
    - eleventh or accessory 951.6
    - twelfth or hypoglossal 951.7
    - newborn 767.7
  - cutaneous sensory
    - lower limb 956.4
    - upper limb 955.5
  - digital (finger) 955.6
    - toe 956.5
  - facial 951.4
    - newborn 767.5
  - femoral 956.1
  - finger 955.9
  - foot and ankle 956.9
  - forearm 955.9
  - glossopharyngeal 951.8
  - hand and wrist 955.9
  - head and neck, superficial 957.0
  - hypoglossal 951.7
  - involving several parts of body 957.8
  - leg (*see also* Injury, nerve, lower limb) 956.9
  - lower limb 956.9
    - multiple 956.8
    - specified site NEC 956.5
  - lumbar plexus 953.5
  - lumbosacral plexus 953.5
  - median 955.1
    - forearm 955.1
    - wrist and hand 955.1
  - multiple (in several parts of body) (sites not classifiable to the same three-digit category) 957.8
  - musculocutaneous 955.4
  - musculospiral 955.3
    - upper arm 955.3
  - oculomotor 951.0
  - olfactory 951.8
  - optic 950.0
  - pelvic girdle 956.9
    - multiple sites 956.8
    - specified site NEC 956.5
  - peripheral 957.9
    - multiple (in several regions) (sites not classifiable to the same three-digit category) 957.8
    - specified site NEC 957.1
  - peroneal 956.3
    - ankle and foot 956.3
    - lower leg 956.3
  - plantar 956.5
  - plexus 957.9
    - celiac 954.1
    - mesenteric, inferior 954.1
    - spinal 953.9
      - brachial 953.4
      - lumbosacral 953.5
      - multiple sites 953.8
    - sympathetic NEC 954.1
  - pneumogastric 951.8
  - radial 955.3
    - wrist and hand 955.3
  - sacral plexus 953.5

Injury – *continued*
- nerve – *continued*
  - sciatic 956.0
    - thigh 956.0
  - shoulder girdle 955.9
    - multiple 955.8
    - specified site NEC 955.7
  - specified site NEC 957.1
  - spinal 953.9
    - plexus - *see* Injury, nerve, plexus, spinal
    - root 953.9
      - cervical 953.0
      - dorsal 953.1
      - lumbar 953.2
      - multiple sites 953.8
      - sacral 953.3
  - splanchnic 954.1
  - sympathetic NEC 954.1
    - cervical 954.0
  - thigh 956.9
  - tibial 956.5
    - ankle and foot 956.2
    - lower leg 956.5
    - posterior 956.2
  - toe 956.9
  - trigeminal 951.2
  - trochlear 951.1
  - trunk, excluding shoulder and pelvic girdles 954.9
    - specified site NEC 954.8
    - sympathetic NEC 954.1
  - ulnar 955.2
    - forearm 955.2
    - wrist (and hand) 955.2
  - upper limb 955.9
    - multiple 955.8
    - specified site NEC 955.7
  - vagus 951.8
  - wrist and hand 955.9
- nervous system, diffuse 957.8
- nose (septum) 959.09
- obstetrical NEC 665.9 [5th]
  - affecting fetus or newborn 763.89
- occipital (region) (scalp) 959.09
  - lobe (*see also* Injury, intracranial) 854.0 [5th]
- optic 950.9
  - chiasm 950.1
  - cortex 950.3
  - nerve 950.0
  - pathways 950.2
- orbit, orbital (region) 921.2
  - penetrating 870.3
    - with foreign body 870.4
- ovary - *see* Injury, internal, ovary
- paint-gun - *see* Wound, open, by site, complicated
- palate (soft) 959.09
- pancreas - *see* Injury, internal, pancreas
- parathyroid (gland) 959.09
- parietal (region) (scalp) 959.09
  - lobe - *see* Injury, intracranial
- pelvic
  - floor 959.19
    - complicating delivery 664.1 [5th]
      - affecting fetus or newborn 763.89
  - joint or ligament, complicating delivery 665.6 [5th]
    - affecting fetus or newborn 763.89
  - organs - *see also* Injury, internal, pelvis
    - with
      - abortion - *see* Abortion, by type, with damage to pelvic organs
      - ectopic pregnancy (*see also* categories 633.0-633.9) 639.2
      - molar pregnancy (*see also* categories 633.0-633.9) 639.2
    - following
      - abortion 639.2

Injury – *continued*
- pelvic – *continued*
  - organs – *continued*
    - following – *continued*
      - ectopic or molar pregnancy 639.2
    - obstetrical trauma 665.5 [5th]
      - affecting fetus or newborn 763.89
- pelvis 959.19
- penis 959.14
  - fracture of corpus cavernosum 959.13
- perineum 959.14
- peritoneum - *see* Injury, internal, peritoneum
- periurethral tissue
  - with
    - abortion - *see* Abortion, by type, with damage to pelvic organs
    - ectopic pregnancy (*see also* categories 633.0-633.9) 639.2
    - molar pregnancy (*see also* categories 630-632) 639.2
  - complicating delivery 665.5 [5th]
    - affecting fetus or newborn 763.89
  - following
    - abortion 639.2
    - ectopic or molar pregnancy 639.2
- phalanges
  - foot 959.7
  - hand 959.5
- pharynx 959.09
- pleura - *see* Injury, internal, pleura
- popliteal space 959.7
- post-cardiac surgery (syndrome) 429.4
- prepuce 959.14
- prostate - *see* Injury, internal, prostate
- pubic region 959.19
- pudenda 959.14
- radiation NEC 990
- radioactive substance or radium NEC 990
- rectovaginal septum 959.14
- rectum - *see* Injury, internal, rectum
- retina 921.3
  - penetrating - *see* Injury, eyeball, penetrating
- retroperitoneal - *see* Injury, internal, retroperitoneum
- roentgen rays NEC 990
- round ligament - *see* Injury, internal, round ligament
- sacral (region) 959.19
  - plexus 953.5
- sacroiliac ligament NEC 959.19
- sacrum 959.19
- salivary ducts or glands 959.09
- scalp 959.09
  - due to birth trauma 767.19
  - fetus or newborn 767.19
- scapular region 959.2
- sclera 921.3
  - penetrating - *see* Injury, eyeball, penetrating
  - superficial 918.2
- scrotum 959.14
- seminal vesicle - *see* Injury, internal, seminal vesicle
- shoulder (and upper arm) 959.2
- sinus
  - cavernous (*see also* Injury, intracranial) 854.0 [5th]
  - nasal 959.09
- skeleton NEC, birth injury 767.3
- skin NEC 959.9
- skull - *see* Fracture, skull, by site
- soft tissue (of external sites) (severe) - *see* Wound, open, by site
- specified site NEC 959.8
- spermatic cord - *see* Injury, internal, spermatic cord
- spinal (cord) 952.9
  - with fracture, vertebra - *see* Fracture, vertebra, by site, with spinal cord injury

Injury – *continued*
- spinal (cord) – *continued*
  - cervical (C_1-C_4) 952.00
    - with
      - anterior cord syndrome 952.02
      - central cord syndrome 952.03
      - complete lesion of cord 952.01
      - incomplete lesion NEC 952.04
      - posterior cord syndrome 952.04
    - C_5-C_7 level 952.05
      - with
        - anterior cord syndrome 952.07
        - central cord syndrome 952.08
        - complete lesion of cord 952.06
        - incomplete lesion NEC 952.09
        - posterior cord syndrome 952.09
      - specified type NEC 952.09
    - specified type NEC 952.04
  - dorsal (D_1-D_6) (T_1-T_6) (thoracic) 952.10
    - with
      - anterior cord syndrome 952.12
      - central cord syndrome 952.13
      - complete lesion of cord 952.11
      - incomplete lesion NEC 952.14
      - posterior cord syndrome 952.14
    - D_7-D_{12} level (T_7-T_{12}) 952.15
      - with
        - anterior cord syndrome 952.17
        - central cord syndrome 952.18
        - complete lesion of cord 952.16
        - incomplete lesion NEC 952.19
        - posterior cord syndrome 952.19
      - specified type NEC 952.19
    - specified type NEC 952.14
  - lumbar 952.2
  - multiple sites 952.8
  - nerve (root) NEC - *see* Injury, nerve, spinal, root
  - plexus 953.9
    - brachial 953.4
    - lumbosacral 953.5
    - multiple sites 953.8
  - sacral 952.3
  - thoracic (*see also* Injury, spinal, dorsal) 952.10
- spleen - *see* Injury, internal, spleen
- stellate ganglion 954.1
- sternal region 959.11
- stomach - *see* Injury, internal, stomach
- subconjunctival 921.1
- subcutaneous 959.9
- subdural - *see* Injury, intracranial
- submaxillary region 959.09
- submental region 959.09
- subungual
  - fingers 959.5
  - toes 959.7

Injury – *continued*
- superficial 919 [4th]

Note *Use the following fourth-digit subdivisions with categories 910-919:*

.0	abrasion or friction burn without mention of infection
.1	abrasion or friction burn, infected
.2	blister without mention of infection
.3	blister, infected
.4	insect bite, nonvenomous, without mention of infection
.5	insect bite, nonvenomous, infected
.6	superficial foreign body (splinter) without major open wound and without mention of infection
.7	superficial foreign body (splinter) without major open wound, infected
.8	other and unspecified superficial injury without mention of infection
.9	other and unspecified superficial injury, infected

For late effects of superficial injury, see category 906.2.

- abdomen, abdominal (muscle) (wall) (and other part(s) of trunk) 911 [4th]
- ankle (and hip, knee, leg, or thigh) 916 [4th]
- anus (and other part(s) of trunk) 911 [4th]
- arm 913 [4th]
  - upper (and shoulder) 912 [4th]
- auditory canal (external) (meatus) (and other part(s) of face, neck, or scalp, except eye) 910 [4th]
- axilla (and upper arm) 912 [4th]
- back (and other part(s) of trunk) 911 [4th]
- breast (and other part(s) of trunk) 911 [4th]
- brow (and other part(s) of face, neck, or scalp, except eye) 910 [4th]
- buttock (and other part(s) of trunk) 911 [4th]
- canthus, eye 918.0
- cheek(s) (and other part(s) of face, neck, or scalp, except eye) 910 [4th]
- chest wall (and other part(s) of trunk) 911 [4th]
- chin (and other part(s) of face, neck, or scalp, except eye) 910 [4th]
- clitoris (and other part(s) of trunk) 911 [4th]
- conjunctiva 918.2
- cornea 918.1
  - due to contact lens 371.82
- costal region (and other part(s) of trunk) 911 [4th]
- ear(s) (auricle) (canal) (drum) (external) (and other part(s) of face, neck, or scalp, except eye) 910 [4th]
- elbow (and forearm) (and wrist) 913 [4th]
- epididymis (and other part(s) of trunk) 911 [4th]
- epigastric region (and other part(s) of trunk) 911 [4th]
- epiglottis (and other part(s) of face, neck, or scalp, except eye) 910 [4th]
- eye(s) (and adnexa) NEC 918.9
- eyelid(s) (and periocular area) 918.0
- face (any part(s), except eye) (and neck or scalp) 910 [4th]
- finger(s) (nail) (any) 915 [4th]
- flank (and other part(s) of trunk) 911 [4th]
- foot (phalanges) (and toe(s)) 917 [4th]
- forearm (and elbow) (and wrist) 913 [4th]
- forehead (and other part(s) of face, neck, or scalp, except eye) 910 [4th]
- globe (eye) 918.9
- groin (and other part(s) of trunk) 911 [4th]
- gums(s) (and other part(s) of face, neck, or scalp, except eye) 910 [4th]
- hand(s) (except fingers alone) 914 [4th]
- head (and other part(s) of face, neck, or scalp, except eye) 910 [4th]
- heel (and foot or toe) 917 [4th]
- hip (and ankle, knee, leg, or thigh) 916 [4th]
- iliac region (and other part(s) of trunk) 911 [4th]
- interscapular region (and other part(s) of trunk) 911 [4th]
- iris 918.9
- knee (and ankle, hip, leg, or thigh) 916 [4th]
- labium (majus) (minus) (and other part(s) of trunk) 911 [4th]
- lacrimal (apparatus) (gland) (sac) 918.0
- leg (lower) (upper) (and ankle, hip, knee, or thigh) 916 [4th]
- lip(s) (and other part(s) of face, neck, or scalp, except eye) 910 [4th]
- lower extremity (except foot) 916 [4th]
- lumbar region (and other part(s) of trunk) 911 [4th]
- malar region (and other part(s) of face, neck, or scalp, except eye) 910 [4th]
- mastoid region (and other part(s) of face, neck, or scalp, except eye) 910 [4th]
- midthoracic region (and other part(s) of trunk) 911 [4th]
- mouth (and other part(s) of face, neck, or scalp, except eye) 910 [4th]
- multiple sites (not classifiable to the same three-digit category) 919 [4th]
- nasal (septum) (and other part(s) of face, neck, or scalp, except eye) 910 [4th]
- neck (and face or scalp, any part(s), except eye) 910 [4th]
- nose (septum) (and other part(s) of face, neck, or scalp, except eye) 910 [4th]
- occipital region (and other part(s) of face, neck, or scalp, except eye) 910 [4th]
- orbital region 918.0
- palate (soft) (and other part(s) of face, neck, or scalp, except eye) 910 [4th]
- parietal region (and other part(s) of face, neck, or scalp, except eye) 910 [4th]
- penis (and other part(s) of trunk) 911 [4th]
- perineum (and other part(s) of trunk) 911 [4th]
- periocular area 918.0
- pharynx (and other part(s) of face, neck, or scalp, except eye) 910 [4th]
- popliteal space (and ankle, hip, leg, or thigh) 916 [4th]
- prepuce (and other part(s) of trunk) 911 [4th]
- pubic region (and other part(s) of trunk) 911 [4th]
- pudenda (and other part(s) of trunk) 911 [4th]
- sacral region (and other part(s) of trunk) 911 [4th]
- salivary (ducts) (glands) (and other part(s) of face, neck, or scalp, except eye) 910 [4th]
- scalp (and other part(s) of face or neck, except eye) 910 [4th]
- scapular region (and upper arm) 912 [4th]
- sclera 918.2
- scrotum (and other part(s) of trunk) 911 [4th]
- shoulder (and upper arm) 912 [4th]
- skin NEC 919 [4th]
- specified site(s) NEC 919 [4th]
- sternal region (and other part(s) of trunk) 911 [4th]
- subconjunctival 918.2
- subcutaneous NEC 919 [4th]
- submaxillary region (and other part(s) of face, neck, or scalp, except eye) 910 [4th]
- submental region (and other part(s) of face, neck, or scalp, except eye) 910 [4th]
- supraclavicular fossa (and other part(s) of face, neck, or scalp, except eye) 910 [4th]
- supraorbital 918.0
- temple (and other part(s) of face, neck, or scalp, except eye) 910 [4th]
- temporal region (and other part(s) of face, neck, or scalp, except eye) 910 [4th]
- testis (and other part(s) of trunk) 911 [4th]
- thigh (and ankle, hip, knee, or leg) 916 [4th]
- thorax, thoracic (external) (and other part(s) of trunk) 911 [4th]
- throat (and other part(s) of face, neck, or scalp, except eye) 910 [4th]
- thumb(s) (nail) 915 [4th]
- toe(s) (nail) (subungual) (and foot) 917 [4th]
- tongue (and other part(s) of face, neck, or scalp, except eye) 910 [4th]
- tooth, teeth (*see also* Abrasion, dental) 521.20
- trunk (any part(s)) 911 [4th]
- tunica vaginalis (and other part(s) of trunk) 911 [4th]
- tympanum, tympanic membrane (and other part(s) of face, neck, or scalp, except eye) 910 [4th]
- upper extremity NEC 913 [4th]
- uvula (and other part(s) of face, neck, or scalp, except eye) 910 [4th]
- vagina (and other part(s) of trunk) 911 [4th]
- vulva (and other part(s) of trunk) 911 [4th]
- wrist (and elbow) (and forearm) 913 [4th]

- supraclavicular fossa 959.19
- supraorbital 959.09
- surgical complication (external or internal site) 998.2
- symphysis pubis 959.19
  - complicating delivery 665.6 [5th]
    - affecting fetus or newborn 763.89
- temple 959.09
- temporal region 959.09
- testis 959.14
- thigh (and hip) 959.6
- thorax, thoracic (external) 959.11
  - cavity - *see* Injury, internal, thorax
  - internal - *see* Injury, internal, intrathoracic organs
- throat 959.09
- thumb(s) (nail) 959.5
- thymus - *see* Injury, internal, thymus
- thyroid (gland) 959.09
- toe (nail) (any) 959.7
- tongue 959.09
- tonsil 959.09
- tooth NEC 873.63
  - complicated 873.73
- trachea - *see* Injury, internal, trachea
- trunk 959.19
- tunica vaginalis 959.14
- tympanum, tympanic membrane 959.09
- ultraviolet rays NEC 990
- ureter - *see* Injury, internal, ureter
- urethra (sphincter) - *see* Injury, internal, urethra
- uterus - *see* Injury, internal, uterus
- uvula 959.09
- vagina 959.14
- vascular - *see* Injury, blood vessel
- vas deferens - *see* Injury, internal, vas deferens
- vein (*see also* Injury, blood vessel, by site) 904.9
- vena cava
  - inferior 902.10
  - superior 901.2
- vesical (sphincter) - *see* Injury, internal, vesical
- viscera (abdominal) - *see* Injury, internal, viscera
  - with fracture, pelvis - *see* Fracture, pelvis
- visual 950.9
  - cortex 950.3
- vitreous (humor) 871.2
- vulva 959.14
- whiplash (cervical spine) 847.0
- wringer - *see* Crush, by site
- wrist (and elbow) (and forearm) 959.3
- x-ray NEC 990

Inoculation - *see also* Vaccination
- complication or reaction - *see* Complication, vaccination

INPH (idiopathic normal pressure hydrocephalus) 331.5

Insanity, insane (*see also* Psychosis) 298.9
- adolescent (*see also* Schizophrenia) 295.9 [5th]
- alternating (*see also* Psychosis, affective, circular) 296.7
- confusional 298.9
  - acute 293.0
  - subacute 293.1
- delusional 298.9
- paralysis, general 094.1
  - progressive 094.1
- paresis, general 094.1
- senile 290.20

Insect
- bite - *see* Injury, superficial, by site
- venomous, poisoning by 989.5

Insemination, artificial V26.1

Insensitivity
- adrenocorticotropin hormone (ACTH) 255.41
- androgen 259.50
  - complete 259.51
  - partial 259.52

Insertion
- cord (umbilical) lateral or velamentous 663.8 [5th]
  - affecting fetus or newborn 762.6
- intrauterine contraceptive device V25.1
- placenta, vicious - *see* Placenta, previa
- subdermal implantable contraceptive V25.5
- velamentous, umbilical cord 663.8 [5th]
  - affecting fetus or newborn 762.6

Insolation 992.0
- meaning sunstroke 992.0

Insomnia, unspecified 780.52
- with sleep apnea, unspecified 780.51
- adjustment 307.41
- alcohol induced 291.82

Injury – Insomnia, unspecified

Insomnia, unspecified – *continued*
- behavioral, of childhood V69.5
- drug induced 292.85
- due to
  - medical condition classified elsewhere 327.01
  - mental disorder 327.02
- fatal familial (FFI) 046.72
- idiopathic 307.42
- nonorganic origin 307.41
  - persistent (primary) 307.42
  - transient 307.41
- organic 327.00
  - other 327.09
- paradoxical 307.42
- primary 307.42
- psychophysiological 307.42
- subjective complaint 307.49

Inspiration
- food or foreign body (*see also* Asphyxia, food or foreign body) 933.1
- mucus (*see also* Asphyxia, mucus) 933.1

Inspissated bile syndrome, newborn 774.4

Instability
- detrusor 596.59
- emotional (excessive) 301.3
- joint (posttraumatic) 718.80
  - ankle 718.87
  - elbow 718.82
  - foot 718.87
  - hand 718.84
  - hip 718.85
  - knee 718.86
  - lumbosacral 724.6
  - multiple sites 718.89
  - pelvic region 718.85
  - sacroiliac 724.6
  - shoulder (region) 718.81
  - specified site NEC 718.88
  - wrist 718.83
- lumbosacral 724.6
- nervous 301.89
- personality (emotional) 301.59
- thyroid, paroxysmal 242.9 [5th]
- urethral 599.83
- vasomotor 780.2

Insufficiency, insufficient
- accommodation 367.4
- adrenal (gland) (acute) (chronic) 255.41
  - medulla 255.5
  - primary 255.41
  - specified site NEC 255.5
- adrenocortical 255.41
- anterior (occlusal) guidance 524.54
- anus 569.49
- aortic (valve) 424.1
  - with
    - mitral (valve) disease 396.1
      - insufficiency, incompetence, or regurgitation 396.3
      - stenosis or obstruction 396.1
    - stenosis or obstruction 424.1
      - with mitral (valve) disease 396.8
  - congenital 746.4
  - rheumatic 395.1
    - with
      - mitral (valve) disease 396.1
        - insufficiency, incompetence, or regurgitation 396.3
        - stenosis or obstruction 396.1
      - stenosis or obstruction 395.2
        - with mitral (valve) disease 396.8
  - specified cause NEC 424.1
  - syphilitic 093.22
- arterial 447.1
  - basilar artery 435.0
  - carotid artery 435.8
  - cerebral 437.1
  - coronary (acute or subacute) 411.89
  - mesenteric 557.1
  - peripheral 443.9
  - precerebral 435.9
  - vertebral artery 435.1

Insufficiency, insufficient – *continued*
- arterial – *continued*
  - vertebrobasilar 435.3
- arteriovenous 459.9
- basilar artery 435.0
- biliary 575.8
- cardiac (*see also* Insufficiency, myocardial) 428.0
  - complicating surgery 997.1
  - due to presence of (cardiac) prosthesis 429.4
  - postoperative 997.1
    - long-term effect of cardiac surgery 429.4
  - specified during or due to a procedure 997.1
    - long-term effect of cardiac surgery 429.4
- cardiorenal (*see also* Hypertension, cardiorenal) 404.90
- cardiovascular (*see also* Disease, cardiovascular) 429.2
  - renal (*see also* Hypertension, cardiorenal) 404.90
- carotid artery 435.8
- cerebral (vascular) 437.9
- cerebrovascular 437.9
  - with transient focal neurological signs and symptoms 435.9
  - acute 437.1
    - with transient focal neurological signs and symptoms 435.9
- circulatory NEC 459.9
  - fetus or newborn 779.89
- convergence 378.83
- coronary (acute or subacute) 411.89
  - chronic or with a stated duration of over 8 weeks 414.8
- corticoadrenal 255.41
- dietary 269.9
- divergence 378.85
- food 994.2
- gastroesophageal 530.89
- gonadal
  - ovary 256.39
  - testis 257.2
- gonadotropic hormone secretion 253.4
- heart - *see also* Insufficiency, myocardial
  - fetus or newborn 779.89
  - valve (*see also* Endocarditis) 424.90
    - congenital NEC 746.89
- hepatic 573.8
- idiopathic autonomic 333.0
- interocclusal distance of teeth (ridge) 524.36
- kidney
  - acute 593.9
  - chronic 585.9
- labyrinth, labyrinthine (function) 386.53
  - bilateral 386.54
  - unilateral 386.53
- lacrimal 375.15
- liver 573.8
- lung (acute) (*see also* Insufficiency, pulmonary) 518.82
  - following trauma, surgery, or shock 518.5
  - newborn 770.89
- mental (congenital) (*see also* Retardation, mental) 319
- mesenteric 557.1
- mitral (valve) 424.0
  - with
    - aortic (valve) disease 396.3
      - insufficiency, incompetence, or regurgitation 396.3
      - stenosis or obstruction 396.2
    - obstruction or stenosis 394.2
      - with aortic valve disease 396.8
  - congenital 746.6

Insufficiency, insufficient – *continued*
- mitral (valve) – *continued*
  - rheumatic 394.1
    - with
      - aortic (valve) disease 396.3
        - insufficiency, incompetence, or regurgitation 396.3
        - stenosis or obstruction 396.2
      - obstruction or stenosis 394.2
        - with aortic valve disease 396.8
    - active or acute 391.1
      - with chorea, rheumatic (Sydenham's) 392.0
  - specified cause, except rheumatic 424.0
- muscle
  - heart - *see* Insufficiency, myocardial
  - ocular (*see also* Strabismus) 378.9
- myocardial, myocardium (with arteriosclerosis) 428.0
  - with rheumatic fever (conditions classifiable to 390)
    - active, acute, or subacute 391.2
      - with chorea 392.0
    - inactive or quiescent (with chorea) 398.0
  - congenital 746.89
  - due to presence of (cardiac) prosthesis 429.4
  - fetus or newborn 779.89
  - following cardiac surgery 429.4
  - hypertensive (*see also* Hypertension, heart) 402.91
    - benign 402.11
    - malignant 402.01
  - postoperative 997.1
    - long-term effect of cardiac surgery 429.4
  - rheumatic 398.0
    - active, acute, or subacute 391.2
      - with chorea (Sydenham's) 392.0
  - syphilitic 093.82
- nourishment 994.2
- organic 799.89
- ovary 256.39
  - postablative 256.2
- pancreatic 577.8
- parathyroid (gland) 252.1
- peripheral vascular (arterial) 443.9
- pituitary (anterior) 253.2
  - posterior 253.5
- placental - *see* Placenta, insufficiency
- platelets 287.5
- prenatal care in current pregnancy V23.7
- progressive pluriglandular 258.9
- pseudocholinesterase 289.89
- pulmonary (acute) 518.82
  - following
    - shock 518.5
    - surgery 518.5
    - trauma 518.5
  - newborn 770.89
  - valve (*see also* Endocarditis, pulmonary) 424.3
    - congenital 746.09
- pyloric 537.0
- renal 593.9
  - acute 593.9
  - chronic 585.9
  - due to a procedure 997.5
- respiratory 786.09
  - acute 518.82
    - following shock, surgery, or trauma 518.5
  - newborn 770.89
- rotation - *see* Malrotation
- suprarenal 255.41
  - medulla 255.5
- tarso-orbital fascia, congenital 743.66
- tear film 375.15
- testis 257.2
- thyroid (gland) (acquired) - *see also* Hypothyroidism
  - congenital 243

Insufficiency, insufficient – *continued*
- tricuspid (*see also* Endocarditis, tricuspid) 397.0
  - congenital 746.89
  - syphilitic 093.23
- urethral sphincter 599.84
- valve, valvular (heart) (*see also* Endocarditis) 424.90
- vascular 459.9
  - intestine NEC 557.9
  - mesenteric 557.1
  - peripheral 443.9
  - renal (*see also* Hypertension, kidney) 403.90
- velopharyngeal
  - acquired 528.9
  - congenital 750.29
- venous (peripheral) 459.81
- ventricular - *see* Insufficiency, myocardial
- vertebral artery 435.1
- vertebrobasilar artery 435.3
- weight gain during pregnancy 646.8 [5th]
- zinc 269.3

Insufflation
- fallopian
  - fertility testing V26.21
  - following sterilization reversal V26.22
- meconium 770.11
  - with respiratory symptoms 770.12

Insular - *see* condition

Insulinoma (M8151/0)
- malignant (M8151/3)
  - pancreas 157.4
  - specified site - *see* Neoplasm, by site, malignant
  - unspecified site 157.4
- pancreas 211.7
- specified site - *see* Neoplasm, by site, benign
- unspecified site 211.7

Insuloma - *see* Insulinoma

Insult
- brain 437.9
  - acute 436
- cerebral 437.9
  - acute 436
- cerebrovascular 437.9
  - acute 436
- vascular NEC 437.9
  - acute 436

Insurance examination (certification) V70.3

Intemperance (*see also* Alcoholism) 303.9 [5th]

Interception of pregnancy (menstrual extraction) V25.3

Interference
- balancing side 524.56
- non-working side 524.56

Intermenstrual
- bleeding 626.6
  - irregular 626.6
  - regular 626.5
- hemorrhage 626.6
  - irregular 626.6
  - regular 626.5
- pain(s) 625.2

Intermittent - *see* condition

Internal - *see* condition

Interproximal wear 521.10

Interruption
- aortic arch 747.11
- bundle of His 426.50
- fallopian tube (for sterilization) V25.2
- phase-shift, sleep cycle 307.45
- repeated REM-sleep 307.48
- sleep
  - due to perceived environmental disturbances 307.48
  - phase-shift, of 24-hour sleep-wake cycle 307.45
  - repeated REM-sleep type 307.48
- vas deferens (for sterilization) V25.2

Intersexuality 752.7

Interstitial - *see* condition

Insomnia, unspecified – Interstitial

Intertrigo 695.89
  labialis 528.5
Intervertebral disc - *see* condition
Intestine, intestinal - *see also* condition
  flu 487.8
Intolerance
  carbohydrate NEC 579.8
  cardiovascular exercise, with pain (at rest) (with less than ordinary activity) (with ordinary activity) V47.2
  cold 780.99
  dissacharide (hereditary) 271.3
  drug
    correct substance properly administered 995.27
    wrong substance given or taken in error 977.9
      specified drug - *see* Table of Drugs and Chemicals
  effort 306.2
  fat NEC 579.8
  foods NEC 579.8
  fructose (hereditary) 271.2
  glucose (-galactose) (congenital) 271.3
  gluten 579.0
  lactose (hereditary) (infantile) 271.3
  lysine (congenital) 270.7
  milk NEC 579.8
  protein (familial) 270.7
  starch NEC 579.8
  sucrose (-isomaltose) (congenital) 271.3
Intoxicated NEC (*see also* Alcoholism) 305.0 5th
Intoxication
  acid 276.2
  acute
    alcoholic 305.0 5th
      with alcoholism 303.0 5th
      hangover effects 305.0 5th
    caffeine 305.9 5th
    hallucinogenic (*see also* Abuse, drugs, nondependent) 305.3 5th
  alcohol (acute) 305.0 5th
    with alcoholism 303.0 5th
    hangover effects 305.0 5th
    idiosyncratic 291.4
    pathological 291.4
  alimentary canal 558.2
  ammonia (hepatic) 572.2
  caffeine 305.9 5th
  chemical - *see also* Table of Drugs and Chemicals
    via placenta or breast milk 760.70
      alcohol 760.71
      anticonvulsants 760.77
      antifungals 760.74
      anti-infective agents 760.74
      antimetabolics 760.78
      cocaine 760.75
      "crack" 760.75
      hallucinogenic agents NEC 760.73
      medicinal agents NEC 760.79
      narcotics 760.72
      obstetric anesthetic or analgesic drug 763.5
      specified agent NEC 760.79
      suspected, affecting management of pregnancy 655.5 5th
  cocaine, through placenta or breast milk 760.75
  delirium
    alcohol 291.0
    drug 292.81
  drug 292.89
    with delirium 292.81
    correct substance properly administered (*see also* Allergy, drug) 995.27
    newborn 779.4
    obstetric anesthetic or sedation 668.9 5th
      affecting fetus or newborn 763.5

Intoxication – *continued*
  drug – *continued*
    overdose or wrong substance given or taken - *see* Table of Drugs and Chemicals
    pathologic 292.2
    specific to newborn 779.4
    via placenta or breast milk 760.70
      alcohol 760.71
      anticonvulsants 760.77
      antifungals 760.74
      anti-infective agents 760.74
      antimetabolics 760.78
      cocaine 760.75
      "crack" 760.75
      hallucinogenic agents 760.73
      medicinal agents NEC 760.79
      narcotics 760.72
      obstetric anesthetic or analgesic drug 763.5
      specified agent NEC 760.79
      suspected, affecting management of pregnancy 655.5 5th
  enteric - *see* Intoxication, intestinal
  fetus or newborn, via placenta or breast milk 760.70
    alcohol 760.71
    anticonvulsants 760.77
    antifungals 760.74
    anti-infective agents 760.74
    antimetabolics 760.78
    cocaine 760.75
    "crack" 760.75
    hallucinogenic agents 760.73
    medicinal agents NEC 760.79
    narcotics 760.72
    obstetric anesthetic or analgesic drug 763.5
    specified agent NEC 760.79
    suspected, affecting management of pregnancy 655.5 5th
  food - *see* Poisoning, food
  gastrointestinal 558.2
  hallucinogenic (acute) 305.3 5th
  hepatocerebral 572.2
  idiosyncratic alcohol 291.4
  intestinal 569.89
    due to putrefaction of food 005.9
  methyl alcohol (*see also* Alcoholism) 305.0 5th
    with alcoholism 303.0 5th
  non-foodborne due to toxins of Clostridium botulinum [C. botulinum] - *see* Botulism
  pathologic 291.4
    drug 292.2
  potassium (K) 276.7
  septic
    with
      abortion - *see* Abortion, by type, with sepsis
      ectopic pregnancy (*see also* categories 633.0-633.9) 639.0
      molar pregnancy (*see also* categories 630-632) 639.0
    during labor 659.3 5th
    following
      abortion 639.0
      ectopic or molar pregnancy 639.0
    generalized - *see* Septicemia
    puerperal, postpartum, childbirth 670.2 5th ▲
  serum (prophylactic) (therapeutic) 999.5
  uremic - *see* Uremia
  water 276.6
Intracranial - *see* condition
Intrahepatic gallbladder 751.69
Intraligamentous - *see also* condition
  pregnancy - *see* Pregnancy, cornual
Intraocular - *see also* condition
  sepsis 360.00
Intrathoracic - *see also* condition
  kidney 753.3
  stomach - *see* Hernia, diaphragm

Intrauterine contraceptive device
  checking V25.42
  insertion V25.1
  in situ V45.51
  management V25.42
  prescription V25.02
    repeat V25.42
  reinsertion V25.42
  removal V25.42
Intraventricular - *see* condition
Intrinsic deformity - *see* Deformity
Intruded tooth 524.34
Intrusion, repetitive, of sleep (due to environmental disturbances) (with atypical polysomnographic features) 307.48
Intumescent, lens (eye) NEC 366.9
  senile 366.12
Intussusception (colon) (enteric) (intestine) (rectum) 560.0
  appendix 543.9
  congenital 751.5
  fallopian tube 620.8
  ileocecal 560.0
  ileocolic 560.0
  ureter (obstruction) 593.4
Invagination
  basilar 756.0
  colon or intestine 560.0
Invalid (since birth) 799.89
Invalidism (chronic) 799.89
Inversion
  albumin-globulin (A-G) ratio 273.8
  bladder 596.8
  cecum (*see also* Intussusception) 560.0
  cervix 622.8
  nipple 611.79
    congenital 757.6
    puerperal, postpartum 676.3 5th
  optic papilla 743.57
  organ or site, congenital NEC - *see* Anomaly, specified type NEC
  sleep rhythm 327.39
    nonorganic origin 307.45
  testis (congenital) 752.51
  uterus (postinfectional) (postpartal, old) 621.7
    chronic 621.7
    complicating delivery 665.2 5th
      affecting fetus or newborn 763.89
  vagina - *see* Prolapse, vagina
Investigation
  allergens V72.7
  clinical research (control) (normal comparison) (participant) V70.7
Inviability - *see* Immaturity
Involuntary movement, abnormal 781.0
Involution, involutional - *see also* condition
  breast, cystic or fibrocystic 610.1
  depression (*see also* Psychosis, affective) 296.2 5th
    recurrent episode 296.3 5th
    single episode 296.2 5th
  melancholia (*see also* Psychosis, affective) 296.2 5th
    recurrent episode 296.3 5th
    single episode 296.2 5th
  ovary, senile 620.3
  paranoid state (reaction) 297.2
  paraphrenia (climacteric) (menopause) 297.2
  psychosis 298.8
  thymus failure 254.8
IQ
  under 20 318.2
  20-34 318.1
  35-49 318.0
  50-70 317
IRDS 769
Irideremia 743.45
Iridis rubeosis 364.42
  diabetic 250.5 5th *[364.42]*
    due to secondary diabetes 249.5 5th *[364.42]*

Iridochoroiditis (panuveitis) 360.12
Iridocyclitis NEC 364.3
  acute 364.00
    primary 364.01
    recurrent 364.02
  chronic 364.10
    in
      lepromatous leprosy 030.0 *[364.11]*
      sarcoidosis 135 *[364.11]*
      tuberculosis (*see also* Tuberculosis) 017.3 5th *[364.11]*
  due to allergy 364.04
  endogenous 364.01
  gonococcal 098.41
  granulomatous 364.10
  herpetic (simplex) 054.44
    zoster 053.22
  hypopyon 364.05
  lens induced 364.23
  nongranulomatous 364.00
  primary 364.01
  recurrent 364.02
  rheumatic 364.10
  secondary 364.04
    infectious 364.03
    noninfectious 364.04
  subacute 364.00
    primary 364.01
    recurrent 364.02
  sympathetic 360.11
  syphilitic (secondary) 091.52
  tuberculous (chronic) (*see also* Tuberculosis) 017.3 5th *[364.11]*
Iridocyclochoroiditis (panuveitis) 360.12
Iridodialysis 364.76
Iridodonesis 364.89
Iridoplegia (complete) (partial) (reflex) 379.49
Iridoschisis 364.52
Iris - *see* condition
Iritis 364.3
  acute 364.00
    primary 364.01
    recurrent 364.02
  chronic 364.10
    in
      sarcoidosis 135 *[364.11]*
      tuberculosis (*see also* Tuberculosis) 017.3 5th *[364.11]*
  diabetic 250.5 5th *[364.42]*
    due to secondary diabetes 249.5 5th *[364.42]*
  due to
    allergy 364.04
    herpes simplex 054.44
    leprosy 030.0 *[364.11]*
  endogenous 364.01
  gonococcal 098.41
  gouty 274.89 *[364.11]*
  granulomatous 364.10
  hypopyon 364.05
  lens induced 364.23
  nongranulomatous 364.00
  papulosa 095.8 *[364.11]*
  primary 364.01
  recurrent 364.02
  rheumatic 364.10
  secondary 364.04
    infectious 364.03
    noninfectious 364.04
  subacute 364.00
    primary 364.01
    recurrent 364.02
  sympathetic 360.11
  syphilitic (secondary) 091.52
    congenital 090.0 *[364.11]*
    late 095.8 *[364.11]*
  tuberculous (*see also* Tuberculosis) 017.3 5th *[364.11]*
  uratic 274.89 *[364.11]*
Iron
  deficiency anemia 280.9
  metabolism disease 275.0
  storage disease 275.0

Iron-miners' lung 503

Irradiated enamel (tooth, teeth) 521.89

Irradiation
- burn - *see* Burn, by site
- effects, adverse 990

Irreducible, irreducibility - *see* condition

Irregular, irregularity
- action, heart 427.9
- alveolar process 525.8
- bleeding NEC 626.4
- breathing 786.09
- colon 569.89
- contour
  - of cornea 743.41
    - acquired 371.70
  - reconstructed breast 612.0
- dentin in pulp 522.3
- eye movements NEC 379.59
- menstruation (cause unknown) 626.4
- periods 626.4
- prostate 602.9
- pupil 364.75
- respiratory 786.09
- septum (nasal) 470
- shape, organ or site, congenital NEC - *see* Distortion
- sleep-wake rhythm (non-24-hour) 327.39
  - nonorganic origin 307.45
- vertebra 733.99

Irritability ~~(nervous)~~ 799.2<u>2</u> ▲
- bladder 596.8
  - neurogenic 596.54
    - with cauda equina syndrome 344.61
- bowel (syndrome) 564.1
- bronchial (*see also* Bronchitis) 490
- cerebral, newborn 779.1
- colon 564.1
  - psychogenic 306.4
- duodenum 564.89
- heart (psychogenic) 306.2
- ileum 564.89
- jejunum 564.89
- myocardium 306.2
- nervousness 799.21 ●
- rectum 564.89
- stomach 536.9
  - psychogenic 306.4
- sympathetic (nervous system) (*see also* Neuropathy, peripheral, autonomic) 337.9
- urethra 599.84
- ventricular (heart) (psychogenic) 306.2

Irritable - <u>(*see also* Irritability) 799.22</u> ▲

Irritation
- anus 569.49
- axillary nerve 353.0
- bladder 596.8
- brachial plexus 353.0
- brain (traumatic) (*see also* Injury, intracranial) 854.0 5th
  - nontraumatic - *see* Encephalitis
- bronchial (*see also* Bronchitis) 490
- cerebral (traumatic) (*see also* Injury, intracranial) 854.0 5th
  - nontraumatic - *see* Encephalitis
- cervical plexus 353.2
- cervix (*see also* Cervicitis) 616.0
- choroid, sympathetic 360.11
- cranial nerve - *see* Disorder, nerve, cranial
- digestive tract 536.9
  - psychogenic 306.4
- gastric 536.9
  - psychogenic 306.4
- gastrointestinal (tract) 536.9
  - functional 536.9
  - psychogenic 306.4
- globe, sympathetic 360.11
- intestinal (bowel) 564.9
- labyrinth 386.50
- lumbosacral plexus 353.1
- meninges (traumatic) (*see also* Injury, intracranial) 854.0 5th
  - nontraumatic - *see* Meningitis
- myocardium 306.2

Irritability – *continued*
- nerve - *see* Disorder, nerve
- nervous 799.2<u>1</u> ▲
- nose 478.19
- penis 607.89
- perineum 709.9
- peripheral
  - autonomic nervous system (*see also* Neuropathy, peripheral, autonomic) 337.9
  - nerve - *see* Disorder, nerve
- peritoneum (*see also* Peritonitis) 567.9
- pharynx 478.29
- plantar nerve 355.6
- spinal (cord) (traumatic) - *see also* Injury, spinal, by site
  - nerve - *see also* Disorder, nerve
    - root NEC 724.9
    - traumatic - *see* Injury, nerve, spinal
  - nontraumatic - *see* Myelitis
- stomach 536.9
  - psychogenic 306.4
- sympathetic nerve NEC (*see also* Neuropathy, peripheral, autonomic) 337.9
- ulnar nerve 354.2
- vagina 623.9

Isambert's disease 012.3 5th

Ischemia, ischemic 459.9
- basilar artery (with transient neurologic deficit) 435.0
- bone NEC 733.40
- bowel (transient) 557.9
  - acute 557.0
  - chronic 557.1
  - due to mesenteric artery insufficiency 557.1
- brain - *see also* Ischemia, cerebral
  - recurrent focal 435.9
- cardiac (*see also* Ischemia, heart) 414.9
- cardiomyopathy 414.8
- carotid artery (with transient neurologic deficit) 435.8
- cerebral (chronic) (generalized) 437.1
  - arteriosclerotic 437.0
  - intermittent (with transient neurologic deficit) 435.9
  - newborn 779.2
  - puerperal, postpartum, childbirth 674.0 5th
  - recurrent focal (with transient neurologic deficit) 435.9
  - transient (with transient neurologic deficit) 435.9
- colon 557.9
  - acute 557.0
  - chronic 557.1
  - due to mesenteric artery insufficiency 557.1
- coronary (chronic) (*see also* Ischemia, heart) 414.9
- heart (chronic or with a stated duration of over 8 weeks) 414.9
  - acute or with a stated duration of 8 weeks or less (*see also* Infarct, myocardium) 410.9 5th
    - without myocardial infarction 411.89
      - with coronary (artery) occlusion 411.81
  - subacute 411.89
- intestine (transient) 557.9
  - acute 557.0
  - chronic 557.1
  - due to mesenteric artery insufficiency 557.1
- kidney 593.81
- labyrinth 386.50
- muscles, leg 728.89

Ischemia, ischemic – *continued*
- myocardium, myocardial (chronic or with a stated duration of over 8 weeks) 414.8
  - acute (*see also* Infarct, myocardium) 410.9 5th
    - without myocardial infarction 411.89
      - with coronary (artery) occlusion 411.81
- renal 593.81
- retina, retinal 362.84
- small bowel 557.9
  - acute 557.0
  - chronic 557.1
  - due to mesenteric artery insufficiency 557.1
- spinal cord 336.1
- subendocardial (*see also* Insufficiency, coronary) 411.89
- vertebral artery (with transient neurologic deficit) 435.1

Ischialgia (*see also* Sciatica) 724.3

Ischiopagus 759.4

Ischium, ischial - *see* condition

Ischomenia 626.8

Ischuria 788.5

Iselin's disease or osteochondrosis 732.5

Islands of
- parotid tissue in
  - lymph nodes 750.26
  - neck structures 750.26
- submaxillary glands in
  - fascia 750.26
  - lymph nodes 750.26
  - neck muscles 750.26

Islet cell tumor, pancreas (M8150/0) 211.7

Isoimmunization NEC (*see also* Incompatibility) 656.2 5th
- anti-E 656.2 5th
- fetus or newborn 773.2
  - ABO blood groups 773.1
  - Rhesus (Rh) factor 773.0

Isolation V07.0
- social V62.4

Isosporosis 007.2

Issue
- medical certificate NEC V68.09
  - cause of death V68.09
  - disability examination V68.01
  - fitness V68.09
  - incapacity V68.09
- repeat prescription NEC V68.1
  - appliance V68.1
  - contraceptive V25.40
    - device NEC V25.49
      - intrauterine V25.42
      - specified type NEC V25.49
    - pill V25.41
  - glasses V68.1
  - medicinal substance V68.1

Itch (*see also* Pruritus) 698.9
- bakers' 692.89
- barbers' 110.0
- bricklayers' 692.89
- cheese 133.8
- clam diggers' 120.3
- coolie 126.9
- copra 133.8
- Cuban 050.1
- dew 126.9
- dhobie 110.3
- eye 379.99
- filarial (*see also* Infestation, filarial) 125.9
- grain 133.8
- grocers' 133.8
- ground 126.9
- harvest 133.8
- jock 110.3
- Malabar 110.9
  - beard 110.0
  - foot 110.4
  - scalp 110.0
- meaning scabies 133.0

Itch – *continued*
- Norwegian 133.0
- perianal 698.0
- poultrymen's 133.8
- sarcoptic 133.0
- scrub 134.1
- seven year V61.10
  - meaning scabies 133.0
- straw 133.8
- swimmers' 120.3
- washerwoman's 692.4
- water 120.3
- winter 698.8

Itsenko-Cushing syndrome (pituitary basophilism) 255.0

Ivemark's syndrome (asplenia with congenital heart disease) 759.0

Ivory bones 756.52

Ixodes 134.8

Ixodiasis 134.8

J

Jaccoud's nodular fibrositis, chronic (Jaccoud's syndrome) 714.4

Jackson's
- membrane 751.4
- paralysis or syndrome 344.89
- veil 751.4

Jacksonian
- epilepsy (*see also* Epilepsy) 345.5 5th
- seizures (focal) (*see also* Epilepsy) 345.5 5th

Jacob's ulcer (M8090/3) - *see* Neoplasm, skin, malignant, by site

Jacquet's dermatitis (diaper dermatitis) 691.0

Jadassohn's
- blue nevus (M8780/0) - *see* Neoplasm, skin, benign
- disease (maculopapular erythroderma) 696.2
- intraepidermal epithelioma (M8096/0) - *see* Neoplasm, skin, benign

Jadassohn-Lewandowski syndrome (pachyonychia congenita) 757.5

Jadassohn-Pellizari's disease (anetoderma) 701.3

Jadassohn-Tièche nevus (M8780/0) - *see* Neoplasm, skin, benign

Jaffe-Lichtenstein (-Uehlinger) syndrome 252.01

Jahnke's syndrome (encephalocutaneous angiomatosis) 759.6

Jakob-Creutzfeldt disease (CJD) (syndrome) 046.19
- with dementia
  - with behavioral disturbance 046.19 *[294.11]*
  - without behavioral disturbance 046.19 *[294.10]*
- familial 046.19
- iatrogenic 046.19
- specified NEC 046.19
- sporadic 046.19
- variant (vCJD) 046.11
  - with dementia
    - with behavioral disturbance 046.11 *[294.11]*
    - without behavioral disturbance 046.11 *[294.10]*

Jaksch (-Luzet) disease or syndrome (pseudoleukemia infantum) 285.8

Jamaican
- neuropathy 349.82
- paraplegic tropical ataxic-spastic syndrome 349.82

Janet's disease (psychasthenia) 300.89

Janiceps 759.4

Jansky-Bielschowsky amaurotic familial idiocy 330.1

- **Japanese**
  - B-type encephalitis 062.0
  - river fever 081.2
  - seven-day fever 100.89
- **Jaundice** (yellow) 782.4
  - acholuric (familial) (splenomegalic) (*see also* Spherocytosis) 282.0
    - acquired 283.9
  - breast milk 774.39
  - catarrhal (acute) 070.1
    - with hepatic coma 070.0
    - chronic 571.9
    - epidemic - *see* Jaundice, epidemic
  - cholestatic (benign) 782.4
  - chronic idiopathic 277.4
  - epidemic (catarrhal) 070.1
    - with hepatic coma 070.0
    - leptospiral 100.0
    - spirochetal 100.0
  - febrile (acute) 070.1
    - with hepatic coma 070.0
    - leptospiral 100.0
    - spirochetal 100.0
  - fetus or newborn 774.6
    - due to or associated with
      - ABO
        - antibodies 773.1
        - incompatibility, maternal/fetal 773.1
        - isoimmunization 773.1
      - absence or deficiency of enzyme system for bilirubin conjugation (congenital) 774.39
      - blood group incompatibility NEC 773.2
      - breast milk inhibitors to conjugation 774.39
        - associated with preterm delivery 774.2
      - bruising 774.1
      - Crigler-Najjar syndrome 277.4 *[774.31]*
      - delayed conjugation 774.30
        - associated with preterm delivery 774.2
        - development 774.39
      - drugs or toxins transmitted from mother 774.1
      - G-6-PD deficiency 282.2 *[774.0]*
      - galactosemia 271.1 *[774.5]*
      - Gilbert's syndrome 277.4 *[774.31]*
      - hepatocellular damage 774.4
      - hereditary hemolytic anemia (*see also* Anemia, hemolytic) 282.9 *[774.0]*
      - hypothyroidism, congenital 243 *[774.31]*
      - incompatibility, maternal/fetal NEC 773.2
      - infection 774.1
      - inspissated bile syndrome 774.4
      - isoimmunization NEC 773.2
      - mucoviscidosis 277.01 *[774.5]*
      - obliteration of bile duct, congenital 751.61 *[774.5]*
      - polycythemia 774.1
      - preterm delivery 774.2
      - red cell defect 282.9 *[774.0]*
      - Rh
        - antibodies 773.0
        - incompatibility, maternal/fetal 773.0
        - isoimmunization 773.0
      - spherocytosis (congenital) 282.0 *[774.0]*
      - swallowed maternal blood 774.1
    - physiological NEC 774.6
  - from injection, inoculation, infusion, or transfusion (blood) (plasma) (serum) (other substance) (onset within 8 months after administration) - *see* Hepatitis, viral
  - Gilbert's (familial nonhemolytic) 277.4
- **Jaundice** – *continued*
  - hematogenous 283.9
  - hemolytic (acquired) 283.9
    - congenital (*see also* Spherocytosis) 282.0
  - hemorrhagic (acute) 100.0
    - leptospiral 100.0
    - newborn 776.0
    - spirochetal 100.0
  - hepatocellular 573.8
  - homologous (serum) - *see* Hepatitis, viral
  - idiopathic, chronic 277.4
  - infectious (acute) (subacute) 070.1
    - with hepatic coma 070.0
    - leptospiral 100.0
    - spirochetal 100.0
  - leptospiral 100.0
  - malignant (*see also* Necrosis, liver) 570
  - newborn (physiological) (*see also* Jaundice, fetus or newborn) 774.6
  - nonhemolytic, congenital familial (Gilbert's) 277.4
  - nuclear, newborn (*see also* Kernicterus of newborn) 774.7
  - obstructive NEC (*see also* Obstruction, biliary) 576.8
  - postimmunization - *see* Hepatitis, viral
  - posttransfusion - *see* Hepatitis, viral
  - regurgitation (*see also* Obstruction, biliary) 576.8
  - serum (homologous) (prophylactic) (therapeutic) - *see* Hepatitis, viral
  - spirochetal (hemorrhagic) 100.0
  - symptomatic 782.4
    - newborn 774.6
- **Jaw** - *see* condition
- **Jaw-blinking** 374.43
  - congenital 742.8
- **Jaw-winking phenomenon or syndrome** 742.8
- **Jealousy**
  - alcoholic 291.5
  - childhood 313.3
  - sibling 313.3
- **Jejunitis** (*see also* Enteritis) 558.9
- **Jejunostomy status** V44.4
- **Jejunum, jejunal** - *see* condition
- **Jensen's disease** 363.05
- **Jericho boil** 085.1
- **Jerks, myoclonic** 333.2
- **Jervell-Lange-Nielsen syndrome** 426.82
- **Jeune's disease or syndrome** (asphyxiating thoracic dystrophy) 756.4
- **Jigger disease** 134.1
- **Job's syndrome (chronic granulomatous disease)** 288.1
- **Jod-Basedow phenomenon** 242.8 5th
- **Johnson-Stevens disease** (erythema multiforme exudativum) 695.13
- **Joint** - *see also* condition
  - Charcôt's 094.0 *[713.5]*
  - false 733.82
  - flail - *see* Flail, joint
  - mice- *see* Loose, body, joint, by site
  - sinus to bone 730.9 5th
  - von Gies' 095.8
- **Jordan's anomaly or syndrome** 288.2
- **Josephs-Diamond-Blackfan anemia** (congenital hypoplastic) 284.01
- **Joubert syndrome** 759.89
- **Jumpers' knee** 727.2
- **Jungle yellow fever** 060.0
- **Jungling's disease** (sarcoidosis) 135
- **Junin virus hemorrhagic fever** 078.7
- **Juvenile** - *see also* condition
  - delinquent 312.9
    - group (*see also* Disturbance, conduct) 312.2 5th
    - neurotic 312.4

K

- **Kabuki syndrome** 759.89
- **Kahler (-Bozzolo) disease** (multiple myeloma) (M9730/3) 203.0 5th
- **Kakergasia** 300.9
- **Kakke** 265.0
- **Kala-azar** (Indian) (infantile) (Mediterranean) (Sudanese) 085.0
- **Kalischer's syndrome** (encephalocutaneous angiomatosis) 759.6
- **Kallmann's syndrome** (hypogonadotropic hypogonadism with anosmia) 253.4
- **Kanner's syndrome** (autism) (*see also* Psychosis, childhood) 299.0 5th
- **Kaolinosis** 502
- **Kaposi's**
  - disease 757.33
    - lichen ruber 696.4
      - acuminatus 696.4
      - moniliformis 697.8
  - xeroderma pigmentosum 757.33
  - sarcoma (M9140/3) 176.9
    - adipose tissue 176.1
    - aponeurosis 176.1
    - artery 176.1
    - associated herpesvirus infection 058.89
    - blood vessel 176.1
    - bursa 176.1
    - connective tissue 176.1
    - external genitalia 176.8
    - fascia 176.1
    - fatty tissue 176.1
    - fibrous tissue 176.1
    - gastrointestinal tract NEC 176.3
    - ligament 176.1
    - lung 176.4
    - lymph
      - gland(s) 176.5
      - node(s) 176.5
    - lymphatic(s) NEC 176.1
    - muscle (skeletal) 176.1
    - oral cavity NEC 176.8
    - palate 176.2
    - scrotum 176.8
    - skin 176.0
    - soft tissue 176.1
    - specified site NEC 176.8
    - subcutaneous tissue 176.1
    - synovia 176.1
    - tendon (sheath) 176.1
    - vein 176.1
    - vessel 176.1
    - viscera NEC 176.9
    - vulva 176.8
  - varicelliform eruption 054.0
    - vaccinia 999.0
- **Kartagener's syndrome or triad** (sinusitis, bronchiectasis, situs inversus) 759.3
- **Kasabach-Merritt syndrome** (capillary hemangioma associated with thrombocytopenic purpura) 287.39
- **Kaschin-Beck disease** (endemic polyarthritis) - *see* Disease, Kaschin-Beck
- **Kast's syndrome** (dyschondroplasia with hemangiomas) 756.4
- **Katatonia**- *see* **Catatonia**
- **Katayama disease or fever** 120.2
- **Kathisophobia** 781.0
- **Kawasaki disease** 446.1
- **Kayser-Fleischer ring** (cornea) (pseudosclerosis) 275.1 *[371.14]*
- **Kaznelson's syndrome** (congenital hypoplastic anemia) 284.01
- **Kearns-Sayre syndrome** 277.87
- **Kedani fever** 081.2
- **Kelis** 701.4
- **Kelly (-Patterson) syndrome** (sideropenic dysphagia) 280.8
- **Keloid, cheloid** 701.4
  - Addison's (morphea) 701.0
  - cornea 371.00
  - Hawkins' 701.4
  - scar 701.4
- **Keloma** 701.4
- **Kenya fever** 082.1
- **Keratectasia** 371.71
  - congenital 743.41
- **Keratinization NEC**
  - alveolar ridge mucosa
    - excessive 528.72
    - minimal 528.71
- **Keratitis** (nodular) (nonulcerative) (simple) (zonular) NEC 370.9
  - with ulceration (*see also* Ulcer, cornea) 370.00
  - actinic 370.24
  - arborescens 054.42
  - areolar 370.22
  - bullosa 370.8
  - deep - *see* Keratitis, interstitial
  - dendritic(a) 054.42
  - desiccation 370.34
  - diffuse interstitial 370.52
  - disciform(is) 054.43
    - varicella 052.7 *[370.44]*
  - epithelialis vernalis 372.13 *[370.32]*
  - exposure 370.34
  - filamentary 370.23
  - gonococcal (congenital) (prenatal) 098.43
  - herpes, herpetic (simplex) NEC 054.43
    - zoster 053.21
  - hypopyon 370.04
  - in
    - chickenpox 052.7 *[370.44]*
    - exanthema (*see also* Exanthem) 057.9 *[370.44]*
    - paravaccinia (*see also* Paravaccinia) 051.9 *[370.44]*
    - smallpox (*see also* Smallpox) 050.9 *[370.44]*
    - vernal conjunctivitis 372.13 *[370.32]*
  - interstitial (nonsyphilitic) 370.50
    - with ulcer (*see also* Ulcer, cornea) 370.00
    - diffuse 370.52
    - herpes, herpetic (simplex) 054.43
      - zoster 053.21
    - syphilitic (congenital) (hereditary) 090.3
    - tuberculous (*see also* Tuberculosis) 017.3 5th *[370.59]*
  - lagophthalmic 370.34
  - macular 370.22
  - neuroparalytic 370.35
  - neurotrophic 370.35
  - nummular 370.22
  - oyster-shuckers' 370.8
  - parenchymatous - *see* Keratitis, interstitial
  - petrificans 370.8
  - phlyctenular 370.31
  - postmeasles 055.71
  - punctata, punctate 370.21
    - leprosa 030.0 *[370.21]*
    - profunda 090.3
    - superficial (Thygeson's) 370.21
  - purulent 370.8
  - pustuliformis profunda 090.3
  - rosacea 695.3 *[370.49]*
  - sclerosing 370.54
  - specified type NEC 370.8
  - stellate 370.22
  - striate 370.22
  - superficial 370.20
    - with conjunctivitis (*see also* Keratoconjunctivitis) 370.40
    - punctate (Thygeson's) 370.21
  - suppurative 370.8
  - syphilitic (congenital) (prenatal) 090.3
  - trachomatous 076.1
    - late effect 139.1
  - tuberculous (phlyctenular) (*see also* Tuberculosis) 017.3 5th *[370.31]*

Japanese – Keratitis

Keratitis – *continued*
- ulcerated (*see also* Ulcer, cornea) 370.00
- vesicular 370.8
- welders' 370.24
- xerotic (*see also* Keratomalacia) 371.45
  - vitamin A deficiency 264.4

Keratoacanthoma 238.2
Keratocele 371.72
Keratoconjunctivitis (*see also* Keratitis) 370.40
- adenovirus type 8 077.1
- epidemic 077.1
- exposure 370.34
- gonococcal 098.43
- herpetic (simplex) 054.43
  - zoster 053.21
- in
  - chickenpox 052.7 *[370.44]*
  - exanthema (*see also* Exanthem) 057.9 *[370.44]*
  - paravaccinia (*see also* Paravaccinia) 051.9 *[370.44]*
  - smallpox (*see also* Smallpox) 050.9 *[370.44]*
- infectious 077.1
- neurotrophic 370.35
- phlyctenular 370.31
- postmeasles 055.71
- shipyard 077.1
- sicca (Sjögren's syndrome) 710.2
  - not in Sjögren's syndrome 370.33
- specified type NEC 370.49
- tuberculous (phlyctenular) (*see also* Tuberculosis) 017.3 5th *[370.31]*

Keratoconus 371.60
- acute hydrops 371.62
- congenital 743.41
- stable 371.61

Keratocyst (dental) 526.0
Keratoderma, keratodermia (congenital) (palmaris et plantaris) (symmetrical) 757.39
- acquired 701.1
- blennorrhagica 701.1
  - gonococcal 098.81
- climacterium 701.1
- eccentrica 757.39
- gonorrheal 098.81
- punctata 701.1
- tylodes, progressive 701.1

Keratodermatocele 371.72
Keratoglobus 371.70
- congenital 743.41
  - associated with buphthalmos 743.22

Keratohemia 371.12
Keratoiritis (*see also* Iridocyclitis) 364.3
- syphilitic 090.3
- tuberculous (*see also* Tuberculosis) 017.3 5th *[364.11]*

Keratolysis exfoliativa (congenital) 757.39
- acquired 695.89
- neonatorum 757.39

Keratoma 701.1
- congenital 757.39
- malignum congenitale 757.1
- palmaris et plantaris hereditarium 757.39
- senile 702.0

Keratomalacia 371.45
- vitamin A deficiency 264.4

Keratomegaly 743.41
Keratomycosis 111.1
- nigricans (palmaris) 111.1

Keratopathy 371.40
- band (*see also* Keratitis) 371.43
- bullous (*see also* Keratitis) 371.23
- degenerative (*see also* Degeneration, cornea) 371.40
  - hereditary (*see also* Dystrophy, cornea) 371.50
- discrete colliquative 371.49

Keratoscleritis, tuberculous (*see also* Tuberculosis) 017.3 5th *[370.31]*
Keratosis 701.1
- actinic 702.0
- arsenical 692.4
- blennorrhagica 701.1
  - gonococcal 098.81
- congenital (any type) 757.39
- ear (middle) (*see also* Cholesteatoma) 385.30
- female genital (external) 629.89
- follicular, vitamin A deficiency 264.8
- follicularis 757.39
  - acquired 701.1
  - congenital (acneiformis) (Siemens') 757.39
  - spinulosa (decalvans) 757.39
  - vitamin A deficiency 264.8
- gonococcal 098.81
- larynx, laryngeal 478.79
- male genital (external) 608.89
- middle ear (*see also* Cholesteatoma) 385.30
- nigricans 701.2
  - congenital 757.39
- obturans 380.21
- oral epithelium
  - residual ridge mucosa
    - excessive 528.72
    - minimal 528.71
- palmaris et plantaris (symmetrical) 757.39
- penile 607.89
- pharyngeus 478.29
- pilaris 757.39
  - acquired 701.1
- punctata (palmaris et plantaris) 701.1
- scrotal 608.89
- seborrheic 702.19
  - inflamed 702.11
- senilis 702.0
- solar 702.0
- suprafollicularis 757.39
- tonsillaris 478.29
- vagina 623.1
- vegetans 757.39
- vitamin A deficiency 264.8

Kerato-uveitis (*see also* Iridocyclitis) 364.3
Keraunoparalysis 994.0
Kerion (celsi) 110.0
Kernicterus of newborn (not due to isoimmunization) 774.7
- due to isoimmunization (conditions classifiable to 773.0-773.2) 773.4

Ketoacidosis 276.2
- diabetic 250.1 5th
  - due to secondary diabetes 249.1 5th

Ketonuria 791.6
- branched-chain, intermittent 270.3

Ketosis 276.2
- diabetic 250.1 5th
  - due to secondary diabetes 249.1 5th

Kidney - *see* condition
Kienböck's
- disease 732.3
  - adult 732.8
- osteochondrosis 732.3

Kimmelstiel (-Wilson) disease or syndrome (intercapillary glomerulosclerosis) 250.4 5th *[581.81]*
- due to secondary diabetes 249.4 5th *[581.81]*

Kink, kinking
- appendix 543.9
- artery 447.1
- cystic duct, congenital 751.61
- hair (acquired) 704.2
- ileum or intestine (*see also* Obstruction, intestine) 560.9
- Lane's (*see also* Obstruction, intestine) 560.9
- organ or site, congenital NEC - *see* Anomaly, specified type NEC, by site
- ureter (pelvic junction) 593.3
  - congenital 753.20
- vein(s) 459.2
  - caval 459.2
  - peripheral 459.2

Kinnier Wilson's disease (hepatolenticular degeneration) 275.1
Kissing
- osteophytes 721.5
- spine 721.5
- vertebra 721.5

Klauder's syndrome (erythema multiforme exudativum) 695.19
Klebs' disease (*see also* Nephritis) 583.9
Klein-Waardenburg syndrome (ptosis-epicanthus) 270.2
Kleine-Levin syndrome 327.13
Kleptomania 312.32
Klinefelter's syndrome 758.7
Klinger's disease 446.4
Klippel's disease 723.8
Klippel-Feil disease or syndrome (brevicollis) 756.16
Klippel-Trenaunay syndrome 759.89
Klumpke (-Déjérine) palsy, paralysis (birth) (newborn) 767.6
Klüver-Bucy (-Terzian) syndrome 310.0
Knee - *see* condition
Knifegrinders' rot (*see also* Tuberculosis) 011.4 5th
Knock-knee (acquired) 736.41
- congenital 755.64

Knot
- intestinal, syndrome (volvulus) 560.2
- umbilical cord (true) 663.2 5th
  - affecting fetus or newborn 762.5

Knots, surfer 919.8
- infected 919.9

Knotting (of)
- hair 704.2
- intestine 560.2

Knuckle pads (Garrod's) 728.79
Köbner's disease (epidermolysis bullosa) 757.39
Koch's
- infection (*see also* Tuberculosis, pulmonary) 011.9 5th
- relapsing fever 087.9

Koch-Weeks conjunctivitis 372.03
Koenig-Wichman disease (pemphigus) 694.4
Köhler's disease (osteochondrosis) 732.5
- first (osteochondrosis juvenilis) 732.5
- second (Freiburg's infarction, metatarsal head) 732.5
- patellar 732.4
- tarsal navicular (bone) (osteoarthrosis juvenilis) 732.5

Köhler-Mouchet disease (osteoarthrosis juvenilis) 732.5
Köhler-Pellegrini-Stieda disease or syndrome (calcification, knee joint) 726.62
Koilonychia 703.8
- congenital 757.5

Kojevnikov's, Kojewnikoff's epilepsy (*see also* Epilepsy) 345.7 5th
König's
- disease (osteochondritis dissecans) 732.7
- syndrome 564.89

Koniophthisis (*see also* Tuberculosis) 011.4 5th
Koplik's spots 055.9
Kopp's asthma 254.8
Korean hemorrhagic fever 078.6
Korsakoff (-Wernicke) disease, psychosis, or syndrome (nonalcoholic) 294.0
- alcoholic 291.1

Korsakov's disease - *see* Korsakoff's disease
Korsakow's disease - *see* Korsakoff's disease
Kostmann's disease or syndrome (infantile genetic agranulocytosis) 288.01
Krabbe's
- disease (leukodystrophy) 330.0
- syndrome
  - congenital muscle hypoplasia 756.89
  - cutaneocerebral angioma 759.6

Kraepelin-Morel disease (*see also* Schizophrenia) 295.9 5th
Kraft-Weber-Dimitri disease 759.6
Kraurosis
- ani 569.49
- penis 607.0
- vagina 623.8
- vulva 624.09

Kreotoxism 005.9
Krukenberg's
- spindle 371.13
- tumor (M8490/6) 198.6

Kufs' disease 330.1
Kugelberg-Welander disease 335.11
Kuhnt-Junius degeneration or disease 362.52
Kulchitsky's cell carcinoma (carcinoid tumor of intestine) 259.2
Kümmell's disease or spondylitis 721.7
Kundrat's disease (lymphosarcoma) 200.1 5th
Kunekune - *see* Dermatophytosis
Kunkel syndrome (lupoid hepatitis) 571.49
Kupffer cell sarcoma (M9124/3) 155.0
Kuru 046.0
Kussmaul's
- coma (diabetic) 250.3 5th
  - due to secondary diabetes 249.3 5th
- disease (polyarteritis nodosa) 446.0
- respiration (air hunger) 786.09

Kwashiorkor (marasmus type) 260
Kyasanur Forest disease 065.2
Kyphoscoliosis, kyphoscoliotic (acquired) (*see also* Scoliosis) 737.30
- congenital 756.19
- due to radiation 737.33
- heart (disease) 416.1
- idiopathic 737.30
  - infantile
    - progressive 737.32
    - resolving 737.31
- late effect of rickets 268.1 *[737.43]*
- specified NEC 737.39
- thoracogenic 737.34
- tuberculous (*see also* Tuberculosis) 015.0 5th *[737.43]*

Kyphosis, kyphotic (acquired) (postural) 737.10
- adolescent postural 737.0
- congenital 756.19
- dorsalis juvenilis 732.0
- due to or associated with
  - Charcôt-Marie-Tooth disease 356.1 *[737.41]*
  - mucopolysaccharidosis 277.5 *[737.41]*
  - neurofibromatosis 237.71 *[737.41]*
  - osteitis
    - deformans 731.0 *[737.41]*
    - fibrosa cystica 252.01 *[737.41]*
  - osteoporosis (*see also* Osteoporosis) 733.0 5th *[737.41]*
  - poliomyelitis (*see also* Poliomyelitis) 138 *[737.41]*
  - radiation 737.11
  - tuberculosis (*see also* Tuberculosis) 015.0 5th *[737.41]*
- Kümmell's 721.7
- late effect of rickets 268.1 *[737.41]*
- Morquio-Brailsford type (spinal) 277.5 *[737.41]*
- pelvis 738.6
- postlaminectomy 737.12
- specified cause NEC 737.19
- syphilitic, congenital 090.5 *[737.41]*
- tuberculous (*see also* Tuberculosis) 015.0 5th *[737.41]*

Kyrle's disease (hyperkeratosis follicularis in cutem penetrans) 701.1

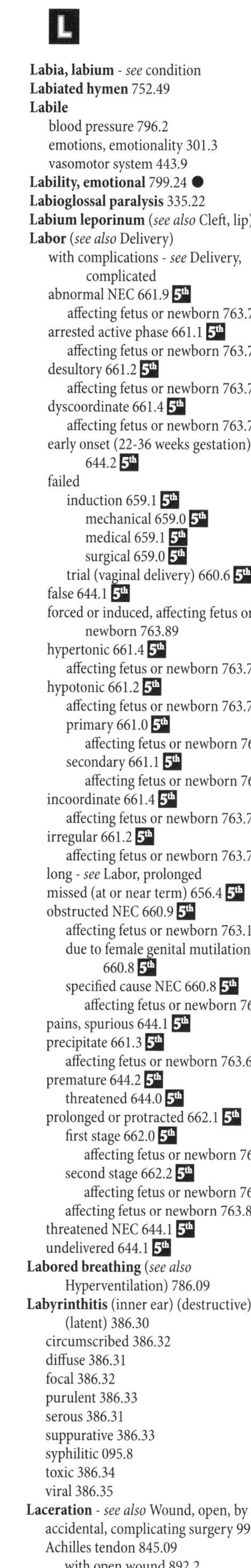

L

- **Labia, labium** - *see* condition
- **Labiated hymen** 752.49
- **Labile**
  - blood pressure 796.2
  - emotions, emotionality 301.3
  - vasomotor system 443.9
- **Lability, emotional** 799.24 ●
- **Labioglossal paralysis** 335.22
- **Labium leporinum** (*see also* Cleft, lip) 749.10
- **Labor** (*see also* Delivery)
  - with complications - *see* Delivery, complicated
  - abnormal NEC 661.9 5th
    - affecting fetus or newborn 763.7
  - arrested active phase 661.1 5th
    - affecting fetus or newborn 763.7
  - desultory 661.2 5th
    - affecting fetus or newborn 763.7
  - dyscoordinate 661.4 5th
    - affecting fetus or newborn 763.7
  - early onset (22-36 weeks gestation) 644.2 5th
  - failed
    - induction 659.1 5th
      - mechanical 659.0 5th
      - medical 659.1 5th
      - surgical 659.0 5th
    - trial (vaginal delivery) 660.6 5th
  - false 644.1 5th
  - forced or induced, affecting fetus or newborn 763.89
  - hypertonic 661.4 5th
    - affecting fetus or newborn 763.7
  - hypotonic 661.2 5th
    - affecting fetus or newborn 763.7
    - primary 661.0 5th
      - affecting fetus or newborn 763.7
    - secondary 661.1 5th
      - affecting fetus or newborn 763.7
  - incoordinate 661.4 5th
    - affecting fetus or newborn 763.7
  - irregular 661.2 5th
    - affecting fetus or newborn 763.7
  - long - *see* Labor, prolonged
  - missed (at or near term) 656.4 5th
  - obstructed NEC 660.9 5th
    - affecting fetus or newborn 763.1
    - due to female genital mutilation 660.8 5th
    - specified cause NEC 660.8 5th
      - affecting fetus or newborn 763.1
  - pains, spurious 644.1 5th
  - precipitate 661.3 5th
    - affecting fetus or newborn 763.6
  - premature 644.2 5th
    - threatened 644.0 5th
  - prolonged or protracted 662.1 5th
    - first stage 662.0 5th
      - affecting fetus or newborn 763.89
    - second stage 662.2 5th
      - affecting fetus or newborn 763.89
    - affecting fetus or newborn 763.89
  - threatened NEC 644.1 5th
  - undelivered 644.1 5th
- **Labored breathing** (*see also* Hyperventilation) 786.09
- **Labyrinthitis** (inner ear) (destructive) (latent) 386.30
  - circumscribed 386.32
  - diffuse 386.31
  - focal 386.32
  - purulent 386.33
  - serous 386.31
  - suppurative 386.33
  - syphilitic 095.8
  - toxic 386.34
  - viral 386.35
- **Laceration** - *see also* Wound, open, by site
  - accidental, complicating surgery 998.2
  - Achilles tendon 845.09
    - with open wound 892.2

Laceration – *continued*

  - anus (sphincter) 879.6
    - with
      - abortion - *see* Abortion, by type, with damage to pelvic organs
      - ectopic pregnancy (*see also* categories 633.0-633.9) 639.2
      - molar pregnancy (*see also* categories 630-632) 639.2
    - complicated 879.7
    - complicating delivery (healed) (old) 654.8 5th
      - with laceration of anal or rectal mucosa 664.3 5th
      - not associated with third-degree perineal laceration 664.6 5th
    - following
      - abortion 639.2
      - ectopic or molar pregnancy 639.2
    - nontraumatic, nonpuerperal (healed) (old) 569.43
  - bladder (urinary)
    - with
      - abortion - *see* Abortion, by type, with damage to pelvic organs
      - ectopic pregnancy (*see also* categories 633.0-633.9) 639.2
      - molar pregnancy (*see also* categories 630-632) 639.2
    - following
      - abortion 639.2
      - ectopic or molar pregnancy 639.2
    - obstetrical trauma 665.5 5th
  - blood vessel - *see* Injury, blood vessel, by site
  - bowel
    - with
      - abortion - *see* Abortion, by type, with damage to pelvic organs
      - ectopic pregnancy (*see also* categories 633.0-633.9) 639.2
      - molar pregnancy (*see also* categories 630-632) 639.2
    - following
      - abortion 639.2
      - ectopic or molar pregnancy 639.2
    - obstetrical trauma 665.5 5th
  - brain (cerebral) (membrane) (with hemorrhage) 851.8 5th

Note *Use the following fifth-digit subclassification with categories 851-854:*

0	unspecified state of consciousness
1	with no loss of consciousness
2	with brief [less than one hour] loss of consciousness
3	with moderate [1-24 hours] loss of consciousness
4	with prolonged [more than 24 hours] loss of consciousness and return to pre-existing conscious level
5	with prolonged [more than 24 hours] loss of consciousness, without return to pre-existing conscious level

Use fifth-digit 5 to designate when a patient is unconscious and dies before regaining consciousness, regardless of the duration of the loss of consciousness

6	with loss of consciousness of unspecified duration
9	with concussion, unspecified

    - with
      - open intracranial wound 851.9 5th
      - skull fracture - *see* Fracture, skull, by site
    - cerebellum 851.6 5th
      - with open intracranial wound 851.7 5th
    - cortex 851.2 5th
      - with open intracranial wound 851.3 5th

Laceration – *continued*

  - brain – *continued*
    - during birth 767.0
    - stem 851.6 5th
      - with open intracranial wound 851.7 5th
  - broad ligament
    - with
      - abortion - *see* Abortion, by type, with damage to pelvic organs
      - ectopic pregnancy (*see also* categories 633.0-633.9) 639.2
      - molar pregnancy (*see also* categories 630-632) 639.2
    - following
      - abortion 639.2
      - ectopic or molar pregnancy 639.2
    - nontraumatic 620.6
    - obstetrical trauma 665.6 5th
    - syndrome (nontraumatic) 620.6
  - capsule, joint - *see* Sprain, by site
  - cardiac - *see* Laceration, heart
  - causing eversion of cervix uteri (old) 622.0
  - central, complicating delivery 664.4 5th
  - cerebellum - *see* Laceration, brain, cerebellum
  - cerebral - *see also* Laceration, brain
    - during birth 767.0
  - cervix (uteri)
    - with
      - abortion - *see* Abortion, by type, with damage to pelvic organs
      - ectopic pregnancy (*see also* categories 633.0-633.9) 639.2
      - molar pregnancy (*see also* categories 630-632) 639.2
    - following
      - abortion 639.2
      - ectopic or molar pregnancy 639.2
    - nonpuerperal, nontraumatic 622.3
    - obstetrical trauma (current) 665.3 5th
    - old (postpartal) 622.3
    - traumatic - *see* Injury, internal, cervix
  - chordae heart 429.5
  - complicated 879.9
  - cornea - *see* Laceration, eyeball
    - superficial 918.1
  - cortex (cerebral) - *see* Laceration, brain, cortex
  - esophagus 530.89
  - eye(s) - *see* Laceration, ocular
  - eyeball NEC 871.4
    - with prolapse or exposure of intraocular tissue 871.1
    - penetrating - *see* Penetrating wound, eyeball
    - specified as without prolapse of intraocular tissue 871.0
  - eyelid NEC 870.8
    - full thickness 870.1
      - involving lacrimal passages 870.2
    - skin (and periocular area) 870.0
      - penetrating - *see* Penetrating wound, orbit
  - fourchette
    - with
      - abortion - *see* Abortion, by type, with damage to pelvic organs
      - ectopic pregnancy (*see also* categories 633.0-633.9) 639.2
      - molar pregnancy (*see also* categories 630-632) 639.2
    - complicating delivery 664.0 5th
    - following
      - abortion 639.2
      - ectopic or molar pregnancy 639.2
  - heart (without penetration of heart chambers) 861.02
    - with
      - open wound into thorax 861.12
      - penetration of heart chambers 861.03
        - with open wound into thorax 861.13

Laceration – *continued*

  - hernial sac - *see* Hernia, by site
  - internal organ (abdomen) (chest) (pelvis) NEC - *see* Injury, internal, by site
  - kidney (parenchyma) 866.02
    - with
      - complete disruption of parenchyma (rupture) 866.03
        - with open wound into cavity 866.13
      - open wound into cavity 866.12
  - labia
    - complicating delivery 664.0 5th
  - ligament - *see also* Sprain, by site
    - with open wound - *see* Wound, open, by site
  - liver 864.05
    - with open wound into cavity 864.15
    - major (disruption of hepatic parenchyma) 864.04
      - with open wound into cavity 864.14
    - minor (capsule only) 864.02
      - with open wound into cavity 864.12
    - moderate (involving parenchyma without major disruption) 864.03
      - with open wound into cavity 864.13
    - multiple 864.04
      - with open wound into cavity 864.14
    - stellate 864.04
      - with open wound into cavity 864.14
  - lung 861.22
    - with open wound into thorax 861.32
  - meninges - *see* Laceration, brain
  - meniscus (knee) (*see also* Tear, meniscus) 836.2
    - old 717.5
    - site other than knee - *see also* Sprain, by site
      - old NEC (*see also* Disorder, cartilage, articular) 718.0 5th
  - muscle - *see also* Sprain, by site
    - with open wound - *see* Wound, open, by site
  - myocardium - *see* Laceration, heart
  - nerve - *see* Injury, nerve, by site
  - ocular NEC (*see also* Laceration, eyeball) 871.4
    - adnexa NEC 870.8
      - penetrating 870.3
        - with foreign body 870.4
  - orbit (eye) 870.8
    - penetrating 870.3
      - with foreign body 870.4
  - pelvic
    - floor (muscles)
      - with
        - abortion - *see* Abortion, by type, with damage to pelvic organs
        - ectopic pregnancy (*see also* categories 633.0-633.9) 639.2
        - molar pregnancy (*see also* categories 630-632) 639.2
      - complicating delivery 664.1 5th
      - following
        - abortion 639.2
        - ectopic or molar pregnancy 639.2
      - nonpuerperal 618.7
      - old (postpartal) 618.7
    - organ NEC
      - with
        - abortion - *see* Abortion, by type, with damage to pelvic organs
        - ectopic pregnancy (*see also* categories 633.0-633.9) 639.2
        - molar pregnancy (*see also* categories 630-632) 639.2

Labia, labium – Laceration

- **Laceration** – *continued*
  - pelvic – *continued*
    - organ NEC – *continued*
      - complicating delivery 665.5 5th
        - affecting fetus or newborn 763.89
      - following
        - abortion 639.2
        - ectopic or molar pregnancy 639.2
      - obstetrical trauma 665.5 5th
  - perineum, perineal (old) (postpartal) 618.7
    - with
      - abortion - *see* Abortion, by type, with damage to pelvic floor
      - ectopic pregnancy (*see also* categories 633.0-633.9) 639.2
      - molar pregnancy (*see also* categories 630-632) 639.2
    - complicating delivery 664.4 5th
      - first degree 664.0 5th
      - second degree 664.1 5th
      - third degree 664.2 5th
      - fourth degree 664.3 5th
      - central 664.4 5th
      - involving
        - anal sphincter (healed) (old) 654.8 5th
          - not associated with third-degree perineal laceration 664.6 5th
        - fourchette 664.0 5th
        - hymen 664.0 5th
        - labia 664.0 5th
        - pelvic floor 664.1 5th
        - perineal muscles 664.1 5th
        - rectovaginal with septum 664.2 5th
          - with anal mucosa 664.3 5th
        - skin 664.0 5th
        - sphincter (anal) (healed) (old) 654.8 5th
          - with anal mucosa 664.3 5th
          - not associated with third-degree perineal laceration 664.6 5th
        - vagina 664.0 5th
        - vaginal muscles 664.1 5th
        - vulva 664.0 5th
      - secondary 674.2
    - following
      - abortion 639.2
      - ectopic or molar pregnancy 639.2
    - male 879.6
      - complicated 879.7
    - muscles, complicating delivery 664.1 5th
    - nonpuerperal, current injury 879.6
      - complicated 879.7
    - secondary (postpartal) 674.2
  - peritoneum
    - with
      - abortion - *see* Abortion, by type, with damage to pelvic organs
      - ectopic pregnancy (*see also* categories 633.0-633.9) 639.2
      - molar pregnancy (*see also* categories 630-632) 639.2
    - following
      - abortion 639.2
      - ectopic or molar pregnancy 639.2
    - obstetrical trauma 665.5 5th
  - periurethral tissue
    - with
      - abortion - *see* Abortion, by type, with damage to pelvic organs
      - ectopic pregnancy (*see also* categories 633.0-633.9) 639.2
      - molar pregnancy (*see also* categories 630-632) 639.2
    - following
      - abortion 639.2
      - ectopic or molar pregnancy 639.2

- **Laceration** – *continued*
  - periurethral tissue – *continued*
    - obstetrical trauma 665.5 5th
  - rectovaginal (septum)
    - with
      - abortion - *see* Abortion, by type, with damage to pelvic organs
      - ectopic pregnancy (*see also* categories 633.0-633.9) 639.2
      - molar pregnancy (*see also* categories 630-632) 639.2
    - complicating delivery 665.4 5th
      - with perineum 664.2 5th
        - involving anal or rectal mucosa 664.3 5th
    - following
      - abortion 639.2
      - ectopic or molar pregnancy 639.2
    - nonpuerperal 623.4
    - old (postpartal) 623.4
  - spinal cord (meninges) - *see also* Injury, spinal, by site
    - due to injury at birth 767.4
    - fetus or newborn 767.4
  - spleen 865.09
    - with
      - disruption of parenchyma (massive) 865.04
        - with open wound into cavity 865.14
      - open wound into cavity 865.19
    - capsule (without disruption of parenchyma) 865.02
      - with open wound into cavity 865.12
    - parenchyma 865.03
      - with open wound into cavity 865.13
      - massive disruption (rupture) 865.04
        - with open wound into cavity 865.14
  - tendon 848.9
    - with open wound - *see* Wound, open, by site
    - Achilles 845.09
      - with open wound 892.2
    - lower limb NEC 844.9
      - with open wound NEC 894.2
    - upper limb NEC 840.9
      - with open wound NEC 884.2
  - tentorium cerebelli - *see* Laceration, brain, cerebellum
  - tongue 873.64
    - complicated 873.74
  - urethra
    - with
      - abortion - *see* Abortion, by type, with damage to pelvic organs
      - ectopic pregnancy (*see also* categories 633.0-633.9) 639.2
      - molar pregnancy (*see also* categories 630-632) 639.2
    - following
      - abortion 639.2
      - ectopic or molar pregnancy 639.2
    - nonpuerperal, nontraumatic 599.84
    - obstetrical trauma 665.5 5th
  - uterus
    - with
      - abortion - *see* Abortion, by type, with damage to pelvic organs
      - ectopic pregnancy (*see also* categories 633.0-633.9) 639.2
      - molar pregnancy (*see also* categories 630-632) 639.2
    - following
      - abortion 639.2
      - ectopic or molar pregnancy 639.2
    - nonpuerperal, nontraumatic 621.8
    - obstetrical trauma NEC 665.5 5th
    - old (postpartal) 621.8
  - vagina
    - with
      - abortion - *see* Abortion, by type, with damage to pelvic organs

- **Laceration** – *continued*
  - vagina – *continued*
    - with – *continued*
      - ectopic pregnancy (*see also* categories 633.0-633.9) 639.2
      - molar pregnancy (*see also* categories 630-632) 639.2
      - perineal involvement, complicating delivery 664.0 5th
    - complicating delivery 665.4 5th
      - first degree 664.0 5th
      - second degree 664.1 5th
      - third degree 664.2 5th
      - fourth degree 664.3 5th
      - high 665.4 5th
      - muscles 664.1 5th
      - sulcus 665.4 5th
      - wall 665.4 5th
    - following
      - abortion 639.2
      - ectopic or molar pregnancy 639.2
    - nonpuerperal, nontraumatic 623.4
    - old (postpartal) 623.4
  - valve, heart - *see* Endocarditis
  - vulva
    - with
      - abortion - *see* Abortion, by type, with damage to pelvic organs
      - ectopic pregnancy (*see also* categories 633.0-633.9) 639.2
      - molar pregnancy (*see also* categories 630-632) 639.2
    - complicating delivery 664.0 5th
    - following
      - abortion 639.2
      - ectopic or molar pregnancy 639.2
    - nonpuerperal, nontraumatic 624.4
    - old (postpartal) 624.4
- **Lachrymal** - *see* condition
- **Lachrymonasal duct** - *see* condition
- **Lack of**
  - adequate intermaxillary vertical dimension 524.36
  - appetite (*see also* Anorexia) 783.0
  - care
    - in home V60.4
    - of adult 995.84
    - of infant (at or after birth) 995.52
  - coordination 781.3
  - development - *see also* Hypoplasia
    - physiological in childhood 783.40
  - education V62.3
  - energy 780.79
  - financial resources V60.2
  - food 994.2
    - in environment V60.89 ▲
  - growth in childhood 783.43
  - heating V60.1
  - housing (permanent) (temporary) V60.0
    - adequate V60.1
  - material resources V60.2
  - medical attention 799.89
  - memory (*see also* Amnesia) 780.93
    - mild, following organic brain damage 310.8 ▲
  - ovulation 628.0
  - person able to render necessary care V60.4
  - physical exercise V69.0
  - physiologic development in childhood 783.40
  - posterior occlusal support 524.57
  - prenatal care in current pregnancy V23.7
  - shelter V60.0
  - sleep V69.4
  - water 994.3
- **Lacrimal** - *see* condition
- **Lacrimation, abnormal** (*see also* Epiphora) 375.20
- **Lacrimonasal duct** - *see* condition
- **Lactation, lactating** (breast) (puerperal) (postpartum)
  - defective 676.4 5th
  - disorder 676.9 5th
    - specified type NEC 676.8 5th

- **Lactation, lactating** – *continued*
  - excessive 676.6 5th
  - failed 676.4 5th
  - mastitis NEC 675.2 5th
  - mother (care and/or examination) V24.1
  - nonpuerperal 611.6
  - suppressed 676.5 5th
- **Lacticemia** 271.3
  - excessive 276.2
- **Lactosuria** 271.3
- **Lacunar skull** 756.0
- **Laennec's cirrhosis** (alcoholic) 571.2
  - nonalcoholic 571.5
- **Lafora's disease** 333.2
- **Lag, lid** (nervous) 374.41
- **Lagleyze-von Hippel disease** (retinocerebral angiomatosis) 759.6
- **Lagophthalmos** (eyelid) (nervous) 374.20
  - cicatricial 374.23
  - keratitis (*see also* Keratitis) 370.34
  - mechanical 374.22
  - paralytic 374.21
- **La grippe** - *see* Influenza
- **Lahore sore** 085.1
- **Lakes, venous** (cerebral) 437.8
- **Laki-Lorand factor deficiency** (*see also* Defect, coagulation) 286.3
- **Lalling** 307.9
- **Lambliasis** 007.1
- **Lame back** 724.5
- **Lancereaux's diabetes** (diabetes mellitus with marked emaciation) 250.8 5th *[261]*
  - due to secondary diabetes 249.8 5th *[261]*
- **Landau-Kleffner syndrome** 345.8 5th
- **Landouzy-Déjérine dystrophy** (fascioscapulohumeral atrophy) 359.1
- **Landry's disease or paralysis** 357.0
- **Landry-Guillain-Barré syndrome** 357.0
- **Lane's**
  - band 751.4
  - disease 569.89
  - kink (*see also* Obstruction, intestine) 560.9
- **Langdon Down's syndrome** (mongolism) 758.0
- **Language abolition** 784.69
- **Lanugo** (persistent) 757.4
- **Laparoscopic surgical procedure converted to open procedure** V64.41
- **Lardaceous**
  - degeneration (any site) 277.39
  - disease 277.39
  - kidney 277.39 *[583.81]*
  - liver 277.39
- **Large**
  - baby (regardless of gestational age) 766.1
    - exceptionally (weight of 4500 grams or more) 766.0
    - of diabetic mother 775.0
  - ear 744.22
  - fetus - *see also* Oversize, fetus
    - causing disproportion 653.5 5th
      - with obstructed labor 660.1 5th
  - for dates
    - fetus or newborn (regardless of gestational age) 766.1
      - affecting management of pregnancy 656.6 5th
      - exceptionally (weight of 4500 grams or more) 766.0
  - physiological cup 743.57
  - stature 783.9
  - waxy liver 277.39
  - white kidney - *see* Nephrosis
- **Larsen's syndrome** (flattened facies and multiple congenital dislocations) 755.8
- **Larsen-Johansson disease** (juvenile osteopathia patellae) 732.4
- **Larva migrans**
  - cutaneous NEC 126.9
    - ancylostoma 126.9
  - of Diptera in vitreous 128.0
  - visceral NEC 128.0

- **Laryngeal** - *see also* condition
  - syncope 786.2
- **Laryngismus** (acute) (infectious) (stridulous) 478.75
  - congenital 748.3
  - diphtheritic 032.3
- **Laryngitis** (acute) (edematous) (fibrinous) (gangrenous) (infective) (infiltrative) (malignant) (membranous) (phlegmonous) (pneumococcal) (pseudomembranous) (septic) (subglottic) (suppurative) (ulcerative) (viral) 464.00
  - with
    - influenza, flu, or grippe 487.1
    - obstruction 464.01
    - tracheitis (*see also* Laryngotracheitis) 464.20
      - with obstruction 464.21
      - acute 464.20
        - with obstruction 464.21
      - chronic 476.1
  - atrophic 476.0
  - borrelia vincentii 101
  - catarrhal 476.0
  - chronic 476.0
    - with tracheitis (chronic) 476.1
    - due to external agent - *see* Condition, respiratory, chronic, due to
  - diphtheritic (membranous) 032.3
  - due to external agent - *see* Inflammation, respiratory, upper, due to
  - H. influenzae 464.00
    - with obstruction 464.01
  - Hemophilus influenzae 464.00
    - with obstruction 464.01
  - hypertrophic 476.0
  - influenzal 487.1
  - pachydermic 478.79
  - sicca 476.0
  - spasmodic 478.75
    - acute 464.00
      - with obstruction 464.01
  - streptococcal 034.0
  - stridulous 478.75
  - syphilitic 095.8
    - congenital 090.5
  - tuberculous (*see also* Tuberculosis, larynx) 012.3 5th
  - Vincent's 101
- **Laryngocele** (congenital) (ventricular) 748.3
- **Laryngofissure** 478.79
  - congenital 748.3
- **Laryngomalacia** (congenital) 748.3
- **Laryngopharyngitis** (acute) 465.0
  - chronic 478.9
    - due to external agent - *see* Condition, respiratory, chronic, due to
  - due to external agent - *see* Inflammation, respiratory, upper, due to
  - septic 034.0
- **Laryngoplegia** (*see also* Paralysis, vocal cord) 478.30
- **Laryngoptosis** 478.79
- **Laryngospasm** 478.75
  - due to external agent - *see* Condition, respiratory, acute, due to
- **Laryngostenosis** 478.74
  - congenital 748.3
- **Laryngotracheitis** (acute) (infectional) (viral) (*see also* Laryngitis) 464.20
  - with obstruction 464.21
  - atrophic 476.1
  - Borrelia vincenti 101
  - catarrhal 476.1
  - chronic 476.1
    - due to external agent - *see* Condition, respiratory, chronic, due to
  - diphtheritic (membranous) 032.3
  - due to external agent - *see* Inflammation, respiratory, upper, due to
  - H. influenzae 464.20
    - with obstruction 464.21
  - hypertrophic 476.1

- **Laryngotracheitis** – *continued*
  - influenzal 487.1
  - pachydermic 478.75
  - sicca 476.1
  - spasmodic 478.75
    - acute 464.20
      - with obstruction 464.21
  - streptococcal 034.0
  - stridulous 478.75
  - syphilitic 095.8
    - congenital 090.5
  - tuberculous (*see also* Tuberculosis, larynx) 012.3 5th
  - Vincent's 101
- **Laryngotracheobronchitis** (*see also* Bronchitis) 490
  - acute 466.0
  - chronic 491.8
  - viral 466.0
- **Laryngotracheobronchopneumonitis** - *see* Pneumonia, broncho-
- **Larynx, laryngeal** - *see* condition
- **Lasègue's disease** (persecution mania) 297.9
- **Lassa fever** 078.89
- **Lassitude** (*see also* Weakness) 780.79
- **Late** - *see also* condition
  - effect(s) (of) - *see also* condition
    - abscess
      - intracranial or intraspinal (conditions classifiable to 324) - *see* category 326
    - adverse effect of drug, medicinal or biological substance 909.5
    - allergic reaction 909.9
    - amputation
      - postoperative (late) 997.60
      - traumatic (injury classifiable to 885-887 and 895-897) 905.9
    - burn (injury classifiable to 948-949) 906.9
      - extremities NEC (injury classifiable to 943 or 945) 906.7
        - hand or wrist (injury classifiable to 944) 906.6
      - eye (injury classifiable to 940) 906.5
      - face, head, and neck (injury classifiable to 941) 906.5
      - specified site NEC (injury classifiable to 942 and 946-947) 906.8
    - cerebrovascular disease (conditions classifiable to 430-437) 438.9
      - with
        - alterations of sensations 438.6
        - aphasia 438.11
        - apraxia 438.81
        - ataxia 438.84
        - cognitive deficits 438.0
        - disturbances of vision 438.7
        - dysarthria 438.13 ●
        - dysphagia 438.82
        - dysphasia 438.12
        - facial droop 438.83
        - facial weakness 438.83
        - fluency disorder 438.14 ●
        - hemiplegia/hemiparesis
          - affecting
            - dominant side 438.21
            - nondomiant side 438.22
            - unspecified side 438.20
        - monoplegia of lower limb
          - affecting
            - dominant side 438.41
            - nondominant side 438.42
            - unspecified side 438.40
        - monoplegia of upper limb
          - affecting
            - dominant side 438.31
            - nondominant side 438.32
            - unspecified side 438.30
        - paralytic syndrome NEC
          - affecting
            - bilateral 438.53
            - dominant side 438.51

- **Late** – *continued*
  - effect(s) (of) – *continued*
    - cerebrovascular disease – *continued*
      - with – *continued*
        - paralytic syndrome – *continued*
          - affecting – *continued*
            - unspecified side 438.50
        - speech and language deficit 438.10
          - specified type NEC 438.19
        - stuttering 438.14 ●
        - vertigo 438.85
      - specified type NEC 438.89
    - childbirth complication(s) 677
    - complication(s) of
      - childbirth 677
      - delivery 677
      - pregnancy 677
      - puerperium 677
      - surgical and medical care (conditions classifiable to 996-999) 909.3
      - trauma (conditions classifiable to 958) 908.6
    - contusion (injury classifiable to 920-924) 906.3
    - crushing (injury classifiable to 925-929) 906.4
    - delivery complication(s) 677
    - dislocation (injury classifiable to 830-839) 905.6
    - encephalitis or encephalomyelitis (conditions classifiable to 323) - *see* category 326
      - in infectious diseases 139.8
        - viral (conditions classifiable to 049.8, 049.9, 062-064) 139.0
    - external cause NEC (conditions classifiable to 995) 909.9
      - certain conditions classifiable to categories 991-994 909.4
    - foreign body in orifice (injury classifiable to 930-939) 908.5
    - fracture (multiple) (injury classifiable to 828-829) 905.5
      - extremity
        - lower (injury classifiable to 821-827) 905.4
          - neck of femur (injury classifiable to 820) 905.3
        - upper (injury classifiable to 810-819) 905.2
      - face and skull (injury classifiable to 800-804) 905.0
      - skull and face (injury classifiable to 800-804) 905.0
      - spine and trunk (injury classifiable to 805 and 807-809) 905.1
        - with spinal cord lesion (injury classifiable to 806) 907.2
    - infection
      - pyogenic, intracranial - *see* category 326
    - infectious diseases (conditions classifiable to 001-136) NEC 139.8
    - injury (injury classifiable to 959) 908.9
      - blood vessel 908.3
        - abdomen and pelvis (injury classifiable to 902) 908.4
        - extremity (injury classifiable to 903-904) 908.3
        - head and neck (injury classifiable to 900) 908.3
          - intracranial (injury classifiable to 850-854) 907.0
            - with skull fracture 905.0
        - thorax (injury classifiable to 901) 908.4

- **Late** – *continued*
  - effect(s) (of) – *continued*
    - injury – *continued*
      - internal organ NEC (injury classifiable to 867 and 869) 908.2
        - abdomen (injury classifiable to 863-866 and 868) 908.1
        - thorax (injury classifiable to 860-862) 908.0
      - intracranial (injury classifiable to 850-854) 907.0
        - with skull fracture (injury classifiable to 800-801 and 803-804) 905.0
      - nerve NEC (injury classifiable to 957) 907.9
        - cranial (injury classifiable to 950-951) 907.1
        - peripheral NEC (injury classifiable to 957) 907.9
          - lower limb and pelvic girdle (injury classifiable to 956) 907.5
          - upper limb and shoulder girdle (injury classifiable to 955) 907.4
        - roots and plexus(es), spinal (injury classifiable to 953) 907.3
        - trunk (injury classifiable to 954) 907.3
      - spinal
        - cord (injury classifiable to 806 and 952) 907.2
        - nerve root(s) and plexus(es) (injury classifiable to 953) 907.3
      - superficial (injury classifiable to 910-919) 906.2
      - tendon (tendon injury classifiable to 840-848, 880-884 with .2, and 890-894 with .2) 905.8
    - meningitis
      - bacterial (conditions classifiable to 320) - *see* category 326
      - unspecified cause (conditions classifiable to 322) - *see* category 326
    - myelitis (*see also* Late, effect(s) (of), encephalitis) - *see* category 326
    - parasitic diseases (conditions classifiable to 001-136 NEC) 139.8
    - phlebitis or thrombophlebitis of intracranial venous sinuses (conditions classifiable to 325) - *see* category 326
    - poisoning due to drug, medicinal or biological substance (conditions classifiable to 960-979) 909.0
    - poliomyelitis, acute (conditions classifiable to 045) 138
    - pregnancy complication(s) 677
    - puerperal complication(s) 677
    - radiation (conditions classifiable to 990) 909.2
    - rickets 268.1
    - sprain and strain without mention of tendon injury (injury classifiable to 840-848, except tendon injury) 905.7
      - tendon involvement 905.8
    - toxic effect of
      - drug, medicinal or biological substance (conditions classifiable to 960-979) 909.0
      - nonmedical substance (conditions classifiable to 980-989) 909.1
    - trachoma (conditions classifiable to 076) 139.1

- **Late** – *continued*
  - effect(s) (of) – *continued*
    - tuberculosis 137.0
      - bones and joints (conditions classifiable to 015) 137.3
      - central nervous system (conditions classifiable to 013) 137.1
      - genitourinary (conditions classifiable to 016) 137.2
      - pulmonary (conditions classifiable to 010-012) 137.0
      - specified organs NEC (conditions classifiable to 014, 017-018) 137.4
    - viral encephalitis (conditions classifiable to 049.8, 049.9, 062-064) 139.0
    - wound, open
      - extremity (injury classifiable to 880-884 and 890-894, except .2) 906.1
        - tendon (injury classifiable to 880-884 with .2 and 890-894 with .2) 905.8
      - head, neck, and trunk (injury classifiable to 870-879) 906.0
  - infant
    - post-term (gestation period over 40 completed weeks to 42 completed weeks) 766.21
    - prolonged gestation (period over 42 completed weeks) 766.22
- **Latent** - *see* condition
- **Lateral** - *see* condition
- **Laterocession** - *see* Lateroversion
- **Lateroflexion** - *see* Lateroversion
- **Lateroversion**
  - cervix - *see* Lateroversion, uterus
  - uterus, uterine (cervix) (postinfectional) (postpartal, old) 621.6
    - congenital 752.3
    - in pregnancy or childbirth 654.4 [5th]
      - affecting fetus or newborn 763.89
- **Lathyrism** 988.2
- **Launois' syndrome** (pituitary gigantism) 253.0
- **Launois-Bensaude's lipomatosis** 272.8
- **Launois-Cleret syndrome** (adiposogenital dystrophy) 253.8
- **Laurence-Moon-Biedl syndrome** (obesity, polydactyly, and mental retardation) 759.89
- **LAV** (disease) (illness) (infection) - *see* Human immunodeficiency virus (disease) (illness) (infection)
- **LAV/HTLV-III** (disease) (illness) (infection) - *see* Human immunodeficiency virus (disease) (illness) (infection)
- **Lawford's syndrome** (encephalocutaneous angiomatosis) 759.6
- **Lax, laxity** - *see also* Relaxation
  - ligament 728.4
  - skin (acquired) 701.8
    - congenital 756.83
- **Laxative habit** (*see also* Abuse, drugs, nondependent) 305.9 [5th]
- **Lazy leukocyte syndrome** 288.09
- **LCAD** (long chain/very long chain acyl CoA dehydrogenase deficiency, VLCAD) 277.85
- **LCHAD** (long chain 3-hydroxyacyl CoA dehydrogenase deficiency) 277.85
- **Lead** - *see also* condition
  - exposure (suspected) to V15.86 ▲
  - incrustation of cornea 371.15
  - poisoning 984.9
    - specified type of lead - *see* Table of Drugs and Chemicals
- **Lead miners' lung** 503
- **Leakage**
  - amniotic fluid 658.1 [5th]
    - with delayed delivery 658.2 [5th]
      - affecting fetus or newborn 761.1
  - bile from drainage tube (T tube) 997.4
- **Leakage** – *continued*
  - blood (microscopic), fetal, into maternal circulation 656.0 [5th]
    - affecting management of pregnancy or puerperium 656.0 [5th]
  - device, implant, or graft - *see* Complications, mechanical
  - spinal fluid at lumbar puncture site 997.09
  - urine, continuous 788.37
- **Leaky heart** - *see* Endocarditis
- **Learning defect, specific NEC** (strephosymbolia) 315.2
- **Leather bottle stomach** (M8142/3) 151.9
- **Leber's**
  - congenital amaurosis 362.76
  - optic atrophy (hereditary) 377.16
- **Lederer's anemia or disease** (acquired infectious hemolytic anemia) 283.19
- **Lederer-Brill syndrome** (acquired infectious hemolytic anemia) 283.19
- **Leeches** (aquatic) (land) 134.2
- **Left-sided neglect** 781.8
- **Leg** - *see* condition
- **Legal investigation** V62.5
- **Legg (-Calvé)-Perthes disease or syndrome** (osteochondrosis, femoral capital) 732.1
- **Legionnaires' disease** 482.84
- **Leigh's disease** 330.8
- **Leiner's disease** (exfoliative dermatitis) 695.89
- **Leiofibromyoma** (M8890/0) - *see also* Leiomyoma
  - uterus (cervix) (corpus) (*see also* Leiomyoma, uterus) 218.9
- **Leiomyoblastoma** (M8891/1) - *see* Neoplasm, connective tissue, uncertain behavior
- **Leiomyofibroma** (M8890/0) - *see also* Neoplasm, connective tissue, benign
  - uterus (cervix) (corpus) (*see also* Leiomyoma, uterus) 218.9
- **Leiomyoma** (M8890/0) - *see also* Neoplasm, connective tissue, benign
  - bizarre (M8893/0) - *see* Neoplasm, connective tissue, benign
  - cellular (M8892/1) - *see* Neoplasm, connective tissue, uncertain behavior
  - epithelioid (M8891/1) - *see* Neoplasm, connective tissue, uncertain behavior
  - prostate (polypoid) 600.20
    - with
      - other lower urinary tract symptoms (LUTS) 600.21
      - urinary
        - obstruction 600.21
        - retention 600.21
  - uterus (cervix) (corpus) 218.9
    - interstitial 218.1
    - intramural 218.1
    - submucous 218.0
    - subperitoneal 218.2
    - subserous 218.2
  - vascular (M8894/0) - *see* Neoplasm, connective tissue, benign
- **Leiomyomatosis** (intravascular) (M8890/1) - *see* Neoplasm, connective tissue, uncertain behavior
- **Leiomyosarcoma** (M8890/3) - *see also* Neoplasm, connective tissue, malignant
  - epithelioid (M8891/3) - *see* Neoplasm, connective tissue, malignant
- **Leishmaniasis** 085.9
  - American 085.5
    - cutaneous 085.4
    - mucocutaneous 085.5
  - Asian desert 085.2
  - Brazilian 085.5
  - cutaneous 085.9
    - acute necrotizing 085.2
    - American 085.4
- **Leishmaniasis** – *continued*
  - cutaneous – *continued*
    - Asian desert 085.2
    - diffuse 085.3
    - dry form 085.1
    - Ethiopian 085.3
    - eyelid 085.5 *[373.6]*
    - late 085.1
    - lepromatous 085.3
    - recurrent 085.1
    - rural 085.2
    - ulcerating 085.1
    - urban 085.1
    - wet form 085.2
    - zoonotic form 085.2
  - dermal - *see also* Leishmaniasis, cutaneous
    - post kala-azar 085.0
  - eyelid 085.5 *[373.6]*
  - infantile 085.0
  - Mediterranean 085.0
  - mucocutaneous (American) 085.5
  - naso-oral 085.5
  - nasopharyngeal 085.5
  - Old World 085.1
  - tegumentaria diffusa 085.4
  - vaccination, prophylactic (against) V05.2
  - visceral (Indian) 085.0
- **Leishmanoid, dermal** - *see also* Leishmaniasis, cutaneous
  - post kala-azar 085.0
- **Leloir's disease** 695.4
- **Lemiere syndrome** 451.89
- **Lenegre's disease** 426.0
- **Lengthening, leg** 736.81
- **Lennox-Gastaut syndrome** 345.0 [5th]
  - with tonic seizures 345.1 [5th]
- **Lennox's syndrome** (*see also* Epilepsy) 345.0 [5th]
- **Lens** - *see* condition
- **Lenticonus** (anterior) (posterior) (congenital) 743.36
- **Lenticular degeneration, progressive** 275.1
- **Lentiglobus** (posterior) (congenital) 743.36
- **Lentigo** (congenital) 709.09
  - juvenile 709.09
  - Maligna (M8742/2) - *see also* Neoplasm, skin, in situ
    - melanoma (M8742/3) - *see* Melanoma
  - senile 709.09
- **Leonine leprosy** 030.0
- **Leontiasis**
  - ossium 733.3
  - syphilitic 095.8
    - congenital 090.5
- **Léopold-Lévi's syndrome** (paroxysmal thyroid instability) 242.9 [5th]
- **Lepore hemoglobin syndrome** 282.49
- **Lepothrix** 039.0
- **Lepra** 030.9
  - Willan's 696.1
- **Leprechaunism** 259.8
- **Lepromatous leprosy** 030.0
- **Leprosy** 030.9
  - anesthetic 030.1
  - beriberi 030.1
  - borderline (group B) (infiltrated) (neuritic) 030.3
  - cornea (*see also* Leprosy, by type) 030.9 *[371.89]*
  - dimorphous (group B) (infiltrated) (lepromatous) (neuritic) (tuberculoid) 030.3
  - eyelid 030.0 *[373.4]*
  - indeterminate (group I) (macular) (neuritic) (uncharacteristic) 030.2
  - leonine 030.0
  - lepromatous (diffuse) (infiltrated) (macular) (neuritic) (nodular) (type L) 030.0
  - macular (early) (neuritic) (simple) 030.2
  - maculoanesthetic 030.1
  - mixed 030.0
  - neuro 030.1
  - nodular 030.0
- **Leprosy** – *continued*
  - primary neuritic 030.3
  - specified type or group NEC 030.8
  - tubercular 030.1
  - tuberculoid (macular) (maculoanesthetic) (major) (minor) (neuritic) (type T) 030.1
- **Leptocytosis, hereditary** 282.49
- **Leptomeningitis** (chronic) (circumscribed) (hemorrhagic) (nonsuppurative) (*see also* Meningitis) 322.9
  - aseptic 047.9
    - adenovirus 049.1
    - Coxsackie virus 047.0
    - ECHO virus 047.1
    - enterovirus 047.9
    - lymphocytic choriomeningitis 049.0
  - epidemic 036.0
  - late effect - *see* category 326
  - meningococcal 036.0
  - pneumococcal 320.1
  - syphilitic 094.2
  - tuberculous (*see also* Tuberculosis, meninges) 013.0 [5th]
- **Leptomeningopathy** (*see also* Meningitis) 322.9
- **Leptospiral** - *see* condition
- **Leptospirochetal** - *see* condition
- **Leptospirosis** 100.9
  - autumnalis 100.89
  - canicula 100.89
  - grippotyphosa 100.89
  - hebdomidis 100.89
  - icterohemorrhagica 100.0
  - nanukayami 100.89
  - pomona 100.89
  - Weil's disease 100.0
- **Leptothricosis** - *see* Actinomycosis
- **Leptothrix infestation** - *see* Actinomycosis
- **Leptotricosis** - *see* Actinomycosis
- **Leptus dermatitis** 133.8
- **Léris pleonosteosis** 756.89
- **Léri-Weill syndrome** 756.59
- **Leriche's syndrome** (aortic bifurcation occlusion) 444.0
- **Lermoyez's syndrome** (*see also* Disease, Ménière's) 386.00
- **Lesbianism** - omit code
  - ego-dystonic 302.0
  - problems with 302.0
- **Lesch-Nyhan syndrome** (hypoxanthine-guanine-phosphoribosyltransferase deficiency) 277.2
- **Lesion(s)**
  - abducens nerve 378.54
  - alveolar process 525.8
  - anorectal 569.49
  - aortic (valve) - *see* Endocarditis, aortic
  - auditory nerve 388.5
  - basal ganglion 333.90
  - bile duct (*see also* Disease, biliary) 576.8
  - bladder 596.9
  - bone 733.90
  - brachial plexus 353.0
  - brain 348.89 ▲
    - congenital 742.9
    - vascular (*see also* Lesion, cerebrovascular) 437.9
      - degenerative 437.1
      - healed or old without residuals V12.54
      - hypertensive 437.2
      - late effect - *see* Late effect(s) (of) cerebrovascular disease
  - buccal 528.9
  - calcified - *see* Calcification
  - canthus 373.9
  - carate - *see* Pinta, lesions
  - cardia 537.89
  - cardiac - *see also* Disease, heart
    - congenital 746.9
    - valvular - *see* Endocarditis
  - cauda equina 344.60
    - with neurogenic bladder 344.61

Lesion(s) – *continued*
- cecum 569.89
- cerebral - *see* Lesion, brain
- cerebrovascular (*see also* Disease, cerebrovascular NEC) 437.9
  - degenerative 437.1
  - healed or old without residuals V12.54
  - hypertensive 437.2
  - specified type NEC 437.8
- cervical root (nerve) NEC 353.2
- chiasmal 377.54
  - associated with
    - inflammatory disorders 377.54
    - neoplasm NEC 377.52
      - pituitary 377.51
    - pituitary disorders 377.51
    - vascular disorders 377.53
- chorda tympani 351.8
- coin, lung 793.1
- colon 569.89
- congenital - *see* Anomaly
- conjunctiva 372.9
- coronary artery (*see also* Ischemia, heart) 414.9
- cranial nerve 352.9
  - first 352.0
  - second 377.49
  - third
    - partial 378.51
    - total 378.52
  - fourth 378.53
  - fifth 350.9
  - sixth 378.54
  - seventh 351.9
  - eighth 388.5
  - ninth 352.2
  - tenth 352.3
  - eleventh 352.4
  - twelfth 352.5
- cystic - *see* Cyst
- degenerative - *see* Degeneration
- dermal (skin) 709.9
- Dieulafoy (hemorrhagic)
  - of
    - duodenum 537.84
    - intestine 569.86
    - stomach 537.84
- duodenum 537.89
  - with obstruction 537.3
- eyelid 373.9
- gasserian ganglion 350.8
- gastric 537.89
- gastroduodenal 537.89
- gastrointestinal 569.89
- glossopharyngeal nerve 352.2
- heart (organic) - *see also* Disease, heart
  - vascular - *see* Disease, cardiovascular
- helix (ear) 709.9
- high grade myelodysplastic syndrome 238.73
- hyperchromic, due to pinta (carate) 103.1
- hyperkeratotic (*see also* Hyperkeratosis) 701.1
- hypoglossal nerve 352.5
- hypopharynx 478.29
- hypothalamic 253.9
- ileocecal coil 569.89
- ileum 569.89
- iliohypogastric nerve 355.79
- ilioinguinal nerve 355.79
- in continuity - *see* Injury, nerve, by site
- inflammatory - *see* Inflammation
- intestine 569.89
- intracerebral - *see* Lesion, brain
- intrachiasmal (optic) (*see also* Lesion, chiasmal) 377.54
- intracranial, space-occupying NEC 784.2
- joint 719.90
  - ankle 719.97
  - elbow 719.92
  - foot 719.97
  - hand 719.94
  - hip 719.95
  - knee 719.96

Lesion(s) – *continued*
- joint – *continued*
  - multiple sites 719.99
  - pelvic region 719.95
  - sacroiliac (old) 724.6
  - shoulder (region) 719.91
  - specified site NEC 719.98
  - wrist 719.93
- keratotic (*see also* Keratosis) 701.1
- kidney (*see also* Disease, renal) 593.9
- laryngeal nerve (recurrent) 352.3
- leonine 030.0
- lip 528.5
- liver 573.8
- low grade myelodysplastic syndrome 238.72
- lumbosacral
  - plexus 353.1
  - root (nerve) NEC 353.4
- lung 518.89
  - coin 793.1
- maxillary sinus 473.0
- mitral - *see* Endocarditis, mitral
- Morel Lavallée - *see* Hematoma, by site ●
- motor cortex 348.89 ▲
- nerve (*see also* Disorder, nerve) 355.9
- nervous system 349.9
  - congenital 742.9
- nonallopathic NEC 739.9
  - in region (of)
    - abdomen 739.9
    - acromioclavicular 739.7
    - cervical, cervicothoracic 739.1
    - costochondral 739.8
    - costovertebral 739.8
    - extremity
      - lower 739.6
      - upper 739.7
    - head 739.0
    - hip 739.5
    - lower extremity 739.6
    - lumbar, lumbosacral 739.3
    - occipitocervical 739.0
    - pelvic 739.5
    - pubic 739.5
    - rib cage 739.8
    - sacral, sacrococcygeal, sacroiliac 739.4
    - sternochondral 739.8
    - sternoclavicular 739.7
    - thoracic, thoracolumbar 739.2
    - upper extremity 739.7
- nose (internal) 478.19
- obstructive - *see* Obstruction
- obturator nerve 355.79
- occlusive
  - artery - *see* Embolism, artery
- organ or site NEC - *see* Disease, by site
- osteolytic 733.90
- paramacular, of retina 363.32
- peptic 537.89
- periodontal, due to traumatic occlusion 523.8
- perirectal 569.49
- peritoneum (granulomatous) 568.89
- pigmented (skin) 709.00
- pinta - *see* Pinta, lesions
- polypoid - *see* Polyp
- prechiasmal (optic) (*see also* Lesion, chiasmal) 377.54
- primary - *see also* Syphilis, primary
  - carate 103.0
  - pinta 103.0
  - yaws 102.0
- pulmonary 518.89
  - valve (*see also* Endocarditis, pulmonary) 424.3
- pylorus 537.89
- radiation NEC 990
- radium NEC 990
- rectosigmoid 569.89
- retina, retinal - *see also* Retinopathy
  - vascular 362.17
- retroperitoneal 568.89

Lesion(s) – *continued*
- romanus 720.1
- sacroiliac (joint) 724.6
- salivary gland 527.8
  - benign lymphoepithelial 527.8
- saphenous nerve 355.79
- secondary - *see* Syphilis, secondary
- sigmoid 569.89
- sinus (accessory) (nasal) (*see also* Sinusitis) 473.9
- skin 709.9
  - suppurative 686.00
- SLAP (superior glenoid labrum) 840.7
- space-occupying, intracranial NEC 784.2
- spinal cord 336.9
  - congenital 742.9
  - traumatic (complete) (incomplete) (transverse) - *see also* Injury, spinal, by site
    - with
      - broken
        - back - *see* Fracture, vertebra, by site, with spinal cord injury
        - neck - *see* Fracture, vertebra, cervical, with spinal cord injury
      - fracture, vertebra - *see* Fracture, vertebra, by site, with spinal cord injury
- spleen 289.50
- stomach 537.89
- superior glenoid labrum (SLAP) 840.7
- syphilitic - *see* Syphilis
- tertiary - *see* Syphilis, tertiary
- thoracic root (nerve) 353.3
- tonsillar fossa 474.9
- tooth, teeth 525.8
  - white spot 521.01
- traumatic NEC (*see also* nature and site of injury) 959.9
- tricuspid (valve) - *see* Endocarditis, tricuspid
- trigeminal nerve 350.9
- ulcerated or ulcerative - *see* Ulcer
- uterus NEC 621.9
- vagina 623.8
- vagus nerve 352.3
- valvular - *see* Endocarditis
- vascular 459.9
  - affecting central nervous system (*see also* Lesion, cerebrovascular) 437.9
  - following trauma (*see also* Injury, blood vessel, by site) 904.9
  - retina 362.17
  - traumatic - *see* Injury, blood vessel, by site
  - umbilical cord 663.6
    - affecting fetus or newborn 762.6
- visual
  - cortex NEC (*see also* Disorder, visual, cortex) 377.73
  - pathway NEC (*see also* Disorder, visual, pathway) 377.63
- warty - *see* Verruca
- white spot, on teeth 521.01
- x-ray NEC 990

Lethargic - *see* condition

Lethargy 780.79

Letterer-Siwe disease (acute histiocytosis X) (M9722/3) 202.5

Leucinosis 270.3

Leucocoria 360.44

Leucosarcoma (M9850/3) 207.8

Leukasmus 270.2

Leukemia, leukemic (congenital) (M9800/3) 208.9 [5th]

> **Note** *Use the following fifth-digit subclassification for categories 203-208:*
>
> **0** without mention of having achieved remission
> failed remission
>
> **1** with remission
>
> **2** in relapse

- acute NEC (M9801/3) 208.0 [5th]
- aleukemic NEC (M9804/3) 208.8 [5th]
  - granulocytic (M9864/3) 205.8 [5th]
- basophilic (M9870/3) 205.1 [5th]
- blast (cell) (M9801/3) 208.0 [5th]
- blastic (M9801/3) 208.0 [5th]
  - granulocytic (M9861/3) 205.0 [5th]
- chronic NEC (M9803/3) 208.1 [5th]
- compound (M9810/3) 207.8 [5th]
- eosinophilic (M9880/3) 205.1 [5th]
- giant cell (M9910/3) 207.2 [5th]
- granulocytic (M9860/3) 205.9 [5th]
  - acute (M9861/3) 205.0 [5th]
  - aleukemic (M9864/3) 205.8 [5th]
  - blastic (M9861/3) 205.0 [5th]
  - chronic (M9863/3) 205.1 [5th]
  - subacute (M9862/3) 205.2 [5th]
  - subleukemic (M9864/3) 205.8 [5th]
- hairy cell (M9940/3) 202.4 [5th]
- hemoblastic (M9801/3) 208.0 [5th]
- histiocytic (M9890/3) 206.9 [5th]
- lymphatic (M9820/3) 204.9 [5th]
  - acute (M9821/3) 204.0 [5th]
  - aleukemic (M9824/3) 204.8 [5th]
  - chronic (M9823/3) 204.1 [5th]
  - subacute (M9822/3) 204.2 [5th]
  - subleukemic (M9824/3) 204.8 [5th]
- lymphoblastic (M9821/3) 204.0 [5th]
- lymphocytic (M9820/3) 204.9 [5th]
  - acute (M9821/3) 204.0 [5th]
  - aleukemic (M9824/3) 204.8 [5th]
  - chronic (M9823/3) 204.1 [5th]
  - granular ●
    - large T-cell 204.8 [5th] ●
  - subacute (M9822/3) 204.2 [5th]
  - subleukemic (M9824/3) 204.8 [5th]
- lymphogenous (M9820/3) - *see* Leukemia, lymphoid
- lymphoid (M9820/3) 204.9 [5th]
  - acute (M9821/3) 204.0 [5th]
  - aleukemic (M9824/3) 204.8 [5th]
  - blastic (M9821/3) 204.0 [5th]
  - chronic (M9823/3) 204.1 [5th]
  - subacute (M9822/3) 204.2 [5th]
  - subleukemic (M9824/3) 204.8 [5th]
- lymphosarcoma cell (M9850/3) 207.8 [5th]
- mast cell (M9900/3) 207.8 [5th]
- megakaryocytic (M9910/3) 207.2 [5th]
- megakaryocytoid (M9910/3) 207.2 [5th]
- mixed (cell) (M9810/3) 207.8 [5th]
- monoblastic (M9891/3) 206.0 [5th]
- monocytic (Schilling-type) (M9890/3) 206.9 [5th]
  - acute (M9891/3) 206.0 [5th]
  - aleukemic (M9894/3) 206.8 [5th]
  - chronic (M9893/3) 206.1 [5th]
  - Naegeli-type (M9863/3) 205.1 [5th]
  - subacute (M9892/3) 206.2 [5th]
  - subleukemic (M9894/3) 206.8 [5th]
- monocytoid (M9890/3) 206.9 [5th]
  - acute (M9891/3) 206.0 [5th]
  - aleukemic (M9894/3) 206.8 [5th]
  - chronic (M9893/3) 206.1 [5th]
  - myelogenous (M9863/3) 205.1 [5th]
  - subacute (M9892/3) 206.2 [5th]
  - subleukemic (M9894/3) 206.8 [5th]
- monomyelocytic (M9860/3) - *see* Leukemia, myelomonocytic
- myeloblastic (M9861/3) 205.0 [5th]
- myelocytic (M9863/3) 205.1 [5th]
  - acute (M9861/3) 205.0 [5th]
- myelogenous (M9860/3) 205.9 [5th]
  - acute (M9861/3) 205.0 [5th]

Leukemia, leukemic – *continued*
  myelogenous – *continued*
    aleukemic (M9864/3) 205.8 [5th]
    chronic (M9863/3) 205.1 [5th]
    monocytoid (M9863/3) 205.1 [5th]
    subacute (M9862/3) 205.2 [5th]
    subleukemic (M9864) 205.8 [5th]
  myeloid (M9860/3) 205.9 [5th]
    acute (M9861/3) 205.0 [5th]
    aleukemic (M9864/3) 205.8 [5th]
    chronic (M9863/3) 205.1 [5th]
    subacute (M9862/3) 205.2 [5th]
    subleukemic (M9864/3) 205.8 [5th]
  myelomonocytic (M9860/3) 205.9 [5th]
    acute (M9861/3) 205.0 [5th]
    chronic (M9863/3) 205.1 [5th]
  Naegeli-type monocytic (M9863/3) 205.1 [5th]
  neutrophilic (M9865/3) 205.1 [5th]
  plasma cell (M9830/3) 203.1 [5th]
  plasmacytic (M9830/3) 203.1 [5th]
  prolymphocytic (M9825/3) - *see* Leukemia, lymphoid
  promyelocytic, acute (M9866/3) 205.0 [5th]
  Schilling-type monocytic (M9890/3) - *see* Leukemia, monocytic
  stem cell (M9801/3) 208.0 [5th]
  subacute NEC (M9802/3) 208.2 [5th]
  subleukemic NEC (M9804/3) 208.8 [5th]
  thrombocytic (M9910/3) 207.2 [5th]
  undifferentiated (M9801/3) 208.0 [5th]
Leukemoid reaction (basophilic) (lymphocytic) (monocytic) (myelocytic) (neutrophilic) 288.62
Leukoaraiosis (hypertensive) 437.1 ●
Leukoariosis - see Leukoaraiosis ●
Leukoclastic vasculitis 446.29
Leukocoria 360.44
Leukocythemia - *see* Leukemia
Leukocytopenia 288.50
Leukocytosis 288.60
  basophilic 288.8
  eosinophilic 288.3
  lymphocytic 288.8
  monocytic 288.8
  neutrophilic 288.8
Leukoderma 709.09
  syphilitic 091.3
    late 095.8
Leukodermia (*see also* Leukoderma) 709.09
Leukodystrophy (cerebral) (globoid cell) (metachromatic) (progressive) (sudanophilic) 330.0
Leukoedema, mouth or tongue 528.79
Leukoencephalitis
  acute hemorrhagic (postinfectious) NEC 136.9 *[323.61]*
    postimmunization or postvaccinal 323.51
  subacute sclerosing 046.2
    van Bogaert's 046.2
  van Bogaert's (sclerosing) 046.2
Leukoencephalopathy (*see also* Encephalitis) 323.9
  acute necrotizing hemorrhagic (postinfectious) 136.9 *[323.61]*
    postimmunization or postvaccinal 323.51
  Binswanger's 290.12 ●
  metachromatic 330.0
  multifocal (progressive) 046.3
  progressive multifocal 046.3
  reversible, posterior 348.5 [5th]
Leukoerythroblastosis 289.9
Leukoerythrosis 289.0
Leukokeratosis (*see also* Leukoplakia) 702.8
  mouth 528.6
  nicotina palati 528.79
  tongue 528.6
Leukokoria 360.44
Leukokraurosis vulva, vulvae 624.09
Leukolymphosarcoma (M9850/3) 207.8 [5th]
Leukoma (cornea) (interfering with central vision) 371.03
  adherent 371.04
Leukomalacia, periventricular 779.7
Leukomelanopathy, hereditary 288.2
Leukonychia (punctata) (striata) 703.8
  congenital 757.5
Leukopathia
  unguium 703.8
    congenital 757.5
Leukopenia 288.50
  basophilic 288.59
  cyclic 288.02
  eosinophilic 288.59
  familial 288.59
  malignant (*see also* Agranulocytosis) 288.09
  periodic 288.02
  transitory neonatal 776.7
Leukopenic - *see* condition
Leukoplakia 702.8
  anus 569.49
  bladder (postinfectional) 596.8
  buccal 528.6
  cervix (uteri) 622.2
  esophagus 530.83
  gingiva 528.6
  kidney (pelvis) 593.89
  larynx 478.79
  lip 528.6
  mouth 528.6
  oral soft tissue (including tongue) (mucosa) 528.6
  palate 528.6
  pelvis (kidney) 593.89
  penis (infectional) 607.0
  rectum 569.49
  syphilitic 095.8
  tongue 528.6
  tonsil 478.29
  ureter (postinfectional) 593.89
  urethra (postinfectional) 599.84
  uterus 621.8
  vagina 623.1
  vesical 596.8
  vocal cords 478.5
  vulva 624.09
Leukopolioencephalopathy 330.0
Leukorrhea (vagina) 623.5
  due to Trichomonas (vaginalis) 131.00
  trichomonal (Trichomonas vaginalis) 131.00
Leukosarcoma (M9850/3) 207.8 [5th]
Leukosis (M9800/3) - *see* Leukemia
Lev's disease or syndrome (acquired complete heart block) 426.0
Levi's syndrome (pituitary dwarfism) 253.3
Levocardia (isolated) 746.87
  with situs inversus 759.3
Levulosuria 271.2
Lewandowski's disease (primary) (*see also* Tuberculosis) 017.0 [5th]
Lewandowski-Lutz disease (epidermodysplasia verruciformis) 078.19
Lewy body dementia 331.82
Lewy body disease 331.82
Leyden's disease (periodic vomiting) 536.2
Leyden-Möbius dystrophy 359.1
Leydig cell
  carcinoma (M8650/3)
    specified site - *see* Neoplasm, by site, malignant
    unspecified site
      female 183.0
      male 186.9
  tumor (M8650/1)
    benign (M8650/0)
      specified site - *see* Neoplasm, by site, benign
      unspecified site
        female 220
        male 222.0
Leydig cell – *continued*
  tumor – *continued*
    malignant (M8650/3)
      specified site - *see* Neoplasm, by site, malignant
      unspecified site
        female 183.0
        male 186.9
    specified site - *see* Neoplasm, by site, uncertain behavior
    unspecified site
      female 236.2
      male 236.4
Leydig-Sertoli cell tumor (M8631/0)
  specified site - *see* Neoplasm, by site, benign
  unspecified site
    female 220
    male 222.0
LGSIL (low grade squamous intraepithelial lesion)
  anus 796.73
  cervix 795.03
  vagina 795.13
Liar, pathologic 301.7
Libman-Sacks disease or syndrome 710.0 *[424.91]*
Lice (infestation) 132.9
  body (pediculus corporis) 132.1
  crab 132.2
  head (pediculus capitis) 132.0
  mixed (classifiable to more than one of the categories 132.0-132.2) 132.3
  pubic (pediculus pubis) 132.2
Lichen 697.9
  albus 701.0
  annularis 695.89
  atrophicus 701.0
  corneus obtusus 698.3
  myxedematous 701.8
  nitidus 697.1
  pilaris 757.39
    acquired 701.1
  planopilaris 697.0
  planus (acute) (chronicus) (hypertrophic) (verrucous) 697.0
    morphoeicus 701.0
    sclerosus (et atrophicus) 701.0
  ruber 696.4
    acuminatus 696.4
    moniliformis 697.8
    obtusus corneus 698.3
    of Wilson 697.0
    planus 697.0
  sclerosus (et atrophicus) 701.0
  scrofulosus (primary) (*see also* Tuberculosis) 017.0 [5th]
  simplex (Vidal's) 698.3
    chronicus 698.3
    circumscriptus 698.3
  spinulosus 757.39
    mycotic 117.9
  striata 697.8
  urticatus 698.2
Lichenification 698.3
  nodular 698.3
Lichenoides tuberculosis (primary) (*see also* Tuberculosis) 017.0 [5th]
Lichtheim's disease or syndrome (subacute combined sclerosis with pernicious anemia) 281.0 *[336.2]*
Lien migrans 289.59
Lientery (*see also* Diarrhea) 787.91
  infectious 009.2
Life circumstance problem NEC V62.89
Li-Fraumeni cancer syndrome V84.01
Ligament - *see* condition
Light-for-dates (infant) 764.0 [5th]
  with signs of fetal malnutrition 764.1 [5th]
  affecting management of pregnancy 656.5 [5th]
Light-headedness 780.4
Lightning (effects) (shock) (stroke) (struck by) 994.0
  burn - *see* Burn, by site
  foot 266.2
Lightwood's disease or syndrome (renal tubular acidosis) 588.89
Lignac's disease (cystinosis) 270.0
Lignac (-de Toni) (-Fanconi) (-Debré) syndrome (cystinosis) 270.0
Lignac (-Fanconi) syndrome (cystinosis) 270.0
Ligneous thyroiditis 245.3
Likoff's syndrome (angina in menopausal women) 413.9
Limb - *see* condition
Limitation of joint motion (*see also* Stiffness, joint) 719.5 [5th]
  sacroiliac 724.6
Limit dextrinosis 271.0
Limited
  cardiac reserve - *see* Disease, heart
  duction, eye NEC 378.63
  mandibular range of motion 524.52
Lindau's disease (retinocerebral angiomatosis) 759.6
Lindau (-von Hippel) disease (angiomatosis retinocerebellosa) 759.6
Linea corneae senilis 371.41
Lines
  Beau's (transverse furrows on fingernails) 703.8
  Harris' 733.91
  Hudson-Stähli 371.11
  Stähli's 371.11
Lingua
  geographical 529.1
  nigra (villosa) 529.3
  plicata 529.5
    congenital 750.13
  tylosis 528.6
Lingual (tongue) - *see also* condition
  thyroid 759.2
Linitis (gastric) 535.4 [5th]
  plastica (M8142/3) 151.9
Lioderma essentialis (cum melanosis et telangiectasia) 757.33
Lip - *see also* condition
  biting 528.9
Lipalgia 272.8
Lipedema - *see* Edema
Lipemia (*see also* Hyperlipidemia) 272.4
  retina, retinalis 272.3
Lipidosis 272.7
  cephalin 272.7
  cerebral (infantile) (juvenile) (late) 330.1
  cerebroretinal 330.1 *[362.71]*
  cerebroside 272.7
  cerebrospinal 272.7
  chemically-induced 272.7
  cholesterol 272.7
  diabetic 250.8 [5th] *[272.7]*
    due to secondary diabetes 249.8 [5th] *[272.7]*
  dystopic (hereditary) 272.7
  glycolipid 272.7
  hepatosplenomegalic 272.3
  hereditary, dystopic 272.7
  sulfatide 330.0
Lipoadenoma (M8324/0 - *see* Neoplasm, by site, benign
Lipoblastoma (M8881/0) - *see* Lipoma, by site
Lipoblastomatosis (M8881/0) - *see* Lipoma, by site
Lipochondrodystrophy 277.5
Lipochrome histiocytosis (familial) 288.1
Lipodystrophia progressiva 272.6
Lipodystrophy (progressive) 272.6
  insulin 272.6
  intestinal 040.2
  mesenteric 567.82
Lipofibroma (M8851/0) - *see* Lipoma, by site
Lipoglycoproteinosis 272.8
Lipogranuloma, sclerosing 709.8

- **Lipogranulomatosis** (disseminated) 272.8
  - kidney 272.8
- **Lipoid** - *see also* condition
  - histiocytosis 272.7
    - essential 272.7
  - nephrosis (*see also* Nephrosis) 581.3
  - proteinosis of Urbach 272.8
- **Lipoidemia** (*see also* Hyperlipidemia) 272.4
- **Lipoidosis** (*see also* Lipidosis) 272.7
- **Lipoma** (M8850/0) 214.9
  - breast (skin) 214.1
  - face 214.0
  - fetal (M8881/0) - *see also* Lipoma, by site
    - fat cell (M8880/0) - *see* Lipoma, by site
  - infiltrating (M8856/0) - *see* Lipoma, by site
  - intra-abdominal 214.3
  - intramuscular (M8856/0) - *see* Lipoma, by site
  - intrathoracic 214.2
  - kidney 214.3
  - mediastinum 214.2
  - muscle 214.8
  - peritoneum 214.3
  - retroperitoneum 214.3
  - skin 214.1
    - face 214.0
  - spermatic cord 214.4
  - spindle cell (M8857/0) - *see* Lipoma, by site
  - stomach 214.3
  - subcutaneous tissue 214.1
    - face 214.0
  - thymus 214.2
  - thyroid gland 214.2
- **Lipomatosis** (dolorosa) 272.8
  - epidural 214.8
  - fetal (M8881/0) - *see* Lipoma, by site
  - Launois-Bensaude's 272.8
- **Lipomyohemangioma** (M8860/0)
  - specified site - *see* Neoplasm, connective tissue, benign
  - unspecified site 223.0
- **Lipomyoma** (M8860/0)
  - specified site - *see* Neoplasm, connective tissue, benign
  - unspecified site 223.0
- **Lipomyxoma** (M8852/0) - *see* Lipoma, by site
- **Lipomyxosarcoma** (M8852/3) - *see* Neoplasm, connective tissue, malignant
- **Lipophagocytosis** 289.89
- **Lipoproteinemia** (alpha) 272.4
  - broad-beta 272.2
  - floating-beta 272.2
  - hyper-pre-beta 272.1
- **Lipoproteinosis** (Rossle-Urbach-Wiethe) 272.8
- **Liposarcoma** (M8850/3) - *see also* Neoplasm, connective tissue, malignant
  - differentiated type (M8851/3) - *see* Neoplasm, connective tissue, malignant
  - embryonal (M8852/3) - *see* Neoplasm, connective tissue, malignant
  - mixed type (M8855/3) - *see* Neoplasm, connective tissue, malignant
  - myxoid (M8852/3) - *see* Neoplasm, connective tissue, malignant
  - pleomorphic (M8854/3) - *see* Neoplasm, connective tissue, malignant
  - round cell (M8853/3) - *see* Neoplasm, connective tissue, malignant
  - well differentiated type (M8851/3) - *see* Neoplasm, connective tissue, malignant
- **Liposynovitis prepatellaris** 272.8
- **Lipping**
  - cervix 622.0
  - spine (*see also* Spondylosis) 721.90
  - vertebra (*see also* Spondylosis) 721.90
- **Lip pits** (mucus), **congenital** 750.25
- **Lipschütz disease or ulcer** 616.50
- **Lipuria** 791.1
  - bilharziasis 120.0
- **Liquefaction, vitreous humor** 379.21
- **Lisping** 307.9
- **Lissauer's paralysis** 094.1
- **Lissencephalia, lissencephaly** 742.2
- **Listerellose** 027.0
- **Listeriose** 027.0
- **Listeriosis** 027.0
  - congenital 771.2
  - fetal 771.2
  - suspected fetal damage affecting management of pregnancy 655.4 5th
- **Listlessness** 780.79
- **Lithemia** 790.6
- **Lithiasis** - *see also* Calculus
  - hepatic (duct) - *see* Choledocholithiasis
  - urinary 592.9
- **Lithopedion** 779.9
  - affecting management of pregnancy 656.8 5th
- **Lithosis** (occupational) 502
  - with tuberculosis - *see* Tuberculosis, pulmonary
- **Lithuria** 791.9
- **Litigation** V62.5
- **Little**
  - league elbow 718.82
  - stroke syndrome 435.9
- **Little's disease** - *see* Palsy, cerebral
- **Littre's**
  - gland - *see* condition
  - hernia - *see* Hernia, Littre's
- **Littritis** (*see also* Urethritis) 597.89
- **Livedo** 782.61
  - annularis 782.61
  - racemose 782.61
  - reticularis 782.61
- **Live flesh** 781.0
- **Liver** - *see also* condition
  - donor V59.6
- **Livida, asphyxia**
  - newborn 768.6
- **Living**
  - alone V60.3
    - with handicapped person V60.4
- **Lloyd's syndrome** 258.1
- **Loa loa** 125.2
- **Loasis** 125.2
- **Lobe, lobar** - *see* condition
- **Lobo's disease or blastomycosis** 116.2
- **Lobomycosis** 116.2
- **Lobotomy syndrome** 310.0
- **Lobstein's disease** (brittle bones and blue sclera) 756.51
- **Lobster-claw hand** 755.58
- **Lobulation** (congenital) - *see also* Anomaly, specified type **NEC**, by site
  - kidney, fetal 753.3
  - liver, abnormal 751.69
  - spleen 759.0
- **Lobule, lobular** - *see* condition
- **Local, localized** - *see* condition
- **Locked bowel or intestine** (*see also* Obstruction, intestine) 560.9
- **Locked-in state** 344.81
- **Locked twins** 660.5 5th
  - affecting fetus or newborn 763.1
- **Locking**
  - joint (*see also* Derangement, joint) 718.90
  - knee 717.9
- **Lockjaw** (*see also* Tetanus) 037
- **Locomotor ataxia** (progressive) 094.0
- **Löffler's**
  - endocarditis 421.0
  - eosinophilia or syndrome 518.3
  - pneumonia 518.3
  - syndrome (eosinophilic pneumonitis) 518.3
- **Löfgren's syndrome** (sarcoidosis) 135
- **Loiasis** 125.2
  - eyelid 125.2 *[373.6]*
- **Loneliness** V62.89
- **Lone star fever** 082.8
- **Long labor** 662.1 5th
  - affecting fetus or newborn 763.89
  - first stage 662.0 5th
  - second stage 662.2 5th
- **Longitudinal stripes or grooves, nails** 703.8
  - congenital 757.5
- **Long-term** (current) **drug use** V58.69
  - antibiotics V58.62
  - anticoagulants V58.61
  - anti-inflammatories, non-steroidal (NSAID) V58.64
  - antiplatelets/antithrombotics V58.63
  - aspirin V58.66
  - high-risk medications NEC V58.69
  - insulin V58.67
  - methadone V58.69
  - opiate analgesic V58.69
  - pain killers V58.69
    - anti-inflammatories, non-steroidal (NSAID) V58.64
    - aspirin V58.66
  - steroids V58.65
  - tamoxifen V07.51 ▲
- **Loop**
  - intestine (*see also* Volvulus) 560.2
  - intrascleral nerve 379.29
  - vascular on papilla (optic) 743.57
- **Loose** - *see also* condition
  - body
    - in tendon sheath 727.82
    - joint 718.10
      - ankle 718.17
      - elbow 718.12
      - foot 718.17
      - hand 718.14
      - hip 718.15
      - knee 717.6
      - multiple sites 718.19
      - pelvic region 718.15
      - prosthetic implant - *see* Complications, mechanical
      - shoulder (region) 718.11
      - specified site NEC 718.18
      - wrist 718.13
  - cartilage (joint) (*see also* Loose, body, joint) 718.1 5th
    - knee 717.6
  - facet (vertebral) 724.9
  - prosthetic implant - *see* Complications, mechanical
  - sesamoid, joint (*see also* Loose, body, joint) 718.1 5th
  - tooth, teeth 525.8
- **Loosening epiphysis** 732.9
- **Looser (-Debray)-Milkman syndrome** (osteomalacia with pseudofractures) 268.2
- **Lop ear** (deformity) 744.29
- **Lorain's disease or syndrome** (pituitary dwarfism) 253.3
- **Lorain-Levi syndrome** (pituitary dwarfism) 253.3
- **Lordosis** (acquired) (postural) 737.20
  - congenital 754.2
  - due to or associated with
    - Charcôt-Marie-Tooth disease 356.1 *[737.42]*
    - mucopolysaccharidosis 277.5 *[737.42]*
    - neurofibromatosis 237.71 *[737.42]*
    - osteitis
      - deformans 731.0 *[737.42]*
      - fibrosa cystica 252.01 *[737.42]*
    - osteoporosis (*see also* Osteoporosis) 733.00 *[737.42]*
    - poliomyelitis (*see also* Poliomyelitis) 138 *[737.42]*
    - tuberculosis (*see also* Tuberculosis) 015.0 5th *[737.42]*
  - late effect of rickets 268.1 *[737.42]*
  - postlaminectomy 737.21
  - postsurgical NEC 737.22
  - rachitic 268.1 *[737.42]*
  - specified NEC 737.29
  - tuberculous (*see also* Tuberculosis) 015.0 5th *[737.42]*
- **Loss**
  - appetite 783.0
    - hysterical 300.11
    - nonorganic origin 307.59
    - psychogenic 307.59
  - blood - *see* Hemorrhage
  - central vision 368.41
  - consciousness 780.09
    - transient 780.2
  - control, sphincter, rectum 787.6
    - nonorganic origin 307.7
  - ear ossicle, partial 385.24
  - elasticity, skin 782.8
  - extremity or member, traumatic, current - *see* Amputation, traumatic
  - fluid (acute) 276.50
    - with
      - hypernatremia 276.0
      - hyponatremia 276.1
    - fetus or newborn 775.5
  - hair 704.00
  - hearing - *see also* Deafness
    - central 389.14
    - conductive (air) 389.00
      - with sensorineural hearing loss 389.20
        - bilateral 389.22
        - unilateral 389.21
      - bilateral 389.06
      - combined types 389.08
      - external ear 389.01
      - inner ear 389.04
      - middle ear 389.03
      - multiple types 389.08
      - tympanic membrane 389.02
      - unilateral 389.05
    - mixed conductive and sensorineural 389.20
      - bilateral 389.22
      - unilateral 389.21
    - mixed type 389.20
      - bilateral 389.22
      - unilateral 389.21
    - nerve
      - bilateral 389.12
      - unilateral 389.13
    - neural
      - bilateral 389.12
      - unilateral 389.13
    - noise-induced 388.12
    - perceptive NEC (*see also* Loss, hearing, sensorineural) 389.10
    - sensorineural 389.10
      - with conductive hearing loss 389.20
        - bilateral 389.22
        - unilateral 389.21
      - asymmetrical 389.16
      - bilateral 389.18
      - central 389.14
      - neural
        - bilateral 389.12
        - unilateral 389.13
      - sensory
        - bilateral 389.11
        - unilateral 389.17
      - unilateral 389.15
    - sensory
      - bilateral 389.11
      - unilateral 389.17
    - specified type NEC 389.8
    - sudden NEC 388.2
  - height 781.91
  - labyrinthine reactivity (unilateral) 386.55
    - bilateral 386.56
  - memory (*see also* Amnesia) 780.93
    - mild, following organic brain damage 310.8 ▲
  - mind (*see also* Psychosis) 298.9
  - occusal vertical dimension 524.37
  - organ or part - *see* Absence, by site, acquired
  - sensation 782.0

Lipogranulomatosis – Loss

Loss – *continued*
- sense of
  - smell (*see also* Disturbance, sensation) 781.1
  - taste (*see also* Disturbance, sensation) 781.1
  - touch (*see also* Disturbance, sensation) 781.1
- sight (acquired) (complete) (congenital) - *see* Blindness
- spinal fluid
  - headache 349.0
- substance of
  - bone (*see also* Osteoporosis) 733.00
  - cartilage 733.99
    - ear 380.32
  - vitreous (humor) 379.26
- tooth, teeth
  - acquired 525.10
    - due to
      - caries 525.13
      - extraction 525.10
      - periodontal disease 525.12
      - specified NEC 525.19
      - trauma 525.11
- vision, visual (*see also* Blindness) 369.9
  - both eyes (*see also* Blindness, both eyes) 369.3
  - complete (*see also* Blindness, both eyes) 369.00
  - one eye 369.8
  - sudden 368.11
  - transient 368.12
- vitreous 379.26
- voice (*see also* Aphonia) 784.41
- weight (cause unknown) 783.21

Lou Gehrig's disease 335.20

Louis-Bar syndrome (ataxia-telangiectasia) 334.8

Louping ill 063.1

Lousiness - *see* Lice

Low
- back syndrome 724.2
- basal metabolic rate (BMR) 794.7
- birthweight 765.1 [5th]
  - extreme (less than 1000 grams) 765.0 [5th]
  - for gestational age 764.0 [5th]
  - status (*see also* Status, low birth weight) V21.30
- bladder compliance 596.52
- blood pressure (*see also* Hypotension) 458.9
  - reading (incidental) (isolated) (nonspecific) 796.3
- cardiac reserve - *see* Disease, heart
- compliance bladder 596.52
- frequency deafness - *see* Disorder, hearing
- function - *see also* Hypofunction
  - kidney (*see also* Disease, renal) 593.9
  - liver 573.9
- hemoglobin 285.9
- implantation, placenta - *see* Placenta, previa
- insertion, placenta - *see* Placenta, previa
- lying
  - kidney 593.0
  - organ or site, congenital - *see* Malposition, congenital
  - placenta - *see* Placenta, previa
- output syndrome (cardiac) (*see also* Failure, heart) 428.9
- platelets (blood) (*see also* Thrombocytopenia) 287.5
- reserve, kidney (*see also* Disease, renal) 593.9
- risk
  - human papillomavirus (HPV) DNA test positive
    - anal 796.79
    - cervical 795.09
    - vaginal 795.19
- salt syndrome 593.9
- tension glaucoma 365.12

Low – *continued*
- vision 369.9
  - both eyes 369.20
  - one eye 369.70

Lowe (-Terrey-MacLachlan) syndrome (oculocerebrorenal dystrophy) 270.8

Lower extremity - *see* condition

Lown (-Ganong)-Levine syndrome (short P-R interval, normal QRS complex, and paroxysmal supraventricular tachycardia) 426.81

LSD reaction (*see also* Abuse, drugs, nondependent) 305.3 [5th]

L-shaped kidney 753.3

Lucas-Championnière disease (fibrinous bronchitis) 466.0

Lucey-Driscoll syndrome (jaundice due to delayed conjugation) 774.30

Ludwig's
- angina 528.3
- disease (submaxillary cellulitis) 528.3

Lues (venerea), **luetic** - *see* Syphilis

Luetscher's syndrome (dehydration) 276.51

Lumbago 724.2
- due to displacement, intervertebral disc 722.10

Lumbalgia 724.2
- due to displacement, intervertebral disc 722.10

Lumbar - *see* condition

Lumbarization, vertebra 756.15

Lumbermen's itch 133.8

Lump - *see also* Mass
- abdominal 789.3 [5th]
- breast 611.72
- chest 786.6
- epigastric 789.3 [5th]
- head 784.2
- kidney 753.3
- liver 789.1
- lung 786.6
- mediastinal 786.6
- neck 784.2
- nose or sinus 784.2
- pelvic 789.3 [5th]
- skin 782.2
- substernal 786.6
- throat 784.2
- umbilicus 789.3 [5th]

Lunacy (*see also* Psychosis) 298.9

Lunatomalacia 732.3

Lung - *see also* condition
- donor V59.8
- drug addict's 417.8
- mainliners' 417.8
- vanishing 492.0

Lupoid (miliary) **of Boeck** 135

Lupus 710.0
- anticoagulant 289.81
- Cazenave's (erythematosus) 695.4
- discoid (local) 695.4
- disseminated 710.0
- erythematodes (discoid) (local) 695.4
- erythematosus (discoid) (local) 695.4
  - disseminated 710.0
  - eyelid 373.34
  - systemic 710.0
    - with
      - encephalitis 710.0 *[323.81]*
      - lung involvement 710.0 *[517.8]*
    - inhibitor (presence of) 286.5
- exedens 017.0 [5th]
- eyelid (*see also* Tuberculosis) 017.0 [5th] *[373.4]*
- Hilliard's 017.0 [5th]
- hydralazine
  - correct substance properly administered 695.4
  - overdose or wrong substance given or taken 972.6
- miliaris disseminatus faciei 017.0 [5th]
- nephritis 710.0 *[583.81]*
  - acute 710.0 *[580.81]*
  - chronic 710.0 *[582.81]*

Lupus – *continued*
- nontuberculous, not disseminated 695.4
- pernio (Besnier) 135
- tuberculous (*see also* Tuberculosis) 017.0 [5th]
  - eyelid (*see also* Tuberculosis) 017.0 [5th] *[373.4]*
- vulgaris 017.0 [5th]

Luschka's joint disease 721.90

Luteinoma (M8610/0) 220

Lutembacher's disease or syndrome (atrial septal defect with mitral stenosis) 745.5

Luteoma (M8610/0) 220

Lutz-Miescher disease (elastosis perforans serpiginosa) 701.1

Lutz-Splendore-de Almeida disease (Brazilian blastomycosis) 116.1

Luxatio
- bulbi due to birth injury 767.8
- coxae congenita (*see also* Dislocation, hip, congenital) 754.30
- erecta - *see* Dislocation, shoulder
- imperfecta - *see* Sprain, by site
- perinealis - *see* Dislocation, hip

Luxation - *see also* Dislocation, by site
- eyeball 360.81
  - due to birth injury 767.8
  - lateral 376.36
- genital organs (external) NEC - *see* Wound, open, genital organs
- globe (eye) 360.81
  - lateral 376.36
- lacrimal gland (postinfectional) 375.16
- lens (old) (partial) 379.32
  - congenital 743.37
    - syphilitic 090.49 *[379.32]*
  - Marfan's disease 090.49
  - spontaneous 379.32
- penis - *see* Wound, open, penis
- scrotum - *see* Wound, open, scrotum
- testis - *see* Wound, open, testis

L-xyloketosuria 271.8

Lycanthropy (*see also* Psychosis) 298.9

Lyell's disease or syndrome (toxic epidermal necrolysis) 695.15
- due to drug
  - correct substance properly administered 695.15
  - overdose or wrong substance given or taken 977.9
    - specified drug - *see* Table of Drugs and Chemicals

Lyme disease 088.81

Lymph
- gland or node - *see* condition
- scrotum (*see also* Infestation, filarial) 125.9

Lymphadenitis 289.3
- with
  - abortion - *see* Abortion, by type, with sepsis
  - ectopic pregnancy (*see also* categories 633.0-633.9) 639.0
  - molar pregnancy (*see also* categories 630-632) 639.0
- acute 683
  - mesenteric 289.2
- any site, except mesenteric 289.3
  - acute 683
  - chronic 289.1
  - mesenteric (acute) (chronic) (nonspecific) (subacute) 289.2
  - subacute 289.1
    - mesenteric 289.2
- breast, puerperal, postpartum 675.2 [5th]
- chancroidal (congenital) 099.0
- chronic 289.1
  - mesenteric 289.2
- dermatopathic 695.89
- due to
  - anthracosis (occupational) 500
  - Brugia (Wuchereria) malayi 125.1
  - diphtheria (toxin) 032.89

Lymphadenitis – *continued*
- due to – *continued*
  - lymphogranuloma venereum 099.1
  - Wuchereria bancrofti 125.0
- following
  - abortion 639.0
  - ectopic or molar pregnancy 639.0
- generalized 289.3
- gonorrheal 098.89
- granulomatous 289.1
- infectional 683
- mesenteric (acute) (chronic) (nonspecific) (subacute) 289.2
  - due to Bacillus typhi 002.0
  - tuberculous (*see also* Tuberculosis) 014.8 [5th]
- mycobacterial 031.8
- purulent 683
- pyogenic 683
- regional 078.3
- septic 683
- streptococcal 683
- subacute, unspecified site 289.1
- suppurative 683
- syphilitic (early) (secondary) 091.4
  - late 095.8
- tuberculous - *see* Tuberculosis, lymph gland
- venereal 099.1

Lymphadenoid goiter 245.2

Lymphadenopathy (general) 785.6
- due to toxoplasmosis (acquired) 130.7
  - congenital (active) 771.2

Lymphadenopathy-associated virus (disease) (illness) (infection) - *see* Human immunodeficiency virus (disease) (illness) (infection)

Lymphadenosis 785.6
- acute 075

Lymphangiectasis 457.1
- conjunctiva 372.89
- postinfectional 457.1
- scrotum 457.1

Lymphangiectatic elephantiasis, nonfilarial 457.1

Lymphangioendothelioma (M9170/0) 228.1
- malignant (M9170/3) - *see* Neoplasm, connective tissue, malignant

Lymphangioma (M9170/0) 228.1
- capillary (M9171/0) 228.1
- cavernous (M9172/0) 228.1
- cystic (M9173/0) 228.1
- malignant (M9170/3) - *see* Neoplasm, connective tissue, malignant

Lymphangiomyoma (M9174/0) 228.1

Lymphangiomyomatosis (M9174/1) - *see* Neoplasm, connective tissue, uncertain behavior

Lymphangiosarcoma (M9170/3) - *see* Neoplasm, connective tissue, malignant

Lymphangitis 457.2
- with
  - abortion - *see* Abortion, by type, with sepsis
  - abscess - *see* Abscess, by site
  - cellulitis - *see* Abscess, by site
  - ectopic pregnancy (*see also* categories 633.0-633.9) 639.0
  - molar pregnancy (*see also* categories 630-632) 639.0
- acute (with abscess or cellulitis) 682.9
  - specified site - *see* Abscess, by site
- breast, puerperal, postpartum 675.2 [5th]
- chancroidal 099.0
- chronic (any site) 457.2
- due to
  - Brugia (Wuchereria) malayi 125.1
  - Wuchereria bancrofti 125.0
- following
  - abortion 639.0
  - ectopic or molar pregnancy 639.0
- gangrenous 457.2

Loss – Lymphangitis

Lymphangitis – *continued*
- penis
  - acute 607.2
  - gonococcal (acute) 098.0
    - chronic or duration of 2 months or more 098.2
- puerperal, postpartum, childbirth 670.8 [5th] ▲
- strumous, tuberculous (*see also* Tuberculosis) 017.2 [5th]
- subacute (any site) 457.2
- tuberculous - *see* Tuberculosis, lymph gland

Lymphatic (vessel) - *see* condition
Lymphatism 254.8
- scrofulous (*see also* Tuberculosis) 017.2 [5th]

Lymphectasia 457.1
Lymphedema (*see also* Elephantiasis) 457.1
- acquired (chronic) 457.1
- chronic hereditary 757.0
- congenital 757.0
- idiopathic hereditary 757.0
- praecox 457.1
- secondary 457.1
- surgical NEC 997.99
  - postmastectomy (syndrome) 457.0

Lymph-hemangioma (M9120/0) - *see* Hemangioma, by site
Lymphoblastic - *see* condition
Lymphoblastoma (diffuse) (M9630/3) 200.1 [5th]
- giant follicular (M9690/3) 202.0 [5th]
- macrofollicular (M9690/3) 202.0 [5th]

Lymphoblastosis, acute benign 075
Lymphocele 457.8
Lymphocythemia 288.51
Lymphocytic - *see also* condition
- chorioencephalitis (acute) (serous) 049.0
- choriomeningitis (acute) (serous) 049.0

Lymphocytoma (diffuse) (malignant) (M9620/3) 200.1 [5th]
Lymphocytomatosis (M9620/3) 200.1 [5th]
Lymphocytopenia 288.51
Lymphocytosis (symptomatic) 288.61
- infectious (acute) 078.89

Lymphoepithelioma (M8082/3) - *see* Neoplasm, by site, malignant
Lymphogranuloma (malignant) (M9650/3) 201.9 [5th]
- inguinale 099.1
- venereal (any site) 099.1
  - with stricture of rectum 099.1
- venereum 099.1

Lymphogranulomatosis (malignant) (M9650/3) 201.9 [5th]
- benign (Boeck's sarcoid) (Schaumann's) 135
- Hodgkin's (M9650/3) 201.9 [5th]

Lymphohistiocytosis, familial hemophagocytic 288.4
Lymphoid - *see* condition
Lympholeukoblastoma (M9850/3) 207.8 [5th]
Lympholeukosarcoma (M9850/3) 207.8 [5th]
Lymphoma (malignant) (M9590/3) 202.8 [5th]

Note *Use the following fifth-digit subclassification with categories 200-202:*

0	unspecified site, extranodal and solid organ sites
1	lymph nodes of head, face, and neck
2	intrathoracic lymph nodes
3	intra-abdominal lymph nodes
4	lymph nodes of axilla and upper limb
5	lymph nodes of inguinal region and lower limb
6	intrapelvic lymph nodes
7	spleen
8	lymph nodes of multiple sites

- benign (M9590/0) - *see* Neoplasm, by site, benign

Lymphoma – *continued*
- Burkitt's type (lymphoblastic) (undifferentiated) (M9750/3) 200.2 [5th]
- Castleman's (mediastinal lymph node hyperplasia) 785.6
- centroblastic-centrocytic
  - diffuse (M9614/3) 202.8 [5th]
  - follicular (M9692/3) 202.0 [5th]
- centroblastic type (diffuse) (M9632/3) 202.8 [5th]
  - follicular (M9697/3) 202.0 [5th]
- centrocytic (M9622/3) 202.8 [5th]
- compound (M9613/3) 200.8 [5th]
- convoluted cell type (lymphoblastic) (M9602/3) 202.8 [5th]
- diffuse NEC (M9590/3) 202.8 [5th]
  - large B cell 202.8 [5th]
- follicular (giant) (M9690/3) 202.0 [5th]
  - center cell (diffuse) (M9615/3) 202.8 [5th]
    - cleaved (diffuse) (M9623/3) 202.8 [5th]
      - follicular (M9695/3) 202.0 [5th]
    - non-cleaved (diffuse) (M9633/3) 202.8 [5th]
      - follicular (M9698/3) 202.0 [5th]
  - centroblastic-centrocytic (M9692/3) 202.0 [5th]
  - centroblastic type (M9697/3) 202.0 [5th]
  - large cell 202.0 [5th] ●
  - lymphocytic
    - intermediate differentiation (M9694/3) 202.0 [5th]
    - poorly differentiated (M9696/3) 202.0 [5th]
  - mixed (cell type) (lymphocytic-histiocytic) (small cell and large cell) (M9691/3) 202.0 [5th]
- germinocytic (M9622/3) 202.8 [5th]
- giant, follicular or follicle (M9690/3) 202.0 [5th]
- histiocytic (diffuse) (M9640/3) 200.0 [5th]
  - nodular (M9642/3) 200.0 [5th]
  - pleomorphic cell type (M9641/3) 200.0 [5th]
- Hodgkin's (M9650/3) (*see also* Disease, Hodgkin's) 201.9 [5th]
- immunoblastic (type) (M9612/3) 200.8 [5th]
- large cell (M9640/3) 200.7 [5th]
  - anaplastic 200.6 [5th]
  - nodular (M9642/3) 202.0 [5th] ▲
  - pleomorphic cell type (M9641/3) 200.0 [5th]
- lymphoblastic (diffuse) (M9630/3) 200.1 [5th]
  - Burkitt's type (M9750/3) 200.2 [5th]
  - convoluted cell type (M9602/3) 202.8 [5th]
- lymphocytic (cell type) (diffuse) (M9620/3) 200.1 [5th]
  - with plasmacytoid differentiation, diffuse (M9611/3) 200.8 [5th]
  - intermediate differentiation (diffuse) (M9621/3) 200.1 [5th]
    - follicular (M9694/3) 202.0 [5th]
    - nodular (M9694/3) 202.0 [5th]
  - nodular (M9690/3) 202.0 [5th]
  - poorly differentiated (diffuse) (M9630/3) 200.1 [5th]
    - follicular (M9696/3) 202.0 [5th]
    - nodular (M9696/3) 202.0 [5th]
  - well differentiated (diffuse) (M9620/3) 200.1 [5th]
    - follicular (M9693/3) 202.0 [5th]
    - nodular (M9693/3) 202.0 [5th]
- lymphocytic-histiocytic, mixed (diffuse) (M9613/3) 200.8 [5th]
  - follicular (M9691/3) 202.0 [5th]
  - nodular (M9691/3) 202.0 [5th]
- lymphoplasmacytoid type (M9611/3) 200.8 [5th]
- lymphosarcoma type (M9610/3) 200.1 [5th]
- macrofollicular (M9690/3) 202.0 [5th]
- mantle cell 200.4 [5th]
- marginal zone 200.3 [5th]
  - extranodal B-cell 200.3 [5th]
  - nodal B-cell 200.3 [5th]
  - splenic B-cell 200.3 [5th]
- mixed cell type (diffuse) (M9613/3) 200.8 [5th]
  - follicular (M9691/3) 202.0 [5th]
  - nodular (M9691/3) 202.0 [5th]
- nodular (M9690/3) 202.0 [5th]
  - histiocytic (M9642/3) 200.0 [5th]
  - lymphocytic (M9690/3) 202.0 [5th]
    - intermediate differentiation (M9694/3) 202.0 [5th]
    - poorly differentiated (M9696/3) 202.0 [5th]
  - mixed (cell type) (lymphocytic-histiocytic) (small cell and large cell) (M9691/3) 202.0 [5th]
- non-Hodgkin's type NEC (M9591/3) 202.8 [5th]
- peripheral T-cell 202.7 [5th]
- primary central nervous system 200.5 [5th]
- reticulum cell (type) (M9640/3) 200.0 [5th]
- small cell and large cell, mixed (diffuse) (M9613/3) 200.8 [5th]
  - follicular (M9691/3) 202.0 [5th]
  - nodular (9691/3) 202.0 [5th]
- stem cell (type) (M9601/3) 202.8 [5th]
- T-cell 202.1 [5th]
  - peripheral 202.7 [5th]
- undifferentiated (cell type) (non-Burkitt's) (M9600/3) 202.8 [5th]
  - Burkitt's type (M9750/3) 200.2 [5th]

Lymphomatosis (M9590/3) - *see also* Lymphoma
- granulomatous 099.1

Lymphopathia
- venereum 099.1
- veneris 099.1

Lymphopenia 288.51
- familial 279.2

Lymphoreticulosis, benign (of inoculation) 078.3
Lymphorrhea 457.8
Lymphosarcoma (M9610/3) 200.1 [5th]
- diffuse (M9610/3) 200.1 [5th]
  - with plasmacytoid differentiation (M9611/3) 200.8 [5th]
  - lymphoplasmacytic (M9611/3) 200.8 [5th]
- follicular (giant) (M9690/3) 202.0 [5th]
  - lymphoblastic (M9696/3) 202.0 [5th]
  - lymphocytic, intermediate differentiation (M9694/3) 202.0 [5th]
  - mixed cell type (M9691/3) 202.0 [5th]
- giant follicular (M9690/3) 202.0 [5th]
- Hodgkin's (M9650/3) 201.9 [5th]
- immunoblastic (M9612/3) 200.8 [5th]
- lymphoblastic (diffuse) (M9630/3) 200.1 [5th]
  - follicular (M9696/3) 202.0 [5th]
  - nodular (M9696/3) 202.0 [5th]
- lymphocytic (diffuse) (M9620/3) 200.1 [5th]
  - intermediate differentiation (diffuse) (M9621/3) 200.1 [5th]
    - follicular (M9694/3) 202.0 [5th]
    - nodular (M9694/3) 202.0 [5th]
- mixed cell type (diffuse) (M9613/3) 200.8 [5th]
  - follicular (M9691/3) 202.0 [5th]
  - nodular (M9691/3) 202.0 [5th]
- nodular (M9690/3) 202.0 [5th]
  - lymphoblastic (M9696/3) 202.0 [5th]
  - lymphocytic, intermediate differentiation (M9694/3) 202.0 [5th]
  - mixed cell type (M9691/3) 202.0 [5th]
- prolymphocytic (M9631/3) 200.1 [5th]
- reticulum cell (M9640/3) 200.0 [5th]

Lymphostasis 457.8
Lypemania (*see also* Melancholia) 296.2 [5th]
Lyssa 071

M

Macacus ear 744.29
Maceration
- fetus (cause not stated) 779.9
- wet feet, tropical (syndrome) 991.4

Machado-Joseph disease 334.8
Machupo virus hemorrhagic fever 078.7
Macleod's syndrome (abnormal transradiancy, one lung) 492.8
Macrocephalia, macrocephaly 756.0
Macrocheilia (congenital) 744.81
Macrochilia (congenital) 744.81
Macrocolon (congenital) 751.3
Macrocornea 743.41
- associated with buphthalmos 743.22

Macrocytic - *see* condition
Macrocytosis 289.89
Macrodactylia, macrodactylism (fingers) (thumbs) 755.57
- toes 755.65

Macrodontia 520.2
Macroencephaly 742.4
Macrogenia 524.05
Macrogenitosomia (female) (male) (praecox) 255.2
Macrogingivae 523.8
Macroglobulinemia (essential) (idiopathic) (monoclonal) (primary) (syndrome) (Waldenström's) 273.3
Macroglossia (congenital) 750.15
- acquired 529.8

Macrognathia, macrognathism (congenital) 524.00
- mandibular 524.02
  - alveolar 524.72
- maxillary 524.01
  - alveolar 524.71

Macrogyria (congenital) 742.4
Macrohydrocephalus (*see also* Hydrocephalus) 331.4
Macromastia (*see also* Hypertrophy, breast) 611.1
Macrophage activation syndrome 288.4
Macropsia 368.14
Macrosigmoid 564.7
- congenital 751.3

Macrospondylitis, acromegalic 253.0
Macrostomia (congenital) 744.83
Macrotia (external ear) (congenital) 744.22
Macula
- cornea, corneal
  - congenital 743.43
    - interfering with vision 743.42
  - interfering with central vision 371.03
  - not interfering with central vision 371.02
- degeneration (*see also* Degeneration, macula) 362.50
  - hereditary (*see also* Dystrophy, retina) 362.70
- edema, cystoid 362.53

Maculae ceruleae 132.1
Macules and papules 709.8
Maculopathy, toxic 362.55
Madarosis 374.55
Madelung's
- deformity (radius) 755.54
- disease (lipomatosis) 272.8
- lipomatosis 272.8

Madness (*see also* Psychosis) 298.9
- myxedema (acute) 293.0
  - subacute 293.1

Madura
- disease (actinomycotic) 039.9
  - mycotic 117.4
- foot (actinomycotic) 039.4
  - mycotic 117.4

Maduromycosis (actinomycotic) 039.9
- mycotic 117.4

Maffucci's syndrome (dyschondroplasia with hemangiomas) 756.4
Magenblase syndrome 306.4

Lymphangitis – Magenblase syndrome

- **Main en griffe** (acquired) 736.06
  - congenital 755.59
- **Maintenance**
  - chemotherapy regimen or treatment V58.11
  - dialysis regimen or treatment
    - extracorporeal (renal) V56.0
    - peritoneal V56.8
    - renal V56.0
  - drug therapy or regimen
    - chemotherapy, antineoplastic V58.11
    - immunotherapy, antineoplastic V58.12
  - external fixation NEC V54.89
  - radiotherapy V58.0
  - traction NEC V54.89
- **Majocchi's**
  - disease (purpura annularis telangiectodes) 709.1
  - granuloma 110.6
- **Major** - *see* condition
- **Mal**
  - cerebral (idiopathic) (*see also* Epilepsy) 345.9 [5th]
  - comital (*see also* Epilepsy) 345.9 [5th]
  - de los pintos (*see also* Pinta) 103.9
  - de Meleda 757.39
  - de mer 994.6
  - lie - *see* Presentation, fetal
  - perforant (*see also* Ulcer, lower extremity) 707.15
- **Malabar itch** 110.9
  - beard 110.0
  - foot 110.4
  - scalp 110.0
- **Malabsorption** 579.9
  - calcium 579.8
  - carbohydrate 579.8
  - disaccharide 271.3
  - drug-induced 579.8
  - due to bacterial overgrowth 579.8
  - fat 579.8
  - folate, congenital 281.2
  - galactose 271.1
  - glucose-galactose (congenital) 271.3
  - intestinal 579.9
  - isomaltose 271.3
  - lactose (hereditary) 271.3
  - methionine 270.4
  - monosaccharide 271.8
  - postgastrectomy 579.3
  - postsurgical 579.3
  - protein 579.8
  - sucrose (-isomaltose) (congenital) 271.3
  - syndrome 579.9
    - postgastrectomy 579.3
    - postsurgical 579.3
- **Malacia, bone** 268.2
  - juvenile (*see also* Rickets) 268.0
  - Kienböck's (juvenile) (lunate) (wrist) 732.3
    - adult 732.8
- **Malacoplakia**
  - bladder 596.8
  - colon 569.89
  - pelvis (kidney) 593.89
  - ureter 593.89
  - urethra 599.84
- **Malacosteon** 268.2
  - juvenile (*see also* Rickets) 268.0
- **Maladaptation** - *see* Maladjustment
- **Maladie de Roger** 745.4
- **Maladjustment**
  - conjugal V61.10
    - involving
      - divorce V61.03
      - estrangement V61.09
  - educational V62.3
  - family V61.9
    - specified circumstance NEC V61.8
  - marital V61.10
    - involving
      - divorce V61.03
      - estrangement V61.09

- **Maladjustment** – *continued*
  - occupational V62.29
    - current military deployment status V62.21
  - simple, adult (*see also* Reaction, adjustment) 309.9
  - situational acute (*see also* Reaction, adjustment) 309.9
  - social V62.4
- **Malaise** 780.79
- **Malakoplakia** - *see* Malacoplakia
- **Malaria, malarial** (fever) 084.6
  - algid 084.9
  - any type, with
    - algid malaria 084.9
    - blackwater fever 084.8
    - fever
      - blackwater 084.8
      - hemoglobinuric (bilious) 084.8
    - hemoglobinuria, malarial 084.8
    - hepatitis 084.9 *[573.2]*
    - nephrosis 084.9 *[581.81]*
    - pernicious complication NEC 084.9
      - cardiac 084.9
      - cerebral 084.9
  - cardiac 084.9
  - carrier (suspected) of V02.9
  - cerebral 084.9
  - complicating pregnancy, childbirth, or puerperium 647.4 [5th]
  - congenital 771.2
  - congestion, congestive 084.6
    - brain 084.9
  - continued 084.0
  - estivo-autumnal 084.0
  - falciparum (malignant tertian) 084.0
  - hematinuria 084.8
  - hematuria 084.8
  - hemoglobinuria 084.8
  - hemorrhagic 084.6
  - induced (therapeutically) 084.7
    - accidental - *see* Malaria, by type
  - liver 084.9 *[573.2]*
  - malariae (quartan) 084.2
  - malignant (tertian) 084.0
  - mixed infections 084.5
  - monkey 084.4
  - ovale 084.3
  - pernicious, acute 084.0
  - Plasmodium, P.
    - falciparum 084.0
    - malariae 084.2
    - ovale 084.3
    - vivax 084.1
  - quartan 084.2
  - quotidian 084.0
  - recurrent 084.6
    - induced (therapeutically) 084.7
      - accidental - *see* Malaria, by type
  - remittent 084.6
  - specified types NEC 084.4
  - spleen 084.6
  - subtertian 084.0
  - tertian (benign) 084.1
    - malignant 084.0
  - tropical 084.0
  - typhoid 084.6
  - vivax (benign tertian) 084.1
- **Malassez's disease** (testicular cyst) 608.89
- **Malassimilation** 579.9
- **Maldescent, testis** 752.51
- **Maldevelopment** - *see also* Anomaly, by site
  - brain 742.9
  - colon 751.5
  - hip (joint) 755.63
    - congenital dislocation (*see also* Dislocation, hip, congenital) 754.30
  - mastoid process 756.0
  - middle ear, except ossicles 744.03
    - ossicles 744.04
  - newborn (not malformation) 764.9 [5th]
  - ossicles, ear 744.04
  - spine 756.10

- **Maldevelopment** – *continued*
  - toe 755.66
- **Male type pelvis** 755.69
  - with disproportion (fetopelvic) 653.2 [5th]
    - affecting fetus or newborn 763.1
    - causing obstructed labor 660.1 [5th]
      - affecting fetus or newborn 763.1
- **Malformation** (congenital) - *see also* Anomaly
  - bone 756.9
  - bursa 756.9
  - Chiari
    - type I 348.4
    - type II (*see also* Spina bifida) 741.0 [5th]
    - type III 742.0
    - type IV 742.2
  - circulatory system NEC 747.9
    - specified type NEC 747.89
  - cochlea 744.05
  - digestive system NEC 751.9
    - lower 751.5
    - specified type NEC 751.8
    - upper 750.9
  - eye 743.9
  - gum 750.9
  - heart NEC 746.9
    - specified type NEC 746.89
    - valve 746.9
  - internal ear 744.05
  - joint NEC 755.9
    - specified type NEC 755.8
  - Mondini's (congenital) (malformation, cochlea) 744.05
  - muscle 756.9
  - nervous system (central) 742.9
  - pelvic organs or tissues
    - in pregnancy or childbirth 654.9 [5th]
      - affecting fetus or newborn 763.89
      - causing obstructed labor 660.2 [5th]
        - affecting fetus or newborn 763.1
  - placenta (*see also* Placenta, abnormal) 656.7 [5th]
  - respiratory organs 748.9
    - specified type NEC 748.8
  - Rieger's 743.44
  - sense organs NEC 742.9
    - specified type NEC 742.8
  - skin 757.9
    - specified type NEC 757.8
  - spinal cord 742.9
  - teeth, tooth NEC 520.9
  - tendon 756.9
  - throat 750.9
  - umbilical cord (complicating delivery) 663.9 [5th]
    - affecting fetus or newborn 762.6
  - umbilicus 759.9
  - urinary system NEC 753.9
    - specified type NEC 753.8
  - venous - *see* Anomaly, vein
- **Malfunction** - *see also* Dysfunction
  - arterial graft 996.1
  - cardiac pacemaker 996.01
  - catheter device - *see* Complications, mechanical, catheter
  - colostomy 569.62
    - valve 569.62
  - cystostomy 997.5
  - device, implant, or graft NEC - *see* Complications, mechanical
  - enteric stoma 569.62
  - enterostomy 569.62
  - esophagostomy 530.87
  - gastroenteric 536.8
  - gastrostomy 536.42
  - ileostomy
    - valve 569.62
  - nephrostomy 997.5
  - pacemaker - *see* Complications, mechanical, pacemaker
  - prosthetic device, internal - *see* Complications, mechanical
  - tracheostomy 519.02

- **Malfunction** – *continued*
  - valve
    - colostomy 569.62
    - ileostomy 569.62
  - vascular graft or shunt 996.1
- **Malgaigne's fracture** (closed) 808.43
  - open 808.53
- **Malherbe's**
  - calcifying epithelioma (M8110/0) - *see* Neoplasm, skin, benign
  - tumor (M8110/0) - *see* Neoplasm, skin, benign
- **Malibu disease** 919.8
  - infected 919.9
- **Malignancy** (M8000/3) - *see* Neoplasm, by site, malignant
- **Malignant** - *see* condition
- **Malingerer, malingering** V65.2
- **Mallet, finger** (acquired) 736.1
  - congenital 755.59
  - late effect of rickets 268.1
- **Malleus** 024
- **Mallory's bodies** 034.1
- **Mallory-Weiss syndrome** 530.7
- **Malnutrition** (calorie) 263.9
  - complicating pregnancy 648.9 [5th]
  - degree
    - first 263.1
    - second 263.0
    - third 262
    - mild 263.1
    - moderate 263.0
    - severe 261
      - protein-calorie 262
  - fetus 764.2 [5th]
    - "light-for-dates" 764.1 [5th]
  - following gastrointestinal surgery 579.3
  - intrauterine or fetal 764.2 [5th]
    - fetus or infant "light-for-dates" 764.1 [5th]
  - lack of care, or neglect (child) (infant) 995.52
    - adult 995.84
  - malignant 260
  - mild 263.1
  - moderate 263.0
  - protein 260
  - protein-calorie 263.9
    - severe 262
    - specified type NEC 263.8
  - severe 261
    - protein-calorie NEC 262
- **Malocclusion** (teeth) 524.4
  - angle's class I 524.21
  - angle's class II 524.22
  - angle's class III 524.23
  - due to
    - abnormal swallowing 524.59
    - accessory teeth (causing crowding) 524.31
    - dentofacial abnormality NEC 524.89
    - impacted teeth (causing crowding) 520.6
    - missing teeth 524.30
    - mouth breathing 524.59
    - sleep postures 524.59
    - supernumerary teeth (causing crowding) 524.31
    - thumb sucking 524.59
    - tongue, lip, or finger habits 524.59
  - temporomandibular (joint) 524.69
- **Malposition**
  - cardiac apex (congenital) 746.87
  - cervix - *see* Malposition, uterus
  - congenital
    - adrenal (gland) 759.1
    - alimentary tract 751.8
      - lower 751.5
      - upper 750.8
    - aorta 747.21
    - appendix 751.5
    - arterial trunk 747.29

Malposition – *continued*
- congenital
  - artery (peripheral) NEC (*see also* Malposition, congenital, peripheral vascular system) 747.60
    - coronary 746.85
    - pulmonary 747.3
  - auditory canal 744.29
    - causing impairment of hearing 744.02
  - auricle (ear) 744.29
    - causing impairment of hearing 744.02
    - cervical 744.43
  - biliary duct or passage 751.69
  - bladder (mucosa) 753.8
    - exteriorized or extroverted 753.5
  - brachial plexus 742.8
  - brain tissue 742.4
  - breast 757.6
  - bronchus 748.3
  - cardiac apex 746.87
  - cecum 751.5
  - clavicle 755.51
  - colon 751.5
  - digestive organ or tract NEC 751.8
    - lower 751.5
    - upper 750.8
  - ear (auricle) (external) 744.29
    - ossicles 744.04
  - endocrine (gland) NEC 759.2
  - epiglottis 748.3
  - Eustachian tube 744.24
  - eye 743.8
  - facial features 744.89
  - fallopian tube 752.19
  - finger(s) 755.59
    - supernumerary 755.01
  - foot 755.67
  - gallbladder 751.69
  - gastrointestinal tract 751.8
  - genitalia, genital organ(s) or tract
    - female 752.89
      - external 752.49
      - internal NEC 752.89
    - male 752.89
      - penis 752.69
      - scrotal transposition 752.81
  - glottis 748.3
  - hand 755.59
  - heart 746.87
    - dextrocardia 746.87
      - with complete transposition of viscera 759.3
  - hepatic duct 751.69
  - hip (joint) (*see also* Dislocation, hip, congenital) 754.30
  - intestine (large) (small) 751.5
    - with anomalous adhesions, fixation, or malrotation 751.4
  - joint NEC 755.8
  - kidney 753.3
  - larynx 748.3
  - limb 755.8
    - lower 755.69
    - upper 755.59
  - liver 751.69
  - lung (lobe) 748.69
  - nail(s) 757.5
  - nerve 742.8
  - nervous system NEC 742.8
  - nose, nasal (septum) 748.1
  - organ or site NEC - *see* Anomaly, specified type NEC, by site
  - ovary 752.0
  - pancreas 751.7
  - parathyroid (gland) 759.2
  - patella 755.64
  - peripheral vascular system 747.60
    - gastrointestinal 747.61
    - lower limb 747.64
    - renal 747.62
    - specified NEC 747.69

Malposition – *continued*
- congenital – *continued*
  - peripheral vascular system – *continued*
    - spinal 747.82
    - upper limb 747.63
  - pituitary (gland) 759.2
  - respiratory organ or system NEC 748.9
  - rib (cage) 756.3
    - supernumerary in cervical region 756.2
  - scapula 755.59
  - shoulder 755.59
  - spinal cord 742.59
  - spine 756.19
  - spleen 759.0
  - sternum 756.3
  - stomach 750.7
  - symphysis pubis 755.69
  - testis (undescended)752.51
  - thymus (gland) 759.2
  - thyroid (gland) (tissue) 759.2
    - cartilage 748.3
  - toe(s) 755.66
    - supernumerary 755.02
  - tongue 750.19
  - trachea 748.3
  - uterus 752.3
  - vein(s) (peripheral) NEC (*see also* Malposition, congenital, peripheral vascular system) 747.60
    - great 747.49
    - portal 747.49
    - pulmonary 747.49
  - vena cava (inferior) (superior) 747.49
- device, implant, or graft - *see* Complications, mechanical
- fetus NEC (*see also* Presentation, fetal) 652.9 [5th]
  - with successful version 652.1 [5th]
  - affecting fetus or newborn 763.1
  - before labor, affecting fetus or newborn 761.7
  - causing obstructed labor 660.0 [5th]
  - in multiple gestation (one fetus or more) 652.6 [5th]
    - with locking 660.5 [5th]
    - causing obstructed labor 660.0 [5th]
- gallbladder (*see also* Disease, gallbladder) 575.8
- gastrointestinal tract 569.89
  - congenital 751.8
- heart (*see also* Malposition, congenital, heart) 746.87
- intestine 569.89
  - congenital 751.5
- pelvic organs or tissues
  - in pregnancy or childbirth 654.4 [5th]
    - affecting fetus or newborn 763.89
    - causing obstructed labor 660.2 [5th]
      - affecting fetus or newborn 763.1
- placenta - *see* Placenta, previa
- stomach 537.89
  - congenital 750.7
- tooth, teeth 524.30
  - with impaction 520.6
- uterus (acquired) (acute) (adherent) (any degree) (asymptomatic) (postinfectional) (postpartal, old) 621.6
  - anteflexion or anteversion (*see also* Anteversion, uterus) 621.6
  - congenital 752.3
  - flexion 621.6
    - lateral (*see also* Lateroversion, uterus) 621.6
  - in pregnancy or childbirth 654.4 [5th]
    - affecting fetus or newborn 763.89
    - causing obstructed labor 660.2 [5th]
      - affecting fetus or newborn 763.1
  - inversion 621.6
  - lateral (flexion) (version) (*see also* Lateroversion, uterus) 621.6

Malposition – *continued*
- uterus – *continued*
  - lateroflexion (*see also* Lateroversion, uterus) 621.6
  - lateroversion (*see also* Lateroversion, uterus) 621.6
  - retroflexion or retroversion (*see also* Retroversion, uterus) 621.6

Malposture 729.90

Malpresentation, fetus (*see also* Presentation, fetal) 652.9 [5th]

Malrotation
- cecum 751.4
- colon 751.4
- intestine 751.4
- kidney 753.3

MALT (mucosa associated lymphoid tissue) 200.3 [5th]

Malta fever (*see also* Brucellosis) 023.9

Maltosuria 271.3

Maltreatment (of)
- adult 995.80
  - emotional 995.82
  - multiple forms 995.85
  - neglect (nutritional) 995.84
  - physical 995.81
  - psychological 995.82
  - sexual 995.83
- child 995.50
  - emotional 995.51
  - multiple forms 995.59
  - neglect (nutritional) 995.52
  - physical 995.54
    - shaken infant syndrome 995.55
  - psychological 995.51
  - sexual 995.53
- spouse (*see also* Maltreatment, adult) 995.80

Malt workers' lung 495.4

Malum coxae senilis 715.25

Malunion, fracture 733.81

Mammillitis (*see also* Mastitis) 611.0
- puerperal, postpartum 675.2 [5th]

Mammitis (*see also* Mastitis) 611.0
- puerperal, postpartum 675.2 [5th]

Mammographic
- calcification 793.89
- calculus 793.89
- microcalcification 793.81

Mammoplasia 611.1

Management
- contraceptive V25.9
  - specified type NEC V25.8
- procreative V26.9
  - specified type NEC V26.89

Mangled NEC (*see also* nature and site of injury) 959.9

Mania (monopolar) (*see also* Psychosis, affective) 296.0 [5th]
- alcoholic (acute) (chronic) 291.9
- Bell's - *see* Mania, chronic
- chronic 296.0 [5th]
  - recurrent episode 296.1 [5th]
  - single episode 296.0 [5th]
- compulsive 300.3
- delirious (acute) 296.0 [5th]
  - recurrent episode 296.1 [5th]
  - single episode 296.0 [5th]
- epileptic (*see also* Epilepsy) 345.4 [5th]
- hysterical 300.10
- inhibited 296.89
- puerperal (after delivery) 296.0 [5th]
  - recurrent episode 296.1 [5th]
  - single episode 296.0 [5th]
- recurrent episode 296.1 [5th]
- senile 290.8
- single episode 296.0 [5th]
- stupor 296.89
- stuporous 296.89
- unproductive 296.89

Manic-depressive insanity, psychosis, reaction, or syndrome (*see also* Psychosis, affective) 296.80
- circular (alternating) 296.7
  - currently
    - depressed 296.5 [5th]
    - episode unspecified 296.7
    - hypomanic, previously depressed 296.4 [5th]
    - manic 296.4 [5th]
  - mixed 296.6 [5th]
- depressed (type), depressive 296.2 [5th]
  - atypical 296.82
  - recurrent episode 296.3 [5th]
  - single episode 296.2 [5th]
- hypomanic 296.0 [5th]
  - recurrent episode 296.1 [5th]
  - single episode 296.0 [5th]
- manic 296.0 [5th]
  - atypical 296.81
  - recurrent episode 296.1 [5th]
  - single episode 296.0 [5th]
- mixed NEC 296.89
- perplexed 296.89
- stuporous 296.89

Manifestations, rheumatoid
- lungs 714.81
- pannus - *see* Arthritis, rheumatoid
- subcutaneous nodules - *see* Arthritis, rheumatoid

Mankowsky's syndrome (familial dysplastic osteopathy) 731.2

Mannoheptulosuria 271.8

Mannosidosis 271.8

Manson's
- disease (schistosomiasis) 120.1
- pyosis (pemphigus contagiosus) 684
- schistosomiasis 120.1

Mansonellosis 125.5

Manual - *see* condition

Maple bark disease 495.6

Maple bark-strippers' lung 495.6

Maple syrup (urine) **disease or syndrome** 270.3

Marable's syndrome (celiac artery compression) 447.4

Marasmus 261
- brain 331.9
- due to malnutrition 261
- intestinal 569.89
- nutritional 261
- senile 797
- tuberculous NEC (*see also* Tuberculosis) 011.9 [5th]

Marble
- bones 756.52
- skin 782.61

Marburg disease (virus) 078.89

March
- foot 733.94
- hemoglobinuria 283.2

Marchand multiple nodular hyperplasia (liver) 571.5

Marchesani (-Weill) syndrome (brachymorphism and ectopia lentis) 759.89

Marchiafava (-Bignami) disease or syndrome 341.8

Marchiafava-Micheli syndrome (paroxysmal nocturnal hemoglobinuria) 283.2

Marcus Gunn's syndrome (jaw-winking syndrome) 742.8

Marfan's
- congenital syphilis 090.49
- disease 090.49
- syndrome (arachnodactyly) 759.82
  - meaning congenital syphilis 090.49
    - with luxation of lens 090.49 *[379.32]*

Marginal
- implantation, placenta - *see* Placenta, previa
- placenta - *see* Placenta, previa

- **Marginal** – *continued*
  - sinus (hemorrhage) (rupture) 641.2 5th
    - affecting fetus or newborn 762.1
- **Marie's**
  - cerebellar ataxia 334.2
  - syndrome (acromegaly) 253.0
- **Marie-Bamberger disease or syndrome** (hypertrophic) (pulmonary) (secondary) 731.2
  - idiopathic (acropachyderma) 757.39
  - primary (acropachyderma) 757.39
- **Marie-Charcôt-Tooth neuropathic atrophy, muscle** 356.1
- **Marie-Strümpell arthritis or disease** (ankylosing spondylitis) 720.0
- **Marihuana, marijuana**
  - abuse (*see also* Abuse, drugs, nondependent) 305.2 5th
  - dependence (*see also* Dependence) 304.3 5th
- **Marion's disease** (bladder neck obstruction) 596.0
- **Marital conflict** V61.10
- **Mark**
  - port wine 757.32
  - raspberry 757.32
  - strawberry 757.32
  - stretch 701.3
  - tattoo 709.09
- **Maroteaux-Lamy syndrome** (mucopolysaccharidosis VI) 277.5
- **Marriage license examination** V70.3
- **Marrow** (bone)
  - arrest 284.9
  - megakaryocytic 287.30
  - poor function 289.9
- **Marseilles fever** 082.1
- **Marsh's disease** (exophthalmic goiter) 242.0 5th
- **Marshall's** (hidrotic) **ectodermal dysplasia** 757.31
- **Marsh fever** (*see also* Malaria) 084.6
- **Martin's disease** 715.27
- **Martin-Albright syndrome** (pseudohypoparathyroidism) 275.49
- **Martorell-Fabre syndrome** (pulseless disease) 446.7
- **Masculinization, female, with adrenal hyperplasia** 255.2
- **Masculinovoblastoma** (M8670/0) 220
- **Masochism** 302.83
- **Masons' lung** 502
- **Mass**
  - abdominal 789.3 5th
  - anus 787.99
  - bone 733.90
  - breast 611.72
  - cheek 784.2
  - chest 786.6
  - cystic - *see* Cyst
  - ear 388.8
  - epigastric 789.3 5th
  - eye 379.92
  - female genital organ 625.8
  - gum 784.2
  - head 784.2
  - intracranial 784.2
  - joint 719.60
    - ankle 719.67
    - elbow 719.62
    - foot 719.67
    - hand 719.64
    - hip 719.65
    - knee 719.66
    - multiple sites 719.69
    - pelvic region 719.65
    - shoulder (region) 719.61
    - specified site NEC 719.68
    - wrist 719.63
  - kidney (*see also* Disease, kidney) 593.9
  - lung 786.6
  - lymph node 785.6
  - malignant (M8000/3) - *see* Neoplasm, by site, malignant
- **Mass** – *continued*
  - mediastinal 786.6
  - mouth 784.2
  - muscle (limb) 729.89
  - neck 784.2
  - nose or sinus 784.2
  - palate 784.2
  - pelvis, pelvic 789.3 5th
  - penis 607.89
  - perineum 625.8
  - rectum 787.99
  - scrotum 608.89
  - skin 782.2
  - specified organ NEC - *see* Disease of specified organ or site
  - splenic 789.2
  - substernal 786.6
    - thyroid (*see also* Goiter) 240.9
  - superficial (localized) 782.2
  - testes 608.89
  - throat 784.2
  - tongue 784.2
  - umbilicus 789.3 5th
  - uterus 625.8
  - vagina 625.8
  - vulva 625.8
- **Massive** - *see* condition
- **Mastalgia** 611.71
  - psychogenic 307.89
- **Mast cell**
  - disease 757.33
    - systemic (M9741/3) 202.6 5th
  - leukemia (M9900/3) 207.8 5th
  - sarcoma (M9742/3) 202.6 5th
  - tumor (M9740/1) 238.5
    - malignant (M9740/3) 202.6 5th
- **Masters-Allen syndrome** 620.6
- **Mastitis** (acute) (adolescent) (diffuse) (interstitial) (lobular) (nonpuerperal) (nonsuppurative) (parenchymatous) (phlegmonous) (simple) (subacute) (suppurative) 611.0
  - chronic (cystic) (fibrocystic) 610.1
  - cystic 610.1
    - Schimmelbusch's type 610.1
  - fibrocystic 610.1
  - infective 611.0
  - lactational 675.2 5th
  - lymphangitis 611.0
  - neonatal (noninfective) 778.7
    - infective 771.5
  - periductal 610.4
  - plasma cell 610.4
  - puerperal, postpartum, (interstitial) (nonpurulent) (parenchymatous) 675.2 5th
    - purulent 675.1 5th
    - stagnation 676.2 5th
  - puerperalis 675.2 5th
  - retromammary 611.0
    - puerperal, postpartum 675.1 5th
  - submammary 611.0
    - puerperal, postpartum 675.1 5th
- **Mastocytoma** (M9740/1) 238.5
  - malignant (M9740/3) 202.6 5th
- **Mastocytosis** 757.33
  - malignant (M9741/3) 202.6 5th
  - systemic (M9741/3) 202.6 5th
- **Mastodynia** 611.71
  - psychogenic 307.89
- **Mastoid** - *see* condition
- **Mastoidalgia** (*see also* Otalgia) 388.70
- **Mastoiditis** (coalescent) (hemorrhagic) (pneumococcal) (streptococcal) (suppurative) 383.9
  - acute or subacute 383.00
    - with
      - Gradenigo's syndrome 383.02
      - petrositis 383.02
      - specified complication NEC 383.02
      - subperiosteal abscess 383.01
  - chronic (necrotic) (recurrent) 383.1
  - tuberculous (*see also* Tuberculosis) 015.6 5th
- **Mastopathy, mastopathia** 611.9
  - chronica cystica 610.1
  - diffuse cystic 610.1
  - estrogenic 611.89
  - ovarian origin 611.89
- **Mastoplasia** 611.1
- **Masturbation** 307.9
- **Maternal condition, affecting fetus or newborn**
  - acute yellow atrophy of liver 760.8
  - albuminuria 760.1
  - anesthesia or analgesia 763.5
  - blood loss 762.1
  - chorioamnionitis 762.7
  - circulatory disease, chronic (conditions classifiable to 390-459, 745-747) 760.3
  - congenital heart disease (conditions classifiable to 745-746) 760.3
  - cortical necrosis of kidney 760.1
  - death 761.6
  - diabetes mellitus 775.0
    - manifest diabetes in the infant 775.1
  - disease NEC 760.9
    - circulatory system, chronic (conditions classifiable to 390-459, 745-747) 760.3
    - genitourinary system (conditions classifiable to 580-599) 760.1
    - respiratory (conditions classifiable to 490-519, 748) 760.3
  - eclampsia 760.0
  - hemorrhage NEC 762.1
  - hepatitis acute, malignant, or subacute 760.8
  - hyperemesis (gravidarum) 761.8
  - hypertension (arising during pregnancy) (conditions classifiable to 642) 760.0
  - infection
    - disease classifiable to 001-136 760.2
    - genital tract NEC 760.8
    - urinary tract 760.1
  - influenza 760.2
    - manifest influenza in the infant 771.2
  - injury (conditions classifiable to 800-996) 760.5
  - malaria 760.2
    - manifest malaria in infant or fetus 771.2
  - malnutrition 760.4
  - necrosis of liver 760.8
  - nephritis (conditions classifiable to 580-583) 760.1
  - nephrosis (conditions classifiable to 581) 760.1
  - noxious substance transmitted via breast milk or placenta 760.70
    - alcohol 760.71
    - anticonvulsants 760.77
    - antifungals 760.74
    - anti-infective agents 760.74
    - antimetabolics 760.78
    - cocaine 760.75
    - "crack" 760.75
    - diethylstilbestrol [DES] 760.76
    - hallucinogenic agents 760.73
    - medicinal agents NEC 760.79
    - narcotics 760.72
    - obstetric anesthetic or analgesic drug 760.72
    - specified agent NEC 760.79
  - nutritional disorder (conditions classifiable to 260-269) 760.4
  - operation unrelated to current delivery (*see also* Newborn, affected by) 760.64
  - pre-eclampsia 760.0
  - pyelitis or pyelonephritis, arising during pregnancy (conditions classifiable to 590) 760.1
  - renal disease or failure 760.1
  - respiratory disease, chronic (conditions classifiable to 490-519, 748) 760.3
- **Maternal condition, affecting fetus or newborn** – *continued*
  - rheumatic heart disease (chronic) (conditions classifiable to 393-398) 760.3
  - rubella (conditions classifiable to 056) 760.2
    - manifest rubella in the infant or fetus 771.0
  - surgery unrelated to current delivery (*see also* Newborn, affected by) 760.64
    - to uterus or pelvic organs 760.64
  - syphilis (conditions classifiable to 090-097) 760.2
    - manifest syphilis in the infant or fetus 090.0
  - thrombophlebitis 760.3
  - toxemia (of pregnancy) 760.0
    - pre-eclamptic 760.0
  - toxoplasmosis (conditions classifiable to 130) 760.2
    - manifest toxoplasmosis in the infant or fetus 771.2
  - transmission of chemical substance through the placenta 760.70
    - alcohol 760.71
    - anticonvulsants 760.77
    - antifungals 760.74
    - anti-infective 760.74
    - antimetabolics 760.78
    - cocaine 760.75
    - "crack" 760.75
    - diethylstilbestrol [DES] 760.76
    - hallucinogenic agents 760.73
    - narcotics 760.72
    - specified substance NEC 760.79
  - uremia 760.1
  - urinary tract conditions (conditions classifiable to 580-599) 760.1
  - vomiting (pernicious) (persistent) (vicious) 761.8
- **Maternity** - *see* Delivery
- **Matheiu's disease** (leptospiral jaundice) 100.0
- **Mauclaire's disease or osteochondrosis** 732.3
- **Maxcy's disease** 081.0
- **Maxilla, maxillary** - *see* condition
- **May (-Hegglin) anomaly or syndrome** 288.2
- **Mayaro fever** 066.3
- **Mazoplasia** 610.8
- **MBD** (minimal brain dysfunction), **child** (*see also* Hyperkinesia) 314.9
- **MCAD** (medium chain acyl CoA dehydrogenase deficiency) 277.85
- **McArdle (-Schmid-Pearson) disease or syndrome** (glycogenosis V) 271.0
- **McCune-Albright syndrome** (osteitis fibrosa disseminata) 756.59
- **MCLS** (mucocutaneous lymph node syndrome) 446.1
- **McQuarrie's syndrome** (idiopathic familial hypoglycemia) 251.2
- **Measles** (black) (hemorrhagic) (suppressed) 055.9
  - with
    - encephalitis 055.0
    - keratitis 055.71
    - keratoconjunctivitis 055.71
    - otitis media 055.2
    - pneumonia 055.1
  - complication 055.8
    - specified type NEC 055.79
  - encephalitis 055.0
  - French 056.9
  - German 056.9
  - keratitis 055.71
  - keratoconjunctivitis 055.71
  - liberty 056.9
  - otitis media 055.2
  - pneumonia 055.1
  - specified complications NEC 055.79
  - vaccination, prophylactic (against) V04.2
- **Meatitis, urethral** (*see also* Urethritis) 597.89

- **Meat poisoning** - *see* Poisoning, food
- **Meatus, meatal** - *see* condition
- **Meat-wrappers' asthma** 506.9
- **Meckel's**
  - diverticulitis 751.0
  - diverticulum (displaced) (hypertrophic) 751.0
- **Meconium**
  - aspiration 770.11
    - with
      - pneumonia 770.12
      - pneumonitis 770.12
      - respiratory symptoms 770.12
    - below vocal cords 770.11
      - with respiratory symptoms 770.12
    - syndrome 770.12
  - delayed passage in newborn 777.1
  - ileus 777.1
    - due to cystic fibrosis 277.01
  - in liquor 792.3
    - noted during delivery 656.8 5th
  - insufflation 770.11
    - with respiratory symptoms 770.12
  - obstruction
    - fetus or newborn 777.1
      - in mucoviscidosis 277.01
  - passage of 792.3
    - noted during delivery 763.84
  - peritonitis 777.6
  - plug syndrome (newborn) NEC 777.1
  - staining 779.84
- **Median** - *see also* condition
  - arcuate ligament syndrome 447.4
  - bar (prostate) 600.90
    - with
      - other lower urinary tract symptoms (LUTS) 600.91
      - urinary
        - obstruction 600.91
        - retention 600.91
  - vesical orifice 600.90
    - with
      - other lower urinary tract symptoms (LUTS) 600.91
      - urinary
        - obstruction 600.91
        - retention 600.91
  - rhomboid glossitis 529.2
- **Mediastinal shift** 793.2
- **Mediastinitis** (acute) (chronic) 519.2
  - actinomycotic 039.8
  - syphilitic 095.8
  - tuberculous (*see also* Tuberculosis) 012.8 5th
- **Mediastinopericarditis** (*see also* Pericarditis) 423.9
  - acute 420.90
  - chronic 423.8
    - rheumatic 393
  - rheumatic, chronic 393
- **Mediastinum, mediastinal** - *see* condition
- **Medical services provided for** - *see* Health, services provided because (of)
- **Medicine poisoning** (by overdose) (wrong substance given or taken in error) 977.9
  - specified drug or substance - *see* Table of Drugs and Chemicals
- **Medin's disease** (poliomyelitis) 045.9 5th
- **Mediterranean**
  - anemia (with other hemoglobinopathy) 282.49
  - disease or syndrome (hemipathic) 282.49
  - fever (*see also* Brucellosis) 023.9
    - familial 277.31
  - kala-azar 085.0
  - leishmaniasis 085.0
  - tick fever 082.1
- **Medulla** - *see* condition
- **Medullary**
  - cystic kidney 753.16
  - sponge kidney 753.17
- **Medullated fibers**
  - optic (nerve) 743.57
- **Medullated fibers** – *continued*
  - retina 362.85
- **Medulloblastoma** (M9470/3)
  - desmoplastic (M9471/3) 191.6
  - specified site - *see* Neoplasm, by site, malignant
  - unspecified site 191.6
- **Medulloepithelioma** (M9501/3) - *see also* Neoplasm, by site, malignant
  - teratoid (M9502/3) - *see* Neoplasm, by site, malignant
- **Medullomyoblastoma** (M9472/3)
  - specified site - *see* Neoplasm, by site, malignant
  - unspecified site 191.6
- **Meekeren-Ehlers-Danlos syndrome** 756.83
- **Megacaryocytic** - *see* condition
- **Megacolon** (acquired) (functional) (not Hirschsprung's disease) 564.7
  - aganglionic 751.3
  - congenital, congenitum 751.3
  - Hirschsprung's (disease) 751.3
  - psychogenic 306.4
  - toxic (*see also* Colitis, ulcerative) 556.9
- **Megaduodenum** 537.3
- **Megaesophagus** (functional) 530.0
  - congenital 750.4
- **Megakaryocytic** - *see* condition
- **Megalencephaly** 742.4
- **Megalerythema** (epidermicum) (infectiosum) 057.0
- **Megalia, cutis et ossium** 757.39
- **Megaloappendix** 751.5
- **Megalocephalus, megalocephaly NEC** 756.0
- **Megalocornea** 743.41
  - associated with buphthalmos 743.22
- **Megalocytic anemia** 281.9
- **Megalodactylia** (fingers) (thumbs) 755.57
  - toes 755.65
- **Megaloduodenum** 751.5
- **Megaloesophagus** (functional) 530.0
  - congenital 750.4
- **Megalogastria** (congenital) 750.7
- **Megalomania** 307.9
- **Megalophthalmos** 743.8
- **Megalopsia** 368.14
- **Megalosplenia** (*see also* Splenomegaly) 789.2
- **Megaloureter** 593.89
  - congenital 753.22
- **Megarectum** 569.49
- **Megasigmoid** 564.7
  - congenital 751.3
- **Megaureter** 593.89
  - congenital 753.22
- **Megrim** 346.9
- **Meibomian**
  - cyst 373.2
    - infected 373.12
  - gland - *see* condition
  - infarct (eyelid) 374.85
  - stye 373.11
- **Meibomitis** 373.12
- **Meige**
  - -Milroy disease (chronic hereditary edema) 757.0
  - syndrome (blepharospasm-oromandibular dystonia) 333.82
- **Melalgia, nutritional** 266.2
- **Melancholia** (*see also* Psychosis, affective) 296.90
  - climacteric 296.2 5th
    - recurrent episode 296.3 5th
    - single episode 296.2 5th
  - hypochondriac 300.7
  - intermittent 296.2 5th
    - recurrent episode 296.3 5th
    - single episode 296.2 5th
  - involutional 296.2 5th
    - recurrent episode 296.3 5th
    - single episode 296.2 5th
  - menopausal 296.2 5th
    - recurrent episode 296.3 5th
    - single episode 296.2 5th
  - puerperal 296.2 5th
- **Melancholia** – *continued*
  - reactive (from emotional stress, psychological trauma) 298.0
  - recurrent 296.3 5th
  - senile 290.21
  - stuporous 296.2 5th
    - recurrent episode 296.3 5th
    - single episode 296.2 5th
- **Melanemia** 275.0
- **Melanoameloblastoma** (M9363/0) - *see* Neoplasm, bone, benign
- **Melanoblastoma** (M8720/3) - *see* Melanoma
- **Melanoblastosis**
  - Block-Sulzberger 757.33
  - cutis linearis sive systematisata 757.33
- **Melanocarcinoma** (M8720/3) - *see* Melanoma
- **Melanocytoma, eyeball** (M8726/0) 224.0
- **Melanoderma, melanodermia** 709.09
  - Addison's (primary adrenal insufficiency) 255.41
- **Melanodontia, infantile** 521.05
- **Melanodontoclasia** 521.05
- **Melanoepithelioma** (M8720/3) - *see* Melanoma
- **Melanoma** (malignant) (M8720/3) 172.9

> **Note** *Except where otherwise indicated, the morphological varieties of melanoma in the list below should be coded by site as for "Melanoma (malignant)." Internal sites should be coded to malignant neoplasm of those sites.*

  - abdominal wall 172.5
  - ala nasi 172.3
  - amelanotic (M8730/3) - *see* Melanoma, by site
  - ankle 172.7
  - anus, anal 154.3
    - canal 154.2
  - arm 172.6
  - auditory canal (external) 172.2
  - auricle (ear) 172.2
  - auricular canal (external) 172.2
  - axilla 172.5
  - axillary fold 172.5
  - back 172.5
  - balloon cell (M8722/3) - *see* Melanoma, by site
  - benign (M8720/0) - *see* Neoplasm, skin, benign
  - breast (female) (male) 172.5
  - brow 172.3
  - buttock 172.5
  - canthus (eye) 172.1
  - cheek (external) 172.3
  - chest wall 172.5
  - chin 172.3
  - choroid 190.6
  - conjunctiva 190.3
  - ear (external) 172.2
  - epithelioid cell (M8771/3) - *see also* Melanoma, by site
    - and spindle cell, mixed (M8775/3) - *see* Melanoma, by site
  - external meatus (ear) 172.2
  - eye 190.9
  - eyebrow 172.3
  - eyelid (lower) (upper) 172.1
  - face NEC 172.3
  - female genital organ (external) NEC 184.4
  - finger 172.6
  - flank 172.5
  - foot 172.7
  - forearm 172.6
  - forehead 172.3
  - foreskin 187.1
  - gluteal region 172.5
  - groin 172.5
  - hand 172.6
  - heel 172.7
  - helix 172.2
  - hip 172.7
- **Melanoma** (malignant) – *continued*
  - in
    - giant pigmented nevus (M8761/3) - *see* Melanoma, by site
    - Hutchinson's melanotic freckle (M8742/3) - *see* Melanoma, by site
    - junctional nevus (M8740/3) - *see* Melanoma, by site
    - precancerous melanosis (M8741/3) - *see* Melanoma, by site
  - in situ - *see* Melanoma, by site
    - skin 172.9
  - interscapular region 172.5
  - iris 190.0
  - jaw 172.3
  - juvenile (M8770/0) - *see* Neoplasm, skin, benign
  - knee 172.7
  - labium
    - majus 184.1
    - minus 184.2
  - lacrimal gland 190.2
  - leg 172.7
  - lip (lower) (upper) 172.0
  - liver 197.7
  - lower limb NEC 172.7
  - male genital organ (external) NEC 187.9
  - meatus, acoustic (external) 172.2
  - meibomian gland 172.1
  - metastatic
    - of or from specified site - *see* Melanoma, by site
    - site not of skin - *see* Neoplasm, by site, malignant, secondary
    - to specified site - *see* Neoplasm, by site, malignant, secondary
    - unspecified site 172.9
  - nail 172.9
    - finger 172.6
    - toe 172.7
  - neck 172.4
  - nodular (M8721/3) - *see* Melanoma, by site
  - nose, external 172.3
  - orbit 190.1
  - penis 187.4
  - perianal skin 172.5
  - perineum 172.5
  - pinna 172.2
  - popliteal (fossa) (space) 172.7
  - prepuce 187.1
  - pubes 172.5
  - pudendum 184.4
  - retina 190.5
  - scalp 172.4
  - scrotum 187.7
  - septum nasal (skin) 172.3
  - shoulder 172.6
  - skin NEC 172.8
    - in situ 172.9
  - spindle cell (M8772/3) - *see also* Melanoma, by site
    - type A (M8773/3) 190.0
    - type B (M8774/3) 190.0
  - submammary fold 172.5
  - superficial spreading (M8743/3) - *see* Melanoma, by site
  - temple 172.3
  - thigh 172.7
  - toe 172.7
  - trunk NEC 172.5
  - umbilicus 172.5
  - upper limb NEC 172.6
  - vagina vault 184.0
  - vulva 184.4
- **Melanoplakia** 528.9
- **Melanosarcoma** (M8720/3) - *see also* Melanoma
  - epithelioid cell (M8771/3) - *see* Melanoma

Meat poisoning – Melanosarcoma

- **Melanosis** 709.09
  - addisonian (primary adrenal insufficiency) 255.41
    - tuberculous (*see also* Tuberculosis) 017.6 5th
  - adrenal 255.41
  - colon 569.89
  - conjunctiva 372.55
    - congenital 743.49
  - corii degenerativa 757.33
  - cornea (presenile) (senile) 371.12
    - congenital 743.43
      - interfering with vision 743.42
    - prenatal 743.43
      - interfering with vision 743.42
  - eye 372.55
    - congenital 743.49
  - jute spinners' 709.09
  - lenticularis progressiva 757.33
  - liver 573.8
  - precancerous (M8741/2) - *see also* Neoplasm, skin, in situ
    - malignant melanoma in (M8741/3) - *see* Melanoma
  - Riehl's 709.09
  - sclera 379.19
    - congenital 743.47
  - suprarenal 255.41
  - tar 709.09
  - toxic 709.09
- **Melanuria** 791.9
- **MELAS syndrome** (mitochondrial encephalopathy, lactic acidosis and stroke-like episodes) 277.87
- **Melasma** 709.09
  - adrenal (gland) 255.41
  - suprarenal (gland) 255.41
- **Melena** 578.1
  - due to
    - swallowed maternal blood 777.3
    - ulcer - *see* Ulcer, by site, with hemorrhage
  - newborn 772.4
    - due to swallowed maternal blood 777.3
- **Meleney's**
  - gangrene (cutaneous) 686.09
  - ulcer (chronic undermining) 686.09
- **Melioidosis** 025
- **Melitensis, febris** 023.0
- **Melitococcosis** 023.0
- **Melkersson (-Rosenthal) syndrome** 351.8
- **Mellitus, diabetes** - *see* Diabetes
- **Melorheostosis** (bone) (leri) 733.99
- **Meloschisis** 744.83
- **Melotia** 744.29
- **Membrana**
  - capsularis lentis posterior 743.39
  - epipapillaris 743.57
- **Membranacea placenta** - *see* Placenta, abnormal
- **Membranaceous uterus** 621.8
- **Membrane, membranous** - *see also* condition
  - folds, congenital - *see* Web
  - Jackson's 751.4
  - over face (causing asphyxia), fetus or newborn 768.9
  - premature rupture - *see* Rupture, membranes, premature
  - pupillary 364.74
    - persistent 743.46
  - retained (complicating delivery) (with hemorrhage) 666.2 5th
    - without hemorrhage 667.1 5th
  - secondary (eye) 366.50
  - unruptured (causing asphyxia) 768.9
  - vitreous humor 379.25
- **Membranitis, fetal** 658.4 5th
  - affecting fetus or newborn 762.7
- **Memory disturbance, loss or lack** (*see also* Amnesia) 780.93
  - mild, following organic brain damage 310.8 ▲
- **MEN** (multiple endocrine neoplasia) **syndromes**
  - type I 258.01
  - type IIA 258.02
  - type IIB 258.03
- **Menadione** (vitamin K) **deficiency** 269.0
- **Menarche, precocious** 259.1
- **Mendacity, pathologic** 301.7
- **Mende's syndrome** (ptosis-epicanthus) 270.2
- **Mendelson's syndrome** (resulting from a procedure) 997.39
  - obstetric 668.0 5th
- **Ménétrier's disease or syndrome** (hypertrophic gastritis) 535.2 5th
- **Ménière's disease, syndrome, or vertigo** 386.00
  - cochlear 386.02
  - cochleovestibular 386.01
  - inactive 386.04
  - in remission 386.04
  - vestibular 386.03
- **Meninges, meningeal** - *see* condition
- **Meningioma** (M9530/0) - *see also* Neoplasm, meninges, benign
  - angioblastic (M9535/0) - *see* Neoplasm, meninges, benign
  - angiomatous (M9534/0) - *see* Neoplasm, meninges, benign
  - endotheliomatous (M9531/0) - *see* Neoplasm, meninges, benign
  - fibroblastic (M9532/0) - *see* Neoplasm, meninges, benign
  - fibrous (M9532/0) - *see* Neoplasm, meninges, benign
  - hemangioblastic (M9535/0) - *see* Neoplasm, meninges, benign
  - hemangiopericytic (M9536/0) - *see* Neoplasm, meninges, benign
  - malignant (M9530/3) - *see* Neoplasm, meninges, malignant
  - meningiothelial (M9531/0) - *see* Neoplasm, meninges, benign
  - meningotheliomatous (M9531/0) - *see* Neoplasm, meninges, benign
  - mixed (M9537/0) - *see* Neoplasm, meninges, benign
  - multiple (M9530/1) 237.6
  - papillary (M9538/1) 237.6
  - psammomatous (M9533/0) - *see* Neoplasm, meninges, benign
  - syncytial (M9531/0) - *see* Neoplasm, meninges, benign
  - transitional (M9537/0) - *see* Neoplasm, meninges, benign
- **Meningiomatosis** (diffuse) (M9530/1) 237.6
- **Meningism** (*see also* Meningismus) 781.6
- **Meningismus** (infectional) (pneumococcal) 781.6
  - due to serum or vaccine 997.09 *[321.8]*
  - influenzal NEC 487.8
- **Meningitis** (basal) (basic) (basilar) (brain) (cerebral) (cervical) (congestive) (diffuse) (hemorrhagic) (infantile) (membranous) (metastatic) (nonspecific) (pontine) (progressive) (simple) (spinal) (subacute) (sympathetica) (toxic) 322.9
  - abacterial NEC (*see also* Meningitis, aseptic) 047.9
  - actinomycotic 039.8 *[320.7]*
  - adenoviral 049.1
  - aerobacter aerogenes 320.82
  - anaerobes (cocci) (gram-negative) (gram-positive) (mixed) (NEC) 320.81
  - arbovirus NEC 066.9 *[321.2]*
    - specified type NEC 066.8 *[321.2]*
  - aseptic (acute) NEC 047.9
    - adenovirus 049.1
    - Coxsackie virus 047.0
    - due to
      - adenovirus 049.1
      - Coxsackie virus 047.0
      - ECHO virus 047.1
      - enterovirus 047.9

Meningitis – *continued*
  - aseptic – *continued*
    - due to – *continued*
      - mumps 072.1
      - poliovirus (*see also* Poliomyelitis) 045.2 5th *[321.2]*
    - ECHO virus 047.1
    - herpes (simplex) virus 054.72
      - zoster 053.0
    - leptospiral 100.81
    - lymphocytic choriomeningitis 049.0
    - noninfective 322.0
  - Bacillus pyocyaneus 320.89
  - bacterial NEC 320.9
    - anaerobic 320.81
    - gram-negative 320.82
      - anaerobic 320.81
  - Bacteroides (fragilis) (oralis) (melaninogenicus) 320.81
  - cancerous (M8000/6) 198.4
  - candidal 112.83
  - carcinomatous (M8010/6) 198.4
  - caseous (*see also* Tuberculosis, meninges) 013.0 5th
  - cerebrospinal (acute) (chronic) (diplococcal) (endemic) (epidemic) (fulminant) (infectious) (malignant) (meningococcal) (sporadic) 036.0
    - carrier (suspected) of V02.59
  - chronic NEC 322.2
  - clear cerebrospinal fluid NEC 322.0
  - Clostridium (haemolyticum) (novyi) NEC 320.81
  - coccidioidomycosis 114.2
  - Coxsackie virus 047.0
  - cryptococcal 117.5 *[321.0]*
  - diplococcal 036.0
    - gram-negative 036.0
    - gram-positive 320.1
  - Diplococcus pneumoniae 320.1
  - due to
    - actinomycosis 039.8 *[320.7]*
    - adenovirus 049.1
    - coccidiomycosis 114.2
    - enterovirus 047.9
      - specified NEC 047.8
    - histoplasmosis (*see also* Histoplasmosis) 115.91
    - Listerosis 027.0 *[320.7]*
    - Lyme disease 088.81 *[320.7]*
    - moniliasis 112.83
    - mumps 072.1
    - neurosyphilis 094.2
    - nonbacterial organisms NEC 321.8
    - oidiomycosis 112.83
    - poliovirus (*see also* Poliomyelitis) 045.2 5th *[321.2]*
    - preventive immunization, inoculation, or vaccination 997.09 *[321.8]*
    - sarcoidosis 135 *[321.4]*
    - sporotrichosis 117.1 *[321.1]*
    - syphilis 094.2
      - acute 091.81
      - congenital 090.42
      - secondary 091.81
    - trypanosomiasis (*see also* Trypanosomiasis) 086.9 *[321.3]*
    - whooping cough 033.9 *[320.7]*
  - E. coli 320.82
  - ECHO virus 047.1
  - endothelial-leukocytic, benign, recurrent 047.9
  - Enterobacter aerogenes 320.82
  - enteroviral 047.9
    - specified type NEC 047.8
  - enterovirus 047.9
    - specified NEC 047.8
  - eosinophilic 322.1
  - epidemic NEC 036.0
  - Escherichia coli (E. coli) 320.82
  - Eubacterium 320.81
  - fibrinopurulent NEC 320.9
    - specified type NEC 320.89

Meningitis – *continued*
  - Friedländer (bacillus) 320.82
  - fungal NEC 117.9 *[321.1]*
  - Fusobacterium 320.81
  - gonococcal 098.82
  - gram-negative bacteria NEC 320.82
    - anaerobic 320.81
    - cocci 036.0
      - specified NEC 320.82
  - gram-negative cocci NEC 036.0
    - specified NEC 320.82
  - gram-positive cocci NEC 320.9
  - H. influenzae 320.0
  - herpes (simplex) virus 054.72
    - zoster 053.0
  - infectious NEC 320.9
  - influenzal 320.0
  - Klebsiella pneumoniae 320.82
  - late effect - *see* Late, effect, meningitis
  - leptospiral (aseptic) 100.81
  - Listerella (monocytogenes) 027.0 *[320.7]*
  - Listeria monocytogenes 027.0 *[320.7]*
  - lymphocytic (acute) (benign) (serous) 049.0
    - choriomeningitis virus 049.0
  - meningococcal (chronic) 036.0
  - Mima polymorpha 320.82
  - Mollaret's 047.9
  - monilial 112.83
  - mumps (virus) 072.1
  - mycotic NEC 117.9 *[321.1]*
  - Neisseria 036.0
  - neurosyphilis 094.2
  - nonbacterial NEC (*see also* Meningitis, aseptic) 047.9
  - nonpyogenic NEC 322.0
  - oidiomycosis 112.83
  - ossificans 349.2
  - Peptococcus 320.81
  - PeptoStreptococcus 320.81
  - pneumococcal 320.1
  - poliovirus (*see also* Poliomyelitis) 045.2 5th *[321.2]*
  - Proprionibacterium 320.81
  - Proteus morganii 320.82
  - Pseudomonas (aeruginosa) (pyocyaneus) 320.82
  - purulent NEC 320.9
    - specified organism NEC 320.89
  - pyogenic NEC 320.9
    - specified organism NEC 320.89
  - Salmonella 003.21
  - septic NEC 320.9
    - specified organism NEC 320.89
  - serosa circumscripta NEC 322.0
  - serous NEC (*see also* Meningitis, aseptic) 047.9
    - lymphocytic 049.0
    - syndrome 348.2
  - Serratia (marcescens) 320.82
  - specified organism NEC 320.89
  - sporadic cerebrospinal 036.0
  - sporotrichosis 117.1 *[321.1]*
  - staphylococcal 320.3
  - sterile 997.09
  - streptococcal (acute) 320.2
  - suppurative 320.9
    - specified organism NEC 320.89
  - syphilitic 094.2
    - acute 091.81
    - congenital 090.42
    - secondary 091.81
  - torula 117.5 *[321.0]*
  - traumatic (complication of injury) 958.8
  - Treponema (denticola) (macrodenticum) 320.81
  - trypanosomiasis 086.1 *[321.3]*
  - tuberculous (*see also* Tuberculosis, meninges) 013.0 5th
  - typhoid 002.0 *[320.7]*
  - Veillonella 320.81
  - Vibrio vulnificus 320.82
  - viral, virus NEC (*see also* Meningitis, aseptic) 047.9

Meningitis – *continued*
- Wallgren's (*see also* Meningitis, aseptic) 047.9

Meningocele (congenital) (spinal) (*see also* Spina bifida) 741.9 [5th]
- acquired (traumatic) 349.2
- cerebral 742.0
- cranial 742.0

Meningocerebritis - *see* Meningoencephalitis

Meningococcemia (acute) (chronic) 036.2

Meningococcus, meningococcal (*see also* condition) 036.9
- adrenalitis, hemorrhagic 036.3
- carditis 036.40
- carrier (suspected) of V02.59
- cerebrospinal fever 036.0
- encephalitis 036.1
- endocarditis 036.42
- exposure to V01.84
- infection NEC 036.9
- meningitis (cerebrospinal) 036.0
- myocarditis 036.43
- optic neuritis 036.81
- pericarditis 036.41
- septicemia (chronic) 036.2

Meningoencephalitis (*see also* Encephalitis) 323.9
- acute NEC 048
- bacterial, purulent, pyogenic, or septic - *see* Meningitis
- chronic NEC 094.1
- diffuse NEC 094.1
- diphasic 063.2
- due to
  - actinomycosis 039.8 *[320.7]*
  - blastomycosis NEC (*see also* Blastomycosis) 116.0 *[323.41]*
  - free-living amebae 136.29
  - Listeria monocytogenes 027.0 *[320.7]*
  - Lyme disease 088.81 *[320.7]*
  - mumps 072.2
  - Naegleria (amebae) (gruberi) (organisms) 136.29
  - rubella 056.01
  - sporotrichosis 117.1 *[321.1]*
  - toxoplasmosis (acquired) 130.0
    - congenital (active) 771.2 *[323.41]*
  - Trypanosoma 086.1 *[323.2]*
- epidemic 036.0
- herpes 054.3
- herpetic 054.3
- H. influenzae 320.0
- infectious (acute) 048
- influenzal 320.0
- late effect - *see* category 326
- Listeria monocytogenes 027.0 *[320.7]*
- lymphocytic (serous) 049.0
- mumps 072.2
- parasitic NEC 123.9 *[323.41]*
- pneumococcal 320.1
- primary amebic 136.29
- rubella 056.01
- serous 048
  - lymphocytic 049.0
- specific 094.2
- staphylococcal 320.3
- streptococcal 320.2
- syphilitic 094.2
- toxic NEC 989.9 *[323.71]*
  - due to
    - carbon (vapor) tetrachloride 987.8 *[323.71]*
    - hydroxyquinoline derivatives poisoning 961.3 *[323.71]*
    - lead 984.9 *[323.71]*
    - mercury 985.0 *[323.71]*
    - thallium 985.8 *[323.71]*
- toxoplasmosis (acquired) 130.0
- trypanosomic 086.1 *[323.2]*
- tuberculous (*see also* Tuberculosis, meninges) 013.0 [5th]
- virus NEC 048

Meningoencephalocele 742.0
- syphilitic 094.89
  - congenital 090.49

Meningoencephalomyelitis (*see also* Meningoencephalitis) 323.9
- acute NEC 048
  - disseminated (postinfectious) 136.9 *[323.61]*
    - postimmunization or postvaccination 323.51
- due to
  - actinomycosis 039.8 *[320.7]*
  - torula 117.5 *[323.41]*
  - toxoplasma or toxoplasmosis (acquired) 130.0
    - congenital (active) 771.2 *[323.41]*
- late effect - *see* category 326

Meningoencephalomyelopathy (*see also* Meningoencephalomyelitis) 349.9

Meningoencephalopathy (*see also* Meningoencephalitis) 348.39

Meningoencephalopoliomyelitis (*see also* Poliomyelitis, bulbar) 045.0 [5th]
- late effect 138

Meningomyelitis (*see also* Meningoencephalitis) 323.9
- blastomycotic NEC (*see also* Blastomycosis) 116.0 *[323.41]*
- due to
  - actinomycosis 039.8 *[320.7]*
  - blastomycosis (*see also* Blastomycosis) 116.0 *[323.41]*
  - Meningococcus 036.0
  - sporotrichosis 117.1 *[323.41]*
  - torula 117.5 *[323.41]*
- late effect - *see* category 326
- lethargic 049.8
- meningococcal 036.0
- syphilitic 094.2
- tuberculous (*see also* Tuberculosis, meninges) 013.0 [5th]

Meningomyelocele (*see also* Spina bifida) 741.9 [5th]
- syphilitic 094.89

Meningomyeloneuritis - *see* Meningoencephalitis

Meningoradiculitis - *see* Meningitis

Meningovascular - *see* condition

Meniscocytosis 282.60

Menkes' syndrome - *see* Syndrome, Menkes'

Menolipsis 626.0

Menometrorrhagia 626.2

Menopause, menopausal (symptoms) (syndrome) 627.2
- arthritis (any site) NEC 716.3 [5th]
- artificial 627.4
- bleeding 627.0
- crisis 627.2
- depression (*see also* Psychosis, affective) 296.2 [5th]
  - agitated 296.2 [5th]
    - recurrent episode 296.3 [5th]
    - single episode 296.2 [5th]
  - psychotic 296.2 [5th]
    - recurrent episode 296.3 [5th]
    - single episode 296.2 [5th]
  - recurrent episode 296.3 [5th]
  - single episode 296.2 [5th]
- melancholia (*see also* Psychosis, affective) 296.2 [5th]
  - recurrent episode 296.3 [5th]
  - single episode 296.2 [5th]
- paranoid state 297.2
- paraphrenia 297.2
- postsurgical 627.4
- premature 256.31
  - postirradiation 256.2
  - postsurgical 256.2
- psychoneurosis 627.2
- psychosis NEC 298.8
- surgical 627.4
- toxic polyarthritis NEC 716.39

Menorrhagia (primary) 626.2
- climacteric 627.0
- menopausal 627.0
- postclimacteric 627.1
- postmenopausal 627.1
- preclimacteric 627.0
- premenopausal 627.0
- puberty (menses retained) 626.3

Menorrhalgia 625.3

Menoschesis 626.8

Menostaxis 626.2

Menses, retention 626.8

Menstrual - *see also* Menstruation
- cycle, irregular 626.4
- disorders NEC 626.9
- extraction V25.3
- fluid, retained 626.8
- molimen 625.4
- period, normal V65.5
- regulation V25.3

Menstruation
- absent 626.0
- anovulatory 628.0
- delayed 626.8
- difficult 625.3
- disorder 626.9
  - psychogenic 306.52
  - specified NEC 626.8
- during pregnancy 640.8 [5th]
- excessive 626.2
- frequent 626.2
- infrequent 626.1
- irregular 626.4
- latent 626.8
- membranous 626.8
- painful (primary) (secondary) 625.3
  - psychogenic 306.52
- passage of clots 626.2
- precocious 626.8
- protracted 626.8
- retained 626.8
- retrograde 626.8
- scanty 626.1
- suppression 626.8
- vicarious (nasal) 625.8

Mentagra (*see also* Sycosis) 704.8

Mental - *see also* condition
- deficiency (*see also* Retardation, mental) 319
- deterioration (*see also* Psychosis) 298.9
- disorder (*see also* Disorder, mental) 300.9
- exhaustion 300.5
- insufficiency (congenital) (*see also* Retardation, mental) 319
- observation without need for further medical care NEC V71.09
- retardation (*see also* Retardation, mental) 319
- subnormality (*see also* Retardation, mental) 319
  - mild 317
  - moderate 318.0
  - profound 318.2
  - severe 318.1
- upset (*see also* Disorder, mental) 300.9

Meralgia paresthetica 355.1

Mercurial - *see* condition

Mercurialism NEC 985.0

Merergasia 300.9

MERRF syndrome (myoclonus with epilepsy and with ragged red fibers) 277.87

Merkel cell tumor - *see* Carcinoma, Merkel cell ~~Neoplasm, by site, malignant~~ ▲

Merocele (*see also* Hernia, femoral) 553.00

Meromelia 755.4
- lower limb 755.30
  - intercalary 755.32
    - femur 755.34
      - tibiofibular (complete) (incomplete) 755.33
    - fibula 755.37
    - metatarsal(s) 755.38
    - tarsal(s) 755.38
    - tibia 755.36
    - tibiofibular 755.35

Meromelia – *continued*
- lower limb – *continued*
  - terminal (complete) (partial) (transverse) 755.31
    - longitudinal 755.32
      - metatarsal(s) 755.38
      - phalange(s) 755.39
      - tarsal(s) 755.38
  - transverse 755.31
- upper limb 755.20
  - intercalary 755.22
    - carpal(s) 755.28
    - humeral 755.24
      - radioulnar (complete) (incomplete) 755.23
    - metacarpal(s) 755.28
    - phalange(s) 755.29
    - radial 755.26
    - radioulnar 755.25
    - ulnar 755.27
  - terminal (complete) (partial) (transverse) 755.21
    - longitudinal 755.22
      - carpal(s) 755.28
      - metacarpal(s) 755.28
      - phalange(s) 755.29
  - transverse 755.21

Merosmia 781.1

Merycism - *see also* Vomiting
- psychogenic 307.53

Merzbacher-Pelizaeus disease 330.0

Mesaortitis - *see* Aortitis

Mesarteritis - *see* Arteritis

Mesencephalitis (*see also* Encephalitis) 323.9
- late effect - *see* category 326

Mesenchymoma (M8990/1) - *see also* Neoplasm, connective tissue, uncertain behavior
- benign (M8990/0) - *see* Neoplasm, connective tissue, benign
- malignant (M8990/3) - *see* Neoplasm, connective tissue, malignant

Mesenteritis
- retractile 567.82
- sclerosing 567.82

Mesentery, mesenteric - *see* condition

Mesiodens, mesiodentes 520.1
- causing crowding 524.31

Mesio-occlusion 524.23

Mesocardia (with asplenia) 746.87

Mesocolon - *see* condition

Mesonephroma (malignant) (M9110/3) - *see also* Neoplasm, by site, malignant
- benign (M9110/0) - *see* Neoplasm, by site, benign

Mesophlebitis - *see* Phlebitis

Mesostromal dysgenesis 743.51

Mesothelioma (malignant) (M9050/3) - *see also* Neoplasm, by site, malignant
- benign (M9050/0) - *see* Neoplasm, by site, benign
- biphasic type (M9053/3) - *see also* Neoplasm, by site, malignant
  - benign (M9053/0) - *see* Neoplasm, by site, benign
- epithelioid (M9052/3) - *see also* Neoplasm, by site, malignant
  - benign (M9052/0) - *see* Neoplasm, by site, benign
- fibrous (M9051/3) - *see also* Neoplasm, by site, malignant
  - benign (M9051/0) - *see* Neoplasm, by site, benign

Metabolic syndrome 277.7

Metabolism disorder 277.9
- specified type NEC 277.89

Metagonimiasis 121.5

Metagonimus infestation (small intestine) 121.5

Metal
- pigmentation (skin) 709.00
- polishers' disease 502

Metalliferous miners' lung 503

Metamorphopsia 368.14

Metaplasia
- bone, in skin 709.3
- breast 611.89
- cervix - omit code
- endometrium (squamous) 621.8
- esophagus 530.85
- intestinal, of gastric mucosa 537.89
- kidney (pelvis) (squamous) (*see also* Disease, renal) 593.89
- myelogenous 289.89
- myeloid 289.89
  - agnogenic 238.76
  - megakaryocytic 238.76
- spleen 289.59
- squamous cell
  - amnion 658.8 5th
  - bladder 596.8
  - cervix - *see* condition
  - trachea 519.19
  - tracheobronchial tree 519.19
  - uterus 621.8
    - cervix - *see* condition

Metastasis, metastatic
- abscess - *see* Abscess
- calcification 275.40
- cancer, neoplasm, or disease
  - from specified site (M8000/3) - *see* Neoplasm, by site, malignant
  - to specified site (M8000/6) - *see* Neoplasm, by site, secondary
- deposits (in) (M8000/6) - *see* Neoplasm, by site, secondary
- mesentery, of neuroendocrine tumor 209.71 ●
- pneumonia 038.8 *[484.8]*
- spread (to) (M8000/6) - *see* Neoplasm, by site, secondary

Metatarsalgia 726.70
- anterior 355.6
- due to Freiberg's disease 732.5
- Morton's 355.6

Metatarsus, metatarsal - *see also* condition
- abductus valgus (congenital) 754.60
- adductus varus (congenital) 754.53
- primus varus 754.52
- valgus (adductus) (congenital) 754.60
- varus (abductus) (congenital) 754.53
  - primus 754.52

Methadone use 304.00

Methemoglobinemia 289.7
- acquired (with sulfhemoglobinemia) 289.7
- congenital 289.7
- enzymatic 289.7
- Hb-M disease 289.7
- hereditary 289.7
- toxic 289.7

Methemoglobinuria (*see also* Hemoglobinuria) 791.2

Methicillin
- resistant staphylococcus aureus (MRSA) 041.12
  - colonization V02.54
  - personal history of V12.04
- susceptible staphylococcus aureus (MSSA) 041.11
  - colonization V02.53

Methioninemia 270.4

Metritis (catarrhal) (septic) (suppurative) (*see also* Endometritis) 615.9
- blennorrhagic 098.16
  - chronic or duration of 2 months or over 098.36
- cervical (*see also* Cervicitis) 616.0
- gonococcal 098.16
  - chronic or duration of 2 months or over 098.36
- hemorrhagic 626.8
- puerperal, postpartum, childbirth 670.1 5th ▲
  - septic 670.2 5th ●
- tuberculous (*see also* Tuberculosis) 016.7 5th

Metropathia hemorrhagica 626.8

Metroperitonitis (*see also* Peritonitis, pelvic, female) 614.5

Metrorrhagia 626.6
- arising during pregnancy - *see* Hemorrhage, pregnancy
- postpartum NEC 666.2 5th
- primary 626.6
- psychogenic 306.59
- puerperal 666.2 5th

Metrorrhexis - *see* Rupture, uterus

Metrosalpingitis (*see also* Salpingo-oophoritis) 614.2

Metrostaxis 626.6

Metrovaginitis (*see also* Endometritis) 615.9
- gonococcal (acute) 098.16
  - chronic or duration of 2 months or over 098.36

Mexican fever - *see* Typhus, Mexican

Meyenburg-Altherr-Uehlinger syndrome 733.99

Meyer-Schwickerath and Weyers syndrome (dysplasia oculodentodigitalis) 759.89

Meynert's amentia (nonalcoholic) 294.0
- alcoholic 291.1

Mibelli's disease 757.39

Mice, joint (*see also* Loose, body, joint) 718.1 5th
- knee 717.6

Micheli-Rietti syndrome (thalassemia minor) 282.49

Michotte's syndrome 721.5

Micrencephalon, micrencephaly 742.1

Microalbuminuria 791.0

Microaneurysm, retina 362.14
- diabetic 250.5 5th *[362.01]*
  - due to secondary diabetes 249.5 5th *[362.01]*

Microangiopathy 443.9
- diabetic (peripheral) 250.7 5th *[443.81]*
  - due to secondary diabetes 249.7 5th *[443.81]*
  - retinal 250.5 5th *[362.01]*
    - due to secondary diabetes 249.5 5th *[362.01]*
- peripheral 443.9
  - diabetic 250.7 5th *[443.81]*
    - due to secondary diabetes 249.7 5th *[443.81]*
- retinal 362.18
  - diabetic 250.5 5th *[362.01]*
    - due to secondary diabetes 249.5 5th *[362.01]*
- thrombotic 446.6
  - Moschcowitz's (thrombotic thrombocytopenic purpura) 446.6

Microcalcification, mammographic 793.81

Microcephalus, microcephalic, microcephaly 742.1
- due to toxoplasmosis (congenital) 771.2

Microcheilia 744.82

Microcolon (congenital) 751.5

Microcornea (congenital) 743.41

Microcytic - *see* condition

Microdeletions NEC 758.33

Microdontia 520.2

Microdrepanocytosis (thalassemia-Hb-S disease) 282.49

Microembolism
- atherothrombotic - *see* Atheroembolism
- retina 362.33

Microencephalon 742.1

Microfilaria streptocerca infestation 125.3

Microgastria (congenital) 750.7

Microgenia 524.06

Microgenitalia (congenital) 752.89
- penis 752.64

Microglioma (M9710/3)
- specified site - *see* Neoplasm, by site, malignant
- unspecified site 191.9

Microglossia (congenital) 750.16

Micrognathia, micrognathism (congenital) 524.00
- mandibular 524.04
  - alveolar 524.74
- maxillary 524.03
  - alveolar 524.73

Microgyria (congenital) 742.2

Microinfarct, heart (*see also* Insufficiency, coronary) 411.89

Microlithiasis, alveolar, pulmonary 516.2

Micromastia 611.82

Micromyelia (congenital) 742.59

Micropenis 752.64

Microphakia (congenital) 743.36

Microphthalmia (congenital) (*see also* Microphthalmos) 743.10

Microphthalmos (congenital) 743.10
- associated with eye and adnexal anomalies NEC 743.12
- due to toxoplasmosis (congenital) 771.2
- isolated 743.11
- simple 743.11
- syndrome 759.89

Micropsia 368.14

Microsporidiosis 136.8

Microsporon furfur infestation 111.0

Microsporosis (*see also* Dermatophytosis) 110.9
- nigra 111.1

Microstomia (congenital) 744.84

Microthelia 757.6

Microthromboembolism - *see* Embolism

Microtia (congenital) (external ear) 744.23

Microtropia 378.34

Micturition
- disorder NEC 788.69
  - psychogenic 306.53
- frequency 788.41
  - psychogenic 306.53
- nocturnal 788.43
- painful 788.1
  - psychogenic 306.53

Middle
- ear - *see* condition
- lobe (right) syndrome 518.0

Midplane - *see* condition

Miescher's disease 709.3
- cheilitis 351.8
- granulomatosis disciformis 709.3

Miescher-Leder syndrome or granulomatosis 709.3

Mieten's syndrome 759.89

Migraine (idiopathic) 346.9 5th

Note *The following fifth digit subclassification is for use with category 346:*

0 without mention of intractable migraine without mention of status migrainosus

1 with intractable migraine, so stated, without mention of status migrainosus

2 without mention of intractable migraine with status migrainosus

3 with intractable migraine, so stated, with status migrainosus

- with aura (acute-onset) (without headache) (prolonged) (typical) 346.0 5th
- without aura 346.1 5th
  - chronic 346.7 5th
  - transformed 346.7 5th
- abdominal (syndrome) 346.2 5th
- allergic (histamine) 346.2 5th
- atypical 346.8 5th
- basilar 346.0 5th
- chronic without aura 346.7 5th
- classic(al) 346.0 5th
- common 346.1 5th
- hemiplegic 346.3 5th
  - familial 346.3 5th
  - sporadic 346.3 5th
- lower-half 339.00

Migraine – *continued*
- menstrual 346.4 5th
- menstrually related 346.4 5th
- ophthalmic 346.8 5th
- ophthalmoplegic 346.2 5th
- premenstrual 346.4 5th
- pure menstrual 346.4 5th
- retinal 346.0 5th
- specified form NEC 346.8 5th
- transformed without aura 346.7 5th
- variant 346.2 5th

Migrant, social V60.0

Migratory, migrating - *see also* condition
- person V60.0
- testis, congenital 752.52

Mikulicz's disease or syndrome (dryness of mouth, absent or decreased lacrimation) 527.1

Milian atrophia blanche 701.3

Miliaria (crystallina) (rubra) (tropicalis) 705.1
- apocrine 705.82

Miliary - *see* condition

Milium (*see also* Cyst, sebaceous) 706.2
- colloid 709.3
- eyelid 374.84

Milk
- crust 690.11
- excess secretion 676.6 5th
- fever, female 672 5th
- poisoning 988.8
- retention 676.2 5th
- sickness 988.8
- spots 423.1

Milkers' nodes 051.1

Milk-leg (deep vessels) 671.4 5th
- complicating pregnancy 671.3 5th
- nonpuerperal 451.19
- puerperal, postpartum, childbirth 671.4 5th

Milkman (-Looser) disease or syndrome (osteomalacia with pseudofractures) 268.2

Milky urine (*see also* Chyluria) 791.1

Millar's asthma (laryngismus stridulus) 478.75

Millard-Gubler paralysis or syndrome 344.89

Millard-Gubler-Foville paralysis 344.89

Miller-Dieker syndrome 758.33

Miller's disease (osteomalacia) 268.2

Miller Fisher's syndrome 357.0

Milles' syndrome (encephalocutaneous angiomatosis) 759.6

Mills' disease 335.29

Millstone makers' asthma or lung 502

Milroy's disease (chronic hereditary edema) 757.0

Miners' - *see also* condition
- asthma 500
- elbow 727.2
- knee 727.2
- lung 500
- nystagmus 300.89
- phthisis (*see also* Tuberculosis) 011.4 5th
- tuberculosis (*see also* Tuberculosis) 011.4 5th

Minkowski-Chauffard syndrome (*see also* Spherocytosis) 282.0

Minor - *see* condition

Minor's disease 336.1

Minot's disease (hemorrhagic disease, newborn) 776.0

Minot-von Willebrand (-Jürgens) disease or syndrome (angiohemophilia) 286.4

Minus (and plus) **hand** (intrinsic) 736.09

Miosis (persistent) (pupil) 379.42

Mirizzi's syndrome (hepatic duct stenosis) (*see also* Obstruction, biliary) 576.2
- with calculus, cholelithiasis, or stones - *see* Choledocholithiasis

Mirror writing 315.09
- secondary to organic lesion 784.69

Misadventure (prophylactic) (therapeutic) (*see also* Complications) 999.9
- administration of insulin 962.3
- infusion - *see* Complications, infusion
- local applications (of fomentations, plasters, etc.) 999.9
  - burn or scald - *see* Burn, by site
- medical care (early) (late) NEC 999.9
  - adverse effect of drugs or chemicals - *see* Table of Drugs and Chemicals
  - burn or scald - *see* Burn, by site
- radiation NEC 990
- radiotherapy NEC 990
- surgical procedure (early) (late) - *see* Complications, surgical procedure
- transfusion - *see* Complications, transfusion
- vaccination or other immunological procedure - *see* Complications, vaccination

Misanthropy 301.7
Miscarriage - *see* Abortion, spontaneous
Mischief, malicious, child (*see also* Disturbance, conduct) 312.0 5th
Misdirection
- aqueous 365.83

Mismanagement, feeding 783.3
Misplaced, misplacement
- kidney (*see also* Disease, renal) 593.0
  - congenital 753.3
- organ or site, congenital NEC - *see* Malposition, congenital

Missed
- abortion 632
- delivery (at or near term) 656.4 5th
- labor (at or near term) 656.4 5th

Misshapen reconstructed breast 612.0
Missing - *see also* Absence
- teeth (acquired) 525.10
  - congenital (*see also* Anodontia) 520.0
  - due to
    - caries 525.13
    - extraction 525.10
    - periodontal disease 525.12
    - specified NEC 525.19
    - trauma 525.11
- vertebrae (congenital) 756.13

Misuse of drugs NEC (*see also* Abuse, drug, nondependent) 305.9 5th
Mitchell's disease (erythromelalgia) 443.82
Mite(s)
- diarrhea 133.8
- grain (itch) 133.8
- hair follicle (itch) 133.8
- in sputum 133.8

Mitochondrial encephalopathy, lactic acidosis and stroke-like episodes (MELAS syndrome) 277.87
Mitochondrial neurogastrointestinal encephalopathy syndrome (MNGIE) 277.87
Mitral - *see* condition
Mittelschmerz 625.2
Mixed - *see* condition
Mljet disease (mal de Meleda) 757.39
Mobile, mobility
- cecum 751.4
- coccyx 733.99
- excessive - *see* Hypermobility
- gallbladder 751.69
- kidney 593.0
  - congenital 753.3
- organ or site, congenital NEC - *see* Malposition, congenital
- spleen 289.59

Mobitz heart block (atrioventricular) 426.10
- type I (Wenckebach's) 426.13
- type II 426.12

Möbius'
- disease 346.2 5th
- syndrome
  - congenital oculofacial paralysis 352.6
  - ophthalmoplegic migraine 346.2 5th

Moeller (-Barlow) disease (infantile scurvy) 267
- glossitis 529.4

Mohr's syndrome (types I and II) 759.89
Mola destruens (M9100/1) 236.1
Molarization, premolars 520.2
Molar pregnancy 631
- hydatidiform (delivered) (undelivered) 630

Mold(s) in vitreous 117.9
Molding, head (during birth) - omit code
Mole (pigmented) (M8720/0) - *see also* Neoplasm, skin, benign
- blood 631
- Breus' 631
- cancerous (M8720/3) - *see* Melanoma
- carneous 631
- destructive (M9100/1) 236.1
- ectopic - *see* Pregnancy, ectopic
- fleshy 631
- hemorrhagic 631
- hydatid, hydatidiform (benign) (complicating pregnancy) (delivered) (undelivered) (*see also* Hydatidiform mole) 630
  - invasive (M9100/1) 236.1
  - malignant (M9100/1) 236.1
  - previous, affecting management of pregnancy V23.1
- invasive (hydatidiform) (M9100/1) 236.1
- malignant
  - meaning
    - malignant hydatidiform mole (9100/1) 236.1
    - melanoma (M8720/3) - *see* Melanoma
- nonpigmented (M8730/0) - *see* Neoplasm, skin, benign
- pregnancy NEC 631
- skin (M8720/0) - *see* Neoplasm, skin, benign
- tubal - *see* Pregnancy, tubal
- vesicular (*see also* Hydatidiform mole) 630

Molimen, molimina (menstrual) 625.4
Mollaret's meningitis 047.9
Mollities (cerebellar) (cerebral) 437.8
- ossium 268.2

Molluscum
- contagiosum 078.0
- epitheliale 078.0
- fibrosum (M8851/0) - *see* Lipoma, by site
- pendulum (M8851/0) - *see* Lipoma, by site

Mönckeberg's arteriosclerosis, degeneration, disease, or sclerosis (*see also* Arteriosclerosis, extremities) 440.20
Monday fever 504
Monday morning dyspnea or asthma 504
Mondini's malformation (cochlea) 744.05
Mondor's disease (thrombophlebitis of breast) 451.89
Mongolian, mongolianism, mongolism, mongoloid 758.0
- spot 757.33

Monilethrix (congenital) 757.4
Monilia infestation - *see* Candidiasis
Monkeypox 059.01
Moniliasis - *see also* Candidiasis
- neonatal 771.7
- vulvovaginitis 112.1

Monoarthritis 716.60
- ankle 716.67
- arm 716.62
  - lower (and wrist) 716.63
  - upper (and elbow) 716.62
- foot (and ankle) 716.67
- forearm (and wrist) 716.63
- hand 716.64
- leg 716.66
  - lower 716.66
  - upper 716.65
- pelvic region (hip) (thigh) 716.65
- shoulder (region) 716.61
- specified site NEC 716.68

Monoblastic - *see* condition
Monochromatism (cone) (rod) 368.54
Monocytic - *see* condition
Monocytopenia 288.59
Monocytosis (symptomatic) 288.63
Monofixation syndrome 378.34
Monomania (*see also* Psychosis) 298.9
Mononeuritis 355.9
- cranial nerve - *see* Disorder, nerve, cranial
- femoral nerve 355.2
- lateral
  - cutaneous nerve of thigh 355.1
  - popliteal nerve 355.3
- lower limb 355.8
  - specified nerve NEC 355.79
- medial popliteal nerve 355.4
- median nerve 354.1
- multiplex 354.5
- plantar nerve 355.6
- posterior tibial nerve 355.5
- radial nerve 354.3
- sciatic nerve 355.0
- ulnar nerve 354.2
- upper limb 354.9
  - specified nerve NEC 354.8
- vestibular 388.5

Mononeuropathy (*see also* Mononeuritis) 355.9
- diabetic NEC 250.6 5th *[355.9]*
  - due to secondary diabetes 249.6 5th *[355.9]*
  - lower limb 250.6 5th *[355.8]*
    - due to secondary diabetes 249.6 5th *[355.8]*
  - upper limb 250.6 5th *[354.9]*
    - due to secondary diabetes 249.6 5th *[354.9]*
- iliohypogastric nerve 355.79
- ilioinguinal nerve 355.79
- obturator nerve 355.79
- saphenous nerve 355.79

Mononucleosis, infectious 075
- with hepatitis 075 *[573.1]*

Monoplegia 344.5
- brain (current episode) (*see also* Paralysis, brain) 437.8
  - fetus or newborn 767.8
- cerebral (current episode) (*see also* Paralysis, brain) 437.8
- congenital or infantile (cerebral) (spastic) (spinal) 343.3
- embolic (current) (*see also* Embolism, brain) 434.1 5th
  - late effect - *see* Late effect(s) (of) cerebrovascular disease
- infantile (cerebral) (spastic) (spinal) 343.3
- lower limb 344.30
  - affecting
    - dominant side 344.31
    - nondominant side 344.32
  - due to late effect of cerebrovascular accident- *see* Late effect(s) (of) cerebrovascular accident
- newborn 767.8
- psychogenic 306.0
  - specified as conversion reaction 300.11
- thrombotic (current) (*see also* Thrombosis, brain) 434.0 5th
  - late effect - *see* Late effect(s) (of) cerebrovascular disease
- transient 781.4
- upper limb 344.40
  - affecting
    - dominant side 344.41
    - nondominant side 344.42
  - due to late effect of cerebrovascular accident- *see* Late effect(s) (of) cerebrovascular accident

Monorchism, monorchidism 752.89
Monteggia's fracture (closed) 813.03
- open 813.13

Mood swings
- brief compensatory 296.99
- rebound 296.99

Moore's syndrome (*see also* Epilepsy) 345.5 5th
Mooren's ulcer (cornea) 370.07
Mooser-Neill reaction 081.0
Mooser bodies 081.0
Moral
- deficiency 301.7
- imbecility 301.7

Morax-Axenfeld conjunctivitis 372.03
Morbilli (*see also* Measles) 055.9
Morbus
- anglicus, anglorum 268.0
- Beigel 111.2
- caducus (*see also* Epilepsy) 345.9 5th
- caeruleus 746.89
- celiacus 579.0
- comitialis (*see also* Epilepsy) 345.9 5th
- cordis - *see also* Disease, heart
  - valvulorum - *see* Endocarditis
- coxae 719.95
  - tuberculous (*see also* Tuberculosis) 015.1 5th
- hemorrhagicus neonatorum 776.0
- maculosus neonatorum 772.6
- renum 593.0
- senilis (*see also* Osteoarthrosis) 715.9 5th

Morel-Kraepelin disease (*see also* Schizophrenia) 295.9 5th
Morel-Moore syndrome (hyperostosis frontalis interna) 733.3
Morel-Morgagni syndrome (hyperostosis frontalis interna) 733.3
Morgagni
- cyst, organ, hydatid, or appendage 752.89
  - fallopian tube 752.11
- disease or syndrome (hyperostosis frontalis interna) 733.3

Morgagni-Adams-Stokes syndrome (syncope with heart block) 426.9
Morgagni-Stewart-Morel syndrome (hyperostosis frontalis interna) 733.3
Moria (*see also* Psychosis) 298.9
Morning sickness 643.0 5th
Moron 317
Morphea (guttate) (linear) 701.0
Morphine dependence (*see also* Dependence) 304.0 5th
Morphinism (*see also* Dependence) 304.0 5th
Morphinomania (*see also* Dependence) 304.0 5th
Morphoea 701.0
Morquio (-Brailsford) (-Ullrich) disease or syndrome (mucopolysaccharidosis IV) 277.5
- kyphosis 277.5

Morris syndrome (testicular feminization) 259.51
Morsus humanus (open wound) - *see also* Wound, open, by site
- skin surface intact - *see* Contusion

Mortification (dry) (moist) (*see also* Gangrene) 785.4
Morton's
- disease 355.6
- foot 355.6
- metatarsalgia (syndrome) 355.6
- neuralgia 355.6
- neuroma 355.6
- syndrome (metatarsalgia) (neuralgia) 355.6
- toe 355.6

Morvan's disease 336.0
Mosaicism, mosaic (chromosomal) 758.9
- autosomal 758.5
- sex 758.81

Moschcowitz's syndrome (thrombotic thrombocytopenic purpura) 446.6
Mother yaw 102.0
Motion sickness (from travel, any vehicle) (from roundabouts or swings) 994.6
Mottled teeth (enamel) (endemic) (nonendemic) 520.3
Mottling enamel (endemic) (nonendemic) (teeth) 520.3

- **Mouchet's disease** 732.5
- **Mould(s)** (in vitreous) 117.9
- **Moulders'**
  - bronchitis 502
  - tuberculosis (*see also* Tuberculosis) 011.4 5th
- **Mounier-Kuhn syndrome** 748.3
  - with
    - acute exacerbation 494.1
    - bronchiectasis 494.0
      - with (acute) exacerbation 494.1
  - acquired 519.19
    - with bronchiectasis 494.0
      - with (acute) exacerbation 494.1
- **Mountain**
  - fever - *see* Fever, mountain
  - sickness 993.2
    - with polycythemia, acquired 289.0
    - acute 289.0
  - tick fever 066.1
- **Mouse, joint** (*see also* Loose, body, joint) 718.1 5th
  - knee 717.6
- **Mouth** - *see* condition
- **Movable**
  - coccyx 724.71
  - kidney (*see also* Disease, renal) 593.0
    - congenital 753.3
  - organ or site, congenital NEC - *see* Malposition, congenital
  - spleen 289.59
- **Movement**
  - abnormal (dystonic) (involuntary) 781.0
  - decreased fetal 655.7 5th
  - paradoxical facial 374.43
- **Moya Moya disease** 437.5
- **Mozart's ear** 744.29
- **MRSA** (methicillin resistant staphylococcus aureus) 041.12
  - colonization V02.54
  - personal history of V12.04
- **MSSA** (methicillin susceptible staphylococcus aureus) 041.11
  - colonization V02.53
- **Mucha's disease** (acute parapsoriasis varioliformis) 696.2
- **Mucha-Haberman syndrome** (acute parapsoriasis varioliformis) 696.2
- **Mu-chain disease** 273.2
- **Mucinosis** (cutaneous) (papular) 701.8
- **Mucocele**
  - appendix 543.9
  - buccal cavity 528.9
  - gallbladder (*see also* Disease, gallbladder) 575.3
  - lacrimal sac 375.43
  - orbit (eye) 376.81
  - salivary gland (any) 527.6
  - sinus (accessory) (nasal) 478.19
  - turbinate (bone) (middle) (nasal) 478.19
  - uterus 621.8
- **Mucocutaneous lymph node syndrome** (acute) (febrile) (infantile) 446.1
- **Mucoenteritis** 564.9
- **Mucolipidosis I, II, III** 272.7
- **Mucopolysaccharidosis** (types 1-6) 277.5
  - cardiopathy 277.5 *[425.7]*
- **Mucormycosis** (lung) 117.7
- **Mucosa associated lymphoid tissue** (MALT) 200.3 5th
- **Mucositis** - *see also* Inflammation, by site 528.00
  - cervix (ulcerative) 616.81
  - due to
    - antineoplastic therapy (ulcerative) 528.01
    - other drugs (ulcerative) 528.02
    - specified NEC 528.09
  - gastrointestinal (ulcerative) 538
  - nasal (ulcerative) 478.11
  - necroticans agranulocytica (*see also* Agranulocytosis) 288.09
  - ulcerative 528.00
  - vagina (ulcerative) 616.81

- **Mucositis** – *continued*
  - vulva (ulcerative) 616.81
- **Mucous** - *see also* condition
  - patches (syphilitic) 091.3
    - congenital 090.0
- **Mucoviscidosis** 277.00
  - with meconium obstruction 277.01
- **Mucus**
  - asphyxia or suffocation (*see also* Asphyxia, mucus) 933.1
    - newborn 770.18
  - in stool 792.1
  - plug (*see also* Asphyxia, mucus) 933.1
    - aspiration, of newborn 770.17
    - tracheobronchial 519.19
      - newborn 770.18
- **Muguet** 112.0
- **Mulberry molars** 090.5
- **Müllerian mixed tumor** (M8950/3) - *see* Neoplasm, by site, malignant
- **Multicystic kidney** 753.19
- **Multilobed placenta** - *see* Placenta, abnormal
- **Multinodular prostate** 600.10
  - with
    - urinary
      - obstruction 600.11
      - retention 600.11
- **Multiparity** V61.5
  - affecting
    - fetus or newborn 763.89
    - management of
      - labor and delivery 659.4 5th
      - pregnancy V23.3
  - requiring contraceptive management (*see also* Contraception) V25.9
- **Multipartita placenta** - *see* Placenta, abnormal
- **Multiple, multiplex** - *see also* condition
  - birth
    - affecting fetus or newborn 761.5
    - healthy liveborn - *see* Newborn, multiple
  - digits (congenital) 755.00
    - fingers 755.01
    - toes 755.02
  - organ or site NEC - *see* Accessory
  - personality 300.14
  - renal arteries 747.62
- **Mumps** 072.9
  - with complication 072.8
    - specified type NEC 072.79
  - encephalitis 072.2
  - hepatitis 072.71
  - meningitis (aseptic) 072.1
  - meningoencephalitis 072.2
  - oophoritis 072.79
  - orchitis 072.0
  - pancreatitis 072.3
  - polyneuropathy 072.72
  - vaccination, prophylactic (against) V04.6
- **Mumu** (*see also* Infestation, filarial) 125.9
- **Münchausen syndrome** 301.51
- **Münchmeyer's disease or syndrome** (exostosis luxurians) 728.11
- **Mural** - *see* condition
- **Murmur** (cardiac) (heart) (nonorganic) (organic) 785.2
  - abdominal 787.5
  - aortic (valve) (*see also* Endocarditis, aortic) 424.1
  - benign - omit code
  - cardiorespiratory 785.2
  - diastolic - *see* condition
  - Flint (*see also* Endocarditis, aortic) 424.1
  - functional - omit code
  - Graham Steell (pulmonic regurgitation) (*see also* Endocarditis, pulmonary) 424.3
  - innocent - omit code
  - insignificant - omit code
  - midsystolic 785.2
  - mitral (valve) - *see* Stenosis
  - physiologic - *see* condition

- **Murmur** – *continued*
  - presystolic, mitral - *see* Insufficiency, mitral
  - pulmonic (valve) (*see also* Endocarditis, pulmonary) 424.3
  - Still's (vibratory) - omit code
  - systolic (valvular) - *see* condition
  - tricuspid (valve) - *see* Endocarditis, tricuspid
  - undiagnosed 785.2
  - valvular - *see* condition
  - vibratory - omit code
- **Murri's disease** (intermittent hemoglobinuria) 283.2
- **Muscae volitantes** 379.24
- **Muscle, muscular** - *see* condition
- **Musculoneuralgia** 729.1
- **Mushrooming hip** 718.95
- **Mushroom workers'** (pickers') **lung** 495.5
- **Mutation**
  - factor V leiden 289.81
  - prothrombin gene 289.81
- **Mutism** (*see also* Aphasia) 784.3
  - akinetic 784.3
  - deaf (acquired) (congenital) 389.7
  - hysterical 300.11
  - selective (elective) 313.23
    - adjustment reaction 309.83
- **Myà's disease** (congenital dilation, colon) 751.3
- **Myalgia** (intercostal) 729.1
  - eosinophilia syndrome 710.5
  - epidemic 074.1
    - cervical 078.89
  - psychogenic 307.89
  - traumatic NEC 959.9
- **Myasthenia** 358.00
  - cordis - *see* Failure, heart
  - gravis 358.00
    - with exacerbation (acute) 358.01
    - in crisis 358.01
    - neonatal 775.2
    - pseudoparalytica 358.00
  - stomach 536.8
    - psychogenic 306.4
  - syndrome
    - in
      - botulism 005.1 *[358.1]*
      - diabetes mellitus 250.6 5th *[358.1]*
        - due to secondary diabetes 249.6 5th *[358.1]*
      - hypothyroidism (*see also* Hypothyroidism) 244.9 *[358.1]*
      - malignant neoplasm NEC 199.1 *[358.1]*
      - pernicious anemia 281.0 *[358.1]*
      - thyrotoxicosis (*see also* Thyrotoxicosis) 242.9 5th *[358.1]*
- **Myasthenic** 728.87
- **Mycelium infection NEC** 117.9
- **Mycetismus** 988.1
- **Mycetoma** (actinomycotic) 039.9
  - bone 039.8
    - mycotic 117.4
  - foot 039.4
    - mycotic 117.4
  - madurae 039.9
    - mycotic 117.4
  - maduromycotic 039.9
    - mycotic 117.4
  - mycotic 117.4
  - nocardial 039.9
- **Mycobacteriosis** - *see* Mycobacterium
- **Mycobacterium, mycobacterial** (infection) 031.9
  - acid-fast (bacilli) 031.9
  - anonymous (*see also* Mycobacterium, atypical) 031.9
  - atypical (acid-fast bacilli) 031.9
    - cutaneous 031.1

- **Mycobacterium, mycobacterial** – *continued*
  - atypical – *continued*
    - pulmonary 031.0
      - tuberculous (*see also* Tuberculosis, pulmonary) 011.9
    - specified site NEC 031.8
  - avium 031.0
    - intracellulare complex bacteremia (MAC) 031.2
  - balnei 031.1
  - Battey 031.0
  - cutaneous 031.1
  - disseminated 031.2
    - avium-intracellulare complex (DMAC) 031.2
  - fortuitum 031.0
  - intracellulare (battey bacillus) 031.0
  - kakerifu 031.8
  - kansasii 031.0
  - kasongo 031.8
  - leprae - *see* Leprosy
  - luciflavum 031.0
  - marinum 031.1
  - pulmonary 031.0
    - tuberculous (*see also* Tuberculosis, pulmonary) 011.9 5th
  - scrofulaceum 031.1
  - tuberculosis (human, bovine) - *see also* Tuberculosis
    - avian type 031.0
  - ulcerans 031.1
  - xenopi 031.0
- **Mycosis, mycotic** 117.9
  - cutaneous NEC 111.9
  - ear 111.8 *[380.15]*
  - fungoides (M9700/3) 202.1 5th
  - mouth 112.0
  - pharynx 117.9
  - skin NEC 111.9
  - stomatitis 112.0
  - systemic NEC 117.9
  - tonsil 117.9
  - vagina, vaginitis 112.1
- **Mydriasis** (persistent) (pupil) 379.43
- **Myelatelia** 742.59
- **Myelinoclasis, perivascular, acute** (postinfectious) NEC 136.9 *[323.61]*
  - postimmunization or postvaccinal 323.51
- **Myelinosis, central pontine** 341.8
- **Myelitis** (ascending) (cerebellar) (childhood) (chronic) (descending) (diffuse) (disseminated) (pressure) (progressive) (spinal cord) (subacute) (*see also* Encephalitis) 323.9
  - acute (transverse) 341.20
    - idiopathic 341.22
    - in conditions classified elsewhere 341.21
  - due to
    - infection classified elsewhere 136.9 *[323.42]*
    - specified cause NEC 323.82
    - vaccination (any) 323.52
    - viral diseases classified elsewhere 323.02
  - herpes simplex 054.74
  - herpes zoster 053.14
  - late effect - *see* category 326
  - optic neuritis in 341.0
  - postchickenpox 052.2
  - postimmunization 323.52
  - postinfectious 136.9 *[323.63]*
  - postvaccinal 323.52
  - postvaricella 052.2
  - syphilitic (transverse) 094.89
  - toxic 989.9 *[323.72]*
  - transverse 323.82
    - acute 341.20
      - idiopathic 341.22
      - in conditions classified elsewhere 341.21
    - idiopathic 341.22
  - tuberculous (*see also* Tuberculosis) 013.6 5th
  - virus 049.9

Mouchet's disease – Myelitis

Myeloblastic - *see* condition
Myelocele (*see also* Spina bifida) 741.9 5th
- with hydrocephalus 741.0 5th

Myelocystocele (*see also* Spina bifida) 741.9 5th
Myelocytic - *see* condition
Myelocytoma 205.1 5th
Myelodysplasia (spinal cord) 742.59
- meaning myelodysplastic syndrome - *see* Syndrome, myelodysplastic

Myeloencephalitis - *see* Encephalitis
Myelofibrosis 289.83
- with myeloid metaplasia 238.76
- idiopathic (chronic) 238.76
- megakaryocytic 238.79
- primary 238.76
- secondary 289.83

Myelogenous - *see* condition
Myeloid - *see* condition
Myelokathexis 288.09
Myeloleukodystrophy 330.0
Myelolipoma (M8870/0) - *see* Neoplasm, by site, benign
Myeloma (multiple) (plasma cell) (plasmacytic) (M9730/3) 203.0 5th
- monostotic (M9731/1) 238.6
- solitary (M9731/1) 238.6

Myelomalacia 336.8
Myelomata, multiple (M9730/3) 203.0 5th
Myelomatosis (M9730/3) 203.0 5th
Myelomeningitis - *see* Meningoencephalitis
Myelomeningocele (spinal cord) (*see also* Spina bifida) 741.9 5th
- fetal, causing fetopelvic disproportion 653.7 5th

Myelo-osteo-musculodysplasia hereditaria 756.89
Myelopathic - *see* condition
Myelopathy (spinal cord) 336.9
- cervical 721.1
- diabetic 250.6 5th *[336.3]*
  - due to secondary diabetes 249.6 5th *[336.3]*
- drug-induced 336.8
- due to or with
  - carbon tetrachloride 987.8 *[323.72]*
  - degeneration or displacement, intervertebral disc 722.70
    - cervical, cervicothoracic 722.71
    - lumbar, lumbosacral 722.73
    - thoracic, thoracolumbar 722.72
  - hydroxyquinoline derivatives 961.3 *[323.72]*
  - infection - *see* Encephalitis
  - intervertebral disc disorder 722.70
    - cervical, cervicothoracic 722.71
    - lumbar, lumbosacral 722.73
    - thoracic, thoracolumbar 722.72
  - lead 984.9 *[323.72]*
  - mercury 985.0 *[323.72]*
  - neoplastic disease (*see also* Neoplasm, by site) 239.9 *[336.3]*
  - pernicious anemia 281.0 *[336.3]*
  - spondylosis 721.91
    - cervical 721.1
    - lumbar, lumbosacral 721.42
    - thoracic 721.41
  - thallium 985.8 *[323.72]*
- lumbar, lumbosacral 721.42
- necrotic (subacute) 336.1
- radiation-induced 336.8
- spondylogenic NEC 721.91
  - cervical 721.1
  - lumbar, lumbosacral 721.42
  - thoracic 721.41
- thoracic 721.41
- toxic NEC 989.9 *[323.72]*
- transverse (*see also* Myelitis) 323.82
- vascular 336.1

Myelophthisis 284.2
Myeloproliferative disease (M9960/1) 238.79
Myeloradiculitis (*see also* Polyneuropathy) 357.0
Myeloradiculodysplasia (spinal) 742.59
Myelosarcoma (M9930/3) 205.3 5th
Myelosclerosis 289.89
- with myeloid metaplasia (M9961/1) 238.76
- disseminated, of nervous system 340
- megakaryocytic (M9961/1) 238.79

Myelosis (M9860/3) (*see also* Leukemia, myeloid) 205.9 5th
- acute (M9861/3) 205.0 5th
- aleukemic (M9864/3) 205.8 5th
- chronic (M9863/3) 205.1 5th
- erythremic (M9840/3) 207.0 5th
  - acute (M9841/3) 207.0 5th
- megakaryocytic (M9920/3) 207.2 5th
- nonleukemic (chronic) 288.8
- subacute (M9862/3) 205.2 5th

Myesthenia - *see* Myasthenia
Myiasis (cavernous) 134.0
- orbit 134.0 *[376.13]*

Myoadenoma, prostate 600.20
- with
  - other lower urinary tract symptoms (LUTS) 600.21
  - urinary
    - obstruction 600.21
    - retention 600.21

Myoblastoma
- granular cell (M9580/0) - *see also* Neoplasm, connective tissue, benign
  - malignant (M9580/3) - *see* Neoplasm, connective tissue, malignant
- tongue (M9580/0) 210.1

Myocardial - *see* condition
Myocardiopathy (congestive) (constrictive) (familial) (hypertrophic nonobstructive) (idiopathic) (infiltrative) (obstructive) (primary) (restrictive) (sporadic) 425.4
- alcoholic 425.5
- amyloid 277.39 *[425.7]*
- beriberi 265.0 *[425.7]*
- cobalt-beer 425.5
- due to
  - amyloidosis 277.39 *[425.7]*
  - beriberi 265.0 *[425.7]*
  - cardiac glycogenosis 271.0 *[425.7]*
  - Chagas' disease 086.0
  - Friedreich's ataxia 334.0 *[425.8]*
  - influenza 487.8 *[425.8]*
  - mucopolysaccharidosis 277.5 *[425.7]*
  - myotonia atrophica 359.21 *[425.8]*
  - progressive muscular dystrophy 359.1 *[425.8]*
  - sarcoidosis 135 *[425.8]*
- glycogen storage 271.0 *[425.7]*
- hypertrophic obstructive 425.1
- metabolic NEC 277.9 *[425.7]*
- nutritional 269.9 *[425.7]*
- obscure (African) 425.2
- peripartum 674.5 5th
- postpartum 674.5 5th
- secondary 425.9
- thyrotoxic (*see also* Thyrotoxicosis) 242.9 5th *[425.7]*
- toxic NEC 425.9

Myocarditis (fibroid) (interstitial) (old) (progressive) (senile) (with arteriosclerosis) 429.0
- with
  - rheumatic fever (conditions classifiable to 390) 398.0
    - active (*see also* Myocarditis, acute, rheumatic) 391.2
    - inactive or quiescent (with chorea) 398.0
- active (nonrheumatic) 422.90
  - rheumatic 391.2
    - with chorea (acute) (rheumatic) (Sydenham's) 392.0
- acute or subacute (interstitial) 422.90
  - due to Streptococcus (beta-hemolytic) 391.2

Myocarditis – *continued*
- acute or subacute – *continued*
  - idiopathic 422.91
  - rheumatic 391.2
    - with chorea (acute) (rheumatic) (Sydenham's) 392.0
  - specified type NEC 422.99
- aseptic of newborn 074.23
- bacterial (acute) 422.92
- chagasic 086.0
- chronic (interstitial) 429.0
- congenital 746.89
- constrictive 425.4
- Coxsackie (virus) 074.23
- diphtheritic 032.82
- due to or in
  - Coxsackie (virus) 074.23
  - diphtheria 032.82
  - epidemic louse-borne typhus 080 *[422.0]*
  - influenza 487.8 *[422.0]*
  - Lyme disease 088.81 *[422.0]*
  - scarlet fever 034.1 *[422.0]*
  - toxoplasmosis (acquired) 130.3
  - tuberculosis (*see also* Tuberculosis) 017.9 5th *[422.0]*
  - typhoid 002.0 *[422.0]*
  - typhus NEC 081.9 *[422.0]*
- eosinophilic 422.91
- epidemic of newborn 074.23
- Fiedler's (acute) (isolated) (subacute) 422.91
- giant cell (acute) (subacute) 422.91
- gonococcal 098.85
- granulomatous (idiopathic) (isolated) (nonspecific) 422.91
- hypertensive (*see also* Hypertension, heart) 402.90
- idiopathic 422.91
  - granulomatous 422.91
- infective 422.92
- influenzal 487.8 *[422.0]*
- isolated (diffuse) (granulomatous) 422.91
- malignant 422.99
- meningococcal 036.43
- nonrheumatic, active 422.90
- parenchymatous 422.90
- pneumococcal (acute) (subacute) 422.92
- rheumatic (chronic) (inactive) (with chorea) 398.0
  - active or acute 391.2
    - with chorea (acute) (rheumatic) (Sydenham's) 392.0
- septic 422.92
- specific (giant cell) (productive) 422.91
- staphylococcal (acute) (subacute) 422.92
- suppurative 422.92
- syphilitic (chronic) 093.82
- toxic 422.93
  - rheumatic (*see also* Myocarditis, acute rheumatic) 391.2
- tuberculous (*see also* Tuberculosis) 017.9 5th *[422.0]*
- typhoid 002.0 *[422.0]*
- valvular - *see* Endocarditis
- viral, except Coxsackie 422.91
  - Coxsackie 074.23
  - of newborn (Coxsackie) 074.23

Myocardium, myocardial - *see* condition
Myocardosis (*see also* Cardiomyopathy) 425.4
Myoclonia (essential) 333.2
- epileptica 345.1 ▲
- Friedreich's 333.2
- massive 333.2

Myoclonic
- epilepsy, familial (progressive) 345.1 ▲
- jerks 333.2

Myoclonus (familial essential) (multifocal) (simplex) 333.2
- with epilepsy and with ragged red fibers (MERRF syndrome) 277.87
- facial 351.8
- massive (infantile) 333.2

Myoclonus – *continued*
- palatal 333.2 ●
- pharyngeal 333.2 ▲

Myocytolysis 429.1 ●
Myodiastasis 728.84
Myoendocarditis - *see also* Endocarditis
- acute or subacute 421.9

Myoepithelioma (M8982/0) - *see* Neoplasm, by site, benign
Myofascitis (acute) 729.1
- low back 724.2

Myofibroma (M8890/0) - *see also* Neoplasm, connective tissue, benign
- uterus (cervix) (corpus) (*see also* Leiomyoma) 218.9

Myofibromatosis
- infantile 759.89

Myofibrosis 728.2
- heart (*see also* Myocarditis) 429.0
- humeroscapular region 726.2
- scapulohumeral 726.2

Myofibrositis (*see also* Myositis) 729.1
- scapulohumeral 726.2

Myogelosis (occupational) 728.89
Myoglobinuria 791.3
Myoglobulinuria, primary 791.3
Myokymia - *see also* Myoclonus
- facial 351.8

Myolipoma (M8860/0)
- specified site - *see* Neoplasm, connective tissue, benign
- unspecified site 223.0

Myoma (M8895/0) - *see also* Neoplasm, connective tissue, benign
- cervix (stump) (uterus) (*see also* Leiomyoma) 218.9
- malignant (M8895/3) - *see* Neoplasm, connective tissue, malignant
- prostate 600.20
  - with
    - other lower urinary tract symptoms (LUTS) 600.21
    - urinary
      - obstruction 600.21
      - retention 600.21
- uterus (cervix) (corpus) (*see also* Leiomyoma) 218.9
  - in pregnancy or childbirth 654.1 5th
    - affecting fetus or newborn 763.89
    - causing obstructed labor 660.2 5th
      - affecting fetus or newborn 763.1

Myomalacia 728.9
- cordis, heart (*see also* Degeneration, myocardial) 429.1

Myometritis (*see also* Endometritis) 615.9
Myometrium - *see* condition
Myonecrosis, clostridial 040.0
Myopathy 359.9
- alcoholic 359.4
- amyloid 277.39 *[359.6]*
- benign, congenital 359.0
- central core 359.0
- centronuclear 359.0
- congenital (benign) 359.0
- critical illness 359.81
- distal 359.1
- due to drugs 359.4
- endocrine 259.9 *[359.5]*
  - specified type NEC 259.8 *[359.5]*
- extraocular muscles 376.82
- facioscapulohumeral 359.1
- in
  - Addison's disease 255.41 *[359.5]*
  - amyloidosis 277.39 *[359.6]*
  - cretinism 243 *[359.5]*
  - Cushing's syndrome 255.0 *[359.5]*
  - disseminated lupus erythematosus 710.0 *[359.6]*
  - giant cell arteritis 446.5 *[359.6]*
  - hyperadrenocorticism NEC 255.3 *[359.5]*
  - hyperparathyroidism 252.01 *[359.5]*
  - hypopituitarism 253.2 *[359.5]*

- **Myopathy** – *continued*
  - in – *continued*
    - hypothyroidism (*see also* Hypothyroidism) 244.9 *[359.5]*
    - malignant neoplasm NEC (M8000/3) 199.1 *[359.6]*
    - myxedema (*see also* Myxedema) 244.9 *[359.5]*
    - polyarteritis nodosa 446.0 *[359.6]*
    - rheumatoid arthritis 714.0 *[359.6]*
    - sarcoidosis 135 *[359.6]*
    - scleroderma 710.1 *[359.6]*
    - Sjögren's disease 710.2 *[359.6]*
    - thyrotoxicosis (*see also* Thyrotoxicosis) 242.9 5th *[359.5]*
  - inflammatory 359.79 ▲
    - immune NEC 359.79 ●
    - specified NEC 359.79 ●
  - intensive care (ICU) 359.81
  - limb-girdle 359.1
  - myotubular 359.0
  - nemaline 359.0
  - necrotizing, acute 359.81
  - ocular 359.1
  - oculopharyngeal 359.1
  - of critical illness 359.81
  - primary 359.89
  - progressive NEC 359.89
  - proximal myotonic (PROMM) 359.21
  - quadriplegic, acute 359.81
  - rod body 359.0
  - scapulohumeral 359.1
  - specified type NEC 359.89
  - toxic 359.4
- **Myopericarditis** (*see also* Pericarditis) 423.9
- **Myopia** (axial) (congenital) (increased curvature or refraction, nucleus of lens) 367.1
  - degenerative, malignant 360.21
  - malignant 360.21
  - progressive high (degenerative) 360.21
- **Myosarcoma** (M8895/3) - *see* Neoplasm, connective tissue, malignant
- **Myosis** (persistent) 379.42
  - stromal (endolymphatic) (M8931/1) 236.0
- **Myositis** 729.1
  - clostridial 040.0
  - due to posture 729.1
  - epidemic 074.1
  - fibrosa or fibrous (chronic) 728.2
    - Volkmann's (complicating trauma) 958.6
  - inclusion body (IBM) 359.71 ●
  - infective 728.0
  - interstitial 728.81
  - multiple - *see* Polymyositis
  - occupational 729.1
  - orbital, chronic 376.12
  - ossificans 728.12
    - circumscribed 728.12
    - progressive 728.11
    - traumatic 728.12
  - progressive fibrosing 728.11
  - purulent 728.0
  - rheumatic 729.1
  - rheumatoid 729.1
  - suppurative 728.0
  - syphilitic 095.6
  - traumatic (old) 729.1
- **Myospasia impulsiva** 307.23
- **Myotonia** (acquisita) (intermittens) 728.85
  - atrophica 359.21
  - congenita 359.22
    - acetazolamide responsive 359.22
    - dominant form 359.22
    - recessive form 359.22
  - drug-induced 359.24
  - dystrophica 359.21
  - fluctuans 359.29
  - levior 359.22 ▲
  - permanens 359.29
- **Myotonic pupil** 379.46
- **Myriapodiasis** 134.1
- **Myringitis**
  - with otitis media - *see* Otitis media
  - acute 384.00
    - specified type NEC 384.09
  - bullosa hemorrhagica 384.01
  - bullous 384.01
  - chronic 384.1
- **Mysophobia** 300.29
- **Mytilotoxism** 988.0
- **Myxadenitis labialis** 528.5
- **Myxedema** (adult) (idiocy) (infantile) (juvenile) (thyroid gland) (*see also* Hypothyroidism) 244.9
  - circumscribed 242.9 5th
  - congenital 243
  - cutis 701.8
  - localized (pretibial) 242.9 5th
  - madness (acute) 293.0
    - subacute 293.1
  - papular 701.8
  - pituitary 244.8
  - postpartum 674.8 5th
  - pretibial 242.9 5th
  - primary 244.9
- **Myxochondrosarcoma** (M9220/3) - *see* Neoplasm, cartilage, malignant
- **Myxofibroma** (M8811/0) - *see also* Neoplasm, connective tissue, benign
  - odontogenic (M9320/0) 213.1
    - upper jaw (bone) 213.0
- **Myxofibrosarcoma** (M8811/3) - *see* Neoplasm, connective tissue, malignant
- **Myxolipoma** (M8852/0) (*see also* Lipoma, by site) 214.9
- **Myxoliposarcoma** (M8852/3) - *see* Neoplasm, connective tissue, malignant
- **Myxoma** (M8840/0) - *see also* Neoplasm, connective tissue, benign
  - odontogenic (M9320/0) 213.1
    - upper jaw (bone) 213.0
- **Myxosarcoma** (M8840/3) - *see* Neoplasm, connective tissue, malignant

N

- **Naegeli's**
  - disease (hereditary hemorrhagic thrombasthenia 287.1
  - leukemia, monocytic (M9863/3) 205.1 5th
  - syndrome (incontinentia pigmenti) 757.33
- **Naffziger's syndrome** 353.0
- **Naga sore** (*see also* Ulcer, skin) 707.9
- **Nägele's pelvis** 738.6
  - with disproportion (fetopelvic) 653.0 5th
    - affecting fetus or newborn 763.1
    - causing obstructed labor 660.1 5th
      - affecting fetus or newborn 763.1
- **Nager-de Reynier syndrome** (dysostosis mandibularis) 756.0
- **Nail** - *see also* condition
  - biting 307.9
  - patella syndrome (hereditary osteoonychodysplasia) 756.89
- **Nanism, nanosomia** (*see also* Dwarfism) 259.4
  - hypophyseal 253.3
  - pituitary 253.3
  - renis, renalis 588.0
- **Nanukayami** 100.89
- **Napkin rash** 691.0
- **Narcissism** 301.81
- **Narcolepsy** 347.00
  - with cataplexy 347.01
  - in conditions classified elsewhere 347.10
    - with cataplexy 347.11
- **Narcosis**
  - carbon dioxide (respiratory) 786.09
  - due to drug
    - correct substance properly administered 780.09
- **Narcosis** – *continued*
  - due to drug – *continued*
    - overdose or wrong substance given or taken 977.9
      - specified drug - *see* Table of Drugs and Chemicals
- **Narcotism** (chronic) (*see also* Dependence) 304.9 5th
  - acute
    - correct substance properly administered 349.82
    - overdose or wrong substance given or taken 967.8
      - specified drug - *see* Table of Drugs and Chemicals
- **NARP** (ataxia and retinitis pigmentosa syndrome) 277.87
- **Narrow**
  - anterior chamber angle 365.02
  - pelvis (inlet) (outlet) - *see* Contraction, pelvis
- **Narrowing**
  - artery NEC 447.1
    - auditory, internal 433.8 5th
    - basilar 433.0 5th
      - with other precerebral artery 433.3 5th
      - bilateral 433.3 5th
    - carotid 433.1 5th
      - with other precerebral artery 433.3 5th
      - bilateral 433.3 5th
    - cerebellar 433.8 5th
    - choroidal 433.8 5th
    - communicating posterior 433.8 5th
    - coronary - *see also* Arteriosclerosis, coronary
      - congenital 746.85
        - due to syphilis 090.5
    - hypophyseal 433.8 5th
    - pontine 433.8 5th
    - precerebral NEC 433.9 5th
      - multiple or bilateral 433.3 5th
      - specified NEC 433.8 5th
    - vertebral 433.2 5th
      - with other precerebral artery 433.3 5th
      - bilateral 433.3 5th
  - auditory canal (external) (*see also* Stricture, ear canal, acquired) 380.50
  - cerebral arteries 437.0
  - cicatricial - *see* Cicatrix
  - congenital - *see* Anomaly, congenital
  - coronary artery - *see* Narrowing, artery, coronary
  - ear, middle 385.22
  - Eustachian tube (*see also* Obstruction, Eustachian tube) 381.60
  - eyelid 374.46
    - congenital 743.62
  - intervertebral disc or space NEC - *see* Degeneration, intervertebral disc
  - joint space, hip 719.85
  - larynx 478.74
  - lids 374.46
    - congenital 743.62
  - mesenteric artery (with gangrene) 557.0
  - palate 524.89
  - palpebral fissure 374.46
  - retinal artery 362.13
  - ureter 593.3
  - urethra (*see also* Stricture, urethra) 598.9
- **Narrowness, abnormal, eyelid** 743.62
- **Nasal** - *see* condition
- **Nasolacrimal** - *see* condition
- **Nasopharyngeal** - *see also* condition
  - bursa 478.29
  - pituitary gland 759.2
  - torticollis 723.5
- **Nasopharyngitis** (acute) (infective) (subacute) 460
  - chronic 472.2
    - due to external agent - *see* Condition, respiratory, chronic, due to
  - due to external agent - *see* Condition, respiratory, due to
  - septic 034.0
  - streptococcal 034.0
  - suppurative (chronic) 472.2
  - ulcerative (chronic) 472.2
- **Nasopharynx, nasopharyngeal** - *see* condition
- **Natal tooth, teeth** 520.6
- **Nausea** (*see also* Vomiting) 787.02
  - with vomiting 787.01
  - epidemic 078.82
  - gravidarum - *see* Hyperemesis, gravidarum
  - marina 994.6
- **Naval** - *see* condition
- **Neapolitan fever** (*see also* Brucellosis) 023.9
- **Near drowning** 994.1
- **Near-syncope** 780.2
- **Nearsightedness** 367.1
- **Nebécourt's syndrome** 253.3
- **Nebula, cornea (eye)** 371.01
  - congenital 743.43
    - interfering with vision 743.42
- **Necator americanus infestation** 126.1
- **Necatoriasis** 126.1
- **Neck** - *see* condition
- **Necrencephalus** (*see also* Softening, brain) 437.8
- **Necrobacillosis** 040.3
- **Necrobiosis** 799.89
  - brain or cerebral (*see also* Softening, brain) 437.8
  - lipoidica 709.3
    - diabeticorum 250.8 5th *[709.3]*
      - due to secondary diabetes 249.8 5th *[709.3]*
- **Necrodermolysis** 695.15
- **Necrolysis, toxic epidermal** 695.15
  - due to drug
    - correct substance properly administered 695.15
    - overdose or wrong substance given or taken 977.9
      - specified drug - *see* Table of Drugs and Chemicals
  - Stevens-Johnson syndrome overlap (SJS-TEN overlap syndrome) 695.14
- **Necrophilia** 302.89
- **Necrosis, necrotic**
  - adrenal (capsule) (gland) 255.8
  - antrum, nasal sinus 478.19
  - aorta (hyaline) (*see also* Aneurysm, aorta) 441.9
    - cystic medial 441.00
      - abdominal 441.02
      - thoracic 441.01
      - thoracoabdominal 441.03
    - ruptured 441.5
  - arteritis 446.0
  - artery 447.5
  - aseptic, bone 733.40
    - femur (head) (neck) 733.42
      - medial condyle 733.43
    - humoral head 733.41
    - jaw 733.45
    - medial femoral condyle 733.43
    - specific site NEC 733.49
    - talus 733.44
  - avascular, bone NEC (*see also* Necrosis, aseptic, bone) 733.40
  - bladder (aseptic) (sphincter) 596.8
  - bone (*see also* Osteomyelitis) 730.1 5th
    - acute 730.0 5th
    - aseptic or avascular 733.40
      - femur (head) (neck) 733.42
        - medial condyle 733.43
      - humoral head 733.41
      - jaw 733.45

- **Necrosis, necrotic** – *continued*
  - bone – *continued*
    - aseptic or avascular – *continued*
      - medial femoral condyle 733.43
      - specified site NEC 733.49
      - talus 733.44
    - ethmoid 478.19
    - ischemic 733.40
    - jaw 526.4
      - aseptic 733.45
    - marrow 289.89
    - Paget's (osteitis deformans) 731.0
    - tuberculous - *see* Tuberculosis, bone
  - brain (softening) (*see also* Softening, brain) 437.8
  - breast (aseptic) (fat) (segmental) 611.3
  - bronchus, bronchi 519.19
  - central nervous system NEC (*see also* Softening, brain) 437.8
  - cerebellar (*see also* Softening, brain) 437.8
  - cerebral (softening) (*see also* Softening, brain) 437.8
  - cerebrospinal (softening) (*see also* Softening, brain) 437.8
  - colon 557.0
  - cornea (*see also* Keratitis) 371.40
  - cortical, kidney 583.6
  - cystic medial (aorta) 441.00
    - abdominal 441.02
    - thoracic 441.01
    - thoracoabdominal 441.03
  - dental 521.09
    - pulp 522.1
  - due to swallowing corrosive substance - *see* Burn, by site
  - ear (ossicle) 385.24
  - esophagus 530.89
  - ethmoid (bone) 478.19
  - eyelid 374.50
  - fat, fatty (generalized) (*see also* Degeneration, fatty) 272.8
    - abdominal wall 567.82
    - breast (aseptic) (segmental) 611.3
    - intestine 569.89
    - localized - *see* Degeneration, by site, fatty
    - mesentery 567.82
    - omentum 567.82
    - pancreas 577.8
    - peritoneum 567.82
    - skin (subcutaneous) 709.3
      - newborn 778.1
  - femur (aseptic) (avascular) 733.42
    - head 733.42
    - medial condyle 733.43
    - neck 733.42
  - gallbladder (*see also* Cholecystitis, acute) 575.0
  - gangrenous 785.4
  - gastric 537.89
  - glottis 478.79
  - heart (myocardium) - *see* Infarct, myocardium
  - hepatic (*see also* Necrosis, liver) 570

- **Necrosis, necrotic** – *continued*
  - hip (aseptic) (avascular) 733.42
  - intestine (acute) (hemorrhagic) (massive) 557.0
  - ischemic 785.4
  - jaw 526.4
    - aseptic 733.45
  - kidney (bilateral) 583.9
    - acute 584.9
    - cortical 583.6
      - acute 584.6
        - with
          - abortion - *see* Abortion, by type, with renal failure
          - ectopic pregnancy (*see also* categories 633.0-633.9) 639.3
          - molar pregnancy (*see also* categories 630-632) 639.3
        - complicating pregnancy 646.2 [5th]
          - affecting fetus or newborn 760.1
        - following labor and delivery 669.3 [5th]
    - medullary (papillary) (*see also* Pyelitis) 590.80
      - in
        - acute renal failure 584.7
        - nephritis, nephropathy 583.7
    - papillary (*see also* Pyelitis) 590.80
      - in
        - acute renal failure 584.7
        - nephritis, nephropathy 583.7
    - tubular 584.5
      - with
        - abortion - *see* Abortion, by type, with renal failure
        - ectopic pregnancy (*see also* categories 633.0-633.9) 639.3
        - molar pregnancy (*see also* categories 630-632) 639.3
      - complicating
        - abortion 639.3
        - ectopic or molar pregnancy 639.3
        - pregnancy 646.2 [5th]
          - affecting fetus or newborn 760.1
      - following labor and delivery 669.3 [5th]
      - traumatic 958.5
  - larynx 478.79
  - liver (acute) (congenital) (diffuse) (massive) (subacute) 570
    - with
      - abortion - *see* Abortion, by type, with specified complication NEC
      - ectopic pregnancy (*see also* categories 633.0-633.9) 639.8

- **Necrosis, necrotic** – *continued*
  - liver – *continued*
    - with – *continued*
      - molar pregnancy (*see also* categories 630-632) 639.8
    - complicating pregnancy 646.7 [5th]
      - affecting fetus or newborn 760.8
    - following
      - abortion 639.8
      - ectopic or molar pregnancy 639.8
    - obstetrical 646.7 [5th]
    - postabortal 639.8
    - puerperal, postpartum 674.8 [5th]
    - toxic 573.3
  - lung 513.0
  - lymphatic gland 683
  - mammary gland 611.3
  - mastoid (chronic) 383.1
  - mesentery 557.0
    - fat 567.82
  - mitral valve - *see* Insufficiency, mitral
  - myocardium, myocardial - *see* Infarct, myocardium
  - nose (septum) 478.19
  - omentum 557.0
    - with mesenteric infarction 557.0
    - fat 567.82
  - orbit, orbital 376.10
  - ossicles, ear (aseptic) 385.24
  - ovary (*see also* Salpingo-oophoritis) 614.2
  - pancreas (aseptic) (duct) (fat) 577.8
    - acute 577.0
    - infective 577.0
  - papillary, kidney (*see also* Pyelitis) 590.80
  - perineum 624.8
  - peritoneum 557.0
    - with mesenteric infarction 557.0
    - fat 567.82
  - pharynx 462
    - in granulocytopenia 288.09
  - phosphorus 983.9
  - pituitary (gland) (postpartum) (Sheehan) 253.2
  - placenta (*see also* Placenta, abnormal) 656.7 [5th]
  - pneumonia 513.0
  - pulmonary 513.0
  - pulp (dental) 522.1
  - pylorus 537.89
  - radiation - *see* Necrosis, by site
  - radium - *see* Necrosis, by site
  - renal - *see* Necrosis, kidney
  - sclera 379.19
  - scrotum 608.89
  - skin or subcutaneous tissue 709.8
    - due to burn-*see* Burn, by site
    - gangrenous 785.4
  - spine, spinal (column) 730.18
    - acute 730.18
    - cord 336.1.
  - spleen 289.59
  - stomach 537.89
  - stomatitis 528.1
  - subcutaneous fat 709.3
    - fetus or newborn 778.1

- **Necrosis, necrotic** – *continued*
  - subendocardial - *see* Infarct, myocardium
  - suprarenal (capsule) (gland) 255.8
  - teeth, tooth 521.09
  - testis 608.89
  - thymus (gland) 254.8
  - tonsil 474.8
  - trachea 519.19
  - tuberculous NEC - *see* Tuberculosis
  - tubular (acute) (anoxic) (toxic) 584.5
    - due to a procedure 997.5
  - umbilical cord, affecting fetus or newborn 762.6
  - vagina 623.8
  - vertebra (lumbar) 730.18
    - acute 730.18
    - tuberculous (*see also* Tuberculosis) 015.0 [5th] *[730.8]* [5th]
  - vesical (aseptic) (bladder) 596.8
  - vulva 624.8
  - x-ray - *see* Necrosis, by site
- **Necrospermia** 606.0
- **Necrotizing angiitis** 446.0
- **Negativism** 301.7
- **Neglect** (child) (newborn) NEC 995.52
  - adult 995.84
  - after or at birth 995.52
  - hemispatial 781.8
  - left-sided 781.8
  - sensory 781.8
  - visuospatial 781.8
- **Negri bodies** 071
  - Neill-Dingwall syndrome (microcephaly and dwarfism) 759.89
- **Neisserian infection** NEC - *see* Gonococcus
- **Nematodiasis** NEC (*see also* Infestation, Nematode) 127.9
  - ancylostoma (*see also* Ancylostomiasis) 126.9
- **Neoformans cryptococcus infection** 117.5
- **Neonatal** - *see also* condition
  - abstinence syndrome 779.5 ●
  - adrenoleukodystrophy 277.86
  - teeth, tooth 520.6
- **Neonatorum** - *see* condition
- **Neoplasia**
  - anal intraepithelial I [AIN I] (histologically confirmed) 569.44
  - anal intraepithelial II [AIN II] (histologically confirmed) 569.44
  - anal intraepithelial III [AIN III] 230.6
    - anal canal 230.5
  - endometrial intraepithelial [EIN] 621.35 ●
  - multiple endocrine [MEN]
    - type I 258.01
    - type IIA 258.02
    - type IIB 258.03
  - vaginal intraepithelial I [VAIN I] 623.0
  - vaginal intraepithelial II [VAIN II] 623.0
  - vaginal intraepithelial III [VAIN III] 233.31
  - vulvar intraepithelial I [VIN I] 624.01
  - vulvar intraepithelial II [VIN II] 624.02
  - vulvar intraepithelial III [VIN III] 233.32

Necrosis, necrotic – Neoplasia

Neoplasm, neoplastic, abdomen, abdominal – Neoplasm, neoplastic, bone

Neoplasm, neoplastic	Malignant					
	Primary	Secondary	Carcinoma in situ	Benign	Uncertain Behavior	Unspecified
Neoplasm, neoplastic	199.1	199.1	234.9	229.9	238.9	239.9

Notes 1. *The list below gives the code numbers for neoplasms by anatomical site. For each site there are six possible code numbers according to whether the neoplasm in question is malignant, benign, in situ, of uncertain behavior, or of unspecified nature. The description of the neoplasm will often indicate which of the six columns is appropriate; e.g., malignant melanoma of skin, benign fibroadenoma of breast, carcinoma in situ of cervix uteri.*

Where such descriptors are not present, the remainder of the Index should be consulted where guidance is given to the appropriate column for each morphological (histological) variety listed; e.g., Mesonephroma – see Neoplasm, malignant; Embryoma – see also Neoplasm, uncertain behavior; Disease, Bowen's – see Neoplasm, skin, in situ. However, the guidance in the Index can be overridden if one of the descriptors mentioned above is present; e.g., malignant adenoma of colon is coded to 153.9 and not to 211.3 as the adjective "malignant" overrides the Index entry "Adenoma – see also Neoplasm, benign."

2. *Sites marked with the sign * (e.g., face NEC*) should be classified to malignant neoplasm of skin of these sites if the variety of neoplasm is a squamous cell carcinoma or an epidermoid carcinoma and to benign neoplasm of skin of these sites if the variety of neoplasm is a papilloma (any type).*

Site	Primary	Secondary	Carcinoma in situ	Benign	Uncertain Behavior	Unspecified
abdomen, abdominal	195.2	198.89	234.8	229.8	238.8	239.89▲
cavity	195.2	198.89	234.8	229.8	238.8	239.89▲
organ	195.2	198.89	234.8	229.8	238.8	239.89▲
viscera	195.2	198.89	234.8	229.8	238.8	239.89▲
wall	173.5	198.2	232.5	216.5	238.2	239.2
connective tissue	171.5	198.89	–	215.5	238.1	239.2
abdominopelvic	195.8	198.89	234.8	229.8	238.8	239.89▲
accessory sinus – *see* Neoplasm, sinus						
acoustic nerve	192.0	198.4	–	225.1	237.9	239.7
acromion (process)	170.4	198.5	–	213.4	238.0	239.2
adenoid (pharynx) (tissue)	147.1	198.89	230.0	210.7	235.1	239.0
adipose tissue (*see also* Neoplasm, connective tissue)	171.9	198.89	–	215.9	238.1	239.2
adnexa (uterine)	183.9	198.82	233.39	221.8	236.3	239.5
adrenal (cortex) (gland) (medulla)	194.0	198.7	234.8	227.0	237.2	239.7
ala nasi (external)	173.3	198.2	232.3	216.3	238.2	239.2
alimentary canal or tract NEC	159.9	197.8	230.9	211.9	235.5	239.0
alveolar	143.9	198.89	230.0	210.4	235.1	239.0
mucosa	143.9	198.89	230.0	210.4	235.1	239.0
lower	143.1	198.89	230.0	210.4	235.1	239.0
upper	143.0	198.89	230.0	210.4	235.1	239.0
ridge or process	170.1	198.5	–	213.1	238.0	239.2
carcinoma	143.9	–	–	–	–	–
lower	143.1	–	–		–	–
upper	143.0	–	–	–	–	–
lower	170.1	198.5	–	213.1	238.0	239.2
mucosa	143.9	198.89	230.0	210.4	235.1	239.0
lower	143.1	198.89	230.0	210.4	235.1	239.0
upper	143.0	198.89	230.0	210.4	235.1	239.0
upper	170.0	198.5	–	213.0	238.0	239.2
sulcus	145.1	198.89	230.0	210.4	235.1	239.0
alveolus	143.9	198.89	230.0	210.4	235.1	239.0
lower	143.1	198.89	230.0	210.4	235.1	239.0
upper	143.0	198.89	230.0	210.4	235.1	239.0
ampulla of Vater	156.2	197.8	230.8	211.5	235.3	239.0
ankle NEC*	195.5	198.89	232.7	229.8	238.8	239.89▲
anorectum, anorectal (junction)	154.8	197.5	230.7	211.4	235.2	239.0
antecubital fossa or space*	195.4	198.89	232.6	229.8	238.8	239.89▲
antrum (Highmore) (maxillary)	160.2	197.3	231.8	212.0	235.9	239.1
pyloric	151.2	197.8	230.2	211.1	235.2	239.0
tympanicum	160.1	197.3	231.8	212.0	235.9	239.1
anus, anal	154.3	197.5	230.6	211.4	235.5	239.0
canal	154.2	197.5	230.5	211.4	235.5	239.0
contiguous sites with rectosigmoid junction or rectum	154.8	–	–	–	–	–
margin	173.5	198.2	232.5	216.5	238.2	239.2
skin	173.5	198.2	232.5	216.5	238.2	239.2
sphincter	154.2	197.5	230.5	211.4	235.5	239.0
aorta (thoracic)	171.4	198.89	–	215.4	238.1	239.2
abdominal	171.5	198.89	–	215.5	238.1	239.2
aortic body	194.6	198.89	–	227.6	237.3	239.7
aponeurosis	171.9	198.89	–	215.9	238.1	239.2
palmar	171.2	198.89	–	215.2	238.1	239.2
plantar	171.3	198.89	–	215.3	238.1	239.2
appendix	153.5	197.5	230.3	211.3	235.2	239.0
arachnoid (cerebral)	192.1	198.4	–	225.2	237.6	239.7
spinal	192.3	198.4	–	225.4	237.6	239.7
areola (female)	174.0	198.81	233.0	217	238.3	239.3
male	175.0	198.81	233.0	217	238.3	239.3
arm NEC*	195.4	198.89	232.6	229.8	238.8	239.89▲
artery – *see* Neoplasm, connective tissue						
aryepiglottic fold	148.2	198.89	230.0	210.8	235.1	239.0
hypopharyngeal aspect	148.2	198.89	230.0	210.8	235.1	239.0
laryngeal aspect	161.1	197.3	231.0	212.1	235.6	239.1
marginal zone	148.2	198.89	230.0	210.8	235.1	239.0
arytenoid (cartilage)	161.3	197.3	231.0	212.1	235.6	239.1
fold – *see* Neoplasm, aryepiglottic						
associated with transplanted organ	199.2	–	–	–	–	–
atlas	170.2	198.5	–	213.2	238.0	239.2
atrium, cardiac	164.1	198.89	–	212.7	238.8	239.89▲
auditory						
canal (external) (skin)	173.2	198.2	232.2	216.2	238.2	239.2
internal	160.1	197.3	231.8	212.0	235.9	239.1
nerve	192.0	198.4	–	225.1	237.9	239.7
tube	160.1	197.3	231.8	212.0	235.9	239.1
opening	147.2	198.89	230.0	210.7	235.1	239.0
auricle, ear	173.2	198.2	232.2	216.2	238.2	239.2
cartilage	171.0	198.89	–	215.0	238.1	239.2
auricular canal (external)	173.2	198.2	232.2	216.2	238.2	239.2
internal	160.1	197.3	231.8	212.0	235.9	239.1
autonomic nerve or nervous system NEC	171.9	198.89	–	215.9	238.1	239.2
axilla, axillary	195.1	198.89	234.8	229.8	238.8	239.89▲
fold	173.5	198.2	232.5	216.5	238.2	239.2
back NEC*	195.8	198.89	232.5	229.8	238.8	239.89▲
Bartholin's gland	184.1	198.82	233.32	221.2	236.3	239.5
basal ganglia	191.0	198.3	–	225.0	237.5	239.6
basis pedunculi	191.7	198.3	–	225.0	237.5	239.6
bile or biliary (tract)	156.9	197.8	230.8	211.5	235.3	239.0
canaliculi (biliferi) (intrahepatic)	155.1	197.8	230.8	211.5	235.3	239.0
canals, interlobular	155.1	197.8	230.8	211.5	235.3	239.0
contiguous sites	156.8	–	–	–	–	–
duct or passage (common) (cystic) (extrahepatic)	156.1	197.8	230.8	211.5	235.3	239.0
contiguous sites with gallbladder	156.8	–	–	–	–	–
interlobular	155.1	197.8	230.8	211.5	235.3	239.0
intrahepatic	155.1	197.8	230.8	211.5	235.3	239.0
and extrahepatic	156.9	197.8	230.8	211.5	235.3	239.0
bladder (urinary)	188.9	198.1	233.7	223.3	236.7	239.4
contiguous sites	188.8	–	–	–	–	–
dome	188.1	198.1	233.7	223.3	236.7	239.4
neck	188.5	198.1	233.7	223.3	236.7	239.4
orifice	188.9	198.1	233.7	223.3	236.7	239.4
ureteric	188.6	198.1	233.7	223.3	236.7	239.4
urethral	188.5	198.1	233.7	223.3	236.7	239.4
sphincter	188.8	198.1	233.7	223.3	236.7	239.4
trigone	188.0	198.1	233.7	223.3	236.7	239.4
urachus	188.7	–	233.7	223.3	236.7	239.4
wall	188.9	198.1	233.7	223.3	236.7	239.4
anterior	188.3	198.1	233.7	223.3	236.7	239.4
lateral	188.2	198.1	233.7	223.3	236.7	239.4
posterior	188.4	198.1	233.7	223.3	236.7	239.4
blood vessel – *see* Neoplasm, connective tissue						

Note *Carcinomas and adenocarcinomas, of any type other than intraosseous or odontogenic, of the sites listed under "Neoplasm, bone" should be considered as constituting metastatic spread from an unspecified primary site and coded to 198.5 for morbidity coding.*

Site	Primary	Secondary	Carcinoma in situ	Benign	Uncertain Behavior	Unspecified
bone (periosteum)	170.9	198.5	–	213.9	238.0	239.2
acetabulum	170.6	198.5	–	213.6	238.0	239.2
acromion (process)	170.4	198.5	–	213.4	238.0	239.2
ankle	170.8	198.5	–	213.8	238.0	239.2
arm NEC	170.4	198.5	–	213.4	238.0	239.2
astragalus	170.8	198.5	–	213.8	238.0	239.2
atlas	170.2	198.5	–	213.2	238.0	239.2
axis	170.2	198.5	–	213.2	238.0	239.2
back NEC	170.2	198.5	–	213.2	238.0	239.2
calcaneus	170.8	198.5	–	213.8	238.0	239.2
calvarium	170.0	198.5	–	213.0	238.0	239.2
carpus (any)	170.5	198.5	–	213.5	238.0	239.2
cartilage NEC	170.9	198.5	–	213.9	238.0	239.2
clavicle	170.3	198.5	–	213.3	238.0	239.2
clivus	170.0	198.5	–	213.0	238.0	239.2

Neoplasm, neoplastic	Malignant					
	Primary	Secondary	Carcinoma in situ	Benign	Uncertain Behavior	Unspecifed
bone (periosteum) – *continued*						
coccygeal vertebra	170.6	198.5	–	213.6	238.0	239.2
coccyx	170.6	198.5	–	213.6	238.0	239.2
costal cartilage	170.3	198.5	–	213.3	238.0	239.2
costovertebral joint	170.3	198.5	–	213.3	238.0	239.2
cranial	170.0	198.5	–	213.0	238.0	239.2
cuboid	170.8	198.5	–	213.8	238.0	239.2
cuneiform	170.9	198.5	–	213.9	238.0	239.2
ankle	170.8	198.5	–	213.8	238.0	239.2
wrist	170.5	198.5	–	213.5	238.0	239.2
digital	170.9	198.5	–	213.9	238.0	239.2
finger	170.5	198.5	–	213.5	238.0	239.2
toe	170.8	198.5	–	213.8	238.0	239.2
elbow	170.4	198.5	–	213.4	238.0	239.2
ethmoid (labyrinth)	170.0	198.5	–	213.0	238.0	239.2
face	170.0	198.5	–	213.0	238.0	239.2
lower jaw	170.1	198.5	–	213.1	238.0	239.2
femur (any part)	170.7	198.5	–	213.7	238.0	239.2
fibula (any part)	170.7	198.5	–	213.7	238.0	239.2
finger (any)	170.5	198.5	–	213.5	238.0	239.2
foot	170.8	198.5	–	213.8	238.0	239.2
forearm	170.4	198.5	–	213.4	238.0	239.2
frontal	170.0	198.5	–	213.0	238.0	239.2
hand	170.5	198.5	–	213.5	238.0	239.2
heel	170.8	198.5	–	213.8	238.0	239.2
hip	170.6	198.5	–	213.6	238.0	239.2
humerus (any part)	170.4	198.5	–	213.4	238.0	239.2
hyoid	170.0	198.5	–	213.0	238.0	239.2
ilium	170.6	198.5	–	213.6	238.0	239.2
innominate	170.6	198.5	–	213.6	238.0	239.2
intervertebral cartilage or disc	170.2	198.5	–	213.2	238.0	239.2
ischium	170.6	198.5	–	213.6	238.0	239.2
jaw (lower)	170.1	198.5	–	213.1	238.0	239.2
upper	170.0	198.5	–	213.0	238.0	239.2
knee	170.7	198.5	–	213.7	238.0	239.2
leg NEC	170.7	198.5	–	213.7	238.0	239.2
limb NEC	170.9	198.5	–	213.9	238.0	239.2
lower (long bones)	170.7	198.5	–	213.7	238.0	239.2
short bones	170.8	198.5	–	213.8	238.0	239.2
upper (long bones)	170.4	198.5	–	213.4	238.0	239.2
short bones	170.5	198.5	–	213.5	238.0	239.2
long	170.9	198.5	–	213.9	238.0	239.2
lower limbs NEC	170.7	198.5	–	213.7	238.0	239.2
upper limbs NEC	170.4	198.5	–	213.4	238.0	239.2
malar	170.0	198.5	–	213.0	238.0	239.2
mandible	170.1	198.5	–	213.1	238.0	239.2
marrow NEC	202.9 5th	198.5	–	–	–	238.79
mastoid	170.0	198.5	–	213.0	238.0	239.2
maxilla, maxillary (superior)	170.0	198.5	–	213.0	238.0	239.2
inferior	170.1	198.5	–	213.1	238.0	239.2
metacarpus (any)	170.5	198.5	–	213.5	238.0	239.2
metatarsus (any)	170.8	198.5	–	213.8	238.0	239.2
navicular (ankle)	170.8	198.5	–	213.8	238.0	239.2
hand	170.5	198.5	–	213.5	238.0	239.2
nose, nasal	170.0	198.5	–	213.0	238.0	239.2
occipital	170.0	198.5	–	213.0	238.0	239.2
orbit	170.0	198.5	–	213.0	238.0	239.2
parietal	170.0	198.5	–	213.0	238.0	239.2
patella	170.8	198.5	–	213.8	238.0	239.2
pelvic	170.6	198.5	–	213.6	238.0	239.2
phalanges	170.9	198.5	–	213.9	238.0	239.2
foot	170.8	198.5	–	213.8	238.0	239.2
hand	170.5	198.5	–	213.5	238.0	239.2
pubic	170.6	198.5	–	213.6	238.0	239.2
radius (any part)	170.4	198.5	–	213.4	238.0	239.2
rib	170.3	198.5	–	213.3	238.0	239.2
sacral vertebra	170.6	198.5	–	213.6	238.0	239.2
sacrum	170.6	198.5	–	213.6	238.0	239.2
scaphoid (of hand)	170.5	198.5	–	213.5	238.0	239.2
of ankle	170.8	198.5	–	213.8	238.0	239.2
scapula (any part)	170.4	198.5	–	213.4	238.0	239.2
sella turcica	170.0	198.5	–	213.0	238.0	239.2
short	170.9	198.5	–	213.9	238.0	239.2
lower limb	170.8	198.5	–	213.8	238.0	239.2
upper limb	170.5	198.5	–	213.5	238.0	239.2
shoulder	170.4	198.5	–	213.4	238.0	239.2
skeleton, skeletal NEC	170.9	198.5	–	213.9	238.0	239.2
skull	170.0	198.5	–	213.0	238.0	239.2
sphenoid	170.0	198.5	–	213.0	238.0	239.2

Neoplasm, neoplastic	Malignant					
	Primary	Secondary	Carcinoma in situ	Benign	Uncertain Behavior	Unspecifed
bone – *continued*						
spine, spinal (column)	170.2	198.5	–	213.2	238.0	239.2
coccyx	170.6	198.5	–	213.6	238.0	239.2
sacrum	170.6	198.5	–	213.6	238.0	239.2
sternum	170.3	198.5	–	213.3	238.0	239.2
tarsus (any)	170.8	198.5	–	213.8	238.0	239.2
temporal	170.0	198.5	–	213.0	238.0	239.2
thumb	170.5	198.5	–	213.5	238.0	239.2
tibia (any part)	170.7	198.5	–	213.7	238.0	239.2
toe (any)	170.8	198.5	–	213.8	238.0	239.2
trapezium	170.5	198.5	–	213.5	238.0	239.2
trapezoid	170.5	198.5	–	213.5	238.0	239.2
turbinate	170.0	198.5	–	213.0	238.0	239.2
ulna (any part)	170.4	198.5	–	213.4	238.0	239.2
unciform	170.5	198.5	–	213.5	238.0	239.2
vertebra (column)	170.2	198.5	–	213.2	238.0	239.2
coccyx	170.6	198.5	–	213.6	238.0	239.2
sacrum	170.6	198.5	–	213.6	238.0	239.2
vomer	170.0	198.5	–	213.0	238.0	239.2
wrist	170.5	198.5	–	213.5	238.0	239.2
xiphoid process	170.3	198.5	–	213.3	238.0	239.2
zygomatic	170.0	198.5	–	213.0	238.0	239.2
book-leaf (mouth)	145.8	198.89	230.0	210.4	235.1	239.0
bowel – *see* Neoplasm, intestine						
brachial plexus	171.2	198.89	–	215.2	238.1	239.2
brain NEC	191.9	198.3	–	225.0	237.5	239.6
basal ganglia	191.0	198.3	–	225.0	237.5	239.6
cerebellopontine angle	191.6	198.3	–	225.0	237.5	239.6
cerebellum NOS	191.6	198.3	–	225.0	237.5	239.6
cerebrum	191.0	198.3	–	225.0	237.5	239.6
choroid plexus	191.5	198.3	–	225.0	237.5	239.6
contiguous sites	191.8	–	–	–	–	–
corpus callosum	191.8	198.3	–	225.0	237.5	239.6
corpus striatum	191.0	198.3	–	225.0	237.5	239.6
cortex (cerebral)	191.0	198.3	–	225.0	237.5	239.6
frontal lobe	191.1	198.3	–	225.0	237.5	239.6
globus pallidus	191.0	198.3	–	225.0	237.5	239.6
hippocampus	191.2	198.3	–	225.0	237.5	239.6
hypothalamus	191.0	198.3	–	225.0	237.5	239.6
internal capsule	191.0	198.3	–	225.0	237.5	239.6
medulla oblongata	191.7	198.3	–	225.0	237.5	239.6
meninges	192.1	198.4	–	225.2	237.6	239.7
midbrain	191.7	198.3	–	225.0	237.5	239.6
occipital lobe	191.4	198.3	–	225.0	237.5	239.6
parietal lobe	191.3	198.3	–	225.0	237.5	239.6
peduncle	191.7	198.3	–	225.0	237.5	239.6
pons	191.7	198.3	–	225.0	237.5	239.6
stem	191.7	198.3	–	225.0	237.5	239.6
tapetum	191.8	198.3	–	225.0	237.5	239.6
temporal lobe	191.2	198.3	–	225.0	237.5	239.6
thalamus	191.0	198.3	–	225.0	237.5	239.6
uncus	191.2	198.3	–	225.0	237.5	239.6
ventricle (floor)	191.5	198.3	–	225.0	237.5	239.6
branchial (cleft) (vestiges)	146.8	198.89	230.0	210.6	235.1	239.0
breast (connective tissue) (female) (glandular tissue) (soft parts)	174.9	198.81	233.0	217	238.3	239.3
areola	174.0	198.81	233.0	217	238.3	239.3
male	175.0	198.81	233.0	217	238.3	239.3
axillary tail	174.6	198.81	233.0	217	238.3	239.3
central portion	174.1	198.81	233.0	217	238.3	239.3
contiguous sites	174.8	–	–	–	–	–
ectopic sites	174.8	198.81	233.0	217	238.3	239.3
inner	174.8	198.81	233.0	217	238.3	239.3
lower	174.8	198.81	233.0	217	238.3	239.3
lower-inner quadrant	174.3	198.81	233.0	217	238.3	239.3
lower-outer quadrant	174.5	198.81	233.0	217	238.3	239.3
male	175.9	198.81	233.0	217	238.3	239.3
areola	175.0	198.81	233.0	217	238.3	239.3
ectopic tissue	175.9	198.81	233.0	217	238.3	239.3
nipple	175.0	198.81	233.0	217	238.3	239.3
mastectomy site (skin)	173.5	198.2	–	–	–	–
specified as breast tissue	174.8	198.81	–	–	–	–
midline	174.8	198.81	233.0	217	238.3	239.3
nipple	174.0	198.81	233.0	217	238.3	239.3
male	175.0	198.81	233.0	217	238.3	239.3
outer	174.8	198.81	233.0	217	238.3	239.3
skin	173.5	198.2	232.5	216.5	238.2	239.2
tail (axillary)	174.6	198.81	233.0	217	238.3	239.3
upper	174.8	198.81	233.0	217	238.3	239.3
upper-inner quadrant	174.2	198.81	233.0	217	238.3	239.3

Neoplasm, neoplastic	Malignant: Primary	Malignant: Secondary	Malignant: Carcinoma in situ	Benign	Uncertain Behavior	Unspecifed
breast – *continued*						
upper-outer quadrant	174.4	198.81	233.0	217	238.3	239.3
broad ligament	183.3	198.82	233.39	221.0	236.3	239.5
bronchiogenic, bronchogenic (lung)	162.9	197.0	231.2	212.3	235.7	239.1
bronchiole	162.9	197.0	231.2	212.3	235.7	239.1
bronchus	162.9	197.0	231.2	212.3	235.7	239.1
carina	162.2	197.0	231.2	212.3	235.7	239.1
contiguous sites with lung or trachea	162.8	–	–	–	–	–
lower lobe of lung	162.5	197.0	231.2	212.3	235.7	239.1
main	162.2	197.0	231.2	212.3	235.7	239.1
middle lobe of lung	162.4	197.0	231.2	212.3	235.7	239.1
upper lobe of lung	162.3	197.0	231.2	212.3	235.7	239.1
brow	173.3	198.2	232.3	216.3	238.2	239.2
buccal (cavity)	145.9	198.89	230.0	210.4	235.1	239.0
commissure	145.0	198.89	230.0	210.4	235.1	239.0
groove (lower) (upper)	145.1	198.89	230.0	210.4	235.1	239.0
mucosa	145.0	198.89	230.0	210.4	235.1	239.0
sulcus (lower) (upper)	145.1	198.89	230.0	210.4	235.1	239.0
bulbourethral gland	189.3	198.1	233.9	223.81	236.99	239.5
bursa – *see* Neoplasm, connective tissue						
buttock NEC*	195.3	198.89	232.5	229.8	238.8	239.89▲
calf*	195.5	198.89	232.7	229.8	238.8	239.89▲
calvarium	170.0	198.5	–	213.0	238.0	239.2
calyx, renal	189.1	198.0	233.9	223.1	236.91	239.5
canal						
anal	154.2	197.5	230.5	211.4	235.5	239.0
auditory (external)	173.2	198.2	232.2	216.2	238.2	239.2
auricular (external)	173.2	198.2	232.2	216.2	238.2	239.2
canaliculi, biliary (biliferi) (intrahepatic)	155.1	197.8	230.8	211.5	235.3	239.0
canthus (eye) (inner) (outer)	173.1	198.2	232.1	216.1	238.2	239.2
capillary – *see* Neoplasm, connective tissue						
caput coli	153.4	197.5	230.3	211.3	235.2	239.0
cardia (gastric)	151.0	197.8	230.2	211.1	235.2	239.0
cardiac orifice (stomach)	151.0	197.8	230.2	211.1	235.2	239.0
cardio-esophageal junction	151.0	197.8	230.2	211.1	235.2	239.0
cardio-esophagus	151.0	197.8	230.2	211.1	235.2	239.0
carina (bronchus)	162.2	197.0	231.2	212.3	235.7	239.1
carotid (artery)	171.0	198.89	–	215.0	238.1	239.2
body	194.5	198.89	–	227.5	237.3	239.7
carpus (any bone)	170.5	198.5	–	213.5	238.0	239.2
cartilage (articular) (joint) NEC – *see also* Neoplasm, bone	170.9	198.5	–	213.9	238.0	239.2
arytenoid	161.3	197.3	231.0	212.1	235.6	239.1
auricular	171.0	198.89	–	215.0	238.1	239.2
bronchi	162.2	197.3	–	212.3	235.7	239.1
connective tissue – *see* Neoplasm, connective tissue						
costal	170.3	198.5	–	213.3	238.0	239.2
cricoid	161.3	197.3	231.0	212.1	235.6	239.1
cuneiform	161.3	197.3	231.0	212.1	235.6	239.1
ear (external)	171.0	198.89	–	215.0	238.1	239.2
ensiform	170.3	198.5	–	213.3	238.0	239.2
epiglottis	161.1	197.3	231.0	212.1	235.6	239.1
anterior surface	146.4	198.89	230.0	210.6	235.1	239.0
eyelid	171.0	198.89	–	215.0	238.1	239.2
intervertebral	170.2	198.5	–	213.2	238.0	239.2
larynx, laryngeal	161.3	197.3	231.0	212.1	235.6	239.1
nose, nasal	160.0	197.3	231.8	212.0	235.9	239.1
pinna	171.0	198.89	–	215.0	238.1	239.2
rib	170.3	198.5	–	213.3	238.0	239.2
semilunar (knee)	170.7	198.5	–	213.7	238.0	239.2
thyroid	161.3	197.3	231.0	212.1	235.6	239.1
trachea	162.0	197.3	231.1	212.2	235.7	239.1
cauda equina	192.2	198.3	–	225.3	237.5	239.7
cavity						
buccal	145.9	198.89	230.0	210.4	235.1	239.0
nasal	160.0	197.3	231.8	212.0	235.9	239.1
oral	145.9	198.89	230.0	210.4	235.1	239.0
peritoneal	158.9	197.6	–	211.8	235.4	239.0
tympanic	160.1	197.3	231.8	212.0	235.9	239.1
cecum	153.4	197.5	230.3	211.3	235.2	239.0
central						
nervous system – *see* Neoplasm, nervous system						
white matter	191.0	198.3	–	225.0	237.5	239.6
cerebellopontine (angle)	191.6	198.3	–	225.0	237.5	239.6
cerebellum, cerebellar	191.6	198.3	–	225.0	237.5	239.6
cerebrum, cerebral (cortex) (hemisphere) (white matter)	191.0	198.3	–	225.0	237.5	239.6
meninges	192.1	198.4	–	225.2	237.6	239.7
peduncle	191.7	198.3	–	225.0	237.5	239.6
ventricle (any)	191.5	198.3	–	225.0	237.5	239.6
cervical region	195.0	198.89	234.8	229.8	238.8	239.89▲
cervix (cervical) (uteri) (uterus)	180.9	198.82	233.1	219.0	236.0	239.5
canal	180.0	198.82	233.1	219.0	236.0	239.5
contiguous sites	180.8	–	–	–	–	–
endocervix (canal) (gland)	180.0	198.82	233.1	219.0	236.0	239.5
exocervix	180.1	198.82	233.1	219.0	236.0	239.5
external os	180.1	198.82	233.1	219.0	236.0	239.5
internal os	180.0	198.82	233.1	219.0	236.0	239.5
nabothian gland	180.0	198.82	233.1	219.0	236.0	239.5
squamocolumnar junction	180.8	198.82	233.1	219.0	236.0	239.5
stump	180.8	198.82	233.1	219.0	236.0	239.5
cheek	195.0	198.89	234.8	229.8	238.8	239.8
external	173.3	198.2	232.3	216.3	238.2	239.2
inner aspect	145.0	198.89	230.0	210.4	235.1	239.0
internal	145.0	198.89	230.0	210.4	235.1	239.0
mucosa	145.0	198.89	230.0	210.4	235.1	239.0
chest (wall) NEC	195.1	198.89	234.8	229.8	238.8	239.89▲
chiasma opticum	192.0	198.4	–	225.1	237.9	239.7
chin	173.3	198.2	232.3	216.3	238.2	239.2
choana	147.3	198.89	230.0	210.7	235.1	239.0
cholangiole	155.1	197.8	230.8	211.5	235.3	239.0
choledochal duct	156.1	197.8	230.8	211.5	235.3	239.0
choroid	190.6	198.4	234.0	224.6	238.8	239.81▲
plexus	191.5	198.3	–	225.0	237.5	239.6
ciliary body	190.0	198.4	234.0	224.0	238.8	239.89▲
clavicle	170.3	198.5	–	213.3	238.0	239.2
clitoris	184.3	198.82	233.32	221.2	236.3	239.5
clivus	170.0	198.5	–	213.0	238.0	239.2
cloacogenic zone	154.8	197.5	230.7	211.4	235.5	239.0
coccygeal						
body or glomus	194.6	198.89	–	227.6	237.3	239.7
vertebra	170.6	198.5	–	213.6	238.0	239.2
coccyx	170.6	198.5	–	213.6	238.0	239.2
colon – *see also* Neoplasm, intestine, large and rectum	154.0	197.5	230.4	211.4	235.2	239.0
column, spinal – *see* Neoplasm, spine						
columnella	173.3	198.2	232.3	216.3	238.2	239.2
commissure						
labial, lip	140.6	198.89	230.0	210.4	235.1	239.0
laryngeal	161.0	197.3	231.0	212.1	235.6	239.1
common (bile) duct	156.1	197.8	230.8	211.5	235.3	239.0
concha	173.2	198.2	232.2	216.2	238.2	239.2
nose	160.0	197.3	231.8	212.0	235.9	239.1
conjunctiva	190.3	198.4	234.0	224.3	238.8	239.89▲

Note *For neoplasms of connective tissue (blood vessel, bursa, fascia, ligament, muscle, peripheral nerves, sympathetic and parasympathetic nerves and ganglia, synovia, tendon, etc.) or of morphological types that indicate connective tissue, code according to the list under "Neoplasm, connective tissue;" for sites that do not appear in this list, code to neoplasm of that site; e.g.,*

liposarcoma, shoulder 171.2
leiomyosarcoma, stomach 151.9
neurofibroma, chest wall 215.4

Morphological types that indicate connective tissue appear in their proper place in the alphabetic index with the instruction "see Neoplasm, connective tissue ...."

Neoplasm, neoplastic	Malignant: Primary	Malignant: Secondary	Malignant: Carcinoma in situ	Benign	Uncertain Behavior	Unspecifed
connective tissue NEC	171.9	198.89	–	215.9	238.1	239.2
abdomen	171.5	198.89	–	215.5	238.1	239.2
abdominal wall	171.5	198.89	–	215.5	238.1	239.2
ankle	171.3	198.89	–	215.3	238.1	239.2
antecubital fossa or space	171.2	198.89	–	215.2	238.1	239.2
arm	171.2	198.89	–	215.2	238.1	239.2
auricle (ear)	171.0	198.89	–	215.0	238.1	239.2
axilla	171.4	198.89	–	215.4	238.1	239.2
back	171.7	198.89	–	215.7	238.1	239.2
breast (female) (*see also* Neoplasm, breast)	174.9	198.81	233.0	217	238.3	239.3
male	175.9	198.81	233.0	217	238.3	239.3
buttock	171.6	198.89	–	215.6	238.1	239.2
calf	171.3	198.89	–	215.3	238.1	239.2
cervical region	171.0	198.89	–	215.0	238.1	239.2
cheek	171.0	198.89	–	215.0	238.1	239.2

Neoplasm, neoplastic	Malignant					
	Primary	Secondary	Carcinoma in situ	Benign	Uncertain Behavior	Unspecified
connective tissue – *continued*						
chest (wall)	171.4	198.89	–	215.4	238.1	239.2
chin	171.0	198.89	–	215.0	238.1	239.2
contiguous sites	171.8	–	–	–	–	–
diaphragm	171.4	198.89	–	215.4	238.1	239.2
ear (external)	171.0	198.89	–	215.0	238.1	239.2
elbow	171.2	198.89	–	215.2	238.1	239.2
extrarectal	171.6	198.89	–	215.6	238.1	239.2
extremity	171.8	198.89	–	215.8	238.1	239.2
lower	171.3	198.89	–	215.3	238.1	239.2
upper	171.2	198.89	–	215.2	238.1	239.2
eyelid	171.0	198.89	–	215.0	238.1	239.2
face	171.0	198.89	–	215.0	238.1	239.2
finger	171.2	198.89	–	215.2	238.1	239.2
flank	171.7	198.89	–	215.7	238.1	239.2
foot	171.3	198.89	–	215.3	238.1	239.2
forearm	171.2	198.89	–	215.2	238.1	239.2
forehead	171.0	198.89	–	215.0	238.1	239.2
gastric	171.5	198.89	–	215.5	238.1	–
gastrointestinal	171.5	198.89	–	215.5	238.1	–
gluteal region	171.6	198.89	–	215.6	238.1	239.2
great vessels NEC	171.4	198.89	–	215.4	238.1	239.2
groin	171.6	198.89	–	215.6	238.1	239.2
hand	171.2	198.89	–	215.2	238.1	239.2
head	171.0	198.89	–	215.0	238.1	239.2
heel	171.3	198.89	–	215.3	238.1	239.2
hip	171.3	198.89	–	215.3	238.1	239.2
hypochondrium	171.5	198.89	–	215.5	238.1	239.2
iliopsoas muscle	171.6	198.89	–	215.5	238.1	239.2
infraclavicular region	171.4	198.89	–	215.4	238.1	239.2
inguinal (canal) (region)	171.6	198.89	–	215.6	238.1	239.2
intestine	171.5	198.89	–	215.5	238.1	–
intrathoracic	171.4	198.89	–	215.4	238.1	239.2
ischorectal fossa	171.6	198.89	–	215.6	238.1	239.2
jaw	143.9	198.89	230.0	210.4	235.1	239.0
knee	171.3	198.89	–	215.3	238.1	239.2
leg	171.3	198.89	–	215.3	238.1	239.2
limb NEC	171.9	198.89	–	215.8	238.1	239.2
lower	171.3	198.89	–	215.3	238.1	239.2
upper	171.2	198.89	–	215.2	238.1	239.2
nates	171.6	198.89	–	215.6	238.1	239.2
neck	171.0	198.89	–	215.0	238.1	239.2
orbit	190.1	198.4	234.0	224.1	238.8	239.89▲
pararectal	171.6	198.89	–	215.6	238.1	239.2
para-urethral	171.6	198.89	–	215.6	238.1	239.2
paravaginal	171.6	198.89	–	215.6	238.1	239.2
pelvis (floor)	171.6	198.89	–	215.6	238.1	239.2
pelvo-abdominal	171.8	198.89	–	215.8	238.1	239.2
perineum	171.6	198.89	–	215.6	238.1	239.2
perirectal (tissue)	171.6	198.89	–	215.6	238.1	239.2
periurethral (tissue)	171.6	198.89	–	215.6	238.1	239.2
popliteal fossa or space	171.3	198.89	–	215.3	238.1	239.2
presacral	171.6	198.89	–	215.6	238.1	239.2
psoas muscle	171.5	198.89	–	215.5	238.1	239.2
pterygoid fossa	171.0	198.89	–	215.0	238.1	239.2
rectovaginal septum or wall	171.6	198.89	–	215.6	238.1	239.2
rectovesical	171.6	198.89	–	215.6	238.1	239.2
retroperitoneum	158.0	197.6	–	211.8	235.4	239.0
sacrococcygeal region	171.6	198.89	–	215.6	238.1	239.2
scalp	171.0	198.89	–	215.0	238.1	239.2
scapular region	171.4	198.89	–	215.4	238.1	239.2
shoulder	171.2	198.89	–	215.2	238.1	239.2
skin (dermis) NEC	173.9	198.2	232.9	216.9	238.2	239.2
stomach	171.5	198.89	–	215.5	238.1	–
submental	171.0	198.89	–	215.0	238.1	239.2
supraclavicular region	171.0	198.89	–	215.0	238.1	239.2
temple	171.0	198.89	–	215.0	238.1	239.2
temporal region	171.0	198.89	–	215.0	238.1	239.2
thigh	171.3	198.89	–	215.3	238.1	239.2
thoracic (duct) (wall)	171.4	198.89	–	215.4	238.1	239.2
thorax	171.4	198.89	–	215.4	238.1	239.2
thumb	171.2	198.89	–	215.2	238.1	239.2
toe	171.3	198.89	–	215.3	238.1	239.2
trunk	171.7	198.89	–	215.7	238.1	239.2
umbilicus	171.5	198.89	–	215.5	238.1	239.2
vesicorectal	171.6	198.89	–	215.6	238.1	239.2
wrist	171.2	198.89	–	215.2	238.1	239.2
conus medullaris	192.2	198.3	–	225.3	237.5	239.7
cord (true) (vocal)	161.0	197.3	231.0	212.1	235.6	239.1
false	161.1	197.3	231.0	212.1	235.6	239.1
spermatic	187.6	198.82	233.6	222.8	236.6	239.5
cord – *continued*						
spinal (cervical) (lumbar) (thoracic)	192.2	198.3	–	225.3	237.5	239.7
cornea (limbus)	190.4	198.4	234.0	224.4	238.8	239.89▲
corpus						
albicans	183.0	198.6	233.39	220	236.2	239.5
callosum, brain	191.8	198.3	–	225.0	237.5	239.6
cavernosum	187.3	198.82	233.5	222.1	236.6	239.5
gastric	151.4	197.8	230.2	211.1	235.2	239.0
penis	187.3	198.82	233.5	222.1	236.6	239.5
striatum, cerebrum	191.0	198.3	–	225.0	237.5	239.6
uteri	182.0	198.82	233.2	219.1	236.0	239.5
isthmus	182.1	198.82	233.2	219.1	236.0	239.5
cortex						
adrenal	194.0	198.7	234.8	227.0	237.2	239.7
cerebral	191.0	198.3	–	225.0	237.5	239.6
costal cartilage	170.3	198.5	–	213.3	238.0	239.2
costovertebral joint	170.3	198.5	–	213.3	238.0	239.2
Cowper's gland	189.3	198.1	233.9	223.81	236.99	239.5
cranial (fossa, any)	191.9	198.3	–	225.0	237.5	239.6
meninges	192.1	198.4	–	225.2	237.6	239.7
nerve (any)	192.0	198.4	–	225.1	237.9	239.7
craniobuccal pouch	194.3	198.89	234.8	227.3	237.0	239.7
craniopharyngeal (duct) (pouch)	194.3	198.89	234.8	227.3	237.0	239.7
cricoid	148.0	198.89	230.0	210.8	235.1	239.0
cartilage	161.3	197.3	231.0	212.1	235.6	239.1
cricopharynx	148.0	198.89	230.0	210.8	235.1	239.0
crypt of Morgagni	154.8	197.5	230.7	211.4	235.2	239.0
crystalline lens	190.0	198.4	234.0	224.0	238.8	239.89▲
cul-de-sac (Douglas')	158.8	197.6	–	211.8	235.4	239.0
cuneiform cartilage	161.3	197.3	231.0	212.1	235.6	239.1
cutaneous – *see* Neoplasm, skin						
cutis – *see* Neoplasm, skin						
cystic (bile) duct (common)	156.1	197.8	230.8	211.5	235.3	239.0
dermis – *see* Neoplasm, skin						
diaphragm	171.4	198.89	–	215.4	238.1	239.2
digestive organs, system, tube, or tract NEC	159.9	197.8	230.9	211.9	235.5	239.0
contiguous sites with peritoneum	159.8	–	–	–	–	–
disc, intervertebral	170.2	198.5	–	213.2	238.0	239.2
disease, generalized	199.0	199.0	234.9	229.9	238.9	199.0
disseminated	199.0	199.0	234.9	229.9	238.9	199.0
Douglas' cul-de-sac or pouch	158.8	197.6	–	211.8	235.4	239.0
duodenojejunal junction	152.8	197.4	230.7	211.2	235.2	239.0
duodenum	152.0	197.4	230.7	211.2	235.2	239.0
dura (cranial) (mater)	192.1	198.4	–	225.2	237.6	239.7
cerebral	192.1	198.4	–	225.2	237.6	239.7
spinal	192.3	198.4	–	225.4	237.6	239.7
ear (external)	173.2	198.2	232.2	216.2	238.2	239.2
auricle or auris	173.2	198.2	232.2	216.2	238.2	239.2
canal, external	173.2	198.2	232.2	216.2	238.2	239.2
cartilage	171.0	198.89	–	215.0	238.1	239.2
external meatus	173.2	198.2	232.2	216.2	238.2	239.2
inner	160.1	197.3	231.8	212.0	235.9	239.89▲
lobule	173.2	198.2	232.2	216.2	238.2	239.2
middle	160.1	197.3	231.8	212.0	235.9	239.89▲
contiguous sites with accessory sinuses or nasal cavities	160.8	–	–	–	–	–
skin	173.2	198.2	232.2	216.2	238.2	239.2
earlobe	173.2	198.2	232.2	216.2	238.2	239.2
ejaculatory duct	187.8	198.82	233.6	222.8	236.6	239.5
elbow NEC*	195.4	198.89	232.6	229.8	238.8	239.89▲
endocardium	164.1	198.89	–	212.7	238.8	239.89▲
endocervix (canal) (gland)	180.0	198.82	233.1	219.0	236.0	239.5
endocrine gland NEC	194.9	198.89	–	227.9	237.4	239.7
pluriglandular NEC	194.8	198.89	234.8	227.8	237.4	239.7
endometrium (gland) (stroma)	182.0	198.82	233.2	219.1	236.0	239.5
ensiform cartilage	170.3	198.5	–	213.3	238.0	239.2
enteric – *see* Neoplasm, intestine						
ependyma (brain)	191.5	198.3	–	225.0	237.5	239.6
epicardium	164.1	198.89	–	212.7	238.8	239.89▲
epididymis	187.5	198.82	233.6	222.3	236.6	239.5
epidural	192.9	198.4	–	225.9	237.9	239.7
epiglottis	161.1	197.3	231.0	212.1	235.6	239.1
anterior aspect or surface	146.4	198.89	230.0	210.6	235.1	239.0
cartilage	161.3	197.3	231.0	212.1	235.6	239.1

Neoplasm, neoplastic	Malignant					
	Primary	Secondary	Carcinoma in situ	Benign	Uncertain Behavior	Unspecified
epiglottis – *continued*						
free border (margin)	146.4	198.89	230.0	210.6	235.1	239.0
junctional region	146.5	198.89	230.0	210.6	235.1	239.0
posterior (laryngeal) surface	161.1	197.3	231.0	212.1	235.6	239.1
suprahyoid portion	161.1	197.3	231.0	212.1	235.6	239.1
esophagogastric junction	151.0	197.8	230.2	211.1	235.2	239.0
esophagus	150.9	197.8	230.1	211.0	235.5	239.0
abdominal	150.2	197.8	230.1	211.0	235.5	239.0
cervical	150.0	197.8	230.1	211.0	235.5	239.0
contiguous sites	150.8	–	–	–	–	–
distal (third)	150.5	197.8	230.1	211.0	235.5	239.0
lower (third)	150.5	197.8	230.1	211.0	235.5	239.0
middle (third)	150.4	197.8	230.1	211.0	235.5	239.0
proximal (third)	150.3	197.8	230.1	211.0	235.5	239.0
specified part NEC	150.8	197.8	230.1	211.0	235.5	239.0
thoracic	150.1	197.8	230.1	211.0	235.5	239.0
upper (third)	150.3	197.8	230.1	211.0	235.5	239.0
ethmoid (sinus)	160.3	197.3	231.8	212.0	235.9	239.1
bone or labyrinth	170.0	198.5	–	213.0	238.0	239.2
Eustachian tube	160.1	197.3	231.8	212.0	235.9	239.1
exocervix	180.1	198.82	233.1	219.0	236.0	239.5
external						
meatus (ear)	173.2	198.2	232.2	216.2	238.2	239.2
os, cervix uteri	180.1	198.82	233.1	219.0	236.0	239.5
extradural	192.9	198.4	–	225.9	237.9	239.7
extrahepatic (bile) duct	156.1	197.8	230.8	211.5	235.3	239.0
contiguous sites with gallbladder	156.8	–	–	–	–	–
extraocular muscle	190.1	198.4	234.0	224.1	238.8	239.89▲
extrarectal	195.3	198.89	234.8	229.8	238.8	239.89▲
extremity*	195.8	198.89	232.8	229.8	238.8	239.89▲
lower*	195.5	198.89	232.7	229.8	238.8	239.89▲
upper*	195.4	198.89	232.6	229.8	238.8	239.89▲
eye NEC	190.9	198.4	234.0	224.9	238.8	239.89▲
contiguous sites	190.8	–	–	–	–	–
specified sites NEC	190.8	198.4	234.0	224.8	238.8	239.89▲
eyeball	190.0	198.4	234.0	224.0	238.8	239.89▲
eyebrow	173.3	198.2	232.3	216.3	238.2	239.2
eyelid (lower) (skin) (upper)	173.1	198.2	232.1	216.1	238.2	239.2
cartilage	171.0	198.89	–	215.0	238.1	239.2
face NEC*	195.0	198.89	232.3	229.8	238.8	239.89▲
Fallopian tube (accessory)	183.2	198.82	233.39	221.0	236.3	239.5
falx (cerebella) (cerebri)	192.1	198.4	–	225.2	237.6	239.7
fascia – *see also* Neoplasm, connective tissue						
palmar	171.2	198.89	–	215.2	238.1	239.2
plantar	171.3	198.89	–	215.3	238.1	239.2
fatty tissue – *see* Neoplasm, connective tissue						
fauces, faucial NEC	146.9	198.89	230.0	210.6	235.1	239.0
pillars	146.2	198.89	230.0	210.6	235.1	239.0
tonsil	146.0	198.89	230.0	210.5	235.1	239.0
femur (any part)	170.7	198.5	–	213.7	238.0	239.2
fetal membrane	181	198.82	233.2	219.8	236.1	239.5
fibrous tissue – *see* Neoplasm, connective tissue						
fibula (any part)	170.7	198.5	–	213.7	238.0	239.2
filum terminale	192.2	198.3	–	225.3	237.5	239.7
finger NEC*	195.4	198.89	232.6	229.8	238.8	239.89▲
flank NEC*	195.8	198.89	232.5	229.8	238.8	239.89▲
follicle, nabothian	180.0	198.82	233.1	219.0	236.0	239.5
foot NEC*	195.5	198.89	232.7	229.8	238.8	239.89▲
forearm NEC*	195.4	198.89	232.6	229.8	238.8	239.89▲
forehead (skin)	173.3	198.2	232.3	216.3	238.2	239.2
foreskin	187.1	198.82	233.5	222.1	236.6	239.5
fornix						
pharyngeal	147.3	198.89	230.0	210.7	235.1	239.0
vagina	184.0	198.82	233.31	221.1	236.3	239.5
fossa (of)						
anterior (cranial)	191.9	198.3	–	225.0	237.5	239.6
cranial	191.9	198.3	–	225.0	237.5	239.6
ischiorectal	195.3	198.89	234.8	229.8	238.8	239.89▲
middle (cranial)	191.9	198.3	–	225.0	237.5	239.6
pituitary	194.3	198.89	234.8	227.3	237.0	239.7
posterior (cranial)	191.9	198.3	–	225.0	237.5	239.6
pterygoid	171.0	198.89	–	215.0	238.1	239.2
pyriform	148.1	198.89	230.0	210.8	235.1	239.0
Rosenmüller	147.2	198.89	230.0	210.7	235.1	239.0
tonsillar	146.1	198.89	230.0	210.6	235.1	239.0
fourchette	184.4	198.82	233.32	221.2	236.3	239.5

Neoplasm, neoplastic	Malignant					
	Primary	Secondary	Carcinoma in situ	Benign	Uncertain Behavior	Unspecified
frenulum						
labii – *see* Neoplasm, lip, internal linguae	141.3	198.89	230.0	210.1	235.1	239.0
frontal						
bone	170.0	198.5	–	213.0	238.0	239.2
lobe, brain	191.1	198.3	–	225.0	237.5	239.6
meninges	192.1	198.4	–	225.2	237.6	239.7
pole	191.1	198.3	–	225.0	237.5	239.6
sinus	160.4	197.3	231.8	212.0	235.9	239.1
fundus						
stomach	151.3	197.8	230.2	211.1	235.2	239.0
uterus	182.0	198.82	233.2	219.1	236.0	239.5
gall duct (extrahepatic)	156.1	197.8	230.8	211.5	235.3	239.0
intrahepatic	155.1	197.8	230.8	211.5	235.3	239.0
gallbladder	156.0	197.8	230.8	211.5	235.3	239.0
contiguous sites with extrahepatic bile ducts	156.8	–	–	–	–	–
ganglia (*see also* Neoplasm, connective tissue)	171.9	198.89	–	215.9	238.1	239.2
basal	191.0	198.3	–	225.0	237.5	239.6
ganglion (*see also* Neoplasm, connective tissue)	171.9	198.89	–	215.9	238.1	239.2
cranial nerve	192.0	198.4	–	225.1	237.9	239.7
Gartner's duct	184.0	198.82	233.31	221.1	236.3	239.5
gastric – *see* Neoplasm, stomach						
gastrocolic	159.8	197.8	230.9	211.9	235.5	239.0
gastroesophageal junction	151.0	197.8	230.2	211.1	235.2	239.0
gastrointestinal (tract) NEC	159.9	197.8	230.9	211.9	235.5	239.0
generalized	199.0	199.0	234.9	229.9	238.9	199.0
genital organ or tract						
female NEC	184.9	198.82	233.39	221.9	236.3	239.5
contiguous sites	184.8	–	–	–	–	–
specified site NEC	184.8	198.82	233.39	221.8	236.3	239.5
male NEC	187.9	198.82	233.6	222.9	236.6	239.5
contiguous sites	187.8	–	–	–	–	–
specified site NEC	187.8	198.82	233.6	222.8	236.6	239.5
genitourinary tract						
female	184.9	198.82	233.39	221.9	236.3	239.5
male	187.9	198.82	233.6	222.9	236.6	239.5
gingiva (alveolar) (marginal)	143.9	198.89	230.0	210.4	235.1	239.0
lower	143.1	198.89	230.0	210.4	235.1	239.0
mandibular	143.1	198.89	230.0	210.4	235.1	239.0
maxillary	143.0	198.89	230.0	210.4	235.1	239.0
upper	143.0	198.89	230.0	210.4	235.1	239.0
gland, glandular (lymphatic) (system) – *see also* Neoplasm, lymph gland						
endocrine NEC	194.9	198.89	–	227.9	237.4	239.7
salivary – *see* Neoplasm, salivary, gland						
glans penis	187.2	198.82	233.5	222.1	236.6	239.5
globus pallidus	191.0	198.3	–	225.0	237.5	239.6
glomus						
coccygeal	194.6	198.89	–	227.6	237.3	239.7
jugularis	194.6	198.89	–	227.6	237.3	239.7
glosso-epiglottic fold(s)	146.4	198.89	230.0	210.6	235.1	239.0
glossopalatine fold	146.2	198.89	230.0	210.6	235.1	239.0
glossopharyngeal sulcus	146.1	198.89	230.0	210.6	235.1	239.0
glottis	161.0	197.3	231.0	212.1	235.6	239.1
gluteal region*	195.3	198.89	232.5	229.8	238.8	239.89▲
great vessels NEC	171.4	198.89	–	215.4	238.1	239.2
groin NEC	195.3	198.89	232.5	229.8	238.8	239.89▲
gum	143.9	198.89	230.0	210.4	235.1	239.0
contiguous sites	143.8	–	–	–	–	–
lower	143.1	198.89	230.0	210.4	235.1	239.0
upper	143.0	198.89	230.0	210.4	235.1	239.0
hand NEC*	195.4	198.89	232.6	229.8	238.8	239.89▲
head NEC*	195.0	198.89	232.4	229.8	238.8	239.89▲
heart	164.1	198.89	–	212.7	238.8	239.89▲
contiguous sites with mediastinum or thymus	164.8	–	–	–	–	–
heel NEC*	195.5	198.89	232.7	229.8	238.8	239.89▲
helix	173.2	198.2	232.2	216.2	238.2	239.2
hematopoietic, hemopoietic tissue NEC	202.8 [5th]	198.89	–	–	–	238.79
hemisphere, cerebral	191.0	198.3	–	225.0	237.5	239.6
hemorrhoidal zone	154.2	197.5	230.5	211.4	235.5	239.0
hepatic	155.2	197.7	230.8	211.5	235.3	239.0
duct (bile)	156.1	197.8	230.8	211.5	235.3	239.0
flexure (colon)	153.0	197.5	230.3	211.3	235.2	239.0
primary	155.0	–	–	–	–	–

Neoplasm, neoplastic	Malignant Primary	Malignant Secondary	Malignant Carcinoma in situ	Benign	Uncertain Behavior	Unspecifed
hilus of lung	162.2	197.0	231.2	212.3	235.7	239.1
hip NEC*	195.5	198.89	232.7	229.8	238.8	239.89▲
hippocampus, brain	191.2	198.3	–	225.0	237.5	239.6
humerus (any part)	170.4	198.5	–	213.4	238.0	239.2
hymen	184.0	198.82	233.31	221.1	236.3	239.5
hypopharynx, hypopharyngeal NEC	148.9	198.89	230.0	210.8	235.1	239.0
contiguous sites	148.8	–	–	–	–	–
postcricoid region	148.0	198.89	230.0	210.8	235.1	239.0
posterior wall	148.3	198.89	230.0	210.8	235.1	239.0
pyriform fossa (sinus)	148.1	198.89	230.0	210.8	235.1	239.0
specified site NEC	148.8	198.89	230.0	210.8	235.1	239.0
wall	148.9	198.89	230.0	210.8	235.1	239.0
posterior	148.3	198.89	230.0	210.8	235.1	239.0
hypophysis	194.3	198.89	234.8	227.3	237.0	239.7
hypothalamus	191.0	198.3	–	225.0	237.5	239.6
ileocecum, ileocecal (coil) (junction) (valve)	153.4	197.5	230.3	211.3	235.2	239.0
ileum	152.2	197.4	230.7	211.2	235.2	239.0
ilium	170.6	198.5	–	213.6	238.0	239.2
immunoproliferative NEC	203.8 5th	–	–	–	–	–
infraclavicular (region)*	195.1	198.89	232.5	229.8	238.8	239.89▲
inguinal (region)*	195.3	198.89	232.5	229.8	238.8	239.89▲
insula	191.0	198.3	–	225.0	237.5	239.6
insular tissue (pancreas)	157.4	197.8	230.9	211.7	235.5	239.0
brain	191.0	198.3	–	225.0	237.5	239.6
interarytenoid fold	148.2	198.89	230.0	210.8	235.1	239.0
hypopharyngeal aspect	148.2	198.89	230.0	210.8	235.1	239.0
laryngeal aspect	161.1	197.3	231.0	212.1	235.6	239.1
marginal zone	148.2	198.89	230.0	210.8	235.1	239.0
interdental papillae	143.9	198.89	230.0	210.4	235.1	239.0
lower	143.1	198.89	230.0	210.4	235.1	239.0
upper	143.0	198.89	230.0	210.4	235.1	239.0
internal						
capsule	191.0	198.3	–	225.0	237.5	239.6
os (cervix)	180.0	198.82	233.1	219.0	236.0	239.5
intervertebral cartilage or disc	170.2	198.5	–	213.2	238.0	239.2
intestine, intestinal	159.0	197.8	230.7	211.9	235.2	239.0
large	153.9	197.5	230.3	211.3	235.2	239.0
appendix	153.5	197.5	230.3	211.3	235.2	239.0
caput coli	153.4	197.5	230.3	211.3	235.2	239.0
cecum	153.4	197.5	230.3	211.3	235.2	239.0
colon	153.9	197.5	230.3	211.3	235.2	239.0
and rectum	154.0	197.5	230.4	211.4	235.2	239.0
ascending	153.6	197.5	230.3	211.3	235.2	239.0
caput	153.4	197.5	230.3	211.3	235.2	239.0
contiguous sites	153.8	–	–	–	–	–
descending	153.2	197.5	230.3	211.3	235.2	239.0
distal	153.2	197.5	230.3	211.3	235.2	239.0
left	153.2	197.5	230.3	211.3	235.2	239.0
pelvic	153.3	197.5	230.3	211.3	235.2	239.0
right	153.6	197.5	230.3	211.3	235.2	239.0
sigmoid (flexure)	153.3	197.5	230.3	211.3	235.2	239.0
transverse	153.1	197.5	230.3	211.3	235.2	239.0
contiguous sites	153.8	–	–	–	–	–
hepatic flexure	153.0	197.5	230.3	211.3	235.2	239.0
ileocecum, ileocecal (coil) (valve)	153.4	197.5	230.3	211.3	235.2	239.0
sigmoid flexure (lower) (upper)	153.3	197.5	230.3	211.3	235.2	239.0
splenic flexure	153.7	197.5	230.3	211.3	235.2	239.0
small	152.9	197.4	230.7	211.2	235.2	239.0
contiguous sites	152.8	–	–	–	–	–
duodenum	152.0	197.4	230.7	211.2	235.2	239.0
ileum	152.2	197.4	230.7	211.2	235.2	239.0
jejunum	152.1	197.4	230.7	211.2	235.2	239.0
tract NEC	159.0	197.8	230.7	211.9	235.2	239.0
intra-abdominal	195.2	198.89	234.8	229.8	238.8	239.89▲
intracranial NEC	191.9	198.3	–	225.0	237.5	239.6
intrahepatic (bile) duct	155.1	197.8	230.8	211.5	235.3	239.0
intraocular	190.0	198.4	234.0	224.0	238.8	239.89▲
intraorbital	190.1	198.4	234.0	224.1	238.8	239.89▲
intrasellar	194.3	198.89	234.8	227.3	237.0	239.7
intrathoracic (cavity) (organs NEC)	195.1	198.89	234.8	229.8	238.8	239.89▲
contiguous sites with respiratory organs	165.8	–	–	–	–	–
iris	190.0	198.4	234.0	224.0	238.8	239.89▲
ischiorectal (fossa)	195.3	198.89	234.8	229.8	238.8	239.89▲
ischium	170.6	198.5	–	213.6	238.0	239.2
island of Reil	191.0	198.3	–	225.0	237.5	239.6
islands or islets of Langerhans	157.4	197.8	230.9	211.7	235.5	239.0
isthmus uteri	182.1	198.82	233.2	219.1	236.0	239.5
jaw	195.0	198.89	234.8	229.8	238.8	239.89▲
bone	170.1	198.5	–	213.1	238.0	239.2
carcinoma	143.9	–	–	–	–	–
lower	143.1	–	–	–	–	–
upper	143.0	–	–	–	–	–
lower	170.1	198.5	–	213.1	238.0	239.2
upper	170.0	198.5	–	213.0	238.0	239.2
carcinoma (any type) (lower) (upper)	195.0	–	–	–	–	–
skin	173.3	198.2	232.3	216.3	238.2	239.2
soft tissues	143.9	198.89	230.0	210.4	235.1	239.0
lower	143.1	198.89	230.0	210.4	235.1	239.0
upper	143.0	198.89	230.0	210.4	235.1	239.0
jejunum	152.1	197.4	230.7	211.2	235.2	239.0
joint NEC (*see also* Neoplasm, bone)	170.9	198.5	–	213.9	238.0	239.2
acromioclavicular	170.4	198.5	–	213.4	238.0	239.2
bursa or synovial membrane – *see* Neoplasm, connective tissue						
costovertebral	170.3	198.5	–	213.3	238.0	239.2
sternocostal	170.3	198.5	–	213.3	238.0	239.2
temporomandibular	170.1	198.5	–	213.1	238.0	239.2
junction						
anorectal	154.8	197.5	230.7	211.4	235.5	239.0
cardioesophageal	151.0	197.8	230.2	211.1	235.2	239.0
esophagogastric	151.0	197.8	230.2	211.1	235.2	239.0
gastroesophageal	151.0	197.8	230.2	211.1	235.2	239.0
hard and soft palate	145.5	198.89	230.0	210.4	235.1	239.0
ileocecal	153.4	197.5	230.3	211.3	235.2	239.0
pelvirectal	154.0	197.5	230.4	211.4	235.2	239.0
pelviureteric	189.1	198.0	233.9	223.1	236.91	239.5
rectosigmoid	154.0	197.5	230.4	211.4	235.2	239.0
squamocolumnar, of cervix	180.8	198.82	233.1	219.0	236.0	239.5
kidney (parenchymal)	189.0	198.0	233.9	223.0	236.91	239.5
calyx	189.1	198.0	233.9	223.1	236.91	239.5
hilus	189.1	198.0	233.9	223.1	236.91	239.5
pelvis	189.1	198.0	233.9	223.1	236.91	239.5
knee NEC*	195.5	198.89	232.7	229.8	238.8	239.8
labia (skin)	184.4	198.82	233.32	221.2	236.3	239.5
majora	184.1	198.82	233.32	221.2	236.3	239.5
minora	184.2	198.82	233.32	221.2	236.3	239.5
labial – *see*, also Neoplasm, lip						
sulcus (lower) (upper)	145.1	198.89	230.0	210.4	235.1	239.0
labium (skin)	184.4	198.82	233.32	221.2	236.3	239.5
majus	184.1	198.82	233.32	221.2	236.3	239.5
minus	184.2	198.82	233.32	221.2	236.3	239.5
lacrimal						
canaliculi	190.7	198.4	234.0	224.7	238.8	239.89▲
duct (nasal)	190.7	198.4	234.0	224.7	238.8	239.89▲
gland	190.2	198.4	234.0	224.2	238.8	239.89▲
punctum	190.7	198.4	234.0	224.7	238.8	239.89▲
sac	190.7	198.4	234.0	224.7	238.8	239.89▲
Langerhans, islands or islets	157.4	197.8	230.9	211.7	235.5	239.0
laryngopharynx	148.9	198.89	230.0	210.8	235.1	239.0
larynx, laryngeal NEC	161.9	197.3	231.0	212.1	235.6	239.1
aryepiglottic fold	161.1	197.3	231.0	212.1	235.6	239.1
cartilage (arytenoid) (cricoid) (cuneiform) (thyroid)	161.3	197.3	231.0	212.1	235.6	239.1
commissure (anterior) (posterior)	161.0	197.3	231.0	212.1	235.6	239.1
contiguous sites	161.8	–	–	–	–	–
extrinsic NEC	161.1	197.3	231.0	212.1	235.6	239.1
meaning hypopharynx	148.9	198.89	230.0	210.8	235.1	239.0
interarytenoid fold	161.1	197.3	231.0	212.1	235.6	239.1
intrinsic	161.0	197.3	231.0	212.1	235.6	239.1
ventricular band	161.1	197.3	231.0	212.1	235.6	239.1
leg NEC*	195.5	198.89	232.7	229.8	238.8	239.89▲
lens, crystalline	190.0	198.4	234.0	224.0	238.8	239.89▲
lid (lower) (upper)	173.1	198.2	232.1	216.1	238.2	239.2
ligament – *see also* Neoplasm, connective tissue						
broad	183.3	198.82	233.39	221.0	236.3	239.5
Mackenrodt's	183.8	198.82	233.39	221.8	236.3	239.5

Neoplasm, neoplastic	Malignant					
	Primary	Secondary	Carcinoma in situ	Benign	Uncertain Behavior	Unspecified
ligament – *continued*						
non-uterine – *see* Neoplasm, connective tissue						
round	183.5	198.82	–	221.0	236.3	239.5
sacro-uterine	183.4	198.82	–	221.0	236.3	239.5
uterine	183.4	198.82	–	221.0	236.3	239.5
utero-ovarian	183.8	198.82	233.39	221.8	236.3	239.5
uterosacral	183.4	198.82	–	221.0	236.3	239.5
limb*	195.8	198.89	232.8	229.8	238.8	239.89▲
lower*	195.5	198.89	232.7	229.8	238.8	239.89▲
upper*	195.4	198.89	232.6	229.8	238.8	239.89▲
limbus of cornea	190.4	198.4	234.0	224.4	238.8	239.89▲
lingual NEC (*see also* Neoplasm, tongue)	141.9	198.89	230.0	210.1	235.1	239.0
lingula, lung	162.3	197.0	231.2	212.3	235.7	239.1
lip (external) (lipstick area) (vermillion border)	140.9	198.89	230.0	210.0	235.1	239.0
buccal aspect – *see* Neoplasm, lip, internal						
commissure	140.6	198.89	230.0	210.4	235.1	239.0
contiguous sites	140.8	–	–	–	–	–
with oral cavity or pharynx	149.8	–	–	–	–	–
frenulum – *see* Neoplasm, lip, internal						
inner aspect – *see* Neoplasm, lip, internal						
internal (buccal) (frenulum) (mucosa) (oral)	140.5	198.89	230.0	210.0	235.1	239.0
lower	140.4	198.89	230.0	210.0	235.1	239.0
upper	140.3	198.89	230.0	210.0	235.1	239.0
lower	140.1	198.89	230.0	210.0	235.1	239.0
internal (buccal) (frenulum) (mucosa) (oral)	140.4	198.89	230.0	210.0	235.1	239.0
mucosa – *see* Neoplasm, lip, internal						
oral aspect – *see* Neoplasm, lip, internal						
skin (commissure) (lower) (upper)	173.0	198.2	232.0	216.0	238.2	239.2
upper	140.0	198.89	230.0	210.0	235.1	239.0
internal (buccal) (frenulum) (mucosa) (oral)	140.3	198.89	230.0	210.0	235.1	239.0
liver	155.2	197.7	230.8	211.5	235.3	239.0
primary	155.0	–	–	–	–	–
lobe						
azygos	162.3	197.0	231.2	212.3	235.7	239.1
frontal	191.1	198.3	–	225.0	237.5	239.6
lower	162.5	197.0	231.2	212.3	235.7	239.1
middle	162.4	197.0	231.2	212.3	235.7	239.1
occipital	191.4	198.3	–	225.0	237.5	239.6
parietal	191.3	198.3	–	225.0	237.5	239.6
temporal	191.2	198.3	–	225.0	237.5	239.6
upper	162.3	197.0	231.2	212.3	235.7	239.1
lumbosacral plexus	171.6	198.4	–	215.6	238.1	239.2
lung	162.9	197.0	231.2	212.3	235.7	239.1
azygos lobe	162.3	197.0	231.2	212.3	235.7	239.1
carina	162.2	197.0	231.2	212.3	235.7	239.1
contiguous sites with bronchus or trachea	162.8	–	–	–	–	–
hilus	162.2	197.0	231.2	212.3	235.7	239.1
linqula	162.3	197.0	231.2	212.3	235.7	239.1
lobe NEC	162.9	197.0	231.2	212.3	235.7	239.1
lower lobe	162.5	197.0	231.2	212.3	235.7	239.1
main bronchus	162.2	197.0	231.2	212.3	235.7	239.1
middle lobe	162.4	197.0	231.2	212.3	235.7	239.1
upper lobe	162.3	197.0	231.2	212.3	235.7	239.1
lymph, lymphatic						
channel NEC (*see also* Neoplasm, connective tissue)	171.9	198.89	–	215.9	238.1	239.2
gland (secondary)	–	196.9	–	229.0	238.8	239.89▲
abdominal	–	196.2	–	229.0	238.8	239.89▲
aortic	–	196.2	–	229.0	238.8	239.89▲
arm	–	196.3	–	229.0	238.8	239.89▲
auricular (anterior) (posterior)	–	196.0	–	229.0	238.8	239.89▲
axilla, axillary	–	196.3	–	229.0	238.8	239.89▲
brachial	–	196.3	–	229.0	238.8	239.89▲

Neoplasm, neoplastic	Malignant					
	Primary	Secondary	Carcinoma in situ	Benign	Uncertain Behavior	Unspecified
lymph, lymphatic – *continued*						
gland – *continued*						
bronchial	–	196.1	–	229.0	238.8	239.89▲
bronchopulmonary	–	196.1	–	229.0	238.8	239.89▲
celiac	–	196.2	–	229.0	238.8	239.89▲
cervical	–	196.0	–	229.0	238.8	239.89▲
cervicofacial	–	196.0	–	229.0	238.8	239.89▲
Cloquet	–	196.5	–	229.0	238.8	239.89▲
colic	–	196.2	–	229.0	238.8	239.89▲
common duct	–	196.2	–	229.0	238.8	239.89▲
cubital	–	196.3	–	229.0	238.8	239.89▲
diaphragmatic	–	196.1	–	229.0	238.8	239.89▲
epigastric, inferior	–	196.6	–	229.0	238.8	239.89▲
epitrochlear	–	196.3	–	229.0	238.8	239.89▲
esophageal	–	196.1	–	229.0	238.8	239.89▲
face	–	196.0	–	229.0	238.8	239.89▲
femoral	–	196.5	–	229.0	238.8	239.89▲
gastric	–	196.2	–	229.0	238.8	239.89▲
groin	–	196.5	–	229.0	238.8	239.89▲
head	–	196.0	–	229.0	238.8	239.89▲
hepatic	–	196.2	–	229.0	238.8	239.89▲
hilar (pulmonary)	–	196.1	–	229.0	238.8	239.89▲
splenic	–	196.2	–	229.0	238.8	239.89▲
hypogastric	–	196.6	–	229.0	238.8	239.89▲
ileocolic	–	196.2	–	229.0	238.8	239.89▲
iliac	–	196.6	–	229.0	238.8	239.89▲
infraclavicular	–	196.3	–	229.0	238.8	239.89▲
inguina, inguinal	–	196.5	–	229.0	238.8	239.89▲
innominate	–	196.1	–	229.0	238.8	239.89▲
intercostal	–	196.1	–	229.0	238.8	239.89▲
intestinal	–	196.2	–	229.0	238.8	239.89▲
intrabdominal	–	196.2	–	229.0	238.8	239.89▲
intrapelvic	–	196.6	–	229.0	238.8	239.89▲
intrathoracic	–	196.1	–	229.0	238.8	239.9
jugular	–	196.0	–	229.0	238.8	239.89▲
leg	–	196.5	–	229.0	238.8	239.89▲
limb						
lower	–	196.5	–	229.0	238.8	239.89▲
upper	–	196.3	–	229.0	238.8	239.89▲
lower limb	–	196.5	–	229.0	238.8	238.9
lumbar	–	196.2	–	229.0	238.8	239.89▲
mandibular	–	196.0	–	229.0	238.8	239.89▲
mediastinal	–	196.1	–	229.0	238.8	239.89▲
mesenteric (inferior) (superior)	–	196.2	–	229.0	238.8	239.89▲
midcolic	–	196.2	–	229.0	238.8	239.89▲
multiple sites in categories 196.0-196.6	–	196.8	–	229.0	238.8	239.89▲
neck	–	196.0	–	229.0	238.8	239.89▲
obturator	–	196.6	–	229.0	238.8	239.89▲
occipital	–	196.0	–	229.0	238.8	239.89▲
pancreatic	–	196.2	–	229.0	238.8	239.89▲
para-aortic	–	196.2	–	229.0	238.8	239.89▲
paracervical	–	196.6	–	229.0	238.8	239.89▲
parametrial	–	196.6	–	229.0	238.8	239.89▲
parasternal	–	196.1	–	229.0	238.8	239.89▲
parotid	–	196.0	–	229.0	238.8	239.89▲
pectoral	–	196.3	–	229.0	238.8	239.89▲
pelvic	–	196.6	–	229.0	238.8	239.89▲
peri-aortic	–	196.2	–	229.0	238.8	239.89▲
peripancreatic	–	196.2	–	229.0	238.8	239.89▲
popliteal	–	196.5	–	229.0	238.8	239.89▲
porta hepatis	–	196.2	–	229.0	238.8	239.89▲
portal	–	196.2	–	229.0	238.8	239.89▲
preauricular	–	196.0	–	229.0	238.8	239.89▲
prelaryngeal	–	196.0	–	229.0	238.8	239.89▲
presymphysial	–	196.6	–	229.0	238.8	239.89▲
pretracheal	–	196.0	–	229.0	238.8	239.89▲
primary (any site) NEC	202.9 5th	–	–	–	–	–
pulmonary (hiler)	–	196.1	–	229.0	238.8	239.89▲
pyloric	–	196.2	–	229.0	238.8	239.89▲
retroperitoneal	–	196.2	–	229.0	238.8	239.89▲
retropharyngeal	–	196.0	–	229.0	238.8	239.89▲
Rosenmüller's	–	196.5	–	229.0	238.8	239.89▲
sacral	–	196.6	–	229.0	238.8	239.89▲
scalene	–	196.0	–	229.0	238.8	239.89▲
site NEC	–	196.9	–	229.0	238.8	239.89▲
splenic (hilar)	–	196.2	–	229.0	238.8	239.89▲
subclavicular	–	196.3	–	229.0	238.8	239.89▲
subinguinal	–	196.5	–	229.0	238.8	239.89▲
sublingual	–	196.0	–	229.0	238.8	239.89▲
submandibular	–	196.0	–	229.0	238.8	239.89▲

Neoplasm, neoplastic	Malignant					
	Primary	Secondary	Carcinoma in situ	Benign	Uncertain Behavior	Unspecified
lymph, lymphatic – *continued*						
gland – *continued*						
submaxillary	–	196.0	–	229.0	238.8	239.89▲
submental	–	196.0	–	229.0	238.8	239.89▲
subscapular	–	196.3	–	229.0	238.8	239.89▲
supraclavicular	–	196.0	–	229.0	238.8	239.89▲
thoracic	–	196.1	–	229.0	238.8	239.89▲
tibial	–	196.5	–	229.0	238.8	239.89▲
tracheal	–	196.1	–	229.0	238.8	239.89▲
tracheobronchial	–	196.1	–	229.0	238.8	239.89▲
upper limb	–	196.3	–	229.0	238.8	239.89▲
Virchow's	–	196.0	–	229.0	238.8	239.89▲
node – *see also* Neoplasm, lymph gland						
primary NEC	202.9 5th	–	–	–	–	–
vessel (*see also* Neoplasm, connective tissue)	171.9	198.89	–	215.9	238.1	239.2
Mackenrodt's ligament	183.8	198.82	233.39	221.8	236.3	239.5
malar	170.0	198.5	–	213.0	238.0	239.2
region – *see* Neoplasm, cheek						
mammary gland – *see* Neoplasm, breast						
mandible	170.1	198.5	–	213.1	238.0	239.2
alveolar						
mucosa	143.1	198.89	230.0	210.4	235.1	239.0
ridge or process	170.1	198.5	–	213.1	238.0	239.2
carcinoma	143.1	–	–	–	–	–
carcinoma	143.1	–	–	–	–	–
marrow (bone) NEC	202.9 5th	198.5	–	–	–	238.79
mastectomy site (skin)	173.5	198.2	–	–	–	–
specified as breast tissue	174.8	198.81	–	–	–	–
mastoid (air cells) (antrum) (cavity)	160.1	197.3	231.8	212.0	235.9	239.1
bone or process	170.0	198.5	–	213.0	238.0	239.2
maxilla, maxillary (superior)	170.0	198.5	–	213.0	238.0	239.2
alveolar						
mucosa	143.0	198.89	230.0	210.4	235.1	239.0
ridge or process	170.0	198.5	–	213.0	238.0	239.2
carcinoma	143.0	–	–	–	–	–
antrum	160.2	197.3	231.8	212.0	235.9	239.1
carcinoma	143.0	–	–	–	–	–
inferior – *see* Neoplasm, mandible						
sinus	160.2	197.3	231.8	212.0	235.9	239.1
meatus						
external (ear)	173.2	198.2	232.2	216.2	238.2	239.2
Meckel's diverticulum	152.3	197.4	230.7	211.2	235.2	239.0
mediastinum, mediastinal	164.9	197.1	–	212.5	235.8	239.89▲
anterior	164.2	197.1	–	212.5	235.8	239.89▲
contiguous sites with heart and thymus	164.8	–	–	–	–	–
posterior	164.3	197.1	–	212.5	235.8	239.89▲
medulla						
adrenal	194.0	198.7	234.8	227.0	237.2	239.7
oblongata	191.7	198.3	–	225.0	237.5	239.6
meibomian gland	173.1	198.2	232.1	216.1	238.2	239.2
melanoma – *see* Melanoma						
meninges (brain) (cerebral) (cranial) (intracranial)	192.1	198.4	–	225.2	237.6	239.7
spinal (cord)	192.3	198.4	–	225.4	237.6	239.7
meniscus, knee joint (lateral) (medial)	170.7	198.5	–	213.7	238.0	239.2
mesentery, mesenteric	158.8	197.6	–	211.8	235.4	239.0
mesoappendix	158.8	197.6	–	211.8	235.4	239.0
mesocolon	158.8	197.6	–	211.8	235.4	239.0
mesopharynx – *see* Neoplasm, oropharynx						
mesosalpinx	183.3	198.82	233.39	221.0	236.3	239.5
mesovarium	183.3	198.82	233.39	221.0	236.3	239.5
metacarpus (any bone)	170.5	198.5	–	213.5	238.0	239.2
metastatic NEC – *see also* Neoplasm, by site, secondary	–	199.1	–	–	–	–
metatarsus (any bone)	170.8	198.5	–	213.8	238.0	239.2
midbrain	191.7	198.3	–	225.0	237.5	239.6
milk duct – *see* Neoplasm, breast						
mons						
pubis	184.4	198.82	233.32	221.2	236.3	239.5
veneris	184.4	198.82	233.32	221.2	236.3	239.5

Neoplasm, neoplastic	Malignant					
	Primary	Secondary	Carcinoma in situ	Benign	Uncertain Behavior	Unspecified
motor tract	192.9	198.4	–	225.9	237.9	239.7
brain	191.9	198.3	–	225.0	237.5	239.6
spinal	192.2	198.3	–	225.3	237.5	239.7
mouth	145.9	198.89	230.0	210.4	235.1	239.0
contiguous sites	145.8	–	–	–	–	–
floor	144.9	198.89	230.0	210.3	235.1	239.0
anterior portion	144.0	198.89	230.0	210.3	235.1	239.0
contiguous sites	144.8	–	–	–	–	–
lateral portion	144.1	198.89	230.0	210.3	235.1	239.0
roof	145.5	198.89	230.0	210.4	235.1	239.0
specified part NEC	145.8	198.89	230.0	210.4	235.1	239.0
vestibule	145.1	198.89	230.0	210.4	235.1	239.0
mucosa						
alveolar (ridge or process)	143.9	198.89	230.0	210.4	235.1	239.0
lower	143.1	198.89	230.0	210.4	235.1	239.0
upper	143.0	198.89	230.0	210.4	235.1	239.0
buccal	145.0	198.89	230.0	210.4	235.1	239.0
cheek	145.0	198.89	230.0	210.4	235.1	239.0
lip – *see* Neoplasm, lip, internal						
nasal	160.0	197.3	231.8	212.0	235.9	239.1
oral	145.0	198.89	230.0	210.4	235.1	239.0
Müllerian duct						
female	184.8	198.82	233.39	221.8	236.3	239.5
male	187.8	198.82	233.6	222.8	236.6	239.5
multiple sites NEC	199.0	199.0	234.9	229.9	238.9	199.0
muscle – *see also* Neoplasm, connective tissue						
extraocular	190.1	198.4	234.0	224.1	238.8	239.89▲
myocardium	164.1	198.89	–	212.7	238.8	239.89▲
myometrium	182.0	198.82	233.2	219.1	236.0	239.5
myopericardium	164.1	198.89	–	212.7	238.8	239.89▲
nabothian gland (follicle)	180.0	198.82	233.1	219.0	236.0	239.5
nail	173.9	198.2	232.9	216.9	238.2	239.2
finger	173.6	198.2	232.6	216.6	238.2	239.2
toe	173.7	198.2	232.7	216.7	238.2	239.2
nares, naris (anterior) (posterior)	160.0	197.3	231.8	212.0	235.9	239.1
nasal – *see* Neoplasm, nose						
nasolabial groove	173.3	198.2	232.3	216.3	238.2	239.2
nasolacrimal duct	190.7	198.4	234.0	224.7	238.8	239.89▲
nasopharynx, nasopharyngeal	147.9	198.89	230.0	210.7	235.1	239.0
contiguous sites	147.8	–	–	–	–	–
floor	147.3	198.89	230.0	210.7	235.1	239.0
roof	147.0	198.89	230.0	210.7	235.1	239.0
specified site NEC	147.8	198.89	230.0	210.7	235.1	239.0
wall	147.9	198.89	230.0	210.7	235.1	239.0
anterior	147.3	198.89	230.0	210.7	235.1	239.0
lateral	147.2	198.89	230.0	210.7	235.1	239.0
posterior	147.1	198.89	230.0	210.7	235.1	239.0
superior	147.0	198.89	230.0	210.7	235.1	239.0
nates	173.5	198.2	232.5	216.5	238.2	239.2
neck NEC*	195.0	198.89	234.8	229.8	238.8	239.89▲
nerve (autonomic) (ganglion) (parasympathetic) (peripheral) (sympathetic) – *see also* Neoplasm, connective tissue						
abducens	192.0	198.4	–	225.1	237.9	239.7
accessory (spinal)	192.0	198.4	–	225.1	237.9	239.7
acoustic	192.0	198.4	–	225.1	237.9	239.7
auditory	192.0	198.4	–	225.1	237.9	239.7
brachial	171.2	198.89	–	215.2	238.1	239.2
cranial (any)	192.0	198.4	–	225.1	237.9	239.7
facial	192.0	198.4	–	225.1	237.9	239.7
femoral	171.3	198.89	–	215.3	238.1	239.2
glossopharyngeal	192.0	198.4	–	225.1	237.9	239.7
hypoglossal	192.0	198.4	–	225.1	237.9	239.7
intercostal	171.4	198.89	–	215.4	238.1	239.2
lumbar	171.7	198.89	–	215.7	238.1	239.2
median	171.2	198.89	–	215.2	238.1	239.2
obturator	171.3	198.89	–	215.3	238.1	239.2
oculomotor	192.0	198.4	–	225.1	237.9	239.7
olfactory	192.0	198.4	–	225.1	237.9	239.7
optic	192.0	198.4	–	225.1	237.9	239.7
peripheral NEC	171.9	198.89	–	215.9	238.1	239.2
radial	171.2	198.89	–	215.2	238.1	239.2
sacral	171.6	198.89	–	215.6	238.1	239.2
sciatic	171.3	198.89	–	215.3	238.1	239.2
spinal NEC	171.9	198.89	–	215.9	238.1	239.2

Neoplasm, neoplastic	Malignant					
	Primary	Secondary	Carcinoma in situ	Benign	Uncertain Behavior	Unspecified
nerve – *continued*						
trigeminal	192.0	198.4	–	225.1	237.9	239.7
trochlear	192.0	198.4	–	225.1	237.9	239.7
ulnar	171.2	198.89	–	215.2	238.1	239.2
vagus	192.0	198.4	–	225.1	237.9	239.7
nervous system (central) NEC	192.9	198.4	–	225.9	237.9	239.7
autonomic NEC	171.9	198.89	–	215.9	238.1	239.2
brain – *see also* Neoplasm, brain membrane or meninges	192.1	198.4	–	225.2	237.6	239.7
contiguous sites	192.8	–	–	–	–	–
parasympathetic NEC	171.9	198.89	–	215.9	238.1	239.2
sympathetic NEC	171.9	198.89	–	215.9	238.1	239.2
nipple (female)	174.0	198.81	233.0	217	238.3	239.3
male	175.0	198.81	233.0	217	238.3	239.3
nose, nasal	195.0	198.89	234.8	229.8	238.8	239.89▲
ala (external)	173.3	198.2	232.3	216.3	238.2	239.2
bone	170.0	198.5	–	213.0	238.0	239.2
cartilage	160.0	197.3	231.8	212.0	235.9	239.1
cavity	160.0	197.3	231.8	212.0	235.9	239.1
contiguous sites with accessory sinuses or middle ear	160.8	–	–	–	–	–
choana	147.3	198.89	230.0	210.7	235.1	239.0
external (skin)	173.3	198.2	232.3	216.3	238.2	239.2
fossil	160.0	197.3	231.8	212.0	235.9	239.1
internal	160.0	197.3	231.8	212.0	235.9	239.1
mucosa	160.0	197.3	231.8	212.0	235.9	239.1
septum	160.0	197.3	231.8	212.0	235.9	239.1
posterior margin	147.3	198.89	230.0	210.7	235.1	239.0
sinus – *see* Neoplasm, sinus						
skin	173.3	198.2	232.3	216.3	238.2	239.2
turbinate (mucosa)	160.0	197.3	231.8	212.0	235.9	239.1
bone	170.0	198.5	–	213.0	238.0	239.2
vestibule	160.0	197.3	231.8	212.0	235.9	239.1
nostril	160.0	197.3	231.8	212.0	235.9	239.1
nucleus pulposus	170.2	198.5	–	213.2	238.0	230.2
occipital						
bone	170.0	198.5	–	213.0	238.0	239.2
lobe or pole, brain	191.4	198.3	–	225.0	237.5	239.6
odontogenic – *see* Neoplasm, jaw bone						
oesophagus – *see* Neoplasm, esophagus						
olfactory nerve or bulb	192.0	198.4	–	225.1	237.9	239.7
olive (brain)	191.7	198.3	–	225.0	237.5	239.6
omentum	158.8	197.6	–	211.8	235.4	239.0
operculum (brain)	191.0	198.3	–	225.0	237.5	239.6
optic nerve, chiasm, or tract	192.0	198.4	–	225.1	237.9	239.7
oral (cavity)	145.9	198.89	230.0	210.4	235.1	239.0
contiguous sites with lip or pharynx	149.8	–	–	–	–	–
ill-defined	149.9	198.89	230.0	210.4	235.1	239.0
mucosa	145.9	198.89	230.0	210.4	235.1	239.0
orbit	190.1	198.4	234.0	224.1	238.8	239.89▲
bone	170.0	198.5	–	213.0	238.0	239.2
eye	190.1	198.4	234.0	224.1	238.8	239.89▲
soft parts	190.1	198.4	234.0	224.1	238.8	239.89▲
organ of Zuckerkandl	194.6	198.89	–	227.6	237.3	239.7
oropharynx	146.9	198.89	230.0	210.6	235.1	239.0
branchial cleft (vestige)	146.8	198.89	230.0	210.6	235.1	239.0
contiguous sites	146.8	–	–	–	–	–
junctional region	146.5	198.89	230.0	210.6	235.1	239.0
lateral wall	146.6	198.89	230.0	210.6	235.1	239.0
pillars of fauces	146.2	198.89	230.0	210.6	235.1	239.0
posterior wall	146.7	198.89	230.0	210.6	235.1	239.0
specified part NEC	146.8	198.89	230.0	210.6	235.1	239.0
vallecula	146.3	198.89	230.0	210.6	235.1	239.0
os						
external	180.1	198.82	233.1	219.0	236.0	239.5
internal	180.0	198.82	233.1	219.0	236.0	239.5
ovary	183.0	198.6	233.39	220	236.2	239.5
oviduct	183.2	198.82	233.39	221.0	236.3	239.5
palate	145.5	198.89	230.0	210.4	235.1	239.0
hard	145.2	198.89	230.0	210.4	235.1	239.0
junction of hard and soft palate	145.5	198.89	230.0	210.4	235.1	239.0
soft	145.3	198.89	230.0	210.4	235.1	239.0
nasopharyngeal surface	147.3	198.89	230.0	210.7	235.1	239.0
posterior surface	147.3	198.89	230.0	210.7	235.1	239.0
superior surface	147.3	198.89	230.0	210.7	235.1	239.0
palatoglossal arch	146.2	198.89	230.0	210.6	235.1	239.0
palatopharyngeal arch	146.2	198.89	230.0	210.6	235.1	239.0
pallium	191.0	198.3	–	225.0	237.5	239.6
palpebra	173.1	198.2	232.1	216.1	238.2	239.2
pancreas	157.9	197.8	230.9	211.6	235.5	239.0
body	157.1	197.8	230.9	211.6	235.5	239.0
contiguous sites	157.8	–	–	–	–	–
duct (of Santorini) (of Wirsung)	157.3	197.8	230.9	211.6	235.5	239.0
ectopic tissue	157.8	197.8	230.9	211.6	235.5	239.0
head	157.0	197.8	230.9	211.6	235.5	239.0
islet cells	157.4	197.8	230.9	211.7	235.5	239.0
neck	157.8	197.8	230.9	211.6	235.5	239.0
tail	157.2	197.8	230.9	211.6	235.5	239.0
para-aortic body	194.6	198.89	–	227.6	237.3	239.7
paraganglion NEC	194.6	198.89	–	227.6	237.3	239.7
parametrium	183.4	198.82	–	221.0	236.3	239.5
paranephric	158.0	197.6	–	211.8	235.4	239.0
pararectal	195.3	198.89	–	229.8	238.8	239.89▲
parasagittal (region)	195.0	198.89	234.8	229.8	238.8	239.89▲
parasellar	192.9	198.4	–	225.9	237.9	239.7
parathyroid (gland)	194.1	198.89	234.8	227.1	237.4	239.7
paraurethral	195.3	198.89	–	229.8	238.8	239.89▲
gland	189.4	198.1	233.9	223.89	236.99	239.5
paravaginal	195.3	198.89	–	229.8	238.8	239.8
parenchyma, kidney	189.0	198.0	233.9	223.0	236.91	239.5
parietal						
bone	170.0	198.5	–	213.0	238.0	239.2
lobe, brain	191.3	198.3	–	225.0	237.5	239.6
paroophoron	183.3	198.82	233.39	221.0	236.3	239.5
parotid (duct) (gland)	142.0	198.89	230.0	210.2	235.0	239.0
parovarium	183.3	198.82	233.39	221.0	236.3	239.5
patella	170.8	198.5	–	213.8	238.0	239.2
peduncle, cerebral	191.7	198.3	–	225.0	237.5	239.6
pelvirectal junction	154.0	197.5	230.4	211.4	235.2	239.0
pelvis, pelvic	195.3	198.89	234.8	229.8	238.8	239.89▲
bone	170.6	198.5	–	213.6	238.0	239.2
floor	195.3	198.89	234.8	229.8	238.8	239.89▲
renal	189.1	198.0	233.9	223.1	236.91	239.5
viscera	195.3	198.89	234.8	229.8	238.8	239.89▲
wall	195.3	198.89	234.8	229.8	238.8	239.89▲
pelvo-abdominal	195.8	198.89	234.8	229.8	238.8	239.89▲
penis	187.4	198.82	233.5	222.1	236.6	239.5
body	187.3	198.82	233.5	222.1	236.6	239.5
corpus (cavernosum)	187.3	198.82	233.5	222.1	236.6	239.5
glans	187.2	198.82	233.5	222.1	236.6	239.5
skin NEC	187.4	198.82	233.5	222.1	236.6	239.5
periadrenal (tissue)	158.0	197.6	–	211.8	235.4	239.0
perianal (skin)	173.5	198.2	232.5	216.5	238.2	239.2
pericardium	164.1	198.89	–	212.7	238.9	239.89▲
perinephric	158.0	197.6	–	211.8	235.4	239.0
perineum	195.3	198.89	234.8	229.8	238.8	239.89▲
periodontal tissue NEC	143.9	198.89	230.0	210.4	235.1	239.0
periosteum – *see* Neoplasm, bone						
peripancreatic	158.0	197.6	–	211.8	235.4	239.0
peripheral nerve NEC	171.9	198.89	–	215.9	238.1	239.2
perirectal (tissue)	195.3	198.89	–	229.8	238.8	239.89▲
perirenal (tissue)	158.0	197.6	–	211.8	235.4	239.0
peritoneum, peritoneal (cavity)	158.9	197.6	–	211.8	235.4	239.0
contiguous sites	158.8	–	–	–	–	–
with digestive organs	159.8	–	–	–	–	–
parietal	158.8	197.6	–	211.8	235.4	239.0
pelvic	158.8	197.6	–	211.8	235.4	239.0
specified part NEC	158.8	197.6	–	211.8	235.4	239.0
peritonsillar (tissue)	195.0	198.89	234.8	229.8	238.8	239.89▲
periurethral tissue	195.3	198.89	–	229.8	238.8	239.89▲
phalanges	170.9	198.5	–	213.9	238.0	239.2
foot	170.8	198.5	–	213.8	238.0	239.2
hand	170.5	198.5	–	213.5	238.0	239.2
pharynx, pharyngeal	149.0	198.89	230.0	210.9	235.1	239.0
bursa	147.1	198.89	230.0	210.7	235.1	239.0
fornix	147.3	198.89	230.0	210.7	235.1	239.0
recess	147.2	198.89	230.0	210.7	235.1	239.0
region	149.0	198.89	230.0	210.9	235.1	239.0
tonsil	147.1	198.89	230.0	210.7	235.1	239.0
wall (lateral) (posterior)	149.0	198.89	230.0	210.9	235.1	239.0
pia mater (cerebral) (cranial)	192.1	198.4	–	225.2	237.6	239.7
spinal	192.3	198.4	–	225.4	237.6	239.7
pillars of fauces	146.2	198.89	230.0	210.6	235.1	239.0
pineal (body) (gland)	194.4	198.89	234.8	227.4	237.1	239.7
pinna (ear) NEC	173.2	198.2	232.2	216.2	238.2	239.2
cartilage	171.0	198.89	–	215.0	238.1	239.2

Neoplasm, neoplastic	Malignant: Primary	Malignant: Secondary	Malignant: Carcinoma in situ	Benign	Uncertain Behavior	Unspecified
piriform fossa or sinus	148.1	198.89	230.0	210.8	235.1	239.0
pituitary (body) (fossa) (gland) (lobe)	194.3	198.89	234.8	227.3	237.0	239.7
placenta	181	198.82	233.2	219.8	236.1	239.5
pleura, pleural (cavity)	163.9	197.2	–	212.4	235.8	239.1
contiguous sites	163.8	–	–	–	–	–
parietal	163.0	197.2	–	212.4	235.8	239.1
visceral	163.1	197.2	–	212.4	235.8	239.1
plexus						
brachial	171.2	198.89	–	215.2	238.1	239.2
cervical	171.0	198.89	–	215.0	238.1	239.2
choroid	191.5	198.3	–	225.0	237.5	239.6
lumbosacral	171.6	198.89	–	215.6	238.1	239.2
sacral	171.6	198.89	–	215.6	238.1	239.2
pluri-endocrine	194.8	198.89	234.8	227.8	237.4	239.7
pole						
frontal	191.1	198.3	–	225.0	237.5	239.6
occipital	191.4	198.3	–	225.0	237.5	239.6
pons (varolii)	191.7	198.3	–	225.0	237.5	239.6
popliteal fossa or space*	195.5	198.89	234.8	229.8	238.8	239.89▲
postcricoid (region)	148.0	198.89	230.0	210.8	235.1	239.0
posterior fossa (cranial)	191.9	198.3	–	225.0	237.5	239.6
postnasal space	147.9	198.89	230.0	210.7	235.1	239.0
prepuce	187.1	198.82	233.5	222.1	236.6	239.5
prepylorus	151.1	197.8	230.2	211.1	235.2	239.0
presacral (region)	195.3	198.89	–	229.8	238.8	239.89▲
prostate (gland)	185	198.82	233.4	222.2	236.5	239.5
utricle	189.3	198.1	233.9	223.81	236.99	239.5
pterygoid fossa	171.0	198.89	–	215.0	238.1	239.2
pubic bone	170.6	198.5	–	213.6	238.0	239.2
pudenda, pudendum (female)	184.4	198.82	233.32	221.2	236.3	239.5
pulmonary	162.9	197.0	231.2	212.3	235.7	239.1
putamen	191.0	198.3	–	225.0	237.5	239.6
pyloric						
antrum	151.2	197.8	230.2	211.1	235.2	239.0
canal	151.1	197.8	230.2	211.1	235.2	239.0
pylorus	151.1	197.8	230.2	211.1	235.2	239.0
pyramid (brain)	191.7	198.3	–	225.0	237.5	239.6
pyriform fossa or sinus	148.1	198.89	230.0	210.8	235.1	239.0
radius (any part)	170.4	198.5	–	213.4	238.0	239.2
Rathke's pouch	194.3	198.89	234.8	227.3	237.0	239.7
rectosigmoid (colon) (junction)	154.0	197.5	230.4	211.4	235.2	239.0
contiguous sites with anus or rectum	154.8	–	–	–	–	–
rectouterine pouch	158.8	197.6	–	211.8	235.4	239.0
rectovaginal septum or wall	195.3	198.89	234.8	229.8	238.8	239.89▲
rectovesical septum	195.3	198.89	234.8	229.8	238.8	239.89▲
rectum (ampulla)	154.1	197.5	230.4	211.4	235.2	239.0
and colon	154.0	197.5	230.4	211.4	235.2	239.0
contiguous sites with anus or rectosigmoid junction	154.8	–	–	–	–	–
renal	189.0	198.0	233.9	223.0	236.91	239.5
calyx	189.1	198.0	233.9	223.1	236.91	239.5
hilus	189.1	198.0	233.9	223.1	236.91	239.5
parenchyma	189.0	198.0	233.9	223.0	236.91	239.5
pelvis	189.1	198.0	233.9	223.1	236.91	239.5
respiratory						
organs or system NEC	165.9	197.3	231.9	212.9	235.9	239.1
contiguous sites with intrathoracic organs	165.8	–	–	–	–	–
specified sites NEC	165.8	197.3	231.8	212.8	235.9	239.1
tract NEC	165.9	197.3	231.9	212.9	235.9	239.1
upper	165.0	197.3	231.9	212.9	235.9	239.1
retina	190.5	198.4	234.0	224.5	238.8	239.81▲
retrobulbar	190.1	198.4	–	224.1	238.8	239.89▲
retrocecal	158.0	197.6	–	211.8	235.4	239.0
retromolar (area) (traingle) (trigone)	145.6	198.89	230.0	210.4	235.1	239.0
retro-orbital	195.0	198.89	234.8	229.8	238.8	239.89▲
retroperitoneal (space) (tissue)	158.0	197.6	–	211.8	235.4	239.0
contiguous sites	158.8	–	–	–	–	–
retroperitoneum	158.0	197.6	–	211.8	235.4	239.0
contiguous sites	158.8	–	–	–	–	–
retropharyngeal	149.0	198.89	230.0	210.9	235.1	239.0
retrovesical (septum)	195.3	198.89	234.8	229.8	238.8	239.89▲
rhinencephalon	191.0	198.3	–	225.0	237.5	239.6
rib	170.3	198.5	–	213.3	238.0	239.2
Rosenmüller's fossa	147.2	198.89	230.0	210.7	235.1	239.0
round ligament	183.5	198.82	–	221.0	236.3	239.5

Neoplasm, neoplastic	Malignant: Primary	Malignant: Secondary	Malignant: Carcinoma in situ	Benign	Uncertain Behavior	Unspecified
sacrococcyx, sacrococcygeal	170.6	198.5	–	213.6	238.0	239.2
region	195.3	198.89	234.8	229.8	238.8	239.89▲
sacrouterine ligament	183.4	198.82	–	221.0	236.3	239.5
sacrum, sacral (vertebra)	170.6	198.5	–	213.6	238.0	239.2
salivary gland or duct (major)	142.9	198.89	230.0	210.2	235.0	239.0
contiguous sites	142.8	–	–	–	–	–
minor NEC	145.9	198.89	230.0	210.4	235.1	239.0
parotid	142.0	198.89	230.0	210.2	235.0	239.0
pluriglandular	142.8	198.89	230.0	210.2	235.0	239.0
sublingual	142.2	198.89	230.0	210.2	235.0	239.0
submandibular	142.1	198.89	230.0	210.2	235.0	239.0
submaxillary	142.1	198.89	230.0	210.2	235.0	239.0
salpinx (uterine)	183.2	198.82	233.39	221.0	236.3	239.5
Santorini's duct	157.3	197.8	230.9	211.6	235.5	239.0
scalp	173.4	198.2	232.4	216.4	238.2	239.2
scapula (any part)	170.4	198.5	–	213.4	238.0	239.2
scapular region	195.1	198.89	234.8	229.8	238.8	239.89▲
scar NEC (*see also* Neoplasm, skin)	173.9	198.2	232.9	216.9	238.2	239.2
sciatic nerve	171.3	198.89	–	215.3	238.1	239.2
sclera	190.0	198.4	234.0	224.0	238.8	239.89▲
scrotum (skin)	187.7	198.82	233.6	222.4	236.6	239.5
sebaceous gland – *see* Neoplasm, skin						
sella turcica	194.3	198.89	234.8	227.3	237.0	239.7
bone	170.0	198.5	–	213.0	238.0	239.2
semilunar cartilage (knee)	170.7	198.5	–	213.7	238.0	239.2
seminal vesicle	187.8	198.82	233.6	222.8	236.6	239.5
septum						
nasal	160.0	197.3	231.8	212.0	235.9	239.1
posterior margin	147.3	198.89	230.0	210.7	235.1	239.0
rectovaginal	195.3	198.89	234.8	229.8	238.8	239.89▲
rectovesical	195.3	198.89	234.8	229.8	238.8	239.89▲
urethrovaginal	184.9	198.82	233.39	221.9	236.3	239.5
vesicovaginal	184.9	198.82	233.39	221.9	236.3	239.5
shoulder NEC*	195.4	198.89	232.6	229.8	238.8	239.89▲
sigmoid flexure (lower) (upper)	153.3	197.5	230.3	211.3	235.2	239.0
sinus (accessory)	160.9	197.3	231.8	212.0	235.9	239.1
bone (any)	170.0	198.5	–	213.0	238.0	239.2
contiguous sites with middle ear or nasal cavities	160.8	–	–	–	–	–
ethmoidal	160.3	197.3	231.8	212.0	235.9	239.1
frontal	160.4	197.3	231.8	212.0	235.9	239.1
maxillary	160.2	197.3	231.8	212.0	235.9	239.1
nasal, paranasal NEC	160.9	197.3	231.8	212.0	235.9	239.1
pyriform	148.1	198.89	230.0	210.8	235.1	239.0
sphenoidal	160.5	197.3	231.8	212.0	235.9	239.1
skeleton, skeletal NEC	170.9	198.5	–	213.9	238.0	239.2
Skene's gland	189.4	198.1	233.9	223.89	236.99	239.5
skin NEC	173.9	198.2	232.9	216.9	238.2	239.2
abdominal wall	173.5	198.2	232.5	216.5	238.2	239.2
ala nasi	173.3	198.2	232.3	216.3	238.2	239.2
ankle	173.7	198.2	232.7	216.7	238.2	239.2
antecubital space	173.6	198.2	232.6	216.6	238.2	239.2
anus	173.5	198.2	232.5	216.5	238.2	239.2
arm	173.6	198.2	232.6	216.6	238.2	239.2
auditory canal (external)	173.2	198.2	232.2	216.2	238.2	239.2
auricle (ear)	173.2	198.2	232.2	216.2	238.2	239.2
auricular canal (external)	173.2	198.2	232.2	216.2	238.2	239.2
axilla, axillary fold	173.5	198.2	232.5	216.5	238.2	239.2
back	173.5	198.2	232.5	216.5	238.2	239.2
breast	173.5	198.2	232.5	216.5	238.2	239.2
brow	173.3	198.2	232.3	216.3	238.2	239.2
buttock	173.5	198.2	232.5	216.5	238.2	239.2
calf	173.7	198.2	232.7	216.7	238.2	239.2
canthus (eye) (inner) (outer)	173.1	198.2	232.1	216.1	238.2	239.2
cervical region	173.4	198.2	232.4	216.4	238.2	239.2
cheek (external)	173.3	198.2	232.3	216.3	238.2	239.2
chest (wall)	173.5	198.2	232.5	216.5	238.2	239.2
chin	173.3	198.2	232.3	216.3	238.2	239.2
clavicular area	173.5	198.2	232.5	216.5	238.2	239.2
clitoris	184.3	198.82	233.32	221.2	236.3	239.5
columnella	173.3	198.2	232.3	216.3	238.2	239.2
concha	173.2	198.2	232.2	216.2	238.2	239.2
contiguous sites	173.8	–	–	–	–	–
ear (external)	173.2	198.2	232.2	216.2	238.2	239.2
elbow	173.6	198.2	232.6	216.6	238.2	239.2
eyebrow	173.3	198.2	232.3	216.3	238.2	239.2
eyelid	173.1	198.2	232.1	216.1	238.2	239.2

Neoplasm, neoplastic	Malignant					
	Primary	Secondary	Carcinoma in situ	Benign	Uncertain Behavior	Unspecified
skin – *continued*						
face NEC	173.3	198.2	232.3	216.3	238.2	239.2
female genital organs (external)	184.4	198.82	233.30	221.2	236.3	239.5
clitoris	184.3	198.82	233.32	221.2	236.3	239.5
labium NEC	184.4	198.82	233.32	221.2	236.3	239.5
majus	184.1	198.82	233.32	221.2	236.3	239.5
minus	184.2	198.82	233.32	221.2	236.3	239.5
pudendum	184.4	198.82	233.32	221.2	236.3	239.5
vulva	184.4	198.82	233.32	221.2	236.3	239.5
finger	173.6	198.2	232.6	216.6	238.2	239.2
flank	173.5	198.2	232.5	216.5	238.2	239.2
foot	173.7	198.2	232.7	216.7	238.2	239.2
forearm	173.6	198.2	232.6	216.6	238.2	239.2
forehead	173.3	198.2	232.3	216.3	238.2	239.2
glabella	173.3	198.2	232.3	216.3	238.2	239.2
gluteal region	173.5	198.2	232.5	216.5	238.2	239.2
groin	173.5	198.2	232.5	216.5	238.2	239.2
hand	173.6	198.2	232.6	216.6	238.2	239.2
head NEC	173.4	198.2	232.4	216.4	238.2	239.2
heel	173.7	198.2	232.7	216.7	238.2	239.2
helix	173.2	198.2	232.2	216.2	238.2	239.2
hip	173.7	198.2	232.7	216.7	238.2	239.2
infraclavicular region	173.5	198.2	232.5	216.5	238.2	239.2
inguinal region	173.5	198.2	232.5	216.5	238.2	239.2
jaw	173.3	198.2	232.3	216.3	238.2	239.2
knee	173.7	198.2	232.7	216.7	238.2	239.2
labia						
majora	184.1	198.82	233.32	221.2	236.3	239.5
minora	184.2	198.82	233.32	221.2	236.3	239.5
leg	173.7	198.2	232.7	216.7	238.2	239.2
lid (lower) (upper)	173.1	198.2	232.1	216.1	238.2	239.2
limb NEC	173.9	198.2	232.9	216.9	238.2	239.5
lower	173.7	198.2	232.7	216.7	238.2	239.2
upper	173.6	198.2	232.6	216.6	238.2	239.2
lip (lower) (upper)	173.0	198.2	232.0	216.0	238.2	239.2
male genital organs	187.9	198.82	233.6	222.9	236.6	239.5
penis	187.4	198.82	233.5	222.1	236.6	239.5
prepuce	187.1	198.82	233.5	222.1	236.6	239.5
scrotum	187.7	198.82	233.6	222.4	236.6	239.5
mastectomy site	173.5	198.2	–	–	–	–
specified as breast tissue	174.8	198.81	–	–	–	–
meatus, acoustic (external)	173.2	198.2	232.2	216.2	238.2	239.2
nates	173.5	198.2	232.5	216.5	238.2	239.2
neck	173.4	198.2	232.4	216.4	238.2	239.2
nose (external)	173.3	198.2	232.3	216.3	238.2	239.2
palm	173.6	198.2	232.6	216.6	238.2	239.2
palpebra	173.1	198.2	232.1	216.1	238.2	239.2
penis NEC	187.4	198.82	233.5	222.1	236.6	239.5
perianal	173.5	198.2	232.5	216.5	238.2	239.2
perineum	173.5	198.2	232.5	216.5	238.2	239.2
pinna	173.2	198.2	232.2	216.2	238.2	239.2
plantar	173.7	198.2	232.7	216.7	238.2	239.2
popliteal fossa or space	173.7	198.2	232.7	216.7	238.2	239.2
prepuce	187.1	198.82	233.5	222.1	236.6	239.5
pubes	173.5	198.2	232.5	216.5	238.2	239.2
sacrococcygeal region	173.5	198.2	232.5	216.5	238.2	239.2
scalp	173.4	198.2	232.4	216.4	238.2	239.2
scapular region	173.5	198.2	232.5	216.5	238.2	239.2
scrotum	187.7	198.82	233.6	222.4	236.6	239.5
shoulder	173.6	198.2	232.6	216.6	238.2	239.2
sole (foot)	173.7	198.2	232.7	216.7	238.2	239.2
specified sites NEC	173.8	198.2	232.8	216.8	232.8	239.2
submammary fold	173.5	198.2	232.5	216.5	238.2	239.2
supraclavicular region	173.4	198.2	232.4	216.4	238.2	239.2
temple	173.3	198.2	232.3	216.3	238.2	239.2
thigh	173.7	198.2	232.7	216.7	238.2	239.2
thoracic wall	173.5	198.2	232.5	216.5	238.2	239.2
thumb	173.6	198.2	232.6	216.6	238.2	239.2
toe	173.7	198.2	232.7	216.7	238.2	239.2
tragus	173.2	198.2	232.2	216.2	238.2	239.2
trunk	173.5	198.2	232.5	216.5	238.2	239.2
umbilicus	173.5	198.2	232.5	216.5	238.2	239.2
vulva	184.4	198.82	233.32	221.2	236.3	239.5
wrist	173.6	198.2	232.6	216.6	238.2	239.2
skull	170.0	198.5	–	213.0	238.0	239.2
soft parts or tissues – *see* Neoplasm, connective tissue						
specified site NEC	195.8	198.89	234.8	229.8	238.8	239.89▲
spermatic cord	187.6	198.82	233.6	222.8	236.6	239.5
sphenoid	160.5	197.3	231.8	212.0	235.9	239.1
bone	170.0	198.5	–	213.0	238.0	239.2
sinus	160.5	197.3	231.8	212.0	235.9	239.1

Neoplasm, neoplastic	Malignant					
	Primary	Secondary	Carcinoma in situ	Benign	Uncertain Behavior	Unspecified
sphincter						
anal	154.2	197.5	230.5	211.4	235.5	239.0
of Oddi	156.1	197.8	230.8	211.5	235.3	239.0
spine, spinal (column)	170.2	198.5	–	213.2	238.0	239.2
bulb	191.7	198.3	–	225.0	237.5	239.6
coccyx	170.6	198.5	–	213.6	238.0	239.2
cord (cervical) (lumbar) (sacral) (thoracic)	192.2	198.3	–	225.3	237.5	239.7
dura mater	192.3	198.4	–	225.4	237.6	239.7
lumbosacral	170.2	198.5	–	213.2	238.0	239.2
membrane	192.3	198.4	–	225.4	237.6	239.7
meninges	192.3	198.4	–	225.4	237.6	239.7
nerve (root)	171.9	198.89	–	215.9	238.1	239.2
pia mater	192.3	198.4	–	225.4	237.6	239.7
root	171.9	198.89	–	215.9	238.1	239.2
sacrum	170.6	198.5	–	213.6	238.0	239.2
spleen, splenic NEC	159.1	197.8	230.9	211.9	235.5	239.0
flexure (colon)	153.7	197.5	230.3	211.3	235.2	239.0
stem, brain	191.7	198.3	–	225.0	237.5	239.6
Stensen's duct	142.0	198.89	230.0	210.2	235.0	239.0
sternum	170.3	198.5	–	213.3	238.0	239.2
stomach	151.9	197.8	230.2	211.1	235.2	239.0
antrum (pyloric)	151.2	197.8	230.2	211.1	235.2	239.0
body	151.4	197.8	230.2	211.1	235.2	239.0
cardia	151.0	197.8	230.2	211.1	235.2	239.0
cardiac orifice	151.0	197.8	230.2	211.1	235.2	239.0
contiguous sites	151.8	–	–	–	–	–
corpus	151.4	197.8	230.2	211.1	235.2	239.0
fundus	151.3	197.8	230.2	211.1	235.2	239.0
greater curvature NEC	151.6	197.8	230.2	211.1	235.2	239.0
lesser curvature NEC	151.5	197.8	230.2	211.1	235.2	239.0
prepylorus	151.1	197.8	230.2	211.1	235.2	239.0
pylorus	151.1	197.8	230.2	211.1	235.2	239.0
wall NEC	151.9	197.8	230.2	211.1	235.2	239.0
anterior NEC	151.8	197.8	230.2	211.1	235.2	239.0
posterior NEC	151.8	197.8	230.2	211.1	235.2	239.0
stroma, endometrial	182.0	198.82	233.2	219.1	236.0	239.5
stump, cervical	180.8	198.82	233.1	219.0	236.0	239.5
subcutaneous (nodule) (tissue) NEC – *see* Neoplasm, connective tissue						
subdural	192.1	198.4	–	225.2	237.6	239.7
subglottis, subglottic	161.2	197.3	231.0	212.1	235.6	239.1
sublingual	144.9	198.89	230.0	210.3	235.1	239.0
gland or duct	142.2	198.89	230.0	210.2	235.0	239.0
submandibular gland	142.1	198.89	230.0	210.2	235.0	239.0
submaxillary gland or duct	142.1	198.89	230.0	210.2	235.0	239.0
submental	195.0	198.89	234.8	229.8	238.8	239.89▲
subpleural	162.9	197.0	–	212.3	235.7	239.1
substernal	164.2	197.1	–	212.5	235.8	239.89▲
sudoriferous, sudoriparous gland, site unspecified	173.9	198.2	232.9	216.9	238.2	239.2
specified site – *see* Neoplasm, skin						
supraclavicular region	195.0	198.89	234.8	229.8	238.8	239.89▲
supraglottis	161.1	197.3	231.0	212.1	235.6	239.1
suprarenal (capsule) (cortex) (gland) (medulla)	194.0	198.7	234.8	227.0	237.2	239.7
suprasellar (region)	191.9	198.3	–	225.0	237.5	239.6
sweat gland (apocrine) (eccrine), site unspecified	173.9	198.2	232.9	216.9	238.2	239.2
specified site – *see* Neoplasm, skin						
sympathetic nerve or nervous system NEC	171.9	198.89	–	215.9	238.1	239.2
symphysis pubis	170.6	198.5	–	213.6	238.0	239.2
synovial membrane – *see* Neoplasm, connective tissue						
tapetum, brain	191.8	198.3	–	225.0	237.5	239.6
tarsus (any bone)	170.8	198.5	–	213.8	238.0	239.2
temple (skin)	173.3	198.2	232.3	216.3	238.2	239.2
temporal						
bone	170.0	198.5	–	213.0	238.0	239.2
lobe or pole	191.2	198.3	–	225.0	237.5	239.6
region	195.0	198.89	234.8	229.8	238.8	239.89▲
skin	173.3	198.2	232.3	216.3	238.2	239.2
tendon (sheath) – *see* Neoplasm, connective tissue						
tentorium (cerebelli)	192.1	198.4	–	225.2	237.6	239.7

Neoplasm, neoplastic	Malignant: Primary	Malignant: Secondary	Malignant: Carcinoma in situ	Benign	Uncertain Behavior	Unspecifed
testis, testes (descended) (scrotal)	186.9	198.82	233.6	222.0	236.4	239.5
ectopic	186.0	198.82	233.6	222.0	236.4	239.5
retained	186.0	198.82	233.6	222.0	236.4	239.5
undescended	186.0	198.82	233.6	222.0	236.4	239.5
thalamus	191.0	198.3	–	225.0	237.5	239.6
thigh NEC*	195.5	198.89	234.8	229.8	238.8	239.89▲
thorax, thoracic (cavity) (organs NEC)	195.1	198.89	234.8	229.8	238.8	239.89▲
duct	171.4	198.89	–	215.4	238.1	239.2
wall NEC	195.1	198.89	234.8	229.8	238.8	239.89▲
throat	149.0	198.89	230.0	210.9	235.1	239.0
thumb NEC*	195.4	198.89	232.6	229.8	238.8	239.89▲
thymus (gland)	164.0	198.89	–	212.6	235.8	239.89▲
contiguous sites with heart and mediastinum	164.8	–	–	–	–	–
thyroglossal duct	193	198.89	234.8	226	237.4	239.7
thyroid (gland)	193	198.89	234.8	226	237.4	239.7
cartilage	161.3	197.3	231.0	212.1	235.6	239.1
tibia (any part)	170.7	198.5	–	213.7	238.0	239.2
toe NEC*	195.5	198.89	232.7	229.8	238.8	239.89▲
tongue	141.9	198.89	230.0	210.1	235.1	239.0
anterior (two-thirds) NEC	141.4	198.89	230.0	210.1	235.1	239.0
dorsal surface	141.1	198.89	230.0	210.1	235.1	239.0
ventral surface	141.3	198.89	230.0	210.1	235.1	239.0
base (dorsal surface)	141.0	198.89	230.0	210.1	235.1	239.0
border (lateral)	141.2	198.89	230.0	210.1	235.1	239.0
contiguous sites	141.8	–	–	–	–	–
dorsal surface NEC	141.1	198.89	230.0	210.1	235.1	239.0
fixed part NEC	141.0	198.89	230.0	210.1	235.1	239.0
foreamen cecum	141.1	198.89	230.0	210.1	235.1	239.0
frenulum linguae	141.3	198.89	230.0	210.1	235.1	239.0
junctional zone	141.5	198.89	230.0	210.1	235.1	239.0
margin (lateral)	141.2	198.89	230.0	210.1	235.1	239.0
midline NEC	141.1	198.89	230.0	210.1	235.1	239.0
mobile part NEC	141.4	198.89	230.0	210.1	235.1	239.0
posterior (third)	141.0	198.89	230.0	210.1	235.1	239.0
root	141.0	198.89	230.0	210.1	235.1	239.0
surface (dorsal)	141.1	198.89	230.0	210.1	235.1	239.0
base	141.0	198.89	230.0	210.1	235.1	239.0
ventral	141.3	198.89	230.0	210.1	235.1	239.0
tip	141.2	198.89	230.0	210.1	235.1	239.0
tonsil	141.6	198.89	230.0	210.1	235.1	239.0
tonsil	146.0	198.89	230.0	210.5	235.1	239.0
fauces, faucial	146.0	198.89	230.0	210.5	235.1	239.0
lingual	141.6	198.89	230.0	210.1	235.1	239.0
palatine	146.0	198.89	230.0	210.5	235.1	239.0
pharyngeal	147.1	198.89	230.0	210.7	235.1	239.0
pillar (anterior) (posterior)	146.2	198.89	230.0	210.6	235.1	239.0
tonsillar fossa	146.1	198.89	230.0	210.6	235.1	239.0
tooth socket NEC	143.9	198.89	230.0	210.4	235.1	239.0
trachea (cartilage) (mucosa)	162.0	197.3	231.1	212.2	235.7	239.1
contiguous sites with bronchus or lung	162.8	–	–	–	–	–
tracheobronchial	162.8	197.3	231.1	212.2	235.7	239.1
contiguous sites with lung	162.8	–	–	–	–	–
tragus	173.2	198.2	232.2	216.2	238.2	239.2
trunk NEC*	195.8	198.89	232.5	229.8	238.8	239.89▲
tubo-ovarian	183.8	198.82	233.39	221.8	236.3	239.5
tunica vaginalis	187.8	198.82	233.6	222.8	236.6	239.5
turbinate (bone)	170.0	198.5	–	213.0	238.0	239.2
nasal	160.0	197.3	231.8	212.0	235.9	239.1
tympanic cavity	160.1	197.3	231.8	212.0	235.9	239.1
ulna (any part)	170.4	198.5	–	213.4	238.0	239.2
umbilicus, umbilical	173.5	198.2	232.5	216.5	238.2	239.2
uncus, brain	191.2	198.3	–	225.0	237.5	239.6
unknown site or unspecified	199.1	199.1	234.9	229.9	238.9	239.9
urachus	188.7	198.1	233.7	223.3	236.7	239.4
ureter, ureteral	189.2	198.1	233.9	223.2	236.91	239.5
orifice (bladder)	188.6	198.1	233.7	223.3	236.7	239.4
ureter-bladder (junction)	188.6	198.1	233.7	223.3	236.7	239.4
urethra, urethral (gland)	189.3	198.1	233.9	223.81	236.99	239.5
orifice, internal	188.5	198.1	233.7	223.3	236.7	239.4
urethrovaginal (septum)	184.9	198.82	233.39	221.9	236.3	239.5
urinary organ or system NEC	189.9	198.1	233.9	223.9	236.99	239.5
bladder – *see* Neoplasm, bladder						
contiguous sites	189.8	–	–	–	–	–
specified sites NEC	189.8	198.1	233.9	223.89	236.99	239.5
utero-ovarian	183.8	198.82	233.39	221.8	236.3	239.5
ligament	183.3	198.82	–	221.0	236.3	239.5
uterosacral ligament	183.4	198.82	–	221.0	236.3	239.5

Neoplasm, neoplastic	Malignant: Primary	Malignant: Secondary	Malignant: Carcinoma in situ	Benign	Uncertain Behavior	Unspecifed
uterus, uteri, uterine	179	198.82	233.2	219.9	236.0	239.5
adnexa NEC	183.9	198.82	233.39	221.8	236.3	239.5
contiguous sites	183.8	–	–	–	–	–
body	182.0	198.82	233.2	219.1	236.0	239.5
contiguous sites	182.8	–	–	–	–	–
cervix	180.9	198.82	233.1	219.0	236.0	239.5
cornu	182.0	198.82	233.2	219.1	236.0	239.5
corpus	182.0	198.82	233.2	219.1	236.0	239.5
endocervix (canal) (gland)	180.0	198.82	233.1	219.0	236.0	239.5
endometrium	182.0	198.82	233.2	219.1	236.0	239.5
exocervix	180.1	198.82	233.1	219.0	236.0	239.5
external os	180.1	198.82	233.1	219.0	236.0	239.5
fundus	182.0	198.82	233.2	219.1	236.0	239.5
internal os	180.0	198.82	233.1	219.0	236.0	239.5
isthmus	182.1	198.82	233.2	219.1	236.0	239.5
ligament	183.4	198.82	–	221.0	236.3	239.5
broad	183.3	198.82	233.39	221.0	236.3	239.5
round	183.5	198.82	–	221.0	236.3	239.5
lower segment	182.1	198.82	233.2	219.1	236.0	239.5
myometrium	182.0	198.82	233.2	219.1	236.0	239.5
squamocolumnar junction	180.8	198.82	233.1	219.0	236.0	239.5
tube	183.2	198.82	233.39	221.0	236.3	239.5
utricle, prostatic	189.3	198.1	233.9	223.81	236.99	239.5
uveal tract	190.0	198.4	234.0	224.0	238.8	239.89▲
uvula	145.4	198.89	230.0	210.4	235.1	239.0
vagina, vaginal (fornix) (vault) (wall)	184.0	198.82	233.31	221.1	236.3	239.5
vaginovesical	184.9	198.82	233.39	221.9	236.3	239.5
septum	184.9	198.82	233.39	221.9	236.3	239.5
vallecula (epigiottis)	146.3	198.89	230.0	210.6	235.1	239.0
vascular – *see* Neoplasm, connective tissue						
vas deferens	187.6	198.82	233.6	222.8	236.6	239.5
Vater's ampulla	156.2	197.8	230.8	211.5	235.3	239.0
vein, venous – *see* Neoplasm, connective tissue						
vena cava (abdominal) (inferior)	171.5	198.89	–	215.5	238.1	239.2
superior	171.4	198.89	–	215.4	238.1	239.2
ventricle (cerebral) (floor) (fourth) (lateral) (third)	191.5	198.3	–	225.0	237.5	239.6
cardiac (left) (right)	164.1	198.89	–	212.7	238.8	239.89▲
ventricular band of larynx	161.1	197.3	231.0	212.1	235.6	239.1
ventriculus – *see* Neoplasm, stomach						
vermillion border – *see* Neoplasm, lip						
vermis, cerebellum	191.6	198.3	–	225.0	237.5	239.6
vertebra (column)	170.2	198.5	–	213.2	238.0	239.2
coccyx	170.6	198.5	–	213.6	238.0	239.2
sacrum	170.6	198.5	–	213.6	238.0	239.2
vesical – *see* Neoplasm, bladder						
vesicle, seminal	187.8	198.82	233.6	222.8	236.6	239.5
vesicocervical tissue	184.9	198.82	233.39	221.9	236.3	239.5
vesicorectal	195.3	198.89	234.8	229.8	238.8	239.89▲
vesicovaginal	184.9	198.82	233.39	221.9	236.3	239.5
septum	184.9	198.82	233.39	221.9	236.3	239.5
vessel (blood) – *see* Neoplasm, connective tissue						
vestibular gland, greater	184.1	198.82	233.32	221.2	236.3	239.5
vestibule						
mouth	145.1	198.89	230.0	210.4	235.1	239.0
nose	160.0	197.3	231.8	212.0	235.9	239.1
Virchow's gland	–	196.0	–	229.0	238.8	239.89▲
viscera NEC	195.8	198.89	234.8	229.8	238.8	239.89▲
vocal cords (true)	161.0	197.3	231.0	212.1	235.6	239.1
false	161.1	197.3	231.0	212.1	235.6	239.1
vomer	170.0	198.5	–	213.0	238.0	239.2
vulva	184.4	198.82	233.32	221.2	236.3	239.5
vulvovaginal gland	184.4	198.82	233.32	221.2	236.3	239.5
Waldeyer's ring	149.1	198.89	230.0	210.9	235.1	239.0
Wharton's duct	142.1	198.89	230.0	210.2	235.0	239.0
white matter (central) (cerebral)	191.0	198.3	–	225.0	237.5	239.6
windpipe	162.0	197.3	231.1	212.2	235.7	239.1
Wirsung's duct	157.3	197.8	230.9	211.6	235.5	239.0
wolffian (body) (duct)						
female	184.8	198.82	233.39	221.8	236.3	239.5
male	187.8	198.82	233.6	222.8	236.6	239.5
womb – *see* Neoplasm, uterus						
wrist NEC*	195.4	198.89	232.6	229.8	238.8	239.89▲
xiphoid process	170.3	198.5	–	213.3	238.0	239.2
Zuckerkandl's organ	194.6	198.89	–	227.6	237.3	239.7

Neovascularization
- choroid 362.16
- ciliary body 364.42
- cornea 370.60
  - deep 370.63
  - localized 370.61
- iris 364.42
- retina 362.16
- subretinal 362.16

Nephralgia 788.0

Nephritis, nephritic (albuminuric) (azotemic) (congenital) (degenerative) (diffuse) (disseminated) (epithelial) (familial) (focal) (granulomatous) (hemorrhagic) (infantile) (nonsuppurative, excretory) (uremic) 583.9
- with
  - edema - *see* Nephrosis
  - lesion of
    - glomerulonephritis
      - hypocomplementemic persistent 583.2
        - with nephrotic syndrome 581.2
        - chronic 582.2
      - lobular 583.2
        - with nephrotic syndrome 581.2
        - chronic 582.2
      - membranoproliferative 583.2
        - with nephrotic syndrome 581.2
        - chronic 582.2
      - membranous 583.1
        - with nephrotic syndrome 581.1
        - chronic 582.1
      - mesangiocapillary 583.2
        - with nephrotic syndrome 581.2
        - chronic 582.2
      - mixed membranous and proliferative 583.2
        - with nephrotic syndrome 581.2
        - chronic 582.2
      - proliferative (diffuse) 583.0
        - with nephrotic syndrome 581.0
        - acute 580.0
        - chronic 582.0
      - rapidly progressive 583.4
        - acute 580.4
        - chronic 582.4
    - interstitial nephritis (diffuse) (focal) 583.89
      - with nephrotic syndrome 581.89
      - acute 580.89
      - chronic 582.89
    - necrotizing glomerulitis 583.4
      - acute 580.4
      - chronic 582.4
    - renal necrosis 583.9
      - cortical 583.6
      - medullary 583.7
    - specified pathology NEC 583.89
      - with nephrotic syndrome 581.89
      - acute 580.89
      - chronic 582.89
  - necrosis, renal 583.9
    - cortical 583.6
    - medullary (papillary) 583.7
  - nephrotic syndrome (*see also* Nephrosis) 581.9
  - papillary necrosis 583.7
  - specified pathology NEC 583.89
- acute 580.9
  - extracapillary with epithelial crescents 580.4
  - hypertensive (*see also* Hypertension, kidney) 403.90
  - necrotizing 580.4
  - poststreptococcal 580.0

Nephritis, nephritic – *continued*
- acute – *continued*
  - proliferative (diffuse) 580.0
  - rapidly progressive 580.4
  - specified pathology NEC 580.89
- amyloid 277.39 *[583.81]*
  - chronic 277.39 *[582.81]*
- arteriolar (*see also* Hypertension, kidney) 403.90
- arteriosclerotic (*see also* Hypertension, kidney) 403.90
- ascending (*see also* Pyelitis) 590.80
- atrophic 582.9
- basement membrane NEC 583.89
  - with pulmonary hemorrhage (Goodpasture's syndrome) 446.21 *[583.81]*
- calculous, calculus 592.0
- cardiac (*see also* Hypertension, kidney) 403.90
- cardiovascular (*see also* Hypertension, kidney) 403.90
- chronic 582.9
  - arteriosclerotic (*see also* Hypertension, kidney) 403.90
  - hypertensive (*see also* Hypertension, kidney) 403.90
- cirrhotic (*see also* Sclerosis, renal) 587
- complicating pregnancy, childbirth, or puerperium 646.2 5th
  - with hypertension 642.1 5th
    - affecting fetus or newborn 760.0
  - affecting fetus or newborn 760.1
- croupous 580.9
- desquamative - *see* Nephrosis
- due to
  - amyloidosis 277.39 *[583.81]*
    - chronic 277.39 *[582.81]*
  - arteriosclerosis (*see also* Hypertension, kidney) 403.90
  - diabetes mellitus 250.4 5th *[583.81]*
    - due to secondary diabetes 249.4 5th *[583.81]*
    - with nephrotic syndrome 250.4 5th *[581.81]*
      - due to secondary diabetes 249.4 5th *[583.81]*
  - diphtheria 032.89 *[580.81]*
  - gonococcal infection (acute) 098.19 *[583.81]*
    - chronic or duration of 2 months or over 098.39 *[583.81]*
  - gout 274.10
  - infectious hepatitis 070.9 *[580.81]*
  - mumps 072.79 *[580.81]*
  - specified kidney pathology NEC 583.89
    - acute 580.89
    - chronic 582.89
  - streptotrichosis 039.8 *[583.81]*
  - subacute bacterial endocarditis 421.0 *[580.81]*
  - systemic lupus erythematosus 710.0 *[583.81]*
    - chronic 710.0 *[582.81]*
  - typhoid fever 002.0 *[580.81]*
- endothelial 582.2
- end state (chronic) (terminal) NEC 585.6
- epimembranous 581.1
- exudative 583.89
  - with nephrotic syndrome 581.89
  - acute 580.89
  - chronic 582.89
- gonococcal (acute) 098.19 *[583.81]*
  - chronic or duration of 2 months or over 098.39 *[583.81]*
- gouty 274.10
- hereditary (Alport's syndrome) 759.89
- hydremic - *see* Nephrosis
- hypertensive (*see also* Hypertension, kidney) 403.90
- hypocomplementemic persistent 583.2
  - with nephrotic syndrome 581.2
  - chronic 582.2
- immune complex NEC 583.89

Nephritis, nephritic – *continued*
- infective (*see also* Pyelitis) 590.80
- interstitial (diffuse) (focal) 583.89
  - with nephrotic syndrome 581.89
  - acute 580.89
  - chronic 582.89
- latent or quiescent - *see* Nephritis, chronic
- lead 984.9
  - specified type of lead - *see* Table of Drugs and Chemicals
- lobular 583.2
  - with nephrotic syndrome 581.2
  - chronic 582.2
- lupus 710.0 *[583.81]*
  - acute 710.0 *[580.81]*
  - chronic 710.0 *[582.81]*
- membranoproliferative 583.2
  - with nephrotic syndrome 581.2
  - chronic 582.2
- membranous 583.1
  - with nephrotic syndrome 581.1
  - chronic 582.1
- mesangiocapillary 583.2
  - with nephrotic syndrome 581.2
  - chronic 582.2
- minimal change 581.3
- mixed membranous and proliferative 583.2
  - with nephrotic syndrome 581.2
  - chronic 582.2
- necrotic, necrotizing 583.4
  - acute 580.4
  - chronic 582.4
- nephrotic - *see* Nephrosis
- old - *see* Nephritis, chronic
- parenchymatous 581.89
- polycystic 753.12
  - adult type (APKD) 753.13
  - autosomal dominant 753.13
  - autosomal recessive 753.14
  - childhood type (CPKD) 753.14
  - infantile type 753.14
- poststreptococcal 580.0
- pregnancy - *see* Nephritis, complicating pregnancy
- proliferative 583.0
  - with nephrotic syndrome 581.0
  - acute 580.0
  - chronic 582.0
- purulent (*see also* Pyelitis) 590.80
- rapidly progressive 583.4
  - acute 580.4
  - chronic 582.4
- salt-losing or salt-wasting (*see also* Disease, renal) 593.9
- saturnine 584.9
  - specified type of lead - *see* Table of Drugs and Chemicals
- septic (*see also* Pyelitis) 590.80
- specified pathology NEC 583.89
  - acute 580.89
  - chronic 582.89
- staphylococcal (*see also* Pyelitis) 590.80
- streptotrichosis 039.8 *[583.81]*
- subacute (*see also* Nephrosis) 581.9
- suppurative (*see also* Pyelitis) 590.80
- syphilitic (late) 095.4
  - congenital 090.5 *[583.81]*
  - early 091.69 *[583.81]*
- terminal (chronic) (end-stage) NEC 585.6
- toxic - *see* Nephritis, acute
- tubal, tubular - *see* Nephrosis, tubular
- tuberculous (*see also* Tuberculosis) 016.0 5th *[583.81]*
- type II (Ellis) - *see* Nephrosis
- vascular - *see also* Hypertension, kidney
- war 580.9

Nephroblastoma (M8960/3) 189.0
- epithelial (M8961/3) 189.0
- mesenchymal (M8962/3) 189.0

Nephrocalcinosis 275.49

Nephrocystitis, pustular (*see also* Pyelitis) 590.80

Nephrolithiasis (congenital) (pelvis) (recurrent) 592.0
- uric acid 274.11

Nephroma (M8960/3) 189.0
- mesoblastic (M8960/1) 236.9 5th

Nephronephritis (*see also* Nephrosis) 581.9

Nephronopthisis 753.16

Nephropathy (*see also* Nephritis) 583.9
- with
  - exudative nephritis 583.89
  - interstitial nephritis (diffuse) (focal) 583.89
  - medullary necrosis 583.7
  - necrosis 583.9
    - cortical 583.6
    - medullary or papillary 583.7
  - papillary necrosis 583.7
  - specified lesion or cause NEC 583.89
- analgesic 583.89
  - with medullary necrosis, acute 584.7
- arteriolar (*see also* Hypertension, kidney) 403.90
- arteriosclerotic (*see also* Hypertension, kidney) 403.90
- complicating pregnancy 646.2 5th
- diabetic 250.4 5th *[583.81]*
  - due to secondary diabetes 249.4 5th *[583.81]*
- gouty 274.10
  - specified type NEC 274.19
- hereditary amyloid 277.31
- hypercalcemic 588.89
- hypertensive (*see also* Hypertension, kidney) 403.90
- hypokalemic (vacuolar) 588.89
- IgA 583.9
- obstructive 593.89
  - congenital 753.20
- phenacetin 584.7
- phosphate-losing 588.0
- potassium depletion 588.89
- proliferative (*see also* Nephritis, proliferative) 583.0
- protein-losing 588.89
- salt-losing or salt-wasting (*see also* Disease, renal) 593.9
- sickle-cell (*see also* Disease, sickle-cell) 282.60 *[583.81]*
- toxic 584.5
- vasomotor 584.5
- water-losing 588.89

Nephroptosis (*see also* Disease, renal) 593.0
- congenital (displaced) 753.3

Nephropyosis (*see also* Abscess, kidney) 590.2

Nephrorrhagia 593.81

Nephrosclerosis (arteriolar) (arteriosclerotic) (chronic) (hyaline) (*see also* Hypertension, kidney) 403.90
- gouty 274.10
- hyperplastic (arteriolar) (*see also* Hypertension, kidney) 403.90
- senile (*see also* Sclerosis, renal) 587

Nephrosis, nephrotic (Epstein's) (syndrome) 581.9
- with
  - lesion of
    - focal glomerulosclerosis 581.1
    - glomerulonephritis
      - endothelial 581.2
      - hypocomplementemic persistent 581.2
      - lobular 581.2
      - membranoproliferative 581.2
      - membranous 581.1
      - mesangiocapillary 581.2
      - minimal change 581.3
      - mixed membranous and proliferative 581.2
      - proliferative 581.0
    - segmental hyalinosis 581.1
    - specified pathology NEC 581.89
- acute - *see* Nephrosis, tubular
- anoxic - *see* Nephrosis, tubular

- **Nephrosis, nephrotic** – *continued*
  - arteriosclerotic (*see also* Hypertension, kidney) 403.90
  - chemical - *see* Nephrosis, tubular
  - cholemic 572.4
  - complicating pregnancy, childbirth, or puerperium - *see* Nephritis, complicating pregnancy
  - diabetic 250.4 5th *[581.81]*
    - due to secondary diabetes 249.4 5th *[583.81]*
  - Finnish type (congenital) 759.89
  - hemoglobinuric - *see* Nephrosis, tubular
  - in
    - amyloidosis 277.39 *[581.81]*
    - diabetes mellitus 250.4 5th *[581.81]*
      - due to secondary diabetes 249.4 5th *[583.81]*
    - epidemic hemorrhagic fever 078.6
    - malaria 084.9 *[581.81]*
    - polyarteritis 446.0 *[581.81]*
    - systemic lupus erythematosus 710.0 *[581.81]*
  - ischemic - *see* Nephrosis, tubular
  - lipoid 581.3
  - lower nephron - *see* Nephrosis, tubular
  - lupoid 710.0 *[581.81]*
  - lupus 710.0 *[581.81]*
  - malarial 084.9 *[581.81]*
  - minimal change 581.3
  - necrotizing - *see* Nephrosis, tubular
  - osmotic (sucrose) 588.89
  - polyarteritic 446.0 *[581.81]*
  - radiation 581.9
  - specified lesion or cause NEC 581.89
  - syphilitic 095.4
  - toxic - *see* Nephrosis, tubular
  - tubular (acute) 584.5
    - due to a procedure 997.5
    - radiation 581.9
- **Nephrosonephritis hemorrhagic** (endemic) 078.6
- **Nephrostomy status** V44.6
  - with complication 997.5
- **Nerve** - *see* condition
- **Nerves** 799.21 ▲
- **Nervous** (*see also* condition) 799.21 ▲
  - breakdown 300.9
  - heart 306.2
  - stomach 306.4
  - tension 799.21 ▲
- **Nervousness** 799.21 ▲
- **Nesidioblastoma** (M8150/0)
  - pancreas 211.7
  - specified site NEC - *see* Neoplasm, by site, benign
  - unspecified site 211.7
- **Netherton's syndrome** (ichthyosiform erythroderma) 757.1
- **Nettle rash** 708.8
- **Nettleship's disease** (urticaria pigmentosa) 757.33
- **Neumann's disease** (pemphigus vegetans) 694.4
- **Neuralgia, neuralgic** (acute) (*see also* Neuritis) 729.2
  - accessory (nerve) 352.4
  - acoustic (nerve) 388.5
  - ankle 355.8
  - anterior crural 355.8
  - anus 787.99
  - arm 723.4
  - auditory (nerve) 388.5
  - axilla 353.0
  - bladder 788.1
  - brachial 723.4
  - brain - *see* Disorder nerve, cranial
  - broad ligament 625.9
  - cerebral - *see* Disorder, nerve, cranial
  - ciliary 339.00
  - cranial nerve - *see also* Disorder, nerve, cranial
    - fifth or trigeminal (*see also* Neuralgia, trigeminal) 350.1
  - ear 388.71
    - middle 352.1
  - facial 351.8
  - finger 354.9
  - flank 355.8
  - foot 355.8
  - forearm 354.9
  - Fothergill's (*see also* Neuralgia, trigeminal) 350.1
    - postherpetic 053.12
  - glossopharyngeal (nerve) 352.1
  - groin 355.8
  - hand 354.9
  - heel 355.8
  - Horton's 339.00
  - Hunt's 053.11
  - hypoglossal (nerve) 352.5
  - iliac region 355.8
  - infraorbital (*see also* Neuralgia, trigeminal) 350.1
  - inguinal 355.8
  - intercostal (nerve) 353.8
    - postherpetic 053.19
  - jaw 352.1
  - kidney 788.0
  - knee 355.8
  - loin 355.8
  - malarial (*see also* Malaria) 084.6
  - mastoid 385.89
  - maxilla 352.1
  - median thenar 354.1
  - metatarsal 355.6
  - middle ear 352.1
  - migrainous 339.00
  - Morton's 355.6
  - nerve, cranial - *see* Disorder, nerve, cranial
  - nose 352.0
  - occipital 723.8
  - olfactory (nerve) 352.0
  - ophthalmic 377.30
    - postherpetic 053.19
  - optic (nerve) 377.30
  - penis 607.9
  - perineum 355.8
  - pleura 511.0
  - postherpetic NEC 053.19
    - geniculate ganglion 053.11
    - ophthalmic 053.19
    - trifacial 053.12
    - trigeminal 053.12
  - pubic region 355.8
  - radial (nerve) 723.4
  - rectum 787.99
  - sacroiliac joint 724.3
  - sciatic (nerve) 724.3
  - scrotum 608.9
  - seminal vesicle 608.9
  - shoulder 354.9
  - sluder's 337.09
  - specified nerve NEC - *see* Disorder, nerve
  - spermatic cord 608.9
  - sphenopalatine (ganglion) 337.09
  - subscapular (nerve) 723.4
  - suprascapular (nerve) 723.4
  - testis 608.89
  - thenar (median) 354.1
  - thigh 355.8
  - tongue 352.5
  - trifacial (nerve) (*see also* Neuralgia, trigeminal) 350.1
  - trigeminal (nerve) 350.1
    - postherpetic 053.12
  - tympanic plexus 388.71
  - ulnar (nerve) 723.4
  - vagus (nerve) 352.3
  - wrist 354.9
  - writers' 300.89
    - organic 333.84
- **Neurapraxia** - *see* Injury, nerve, by site
- **Neurasthenia** 300.5
  - cardiac 306.2
  - gastric 306.4
  - heart 306.2
  - postfebrile 780.79
  - postviral 780.79
- **Neurilemmoma** (M9560/0) - *see also* Neoplasm, connective tissue, benign
  - acoustic (nerve) 225.1
  - malignant (M9560/3) - *see also* Neoplasm, connective tissue, malignant
    - acoustic (nerve) 192.0
- **Neurilemmosarcoma** (M9560/3) - *see* Neoplasm, connective tissue, malignant
- **Neurilemoma** - *see* Neurilemmoma
- **Neurinoma** (M9560/0) - *see* Neurilemmoma
- **Neurinomatosis** (M9560/1) - *see also* Neoplasm, connective tissue, uncertain behavior
  - centralis 759.5
- **Neuritis** (*see also* Neuralgia) 729.2
  - abducens (nerve) 378.54
  - accessory (nerve) 352.4
  - acoustic (nerve) 388.5
    - syphilitic 094.86
  - alcoholic 357.5
    - with psychosis 291.1
  - amyloid, any site 277.39 *[357.4]*
  - anterior crural 355.8
  - arising during pregnancy 646.4 5th
  - arm 723.4
  - ascending 355.2
  - auditory (nerve) 388.5
  - brachial (nerve) NEC 723.4
    - due to displacement, intervertebral disc 722.0
  - cervical 723.4
  - chest (wall) 353.8
  - costal region 353.8
  - cranial nerve - *see also* Disorder, nerve, cranial
    - first or olfactory 352.0
    - second or optic 377.30
    - third or oculomotor 378.52
    - fourth or trochlear 378.53
    - fifth or trigeminal (*see also* Neuralgia, trigeminal) 350.1
    - sixth or abducens 378.54
    - seventh or facial 351.8
      - newborn 767.5
    - eighth or acoustic 388.5
    - ninth or glossopharyngeal 352.1
    - tenth or vagus 352.3
    - eleventh or accessory 352.4
    - twelfth or hypoglossal 352.5
  - Déjérine-Sottas 356.0
  - diabetic 250.6 5th *[357.2]*
    - due to secondary diabetes 249.6 5th *[357.2]*
  - diphtheritic 032.89 *[357.4]*
  - due to
    - beriberi 265.0 *[357.4]*
    - displacement, prolapse, protrusion, or rupture of intervertebral disc 722.2
      - cervical 722.0
      - lumbar, lumbosacral 722.10
      - thoracic, thoracolumbar 722.11
    - herniation, nucleus pulposus 722.2
      - cervical 722.0
      - lumbar, lumbosacral 722.10
      - thoracic, thoracolumbar 722.11
  - endemic 265.0 *[357.4]*
  - facial (nerve) 351.8
    - newborn 767.5
  - general - *see* Polyneuropathy
  - geniculate ganglion 351.1
    - due to herpes 053.11
  - glossopharyngeal (nerve) 352.1
  - gouty 274.89 *[357.4]*
  - hypoglossal (nerve) 352.5
  - ilioinguinal (nerve) 355.8
  - in diseases classified elsewhere - *see* Polyneuropathy, in
  - infectious (multiple) 357.0
  - intercostal (nerve) 353.8
  - interstitial hypertrophic progressive NEC 356.9
  - leg 355.8
  - lumbosacral NEC 724.4
  - median (nerve) 354.1
    - thenar 354.1
  - multiple (acute) (infective) 356.9
    - endemic 265.0 *[357.4]*
  - multiplex endemica 265.0 *[357.4]*
  - nerve root (*see also* Radiculitis) 729.2
  - oculomotor (nerve) 378.52
  - olfactory (nerve) 352.0
  - optic (nerve) 377.30
    - in myelitis 341.0
    - meningococcal 036.81
  - pelvic 355.8
  - peripheral (nerve) - *see also* Neuropathy, peripheral
    - complicating pregnancy or puerperium 646.4 5th
    - specified nerve NEC - *see* Mononeuritis
  - pneumogastric (nerve) 352.3
  - postchickenpox 052.7
  - postherpetic 053.19
  - progressive hypertrophic interstitial NEC 356.9
  - puerperal, postpartum 646.4 5th
  - radial (nerve) 723.4
  - retrobulbar 377.32
    - syphilitic 094.85
  - rheumatic (chronic) 729.2
  - sacral region 355.8
  - sciatic (nerve) 724.3
    - due to displacement of intervertebral disc 722.10
  - serum 999.5
  - specified nerve NEC - *see* Disorder, nerve
  - spinal (nerve) 355.9
    - root (*see also* Radiculitis) 729.2
  - subscapular (nerve) 723.4
  - suprascapular (nerve) 723.4
  - syphilitic 095.8
  - thenar (median) 354.1
  - thoracic NEC 724.4
  - toxic NEC 357.7
  - trochlear (nerve) 378.53
  - ulnar (nerve) 723.4
  - vagus (nerve) 352.3
- **Neuroangiomatosis, encephalofacial** 759.6
- **Neuroastrocytoma** (M9505/1) - *see* Neoplasm, by site, uncertain behavior
- **Neuro-avitaminosis** 269.2
- **Neuroblastoma** (M9500/3)
  - olfactory (M9522/3) 160.0
  - specified site - *see* Neoplasm, by site, malignant
  - unspecified site 194.0
- **Neurochorioretinitis** (*see also* Chorioretinitis) 363.20
- **Neurocirculatory asthenia** 306.2
- **Neurocytoma** (M9506/0) - *see* Neoplasm, by site, benign
- **Neurodermatitis** (circumscribed) (circumscripta) (local) 698.3
  - atopic 691.8
  - diffuse (Brocq) 691.8
  - disseminated 691.8
  - nodulosa 698.3
- **Neuroencephalomyelopathy, optic** 341.0
- **Neuroendocrine tumor** - *see* Tumor, neuroendocrine
- **Neuroepithelioma** (M9503/3) - *see also* Neoplasm, by site, malignant
  - olfactory (M9521/3) 160.0
- **Neurofibroma** (M9540/0) - *see also* Neoplasm, connective tissue, benign
  - melanotic (M9541/0) - *see* Neoplasm, connective tissue, benign
  - multiple (M9540/1) 237.70
    - type 1 237.71
    - type 2 237.72
  - plexiform (M9550/0) - *see* Neoplasm, connective tissue, benign

Neurofibromatosis – Neutropenia, neutropenic

Neurofibromatosis (multiple) (M9540/1) 237.70
- acoustic 237.72
- malignant (M9540/3) - *see* Neoplasm, connective tissue, malignant
- type 1 237.71
- type 2 237.72
- von Recklinghausen's 237.71

Neurofibrosarcoma (M9540/3) - *see* Neoplasm, connective tissue, malignant

Neurogenic - *see also* condition
- bladder (atonic) (automatic) (autonomic) (flaccid) (hypertonic) (hypotonic) (inertia) (infranuclear) (irritable) (motor) (nonreflex) (nuclear) (paralysis) (reflex) (sensory) (spastic) (supranuclear) (uninhibited) 596.54
  - with cauda equina syndrome 344.61
- bowel 564.81
- heart 306.2

Neuroglioma (M9505/1) - *see* Neoplasm, by site, uncertain behavior

Neurolabyrinthitis (of Dix and Hallpike) 386.12

Neurolathyrism 988.2

Neuroleprosy 030.1

Neuroleptic malignant syndrome 333.92

Neurolipomatosis 272.8

Neuroma (M9570/0) - *see also* Neoplasm, connective tissue, benign
- acoustic (nerve) (M9560/0) 225.1
- amputation (traumatic) - *see also* Injury, nerve, by site
  - surgical complication (late) 997.61
- appendix 211.3
- auditory nerve 225.1
- digital 355.6
  - toe 355.6
- interdigital (toe) 355.6
- intermetatarsal 355.6
- Morton's 355.6
- multiple 237.70
  - type 1 237.71
  - type 2 237.72
- nonneoplastic 355.9
  - arm NEC 354.9
  - leg NEC 355.8
  - lower extremity NEC 355.8
  - specified site NEC - *see* Mononeuritis, by site
  - upper extremity NEC 354.9
- optic (nerve) 225.1
- plantar 355.6
- plexiform (M9550/0) - *see* Neoplasm, connective tissue, benign
- surgical (nonneoplastic) 355.9
  - arm NEC 354.9
  - leg NEC 355.8
  - lower extremity NEC 355.8
  - upper extremity NEC 354.9
- traumatic - *see also* Injury, nerve, by site oldsee Neuroma, nonneoplastic

Neuromyalgia 729.1

Neuromyasthenia (epidemic) 049.8

Neuromyelitis 341.8
- ascending 357.0
- optica 341.0

Neuromyopathy NEC 358.9

Neuromyositis 729.1

Neuronevus (M8725/0) - *see* Neoplasm, skin, benign

Neuronitis 357.0
- ascending (acute) 355.2
- vestibular 386.12

Neuroparalytic - *see* condition

Neuropathy, neuropathic (*see also* Disorder, nerve) 355.9
- acute motor 357.82
- alcoholic 357.5
  - with psychosis 291.1
- arm NEC 354.9

Neuropathy, neuropathic – *continued*
- ataxia and retinitis pigmentosa (NARP syndrome) 277.87
- autonomic (peripheral) - *see* Neuropathy, peripheral, autonomic
- axillary nerve 353.0
- brachial plexus 353.0
- cervical plexus 353.2
- chronic
  - progressive segmentally demyelinating 357.89
  - relapsing demyelinating 357.89
- congenital sensory 356.2
- Déjérine-Sottas 356.0
- diabetic 250.6 5th *[357.2]*
  - autonomic (peripheral) 250.6 5th *[337.1]* ●
  - due to secondary diabetes 249.6 5th *[357.2]*
    - autonomic (peripheral) 249.6 5th *[337.1]* ●
- entrapment 355.9
  - iliohypogastric nerve 355.79
  - ilioinguinal nerve 355.79
  - lateral cutaneous nerve of thigh 355.1
  - median nerve 354.0
  - obturator nerve 355.79
  - peroneal nerve 355.3
  - posterior tibial nerve 355.5
  - saphenous nerve 355.79
  - ulnar nerve 354.2
- facial nerve 351.9
- hereditary 356.9
  - peripheral 356.0
  - sensory (radicular) 356.2
- hypertrophic
  - Charcôt-Marie-Tooth 356.1
  - Déjérine-Sottas 356.0
  - interstitial 356.9
  - Refsum 356.3
- intercostal nerve 354.8
- ischemic - *see* Disorder, nerve
- Jamaican (ginger) 357.7
- leg NEC 355.8
- lower extremity NEC 355.8
- lumbar plexus 353.1
- median nerve 354.1
- motor
  - acute 357.82
- multiple (acute) (chronic) (*see also* Polyneuropathy) 356.9
- optic 377.39
  - ischemic 377.41
  - nutritional 377.33
  - toxic 377.34
- peripheral (nerve) (*see also* Polyneuropathy) 356.9
  - arm NEC 354.9
  - autonomic 337.9
    - amyloid 277.39 *[337.1]*
    - idiopathic 337.00
    - in
      - amyloidosis 277.39 *[337.1]*
      - diabetes (mellitus) 250.6 5th *[337.1]*
        - due to secondary diabetes 249.6 5th *[337.1]*
      - diseases classified elsewhere 337.1
      - gout 274.89 *[337.1]*
      - hyperthyroidism 242.9 5th *[337.1]*
  - due to
    - antitetanus serum 357.6
    - arsenic 357.7
    - drugs 357.6
    - lead 357.7
    - organophosphate compounds 357.7
    - toxic agent NEC 357.7
  - hereditary 356.0
  - idiopathic 356.9
    - progressive 356.4
    - specified type NEC 356.8

Neuropathy, neuropathic – *continued*
- peripheral (nerve) – *continued*
  - in diseases classified elsewhere - *see* Polyneuropathy, in
  - leg NEC 355.8
  - lower extremity NEC 355.8
  - upper extremity NEC 354.9
- plantar nerves 355.6
- progressive ~~hypertrophic interstitial 356.9~~ ▲
  - hypertrophic interstitial 356.9 ●
  - inflammatory 357.89 ●
- radicular NEC 729.2
  - brachial 723.4
  - cervical NEC 723.4
  - hereditary sensory 356.2
  - lumbar 724.4
  - lumbosacral 724.4
  - thoracic NEC 724.4
- sacral plexus 353.1
- sciatic 355.0
- spinal nerve NEC 355.9
  - root (*see also* Radiculitis) 729.2
- toxic 357.7
- trigeminal sensory 350.8
- ulnar nerve 354.2
- upper extremity NEC 354.9
- uremic 585.9 *[357.4]*
- vitamin B_{12} 266.2 *[357.4]*
  - with anemia (pernicious) 281.0 *[357.4]*
    - due to dietary deficiency 281.1 *[357.4]*

Neurophthisis - *see also* Disorder, nerve
- peripheral 356.9
- diabetic 250.6 5th *[357.2]*
  - due to secondary diabetes 249.6 5th *[357.2]*

Neuropraxia - *see* Injury, nerve

Neuroretinitis 363.05
- syphilitic 094.85

Neurosarcoma (M9540/3) - *see* Neoplasm, connective tissue, malignant

Neurosclerosis - *see* Disorder, nerve

Neurosis, neurotic 300.9
- accident 300.16
- anancastic, anankastic 300.3
- anxiety (state) 300.00
  - generalized 300.02
- panic type 300.01
- asthenic 300.5
- bladder 306.53
- cardiac (reflex) 306.2
- cardiovascular 306.2
- climacteric, unspecified type 627.2
- colon 306.4
- compensation 300.16
- compulsive, compulsion 300.3
- conversion 300.11
- craft 300.89
- cutaneous 306.3
- depersonalization 300.6
- depressive (reaction) (type) 300.4
- endocrine 306.6
- environmental 300.89
- fatigue 300.5
- functional (*see also* Disorder, psychosomatic) 306.9
- gastric 306.4
- gastrointestinal 306.4
- genitourinary 306.50
- heart 306.2
- hypochondriacal 300.7
- hysterical 300.10
  - conversion type 300.11
  - dissociative type 300.15
- impulsive 300.3
- incoordination 306.0
  - larynx 306.1
  - vocal cord 306.1
- intestine 306.4
- larynx 306.1
  - hysterical 300.11
  - sensory 306.1
- menopause, unspecified type 627.2

Neurosis, neurotic – *continued*
- mixed NEC 300.89
- musculoskeletal 306.0
- obsessional 300.3
  - phobia 300.3
- obsessive-compulsive 300.3
- occupational 300.89
- ocular 306.7
- oral 307.0
- organ (*see also* Disorder, psychosomatic) 306.9
- pharynx 306.1
- phobic 300.20
- posttraumatic (acute) (situational) 309.81
  - chronic 309.81
- psychasthenic (type) 300.89
- railroad 300.16
- rectum 306.4
- respiratory 306.1
- rumination 306.4
- senile 300.89
- sexual 302.70
- situational 300.89
- specified type NEC 300.89
- state 300.9
  - with depersonalization episode 300.6
- stomach 306.4
- vasomotor 306.2
- visceral 306.4
- war 300.16

Neurospongioblastosis diffusa 759.5

Neurosyphilis (arrested) (early) (inactive) (late) (latent) (recurrent) 094.9
- with ataxia (cerebellar) (locomotor) (spastic) (spinal) 094.0
- acute meningitis 094.2
- aneurysm 094.89
- arachnoid (adhesive) 094.2
- arteritis (any artery) 094.89
- asymptomatic 094.3
- congenital 090.40
- dura (mater) 094.89
- general paresis 094.1
- gumma 094.9
- hemorrhagic 094.9
- juvenile (asymptomatic) (meningeal) 090.40
- leptomeninges (aseptic) 094.2
- meningeal 094.2
- meninges (adhesive) 094.2
- meningovascular (diffuse) 094.2
- optic atrophy 094.84
- parenchymatous (degenerative) 094.1
- paresis (*see also* Paresis, general) 094.1
- paretic (*see also* Paresis, general) 094.1
- relapse 094.9
- remission in (sustained) 094.9
- serological 094.3
- specified nature or site NEC 094.89
- tabes (dorsalis) 094.0
  - juvenile 090.40
- tabetic 094.0
  - juvenile 090.40
- taboparesis 094.1
  - juvenile 090.40
- thrombosis 094.89
- vascular 094.89

Neurotic (*see also* Neurosis) 300.9
- excoriation 698.4
  - psychogenic 306.3

Neurotmesis - *see* Injury, nerve, by site

Neurotoxemia - *see* Toxemia

Neutro-occlusion 524.21

Neutropenia, neutropenic (idiopathic) (pernicious) (primary) 288.00
- chronic 288.09
  - hypoplastic 288.09
- congenital (nontransient) 288.01
- cyclic 288.02
- drug induced 288.03
- due to infection 288.04
- fever 288.00
- genetic 288.01

- **Nomadism** V60.0
- **Non-adherence**
  - artificial skin graft 996.55
  - decellularized allodermis graft 996.55
- **Non-autoimmune hemolytic anemia NEC** 283.10
- **Nonclosure** - *see also* Imperfect, closure
  - ductus
    - arteriosus 747.0
    - Botalli 747.0
  - Eustachian valve 746.89
  - foramen
    - Botalli 745.5
    - ovale 745.5
- **Noncompliance with medical treatment** V15.81
  - renal dialysis V45.12
- **Nondescent** (congenital) - *see also* Malposition, congenital
  - cecum 751.4
  - colon 751.4
  - testis 752.51
- **Nondevelopment**
  - brain 742.1
    - specified part 742.2
  - heart 746.89
  - organ or site, congenital NEC - *see* Hypoplasia
- **Nonengagement**
  - head NEC 652.5 5th
    - in labor 660.1 5th
      - affecting fetus or newborn 763.1
- **Nonexanthematous tick fever** 066.1
- **Nonexpansion, lung** (newborn) **NEC** 770.4
- **Nonfunctioning**
  - cystic duct (*see also* Disease, gallbladder) 575.8
  - gallbladder (*see also* Disease, gallbladder) 575.8
  - kidney (*see also* Disease, renal) 593.9
  - labyrinth 386.58
- **Nonhealing**
  - stump (surgical) 997.69
  - wound, surgical 998.83
- **Nonimplantation of ovum, causing infertility** 628.3
- **Noninsufflation, fallopian tube** 628.2
- **Nonne-Milroy-Meige syndrome** (chronic hereditary edema) 757.0
- **Nonovulation** 628.0
- **Nonpatent fallopian tube** 628.2
- **Nonpneumatization, lung NEC** 770.4
- **Nonreflex bladder** 596.54
  - with cauda equina 344.61
- **Nonretention of food** - *see* Vomiting
- **Nonrotation** - *see* Malrotation
- **Nonsecretion, urine** (*see also* Anuria) 788.5
  - newborn 753.3
- **Nonunion**
  - fracture 733.82
  - organ or site, congenital NEC - *see* Imperfect, closure
  - symphysis pubis, congenital 755.69
  - top sacrum, congenital 756.19
- **Nonviability** 765.0 5th
- **Nonvisualization, gallbladder** 793.3
- **Nonvitalized tooth** 522.9
- **Non-working side interference** 524.56
- **Normal**
  - delivery - *see* category 650
  - menses V65.5
  - state (feared complaint unfounded) V65.5
- **Normoblastosis** 289.89
- **Normocytic anemia** (infectional) 285.9
  - due to blood loss (chronic) 280.0
    - acute 285.1
- **Norrie's disease** (congenital) (progressive oculoacousticocerebral degeneration) 743.8
- **North American blastomycosis** 116.0
- **Norwegian itch** 133.0
- **Nose, nasal** - *see* condition
- **Nosebleed** 784.7
- **Nosomania** 298.9
- **Nosophobia** 300.29
- **Nostalgia** 309.89
- **Notch of iris** 743.46
- **Notched lip, congenital** (*see also* Cleft, lip) 749.10
- **Notching nose, congenital** (tip) 748.1
- **Nothnagel's**
  - syndrome 378.52
  - vasomotor acroparesthesia 443.89
- **Novy's relapsing fever** (American) 087.1
- **Noxious**
  - foodstuffs, poisoning by
    - fish 988.0
    - fungi 988.1
    - mushrooms 988.1
    - plants (food) 988.2
    - shellfish 988.0
    - specified type NEC 988.8
    - toadstool 988.1
  - substances transmitted through placenta or breast milk (affecting fetus or newborn) 760.70
    - acetretin 760.78
    - alcohol 760.71
    - aminopterin 760.78
    - antiandrogens 760.79
    - anticonvulsant 760.77
    - antifungal 760.74
    - anti-infective agents 760.74
    - antimetabolic 760.78
    - atorvastatin 760.78
    - carbamazepine 760.77
    - cocaine 760.75
    - "crack" 760.75
    - diethylstilbestrol (DES) 760.76
    - divalproex sodium 760.77
    - endocrine disrupting chemicals 760.79
    - estrogens 760.79
    - etretinate 760.78
    - fluconazole 760.74
    - fluvastatin 760.78
    - hallucinogenic agents NEC 760.73
    - hormones 760.79
    - lithium 760.79
    - lovastatin 760.78
    - medicinal agents NEC 760.79
    - methotrexate 760.78
    - misoprostil 760.79
    - narcotics 760.72
    - obstetric anesthetic or analgesic 763.5
    - phenobarbital 760.77
    - phenytoin 760.77
    - pravastatin 760.78
    - progestins 760.79
    - retinoic acid 760.78
    - simvastatin 760.78
    - solvents 760.79
    - specified agent NEC 760.79
    - statins 760.78
    - suspected, affecting management of pregnancy 655.5 5th
    - tetracycline 760.74
    - thalidomide 760.79
    - trimethadione 760.77
    - valproate 760.77
    - valproic acid 760.77
    - vitamin A 760.78
- **NPDH** (new persistent daily headache) 339.42
- **Nuchal hitch** (arm) 652.8 5th
- **Nucleus pulposus** - *see* condition
- **Numbness** 782.0
- **Nuns' knee** 727.2
- **Nursemaid's**
  - elbow 832.2 ▲
  - shoulder 831.0 5th
- **Nutmeg liver** 573.8
- **Nutrition, deficient or insufficient** (particular kind of food) 269.9
  - due to
    - insufficient food 994.2
    - lack of
      - care (child) (infant) 995.52
        - adult 995.84
      - food 994.2
- **Nyctalopia** (*see also* Blindness, night) 368.60
  - vitamin A deficiency 264.5
- **Nycturia** 788.43
  - psychogenic 306.53
- **Nymphomania** 302.89
- **Nystagmus** 379.50
  - associated with vestibular system disorders 379.54
  - benign paroxysmal positional 386.11
  - central positional 386.2
  - congenital 379.51
  - deprivation 379.53
  - dissociated 379.55
  - latent 379.52
  - miners' 300.89
  - positional
    - benign paroxysmal 386.11
    - central 386.2
  - specified NEC 379.56
  - vestibular 379.54
  - visual deprivation 379.53

O

- **Oasthouse urine disease** 270.2
- **Obermeyer's relapsing fever** (European) 087.0
- **Obesity** (constitutional) (exogenous) (familial) (nutritional) (simple) 278.00
  - adrenal 255.8
  - complicating pregnancy, childbirth, or puerperium 649.1 5th
  - due to hyperalimentation 278.00
  - endocrine NEC 259.9
  - endogenous 259.9
  - Fröhlich's (adiposogenital dystrophy) 253.8
  - glandular NEC 259.9
  - hypothyroid (*see also* Hypothyroidism) 244.9
  - morbid 278.01
  - of pregnancy 649.1 5th
  - pituitary 253.8
  - severe 278.01
  - thyroid (*see also* Hypothyroidism) 244.9
- **Oblique** - *see also* condition
  - lie before labor, affecting fetus or newborn 761.7
- **Obliquity, pelvis** 738.6
- **Obliteration**
  - abdominal aorta 446.7
  - appendix (lumen) 543.9
  - artery 447.1
  - ascending aorta 446.7
  - bile ducts 576.8
    - with calculus, choledocholithiasis, or stones - *see* Choledocholithiasis
    - congenital 751.61
      - jaundice from 751.61 *[774.5]*
  - common duct 576.8
    - with calculus, choledocholithiasis, or stones - *see* Choledocholithiasis
    - congenital 751.61
  - cystic duct 575.8
    - with calculus, choledocholithiasis, or stones - *see* Choledocholithiasis
  - disease, arteriolar 447.1
  - endometrium 621.8
  - eye, anterior chamber 360.34
  - fallopian tube 628.2
  - lymphatic vessel 457.1
    - postmastectomy 457.0
  - organ or site, congenital NEC - *see* Atresia
  - placental blood vessels - *see* Placenta, abnormal
  - supra-aortic branches 446.7
  - ureter 593.89
  - urethra 599.84
  - vein 459.9
  - vestibule (oral) 525.8
- **Observation** (for) V71.9
  - without need for further medical care V71.9
  - accident NEC V71.4
    - at work V71.3
  - criminal assault V71.6
  - deleterious agent ingestion V71.89
  - disease V71.9
    - cardiovascular V71.7
    - heart V71.7
    - mental V71.09
    - specified condition NEC V71.89
  - foreign body ingestion V71.89
  - growth and development variations V21.8
  - injuries (accidental) V71.4
    - inflicted NEC V71.6
      - during alleged rape or seduction V71.5
  - malignant neoplasm, suspected V71.1
  - postpartum
    - immediately after delivery V24.0
    - routine follow-up V24.2
  - pregnancy
    - high-risk V23.9
      - specified problem NEC V23.89
    - normal (without complication) V22.1
      - with nonobstetric complication V22.2
      - first V22.0
  - rape or seduction, alleged V71.5
    - injury during V71.5
  - suicide attempt, alleged V71.89
  - suspected (undiagnosed) (unproven)
    - abuse V71.81
    - cardiovascular disease V71.7
    - child or wife battering victim V71.6
    - concussion (cerebral) V71.6
    - condition NEC V71.89
      - infant - *see* Observation, suspected, condition, newborn
      - maternal and fetal
        - amniotic cavity and membrane problem V89.01
        - cervical shortening V89.05
        - fetal anomaly V89.03
        - fetal growth problem V89.04
        - oligohydramnios V89.01
        - other specified problem NEC V89.09
        - placental problem V89.02
        - polyhydramnios V89.01
      - newborn V29.9
        - cardiovascular disease V29.8
        - congenital anomaly V29.8
        - genetic V29.3
        - infectious V29.0
        - ingestion foreign object V29.8
        - injury V29.8
        - metabolic V29.3
        - neoplasm V29.8
        - neurological V29.1
        - poison, poisoning V29.8
        - respiratory V29.2
        - specified NEC V29.8
    - exposure
      - anthrax V71.82
      - biologic agent NEC V71.83
      - SARS V71.83
    - infectious disease not requiring isolation V71.89
    - malignant neoplasm V71.1
    - mental disorder V71.09
    - neglect V71.81
    - neoplasm
      - benign V71.89
      - malignant V71.1
    - specified condition NEC V71.89
    - tuberculosis V71.2
  - tuberculosis, suspected V71.2
- **Obsession, obsessional** 300.3
  - ideas and mental images 300.3
  - impulses 300.3
  - neurosis 300.3
  - phobia 300.3

Nomadism – Obsession, obsessional

- **Obsession, obsessional** – *continued*
  - psychasthenia 300.3
  - ruminations 300.3
  - state 300.3
  - syndrome 300.3
- **Obsessive-compulsive** 300.3
  - neurosis 300.3
  - personality 301.4
  - reaction 300.3
- **Obstetrical trauma** NEC (complicating delivery) 665.9 [5th]
  - with
    - abortion - *see* Abortion, by type, with damage to pelvic organs
    - ectopic pregnancy (*see also* categories 633.0-633.9) 639.2
    - molar pregnancy (*see also* categories 630-632) 639.2
  - affecting fetus or newborn 763.89
  - following
    - abortion 639.2
    - ectopic or molar pregnancy 639.2
- **Obstipation** (*see also* Constipation) 564.00
  - psychogenic 306.4
- **Obstruction, obstructed, obstructive**
  - airway NEC 519.8
    - with
      - allergic alveolitis NEC 495.9
      - asthma NEC (*see also* Asthma) 493.9 [5th]
      - bronchiectasis 494.0
        - with acute exacerbation 494.1
      - bronchitis (*see also* Bronchitis, with, obstruction) 491.20
      - emphysema NEC 492.8
    - chronic 496
      - with
        - allergic alveolitis NEC 495.5
        - asthma NEC (*see also* Asthma) 493.2 [5th]
        - bronchiectasis 494.0
          - with acute exacerbation 494.1
        - bronchitis (chronic) (*see also* Bronchitis, chronic, obstructive) 491.20
        - emphysema NEC 492.8
    - due to
      - bronchospasm 519.11
      - foreign body 934.9
      - inhalation of fumes or vapors 506.9
      - laryngospasm 478.75
  - alimentary canal (*see also* Obstruction, intestine) 560.9
  - ampulla of Vater 576.2
    - with calculus, cholelithiasis, or stones - *see* Choledocholithiasis
  - aortic (heart) (valve) (*see also* Stenosis, aortic) 424.1
    - rheumatic (*see also* Stenosis, aortic, rheumatic) 395.0
  - aortoiliac 444.0
  - aqueduct of Sylvius 331.4
    - congenital 742.3
      - with spina bifida (*see also* Spina bifida) 741.0 [5th]
  - Arnold-Chiari (*see also* Spina bifida) 741.0 [5th]
  - artery (*see also* Embolism, artery) 444.9
    - basilar (complete) (partial) (*see also* Occlusion, artery, basilar) 433.0 [5th]
    - carotid (complete) (partial) (*see also* Occlusion, artery, carotid) 433.1 [5th]
    - precerebral - *see* Occlusion, artery, precerebral NEC
    - retinal (central) (*see also* Occlusion, retina) 362.30
    - vertebral (complete) (partial) (*see also* Occlusion, artery, vertebral) 433.2 [5th]
  - asthma (chronic) (with obstructive pulmonary disease) 493.2 [5th]

- **Obstruction, obstructed, obstructive** – *continued*
  - band (intestinal) 560.81
  - bile duct or passage (*see also* Obstruction, biliary) 576.2
    - congenital 751.61
      - jaundice from 751.61 *[774.5]*
  - biliary (duct) (tract) 576.2
    - with calculus 574.51
      - with cholecystitis (chronic) 574.41
        - acute 574.31
    - congenital 751.61
      - jaundice from 751.61 *[774.5]*
    - gallbladder 575.2
      - with calculus 574.21
        - with cholecystitis (chronic) 574.11
          - acute 574.01
  - bladder neck (acquired) 596.0
    - congenital 753.6
  - bowel (*see also* Obstruction, intestine) 560.9
  - bronchus 519.19
  - canal, ear (*see also* Stricture, ear canal, acquired) 380.50
  - cardia 537.89
  - caval veins (inferior) (superior) 459.2
  - cecum (*see also* Obstruction, intestine) 560.9
  - circulatory 459.9
  - colon (*see also* Obstruction, intestine) 560.9
    - sympathicotonic 560.89
  - common duct (*see also* Obstruction, biliary) 576.2
    - congenital 751.61
  - coronary (artery) (heart) - (*see also* Arteriosclerosis, coronary)
    - acute (*see also* Infarct, myocardium) 410.9 [5th]
      - without myocardial infarction 411.81
  - cystic duct (*see also* Obstruction, gallbladder) 575.2
    - congenital 751.61
  - device, implant, or graft - *see* Complications, due to (presence of) any device, implant, or graft classified to 996.0-996.5 NEC
  - due to foreign body accidentally left in operation wound 998.4
  - duodenum 537.3
    - congenital 751.1
    - due to
      - compression NEC 537.3
      - cyst 537.3
      - intrinsic lesion or disease NEC 537.3
      - scarring 537.3
      - torsion 537.3
      - ulcer 532.91
      - volvulus 537.3
  - ejaculatory duct 608.89
  - endocardium 424.90
    - arteriosclerotic 424.99
    - specified cause, except rheumatic 424.99
  - esophagus 530.3
  - Eustachian tube (complete) (partial) 381.60
    - cartilaginous
      - extrinsic 381.63
      - intrinsic 381.62
    - due to
      - cholesteatoma 381.61
      - osseous lesion NEC 381.61
      - polyp 381.61
    - osseous 381.61
  - fallopian tube (bilateral) 628.2
  - fecal 560.39
    - with hernia - *see also* Hernia, by site, with obstruction
      - gangrenous - *see* Hernia, by site, with gangrene

- **Obstruction, obstructed, obstructive** – *continued*
  - foramen of Monro (congenital) 742.3
    - with spina bifida (*see also* Spina bifida) 741.0 [5th]
  - foreign body - *see* Foreign body
  - gallbladder 575.2
    - with calculus, cholelithiasis, or stones 574.21
      - with cholecystitis (chronic) 574.11
        - acute 574.01
    - congenital 751.69
      - jaundice from 751.69 *[774.5]*
  - gastric outlet 537.0
  - gastrointestinal (*see also* Obstruction, intestine) 560.9
  - glottis 478.79
  - hepatic 573.8
    - duct (*see also* Obstruction, biliary) 576.2
      - congenital 751.61
  - icterus (*see also* Obstruction, biliary) 576.8
    - congenital 751.61
  - ileocecal coil (*see also* Obstruction, intestine) 560.9
  - ileum (*see also* Obstruction, intestine) 560.9
  - iliofemoral (artery) 444.81
  - internal anastomosis - *see* Complications, mechanical, graft
  - intestine (mechanical) (neurogenic) (paroxysmal) (postinfectional) (reflex) 560.9
    - with
      - adhesions (intestinal) (peritoneal) 560.81
      - hernia - *see also* Hernia, by site, with obstruction
        - gangrenous - *see* Hernia, by site, with gangrene
    - adynamic (*see also* Ileus) 560.1
    - by gallstone 560.31
    - congenital or infantile (small) 751.1
      - large 751.2
    - due to
      - Ascaris lumbricoides 127.0
      - mural thickening 560.89
      - procedure 997.4
        - involving urinary tract 997.5
    - impaction 560.39
    - infantile - *see* Obstruction, intestine, congenital
    - newborn
      - due to
        - fecaliths 777.1
        - inspissated milk 777.2
        - meconium (plug) 777.1
          - in mucoviscidosis 277.01
      - transitory 777.4
    - specified cause NEC 560.89
    - transitory, newborn 777.4
    - volvulus 560.2
  - intracardiac ball valve prosthesis 996.02
  - jaundice (*see also* Obstruction, biliary) 576.8
    - congenital 751.61
  - jejunum (*see also* Obstruction, intestine) 560.9
  - kidney 593.89
  - labor 660.9 [5th]
    - affecting fetus or newborn 763.1
    - by
      - bony pelvis (conditions classifiable to 653.0-653.9) 660.1 [5th]
      - deep transverse arrest 660.3 [5th]
      - impacted shoulder 660.4 [5th]
      - locked twins 660.5 [5th]
      - malposition (fetus) (conditions classifiable to 652.0-652.9) 660.0 [5th]
        - head during labor 660.3 [5th]
      - persistent occipitoposterior position 660.3 [5th]

- **Obstruction, obstructed, obstructive** – *continued*
  - labor – *continued*
    - by – *continued*
      - soft tissue, pelvic (conditions classifiable to 654.0-654.9) 660.2 [5th]
  - lacrimal
    - canaliculi 375.53
    - congenital 743.65
    - punctum 375.52
    - sac 375.54
  - lacrimonasal duct 375.56
    - congenital 743.65
    - neonatal 375.55
  - lacteal, with steatorrhea 579.2
  - laryngitis (*see also* Laryngitis) 464.01
  - larynx 478.79
    - congenital 748.3
  - liver 573.8
    - cirrhotic (*see also* Cirrhosis, liver) 571.5
  - lung 518.89
    - with
      - asthma - *see* Asthma
      - bronchitis (chronic) 491.20
      - emphysema NEC 492.8
    - airway, chronic 496
    - chronic NEC 496
      - with
        - asthma (chronic) (obstructive) 493.2 [5th]
    - disease, chronic 496
      - with
        - asthma (chronic) (obstructive) 493.2 [5th]
    - emphysematous 492.8
  - lymphatic 457.1
  - meconium
    - fetus or newborn 777.1
      - in mucoviscidosis 277.01
    - newborn due to fecaliths 777.1
  - mediastinum 519.3
  - mitral (rheumatic) - *see* Stenosis, mitral
  - nasal 478.19
    - duct 375.56
      - neonatal 375.55
    - sinus - *see* Sinusitis
  - nasolacrimal duct 375.56
    - congenital 743.65
    - neonatal 375.55
  - nasopharynx 478.29
  - nose 478.19
  - organ or site, congenital NEC - *see* Atresia
  - pancreatic duct 577.8
  - parotid gland 527.8
  - pelviureteral junction (*see also* Obstruction, ureter) 593.4
  - pharynx 478.29
  - portal (circulation) (vein) 452
  - prostate 600.90
    - with
      - other lower urinary tract symptoms (LUTS) 600.91
      - urinary
        - obstruction 600.91
        - retention 600.91
    - valve (urinary) 596.0
  - pulmonary
    - valve (heart) (*see also* Endocarditis, pulmonary) 424.3
    - vein, isolated 747.49
  - pyemic - *see* Septicemia
  - pylorus (acquired) 537.0
    - congenital 750.5
    - infantile 750.5
  - rectosigmoid (*see also* Obstruction, intestine) 560.9
  - rectum 569.49
  - renal 593.89
  - respiratory 519.8
    - chronic 496
  - retinal (artery) (vein) (central) (*see also* Occlusion, retina) 362.30

Obsession, obsessional – Obstruction, obstructed, obstructive

- **Obstruction, obstructed, obstructive** – *continued*
  - salivary duct (any) 527.8
    - with calculus 527.5
  - sigmoid (*see also* Obstruction, intestine) 560.9
  - sinus (accessory) (nasal) (*see also* Sinusitis) 473.9
  - Stensen's duct 527.8
  - stomach 537.89
    - acute 536.1
    - congenital 750.7
  - submaxillary gland 527.8
    - with calculus 527.5
  - thoracic duct 457.1
  - thrombotic - *see* Thrombosis
  - tooth eruption 520.6
  - trachea 519.19
  - tracheostomy airway 519.09
  - tricuspid - *see* Endocarditis, tricuspid
  - upper respiratory, congenital 748.8
  - ureter (functional) 593.4
    - congenital 753.20
    - due to calculus 592.1
  - ureteropelvic junction, congenital 753.21
  - ureterovesical junction, congenital 753.22
  - urethra 599.60
    - congenital 753.6
  - urinary (moderate) 599.60
    - organ or tract (lower) 599.60
      - due to
        - benign prostatic hypertrophy (BPH) - *see* category 600
      - specified NEC 599.69
        - due to
          - benign prostatic hypertrophy (BPH) - *see* category 600
    - prostatic valve 596.0
    - specified NEC 599.69
      - due to
        - benign prostatic hypertrophy (BPH) - *see* category 600
  - uropathy 599.60
  - uterus 621.8
  - vagina 623.2
  - valvular - *see* Endocarditis
  - vascular graft or shunt 996.1
    - atherosclerosis - *see* Arteriosclerosis, coronary
    - embolism 996.74
    - occlusion NEC 996.74
    - thrombus 996.74
  - vein, venous 459.2
    - caval (inferior) (superior) 459.2
    - thrombotic - *see* Thrombosis
  - vena cava ~~(inferior) (superior) 459.2~~ ▲
    - inferior 453.2 ●
    - superior ●
      - acute 453.87 ●
      - chronic 453.77 ●
  - ventricular shunt 996.2
  - vesical 596.0
  - vesicourethral orifice 596.0
  - vessel NEC 459.9
- **Obturator** - *see* condition
- **Occlusal**
  - plane deviation 524.76
  - wear, teeth 521.10
- **Occlusion**
  - anus 569.49
    - congenital 751.2
    - infantile 751.2
  - aortoiliac (chronic) 444.0
  - aqueduct of Sylvius 331.4
    - congenital 742.3
      - with spina bifida (*see also* Spina bifida) 741.0 5th
  - arteries of extremities, lower 444.22
    - without thrombus or embolus (*see also* Arteriosclerosis, extremities) 440.20
    - due to stricture or stenosis 447.1

- **Occlusion** – *continued*
  - arteries of extremities, lower – *continued*
    - upper 444.21
      - without thrombus or embolus (*see also* Arteriosclerosis, extremities) 440.20
      - due to stricture or stenosis 447.1
  - artery NEC (*see also* Embolism, artery) 444.9
    - auditory, internal 433.8 5th
    - basilar 433.0 5th
      - with other precerebral artery 433.3 5th
      - bilateral 433.3 5th
    - brain or cerebral (*see also* Infarct, brain) 434.9 5th
    - carotid 433.1 5th
      - with other precerebral artery 433.3 5th
      - bilateral 433.3 5th
    - cerebellar (anterior inferior) (posterior inferior) (superior) 433.8 5th
    - cerebral (*see also* Infarct, brain) 434.9 5th
    - choroidal (anterior) 433.8 5th
    - chronic total
      - coronary 414.2
      - extremity(ies) 440.4
    - communicating posterior 433.8 5th
    - complete
      - coronary 414.2
      - extremity(ies) 440.4
    - coronary (thrombotic) (*see also* Infarct, myocardium) 410.9 5th
      - acute 410.9 5th
        - without myocardial infarction 411.81
      - chronic total 414.2
      - complete 414.2
      - healed or old 412
      - total 414.2
    - extremity(ies)
      - chronic total 440.4
      - complete 440.4
      - total 440.4
    - hypophyseal 433.8 5th
    - iliac 444.81
    - mesenteric (embolic) (thrombotic) (with gangrene) 557.0
    - pontine 433.8 5th
    - precerebral NEC 433.9 5th
      - late effect - *see* Late effect(s) (of) cerebrovascular disease
      - multiple or bilateral 433.3 5th
      - puerperal, postpartum, childbirth 674.0 5th
      - specified NEC 433.8 5th
    - renal 593.81
    - retinal - *see* Occlusion, retina, artery
    - spinal 433.8 5th
    - vertebral 433.2 5th
      - with other precerebral artery 433.3 5th
      - bilateral 433.3 5th
  - basilar (artery) - *see* Occlusion, artery, basilar
  - bile duct (any) (*see also* Obstruction, biliary) 576.2
  - bowel (*see also* Obstruction, intestine) 560.9
  - brain (artery) (vascular) (*see also* Infarct, brain) 434.9 5th
  - breast (duct) 611.89
  - carotid (artery) (common) (internal) - *see* Occlusion, artery, carotid
  - cerebellar (anterior inferior) (artery) (posterior inferior) (superior) 433.8 5th
  - cerebral (artery) (*see also* Infarct, brain) 434.9 5th
  - cerebrovascular (*see also* Infarct, brain) 434.9 5th
    - diffuse 437.0

- **Occlusion** – *continued*
  - cervical canal (*see also* Stricture, cervix) 622.4
    - by falciparum malaria 084.0
  - cervix (uteri) (*see also* Stricture, cervix) 622.4
  - choanal 748.0
  - choroidal (artery) 433.8 5th
  - colon (*see also* Obstruction, intestine) 560.9
  - communicating posterior artery 433.8 5th
  - coronary (artery) (thrombotic) (*see also* Infarct, myocardium) 410.9 5th
    - acute 410.9 5th
      - without myocardial infarction 411.81
    - healed or old 412
  - cystic duct (*see also* Obstruction, gallbladder) 575.2
    - congenital 751.69
  - embolic - *see* Embolism
  - disto
    - division I 524.22
    - division II 524.22
  - fallopian tube 628.2
    - congenital 752.19
  - gallbladder (*see also* Obstruction, gallbladder) 575.2
    - congenital 751.69
      - jaundice from 751.69 *[744.5]*
  - gingiva, traumatic 523.8
  - hymen 623.3
    - congenital 752.42
  - hypophyseal (artery) 433.8 5th
  - iliac (artery) 444.81
  - intestine (*see also* Obstruction, intestine) 560.9
  - kidney 593.89
  - lacrimal apparatus - *see* Stenosis, lacrimal
  - lung 518.89
  - lymph or lymphatic channel 457.1
  - mammary duct 611.89
  - mesenteric artery (embolic) (thrombotic) (with gangrene) 557.0
  - nose 478.19
    - congenital 748.0
  - organ or site, congenital NEC - *see* Atresia
  - oviduct 628.2
    - congenital 752.19
  - periodontal, traumatic 523.8
  - peripheral arteries (lower extremity) 444.22
    - without thrombus or embolus (*see also* Arteriosclerosis, extremities) 440.20
    - due to stricture or stenosis 447.1
    - upper extremity 444.21
      - without thrombus or embolus (*see also* Arteriosclerosis, extremities) 440.20
      - due to stricture or stenosis 447.1
  - pontine (artery) 433.8 5th
  - posterior lingual, of mandibular teeth 524.29
  - precerebral artery - *see* Occlusion, artery, precerebral NEC
  - puncta lacrimalia 375.52
  - pupil 364.74
  - pylorus (*see also* Stricture, pylorus) 537.0
  - renal artery 593.81
  - retina, retinal (vascular) 362.30
    - artery, arterial 362.30
      - branch 362.32
      - central (total) 362.31
      - partial 362.33
      - transient 362.34
      - tributary 362.32
    - vein 362.30
      - branch 362.36
      - central (total) 362.35
      - incipient 362.37
      - partial 362.37
      - tributary 362.36
  - spinal artery 433.8 5th

- **Occlusion** – *continued*
  - stent
    - coronary 996.72
  - teeth (mandibular) (posterior lingual) 524.29
  - thoracic duct 457.1
  - tubal 628.2
  - ureter (complete) (partial) 593.4
    - congenital 753.29
  - urethra (*see also* Stricture, urethra) 598.9
    - congenital 753.6
  - uterus 621.8
  - vagina 623.2
  - vascular NEC 459.9
  - vein - *see* Thrombosis
  - vena cava ~~(inferior) (superior) 459.2~~ ▲
    - inferior 453.2 ●
    - superior ●
      - acute 453.87 ●
      - chronic 453.77 ●
  - ventricle (brain) NEC 331.4
  - vertebral (artery) - *see* Occlusion, artery, vertebral
  - vessel (blood) NEC 459.9
  - vulva 624.8
- **Occlusio pupillae** 364.74
- **Occupational**
  - problems NEC V62.29
  - therapy V57.21
- **Ochlophobia** 300.29
- **Ochronosis** (alkaptonuric) (congenital) (endogenous) 270.2
  - with chloasma of eyelid 270.2
- **Ocular muscle** - *see also* condition
  - myopathy 359.1
  - torticollis 781.93
- **Oculoauriculovertebral dysplasia** 756.0
- **Oculogyric**
  - crisis or disturbance 378.87
    - psychogenic 306.7
- **Oculomotor syndrome** 378.81
- **Oddi's sphincter spasm** 576.5
- **Odelberg's disease** (juvenile osteochondrosis) 732.1
- **Odontalgia** 525.9
- **Odontoameloblastoma** (M9311/0) 213.1
  - upper jaw (bone) 213.0
- **Odontoclasia** 521.05
- **Odontoclasis** 873.63
  - complicated 873.73
- **Odontodysplasia, regional** 520.4
- **Odontogenesis imperfecta** 520.5
- **Odontoma** (M9280/0) 213.1
  - ameloblastic (M9311/0) 213.1
    - upper jaw (bone) 213.0
  - calcified (M9280/0) 213.1
    - upper jaw (bone) 213.0
  - complex (M9282/0) 213.1
    - upper jaw (bone) 213.0
  - compound (M9281/0) 213.1
    - upper jaw (bone) 213.0
  - fibroameloblastic (M9290/0) 213.1
    - upper jaw (bone) 213.0
  - follicular 526.0
    - upper jaw (bone) 213.0
- **Odontomyelitis** (closed) (open) 522.0
- **Odontonecrosis** 521.09
- **Odontorrhagia** 525.8
- **Odontosarcoma, ameloblastic** (M9290/3) 170.1
  - upper jaw (bone) 170.0
- **Odynophagia** 787.20
- **Oesophagostomiasis** 127.7
- **Oesophagostomum infestation** 127.7
- **Oestriasis** 134.0
- **Ogilvie's syndrome** (sympathicotonic colon obstruction) 560.89
- **Oguchi's disease** (retina) 368.61
- **Ohara's disease** (*see also* Tularemia) 021.9
- **Oidiomycosis** (*see also* Candidiasis) 112.9
- **Oidiomycotic meningitis** 112.83
- **Oidium albicans infection** (*see also* Candidiasis) 112.9

- **Old age** 797
  - dementia (of) 290.0
- **Olfactory** - *see* condition
- **Oligemia** 285.9
- **Oligergasia** (*see also* Retardation, mental) 319
- **Oligoamnios** 658.0 5th
  - affecting fetus or newborn 761.2
- **Oligoastrocytoma, mixed** (M9382/3)
  - specified site - *see* Neoplasm, by site, malignant
  - unspecified site 191.9
- **Oligocythemia** 285.9
- **Oligodendroblastoma** (M9460/3)
  - specified site - *see* Neoplasm, by site, malignant
  - unspecified site 191.9
- **Oligodendroglioma** (M9450/3)
  - anaplastic type (M9451/3)
    - specified site - *see* Neoplasm, by site, malignant
    - unspecified site 191.9
  - specified site - *see* Neoplasm, by site, malignant
  - unspecified site 191.9
- **Oligodendroma** - *see* Oligodendroglioma
- **Oligodontia** (*see also* Anodontia) 520.0
- **Oligoencephalon** 742.1
- **Oligohydramnios** 658.0 5th
  - affecting fetus or newborn 761.2
  - due to premature rupture of membranes 658.1 5th
    - affecting fetus or newborn 761.2
- **Oligohydrosis** 705.0
- **Oligomenorrhea** 626.1
- **Oligophrenia** (*see also* Retardation, mental) 319
  - phenylpyruvic 270.1
- **Oligospermia** 606.1
- **Oligotrichia** 704.09
  - congenita 757.4
- **Oliguria** 788.5
  - with
    - abortion - *see* Abortion, by type, with renal failure
    - ectopic pregnancy (*see also* categories 633.0-633.9) 639.3
    - molar pregnancy (*see also* categories 630-632) 639.3
  - complicating
    - abortion 639.3
    - ectopic or molar pregnancy 639.3
    - pregnancy 646.2 5th
      - with hypertension - *see* Toxemia, of pregnancy
  - due to a procedure 997.5
  - following labor and delivery 669.3 5th
  - heart or cardiac - *see* Failure, heart
  - puerperal, postpartum 669.3 5th
  - specified due to a procedure 997.5
- **Ollier's disease** (chondrodysplasia) 756.4
- **Omentitis** (*see also* Peritonitis) 567.9
- **Omentocele** (*see also* Hernia, omental) 553.8
- **Omentum, omental** - *see* condition
- **Omphalitis** (congenital) (newborn) 771.4
  - not of newborn 686.9
  - tetanus 771.3
- **Omphalocele** 756.72 ▲
- **Omphalomesenteric duct, persistent** 751.0
- **Omphalorrhagia, newborn** 772.3
- **Omsk hemorrhagic fever** 065.1
- **Onanism** 307.9
- **Onchocerciasis** 125.3
  - eye 125.3 *[360.13]*
- **Onchocercosis** 125.3
- **Oncocytoma** (M8290/0) - *see* Neoplasm, by site, benign
- **Ondine's curse** 348.89 ▲
- **Oneirophrenia** (*see also* Schizophrenia) 295.4 5th
- **Onychauxis** 703.8
  - congenital 757.5
- **Onychia** (with lymphangitis) 681.9
  - dermatophytic 110.1
- **Onychia** – *continued*
  - finger 681.02
  - toe 681.11
- **Onychitis** (with lymphangitis) 681.9
  - finger 681.02
  - toe 681.11
- **Onychocryptosis** 703.0
- **Onychodystrophy** 703.8
  - congenital 757.5
- **Onychogryphosis** 703.8
- **Onychogryposis** 703.8
- **Onycholysis** 703.8
- **Onychomadesis** 703.8
- **Onychomalacia** 703.8
- **Onychomycosis** 110.1
  - finger 110.1
  - toe 110.1
- **Onycho-osteodysplasia** 756.89
- **Onychophagy** 307.9
- **Onychoptosis** 703.8
- **Onychorrhexis** 703.8
  - congenital 757.5
- **Onychoschizia** 703.8
- **Onychotrophia** (*see also* Atrophy, nail) 703.8
- **O'Nyong Nyong fever** 066.3
- **Onyxis** (finger) (toe) 703.0
- **Onyxitis** (with lymphangitis) 681.9
  - finger 681.02
  - toe 681.11
- **Oocyte** (egg) (ovum)
  - donor V59.70
    - over age 35 V59.73
      - anonymous recipient V59.73
      - designated recipient V59.74
    - under age 35 V59.71
      - anonymous recipient V59.71
      - designated recipient V59.72
- **Oophoritis** (cystic) (infectional) (interstitial) (*see also* Salpingo-oophoritis) 614.2
  - complicating pregnancy 646.6 5th
  - fetal (acute) 752.0
  - gonococcal (acute) 098.19
    - chronic or duration of 2 months or over 098.39
  - tuberculous (*see also* Tuberculosis) 016.6 5th
- **Opacity, opacities**
  - cornea 371.00
    - central 371.03
    - congenital 743.43
      - interfering with vision 743.42
    - degenerative (*see also* Degeneration, cornea) 371.40
    - hereditary (*see also* Dystrophy, cornea) 371.50
    - inflammatory (*see also* Keratitis) 370.9
    - late effect of trachoma (healed) 139.1
    - minor 371.01
    - peripheral 371.02
  - enamel (fluoride) (nonfluoride) (teeth) 520.3
  - lens (*see also* Cataract) 366.9
  - snowball 379.22
  - vitreous (humor) 379.24
    - congenital 743.51
- **Opalescent dentin** (hereditary) 520.5
- **Open, opening**
  - abnormal, organ or site, congenital - *see* Imperfect, closure
  - angle with
    - borderline intraocular pressure 365.01
    - cupping of discs 365.01
  - bite
    - anterior 524.24
    - posterior 524.25
  - false - *see* Imperfect, closure
  - margin on tooth restoration 525.61
  - restoration margins 525.61
  - wound - *see* Wound, open, by site
- **Operation**
  - causing mutilation of fetus 763.89
  - destructive, on live fetus, to facilitate birth 763.89
  - for delivery, fetus or newborn 763.89
- **Operation** – *continued*
  - maternal, unrelated to current delivery, affecting fetus or newborn (*see also* Newborn, affected by) 760.64
- **Operational fatigue** 300.89
- **Operative** - *see* condition
- **Operculitis** (chronic) 523.40
  - acute 523.30
- **Operculum, retina** 361.32
  - with detachment 361.01
- **Ophiasis** 704.01
- **Ophthalmia** (*see also* Conjunctivitis) 372.30
  - actinic rays 370.24
  - allergic (acute) 372.05
    - chronic 372.14
- **Ophthalmia** – *continued*
  - blennorrhagic (neonatorum) 098.40
  - catarrhal 372.03
  - diphtheritic 032.81
  - Egyptian 076.1
  - electric, electrica 370.24
  - gonococcal (neonatorum) 098.40
  - metastatic 360.11
  - migraine 346.8 5th
  - neonatorum, newborn 771.6
    - gonococcal 098.40
  - nodosa 360.14
  - phlyctenular 370.31
    - with ulcer (*see also* Ulcer, cornea) 370.00
  - sympathetic 360.11
- **Ophthalmitis** - *see* Ophthalmia
- **Ophthalmocele** (congenital) 743.66
- **Ophthalmoneuromyelitis** 341.0
- **Ophthalmopathy, infiltrative with thyrotoxicosis** 242.0 5th
- **Ophthalmoplegia** (*see also* Strabismus) 378.9
  - anterior internuclear 378.86
  - ataxia-areflexia syndrome 357.0
  - bilateral 378.9
  - diabetic 250.5 5th *[378.86]*
    - due to secondary diabetes 249.5 5th *[378.86]*
  - exophthalmic 242.0 5th *[376.22]*
  - external 378.55
    - progressive 378.72
    - total 378.56
  - internal (complete) (total) 367.52
  - internuclear 378.86
  - migraine 346.2 5th
  - painful 378.55
  - Parinaud's 378.81
  - progressive external 378.72
  - supranuclear, progressive 333.0
  - total (external) 378.56
    - internal 367.52
  - unilateral 378.9
- **Opisthognathism** 524.00
- **Opisthorchiasis** (felineus) (tenuicollis) (viverrini) 121.0
- **Opisthotonos, opisthotonus** 781.0
- **Opitz's disease** (congestive splenomegaly) 289.51
- **Opiumism** (*see also* Dependence) 304.0 5th
- **Oppenheim's disease** 358.8
- **Oppenheim-Urbach disease or syndrome** (necrobiosis lipoidica diabeticorum) 250.8 5th *[709.3]*
  - due to secondary diabetes 249.8 5th *[709.3]*
- **Opsoclonia** 379.59
- **Optic nerve** - *see* condition
- **Orbit** - *see* condition
- **Orchioblastoma** (M9071/3) 186.9
- **Orchitis** (nonspecific) (septic) 604.90
  - with abscess 604.0
  - blennorrhagic (acute) 098.13
    - chronic or duration of 2 months or over 098.33
  - diphtheritic 032.89 *[604.91]*
  - filarial 125.9 *[604.91]*
  - gangrenous 604.99
- **Orchitis** – *continued*
  - gonococcal (acute) 098.13
    - chronic or duration of 2 months or over 098.33
  - mumps 072.0
  - parotidea 072.0
  - suppurative 604.99
  - syphilitic 095.8 *[604.91]*
  - tuberculous (*see also* Tuberculosis) 016.5 5th *[608.81]*
- **Orf** 051.2
- **Organic** - *see also* condition
  - heart - *see* Disease, heart
  - insufficiency 799.89
- **Oriental**
  - bilharziasis 120.2
  - schistosomiasis 120.2
  - sore 085.1
- **Orientation**
  - ego-dystonic sexual 302.0
- **Orifice** - *see* condition
- **Origin, both great vessels from right ventricle** 745.11
- **Ormond's disease or syndrome** 593.4
- **Ornithosis** 073.9
  - with
    - complication 073.8
      - specified NEC 073.7
    - pneumonia 073.0
    - pneumonitis (lobular) 073.0
- **Orodigitofacial dysostosis** 759.89
- **Oropouche fever** 066.3
- **Orotaciduria, oroticaciduria** (congenital) (hereditary) (pyrimidine deficiency) 281.4
- **Oroya fever** 088.0
- **Orthodontics** V58.5
  - adjustment V53.4
  - aftercare V58.5
  - fitting V53.4
- **Orthopnea** 786.02
- **Os, uterus** - *see* condition
- **Osgood-Schlatter**
  - disease 732.4
  - osteochondrosis 732.4
- **Osler's**
  - disease (M9950/1) (polycythemia vera) 238.4
  - nodes 421.0
- **Osler-Rendu disease** (familial hemorrhagic telangiectasia) 448.0
- **Osler-Vaquez disease** (M9950/1) (polycythemia vera) 238.4
- **Osler-Weber-Rendu syndrome** (familial hemorrhagic telangiectasia) 448.0
- **Osmidrosis** 705.89
- **Osseous** - *see* condition
- **Ossification**
  - artery - *see* Arteriosclerosis
  - auricle (ear) 380.39
  - bronchus 519.19
  - cardiac (*see also* Degeneration, myocardial) 429.1
  - cartilage (senile) 733.99
  - coronary - *see* Arteriosclerosis, coronary
  - diaphragm 728.10
  - ear 380.39
    - middle (*see also* Otosclerosis) 387.9
  - falx cerebri 349.2
  - fascia 728.10
  - fontanel
    - defective or delayed 756.0
    - premature 756.0
  - heart (*see also* Degeneration, myocardial) 429.1
    - valve - *see* Endocarditis
  - larynx 478.79
  - ligament
    - posterior longitudinal 724.8
      - cervical 723.7
  - meninges (cerebral) 349.2
    - spinal 336.8
  - multiple, eccentric centers 733.99

- **Ossification** – *continued*
  - muscle 728.10
    - heterotopic, postoperative 728.13
  - myocardium, myocardial (*see also* Degeneration, myocardial) 429.1
  - penis 607.81
  - periarticular 728.89
  - sclera 379.16
  - tendon 727.82
  - trachea 519.19
  - tympanic membrane (*see also* Tympanosclerosis) 385.00
  - vitreous (humor) 360.44
- **Osteitis** (*see also* Osteomyelitis) 730.2 [5th]
  - acute 730.0 [5th]
  - alveolar 526.5
  - chronic 730.1 [5th]
  - condensans (ilii) 733.5
  - deformans (Paget's) 731.0
    - due to or associated with malignant neoplasm (*see also* Neoplasm, bone, malignant) 170.9 *[731.1]*
  - due to yaws 102.6
  - fibrosa NEC 733.29
    - cystica (generalisata) 252.01
    - disseminata 756.59
    - osteoplastica 252.01
  - fragilitans 756.51
  - Garré's (sclerosing) 730.1 [5th]
  - infectious (acute) (subacute) 730.0 [5th]
    - chronic or old 730.1 [5th]
  - jaw (acute) (chronic) (lower) (neonatal) (suppurative) (upper) 526.4
  - parathyroid 252.01
  - petrous bone (*see also* Petrositis) 383.20
  - pubis 733.5
  - sclerotic, nonsuppurative 730.1 [5th]
  - syphilitic 095.5
  - tuberculosa
    - cystica (of Jüngling) 135
    - multiplex cystoides 135
- **Osteoarthritica spondylitis** (spine) (*see also* Spondylosis) 721.90
- **Osteoarthritis** (*see also* Osteoarthrosis) 715.9 [5th]
  - distal interphalangeal 715.9 [5th]
  - hyperplastic 731.2
  - interspinalis (*see also* Spondylosis) 721.90
  - spine, spinal NEC (*see also* Spondylosis) 721.90
- **Osteoarthropathy** (*see also* Osteoarthrosis) 715.9 [5th]
  - chronic idiopathic hypertrophic 757.39
  - familial idiopathic 757.39
  - hypertrophic pulmonary 731.2
    - secondary 731.2
  - idiopathic hypertrophic 757.39
  - primary hypertrophic 731.2
  - pulmonary hypertrophic 731.2
  - secondary hypertrophic 731.2
- **Osteoarthrosis** (degenerative) (hypertrophic) (rheumatoid) 715.9 [5th]

Note *Use the following fifth-digit subclassification with category 715:*

0	site unspecified
1	shoulder region
2	upper arm
3	forearm
4	hand
5	pelvic region and thigh
6	lower leg
7	ankle and foot
8	other specified sites except spine
9	multiple sites

  - Deformans alkaptonurica 270.2
  - generalized 715.09
  - juvenilis (Köhler's) 732.5
  - localized 715.3 [5th]
    - idiopathic 715.1 [5th]
    - primary 715.1 [5th]
    - secondary 715.2 [5th]
- **Osteoarthrosis** – *continued*
  - multiple sites, not specified as generalized 715.89
  - polyarticular 715.09
  - spine (*see also* Spondylosis) 721.90
  - temporomandibular joint 524.69
- **Osteoblastoma** (M9200/0) - *see* Neoplasm, bone, benign
- **Osteochondritis** (*see also* Osteochondrosis) 732.9
  - dissecans 732.7
    - hip 732.7
  - ischiopubica 732.1
  - multiple 756.59
  - syphilitic (congenital) 090.0
- **Osteochondrodermodysplasia** 756.59
- **Osteochondrodystrophy** 277.5
  - deformans 277.5
- **Osteochondrodystrophy** – *continued*
  - familial 277.5
  - fetalis 756.4
- **Osteochondrolysis** 732.7
- **Osteochondroma** (M9210/0) - *see also* Neoplasm, bone, benign
  - multiple, congenital 756.4
- **Osteochondromatosis** (M9210/1) 238.0
  - synovial 727.82
- **Osteochondromyxosarcoma** (M9180/3) - *see* Neoplasm, bone, malignant
- **Osteochondropathy NEC** 732.9
- **Osteochondrosarcoma** (M9180/3) - *see* Neoplasm, bone, malignant
- **Osteochondrosis** 732.9
  - acetabulum 732.1
  - adult spine 732.8
  - astragalus 732.5
  - Blount's 732.4
  - Buchanan's (juvenile osteochondrosis of iliac crest) 732.1
  - Buchman's (juvenile osteochondrosis) 732.1
  - Burns' 732.3
  - calcaneus 732.5
  - capitular epiphysis (femur) 732.1
  - carpal
    - lunate (wrist) 732.3
    - scaphoid 732.3
  - coxae juvenilis 732.1
  - deformans juvenilis (coxae) (hip) 732.1
    - Scheuermann's 732.0
    - spine 732.0
    - tibia 732.4
    - vertebra 732.0
  - Diaz's (astragalus) 732.5
  - dissecans (knee) (shoulder) 732.7
  - femoral capital epiphysis 732.1
  - femur (head) (juvenile) 732.1
  - foot (juvenile) 732.5
  - Freiberg's (disease) (second metatarsal) 732.5
  - Haas' 732.3
  - Haglund's (os tibiale externum) 732.5
  - hand (juvenile) 732.3
  - head of
    - femur 732.1
    - humerus (juvenile) 732.3
  - hip (juvenile) 732.1
  - humerus (juvenile) 732.3
  - iliac crest (juvenile) 732.1
  - ilium (juvenile) 732.1
  - ischiopubic synchondrosis 732.1
  - Iselin's (osteochondrosis fifth metatarsal) 732.5
  - juvenile, juvenilis 732.6
    - arm 732.3
    - capital femoral epiphysis 732.1
    - capitellum humeri 732.3
    - capitular epiphysis 732.1
    - carpal scaphoid 732.3
    - clavicle, sternal epiphysis 732.6
    - coxae 732.1
    - deformans 732.1
    - foot 732.5
    - hand 732.3
- **Osteochondrosis** – *continued*
  - juvenile, juvenilis – *continued*
    - hip and pelvis 732.1
    - lower extremity, except foot 732.4
    - lunate, wrist 732.3
    - medial cuneiform bone 732.5
    - metatarsal (head) 732.5
    - metatarsophalangeal 732.5
    - navicular, ankle 732.5
    - patella 732.4
    - primary patellar center (of Köhler) 732.4
    - specified site NEC 732.6
    - spine 732.0
    - tarsal scaphoid 732.5
    - tibia (epiphysis) (tuberosity) 732.4
    - upper extremity 732.3
    - vertebra (body) (Calvé) 732.0
      - epiphyseal plates (of Scheuermann) 732.0
  - Kienböck's (disease) 732.3
  - Köhler's (disease) (navicular, ankle) 732.5
    - patellar 732.4
    - tarsal navicular 732.5
  - Legg-Calvé-Perthes (disease) 732.1
  - lower extremity (juvenile) 732.4
  - lunate bone 732.3
  - Mauclaire's 732.3
  - metacarpal heads (of Mauclaire) 732.3
  - metatarsal (fifth) (head) (second) 732.5
  - navicular, ankle 732.5
  - os calcis 732.5
  - Osgood-Schlatter 732.4
  - os tibiale externum 732.5
  - Panner's 732.3
  - patella (juvenile) 732.4
  - patellar center
    - primary (of Köhler) 732.4
    - secondary (of Sinding-Larsen) 732.4
  - pelvis (juvenile) 732.1
  - Pierson's 732.1
  - radial head (juvenile) 732.3
  - Scheuermann's 732.0
  - Sever's (calcaneum) 732.5
  - Sinding-Larsen (secondary patellar center) 732.4
  - spine (juvenile) 732.0
    - adult 732.8
  - symphysis pubis (of Pierson) (juvenile) 732.1
  - syphilitic (congenital) 090.0
  - tarsal (navicular) (scaphoid) 732.5
  - tibia (proximal) (tubercle) 732.4
  - tuberculous - *see* Tuberculosis, bone
  - ulna 732.3
  - upper extremity (juvenile) 732.3
  - van Neck's (juvenile osteochondrosis) 732.1
  - vertebral (juvenile) 732.0
    - adult 732.8
- **Osteoclastoma** (M9250/1) 238.0
  - malignant (M9250/3) - *see* Neoplasm, bone, malignant
- **Osteocopic pain** 733.90
- **Osteodynia** 733.90
- **Osteodystrophy**
  - azotemic 588.0
  - chronica deformans hypertrophica 731.0
  - congenital 756.50
    - specified type NEC 756.59
  - deformans 731.0
  - fibrosa localisata 731.0
  - parathyroid 252.01
  - renal 588.0
- **Osteofibroma** (M9262/0) - *see* Neoplasm, bone, benign
- **Osteofibrosarcoma** (M9182/3) - *see* Neoplasm, bone, malignant
- **Osteogenesis imperfecta** 756.51
- **Osteogenic** - *see* condition
- **Osteoma** (M9180/0) - *see also* Neoplasm, bone, benign
  - osteoid (M9191/0) - *see also* Neoplasm, bone, benign
    - giant (M9200/0) - *see* Neoplasm, bone, benign
- **Osteomalacia** 268.2
  - chronica deformans hypertrophica 731.0
  - due to vitamin D deficiency 268.2
  - infantile (*see also* Rickets) 268.0
  - juvenile (*see also* Rickets) 268.0
  - pelvis 268.2
  - vitamin D-resistant 275.3
- **Osteomalacic bone** 268.2
- **Osteomalacosis** 268.2
- **Osteomyelitis** (general) (infective) (localized) (neonatal) (purulent) (pyogenic) (septic) (staphylococcal) (streptococcal) (suppurative) (with periostitis) 730.2 [5th]

Note *Use the following fifth-digit subclassification with category 730:*

0	site unspecified
1	shoulder region
2	upper arm
3	forearm
4	hand
5	pelvic region and thigh
6	lower leg
7	ankle and foot
8	other specified sites
9	multiple sites

  - acute or subacute 730.0 [5th]
  - chronic or old 730.1 [5th]
  - due to or associated with
    - diabetes mellitus 250.8 [5th] *[731.8]*
      - due to secondary diabetes 249.8 [5th] *[731.8]*
    - tuberculosis (*see also* Tuberculosis, bone) 015.9 [5th] *[730.8]* [5th]
      - limb bones 015.5 [5th] *[730.8]* [5th]
      - specified bones NEC 015.7 [5th] *[730.8]* [5th]
      - spine 015.0 [5th] *[730.8]* [5th]
    - typhoid 002.0 *[730.8]* [5th]
  - Garré's 730.1
  - jaw (acute) (chronic) (lower) (neonatal) (suppurative) (upper) 526.4
  - nonsuppurating 730.1 [5th]
  - orbital 376.03
  - petrous bone (*see also* Petrositis) 383.20
  - Salmonella 003.24
  - sclerosing, nonsuppurative 730.1 [5th]
  - sicca 730.1 [5th]
  - syphilitic 095.5
    - congenital 090.0 *[730.8]* [5th]
  - tuberculous - *see* Tuberculosis, bone
  - typhoid 002.0 *[730.8]* [5th]
- **Osteomyelofibrosis** 289.89
- **Osteomyelosclerosis** 289.89
- **Osteonecrosis** 733.40
  - meaning osteomyelitis 730.1 [5th]
- **Osteo-onycho-arthro dysplasia** 756.89
- **Osteo-onychodysplasia, hereditary** 756.89
- **Osteopathia**
  - condensans disseminata 756.53
  - hyperostotica multiplex infantilis 756.59
  - hypertrophica toxica 731.2
  - striata 756.4
- **Osteopathy resulting from poliomyelitis** (*see also* Poliomyelitis) 045.9 [5th] *[730.7]* [5th]
  - familial dysplastic 731.2
- **Osteopecilia** 756.53
- **Osteopenia** 733.90
  - borderline 733.90
- **Osteoperiostitis** (*see also* Osteomyelitis) 730.2 [5th]
  - ossificans toxica 731.2
  - toxica ossificans 731.2
- **Osteopetrosis** (familial) 756.52

- **Overnutrition** (*see also* Hyperalimentation) 783.6
- **Overproduction** - *see also* Hypersecretion
  - ACTH 255.3
  - cortisol 255.0
  - growth hormone 253.0
  - thyroid-stimulating hormone (TSH) 242.8 5th
- **Overriding**
  - aorta 747.21
  - finger (acquired) 736.29
    - congenital 755.59
  - toe (acquired) 735.8
    - congenital 755.66
- **Oversize**
  - fetus (weight of 4500 grams or more) 766.0
    - affecting management of pregnancy 656.6 5th
    - causing disproportion 653.5 5th
      - with obstructed labor 660.1 5th
        - affecting fetus or newborn 763.1
- **Overstimulation, ovarian** 256.1
- **Overstrained** 780.79
  - heart - *see* Hypertrophy, cardiac
- **Overweight** (*see also* Obesity) 278.02
- **Overwork** 780.79
- **Oviduct** - *see* condition
- **Ovotestis** 752.7
- **Ovulation** (cycle)
  - failure or lack of 628.0
  - pain 625.2
- **Ovum**
  - blighted 631
  - donor V59.70
    - over age 35 V59.73
      - anonymous recipient V59.73
      - designated recipient V59.74
    - under age 35 V59.71
      - anonymous recipient V59.71
      - designated recipient V59.72
  - dropsical 631
  - pathologic 631
- **Owren's disease or syndrome** (parahemophilia) (*see also* Defect, coagulation) 286.3
- **Oxalosis** 271.8
- **Oxaluria** 271.8
- **Ox heart** - *see* Hypertrophy, cardiac
- **OX syndrome** 758.6
- **Oxycephaly, oxycephalic** 756.0
  - syphilitic, congenital 090.0
- **Oxyuriasis** 127.4
- **Oxyuris vermicularis** (infestation) 127.4
- **Ozena** 472.0

P

- **Pacemaker syndrome** 429.4
- **Pachyderma, pachydermia** 701.8
  - laryngis 478.5
  - laryngitis 478.79
  - larynx (verrucosa) 478.79
- **Pachydermatitis** 701.8
- **Pachydermatocele** (congenital) 757.39
  - acquired 701.8
- **Pachydermatosis** 701.8
- **Pachydermoperiostitis**
  - secondary 731.2
- **Pachydermoperiostosis**
  - primary idiopathic 757.39
  - secondary 731.2
- **Pachymeningitis** (adhesive) (basal) (brain) (cerebral) (cervical) (chronic) (circumscribed) (external) (fibrous) (hemorrhagic) (hypertrophic) (internal) (purulent) (spinal) (suppurative) (*see also* Meningitis) 322.9
  - gonococcal 098.82
- **Pachyonychia** (congenital) 757.5
  - acquired 703.8
- **Pachyperiosteodermia**
  - primary or idiopathic 757.39
  - secondary 731.2
- **Pachyperiostosis**
  - primary or idiopathic 757.39
  - secondary 731.2
- **Pacinian tumor** (M9507/0) - *see* Neoplasm, skin, benign
- **Pads, knuckle or Garrod's** 728.79
- **Paget's disease** (osteitis deformans) 731.0
  - with infiltrating duct carcinoma of the breast (M8541/3) - *see* Neoplasm, breast, malignant
  - bone 731.0
    - osteosarcoma in (M9184/3) - *see* Neoplasm, bone, malignant
  - breast (M8540/3) 174.0
- **Paget's disease** – *continued*
  - extramammary (M8542/3) - *see also* Neoplasm, skin, malignant
    - anus 154.3
      - skin 173.5
  - malignant (M8540/3)
    - breast 174.0
    - specified site NEC (M8542/3) - *see* Neoplasm, skin, malignant
    - unspecified site 174.0
  - mammary (M8540/3) 174.0
  - necrosis of bone 731.0
  - nipple (M8540/3) 174.0
  - osteitis deformans 731.0
- **Paget-Schroetter syndrome** (intermittent venous claudication) 453.89 ▲
- **Pain(s)** (*see also* Painful) 780.96
  - abdominal 789.0 5th
  - acute 338.19
    - due to trauma 338.11
    - postoperative 338.18
      - post-thoracotomy 338.12
  - adnexa (uteri) 625.9
  - alimentary, due to vascular insufficiency 557.9
  - anginoid (*see also* Pain, precordial) 786.51
  - anus 569.42
  - arch 729.5
  - arm 729.5
  - axillary 729.5
  - back (postural) 724.5
    - low 724.2
    - psychogenic 307.89
  - bile duct 576.9
  - bladder 788.99
  - bone 733.90
  - breast 611.71
    - psychogenic 307.89
  - broad ligament 625.9
  - cancer associated 338.3
  - cartilage NEC 733.90
  - cecum 789.0 5th
  - cervicobrachial 723.3
  - chest (central) 786.50
    - atypical 786.59
    - midsternal 786.51
    - musculoskeletal 786.59
    - noncardiac 786.59
    - substernal 786.51
    - wall (anterior) 786.52
  - chronic 338.29
    - associated with significant psychosocial dysfunction 338.4
    - due to trauma 338.21
    - postoperative 338.28
      - post-thoracotomy 338.22
    - syndrome 338.4
  - coccyx 724.79
  - colon 789.0 5th
  - common duct 576.9
  - coronary - *see* Angina
  - costochondral 786.52
  - diaphragm 786.52
- **Pain(s)** – *continued*
  - due to (presence of) any device, implant, or graft classifiable to 996.0-996.5 - *see* Complications, due to (presence of) any device, implant, or graft classified to 996.0-996.5 NEC
  - malignancy (primary) (secondary) 338.3
  - ear (*see also* Otalgia) 388.70
  - epigastric, epigastrium 789.06
  - extremity (lower) (upper) 729.5
  - eye 379.91
  - face, facial 784.0
    - atypical 350.2
    - nerve 351.8
  - false (labor) 644.1 5th
  - female genital organ NEC 625.9
    - psychogenic 307.89
  - finger 729.5
  - flank 789.0 5th
  - foot 729.5
  - gallbladder 575.9
  - gas (intestinal) 787.3
  - gastric 536.8
  - generalized 780.96
  - genital organ
    - female 625.9
    - male 608.9
    - psychogenic 307.89
  - groin 789.0 5th
  - growing 781.99
  - hand 729.5
  - head (*see also* Headache) 784.0
  - heart (*see also* Pain, precordial) 786.51
  - infraorbital (*see also* Neuralgia, trigeminal) 350.1
  - intermenstrual 625.2
  - jaw 526.9
  - joint 719.40
    - ankle 719.47
    - elbow 719.42
    - foot 719.47
    - hand 719.44
    - hip 719.45
    - knee 719.46
    - multiple sites 719.49
    - pelvic region 719.45
    - psychogenic 307.89
    - shoulder (region) 719.41
    - specified site NEC 719.48
    - wrist 719.43
  - kidney 788.0
  - labor, false or spurious 644.1 5th
  - laryngeal 784.1
  - leg 729.5
  - limb 729.5
  - low back 724.2
  - lumbar region 724.2
  - mastoid (*see also* Otalgia) 388.70
  - maxilla 526.9
  - menstrual 625.3
  - metacarpophalangeal (joint) 719.44
  - metatarsophalangeal (joint) 719.47
  - mouth 528.9
  - muscle 729.1
    - intercostal 786.59
  - musculoskeletal (*see also* Pain, by site) 729.1
  - nasal 478.19
  - nasopharynx 478.29
  - neck NEC 723.1
    - psychogenic 307.89
  - nerve NEC 729.2
  - neoplasm related (acute) (chronic) 338.3
  - neuromuscular 729.1
  - nose 478.19
  - ocular 379.91
  - ophthalmic 379.91
  - orbital region 379.91
  - osteocopic 733.90
  - ovary 625.9
    - psychogenic 307.89
  - over heart (*see also* Pain, precordial) 786.51
- **Pain(s)** – *continued*
  - ovulation 625.2
  - pelvic (female) 625.9
    - male NEC 789.0 5th
      - psychogenic 307.89
    - psychogenic 307.89
  - penis 607.9
    - psychogenic 307.89
  - pericardial (*see also* Pain, precordial) 786.51
  - perineum
    - female 625.9
    - male 608.9
  - pharynx 478.29
  - pleura, pleural, pleuritic 786.52
  - postoperative 338.18
    - acute 338.18
    - chronic 338.28
  - post-thoracotomy 338.12
    - acute 338.12
    - chronic 338.22
  - preauricular 388.70
  - precordial (region) 786.51
    - psychogenic 307.89
  - premenstrual 625.4
  - psychogenic 307.80
    - cardiovascular system 307.89
    - gastrointestinal system 307.89
    - genitourinary system 307.89
    - heart 307.89
    - musculoskeletal system 307.89
    - respiratory system 307.89
    - skin 306.3
  - radicular (spinal) (*see also* Radiculitis) 729.2
  - rectum 569.42
  - respiration 786.52
  - retrosternal 786.51
  - rheumatic NEC 729.0
    - muscular 729.1
  - rib 786.50
  - root (spinal) (*see also* Radiculitis) 729.2
  - round ligament (stretch) 625.9
  - sacroiliac 724.6
  - sciatic 724.3
  - scrotum 608.9
    - psychogenic 307.89
  - seminal vesicle 608.9
  - sinus 478.19
  - skin 782.0
  - spermatic cord 608.9
  - spinal root (*see also* Radiculitis) 729.2
  - stomach 536.8
    - psychogenic 307.89
  - substernal 786.51
  - temporomandibular (joint) 524.62
  - temporomaxillary joint 524.62
  - testis 608.9
    - psychogenic 307.89
  - thoracic spine 724.1
    - with radicular and visceral pain 724.4
  - throat 784.1
  - tibia 733.90
  - toe 729.5
  - tongue 529.6
  - tooth 525.9
  - tumor associated 338.3
  - trigeminal (*see also* Neuralgia, trigeminal) 350.1
  - umbilicus 789.05
  - ureter 788.0
  - urinary (organ) (system) 788.0
  - uterus 625.9
    - psychogenic 307.89
  - vagina 625.9
  - vertebrogenic (syndrome) 724.5
  - vesical 788.99
  - vulva 625.9
  - xiphoid 733.90
- **Painful** - *see also* Pain
  - arc syndrome 726.19
  - coitus
    - female 625.0
    - male 608.89

- **Painful** – *continued*
  - coitus – *continued*
    - psychogenic 302.76
  - ejaculation (semen) 608.89
    - psychogenic 302.79
  - erection 607.3
  - feet syndrome 266.2
  - menstruation 625.3
    - psychogenic 306.52
  - micturition 788.1
  - ophthalmoplegia 378.55
  - respiration 786.52
  - scar NEC 709.2
  - total hip replacement 996.77
  - total knee replacement 996.77
  - urination 788.1
  - wire sutures 998.89
- **Painters' colic** 984.9
  - specified type of lead - *see* Table of Drugs and Chemicals
- **Palate** - *see* condition
- **Palatoplegia** 528.9
- **Palatoschisis** (*see also* Cleft, palate) 749.00
- **Palilalia** 784.69
- **Palindromic arthritis** (*see also* Rheumatism, palindromic) 719.3 [5th]
- **Palliative care** V66.7
- **Pallor** 782.61
  - temporal, optic disc 377.15
- **Palmar** - *see also* condition
  - fascia - *see* condition
- **Palpable**
  - cecum 569.89
  - kidney 593.89
  - liver 573.9
  - lymph nodes 785.6
  - ovary 620.8
  - prostate 602.9
  - spleen (*see also* Splenomegaly) 789.2
  - uterus 625.8
- **Palpitation** (heart) 785.1
  - psychogenic 306.2
- **Palsy** (*see also* Paralysis) 344.9
  - atrophic diffuse 335.20
  - Bell's 351.0
    - newborn 767.5
  - birth 767.7
  - brachial plexus 353.0
    - fetus or newborn 767.6
  - brain - *see also* Palsy, cerebral
    - noncongenital or noninfantile 344.89
      - late effect - *see* Late effect(s) (of) cerebrovascular disease
    - syphilitic 094.89
      - congenital 090.49
  - bulbar (chronic) (progressive) 335.22
    - pseudo NEC 335.23
    - supranuclear NEC 344.89
  - cerebral (congenital) (infantile) (spastic) 343.9
    - athetoid 333.71
    - diplegic 343.0
      - late effect - *see* Late effect(s) (of) cerebrovascular disease
    - hemiplegic 343.1
    - monoplegic 343.3
    - noncongenital or noninfantile 437.8
      - late effect - *see* Late effect(s) (of) cerebrovascular disease
    - paraplegic 343.0
    - quadriplegic 343.2
    - spastic, not congenital or infantile 344.89
    - syphilitic 094.89
      - congenital 090.49
    - tetraplegic 343.2
  - cranial nerve - *see also* Disorder, nerve, cranial
    - multiple 352.6
  - creeping 335.21
  - divers' 993.3
  - Erb's (birth injury) 767.6
  - facial 351.0
    - newborn 767.5
- **Palsy** – *continued*
  - glossopharyngeal 352.2
  - Klumpke (-Déjérine) 767.6
  - lead 984.9
    - specified type of lead - *see* Table of Drugs and Chemicals
  - median nerve (tardy) 354.0
  - peroneal nerve (acute) (tardy) 355.3
  - progressive supranuclear 333.0
  - pseudobulbar NEC 335.23
  - radial nerve (acute) 354.3
  - seventh nerve 351.0
    - newborn 767.5
  - shaking (*see also* Parkinsonism) 332.0
  - spastic (cerebral) (spinal) 343.9
    - hemiplegic 343.1
  - specified nerve NEC - *see* Disorder, nerve
  - supranuclear NEC 356.8
    - progressive 333.0
  - ulnar nerve (tardy) 354.2
  - wasting 335.21
- **Paltauf-Sternberg disease** 201.9 [5th]
- **Paludism** - *see* Malaria
- **Panama fever** 084.0
- **Panaris** (with lymphangitis) 681.9
  - finger 681.02
  - toe 681.11
- **Panaritium** (with lymphangitis) 681.9
  - finger 681.02
  - toe 681.11
- **Panarteritis** (nodosa) 446.0
  - brain or cerebral 437.4
- **Pancake heart** 793.2
  - with cor pulmonale (chronic) 416.9
- **Pancarditis** (acute) (chronic) 429.89
  - with
    - rheumatic
      - fever (active) (acute) (chronic) (subacute) 391.8
        - inactive or quiescent 398.99
  - rheumatic, acute 391.8
    - chronic or inactive 398.99
- **Pancoast's syndrome or tumor** (carcinoma, pulmonary apex) (M8010/3) 162.3
- **Pancoast-Tobias syndrome** (M8010/3) (carcinoma, pulmonary apex) 162.3
- **Pancolitis** 556.6
- **Pancreas, pancreatic** - *see* condition
- **Pancreatitis** 577.0
  - acute (edematous) (hemorrhagic) (recurrent) 577.0
  - annular 577.0
  - apoplectic 577.0
  - calcereous 577.0
  - chronic (infectious) 577.1
    - recurrent 577.1
  - cystic 577.2
  - fibrous 577.8
  - gangrenous 577.0
  - hemorrhagic (acute) 577.0
  - interstitial (chronic) 577.1
    - acute 577.0
  - malignant 577.0
  - mumps 072.3
  - painless 577.1
  - recurrent 577.1
  - relapsing 577.1
  - subacute 577.0
  - suppurative 577.0
  - syphilitic 095.8
- **Pancreatolithiasis** 577.8
- **Pancytolysis** 289.9
- **Pancytopenia** (acquired) 284.1
  - with malformations 284.09
  - congenital 284.09
- **Panencephalitis** - *see also* Encephalitis
  - subacute, sclerosing 046.2
- **Panhematopenia** 284.81
  - congenital 284.09
  - constitutional 284.09
  - splenic, primary 289.4
- **Panhemocytopenia** 284.81
  - congenital 284.09
  - constitutional 284.09
- **Panhypogonadism** 257.2
- **Panhypopituitarism** 253.2
  - prepubertal 253.3
- **Panic** (attack) (state) 300.01
  - reaction to exceptional stress (transient) 308.0
- **Panmyelopathy, familial constitutional** 284.09
- **Panmyelophthisis** 284.2
  - acquired (secondary) 284.81
  - congenital 284.2
  - idiopathic 284.9
- **Panmyelosis** (acute) (M9951/1) 238.79
- **Panner's disease** 732.3
  - capitellum humeri 732.3
  - head of humerus 732.3
  - tarsal navicular (bone) (osteochondrosis) 732.5
- **Panneuritis endemica** 265.0 *[357.4]*
- **Panniculitis** 729.30
  - back 724.8
  - knee 729.31
  - mesenteric 567.82
  - neck 723.6
  - nodular, nonsuppurative 729.30
  - sacral 724.8
  - specified site NEC 729.39
- **Panniculus adiposus** (abdominal) 278.1
- **Pannus** (corneal) 370.62
  - abdominal (symptomatic) 278.1
  - allergic eczematous 370.62
  - degenerativus 370.62
  - keratic 370.62
  - rheumatoid - *see* Arthritis, rheumatoid
  - trachomatosus, trachomatous (active) 076.1 *[370.62]*
    - late effect 139.1
- **Panophthalmitis** 360.02
- **Panotitis** - *see* Otitis media
- **Pansinusitis** (chronic) (hyperplastic) (nonpurulent) (purulent) 473.8
  - acute 461.8
  - due to fungus NEC 117.9
  - tuberculous (*see also* Tuberculosis) 012.8 [5th]
- **Panuveitis** 360.12
  - sympathetic 360.11
- **Panvalvular disease** - *see* Endocarditis, mitral
- **Papageienkrankheit** 073.9
- **Papanicolaou smear**
  - anus 796.70
    - with
      - atypical squamous cells
        - cannot exclude high grade squamous intraepithelial lesion (ASC-H) 796.72
        - of undetermined significance (ASC-US) 796.71
      - cytologic evidence of malignancy 796.76
      - high grade squamous intraepithelial lesion (HGSIL) 796.74
      - low grade squamous intraepithelial lesion (LGSIL) 796.73
    - glandular 796.70
    - specified finding NEC 796.79
    - unsatisfactory cytology 796.78
  - cervix (screening test) V76.2
    - as part of gynecological examination V72.31
    - for suspected malignant neoplasm V76.2
      - no disease found V71.1
    - inadequate cytology sample 795.08
    - nonspecific abnormal finding 795.00
      - with
        - atypical squamous cells
          - cannot exclude high grade squamous intraepithelial lesion (ASC-H) 795.02
- **Papanicolaou smear** – *continued*
  - cervix – *continued*
    - nonspecific abnormal finding – *continued*
      - with – *continued*
        - atypical squamous cells – *continued*
          - of undetermined significance (ASC-US) 795.01
        - cytologic evidence of malignancy 795.06
        - high grade squamous intraepithelial lesion (HGSIL) 795.04
        - low grade squamous intraepithelial lesion (LGSIL) 795.03
    - nonspecific finding NEC 795.09
    - to confirm findings of recent normal smear following initial abnormal smear V72.32
    - satisfactory smear but lacking transformation zone 795.07
    - unsatisfactory cervical cytology 795.08
  - other specified site - *see also* Screening, malignant neoplasm
    - for suspected malignant neoplasm - *see also* Screening, malignant neoplasm
      - no disease found V71.1
    - nonspecific abnormal finding 796.9
  - vagina V76.47
    - with
      - atypical squamous cells
        - cannot exclude high grade squamous intraepithelial lesion (ASC-H) 795.12
        - of undetermined significance (ASC-US) 795.11
      - cytologic evidence of malignancy 795.16
      - high grade squamous intraepithelial lesion (HGSIL) 795.14
      - low grade squamous intraepithelial lesion (LGSIL) 795.13
    - abnormal NEC 795.19
    - following hysterectomy for malignant condition V67.01
    - inadequate cytology sample 795.18
    - unsatisfactory cytology 795.18
- **Papilledema** 377.00
  - associated with
    - decreased ocular pressure 377.02
    - increased intracranial pressure 377.01
    - retinal disorder 377.03
  - choked disc 377.00
  - infectional 377.00
- **Papillitis** 377.31
  - anus 569.49
  - chronic lingual 529.4
  - necrotizing, kidney 584.7
  - optic 377.31
  - rectum 569.49
  - renal, necrotizing 584.7
  - tongue 529.0
- **Papilloma** (M8050/0) - *see also* Neoplasm, by site, benign

Note *Except where otherwise indicated, the morphological varieties of papilloma in the list below should be coded by site as for "Neoplasm, benign".*

- acuminatum (female) (male) 078.11
- bladder (urinary) (transitional cell) (M8120/1) 236.7
  - benign (M8120/0) 223.3
- choroid plexus (M9390/0) 225.0
  - anaplastic type (M9390/3) 191.5
  - malignant (M9390/3) 191.5
- ductal (M8503/0)
- dyskeratotic (M8052/0)
- epidermoid (M8052/0)
- hyperkeratotic (M8052/0)

- **Papilloma** – *continued*
  - intracystic (M8504/0)
  - intraductal (M8503/0)
  - inverted (M8053/0)
  - keratotic (M8052/0)
  - parakeratotic (M8052/0)
  - pinta (primary) 103.0
  - renal pelvis (transitional cell) (M8120/1) 236.99
    - benign (M8120/0) 223.1
  - Schneiderian (M8121/0)
    - specified site - *see* Neoplasm, by site, benign
    - unspecified site 212.0
  - serous surface (M8461/0)
    - borderline malignancy (M8461/1)
      - specified site - *see* Neoplasm, by site, uncertain behavior
      - unspecified site 236.2
    - specified site - *see* Neoplasm, by site, benign
    - unspecified site 220
  - squamous (cell) (M8052/0)
  - transitional (cell) (M8120/0)
    - bladder (urinary) (M8120/1) 236.7
    - inverted type (M8121/1) - *see* Neoplasm, by site, uncertain behavior
    - renal pelvis (M8120/1) 236.91
    - ureter (M8120/1) 236.91
  - ureter (transitional cell) (M8120/1) 236.91
    - benign (M8120/0) 223.2
  - urothelial (M8120/1) - *see* Neoplasm, by site, uncertain behavior
  - verrucous (M8051/0)
  - villous (M8261/1) - *see* Neoplasm, by site, uncertain behavior
  - yaws, plantar or palmar 102.1
- **Papillomata, multiple, of yaws** 102.1
- **Papillomatosis** (M8060/0) - *see also* Neoplasm, by site, benign
  - confluent and reticulate 701.8
  - cutaneous 701.8
  - ductal, breast 610.1
  - Gougerot-Carteaud (confluent reticulate) 701.8
  - intraductal (diffuse) (M8505/0) - *see* Neoplasm, by site, benign
  - subareolar duct (M8506/0) 217
- **Papillon-Léage and Psaume syndrome** (orodigitofacial dysostosis) 759.89
- **Papule** 709.8
  - carate (primary) 103.0
  - fibrous, of nose (M8724/0) 216.3
  - pinta (primary) 103.0
- **Papulosis, malignant** 447.8
- **Papyraceous fetus** 779.89
  - complicating pregnancy 646.0 [5th]
- **Paracephalus** 759.7
- **Parachute mitral valve** 746.5
- **Paracoccidioidomycosis** 116.1
  - mucocutaneous-lymphangitic 116.1
  - pulmonary 116.1
  - visceral 116.1
- **Paracoccidiomycosis** - *see* Paracoccidioidomycosis
- **Paracusis** 388.40
- **Paradentosis** 523.5
- **Paradoxical facial movements** 374.43
- **Paraffinoma** 999.9
- **Paraganglioma** (M8680/1)
  - adrenal (M8700/0) 227.0
    - malignant (M8700/3) 194.0
  - aortic body (M8691/1) 237.3
    - malignant (M8691/3) 194.6
  - carotid body (M8692/1) 237.3
    - malignant (M8692/3) 194.5
  - chromaffin (M8700/0) - *see also* Neoplasm, by site, benign
    - malignant (M8700/3) - *see* Neoplasm, by site, malignant
- **Paraganglioma** – *continued*
  - extra-adrenal (M8693/1)
    - malignant (M8693/3)
      - specified site - *see* Neoplasm, by site, malignant
      - unspecified site 194.6
    - specified site - *see* Neoplasm, by site, uncertain behavior
    - unspecified site 237.3
  - glomus jugulare (M8690/1) 237.3
    - malignant (M8690/3) 194.6
  - jugular (M8690/1) 237.3
  - malignant (M8680/3)
    - specified site - *see* Neoplasm, by site, malignant
    - unspecified site 194.6
  - nonchromaffin (M8693/1)
    - malignant (M8693/3)
      - specified site - *see* Neoplasm, by site, malignant
      - unspecified site 194.6
    - specified site - *see* Neoplasm, by site, uncertain behavior
    - unspecified site 237.3
  - parasympathetic (M8682/1)
    - specified site - *see* Neoplasm, by site, uncertain behavior
    - unspecified site 237.3
  - specified site - *see* Neoplasm, by site, uncertain behavior
  - sympathetic (M8681/1)
    - specified site - *see* Neoplasm, by site, uncertain behavior
    - unspecified site 237.3
  - unspecified site 237.3
- **Parageusia** 781.1
  - psychogenic 306.7
- **Paragonimiasis** 121.2
- **Paragranuloma, Hodgkin's** (M9660/3) 201.0 [5th]
- **Parahemophilia** (*see also* Defect, coagulation) 286.3
- **Parakeratosis** 690.8
  - psoriasiformis 696.2
  - variegata 696.2
- **Paralysis, paralytic** (complete) (incomplete) 344.9
  - with
    - broken
      - back - *see* Fracture, vertebra, by site, with spinal cord injury
      - neck - *see* Fracture, vertebra, cervical, with spinal cord injury
    - fracture, vertebra - *see* Fracture, vertebra, by site, with spinal cord injury
    - syphilis 094.89
  - abdomen and back muscles 355.9
  - abdominal muscles 355.9
  - abducens (nerve) 378.54
  - abductor 355.9
    - lower extremity 355.8
    - upper extremity 354.9
  - accessory nerve 352.4
  - accommodation 367.51
    - hysterical 300.11
  - acoustic nerve 388.5
  - agitans 332.0
    - arteriosclerotic 332.0
  - alternating 344.89
    - oculomotor 344.89
  - amyotrophic 335.20
  - ankle 355.8
  - anterior serratus 355.9
  - anus (sphincter) 569.49
  - apoplectic (current episode) (*see also* Disease, cerebrovascular, acute) 436
    - late effect - *see* Late effect(s) (of) cerebrovascular disease
  - arm 344.40
    - affecting
      - dominant side 344.41
      - nondominant side 344.42
- **Paralysis, paralytic** – *continued*
  - arm – *continued*
    - both 344.2
    - hysterical 300.11
    - late effect - *see* Late effect(s) (of) cerebrovascular disease
    - psychogenic 306.0
    - transient 781.4
      - traumatic NEC (*see also* Injury, nerve, upper limb) 955.9
  - arteriosclerotic (current episode) 437.0
    - late effect - *see* Late effect(s) (of) cerebrovascular disease
  - ascending (spinal), acute 357.0
  - associated, nuclear 344.89
  - asthenic bulbar 358.00
  - ataxic NEC 334.9
    - general 094.1
  - athetoid 333.71
  - atrophic 356.9
    - infantile, acute (*see also* Poliomyelitis, with paralysis) 045.1
    - muscle NEC 355.9
    - progressive 335.21
    - spinal (acute) (*see also* Poliomyelitis, with paralysis) 045.1
  - attack (*see also* Disease, cerebrovascular, acute) 436
  - axillary 353.0
  - Babinski-Nageotte's 344.89
  - Bell's 351.0
    - newborn 767.5
  - Benedikt's 344.89
  - birth (injury) 767.7
    - brain 767.0
    - intracranial 767.0
    - spinal cord 767.4
  - bladder (sphincter) 596.53
    - neurogenic 596.54
      - with cauda equina syndrome 344.61
    - puerperal, postpartum, childbirth 665.5
    - sensory 596.54
      - with cauda equina 344.61
    - spastic 596.54
      - with cauda equina 344.61
  - bowel, colon, or intestine (*see also* Ileus) 560.1
  - brachial plexus 353.0
    - due to birth injury 767.6
    - newborn 767.6
  - brain
    - congenital - *see* Palsy, cerebral
    - current episode 437.8
    - diplegia 344.2
      - late effect - *see* Late effect(s) (of) cerebrovascular disease
    - hemiplegia 342.9
      - late effect - *see* Late effect(s) (of) cerebrovascular disease
    - infantile - *see* Palsy, cerebral
    - monoplegia - *see also* Monoplegia
      - late effect - *see* Late effect(s) (of) cerebrovascular disease
    - paraplegia 344.1
    - quadriplegia - *see* Quadriplegia
    - syphilitic, congenital 090.49
    - triplegia 344.89
  - bronchi 519.19
  - Brown-Séquard's 344.89
  - bulbar (chronic) (progressive) 335.22
    - infantile (*see also* Poliomyelitis, bulbar) 045.0 [5th]
    - poliomyelitic (*see also* Poliomyelitis, bulbar) 045.0 [5th]
    - pseudo 335.23
    - supranuclear 344.89
  - bulbospinal 358.00
  - cardiac (*see also* Failure, heart) 428.9
  - cerebral
    - current episode 437.8
    - spastic, infantile - *see* Palsy, cerebral
  - cerebrocerebellar 437.8
    - diplegic infantile 343.0
- **Paralysis, paralytic** – *continued*
  - cervical
    - plexus 353.2
    - sympathetic NEC 337.09
  - Céstan-Chenais 344.89
  - Charcôt-Marie-Tooth type 356.1
  - childhood - *see* Palsy, cerebral
  - Clark's 343.9
  - colon (*see also* Ileus) 560.1
  - compressed air 993.3
  - compression
    - arm NEC 354.9
    - cerebral - *see* Paralysis, brain
    - leg NEC 355.8
    - lower extremity NEC 355.8
    - upper extremity NEC 354.9
  - congenital (cerebral) (spastic) (spinal) - *see* Palsy, cerebral
  - conjugate movement (of eye) 378.81
    - cortical (nuclear) (supranuclear) 378.81
  - convergence 378.83
  - cordis (*see also* Failure, heart) 428.9
  - cortical (*see also* Paralysis, brain) 437.8
  - cranial or cerebral nerve (*see also* Disorder, nerve, cranial) 352.9
  - creeping 335.21
  - crossed leg 344.89
  - crutch 953.4
  - deglutition 784.99
    - hysterical 300.11
  - dementia 094.1
  - descending (spinal) NEC 335.9
  - diaphragm (flaccid) 519.4
    - due to accidental section of phrenic nerve during procedure 998.2
  - digestive organs NEC 564.89
  - diplegic - *see* Diplegia
  - divergence (nuclear) 378.85
  - divers' 993.3
  - Duchenne's 335.22
  - due to intracranial or spinal birth injury - *see* Palsy, cerebral
  - embolic (current episode) (*see also* Embolism, brain) 434.1 [5th]
    - late effect - *see* Late effect(s) (of) cerebrovascular disease
  - enteric (*see also* Ileus) 560.1
    - with hernia - *see* Hernia, by site, with obstruction
  - Erb's syphilitic spastic spinal 094.89
  - Erb (-Duchenne) (birth) (newborn) 767.6
  - esophagus 530.89
  - essential, infancy (*see also* Poliomyelitis) 045.9 [5th]
  - extremity
    - lower - *see* Paralysis, leg
    - spastic (hereditary) 343.3
      - noncongenital or noninfantile 344.1
    - transient (cause unknown) 781.4
    - upper - *see* Paralysis, arm
  - eye muscle (extrinsic) 378.55
    - intrinsic 367.51
  - facial (nerve) 351.0
    - birth injury 767.5
    - congenital 767.5
    - following operation NEC 998.2
    - newborn 767.5
  - familial 359.3
    - periodic 359.3
    - spastic 334.1
  - fauces 478.29
  - finger NEC 354.9
  - foot NEC 355.8
  - gait 781.2
  - gastric nerve 352.3
  - gaze 378.81
  - general 094.1
    - ataxic 094.1
    - insane 094.1
    - juvenile 090.40
    - progressive 094.1
    - tabetic 094.1
  - glossopharyngeal (nerve) 352.2

[4th] Fourth Digit Required [5th] Fifth Digit Required | *[code]* Manifestation Code | ● New Line ▲ Revised Line <u>text</u> New Text ~~text~~ Deleted text

Paralysis, paralytic – *continued*
- glottis (*see also* Paralysis, vocal cord) 478.30
- gluteal 353.4
- Gubler (-Millard) 344.89
- hand 354.9
  - hysterical 300.11
  - psychogenic 306.0
- heart (*see also* Failure, heart) 428.9
- hemifacial, progressive 349.89
- hemiplegic - *see* Hemiplegia
- hyperkalemic periodic (familial) 359.3
- hypertensive (current episode) 437.8
- hypoglossal (nerve) 352.5
- hypokalemic periodic 359.3
- Hyrtl's sphincter (rectum) 569.49
- hysterical 300.11
- ileus (*see also* Ileus) 560.1
- infantile (*see also* Poliomyelitis) 045.9 [5th]
  - atrophic acute 045.1 [5th]
  - bulbar 045.0 [5th]
  - cerebral - *see* Palsy, cerebral
  - paralytic 045.1 [5th]
  - progressive acute 045.9 [5th]
  - spastic - *see* Palsy, cerebral
  - spinal 045.9 [5th]
- infective (*see also* Poliomyelitis) 045.9 [5th]
- inferior nuclear 344.9
- insane, general or progressive 094.1
- internuclear 378.86
- interosseous 355.9
- intestine (*see also* Ileus) 560.1
- intracranial (current episode) (*see also* Paralysis, brain) 437.8
  - due to birth injury 767.0
- iris 379.49
  - due to diphtheria (toxin) 032.81 *[379.49]*
- ischemic, Volkmann's (complicating trauma) 958.6
- isolated sleep, recurrent 327.43
- Jackson's 344.89
- jake 357.7
- Jamaica ginger (jake) 357.7
- juvenile general 090.40
- Klumpke (-Déjérine) (birth) (newborn) 767.6
- labioglossal (laryngeal) (pharyngeal) 335.22
- Landry's 357.0
- laryngeal nerve (recurrent) (superior) (*see also* Paralysis, vocal cord) 478.30
- larynx (*see also* Paralysis, vocal cord) 478.30
  - due to diphtheria (toxin) 032.3
- late effect
  - due to
    - birth injury, brain or spinal (cord) - *see* Palsy, cerebral
    - edema, brain or cerebral - *see* Paralysis, brain
    - lesion
      - late effect - *see* Late effect(s) (of) cerebrovascular disease
      - spinal (cord) - *see* Paralysis, spinal
- lateral 335.24
- lead 984.9
  - specified type of lead - *see* Table of Drugs and Chemicals
- left side - *see* Hemiplegia
- leg 344.30
  - affecting
    - dominant side 344.31
    - nondominant side 344.32
  - both (*see also* Paraplegia) 344.1
  - crossed 344.89
  - hysterical 300.11
  - psychogenic 306.0
  - transient or transitory 781.4
    - traumatic NEC (*see also* Injury, nerve, lower limb) 956.9
- levator palpebrae superioris 374.31

Paralysis, paralytic – *continued*
- limb NEC 344.5
  - all four - *see* Quadriplegia
  - quadriplegia - *see* Quadriplegia
- lip 528.5
- Lissauer's 094.1
- local 355.9
- lower limb - *see also* Paralysis, leg
  - both (*see also* Paraplegia) 344.1
- lung 518.89
  - newborn 770.89
- median nerve 354.1
- medullary (tegmental) 344.89
- mesencephalic NEC 344.89
  - tegmental 344.89
- middle alternating 344.89
- Millard-Gubler-Foville 344.89
- monoplegic - *see* Monoplegia
- motor NEC 344.9
  - cerebral - *see* Paralysis, brain
  - spinal - *see* Paralysis, spinal
- multiple
  - cerebral - *see* Paralysis, brain
  - spinal - *see* Paralysis, spinal
- muscle (flaccid) 359.9
  - due to nerve lesion NEC 355.9
  - eye (extrinsic) 378.55
    - intrinsic 367.51
    - oblique 378.51
  - iris sphincter 364.89
  - ischemic (complicating trauma) (Volkmann's) 958.6
  - pseudohypertrophic 359.1
- muscular (atrophic) 359.9
  - progressive 335.21
- musculocutaneous nerve 354.9
- musculospiral 354.9
- nerve - *see also* Disorder, nerve
  - third or oculomotor (partial) 378.51
    - total 378.52
  - fourth or trochlear 378.53
  - sixth or abducens 378.54
  - seventh or facial 351.0
    - birth injury 767.5
    - due to
      - injection NEC 999.9
      - operation NEC 997.09
    - newborn 767.5
  - accessory 352.4
  - auditory 388.5
  - birth injury 767.7
  - cranial or cerebral (*see also* Disorder, nerve, cranial) 352.9
  - facial 351.0
    - birth injury 767.5
    - newborn 767.5
  - laryngeal (*see also* Paralysis, vocal cord) 478.30
  - newborn 767.7
  - phrenic 354.8
    - newborn 767.7
  - radial 354.3
    - birth injury 767.6
    - newborn 767.6
  - syphilitic 094.89
  - traumatic NEC (*see also* Injury, nerve, by site) 957.9
  - trigeminal 350.9
  - ulnar 354.2
- newborn NEC 767.0
- normokalemic periodic 359.3
- obstetrical, newborn 767.7
- ocular 378.9
- oculofacial, congenital 352.6
- oculomotor (nerve) (partial) 378.51
  - alternating 344.89
  - external bilateral 378.55
  - total 378.52
- olfactory nerve 352.0
- palate 528.9
- palatopharyngolaryngeal 352.6
- paratrigeminal 350.9

Paralysis, paralytic – *continued*
- periodic (familial) (hyperkalemic) (hypokalemic) (normokalemic) (potassium sensitive) (secondary) 359.3
- peripheral
  - autonomic nervous system - *see* Neuropathy, peripheral, autonomic
  - nerve NEC 355.9
- peroneal (nerve) 355.3
- pharynx 478.29
- phrenic nerve 354.8
- plantar nerves 355.6
- pneumogastric nerve 352.3
- poliomyelitis (current) (*see also* Poliomyelitis, with paralysis) 045.1 [5th]
  - bulbar 045.0 [5th]
- popliteal nerve 355.3
- pressure (*see also* Neuropathy, entrapment) 355.9
- progressive 335.21
  - atrophic 335.21
  - bulbar 335.22
  - general 094.1
  - hemifacial 349.89
  - infantile, acute (*see also* Poliomyelitis) 045.9 [5th]
  - multiple 335.20
- pseudobulbar 335.23
- pseudohypertrophic 359.1
  - muscle 359.1
- psychogenic 306.0
- pupil, pupillary 379.49
- quadriceps 355.8
- quadriplegic (*see also* Quadriplegia) 344.0 [5th]
- radial nerve 354.3
  - birth injury 767.6
- rectum (sphincter) 569.49
- rectus muscle (eye) 378.55
- recurrent
  - isolated sleep 327.43
  - laryngeal nerve (*see also* Paralysis, vocal cord) 478.30
- respiratory (muscle) (system) (tract) 786.09
  - center NEC 344.89
    - fetus or newborn 770.87
  - congenital 768.9
  - newborn 768.9
- right side - *see* Hemiplegia
- Saturday night 354.3
- saturnine 984.9
  - specified type of lead - *see* Table of Drugs and Chemicals
- sciatic nerve 355.0
- secondary - *see* Paralysis, late effect
- seizure (cerebral) (current episode) (*see also* Disease, cerebrovascular, acute) 436
  - late effect - *see* Late effect(s) (of) cerebrovascular disease
- senile NEC 344.9
- serratus magnus 355.9
- shaking (*see also* Parkinsonism) 332.0
- shock (*see also* Disease, cerebrovascular, acute) 436
  - late effect - *see* Late effect(s) (of) cerebrovascular disease
- shoulder 354.9
- soft palate 528.9
- spasmodic - *see* Paralysis, spastic
- spastic 344.9
  - cerebral infantile - *see* Palsy, cerebral
  - congenital (cerebral) - *see* Palsy, cerebral
  - familial 334.1
  - hereditary 334.1
  - infantile 343.9
  - noncongenital or noninfantile, cerebral 344.9

Paralysis, paralytic – *continued*
- spastic – *continued*
  - syphilitic 094.0
    - spinal 094.89
- sphincter, bladder (*see also* Paralysis, bladder) 596.53
- spinal (cord) NEC 344.1
  - accessory nerve 352.4
  - acute (*see also* Poliomyelitis) 045.9 [5th]
  - ascending acute 357.0
  - atrophic (acute) (*see also* Poliomyelitis, with paralysis) 045.1 [5th]
    - spastic, syphilitic 094.89
  - congenital NEC 343.9
  - hemiplegic - *see* Hemiplegia
  - hereditary 336.8
  - infantile (*see also* Poliomyelitis) 045.9 [5th]
  - late effect NEC 344.89
  - monoplegic - *see* Monoplegia
  - nerve 355.9
  - progressive 335.10
  - quadriplegic - *see* Quadriplegia
  - spastic NEC 343.9
  - traumatic - *see* Injury, spinal, by site
- sternomastoid 352.4
- stomach 536.3
  - diabetic 250.6 [5th] *[536.3]*
    - due to secondary diabetes 249.6 [5th] *[536.3]*
  - nerve (nondiabetic) 352.3
- stroke (current episode) - *see* Infarct, brain
  - late effect - *see* Late effect(s) (of) cerebrovascular disease
- subscapularis 354.8
- superior nuclear NEC 334.9
- supranuclear 356.8
- sympathetic
  - cervical NEC 337.09
  - nerve NEC (*see also* Neuropathy, peripheral, autonomic) 337.9
  - nervous system - *see* Neuropathy, peripheral, autonomic
- syndrome 344.9
  - specified NEC 344.89
- syphilitic spastic spinal (Erb's) 094.89
- tabetic general 094.1
- thigh 355.8
- throat 478.29
  - diphtheritic 032.0
  - muscle 478.29
- thrombotic (current episode) (*see also* Thrombosis, brain) 434.0 [5th]
  - late effect - *see* Late effect(s) (of) cerebrovascular disease
- thumb NEC 354.9
- tick (-bite) 989.5
- Todd's (postepileptic transitory paralysis) 344.89
- toe 355.6
- tongue 529.8
- transient
  - arm or leg NEC 781.4
  - traumatic NEC (*see also* Injury, nerve, by site) 957.9
- trapezius 352.4
- traumatic, transient NEC (*see also* Injury, nerve, by site) 957.9
- trembling (*see also* Parkinsonism) 332.0
- triceps brachii 354.9
- trigeminal nerve 350.9
- trochlear nerve 378.53
- ulnar nerve 354.2
- upper limb - *see also* Paralysis, arm
  - both (*see also* Diplegia) 344.2
- uremic - *see* Uremia
- uveoparotitic 135
- uvula 528.9
  - hysterical 300.11
  - postdiphtheritic 032.0
- vagus nerve 352.3
- vasomotor NEC 337.9
- velum palati 528.9
- vesical (*see also* Paralysis, bladder) 596.53

Paralysis, paralytic – Paterson (-Brown) (-Kelly) syndrome

- **Paralysis, paralytic** – *continued*
  - vestibular nerve 388.5
  - visual field, psychic 368.16
  - vocal cord 478.30
    - bilateral (partial) 478.33
      - complete 478.34
    - complete (bilateral) 478.34
    - unilateral (partial) 478.31
      - complete 478.32
  - Volkmann's (complicating trauma) 958.6
  - wasting 335.21
  - Weber's 344.89
  - wrist NEC 354.9
- **Paramedial orifice, urethrovesical** 753.8
- **Paramenia** 626.9
- **Parametritis** (chronic) (*see also* Disease, pelvis, inflammatory) 614.4
  - acute 614.3
  - puerperal, postpartum, childbirth 670.8 5th ▲
- **Parametrium, parametric** - *see* condition
- **Paramnesia** (*see also* Amnesia) 780.93
- **Paramolar** 520.1
  - causing crowding 524.31
- **Paramyloidosis** 277.30
- **Paramyoclonus multiplex** 333.2
- **Paramyotonia** 359.29
  - congenita (of von Eulenburg) 359.29
- **Paraneoplastic syndrome**- *see* condition
- **Parangi** (*see also* Yaws) 102.9
- **Paranoia** 297.1
  - alcoholic 291.5
  - querulans 297.8
  - senile 290.20
- **Paranoid**
  - dementia (*see also* Schizophrenia) 295.3 5th
    - praecox (acute) 295.3 5th
    - senile 290.20
  - personality 301.0
  - psychosis 297.9
    - alcoholic 291.5
    - climacteric 297.2
    - drug-induced 292.11
    - involutional 297.2
    - menopausal 297.2
    - protracted reactive 298.4
    - psychogenic 298.4
      - acute 298.3
    - senile 290.20
  - reaction (chronic) 297.9
    - acute 298.3
  - schizophrenia (acute) (*see also* Schizophrenia) 295.3 5th
  - state 297.9
    - alcohol-induced 291.5
    - climacteric 297.2
    - drug-induced 292.11
    - due to or associated with
      - arteriosclerosis (cerebrovascular) 290.42
      - presenile brain disease 290.12
      - senile brain disease 290.20
    - involutional 297.2
    - menopausal 297.2
    - senile 290.20
    - simple 297.0
    - specified type NEC 297.8
  - tendencies 301.0
  - traits 301.0
  - trends 301.0
  - type, psychopathic personality 301.0
- **Paraparesis** (*see also* Paraplegia) 344.1
- **Paraphasia** 784.3
- **Paraphilia** (*see also* Deviation, sexual) 302.9
- **Paraphimosis** (congenital) 605
  - chancroidal 099.0
- **Paraphrenia, paraphrenic** (late) 297.2
  - climacteric 297.2
  - dementia (*see also* Schizophrenia) 295.3 5th
  - involutional 297.2
  - menopausal 297.2
- **Paraphrenia, paraphrenic** – *continued*
  - schizophrenia (acute) (*see also* Schizophrenia) 295.3 5th
- **Paraplegia** 344.1
  - with
    - broken back - *see* Fracture, vertebra, by site, with spinal cord injury
    - fracture, vertebra - *see* Fracture, vertebra, by site, with spinal cord injury
  - ataxic - *see* Degeneration, combined, spinal cord
  - brain (current episode) (*see also* Paralysis, brain) 437.8
  - cerebral (current episode) (*see also* Paralysis, brain) 437.8
  - congenital or infantile (cerebral) (spastic) (spinal) 343.0
  - cortical - *see* Paralysis, brain
  - familial spastic 334.1
  - functional (hysterical) 300.11
  - hysterical 300.11
  - infantile 343.0
  - late effect 344.1
  - Pott's (*see also* Tuberculosis) 015.0 5th *[730.88]*
  - psychogenic 306.0
  - spastic
    - Erb's spinal 094.89
    - hereditary 334.1
    - not infantile or congenital 344.1
  - spinal (cord)
    - traumatic NEC - *see* Injury, spinal, by site
  - syphilitic (spastic) 094.89
  - traumatic NEC - *see* Injury, spinal, by site
- **Paraproteinemia** 273.2
  - benign (familial) 273.1
- **Paraproteinemia** – *continued*
  - monoclonal 273.1
  - secondary to malignant or inflammatory disease 273.1
- **Parapsoriasis** 696.2
  - en plaques 696.2
  - guttata 696.2
  - lichenoides chronica 696.2
  - retiformis 696.2
  - varioliformis (acuta) 696.2
- **Parascarlatina** 057.8
- **Parasitic** - *see also* condition
  - disease NEC (*see also* Infestation, parasitic) 136.9
    - contact V01.89
    - exposure to V01.89
    - intestinal NEC 129
    - skin NEC 134.9
  - stomatitis 112.0
  - sycosis 110.0
    - beard 110.0
    - scalp 110.0
  - twin 759.4
- **Parasitism** NEC 136.9
  - intestinal NEC 129
  - skin NEC 134.9
  - specified - *see* Infestation
- **Parasitophobia** 300.29
- **Parasomnia** 307.47
  - alcohol induced 291.82
  - drug induced 292.85
  - nonorganic origin 307.47
  - organic 327.40
    - in conditions classified elsewhere 327.44
    - other 327.49
- **Paraspadias** 752.69
- **Paraspasm facialis** 351.8
- **Parathyroid gland** - *see* condition
- **Parathyroiditis** (autoimmune) 252.1
- **Parathyroprival tetany** 252.1
- **Paratrachoma** 077.0
- **Paratyphilitis** (*see also* Appendicitis) 541
- **Paratyphoid** (fever) - *see* Fever, paratyphoid
- **Paratyphus** - *see* Fever, paratyphoid
- **Paraurethral duct** 753.8
- **Para-urethritis** 597.89
  - gonococcal (acute) 098.0
    - chronic or duration of 2 months or over 098.2
- **Paravaccinia** NEC 051.9
  - milkers' node 051.1
- **Paravaginitis** (*see also* Vaginitis) 616.10
- **Parencephalitis** (*see also* Encephalitis) 323.9
  - late effect - *see* category 326
- **Parergasia** 298.9
- **Paresis** (*see also* Paralysis) 344.9
  - accommodation 367.51
  - bladder (spastic) (sphincter) (*see also* Paralysis, bladder) 596.53
    - tabetic 094.0
  - bowel, colon, or intestine (*see also* Ileus) 560.1
  - brain or cerebral - *see* Paralysis, brain
  - extrinsic muscle, eye 378.55
  - general 094.1
    - arrested 094.1
    - brain 094.1
    - cerebral 094.1
    - insane 094.1
    - juvenile 090.40
      - remission 090.49
    - progressive 094.1
    - remission (sustained) 094.1
    - tabetic 094.1
  - heart (*see also* Failure, heart) 428.9
  - infantile (*see also* Poliomyelitis) 045.9 5th
  - insane 094.1
  - juvenile 090.40
  - late effect - *see* Paralysis, late effect
  - luetic (general) 094.1
  - peripheral progressive 356.9
  - pseudohypertrophic 359.1
  - senile NEC 344.9
  - stomach 536.3
    - diabetic 250.6 5th *[536.3]*
      - due to secondary diabetes 249.6 5th *[536.3]*
  - syphilitic (general) 094.1
    - congenital 090.40
  - transient, limb 781.4
  - vesical (sphincter) NEC 596.53
- **Paresthesia** (*see also* Disturbance, sensation) 782.0
  - Berger's (paresthesia of lower limb) 782.0
  - Bernhardt 355.1
  - Magnan's 782.0
- **Paretic** - *see* condition
- **Parinaud's**
  - conjunctivitis 372.02
  - oculoglandular syndrome 372.02
  - ophthalmoplegia 378.81
  - syndrome (paralysis of conjugate upward gaze) 378.81
- **Parkes Weber and Dimitri syndrome** (encephalocutaneous angiomatosis) 759.6
- **Parkinson's disease, syndrome, or tremor** - *see* Parkinsonism
- **Parkinsonism** (arteriosclerotic) (idiopathic) (primary) 332.0
  - associated with orthostatic hypotension (idiopathic) (symptomatic) 333.0
  - due to drugs 332.1
  - neuroleptic-induced 332.1
  - secondary 332.1
  - syphilitic 094.82
- **Parodontitis** 523.40
- **Parodontosis** 523.5
- **Paronychia** (with lymphangitis) 681.9
  - candidal (chronic) 112.3
  - chronic 681.9
    - candidal 112.3
    - finger 681.02
    - toe 681.11
  - finger 681.02
  - toe 681.11
  - tuberculous (primary) (*see also* Tuberculosis) 017.0 5th
- **Parorexia** NEC 307.52
  - hysterical 300.11
- **Parosmia** 781.1
  - psychogenic 306.7
- **Parotid gland** - *see* condition
- **Parotiditis** (*see also* Parotitis) 527.2
  - epidemic 072.9
  - infectious 072.9
- **Parotitis** 527.2
  - allergic 527.2
  - chronic 527.2
  - epidemic (*see also* Mumps) 072.9
  - infectious (*see also* Mumps) 072.9
  - noninfectious 527.2
  - nonspecific toxic 527.2
  - not mumps 527.2
  - postoperative 527.2
  - purulent 527.2
  - septic 527.2
  - suppurative (acute) 527.2
  - surgical 527.2
  - toxic 527.2
- **Paroxysmal** - *see also* condition
  - dyspnea (nocturnal) 786.09
- **Parrot's disease** (syphilitic osteochondritis) 090.0
- **Parrot fever** 073.9
- **Parry's disease or syndrome** (exophthalmic goiter) 242.0 5th
- **Parry-Romberg syndrome** 349.89
- **Parson's disease** (exophthalmic goiter) 242.0 5th
- **Parsonage-Aldren-Turner syndrome** 353.5
- **Parsonage-Turner syndrome** 353.5
- **Pars planitis** 363.21
- **Particolored infant** 757.39
- **Parturition** - *see* **Delivery**
- **Parvovirus** 079.83
  - B19 079.83
  - human 079.83
- **Passage**
  - false, urethra 599.4
  - meconium noted during delivery 763.84
  - of sounds or bougies (*see also* Attention to artificial opening) V55.9
- **Passive** - *see* condition
- **Pasteurella septica** 027.2
- **Pasteurellosis** (*see also* Infection, Pasteurella) 027.2
- **PAT** (paroxysmal atrial tachycardia) 427.0
- **Patau's syndrome** (trisomy D_1) 758.1
- **Patch**
  - herald 696.3
- **Patches**
  - mucous (syphilitic) 091.3
    - congenital 090.0
  - smokers' (mouth) 528.6
- **Patellar** - *see* condition
- **Patellofemoral syndrome** 719.46
- **Patent** - *see also* Imperfect closure
  - atrioventricular ostium 745.69
  - canal of Nuck 752.41
  - cervix 622.5
    - complicating pregnancy 654.5 5th
      - affecting fetus or newborn 761.0
  - ductus arteriosus or Botalli 747.0
  - Eustachian
    - tube 381.7
    - valve 746.89
  - foramen
    - Botalli 745.5
    - ovale 745.5
  - interauricular septum 745.5
  - interventricular septum 745.4
  - omphalomesenteric duct 751.0
  - os (uteri) - *see* Patent, cervix
  - ostium secundum 745.5
  - urachus 753.7
  - vitelline duct 751.0
- **Paternity testing** V70.4
- **Paterson's syndrome** (sideropenic dysphagia) 280.8
- **Paterson (-Brown) (-Kelly) syndrome** (sideropenic dysphagia) 280.8

4th Fourth Digit Required 5th Fifth Digit Required | *[code]* Manifestation Code | ● New Line ▲ Revised Line text New Text ~~text~~ Deleted text

- **Paterson-Kelly syndrome or web** (sideropenic dysphagia) 280.8
- **Pathologic, pathological** - *see also* condition
  - asphyxia 799.01
  - drunkenness 291.4
  - emotionality 301.3
  - fracture - *see* Fracture, pathologic
  - liar 301.7
  - personality 301.9
  - resorption, tooth 521.40
    - external 521.42
    - internal 521.41
    - specified NEC 521.49
  - sexuality (*see also* Deviation, sexual) 302.9
- **Pathology** (of) - *see also* Disease
  - periradicular, associated with previous endodontic treatment 526.69
- **Patterned motor discharge, idiopathic** (*see also* Epilepsy) 345.5 [5th]
- **Patulous** - *see also* Patent
  - anus 569.49
  - Eustachian tube 381.7
- **Pause, sinoatrial** 427.81
- **Pavor nocturnus** 307.46
- **Pavy's disease** 593.6
- **Paxton's disease** (white piedra) 111.2
- **Payr's disease or syndrome** (splenic flexure syndrome) 569.89
- **PBA** (pseudobulbar affect) 310.8
- **Pearls**
  - Elschnig 366.51
  - enamel 520.2
- **Pearl-workers' disease** (chronic osteomyelitis) (*see also* Osteomyelitis) 730.1 [5th]
- **Pectenitis** 569.49
- **Pectenosis** 569.49
- **Pectoral** - *see* condition
- **Pectus**
  - carinatum (congenital) 754.82
    - acquired 738.3
    - rachitic (*see also* Rickets) 268.0
  - excavatum (congenital) 754.81
    - acquired 738.3
    - rachitic (*see also* Rickets) 268.0
  - recurvatum (congenital) 754.81
    - acquired 738.3
- **Pedatrophia** 261
- **Pederosis** 302.2
- **Pediculosis** (infestation) 132.9
  - capitis (head louse) (any site) 132.0
  - corporis (body louse) (any site) 132.1
  - eyelid 132.0 *[373.6]*
  - mixed (classifiable to more than one category in 132.0-132.2) 132.3
  - pubis (pubic louse) (any site) 132.2
  - vestimenti 132.1
  - vulvae 132.2
- **Pediculus** (infestation) - *see* Pediculosis
- **Pedophilia** 302.2
- **Peg-shaped teeth** 520.2
- **Pel's crisis** 094.0
- **Pel-Ebstein disease** - *see* Disease, Hodgkin's
- **Pelade** 704.01
- **Pelger-Huët anomaly or syndrome** (hereditary hyposegmentation) 288.2
- **Peliosis** (rheumatica) 287.0
- **Pelizaeus-Merzbacher**
  - disease 330.0
  - sclerosis, diffuse cerebral 330.0
- **Pellagra** (alcoholic or with alcoholism) 265.2
  - with polyneuropathy 265.2 *[357.4]*
- **Pellagra-cerebellar-ataxia-renal aminoaciduria syndrome** 270.0
- **Pellegrini's disease** (calcification, knee joint) 726.62
- **Pellegrini (-Stieda) disease or syndrome** (calcification, knee joint) 726.62
- **Pellizzi's syndrome** (pineal) 259.8
- **Pelvic** - *see also* condition
  - congestion-fibrosis syndrome 625.5
  - kidney 753.3
- **Pelvioectasis** 591
- **Pelviolithiasis** 592.0
- **Pelviperitonitis**
  - female (*see also* Peritonitis, pelvic, female) 614.5
  - male (*see also* Peritonitis) 567.21
- **Pelvis, pelvic** - *see also* condition or type
  - infantile 738.6
  - Nägele's 738.6
  - obliquity 738.6
  - Robert's 755.69
- **Pemphigoid** 694.5
  - benign, mucous membrane 694.60
    - with ocular involvement 694.61
  - bullous 694.5
  - cicatricial 694.60
    - with ocular involvement 694.61
  - juvenile 694.2
- **Pemphigus** 694.4
  - benign 694.5
    - chronic familial 757.39
  - Brazilian 694.4
  - circinatus 694.0
  - congenital, traumatic 757.39
  - conjunctiva 694.61
  - contagiosus 684
  - erythematodes 694.4
  - erythematosus 694.4
  - foliaceus 694.4
  - frambesiodes 694.4
  - gangrenous (*see also* Gangrene) 785.4
  - malignant 694.4
  - neonatorum, newborn 684
  - ocular 694.61
  - papillaris 694.4
  - seborrheic 694.4
  - South American 694.4
  - syphilitic (congenital) 090.0
  - vegetans 694.4
  - vulgaris 694.4
  - wildfire 694.4
- **Pendred's syndrome** (familial goiter with deaf-mutism) 243
- **Pendulous**
  - abdomen 701.9
    - in pregnancy or childbirth 654.4 [5th]
      - affecting fetus or newborn 763.89
  - breast 611.89
- **Penetrating wound** - *see also* Wound, open, by site
  - with internal injury - *see* Injury, internal, by site, with open wound
  - eyeball 871.7
    - with foreign body (nonmagnetic) 871.6
      - magnetic 871.5
  - ocular (*see also* Penetrating wound, eyeball) 871.7
    - adnexa 870.3
      - with foreign body 870.4
  - orbit 870.3
    - with foreign body 870.4
- **Penetration, pregnant uterus by instrument**
  - with
    - abortion - *see* Abortion, by type, with damage to pelvic organs
    - ectopic pregnancy (*see also* categories 633.0-633.9) 639.2
    - molar pregnancy (*see also* categories 630-632) 639.2
  - complication of delivery 665.1 [5th]
    - affecting fetus or newborn 763.89
  - following
    - abortion 639.2
    - ectopic or molar pregnancy 639.2
- **Penfield's syndrome** (*see also* Epilepsy) 345.5 [5th]
- **Penicilliosis of lung** 117.3
- **Penis** - *see* condition
- **Penitis** 607.2
- **Penta X syndrome** 758.81
- **Pentalogy** (of Fallot) 745.2
- **Pentosuria** (benign) (essential) 271.8
- **Peptic acid disease** 536.8
- **Peregrinating patient** V65.2
- **Perforated** - *see* Perforation
- **Perforation, perforative** (nontraumatic)
  - antrum (*see also* Sinusitis, maxillary) 473.0
  - appendix 540.0
    - with peritoneal abscess 540.1
  - atrial septum, multiple 745.5
  - attic, ear 384.22
    - healed 384.81
  - bile duct, except cystic (*see also* Disease, biliary) 576.3
    - cystic 575.4
  - bladder (urinary) 596.6
    - with
      - abortion - *see* Abortion, by type, with damage to pelvic organs
      - ectopic pregnancy (*see also* categories 633.0-633.9) 639.2
      - molar pregnancy (*see also* categories 630-632) 639.2
    - following
      - abortion 639.2
      - ectopic or molar pregnancy 639.2
    - obstetrical trauma 665.5 [5th]
  - bowel 569.83
    - with
      - abortion - *see* Abortion, by type, with damage to pelvic organs
      - ectopic pregnancy (*see also* categories 633.0-633.9) 639.2
      - molar pregnancy (*see also* categories 630-632) 639.2
    - fetus or newborn 777.6
    - following
      - abortion 639.2
      - ectopic or molar pregnancy 639.2
    - obstetrical trauma 665.5 [5th]
  - broad ligament
    - with
      - abortion - *see* Abortion, by type, with damage to pelvic organs
      - ectopic pregnancy (*see also* categories 633.0-633.9) 639.2
      - molar pregnancy (*see also* categories 630-632) 639.2
    - following
      - abortion 639.2
      - ectopic or molar pregnancy 639.2
    - obstetrical trauma 665.6 [5th]
  - by
    - device, implant, or graft - *see* Complications, mechanical
    - foreign body left accidentally in operation wound 998.4
    - instrument (any) during a procedure, accidental 998.2
  - cecum 540.0
    - with peritoneal abscess 540.1
  - cervix (uteri) - *see also* Injury, internal, cervix
    - with
      - abortion - *see* Abortion, by type, with damage to pelvic organs
      - ectopic pregnancy (*see also* categories 633.0-633.9) 639.2
      - molar pregnancy (*see also* categories 630-632) 639.2
    - following
      - abortion 639.2
      - ectopic or molar pregnancy 639.2
    - obstetrical trauma 665.3 [5th]
  - colon 569.83
  - common duct (bile) 576.3
  - cornea (*see also* Ulcer, cornea) 370.00
    - due to ulceration 370.06
  - cystic duct 575.4
  - diverticulum (*see also* Diverticula) 562.10
    - small intestine 562.00
  - duodenum, duodenal (ulcer) - *see* Ulcer, duodenum, with perforation
  - ear drum - *see* Perforation, tympanum
  - enteritis - *see* Enteritis
  - esophagus 530.4
  - ethmoidal sinus (*see also* Sinusitis, ethmoidal) 473.2
- **Perforation, perforative** – *continued*
  - foreign body (external site) - *see also* Wound, open, by site, complicated
    - internal site, by ingested object - *see* Foreign body
  - frontal sinus (*see also* Sinusitis, frontal) 473.1
  - gallbladder or duct (*see also* Disease, gallbladder) 575.4
  - gastric (ulcer) - *see* Ulcer, stomach, with perforation
  - heart valve - *see* Endocarditis
  - ileum (*see also* Perforation, intestine) 569.83
  - instrumental
    - external - *see* Wound, open, by site
    - pregnant uterus, complicating delivery 665.9 [5th]
    - surgical (accidental) (blood vessel) (nerve) (organ) 998.2
  - intestine 569.83
    - with
      - abortion - *see* Abortion, by type, with damage to pelvic organs
      - ectopic pregnancy (*see also* categories 633.0-633.9) 639.2
      - molar pregnancy (*see also* categories 630-632) 639.2
    - fetus or newborn 777.6
    - obstetrical trauma 665.5 [5th]
    - ulcerative NEC 569.83
  - jejunum, jejunal 569.83
    - ulcer - *see* Ulcer, gastrojejunal, with perforation
  - mastoid (antrum) (cell) 383.89
  - maxillary sinus (*see also* Sinusitis, maxillary) 473.0
  - membrana tympani - *see* Perforation, tympanum
  - nasal
    - septum 478.19
      - congenital 748.1
      - syphilitic 095.8
    - sinus (*see also* Sinusitis) 473.9
      - congenital 748.1
  - palate (hard) 526.89
    - soft 528.9
      - syphilitic 095.8
    - syphilitic 095.8
  - palatine vault 526.89
    - syphilitic 095.8
      - congenital 090.5
  - pelvic
    - floor
      - with
        - abortion - *see* Abortion, by type, with damage to pelvic organs
        - ectopic pregnancy (*see also* categories 633.0-633.9) 639.2
        - molar pregnancy (*see also* categories 630-632) 639.2
      - obstetrical trauma 664.1 [5th]
    - organ
      - with
        - abortion - *see* Abortion, by type, with damage to pelvic organs
        - ectopic pregnancy (*see also* categories 633.0-633.9) 639.2
        - molar pregnancy (*see also* categories 630-632) 639.2
      - following
        - abortion 639.2
        - ectopic or molar pregnancy 639.2
      - obstetrical trauma 665.5 [5th]
  - perineum - *see* Laceration, perineum
  - periurethral tissue
    - with
      - abortion - *see* Abortion, by type, with damage to pelvic organs

Paterson-Kelly syndrome or web – Perforation, perforative

Perforation, perforative – *continued*
- periurethral tissue – *continued*
  - with – *continued*
    - ectopic pregnancy (*see also* categories 630-632) 639.2
    - molar pregnancy (*see also* categories 630-632) 639.2
- pharynx 478.29
- pylorus, pyloric (ulcer) - *see* Ulcer, stomach, with perforation
- rectum 569.49
- root canal space 526.61
- sigmoid 569.83
- sinus (accessory) (chronic) (nasal) (*see also* Sinusitis) 473.9
- sphenoidal sinus (*see also* Sinusitis, sphenoidal) 473.3
- stomach (due to ulcer) - *see* Ulcer, stomach, with perforation
- surgical (accidental) (by instrument) (blood vessel) (nerve) (organ) 998.2
- traumatic
  - external - *see* Wound, open, by site
  - eye (*see also* Penetrating wound, ocular) 871.7
  - internal organ - *see* Injury, internal, by site
- tympanum (membrane) (persistent posttraumatic) (postinflammatory) 384.20
  - with
    - otitis media- *see* Otitis media
  - attic 384.22
  - central 384.21
  - healed 384.81
  - marginal NEC 384.23
  - multiple 384.24
  - pars flaccida 384.22
  - total 384.25
  - traumatic - *see* Wound, open, ear, drum
- typhoid, gastrointestinal 002.0
- ulcer - *see* Ulcer, by site, with perforation
- ureter 593.89
- urethra
  - with
    - abortion - *see* Abortion, by type, with damage to pelvic organs
    - ectopic pregnancy (*see also* categories 633.0-633.9) 639.2
    - molar pregnancy (*see also* categories 630-632) 639.2
  - following
    - abortion 639.2
    - ectopic or molar pregnancy 639.2
  - obstetrical trauma 665.5 5th
- uterus - *see also* Injury, internal, uterus
  - with
    - abortion - *see* Abortion, by type, with damage to pelvic organs
    - ectopic pregnancy (*see also* categories 633.0-633.9) 639.2
    - molar pregnancy (*see also* categories 630-632) 639.2
  - by intrauterine contraceptive device 996.32
  - following
    - abortion 639.2
    - ectopic or molar pregnancy 639.2
  - obstetrical trauma - *see* Injury, internal, uterus, obstetrical trauma
- uvula 528.9
  - syphilitic 095.8
- vagina - *see* Laceration, vagina
- viscus NEC 799.89
  - traumatic 868.00
    - with open wound into cavity 868.10

Periadenitis mucosa necrotica recurrens 528.2

Periangiitis 446.0

Periantritis 535.4 5th

Periappendicitis (acute) (*see also* Appendicitis) 541

Periarteritis (disseminated) (infectious) (necrotizing) (nodosa) 446.0

Periarthritis (joint) 726.90
- Duplay's 726.2
- gonococcal 098.50
- humeroscapularis 726.2
- scapulohumeral 726.2
- shoulder 726.2
- wrist 726.4

Periarthrosis (angioneural) - *see* Periarthritis

Peribronchitis 491.9
- tuberculous (*see also* Tuberculosis) 011.3 5th

Pericapsulitis, adhesive (shoulder) 726.0

Pericarditis (granular) (with decompensation) (with effusion) 423.9
- with
  - rheumatic fever (conditions classifiable to 390)
    - active (*see also* Pericarditis, rheumatic) 391.0
    - inactive or quiescent 393
- actinomycotic 039.8 *[420.0]*
- acute (nonrheumatic) 420.90
  - with chorea (acute) (rheumatic) (Sydenham's) 392.0
  - bacterial 420.99
  - benign 420.91
  - hemorrhagic 420.90
  - idiopathic 420.91
  - infective 420.90
  - nonspecific 420.91
  - rheumatic 391.0
    - with chorea (acute) (rheumatic) (Sydenham's) 392.0
  - sicca 420.90
  - viral 420.91
- adhesive or adherent (external) (internal) 423.1
  - acute - *see* Pericarditis, acute
  - rheumatic (external) (internal) 393
- amebic 006.8 *[420.0]*
- bacterial (acute) (subacute) (with serous or seropurulent effusion) 420.99
- calcareous 423.2
- cholesterol (chronic) 423.8
  - acute 420.90
- chronic (nonrheumatic) 423.8
  - rheumatic 393
- constrictive 423.2
- Coxsackie 074.21
- due to
  - actinomycosis 039.8 *[420.0]*
  - amebiasis 006.8 *[420.0]*
  - Coxsackie (virus) 074.21
  - histoplasmosis (*see also* Histoplasmosis) 115.93
  - nocardiosis 039.8 *[420.0]*
  - tuberculosis (*see also* Tuberculosis) 017.9 5th *[420.0]*
- fibrinocaseous (*see also* Tuberculosis) 017.9 5th *[420.0]*
- fibrinopurulent 420.99
- fibrinous - *see* Pericarditis, rheumatic
- fibropurulent 420.99
- fibrous 423.1
- gonococcal 098.83
- hemorrhagic 423.0
- idiopathic (acute) 420.91
- infective (acute) 420.90
- meningococcal 036.41
- neoplastic (chronic) 423.8
  - acute 420.90
- nonspecific 420.91
- obliterans, obliterating 423.1
- plastic 423.1
- pneumococcal (acute) 420.99
- postinfarction 411.0
- purulent (acute) 420.99
- rheumatic (active) (acute) (with effusion) (with pneumonia) 391.0
  - with chorea (acute) (rheumatic) (Sydenham's) 392.0
  - chronic or inactive (with chorea) 393
- septic (acute) 420.99
- serofibrinous - *see* Pericarditis, rheumatic
- staphylococcal (acute) 420.99
- streptococcal (acute) 420.99
- suppurative (acute) 420.99
- syphilitic 093.81
- tuberculous (acute) (chronic) (*see also* Tuberculosis) 017.9 5th *[420.0]*
- uremic 585.9 *[420.0]*
- viral (acute) 420.91

Pericardium, pericardial - *see* condition

Pericellulitis (*see also* Cellulitis) 682.9

Pericementitis 523.40
- acute 523.30
- chronic (suppurative) 523.40

Pericholecystitis (*see also* Cholecystitis) 575.10

Perichondritis
- auricle 380.00
  - acute 380.01
  - chronic 380.02
- bronchus 491.9
- ear (external) 380.00
  - acute 380.01
  - chronic 380.02
- larynx 478.71
  - syphilitic 095.8
  - typhoid 002.0 *[478.71]*
- nose 478.19
- pinna 380.00
  - acute 380.01
  - chronic 380.02
- trachea 478.9

Periclasia 523.5

Pericolitis 569.89

Pericoronitis (chronic) 523.40
- acute 523.33

Pericystitis (*see also* Cystitis) 595.9

Pericytoma (M9150/1) - *see also* Neoplasm, connective tissue, uncertain behavior
- benign (M9150/0) - *see* Neoplasm, connective tissue, benign
- malignant (M9150/3) - *see* Neoplasm, connective tissue, malignant

Peridacryocystitis, acute 375.32

Peridiverticulitis (*see also* Diverticulitis) 562.11

Periduodenitis 535.6 5th

Periendocarditis (*see also* Endocarditis) 424.90
- acute or subacute 421.9

Periepididymitis (*see also* Epididymitis) 604.90

Perifolliculitis (abscedens) 704.8
- capitis, abscedens et suffodiens 704.8
- dissecting, scalp 704.8
- scalp 704.8
- superficial pustular 704.8

Perigastritis (acute) 535.0 5th

Perigastrojejunitis (acute) 535.0 5th

Perihepatitis (acute) 573.3
- chlamydial 099.56
- gonococcal 098.86

Peri-ileitis (subacute) 569.89

Perilabyrinthitis (acute) - *see* Labyrinthitis

Perimeningitis - *see* Meningitis

Perimetritis (*see also* Endometritis) 615.9

Perimetrosalpingitis (*see also* Salpingo-oophoritis) 614.2

Perineocele 618.05

Perinephric - *see* condition

Perinephritic - *see* condition

Perinephritis (*see also* Infection, kidney) 590.9
- purulent (*see also* Abscess, kidney) 590.2

Perineum, perineal - *see* condition

Perineuritis NEC 729.2

Periodic - *see also* condition
- disease (familial) 277.31
- edema 995.1
  - hereditary 277.6
- fever 277.31
- headache syndromes in child or adolescent 346.2 5th
- limb movement disorder 327.51
- paralysis (familial) 359.3
- peritonitis 277.31
- polyserositis 277.31
- somnolence (*see also* Narcolepsy) 347.00

Periodontal
- cyst 522.8
- pocket 523.8

Periodontitis (chronic) (complex) (compound) (simplex) 523.40
- acute 523.33
- apical 522.6
  - acute (pulpal origin) 522.4
- aggressive 523.30
  - generalized 523.32
  - localized 523.31
- generalized 523.42
- localized 523.41

Periodontoclasia 523.5

Periodontosis 523.5

Periods - *see also* Menstruation
- heavy 626.2
- irregular 626.4

Perionychia (with lymphangitis) 681.9
- finger 681.02
- toe 681.11

Perioophoritis (*see also* Salpingo-oophoritis) 614.2

Periorchitis (*see also* Orchitis) 604.90

Periosteum, periosteal - *see* condition

Periostitis (circumscribed) (diffuse) (infective) 730.3 5th

Note *Use the following fifth-digit subclassification with category 730:*

0	site unspecified
1	shoulder region
2	upper arm
3	forearm
4	hand
5	pelvic region and thigh
6	lower leg
7	ankle and foot
8	other specified sites
9	multiple sites

- with osteomyelitis (*see also* Osteomyelitis) 730.2 5th
  - acute or subacute 730.0 5th
  - chronic or old 730.1 5th
- albuminosa, albuminosus 730.3 5th
- alveolar 526.5
- alveolodental 526.5
- dental 526.5
- gonorrheal 098.89
- hyperplastica, generalized 731.2
- jaw (lower) (upper) 526.4
- monomelic 733.99
- orbital 376.02
- syphilitic 095.5
  - congenital 090.0 *[730.8]* 5th
  - secondary 091.61
- tuberculous (*see also* Tuberculosis, bone) 015.9 5th *[730.8]* 5th
- yaws (early) (hypertrophic) (late) 102.6

Periostosis (*see also* Periostitis) 730.3 5th
- with osteomyelitis (*see also* Osteomyelitis) 730.2 5th
  - acute or subacute 730.0 5th
  - chronic or old 730.1 5th
- hyperplastic 756.59

Peripartum cardiomyopathy 674.5 5th

Periphlebitis (*see also* Phlebitis) 451.9
- lower extremity 451.2
  - deep (vessels) 451.19
  - superficial (vessels) 451.0
- portal 572.1
- retina 362.18
- superficial (vessels) 451.0

Perforation, perforative – Periphlebitis

Periphlebitis – *continued*
  tuberculous (*see also* Tuberculosis) 017.9 [5th]
    retina 017.3 [5th] *[362.18]*
Peripneumonia - *see* Pneumonia
Periproctitis 569.49
Periprostatitis (*see also* Prostatitis) 601.9
Perirectal - *see* condition
Perirenal - *see* condition
Perisalpingitis (*see also* Salpingo-oophoritis) 614.2
Perisigmoiditis 569.89
Perisplenitis (infectional) 289.59
Perispondylitis - *see* Spondylitis
Peristalsis reversed or visible 787.4
Peritendinitis (*see also* Tenosynovitis) 726.90
  adhesive (shoulder) 726.0
Perithelioma (M9150/1) - *see* Pericytoma
Peritoneum, peritoneal - *see also* condition
  equilibration test V56.32
Peritonitis (acute) (adhesive) (fibrinous) (hemorrhagic) (idiopathic) (localized) (perforative) (primary) (with adhesions) (with effusion) 567.9
  with or following
    abortion - *see* Abortion, by type, with sepsis
    abscess 567.21
    appendicitis 540.0
      with peritoneal abscess 540.1
    ectopic pregnancy (*see also* categories 633.0-633.9) 639.0
    molar pregnancy (*see also* categories 630-632) 639.0
  aseptic 998.7
  bacterial 567.29
    spontaneous 567.23
  bile, biliary 567.81
  chemical 998.7
  chlamydial 099.56
  chronic proliferative 567.89
  congenital NEC 777.6
  diaphragmatic 567.22
  diffuse NEC 567.29
  diphtheritic 032.83
  disseminated NEC 567.29
  due to
    bile 567.81
    foreign
      body or object accidentally left during a procedure (instrument) (sponge) (swab) 998.4
      substance accidentally left during a procedure (chemical) (powder) (talc) 998.7
    talc 998.7
    urine 567.89
  fibrinopurulent 567.29
  fibrinous 567.29
  fibrocaseous (*see also* Tuberculosis) 014.0 [5th]
  fibropurulent 567.29
  general, generalized (acute) 567.21
  gonococcal 098.86
  in infective disease NEC 136.9 *[567.0]*
  meconium (newborn) 777.6
  pancreatic 577.8
  paroxysmal, benign 277.31
  pelvic
    female (acute) 614.5
      chronic NEC 614.7
        with adhesions 614.6
      puerperal, postpartum, childbirth 670.8 [5th] ▲
    male (acute) 567.21
  periodic (familial) 277.31
  phlegmonous 567.29
  pneumococcal 567.1
  postabortal 639.0
  proliferative, chronic 567.89
  puerperal, postpartum, childbirth 670.8 [5th] ▲
  purulent 567.29

Peritonitis – *continued*
  septic 567.29
  spontaneous bacterial 567.23
  staphylococcal 567.29
  streptococcal 567.29
  subdiaphragmatic 567.29
  subphrenic 567.29
  suppurative 567.29
  syphilitic 095.2
    congenital 090.0 *[567.0]*
  talc 998.7
  tuberculous (*see also* Tuberculosis) 014.0 [5th]
  urine 567.89
Peritonsillar - *see* condition
Peritonsillitis 475
Perityphlitis (*see also* Appendicitis) 541
Periureteritis 593.89
Periurethral - *see* condition
Periurethritis (gangrenous) 597.89
Periuterine - *see* condition
Perivaginitis (*see also* Vaginitis) 616.10
Perivasculitis, retinal 362.18
Perivasitis (chronic) 608.4
Periventricular leukomalacia 779.7
Perivesiculitis (seminal) (*see also* Vesiculitis) 608.0
Perlèche 686.8
  due to
    moniliasis 112.0
    riboflavin deficiency 266.0
Pernicious - *see* condition
Pernio, perniosis 991.5
Persecution
  delusion 297.9
  social V62.4
Perseveration (tonic) 784.69
Persistence, persistent (congenital) 759.89
  anal membrane 751.2
  arteria stapedia 744.04
  atrioventricular canal 745.69
  bloody ejaculate 792.2
  branchial cleft 744.41
  bulbus cordis in left ventricle 745.8
  canal of Cloquet 743.51
  capsule (opaque) 743.51
  cilioretinal artery or vein 743.51
  cloaca 751.5
  communication - *see* Fistula, congenital
  convolutions
    aortic arch 747.21
    fallopian tube 752.19
    oviduct 752.19
    uterine tube 752.19
  double aortic arch 747.21
  ductus
    arteriosus 747.0
    Botalli 747.0
  fetal
    circulation 747.83
    form of cervix (uteri) 752.49
    hemoglobin (hereditary) ("Swiss variety") 282.7
    pulmonary hypertension 747.83
  foramen
    Botalli 745.5
    ovale 745.5
  Gartner's duct 752.41
  hemoglobin, fetal (hereditary) (HPFH) 282.7
  hyaloid
    artery (generally incomplete) 743.51
    system 743.51
  hymen (tag)
    in pregnancy or childbirth 654.8 [5th]
      causing obstructed labor 660.2 [5th]
  lanugo 757.4
  left
    posterior cardinal vein 747.49
    root with right arch of aorta 747.21
    superior vena cava 747.49
  Meckel's diverticulum 751.0
  mesonephric duct 752.89
    fallopian tube 752.11

Persistence, persistent – *continued*
  mucosal disease (middle ear) (with posterior or superior marginal perforation of ear drum) 382.2
  nail(s), anomalous 757.5
  occiput, anterior or posterior 660.3 [5th]
    fetus or newborn 763.1
  omphalomesenteric duct 751.0
  organ or site NEC - *see* Anomaly, specified type NEC
  ostium
    atrioventriculare commune 745.69
    primum 745.61
    secundum 745.5
  ovarian rests in fallopian tube 752.19
  pancreatic tissue in intestinal tract 751.5
  primary (deciduous)
    teeth 520.6
    vitreous hyperplasia 743.51
  pulmonary hypertension 747.83
  pupillary membrane 743.46
    iris 743.46
    Rhesus (Rh) titer 999.7
  right aortic arch 747.21
  sinus
    urogenitalis 752.89
    venosus with imperfect incorporation in right auricle 747.49
  thymus (gland) 254.8
    hyperplasia 254.0
  thyroglossal duct 759.2
  thyrolingual duct 759.2
  truncus arteriosus or communis 745.0
  tunica vasculosa lentis 743.39
  umbilical sinus 753.7
  urachus 753.7
  vegetative state 780.03
  vitelline duct 751.0
  wolffian duct 752.89
Person (with)
  admitted for clinical research, as participant or control subject V70.7
  affected by
    family member
      currently on deployment (military) V61.01
      returned from deployment (military) (current or past conflict) V61.02
  awaiting admission to adequate facility elsewhere V63.2
    undergoing social agency investigation V63.8
  concern (normal) about sick person in family V61.49
  consulting on behalf of another V65.19
    pediatric ~~pre-birth visit for expectant mother V65.11~~ ▲
      pre-adoption visit for adoptive parents V65.11 ●
      pre-birth visit for expectant parents V65.11 ●
  currently deployed in theater or in support of military war, peacekeeping and humanitarian operations V62.21
  feared
    complaint in whom no diagnosis was made V65.5
    condition not demonstrated V65.5
  feigning illness V65.2
  healthy, accompanying sick person V65.0
  history of military war, peacekeeping and humanitarian deployment (current or past conflict) V62.22
  living (in)
    alone V60.3
    boarding school V60.6
    residence remote from hospital or medical care facility V63.0
    residential institution V60.6
    without
      adequate
        financial resources V60.2
        housing (heating) (space) V60.1

Person (with) – *continued*
  living – *continued*
    without – *continued*
      housing (permanent) (temporary) V60.0
      material resources V60.2
      person able to render necessary care V60.4
      shelter V60.0
  medical services in home not available V63.1
  on waiting list V63.2
    undergoing social agency investigation V63.8
  sick or handicapped in family V61.49
  "worried well" V65.5
Personality
  affective 301.10
  aggressive 301.3
  amoral 301.7
  anancastic, anankastic 301.4
  antisocial 301.7
  asocial 301.7
  asthenic 301.6
  avoidant 301.82
  borderline 301.83
  change 310.1
  compulsive 301.4
  cycloid 301.13
  cyclothymic 301.13
  dependent 301.6
  depressive (chronic) 301.12
  disorder, disturbance NEC 301.9
    with
      antisocial disturbance 301.7
      pattern disturbance NEC 301.9
      sociopathic disturbance 301.7
      trait disturbance 301.9
  dual 300.14
  dyssocial 301.7
  eccentric 301.89
  "haltlose" type 301.89
  emotionally unstable 301.59
  epileptoid 301.3
  explosive 301.3
  fanatic 301.0
  histrionic 301.50
  hyperthymic 301.11
  hypomanic 301.11
  hypothymic 301.12
  hysterical 301.50
  immature 301.89
  inadequate 301.6
  labile 301.59
  masochistic 301.89
  morally defective 301.7
  multiple 300.14
  narcissistic 301.81
  obsessional 301.4
  obsessive-compulsive 301.4
  overconscientious 301.4
  paranoid 301.0
  passive (-dependent) 301.6
  passive-aggressive 301.84
  pathologic NEC 301.9
  pattern defect or disturbance 301.9
  pseudosocial 301.7
  psychoinfantile 301.59
  psychoneurotic NEC 301.89
  psychopathic 301.9
    with
      amoral trend 301.7
      antisocial trend 301.7
      asocial trend 301.7
      pathologic sexuality (*see also* Deviation, sexual) 302.9
    mixed types 301.9
  schizoid 301.20
    introverted 301.21
    schizotypal 301.22
  type A 301.4
  unstable (emotional) 301.59
Perthes' disease (capital femoral osteochondrosis) 732.1

Periphlebitis – Perthes' disease

- **Pertussis** (*see also* Whooping cough) 033.9
  - vaccination, prophylactic (against) V03.6
- **Peruvian wart** 088.0
- **Perversion, perverted**
  - appetite 307.52
    - hysterical 300.11
  - function
    - pineal gland 259.8
    - pituitary gland 253.9
      - anterior lobe
        - deficient 253.2
        - excessive 253.1
      - posterior lobe 253.6
    - placenta - *see* Placenta, abnormal
  - sense of smell or taste 781.1
    - psychogenic 306.7
  - sexual (*see also* Deviation, sexual) 302.9
- **Pervious, congenital** - *see also* Imperfect, closure
  - ductus arteriosus 747.0
- **Pes** (congenital) (*see also* Talipes) 754.70
  - abductus (congenital) 754.60
    - acquired 736.79
  - acquired NEC 736.79
    - planus 734
  - adductus (congenital) 754.79
    - acquired 736.79
  - cavus 754.71
    - acquired 736.73
  - planovalgus (congenital) 754.69
    - acquired 736.79
  - planus (acquired) (any degree) 734
    - congenital 754.61
    - rachitic 268.1
  - valgus (congenital) 754.61
    - acquired 736.79
  - varus (congenital) 754.50
    - acquired 736.79
- **Pest** (*see also* Plague) 020.9
- **Pestis** (*see also* Plague) 020.9
  - bubonica 020.0
  - fulminans 020.0
  - minor 020.8
  - pneumonica - *see* Plague, pneumonic
- **Petechia, petechiae** 782.7
  - fetus or newborn 772.6
- **Petechial**
  - fever 036.0
  - typhus 081.9
- **Petges-Cléjat or Petges-Clégat syndrome** (poikilodermatomyositis) 710.3
- **Petit's**
  - disease (*see also* Hernia, lumbar) 553.8
- **Petit mal** (idiopathic) (*see also* Epilepsy) 345.0 5th
  - status 345.2
- **Petrellidosis** 117.6
- **Petrositis** 383.20
  - acute 383.21
  - chronic 383.22
- **Peutz-Jeghers disease or syndrome** 759.6
- **Peyronie's disease** 607.85
- **Pfeiffer's disease** 075
- **Phacentocele** 379.32
  - traumatic 921.3
- **Phacoanaphylaxis** 360.19
- **Phacocele** (old) 379.32
  - traumatic 921.3
- **Phaehyphomycosis** 117.8
- **Phagedena** (dry) (moist) (*see also* Gangrene) 785.4
  - arteriosclerotic 440.24
  - geometric 686.09
  - penis 607.89
  - senile 440.24
  - sloughing 785.4
  - tropical (*see also* Ulcer, skin) 707.9
  - vulva 616.50
- **Phagedenic** - *see also* condition
  - abscess - *see also* Abscess
    - chancroid 099.0
  - bubo NEC 099.8
  - chancre 099.0
  - ulcer (tropical) (*see also* Ulcer, skin) 707.9
- **Phagomania** 307.52
- **Phakoma** 362.89
- **Phantom limb** (syndrome) 353.6
- **Pharyngeal** - *see also* condition
  - arch remnant 744.41
  - pouch syndrome 279.11
- **Pharyngitis** (acute) (catarrhal) (gangrenous) (infective) (malignant) (membranous) (phlegmonous) (pneumococcal) (pseudomembranous) (simple) (staphylococcal) (subacute) (suppurative) (ulcerative) (viral) 462
  - with influenza, flu, or grippe 487.1
  - aphthous 074.0
  - atrophic 472.1
  - chlamydial 099.51
  - chronic 472.1
  - Coxsackie virus 074.0
  - diphtheritic (membranous) 032.0
  - follicular 472.1
  - fusospirochetal 101
  - gonococcal 098.6
  - granular (chronic) 472.1
  - herpetic 054.79
  - hypertrophic 472.1
  - infectional, chronic 472.1
  - influenzal 487.1
  - lymphonodular, acute 074.8
  - septic 034.0
  - streptococcal 034.0
  - tuberculous (*see also* Tuberculosis) 012.8 5th
  - vesicular 074.0
- **Pharyngoconjunctival fever** 077.2
- **Pharyngoconjunctivitis, viral** 077.2
- **Pharyngolaryngitis** (acute) 465.0
  - chronic 478.9
  - septic 034.0
- **Pharyngoplegia** 478.29
- **Pharyngotonsillitis** 465.8
  - tuberculous 012.8 5th
- **Pharyngotracheitis** (acute) 465.8
  - chronic 478.9
- **Pharynx, pharyngeal** - *see* condition
- **Phase of life problem NEC** V62.89
- **Phenomenon**
  - Arthus 995.21
  - flashback (drug) 292.89
  - jaw-winking 742.8
  - Jod-Basedow 242.8 5th
  - L. E. cell 710.0
  - lupus erythematosus cell 710.0
  - Pelger-Huët (hereditary hyposegmentation) 288.2
  - Raynaud's (paroxysmal digital cyanosis) (secondary) 443.0
  - Reilly's (*see also* Neuropathy, peripheral, autonomic) 337.9
  - vasomotor 780.2
  - vasospastic 443.9
  - vasovagal 780.2
  - Wenckebach's, heart block (second degree) 426.13
- **Phenylketonuria** (PKU) 270.1
- **Phenylpyruvicaciduria** 270.1
- **Pheochromoblastoma** (M8700/3)
  - specified site - *see* Neoplasm, by site, malignant
  - unspecified site 194.0
- **Pheochromocytoma** (M8700/0)
  - malignant (M8700/3)
    - specified site - *see* Neoplasm, by site, malignant
    - unspecified site 194.0
  - specified site - *see* Neoplasm, by site, benign
  - unspecified site 227.0
- **Phimosis** (congenital) 605
  - chancroidal 099.0
  - due to infection 605
- **Phlebectasia** (*see also* Varicose, vein) 454.9
  - congenital NEC 747.60
- **Phlebectasia** – *continued*
  - esophagus (*see also* Varix, esophagus) 456.1
    - with hemorrhage (*see also* Varix, esophagus, bleeding) 456.0
- **Phlebitis** (infective) (pyemic) (septic) (suppurative) 451.9
  - antecubital vein 451.82
  - arm NEC 451.84
    - axillary vein 451.89
    - basilic vein 451.82
    - deep 451.83
    - superficial 451.82
  - axillary vein 451.89
  - basilic vein 451.82
  - blue 451.9
  - brachial vein 451.83
  - breast, superficial 451.89
  - cavernous (venous) sinus - *see* Phlebitis, intracranial sinus
  - cephalic vein 451.82
  - cerebral (venous) sinus - *see* Phlebitis, intracranial sinus
  - chest wall, superficial 451.89
  - complicating pregnancy or puerperium 671.2 5th ▲
    - affecting fetus or newborn 760.3
  - cranial (venous) sinus - *see* Phlebitis, intracranial sinus
  - deep (vessels) 451.19
    - femoral vein 451.11
    - specified vessel NEC 451.19
  - due to implanted device - *see* Complications, due to (presence of) any device, implant, or graft classified to 996.0-996.5 NEC
  - during or resulting from a procedure 997.2
  - femoral vein (deep) (superficial) 451.11
  - femoropopliteal 451.19
  - following infusion, perfusion, or transfusion 999.2
  - gouty 274.89 *[451.9]*
  - hepatic veins 451.89
  - iliac vein 451.81
  - iliofemoral 451.11
  - intracranial sinus (any) (venous) 325
    - late effect - *see* category 326
    - nonpyogenic 437.6
      - in pregnancy or puerperium 671.5 5th
  - jugular vein 451.89
  - lateral (venous) sinus - *see* Phlebitis, intracranial sinus
  - leg 451.2
    - deep (vessels) 451.19
      - specified vessel NEC 451.19
    - superficial (vessels) 451.0
      - femoral vein 451.11
  - longitudinal sinus - *see* Phlebitis, intracranial sinus
  - lower extremity 451.2
    - deep (vessels) 451.19
      - specified vessel NEC 451.19
    - superficial (vessels) 451.0
      - femoral vein 451.11
  - migrans, migrating (superficial) 453.1
  - pelvic
    - with
      - abortion - *see* Abortion, by type, with sepsis
      - ectopic pregnancy (*see also* categories 633.0-633.9) 639.0
      - molar pregnancy (*see also* categories 630-632) 639.0
    - following
      - abortion 639.0
      - ectopic or molar pregnancy 639.0
    - puerperal, postpartum 671.4 5th
  - popliteal vein 451.19
  - portal (vein) 572.1
  - postoperative 997.2
  - pregnancy 671.2 5th ▲
    - deep 671.3 5th
    - specified type NEC 671.5 5th
- **Phlebitis** – *continued*
    - superficial 671.2 5th
  - puerperal, postpartum, childbirth 671.2 5th ▲
    - deep 671.4 5th
    - lower extremities 671.2 5th
    - pelvis 671.4 5th
    - specified site NEC 671.5 5th
      - superficial 671.2 5th
  - radial vein 451.83
  - retina 362.18
  - saphenous (great) (long) 451.0
    - accessory or small 451.0
  - sinus (meninges) - *see* Phlebitis, intracranial sinus
  - specified site NEC 451.89
  - subclavian vein 451.89
  - syphilitic 093.89
  - tibial vein 451.19
  - ulcer, ulcerative 451.9
    - leg 451.2
      - deep (vessels) 451.19
        - specified vessel NEC 451.19
      - superficial (vessels) 451.0
        - femoral vein 451.11
    - lower extremity 451.2
      - deep (vessels) 451.19
        - femoral vein 451.11
        - specified vessel NEC 451.19
      - superficial (vessels) 451.0
  - ulnar vein 451.83
  - umbilicus 451.89
  - upper extremity - *see* Phlebitis, arm
    - deep (veins) 451.83
      - brachial vein 451.83
      - radial vein 451.83
      - ulnar vein 451.83
    - superficial (veins) 451.82
      - antecubital vein 451.82
      - basilic vein 451.82
      - cephalic vein 451.82
  - uterus (septic) (*see also* Endometritis) 615.9
  - varicose (leg) (lower extremity) (*see also* Varicose, vein) 454.1
- **Phlebofibrosis** 459.89
- **Phleboliths** 459.89
- **Phlebosclerosis** 459.89
- **Phlebothrombosis** - *see* Thrombosis
- **Phlebotomus fever** 066.0
- **Phlegm, choked on** 933.1
- **Phlegmasia**
  - alba dolens (deep vessels) 451.19
    - complicating pregnancy 671.3 5th
    - nonpuerperal 451.19
    - puerperal, postpartum, childbirth 671.4 5th
  - cerulea dolens 451.19
- **Phlegmon** (*see also* Abscess) 682.9
  - erysipelatous (*see also* Erysipelas) 035
  - iliac 682.2
    - fossa 540.1
  - throat 478.29
- **Phlegmonous** - *see* condition
- **Phlyctenulosis** (allergic) (keratoconjunctivitis) (nontuberculous) 370.31
  - cornea 370.31
    - with ulcer (*see also* Ulcer, cornea) 370.00
  - tuberculous (*see also* Tuberculosis) 017.3 5th *[370.31]*
- **Phobia, phobic** (reaction) 300.20
  - animal 300.29
  - isolated NEC 300.29
  - obsessional 300.3
  - simple NEC 300.29
  - social 300.23
  - specified NEC 300.29
  - state 300.20
- **Phocas' disease** 610.1
- **Phocomelia** 755.4
  - lower limb 755.32
    - complete 755.33

Pertussis – Phocomelia

- **Phocomelia** – *continued*
  - lower limb – *continued*
    - distal 755.35
    - proximal 755.34
  - upper limb 755.22
    - complete 755.23
    - distal 755.25
    - proximal 755.24
- **Phoria** (*see also* Heterophoria) 378.40
- **Phosphate-losing tubular disorder** 588.0
- **Phosphatemia** 275.3
- **Phosphaturia** 275.3
- **Photoallergic response** 692.72
- **Photocoproporphyria** 277.1
- **Photodermatitis** (sun) 692.72
  - light other than sun 692.82
- **Photokeratitis** 370.24
- **Photo-ophthalmia** 370.24
- **Photophobia** 368.13
- **Photopsia** 368.15
- **Photoretinitis** 363.31
- **Photoretinopathy** 363.31
- **Photosensitiveness** (sun) 692.72
  - light other than sun 692.82
- **Photosensitization skin** (sun) 692.72
  - light other than sun 692.82
- **Phototoxic response** 692.72
- **Phrenitis** 323.9
- **Phrynoderma** 264.8
- **Phthiriasis** (pubis) (any site) 132.2
  - with any infestation classifiable to 132.0 and 132.1 132.3
- **Phthirus infestation** - *see* Phthiriasis
- **Phthisis** (*see also* Tuberculosis) 011.9 5th
  - bulbi (infectional) 360.41
  - colliers' 011.4 5th
  - cornea 371.05
  - eyeball (due to infection) 360.41
  - millstone makers' 011.4 5th
  - miners' 011.4 5th
  - potters' 011.4 5th
  - sandblasters' 011.4 5th
  - stonemasons' 011.4 5th
- **Phycomycosis** 117.7
- **Physalopteriasis** 127.7
- **Physical therapy** NEC V57.1
  - breathing exercises V57.0
- **Physiological cup, optic papilla**
  - borderline, glaucoma suspect 365.00
  - enlarged 377.14
  - glaucomatous 377.14
- **Phytobezoar** 938
  - intestine 936
  - stomach 935.2
- **Pian** (*see also* Yaws) 102.9
- **Pianoma** 102.1
- **Piarhemia, piarrhemia** (*see also* Hyperlipemia) 272.4
  - bilharziasis 120.9
- **Pica** 307.52
  - hysterical 300.11
- **Pick's**
  - cerebral atrophy 331.11
    - with dementia
      - with behavioral disturbance 331.11 *[294.11]*
      - without behavioral disturbance 331.11 *[294.10]*
  - disease
    - brain 331.11
      - dementia in
        - with behavioral disturbance 331.11 *[294.11]*
        - without behavioral disturbance 331.11 *[294.10]*
    - lipid histiocytosis 272.7
    - liver (pericardial pseudocirrhosis of liver) 423.2
    - pericardium (pericardial pseudocirrhosis of liver) 423.2
    - polyserositis (pericardial pseudocirrhosis of liver) 423.2
- **Pick's** – *continued*
  - syndrome
    - heart (pericardial pseudocirrhosis of liver) 423.2
    - liver (pericardial pseudocirrhosis of liver) 423.2
  - tubular adenoma (M8640/0)
    - specified site - *see* Neoplasm, by site, benign
    - unspecified site
      - female 220
      - male 222.0
- **Pick-Herxheimer syndrome** (diffuse idiopathic cutaneous atrophy) 701.8
- **Pick-Niemann disease** (lipid histiocytosis) 272.7
- **Pickwickian syndrome** (cardiopulmonary obesity) 278.8
- **Piebaldism, classic** 709.09
- **Piedra** 111.2
  - beard 111.2
    - black 111.3
    - white 111.2
  - black 111.3
  - scalp 111.3
    - black 111.3
    - white 111.2
  - white 111.2
- **Pierre Marie's syndrome** (pulmonary hypertrophic osteoarthropathy) 731.2
- **Pierre Marie-Bamberger syndrome** (hypertrophic pulmonary osteoarthropathy) 731.2
- **Pierre Mauriac's syndrome** (diabetes-dwarfism-obesity) 258.1
- **Pierre Robin deformity or syndrome** (congenital) 756.0
- **Pierson's disease or osteochondrosis** 732.1
- **Pigeon**
  - breast or chest (acquired) 738.3
    - congenital 754.82
    - rachitic (*see also* Rickets) 268.0
  - breeders' disease or lung 495.2
  - fanciers' disease or lung 495.2
  - toe 735.8
- **Pigmentation** (abnormal) 709.00
  - anomalies NEC 709.00
    - congenital 757.33
    - specified NEC 709.09
  - conjunctiva 372.55
  - cornea 371.10
    - anterior 371.11
    - posterior 371.13
    - stromal 371.12
  - lids (congenital) 757.33
    - acquired 374.52
  - limbus corneae 371.10
  - metals 709.00
  - optic papilla, congenital 743.57
  - retina (congenital) (grouped) (nevoid) 743.53
    - acquired 362.74
  - scrotum, congenital 757.33
- **Piles** - *see* Hemorrhoids
- **Pili**
  - annulati or torti (congenital) 757.4
  - incarnati 704.8
- **Pill roller hand** (intrinsic) 736.09
- **Pilomatrixoma** (M8110/0) - *see* Neoplasm, skin, benign
- **Pilonidal** - *see* condition
- **Pimple** 709.8
- **PIN I** (prostatic intraepithelial neoplasia I) 602.3
- **PIN II** (prostatic intraepithelial neoplasia II) 602.3
- **PIN III** (prostatic intraepithelial neoplasia III) 233.4
- **Pinched nerve** - *see* Neuropathy, entrapment
- **Pineal body or gland** - *see* condition
- **Pinealoblastoma** (M9362/3) 194.4
- **Pinealoma** (M9360/1) 237.1
  - malignant (M9360/3) 194.4
- **Pineoblastoma** (M9362/3) 194.4
- **Pineocytoma** (M9361/1) 237.1
- **Pinguecula** 372.51
- **Pingueculitis** 372.34
- **Pinhole meatus** (*see also* Stricture, urethra) 598.9
- **Pink**
  - disease 985.0
  - eye 372.03
  - puffer 492.8
- **Pinkus' disease** (lichen nitidus) 697.1
- **Pinpoint**
  - meatus (*see also* Stricture, urethra) 598.9
  - os (uteri) (*see also* Stricture, cervix) 622.4
- **Pinselhaare** (congenital) 757.4
- **Pinta** 103.9
  - cardiovascular lesions 103.2
  - chancre (primary) 103.0
  - erythematous plaques 103.1
  - hyperchromic lesions 103.1
  - hyperkeratosis 103.1
  - lesions 103.9
    - cardiovascular 103.2
    - hyperchromic 103.1
    - intermediate 103.1
    - late 103.2
    - mixed 103.3
    - primary 103.0
    - skin (achromic) (cicatricial) (dyschromic) 103.2
      - hyperchromic 103.1
      - mixed (achromic and hyperchromic) 103.3
  - papule (primary) 103.0
  - skin lesions (achromic) (cicatricial) (dyschromic) 103.2
    - hyperchromic 103.1
    - mixed (achromic and hyperchromic) 103.3
  - vitiligo 103.2
- **Pintid** 103.0
- **Pinworms** (disease) (infection) (infestation) 127.4
- **Piry fever** 066.8
- **Pistol wound** - *see* Gunshot wound
- **Pit, lip** (mucus), **congenital** 750.25
- **Pitchers' elbow** 718.82
- **Pithecoid pelvis** 755.69
  - with disproportion (fetopelvic) 653.2 5th
    - affecting fetus or newborn 763.1
    - causing obstructed labor 660.1 5th
- **Pithiatism** 300.11
- **Pitted** - *see also* Pitting
  - teeth 520.4
- **Pitting** (edema) (*see also* Edema) 782.3
  - lip 782.3
  - nail 703.8
    - congenital 757.5
- **Pituitary gland** - *see* condition
- **Pituitary snuff-takers' disease** 495.8
- **Pityriasis** 696.5
  - alba 696.5
  - capitis 690.11
  - circinata (et maculata) 696.3
  - Hebra's (exfoliative dermatitis) 695.89
  - lichenoides et varioliformis 696.2
  - maculata (et circinata) 696.3
  - nigra 111.1
  - pilaris 757.39
    - acquired 701.1
    - Hebra's 696.4
  - rosea 696.3
  - rotunda 696.3
  - rubra (Hebra) 695.89
    - pilaris 696.4
  - sicca 690.18
  - simplex 690.18
  - specified type NEC 696.5
  - streptogenes 696.5
  - versicolor 111.0
    - scrotal 111.0
- **Placenta, placental**
  - ablatio 641.2 5th
    - affecting fetus or newborn 762.1
- **Placenta, placental** – *continued*
  - abnormal, abnormality 656.7 5th
    - with hemorrhage 641.8 5th
      - affecting fetus or newborn 762.1
    - affecting fetus or newborn 762.2
  - abruptio 641.2 5th
    - affecting fetus or newborn 762.1
  - accessory lobe - *see* Placenta, abnormal
  - accreta (without hemorrhage) 667.0 5th
    - with hemorrhage 666.0 5th
  - adherent (without hemorrhage) 667.0 5th
    - with hemorrhage 666.0 5th
  - apoplexy - *see* Placenta, separation
  - battledore - *see* Placenta, abnormal
  - bilobate - *see* Placenta, abnormal
  - bipartita - *see* Placenta, abnormal
  - carneous mole 631
  - centralis - *see* Placenta, previa
  - circumvallata - *see* Placenta, abnormal
  - cyst (amniotic) - *see* Placenta, abnormal
  - deficiency - *see* Placenta, insufficiency
  - degeneration - *see* Placenta, insufficiency
  - detachment (partial) (premature) (with hemorrhage) 641.2 5th
    - affecting fetus or newborn 762.1
  - dimidiata - *see* Placenta, abnormal
  - disease 656.7 5th
    - affecting fetus or newborn 762.2
  - duplex - *see* Placenta, abnormal
  - dysfunction - *see* Placenta, insufficiency
  - fenestrata - *see* Placenta, abnormal
  - fibrosis - *see* Placenta, abnormal
  - fleshy mole 631
  - hematoma - *see* Placenta, abnormal
  - hemorrhage NEC - *see* Placenta, separation
  - hormone disturbance or malfunction - *see* Placenta, abnormal
  - hyperplasia - *see* Placenta, abnormal
  - increta (without hemorrhage) 667.0 5th
    - with hemorrhage 666.0 5th
  - infarction 656.7 5th
    - affecting fetus or newborn 762.2
  - insertion, vicious - *see* Placenta, previa
  - insufficiency
    - affecting
      - fetus or newborn 762.2
      - management of pregnancy 656.5 5th
  - lateral - *see* Placenta, previa
  - low implantation or insertion - *see* Placenta, previa
  - low-lying - *see* Placenta, previa
  - malformation - *see* Placenta, abnormal
  - malposition - *see* Placenta, previa
  - marginalis, marginata - *see* Placenta, previa
  - marginal sinus (hemorrhage) (rupture) 641.2 5th
    - affecting fetus or newborn 762.1
  - membranacea - *see* Placenta, abnormal
  - multilobed - *see* Placenta, abnormal
  - multipartita - *see* Placenta, abnormal
  - necrosis - *see* Placenta, abnormal
  - percreta (without hemorrhage) 667.0 5th
    - with hemorrhage 666.0 5th
  - polyp 674.4 5th
  - previa (central) (centralis) (complete) (lateral) (marginal) (marginalis) (partial) (partialis) (total) (with hemorrhage) 641.1 5th
    - affecting fetus or newborn 762.0
    - noted
      - before labor, without hemorrhage (with cesarean delivery) 641.0 5th
      - during pregnancy (without hemorrhage) 641.0 5th
    - without hemorrhage (before labor and delivery) (during pregnancy) 641.0 5th
  - retention (with hemorrhage) 666.0 5th
    - fragments, complicating puerperium (delayed hemorrhage) 666.2 5th
      - without hemorrhage 667.1 5th

- **Placenta, placental** – *continued*
  - retention (with hemorrhage) – *continued*
    - postpartum, puerperal 666.2 5th
      - without hemorrhage 667.0 5th
  - separation (normally implanted) (partial) (premature) (with hemorrhage) 641.2 5th
    - affecting fetus or newborn 762.1
  - septuplex - *see* Placenta, abnormal
  - small - *see* Placenta, insufficiency
  - softening (premature) - *see* Placenta, abnormal
  - spuria - *see* Placenta, abnormal
  - succenturiata - *see* Placenta, abnormal
  - syphilitic 095.8
  - transfusion syndromes 762.3
  - transmission of chemical substance - *see* Absorption, chemical, through placenta
  - trapped (with hemorrhage) 666.0 5th
    - without hemorrhage 667.0 5th
  - trilobate - *see* Placenta, abnormal
  - tripartita - *see* Placenta, abnormal
  - triplex - *see* Placenta, abnormal
  - varicose vessel - *see* Placenta, abnormal
  - vicious insertion - *see* Placenta, previa
- **Placentitis**
  - affecting fetus or newborn 762.7
  - complicating pregnancy 658.4 5th
- **Plagiocephaly** (skull) 754.0
- **Plague** 020.9
  - abortive 020.8
  - ambulatory 020.8
  - bubonic 020.0
  - cellulocutaneous 020.1
  - lymphatic gland 020.0
  - pneumonic 020.5
    - primary 020.3
    - secondary 020.4
  - pulmonary - *see* Plague, pneumonic
  - pulmonic - *see* Plague, pneumonic
  - septicemic 020.2
  - tonsillar 020.9
    - septicemic 020.2
  - vaccination, prophylactic (against) V03.3
- **Planning, family** V25.09
  - contraception V25.9
  - natural
    - procreative V26.41
    - to avoid pregnancy V25.04
  - procreation V26.49
    - natural V26.41
- **Plaque**
  - artery, arterial - *see* Arteriosclerosis
  - calcareous - *see* Calcification
  - Hollenhorst's (retinal) 362.33
  - tongue 528.6
- **Plasma cell myeloma** 203.0 5th
- **Plasmacytoma, plasmocytoma** (solitary) (M9731/1) 238.6
  - benign (M9731/0) - *see* Neoplasm, by site, benign
  - malignant (M9731/3) 203.8 5th
- **Plasmacytopenia** 288.59
- **Plasmacytosis** 288.64
- **Plaster ulcer** (*see also* Ulcer, pressure) 707.00
- **Plateau iris syndrome** 364.82
- **Platybasia** 756.0
- **Platyonychia** (congenital) 757.5
  - acquired 703.8
- **Platypelloid pelvis** 738.6
  - with disproportion (fetopelvic) 653.2
    - affecting fetus or newborn 763.1
    - causing obstructed labor 660.1
      - affecting fetus or newborn 763.1
  - congenital 755.69
- **Platyspondylia** 756.19
- **Plethora** 782.62
  - newborn 776.4
- **Pleura, pleural** - *see* condition
- **Pleuralgia** 786.52
- **Pleurisy** (acute) (adhesive) (chronic) (costal) (diaphragmatic) (double) (dry) (fetid) (fibrinous) (fibrous) (interlobar) (latent) (lung) (old) (plastic) (primary) (residual) (sicca) (sterile) (subacute) (unresolved) (with adherent pleura) 511.0
  - with
    - effusion (without mention of cause) 511.9
      - bacterial, nontuberculous 511.1
      - nontuberculous NEC 511.9
        - bacterial 511.1
      - pneumococcal 511.1
      - specified type NEC 511.89
      - staphylococcal 511.1
      - streptococcal 511.1
      - tuberculous (*see also* Tuberculosis, pleura) 012.0 5th
        - primary, progressive 010.1 5th
    - influenza, flu, or grippe 487.1
    - tuberculosis - *see* Pleurisy, tuberculous
  - encysted 511.89
  - exudative (*see also* Pleurisy, with effusion) 511.9
    - bacterial, nontuberculous 511.1
  - fibrinopurulent 510.9
    - with fistula 510.0
  - fibropurulent 510.9
    - with fistula 510.0
  - hemorrhagic 511.89
  - influenzal 487.1
  - pneumococcal 511.0
    - with effusion 511.1
  - purulent 510.9
    - with fistula 510.0
  - septic 510.9
    - with fistula 510.0
  - serofibrinous (*see also* Pleurisy, with effusion) 511.9
    - bacterial, nontuberculous 511.1
  - seropurulent 510.9
    - with fistula 510.0
  - serous (*see also* Pleurisy, with effusion) 511.9
    - bacterial, nontuberculous 511.1
  - staphylococcal 511.0
    - with effusion 511.1
  - streptococcal 511.0
    - with effusion 511.1
  - suppurative 510.9
    - with fistula 510.0
  - traumatic (post) (current) 862.29
    - with open wound into cavity 862.39
  - tuberculous (with effusion) (*see also* Tuberculosis, pleura) 012.0 5th
    - primary, progressive 010.1 5th
- **Pleuritis sicca** - *see* Pleurisy
- **Pleurobronchopneumonia** (*see also* Pneumonia, broncho-) 485
- **Pleurodynia** 786.52
  - epidemic 074.1
  - viral 074.1
- **Pleurohepatitis** 573.8
- **Pleuropericarditis** (*see also* Pericarditis) 423.9
  - acute 420.90
- **Pleuropneumonia** (acute) (bilateral) (double) (septic) (*see also* Pneumonia) 486
  - chronic (*see also* Fibrosis, lung) 515
- **Pleurorrhea** (*see also* Hydrothorax) 511.89
- **Plexitis, brachial** 353.0
- **Plica**
  - knee 727.83
  - polonica 132.0
  - tonsil 474.8
- **Plicae dysphonia ventricularis** 784.49
- **Plicated tongue** 529.5
  - congenital 750.13
- **Plug**
  - bronchus NEC 519.19
  - meconium (newborn) NEC 777.1
  - mucus - *see* Mucus, plug
- **Plumbism** 984.9
  - specified type of lead - *see* Table of Drugs and Chemicals
- **Plummer's disease** (toxic nodular goiter) 242.3 5th
- **Plummer-Vinson syndrome** (sideropenic dysphagia) 280.8
- **Pluricarential syndrome of infancy** 260
- **Plurideficiency syndrome of infancy** 260
- **Plus** (and minus) **hand** (intrinsic) 736.09
- **PMDD** (premenstrual dysphoric disorder) 625.4
- **PMS** 625.4
- **Pneumathemia** - *see* Air, embolism, by type
- **Pneumatic drill or hammer disease** 994.9
- **Pneumatocele** (lung) 518.89
  - intracranial 348.89 ▲
  - tension 492.0
- **Pneumatosis**
  - cystoides intestinalis 569.89
  - peritonei 568.89
  - pulmonum 492.8
- **Pneumaturia** 599.84
- **Pneumoblastoma** (M8981/3) - *see* Neoplasm, lung, malignant
- **Pneumocephalus** 348.89 ▲
- **Pneumococcemia** 038.2
- **Pneumococcus, pneumococcal** - *see* condition
- **Pneumoconiosis** (due to) (inhalation of) 505
  - aluminum 503
  - asbestos 501
  - bagasse 495.1
  - bauxite 503
  - beryllium 503
  - carbon electrode makers' 503
  - coal
    - miners' (simple) 500
    - workers' (simple) 500
  - cotton dust 504
  - diatomite fibrosis 502
  - dust NEC 504
    - inorganic 503
    - lime 502
    - marble 502
    - organic NEC 504
  - fumes or vapors (from silo) 506.9
  - graphite 503
  - hard metal 503
  - mica 502
  - moldy hay 495.0
  - rheumatoid 714.81
  - silica NEC 502
    - and carbon 500
  - silicate NEC 502
  - talc 502
- **Pneumocystis carinii pneumonia** 136.3
- **Pneumocystis jiroveci pneumonia** 136.3
- **Pneumocystosis** 136.3
  - with pneumonia 136.3
- **Pneumoenteritis** 025
- **Pneumohemopericardium** (*see also* Pericarditis) 423.9
- **Pneumohemothorax** (*see also* Hemothorax) 511.89
  - traumatic 860.4
    - with open wound into thorax 860.5
- **Pneumohydropericardium** (*see also* Pericarditis) 423.9
- **Pneumohydrothorax** (*see also* Hydrothorax) 511.89
- **Pneumomediastinum** 518.1
  - congenital 770.2
  - fetus or newborn 770.2
- **Pneumomycosis** 117.9
- **Pneumonia** (acute) (Alpenstich) (benign) (bilateral) (brain) (cerebral) (circumscribed) (congestive) (creeping) (delayed resolution) (double) (epidemic) (fever) (flash) (fulminant) (fungoid) (granulomatous) (hemorrhagic) (incipient) (infantile) (infectious) (infiltration) (insular) (intermittent) (latent) (lobe) (migratory) (newborn) (organized) (overwhelming) (primary) (progressive) (pseudolobar) (purulent) (resolved) (secondary) (senile) (septic) (suppurative) (terminal) (true) (unresolved) (vesicular) 486
  - with influenza, flu, or grippe 487.0
  - adenoviral 480.0
  - adynamic 514
  - alba 090.0
  - allergic 518.3
  - alveolar - *see* Pneumonia, lobar
  - anaerobes 482.81
  - anthrax 022.1 *[484.5]*
  - apex, apical - *see* Pneumonia, lobar
  - ascaris 127.0 *[484.8]*
  - aspiration 507.0
    - due to
      - aspiration of microorganisms
        - bacterial 482.9
          - specified type NEC 482.89
        - specified organism NEC 483.8
          - bacterial NEC 482.89
        - viral 480.9
          - specified type NEC 480.8
      - food (regurgitated) 507.0
      - gastric secretions 507.0
      - milk 507.0
      - oils, essences 507.1
      - solids, liquids NEC 507.8
      - vomitus 507.0
    - fetal 770.18
      - due to
        - blood 770.16
        - clear amniotic fluid 770.14
        - meconium 770.12
        - postnatal stomach contents 770.86
    - newborn 770.18
      - due to
        - blood 770.16
        - clear amniotic fluid 770.14
        - meconium 770.12
        - postnatal stomach contents 770.86
  - asthenic 514
  - atypical (disseminated) (focal) (primary) 486
    - with influenza 487.0
  - bacillus 482.9
    - specified type NEC 482.89
  - bacterial 482.9
    - specified type NEC 482.89
  - Bacteroides (fragilis) (oralis) (melaninogenicus) 482.81
  - basal, basic, basilar - *see* Pneumonia, lobar
  - bronchiolitis obliterans organized (BOOP) 516.8
  - broncho-, bronchial (confluent) (croupous) (diffuse) (disseminated) (hemorrhagic) (involving lobes) (lobar) (terminal) 485
    - with influenza 487.0
    - allergic 518.3
    - aspiration (*see also* Pneumonia, aspiration) 507.0
    - bacterial 482.9
      - specified type NEC 482.89
    - capillary 466.19
      - with bronchospasm or obstruction 466.19
    - chronic (*see also* Fibrosis, lung) 515
    - congenital (infective) 770.0
    - diplococcal 481
    - Eaton's agent 483.0

- **Pneumonia** – *continued*
  - broncho-, bronchial – *continued*
    - Escherichia coli (E. coli) 482.82
    - Friedländer's bacillus 482.0
    - Hemophilus influenzae 482.2
    - hiberno-vernal 083.0 *[484.8]*
    - hypostatic 514
    - influenzal 487.0
    - inhalation (*see also* Pneumonia, aspiration) 507.0
      - due to fumes or vapors (chemical) 506.0
    - Klebsiella 482.0
    - lipid 507.1
      - endogenous 516.8
    - Mycoplasma (pneumoniae) 483.0
    - ornithosis 073.0
    - pleuropneumonia-like organisms (PPLO) 483.0
    - pneumococcal 481
    - Proteus 482.83
    - Pseudomonas 482.1
    - specified organism NEC 483.8
      - bacterial NEC 482.89
    - staphylococcal 482.40
      - aureus 482.41
        - methicillin
          - resistant (MRSA) 482.42
          - susceptible (MSSA) 482.41
      - specified type NEC 482.49
    - streptococcal - *see* Pneumonia, streptococcal
    - typhoid 002.0 *[484.8]*
    - viral, virus (*see also* Pneumonia, viral) 480.9
  - Butyrivibrio (fibriosolvens) 482.81
  - Candida 112.4
  - capillary 466.19
    - with bronchospasm or obstruction 466.19
  - caseous (*see also* Tuberculosis) 011.6 [5th]
  - catarrhal - *see* Pneumonia, broncho-
  - central - *see* Pneumonia, lobar
  - Chlamydia, chlamydial 483.1
    - pneumoniae 483.1
    - psittaci 073.0
    - specified type NEC 483.1
    - trachomatis 483.1
  - cholesterol 516.8
  - chronic (*see also* Fibrosis, lung) 515
  - cirrhotic (chronic) (*see also* Fibrosis, lung) 515
  - Clostridium (haemolyticum) (novyi) NEC 482.81
  - confluent - *see* Pneumonia, broncho-
  - congenital (infective) 770.0
    - aspiration 770.18
  - croupous - *see* Pneumonia, lobar
  - cytomegalic inclusion 078.5 *[484.1]*
  - deglutition (*see also* Pneumonia, aspiration) 507.0
  - desquamative interstitial 516.8
  - diffuse - *see* Pneumonia, broncho-
  - diplococcal, diplococcus (broncho-) (lobar) 481
  - disseminated (focal) - *see* Pneumonia, broncho-
  - due to
    - adenovirus 480.0
    - anaerobes 482.81
    - Bacterium anitratum 482.83
    - Chlamydia, chlamydial 483.1
      - pneumoniae 483.1
      - psittaci 073.0
      - specified type NEC 483.1
      - trachomatis 483.1
    - coccidioidomycosis 114.0
    - Diplococcus (pneumoniae) 481
    - Eaton's agent 483.0
    - Escherichia coli (E. coli) 482.82
    - Friedländer's bacillus 482.0
    - fumes or vapors (chemical) (inhalation) 506.0

- **Pneumonia** – *continued*
  - due to – *continued*
    - fungus NEC 117.9 *[484.7]*
      - coccidioidomycosis 114.0
    - Hemophilus influenzae (H. influenzae) 482.2
    - Herellea 482.83
    - influenza 487.0
    - Klebsiella pneumoniae 482.0
    - Mycoplasma (pneumoniae) 483.0
    - parainfluenza virus 480.2
    - pleuropneumonia-like organism (PPLO) 483.0
    - Pneumococcus 481
    - Pneumocystis carinii 136.3
    - Pneumocystis jiroveci 136.3
    - Proteus 482.83
    - Pseudomonas 482.1
    - respiratory syncytial virus 480.1
    - rickettsia 083.9 *[484.8]*
    - SARS-associated coronavirus 480.3
    - specified
      - bacteria NEC 482.89
      - organism NEC 483.8
      - virus NEC 480.8
    - Staphylococcus 482.40
      - aureus 482.41
        - methicillin
          - resistant (MRSA) 482.42
          - susceptible (MSSA) 482.41
      - specified type NEC 482.49
    - Streptococcus - *see also* Pneumonia, streptococcal
      - pneumoniae 481
    - virus (*see also* Pneumonia, viral) 480.9
      - SARS-associated coronavirus 480.3
  - Eaton's agent 483.0
  - embolic, embolism (*see* Embolism, pulmonary)
  - eosinophilic 518.3
  - Escherichia coli (E. coli) 482.82
  - Eubacterium 482.81
  - fibrinous - *see* Pneumonia, lobar
  - fibroid (chronic) (*see also* Fibrosis, lung) 515
  - fibrous (*see also* Fibrosis, lung) 515
  - Friedländer's bacillus 482.0
  - fusobacterium (nucleatum) 482.81
  - gangrenous 513.0
  - giant cell (*see also* Pneumonia, viral) 480.9
  - gram-negative bacteria NEC 482.83
    - anaerobic 482.81
  - grippal 487.0
  - Hemophilus influenzae (bronchial) (lobar) 482.2
  - hypostatic (broncho-) (lobar) 514
  - in
    - actinomycosis 039.1
    - anthrax 022.1 *[484.5]*
    - aspergillosis 117.3 *[484.6]*
    - candidiasis 112.4
    - coccidioidomycosis 114.0
    - cytomegalic inclusion disease 078.5 *[484.1]*
    - histoplasmosis (*see also* Histoplasmosis) 115.95
    - infectious disease NEC 136.9 *[484.8]*
    - measles 055.1
    - mycosis, systemic NEC 117.9 *[484.7]*
    - nocardiasis, nocardiosis 039.1
    - ornithosis 073.0
    - pneumocystosis 136.3
    - psittacosis 073.0
    - Q fever 083.0 *[484.8]*
    - salmonellosis 003.22
    - toxoplasmosis 130.4
    - tularemia 021.2
    - typhoid (fever) 002.0 *[484.8]*
    - varicella 052.1
    - whooping cough (*see also* Whooping cough) 033.9 *[484.3]*
  - infective, acquired prenatally 770.0
  - influenzal (broncho) (lobar) (virus) 487.0

- **Pneumonia** – *continued*
  - inhalation (*see also* Pneumonia, aspiration) 507.0
    - fumes or vapors (chemical) 506.0
  - interstitial 516.8
    - with influenzal 487.0
    - acute 136.3
    - chronic (*see also* Fibrosis, lung) 515
    - desquamative 516.8
    - hypostatic 514
    - lipoid 507.1
    - lymphoid 516.8
    - plasma cell 136.3
    - Pseudomonas 482.1
  - intrauterine (infective) 770.0
    - aspiration 770.18
      - blood 770.16
      - clear amniotic fluid 770.14
      - meconium 770.12
      - postnatal stomach contents 770.86
  - Klebsiella pneumoniae 482.0
  - Legionnaires' 482.84
  - lipid, lipoid (exogenous) (interstitial) 507.1
    - endogenous 516.8
  - lobar (diplococcal) (disseminated) (double) (interstitial) (pneumococcal, any type) 481
    - with influenza 487.0
    - bacterial 482.9
      - specified type NEC 482.89
    - chronic (*see also* Fibrosis, lung) 515
    - Escherichia coli (E. coli) 482.82
    - Friedländer's bacillus 482.0
    - Hemophilus influenzae (H. influenzae) 482.2
    - hypostatic 514
    - influenzal 487.0
    - Klebsiella 482.0
    - ornithosis 073.0
    - Proteus 482.83
    - Pseudomonas 482.1
    - psittacosis 073.0
    - specified organism NEC 483.8
      - bacterial NEC 482.89
    - staphylococcal 482.40
      - aureus 482.41
        - methicillin
          - resistant (MRSA) 482.42
          - susceptible (MSSA) 482.41
      - specified type NEC 482.49
    - streptococcal - *see* Pneumonia, streptococcal
    - viral, virus (*see also* Pneumonia, viral) 480.9
  - lobular (confluent) - *see* Pneumonia, broncho-
  - Löffler's 518.3
  - massive - *see* Pneumonia, lobar
  - meconium aspiration 770.12
  - metastatic NEC 038.8 *[484.8]*
  - methicillin resistant Staphylococcus aureus (MRSA) 482.42
  - methicillin susceptible Staphylococcus aureus (MSSA) 482.41
  - MRSA (methicillin resistant Staphylococcus aureus) 482.42
  - MSSA (methicillin susceptible Staphylococcus aureus) 482.41
  - Mycoplasma (pneumoniae) 483.0
  - necrotic 513.0
  - nitrogen dioxide 506.9
  - orthostatic 514
  - parainfluenza virus 480.2
  - parenchymatous (*see also* Fibrosis, lung) 515
  - passive 514
  - patchy - *see* Pneumonia, broncho
  - Peptococcus 482.81
  - Peptostreptococcus 482.81
  - plasma cell 136.3
  - pleurolobar - *see* Pneumonia, lobar
  - pleuropneumonia-like organism (PPLO) 483.0

- **Pneumonia** – *continued*
  - pneumococcal (broncho) (lobar) 481
  - Pneumocystis (carinii) (jiroveci) 136.3
  - postinfectional NEC 136.9 *[484.8]*
  - postmeasles 055.1
  - postoperative 997.39
  - primary atypical 486
  - Proprionibacterium 482.81
  - Proteus 482.83
  - Pseudomonas 482.1
  - psittacosis 073.0
  - radiation 508.0
  - respiratory syncytial virus 480.1
  - resulting from a procedure 997.39
  - rheumatic 390 *[517.1]*
  - Salmonella 003.22
  - SARS-associated coronavirus 480.3
  - segmented, segmental - *see* Pneumonia, broncho-
  - Serratia (marcascens) 482.83
  - specified
    - bacteria NEC 482.89
    - organism NEC 483.8
    - virus NEC 480.8
  - spirochetal 104.8 [484.]
  - staphylococcal (broncho) (lobar) 482.40
    - aureus 482.41
      - methicillin
        - resistant 482.42
        - susceptible (MSSA) 482.41
    - specified type NEC 482.49
  - static, stasis 514
  - streptococcal (broncho) (lobar) NEC 482.30
    - Group
      - A 482.31
      - B 482.32
      - specified NEC 482.39
    - pneumoniae 481
    - specified type NEC 482.39
  - Streptococcus pneumoniae 481
  - traumatic (complication) (early) (secondary) 958.8
  - tuberculous (any) (*see also* Tuberculosis) 011.6 [5th]
  - tularemic 021.2
  - TWAR agent 483.1
  - varicella 052.1
  - Veillonella 482.81
  - ventilator associated 997.31
  - viral, virus (broncho) (interstitial) (lobar) 480.9
    - with influenza, flu, or grippe 487.0
    - adenoviral 480.0
    - parainfluenza 480.2
    - respiratory syncytial 480.1
    - SARS-associated coronavirus 480.3
    - specified type NEC 480.8
  - white (congenital) 090.0
- **Pneumonic** - *see* condition
- **Pneumonitis** (acute) (primary) (*see also* Pneumonia) 486
  - allergic 495.9
    - specified type NEC 495.8
  - aspiration 507.0
    - due to fumes or gases 506.0
    - fetal 770.18
      - due to
        - blood 770.16
        - clear amniotic fluid 770.14
        - meconium 770.12
        - postnatal stomach contents 770.86
    - newborn 770.18
      - due to
        - blood 770.16
        - clear amniotic fluid 770.14
        - meconium 770.12
        - postnatal stomach contents 770.86
    - obstetric 668.0 [5th]
  - chemical 506.0
    - due to fumes or gases 506.0
  - cholesterol 516.8

- **Pneumonitis** – *continued*
  - chronic (*see also* Fibrosis, lung) 515
  - congenital rubella 771.0
  - crack 506.0
  - due to
    - crack (cocaine) 506.0
    - fumes or vapors 506.0
    - inhalation
      - food (regurgitated), milk, vomitus 507.0
      - oils, essences 507.1
      - saliva 507.0
      - solids, liquids NEC 507.8
    - toxoplasmosis (acquired) 130.4
      - congenital (active) 771.2 *[484.8]*
  - eosinophilic 518.3
  - fetal aspiration 770.18
    - due to
      - blood 770.16
      - clear amniotic fluid 770.14
      - meconium 770.12
      - postnatal stomach contents 770.86
  - hypersensitivity 495.9
  - interstitial (chronic) (*see also* Fibrosis, lung) 515
    - lymphoid 516.8
  - lymphoid, interstitial 516.8
  - meconium aspiration 770.12
  - postanesthetic
    - correct substance properly administered 507.0
    - obstetric 668.0 5th
    - overdose or wrong substance given 968.4
      - specified anesthetic - *see* Table of Drugs and Chemicals
  - postoperative 997.39
    - obstetric 668.0 5th
  - radiation 508.0
  - rubella, congenital 771.0
  - "ventilation" 495.7
  - ventilator associated 997.31 ▲
  - wood-dust 495.8
- **Pneumonoconiosis** - *see* Pneumoconiosis
- **Pneumoparotid** 527.8
- **Pneumopathy** NEC 518.89
  - alveolar 516.9
    - specified NEC 516.8
  - due to dust NEC 504
  - parietoalveolar 516.9
    - specified condition NEC 516.8
- **Pneumopericarditis** (*see also* Pericarditis) 423.9
  - acute 420.90
- **Pneumopericardium** - *see also* Pericarditis
  - congenital 770.2
  - fetus or newborn 770.2
  - traumatic (post) (*see also* Pneumothorax, traumatic) 860.0
    - with open wound into thorax 860.1
- **Pneumoperitoneum** 568.89
  - fetus or newborn 770.2
- **Pneumophagia** (psychogenic) 306.4
- **Pneumopleurisy, pneumopleuritis** (*see also* Pneumonia) 486
- **Pneumopyopericardium** 420.99
- **Pneumopyothorax** (*see also* Pyopneumothorax) 510.9
  - with fistula 510.0
- **Pneumorrhagia** 786.3
  - newborn 770.3
  - tuberculous (*see also* Tuberculosis, pulmonary) 011.9 5th
- **Pneumosiderosis** (occupational) 503
- **Pneumothorax** (acute) (chronic) 512.8
  - congenital 770.2
  - due to operative injury of chest wall or lung 512.1
    - accidental puncture or laceration 512.1
  - fetus or newborn 770.2
  - iatrogenic 512.1
  - postoperative 512.1
  - spontaneous 512.8
    - fetus or newborn 770.2
- **Pneumothorax** – *continued*
  - spontaneous – *continued*
    - tension 512.0
  - sucking 512.8
    - iatrogenic 512.1
    - postoperative 512.1
  - tense valvular, infectional 512.0
  - tension 512.0
    - iatrogenic 512.1
    - postoperative 512.1
    - spontaneous 512.0
  - traumatic 860.0
    - with
      - hemothorax 860.4
        - with open wound into thorax 860.5
      - open wound into thorax 860.1
  - tuberculous (*see also* Tuberculosis) 011.7 5th
- **Pocket(s)**
  - endocardial (*see also* Endocarditis) 424.90
  - periodontal 523.8
- **Podagra** 274.01 ▲
- **Podencephalus** 759.89
- **Poikilocytosis** 790.09
- **Poikiloderma** 709.09
  - Civatte's 709.09
  - congenital 757.33
  - vasculare atrophicans 696.2
- **Poikilodermatomyositis** 710.3
- **Pointed ear** 744.29
- **Poise imperfect** 729.90
- **Poisoned** - *see* Poisoning
- **Poisoning** (acute) - *see also* Table of Drugs and Chemicals
  - Bacillus, B.
    - aertrycke (*see also* Infection, Salmonella) 003.9
    - botulinus 005.1
    - cholerae (suis) (*see also* Infection, Salmonella) 003.9
    - paratyphosus (*see also* Infection, Salmonella) 003.9
    - suipestifer (*see also* Infection, Salmonella) 003.9
  - bacterial toxins NEC 005.9
  - berries, noxious 988.2
  - blood (general) - *see* Septicemia
  - botulism 005.1
  - bread, moldy, mouldy - *see* Poisoning, food
  - Ciguatera 988.0
  - damaged meat - *see* Poisoning, food
  - death-cap (Amanita phalloides) (Amanita verna) 988.1
  - decomposed food - *see* Poisoning, food
  - diseased food - *see* Poisoning, food
  - drug - *see* Table of Drugs and Chemicals
  - epidemic, fish, meat, or other food - *see* Poisoning, food
  - fava bean 282.2
  - fish (bacterial) - *see also* Poisoning, food
    - noxious 988.0
  - food (acute) (bacterial) (diseased) (infected) NEC 005.9
    - due to
      - bacillus
        - aertrycke (*see also* Poisoning, food, due to Salmonella) 003.9
        - botulinus 005.1
        - cereus 005.89
        - choleraesuis (*see also* Poisoning, food, due to Salmonella) 003.9
        - paratyphosus (*see also* Poisoning, food, due to Salmonella) 003.9
        - suipestifer (*see also* Poisoning, food, due to Salmonella) 003.9
      - Clostridium 005.3
        - botulinum 005.1
        - perfringens 005.2
- **Poisoning** – *continued*
  - food – *continued*
    - due to – *continued*
      - Clostridium – *continued*
        - welchii 005.2
      - Salmonella (aertrycke) (callinarum) (choleraesuis) (enteritidis) (paratyphi) (suipestifer) 003.9
        - with
          - gastroenteritis 003.0
          - localized infection(s) (*see also* Infection, Salmonella) 003.20
          - septicemia 003.1
          - specified manifestation NEC 003.8
      - specified bacterium NEC 005.89
      - Staphylococcus 005.0
      - Streptococcus 005.89
      - Vibrio parahaemolyticus 005.4
      - Vibrio vulnificus 005.81
    - noxious or naturally toxic 988.0
      - berries 988.2
      - fish 988.0
      - mushroom 988.1
      - plants NEC 988.2
  - ice cream - *see* Poisoning, food
  - ichthyotoxism (bacterial) 005.9
  - kreotoxism, food 005.9
  - malarial - *see* Malaria
  - meat - *see* Poisoning, food
  - mushroom (noxious) 988.1
  - mussel - *see also* Poisoning, food
    - noxious 988.0
  - noxious foodstuffs (*see also* Poisoning, food, noxious) 988.9
    - specified type NEC 988.8
  - plants, noxious 988.2
  - pork - *see also* Poisoning, food
    - specified NEC 988.8
    - Trichinosis 124
  - ptomaine - *see* Poisoning, food
  - putrefaction, food - *see* Poisoning, food
  - radiation 508.0
  - Salmonella (*see also* Infection, Salmonella) 003.9
  - sausage - *see also* Poisoning, food
    - Trichinosis 124
  - saxitoxin 988.0
  - shellfish - *see also* Poisoning, food
    - noxious (amnesic) (azaspiracid) (diarrheic) (neurotoxic) (paralytic) 988.0
  - Staphylococcus, food 005.0
  - toxic, from disease NEC 799.89
  - truffles - *see* Poisoning, food
  - uremic - *see* Uremia
  - uric acid 274.9
  - water 276.6
- **Poison ivy, oak, sumac or other plant dermatitis** 692.6
- **Poker spine** 720.0
- **Policeman's disease** 729.2
- **Polioencephalitis** (acute) (bulbar) (*see also* Poliomyelitis, bulbar) 045.0 5th
  - inferior 335.22
  - influenzal 487.8
  - superior hemorrhagic (acute) (Wernicke's) 265.1
  - Wernicke's (superior hemorrhagic) 265.1
- **Polioencephalomyelitis** (acute) (anterior) (bulbar) (*see also* Polioencephalitis) 045.0 5th
- **Polioencephalopathy, superior hemorrhagic** 265.1
  - with
    - beriberi 265.0
    - pellagra 265.2
- **Poliomeningoencephalitis** - *see* Meningoencephalitis
- **Poliomyelitis** (acute) (anterior) (epidemic) 045.9 5th

Note *Use the following fifth-digit subclassification with category 045:*

0	poliovirus, unspecified type
1	poliovirus, type I
2	poliovirus, type II
3	poliovirus, type III

  - with
    - paralysis 045.1 5th
      - bulbar 045.0 5th
  - abortive 045.2 5th
  - ascending 045.9 5th
    - progressive 045.9 5th
  - bulbar 045.0 5th
  - cerebral 045.0 5th
  - chronic 335.21
  - congenital 771.2
  - contact V01.2
  - deformities 138
  - exposure to V01.2
  - late effect 138
  - nonepidemic 045.9 5th
  - nonparalytic 045.2 5th
  - old with deformity 138
  - posterior, acute 053.19
  - residual 138
  - sequelae 138
  - spinal, acute 045.9 5th
  - syphilitic (chronic) 094.89
  - vaccination, prophylactic (against) V04.0
- **Poliosis** (eyebrow) (eyelashes) 704.3
  - circumscripta (congenital) 757.4
    - acquired 704.3
  - congenital 757.4
- **Pollakiuria** 788.41
  - psychogenic 306.53
- **Pollinosis** 477.0
- **Pollitzer's disease** (hidradenitis suppurativa) 705.83
- **Polyadenitis** (*see also* Adenitis) 289.3
  - malignant 020.0
- **Polyalgia** 729.99 ▲
- **Polyangiitis** (essential) 446.0
- **Polyarteritis** (nodosa) (renal) 446.0
- **Polyarthralgia** 719.49
  - psychogenic 306.0
- **Polyarthritis, polyarthropathy** NEC 716.59
  - due to or associated with other specified conditions - *see* Arthritis, due to or associated with
  - endemic (*see also* Disease, Kaschin-Beck) 716.0 5th
  - inflammatory 714.9
    - specified type NEC 714.89
  - juvenile (chronic) 714.30
    - acute 714.31
  - migratory - *see* Fever, rheumatic
  - rheumatic 714.0
    - fever (acute) - *see* Fever, rheumatic
- **Polycarential syndrome of infancy** 260
- **Polychondritis** (atrophic) (chronic) (relapsing) 733.99
- **Polycoria** 743.46
- **Polycystic** (congenital) (disease) 759.89
  - degeneration, kidney - *see* Polycystic, kidney
  - kidney (congenital) 753.12
    - adult type (APKD) 753.13
    - autosomal dominant 753.13
    - autosomal recessive 753.14
    - childhood type (CPKD) 753.14
    - infantile type 753.14
  - liver 751.62
  - lung 518.89
    - congenital 748.4
  - ovary, ovaries 256.4
  - spleen 759.0
- **Polycythemia** (primary) (rubra) (vera) (M9950/1) 238.4
  - acquired 289.0

Pneumonitis – Polycythemia

Polycythemia – *continued*
  benign 289.0
    familial 289.6
  due to
    donor twin 776.4
    fall in plasma volume 289.0
    high altitude 289.0
    maternal-fetal transfusion 776.4
    stress 289.0
  emotional 289.0
  erythropoietin 289.0
  familial (benign) 289.6
  Gaisböck's (hypertonica) 289.0
  high altitude 289.0
  hypertonica 289.0
  hypoxemic 289.0
  neonatorum 776.4
  nephrogenous 289.0
  relative 289.0
  secondary 289.0
  spurious 289.0
  stress 289.0
Polycytosis cryptogenica 289.0
Polydactylism, polydactyly 755.00
  fingers 755.01
  toes 755.02
Polydipsia 783.5
Polydystrophic oligophrenia 277.5
Polyembryoma (M9072/3) - *see* Neoplasm, by site, malignant
Polygalactia 676.6 [5th]
Polyglandular
  deficiency 258.9
  dyscrasia 258.9
  dysfunction 258.9
  syndrome 258.8
Polyhydramnios (*see also* Hydramnios) 657
Polymastia 757.6
Polymenorrhea 626.2
Polymicrogyria 742.2
Polymyalgia 725
  arteritica 446.5
  rheumatica 725
Polymyositis (acute) (chronic) (hemorrhagic) 710.4
  with involvement of
    lung 710.4 *[517.8]*
    skin 710.3
  ossificans (generalisata) (progressiva) 728.19
  Wagner's (dermatomyositis) 710.3
Polyneuritis, polyneuritic (*see also* Polyneuropathy) 356.9
  alcoholic 357.5
    with psychosis 291.1
  cranialis 352.6
  demyelinating, chronic inflammatory (CIDP) 357.81
  diabetic 250.6 [5th] *[357.2]*
    due to secondary diabetes 249.6 [5th] *[357.2]*
  due to lack of vitamin NEC 269.2 *[357.4]*
  endemic 265.0 *[357.4]*
  erythredema 985.0
  febrile 357.0
  hereditary ataxic 356.3
  idiopathic, acute 357.0
  infective (acute) 357.0
  nutritional 269.9 *[357.4]*
  postinfectious 357.0
Polyneuropathy (peripheral) 356.9
  alcoholic 357.5
  amyloid 277.39 *[357.4]*
  arsenical 357.7
  critical illness 357.82
  demyelinating, chronic inflammatory (CIDP) 357.81
  diabetic 250.6 [5th] *[357.2]*
    due to secondary diabetes 249.6 [5th] *[357.2]*
  due to
    antitetanus serum 357.6
    arsenic 357.7

Polyneuropathy – *continued*
  due to – *continued*
    drug or medicinal substance 357.6
      correct substance properly administered 357.6
      overdose or wrong substance given or taken 977.9
        specified drug - *see* Table of Drugs and Chemicals
    lack of vitamin NEC 269.2 *[357.4]*
    lead 357.7
    organophosphate compounds 357.7
    pellagra 265.2 *[357.4]*
    porphyria 277.1 *[357.4]*
    serum 357.6
    toxic agent NEC 357.7
  hereditary 356.0
  idiopathic 356.9
    progressive 356.4
  in
    amyloidosis 277.39 *[357.4]*
    avitaminosis 269.2 *[357.4]*
      specified NEC 269.1 *[357.4]*
    beriberi 265.0 *[357.4]*
    collagen vascular disease NEC 710.9 *[357.1]*
    deficiency
      B-complex NEC 266.2 *[357.4]*
      vitamin B 266.9 *[357.4]*
      vitamin B_6 266.1 *[357.4]*
    diabetes 250.6 [5th] *[357.2]*
      due to secondary diabetes 249.6 [5th] *[357.2]*
    diphtheria (*see also* Diphtheria) 032.89 *[357.4]*
    disseminated lupus erythematosus 710.0 *[357.1]*
    herpes zoster 053.13
    hypoglycemia 251.2 *[357.4]*
    malignant neoplasm (M8000/3) NEC 199.1 *[357.3]*
    mumps 072.72
    pellagra 265.2 *[357.4]*
    polyarteritis nodosa 446.0 *[357.1]*
    porphyria 277.1 *[357.4]*
    rheumatoid arthritis 714.0 *[357.1]*
    sarcoidosis 135 *[357.4]*
    uremia 585.9 *[357.4]*
  lead 357.7
  nutritional 269.9 *[357.4]*
    specified NEC 269.8 *[357.4]*
  postherpetic 053.13
  progressive 356.4
  sensory (hereditary) 356.2
  specified NEC 356.8
Polyonychia 757.5
Polyopia 368.2
  refractive 368.15
Polyorchism, polyorchidism (three testes) 752.89
Polyorrhymenitis (peritoneal) (*see also* Polyserositis) 568.82
  pericardial 423.2
Polyostotic fibrous dysplasia 756.54
Polyotia 744.1
Polyp, polypus

Note *Polyps of organs or sites that do not appear in the list below should be coded to the residual category for diseases of the organ or site concerned.*

  accessory sinus 471.8
  adenoid tissue 471.0
  adenomatous (M8210/0) - *see also* Neoplasm, by site, benign
    adenocarcinoma in (M8210/3) - *see* Neoplasm, by site, malignant
    carcinoma in (M8210/3) - *see* Neoplasm, by site, malignant
    multiple (M8221/0) - *see* Neoplasm, by site, benign
  antrum 471.8

Polyp, polypus – *continued*
  anus, anal (canal) (nonadenomatous) 569.0
    adenomatous 211.4
  Bartholin's gland 624.6
  bladder (M8120/1) 236.7
  broad ligament 620.8
  cervix (uteri) 622.7
    adenomatous 219.0
    in pregnancy or childbirth 654.6 [5th]
      affecting fetus or newborn 763.89
      causing obstructed labor 660.2 [5th]
    mucous 622.7
    nonneoplastic 622.7
  choanal 471.0
  cholesterol 575.6
  clitoris 624.6
  colon (M8210/0) (*see also* Polyp, adenomatous) 211.3
  corpus uteri 621.0
  dental 522.0
  ear (middle) 385.30
  endometrium 621.0
  ethmoidal (sinus) 471.8
  fallopian tube 620.8
  female genital organs NEC 624.8
  frontal (sinus) 471.8
  gallbladder 575.6
  gingiva 523.8
  gum 523.8
  labia 624.6
  larynx (mucous) 478.4
  malignant (M8000/3) - *see* Neoplasm, by site, malignant
  maxillary (sinus) 471.8
  middle ear 385.30
  myometrium 621.0
  nares
    anterior 471.9
    posterior 471.0
  nasal (mucous) 471.9
    cavity 471.0
    septum 471.9
  nasopharyngeal 471.0
  neoplastic (M8210/0) - *see* Neoplasm, by site, benign
  nose (mucous) 471.9
  oviduct 620.8
  paratubal 620.8
  pharynx 478.29
    congenital 750.29
  placenta, placental 674.4 [5th]
  prostate 600.20
    with
      other lower urinary tract symptoms (LUTS) 600.21
      urinary
        obstruction 600.21
        retention 600.21
  pudenda 624.6
  pulp (dental) 522.0
  rectosigmoid 211.4
  rectum (nonadenomatous) 569.0
    adenomatous 211.4
  septum (nasal) 471.9
  sinus (accessory) (ethmoidal) (frontal) (maxillary) (sphenoidal) 471.8
  sphenoidal (sinus) 471.8
  stomach (M8210/0) 211.1
  tube, fallopian 620.8
  turbinate, mucous membrane 471.8
  ureter 593.89
  urethra 599.3
  uterine
    ligament 620.8
    tube 620.8
  uterus (body) (corpus) (mucous) 621.0
    in pregnancy or childbirth 654.1 [5th]
      affecting fetus or newborn 763.89
      causing obstructed labor 660.2 [5th]
  vagina 623.7
  vocal cord (mucous) 478.4
  vulva 624.6
Polyphagia 783.6

Polypoid - *see* condition
Polyposis - *see also* Polyp
  coli (adenomatous) (M8220/0) 211.3
    adenocarcinoma in (M8220/3) 153.9
    carcinoma in (M8220/3) 153.9
  familial (M8220/0) 211.3
  intestinal (adenomatous) (M8220/0) 211.3
  multiple (M8221/0) - *see* Neoplasm, by site, benign
Polyradiculitis (acute) 357.0
Polyradiculoneuropathy (acute) (segmentally demyelinating) 357.0
Polysarcia 278.00
Polyserositis (peritoneal) 568.82
  due to pericarditis 423.2
  paroxysmal (familial) 277.31
  pericardial 423.2
  periodic (familial) 277.31
  pleural - *see* Pleurisy
  recurrent 277.31
  tuberculous (*see also* Tuberculosis, polyserositis) 018.9 [5th]
Polysialia 527.7
Polysplenia syndrome 759.0
Polythelia 757.6
Polytrichia (*see also* Hypertrichosis) 704.1
Polyunguia (congenital) 757.5
  acquired 703.8
Polyuria 788.42
Pompe's disease (glycogenosis II) 271.0
Pompholyx 705.81
Poncet's disease (tuberculous rheumatism) (*see also* Tuberculosis) 015.9 [5th]
Pond fracture - *see* Fracture, skull, vault
Ponos 085.0
Pons, pontine - *see* condition
Poor
  aesthetics of existing restoration of tooth 525.67
  contractions, labor 661.2 [5th]
    affecting fetus or newborn 763.7
  fetal growth NEC 764.9
    affecting management of pregnancy 656.5 [5th]
  incorporation
    artificial skin graft 996.55
    decellularized allodermis graft 996.55
  obstetrical history V13.29
    affecting management of current pregnancy V23.49
      pre-term labor V23.41
    pre-term labor V13.21
  sucking reflex (newborn) 796.1
  vision NEC 369.9
Poradenitis, nostras 099.1
Porencephaly (congenital) (developmental) (true) 742.4
  acquired 348.0
  nondevelopmental 348.0
  traumatic (post) 310.2
Porocephaliasis 134.1
Porokeratosis 757.39
  disseminated superficial actinic (DSAP) 692.75
Poroma, eccrine (M8402/0) - *see* Neoplasm, skin, benign
Porphyria (acute) (congenital) (constitutional) (erythropoietic) (familial) (hepatica) (idiopathic) (idiosyncratic) (intermittent) (latent) (mixed hepatic) (photosensitive) (South African genetic) (Swedish) 277.1
  acquired 277.1
  cutaneatarda
    hereditaria 277.1
    symptomatica 277.1
  due to drugs
    correct substance properly administered 277.1
    overdose or wrong substance given or taken 977.9
      specified drug - *see* Table of Drugs and Chemicals

Polycythemia – Porphyria

- **Porphyria** – *continued*
  - secondary 277.1
  - toxic NEC 277.1
  - variegata 277.1
- **Porphyrinuria** (acquired) (congenital) (secondary) 277.1
- **Porphyruria** (acquired) (congenital) 277.1
- **Portal** - *see* condition
- **Port wine nevus or mark** 757.32
- **Posadas-Wernicke disease** 114.9
- **Position**
  - fetus, abnormal (*see also* Presentation, fetal) 652.9 [5th]
  - teeth, faulty (*see also* Anomaly, position tooth) 524.30
- **Positive**
  - culture (nonspecific) 795.39
    - AIDS virus V08
    - blood 790.7
    - HIV V08
    - human immunodeficiency virus V08
    - nose 795.39
      - Staphylococcus - *see* Carrier (suspected) of, Staphylococcus
    - skin lesion NEC 795.39
    - spinal fluid 792.0
    - sputum 795.39
    - stool 792.1
    - throat 795.39
    - urine 791.9
    - wound 795.39
  - findings, anthrax 795.31
  - HIV V08
  - human immunodeficiency virus (HIV) V08
  - PPD 795.5
  - serology
    - AIDS virus V08
      - inconclusive 795.71
    - HIV V08
      - inconclusive 795.71
    - human immunodeficiency virus V08
      - inconclusive 795.71
    - syphilis 097.1
      - with signs or symptoms - *see* Syphilis, by site and stage
      - false 795.6
  - skin test 795.7 [5th]
    - tuberculin (without active tuberculosis) 795.5
  - VDRL 097.1
    - with signs or symptoms - *see* Syphilis, by site and stage
    - false 795.6
  - Wassermann reaction 097.1
    - false 795.6
- **Postcardiotomy syndrome** 429.4
- **Postcaval ureter** 753.4
- **Postcholecystectomy syndrome** 576.0
- **Postclimacteric bleeding** 627.1
- **Postcommissurotomy syndrome** 429.4
- **Postconcussional syndrome** 310.2
- **Postcontusional syndrome** 310.2
- **Postcricoid region** - *see* condition
- **Post-dates** (pregnancy) - *see* Pregnancy
- **Postencephalitic** - *see also* condition
  - syndrome 310.8
- **Posterior** - *see* condition
- **Posterolateral sclerosis** (spinal cord) - *see* Degeneration, combined
- **Postexanthematous** - *see* condition
- **Postfebrile** - *see* condition
- **Postgastrectomy dumping syndrome** 564.2
- **Posthemiplegic chorea** 344.89
- **Posthemorrhagic anemia** (chronic) 280.0
  - acute 285.1
  - newborn 776.5
- **Posthepatitis syndrome** 780.79
- **Postherpetic neuralgia** (intercostal) (syndrome) (zoster) 053.19
  - geniculate ganglion 053.11
  - ophthalmica 053.19
  - trigeminal 053.12
- **Posthitis** 607.1
- **Postimmunization complication or reaction** - *see* Complications, vaccination
- **Postinfectious** - *see* condition
- **Postinfluenzal syndrome** 780.79
- **Postlaminectomy syndrome** 722.80
  - cervical, cervicothoracic 722.81
  - kyphosis 737.12
  - lumbar, lumbosacral 722.83
  - thoracic, thoracolumbar 722.82
- **Postleukotomy syndrome** 310.0
- **Postlobectomy syndrome** 310.0
- **Postmastectomy lymphedema** (syndrome) 457.0
- **Postmaturity, postmature** (fetus or newborn) (gestation period over 42 completed weeks) 766.22
  - affecting management of pregnancy
    - post-term pregnancy 645.1 [5th]
    - prolonged pregnancy 645.2 [5th]
  - syndrome 766.22
- **Postmeasles** - *see also* condition
  - complication 055.8
    - specified NEC 055.79
- **Postmenopausal**
  - endometrium (atrophic) 627.8
    - suppurative (*see also* Endometritis) 615.9
  - hormone replacement therapy V07.4
  - status (age related) (natural) V49.81
- **Postnasal drip** 784.91
- **Postnatal** - *see* condition
- **Postoperative** - *see also* condition
  - confusion state 293.9
  - psychosis 293.9
  - status NEC (*see also* Status (post)) V45.89
- **Postpancreatectomy hyperglycemia** 251.3
- **Postpartum** - *see also* condition
  - anemia 648.2 [5th]
  - cardiomyopathy 674.5 [5th]
  - observation
    - immediately after delivery V24.0
    - routine follow-up V24.2
- **Postperfusion syndrome** NEC 999.89
  - bone marrow 996.85
- **Postpoliomyelitic** - *see* condition
- **Postsurgery status NEC** (*see also* Status (post)) V45.89
- **Post-term** (pregnancy) 645.1
  - infant (gestation period over 40 completed weeks to 42 completed weeks) 766.21
- **Post-transplant lymphoproliferative disorder** (PTLD) 238.77
- **Posttraumatic** - *see* condition
- **Posttraumatic brain syndrome, nonpsychotic** 310.2
- **Post-Traumatic Stress Disorder** (PTSD) 309.81
- **Post-typhoid abscess** 002.0
- **Postures, hysterical** 300.11
- **Postvaccinal reaction or complication** - *see* Complications, vaccination
- **Postvagotomy syndrome** 564.2
- **Postvalvulotomy syndrome** 429.4
- **Postvasectomy sperm count** V25.8
- **Potain's disease** (pulmonary edema) 514
- **Potain's syndrome** (gastrectasis with dyspepsia) 536.1
- **Pott's**
  - curvature (spinal) (*see also* Tuberculosis) 015.0 [5th] *[737.43]*
  - disease or paraplegia (*see also* Tuberculosis) 015.0 [5th] *[730.88]*
  - fracture (closed) 824.4
    - open 824.5
  - gangrene 440.24
  - osteomyelitis (*see also* Tuberculosis) 015.0 [5th] *[730.88]*
  - spinal curvature (*see also* Tuberculosis) 015.0 [5th] *[737.43]*
  - tumor, puffy (*see also* Osteomyelitis) 730.2 [5th]
- **Potter's**
  - asthma 502
  - disease 753.0
  - facies 754.0
  - lung 502
  - syndrome (with renal agenesis) 753.0
- **Pouch**
  - bronchus 748.3
  - Douglas' - *see* condition
  - esophagus, esophageal (congenital) 750.4
    - acquired 530.6
  - gastric 537.1
  - Hartmann's (abnormal sacculation of gallbladder neck) 575.8
    - of intestine V44.3
      - attention to V55.3
  - pharynx, pharyngeal (congenital) 750.27
- **Pouchitis** 569.71 ●
- **Poulet's disease** 714.2
- **Poultrymen's itch** 133.8
- **Poverty** V60.2
- **PPE** (palmar plantar erythrodysesthesia) 693.0
- **Prader-Labhart-Willi-Fanconi syndrome** (hypogenital dystrophy with diabetic tendency) 759.81
- **Prader-Willi syndrome** (hypogenital dystrophy with diabetic tendency) 759.81
- **Preachers' voice** 784.49
- **Pre-AIDS** - *see* Human immunodeficiency virus (disease) (illness) (infection)
- **Preauricular appendage** 744.1
- **Prebetalipoproteinemia** (acquired) (essential) (familial) (hereditary) (primary) (secondary) 272.1
  - with chylomicronemia 272.3
- **Precipitate labor** 661.3 [5th]
  - affecting fetus or newborn 763.6
- **Preclimacteric bleeding** 627.0
  - menorrhagia 627.0
- **Precocious**
  - adrenarche 259.1
  - menarche 259.1
  - menstruation 626.8
  - pubarche 259.1
  - puberty NEC 259.1
  - sexual development NEC 259.1
  - thelarche 259.1
- **Precocity, sexual** (constitutional) (cryptogenic) (female) (idiopathic) (male) NEC 259.1
  - with adrenal hyperplasia 255.2
- **Precordial pain** 786.51
  - psychogenic 307.89
- **Predeciduous teeth** 520.2
- **Prediabetes, prediabetic** 790.29
  - complicating pregnancy, childbirth, or puerperium 648.8 [5th]
    - fetus or newborn 775.89
- **Predislocation status of hip, at birth** (*see also* Subluxation, congenital, hip) 754.32
- **Pre-eclampsia** (mild) 642.4 [5th]
  - with pre-existing hypertension 642.7 [5th]
  - affecting fetus or newborn 760.0
  - severe 642.5 [5th]
  - superimposed on pre-existing hypertensive disease 642.7 [5th]
- **Preeruptive color change, teeth, tooth** 520.8
- **Preexcitation** 426.7
  - atrioventricular conduction 426.7
  - ventricular 426.7
- **Preglaucoma** 365.00
- **Pregnancy** (single) (uterine) (without sickness) V22.2

Note *Use the following fifth-digit subclassification with categories 640-649, 651-679:* ▲

0	unspecified as to episode of care
1	delivered, with or without mention of antepartum condition
2	delivered, with mention of postpartum complication
3	antepartum condition or complication
4	postpartum condition or complication

  - abdominal (ectopic) 633.00
    - with intrauterine pregnancy 633.01
    - affecting fetus or newborn 761.4
  - abnormal NEC 646.9 [5th]
  - ampullar - *see* Pregnancy, tubal
  - broad ligament - *see* Pregnancy, cornual
  - cervical - *see* Pregnancy, cornual
  - chemical 631 ●
  - combined (extrauterine and intrauterine) - *see* Pregnancy, cornual
  - complicated (by) 646.9
    - abnormal, abnormality NEC 646.9 [5th]
      - cervix 654.6 [5th]
      - cord (umbilical) 663.9 [5th]
      - glucose tolerance (conditions classifiable to 790.21-790.29) 648.8 [5th]
      - pelvic organs or tissues NEC 654.9 [5th]
      - pelvis (bony) 653.0 [5th]
      - perineum or vulva 654.8 [5th]
      - placenta, placental (vessel) 656.7 [5th]
      - position
        - cervix 654.4 [5th]
        - placenta 641.1 [5th]
          - without hemorrhage 641.0 [5th]
        - uterus 654.4 [5th]
      - size, fetus 653.5 [5th]
      - uterus (congenital) 654.0 [5th]
    - abscess or cellulitis
      - bladder 646.6 [5th]
      - genitourinary tract (conditions classifiable to 590, 595, 597, 599.0, 614.0-614.5, 614.7-614.9, 615) 646.6 [5th]
      - kidney 646.6 [5th]
      - urinary tract NEC 646.6 [5th]
    - adhesion, pelvic peritoneal 648.9 [5th]
    - air embolism 673.0 [5th]
    - albuminuria 646.2 [5th]
      - with hypertension - *see* Toxemia, of pregnancy
    - amnionitis 658.4 [5th]
    - amniotic fluid embolism 673.1 [5th]
    - anemia (conditions classifiable to 280-285) 648.2 [5th]
    - appendicitis 648.9 [5th]
    - atrophy, yellow (acute) (liver) (subacute) 646.7 [5th]
    - bacilluria, asymptomatic 646.5 [5th]
    - bacteriuria, asymptomatic 646.5 [5th]
    - bariatric surgery status 649.2 [5th]
    - bicornis or bicornuate uterus 654.0 [5th]
    - biliary problems 646.8 [5th]
    - bone and joint disorders (conditions classifiable to 720-724 or conditions affecting lower limbs classifiable to 711-719, 725-738) 648.7 [5th]
    - breech presentation (buttocks) (complete) (frank) 652.2 [5th]
      - with successful version 652.1 [5th]
    - cardiovascular disease (conditions classifiable to 390-398, 410-429) 648.6 [5th]
      - congenital (conditions classifiable to 745-747) 648.5 [5th]

- **Pregnancy** – *continued*
  - complicated (by) – *continued*
    - cerebrovascular disorders (conditions classifiable to 430-434, 436-437) 674.0 5th
    - cervicitis (conditions classifiable to 616.0) 646.6 5th
    - chloasma (gravidarum) 646.8 5th
    - cholelithiasis 646.8 5th
    - chorea (gravidarum) - *see* Eclampsia, pregnancy
    - coagulation defect 649.3 5th
    - conjoined twins 678.1 5th
    - contraction, pelvis (general) 653.1 5th
      - inlet 653.2 5th
      - outlet 653.3 5th
    - convulsions (eclamptic) (uremic) 642.6 5th
      - with pre-existing hypertension 642.7 5th
    - current disease or condition (nonobstetric)
      - abnormal glucose tolerance 648.8 5th
      - anemia 648.2 5th
      - bone and joint (lower limb) 648.7 5th
      - cardiovascular 648.6 5th
        - congenital 648.5 5th
      - cerebrovascular 674.0 5th
      - diabetes (conditions classifiable to 249 and 250) 648.0 5th
      - drug dependence 648.3 5th
      - female genital mutilation 648.9 5th
      - genital organ or tract 646.6 5th
      - gonorrheal 647.1 5th
      - hypertensive 642.2 5th
        - chronic kidney 642.2 5th
        - renal 642.1 5th
      - infectious 647.9 5th
        - specified type NEC 647.8 5th
      - liver 646.7 5th
      - malarial 647.4 5th
      - nutritional deficiency 648.9 5th
      - parasitic NEC 647.8 5th
      - periodontal disease 648.9 5th
      - renal 646.2 5th
        - hypertensive 642.1 5th
      - rubella 647.5 5th
      - specified condition NEC 648.9 5th
      - syphilitic 647.0 5th
      - thyroid 648.1 5th
      - tuberculous 647.3 5th
      - urinary 646.6 5th
      - venereal 647.2 5th
      - viral NEC 647.6 5th
    - cystitis 646.6 5th
    - cystocele 654.4 5th
    - death of fetus (near term) 656.4 5th
      - early pregnancy (before 22 completed weeks gestation) 632
    - deciduitis 646.6 5th
    - decreased fetal movements 655.7 5th
    - diabetes (mellitus) (conditions classifiable to 249 and 250) 648.0 5th
    - disorders of liver 646.7 5th
    - displacement, uterus NEC 654.4 5th
    - disproportion - *see* Disproportion
    - double uterus 654.0 5th
    - drug dependence (conditions classifiable to 304) 648.3 5th
    - dysplasia, cervix 654.6 5th
    - early onset of delivery (spontaneous) 644.2 5th
    - eclampsia, eclamptic (coma) (convulsions) (delirium) (nephritis) (uremia) 642.6 5th
      - with pre-existing hypertension 642.7 5th
    - edema 646.1 5th
      - with hypertension - *see* Toxemia, of pregnancy

- **Pregnancy** – *continued*
  - complicated (by) – *continued*
    - effusion, amniotic fluid 658.1 5th
      - delayed delivery following 658.2 5th
    - embolism
      - air 673.0 5th
      - amniotic fluid 673.1 5th
      - blood-clot 673.2 5th
      - cerebral 674.0 5th
      - pulmonary NEC 673.2 5th
      - pyemic 673.3 5th
      - septic 673.3 5th
    - emesis (gravidarum) - *see* Pregnancy, complicated, vomiting
    - endometritis (conditions classifiable to 615.0-615.9) 670.1 5th ▲
      - decidual 646.6 5th
    - epilepsy 649.4 5th
    - excessive weight gain NEC 646.1 5th
    - face presentation 652.4 5th
    - failure, fetal head to enter pelvic brim 652.5 5th
    - false labor (pains) 644.1 5th
    - fatigue 646.8 5th
    - fatty metamorphosis of liver 646.7 5th
    - female genital mutilation 648.9 5th
    - fetal
      - anemia 678.0 5th ●
      - complications from in utero procedure 679.1 5th ●
      - conjoined twins 678.1 5th
      - death (near term) 656.4 5th
        - early (before 22 completed weeks gestation) 632
      - deformity 653.7 5th
      - distress 656.8 5th
      - hematologic conditions 678.0 5th ●
      - reduction of multiple fetuses reduced to single fetus 651.7 5th
      - thrombocytopenia 678.0 5th ●
      - twin to twin transfusion 678.0 5th ●
    - fibroid (tumor) (uterus) 654.1 5th
    - footling presentation 652.8 5th
      - with successful version 652.1 5th
    - gallbladder disease 646.8 5th
    - gastric banding status 649.2 5th
    - gastric bypass status for obesity 649.2 5th
    - goiter 648.1 5th
    - gonococcal infection (conditions classifiable to 098) 647.1 5th
    - gonorrhea (conditions classifiable to 098) 647.1 5th
    - hypertensive heart and chronic kidney disease 642.2 5th
    - hemorrhage 641.9 5th
      - accidental 641.2 5th
      - before 22 completed weeks gestation NEC 640.9 5th
      - cerebrovascular 674.0 5th
      - due to
        - afibrinogenemia or other coagulation defect (conditions classifiable to 286.0-286.9) 641.3 5th
        - leiomyoma, uterine 641.8 5th
        - marginal sinus (rupture) 641.2 5th
        - premature separation, placenta 641.2 5th
        - trauma 641.8 5th
      - early (before 22 completed weeks gestation) 640.9 5th
      - threatened abortion 640.0 5th
      - unavoidable 641.1 5th
    - hepatitis (acute) (malignant) (subacute) 646.7 5th
      - viral 647.6 5th
    - herniation of uterus 654.4 5th
    - high head at term 652.5 5th
    - hydatidiform mole (delivered) (undelivered) 630

- **Pregnancy** – *continued*
  - complicated (by) – *continued*
    - hydramnios 657 5th
    - hydrocephalic fetus 653.6 5th
    - hydrops amnii 657 5th
    - hydrorrhea 658.1 5th
    - hyperemesis (gravidarum) - *see* Hyperemesis, gravidarum
    - hypertension - *see* Hypertension, complicating pregnancy
    - hypertensive
      - chronic kidney disease 642.2 5th
      - heart and chronic kidney disease 642.2 5th
      - heart and renal disease 642.2 5th
      - heart disease 642.2 5th
      - renal disease 642.2 5th
    - hyperthyroidism 648.1 5th
    - hypothyroidism 648.1 5th
    - hysteralgia 646.8 5th
    - icterus gravis 646.7 5th
    - incarceration, uterus 654.3 5th
    - incompetent cervix (os) 654.5 5th
    - infection 647.9 5th
      - amniotic fluid 658.4 5th
      - bladder 646.6 5th
      - genital organ (conditions classifiable to 614.0-614.5, 614.7-614.9, 615) 646.6 5th
      - kidney (conditions classifiable to 590.0-590.9) 646.6 5th
      - urinary (tract) 646.6 5th
        - asymptomatic 646.5 5th
    - infective and parasitic diseases NEC 647.8 5th
    - inflammation
      - bladder 646.6 5th
      - genital organ (conditions classifiable to 614.0-614.5, 614.7-614.9, 615) 646.6 5th
      - urinary tract NEC 646.6 5th
    - injury 648.9 5th
      - obstetrical NEC 665.9 5th
    - insufficient weight gain 646.8 5th
    - intrauterine fetal death (near term) NEC 656.4 5th
      - early (before 22 completed weeks gestation) 632
    - malaria (conditions classifiable to 084) 647.4 5th
    - malformation, uterus (congenital) 654.0 5th
    - malnutrition (conditions classifiable to 260-269) 648.9 5th
    - malposition
      - fetus - *see* Pregnancy, complicated, malpresentation
      - uterus or cervix 654.4 5th
    - malpresentation 652.9 5th
      - with successful version 652.1 5th
      - in multiple gestation 652.6 5th
      - specified type NEC 652.8 5th
    - marginal sinus hemorrhage or rupture 641.2 5th
    - maternal complications from in utero procedure 679.0 5th ●
    - maternal drug abuse 648.4 5th
    - maternal obesity syndrome 646.1 5th
    - menstruation 640.8 5th
    - mental disorders (conditions classifiable to 290-303, 305.0, 305.2-305.9, 306-316, 317-319) 648.4 5th
    - mentum presentation 652.4 5th
    - missed
      - abortion 632
      - delivery (at or near term) 656.4 5th
      - labor (at or near term) 656.4 5th
    - necrosis
      - genital organ or tract (conditions classifiable to 614.0-614.5, 614.7-614.9, 615) 646.6 5th
      - liver (conditions classifiable to 570) 646.7 5th

- **Pregnancy** – *continued*
  - complicated (by) – *continued*
    - necrosis – *continued*
      - renal, cortical 646.2 5th
    - nephritis or nephrosis (conditions classifiable to 580-589) 646.2 5th
      - with hypertension 642.1 5th
    - nephropathy NEC 646.2 5th
    - neuritis (peripheral) 646.4 5th
    - nutritional deficiency (conditions classifiable to 260-269) 648.9 5th
    - obesity 649.1 5th
      - surgery status 649.2 5th
    - oblique lie or presentation 652.3 5th
      - with successful version 652.1 5th
    - obstetrical trauma NEC 665.9 5th
    - oligohydramnios NEC 658.0 5th
    - onset of contractions before 37 weeks 644.0 5th
    - oversize fetus 653.5 5th
    - papyraceous fetus 646.0 5th
    - patent cervix 654.5 5th
    - pelvic inflammatory disease (conditions classifiable to 614.0-614.5, 614.7-614.9, 615) 646.6 5th
    - pelvic peritoneal adhesion 648.9 5th
    - placenta, placental
      - abnormality 656.7 5th
      - abruptio or ablatio 641.2 5th
      - detachment 641.2 5th
      - disease 656.7 5th
      - infarct 656.7 5th
      - low implantation 641.1 5th
        - without hemorrhage 641.0 5th
      - malformation 656.7 5th
      - malposition 641.1 5th
        - without hemorrhage 641.0 5th
      - marginal sinus hemorrhage 641.2 5th
      - previa 641.1 5th
        - without hemorrhage 641.0 5th
      - separation (premature) (undelivered) 641.2 5th
    - placentitis 658.4 5th
    - polyhydramnios 657 5th
    - postmaturity
      - post-term 645.1 5th
      - prolonged 645.2 5th
    - prediabetes 648.8 5th
    - pre-eclampsia (mild) 642.4 5th
      - severe 642.5 5th
      - superimposed on pre-existing hypertensive disease 642.7 5th
    - premature rupture of membranes 658.1 5th
      - with delayed delivery 658.2 5th
    - previous
      - infertility V23.0
      - in utero procedure during previous pregnancy V23.86
      - nonobstetric condition V23.89
      - poor obstetrical history V23.49
      - premature delivery V23.41
      - trophoblastic disease (conditions classifiable to 630) V23.1
    - prolapse, uterus 654.4 5th
    - proteinuria (gestational) 646.2 5th
      - with hypertension - *see* Toxemia, of pregnancy
    - pruritus (neurogenic) 646.8 5th
    - psychosis or psychoneurosis 648.4 5th
    - ptyalism 646.8 5th
    - pyelitis (conditions classifiable to 590.0-590.9) 646.6 5th
    - renal disease or failure NEC 646.2 5th
      - with secondary hypertension 642.1 5th
      - hypertensive 642.2 5th
    - retention, retained dead ovum 631
    - retroversion, uterus 654.3 5th
    - Rh immunization, incompatibility, or sensitization 656.1 5th

- **Pregnancy** – *continued*
  - complicated (by) – *continued*
    - rubella (conditions classifiable to 056) 647.5 [5th]
    - rupture
      - amnion (premature) 658.1 [5th]
        - with delayed delivery 658.2 [5th]
      - marginal sinus (hemorrhage) 641.2 [5th]
      - membranes (premature) 658.1 [5th]
        - with delayed delivery 658.2 [5th]
      - uterus (before onset of labor) 665.0 [5th]
    - salivation (excessive) 646.8 [5th]
    - salpingo-oophoritis (conditions classifiable to 614.0-614.2) 646.6 [5th]
    - septicemia (conditions classifiable to 038.0-038.9) 647.8 [5th]
      - postpartum 670.2 [5th] ▲
      - puerperal 670.2 [5th] ▲
    - smoking 649.0 [5th]
    - spasms, uterus (abnormal) 646.8 [5th]
    - specified condition NEC 646.8 [5th]
    - spotting 649.5 [5th]
    - spurious labor pains 644.1 [5th]
    - status post
      - bariatric surgery 649.2 [5th]
      - gastric banding 649.2 [5th]
      - gastric bypass for obesity 649.2 [5th]
      - obesity surgery 649.2 [5th]
    - superfecundation 651.9 [5th]
    - superfetation 651.9 [5th]
    - syphilis (conditions classifiable to 090-097) 647.0 [5th]
    - threatened
      - abortion 640.0 [5th]
      - premature delivery 644.2 [5th]
      - premature labor 644.0 [5th]
    - thrombophlebitis (superficial) 671.2 [5th]
      - deep 671.3 [5th]
      - septic 670.3 [5th] ●
    - thrombosis 671.2 [5th] ▲
      - venous (superficial) 671.2 [5th]
        - deep 671.3 [5th]
    - thyroid dysfunction (conditions classifiable to 240-246) 648.1 [5th]
    - thyroiditis 648.1 [5th]
    - thyrotoxicosis 648.1 [5th]
    - tobacco use disorder 649.0 [5th]
    - torsion of uterus 654.4 [5th]
    - toxemia - *see* Toxemia, of pregnancy
    - transverse lie or presentation 652.3 [5th]
      - with successful version 652.1 [5th]
    - trauma 648.9 [5th]
      - obstetrical 665.9 [5th]
    - tuberculosis (conditions classifiable to 010-018) 647.3 [5th]
    - tumor
      - cervix 654.6 [5th]
      - ovary 654.4 [5th]
      - pelvic organs or tissue NEC 654.4 [5th]
      - uterus (body) 654.1 [5th]
        - cervix 654.6 [5th]
      - vagina 654.7 [5th]
      - vulva 654.8 [5th]
    - unstable lie 652.0 [5th]
    - uremia - *see* Pregnancy, complicated, renal disease
    - urethritis 646.6 [5th]
    - vaginitis or vulvitis (conditions classifiable to 616.1) 646.6 [5th]
    - varicose
      - placental vessels 656.7 [5th]
      - veins (legs) 671.0 [5th]
        - perineum 671.1 [5th]
        - vulva 671.1 [5th]
    - varicosity, labia or vulva 671.1 [5th]
    - venereal disease NEC (conditions classifiable to 099) 647.2 [5th]
    - venous complication 671.9 [5th] ●

- **Pregnancy** – *continued*
  - complicated (by) – *continued*
    - viral disease NEC (conditions classifiable to 042, 050-055, 057-079, 795.05, 795.15, 796.75) 647.6 [5th]
    - vomiting (incoercible) (pernicious) (persistent) (uncontrollable) (vicious) 643.9 [5th]
      - due to organic disease or other cause 643.8 [5th]
      - early - *see* Hyperemesis, gravidarum
      - late (after 22 completed weeks gestation) 643.2 [5th]
    - young maternal age 659.8 [5th]
  - complications NEC 646.9 [5th]
  - cornual 633.80
    - with intrauterine pregnancy 633.81
    - affecting fetus or newborn 761.4
  - death, maternal NEC 646.9 [5th]
  - delivered - *see* Delivery
  - ectopic (ruptured) NEC 633.90
    - with intrauterine pregnancy 633.91
    - abdominal - *see* Pregnancy, abdominal
    - affecting fetus or newborn 761.4
    - combined (extrauterine and intrauterine) - *see* Pregnancy, cornual
    - ovarian - *see* Pregnancy, ovarian
    - specified type NEC 633.80
      - with intrauterine pregnancy 633.81
      - affecting fetus or newborn 761.4
    - tubal - *see* Pregnancy, tubal
  - examination, pregnancy
    - negative result V72.41
    - not confirmed V72.40
    - positive result V72.42
  - extrauterine - *see* Pregnancy, ectopic
  - fallopian - *see* Pregnancy, tubal
  - false 300.11
    - labor (pains) 644.1 [5th]
  - fatigue 646.8 [5th]
  - illegitimate V61.6
  - incidental finding V22.2
  - in double uterus 654.0 [5th]
  - interstitial - *see* Pregnancy, cornual
  - intraligamentous - *see* Pregnancy, cornual
  - intramural - *see* Pregnancy, cornual
  - intraperitoneal - *see* Pregnancy, abdominal
  - isthmian - *see* Pregnancy, tubal
  - management affected by
    - abnormal, abnormality
      - fetus (suspected) 655.9 [5th]
        - specified NEC 655.8 [5th]
      - placenta 656.7 [5th]
    - advanced maternal age NEC 659.6 [5th]
      - multigravida 659.6 [5th]
      - primigravida 659.5 [5th]
    - antibodies (maternal)
      - anti-c 656.1 [5th]
      - anti-d 656.1 [5th]
      - anti-e 656.1 [5th]
      - blood group (ABO) 656.2 [5th]
        - Rh(esus) 656.1 [5th]
    - appendicitis 648.9 [5th]
    - bariatric surgery status 649.2 [5th]
    - coagulation defect 649.3 [5th]
    - elderly multigravida 659.6 [5th]
    - elderly primigravida 659.5 [5th]
    - epilepsy 649.4 [5th]
    - fetal (suspected)
      - abnormality 655.9 [5th]
        - abdominal 655.8 [5th]
        - acid-base balance 656.8 [5th]
        - cardiovascular 655.8 [5th]
        - facial 655.8 [5th]
        - gastrointestinal 655.8 [5th]
        - genitourinary 655.8 [5th]
        - heart rate or rhythm 659.7 [5th]
        - limb 655.8 [5th]
        - specified NEC 655.8 [5th]
      - acidemia 656.3 [5th]
      - anencephaly 655.0 [5th]
      - aneuploidy 655.1 [5th]

- **Pregnancy** – *continued*
  - management affected by – *continued*
    - fetal (suspected) – *continued*
      - bradycardia 659.7 [5th]
      - central nervous system malformation 655.0 [5th]
      - chromosomal abnormalities (conditions classifiable to 758.0-758.9) 655.1 [5th]
      - damage from
        - drugs 655.5 [5th]
          - obstetric, anesthetic, or sedative 655.5 [5th]
        - environmental toxins 655.8 [5th]
        - intrauterine contraceptive device 655.8 [5th]
        - maternal
          - alcohol addiction 655.4 [5th]
          - disease NEC 655.4 [5th]
          - drug use 655.5 [5th]
          - listeriosis 655.4 [5th]
          - rubella 655.3 [5th]
          - toxoplasmosis 655.4 [5th]
          - viral infection 655.3 [5th]
        - radiation 655.6 [5th]
      - death (near term) 656.4 [5th]
        - early (before 22 completed weeks gestation) 632
      - distress 656.8 [5th]
      - excessive growth 656.6 [5th]
      - growth retardation 656.5 [5th]
      - hereditary disease 655.2 [5th]
      - hydrocephalus 655.0 [5th]
      - intrauterine death 656.4 [5th]
      - poor growth 656.5 [5th]
      - spina bifida (with myelomeningocele) 655.0 [5th]
    - fetal-maternal hemorrhage 656.0 [5th]
    - gastric banding status 649.2 [5th]
    - gastric bypass status for obesity 649.2 [5th]
    - hereditary disease in family (possibly) affecting fetus 655.2 [5th]
    - incompatibility, blood groups (ABO) 656.2 [5th]
      - Rh(esus) 656.1 [5th]
    - insufficient prenatal care V23.7
    - intrauterine death 656.4 [5th]
    - isoimmunization (ABO) 656.2 [5th]
      - Rh(esus) 656.1 [5th]
    - large-for-dates fetus 656.6 [5th]
    - light-for-dates fetus 656.5 [5th]
    - meconium in liquor 656.8 [5th]
    - mental disorder (conditions classifiable to 290-303, 305.0, 305.2-305.9, 306-316, 317-319) 648.4 [5th]
    - multiparity (grand) 659.4 [5th]
    - obesity 649.1 [5th]
      - surgery status 649.2 [5th]
    - poor obstetric history V23.49
      - pre-term labor V23.41
    - postmaturity
      - post-term 645.1 [5th]
      - prolonged 645.2 [5th]
    - post-term pregnancy 645.1 [5th]
    - previous
      - abortion V23.2
        - habitual 646.3 [5th]
      - cesarean delivery 654.2 [5th]
      - difficult delivery V23.49
      - forceps delivery V23.49
      - habitual abortions 646.3 [5th]
      - hemorrhage, antepartum or postpartum V23.49
      - hydatidiform mole V23.1
      - infertility V23.0
      - in utero procedure during previous pregnancy V23.86
      - malignancy NEC V23.89
      - nonobstetrical conditions V23.89
      - premature delivery V23.41
      - trophoblastic disease (conditions in 630) V23.1
      - vesicular mole V23.1

- **Pregnancy** – *continued*
  - management affected by – *continued*
    - prolonged pregnancy 645.2 [5th]
    - small-for-dates fetus 656.5 [5th]
    - smoking 649.0 [5th]
    - spotting 649.5 [5th]
    - suspected conditions not found
      - amniotic cavity and membrane problem V89.01
      - cervical shortening V89.05
      - fetal anomaly V89.03
      - fetal growth problem V89.04
      - oligohydramnios V89.01
      - other specified problem NEC V89.09
      - placental problem V89.02
      - polyhydramnios V89.01
    - tobacco use disorder 649.0 [5th]
    - venous complication 671.9 [5th] ●
    - young maternal age 659.8 [5th]
  - maternal death NEC 646.9 [5th]
  - mesometric (mural) - *see* Pregnancy, cornual
  - molar 631
    - hydatidiform (*see also* Hydatidiform mole) 630
      - previous, affecting management of pregnancy V23.1
    - previous, affecting management of pregnancy V23.49
  - multiple NEC 651.9 [5th]
    - with fetal loss and retention of one or more fetus(es) 651.6 [5th]
    - affecting fetus or newborn 761.5
    - following (elective) fetal reduction 651.7 [5th]
    - specified type NEC 651.8 [5th]
      - with fetal loss and retention of one or more fetus(es) 651.6 [5th]
      - following (elective) fetal reduction 651.7 [5th]
  - mural - *see* Pregnancy, cornual
  - observation NEC V22.1
    - first pregnancy V22.0
    - high-risk V23.9
      - specified problem NEC V23.89
  - ovarian 633.20
    - with intrauterine pregnancy 633.21
    - affecting fetus or newborn 761.4
  - possible, not (yet) confirmed V72.40
  - postmature
    - post-term 645.1 [5th]
    - prolonged 645.2 [5th]
  - post-term 645.1 [5th]
  - prenatal care only V22.1
    - first pregnancy V22.0
    - high-risk V23.9
      - specified problem NEC V23.89
  - prolonged 645.2 [5th]
  - quadruplet NEC 651.2 [5th]
    - with fetal loss and retention of one or more fetus(es) 651.5 [5th]
    - affecting fetus or newborn 761.5
    - following (elective) fetal reduction 651.7 [5th]
  - quintuplet NEC 651.8 [5th]
    - with fetal loss and retention of one or more fetus(es) 651.6 [5th]
    - affecting fetus or newborn 761.5
    - following (elective) fetal reduction 651.7 [5th]
  - resulting from
    - assisted reproductive technology V23.85
    - in vitro fertilization V23.85
  - sextuplet NEC 651.8 [5th]
    - with fetal loss and retention of one or more fetus(es) 651.6 [5th]
    - affecting fetus or newborn 761.5
    - following (elective) fetal reduction 651.7 [5th]
  - spurious 300.11

- **Pregnancy** – *continued*
  - superfecundation NEC 651.9 [5th]
    - with fetal loss and retention of one or more fetus(es) 651.6 [5th]
    - following (elective) fetal reduction 651.7 [5th]
  - superfetation NEC 651.9 [5th]
    - with fetal loss and retention of one or more fetus(es) 651.6 [5th]
    - following (elective) fetal reduction 651.7 [5th]
  - supervision (of) (for) - *see also* Pregnancy, management affected by
    - elderly
      - multigravida V23.82
      - primigravida V23.81
    - high-risk V23.9
      - insufficient prenatal care V23.7
      - specified problem NEC V23.89
    - multiparity V23.3
    - normal NEC V22.1
      - first V22.0
    - poor
      - obstetric history V23.49
        - pre-term labor V23.41
      - reproductive history V23.5
    - previous
      - abortion V23.2
      - hydatidiform mole V23.1
      - infertility V23.0
      - neonatal death V23.5
      - stillbirth V23.5
      - trophoblastic disease V23.1
      - vesicular mole V23.1
    - specified problem NEC V23.89
    - young
      - multigravida V23.84
      - primigravida V23.83
  - triplet NEC 651.1 [5th]
    - with fetal loss and retention of one or more fetus(es) 651.4 [5th]
    - affecting fetus or newborn 761.5
    - following (elective) fetal reduction 651.7 [5th]
  - tubal (with rupture) 633.10
    - with intrauterine pregnancy 633.11
    - affecting fetus or newborn 761.4
  - twin NEC 651.0 [5th]
    - with fetal loss and retention of one fetus 651.3 [5th]
    - affecting fetus or newborn 761.5
    - conjoined 678.1 [5th]
    - following (elective) fetal reduction 651.7 [5th]
  - unconfirmed V72.40
  - undelivered (no other diagnosis) V22.2
    - with false labor 644.1 [5th]
    - high-risk V23.9
      - specified problem NEC V23.89
  - unwanted NEC V61.7
- **Pregnant uterus** - *see* condition
- **Preiser's disease** (osteoporosis) 733.09
- **Prekwashiorkor** 260
- **Preleukemia** 238.75
- **Preluxation of hip, congenital** (*see also* Subluxation, congenital, hip) 754.32
- **Premature** - *see also* condition
  - beats (nodal) 427.60
    - atrial 427.61
    - auricular 427.61
    - postoperative 997.1
    - specified type NEC 427.69
    - supraventricular 427.61
    - ventricular 427.69
  - birth NEC 765.1 [5th]
  - closure
    - cranial suture 756.0
    - fontanel 756.0
    - foramen ovale 745.8
  - contractions 427.60
    - atrial 427.61
    - auricular 427.61
    - auriculoventricular 427.61
    - heart (extrasystole) 427.60

- **Premature** – *continued*
  - contractions – *continued*
    - junctional 427.60
    - nodal 427.60
    - postoperative 997.1
    - ventricular 427.69
  - ejaculation 302.75
  - infant NEC 765.1 [5th]
    - excessive 765.0 [5th]
    - light-for-dates - *see* Light-for-dates
  - labor 644.2 [5th]
    - threatened 644.0 [5th]
  - lungs 770.4
  - menopause 256.31
  - puberty 259.1
  - rupture of membranes or amnion 658.1 [5th]
    - affecting fetus or newborn 761.1
    - delayed delivery following 658.2 [5th]
  - senility (syndrome) 259.8
  - separation, placenta (partial) - *see* Placenta, separation
  - ventricular systole 427.69
- **Prematurity** NEC 765.1 [5th]
  - extreme 765.0 [5th]
- **Premenstrual syndrome** 625.4
- **Premenstrual tension** 625.4
- **Premolarization, cuspids** 520.2
- **Premyeloma** 273.1
- **Prenatal**
  - care, normal pregnancy V22.1
    - first V22.0
  - death, cause unknown - *see* Death, fetus
  - screening - *see* Antenatal, screening
  - teeth 520.6
- **Prepartum** - *see* condition
- **Preponderance, left or right ventricular** 429.3
- **Prepuce** - *see* condition
- **PRES** (posterior reversible encephalopathy syndrome) 348.39
- **Presbycardia** 797
  - hypertensive (*see also* Hypertension, heart) 402.90
- **Presbycusis** 388.01
- **Presbyesophagus** 530.89
- **Presbyophrenia** 310.1
- **Presbyopia** 367.4
- **Prescription of contraceptives** NEC V25.02
  - diaphragm V25.02
  - oral (pill) V25.01
    - emergency V25.03
    - postcoital V25.03
    - repeat V25.41
  - repeat V25.40
    - oral (pill) V25.41
- **Presenile** - *see also* condition
  - aging 259.8
  - dementia (*see also* Dementia, presenile) 290.10
- **Presenility** 259.8
- **Presentation, fetal**
  - abnormal 652.9 [5th]
    - with successful version 652.1 [5th]
    - before labor, affecting fetus or newborn 761.7
    - causing obstructed labor 660.0 [5th]
      - affecting fetus or newborn, any, except breech 763.1
    - in multiple gestation (one or more) 652.6 [5th]
    - specified NEC 652.8 [5th]
  - arm 652.7 [5th]
    - causing obstructed labor 660.0 [5th]
  - breech (buttocks) (complete) (frank) 652.2 [5th]
    - with successful version 652.1 [5th]
      - before labor, affecting fetus or newborn 761.7
    - before labor, affecting fetus or newborn 761.7
  - brow 652.4 [5th]
    - causing obstructed labor 660.0 [5th]
  - buttocks 652.2 [5th]

- **Presentation, fetal** – *continued*
  - chin 652.4 [5th]
  - complete 652.2 [5th]
  - compound 652.8 [5th]
  - cord 663.0 [5th]
  - extended head 652.4 [5th]
  - face 652.4 [5th]
    - to pubes 652.8 [5th]
  - footling 652.8 [5th]
  - frank 652.2 [5th]
  - hand, leg, or foot NEC 652.8 [5th]
  - incomplete 652.8 [5th]
  - mentum 652.4 [5th]
  - multiple gestation (one fetus or more) 652.6 [5th]
  - oblique 652.3 [5th]
    - with successful version 652.1 [5th]
  - shoulder 652.8 [5th]
    - affecting fetus or newborn 763.1
  - transverse 652.3 [5th]
    - with successful version 652.1 [5th]
  - umbilical cord 663.0 [5th]
  - unstable 652.0 [5th]
- **Prespondylolisthesis** (congenital) (lumbosacral) 756.11
- **Pressure**
  - area, skin ulcer (*see also* Ulcer, pressure) 707.00
  - atrophy, spine 733.99
  - birth, fetus or newborn NEC 767.9
  - brachial plexus 353.0
  - brain 348.4
    - injury at birth 767.0
  - cerebral - *see* Pressure, brain
  - chest 786.59
  - cone, tentorial 348.4
    - injury at birth 767.0
  - funis - *see* Compression, umbilical cord
  - hyposystolic (*see also* Hypotension) 458.9
  - increased
    - intracranial 781.99
      - due to
        - benign intracranial hypertension 348.2
        - hydrocephalus -*see* hydrocephalus
      - injury at birth 767.8
    - intraocular 365.00
  - lumbosacral plexus 353.1
  - mediastinum 519.3
  - necrosis (chronic) (skin) (*see also* Decubitus) 707.00
  - nerve - *see* Compression, nerve
  - paralysis (*see also* Neuropathy, entrapment) 355.9
  - pre-ulcer skin changes limited to persistent focal erythema (*see also* Ulcer, pressure) 707.21
  - sore (chronic) (*see also* Ulcer, pressure) 707.00
  - spinal cord 336.9
  - ulcer (chronic) (*see also* Ulcer, pressure) 707.00
  - umbilical cord - *see* Compression, umbilical cord
  - venous, increased 459.89
- **Pre-syncope** 780.2
- **Preterm infant** NEC 765.1 [5th]
  - extreme 765.0 [5th]
- **Priapism** (penis) 607.3
- **Prickling sensation** (*see also* Disturbance, sensation) 782.0
- **Prickly heat** 705.1
- **Primary** - *see* condition
- **Primigravida, elderly**
  - affecting
    - fetus or newborn 763.89
    - management of pregnancy, labor, and delivery 659.5 [5th]
- **Primipara, old**
  - affecting
    - fetus or newborn 763.89

- **Primipara, old** – *continued*
  - affecting – *continued*
    - management of pregnancy, labor, and delivery 659.5 [5th]
- **Primula dermatitis** 692.6
- **Primus varus** (bilateral) (metatarsus) 754.52
- **PRIND** (prolonged reversible ischemic neurologic deficit) 434.91
  - history of (personal) V12.54
- **Pringle's disease** (tuberous sclerosis) 759.5
- **Prinzmetal's angina** 413.1
- **Prinzmetal-Massumi syndrome** (anterior chest wall) 786.52
- **Prizefighter ear** 738.7
- **Problem** (with) V49.9
  - academic V62.3
  - acculturation V62.4
  - adopted child V61.24 ▲
  - aged
    - in-law V61.3
    - parent V61.3
    - person NEC V61.8
  - alcoholism in family V61.41
  - anger reaction (*see also* Disturbance, conduct) 312.0 [5th]
  - behavior, child 312.9
  - behavioral V40.9
    - specified NEC V40.3
  - betting V69.3
  - biological child V61.23 ●
  - cardiorespiratory NEC V47.2
  - care of sick or handicapped person in family or household V61.49
  - career choice V62.29
  - communication V40.1
  - conscience regarding medical care V62.6
  - delinquency (juvenile) 312.9
  - diet, inappropriate V69.1
  - digestive NEC V47.3
  - ear NEC V41.3
  - eating habits, inappropriate V69.1
  - economic V60.2
    - affecting care V60.9
      - specified type NEC V60.89 ▲
  - educational V62.3
  - enuresis, child 307.6
  - exercise, lack of V69.0
  - eye NEC V41.1
  - family V61.9
    - specified circumstance NEC V61.8
  - fear reaction, child 313.0
  - feeding (elderly) (infant) 783.3
    - newborn 779.31 ▲
    - nonorganic 307.59
  - fetal, affecting management of pregnancy 656.9 [5th]
    - specified type NEC 656.8 [5th]
  - financial V60.2
  - foster child V61.29
    - ~~specified NEC V41.8~~
  - functional V41.9
    - specified type NEC V41.8
  - gambling V69.3
  - genital NEC V47.5
  - head V48.9
    - deficiency V48.0
    - disfigurement V48.6
    - mechanical V48.2
    - motor V48.2
    - movement of V48.2
    - sensory V48.4
    - specified condition NEC V48.8
  - hearing V41.2
  - high-risk sexual behavior V69.2
  - identity 313.82
  - influencing health status NEC V49.89
  - internal organ NEC V47.9
    - deficiency V47.0
    - mechanical or motor V47.1
  - interpersonal NEC V62.81
  - jealousy, child 313.3
  - learning V40.0
  - legal V62.5
  - life circumstance NEC V62.89

Pregnancy – Problem

Problem (with) – *continued*
lifestyle V69.9
specified NEC V69.8
limb V49.9
deficiency V49.0
disfigurement V49.4
mechanical V49.1
motor V49.2
movement, involving
musculoskeletal system V49.1
nervous system V49.2
sensory V49.3
specified condition NEC V49.5
litigation V62.5
living alone V60.3
loneliness NEC V62.89
marital V61.10
involving
divorce V61.03
estrangement V61.09
psychosexual disorder 302.9
sexual function V41.7
relationship V61.10
mastication V41.6
medical care, within family V61.49
mental V40.9
specified NEC V40.2
mental hygiene, adult V40.9
multiparity V61.5
nail biting, child 307.9
neck V48.9
deficiency V48.1
disfigurement V48.7
mechanical V48.3
motor V48.3
movement V48.3
sensory V48.5
specified condition NEC V48.8
neurological NEC 781.99
none (feared complaint unfounded) V65.5
occupational V62.29
parent-child V61.20
adopted child V61.24 ●
biological child V61.23 ●
foster child V61.25 ●
relationship V61.20
partner V61.10
relationship V61.10
personal NEC V62.89
interpersonal conflict NEC V62.81
personality (*see also* Disorder, personality) 301.9
phase of life V62.89
placenta, affecting management of pregnancy 656.9 [5th]
specified type NEC 656.8 [5th]
poverty V60.2
presence of sick or handicapped person in family or household V61.49
psychiatric 300.9
psychosocial V62.9
specified type NEC V62.89
relational NEC V62.81
relationship, childhood 313.3
religious or spiritual belief
other than medical care V62.89
regarding medical care V62.6
self-damaging behavior V69.8
sexual
behavior, high-risk V69.2
function NEC V41.7
sibling
relational V61.8
relationship V61.8
sight V41.0
sleep, lack of V69.4
sleep disorder, child 307.40
smell V41.5
speech V40.1
spite reaction, child (*see also* Disturbance, conduct) 312.0 [5th]
spoiled child reaction (*see also* Disturbance, conduct) 312.1 [5th]
substance abuse in family V61.42 ●

Problem (with) – *continued*
swallowing V41.6
tantrum, child (*see also* Disturbance, conduct) 312.1 [5th]
taste V41.5
thumb sucking, child 307.9
tic (child) 307.21
trunk V48.9
deficiency V48.1
disfigurement V48.7
mechanical V48.3
motor V48.3
movement V48.3
sensory V48.5
specified condition NEC V48.8
unemployment V62.0
urinary NEC V47.4
voice production V41.4
Procedure (surgical) **not done** NEC V64.3
because of
contraindication V64.1
patient's decision V64.2
for reasons of conscience or religion V62.6
specified reason NEC V64.3
Procidentia
anus (sphincter) 569.1
rectum (sphincter) 569.1
stomach 537.89
uteri 618.1
Proctalgia 569.42
fugax 564.6
spasmodic 564.6
psychogenic 307.89
Proctitis 569.49
amebic 006.8
chlamydial 099.52
gonococcal 098.7
granulomatous 555.1
idiopathic 556.2
with ulcerative sigmoiditis 556.3
tuberculous (*see also* Tuberculosis) 014.8 [5th]
ulcerative (chronic) (nonspecific) 556.2
with ulcerative sigmoiditis 556.3
Proctocele
female (without uterine prolapse) 618.04
with uterine prolapse 618.4
complete 618.3
incomplete 618.2
male 569.49
Proctocolitis, idiopathic 556.2
with ulcerative sigmoiditis 556.3
Proctoptosis 569.1
Proctosigmoiditis 569.89
ulcerative (chronic) 556.3
Proctospasm 564.6
psychogenic 306.4
Prodromal-AIDS - *see* Human immunodeficiency virus (disease) (illness) (infection)
Profichet's disease or syndrome 729.90
Progeria (adultorum) (syndrome) 259.8
Prognathism (mandibular) (maxillary) 524.00
Progonoma (melanotic) (M9363/0) - *see* Neoplasm, by site, benign
Progressive - *see* condition
Prolapse, prolapsed
anus, anal (canal) (sphincter) 569.1
arm or hand, complicating delivery 652.7 [5th]
causing obstructed labor 660.0 [5th]
affecting fetus or newborn 763.1
fetus or newborn 763.1
bladder (acquired) (mucosa) (sphincter)
congenital (female) (male) 756.71
female (*see also* Cystocele, female) 618.01
male 596.8
breast implant (prosthetic) 996.54
cecostomy 569.69
cecum 569.89

Prolapse, prolapsed – *continued*
cervix, cervical (hypertrophied) 618.1
anterior lip, obstructing labor 660.2 [5th]
affecting fetus or newborn 763.1
congenital 752.49
postpartal (old) 618.1
stump 618.84
ciliary body 871.1
colon (pedunculated) 569.89
colostomy 569.69
conjunctiva 372.73
cord - *see* Prolapse, umbilical cord
disc (intervertebral) - *see* Displacement, intervertebral disc
duodenum 537.89
eye implant (orbital) 996.59
lens (ocular) 996.53
fallopian tube 620.4
fetal extremity, complicating delivery 652.8 [5th]
causing obstructed labor 660.0 [5th]
fetus or newborn 763.1
funis - *see* Prolapse, umbilical cord
gastric (mucosa) 537.89
genital, female 618.9
specified NEC 618.89
globe 360.81
ileostomy bud 569.69
intervertebral disc - *see* Displacement, intervertebral disc
intestine (small) 569.89
iris 364.89
traumatic 871.1
kidney (*see also* Disease, renal) 593.0
congenital 753.3
laryngeal muscles or ventricle 478.79
leg, complicating delivery 652.8 [5th]
causing obstructed labor 660.0 [5th]
fetus or newborn 763.1
liver 573.8
meatus urinarius 599.5
mitral valve 424.0
ocular lens implant 996.53
organ or site, congenital NEC - *see* Malposition, congenital
ovary 620.4
pelvic (floor), female 618.89
perineum, female 618.89
pregnant uterus 654.4 [5th]
rectum (mucosa) (sphincter) 569.1
due to Trichuris trichiuria 127.3
spleen 289.59
stomach 537.89
umbilical cord
affecting fetus or newborn 762.4
complicating delivery 663.0 [5th]
ureter 593.89
with obstruction 593.4
ureterovesical orifice 593.89
urethra (acquired) (infected) (mucosa) 599.5
congenital 753.8
uterovaginal 618.4
complete 618.3
incomplete 618.2
specified NEC 618.89
uterus (first degree) (second degree) (third degree) (complete) (without vaginal wall prolapse) 618.1
with mention of vaginal wall prolapse - *see* Prolapse, uterovaginal
congenital 752.3
in pregnancy or childbirth 654.4 [5th]
affecting fetus or newborn 763.1
causing obstructed labor 660.2 [5th]
affecting fetus or newborn 763.1
postpartal (old) 618.1
uveal 871.1
vagina (anterior) (posterior) (vault) (wall) (without uterine prolapse) 618.00
with uterine prolapse 618.4
complete 618.3
incomplete 618.2
paravaginal 618.02

Prolapse, prolapsed – *continued*
vagina – *continued*
posthysterectomy 618.5
specified NEC 618.09
vitreous (humor) 379.26
traumatic 871.1
womb - *see* Prolapse, uterus
Prolapsus, female 618.9
Proliferative - *see* condition
Prolinemia 270.8
Prolinuria 270.8
Prolonged, prolongation
bleeding time (*see also* Defect, coagulation) 790.92
"idiopathic" (in von Willebrand's disease) 286.4
coagulation time (*see also* Defect, coagulation) 790.92
gestation syndrome 766.22
labor 662.1 [5th]
first stage 662.0 [5th]
second stage 662.2 [5th]
affecting fetus or newborn 763.89
PR interval 426.11
pregnancy 645.2 [5th]
prothrombin time (*see also* Defect, coagulation) 790.92
QT interval 794.31
syndrome 426.82
rupture of membranes (24 hours or more prior to onset of labor) 658.2 [5th]
uterine contractions in labor 661.4 [5th]
affecting fetus or newborn 763.7
Prominauris 744.29
Prominence
auricle (ear) (congenital) 744.29
acquired 380.32
ischial spine or sacral promontory
with disproportion (fetopelvic) 653.3 [5th]
affecting fetus or newborn 763.1
causing obstructed labor 660.1 [5th]
affecting fetus or newborn 763.1
nose (congenital) 748.1
acquired 738.0
PROMM (proximal myotonic myotonia) 359.21
Pronation
ankle 736.79
foot 736.79
congenital 755.67
Prophylactic
administration of
agents affecting estrogen receptors and estrogen levels NEC V07.59
anastrozole (Arimidex) V07.52
antibiotics V07.39
antitoxin, any V07.2
antivenin V07.2
aromatase inhibitors V07.52
chemotherapeutic agent NEC V07.39
fluoride V07.31
diphtheria antitoxin V07.2
drug V07.39
estrogen receptor downregulators V07.59
exemestane (Aromasin) V07.52 ▲
fulvestrant (Faslodex) V07.59
gamma globulin V07.2
gonadotropin-releasing hormone (GnRH) agonist V07.59
goserelin acetate (Zoladex) V07.59
immune sera (gamma globulin) V07.2
letrozole (Femara) V07.52
leuprolide acetate (leuprorelin) (Lupron) V07.59
megestrol acetate (Megace) V07.59
raloxifene (Evista) V07.51
RhoGAM V07.2
selective estrogen receptor modulators (SERMs) V07.51
tamoxifen (Nolvadex) V07.51
tetanus antitoxin V07.2
toremifene (Fareston) V07.51

Problem – Prophylactic

[4th] Fourth Digit Required | [5th] Fifth Digit Required | *[code]* Manifestation Code | ● New Line | ▲ Revised Line | text New Text | ~~text~~ Deleted text

Prophylactic – *continued*
- chemotherapy NEC V07.39
  - fluoride V07.31
- hormone replacement (postmenopausal) V07.4
- immunotherapy V07.2
- measure V07.9
  - specified type NEC V07.8
- medication V07.39
- postmenopausal hormone replacement V07.4
- sterilization V25.2

Proptosis (ocular) (*see also* Exophthalmos) 376.30
- thyroid 242.0 5th

Propulsion
- eyeball 360.81

Prosecution, anxiety concerning V62.5

Prosopagnosia 368.16

Prostate, prostatic - *see* condition

Prostatism 600.90
- with
  - other lower urinary tract symptoms (LUTS) 600.91
  - urinary
    - obstruction 600.91
    - retention 600.91

Prostatitis (congestive) (suppurative) 601.9
- acute 601.0
- cavitary 601.8
- chlamydial 099.54
- chronic 601.1
- diverticular 601.8
- due to Trichomonas (vaginalis) 131.03
- fibrous 600.90
  - with
    - other lower urinary tract symptoms (LUTS) 600.91
    - urinary
      - obstruction 600.91
      - retention 600.91
- gonococcal (acute) 098.12
  - chronic or duration of 2 months or over 098.32
- granulomatous 601.8
- hypertrophic 600.00
  - with
    - other lower urinary tract symptoms (LUTS) 600.01
    - urinary
      - obstruction 600.01
      - retention 600.01
- specified type NEC 601.8
- subacute 601.1
- trichomonal 131.03
- tuberculous (*see also* Tuberculosis) 016.5 5th *[601.4]*

Prostatocystitis 601.3

Prostatorrhea 602.8

Prostatoseminovesiculitis, trichomonal 131.03

Prostration 780.79
- heat 992.5
  - anhydrotic 992.3
  - due to
    - salt (and water) depletion 992.4
    - water depletion 992.3
- nervous 300.5
- newborn 779.89
- senile 797

Protanomaly 368.51

Protanopia (anomalous trichromat) (complete) (incomplete) 368.51

Protection (against) (from) - *see* Prophylactic

Protein
- deficiency 260
- malnutrition 260
- sickness (prophylactic) (therapeutic) 999.5

Proteinemia 790.99

Proteinosis
- alveolar, lung or pulmonary 516.0
- lipid 272.8
- lipoid (of Urbach) 272.8

Proteinuria (*see also* Albuminuria) 791.0
- Bence-Jones NEC 791.0
- gestational 646.2 5th
  - with hypertension - *see* Toxemia, of pregnancy
- orthostatic 593.6
- postural 593.6

Proteolysis, pathologic 286.6

Protocoproporphyria 277.1

Protoporphyria (erythrohepatic) (erythropoietic) 277.1

Protrusio acetabuli 718.65

Protrusion
- acetabulum (into pelvis) 718.65
- device, implant, or graft - *see* Complications, mechanical
- ear, congenital 744.29
- intervertebral disc - *see* Displacement, intervertebral disc
- nucleus pulposus - *see* Displacement, intervertebral disc

Proud flesh 701.5

Prune belly (syndrome) 756.71

Prurigo (ferox) (gravis) (Hebra's) (hebrae) (mitis) (simplex) 698.2
- agria 698.3
- asthma syndrome 691.8
- Besnier's (atopic dermatitis) (infantile eczema) 691.8
- eczematodes allergicum 691.8
- estivalis (Hutchinson's) 692.72
- Hutchinson's 692.72
- nodularis 698.3
- psychogenic 306.3

Pruritus, pruritic 698.9
- ani 698.0
  - psychogenic 306.3
- conditions NEC 698.9
  - psychogenic 306.3
- due to Onchocerca volvulus 125.3
- ear 698.9
- essential 698.9
- genital organ(s) 698.1
  - psychogenic 306.3
- gravidarum 646.8 5th
- hiemalis 698.8
- neurogenic (any site) 306.3
- perianal 698.0
- psychogenic (any site) 306.3
- scrotum 698.1
  - psychogenic 306.3
- senile, senilis 698.8
- Trichomonas 131.9
- vulva, vulvae 698.1
  - psychogenic 306.3

Psammocarcinoma (M8140/3) - *see* Neoplasm, by site, malignant

Pseudarthrosis, pseudoarthrosis (bone) 733.82
- joint following fusion V45.4

Pseudoacanthosis
- nigricans 701.8

Pseudoaneurysm - *see* Aneurysm

Pseudoangina (pectoris) - *see* Angina

Pseudoangioma 452

Pseudo-Argyll-Robertson pupil 379.45

Pseudoarteriosus 747.89

Pseudoarthrosis - *see* Pseudarthrosis

Pseudoataxia 799.89

Pseudobulbar affect (PBA) 310.8

Pseudobursa 727.89

Pseudocholera 025

Pseudochromidrosis 705.89

Pseudocirrhosis, liver, pericardial 423.2

Pseudocoarctation 747.21

Pseudocowpox 051.1

Pseudocoxalgia 732.1

Pseudocroup 478.75

Pseudocyesis 300.11

Pseudocyst
- lung 518.89
- pancreas 577.2
- retina 361.19

Pseudodementia 300.16

Pseudoelephantiasis neuroarthritica 757.0

Pseudoemphysema 518.89

Pseudoencephalitis
- superior (acute) hemorrhagic 265.1

Pseudoerosion cervix, congenital 752.49

Pseudoexfoliation, lens capsule 366.11

Pseudofracture (idiopathic) (multiple) (spontaneous) (symmetrical) 268.2

Pseudoglanders 025

Pseudoglioma 360.44

Pseudogout - *see* Chondrocalcinosis

Pseudohallucination 780.1

Pseudohemianesthesia 782.0

Pseudohemophilia (Bernuth's) (hereditary) (type B) 286.4
- type A 287.8
- vascular 287.8

Pseudohermaphroditism 752.7
- with chromosomal anomaly - *see* Anomaly, chromosomal
- adrenal 255.2
- female (without adrenocortical disorder) 752.7
  - with adrenocortical disorder 255.2
  - adrenal 255.2
- male (without gonadal disorder) 752.7
  - with
    - adrenocortical disorder 255.2
    - cleft scrotum 752.7
    - feminizing testis 259.51
    - gonadal disorder 257.9
  - adrenal 255.2

Pseudohole, macula 362.54

Pseudo-Hurler's disease (mucolipidosis III) 272.7

Pseudohydrocephalus 348.2

Pseudohypertrophic muscular dystrophy (Erb's) 359.1

Pseudohypertrophy, muscle 359.1

Pseudohypoparathyroidism 275.49

Pseudoinfluenza 487.1

Pseudoinsomnia 307.49

Pseudoleukemia 288.8
- infantile 285.8

Pseudomembranous - *see* condition

Pseudomeningocele (cerebral) (infective) 349.2
- postprocedural 997.01
- spinal 349.2

Pseudomenstruation 626.8

Pseudomucinous
- cyst (ovary) (M8470/0) 220
- peritoneum 568.89

Pseudomyeloma 273.1

Pseudomyxoma peritonei (M8480/6) 197.6

Pseudoneuritis optic (nerve) 377.24
- papilla 377.24
  - congenital 743.57

Pseudoneuroma - *see* Injury, nerve, by site

Pseudo-obstruction
- intestine (chronic) (idiopathic) (intermittent secondary) (primary) 564.89
  - acute 560.89

Pseudopapilledema 377.24

Pseudoparalysis
- arm or leg 781.4
- atonic, congenital 358.8

Pseudopelade 704.09

Pseudophakia V43.1

Pseudopolycythemia 289.0

Pseudopolyposis, colon 556.4

Pseudoporencephaly 348.0

Pseudopseudohypoparathyroidism 275.49

Pseudopsychosis 300.16

Pseudopterygium 372.52

Pseudoptosis (eyelid) 374.34

Pseudorabies 078.89

Pseudoretinitis, pigmentosa 362.65

Pseudorickets 588.0
- senile (Pozzi's) 731.0

Pseudorubella 057.8

Pseudoscarlatina 057.8

Pseudosclerema 778.1

Pseudosclerosis (brain)
- Jakob's 046.19
- of Westphal (-Strümpell) (hepatolenticular degeneration) 275.1
- spastic 046.19
  - with dementia
    - with behavioral disturbance 046.19 *[294.11]*
    - without behavioral disturbance 046.19 *[294.10]*

Pseudoseizure 780.39
- non-psychiatric 780.39
- psychiatric 300.11

Pseudotabes 799.89
- diabetic 250.6 5th *[337.1]*
  - due to secondary diabetes 249.6 5th *[337.1]*

Pseudotetanus (*see also* Convulsions) 780.39

Pseudotetany 781.7
- hysterical 300.11

Pseudothalassemia 285.0

Pseudotrichinosis 710.3

Pseudotruncus arteriosus 747.29

Pseudotuberculosis, pasteurella (infection) 027.2

Pseudotumor
- cerebri 348.2
- orbit (inflammatory) 376.11

Pseudo-Turner's syndrome 759.89

Pseudoxanthoma elasticum 757.39

Psilosis (sprue) (tropical) 579.1
- Monilia 112.89
- nontropical 579.0
- not sprue 704.00

Psittacosis 073.9

Psoitis 728.89

Psora NEC 696.1

Psoriasis 696.1
- any type, except arthropathic 696.1
- arthritic, arthropathic 696.0
- buccal 528.6
- flexural 696.1
- follicularis 696.1
- guttate 696.1
- inverse 696.1
- mouth 528.6
- nummularis 696.1
- psychogenic 316 *[696.1]*
- punctata 696.1
- pustular 696.1
- rupioides 696.1
- vulgaris 696.1

Psorospermiasis 136.4

Psorospermosis 136.4
- follicularis (vegetans) 757.39

Psychalgia 307.80

Psychasthenia 300.89
- compulsive 300.3
- mixed compulsive states 300.3
- obsession 300.3

Psychiatric disorder or problem NEC 300.9

Psychogenic - *see also* condition
- factors associated with physical conditions 316

Psychoneurosis, psychoneurotic (*see also* Neurosis) 300.9
- anxiety (state) 300.00
- climacteric 627.2
- compensation 300.16
- compulsion 300.3
- conversion hysteria 300.11
- depersonalization 300.6
- depressive type 300.4
- dissociative hysteria 300.15
- hypochondriacal 300.7
- hysteria 300.10
  - conversion type 300.11
  - dissociative type 300.15
- mixed NEC 300.89
- neurasthenic 300.5
- obsessional 300.3
- obsessive-compulsive 300.3
- occupational 300.89
- personality NEC 301.89

Psychoneurosis, psychoneurotic – *continued*
- phobia 300.20
- senile NEC 300.89

Psychopathic - *see also* condition
- constitution, posttraumatic 310.2
  - with psychosis 293.9
- personality 301.9
  - amoral trends 301.7
  - antisocial trends 301.7
  - asocial trends 301.7
  - mixed types 301.7
- state 301.9

Psychopathy, sexual (*see also* Deviation, sexual) 302.9

Psychophysiologic, psychophysiological condition - *see* Reaction, psychophysiologic

Psychose passionelle 297.8

Psychosexual identity disorder 302.6
- adult-life 302.85
- childhood 302.6

Psychosis 298.9
- acute hysterical 298.1
- affecting management of pregnancy, childbirth, or puerperium 648.4 5th
- affective (*see also* Disorder, mood) 296.90

Note *Use the following fifth-digit subclassification with categories 296.0-296.6:*

0	unspecified
1	mild
2	moderate
3	severe, without mention of psychotic behavior
4	severe, specified as with psychotic behavior
5	in partial or unspecified remission
6	in full remission

  - drug-induced 292.84
  - due to or associated with physical condition 293.9
  - involutional 293.83
    - recurrent episode 296.3 5th
    - single episode 296.2 5th
  - manic-depressive 296.80
    - circular (alternating) 296.7
      - currently depressed 296.5 5th
      - currently manic 296.4 5th
    - depressed type 296.2 5th
      - atypical 296.82
      - recurrent episode 296.3 5th
      - single episode 296.2 5th
    - manic 296.0 5th
      - atypical 296.81
      - recurrent episode 296.1 5th
      - single episode 296.0 5th
    - mixed type NEC 296.89
    - specified type NEC 296.89
  - senile 290.21
  - specified type NEC 296.99
- alcoholic 291.9
  - with
    - anxiety 291.89
    - delirium tremens 291.0
    - delusions 291.5
    - dementia 291.2
    - hallucinosis 291.3
    - jealousy 291.5
    - mood disturbance 291.89
    - paranoia 291.5
    - persisting amnesia 291.1
    - sexual dysfunction 291.89
    - sleep disturbance 291.89
  - amnestic confabulatory 291.1
  - delirium tremens 291.0
  - hallucinosis 291.3
  - Korsakoff's, Korsakov's, Korsakow's 291.1
  - paranoid type 291.5
  - pathological intoxication 291.4
  - polyneuritic 291.1

Psychosis – *continued*
- alcoholic – *continued*
  - specified type NEC 291.89
- alternating (*see also* Psychosis, manic-depressive, circular) 296.7
- anergastic (*see also* Psychosis, organic) 294.9
- arteriosclerotic 290.40
  - with
    - acute confusional state 290.41
    - delirium 290.41
    - delusions 290.42
    - depressed mood 290.43
  - depressed type 290.43
  - paranoid type 290.42
  - simple type 290.40
  - uncomplicated 290.40
- atypical 298.9
  - depressive 296.82
  - manic 296.81
- borderline (schizophrenia) (*see also* Schizophrenia) 295.5 5th
  - of childhood (*see also* Psychosis, childhood) 299.8 5th
  - prepubertal 299.8 5th
- brief reactive 298.8 5th
- childhood, with origin specific to 299.9 5th

Note *Use the following fifth-digit subclassification with category 299:*

0	current or active state
1	residual state

  - atypical 299.8 5th
  - specified type NEC 299.8 5th
- circular (*see also* Psychosis, manic-depressive, circular) 296.7
- climacteric (*see also* Psychosis, involutional) 298.8
- confusional 298.9
  - acute 293.0
  - reactive 298.2
  - subacute 293.1
- depressive (*see also* Psychosis, affective) 296.2 5th
  - atypical 296.82
  - involutional 296.2 5th
    - with hypomania (bipolar II) 296.89
    - recurrent episode 296.3 5th
    - single episode 296.2 5th
  - psychogenic 298.0
  - reactive (emotional stress) (psychological trauma) 298.0
  - recurrent episode 296.3 5th
    - with hypomania (bipolar II) 296.89
  - single episode 296.2 5th
- disintegrative, childhood (*see also* Psychosis, childhood) 299.1 5th
- drug 292.9
  - with
    - affective syndrome 292.84
    - amnestic syndrome 292.83
    - anxiety 292.89
    - delirium 292.81
      - withdrawal 292.0
    - delusions 292.11
    - dementia 292.82
    - depressive state 292.84
    - hallucinations 292.12
    - hallucinosis 292.12
    - mood disorder 292.84
    - mood disturbance 292.84
    - organic personality syndrome NEC 292.89
    - sexual dysfunction 292.89
    - sleep disturbance 292.89
    - withdrawal syndrome (and delirium) 292.0
  - affective syndrome 292.84
  - delusions 292.11
  - hallucinatory state 292.12
  - hallucinosis 292.12
  - paranoid state 292.11
  - specified type NEC 292.89

Psychosis – *continued*
- drug – *continued*
  - withdrawal syndrome (and delirium) 292.0
- due to or associated with physical condition (*see also* Psychosis, organic) 294.9
- epileptic NEC 293.9
- excitation (psychogenic) (reactive) 298.1
- exhaustive (*see also* Reaction, stress, acute) 308.9
- hypomanic (*see also* Psychosis, affective) 296.0 5th
  - recurrent episode 296.1 5th
  - single episode 296.0 5th
- hysterical 298.8
  - acute 298.1
- in
  - conditions classified elsewhere
    - with
      - delusions 293.81
      - hallucinations 293.82
  - pregnancy, childbirth, or puerperium 648.4 5th
- incipient 298.8
  - schizophrenic (*see also* Schizophrenia) 295.5 5th
- induced 297.3
- infantile (*see also* Psychosis, childhood) 299.0 5th
- infective 293.9
  - acute 293.0
  - subacute 293.1
- interactional (childhood) (*see also* Psychosis, childhood) 299.1 5th
- involutional 298.8
  - depressive (*see also* Psychosis, affective) 296.2 5th
    - recurrent episode 296.3 5th
    - single episode 296.2 5th
  - melancholic 296.2 5th
    - recurrent episode 296.3 5th
    - single episode 296.2 5th
  - paranoid state 297.2
  - paraphrenia 297.2
- Korsakoff's, Korakov's, Korsakow's (nonalcoholic) 294.0
  - alcoholic 291.1
- mania (phase) (*see also* Psychosis, affective) 296.0 5th
  - recurrent episode 296.1 5th
  - single episode 296.0 5th
- manic (*see also* Psychosis, affective) 296.0 5th
  - atypical 296.81
  - recurrent episode 296.1 5th
  - single episode 296.0 5th
- manic-depressive 296.80
  - circular 296.7
    - currently
      - depressed 296.5 5th
      - manic 296.4 5th
    - mixed 296.6 5th
  - depressive 296.2 5th
    - recurrent episode 296.3 5th
      - with hypomania (bipolar II) 296.89
    - single episode 296.2 5th
  - hypomanic 296.0 5th
    - recurrent episode 296.1 5th
    - single episode 296.0 5th
  - manic 296.0 5th
    - atypical 296.81
    - recurrent episode 296.1 5th
    - single episode 296.0 5th
  - mixed NEC 296.89
  - perplexed 296.89
  - stuporous 296.89
- menopausal (*see also* Psychosis, involutional) 298.8
- mixed schizophrenic and affective (*see also* Schizophrenia) 295.7 5th
- multi-infarct (cerebrovascular) (*see also* Psychosis, arteriosclerotic) 290.40

Psychosis – *continued*
- organic NEC 294.9
  - due to or associated with
    - addiction
      - alcohol (*see also* Psychosis, alcoholic) 291.9
      - drug (*see also* Psychosis, drug) 292.9
    - alcohol intoxication, acute (*see also* Psychosis, alcoholic) 291.9
    - alcoholism (*see also* Psychosis, alcoholic) 291.9
    - arteriosclerosis (cerebral) (*see also* Psychosis, arteriosclerotic) 290.40
    - cerebrovascular disease
      - acute (psychosis) 293.0
      - arteriosclerotic (*see also* Psychosis, arteriosclerotic) 290.40
    - childbirth - *see* Psychosis, puerperal
    - dependence
      - alcohol (*see also* Psychosis, alcoholic) 291.9
      - drug 292.9
    - disease
      - alcoholic liver (*see also* Psychosis, alcoholic) 291.9
      - brain
        - arteriosclerotic (*see also* Psychosis, arteriosclerotic) 290.40
      - cerebrovascular
        - acute (psychosis) 293.0
        - arteriosclerotic (*see also* Psychosis, arteriosclerotic) 290.40
      - endocrine or metabolic 293.9
        - acute (psychosis) 293.0
        - subacute (psychosis) 293.1
      - Jakob-Creutzfeldt 046.19
        - with behavioral disturbance 046.19 *[294.11]*
        - without behavioral disturbance 046.19 *[294.10]*
        - familial 046.19
        - iatrogenic 046.19
        - specified NEC 046.19
        - sporadic 046.19
        - variant 046.11
          - with dementia
            - with behavioral disturbance 046.11 *[294.11]*
            - without behavioral disturbance 046.11 *[294.10]*
      - liver, alcoholic (*see also* Psychosis, alcoholic) 291.9
    - disorder
      - cerebrovascular
        - acute (psychosis) 293.0
      - endocrine or metabolic 293.9
        - acute (psychosis) 293.0
        - subacute (psychosis) 293.1
    - epilepsy
      - with behavioral disturbance 345.9 5th *[294.11]*
      - without behavioral disturbance 345.9 5th *[294.10]*
      - transient (acute) 293.0
    - Huntington's chorea
      - with behavioral disturbance 333.4 *[294.11]*
      - without behavioral disturbance 333.4 *[294.10]*
    - infection
      - brain 293.9
        - acute (psychosis) 293.0

- **Psychosis** – *continued*
  - organic – *continued*
    - due to or associated with – *continued*
      - infection – *continued*
        - brain – *continued*
          - chronic 294.8
          - subacute (psychosis) 293.1
        - intracranial NEC 293.9
          - acute (psychosis) 293.0
          - chronic 294.8
          - subacute (psychosis) 293.1
      - intoxication
        - alcoholic (acute) (*see also* Psychosis, alcoholic) 291.9
          - pathological 291.4
        - drug (*see also* Psychosis, drug) 292.9
      - ischemia
        - cerebrovascular (generalized) (*see also* Psychosis, arteriosclerotic) 290.40
      - Jakob-Creutzfeldt disease (syndrome) 046.19
        - with behavioral disturbance 046.19 *[294.11]*
        - without behavioral disturbance 046.19 *[294.10]*
        - variant 046.11
          - with dementia
            - with behavioral disturbance 046.11 *[294.11]*
            - without behavioral disturbance 046.11 *[294.10]*
      - multiple sclerosis
        - with behavioral disturbance 340 *[294.11]*
        - without behavioral disturbance 340 *[294.10]*
      - physical condition NEC 293.9
        - with
          - delusions 293.81
          - hallucinations 293.82
      - presenility 290.10
      - puerperium - *see* Psychosis, puerperal
      - sclerosis, multiple
        - with behavioral disturbance 340 *[294.11]*
        - without behavioral disturbance 340 *[294.10]*
      - senility 290.20
      - status epilepticus
        - with behavioral disturbance 345.3 *[294.11]*
        - without behavioral disturbance 345.3 *[294.10]*
      - trauma
        - brain (birth) (from electrical current) (surgical) 293.9
          - acute (psychosis) 293.0
          - chronic 294.8
          - subacute (psychosis) 293.1
      - unspecified physical condition 293.9
        - with
          - delusions 293.81
          - hallucinations 293.82
    - infective 293.9
      - acute (psychosis) 293.0
      - subacute 293.1
    - posttraumatic 293.9
      - acute 293.0
      - subacute 293.1
    - specified type NEC 294.8
    - transient 293.9
      - with
        - anxiety 293.84
        - delusions 293.81
        - depression 293.83
        - hallucinations 293.82
      - depressive type 293.83
      - hallucinatory type 293.82
      - paranoid type 293.81
      - specified type NEC 293.89
  - paranoic 297.1
  - paranoid (chronic) 297.9
    - alcoholic 291.5
    - chronic 297.1
    - climacteric 297.2
    - involutional 297.2
    - menopausal 297.2
    - protracted reactive 298.4
    - psychogenic 298.4
      - acute 298.3
    - schizophrenic (*see also* Schizophrenia) 295.3 5th
    - senile 290.20
  - paroxysmal 298.9
    - senile 290.20
  - polyneuritic, alcoholic 291.1
  - postoperative 293.9
  - postpartum - *see* Psychosis, puerperal
  - prepsychotic (*see also* Schizophrenia) 295.5 5th
  - presbyophrenic (type) 290.8
  - presenile (*see also* Dementia, presenile) 290.10
  - prison 300.16
  - psychogenic 298.8
    - depressive 298.0
    - paranoid 298.4
      - acute 298.3
  - puerperal
    - specified type - *see* categories 295-298
    - unspecified type 293.89
      - acute 293.0
      - chronic 293.89
      - subacute 293.1
  - reactive (emotional stress) (psychological trauma) 298.8
    - brief 298.8
    - confusion 298.2
    - depressive 298.0
    - excitation 298.1
  - schizo-affective (depressed) (excited) (*see also* Schizophrenia) 295.7 5th
  - schizophrenia, schizophrenic (*see also* Schizophrenia) 295.9 5th
    - borderline type 295.5 5th
      - of childhood (*see also* Psychosis, childhood) 299.8 5th
    - catatonic (excited) (withdrawn) 295.2 5th
    - childhood type (*see also* Psychosis, childhood) 299.9 5th
    - hebephrenic 295.1 5th
    - incipient 295.5 5th
    - latent 295.5 5th
    - paranoid 295.3 5th
    - prepsychotic 295.5 5th
    - prodromal 295.5 5th
    - pseudoneurotic 295.5 5th
    - pseudopsychopathic 295.5 5th
    - schizophreniform 295.4 5th
    - simple 295.0 5th
    - undifferentiated type 295.9 5th
  - schizophreniform 295.4 5th
  - senile NEC 290.20
    - with
      - delusional features 290.20
      - depressive features 290.21
    - depressed type 290.21
    - paranoid type 290.20
    - simple deterioration 290.20
    - specified type - *see* categories 295-298
  - shared 297.3
  - situational (reactive) 298.8
  - symbiotic (childhood) (*see also* Psychosis, childhood) 299.1 5th
  - toxic (acute) 293.9
- **Psychotic** (*see also* condition) 298.9
  - episode 298.9
    - due to or associated with physical conditions (*see also* Psychosis, organic) 293.9
- **Pterygium** (eye) 372.40
  - central 372.43
  - colli 744.5
  - double 372.44
  - peripheral (stationary) 372.41
    - progressive 372.42
  - recurrent 372.45
- **Ptilosis** 374.55
- **PTLD** (post-transplant lymphoproliferative disorder) 238.77
- **Ptomaine** (poisoning) (*see also* Poisoning, food) 005.9
- **Ptosis** (adiposa) 374.30
  - breast 611.81
  - cecum 569.89
  - colon 569.89
  - congenital (eyelid) 743.61
    - specified site NEC - *see* Anomaly, specified type NEC
  - epicanthus syndrome 270.2
  - eyelid 374.30
    - congenital 743.61
    - mechanical 374.33
    - myogenic 374.32
    - paralytic 374.31
  - gastric 537.5
  - intestine 569.89
  - kidney (*see also* Disease, renal) 593.0
    - congenital 753.3
  - liver 573.8
  - renal (*see also* Disease, renal) 593.0
    - congenital 753.3
  - splanchnic 569.89
  - spleen 289.59
  - stomach 537.5
  - viscera 569.89
- **PTSD** (Post-Traumatic Stress Disorder) 309.81
- **Ptyalism** 527.7
  - hysterical 300.11
  - periodic 527.2
  - pregnancy 646.8 5th
  - psychogenic 306.4
- **Ptyalolithiasis** 527.5
- **Pubalgia** 848.8
- **Pubarche, precocious** 259.1
- **Pubertas praecox** 259.1
- **Puberty** V21.1
  - abnormal 259.9
  - bleeding 626.3
  - delayed 259.0
  - precocious (constitutional) (cryptogenic) (idiopathic) NEC 259.1
    - due to
      - adrenal
        - cortical hyperfunction 255.2
        - hyperplasia 255.2
      - cortical hyperfunction 255.2
      - ovarian hyperfunction 256.1
        - estrogen 256.0
      - pineal tumor 259.8
      - testicular hyperfunction 257.0
  - premature 259.1
    - due to
      - adrenal cortical hyperfunction 255.2
      - pineal tumor 259.8
      - pituitary (anterior) hyperfunction 253.1
- **Puckering, macula** 362.56
- **Pudenda, pudendum** - *see* condition
- **Puente's disease** (simple glandular cheilitis) 528.5
- **Puerperal**
  - abscess
    - areola 675.1 5th
    - Bartholin's gland 646.6 5th
    - breast 675.1 5th
    - cervix (uteri) 670.8 5th ▲
    - fallopian tube 670.8 5th ▲
    - genital organ 670.8 5th ▲
    - kidney 646.6 5th
    - mammary 675.1 5th
    - mesosalpinx 670.8 5th ▲
    - nabothian 646.6 5th
    - nipple 675.0 5th
    - ovary, ovarian 670.8 5th ▲
    - oviduct 670.8 5th ▲
    - parametric 670.8 5th ▲
    - para-uterine 670.8 5th ▲
    - pelvic 670.8 5th ▲
    - perimetric 670.8 5th ▲
    - periuterine 670.8 5th ▲
    - retro-uterine 670.8 5th ▲
    - subareolar 675.1 5th
    - suprapelvic 670.8 5th ▲
    - tubal (ruptured) 670.8 5th ▲
    - tubo-ovarian 670.8 5th ▲
    - urinary tract NEC 646.6 5th
    - uterine, uterus 670.8 5th ▲
    - vagina (wall) 646.6 5th
    - vaginorectal 646.6 5th
    - vulvovaginal gland 646.6 5th
  - accident 674.9 5th
  - adnexitis 670.8 5th ▲
  - afibrinogenemia, or other coagulation defect 666.3 5th
  - albuminuria (acute) (subacute) 646.2 5th
    - pre-eclamptic 642.4 5th
  - anemia (conditions classifiable to 280-285) 648.2 5th
  - anuria 669.3 5th
  - apoplexy 674.0 5th
  - asymptomatic bacteriuria 646.5 5th
  - atrophy, breast 676.3 5th
  - blood dyscrasia 666.3 5th
  - caked breast 676.2 5th
  - cardiomyopathy 674.5 5th
  - cellulitis - *see* Puerperal, abscess
  - cerebrovascular disorder (conditions classifiable to 430-434, 436-437) 674.0 5th
  - cervicitis (conditions classifiable to 616.0) 646.6 5th
  - coagulopathy (any) 666.3 5th
  - complications 674.9 5th
    - specified type NEC 674.8 5th
  - convulsions (eclamptic) (uremic) 642.6 5th
    - with pre-existing hypertension 642.7 5th
  - cracked nipple 676.1 5th
  - cystitis 646.6 5th
  - cystopyelitis 646.6 5th
  - deciduitis (acute) 670.8 5th ▲
  - delirium NEC 293.9
  - diabetes (mellitus) (conditions classifiable to 249 and 250) 648.0 5th
  - disease 674.9 5th
    - breast NEC 676.3 5th
    - cerebrovascular (acute) 674.0 5th
    - nonobstetric NEC (*see also* Pregnancy, complicated, current disease or condition) 648.9 5th
    - pelvis inflammatory 670.8 5th ▲
    - renal NEC 646.2 5th
    - tubo-ovarian 670.8 5th ▲
    - Valsuani's (progressive pernicious anemia) 648.2 5th
  - disorder
    - lactation 676.9 5th
      - specified type NEC 676.8 5th
    - nonobstetric NEC (*see also* Pregnancy, complicated, current disease or condition) 648.9 5th
  - disruption
    - cesarean wound 674.1 5th
    - episiotomy wound 674.2 5th
    - perineal laceration wound 674.2 5th
  - drug dependence (conditions classifiable to 304) 648.3 5th

- **Puerperal** – *continued*
  - eclampsia 642.6 5th
    - with pre-existing hypertension 642.7 5th
  - embolism (pulmonary) 673.2 5th
    - air 673.0 5th
    - amniotic fluid 673.1 5th
    - blood clot 673.2 5th
    - brain or cerebral 674.0 5th
    - cardiac 674.8 5th
    - fat 673.8 5th
    - intracranial sinus (venous) 671.5 5th
    - pyemic 673.3 5th
    - septic 673.3 5th
    - spinal cord 671.5 5th
  - endometritis (conditions classifiable to 615.0-615.9) 670.1 5th ▲
  - endophlebitis - *see* Puerperal, phlebitis
  - endotrachelitis 646.6 5th
  - engorgement, breasts 676.2 5th
  - erysipelas 670.8 5th ▲
  - failure
    - lactation 676.4 5th
    - renal, acute 669.3 5th
  - fever 670 5th
    - meaning sepsis 670.2 5th ▲
    - meaning pyrexia (of unknown origin) 672 5th
  - fissure, nipple 676.1 5th
  - fistula
    - breast 675.1 5th
    - mammary gland 675.1 5th
    - nipple 675.0 5th
  - galactophoritis 675.2 5th
  - galactorrhea 676.6 5th
  - gangrene
    - gas 670.8 5th ▲
      - with sepsis 670.2 5th ●
    - uterus 670.8 5th ▲
  - gonorrhea (conditions classifiable to 098) 647.1 5th
  - hematoma, subdural 674.0 5th
  - hematosalpinx, infectional 670.8 5th ▲
  - hemiplegia, cerebral 674.0 5th
  - hemorrhage 666.1 5th
    - brain 674.0 5th
    - bulbar 674.0 5th
    - cerebellar 674.0 5th
    - cerebral 674.0 5th
    - cortical 674.0 5th
    - delayed (after 24 hours) (uterine) 666.2 5th
    - extradural 674.0 5th
    - internal capsule 674.0 5th
    - intracranial 674.0 5th
    - intrapontine 674.0 5th
    - meningeal 674.0 5th
    - pontine 674.0 5th
    - subarachnoid 674.0 5th
    - subcortical 674.0 5th
    - subdural 674.0 5th
    - uterine, delayed 666.2 5th
    - ventricular 674.0 5th
  - hemorrhoids 671.8 5th
  - hepatorenal syndrome 674.8 5th
  - hypertrophy
    - breast 676.3 5th
    - mammary gland 676.3 5th
  - induration breast (fibrous) 676.3 5th
  - infarction
    - lung - *see* Puerperal, embolism
    - pulmonary - *see* Puerperal, embolism
  - infection
    - Bartholin's gland 646.6 5th
    - breast 675.2 5th
      - with nipple 675.9 5th
        - specified type NEC 675.8 5th
    - cervix 646.6 5th
    - endocervix 646.6 5th
    - fallopian tube 670.8 5th ▲
    - generalized 670.0 5th ▲
    - genital tract (major) 670.0 5th ▲
      - minor or localized 646.6 5th
    - kidney (bacillus coli) 646.6 5th

- **Puerperal** – *continued*
  - infection – *continued*
    - mammary gland 675.2 5th
      - with nipple 675.9 5th
        - specified type NEC 675.8 5th
    - nipple 675.0 5th
      - with breast 675.9 5th
        - specified type NEC 675.8 5th
    - ovary 670.8 5th ▲
    - pelvic 670.8 5th ▲
    - peritoneum 670.8 5th ▲
    - renal 646.6 5th
    - tubo-ovarian 670.8 5th ▲
    - urinary (tract) NEC 646.6 5th
      - asymptomatic 646.5 5th
    - uterus, uterine 670.8 5th ▲
    - vagina 646.6 5th
  - inflammation - *see also* Puerperal, infection
    - areola 675.1 5th
    - Bartholin's gland 646.6 5th
    - breast 675.2 5th
    - broad ligament 670.8 5th ▲
    - cervix (uteri) 646.6 5th
    - fallopian tube 670.8 5th ▲
    - genital organs 670.8 5th ▲
      - localized 646.6 5th
    - mammary gland 675.2 5th
    - nipple 675.0 5th
    - ovary 670.8 5th ▲
    - oviduct 670.8 5th ▲
    - pelvis 670.8 5th ▲
    - periuterine 670.8 5th ▲
    - tubal 670.8 5th ▲
    - vagina 646.6 5th
    - vein - *see* Puerperal, phlebitis
  - inversion, nipple 676.3 5th
  - ischemia, cerebral 674.0 5th
  - lymphangitis 670.8 5th ▲
    - breast 675.2 5th
  - malaria (conditions classifiable to 084) 647.4 5th
  - malnutrition 648.9 5th
  - mammillitis 675.0 5th
  - mammitis 675.2 5th
  - mania 296.0 5th
    - recurrent episode 296.1 5th
    - single episode 296.0 5th
  - mastitis 675.2 5th
    - purulent 675.1 5th
    - retromammary 675.1 5th
    - submammary 675.1 5th
  - melancholia 296.2 5th
    - recurrent episode 296.3 5th
    - single episode 296.2 5th
  - mental disorder (conditions classifiable to 290-303, 305.0, 305.2-305.9, 306-316, 317-319) 648.4 5th
  - metritis ~~(septic)~~ (suppurative) 670.1 5th ▲
    - septic 670.2 5th ●
  - metroperitonitis 670.8 5th ▲
  - metrorrhagia 666.2 5th
  - metrosalpingitis 670.8 5th ▲
  - metrovaginitis 670.8 5th ▲
  - milk leg 671.4 5th
  - monoplegia, cerebral 674.0 5th
  - necrosis
    - kidney, tubular 669.3 5th
    - liver (acute) (subacute) (conditions classifiable to 570) 674.8 5th
    - ovary 670.8 5th ▲
    - renal cortex 669.3 5th
  - nephritis or nephrosis (conditions classifiable to 580-589) 646.2 5th
    - with hypertension 642.1 5th
  - nutritional deficiency (conditions classifiable to 260-269) 648.9 5th
  - occlusion, precerebral artery 674.0 5th
  - oliguria 669.3 5th
  - oophoritis 670.8 5th ▲
  - ovaritis 670.8 5th ▲
  - paralysis
    - bladder (sphincter) 665.5 5th

- **Puerperal** – *continued*
  - paralysis – *continued*
    - cerebral 674.0 5th
  - paralytic stroke 674.0 5th
  - parametritis 670.8 5th ▲
  - paravaginitis 646.6 5th
  - pelviperitonitis 670 5th
  - perimetritis 670.8 5th ▲
  - perimetrosalpingitis 670.8 5th ▲
  - perinephritis 646.6 5th
  - perioophoritis 670.8 5th ▲
  - periphlebitis - *see* Puerperal, phlebitis
  - perisalpingitis 670.8 5th ▲
  - peritoneal infection 670.8 5th ▲
  - peritonitis (pelvic) 670.8 5th ▲
  - perivaginitis 646.6 5th
  - phlebitis 671.2 5th ▲
    - deep 671.4 5th
    - intracranial sinus (venous) 671.5 5th
    - pelvic 671.4 5th
    - specified site NEC 671.5 5th
    - superficial 671.2 5th
  - phlegmasia alba dolens 671.4 5th
  - placental polyp 674.4 5th
  - pneumonia, embolic - *see* Puerperal, embolism
  - prediabetes 648.8 5th
  - pre-eclampsia (mild) 642.4 5th
    - with pre-existing hypertension 642.7 5th
    - severe 642.5 5th
  - psychosis, unspecified (*see also* Psychosis, puerperal) 293.89
  - pyelitis 646.6 5th
  - pyelocystitis 646.6 5th
  - pyelohydronephrosis 646.6 5th
  - pyelonephritis 646.6 5th
  - pyelonephrosis 646.6 5th
  - pyemia 670.2 5th ▲
  - pyocystitis 646.6 5th
  - pyohemia 670.2 5th ▲
  - pyometra 670.8 5th ▲
  - pyonephritis 646.6 5th
  - pyonephrosis 646.6 5th
  - pyo-oophoritis 670.8 5th ▲
  - pyosalpingitis 670.8 5th ▲
  - pyosalpinx 670.8 5th ▲
  - pyrexia (of unknown origin) 672 5th
  - renal
    - disease NEC 646.2 5th
    - failure, acute 669.3 5th
  - retention
    - decidua (fragments) (with delayed hemorrhage) 666.2 5th
      - without hemorrhage 667.1 5th
    - placenta (fragments) (with delayed hemorrhage) 666.2 5th
      - without hemorrhage 667.1 5th
    - secundines (fragments) (with delayed hemorrhage) 666.2 5th
      - without hemorrhage 667.1 5th
  - retracted nipple 676.0 5th
  - rubella (conditions classifiable to 056) 647.5 5th
  - salpingitis 670 5th
  - salpingo-oophoritis 670.8 5th ▲
  - salpingo-ovaritis 670.8 5th ▲
  - salpingoperitonitis 670.8 5th ▲
  - sapremia 670.2 5th ▲
  - secondary perineal tear 674.2 5th
  - sepsis (pelvic) 670.2 5th ▲
  - septicemia 670.2 5th ▲
  - subinvolution (uterus) 674.8 5th
  - sudden death (cause unknown) 674.9 5th
  - suppuration - *see* Puerperal, abscess
  - syphilis (conditions classifiable to 090-097) 647.0 5th
  - tetanus 670.8 5th ▲
  - thelitis 675.0 5th
  - thrombocytopenia 666.3 5th
  - thrombophlebitis (superficial) 671.2 5th
    - deep 671.4 5th
    - pelvic 671.4 5th
    - septic 670.3 5th ●

- **Puerperal** – *continued*
  - thrombophlebitis – *continued*
    - specified site NEC 671.5 5th
  - thrombosis (venous) - *see* Thrombosis, puerperal
  - thyroid dysfunction (conditions classifiable to 240-246) 648.1 5th
  - toxemia (*see also* Toxemia, of pregnancy) 642.4 5th
    - eclamptic 642.6 5th
      - with pre-existing hypertension 642.7 5th
    - pre-eclamptic (mild) 642.4 5th
      - with
        - convulsions 642.6 5th
        - pre-existing hypertension 642.7 5th
    - severe 642.5 5th
  - tuberculosis (conditions classifiable to 010-018) 647.3 5th
  - uremia 669.3 5th
  - vaginitis (conditions classifiable to 616.1) 646.6 5th
  - varicose veins (legs) 671.0 5th
    - vulva or perineum 671.1 5th
  - venous complication 671.9 5th ●
  - vulvitis (conditions classifiable to 616.1) 646.6 5th
  - vulvovaginitis (conditions classifiable to 616.1) 646.6 5th
  - white leg 671.4 5th
- **Pulled muscle** - *see* Sprain, by site
- **Pulmolithiasis** 518.89
- **Pulmonary** - *see* condition
- **Pulmonitis** (unknown etiology) 486
- **Pulpitis** (acute) (anachoretic) (chronic) (hyperplastic) (putrescent) (suppurative) (ulcerative) 522.0
- **Pulpless tooth** 522.9
- **Pulse**
  - alternating 427.89
    - psychogenic 306.2
  - bigeminal 427.89
  - fast 785.0
  - feeble, rapid, due to shock following injury 958.4
  - rapid 785.0
  - slow 427.89
  - strong 785.9
  - trigeminal 427.89
  - water-hammer (*see also* Insufficiency, aortic) 424.1
  - weak 785.9
- **Pulseless disease** 446.7
- **Pulsus**
  - alternans or trigeminy 427.89
    - psychogenic 306.2
- **Punch drunk** 310.2
- **Puncta lacrimalia occlusion** 375.52
- **Punctiform hymen** 752.49
- **Puncture** (traumatic) - *see also* Wound, open, by site
  - accidental, complicating surgery 998.2
  - bladder, nontraumatic 596.6
  - by
    - device, implant, or graft - *see* Complications, mechanical
    - foreign body
      - internal organs - *see also* Injury, internal, by site
        - by ingested object - *see* Foreign body
      - left accidentally in operation wound 998.4
    - instrument (any) during a procedure, accidental 998.2
  - internal organs, abdomen, chest, or pelvis - *see* Injury, internal, by site
  - kidney, nontraumatic 593.89
- **Pupil** - *see* condition
- **Pupillary membrane** 364.74
  - persistent 743.46
- **Pupillotonia** 379.46
  - pseudotabetic 379.46

Puerperal – Pupillotonia

- **Purpura** 287.2
  - abdominal 287.0
  - allergic 287.0
  - anaphylactoid 287.0
  - annularis telangiectodes 709.1
  - arthritic 287.0
  - autoerythrocyte sensitization 287.2
  - autoimmune 287.0
  - bacterial 287.0
  - Bateman's (senile) 287.2
  - capillary fragility (hereditary) (idiopathic) 287.8
  - cryoglobulinemic 273.2
  - devil's pinches 287.2
  - fibrinolytic (*see also* Fibrinolysis) 286.6
  - fulminans, fulminous 286.6
  - gangrenous 287.0
  - hemorrhagic (*see also* Purpura, thrombocytopenic) 287.39
    - nodular 272.7
    - nonthrombocytopenic 287.0
    - thrombocytopenic 287.39
  - Henoch's (purpura nervosa) 287.0
  - Henoch-Schönlein (allergic) 287.0
  - hypergammaglobulinemic (benign primary) (Waldenström's) 273.0
  - idiopathic 287.31
    - nonthrombocytopenic 287.0
    - thrombocytopenic 287.31
  - immune thrombocytopenic 287.31
  - infectious 287.0
  - malignant 287.0
  - neonatorum 772.6
  - nervosa 287.0
  - newborn NEC 772.6
  - nonthrombocytopenic 287.2
    - hemorrhagic 287.0
    - idiopathic 287.0
  - nonthrombopenic 287.2
  - peliosis rheumatica 287.0
  - pigmentaria, progressiva 709.09
  - posttransfusion 287.4
  - primary 287.0
  - primitive 287.0
  - red cell membrane sensitivity 287.2
  - rheumatica 287.0
  - Schönlein (-Henoch) (allergic) 287.0
  - scorbutic 267
  - senile 287.2
  - simplex 287.2
  - symptomatica 287.0
  - telangiectasia annularis 709.1
  - thrombocytopenic (*see also* Thrombocytopenia) 287.30
    - congenital 287.33
    - essential 287.30
    - hereditary 287.31
    - idiopathic 287.31
    - immune 287.31
    - neonatal, transitory (*see also* Thrombocytopenia, neonatal transitory) 776.1
    - primary 287.30
    - puerperal, postpartum 666.3 [5th]
    - thrombotic 446.6
  - thrombohemolytic (*see also* Fibrinolysis) 286.6
  - thrombopenic (*see also* Thrombocytopenia) 287.30
    - congenital 287.33
    - essential 287.30
  - thrombotic 446.6
    - thrombocytic 446.6
    - thrombocytopenic 446.6
  - toxic 287.0
  - variolosa 050.0
  - vascular 287.0
  - visceral symptoms 287.0
  - Werlhof's (*see also* Purpura, thrombocytopenic) 287.39
- **Purpuric spots** 782.7
- **Purulent** - *see* condition
- **Pus**
  - absorption, general - *see* Septicemia
  - in
    - stool 792.1
    - urine 791.9
  - tube (rupture) (*see also* Salpingo-oophoritis) 614.2
- **Pustular rash** 782.1
- **Pustule** 686.9
  - malignant 022.0
  - nonmalignant 686.9
- **Putnam's disease** (subacute combined sclerosis with pernicious anemia) 281.0 *[336.2]*
- **Putnam-Dana syndrome** (subacute combined sclerosis with pernicious anemia) 281.0 *[336.2]*
- **Putrefaction, intestinal** 569.89
- **Putrescent pulp** (dental) 522.1
- **Pyarthritis** - *see* Pyarthrosis
- **Pyarthrosis** (*see also* Arthritis, pyogenic) 711.0 [5th]
  - tuberculous - *see* Tuberculosis, joint
- **Pycnoepilepsy, pycnolepsy** (idiopathic) (*see also* Epilepsy) 345.0 [5th]
- **Pyelectasia** 593.89
- **Pyelectasis** 593.89
- **Pyelitis** (congenital) (uremic) 590.80
  - with
    - abortion - *see* Abortion, by type, with specified complication NEC
    - contracted kidney 590.00
    - ectopic pregnancy (*see also* categories 633.0-633.9) 639.8
    - molar pregnancy (*see also* categories 630-632) 639.8
  - acute 590.10
    - with renal medullary necrosis 590.11
  - chronic 590.00
    - with
      - renal medullary necrosis 590.01
  - complicating pregnancy, childbirth, or puerperium 646.6
    - affecting fetus or newborn 760.1
  - cystica 590.3
  - following
    - abortion 639.8
    - ectopic or molar pregnancy 639.8
  - gonococcal 098.19
    - chronic or duration of 2 months or over 098.39
  - tuberculous (*see also* Tuberculosis) 016.0 [5th] *[590.81]*
- **Pyelocaliectasis** 593.89
- **Pyelocystitis** (*see also* Pyelitis) 590.80
- **Pyelohydronephrosis** 591
- **Pyelonephritis** (*see also* Pyelitis) 590.80
  - acute 590.10
    - with renal medullary necrosis 590.11
  - chronic 590.00
  - syphilitic (late) 095.4
  - tuberculous (*see also* Tuberculosis) 016.0 [5th] *[590.81]*
- **Pyelonephrosis** (*see also* Pyelitis) 590.80
  - chronic 590.00
- **Pyelophlebitis** 451.89
- **Pyelo-ureteritis cystica** 590.3
- **Pyemia, pyemic** (purulent) (*see also* Septicemia) 038.9
  - abscess - *see* Abscess
  - arthritis (*see also* Arthritis, pyogenic) 711.0 [5th]
  - Bacillus coli 038.42
  - embolism (*see also* Septicemia) 415.12
  - fever 038.9
  - infection 038.9
  - joint (*see also* Arthritis, pyogenic) 711.0 [5th]
  - liver 572.1
  - meningococcal 036.2
  - newborn 771.81
  - phlebitis - *see* Phlebitis
  - pneumococcal 038.2
  - portal 572.1
  - postvaccinal 999.39
  - puerperal 670.2 [5th] ●
  - specified organism NEC 038.8
  - staphylococcal 038.10
    - aureus 038.11
      - methicillin
        - resistant 038.12
        - susceptible 038.11
    - specified organism NEC 038.19
  - streptococcal 038.0
  - tuberculous - *see* Tuberculosis, miliary
- **Pygopagus** 759.4
- **Pykno-epilepsy, pyknolepsy** (idiopathic) (*see also* Epilepsy) 345.0 [5th]
- **Pyle (-Cohn) disease** (craniometaphyseal dysplasia) 756.89
- **Pylephlebitis** (suppurative) 572.1
- **Pylethrombophlebitis** 572.1
- **Pylethrombosis** 572.1
- **Pyloritis** (*see also* Gastritis) 535.5 [5th]
- **Pylorospasm** (reflex) 537.81
  - congenital or infantile 750.5
  - neurotic 306.4
  - newborn 750.5
  - psychogenic 306.4
- **Pylorus, pyloric** - *see* condition
- **Pyoarthrosis** - *see* Pyarthrosis
- **Pyocele**
  - mastoid 383.00
  - sinus (accessory) (nasal) (*see also* Sinusitis) 473.9
  - turbinate (bone) 473.9
  - urethra (*see also* Urethritis) 597.0
- **Pyococcal dermatitis** 686.00
- **Pyococcide, skin** 686.00
- **Pyocolpos** (*see also* Vaginitis) 616.10
- **Pyocyaneus dermatitis** 686.09
- **Pyocystitis** (*see also* Cystitis) 595.9
- **Pyoderma, pyodermia** 686.00
  - gangrenosum 686.01
  - specified type NEC 686.09
  - vegetans 686.8
- **Pyodermatitis** 686.00
  - vegetans 686.8
- **Pyogenic** - *see* condition
- **Pyohemia** - *see* Septicemia
- **Pyohydronephrosis** (*see also* Pyelitis) 590.80
- **Pyometra** 615.9
- **Pyometritis** (*see also* Endometritis) 615.9
- **Pyometrium** (*see also* Endometritis) 615.9
- **Pyomyositis** 728.0
  - ossificans 728.19
  - tropical (bungpagga) 040.81
- **Pyonephritis** (*see also* Pyelitis) 590.80
  - chronic 590.00
- **Pyonephrosis** (congenital) (*see also* Pyelitis) 590.80
  - acute 590.10
- **Pyo-oophoritis** (*see also* Salpingo-oophoritis) 614.2
- **Pyo-ovarium** (*see also* Salpingo-oophoritis) 614.2
- **Pyopericarditis** 420.99
- **Pyopericardium** 420.99
- **Pyophlebitis** - *see* Phlebitis
- **Pyopneumopericardium** 420.99
- **Pyopneumothorax** (infectional) 510.9
  - with fistula 510.0
  - subdiaphragmatic (*see also* Peritonitis) 567.29
  - subphrenic (*see also* Peritonitis) 567.29
  - tuberculous (*see also* Tuberculosis, pleura) 012.0 [5th]
- **Pyorrhea** (alveolar) (alveolaris) 523.40
  - degenerative 523.5
- **Pyosalpingitis** (*see also* Salpingo-oophoritis) 614.2
- **Pyosalpinx** (*see also* Salpingo-oophoritis) 614.2
- **Pyosepticemia** - *see* Septicemia
- **Pyosis**
  - Corlett's (impetigo) 684
  - Manson's (pemphigus contagiosus) 684
- **Pyothorax** 510.9
  - with fistula 510.0
  - tuberculous (*see also* Tuberculosis, pleura) 012.0 [5th]
- **Pyoureter** 593.89
  - tuberculous (*see also* Tuberculosis) 016.2 [5th]
- **Pyramidopallidonigral syndrome** 332.0
- **Pyrexia** (of unknown origin) (P.U.O.) 780.60
  - atmospheric 992.0
  - during labor 659.2 [5th]
  - environmentally-induced newborn 778.4
  - heat 992.0
  - newborn, environmentally-induced 778.4
  - puerperal 672 [5th]
- **Pyroglobulinemia** 273.8
- **Pyromania** 312.33
- **Pyrosis** 787.1
- **Pyrroloporphyria** 277.1
- **Pyuria** (bacterial) 791.9

Q

- **Q fever** 083.0
  - with pneumonia 083.0 *[484.8]*
- **Quadricuspid aortic valve** 746.89
- **Quadrilateral fever** 083.0
- **Quadriparesis** - *see* Quadriplegia
  - meaning muscle weakness 728.87
- **Quadriplegia** 344.00
  - with fracture, vertebra (process) - *see* Fracture, vertebra, cervical, with spinal cord injury
  - brain (current episode) 437.8
  - C_1-C_4
    - complete 344.01
    - incomplete 344.02
  - C_5-C_7
    - complete 344.03
    - incomplete 344.04
  - cerebral (current episode) 437.8
  - congenital or infantile (cerebral) (spastic) (spinal) 343.2
  - cortical 437.8
  - embolic (current episode) (*see also* Embolism, brain) 434.1 [5th]
  - functional 780.72
  - infantile (cerebral) (spastic) (spinal) 343.2
  - newborn NEC 767.0
  - specified NEC 344.09
  - thrombotic (current episode) (*see also* Thrombosis, brain) 434.0 [5th]
  - traumatic - *see* Injury, spinal, cervical
- **Quadruplet**
  - affected by maternal complications of pregnancy 761.5
  - healthy liveborn - *see* Newborn, multiple
  - pregnancy (complicating delivery) NEC 651.8 [5th]
    - with fetal loss and retention of one or more fetus(es) 651.5 [5th]
    - following (elective) fetal reduction 651.7 [5th]
- **Quarrelsomeness** 301.3
- **Quartan**
  - fever 084.2
  - malaria (fever) 084.2
- **Queensland fever** 083.0
  - coastal 083.0
  - seven-day 100.89
- **Quervain's disease** 727.04
  - thyroid (subacute granulomatous thyroiditis) 245.1
- **Queyrat's erythroplasia** (M8080/2)
  - specified site - *see* Neoplasm, skin, in situ
  - unspecified site 233.5
- **Quincke's disease or edema** - *see* Edema, angioneurotic
- **Quinquaud's disease** (acne decalvans) 704.09
- **Quinsy** (gangrenous) 475
- **Quintan fever** 083.1

Purpura – Quintan fever

- **Quintuplet**
  - affected by maternal complications of pregnancy 761.5
  - healthy liveborn - *see* Newborn, multiple
  - pregnancy (complicating delivery) NEC 651.2 5th
    - with fetal loss and retention of one or more fetus(es) 651.6 5th
    - following (elective) fetal reduction 651.7 5th
- **Quotidian**
  - fever 084.0
    - malaria (fever) 084.0

R

- **Rabbia** 071
- **Rabbit fever** (*see also* Tularemia) 021.9
- **Rabies** 071
  - contact V01.5
  - exposure to V01.5
  - inoculation V04.5
    - reaction - *see* Complications, vaccination
  - vaccination, prophylactic (against) V04.5
- **Rachischisis** (*see also* Spina bifida) 741.9 5th
- **Rachitic** - *see also* condition
  - deformities of spine 268.1
  - pelvis 268.1
    - with disproportion (fetopelvic) 653.2 5th
      - affecting fetus or newborn 763.1
      - causing obstructed labor 660.1 5th
        - affecting fetus or newborn 763.1
- **Rachitis, rachitism** - *see also* Rickets
  - acute 268.0
  - fetalis 756.4
  - renalis 588.0
  - tarda 268.0
- **Racket nail** 757.5
- **Radial nerve** - *see* condition
- **Radiation effects or sickness** - *see also* Effect, adverse, radiation
  - cataract 366.46
  - dermatitis 692.82
    - sunburn (*see also* Sunburn) 692.71
- **Radiculitis** (pressure) (vertebrogenic) 729.2
  - accessory nerve 723.4
  - anterior crural 724.4
  - arm 723.4
  - brachial 723.4
  - cervical NEC 723.4
  - due to displacement of intervertebral disc - *see* Neuritis, due to, displacement intervertebral disc
  - leg 724.4
  - lumbar NEC 724.4
  - lumbosacral 724.4
  - rheumatic 729.2
  - syphilitic 094.89
  - thoracic (with visceral pain) 724.4
- **Radiculomyelitis** 357.0
  - toxic, due to
    - Clostridium tetani 037
    - corynebacterium diphtheriae 032.89
- **Radiculopathy** (*see also* Radiculitis) 729.2
- **Radioactive substances, adverse effect** - *see* Effect, adverse, radioactive substance
- **Radiodermal burns** (acute) (chronic) (occupational) - *see* Burn, by site
- **Radiodermatitis** 692.82
- **Radionecrosis** - *see* Effect, adverse, radiation
- **Radiotherapy session** V58.0
- **Radium, adverse effect** - *see* Effect, adverse, radioactive substance
- **Raeder-Harbitz syndrome** (pulseless disease) 446.7
- **Rage** (*see also* Disturbance, conduct) 312.0 5th
  - meaning rabies 071
- **Rag sorters' disease** 022.1
- **Raillietiniasis** 123.8
- **Railroad neurosis** 300.16
- **Railway spine** 300.16
- **Raised** - *see* Elevation
- **Raiva** 071
- **Rake teeth, tooth** 524.39
- **Rales** 786.7
- **Ramifying renal pelvis** 753.3
- **Ramsay Hunt syndrome** (herpetic geniculate ganglionitis) 053.11
  - meaning dyssynergia cerebellaris myoclonica 334.2
- **Ranke's primary infiltration** (*see also* Tuberculosis) 010.0 5th
- **Ranula** 527.6
  - congenital 750.26
- **Rape**
  - adult 995.83
  - alleged, observation or examination V71.5
  - child 995.53
- **Rapid**
  - feeble pulse, due to shock, following injury 958.4
  - heart (beat) 785.0
    - psychogenic 306.2
  - respiration 786.06
    - psychogenic 306.1
  - second stage (delivery) 661.3 5th
    - affecting fetus or newborn 763.6
  - time-zone change syndrome 327.35
- **Rarefaction, bone** 733.99
- **Rash** 782.1
  - canker 034.1
  - diaper 691.0
  - drug (internal use) 693.0
    - contact 692.3
  - ECHO 9 virus 078.89
  - enema 692.89
  - food (*see also* Allergy, food) 693.1
  - heat 705.1
  - napkin 691.0
  - nettle 708.8
  - pustular 782.1
  - rose 782.1
    - epidemic 056.9
    - of infants 057.8
  - scarlet 034.1
  - serum (prophylactic) (therapeutic) 999.5
  - toxic 782.1
  - wandering tongue 529.1
- **Rasmussen's aneurysm** (*see also* Tuberculosis) 011.2 5th
- **Rat-bite fever** 026.9
  - due to Streptobacillus moniliformis 026.1
  - spirochetal (morsus muris) 026.0
- **Rathke's pouch tumor** (M9350/1) 237.0
- **Raymond (-Céstan) syndrome** 433.8 5th
- **Raynaud's**
  - disease or syndrome (paroxysmal digital cyanosis) 443.0
  - gangrene (symmetric) 443.0 *[785.4]*
  - phenomenon (paroxysmal digital cyanosis) (secondary) 443.0
- **RDS** 769
- **Reaction**
  - acute situational maladjustment (*see also* Reaction, adjustment) 309.9
  - adaptation (*see also* Reaction, adjustment) 309.9
  - adjustment 309.9
    - with
      - anxious mood 309.24
        - with depressed mood 309.28
      - conduct disturbance 309.3
        - combined with disturbance of emotions 309.4
      - depressed mood 309.0
        - brief 309.0
          - with anxious mood 309.28
        - prolonged 309.1
      - elective mutism 309.83
      - mixed emotions and conduct 309.4
      - mutism, elective 309.83
      - physical symptoms 309.82

Reaction – *continued*

  - adjustment – *continued*
    - with – *continued*
      - predominant disturbance (of)
        - conduct 309.3
        - emotions NEC 309.29
          - mixed 309.28
        - mixed, emotions and conduct 309.4
      - specified type NEC 309.89
      - specific academic or work inhibition 309.23
      - withdrawal 309.83
    - depressive 309.0
      - with conduct disturbance 309.4
      - brief 309.0
      - prolonged 309.1
    - specified type NEC 309.89
  - adverse food NEC 995.7
  - affective (*see also* Psychosis, affective) 296.90
    - specified type NEC 296.99
  - aggressive 301.3
    - unsocialized (*see also* Disturbance, conduct) 312.0 5th
  - allergic (*see also* Allergy) 995.3
    - drug, medicinal substance, and biological - *see* Allergy, drug
    - food - *see* Allergy, food
    - serum 999.5
  - anaphylactic - *see* Shock, anaphylactic
  - anesthesia - *see* Anesthesia, complication
  - anger 312.0 5th
  - antisocial 301.7
  - antitoxin (prophylactic) (therapeutic) - *see* Complications, vaccination
  - anxiety 300.00
  - Arthus 995.21
  - asthenic 300.5
  - compulsive 300.3
  - conversion (anesthetic) (autonomic) (hyperkinetic) (mixed paralytic) (paresthetic) 300.11
  - deoxyribonuclease (DNA) (DNase) hypersensitivity NEC 287.2
  - depressive 300.4
    - acute 309.0
    - affective (*see also* Psychosis, affective) 296.2 5th
      - recurrent episode 296.3 5th
      - single episode 296.2 5th
    - brief 309.0
    - manic (*see also* Psychosis, affective) 296.80
    - neurotic 300.4
    - psychoneurotic 300.4
    - psychotic 298.0
  - dissociative 300.15
  - drug NEC (*see also* Table of Drugs and Chemicals) 995.20
    - allergic - *see also* Allergy, drug 995.27
    - correct substance properly administered 995.20
    - obstetric anesthetic or analgesic NEC 668.9 5th
      - affecting fetus or newborn 763.5
      - specified drug - *see* Table of Drugs and Chemicals
    - overdose or poisoning 977.9
      - specified drug - *see* Table of Drugs and Chemicals
    - specific to newborn 779.4
    - transmitted via placenta or breast milk - *see* Absorption, drug, through placenta
    - withdrawal NEC 292.0
      - infant of dependent mother 779.5
    - wrong substance given or taken in error 977.9
      - specified drug - *see* Table of Drugs and Chemicals
  - dyssocial 301.7
  - dystonic, acute, due to drugs 333.72
  - erysipeloid 027.1

Reaction – *continued*

  - fear 300.20
    - child 313.0
  - fluid loss, cerebrospinal 349.0
  - food - *see also* Allergy, food
    - adverse NEC 995.7
    - anaphylactic shock - *see* Anaphylactic shock, due to, food
  - foreign
    - body NEC 728.82
      - in operative wound (inadvertently left) 998.4
        - due to surgical material intentionally left - *see* Complications, due to (presence of) any device, implant, or graft classified to 996.0-996.5 NEC
    - substance accidentally left during a procedure (chemical) (powder) (talc) 998.7
      - body or object (instrument) (sponge) (swab) 998.4
  - graft-versus-host (GVH) 279.50
  - grief (acute) (brief) 309.0
    - prolonged 309.1
  - gross stress (*see also* Reaction, stress, acute) 308.9
  - group delinquent (*see also* Disturbance, conduct) 312.2 5th
  - Herxheimer's 995.0
  - hyperkinetic (*see also* Hyperkinesia) 314.9
  - hypochondriacal 300.7
  - hypoglycemic, due to insulin 251.0
    - therapeutic misadventure 962.3
  - hypomanic (*see also* Psychosis, affective) 296.0 5th
    - recurrent episode 296.1 5th
    - single episode 296.0 5th
  - hysterical 300.10
    - conversion type 300.11
    - dissociative 300.15
  - id (bacterial cause) 692.89
  - immaturity NEC 301.89
    - aggressive 301.3
    - emotional instability 301.59
  - immunization - *see* Complications, vaccination
  - incompatibility
    - blood group ~~(ABO) (infusion) (transfusion) 999.6~~ ▲
      - ABO 999.6 ●
      - minor blood group 999.89 ●
    - Rh (factor) (infusion) (transfusion) 999.7
  - inflammatory - *see* Infection
  - infusion - *see* Complications, infusion
  - inoculation (immune serum) - *see* Complications, vaccination
  - insulin 995.23
  - involutional
    - paranoid 297.2
    - psychotic (*see also* Psychosis, affective, depressive) 296.2 5th
  - leukemoid (basophilic) (lymphocytic) (monocytic) (myelocytic)(neutrophilic) 288.62
  - LSD (*see also* Abuse, drugs, nondependent) 305.3 5th
  - lumbar puncture 349.0
  - manic-depressive (*see also* Psychosis, affective) 296.80
    - depressed 296.2 5th
      - recurrent episode 296.3 5th
      - single episode 296.2 5th
    - hypomanic 296.0 5th
  - neurasthenic 300.5
  - neurogenic (*see also* Neurosis) 300.9
  - neurotic NEC 300.9
  - neurotic-depressive 300.4
  - nitritoid - *see* Crisis, nitritoid
  - obsessive-compulsive 300.3
  - organic 293.9
    - acute 293.0

4th Fourth Digit Required | 5th Fifth Digit Required | *[code]* Manifestation Code | ● New Line | ▲ Revised Line | text New Text | ~~text~~ Deleted text

- **Reaction** – *continued*
  - organic – *continued*
    - subacute 293.1
  - overanxious, child or adolescent 313.0
  - paranoid (chronic) 297.9
    - acute 298.3
    - climacteric 297.2
    - involutional 297.2
    - menopausal 297.2
    - senile 290.20
    - simple 297.0
  - passive
    - aggressive 301.84
    - dependency 301.6
  - personality (*see also* Disorder, personality) 301.9
  - phobic 300.20
  - postradiation - *see* Effect, adverse, radiation
  - psychogenic NEC 300.9
  - psychoneurotic (*see also* Neurosis) 300.9
    - anxiety 300.00
    - compulsive 300.3
    - conversion 300.11
    - depersonalization 300.6
    - depressive 300.4
    - dissociative 300.15
    - hypochondriacal 300.7
    - hysterical 300.10
      - conversion type 300.11
      - dissociative type 300.15
    - neurasthenic 300.5
    - obsessive 300.3
    - obsessive-compulsive 300.3
    - phobic 300.20
    - tension state 300.9
  - psychophysiologic NEC (*see also* Disorder, psychosomatic) 306.9
    - cardiovascular 306.2
    - digestive 306.4
    - endocrine 306.6
    - gastrointestinal 306.4
    - genitourinary 306.50
    - heart 306.2
    - hemic 306.8
    - intestinal (large) (small) 306.4
    - laryngeal 306.1
    - lymphatic 306.8
    - musculoskeletal 306.0
    - pharyngeal 306.1
    - respiratory 306.1
    - skin 306.3
    - special sense organs 306.7
  - psychosomatic (*see also* Disorder, psychosomatic) 306.9
  - psychotic (*see also* Psychosis) 298.9
    - depressive 298.0
    - due to or associated with physical condition (*see also* Psychosis, organic) 293.9
    - involutional (*see also* Psychosis, affective) 296.2 [5th]
      - recurrent episode 296.3 [5th]
      - single episode 296.2 [5th]
  - pupillary (myotonic) (tonic) 379.46
  - radiation - *see* Effect, adverse, radiation
  - runaway - *see also* Disturbance, conduct
    - socialized 312.2 [5th]
    - undersocialized, unsocialized 312.1 [5th]
  - scarlet fever toxin - *see* Complications, vaccination
  - schizophrenic (*see also* Schizophrenia) 295.9 [5th]
    - latent 295.5 [5th]
  - serological for syphilis - *see* Serology for syphilis
  - serum (prophylactic) (therapeutic) 999.5
    - immediate 999.4
  - situational (*see also* Reaction, adjustment) 309.9
    - acute, to stress 308.3
    - adjustment (*see also* Reaction, adjustment) 309.9
  - somatization (*see also* Disorder, psychosomatic) 306.9
  - spinal puncture 349.0
  - spite, child (*see also* Disturbance, conduct) 312.0 [5th]
  - stress, acute 308.9
    - with predominant disturbance (of)
      - consciousness 308.1
      - emotions 308.0
      - mixed 308.4
      - psychomotor 308.2
      - specified type NEC 308.3
    - bone or cartilage - *see* Fracture, stress
  - surgical procedure - *see* Complications, surgical procedure
  - tetanus antitoxin - *see* Complications, vaccination
  - toxin-antitoxin - *see* Complications, vaccination
  - transfusion (blood) (bone marrow) (lymphocytes) (allergic) - *see* Complications, transfusion
  - tuberculin skin test, nonspecific (without active tuberculosis) 795.5
    - positive (without active tuberculosis) 795.5
  - ultraviolet - *see* Effect, adverse, ultraviolet
  - undersocialized, unsocialized - *see also* Disturbance, conduct
    - aggressive (type) 312.0 [5th]
    - unaggressive (type) 312.1 [5th]
  - vaccination (any) - *see* Complications, vaccination
  - white graft (skin) 996.52
  - withdrawing, child or adolescent 313.22
  - x-ray - *see* Effect, adverse, x-rays
- **Reactive depression** (*see also* Reaction, depressive) 300.4
  - neurotic 300.4
  - psychoneurotic 300.4
  - psychotic 298.0
- **Rebound tenderness** 789.6 [5th]
- **Recalcitrant patient** V15.81
- **Recanalization, thrombus** - *see* Thrombosis
- **Recession, receding**
  - chamber angle (eye) 364.77
  - chin 524.06
  - gingival (postinfective) (postoperative) 523.20
    - generalized 523.25
    - localized 523.24
    - minimal 523.21
    - moderate 523.22
    - severe 523.23
- **Recklinghausen's disease** (M9540/1) 237.71
  - bones (osteitis fibrosa cystica) 252.01
- **Recklinghausen-Applebaum disease** (hemochromatosis) 275.0
- **Reclus' disease** (cystic) 610.1
- **Recrudescent typhus** (fever) 081.1
- **Recruitment, auditory** 388.44
- **Rectalgia** 569.42
- **Rectitis** 569.49
- **Rectocele**
  - female (without uterine prolapse) 618.04
    - with uterine prolapse 618.4
      - complete 618.3
      - incomplete 618.2
  - in pregnancy or childbirth 654.4 [5th]
    - causing obstructed labor 660.2 [5th]
      - affecting fetus or newborn 763.1
  - male 569.49
  - vagina, vaginal (outlet) 618.04
- **Rectosigmoiditis** 569.89
  - ulcerative (chronic) 556.3
- **Rectosigmoid junction** - *see* condition
- **Rectourethral** - *see* condition
- **Rectovaginal** - *see* condition
- **Rectovesical** - *see* condition
- **Rectum, rectal** - *see* condition
- **Recurrent** - *see* condition
- **Red bugs** 133.8
- **Red cedar asthma** 495.8
- **Redness**
  - conjunctiva 379.93
  - eye 379.93
  - nose 478.19
- **Reduced ventilatory or vital capacity** 794.2
- **Reduction**
  - function
    - kidney (*see also* Disease, renal) 593.9
    - liver 573.8
  - ventilatory capacity 794.2
  - vital capacity 794.2
- **Redundant, redundancy**
  - abdomen 701.9
  - anus 751.5
  - cardia 537.89
  - clitoris 624.2
  - colon (congenital) 751.5
  - foreskin (congenital) 605
  - intestine 751.5
  - labia 624.3
  - organ or site, congenital NEC - *see* Accessory
  - panniculus (abdominal) 278.1
  - prepuce (congenital) 605
  - pylorus 537.89
  - rectum 751.5
  - scrotum 608.89
  - sigmoid 751.5
  - skin (of face) 701.9
    - eyelids 374.30
  - stomach 537.89
  - uvula 528.9
  - vagina 623.8
- **Reduplication** - *see* Duplication
- **Referral**
  - adoption (agency) V68.89
  - nursing care V63.8
  - patient without examination or treatment V68.81
  - social services V63.8
- **Reflex** - *see also* condition
  - blink, deficient 374.45
  - hyperactive gag 478.29
  - neurogenic bladder NEC 596.54
    - atonic 596.54
      - with cauda equina syndrome 344.61
  - vasoconstriction 443.9
  - vasovagal 780.2
- **Reflux** 530.81
  - acid 530.81
  - esophageal 530.81
    - with esophagitis 530.11
  - esophagitis 530.11
  - gastroesophageal 530.81
  - mitral - *see* Insufficiency, mitral
  - ureteral - *see* Reflux, vesicoureteral
  - vesicoureteral 593.70
    - with
      - reflux nephropathy 593.73
        - bilateral 593.72
        - unilateral 593.71
- **Reformed gallbladder** 576.0
- **Reforming, artificial openings** (*see also* Attention to, artificial, opening) V55.9
- **Refractive error** (*see also* Error, refractive) 367.9
- **Refsum's disease or syndrome** (heredopathia atactica polyneuritiformis) 356.3
- **Refusal of**
  - food 307.59
    - hysterical 300.11
  - treatment because of, due to
    - patient's decision NEC V64.2
    - reason of conscience or religion V62.6
- **Regaud**
  - tumor (M8082/3) - *see* Neoplasm, nasopharynx, malignant
  - type carcinoma (M8082/3) - *see* Neoplasm, nasopharynx, malignant
- **Regional** - *see* condition
- **Regulation feeding** (elderly) (infant) 783.3
  - newborn 779.31 ▲
- **Regurgitated**
  - food, choked on 933.1
- **Regurgitated** – *continued*
  - stomach contents, choked on 933.1
- **Regurgitation** 787.03
  - aortic (valve) (*see also* Insufficiency, aortic) 424.1
    - congenital 746.4
    - syphilitic 093.22
  - food - *see also* Vomiting
    - with reswallowing - *see* Rumination
    - newborn 779.33 ▲
  - gastric contents - *see* Vomiting
  - heart - *see* Endocarditis
  - mitral (valve) - *see also* Insufficiency, mitral
    - congenital 746.6
  - myocardial - *see* Endocarditis
  - pulmonary (heart) (valve) (*see also* Endocarditis, pulmonary) 424.3
  - stomach - *see* Vomiting
  - tricuspid - *see* Endocarditis, tricuspid
  - valve, valvular - *see* Endocarditis
  - vesicoureteral - *see* Reflux, vesicoureteral
- **Rehabilitation** V57.9
  - multiple types V57.89
  - occupational V57.21
  - specified type NEC V57.89
  - speech(-language) V57.3 ▲
  - vocational V57.22
- **Reichmann's disease or syndrome** (gastrosuccorrhea) 536.8
- **Reifenstein's syndrome** (hereditary familial hypogonadism, male) 259.52
- **Reilly's syndrome or phenomenon** (*see also* Neuropathy, peripheral, autonomic) 337.9
- **Reimann's periodic disease** 277.31
- **Reinsertion, contraceptive device** V25.42
- **Reiter's disease, syndrome, or urethritis** 099.3 *[711.1]* [5th]
- **Rejection**
  - food, hysterical 300.11
  - transplant 996.80
    - bone marrow 996.85
    - corneal 996.51
    - organ (immune or nonimmune cause) 996.80
      - bone marrow 996.85
      - heart 996.83
      - intestines 996.87
      - kidney 996.81
      - liver 996.82
      - lung 996.84
      - pancreas 996.86
      - specified NEC 996.89
    - skin 996.52
      - artificial 996.55
      - decellularized allodermis 996.55
- **Relapsing fever** 087.9
  - Carter's (Asiatic) 087.0
  - Dutton's (West African) 087.1
  - Koch's 087.9
  - louse-borne (epidemic) 087.0
  - Novy's (American) 087.1
  - Obermeyer's (European) 087.0
  - Spirillum 087.9
  - tick-borne (endemic) 087.1
- **Relaxation**
  - anus (sphincter) 569.49
    - due to hysteria 300.11
  - arch (foot) 734
    - congenital 754.61
  - back ligaments 728.4
  - bladder (sphincter) 596.59
  - cardio-esophageal 530.89
  - cervix (*see also* Incompetency, cervix) 622.5
  - diaphragm 519.4
  - inguinal rings - *see* Hernia, inguinal
  - joint (capsule) (ligament) (paralytic) (*see also* Derangement, joint) 718.90
    - congenital 755.8
  - lumbosacral joint 724.6
  - pelvic floor 618.89
  - pelvis 618.89

- **Relaxation** – *continued*
  - perineum 618.89
  - posture 729.90
  - rectum (sphincter) 569.49
  - sacroiliac (joint) 724.6
  - scrotum 608.89
  - urethra (sphincter) 599.84
  - uterus (outlet) 618.89
  - vagina (outlet) 618.89
  - vesical 596.59
- **Remains**
  - canal of Cloquet 743.51
  - capsule (opaque) 743.51
- **Remittent fever** (malarial) 084.6
- **Remnant**
  - canal of Cloquet 743.51
  - capsule (opaque) 743.51
  - cervix, cervical stump (acquired) (postoperative) 622.8
  - cystic duct, postcholecystectomy 576.0
  - fingernail 703.8
    - congenital 757.5
  - meniscus, knee 717.5
  - thyroglossal duct 759.2
  - tonsil 474.8
    - infected 474.00
  - urachus 753.7
- **Remote effect of cancer**- *see* condition
- **Removal** (of)
  - catheter (urinary) (indwelling) V53.6
    - from artificial opening - *see* Attention to, artificial, opening
    - non-vascular V58.82
    - vascular V58.81
  - cerebral ventricle (communicating) shunt V53.01
  - device - *see also* Fitting (of)
    - contraceptive V25.42
    - fixation
      - external V54.89
      - internal V54.01
    - traction V54.89
  - drains V58.49
  - dressing
    - wound V58.30
      - nonsurgical V58.30
      - surgical V58.31
  - ileostomy V55.2
  - Kirschner wire V54.89
  - non-vascular catheter V58.82
  - pin V54.01
  - plaster cast V54.89
  - plate (fracture) V54.01
  - rod V54.01
  - screw V54.01
  - splint, external V54.89
  - staples V58.32
  - subdermal implantable contraceptive V25.43
  - sutures V58.32
  - traction device, external V54.89
  - vascular catheter V58.81
  - wound packing V58.30
    - nonsurgical V58.30
    - surgical V58.31
- **Ren**
  - arcuatus 753.3
  - mobile, mobilis (*see also* Disease, renal) 593.0
    - congenital 753.3
    - unguliformis 753.3
- **Renal** - *see also* condition
  - glomerulohyalinosis-diabetic syndrome 250.4 5th *[581.81]*
    - due to secondary diabetes 249.4 5th *[581.81]*
- **Rendu-Osler-Weber disease or syndrome** (familial hemorrhagic telangiectasia) 448.0
- **Reninoma** (M8361/1) 236.91
- **Rénon-Delille syndrome** 253.8
- **Repair**
  - pelvic floor, previous, in pregnancy or childbirth 654.4 5th
    - affecting fetus or newborn 763.89
  - scarred tissue V51.8
- **Replacement by artificial or mechanical device or prosthesis of** (*see also* Fitting (of))
  - artificial skin V43.83
  - bladder V43.5
  - blood vessel V43.4
  - breast V43.82
  - eye globe V43.0
  - heart
    - with
      - assist device V43.21
      - fully implantable artificial heart V43.22
    - valve V43.3
  - intestine V43.89
  - joint V43.60
    - ankle V43.66
    - elbow V43.62
    - finger V43.69
    - hip (partial) (total) V43.64
    - knee V43.65
    - shoulder V43.61
    - specified NEC V43.69
    - wrist V43.63
  - kidney V43.89
  - larynx V43.81
  - lens V43.1
  - limb(s) V43.7
  - liver V43.89
  - lung V43.89
  - organ NEC V43.89
  - pancreas V43.89
  - skin (artificial) V43.83
  - tissue NEC V43.89
- **Reprogramming**
  - cardiac pacemaker V53.31
- **Request for expert evidence** V68.2
- **Reserve, decreased or low**
  - cardiac - *see* Disease, heart
    - kidney (*see also* Disease, renal) 593.9
- **Residual** - *see also* condition
  - bladder 596.8
  - foreign body - *see* Retention, foreign body
  - state, schizophrenic (*see also* Schizophrenia) 295.6 5th
  - urine 788.69
- **Resistance, resistant** (to)
  - activated protein C 289.81

Note *Use the following subclassification for categories V09.5, V09.7, V09.8, V09.9*

0 without mention of resistance to multiple drugs

1 with resistance to multiple drugs

V09.5 quinolones and fluoroquinolones

V09.7 antimycobacterial agents

V09.8 specified drugs NEC

V09.9 unspecified drugs

- **Resistance, resistant** (to) – *continued*
  - drugs by microorganisms V09.90
    - Amikacin V09.4
    - aminoglycosides V09.4
    - Amodiaquine V09.5 5th
    - Amoxicillin V09.0
    - Ampicillin V09.0
    - antimycobacterial agents V09.7 5th
    - Azithromycin V09.2
    - Azlocillin V09.0
    - Aztreonam V09.1
    - B-lactam antibiotics V09.1
    - Bacampicillin V09.0
    - Bacitracin V09.8 5th
    - Benznidazole V09.8 5th
    - Capreomycin V09.7 5th
    - Carbenicillin V09.0
    - Cefaclor V09.1
    - Cefadroxil V09.1
    - Cefamandole V09.1
    - Cefatetan V09.1
    - Cefazolin V09.1
    - Cefixime V09.1
    - Cefonicid V09.1
    - Cefoperazone V09.1
    - Ceforanide V09.1
    - Cefotaxime V09.1
    - Cefoxitin V09.1
    - Ceftazidine V09.1
    - Ceftizoxime V09.1
    - Ceftriaxone V09.1
    - Cefuroxime V09.1
    - Cephalexin V09.1
    - Cephaloglycin V09.1
    - Cephaloridine V09.1
    - cephalosporins V09.1
    - Cephalothin V09.1
    - Cephapirin V09.1
    - Cephradine V09.1
    - Chloramphenicol V09.8 5th
    - Chloraquine V09.5 5th
    - Chlorguanide V09.8 5th
    - Chlorproguanil V09.8 5th
    - Chlortetracyline V09.3
    - Cinoxacin V09.5 5th
    - Ciprofloxacin V09.5 5th
    - Clarithromycin V09.2
    - Clindamycin V09.8 5th
    - Clioquinol V09.5 5th
    - Clofazimine V09.7 5th
    - Cloxacillin V09.0
    - Cyclacillin V09.0
    - Cycloserine V09.7
    - Dapsone [Dz] V09.7 5th
    - Demeclocycline V09.3
    - Dicloxacillin V09.0
    - Doxycycline V09.3
    - Enoxacin V09.5 5th
    - Erythromycin V09.2
    - Ethambutol [EMB] V09.7 5th
    - Ethionamide [ETA] V09.7 5th
    - fluoroquinolones NEC V09.5 5th
    - Gentamicin V09.4
    - Halofantrine V09.8 5th
    - Imipenem V09.1
    - Iodoquinol V09.5 5th
    - Isoniazid [INH] V09.7 5th
    - Kanamycin V09.4
    - macrolides V09.2
    - Mafenide V09.6
    - MDRO (multiple drug resistant organisms) NOS V09.91
    - Mefloquine V09.8 5th
    - Melassoprol V09.8 5th
    - Methicillin - *see* Infection, Methicillin
    - Methacycline V09.3
    - Methenamine V09.8 5th
    - Metronidazole V09.8 5th
    - Mezlocillin V09.0
    - Minocycline V09.3
    - multiple drug resistant organisms NOS V09.91
    - Nafcillin V09.0
    - Nalidixic acid V09.5 5th
    - Natamycin V09.2
    - Neomycin V09.4
    - Netilmicin V09.4
    - Nimorazole V09.8 5th
    - Nitrofurantoin V09.8 5th
    - Nitrofurtimox V09.8 5th
    - Norfloxacin V09.5 5th
    - Nystatin V09.2
    - Ofloxacin V09.5 5th
    - Oleandomycin V09.2
    - Oxacillin V09.0
    - Oxytetracycline V09.3
    - Para-amino salicyclic acid [PAS] V09.7 5th
    - Paromomycin V09.4
    - Penicillin (G) (V) (Vk) V09.0
    - penicillins V09.0
    - Pentamidine V09.8 5th
    - Piperacillin V09.0
    - Primaquine V09.5 5th
    - Proguanil V09.8 5th
    - Pyrazinamide [PZA] V09.7 5th
    - Pyrimethamine/Sulfalene V09.8 5th
    - Pyrimethamine/Sulfodoxine V09.8 5th
    - Quinacrine V09.5 5th
    - Quinidine V09.8 5th
    - Quinine V09.8 5th
    - quinolones V09.5 5th
    - Rifabutin V09.7 5th
    - Rifampin [Rif] V09.7 5th
    - Rifamycin V09.7 5th
    - Rolitetracycline V09.3
    - specified drug(s) NEC V09.8 5th
    - Spectinomycin V09.8 5th
    - Spiramycin V09.2
    - Streptomycin [Sm] V09.4
    - Sulfacetamide V09.6
    - Sulfacytine V09.6
    - Sulfadiazine V09.6
    - Sulfadoxine V09.6
    - Sulfamethoxazole V09.6
    - Sulfapyridine V09.6
    - Sulfasalizine V09.6
    - Sulfasoxazole V09.6
    - sulfonamides V09.6
    - Sulfoxone V09.7 5th
    - Tetracycline V09.3
    - tetracyclines V09.3
    - Thiamphenicol V09.8 5th
    - Ticarcillin V09.0
    - Tinidazole V09.8 5th
    - Tobramycin V09.4
    - Triamphenicol V09.8 5th
    - Trimethoprim V09.8 5th
    - Vancomycin V09.8 5th
  - insulin 277.7
  - thyroid hormone 246.8
- **Resorption**
  - biliary 576.8
    - purulent or putrid (*see also* Cholecystitis) 576.8
  - dental (roots) 521.40
    - alveoli 525.8
    - pathological
      - external 521.42
      - internal 521.41
      - specified NEC 521.49
  - septic - *see* Septicemia
  - teeth (roots) 521.40
    - pathological
      - external 521.42
      - internal 521.41
      - specified NEC 521.49
- **Respiration**
  - asymmetrical 786.09
  - bronchial 786.09
  - Cheyne-Stokes (periodic respiration) 786.04
  - decreased, due to shock following injury 958.4
  - disorder of 786.00
    - psychogenic 306.1
    - specified NEC 786.09
  - failure 518.81
    - acute 518.81
    - acute and chronic 518.84
    - chronic 518.83
    - newborn 770.84
  - insufficiency 786.09
    - acute 518.82
    - newborn NEC 770.89
  - Kussmaul (air hunger) 786.09
  - painful 786.52
  - periodic 786.09
    - high altitude 327.22
  - poor 786.09
    - newborn NEC 770.89
  - sighing 786.7
    - psychogenic 306.1
  - wheezing 786.07

- **Respiratory** - *see also* condition
  - distress 786.09
    - acute 518.82
    - fetus or newborn NEC 770.89
    - syndrome (newborn) 769
      - adult (following shock, surgery, or trauma) 518.5
        - specified NEC 518.82
  - failure 518.81
    - acute 518.81
    - acute and chronic 518.84
    - chronic 518.83
- **Respiratory syncytial virus** (RSV) 079.6
  - bronchiolitis 466.11
  - pneumonia 480.1
  - vaccination, prophylactic (against) V04.82
- **Response**
  - photoallergic 692.72
  - phototoxic 692.72
- **Rest, rests**
  - mesonephric duct 752.89
    - fallopian tube 752.11
  - ovarian, in fallopian tubes 752.19
  - wolffian duct 752.89
- **Restless legs syndrome** (RLS) 333.94
- **Restlessness** 799.29 ▲
- **Restoration of organ continuity from previous sterilization** (tuboplasty) (vasoplasty) V26.0
- **Restriction of housing space** V60.1
- **Restzustand, schizophrenic** (*see also* Schizophrenia) 295.6 [5th]
- **Retained** - *see* Retention
- **Retardation**
  - development, developmental, specific (*see also* Disorder, development, specific) 315.9
    - learning, specific 315.2
      - arithmetical 315.1
      - language (skills) 315.31
        - expressive 315.31
        - mixed receptive-expressive 315.32
      - mathematics 315.1
      - reading 315.00
        - phonological 315.39
      - written expression 315.2
    - motor 315.4
  - endochondral bone growth 733.91
  - growth (physical) in childhood 783.43
    - due to malnutrition 263.2
    - fetal (intrauterine) 764.9
      - affecting management of pregnancy 656.5 [5th]
  - intrauterine growth 764.9
    - affecting management of pregnancy 656.5 [5th]
  - mental 319
    - borderline V62.89
    - mild, IQ 50-70 317
    - moderate, IQ 35-49 318.0
    - profound, IQ under 20 318.2
    - severe, IQ 20-34 318.1
  - motor, specific 315.4
  - physical 783.43
    - child 783.43
    - due to malnutrition 263.2
    - fetus (intrauterine) 764.9 [5th]
      - affecting management of pregnancy 656.5 [5th]
  - psychomotor NEC 307.9
  - reading 315.00
- **Retching** - *see* Vomiting
- **Retention, retained**
  - bladder (*see also* Retention, urine) 788.20
    - psychogenic 306.53
  - carbon dioxide 276.2
  - cholelithiasis 997.4
  - cyst - *see* Cyst

- **Retention, retained** – *continued*
  - dead
    - fetus (after 22 completed weeks gestation) 656.4 [5th]
      - early fetal death (before 22 completed weeks gestation) 632
    - ovum 631
  - decidua (following delivery) (fragments) (with hemorrhage) 666.2 [5th]
    - without hemorrhage 667.1 [5th]
  - deciduous tooth 520.6
  - dental root 525.3
  - fecal (*see also* Constipation) 564.00
  - fluid 276.6
  - foreign body - *see also* Foreign body, retained
    - bone 733.99
    - current trauma - *see* Foreign body, by site or type
    - middle ear 385.83
    - muscle 729.6
    - soft tissue NEC 729.6
  - gallstones 997.4
  - gastric 536.8
  - membranes (following delivery) (with hemorrhage) 666.2 [5th]
    - with abortion - *see* Abortion, by type
    - without hemorrhage 667.1 [5th]
  - menses 626.8
  - milk (puerperal) 676.2 [5th]
  - nitrogen, extrarenal 788.99
  - placenta (total) (with hemorrhage) 666.0 [5th]
    - with abortion - *see* Abortion, by type
    - portions or fragments 666.2 [5th]
      - without hemorrhage 667.1 [5th]
    - without hemorrhage 667.0 [5th]
  - products of conception
    - early pregnancy (fetal death before 22 completed weeks gestation) 632
    - following
      - abortion - *see* Abortion, by type
      - delivery 666.2 [5th]
        - with hemorrhage 666.2 [5th]
        - without hemorrhage 667.1 [5th]
  - secundines (following delivery) (with hemorrhage) 666.2 [5th]
    - with abortion - *see* Abortion, by type
    - complicating puerperium (delayed hemorrhage) 666.2 [5th]
    - without hemorrhage 667.1 [5th]
  - smegma, clitoris 624.8
  - urine NEC 788.20
    - bladder, incomplete emptying 788.21
      - due to
        - benign prostatic hypertrophy (BPH) - *see* category 600
    - due to
      - benign prostatic hypertrophy (BPH) - *see* category 600
    - psychogenic 306.53
    - specified NEC 788.29
  - water (in tissue) (*see also* Edema) 782.3
- **Reticulation, dust** (occupational) 504
- **Reticulocytosis NEC** 790.99
- **Reticuloendotheliosis**
  - acute infantile (M9722/3) 202.5 [5th]
  - leukemic (M9940/3) 202.4 [5th]
  - malignant (M9720/3) 202.3 [5th]
  - nonlipid (M9722/3) 202.5 [5th]
- **Reticulohistiocytoma** (giant cell) 277.89
- **Reticulohistiocytosis, multicentric** 272.8
- **Reticulolymphosarcoma** (diffuse) (M9613/3) 200.8 [5th]
  - follicular (M9691/3) 202.0 [5th]
  - nodular (M9691/3) 202.0 [5th]
- **Reticulosarcoma** (M9640/3) 200.0 [5th]
  - nodular (M9642/3) 200.0 [5th]
  - pleomorphic cell type (M9641/3) 200.0 [5th]
- **Reticulosis** (skin)
  - acute of infancy (M9722/3) 202.5 [5th]
  - familial hemophagocytic 288.4
  - histiocytic medullary (M9721/3) 202.3 [5th]

- **Reticulosis** (skin) – *continued*
  - lipomelanotic 695.89
  - malignant (M9720/3) 202.3 [5th]
  - Sezary's (M9701/3) 202.2 [5th]
- **Retina, retinal** - *see* condition
- **Retinitis** (*see also* Chorioretinitis) 363.20
  - albuminurica 585.9 *[363.10]*
  - arteriosclerotic 440.8 *[362.13]*
- **Retinitis** – *continued*
  - central angiospastic 362.41
  - Coat's 362.12
  - diabetic 250.5 [5th] *[362.01]*
    - due to secondary diabetes 249.5 [5th] *[362.01]*
  - disciformis 362.52
  - disseminated 363.10
    - metastatic 363.14
    - neurosyphilitic 094.83
    - pigment epitheliopathy 363.15
  - exudative 362.12
  - focal 363.00
    - in histoplasmosis 115.92
      - capsulatum 115.02
      - duboisii 115.12
    - juxtapapillary 363.05
    - macular 363.06
    - paramacular 363.06
    - peripheral 363.08
    - posterior pole NEC 363.07
  - gravidarum 646.8 [5th]
  - hemorrhagica externa 362.12
  - juxtapapillary (Jensen's) 363.05
  - luetic - *see* Retinitis, syphilitic
  - metastatic 363.14
  - pigmentosa 362.74
  - proliferans 362.29
  - proliferating 362.29
  - punctata albescens 362.76
  - renal 585.9 *[363.13]*
  - syphilitic (secondary) 091.51
    - congenital 090.0 *[363.13]*
    - early 091.51
    - late 095.8 *[363.13]*
  - syphilitica, central, recurrent 095.8 *[363.13]*
  - tuberculous (*see also* Tuberculous) 017.3 [5th] *[363.13]*
- **Retinoblastoma** (M9510/3) 190.5
  - differentiated type (M9511/3) 190.5
  - undifferentiated type (M9512/3) 190.5
- **Retinochoroiditis** (*see also* Chorioretinitis) 363.20
  - central angiospastic 362.41
  - disseminated 363.10
    - metastatic 363.14
    - neurosyphilitic 094.83
    - pigment epitheliopathy 363.15
    - syphilitic 094.83
  - due to toxoplasmosis (acquired) (focal) 130.2
  - focal 363.00
    - in histoplasmosis 115.92
      - capsulatum 115.02
      - duboisii 115.12
    - juxtapapillary (Jensen's) 363.05
    - macular 363.06
    - paramacular 363.06
    - peripheral 363.08
    - posterior pole NEC 363.07
  - juxtapapillaris 363.05
  - syphilitic (disseminated) 094.83
- **Retinopathy** (background) 362.10
  - arteriosclerotic 440.8 *[362.13]*
  - atherosclerotic 440.8 *[362.13]*
  - central serous 362.41
  - circinate 362.10
  - Coat's 362.12
  - diabetic 250.5 [5th] *[362.01]*
    - due to secondary diabetes 249.5 [5th] *[362.01]*
    - nonproliferative 250.5 [5th] *[362.03]*
      - due to secondary diabetes 249.5 [5th] *[362.03]*

- **Retinopathy** (background) – *continued*
  - diabetic – *continued*
    - nonproliferative – *continued*
      - mild 250.5 [5th] *[362.04]*
        - due to secondary diabetes 249.5 [5th] *[362.04]*
      - moderate 250.5 [5th] *[362.05]*
        - due to secondary diabetes 249.5 [5th] *[362.05]*
      - severe 250.5 [5th] *[362.06]*
        - due to secondary diabetes 249.5 [5th] *[362.06]*
    - proliferative 250.5 [5th] *[362.02]*
      - due to secondary diabetes 249.5 [5th] *[362.02]*
  - exudative 362.12
  - hypertensive 362.11
  - nonproliferative
    - diabetic 250.5 [5th] *[362.03]*
      - due to secondary diabetes 249.5 [5th] *[362.03]*
      - mild 250.5 [5th] *[362.04]*
        - due to secondary diabetes 249.5 [5th] *[362.04]*
      - moderate 250.5 [5th] *[362.05]*
        - due to secondary diabetes 249.5 [5th] *[362.05]*
      - severe 250.5 [5th] *[362.06]*
        - due to secondary diabetes 249.5 [5th] *[362.06]*
  - of prematurity 362.20
    - cicatricial 362.21
    - stage
      - 0 362.22
      - 1 362.23
      - 2 362.24
      - 3 362.25
      - 4 362.26
      - 5 362.27
  - pigmentary, congenital 362.74
  - proliferative 362.29
    - diabetic 250.5 [5th] *[362.02]*
      - due to secondary diabetes 249.5 [5th] *[362.02]*
    - sickle-cell 282.60 *[362.29]*
  - solar 363.31
- **Retinoschisis** 361.10
  - bullous 361.12
  - congenital 743.56
  - flat 361.11
  - juvenile 362.73
- **Retractile testis** 752.52
- **Retraction**
  - cervix *see* Retraction, uterus
  - drum (membrane) 384.82
  - eyelid 374.41
  - finger 736.29
  - head 781.0
  - lid 374.41
  - lung 518.89
  - mediastinum 519.3
  - nipple 611.79
    - congenital 757.6
    - puerperal, postpartum 676.0 [5th]
  - palmar fascia 728.6
  - pleura (*see also* Pleurisy) 511.0
  - ring, uterus (Bandl's) (pathological) 661.4 [5th]
    - affecting fetus or newborn 763.7
  - sternum (congenital) 756.3
    - acquired 738.3
    - during respiration 786.9
  - substernal 738.3
  - supraclavicular 738.8
  - syndrome (Duane's) 378.71
  - uterus 621.6
  - valve (heart) - *see* Endocarditis
- **Retrobulbar** - *see* condition
- **Retrocaval ureter** 753.4
- **Retrocecal** - *see also* condition
  - appendix (congenital) 751.5
- **Retrocession** - *see* Retroversion
- **Retrodisplacement** - *see* Retroversion
- **Retroflection, retroflexion** - *see* Retroversion

Retrognathia, retrognathism (mandibular) (maxillary) 524.10
Retrograde
  ejaculation 608.87
  menstruation 626.8
Retroiliac ureter 753.4
Retroperineal - *see* condition
Retroperitoneal - *see* condition
Retroperitonitis 567.39
Retropharyngeal - *see* condition
Retroplacental - *see* condition
Retroposition - *see* Retroversion
Retrosternal thyroid (congenital) 759.2
Retroversion, retroverted
  cervix - *see* Retroversion, uterus
  female NEC (*see also* Retroversion, uterus) 621.6
  iris 364.70
  testis (congenital) 752.51
  uterus, uterine (acquired) (acute) (adherent) (any degree) (asymptomatic) (cervix) (postinfectional) (postpartal, old) 621.6
    congenital 752.3
    in pregnancy or childbirth 654.3 [5th]
      affecting fetus or newborn 763.89
      causing obstructed labor 660.2 [5th]
        affecting fetus or newborn 763.1
Retrusion, premaxilla (developmental) 524.04
Rett's syndrome 330.8
Reverse, reversed
  peristalsis 787.4
Reye's syndrome 331.81
Reye-Sheehan syndrome (postpartum pituitary necrosis) 253.2
Rh (factor)
  hemolytic disease 773.0
  incompatibility, immunization, or sensitization
    affecting management of pregnancy 656.1 [5th]
    fetus or newborn 773.0
    transfusion reaction 999.7
  negative mother, affecting fetus or newborn 773.0
  titer elevated 999.7
  transfusion reaction 999.7
Rhabdomyolysis (idiopathic) 728.88
Rhabdomyoma (M8900/0) - *see also* Neoplasm, connective tissue, benign
  adult (M8904/0) - *see* Neoplasm, connective tissue, benign
  fetal (M8903/0) - *see* Neoplasm, connective tissue, benign
  glycogenic (M8904/0) - *see* Neoplasm, connective tissue, benign
Rhabdomyosarcoma (M8900/3) - *see also* Neoplasm connective tissue, malignant
  alveolar (M8920/3) - *see* Neoplasm, connective tissue, malignant
  embryonal (M8910/3) - *see* Neoplasm, connective tissue, malignant
  mixed type (M8902/3) - *see* Neoplasm, connective tissue, malignant
  pleomorphic (M8901/3) - *see* Neoplasm, connective tissue, malignant
Rhabdosarcoma (M8900/3) - *see* Rhabdomyosarcoma
Rhesus (factor) (Rh) **incompatibility** - *see* Rh, incompatibility
Rheumaticosis - *see* Rheumatism
Rheumatism, rheumatic (acute NEC) 729.0
  adherent pericardium 393
  arthritis
    acute or subacute - *see* Fever, rheumatic
    chronic 714.0
      spine 720.0
  articular (chronic) NEC (*see also* Arthritis) 716.9 [5th]
    acute or subacute - *see* Fever, rheumatic

Rheumatism, rheumatic – *continued*
  back 724.9
  blennorrhagic 098.59
  carditis - *see* Disease, heart, rheumatic
  cerebral - *see* Fever, rheumatic
  chorea (acute) - *see* Chorea, rheumatic
  chronic NEC 729.0
  coronary arteritis 391.9
    chronic 398.99
  degeneration, myocardium (*see also* Degeneration, myocardium, with rheumatic fever) 398.0
  desert 114.0
  febrile - *see* Fever, rheumatic
  fever - *see* Fever, rheumatic
  gonococcal 098.59
  gout 274.0<u>0</u> ▲
  heart
    disease (*see also* Disease, heart, rheumatic) 398.90
    failure (chronic) (congestive) (inactive) 398.91
  hemopericardium - *see* Rheumatic, pericarditis
  hydropericardium - *see* Rheumatic, pericarditis
  inflammatory (acute) (chronic) (subacute) - *see* Fever, rheumatic
  intercostal 729.0
    meaning Tietze's disease 733.6
  joint (chronic) NEC (*see also* Arthritis) 716.9 [5th]
    acute - *see* Fever, rheumatic
  mediastinopericarditis - *see* Rheumatic, pericarditis
  muscular 729.0
  myocardial degeneration (*see also* Degeneration, myocardium, with rheumatic fever) 398.0
  myocarditis (chronic) (inactive) (with chorea) 398.0
    active or acute 391.2
      with chorea (acute) (rheumatic) (Sydenham's) 392.0
  myositis 729.1
  neck 724.9
  neuralgic 729.0
  neuritis (acute) (chronic) 729.2
  neuromuscular 729.0
  nodose - *see* Arthritis, nodosa
  nonarticular 729.0
  palindromic 719.30
    ankle 719.37
    elbow 719.32
    foot 719.37
    hand 719.34
    hip 719.35
    knee 719.36
    multiple sites 719.39
    pelvic region 719.35
    shoulder (region) 719.31
    specified site NEC 719.38
    wrist 719.33
  pancarditis, acute 391.8
    with chorea (acute) (rheumatic) (Sydenham's) 392.0
    chronic or inactive 398.99
  pericarditis (active) (acute) (with effusion) (with pneumonia) 391.0
    with chorea (acute) (rheumatic) (Sydenham's) 392.0
    chronic or inactive 393
  pericardium - *see* Rheumatic, pericarditis
  pleuropericarditis - *see* Rheumatic, pericarditis
  pneumonia 390 *[517.1]*
  pneumonitis 390 *[517.1]*
  pneumopericarditis - *see* Rheumatic, pericarditis
  polyarthritis
    acute or subacute - *see* Fever, rheumatic
    chronic 714.0

Rheumatism, rheumatic – *continued*
  polyarticular NEC (*see also* Arthritis) 716.9 [5th]
  psychogenic 306.0
  radiculitis 729.2
  sciatic 724.3
  septic - *see* Fever, rheumatic
  spine 724.9
  subacute NEC 729.0
  torticollis 723.5
  tuberculous NEC (*see also* Tuberculosis) 015.9 [5th]
  typhoid fever 002.0
Rheumatoid - *see also* condition
  lungs 714.81
Rhinitis (atrophic) (catarrhal) (chronic) (croupous) (fibrinous) (hyperplastic) (hypertrophic) (membranous) (purulent) (suppurative) (ulcerative) 472.0
  with
    hay fever (*see also* Fever, hay) 477.9
      with asthma (bronchial) 493.0 [5th]
    sore throat - *see* Nasopharyngitis
  acute 460
  allergic (nonseasonal) (seasonal) (*see also* Fever, hay) 477.9
    with asthma (*see also* Asthma) 493.0 [5th]
    due to food 477.1
  granulomatous 472.0
  infective 460
  obstructive 472.0
  pneumococcal 460
  syphilitic 095.8
    congenital 090.0
  tuberculous (*see also* Tuberculosis) 012.8 [5th]
  vasomotor (*see also* Fever, hay) 477.9
Rhinoantritis (chronic) 473.0
  acute 461.0
Rhinodacryolith 375.57
Rhinolalia (aperta) (clausa) (open) 784.4<u>3</u> ▲
Rhinolith 478.19
  nasal sinus (*see also* Sinusitis) 473.9
Rhinomegaly 478.19
Rhinopharyngitis (acute) (subacute) (*see also* Nasopharyngitis) 460
  chronic 472.2
  destructive ulcerating 102.5
  mutilans 102.5
Rhinophyma 695.3
Rhinorrhea 478.19
  cerebrospinal (fluid) 349.81
  paroxysmal (*see also* Fever, hay) 477.9
  spasmodic (*see also* Fever, hay) 477.9
Rhinosalpingitis 381.50
  acute 381.51
  chronic 381.52
Rhinoscleroma 040.1
Rhinosporidiosis 117.0
Rhinovirus infection 079.3
Rhizomelic chrondrodysplasia punctata 277.86
Rhizomelique, pseudopolyarthritic 446.5
Rhoads and Bomford anemia (refractory) 238.72
Rhus
  diversiloba dermatitis 692.6
  radicans dermatitis 692.6
  toxicodendron dermatitis 692.6
  venenata dermatitis 692.6
  verniciflua dermatitis 692.6
Rhythm
  atrioventricular nodal 427.89
  disorder 427.9
    coronary sinus 427.89
    ectopic 427.89
    nodal 427.89
  escape 427.89
  heart, abnormal 427.9
    fetus or newborn - *see* Abnormal, heart rate

Rhythm – *continued*
  idioventricular 426.89
    accelerated 427.89
  nodal 427.89
  sleep, inversion 327.39
    nonorganic origin 307.45
Rhytidosis facialis 701.8
Rib - *see also* condition
  cervical 756.2
Riboflavin deficiency 266.0
Rice bodies (*see also* Loose, body, joint) 718.1 [5th]
  knee 717.6
Richter's hernia - *see* Hernia, Richter's
Ricinism 988.2
Rickets (active) (acute) (adolescent) (adult) (chest wall) (congenital) (current) (infantile) (intestinal) 268.0
  celiac 579.0
  fetal 756.4
  hemorrhagic 267
  hypophosphatemic with nephrotic-glycosuric dwarfism 270.0
  kidney 588.0
  late effect 268.1
  renal 588.0
  scurvy 267
  vitamin D-resistant 275.3
Rickettsial disease 083.9
  specified type NEC 083.8
Rickettsialpox 083.2
Rickettsiosis NEC 083.9
  specified type NEC 083.8
  tick-borne 082.9
    specified type NEC 082.8
  vesicular 083.2
Ricord's chancre 091.0
Riddoch's syndrome (visual disorientation) 368.16
Rider's
  bone 733.99
  chancre 091.0
Ridge, alveolus - *see also* condition
  edentulous
    atrophy 525.20
      mandible 525.20
        minimal 525.21
        moderate 525.22
        severe 525.23
      maxilla 525.20
        minimal 525.24
        moderate 525.25
        severe 525.26
  flabby 525.20
Ridged ear 744.29
Riedel's
  disease (ligneous thyroiditis) 245.3
  lobe, liver 751.69
  struma (ligneous thyroiditis) 245.3
  thyroiditis (ligneous) 245.3
Rieger's anomaly or syndrome (mesodermal dysgenesis, anterior ocular segment) 743.44
Riehl's melanosis 709.09
Rietti-Greppi-Micheli anemia or syndrome 282.49
Rieux's hernia - *see* Hernia, Rieux's
Rift Valley fever 066.3
Riga's disease (cachectic aphthae) 529.0
Riga-Fede disease (cachectic aphthae) 529.0
Riggs' disease (compound periodontitis) 523.40
Right middle lobe syndrome 518.0
Rigid, rigidity - *see also* condition
  abdominal 789.4 [5th]
  articular, multiple congenital 754.89
  back 724.8
  cervix uteri
    in pregnancy or childbirth 654.6 [5th]
      affecting fetus or newborn 763.89
      causing obstructed labor 660.2 [5th]
        affecting fetus or newborn 763.1
  hymen (acquired) (congenital) 623.3
  nuchal 781.6

[4th] Fourth Digit Required [5th] Fifth Digit Required | *[code]* Manifestation Code | ● New Line ▲ Revised Line <u>text</u> New Text ~~text~~ Deleted text

Retrognathia, retrognathism – Rigid, rigidity

- **Rigid, rigidity** – *continued*
  - pelvic floor
    - in pregnancy or childbirth 654.4 5th
      - affecting fetus or newborn 763.89
      - causing obstructed labor 660.2 5th
        - affecting fetus or newborn 763.1
  - perineum or vulva
    - in pregnancy or childbirth 654.8 5th
      - affecting fetus or newborn 763.89
      - causing obstructed labor 660.2 5th
        - affecting fetus or newborn 763.1
  - spine 724.8
  - vagina
    - in pregnancy or childbirth 654.7 5th
      - affecting fetus or newborn 763.89
      - causing obstructed labor 660.2 5th
        - affecting fetus or newborn 763.1
- **Rigors** 780.99
- **Riley-Day syndrome** (familial dysautonomia) 742.8
- **RIND** (reversible ischemic neurological deficit) 434.91
  - history of (personal) V12.54
- **Ring(s)**
  - aorta 747.21
  - Bandl's, complicating delivery 661.4 5th
    - affecting fetus or newborn 763.7
  - contraction, complicating delivery 661.4 5th
    - affecting fetus or newborn 763.7
  - esophageal (congenital) 750.3
  - Fleischer (-Kayser) (cornea) 275.1 *[371.14]*
  - hymenal, tight (acquired) (congenital) 623.3
  - Kayser-Fleischer (cornea) 275.1 *[371.14]*
  - retraction, uterus, pathological 661.4 5th
    - affecting fetus or newborn 763.7
  - Schatzki's (esophagus) (congenital) (lower) 750.3
    - acquired 530.3
  - Soemmering's 366.51
  - trachea, abnormal 748.3
  - vascular (congenital) 747.21
  - Vossius' 921.3
    - late effect 366.21
- **Ringed hair** (congenital) 757.4
- **Ringing in the ear** (*see also* Tinnitus) 388.30
- **Ringworm** 110.9
  - beard 110.0
  - body 110.5
  - Burmese 110.9
  - corporeal 110.5
  - foot 110.4
  - groin 110.3
  - hand 110.2
  - honeycomb 110.0
  - nails 110.1
  - perianal (area) 110.3
  - scalp 110.0
  - specified site NEC 110.8
  - Tokelau 110.5
- **Rise, venous pressure** 459.89
- **Risk**
  - factor-*see* Problem
  - falling V15.88
  - suicidal 300.9
- **Ritter's disease** (dermatitis exfoliativa neonatorum) 695.81
- **Rivalry, sibling** 313.3
- **Rivalta's disease** (cervicofacial actinomycosis) 039.3
- **River blindness** 125.3 *[360.13]*
- **Robert's pelvis** 755.69
  - with disproportion (fetopelvic) 653.0 5th
    - affecting fetus or newborn 763.1
    - causing obstructed labor 660.1 5th
      - affecting fetus or newborn 763.1
- **Robin's syndrome** 756.0
- **Robinson's** (hidrotic) **ectodermal dysplasia** 757.31
- **Robles' disease** (onchocerciasis) 125.3 *[360.13]*
- **Rochalimea** - *see* Rickettsial disease
- **Rocky Mountain fever** (spotted) 082.0
- **Rodent ulcer** (M8090/3) - *see also* Neoplasm, skin, malignant
  - cornea 370.07
- **Roentgen ray, adverse effect** - *see* Effect, adverse, x-ray
- **Roetheln** 056.9
- **Roger's disease** (congenital interventricular septal defect) 745.4
- **Rokitansky's**
  - disease (*see also* Necrosis, liver) 570
  - tumor 620.2
- **Rokitansky-Aschoff sinuses** (mucosal outpouching of gallbladder) (*see also* Disease, gallbladder) 575.8
- **Rokitansky-Kuster-Hauser syndrome** (congenital absence vagina) 752.49
- **Rollet's chancre** (syphilitic) 091.0
- **Rolling of head** 781.0
- **Romano-Ward syndrome** (prolonged QT interval syndrome) 426.82
- **Romanus lesion** 720.1
- **Romberg's disease or syndrome** 349.89
- **Roof, mouth** - *see* condition
- **Rosacea** 695.3
  - acne 695.3
  - keratitis 695.3 *[370.49]*
- **Rosary, rachitic** 268.0
- **Rose**
  - cold 477.0
  - fever 477.0
  - rash 782.1
    - epidemic 056.9
    - of infants 057.8
- **Rosen-Castleman-Liebow syndrome** (pulmonary proteinosis) 516.0
- **Rosenbach's erysipelatoid or erysipeloid** 027.1
- **Rosenthal's disease** (factor XI deficiency) 286.2
- **Roseola** 057.8
  - infantum, infantilis (*see also* Exanthem subitum) 058.10
- **Rossbach's disease** (hyperchlorhydria) 536.8
  - psychogenic 306.4
- **Rossle-Urbach-Wiethe lipoproteinosis** 272.8
- **Ross river fever** 066.3
- **Rostan's asthma** (cardiac) (*see also* Failure, ventricular, left) 428.1
- **Rot**
  - Barcoo (*see also* Ulcer, skin) 707.9
  - knife-grinders' (*see also* Tuberculosis) 011.4 5th
- **Rot-Bernhardt disease** 355.1
- **Rotation**
  - anomalous, incomplete or insufficient - *see* Malrotation
  - cecum (congenital) 751.4
  - colon (congenital) 751.4
  - manual, affecting fetus or newborn 763.89
  - spine, incomplete or insufficient 737.8
  - tooth, teeth 524.35
  - vertebra, incomplete or insufficient 737.8
- **Röteln** 056.9
- **Roth's disease or meralgia** 355.1
- **Roth-Bernhardt disease or syndrome** 355.1
- **Rothmund (-Thomson) syndrome** 757.33
- **Rotor's disease or syndrome** (idiopathic hyperbilirubinemia) 277.4
- **Rotundum ulcus** - *see* Ulcer, stomach
- **Round**
  - back (with wedging of vertebrae) 737.10
    - late effect of rickets 268.1
  - hole, retina 361.31
    - with detachment 361.01
  - ulcer (stomach) - *see* Ulcer, stomach
  - worms (infestation) (large) NEC 127.0
- **Roussy-Lévy syndrome** 334.3
- **Routine postpartum follow-up** V24.2
- **Roy (-Jutras) syndrome** (acropachyderma) 757.39
- **Rubella** (German measles) 056.9
  - complicating pregnancy, childbirth, or puerperium 647.5 5th
  - complication 056.8
    - neurological 056.00
      - encephalomyelitis 056.01
      - specified type NEC 056.09
    - specified type NEC 056.79
  - congenital 771.0
  - contact V01.4
  - exposure to V01.4
  - maternal
    - with suspected fetal damage affecting management of pregnancy 655.3 5th
    - affecting fetus or newborn 760.2
      - manifest rubella in infant 771.0
  - specified complications NEC 056.79
  - vaccination, prophylactic (against) V04.3
- **Rubeola** (measles) (*see also* Measles) 055.9
  - complicated 055.8
  - meaning rubella (*see also* Rubella) 056.9
  - scarlatinosis 057.8
- **Rubeosis iridis** 364.42
  - diabetica 250.5 5th *[364.42]*
    - due to secondary diabetes 249.5 5th *[364.42]*
- **Rubinstein-Taybi's syndrome** (brachydactylia, short stature and mental retardation) 759.89
- **Rud's syndrome** (mental deficiency, epilepsy, and infantilism) 759.89
- **Rudimentary** (congenital) - *see also* Agenesis
  - arm 755.22
  - bone 756.9
  - cervix uteri 752.49
  - eye (*see also* Microphthalmos) 743.10
  - fallopian tube 752.19
  - leg 755.32
  - lobule of ear 744.21
  - patella 755.64
  - respiratory organs in thoracopagus 759.4
  - tracheal bronchus 748.3
  - uterine horn 752.3
  - uterus 752.3
    - in male 752.7
    - solid or with cavity 752.3
  - vagina 752.49
- **Ruiter-Pompen (-Wyers) syndrome** (angiokeratoma corporis diffusum) 272.7
- **Ruled out condition** (*see also* Observation, suspected) V71.9
- **Rumination** - *see also* Vomiting
  - disorder 307.53
  - neurotic 300.3
  - obsessional 300.3
  - psychogenic 307.53
- **Runaway reaction** - *see also* Disturbance, conduct
  - socialized 312.2 5th
  - undersocialized, unsocialized 312.1 5th
- **Runeberg's disease** (progressive pernicious anemia) 281.0
- **Runge's syndrome** (postmaturity) 766.22
- **Runny nose** 784.99
- **Rupia** 091.3
  - congenital 090.0
  - tertiary 095.9
- **Rupture, ruptured** 553.9
  - abdominal viscera NEC 799.89
    - obstetrical trauma 665.5 5th
  - abscess (spontaneous) - *see* Abscess, by site
  - amnion - *see* Rupture, membranes
  - aneurysm - *see* Aneurysm
  - anus (sphincter) - *see* Laceration, anus
  - aorta, aortic 441.5
    - abdominal 441.3
    - arch 441.1
    - ascending 441.1
    - descending 441.5
      - abdominal 441.3
      - thoracic 441.1
- **Rupture, ruptured** – *continued*
  - aorta, aortic – *continued*
    - syphilitic 093.0
    - thoracoabdominal 441.6
    - thorax, thoracic 441.1
    - transverse 441.1
    - traumatic (thoracic) 901.0
      - abdominal 902.0
    - valve or cusp (*see also* Endocarditis, aortic) 424.1
  - appendix (with peritonitis) 540.0
    - with peritoneal abscess 540.1
    - traumatic - *see* Injury, internal, gastrointestinal tract
  - arteriovenous fistula, brain (congenital) 430
  - artery 447.2
    - brain (*see also* Hemorrhage, brain) 431
    - coronary (*see also* Infarct, myocardium) 410.9 5th
    - heart (*see also* Infarct, myocardium) 410.9 5th
    - pulmonary 417.8
    - traumatic (complication) (*see also* Injury, blood vessel, by site) 904.9
  - bile duct, except cystic (*see also* Disease, biliary) 576.3
    - cystic 575.4
    - traumatic - *see* Injury, internal, intra-abdominal
  - bladder (sphincter) 596.6
    - with
      - abortion - *see* Abortion, by type, with damage to pelvic organs
      - ectopic pregnancy (*see also* categories 633.0-633.9) 639.2
      - molar pregnancy (*see also* categories 630-632) 639.2
    - following
      - abortion 639.2
      - ectopic or molar pregnancy 639.2
    - nontraumatic 596.6
    - obstetrical trauma 665.5 5th
    - spontaneous 596.6
    - traumatic - *see* Injury, internal, bladder
  - blood vessel (*see also* Hemorrhage) 459.0
    - brain (*see also* Hemorrhage, brain) 431
    - heart (*see also* Infarct, myocardium) 410.9 5th
    - traumatic (complication) (*see also* Injury, blood vessel, by site) 904.9
  - bone - *see* Fracture, by site
  - bowel 569.89
    - traumatic - *see* Injury, internal, intestine
  - Bowman's membrane 371.31
  - brain
    - aneurysm (congenital) (*see also* Hemorrhage, subarachnoid) 430
      - late effect - *see* Late effect(s) (of) cerebrovascular disease
      - syphilitic 094.87
    - hemorrhagic (*see also* Hemorrhage, brain) 431
    - injury at birth 767.0
    - syphilitic 094.89
  - capillaries 448.9
  - cardiac (*see also* Infarct, myocardium) 410.9 5th
  - cartilage (articular) (current) - *see also* Sprain, by site
    - knee - *see* Tear, meniscus
    - semilunar - *see* Tear, meniscus
  - cecum (with peritonitis) 540.0
    - with peritoneal abscess 540.1
    - traumatic 863.89
      - with open wound into cavity 863.99
  - cerebral aneurysm (congenital) (*see also* Hemorrhage, subarachnoid) 430
    - late effect - *see* Late effect(s) (of) cerebrovascular disease

Rupture, ruptured – *continued*
- cervix (uteri)
  - with
    - abortion - *see* Abortion, by type, with damage to pelvic organs
    - ectopic pregnancy (*see also* categories 633.0-633.9) 639.2
    - molar pregnancy (*see also* categories 630-632) 639.2
  - following
    - abortion 639.2
    - ectopic or molar pregnancy 639.2
  - obstetrical trauma 665.3 5th
  - traumatic - *see* Injury, internal, cervix
- chordae tendineae 429.5
- choroid (direct) (indirect) (traumatic) 363.63
- circle of Willis (*see also* Hemorrhage, subarachnoid) 430
  - late effect - *see* Late effect(s) (of) cerebrovascular disease
- colon 569.89
  - traumatic - *see* Injury, internal, colon
- cornea (traumatic) - *see also* Rupture, eye
  - due to ulcer 370.00
- coronary (artery) (thrombotic) (*see also* Infarct, myocardium) 410.9 5th
- corpus luteum (infected) (ovary) 620.1
- cyst - *see* Cyst
- cystic duct (*see also* Disease, gallbladder) 575.4
- Descemet's membrane 371.33
  - traumatic - *see* Rupture, eye
- diaphragm - *see also* Hernia, diaphragm
  - traumatic - *see* Injury, internal, diaphragm
- diverticulum
  - bladder 596.3
  - intestine (large) (*see also* Diverticula) 562.10
    - small 562.00
- duodenal stump 537.89
- duodenum (ulcer) - *see* Ulcer, duodenum, with perforation
- ear drum (*see also* Perforation, tympanum) 384.20
  - with otitis media - *see* Otitis media
  - traumatic - *see* Wound, open, ear
- esophagus 530.4
  - traumatic 862.22
    - with open wound into cavity 862.32
    - cervical region - *see* Wound, open, esophagus
- eye (without prolapse of intraocular tissue) 871.0
  - with
    - exposure of intraocular tissue 871.1
    - partial loss of intraocular tissue 871.2
    - prolapse of intraocular tissue 871.1
  - due to burn 940.5
- fallopian tube 620.8
  - due to pregnancy - *see* Pregnancy, tubal
  - traumatic - *see* Injury, internal, fallopian tube
- fontanel 767.3
- free wall (ventricle) (*see also* Infarct, myocardium) 410.9 5th
- gallbladder or duct (*see also* Disease, gallbladder) 575.4
  - traumatic - *see* Injury, internal, gallbladder
- gastric (*see also* Rupture, stomach) 537.89
  - vessel 459.0
- globe (eye) (traumatic) - *see* Rupture, eye
- graafian follicle (hematoma) 620.0
- heart (auricle) (ventricle) (*see also* Infarct, myocardium) 410.9
  - infectional 422.90
  - traumatic - *see* Rupture, myocardium, traumatic
- hymen 623.8
- internal
  - organ, traumatic - *see also* Injury, internal, by site
    - heart - *see* Rupture, myocardium, traumatic
    - kidney - *see* Rupture, kidney
    - liver - *see* Rupture, liver
    - spleen - *see* Rupture, spleen, traumatic
  - semilunar cartilage - *see* Tear, meniscus
- intervertebral disc - *see* Displacement, intervertebral disc
  - traumatic (current) - *see* Dislocation, vertebra
- intestine 569.89
  - traumatic - *see* Injury, internal, intestine
- intracranial, birth injury 767.0
- iris 364.76
  - traumatic - *see* Rupture, eye
- joint capsule - *see* Sprain, by site
- kidney (traumatic) 866.03
  - with open wound into cavity 866.13
  - due to birth injury 767.8
  - nontraumatic 593.89
- lacrimal apparatus (traumatic) 870.2
- lens (traumatic) 366.20
- ligament - *see also* Sprain, by site
  - with open wound - *see* Wound, open, by site
  - old (*see also* Disorder, cartilage, articular) 718.0 5th
- liver (traumatic) 864.04
  - with open wound into cavity 864.14
  - due to birth injury 767.8
  - nontraumatic 573.8
- lymphatic (node) (vessel) 457.8
- marginal sinus (placental) (with hemorrhage) 641.2 5th
  - affecting fetus or newborn 762.1
- meaning hernia - *see* Hernia
- membrana tympani (*see also* Perforation, tympanum) 384.20
  - with otitis media - *see* Otitis media
  - traumatic - *see* Wound, open, ear
- membranes (spontaneous)
  - artificial
    - delayed delivery following 658.3 5th
      - affecting fetus or newborn 761.1
    - fetus or newborn 761.1
  - delayed delivery following 658.2 5th
    - affecting fetus or newborn 761.1
  - premature (less than 24 hours prior to onset of labor) 658.1 5th
    - affecting fetus or newborn 761.1
    - delayed delivery following 658.2 5th
      - affecting fetus or newborn 761.1
- meningeal artery (*see also* Hemorrhage, subarachnoid) 430
  - late effect - *see* Late effect(s) (of) cerebrovascular disease
- meniscus (knee) - *see also* Tear, meniscus
  - old (*see also* Derangement, meniscus) 717.5
    - site other than knee - *see* Disorder, cartilage, articular
  - site other than knee - *see* Sprain, by site
- mesentery 568.89
  - traumatic - *see* Injury, internal, mesentery
- mitral - *see* Insufficiency, mitral
- muscle (traumatic) NEC - *see also* Sprain, by site
  - with open wound - *see* Wound, open, by site
  - nontraumatic 728.83
- musculotendinous cuff (nontraumatic) (shoulder) 840.4
- mycotic aneurysm, causing cerebral hemorrhage (*see also* Hemorrhage, subarachnoid) 430
  - late effect - *see* Late effect(s) (of) cerebrovascular disease
- myocardium, myocardial (*see also* Infarct, myocardium) 410.9 5th
  - traumatic 861.03
    - with open wound into thorax 861.13
- nontraumatic (meaning hernia) (*see also* Hernia, by site) 553.9
- obstructed (*see also* Hernia, by site, with obstruction) 552.9
  - gangrenous (*see also* Hernia, by site, with gangrene) 551.9
- operation wound (*see also* Dehiscence) 998.32
  - internal 998.31
- ovary, ovarian 620.8
  - corpus luteum 620.1
  - follicle (graafian) 620.0
- oviduct 620.8
  - due to pregnancy - *see* Pregnancy, tubal
- pancreas 577.8
  - traumatic - *see* Injury, internal, pancreas
- papillary muscle (ventricular) 429.6
- pelvic
  - floor, complicating delivery 664.1 5th
  - organ NEC - *see* Injury, pelvic, organs
- penis (traumatic) - *see* Wound, open, penis
- perineum 624.8
  - during delivery (*see also* Laceration, perineum, complicating delivery) 664.4 5th
- pharynx (nontraumatic) (spontaneous) 478.29
- pregnant uterus (before onset of labor) 665.0 5th
- prostate (traumatic) - *see* Injury, internal, prostate
- pulmonary
  - artery 417.8
  - valve (heart) (*see also* Endocarditis, pulmonary) 424.3
  - vein 417.8
  - vessel 417.8
- pupil, sphincter 364.75
- pus tube (*see also* Salpingo-oophoritis) 614.2
- pyosalpinx (*see also* Salpingo-oophoritis) 614.2
- rectum 569.49
  - traumatic - *see* Injury, internal, rectum
- retina, retinal (traumatic) (without detachment) 361.30
  - with detachment (*see also* Detachment, retina, with retinal defect) 361.00
- rotator cuff (capsule) (traumatic) 840.4
  - nontraumatic, complete 727.61
- sclera 871.0
- semilunar cartilage, knee (*see also* Tear, meniscus) 836.2
  - old (*see also* Derangement, meniscus) 717.5
- septum (cardiac) 410.8 5th
- sigmoid 569.89
  - traumatic - *see* Injury, internal, colon, sigmoid
- sinus of Valsalva 747.29
- spinal cord - *see also* Injury, spinal, by site
  - due to injury at birth 767.4
  - fetus or newborn 767.4
  - syphilitic 094.89
  - traumatic - *see also* Injury, spinal, by site
    - with fracture - *see* Fracture, vertebra, by site, with spinal cord injury
- spleen 289.59
  - congenital 767.8
  - due to injury at birth 767.8
  - malarial 084.9
  - nontraumatic 289.59
  - spontaneous 289.59
  - traumatic 865.04
    - with open wound into cavity 865.14
- splenic vein 459.0
- stomach 537.89
  - due to injury at birth 767.8
  - traumatic - *see* Injury, internal, stomach
  - ulcer - *see* Ulcer, stomach, with perforation
- synovium 727.50
  - specified site NEC 727.59
- tendon (traumatic) - *see also* Sprain, by site
  - with open wound - *see* Wound, open, by site
  - Achilles 845.09
    - nontraumatic 727.67
  - ankle 845.09
    - nontraumatic 727.68
  - biceps (long bead) 840.8
    - nontraumatic 727.62
  - foot 845.10
    - interphalangeal (joint) 845.13
    - metatarsophalangeal (joint) 845.12
    - nontraumatic 727.68
    - specified site NEC 845.19
    - tarsometatarsal (joint) 845.11
  - hand 842.10
    - carpometacarpal (joint) 842.11
    - interphalangeal (joint) 842.13
    - metacarpophalangeal (joint) 842.12
    - nontraumatic 727.63
      - extensors 727.63
      - flexors 727.64
    - specified site NEC 842.19
  - nontraumatic 727.60
    - specified site NEC 727.69
  - patellar 844.8
    - nontraumatic 727.66
  - quadriceps 844.8
    - nontraumatic 727.65
  - rotator cuff (capsule) 840.4
    - nontraumatic, complete 727.61
  - wrist 842.00
    - carpal (joint) 842.01
    - nontraumatic 727.63
      - extensors 727.63
      - flexors 727.64
    - radiocarpal (joint) (ligament) 842.02
    - radioulnar (joint), distal 842.09
    - specified site NEC 842.09
- testis (traumatic) 878.2
  - complicated 878.3
  - due to syphilis 095.8
- thoracic duct 457.8
- tonsil 474.8
- traumatic
  - with open wound - *see* Wound, open, by site
  - aorta - *see* Rupture, aorta, traumatic
  - ear drum - *see* Wound, open, ear, drum
  - external site - *see* Wound, open, by site
  - eye 871.2
  - globe (eye) - *see* Wound, open, eyeball
  - internal organ (abdomen, chest, or pelvis) - *see also* Injury, internal, by site
    - heart - *see* Rupture, myocardium, traumatic
    - kidney - *see* Rupture, kidney
    - liver - *see* Rupture, liver
    - spleen - *see* Rupture, spleen, traumatic
  - ligament, muscle, or tendon - *see also* Sprain, by site
    - with open wound - *see* Wound, open, by site

- **Rupture, ruptured** – *continued*
  - traumatic – *continued*
    - meaning hernia - *see* Hernia
  - tricuspid (heart) (valve) - *see* Endocarditis, tricuspid
  - tube, tubal 620.8
    - abscess (*see also* Salpingo-oophoritis) 614.2
    - due to pregnancy - *see* Pregnancy, tubal
  - tympanum, tympanic (membrane) (*see also* Perforation, tympanum) 384.20
    - with otitis media - *see* Otitis media
    - traumatic - *see* Wound, open, ear, drum
  - umbilical cord 663.8 5th
    - fetus or newborn 772.0
  - ureter (traumatic) (*see also* Injury, internal, ureter) 867.2
    - nontraumatic 593.89
  - urethra 599.84
    - with
      - abortion - *see* Abortion, by type, with damage to pelvic organs
      - ectopic pregnancy (*see also* categories 633.0-633.9) 639.2
      - molar pregnancy (*see also* categories 630-632) 639.2
    - following
      - abortion 639.2
      - ectopic or molar pregnancy 639.2
    - obstetrical trauma 665.5 5th
    - traumatic - *see* Injury, internal urethra
  - uterosacral ligament 620.8
  - uterus (traumatic) - *see also* Injury, internal uterus
    - affecting fetus or newborn 763.89
    - during labor 665.1 5th
    - nonpuerperal, nontraumatic 621.8
    - nontraumatic 621.8
    - pregnant (during labor) 665.1 5th
      - before labor 665.0 5th
  - vagina 878.6
    - complicated 878.7
    - complicating delivery - *see* Laceration, vagina, complicating delivery
  - valve, valvular (heart) - *see* Endocarditis
  - varicose vein - *see* Varicose, vein
  - varix - *see* Varix
  - vena cava 459.0
  - ventricle (free wall) (left) (*see also* Infarct, myocardium) 410.9 5th
  - vesical (urinary) 596.6
    - traumatic - *see* Injury, internal, bladder
  - vessel (blood) 459.0
    - pulmonary 417.8
  - viscus 799.89
  - vulva 878.4
    - complicated 878.5
    - complicating delivery 664.0 5th
- **Russell's dwarf** (uterine dwarfism and craniofacial dysostosis) 759.89
- **Russell's dysentery** 004.8
- **Russell (-Silver) syndrome** (congenital hemihypertrophy and short stature) 759.89
- **Russian spring-summer type encephalitis** 063.0
- **Rust's disease** (tuberculous spondylitis) 015.0 5th *[720.81]*
- **Rustitskii's disease** (multiple myeloma) (M9730/3) 203.0 5th
- **Ruysch's disease** (Hirschsprung's disease) 751.3
- **Rytand-Lipsitch syndrome** (complete atrioventricular block) 426.0

S

- **Saber**
  - shin 090.5
  - tibia 090.5
- **Sac, lacrimal** - *see* condition
- **Saccharomyces infection** (*see also* Candidiasis) 112.9
- **Saccharopinuria** 270.7
- **Saccular** - *see* condition
- **Sacculation**
  - aorta (nonsyphilitic) (*see also* Aneurysm, aorta) 441.9
    - ruptured 441.5
    - syphilitic 093.0
  - bladder 596.3
  - colon 569.89
  - intralaryngeal (congenital) (ventricular) 748.3
  - larynx (congenital) (ventricular) 748.3
  - organ or site, congenital - *see* Distortion
  - pregnant uterus, complicating delivery 654.4 5th
    - affecting fetus or newborn 763.1
      - causing obstructed labor 660.2 5th
        - affecting fetus or newborn 763.1
  - rectosigmoid 569.89
  - sigmoid 569.89
  - ureter 593.89
  - urethra 599.2
  - vesical 596.3
- **Sachs (-Tay) disease** (amaurotic familial idiocy) 330.1
- **Sacks-Libman disease** 710.0 *[424.91]*
- **Sacralgia** 724.6
- **Sacralization**
  - fifth lumbar vertebra 756.15
  - incomplete (vertebra) 756.15
- **Sacrodynia** 724.6
- **Sacroiliac joint** - *see* condition
- **Sacroiliitis NEC** 720.2
- **Sacrum** - *see* condition
- **Saddle**
  - back 737.8
  - embolus, aorta 444.0
  - nose 738.0
    - congenital 754.0
    - due to syphilis 090.5
- **Sadism** (sexual) 302.84
- **Saemisch's ulcer** 370.04
- **Saenger's syndrome** 379.46
- **Sago spleen** 277.39
- **Sailors' skin** 692.74
- **Saint**
  - Anthony's fire (*see also* Erysipelas) 035
  - Guy's dance - *see* Chorea
  - Louis-type encephalitis 062.3
  - triad (*see also* Hernia, diaphragm) 553.3
  - Vitus' dance - *see* Chorea
- **Salicylism**
  - correct substance properly administered 535.4 5th
  - overdose or wrong substance given or taken 965.1
- **Salivary duct or gland** - *see also* condition
  - virus disease 078.5
- **Salivation** (excessive) (*see also* Ptyalism) 527.7
- **Salmonella** (aertrycke) (choleraesuis) (enteritidis) (gallinarum) (suipestifer) (typhimurium) (*see also* Infection, Salmonella) 003.9
  - arthritis 003.23
  - carrier (suspected) of V02.3
  - meningitis 003.21
  - osteomyelitis 003.24
  - pneumonia 003.22
  - septicemia 003.1
  - typhosa 002.0
    - carrier (suspected) of V02.1
- **Salmonellosis** 003.0
  - with pneumonia 003.22
- **Salpingitis** (catarrhal) (fallopian tube) (nodular) (pseudofollicular) (purulent) (septic) (*see also* Salpingo-oophoritis) 614.2
  - ear 381.50
    - acute 381.51
    - chronic 381.52
- **Salpingitis** – *continued*
  - Eustachian (tube) 381.50
    - acute 381.51
    - chronic 381.52
  - follicularis 614.1
  - gonococcal (chronic) 098.37
    - acute 098.17
  - interstitial, chronic 614.1
  - isthmica nodosa 614.1
  - old - *see* Salpingo-oophoritis, chronic
  - puerperal, postpartum, childbirth 670.8 5th ▲
  - specific (chronic) 098.37
    - acute 098.17
  - tuberculous (acute) (chronic) (*see also* Tuberculosis) 016.6 5th
  - venereal (chronic) 098.37
    - acute 098.17
- **Salpingocele** 620.4
- **Salpingo-oophoritis** (catarrhal) (purulent) (ruptured) (septic) (suppurative) 614.2
  - acute 614.0
    - with
      - abortion - *see* Abortion, by type, with sepsis
      - ectopic pregnancy (*see also* categories 633.0-633.9) 639.0
      - molar pregnancy (*see also* categories 630-632) 639.0
    - following
      - abortion 639.0
      - ectopic or molar pregnancy 639.0
    - gonococcal 098.17
    - puerperal, postpartum, childbirth 670.8 5th ▲
    - tuberculous (*see also* Tuberculosis) 016.6 5th
  - chronic 614.1
    - gonococcal 098.37
    - tuberculous (*see also* Tuberculosis) 016.6 5th
  - complicating pregnancy 646.6 5th
    - affecting fetus or newborn 760.8
  - gonococcal (chronic) 098.37
    - acute 098.17
  - old - *see* Salpingo-oophoritis, chronic
  - puerperal 670.8 5th ▲
  - specific - *see* Salpingo-oophoritis, gonococcal
  - subacute (*see also* Salpingo-oophoritis, acute) 614.0
  - tuberculous (acute) (chronic) (*see also* Tuberculosis) 016.6 5th
  - venereal - *see* Salpingo-oophoritis, gonococcal
- **Salpingo-ovaritis** (*see also* Salpingo-oophoritis) 614.2
- **Salpingoperitonitis** (*see also* Salpingo-oophoritis) 614.2
- **Salt-losing**
  - nephritis (*see also* Disease, renal) 593.9
  - syndrome (*see also* Disease, renal) 593.9
- **Salt-rheum** (*see also* Eczema) 692.9
- **Salzmann's nodular dystrophy** 371.46
- **Sampling**
  - chorionic villus V28.89
- **Sampson's cyst or tumor** 617.1
- **Sandblasters'**
  - asthma 502
  - lung 502
- **Sander's disease** (paranoia) 297.1
- **Sandfly fever** 066.0
- **Sandhoff's disease** 330.1
- **Sanfilippo's syndrome** (mucopolysaccharidosis III) 277.5
- **Sanger-Brown's ataxia** 334.2
- **San Joaquin Valley fever** 114.0
- **Sao Paulo fever or typhus** 082.0
- **Saponification, mesenteric** 567.89
- **Sapremia** - *see* Septicemia
- **Sarcocele** (benign)
  - syphilitic 095.8
    - congenital 090.5
- **Sarcoepiplocele** (*see also* Hernia) 553.9
- **Sarcoepiplomphalocele** (*see also* Hernia, umbilicus) 553.1
- **Sarcoid** (any site) 135
  - with lung involvement 135 *[517.8]*
  - Boeck's 135
  - Darier-Roussy 135
  - Spiegler-Fendt 686.8
- **Sarcoidosis** 135
  - cardiac 135 *[425.8]*
  - lung 135 *[517.8]*
- **Sarcoma** (M8800/3) - *see also* Neoplasm, connective tissue, malignant
  - alveolar soft part (M9581/3) - *see* Neoplasm, connective tissue, malignant
  - ameloblastic (M9330/3) 170.1
    - upper jaw (bone) 170.0
  - botryoid (M8910/3) - *see* Neoplasm, connective tissue, malignant
  - botryoides (M8910/3) - *see* Neoplasm, connective tissue, malignant
  - cerebellar (M9480/3) 191.6
    - circumscribed (arachnoidal) (M9471/3) 191.6
  - circumscribed (arachnoidal) cerebellar (M9471/3) 191.6
  - clear cell, of tendons and aponeuroses (M9044/3) - *see* Neoplasm, connective tissue, malignant
  - embryonal (M8991/3) - *see* Neoplasm, connective tissue, malignant
  - endometrial (stromal) (M8930/3) 182.0
    - isthmus 182.1
  - endothelial (M9130/3) - *see also* Neoplasm, connective tissue, malignant
    - bone (M9260/3) - *see* Neoplasm, bone, malignant
  - epithelioid cell (M8804/3) - *see* Neoplasm, connective tissue, malignant
  - Ewing's (M9260/3) - *see* Neoplasm, bone, malignant
  - follicular dendritic cell 202.9 5th
  - germinoblastic (diffuse) (M9632/3) 202.8 5th
    - follicular (M9697/3) 202.0 5th
  - giant cell (M8802/3) - *see also* Neoplasm, connective tissue, malignant
    - bone (M9250/3) - *see* Neoplasm, bone, malignant
  - glomoid (M8710/3) - *see* Neoplasm, connective tissue, malignant
  - granulocytic (M9930/3) 205.3 5th
  - hemangioendothelial (M9130/3) - *see* Neoplasm, connective tissue, malignant
  - hemorrhagic, multiple (M9140/3) - *see* Kaposi's, sarcoma
  - Hodgkin's (M9662/3) 201.2 5th
  - immunoblastic (M9612/3) 200.8 5th
  - interdigitating dendritic cell 202.9 5th
  - Kaposi's (M9140/3) - *see* Kaposi's, sarcoma
  - Kupffer cell (M9124/3) 155.0
  - Langerhans cell 202.9 5th
  - leptomeningeal (M9530/3) - *see* Neoplasm, meninges, malignant
  - lymphangioendothelial (M9170/3) - *see* Neoplasm, connective tissue, malignant
  - lymphoblastic (M9630/3) 200.1 5th
  - lymphocytic (M9620/3) 200.1 5th
  - mast cell (M9740/3) 202.6 5th
  - melanotic (M8720/3) - *see* Melanoma
  - meningeal (M9530/3) - *see* Neoplasm, meninges, malignant
  - meningothelial (M9530/3) - *see* Neoplasm, meninges, malignant
  - mesenchymal (M8800/3) - *see also* Neoplasm, connective tissue, malignant
    - mixed (M8990/3) - *see* Neoplasm, connective tissue, malignant
  - mesothelial (M9050/3) - *see* Neoplasm, by site, malignant

Rupture, ruptured – Sarcoma

Sarcoma – *continued*
- monstrocellular (M9481/3)
  - specified site - *see* Neoplasm, by site, malignant
  - unspecified site 191.9
- myeloid (M9930/3) 205.3 [5th]
- neurogenic (M9540/3) - *see* Neoplasm, connective tissue, malignant
- odontogenic (M9270/3) 170.1
  - upper jaw (bone) 170.0
- osteoblastic (M9180/3) - *see* Neoplasm, bone, malignant
- osteogenic (M9180/3) - *see also* Neoplasm, bone, malignant
  - juxtacortical (M9190/3) - *see* Neoplasm, bone, malignant
  - periosteal (M9190/3) - *see* Neoplasm, bone, malignant
- periosteal (M8812/3) - *see also* Neoplasm, bone, malignant
  - osteogenic (M9190/3) - *see* Neoplasm, bone, malignant
- plasma cell (M9731/3) 203.8 [5th]
- pleomorphic cell (M8802/3) - *see* Neoplasm, connective tissue, malignant
- reticuloendothelial (M9720/3) 202.3 [5th]
- reticulum cell (M9640/3) 200.0 [5th]
  - nodular (M9642/3) 200.0 [5th]
  - pleomorphic cell type (M9641/3) 200.0 [5th]
- round cell (M8803/3) - *see* Neoplasm, connective tissue, malignant
- small cell (M8803/3) - *see* Neoplasm, connective tissue, malignant
- spindle cell (M8801/3) - *see* Neoplasm, connective tissue, malignant
- stromal (endometrial) (M8930/3) 182.0
  - isthmus 182.1
- synovial (M9040/3) - *see also* Neoplasm, connective tissue, malignant
  - biphasic type (M9043/3) - *see* Neoplasm, connective tissue, malignant
  - epithelioid cell type (M9042/3) - *see* Neoplasm, connective tissue, malignant
  - spindle cell type (M9041/3) - *see* Neoplasm, connective tissue, malignant

Sarcomatosis
- meningeal (M9539/3) - *see* Neoplasm, meninges, malignant
- specified site NEC (M8800/3) - *see* Neoplasm, connective tissue, malignant
- unspecified site (M8800/6) 171.9

Sarcosinemia 270.8

Sarcosporidiosis 136.5

Satiety, early 780.94

Satisfactory smear but lacking transformation zone
- anal 796.77
- cervical 795.07

Saturnine - *see* condition

Saturnism 984.9
- specified type of lead - *see* Table of Drugs and Chemicals

Satyriasis 302.89

Sauriasis - *see* Ichthyosis

Sauriderma 757.39

Sauriosis - *see* Ichthyosis

Savill's disease (epidemic exfoliative dermatitis) 695.89

SBE (subacute bacterial endocarditis) 421.0

Scabies (any site) 133.0

Scabs 782.8

Scaglietti-Dagnini syndrome (acromegalic macrospondylitis) 253.0

Scald, scalded - *see also* Burn, by site
- skin syndrome 695.81

Scalenus anticus (anterior) **syndrome** 353.0

Scales 782.8

Scalp - *see* condition

Scaphocephaly 756.0

Scaphoiditis, tarsal 732.5

Scapulalgia 733.90

Scapulohumeral myopathy 359.1

Scar, scarring (*see also* Cicatrix) 709.2
- adherent 709.2
- atrophic 709.2
- cervix
  - in pregnancy or childbirth 654.6 [5th]
    - affecting fetus or newborn 763.89
    - causing obstructed labor 660.2 [5th]
      - affecting fetus or newborn 763.1
- cheloid 701.4
- chorioretinal 363.30
  - disseminated 363.35
  - macular 363.32
  - peripheral 363.34
  - posterior pole NEC 363.33
- choroid (*see also* Scar, chorioretinal) 363.30
- compression, pericardial 423.9
- congenital 757.39
- conjunctiva 372.64
- cornea 371.00
  - xerophthalmic 264.6
- due to previous cesarean delivery, complicating pregnancy or childbirth 654.2 [5th]
  - affecting fetus or newborn 763.89
- duodenal (bulb) (cap) 537.3
- hypertrophic 701.4
- keloid 701.4
- labia 624.4
- lung (base) 518.89
- macula 363.32
  - disseminated 363.35
  - peripheral 363.34
- muscle 728.89
- myocardium, myocardial 412
- painful 709.2
- papillary muscle 429.81
- posterior pole NEC 363.33
  - macular - *see* Scar, macula
- postnecrotic (hepatic) (liver) 571.9
- psychic V15.49
- retina (*see also* Scar, chorioretinal) 363.30
- trachea 478.9
- uterus 621.8
  - in pregnancy or childbirth NEC 654.9 [5th]
    - affecting fetus or newborn 763.89
    - from previous cesarean delivery 654.2 [5th]
- vulva 624.4

Scarabiasis 134.1

Scarlatina 034.1
- anginosa 034.1
- maligna 034.1
- myocarditis, acute 034.1 *[422.0]*
  - old (*see also* Myocarditis) 429.0
- otitis media 034.1 *[382.02]*
- ulcerosa 034.1

Scarlatinella 057.8

Scarlet fever (albuminuria) (angina) (convulsions) (lesions of lid) (rash) 034.1

Schamberg's disease, dermatitis, or dermatosis (progressive pigmentary dermatosis) 709.09

Schatzki's ring (esophagus) (lower) (congenital) 750.3
- acquired 530.3

Schaufenster krankheit 413.9

Schaumann's
- benign lymphogranulomatosis 135
- disease (sarcoidosis) 135
- syndrome (sarcoidosis) 135

Scheie's syndrome (mucopolysaccharidosis IS) 277.5

Schenck's disease (sporotrichosis) 117.1

Scheuermann's disease or osteochondrosis 732.0

Scheuthauer-Marie-Sainton syndrome (cleidocranialis dysostosis) 755.59

Schilder (-Flatau) disease 341.1

Schilling-type monocytic leukemia (M9890/3) 206.9 [5th]

Schimmelbusch's disease, cystic mastitis, or hyperplasia 610.1

Schirmer's syndrome (encephalocutaneous angiomatosis) 759.6

Schistocelia 756.79

Schistoglossia 750.13

Schistosoma infestation - *see* Infestation, Schistosoma

Schistosomiasis 120.9
- Asiatic 120.2
- bladder 120.0
- chestermani 120.8
- colon 120.1
- cutaneous 120.3
- due to
  - S. hematobium 120.0
  - S. japonicum 120.2
  - S. mansoni 120.1
  - S. mattheii 120.8
- eastern 120.2
- genitourinary tract 120.0
- intestinal 120.1
- lung 120.2
- Manson's (intestinal) 120.1
- Oriental 120.2
- pulmonary 120.2
- specified type NEC 120.8
- vesical 120.0

Schizencephaly 742.4

Schizo-affective psychosis (*see also* Schizophrenia) 295.7 [5th]

Schizodontia 520.2

Schizoid personality 301.20
- introverted 301.21
- schizotypal 301.22

Schizophrenia, schizophrenic (reaction) 295.9 [5th]

Note *Use the following fifth-digit subclassification with category 295:*

0	unspecified
1	subchronic
2	chronic
3	subchronic with acute exacerbation
4	chronic with acute exacerbation
5	in remission

- acute (attack) NEC 295.8 [5th]
  - episode 295.4 [5th]
- atypical form 295.8 [5th]
- borderline 295.5 [5th]
- catalepsy 295.2 [5th]
- catatonic (type) (acute) (excited) (withdrawn) 295.2 [5th]
- childhood (type) (*see also* Psychosis, childhood) 299.9 [5th]
- chronic NEC 295.6 [5th]
- coenesthesiopathic 295.8 [5th]
- cyclic (type) 295.7 [5th]
- disorganized (type) 295.1 [5th]
- flexibilitas cerea 295.2 [5th]
- hebephrenic (type) (acute) 295.1 [5th]
- incipient 295.5 [5th]
- latent 295.5 [5th]
- paranoid (type) (acute) 295.3 [5th]
- paraphrenic (acute) 295.3 [5th]
- prepsychotic 295.5 [5th]
- primary (acute) 295.0 [5th]
- prodromal 295.5 [5th]
- pseudoneurotic 295.5 [5th]
- pseudopsychopathic 295.5 [5th]
- reaction 295.9 [5th]
- residual type (state) 295.6 [5th]
- restzustand 295.6 [5th]
- schizo-affective (type) (depressed) (excited) 295.7 [5th]
- schizophreniform type 295.4 [5th]
- simple (type) (acute) 295.0 [5th]
- simplex (acute) 295.0 [5th]
- specified type NEC 295.8 [5th]

Schizophrenia, schizophrenic – *continued*
- syndrome of childhood NEC (*see also* Psychosis, childhood) 299.9 [5th]
- undifferentiated type 295.9 [5th]
  - acute 295.8 [5th]
  - chronic 295.6 [5th]

Schizothymia 301.20
- introverted 301.21
- schizotypal 301.22

Schlafkrankheit 086.5

Schlatter's tibia (osteochondrosis) 732.4

Schlatter-Osgood disease (osteochondrosis, tibial tubercle) 732.4

Schloffer's tumor (*see also* Peritonitis) 567.29

Schmidt's syndrome
- sphallo-pharyngo-laryngeal hemiplegia 352.6
- thyroid-adrenocortical insufficiency 258.1
- vagoaccessory 352.6

Schmincke
- carcinoma (M8082/3) - *see* Neoplasm, nasopharynx, malignant
- tumor (M8082/3) - *see* Neoplasm, nasopharynx, malignant

Schmitz (-Stutzer) dysentery 004.0

Schmorl's disease or nodes 722.30
- lumbar, lumbosacral 722.32
- specified region NEC 722.39
- thoracic, thoracolumbar 722.31

Schneider's syndrome 047.9

Schneiderian
- carcinoma (M8121/3)
  - specified site - *see* Neoplasm, by site, malignant
  - unspecified site 160.0
- papilloma (M8121/0)
  - specified site - *see* Neoplasm, by site, benign
  - unspecified site 212.0

Schnitzler syndrome 273.1

Schoffer's tumor (*see also* Peritonitis) 567.29

Scholte's syndrome (malignant carcinoid) 259.2

Scholz's disease 330.0

Scholz (-Bielschowsky-Henneberg) syndrome 330.0

Schönlein (-Henoch) disease (primary) (purpura) (rheumatic) 287.0

School examination V70.3
- following surgery V67.09 ●

Schottmüller's disease (*see also* Fever, paratyphoid) 002.9

Schroeder's syndrome (endocrine-hypertensive) 255.3

Schüller-Christian disease or syndrome (chronic histiocytosis X) 277.89

Schultz's disease or syndrome (agranulocytosis) 288.09

Schultze's acroparesthesia, simple 443.89

Schwalbe-Ziehen-Oppenheimer disease 333.6

Schwannoma (M9560/0) - *see also* Neoplasm, connective tissues, benign
- malignant (M9560/3) - *see* Neoplasm, connective tissue, malignant

Schwartz (-Jampel) syndrome 359.23

Schwartz-Bartter syndrome (inappropriate secretion of antidiuretic hormone) 253.6

Schweninger-Buzzi disease (macular atrophy) 701.3

Sciatic - *see* condition

Sciatica (infectional) 724.3
- due to
  - displacement of intervertebral disc 722.10
  - herniation, nucleus pulposus 722.10
- wallet 724.3

Scimitar syndrome (anomalous venous drainage, right lung to inferior vena cava) 747.49

Sclera - *see* condition

Sclerectasia 379.11

- **Scleredema**
  - adultorum 710.1
  - Buschke's 710.1
  - newborn 778.1
- **Sclerema**
  - adiposum (newborn) 778.1
  - adultorum 710.1
  - edematosum (newborn) 778.1
  - neonatorum 778.1
  - newborn 778.1
- **Scleriasis** - *see* Scleroderma
- **Scleritis** 379.00
  - with corneal involvement 379.05
  - anterior (annular) (localized) 379.03
  - brawny 379.06
  - granulomatous 379.09
  - posterior 379.07
  - specified NEC 379.09
  - suppurative 379.09
  - syphilitic 095.0
  - tuberculous (nodular) (*see also* Tuberculosis) 017.3 [5th] *[379.09]*
- **Sclerochoroiditis** (*see also* Scleritis) 379.00
- **Scleroconjunctivitis** (*see also* Scleritis) 379.00
- **Sclerocystic ovary** (syndrome) 256.4
- **Sclerodactylia** 701.0
- **Scleroderma, sclerodermia** (acrosclerotic) (diffuse) (generalized) (progressive) (pulmonary) 710.1
  - circumscribed 701.0
  - linear 701.0
  - localized (linear) 701.0
  - newborn 778.1
- **Sclerokeratitis** 379.05
  - meaning sclerosing keratitis 370.54
  - tuberculous (*see also* Tuberculosis) 017.3 [5th] *[379.09]*
- **Scleroma, trachea** 040.1
- **Scleromalacia**
  - multiple 731.0
  - perforans 379.04
- **Scleromyxedema** 701.8
- **Scleroperikeratitis** 379.05
- **Sclerose en plaques** 340
- **Sclerosis, sclerotic**
  - adrenal (gland) 255.8
  - Alzheimer's 331.0
    - with dementia - *see* Alzheimer's, dementia
  - amyotrophic (lateral) 335.20
  - annularis fibrosi
    - aortic 424.1
    - mitral 424.0
  - aorta, aortic 440.0
    - valve (*see also* Endocarditis, aortic) 424.1
  - artery, arterial, arteriolar, arteriovascular - *see* Arteriosclerosis
  - ascending multiple 340
  - Baló's (concentric) 341.1
  - basilar - *see* Sclerosis, brain
  - bone (localized) NEC 733.99
  - brain (general) (lobular) 348.89 ▲
    - Alzheimer's - *see* Alzheimer's, dementia
    - artery, arterial 437.0
    - atrophic lobar 331.0
      - with dementia
        - with behavioral disturbance 331.0 *[294.11]*
        - without behavioral disturbance 331.0 *[294.10]*
    - diffuse 341.1
      - familial (chronic) (infantile) 330.0
      - infantile (chronic) (familial) 330.0
      - Pelizaeus-Merzbacher type 330.0
    - disseminated 340
    - hereditary 334.2
    - hippocampal 348.81 ●
    - infantile (degenerative) (diffuse) 330.0
    - insular 340
    - Krabbe's 330.0
    - mesial temporal 348.81 ●
    - miliary 340

Sclerosis, sclerotic – *continued*
  - brain – *continued*
    - multiple 340
    - Pelizaeus-Merzbacher 330.0
    - progressive familial 330.0
    - senile 437.0
    - temporal 348.81 ●
      - mesial 348.81 ●
    - tuberous 759.5
  - bulbar, progressive 340
  - bundle of His 426.50
    - left 426.3
    - right 426.4
  - cardiac - *see* Arteriosclerosis, coronary
  - cardiorenal (*see also* Hypertension, cardiorenal) 404.90
  - cardiovascular (*see also* Disease, cardiovascular) 429.2
    - renal (*see also* Hypertension, cardiorenal) 404.90
  - centrolobar, familial 330.0
  - cerebellar - *see* Sclerosis, brain
  - cerebral - *see* Sclerosis, brain
  - cerebrospinal 340
    - disseminated 340
    - multiple 340
  - cerebrovascular 437.0
  - choroid 363.40
    - diffuse 363.56
  - combined (spinal cord) - *see also* Degeneration, combined
    - multiple 340
  - concentric, Balo's 341.1
  - cornea 370.54
  - coronary (artery) - *see* Arteriosclerosis, coronary
  - corpus cavernosum
    - female 624.8
    - male 607.89
  - Dewitzky's
    - aortic 424.1
    - mitral 424.0
  - diffuse NEC 341.1
  - disease, heart - *see* Arteriosclerosis, coronary
  - disseminated 340
  - dorsal 340
  - dorsolateral (spinal cord) - *see* Degeneration, combined
  - endometrium 621.8
  - extrapyramidal 333.90
  - eye, nuclear (senile) 366.16
  - Friedreich's (spinal cord) 334.0
  - funicular (spermatic cord) 608.89
  - gastritis 535.4 [5th]
  - general (vascular) - *see* Arteriosclerosis
  - gland (lymphatic) 457.8
  - hepatic 571.9
  - hereditary
    - cerebellar 334.2
    - spinal 334.0
  - hippocampal 348.81 ●
  - idiopathic cortical (Garre's) (*see also* Osteomyelitis) 730.1 [5th]
  - ilium, piriform 733.5
  - insular 340
    - pancreas 251.8
  - Islands of Langerhans 251.8
  - kidney - *see* Sclerosis, renal
  - larynx 478.79
  - lateral 335.24
    - amyotrophic 335.20
    - descending 335.24
    - primary 335.24
    - spinal 335.24
  - liver 571.9
  - lobar, atrophic (of brain) 331.0
    - with dementia
      - with behavioral disturbance 331.0 *[294.11]*
      - without behavioral disturbance 331.0 *[294.10]*
  - lung (*see also* Fibrosis, lung) 515
  - mastoid 383.1

Sclerosis, sclerotic – *continued*
  - mesial temporal 348.81 ●
  - mitral - *see* Endocarditis, mitral
  - Mönckeberg's (medial) (*see also* Arteriosclerosis, extremities) 440.20
  - multiple (brain stem) (cerebral) (generalized) (spinal cord) 340
  - myocardium, myocardial - *see* Arteriosclerosis, coronary
  - nuclear (senile), eye 366.16
  - ovary 620.8
  - pancreas 577.8
  - penis 607.89
  - peripheral arteries (*see also* Arteriosclerosis, extremities) 440.20
  - plaques 340
  - pluriglandular 258.8
  - polyglandular 258.8
  - posterior (spinal cord) (syphilitic) 094.0
  - posterolateral (spinal cord) - *see* Degeneration, combined
  - prepuce 607.89
  - primary lateral 335.24
  - progressive systemic 710.1
  - pulmonary (*see also* Fibrosis, lung) 515
    - artery 416.0
    - valve (heart) (*see also* Endocarditis, pulmonary) 424.3
  - renal 587
    - with
      - cystine storage disease 270.0
      - hypertension (*see also* Hypertension, kidney) 403.90
      - hypertensive heart disease (conditions classifiable to 402) (*see also* Hypertension, cardiorenal) 404.90
    - arteriolar (hyaline) (*see also* Hypertension, kidney) 403.90
      - hyperplastic (*see also* Hypertension, kidney) 403.90
  - retina (senile) (vascular) 362.17
  - rheumatic
    - aortic valve 395.9
    - mitral valve 394.9
  - Schilder's 341.1
  - senile - *see* Arteriosclerosis
  - spinal (cord) (general) (progressive) (transverse) 336.8
    - ascending 357.0
    - combined - *see also* Degeneration, combined
      - multiple 340
      - syphilitic 094.89
    - disseminated 340
    - dorsolateral - *see* Degeneration, combined
    - hereditary (Friedreich's) (mixed form) 334.0
    - lateral (amyotrophic) 335.24
    - multiple 340
    - posterior (syphilitic) 094.0
  - stomach 537.89
  - subendocardial, congenital 425.3
  - systemic (progressive) 710.1
    - with lung involvement 710.1 *[517.2]*
  - temporal 348.81 ●
    - mesial 348.81 ●
  - tricuspid (heart) (valve) - *see* Endocarditis, tricuspid
  - tuberous (brain) 759.5
  - tympanic membrane (*see also* Tympanosclerosis) 385.00
  - valve, valvular (heart) - *see* Endocarditis
  - vascular - *see* Arteriosclerosis
  - vein 459.89
- **Sclerotenonitis** 379.07
- **Sclerotitis** (*see also* Scleritis) 379.00
  - syphilitic 095.0
  - tuberculous (*see also* Tuberculosis) 017.3 [5th] *[379.09]*
- **Scoliosis** (acquired) (postural) 737.30
  - congenital 754.2

Scoliosis – *continued*
  - due to or associated with
    - Charcôt-Marie-Tooth disease 356.1 *[737.43]*
    - mucopolysaccharidosis 277.5 *[737.43]*
    - neurofibromatosis 237.71 *[737.43]*
    - osteitis
      - deformans 731.0 *[737.43]*
      - fibrosa cystica 252.01 *[737.43]*
    - osteoporosis (*see also* Osteoporosis) 733.00 *[737.43]*
    - poliomyelitis 138 *[737.43]*
    - radiation 737.33
    - tuberculosis (*see also* Tuberculosis) 015.0 [5th] *[737.43]*
  - idiopathic 737.30
    - infantile
      - progressive 737.32
      - resolving 737.31
  - paralytic 737.39
  - rachitic 268.1
  - sciatic 724.3
  - specified NEC 737.39
  - thoracogenic 737.34
  - tuberculous (*see also* Tuberculosis) 015.0 [5th] *[737.43]*
- **Scoliotic pelvis** 738.6
  - with disproportion (fetopelvic) 653.0 [5th]
    - affecting fetus or newborn 763.1
    - causing obstructed labor 660.1 [5th]
      - affecting fetus or newborn 763.1
- **Scorbutus, scorbutic** 267
  - anemia 281.8
- **Scotoma** (ring) 368.44
  - arcuate 368.43
  - Bjerrum 368.43
  - blind spot area 368.42
  - central 368.41
  - centrocecal 368.41
  - paracecal 368.42
  - paracentral 368.41
  - scintillating 368.12
  - Seidel 368.43
- **Scratch** - *see* Injury, superficial, by site
- **Scratchy throat** 784.99
- **Screening** (for) V82.9
  - alcoholism V79.1
  - anemia, deficiency NEC V78.1
    - iron V78.0
  - anomaly, congenital V82.89
  - antenatal, of mother V28.9
    - alphafetoprotein levels, raised V28.1
    - based on amniocentesis V28.2
      - chromosomal anomalies V28.0
      - raised alphafetoprotein levels V28.1
    - fetal growth retardation using ultrasonics V28.4
    - genomic V28.89
    - isoimmunization V28.5
    - malformations using ultrasonics V28.3
    - proteomic V28.89
    - raised alphafetoprotein levels V28.1
    - risk
      - pre-term labor V28.82
    - specified condition NEC V28.89
    - Streptococcus B V28.6
  - arterial hypertension V81.1
  - arthropod-borne viral disease NEC V73.5
  - asymptomatic bacteriuria V81.5
  - bacterial
    - and spirochetal sexually transmitted diseases V74.5
    - conjunctivitis V74.4
    - disease V74.9
      - sexually transmitted V74.5
      - specified condition NEC V74.8
  - bacteriuria, asymptomatic V81.5
  - blood disorder NEC V78.9
    - specified type NEC V78.8
  - bronchitis, chronic V81.3
  - brucellosis V74.8
  - cancer - *see* Screening, malignant neoplasm
  - cardiovascular disease NEC V81.2

- **Screening** (for) – *continued*
  - cataract V80.2
  - Chagas' disease V75.3
  - chemical poisoning V82.5
  - cholera V74.0
  - cholesterol level V77.91
  - chromosomal
    - anomalies
      - by amniocentesis, antenatal V28.0
      - maternal postnatal V82.4
    - athletes V70.3
  - condition
    - cardiovascular NEC V81.2
    - eye NEC V80.2
    - genitourinary NEC V81.6
    - neurological <u>NEC</u> V80.0<u>9</u> ▲
    - respiratory NEC V81.4
    - skin V82.0
    - specified NEC V82.89
  - congenital
    - anomaly V82.89
      - eye V80.2
    - dislocation of hip V82.3
    - eye condition or disease V80.2
  - conjunctivitis, bacterial V74.4
  - contamination NEC (*see also* Poisoning) V82.5
  - coronary artery disease V81.0
  - cystic fibrosis V77.6
  - deficiency anemia NEC V78.1
    - iron V78.0
  - dengue fever V73.5
  - depression V79.0
  - developmental handicap V79.9
    - in early childhood V79.3
    - specified type NEC V79.8
  - diabetes mellitus V77.1
  - diphtheria V74.3
  - disease or disorder V82.9
    - bacterial V74.9
      - specified NEC V74.8
    - blood V78.9
      - specified type NEC V78.8
    - blood-forming organ V78.9
      - specified type NEC V78.8
    - cardiovascular NEC V81.2
      - hypertensive V81.1
      - ischemic V81.0
    - Chagas' V75.3
    - chlamydial V73.98
      - specified NEC V73.88
    - ear NEC V80.3
    - endocrine NEC V77.99
    - eye NEC V80.2
    - genitourinary NEC V81.6
    - heart NEC V81.2
      - hypertensive V81.1
      - ischemic V81.0
    - HPV (human papillomavirus) V73.81
    - human papillomavirus (HPV) V73.81
    - immunity NEC V77.99
    - infectious NEC V75.9
    - lipoid NEC V77.91
    - mental V79.9
      - specified type NEC V79.8
    - metabolic NEC V77.99
      - inborn NEC V77.7
    - neurological <u>NEC</u> V80.0<u>9</u> ▲
    - nutritional NEC V77.99
    - rheumatic NEC V82.2
    - rickettsial V75.0
    - sexually transmitted V74.5
      - bacterial V74.5
      - spirochetal V74.5
    - sickle-cell V78.2
      - trait V78.2
    - specified type NEC V82.89
    - thyroid V77.0
    - vascular NEC V81.2
      - ischemic V81.0
    - venereal V74.5
    - viral V73.99
      - arthropod-borne NEC V73.5
      - specified type NEC V73.89
  - dislocation of hip, congenital V82.3
  - drugs in athletes V70.3
  - elevated titer V82.9
  - emphysema (chronic) V81.3
  - encephalitis, viral (mosquito or tick borne) V73.5
  - endocrine disorder NEC V77.99
  - eye disorder NEC V80.2
    - congenital V80.2
  - fever
    - dengue V73.5
    - hemorrhagic V73.5
    - yellow V73.4
  - filariasis V75.6
  - galactosemia V77.4
  - genetic V82.79
    - disease carrier status V82.71
  - genitourinary condition NEC V81.6
  - glaucoma V80.1
  - gonorrhea V74.5
  - gout V77.5
  - Hansen's disease V74.2
  - heart disease NEC V81.2
    - hypertensive V81.1
    - ischemic V81.0
  - heavy metal poisoning V82.5
  - helminthiasis, intestinal V75.7
  - hematopoietic malignancy V76.89
  - hemoglobinopathies NEC V78.3
  - hemorrhagic fever V73.5
  - Hodgkin's disease V76.89
  - hormones in athletes V70.3
  - HPV (human papillomavirus) V73.81
  - human papillomavirus (HPV) V73.81
  - hypercholesterolemia V77.91
  - hyperlipdemia V77.91
  - hypertension V81.1
  - immunity disorder NEC V77.99
  - inborn errors of metabolism NEC V77.7
  - infection
    - bacterial V74.9
      - specified type NEC V74.8
    - mycotic V75.4
    - parasitic NEC V75.8
  - infectious disease V75.9
    - specified type NEC V75.8
  - ingestion of radioactive substance V82.5
  - intestinal helminthiasis V75.7
  - iron deficiency anemia V78.0
  - ischemic heart disease V81.0
  - lead poisoning V82.5
  - leishmaniasis V75.2
  - leprosy V74.2
  - leptospirosis V74.8
  - leukemia V76.89
  - lipoid disorder NEC V77.91
  - lymphoma V76.89
  - malaria V75.1
  - malignant neoplasm (of) V76.9
    - bladder V76.3
    - blood V76.89
    - breast V76.10
      - mammogram NEC V76.12
        - for high-risk patient V76.11
      - specified type NEC V76.19
    - cervix V76.2
    - colon V76.51
    - colorectal V76.51
    - hematopoietic system V76.89
    - intestine V76.50
      - colon V76.51
      - small V76.52
    - lung V76.0
    - lymph (glands) V76.89
    - nervous system V76.81
    - oral cavity V76.42
    - other specified neoplasm NEC V76.89
    - ovary V76.46
    - prostate V76.44
    - rectum V76.41
    - respiratory organs V76.0
    - skin V76.43
    - specified sites NEC V76.49
    - testis V76.45
    - vagina V76.47
      - following hysterectomy for malignant condition V67.01
  - malnutrition V77.2
  - mammogram NEC V76.12
    - for high-risk patient V76.11
  - maternal postnatal chromosomal anomalies V82.4
  - measles V73.2
  - mental
    - disorder V79.9
      - specified type NEC V79.8
    - retardation V79.2
  - metabolic disorder NEC V77.99
  - metabolic errors, inborn V77.7
  - mucoviscidosis V77.6
  - multiphasic V82.6
  - mycosis V75.4
  - mycotic infection V75.4
  - nephropathy V81.5
  - neurological condition <u>NEC</u> V80.0<u>9</u> ▲
  - nutritional disorder NEC V77.99
  - obesity V77.8
  - osteoporosis V82.81
  - parasitic infection NEC V75.8
  - phenylketonuria V77.3
  - plague V74.8
  - poisoning
    - chemical NEC V82.5
    - contaminated water supply V82.5
    - heavy metal V82.5
  - poliomyelitis V73.0
  - postnatal chromosomal anomalies, maternal V82.4
  - prenatal - *see* Screening, antenatal
  - pulmonary tuberculosis V74.1
  - radiation exposure V82.5
  - renal disease V81.5
  - respiratory condition NEC V81.4
  - rheumatic disorder NEC V82.2
  - rheumatoid arthritis V82.1
  - rickettsial disease V75.0
  - rubella V73.3
  - schistosomiasis V75.5
  - senile macular lesions of eye V80.2
  - sexually transmitted diseases V74.5
    - bacterial V74.5
    - spirochetal V74.5
  - sickle-cell anemia, disease, or trait V78.2
  - skin condition V82.0
  - sleeping sickness V75.3
  - smallpox V73.1
  - special V82.9
    - specified condition NEC V82.89
  - specified type NEC V82.89
  - spirochetal disease V74.9
    - sexually transmitted V74.5
    - specified type NEC V74.8
  - stimulants in athletes V70.3
  - syphilis V74.5
  - tetanus V74.8
  - thyroid disorder V77.0
  - trachoma V73.6
  - traumatic brain injury V80.01 ●
  - trypanosomiasis V75.3
  - tuberculosis, pulmonary V74.1
  - venereal disease V74.5
  - viral encephalitis
    - mosquito-borne V73.5
    - tick-borne V73.5
  - whooping cough V74.8
  - worms, intestinal V75.7
  - yaws V74.6
  - yellow fever V73.4
- **Scrofula** (*see also* Tuberculosis) 017.2 [5th]
- **Scrofulide** (primary) (*see also* Tuberculosis) 017.0 [5th]
- **Scrofuloderma, scrofulodermia** (any site) (primary) (*see also* Tuberculosis) 017.0 [5th]
- **Scrofulosis** (universal) (*see also* Tuberculosis) 017.2 [5th]
- **Scrofulosis lichen** (primary) (*see also* Tuberculosis) 017.0 [5th]
- **Scrofulous** - *see* condition
- **Scrotal tongue** 529.5
  - congenital 750.13
- **Scrotum** - *see* condition
- **Scurvy** (gum) (infantile) (rickets) (scorbutic) 267
- **Sea-blue histiocyte syndrome** 272.7
- **Seabright-Bantam syndrome** (pseudohypoparathyroidism) 275.49
- **Sealpox** 059.12
- **Seasickness** 994.6
- **Seatworm** 127.4
- **Sebaceous**
  - cyst (*see also* Cyst, sebaceous) 706.2
  - gland disease NEC 706.9
- **Sebocystomatosis** 706.2
- **Seborrhea, seborrheic** 706.3
  - adiposa 706.3
  - capitis 690.11
  - congestiva 695.4
  - corporis 706.3
  - dermatitis 690.10
    - infantile 690.12
  - diathesis in infants 695.89
  - eczema 690.18
    - infantile 690.12
  - keratosis 702.19
    - inflamed 702.11
  - nigricans 759.89
  - sicca 690.18
  - wart 702.19
    - inflamed 702.11
- **Seckel's syndrome** 759.89
- **Seclusion pupil** 364.74
- **Seclusiveness, child** 313.22
- **Secondary** - *see also* condition
  - neoplasm - *see* Neoplasm, by site, malignant, secondary
- **Secretan's disease or syndrome** (posttraumatic edema) 782.3
- **Secretion**
  - antidiuretic hormone, inappropriate (syndrome) 253.6
  - catecholamine, by pheochromocytoma 255.6
  - hormone
    - antidiuretic, inappropriate (syndrome) 253.6
    - by
      - carcinoid tumor 259.2
      - pheochromocytoma 255.6
    - ectopic NEC 259.3
  - urinary
    - excessive 788.42
    - suppression 788.5
- **Section**
  - cesarean
    - affecting fetus or newborn 763.4
    - post mortem, affecting fetus or newborn 761.6
    - previous, in pregnancy or childbirth 654.2 [5th]
      - affecting fetus or newborn 763.89
  - nerve, traumatic - *see* Injury, nerve, by site
- **Seeligmann's syndrome** (ichthyosis congenita) 757.1
- **Segmentation, incomplete** (congenital) - *see also* Fusion
  - bone NEC 756.9
  - lumbosacral (joint) 756.15
  - vertebra 756.15
    - lumbosacral 756.15
- **Seizure(s)** 780.39
  - akinetic (idiopathic) (*see also* Epilepsy) 345.0 [5th]
    - psychomotor 345.4 [5th]
  - apoplexy, apoplectic (*see also* Disease, cerebrovascular, acute) 436
  - atonic (*see also* Epilepsy) 345.0 [5th]
  - autonomic 300.11

Screening – Seizure(s)

[4th] Fourth Digit Required [5th] Fifth Digit Required | *[code]* Manifestation Code | ● New Line ▲ Revised Line <u>text</u> New Text ~~text~~ Deleted text

Seizure(s) – *continued*
- brain or cerebral (*see also* Disease, cerebrovascular, acute) 436
- convulsive (*see also* Convulsions) 780.39
- cortical (focal) (motor) (*see also* Epilepsy) 345.5 5th
- disorder (*see also* Epilepsy) 345.9 5th ●
- due to stroke 438.89
- epilepsy, epileptic (cryptogenic) (*see also* Epilepsy) 345.9 5th
- epileptiform, epileptoid 780.39
  - focal (*see also* Epilepsy) 345.5 5th
- febrile (simple) 780.31
  - with status epilepticus 345.3
  - atypical 780.32
  - complex 780.32
  - complicated 780.32
- heart - *see* Disease, heart
- hysterical 300.11
- Jacksonian (focal) (*see also* Epilepsy) 345.5 5th
  - motor type 345.5 5th
  - sensory type 345.5 5th
- migraine triggered 346.0 5th
- newborn 779.0
- paralysis (*see also* Disease, cerebrovascular, acute) 436
- recurrent 345.9 5th
  - epileptic - *see* Epilepsy
- repetitive 780.39
  - epileptic - *see* Epilepsy
- salaam (*see also* Epilepsy) 345.6 5th
- uncinate (*see also* Epilepsy) 345.4 5th

Self-mutilation 300.9

Semicoma 780.09

Semiconsciousness 780.09

Seminal
- vesicle - *see* condition
- vesiculitis (*see also* Vesiculitis) 608.0

Seminoma (M9061/3)
- anaplastic type (M9062/3)
  - specified site - *see* Neoplasm, by site, malignant
  - unspecified site 186.9
- specified site - *see* Neoplasm, by site, malignant
- spermatocytic (M9063/3)
  - specified site - *see* Neoplasm, by site, malignant
  - unspecified site 186.9
- unspecified site 186.9

Semliki Forest encephalitis 062.8

Senear-Usher disease or syndrome (pemphigus erythematosus) 694.4

Senecio jacobae dermatitis 692.6

Senectus 797

Senescence 797

Senile (*see also* condition) 797
- cervix (atrophic) 622.8
- degenerative atrophy, skin 701.3
- endometrium (atrophic) 621.8
- fallopian tube (atrophic) 620.3
- heart (failure) 797
- lung 492.8
- ovary (atrophic) 620.3
- syndrome 259.8
- vagina, vaginitis (atrophic) 627.3
- wart 702.0

Senility 797
- with
  - acute confusional state 290.3
  - delirium 290.3
  - mental changes 290.9
  - psychosis NEC (*see also* Psychosis, senile) 290.20
- premature (syndrome) 259.8

Sensation
- burning (*see also* Disturbance, sensation) 782.0
  - tongue 529.6
- choking 784.99
- loss of (*see also* Disturbance, sensation) 782.0

Sensation – *continued*
- prickling (*see also* Disturbance, sensation) 782.0
- tingling (*see also* Disturbance, sensation) 782.0

Sense loss (touch) (*see also* Disturbance, sensation) 782.0
- smell 781.1
- taste 781.1

Sensibility disturbance NEC (cortical) (deep) (vibratory) (*see also* Disturbance, sensation) 782.0

Sensitive dentine 521.89

Sensitiver Beziehungswahn 297.8

Sensitivity, sensitization - *see also* Allergy
- autoerythrocyte 287.2
- carotid sinus 337.01
- child (excessive) 313.21
- cold, autoimmune 283.0

Sensitivity, sensitization – *continued*
- methemoglobin 289.7
- suxamethonium 289.89
- tuberculin, without clinical or radiological symptoms 795.5

Sensory
- extinction 781.8
- neglect 781.8

Separation
- acromioclavicular - *see* Dislocation, acromioclavicular
- anxiety, abnormal 309.21
- apophysis, traumatic - *see* Fracture, by site
- choroid 363.70
  - hemorrhagic 363.72
  - serous 363.71
- costochondral (simple) (traumatic) - *see* Dislocation, costochondral
- delayed
  - umbilical cord 779.83
- epiphysis, epiphyseal
  - nontraumatic 732.9
    - upper femoral 732.2
  - traumatic - *see* Fracture, by site
- fracture - *see* Fracture, by site
- infundibulum cardiac from right ventricle by a partition 746.83
- joint (current) (traumatic) - *see* Dislocation, by site
- placenta (normally implanted) - *see* Placenta, separation
- pubic bone, obstetrical trauma 665.6 5th
- retina, retinal (*see also* Detachment, retina) 361.9
  - layers 362.40
    - sensory (*see also* Retinoschisis) 361.10
  - pigment epithelium (exudative) 362.42
    - hemorrhagic 362.43
- sternoclavicular (traumatic) - *see* Dislocation, sternoclavicular
- symphysis pubis, obstetrical trauma 665.6 5th
- tracheal ring, incomplete (congenital) 748.3

Sepsis (generalized) 995.91
- with
  - abortion - *see* Abortion, by type, with sepsis
  - acute organ dysfunction 995.92
  - ectopic pregnancy (*see also* categories 633.0-633.9) 639.0
  - molar pregnancy (*see also* categories 630-632) 639.0
  - multiple organ dysfunction (MOD) 995.92
- buccal 528.3
- complicating labor 659.3 5th
- dental (pulpal origin) 522.4
- female genital organ NEC 614.9
- fetus (intrauterine) 771.81
- following
  - abortion 639.0
  - ectopic or molar pregnancy 639.0

Sepsis – *continued*
- following – *continued*
  - infusion, perfusion, or transfusion 999.39
- Friedländer's 038.49
- intraocular 360.00
- localized
  - in operation wound 998.59
  - skin (*see also* Abscess) 682.9
- malleus 024
- nadir 038.9
- newborn (organism unspecified) NEC 771.81
- oral 528.3
- puerperal, postpartum, childbirth (pelvic) 670.2 5th ▲
- resulting from infusion, injection, transfusion, or vaccination 999.39
- severe 995.92
- skin, localized (*see also* Abscess) 682.9
- umbilical (newborn) (organism unspecified) 771.89
  - tetanus 771.3
- urinary 599.0
  - meaning sepsis 995.91
  - meaning urinary tract infection 599.0

Septate - *see also* Septum

Septic - *see also* condition
- adenoids 474.01
  - and tonsils 474.02
- arm (with lymphangitis) 682.3
- embolus - *see* Embolism
- finger (with lymphangitis) 681.00
- foot (with lymphangitis) 682.7
- gallbladder (*see also* Cholecystitis) 575.8
- hand (with lymphangitis) 682.4
- joint (*see also* Arthritis, septic) 711.0 5th
- kidney (*see also* Infection, kidney) 590.9
- leg (with lymphangitis) 682.6
- mouth 528.3
- nail 681.9
  - finger 681.02
  - toe 681.11
- shock (endotoxic) 785.52
- sore (*see also* Abscess) 682.9
  - throat 034.0
    - milk-borne 034.0
    - streptococcal 034.0
- spleen (acute) 289.59
- teeth (pulpal origin) 522.4
- throat 034.0
- thrombus - *see* Thrombosis
- toe (with lymphangitis) 681.10
- tonsils 474.00
  - and adenoids 474.02
- umbilical cord (newborn) (organism unspecified) 771.89
- uterus (*see also* Endometritis) 615.9

Septicemia, septicemic (generalized) (suppurative) 038.9
- with
  - abortion - *see* Abortion, by type, with sepsis
  - ectopic pregnancy (*see also* categories 633.0-633.9) 639.0
  - molar pregnancy (*see also* categories 630-632) 639.0
- Aerobacter aerogenes 038.49
- anaerobic 038.3
- anthrax 022.3
- Bacillus coli 038.42
- Bacteroides 038.3
- Clostridium 038.3
- complicating labor 659.3 5th
- cryptogenic 038.9
- enteric gram-negative bacilli 038.40
- Enterobacter aerogenes 038.49
- Erysipelothrix (insidiosa) (rhusiopathiae) 027.1
- Escherichia coli 038.42
- following
  - abortion 639.0
  - ectopic or molar pregnancy 639.0

Septicemia, septicemic – *continued*
- following – *continued*
  - infusion, injection, transfusion, or vaccination 999.39
- Friedländer's (bacillus) 038.49
- gangrenous 038.9
- gonococcal 098.89
- gram-negative (organism) 038.40
  - anaerobic 038.3
- Hemophilus influenzae 038.41
- herpes (simplex) 054.5
- herpetic 054.5
- Listeria monocytogenes 027.0
- meningeal - *see* Meningitis
- meningococcal (chronic) (fulminating) 036.2
- methicillin
  - resistant Staphylococcus aureus (MRSA) 038.12
  - susceptible Staphylococcus aureus (MSSA) 038.11
- MRSA (methicillin resistant Staphylococcus aureus) 038.12
- MSSA (methicillin susceptible Staphylococcus aureus) 038.11
- navel, newborn (organism unspecified) 771.89
- newborn (organism unspecified) 771.81
- plague 020.2
- pneumococcal 038.2
- postabortal 639.0
- postoperative 998.59
- Proteus vulgaris 038.49
- Pseudomonas (aeruginosa) 038.43
- puerperal, postpartum 670.2 5th ▲
- Salmonella (aertrycke) (callinarum) (choleraesuis) (enteritidis) (suipestifer) 003.1
- Serratia 038.44
- Shigella (*see also* Dysentery, bacillary) 004.9
- specified organism NEC 038.8
- staphylococcal 038.10
  - aureus 038.11
    - methicillin
      - resistant (MRSA) 038.12
      - susceptible (MSSA) 038.11
  - specified organism NEC 038.19
- streptococcal (anaerobic) 038.0
- Streptococcus pneumoniae 038.2
- suipestifer 003.1
- umbilicus, newborn (organism unspecified) 771.89
- viral 079.99
- Yersinia enterocolitica 038.49

Septum, septate (congenital) - *see also* Anomaly, specified type NEC
- anal 751.2
- aqueduct of Sylvius 742.3
  - with spina bifida (*see also* Spina bifida) 741.0 5th
- hymen 752.49
- uterus (*see also* Double, uterus) 752.2
- vagina 752.49
  - in pregnancy or childbirth 654.7 5th
    - affecting fetus or newborn 763.89
    - causing obstructed labor 660.2 5th
      - affecting fetus or newborn 763.1

Sequestration
- lung (congenital) (extralobar) (intralobar) 748.5
- orbit 376.10
- pulmonary artery (congenital) 747.3
- splenic 289.52

Sequestrum
- bone (*see also* Osteomyelitis) 730.1 5th
  - jaw 526.4
- dental 525.8
- jaw bone 526.4
- sinus (accessory) (nasal) (*see also* Sinusitis) 473.9
  - maxillary 473.0

Sequoiosis asthma 495.8

Seizure(s) – Sequoiosis asthma

Serology for syphilis – Short, shortening, shortness

- **Sleep** – *continued*
  - paroxysmal (*see also* Narcolepsy) 347.00
  - related movement disorder, unspecified 780.58
  - rhythm inversion 327.39
    - nonorganic origin 307.45
  - walking 307.46
    - hysterical 300.13
- **Sleeping sickness** 086.5
  - late effect 139.8
- **Sleeplessness** (*see also* Insomnia) 780.52
  - menopausal 627.2
  - nonorganic origin 307.41
- **Slipped, slipping**
  - epiphysis (postinfectional) 732.9
    - traumatic (old) 732.9
      - current - *see* Fracture, by site
    - upper femoral (nontraumatic) 732.2
  - intervertebral disc - *see* Displacement, intervertebral disc
  - ligature, umbilical 772.3
  - patella 717.89
  - rib 733.99
  - sacroiliac joint 724.6
  - tendon 727.9
  - ulnar nerve, nontraumatic 354.2
  - vertebra NEC (*see also* Spondylolisthesis) 756.12
- **Slocumb's syndrome** 255.3
- **Sloughing** (multiple) (skin) 686.9
  - abscess - *see* Abscess, by site
  - appendix 543.9
  - bladder 596.8
  - fascia 728.9
  - graft - *see* Complications, graft
  - phagedena (*see also* Gangrene) 785.4
  - reattached extremity (*see also* Complications, reattached extremity) 996.90
  - rectum 569.49
  - scrotum 608.89
  - tendon 727.9
  - transplanted organ (*see also* Rejection, transplant, organ, by site) 996.80
  - ulcer (*see also* Ulcer, skin) 707.9
- **Slow**
  - feeding newborn 779.31 ▲
  - fetal, growth NEC 764.9 [5th]
    - affecting management of pregnancy 656.5 [5th]
- **Slowing**
  - heart 427.89
  - urinary stream 788.62
- **Sluder's neuralgia or syndrome** 337.09
- **Slurred, slurring, speech** 784.59 ▲
- **Small, smallness**
  - cardia reserve - *see* Disease, heart
  - for dates
    - fetus or newborn 764.0 [5th]
      - with malnutrition 764.1
        - affecting management of pregnancy 656.5 [5th]
  - infant, term 764.0 [5th]
    - with malnutrition 764.1 [5th]
    - affecting management of pregnancy 656.5 [5th]
  - introitus, vagina 623.3
  - kidney, unknown cause 589.9
    - bilateral 589.1
    - unilateral 589.0
  - ovary 620.8
  - pelvis
    - with disproportion (fetopelvic) 653.1 [5th]
      - affecting fetus or newborn 763.1
    - causing obstructed labor 660.1 [5th]
      - affecting fetus or newborn 763.1
  - placenta - *see* Placenta, insufficiency
  - uterus 621.8
  - white kidney 582.9
- **Small-for-dates** (*see also* Light-for-dates) 764.0 [5th]
  - affecting management of pregnancy 656.5 [5th]
- **Smallpox** 050.9
  - contact V01.3
  - exposure to V01.3
  - hemorrhagic (pustular) 050.0
  - malignant 050.0
  - modified 050.2
  - vaccination
    - complications - *see* Complications, vaccination
    - prophylactic (against) V04.1
- **Smith's fracture** (separation) (closed) 813.41
  - open 813.51
- **Smith-Lemli-Opitz syndrome** (cerebrohepatorenal syndrome) 759.89
- **Smith-Magenis syndrome** 758.33
- **Smith-Strang disease** (oasthouse urine) 270.2
- **Smokers'**
  - bronchitis 491.0
  - cough 491.0
  - syndrome (*see also* Abuse, drugs, nondependent) 305.1
  - throat 472.1
  - tongue 528.6
- **Smoking complicating pregnancy, childbirth, or the puerperium** 649.0 [5th]
- **Smothering spells** 786.09
- **Snaggle teeth, tooth** 524.39
- **Snapping**
  - finger 727.05
  - hip 719.65
  - jaw 524.69
    - temporomandibular joint sounds on opening or closing 524.64
  - knee 717.9
  - thumb 727.05
- **Sneddon-Wilkinson disease or syndrome** (subcorneal pustular dermatosis) 694.1
- **Sneezing** 784.99
  - intractable 478.19
- **Sniffing**
  - cocaine (*see also* Dependence) 304.2 [5th]
  - ether (*see also* Dependence) 304.6 [5th]
  - glue (airplane) (*see also* Dependence) 304.6 [5th]
- **Snoring** 786.09
- **Snow blindness** 370.24
- **Snuffles** (nonsyphilitic) 460
  - syphilitic (infant) 090.0
- **Social migrant** V60.0
- **Sodoku** 026.0
- **Soemmering's ring** 366.51
- **Soft** - *see also* condition
  - enlarged prostate 600.00
    - with
      - other lower urinary tract symptoms (LUTS) 600.01
      - urinary
        - obstruction 600.01
        - retention 600.01
  - nails 703.8
- **Softening**
  - bone 268.2
  - brain (necrotic) (progressive) 434.9 [5th]
    - arteriosclerotic 437.0
    - congenital 742.4
    - embolic (*see also* Embolism, brain) 434.1 [5th]
    - hemorrhagic (*see also* Hemorrhage, brain) 431
    - occlusive 434.9 [5th]
    - thrombotic (*see also* Thrombosis, brain) 434.0 [5th]
  - cartilage 733.92
  - cerebellar - *see* Softening, brain
  - cerebral - *see* Softening, brain
  - cerebrospinal - *see* Softening, brain
  - myocardial, heart (*see also* Degeneration, myocardial) 429.1
  - nails 703.8
  - spinal cord 336.8
  - stomach 537.89
- **Solar fever** 061
- **Soldier's**
  - heart 306.2
  - patches 423.1
- **Solitary**
  - cyst
    - bone 733.21
    - kidney 593.2
  - kidney (congenital) 753.0
  - tubercle, brain (*see also* Tuberculosis, brain) 013.2 [5th]
  - ulcer, bladder 596.8
- **Somatization reaction, somatic reaction** (*see also* Disorder, psychosomatic) 306.9
  - disorder 300.81
- **Somatoform disorder** 300.82
  - atypical 300.82
  - severe 300.81
  - undifferentiated 300.82
- **Somnambulism** 307.46
  - hysterical 300.13
- **Somnolence** 780.09
  - nonorganic origin 307.43
  - periodic 349.89
- **Sonne dysentery** 004.3
- **Soor** 112.0
- **Sore**
  - Delhi 085.1
  - desert (*see also* Ulcer, skin) 707.9
  - eye 379.99
  - Lahore 085.1
  - mouth 528.9
    - canker 528.2
    - due to dentures 528.9
  - muscle 729.1
  - naga (*see also* Ulcer, skin) 707.9
  - oriental 085.1
  - pressure (*see also* Ulcer, pressure) 707.00
    - with gangrene (*see also* Ulcer, pressure) 707.00 *[785.4]*
  - skin NEC 709.9
  - soft 099.0
  - throat 462
    - with influenza, flu, or grippe 487.1
    - acute 462
    - chronic 472.1
    - clergyman's 784.49
    - Coxsackie (virus) 074.0
    - diphtheritic 032.0
    - epidemic 034.0
    - gangrenous 462
    - herpetic 054.79
    - influenzal 487.1
    - malignant 462
    - purulent 462
    - putrid 462
    - septic 034.0
    - streptococcal (ulcerative) 034.0
    - ulcerated 462
    - viral NEC 462
      - Coxsackie 074.0
  - tropical (*see also* Ulcer, skin) 707.9
  - veldt (*see also* Ulcer, skin) 707.9
- **Sotos' syndrome** (cerebral gigantism) 253.0
- **Sounds**
  - friction, pleural 786.7
  - succussion, chest 786.7
  - temporomandibular joint
    - on opening or closing 524.64
- **South African cardiomyopathy syndrome** 425.2
- **South American**
  - blastomycosis 116.1
  - trypanosomiasis - *see* Trypanosomiasis
- **Southeast Asian hemorrhagic fever** 065.4
- **Spacing, teeth, abnormal** 524.30
  - excessive 524.32
- **Spade-like hand** (congenital) 754.89
- **Spading nail** 703.8
  - congenital 757.5
- **Spanemia** 285.9
- **Spanish collar** 605
- **Sparganosis** 123.5
- **Spasm, spastic, spasticity** (*see also* condition) 781.0
  - accommodation 367.53
  - ampulla of Vater (*see also* Disease, gallbladder) 576.8
  - anus, ani (sphincter) (reflex) 564.6
    - psychogenic 306.4
  - artery NEC 443.9
    - basilar 435.0
    - carotid 435.8
    - cerebral 435.9
      - specified artery NEC 435.8
    - retinal (*see also* Occlusion, retinal, artery) 362.30
    - vertebral 435.1
    - vertebrobasilar 435.3
  - Bell's 351.0
  - bladder (sphincter, external or internal) 596.8
  - bowel 564.9
    - psychogenic 306.4
  - bronchus, bronchiole 519.11
  - cardia 530.0
  - cardiac - *see* Angina
  - carpopedal (*see also* Tetany) 781.7
  - cecum 564.9
    - psychogenic 306.4
  - cerebral (arteries) (vascular) 435.9
    - specified artery NEC 435.8
  - cerebrovascular 435.9
  - cervix, complicating delivery 661.4 [5th]
    - affecting fetus or newborn 763.7
  - ciliary body (of accommodation) 367.53
  - colon 564.1
    - psychogenic 306.4
  - common duct (*see also* Disease, biliary) 576.8
  - compulsive 307.22
  - conjugate 378.82
  - convergence 378.84
  - coronary (artery) - *see* Angina
  - diaphragm (reflex) 786.8
    - psychogenic 306.1
  - duodenum, duodenal (bulb) 564.89
  - esophagus (diffuse) 530.5
    - psychogenic 306.4
  - facial 351.8
  - fallopian tube 620.8
  - gait 781.2
  - gastrointestinal (tract) 536.8
    - psychogenic 306.4
  - glottis 478.75
    - hysterical 300.11
    - psychogenic 306.1
      - specified as conversion reaction 300.11
    - reflex through recurrent laryngeal nerve 478.75
  - habit 307.20
    - chronic 307.22
    - transient (of childhood) 307.21
  - heart - *see* Angina
  - hourglass - *see* Contraction, hourglass
  - hysterical 300.11
  - infantile (*see also* Epilepsy) 345.6
  - internal oblique, eye 378.51
  - intestinal 564.9
    - psychogenic 306.4
  - larynx, laryngeal 478.75
    - hysterical 300.11
    - psychogenic 306.1
      - specified as conversion reaction 300.11
  - levator palpebrae superioris 333.81
  - lightning (*see also* Epilepsy) 345.6
  - mobile 781.0
  - muscle 728.85
    - back 724.8
    - psychogenic 306.0
  - nerve, trigeminal 350.1
  - nervous 306.0
  - nodding 307.3
    - infantile (*see also* Epilepsy) 345.6 [5th]
  - occupational 300.89

Spasm, spastic, spasticity – *continued*
- oculogyric 378.87
- ophthalmic artery 362.30
- orbicularis 781.0
- perineal 625.8
- peroneo-extensor (*see also* Flat, foot) 734
- pharynx (reflex) 478.29
  - hysterical 300.11
  - psychogenic 306.1
    - specified as conversion reaction 300.11
- pregnant uterus, complicating delivery 661.4 [5th]
- psychogenic 306.0
- pylorus 537.81
  - adult hypertrophic 537.0
  - congenital or infantile 750.5
  - psychogenic 306.4
- rectum (sphincter) 564.6
  - psychogenic 306.4
- retinal artery NEC (*see also* Occlusion, retina, artery) 362.30
- sacroiliac 724.6
- salaam (infantile) (*see also* Epilepsy) 345.6 [5th]
- saltatory 781.0
- sigmoid 564.9
  - psychogenic 306.4
- sphincter of Oddi (*see also* Disease, gallbladder) 576.5
- stomach 536.8
  - neurotic 306.4
- throat 478.29
  - hysterical 300.11
  - psychogenic 306.1
    - specified as conversion reaction 300.11
- tic 307.20
  - chronic 307.22
  - transient (of childhood) 307.21
- tongue 529.8
- torsion 333.6
- trigeminal nerve 350.1
  - postherpetic 053.12
- ureter 593.89
- urethra (sphincter) 599.84
- uterus 625.8
  - complicating labor 661.4 [5th]
    - affecting fetus or newborn 763.7
- vagina 625.1
  - psychogenic 306.51
- vascular NEC 443.9
- vasomotor NEC 443.9
- vein NEC 459.89
- vesical (sphincter, external or internal) 596.8
- viscera 789.0 [5th]

Spasmodic - *see* condition
Spasmophilia (*see also* Tetany) 781.7
Spasmus nutans 307.3
Spastic - *see also* Spasm
- child 343.9

Spasticity - *see also* Spasm
- cerebral, child 343.9

Speakers' throat 784.49
Specific, specified - *see* condition
Speech
- defect, disorder, disturbance, impediment NEC 784.59 ▲
  - psychogenic 307.9
- (language) therapy V57.3 ▲

Spells 780.39
- breath-holding 786.9

Spencer's disease (epidemic vomiting) 078.82
Spens' syndrome (syncope with heart block) 426.9
Spermatic cord - *see* condition
Spermatocele 608.1
- congenital 752.89

Spermatocystitis 608.4
Spermatocytoma (M9063/3)
- specified site - *see* Neoplasm, by site, malignant
- unspecified site 186.9

Spermatorrhea 608.89
Sperm counts
- fertility testing V26.21
- following sterilization reversal V26.22
- postvasectomy V25.8

Sphacelus (*see also* Gangrene) 785.4
Sphenoidal - *see* condition
Sphenoiditis (chronic) (*see also* Sinusitis, sphenoidal) 473.3
Sphenopalatine ganglion neuralgia 337.09
Sphericity, increased, lens 743.36
Spherocytosis (congenital) (familial) (hereditary) 282.0
- hemoglobin disease 282.7
- sickle-cell (disease) 282.60

Spherophakia 743.36
Sphincter - *see* condition
Sphincteritis, sphincter of Oddi (*see also* Cholecystitis) 576.8
Sphingolipidosis 272.7
Sphingolipodystrophy 272.7
Sphingomyelinosis 272.7
Spicule tooth 520.2
Spider
- finger 755.59
- nevus 448.1
- vascular 448.1

Spiegler-Fendt sarcoid 686.8
Spielmeyer-Stock disease 330.1
Spielmeyer-Vogt disease 330.1
Spina bifida (aperta) 741.9 [5th]

Note *Use the following fifth-digit subclassification with category 741:*

0	unspecified region
1	cervical region
2	dorsal [thoracic] region
3	lumbar region

- with hydrocephalus 741.0 [5th]
- fetal (suspected), affecting management of pregnancy 655.0 [5th]
- occulta 756.17

Spindle, Krukenberg's 371.13
Spine, spinal - *see* condition
Spiradenoma (eccrine) (M8403/0) - *see* Neoplasm, skin, benign
Spirillosis NEC (*see also* Fever, relapsing) 087.9
Spirillum minus 026.0
Spirillum obermeieri infection 087.0
Spirochetal - *see* condition
Spirochetosis 104.9
- arthritic, arthritica 104.9 *[711.8]* [5th]
- bronchopulmonary 104.8
- icterohemorrhagica 100.0
- lung 104.8

Spitting blood (*see also* Hemoptysis) 786.3
Splanchnomegaly 569.89
Splanchnoptosis 569.89
Spleen, splenic - *see also* condition
- agenesis 759.0
- flexure syndrome 569.89
- neutropenia syndrome 289.53
- sequestration syndrome 289.52

Splenectasis (*see also* Splenomegaly) 789.2
Splenitis (interstitial) (malignant) (nonspecific) 289.59
- malarial (*see also* Malaria) 084.6
- tuberculous (*see also* Tuberculosis) 017.7 [5th]

Splenocele 289.59
Splenomegalia - *see* Splenomegaly
Splenomegalic - *see* condition
Splenomegaly 789.2
- Bengal 789.2
- cirrhotic 289.51
- congenital 759.0
- congestive, chronic 289.51
- cryptogenic 789.2

Splenomegaly – *continued*
- Egyptian 120.1
- Gaucher's (cerebroside lipidosis) 272.7
- idiopathic 789.2
- malarial (*see also* Malaria) 084.6
- neutropenic 289.53
- Niemann-Pick (lipid histiocytosis) 272.7
- siderotic 289.51
- syphilitic 095.8
  - congenital 090.0
- tropical (Bengal) (idiopathic) 789.2

Splenopathy 289.50
Splenopneumonia - *see* Pneumonia
Splenoptosis 289.59
Splinter - *see* Injury, superficial, by site
Split, splitting
- heart sounds 427.89
- lip, congenital (*see also* Cleft, lip) 749.10
- nails 703.8
- urinary stream 788.61

Spoiled child reaction (*see also* Disturbance, conduct) 312.1 [5th]
Spondylarthritis (*see also* Spondylosis) 721.90
Spondylarthrosis (*see also* Spondylosis) 721.90
Spondylitis 720.9
- ankylopoietica 720.0
- ankylosing (chronic) 720.0
- atrophic 720.9
  - ligamentous 720.9
- chronic (traumatic) (*see also* Spondylosis) 721.90
- deformans (chronic) (*see also* Spondylosis) 721.90
- gonococcal 098.53
- gouty 274.00 ▲
- hypertrophic (*see also* Spondylosis) 721.90
- infectious NEC 720.9
- juvenile (adolescent) 720.0
- Kummell's 721.7
- Marie-Strümpell (ankylosing) 720.0
- muscularis 720.9
- ossificans ligamentosa 721.6
- osteoarthritica (*see also* Spondylosis) 721.90
- posttraumatic 721.7
- proliferative 720.0
- rheumatoid 720.0
- rhizomelica 720.0
- sacroiliac NEC 720.2
- senescent (*see also* Spondylosis) 721.90
- senile (*see also* Spondylosis) 721.90
- static (*see also* Spondylosis) 721.90
- traumatic (chronic) (*see also* Spondylosis) 721.90
- tuberculous (*see also* Tuberculosis) 015.0 [5th] *[720.81]*
- typhosa 002.0 *[720.81]*

Spondyloarthrosis (*see also* Spondylosis) 721.90
Spondylolisthesis (congenital) (lumbosacral) 756.12
- with disproportion (fetopelvic) 653.3 [5th]
  - affecting fetus or newborn 763.1
  - causing obstructed labor 660.1 [5th]
    - affecting fetus or newborn 763.1
- acquired 738.4
- degenerative 738.4
- traumatic 738.4
  - acute (lumbar) - *see* Fracture, vertebra, lumbar
    - site other than lumbosacral - *see* Fracture, vertebra, by site

Spondylolysis (congenital) 756.11
- acquired 738.4
- cervical 756.19
- lumbosacral region 756.11
  - with disproportion (fetopelvic) 653.3 [5th]
    - affecting fetus or newborn 763.1
    - causing obstructed labor 660.1 [5th]
      - affecting fetus or newborn 763.1

Spondylopathy
- inflammatory 720.9
  - specified type NEC 720.89
- traumatic 721.7

Spondylose rhizomelique 720.0
Spondylosis 721.90
- with
  - disproportion 653.3 [5th]
    - affecting fetus or newborn 763.1
    - causing obstructed labor 660.1 [5th]
      - affecting fetus or newborn 763.1
  - myelopathy NEC 721.91
- cervical, cervicodorsal 721.0
  - with myelopathy 721.1
- inflammatory 720.9
- lumbar, lumbosacral 721.3
  - with myelopathy 721.42
- sacral 721.3
  - with myelopathy 721.42
- thoracic 721.2
  - with myelopathy 721.41

Spondylosis – *continued*
- traumatic 721.7

Sponge
- divers' disease 989.5
- inadvertently left in operation wound 998.4
- kidney (medullary) 753.17

Spongioblastoma (M9422/3)
- multiforme (M9440/3)
  - specified site - *see* Neoplasm, by site, malignant
  - unspecified site 191.9
- polare (M9423/3)
  - specified site - *see* Neoplasm, by site, malignant
  - unspecified site 191.9
- primitive polar (M9443/3)
  - specified site - *see* Neoplasm, by site, malignant
  - unspecified site 191.9
- specified site - *see* Neoplasm, by site, malignant
- unspecified site 191.9

Spongiocytoma (M9400/3)
- specified site - *see* Neoplasm, by site, malignant
- unspecified site 191.9

Spongioneuroblastoma (M9504/3) - *see* Neoplasm, by site, malignant
Spontaneous - *see also* condition
- fracture - *see* Fracture, pathologic

Spoon nail 703.8
- congenital 757.5

Sporadic - *see* condition
Sporotrichosis (bones) (cutaneous) (disseminated) (epidermal) (lymphatic) (lymphocutaneous) (mucous membranes) (pulmonary) (skeletal) (visceral) 117.1
Sporotrichum schenckii infection 117.1
Spots, spotting
- atrophic (skin) 701.3
- Bitôt's (in the young child) 264.1
- café au lait 709.09
- cayenne pepper 448.1
- complicating pregnancy 649.5 [5th]
- cotton wool (retina) 362.83
- de Morgan's (senile angiomas) 448.1
- Fúchs' black (myopic) 360.21
- intermenstrual
  - irregular 626.6
  - regular 626.5
- interpalpebral 372.53
- Koplik's 055.9
- liver 709.09
- Mongolian (pigmented) 757.33
- of pregnancy 649.5 [5th]
- purpuric 782.7
- ruby 448.1

Spotted fever - *see* Fever, spotted
Sprain, strain (joint) (ligament) (muscle) (tendon) 848.9
- abdominal wall (muscle) 848.8

Sprain, strain – *continued*
- Achilles tendon 845.09
- acromioclavicular 840.0
- ankle 845.00
  - and foot 845.00
- anterior longitudinal, cervical 847.0
- arm 840.9
  - upper 840.9
    - and shoulder 840.9
- astragalus 845.00
- atlanto-axial 847.0
- atlanto-occipital 847.0
- atlas 847.0
- axis 847.0
- back (*see also* Sprain, spine) 847.9
- breast bone 848.40
- broad ligaments - *see* Injury, internal, broad ligament
- calcaneofibular 845.02
- carpal 842.01
- carpometacarpal 842.11
- cartilage
  - costal, without mention of injury to sternum 848.3
    - involving sternum 848.42
  - ear 848.8
  - knee 844.9
    - with current tear (*see also* Tear, meniscus) 836.2
  - semilunar (knee) 844.8
    - with current tear (*see also* Tear, meniscus) 836.2
  - septal, nose 848.0
  - thyroid region 848.2
  - xiphoid 848.49
- cervical, cervicodorsal, cervicothoracic 847.0
- chondrocostal, without mention of injury to sternum 848.3
  - involving sternum 848.42
- chondrosternal 848.42
- chronic (joint) - *see* Derangement, joint
- clavicle 840.9
- coccyx 847.4
- collar bone 840.9
- collateral, knee (medial) (tibial) 844.1
  - lateral (fibular) 844.0
  - recurrent or old 717.89
    - lateral 717.81
    - medial 717.82
- coracoacromial 840.8
- coracoclavicular 840.1
- coracohumeral 840.2
- coracoid (process) 840.9
- coronary, knee 844.8
- costal cartilage, without mention of injury to sternum 848.3
  - involving sternum 848.42
- cricoarytenoid articulation 848.2
- cricothyroid articulation 848.2
- cruciate
  - knee 844.2
  - old 717.89
    - anterior 717.83
    - posterior 717.84
- deltoid
  - ankle 845.01
  - shoulder 840.8
- dorsal (spine) 847.1
- ear cartilage 848.8
- elbow 841.9
  - and forearm 841.9
  - specified site NEC 841.8
- femur (proximal end) 843.9
  - distal end 844.9
- fibula (proximal end) 844.9
  - distal end 845.00
- fibulocalcaneal 845.02
- finger(s) 842.10
- foot 845.10
  - and ankle 845.00
- forearm 841.9
  - and elbow 841.9
  - specified site NEC 841.8

Sprain, strain – *continued*
- glenoid (shoulder) - (*see also* SLAP lesion) 840.8
- hand 842.10
- hip 843.9
  - and thigh 843.9
- humerus (proximal end) 840.9
  - distal end 841.9
- iliofemoral 843.0
- infraspinatus 840.3
- innominate
  - acetabulum 843.9
  - pubic junction 848.5
  - sacral junction 846.1
- internal
  - collateral, ankle 845.01
  - semilunar cartilage 844.8
    - with current tear (*see also* Tear, meniscus) 836.2
  - old 717.5
- interphalangeal
  - finger 842.13
  - toe 845.13
- ischiocapsular 843.1
- jaw (cartilage) (meniscus) 848.1
  - old 524.69
- knee 844.9
  - and leg 844.9
  - old 717.5
    - collateral
      - lateral 717.81
      - medial 717.82
    - cruciate
      - anterior 717.83
      - posterior 717.84
- late effect - *see* Late, effects (of), sprain
- lateral collateral, knee 844.0
  - old 717.81
- leg 844.9
  - and knee 844.9
- ligamentum teres femoris 843.8
- low back 846.9
- lumbar (spine) 847.2
- lumbosacral 846.0
  - chronic or old 724.6
- mandible 848.1
  - old 524.69
- maxilla 848.1
- medial collateral, knee 844.1
  - old 717.82
- meniscus
  - jaw 848.1
    - old 524.69
  - knee 844.8
    - with current tear (*see also* Tear, meniscus) 836.2
    - old 717.5
  - mandible 848.1
    - old 524.69
  - specified site NEC 848.8
- metacarpal 842.10
  - distal 842.12
  - proximal 842.11
- metacarpophalangeal 842.12
- metatarsal 845.10
- metatarsophalangeal 845.12
- midcarpal 842.19
- midtarsal 845.19
- multiple sites, except fingers alone or toes alone 848.8
- neck 847.0
- nose (septal cartilage) 848.0
- occiput from atlas 847.0
- old - *see* Derangement, joint
- orbicular, hip 843.8
- patella(r) 844.8
  - old 717.89
- pelvis 848.5
- phalanx
  - finger 842.10
  - toe 845.10
- radiocarpal 842.02
- radiohumeral 841.2

Sprain, strain – *continued*
- radioulnar 841.9
  - distal 842.09
- radius, radial (proximal end) 841.9
  - and ulna 841.9
    - distal 842.09
  - collateral 841.0
  - distal end 842.00
- recurrent - *see* Sprain, by site
- rib (cage), without mention of injury to sternum 848.3
  - involving sternum 848.42
- rotator cuff (capsule) 840.4
- round ligament - *see also* Injury, internal, round ligament
  - femur 843.8
- sacral (spine) 847.3
- sacrococcygeal 847.3
- sacroiliac (region) 846.9
  - chronic or old 724.6
  - ligament 846.1
  - specified site NEC 846.8
- sacrospinatus 846.2
- sacrospinous 846.2
- sacrotuberous 846.3
- scaphoid bone, ankle 845.00
- scapula(r) 840.9
- semilunar cartilage (knee) 844.8
  - with current tear (*see also* Tear, meniscus) 836.2
  - old 717.5
- septal cartilage (nose) 848.0
- shoulder 840.9
  - and arm, upper 840.9
  - blade 840.9
- specified site NEC 848.8
- spine 847.9
  - cervical 847.0
  - coccyx 847.4
  - dorsal 847.1
  - lumbar 847.2
  - lumbosacral 846.0
    - chronic or old 724.6
  - sacral 847.3
  - sacroiliac (*see also* Sprain, sacroiliac) 846.9
    - chronic or old 724.6
  - thoracic 847.1
- sternoclavicular 848.41
- sternum 848.40
- subglenoid - (*see also* SLAP lesion) 840.8
- subscapularis 840.5
- supraspinatus 840.6
- symphysis
  - jaw 848.1
    - old 524.69
  - mandibular 848.1
    - old 524.69
  - pubis 848.5
- talofibular 845.09
- tarsal 845.10
- tarsometatarsal 845.11
- temporomandibular 848.1
  - old 524.69
- teres
  - ligamentum femoris 843.8
  - major or minor 840.8
- thigh (proximal end) 843.9
  - and hip 843.9
  - distal end 844.9
- thoracic (spine) 847.1
- thorax 848.8
- thumb 842.10
- thyroid cartilage or region 848.2
- tibia (proximal end) 844.9
  - distal end 845.00
- tibiofibular
  - distal 845.03
  - superior 844.3
- toe(s) 845.10
- trachea 848.8
- trapezoid 840.8
- ulna, ulnar (proximal end) 841.9
  - collateral 841.1

Sprain, strain – *continued*
- ulna, ulnar – *continued*
  - distal end 842.00
- ulnohumeral 841.3
- vertebrae (*see also* Sprain, spine) 847.9
  - cervical, cervicodorsal, cervicothoracic 847.0
- wrist (cuneiform) (scaphoid) (semilunar) 842.00
- xiphoid cartilage 848.49

Sprengel's deformity (congenital) 755.52

Spring fever 309.23

Sprue 579.1
- celiac 579.0
- idiopathic 579.0
- meaning thrush 112.0
- nontropical 579.0
- tropical 579.1

Spur - *see also* Exostosis
- bone 726.91
  - calcaneal 726.73
- calcaneal 726.73
- iliac crest 726.5
- nose (septum) 478.19
  - bone 726.91
- septal 478.19

Spuria placenta - *see* Placenta, abnormal

Spurway's syndrome (brittle bones and blue sclera) 756.51

Sputum, abnormal (amount) (color) (excessive) (odor) (purulent) 786.4
- bloody 786.3

Squamous - *see also* condition
- cell metaplasia
  - bladder 596.8
  - cervix - *see* condition
- epithelium in
  - cervical canal (congenital) 752.49
  - uterine mucosa (congenital) 752.3
- metaplasia
  - bladder 596.8
  - cervix - *see* condition

Squashed nose 738.0
- congenital 754.0

Squeeze, divers' 993.3

Squint (*see also* Strabismus) 378.9
- accommodative (*see also* Esotropia) 378.00
- concomitant (*see also* Heterotropia) 378.30

Stab - *see also* Wound, open, by site
- internal organs - *see* Injury, internal, by site, with open wound

Staggering gait 781.2
- hysterical 300.11

Staghorn calculus 592.0

Stähl's
- ear 744.29
- pigment line (cornea) 371.11

Stahli's pigment lines (cornea) 371.11

Stain, staining
- meconium 779.84
- port wine 757.32
- tooth, teeth (hard tissues) 521.7
  - due to
    - accretions 523.6
    - deposits (betel) (black) (green) (materia alba) (orange) (tobacco) 523.6
    - metals (copper) (silver) 521.7
    - nicotine 523.6
    - pulpal bleeding 521.7
    - tobacco 523.6

Stammering 307.0

Standstill
- atrial 426.6
- auricular 426.6
- cardiac (*see also* Arrest, cardiac) 427.5
- sinoatrial 426.6
- sinus 426.6
- ventricular (*see also* Arrest, cardiac) 427.5

Stannosis 503

Stanton's disease (melioidosis) 025

Staphylitis (acute) (catarrhal) (chronic) (gangrenous) (membranous) (suppurative) (ulcerative) 528.3

- **Staphylococcemia** 038.10
  - aureus 038.11
  - specified organism NEC 038.19
- **Staphylococcus, staphylococcal** - *see* condition
- **Staphyloderma** (skin) 686.00
- **Staphyloma** 379.11
  - anterior, localized 379.14
  - ciliary 379.11
  - cornea 371.73
  - equatorial 379.13
  - posterior 379.12
  - posticum 379.12
  - ring 379.15
  - sclera NEC 379.11
- **Starch eating** 307.52
- **Stargardt's disease** 362.75
- **Starvation** (inanition) (due to lack of food) 994.2
  - edema 262
  - voluntary NEC 307.1
- **Stasis**
  - bile (duct) (*see also* Disease, biliary) 576.8
  - bronchus (*see also* Bronchitis) 490
  - cardiac (*see also* Failure, heart) 428.0
  - cecum 564.89
  - colon 564.89
  - dermatitis (*see also* Varix, with stasis dermatitis) 454.1
  - duodenal 536.8
  - eczema (*see also* Varix, with stasis dermatitis) 454.1
  - edema (*see also* Hypertension, venous) 459.30
  - foot 991.4
  - gastric 536.3
  - ileocecal coil 564.89
  - ileum 564.89
  - intestinal 564.89
  - jejunum 564.89
  - kidney 586
  - liver 571.9
    - cirrhotic - *see* Cirrhosis, liver
  - lymphatic 457.8
  - pneumonia 514
  - portal 571.9
  - pulmonary 514
  - rectal 564.89
  - renal 586
    - tubular 584.5
  - stomach 536.3
  - ulcer
    - with varicose veins 454.0
    - without varicose veins 459.81
  - urine NEC (*see also* Retention, urine) 788.20
  - venous 459.81
- **State**
  - affective and paranoid, mixed, organic psychotic 294.8
  - agitated 307.9
    - acute reaction to stress 308.2
  - anxiety (neurotic) (*see also* Anxiety) 300.00
    - specified type NEC 300.09
  - apprehension (*see also* Anxiety) 300.00
    - specified type NEC 300.09
  - climacteric, female 627.2
    - following induced menopause 627.4
  - clouded
    - epileptic (*see also* Epilepsy) 345.9 [5th]
    - paroxysmal (idiopathic) (*see also* Epilepsy) 345.9 [5th]
  - compulsive (mixed) (with obsession) 300.3
  - confusional 298.9
    - acute 293.0
      - with
        - arteriosclerotic dementia 290.41
        - presenile brain disease 290.11
        - senility 290.3
      - alcoholic 291.0
      - drug-induced 292.81
    - epileptic 293.0
    - postoperative 293.9

State – *continued*

  - confusional – *continued*
    - reactive (emotional stress) (psychological trauma) 298.2
    - subacute 293.1
  - constitutional psychopathic 301.9
  - convulsive (*see also* Convulsions) 780.39
  - depressive NEC 311
    - induced by drug 292.84
    - neurotic 300.4
  - dissociative 300.15
  - hallucinatory 780.1
    - induced by drug 292.12
  - hypercoagulable (primary) 289.81
    - secondary 289.82
  - hyperdynamic beta-adrenergic circulatory 429.82
  - locked-in 344.81
  - menopausal 627.2
    - artificial 627.4
    - following induced menopause 627.4
  - neurotic NEC 300.9
    - with depersonalization episode 300.6
  - obsessional 300.3
  - oneiroid (*see also* Schizophrenia) 295.4 [5th]
  - panic 300.01
  - paranoid 297.9
    - alcohol-induced 291.5
    - arteriosclerotic 290.42
    - climacteric 297.2
    - drug-induced 292.11
    - in
      - presenile brain disease 290.12
      - senile brain disease 290.20
    - involutional 297.2
    - menopausal 297.2
    - senile 290.20
    - simple 297.0
  - postleukotomy 310.0
  - pregnant (*see also* Pregnancy) V22.2
  - psychogenic, twilight 298.2
  - psychotic, organic (*see also* Psychosis, organic) 294.9
    - mixed paranoid and affective 294.8
    - senile or presenile NEC 290.9
    - transient NEC 293.9
      - with
        - anxiety 293.84
        - delusions 293.81
        - depression 293.83
        - hallucinations 293.82
  - residual schizophrenic (*see also* Schizophrenia) 295.6 [5th]
  - tension (*see also* Anxiety) 300.9
  - transient organic psychotic 293.9
    - anxiety type 293.84
    - depressive type 293.83
    - hallucinatory type 293.83
    - paranoid type 293.81
    - specified type NEC 293.89
  - twilight
    - epileptic 293.0
    - psychogenic 298.2
  - vegetative (persistent) 780.03
- **Status** (post)
  - absence
    - epileptic (*see also* Epilepsy) 345.2
    - of organ, acquired (postsurgical) - *see* Absence, by site, acquired
  - administration of tPA (rtPA) in a different institution within the last 24 hours prior to admission to facility V45.88
  - anastomosis of intestine (for bypass) V45.3
  - anginosus 413.9
  - angioplasty, percutaneous transluminal coronary V45.82
  - ankle prosthesis V43.66
  - aortocoronary bypass or shunt V45.81
  - arthrodesis V45.4
  - artificially induced condition NEC V45.89
  - artificial opening (of) V44.9
    - gastrointestinal tract NEC V44.4
    - specified site NEC V44.8

Status (post) – *continued*

  - artificial opening (of) – *continued*
    - urinary tract NEC V44.6
    - vagina V44.7
  - aspirator V46.0
  - asthmaticus (*see also* Asthma) 493.9 [5th]
  - awaiting organ transplant V49.83
  - bariatric surgery V45.86
    - complicating pregnancy, childbirth, or the puerperium 649.2 [5th]
  - bed confinement V49.84
  - breast
    - correction V43.82
    - implant removal V45.83
    - reconstruction V43.82
  - cardiac
    - device (in situ) V45.00
      - carotid sinus V45.09
        - fitting or adjustment V53.39
      - defibrillator, automatic implantable V45.02
      - pacemaker V45.01
        - fitting or adjustment V53.31
  - carotid sinus stimulator V45.09
  - cataract extraction V45.61
  - chemotherapy V66.2
    - current V58.69
  - circumcision, female 629.20
  - clitorectomy (female genital mutilation type I) 629.21
    - with excision of labia minora (female genital mutilation type II 629.22
  - colonization - *see* Carrier (suspected) of
  - colostomy V44.3
  - contraceptive device V45.59
    - intrauterine V45.51
    - subdermal V45.52
  - convulsivus idiopathicus (*see also* Epilepsy) 345.3
  - coronary artery bypass or shunt V45.81
  - ~~current military deployment status V62.21~~
  - cutting
    - female genital 629.20
      - specified NEC 629.29
      - type I 629.21
      - type II 629.22
      - type III 629.23
      - type IV 629.29
  - cystostomy V44.50
    - appendico-vesicostomy V44.52
    - cutaneous-vesicostomy V44.51
    - specifed type NEC V44.59
  - defibrillator, automatic implantable cardiac V45.02
  - delinquent immunization V15.83 ●
  - dental crowns V45.84
  - dental fillings V45.84
  - dental restoration V45.84
  - dental sealant V49.82
  - dialysis (hemo) (peritoneal) V45.11
  - donor V59.9
  - drug therapy or regimen V67.59
    - high-risk medication NEC V67.51
  - elbow prosthesis V43.62
  - enterostomy V44.4
  - epileptic, epilepticus (absence) (grand mal) (*see also* Epilepsy) 345.3 [5th]
    - focal motor 345.7 [5th]
    - partial 345.7 [5th]
    - petit mal 345.2
    - psychomotor 345.7 [5th]
    - temporal lobe 345.7 [5th]
  - estrogen receptor
    - negative [ER-] V86.1
    - positive [ER+] V86.0
  - eye (adnexa) surgery V45.69
  - female genital
    - cutting 629.20
      - specified NEC 629.29
      - type I 629.21
      - type II 629.22
      - type III 629.23
      - type IV 629.29

Status (post) – *continued*

  - female genital – *continued*
    - mutilation 629.20
      - type I 629.21
      - type II 629.22
      - type III 629.23
      - type IV 629.29
  - filtering bleb (eye) (postglaucoma) V45.69
    - with rupture or complication 997.99
    - postcataract extraction (complication) 997.99
  - finger joint prosthesis V43.69
  - foster care V60.81 ●
  - gastric
    - banding V45.86
      - complicating pregnancy, childbirth, or the puerperium 649.2 [5th]
    - bypass for obesity V45.86
      - complicating pregnancy, childbirth, or the puerperium 649.2 [5th]
  - gastrostomy V44.1
  - grand mal 345.3
  - heart valve prosthesis V43.3
  - hemodialysis V45.11
  - hip prosthesis (joint) (partial) (total) V43.64
  - hysterectomy V88.01
    - partial with remaining cervical stump V88.02
    - total V88.01
  - ileostomy V44.2
  - infibulation (female genital mutilation type III) 629.23
  - insulin pump V45.85
  - intestinal bypass V45.3
  - intrauterine contraceptive device V45.51
  - jejunostomy V44.4
  - knee joint prosthesis V43.65
  - lacunaris 437.8
  - lacunosis 437.8
  - lapsed immunization schedule V15.83 ●
  - low birth weight V21.30
    - less than 500 grams V21.31
    - 500-999 grams V21.32
    - 1000-1499 grams V21.33
    - 1500-1999 grams V21.34
    - 2000-2500 grams V21.35
  - lymphaticus 254.8
  - malignant neoplasm, ablated or excised - *see* History, malignant neoplasm
  - marmoratus 333.79
  - military deployment V62.22 ●
  - mutilation, female 629.20
    - type I 629.21
    - type II 629.22
    - type III 629.23
    - type IV 629.29
  - nephrostomy V44.6
  - neuropacemaker NEC V45.89
    - brain V45.89
    - carotid sinus V45.09
    - neurologic NEC V45.89
  - obesity surgery V45.86
    - complicating pregnancy, childbirth, or the puerperium 649.2 [5th]
  - organ replacement
    - by artificial or mechanical device or prosthesis of
      - artery V43.4
      - artificial skin V43.83
      - bladder V43.5
      - blood vessel V43.4
      - breast V43.82
      - eye globe V43.0
      - heart
        - assist device V43.21
        - fully implantable artificial heart V43.22
        - valve V43.3
      - intestine V43.89
      - joint V43.60
        - ankle V43.66
        - elbow V43.62
        - finger V43.69

Staphylococcemia – Status

- **Status** (post) – *continued*
  - organ replacement – *continued*
    - by artificial or mechanical device or prosthesis of – *continued*
      - joint – *continued*
        - hip (partial) (total) V43.64
        - knee V43.65
        - shoulder V43.61
        - specified NEC V43.69
        - wrist V43.63
      - kidney V43.89
      - larynx V43.81
      - lens V43.1
      - limb(s) V43.7
      - liver V43.89
      - lung V43.89
      - organ NEC V43.89
      - pancreas V43.89
      - skin (artificial) V43.83
      - tissue NEC V43.89
      - vein V43.4
    - by organ transplant (heterologous) (homologous) - *see* Status, transplant
  - pacemaker
    - brain V45.89
    - cardiac V45.01
    - carotid sinus V45.09
    - neurologic NEC V45.89
    - specified site NEC V45.89
  - percutaneous transluminal coronary angioplasty V45.82
  - peritoneal dialysis V45.11
  - petit mal 345.2
  - postcommotio cerebri 310.2
  - postmenopausal (age related) (natural) V49.81
  - postoperative NEC V45.89
  - postpartum NEC V24.2
    - care immediately following delivery V24.0
    - routine follow-up V24.2
  - postsurgical NEC V45.89
  - renal dialysis V45.11
    - noncompliance V45.12
  - respirator [ventilator]V46.11
    - encounter
      - during
        - mechanical failure V46.14
        - power failure V46.12
      - for weaning V46.13
  - reversed jejunal transposition (for bypass) V45.3
  - sex reassignment surgery (*see also* Trans-sexualism) 302.50 ▲
  - shoulder prosthesis V43.61
  - shunt
    - aortocoronary bypass V45.81
    - arteriovenous (for dialysis) V45.11
    - cerebrospinal fluid V45.2
    - vascular NEC V45.89
      - aortocoronary (bypass) V45.81
    - ventricular (communicating) (for drainage) V45.2
  - sterilization
    - tubal ligation V26.51
    - vasectomy V26.52
  - subdermal contraceptive device V45.52
  - thymicolymphaticus 254.8
  - thymicus 254.8
  - thymolymphaticus 254.8
  - tooth extraction 525.10
  - tracheostomy V44.0
  - transplant
    - blood vessel V42.89
    - bone V42.4
      - marrow V42.81
    - cornea V42.5
    - heart V42.1
      - valve V42.2
    - intestine V42.84
    - kidney V42.0
    - liver V42.7
    - lung V42.6
- **Status** (post) – *continued*
  - transplant – *continued*
    - organ V42.9
      - removal (due to complication, failure, rejection or infection) V45.87
      - specified site NEC V42.89
    - pancreas V42.83
    - peripheral stem cells V42.82
    - skin V42.3
    - stem cells, peripheral V42.82
    - tissue V42.9
      - specified type NEC V42.89
    - vessel, blood V42.89
  - tubal ligation V26.51
  - underimmunization V15.83 ●
  - ureterostomy V44.6
  - urethrostomy V44.6
  - vagina, artificial V44.7
  - vascular shunt NEC V45.89
    - aortocoronary (bypass) V45.81
  - vasectomy V26.52
  - ventilator [respirator] V46.11
    - encounter
      - during
        - mechanical failure V46.14
        - power failure V46.12
      - for weaning V46.13
  - wheelchair confinement V46.3
  - wrist prosthesis V43.63
- **Stave fracture** - *see* Fracture, metacarpus, metacarpal bone(s)
- **Steal**
  - subclavian artery 435.2
  - vertebral artery 435.1
- **Stealing, solitary, child problem** (*see also* Disturbance, conduct) 312.1 5th
- **Steam burn** - *see* Burn, by site
- **Steatocystoma multiplex** 706.2
- **Steatoma** (infected) 706.2
  - eyelid (cystic) 374.84
    - infected 373.13
- **Steatorrhea** (chronic) 579.8
  - with lacteal obstruction 579.2
  - idiopathic 579.0
    - adult 579.0
    - infantile 579.0
  - pancreatic 579.4
  - primary 579.0
  - secondary 579.8
  - specified cause NEC 579.8
  - tropical 579.1
- **Steatosis** 272.8
  - heart (*see also* Degeneration, myocardial) 429.1
  - kidney 593.89
  - liver 571.8
- **Steele-Richardson (-Olszewski) Syndrome** 333.0
- **Stein's syndrome** (polycystic ovary) 256.4
- **Stein-Leventhal syndrome** (polycystic ovary) 256.4
- **Steinbrocker's syndrome** (*see also* Neuropathy, peripheral, autonomic) 337.9
- **Steinert's disease** 359.21
- **STEMI** (ST elevation myocardial infarction) (*see also* - Infarct, myocardium, ST elevation) 410.9 5th
- **Stenocardia** (*see also* Angina) 413.9
- **Stenocephaly** 756.0
- **Stenosis** (cicatricial) - *see also* Stricture
  - ampulla of Vater 576.2
    - with calculus, cholelithiasis, or stones - *see* Choledocholithiasis
  - anus, anal (canal) (sphincter) 569.2
    - congenital 751.2
  - aorta (ascending) 747.22
    - arch 747.10
    - arteriosclerotic 440.0
    - calcified 440.0
- **Stenosis** – *continued*
  - aortic (valve) 424.1
    - with
      - mitral (valve)
        - insufficiency or incompetence 396.2
        - stenosis or obstruction 396.0
    - atypical 396.0
    - congenital 746.3
    - rheumatic 395.0
      - with
        - insufficiency, incompetency or regurgitation 395.2
          - with mitral (valve) disease 396.8
        - mitral (valve)
          - disease (stenosis) 396.0
          - insufficiency or incompetence 396.2
          - stenosis or obstruction 396.0
    - specified cause, except rheumatic 424.1
    - syphilitic 093.22
  - aqueduct of Sylvius (congenital) 742.3
    - with spina bifida (*see also* Spina bifida) 741.0 5th
    - acquired 331.4
  - artery NEC (*see also* Arteriosclerosis) 447.1
    - basilar - *see* Narrowing, artery, basilar
    - carotid (common) (internal) - *see* Narrowing, artery, carotid
    - celiac 447.4
    - cerebral 437.0
      - due to
        - embolism (*see also* Embolism, brain) 434.1 5th
        - thrombus (*see also* Thrombosis, brain) 434.0 5th
    - extremities 440.20
    - precerebral - *see* Narrowing, artery, precerebral
    - pulmonary (congenital) 747.3
      - acquired 417.8
    - renal 440.1
    - vertebral - *see* Narrowing, artery, vertebral
  - bile duct or biliary passage (*see also* Obstruction, biliary) 576.2
    - congenital 751.61
  - bladder neck (acquired) 596.0
    - congenital 753.6
  - brain 348.89 ▲
  - bronchus 519.19
    - syphilitic 095.8
  - cardia (stomach) 537.89
    - congenital 750.7
  - cardiovascular (*see also* Disease, cardiovascular) 429.2
  - carotid artery - *see* Narrowing, artery, carotid
  - cervix, cervical (canal) 622.4
    - congenital 752.49
    - in pregnancy or childbirth 654.6 5th
      - affecting fetus or newborn 763.89
      - causing obstructed labor 660.2 5th
        - affecting fetus or newborn 763.1
  - colon (*see also* Obstruction, intestine) 560.9
    - congenital 751.2
  - colostomy 569.62
  - common bile duct (*see also* Obstruction, biliary) 576.2
    - congenital 751.61
  - coronary (artery) - *see* Arteriosclerosis, coronary
  - cystic duct (*see also* Obstruction, gallbladder) 575.2
    - congenital 751.61
  - due to (presence of) any device, implant, or graft classifiable to 996.0-996.5 - *see* Complications, due to (presence of) any device, implant, or graft classified to 996.0-996.5 NEC
- **Stenosis** – *continued*
  - duodenum 537.3
    - congenital 751.1
  - ejaculatory duct NEC 608.89
  - endocervical os - *see* Stenosis, cervix
  - enterostomy 569.62
  - esophagostomy 530.87
  - esophagus 530.3
    - congenital 750.3
    - syphilitic 095.8
      - congenital 090.5
  - external ear canal 380.50
    - secondary to
      - inflammation 380.53
      - surgery 380.52
      - trauma 380.51
  - gallbladder (*see also* Obstruction, gallbladder) 575.2
  - glottis 478.74
  - heart valve (acquired) - *see also* Endocarditis
    - congenital NEC 746.89
      - aortic 746.3
      - mitral 746.5
      - pulmonary 746.02
      - tricuspid 746.1
  - hepatic duct (*see also* Obstruction, biliary) 576.2
  - hymen 623.3
  - hypertrophic subaortic (idiopathic) 425.1
  - infundibulum cardiac 746.83
  - intestine (*see also* Obstruction, intestine) 560.9
    - congenital (small) 751.1
      - large 751.2
  - lacrimal
    - canaliculi 375.53
    - duct 375.56
      - congenital 743.65
    - punctum 375.52
      - congenital 743.65
    - sac 375.54
      - congenital 743.65
  - lacrimonasal duct 375.56
    - congenital 743.65
    - neonatal 375.55
  - larynx 478.74
    - congenital 748.3
    - syphilitic 095.8
      - congenital 090.5
  - mitral (valve) (chronic) (inactive) 394.0
    - with
      - aortic (valve)
        - disease (insufficiency) 396.1
        - insufficiency or incompetence 396.1
        - stenosis or obstruction 396.0
      - incompetency, insufficiency or regurgitation 394.2
        - with aortic valve disease 396.8
    - active or acute 391.1
      - with chorea (acute) (rheumatic) (Sydenham's) 392.0
    - congenital 746.5
    - specified cause, except rheumatic 424.0
    - syphilitic 093.21
  - myocardium, myocardial (*see also* Degeneration, myocardial) 429.1
    - hypertrophic subaortic (idiopathic) 425.1
  - nares (anterior) (posterior) 478.19
    - congenital 748.0
  - nasal duct 375.56
    - congenital 743.65
  - nasolacrimal duct 375.56
    - congenital 743.65
    - neonatal 375.55
  - organ or site, congenital NEC - *see* Atresia
  - papilla of Vater 576.2
    - with calculus, cholelithiasis, or stones - *see* Choledocholithiasis

- **Stenosis** – *continued*
  - pulmonary (artery) (congenital) 747.3
    - with ventricular septal defect, dextraposition of aorta and hypertrophy of right ventricle 745.2
    - acquired 417.8
    - infundibular 746.83
    - in tetralogy of Fallot 745.2
    - subvalvular 746.83
    - valve (*see also* Endocarditis, pulmonary) 424.3
      - congenital 746.02
    - vein 747.49
      - acquired 417.8
    - vessel NEC 417.8
  - pulmonic (congenital) 746.02
    - infundibular 746.83
    - subvalvular 746.83
  - pylorus (hypertrophic) 537.0
    - adult 537.0
    - congenital 750.5
    - infantile 750.5
  - rectum (sphincter) (*see also* Stricture, rectum) 569.2
  - renal artery 440.1
  - salivary duct (any) 527.8
  - sphincter of Oddi (*see also* Obstruction, biliary) 576.2
  - spinal 724.00
    - cervical 723.0
    - lumbar, lumbosacral 724.02
    - nerve (root) NEC 724.9
    - specified region NEC 724.09
    - thoracic, thoracolumbar 724.01
  - stomach, hourglass 537.6
  - subaortic 746.81
    - hypertrophic (idiopathic) 425.1
  - supra (valvular)-aortic 747.22
  - trachea 519.19
    - congenital 748.3
    - syphilitic 095.8
    - tuberculous (*see also* Tuberculosis) 012.8 [5th]
  - tracheostomy 519.02
  - tricuspid (valve) (*see also* Endocarditis, tricuspid) 397.0
    - congenital 746.1
    - nonrheumatic 424.2
  - tubal 628.2
  - ureter (*see also* Stricture, ureter) 593.3
    - congenital 753.29
  - urethra (*see also* Stricture, urethra) 598.9
  - vagina 623.2
    - congenital 752.49
    - in pregnancy or childbirth 654.7 [5th]
      - affecting fetus or newborn 763.89
      - causing obstructed labor 660.2 [5th]
        - affecting fetus or newborn 763.1
  - valve (cardiac) (heart) (*see also* Endocarditis) 424.90
    - congenital NEC 746.89
      - aortic 746.3
      - mitral 746.5
      - pulmonary 746.02
      - tricuspid 746.1
      - urethra 753.6
  - valvular (*see also* Endocarditis) 424.90
    - congenital NEC 746.89
      - urethra 753.6
  - vascular graft or shunt 996.1
    - atherosclerosis - *see* Arteriosclerosis, extremities
    - embolism 996.74
    - occlusion NEC 996.74
    - thrombus 996.74
  - vena cava (inferior) (superior) 459.2
    - congenital 747.49
  - ventricular shunt 996.2
  - vulva 624.8
- **Stercolith** (*see also* Fecalith) 560.39
  - appendix 543.9
- **Stercoraceous, stercoral ulcer** 569.82
  - anus or rectum 569.41
- **Stereopsis, defective**
  - with fusion 368.33
  - without fusion 368.32
- **Stereotypies NEC** 307.3
- **Sterility**
  - female - *see* Infertility, female
  - male (*see also* Infertility, male) 606.9
- **Sterilization, admission for** V25.2
  - status
    - tubal ligation V26.51
    - vasectomy V26.52
- **Sternalgia** (*see also* Angina) 413.9
- **Sternopagus** 759.4
- **Sternum bifidum** 756.3
- **Sternutation** 784.99
- **Steroid**
  - effects (adverse) (iatrogenic)
    - cushingoid
      - correct substance properly administered 255.0
      - overdose or wrong substance given or taken 962.0
    - diabetes - *see* Diabetes, secondary
      - correct substance properly administered 251.8
- **Steroid** – *continued*
  - effects – *continued*
    - diabetes – *continued*
      - overdose or wrong substance given or taken 962.0
    - due to
      - correct substance properly administered 255.8
      - overdose or wrong substance given or taken 962.0
    - fever
      - correct substance properly administered 780.60
      - overdose or wrong substance given or taken 962.0
    - withdrawal
      - correct substance properly administered 255.41
      - overdose or wrong substance given or taken 962.0
  - responder 365.03
- **Stevens-Johnson disease or syndrome** (erythema multiforme exudativum) 695.13
  - toxic epidermal necrolysis overlap (SJS-TEN overlap syndrome) 695.14
- **Stewart-Morel syndrome** (hyperostosis frontalis interna) 733.3
- **Sticker's disease** (erythema infectiosum) 057.0
- **Stickler syndrome** 759.89
- **Sticky eye** 372.03
- **Stieda's disease** (calcification, knee joint) 726.62
- **Stiff**
  - back 724.8
  - neck (*see also* Torticollis) 723.5
- **Stiff-baby** 759.89
- **Stiff-man syndrome** 333.91
- **Stiffness, joint** NEC 719.50
  - ankle 719.57
  - back 724.8
  - elbow 719.52
  - finger 719.54
  - hip 719.55
  - knee 719.56
  - multiple sites 719.59
  - sacroiliac 724.6
  - shoulder 719.51
  - specified site NEC 719.58
  - spine 724.9
  - surgical fusion V45.4
  - wrist 719.53
- **Stigmata, congenital syphilis** 090.5
- **Still's disease or syndrome** 714.30
  - adult onset 714.2
- **Still-Felty syndrome** (rheumatoid arthritis with splenomegaly and leukopenia) 714.1
- **Stillbirth, stillborn NEC** 779.9
- **Stiller's disease** (asthenia) 780.79
- **Stilling-Türk-Duane syndrome** (ocular retraction syndrome) 378.71
- **Stimulation, ovary** 256.1
- **Sting** (animal) (bee) (fish) (insect) (jellyfish) (Portuguese man-o-war) (wasp) (venomous) 989.5
  - anaphylactic shock or reaction 989.5
  - plant 692.6
- **Stippled epiphyses** 756.59
- **Stitch**
  - abscess 998.59
  - burst (in external operation wound) (*see also* Dehiscence) 998.32
    - internal 998.31
  - in back 724.5
- **Stojano's** (subcostal) **syndrome** 098.86
- **Stokes' disease** (exophthalmic goiter) 242.0 [5th]
- **Stokes-Adams syndrome** (syncope with heart block) 426.9
- **Stokvis' (-Talma) disease** (enterogenous cyanosis) 289.7
- **Stomach** - *see* condition
- **Stoma malfunction**
  - colostomy 569.62
  - cystostomy 997.5
  - enterostomy 569.62
  - esophagostomy 530.87
  - gastrostomy 536.42
  - ileostomy 569.62
  - nephrostomy 997.5
  - tracheostomy 519.02
  - ureterostomy 997.5
- **Stomatitis** 528.00
  - angular 528.5
    - due to dietary or vitamin deficiency 266.0
  - aphthous 528.2
  - bovine 059.11
  - candidal 112.0
  - catarrhal 528.00
  - denture 528.9
  - diphtheritic (membranous) 032.0
  - due to
    - dietary deficiency 266.0
    - thrush 112.0
    - vitamin deficiency 266.0
  - epidemic 078.4
  - epizootic 078.4
  - follicular 528.00
  - gangrenous 528.1
  - herpetic 054.2
  - herpetiformis 528.2
  - malignant 528.00
  - membranous acute 528.00
  - monilial 112.0
  - mycotic 112.0
  - necrotic 528.1
    - ulcerative 101
  - necrotizing ulcerative 101
  - parasitic 112.0
  - septic 528.00
  - specified NEC 528.09
  - spirochetal 101
  - suppurative (acute) 528.00
  - ulcerative 528.00
    - necrotizing 101
  - ulceromembranous 101
  - vesicular 528.00
    - with exanthem 074.3
  - Vincent's 101
- **Stomatocytosis** 282.8
- **Stomatomycosis** 112.0
- **Stomatorrhagia** 528.9
- **Stone(s)** - *see also* Calculus
  - bladder 594.1
    - diverticulum 594.0
  - cystine 270.0
  - heart syndrome (*see also* Failure, ventricular, left) 428.1
  - kidney 592.0
  - prostate 602.0
- **Stone(s)** – *continued*
  - pulp (dental) 522.2
  - renal 592.0
  - salivary duct or gland (any) 527.5
  - ureter 592.1
  - urethra (impacted) 594.2
  - urinary (duct) (impacted) (passage) 592.9
    - bladder 594.1
      - diverticulum 594.0
    - lower tract NEC 594.9
    - specified site 594.8
  - xanthine 277.2
- **Stonecutters' lung** 502
  - tuberculous (*see also* Tuberculosis) 011.4 [5th]
- **Stonemasons'**
  - asthma, disease, or lung 502
    - tuberculous (*see also* Tuberculosis) 011.4 [5th]
  - phthisis (*see also* Tuberculosis) 011.4 [5th]
- **Stoppage**
  - bowel (*see also* Obstruction, intestine) 560.9
  - heart (*see also* Arrest, cardiac) 427.5
  - intestine (*see also* Obstruction, intestine) 560.9
- **Stoppage** – *continued*
  - urine NEC (*see also* Retention, urine) 788.20
- **Storm, thyroid** (apathetic) (*see also* Thyrotoxicosis) 242.9 [5th]
- **Strabismus** (alternating) (congenital) (nonparalytic) 378.9
  - concomitant (*see also* Heterotropia) 378.30
    - convergent (*see also* Esotropia) 378.00
    - divergent (*see also* Exotropia) 378.10
  - convergent (*see also* Esotropia) 378.00
  - divergent (*see also* Exotropia) 378.10
  - due to adhesions, scars - *see* Strabismus, mechanical
  - in neuromuscular disorder NEC 378.73
    - intermittent 378.20
      - vertical 378.31
  - latent 378.40
    - convergent (esophoria) 378.41
    - divergent (exophoria) 378.42
    - vertical 378.43
  - mechanical 378.60
    - due to
      - Brown's tendon sheath syndrome 378.61
      - specified musculofascial disorder NEC 378.62
  - paralytic 378.50
    - third or oculomotor nerve (partial) 378.51
      - total 378.52
    - fourth or trochlear nerve 378.53
    - sixth or abducens nerve 378.54
  - specified type NEC 378.73
  - vertical (hypertropia) 378.31
- **Strain** - *see also* Sprain, by site
  - eye NEC 368.13
  - heart - *see* Disease, heart
  - meaning gonorrhea - *see* Gonorrhea
  - on urination 788.65
  - physical NEC V62.89
  - postural 729.90
  - psychological NEC V62.89
- **Strands**
  - conjunctiva 372.62
  - vitreous humor 379.25
- **Strangulation, strangulated** 994.7
  - appendix 543.9
  - asphyxiation or suffocation by 994.7
  - bladder neck 596.0
  - bowel - *see* Strangulation, intestine
  - colon - *see* Strangulation, intestine
  - cord (umbilical) - *see* Compression, umbilical cord
  - due to birth injury 767.8
  - food or foreign body (*see also* Asphyxia, food) 933.1

Stenosis – Strangulation, strangulated

- **Supernumerary** (congenital) – *continued*
  - bone 756.9
  - breast 757.6
  - carpal bones 755.56
  - cusps, heart valve NEC 746.89
    - mitral 746.5
    - pulmonary 746.09
  - digit(s) 755.00
    - finger 755.01
    - toe 755.02
  - ear (lobule) 744.1
  - fallopian tube 752.19
  - finger 755.01
  - hymen 752.49
  - kidney 753.3
  - lacrimal glands 743.64
  - lacrimonasal duct 743.65
  - lobule (ear) 744.1
  - mitral cusps 746.5
  - muscle 756.82
  - nipples 757.6
  - organ or site NEC - *see* Accessory
  - ossicles, auditory 744.04
  - ovary 752.0
  - oviduct 752.19
  - pulmonic cusps 746.09
  - rib 756.3
    - cervical or first 756.2
      - syndrome 756.2
  - roots (of teeth) 520.2
  - spinal vertebra 756.19
  - spleen 759.0
  - tarsal bones 755.67
  - teeth 520.1
    - causing crowding 524.31
  - testis 752.89
  - thumb 755.01
  - toe 755.02
  - uterus 752.2
  - vagina 752.49
  - vertebra 756.19
- **Supervision** (of)
  - contraceptive method previously prescribed V25.40
    - intrauterine device V25.42
    - oral contraceptive (pill) V25.41
    - specified type NEC V25.49
    - subdermal implantable contraceptive V25.43
  - dietary (for) V65.3
    - allergy (food) V65.3
    - colitis V65.3
    - diabetes mellitus V65.3
    - food allergy intolerance V65.3
    - gastritis V65.3
    - hypercholesterolemia V65.3
    - hypoglycemia V65.3
    - intolerance (food) V65.3
    - obesity V65.3
    - specified NEC V65.3
  - lactation V24.1
  - newborn health ●
    - 8 to 28 days old V20.32 ●
    - under 8 days old V20.31 ●
  - pregnancy - *see* Pregnancy, supervision of
- **Supplemental teeth** 520.1
  - causing crowding 524.31
- **Suppression**
  - binocular vision 368.31
  - lactation 676.5 [5th]
  - menstruation 626.8
  - ovarian secretion 256.39
  - renal 586
  - urinary secretion 788.5
  - urine 788.5
- **Suppuration, suppurative** - *see also* condition
  - accessory sinus (chronic) (*see also* Sinusitis) 473.9
  - adrenal gland 255.8
  - antrum (chronic) (*see also* Sinusitis, maxillary) 473.0
  - bladder (*see also* Cystitis) 595.89
  - bowel 569.89
- **Suppuration, suppurative** – *continued*
  - brain 324.0
    - late effect 326
  - breast 611.0
    - puerperal, postpartum 675.1 [5th]
  - dental periosteum 526.5
  - diffuse (skin) 686.00
  - ear (middle) (*see also* Otitis media) 382.4
    - external (*see also* Otitis, externa) 380.10
    - internal 386.33
  - ethmoidal (sinus) (chronic) (*see also* Sinusitis, ethmoidal) 473.2
  - fallopian tube (*see also* Salpingo-oophoritis) 614.2
  - frontal (sinus) (chronic) (*see also* Sinusitis, frontal) 473.1
  - gallbladder (*see also* Cholecystitis, acute) 575.0
  - gum 523.30
  - hernial sac - *see* Hernia, by site
  - intestine 569.89
  - joint (*see also* Arthritis, suppurative) 711.0 [5th]
  - labyrinthine 386.33
  - lung 513.0
  - mammary gland 611.0
    - puerperal, postpartum 675.1 [5th]
  - maxilla, maxillary 526.4
    - sinus (chronic) (*see also* Sinusitis, maxillary) 473.0
  - muscle 728.0
  - nasal sinus (chronic) (*see also* Sinusitis) 473.9
  - pancreas 577.0
  - parotid gland 527.2
  - pelvis, pelvic
    - female (*see also* Disease, pelvis, inflammatory) 614.4
      - acute 614.3
    - male (*see also* Peritonitis) 567.21
  - pericranial (*see also* Osteomyelitis) 730.2 [5th]
  - salivary duct or gland (any) 527.2
  - sinus (nasal) (*see also* Sinusitis) 473.9
  - sphenoidal (sinus) (chronic) (*see also* Sinusitis, sphenoidal) 473.3
  - thymus (gland) 254.1
  - thyroid (gland) 245.0
  - tonsil 474.8
  - uterus (*see also* Endometritis) 615.9
  - vagina 616.10
  - wound - *see also* Wound, open, by site, complicated
    - dislocation - *see* Dislocation, by site, compound
    - fracture - *see* Fracture, by site, open
    - scratch or other superficial injury - *see* Injury, superficial, by site
- **Supraeruption, teeth** 524.34
- **Supraglottitis** 464.50
  - with obstruction 464.51
- **Suprapubic drainage** 596.8
- **Suprarenal** (gland) - *see* condition
- **Suprascapular nerve** - *see* condition
- **Suprasellar** - *see* condition
- **Supraspinatus syndrome** 726.10
- **Surfer knots** 919.8
  - infected 919.9
- **Surgery**
  - cosmetic NEC V50.1
    - breast reconstruction following mastectomy V51.0
    - following healed injury or operation V51.8
    - hair transplant V50.0
  - elective V50.9
    - breast
      - augmentation or reduction V50.1
      - reconstruction following mastectomy V51.0
    - circumcision, ritual or routine (in absence of medical indication) V50.2
- **Surgery** – *continued*
  - elective – *continued*
    - cosmetic NEC V50.1
    - ear piercing V50.3
    - face-lift V50.1
    - following healed injury or operation V51.8
    - hair transplant V50.0
  - not done because of
    - contraindication V64.1
    - patient's decision V64.2
    - specified reason NEC V64.3
  - plastic
    - breast
      - augmentation or reduction V50.1
      - reconstruction following mastectomy V51.0
    - cosmetic V50.1
    - face-lift V50.1
    - following healed injury or operation V51.8
    - repair of scarred tissue (following healed injury or operation) V51.8
    - specified type NEC V50.8
  - previous, in pregnancy or childbirth
    - cervix 654.6 [5th]
      - affecting fetus or newborn (*see also* Newborn, affected by) 760.63
      - causing obstructed labor 660.2 [5th]
        - affecting fetus or newborn 763.1
    - pelvic soft tissues NEC 654.9 [5th]
      - affecting fetus or newborn (*see also* Newborn, affected by) 760.63
      - causing obstructed labor 660.2 [5th]
        - affecting fetus or newborn 763.1
    - perineum or vulva 654.8 [5th]
    - uterus NEC 654.9 [5th]
      - affecting fetus or newborn (*see also* Newborn, affected by) 760.63
      - causing obstructed labor 660.2 [5th]
        - affecting fetus or newborn 763.1
      - from previous cesarean delivery 654.2 [5th]
    - vagina 654.7 [5th]
- **Surgical**
  - abortion - *see* Abortion, legal
  - emphysema 998.81
  - kidney (*see also* Pyelitis) 590.80
  - operation NEC 799.9
  - procedures, complication or misadventure - *see* Complications, surgical procedure
  - shock 998.0
- **Survey**
  - fetal anatomic V28.81
- **Susceptibility**
  - genetic
    - to
      - MEN (multiple endocrine neoplasia) V84.81
      - neoplasia
        - multiple endocrine [MEN] V84.81
      - neoplasm
        - malignant, of
          - breast V84.01
          - endometrium V84.04
          - other V84.09
          - ovary V84.02
          - prostate V84.03
      - specified disease NEC V84.89
- **Suspected condition, ruled out** (*see also* Observation, suspected) V71.9
  - specified condition NEC V71.89
- **Suspended uterus, in pregnancy or childbirth** 654.4 [5th]
  - affecting fetus or newborn 763.89
  - causing obstructed labor 660.2 [5th]
    - affecting fetus or newborn 763.1
- **Sutton's disease** 709.09
- **Sutton and Gull's disease** (arteriolar nephrosclerosis) (*see also* Hypertension, kidney) 403.90
- **Suture** – *continued*
  - burst (in external operation wound) (*see also* Dehiscence) 998.32
    - internal 998.31
  - inadvertently left in operation wound 998.4
  - removal V58.32
  - Shirodkar, in pregnancy (with or without cervical incompetence) 654.5 [5th]
- **Swab inadvertently left in operation wound** 998.4
- **Swallowed, swallowing**
  - difficulty (*see also* Dysphagia) 787.20
  - foreign body NEC (*see also* Foreign body) 938
- **Swamp fever** 100.89
- **Swan neck hand** (intrinsic) 736.09
- **Sweat(s), sweating**
  - disease or sickness 078.2
  - excessive (*see also* Hyperhidrosis) 780.8
  - fetid 705.89
  - fever 078.2
  - gland disease 705.9
    - specified type NEC 705.89
  - miliary 078.2
  - night 780.8
- **Sweeley-Klionsky disease** (angiokeratoma corporis diffusum) 272.7
- **Sweet's syndrome** (acute febrile neutrophilic dermatosis) 695.89
- **Swelling** 782.3
  - abdominal (not referable to specific organ) 789.3 [5th]
  - adrenal gland, cloudy 255.8
  - ankle 719.07
  - anus 787.99
  - arm 729.81
  - breast 611.72
  - Calabar 125.2
  - cervical gland 785.6
  - cheek 784.2
  - chest 786.6
  - ear 388.8
  - epigastric 789.3 [5th]
  - extremity (lower) (upper) 729.81
  - eye 379.92
  - female genital organ 625.8
  - finger 729.81
  - foot 729.81
  - glands 785.6
  - gum 784.2
  - hand 729.81
  - head 784.2
  - inflammatory - *see* Inflammation
  - joint (*see also* Effusion, joint) 719.0 [5th]
    - tuberculous - *see* Tuberculosis, joint
  - kidney, cloudy 593.89
  - leg 729.81
  - limb 729.81
  - liver 573.8
  - lung 786.6
  - lymph nodes 785.6
  - mediastinal 786.6
  - mouth 784.2
  - muscle (limb) 729.81
  - neck 784.2
  - nose or sinus 784.2
  - palate 784.2
  - pelvis 789.3 [5th]
  - penis 607.83
  - perineum 625.8
  - rectum 787.99
  - scrotum 608.86
  - skin 782.2
  - splenic (*see also* Splenomegaly) 789.2
  - substernal 786.6
  - superficial, localized (skin) 782.2
  - testicle 608.86
  - throat 784.2
  - toe 729.81
  - tongue 784.2
  - tubular (*see also* Disease, renal) 593.9
  - umbilicus 789.3 [5th]
  - uterus 625.8

- **Swelling** 782.3
  - vagina 625.8
  - vulva 625.8
  - wandering, due to Gnathostoma (spinigerum) 128.1
  - white - *see* Tuberculosis, arthritis
- **Swift's disease** 985.0
- **Swimmers'**
  - ear (acute) 380.12
  - itch 120.3
- **Swimming in the head** 780.4
- **Swollen** - *see also* Swelling
  - glands 785.6
- **Swyer-James syndrome** (unilateral hyperlucent lung) 492.8
- **Swyer's syndrome** (XY pure gonadal dysgenesis) 752.7
- **Sycosis** 704.8
  - barbae (not parasitic) 704.8
  - contagiosa 110.0
  - lupoid 704.8
  - mycotic 110.0
  - parasitic 110.0
  - vulgaris 704.8
- **Sydenham's chorea** - *see* Chorea, Sydenham's
- **Sylvatic yellow fever** 060.0
- **Sylvest's disease** (epidemic pleurodynia) 074.1
- **Symblepharon** 372.63
  - congenital 743.62
- **Symonds' syndrome** 348.2
- **Sympathetic** - *see* condition
- **Sympatheticotonia** (*see also* Neuropathy, peripheral, autonomic) 337.9
- **Sympathicoblastoma** (M9500/3)
  - specified site - *see* Neoplasm, by site, malignant
  - unspecified site 194.0
- **Sympathicogonioma** (M9500/3) - *see* Sympathicoblastoma
- **Sympathoblastoma** (M9500/3) - *see* Sympathicoblastoma
- **Sympathogonioma** (M9500/3) - *see* Sympathicoblastoma
- **Symphalangy** (*see also* Syndactylism) 755.10
- **Symptoms, specified** (general) NEC 780.99
  - abdomen NEC 789.9
  - bone NEC 733.90
  - breast NEC 611.79
  - cardiac NEC 785.9
  - cardiovascular NEC 785.9
  - chest NEC 786.9
  - development NEC 783.9
  - digestive system NEC 787.99
  - emotional state NEC 799.29 ●
  - eye NEC 379.99
  - gastrointestinal tract NEC 787.99
  - genital organs NEC
    - female 625.9
    - male 608.9
  - head and neck NEC 784.99
  - heart NEC 785.9
  - joint NEC 719.60
    - ankle 719.67
    - elbow 719.62
    - foot 719.67
    - hand 719.64
    - hip 719.65
    - knee 719.66
    - multiple sites 719.69
    - pelvic region 719.65
    - shoulder (region) 719.61
    - specified site NEC 719.68
    - wrist 719.63
  - larynx NEC 784.99
  - limbs NEC 729.89
  - lymphatic system NEC 785.9
  - menopausal 627.2
  - metabolism NEC 783.9
  - mouth NEC 528.9
  - muscle NEC 728.9
  - musculoskeletal NEC 781.99
    - limbs NEC 729.89
  - nervous system NEC 781.99

Symptoms, specified – *continued*

  - neurotic NEC 300.9
  - nutrition, metabolism, and development NEC 783.9
  - pelvis NEC 789.9
    - female 625.9
  - peritoneum NEC 789.9
  - respiratory system NEC 786.9
  - skin and integument NEC 782.9
  - subcutaneous tissue NEC 782.9
  - throat NEC 784.99
  - tonsil NEC 784.99
  - urinary system NEC 788.99
  - vascular NEC 785.9
- **Sympus** 759.89
- **Synarthrosis** 719.80
  - ankle 719.87
  - elbow 719.82
  - foot 719.87
  - hand 719.84
  - hip 719.85
  - knee 719.86
  - multiple sites 719.89
  - pelvic region 719.85
  - shoulder (region) 719.81
  - specified site NEC 719.88
  - wrist 719.83
- **Syncephalus** 759.4
- **Synchondrosis** 756.9
  - abnormal (congenital) 756.9
  - ischiopubic (van Neck's) 732.1
- **Synchysis** (senile) (vitreous humor) 379.21
  - scintillans 379.22
- **Syncope** (near) (pre-) 780.2
  - anginosa 413.9
  - bradycardia 427.89
  - cardiac 780.2
  - carotid sinus 337.01
  - complicating delivery 669.2 [5th]
  - due to lumbar puncture 349.0
  - fatal 798.1
  - heart 780.2
  - heat 992.1
  - laryngeal 786.2
  - tussive 786.2
  - vasoconstriction 780.2
  - vasodepressor 780.2
  - vasomotor 780.2
  - vasovagal 780.2
- **Syncytial infarct** - *see* Placenta, abnormal
- **Syndactylism, syndactyly** (multiple sites) 755.10
  - fingers (without fusion of bone) 755.11
    - with fusion of bone 755.12
  - toes (without fusion of bone) 755.13
    - with fusion of bone 755.14
- **Syndrome** - *see also* Disease
  - 5q minus 238.74
  - abdominal
    - acute 789.0 [5th]
    - migraine 346.2 [5th]
    - muscle deficiency 756.79
  - Abercrombie's (amyloid degeneration) 277.39
  - abnormal innervation 374.43
  - abstinence
    - alcohol 291.81
    - drug 292.0
    - neonatal 779.5 ●
  - Abt-Letterer-Siwe (acute histiocytosis X) (M9722/3) 202.5 [5th]
  - Achard-Thiers (adrenogenital) 255.2
  - acid pulmonary aspiration 997.39
    - obstetric (Mendelson's) 668.0 [5th]
  - acquired immune deficiency 042
  - acquired immunodeficiency 042
  - acrocephalosyndactylism 755.55
  - acute abdominal 789.0 [5th]
  - acute chest 517.3
  - acute coronary 411.1
  - Adair-Dighton (brittle bones and blue sclera, deafness) 756.51
  - Adams-Stokes (-Morgagni) (syncope with heart block) 426.9

Syndrome – *continued*

  - Addisonian 255.41
  - Adie (-Holmes) (pupil) 379.46
  - adiposogenital 253.8
  - adrenal
    - hemorrhage 036.3
    - meningococcic 036.3
  - adrenocortical 255.3
  - adrenogenital (acquired) (congenital) 255.2
    - feminizing 255.2
    - iatrogenic 760.79
    - virilism (acquired) (congenital) 255.2
  - affective organic NEC 293.89
    - drug-induced 292.84
  - afferent loop NEC 537.89
  - African macroglobulinemia 273.3
  - Ahumada-Del Castillo (nonpuerperal galactorrhea and amenorrhea) 253.1
  - air blast concussion - *see* Injury, internal, by site
  - Alagille 759.89
  - Albright (-Martin) (pseudohypoparathyroidism) 275.49
  - Albright-McCune-Sternberg (osteitis fibrosa disseminata) 756.59
  - alcohol withdrawal 291.81
  - Alder's (leukocyte granulation anomaly) 288.2
  - Aldrich (-Wiskott) (eczema-thrombocytopenia) 279.12
  - Alibert-Bazin (mycosis fungoides) (M9700/3) 202.1 [5th]
  - Alice in Wonderland 293.89
  - alien hand 781.8
  - Allen-Masters 620.6
  - Alligator baby (ichthyosis congenita) 757.1
  - Alport's (hereditary hematuria-nephropathy-deafness) 759.89
  - Alvarez (transient cerebral ischemia) 435.9
  - alveolar capillary block 516.3
  - Alzheimer's 331.0
    - with dementia - *see* Alzheimer's, dementia
  - amnestic (confabulatory) 294.0
    - alcohol-induced persisting 291.1
    - drug-induced 292.83
    - posttraumatic 294.0
  - amotivational 292.89
  - amyostatic 275.1
  - amyotrophic lateral sclerosis 335.20
  - androgen insensitivity 259.51
    - partial 259.52
  - Angelman 759.89
  - angina (*see also* Angina) 413.9
  - ankyloglossia superior 750.0
  - anterior
    - chest wall 786.52
    - compartment (tibial) 958.8
    - spinal artery 433.8 [5th]
      - compression 721.1
    - tibial (compartment) 958.8
  - antibody deficiency 279.00
    - agammaglobulinemic 279.00
    - congenital 279.04
    - hypogammaglobulinemic 279.00
  - anticardiolipin antibody 289.81
  - antimongolism 758.39
  - antiphospholipid antibody 289.81
  - Anton (-Babinski) (hemiasomatognosia) 307.9
  - anxiety (*see also* Anxiety) 300.00
    - organic 293.84
  - aortic
    - arch 446.7
    - bifurcation (occlusion) 444.0
    - ring 747.21
  - Apert's (acrocephalosyndactyly) 755.55
  - Apert-Gallais (adrenogenital) 255.2
  - aphasia-apraxia-alexia 784.69
  - apical ballooning 429.83

Syndrome – *continued*

  - "approximate answers" 300.16
  - arcuate ligament (-celiac axis) 447.4
  - arcus aortae 446.7
  - arc welders' 370.24
  - argentaffin, argintaffinoma 259.2
  - Argonz-Del Castillo (nonpuerperal galactorrhea and amenorrhea) 253.1
  - Argyll Robertson's (syphilitic) 094.89
    - nonsyphilitic 379.45
  - arm-shoulder (*see also* Neuropathy, peripheral, autonomic) 337.9
  - Armenian 277.31
  - Arnold-Chiari (*see also* Spina bifida) 741.0 [5th]
    - type I 348.4
    - type II 741.0 [5th]
    - type III 742.0
    - type IV 742.2
  - Arrillaga-Ayerza (pulmonary artery sclerosis with pulmonary hypertension) 416.0
  - arteriomesenteric duodenum occlusion 537.89
  - arteriovenous steal 996.73
  - arteritis, young female (obliterative brachiocephalic) 446.7
  - aseptic meningitis - *see* Meningitis, aseptic
  - Asherman's 621.5
  - Asperger's 299.8 [5th]
  - asphyctic (*see also* Anxiety) 300.00
  - aspiration, of newborn (massive) 770.18
    - meconium 770.12
  - ataxia-telangiectasia 334.8
  - Audry's (acropachyderma) 757.39
  - auriculotemporal 350.8
  - autoimmune lymphoproliferative (ALPS) 279.41 ●
  - autosomal - *see also* Abnormal, autosomes NEC
    - deletion 758.39
      - 5p 758.31
      - 22q11.2 758.32
  - Avellis' 344.89
  - Axenfeld's 743.44
  - Ayerza (-Arrillaga) (pulmonary artery sclerosis with pulmonary hypertension) 416.0
  - Baader's (erythema multiforme exudativum) 695.19
  - Baastrup's 721.5
  - Babinski (-Vaquez) (cardiovascular syphilis) 093.89
  - Babinski-Fröhlich (adiposogenital dystrophy) 253.8
  - Babinski-Nageotte 344.89
  - Bagratuni's (temporal arteritis) 446.5
  - Bakwin-Krida (craniometaphyseal dysplasia) 756.89
  - Balint's (psychic paralysis of visual disorientation) 368.16
  - Ballantyne (-Runge) (postmaturity) 766.22
  - ballooning posterior leaflet 424.0
  - Banti's - *see* Cirrhosis, liver
  - Bard-Pic's (carcinoma, head of pancreas) 157.0
  - Bardet-Biedl (obesity, polydactyly, and mental retardation) 759.89
  - Barlow's (mitral valve prolapse) 424.0
  - Barlow (-Möller) (infantile scurvy) 267
  - Baron Munchausen's 301.51
  - Barré-Guillain 357.0
  - Barré-Liéou (posterior cervical sympathetic) 723.2
  - Barrett's (chronic peptic ulcer of esophagus) 530.85
  - Bársony-Pólgar (corkscrew esophagus) 530.5
  - Bársony-Teschendorf (corkscrew esophagus) 530.5
  - Barth 759.89

Swelling – Symdrome

- **Syndrome** – *continued*
  - Bartter's (secondary hyperaldosteronism with juxtaglomerular hyperplasia) 255.13
  - Basedow's (exophthalmic goiter) 242.0 5th
  - basal cell nevus 759.89 ●
  - basilar artery 435.0
  - basofrontal 377.04
  - Bassen-Kornzweig (abetalipoproteinemia) 272.5
  - Batten-Steinert 359.21
  - battered
    - adult 995.81
    - baby or child 995.54
    - spouse 995.81
  - Baumgarten-Cruveilhier (cirrhosis of liver) 571.5
  - Beals 759.82
  - Bearn-Kunkel (-Slater) (lupoid hepatitis) 571.49
  - Beau's (*see also* Degeneration, myocardial) 429.1
  - Bechterew-Strümpell-Marie (ankylosing spondylitis) 720.0
  - Beck's (anterior spinal artery occlusion) 433.8 5th
  - Beckwith (-Wiedemann) 759.89
  - Behçet's 136.1
  - Bekhterev-Strümpell-Marie (ankylosing spondylitis) 720.0
  - Benedikt's 344.89
  - Béquez César (-Steinbrinck-Chédiak-Higashi) (congenital gigantism of peroxidase granules) 288.2
  - Bernard-Horner (*see also* Neuropathy, peripheral, autonomic) 337.9
  - Bernard-Sergent (acute adrenocortical insufficiency) 255.41
  - Bernhardt-Roth 355.1
  - Bernheim's (*see also* Failure, heart) 428.0
  - Bertolotti's (sacralization of fifth lumbar vertebra) 756.15
  - Besnier-Boeck-Schaumann (sarcoidosis) 135
  - Bianchi's (aphasia-apraxia-alexia syndrome) 784.69
  - Biedl-Bardet (obesity, polydactyly, and mental retardation) 759.89
  - Biemond's (obesity, polydactyly, and mental retardation) 759.89
  - big spleen 289.4
  - bilateral polycystic ovarian 256.4
  - Bing-Horton's 339.00
  - Biörck (-Thorson) (malignant carcinoid) 259.2
  - Birt-Hogg-Dube 759.89
  - Blackfan-Diamond (congenital hypoplastic anemia) 284.01
  - black lung 500
  - black widow spider bite 989.5
  - bladder neck (*see also* Incontinence, urine) 788.30
  - blast (concussion) - *see* Blast, injury
  - blind loop (postoperative) 579.2
  - Block-Siemens (incontinentia pigmenti) 757.33
  - Bloch-Sulzberger (incontinentia pigmenti) 757.33
  - Bloom (-Machacek) (-Torre) 757.39
  - Blount-Barber (tibia vara) 732.4
  - blue
    - bloater 491.20
      - with
        - acute bronchitis 491.22
        - exacerbation (acute) 491.21
    - diaper 270.0
    - drum 381.02
    - sclera 756.51
    - toe 445.02
  - Boder-Sedgwick (ataxia-telangiectasia) 334.8
  - Boerhaave's (spontaneous esophageal rupture) 530.4
  - Bonnevie-Ullrich 758.6
  - Bonnier's 386.19
  - Borjeson-Forssman-Lehmann 759.89
  - Bouillaud's (rheumatic heart disease) 391.9
  - Bourneville (-Pringle) (tuberous sclerosis) 759.5
  - Bouveret (-Hoffmann) (paroxysmal tachycardia) 427.2
  - brachial plexus 353.0
  - Brachman-de Lange (Amsterdam dwarf, mental retardation, and brachycephaly) 759.89
  - bradycardia-tachycardia 427.81
  - Brailsford-Morquio (dystrophy) (mucopolysaccharidosis IV) 277.5
  - brain (acute) (chronic) (nonpsychotic) (organic) (with behavioral reaction) (with neurotic reaction) 310.9
    - with
      - presenile brain disease (*see also* Dementia, presenile) 290.10
      - psychosis, psychotic reaction (*see also* Psychosis, organic) 294.9
    - chronic alcoholic 291.2
    - congenital (*see also* Retardation, mental) 319
    - postcontusional 310.2
    - posttraumatic
      - nonpsychotic 310.2
      - psychotic 293.9
        - acute 293.0
        - chronic (*see also* Psychosis, organic) 294.8
        - subacute 293.1
    - psycho-organic (*see also* Syndrome, psycho-organic) 310.9
    - psychotic (*see also* Psychosis, organic) 294.9
    - senile (*see also* Dementia, senile) 290.0
  - branchial arch 744.41
  - Brandt's (acrodermatitis enteropathica) 686.8
  - Brennemann's 289.2
  - Briquet's 300.81
  - Brissaud-Meige (infantile myxedema) 244.9
  - broad ligament laceration 620.6
  - Brock's (atelectasis due to enlarged lymph nodes) 518.0
  - broken heart 429.83
  - Brown's tendon sheath 378.61
  - Brown-Séquard 344.89
  - brown spot 756.59
  - Brugada 746.89
  - Brugsch's (acropachyderma) 757.39
  - bubbly lung 770.7
  - Buchem's (hyperostosis corticalis) 733.3
  - Budd-Chiari (hepatic vein thrombosis) 453.0
  - Büdinger-Ludloff-Läwen 717.89
  - bulbar 335.22
    - lateral (*see also* Disease, cerebrovascular, acute) 436
  - Bullis fever 082.8
  - bundle of Kent (anomalous atrioventricular excitation) 426.7
  - Bürger-Grutz (essential familial hyperlipemia) 272.3
  - Burke's (pancreatic insufficiency and chronic neutropenia) 577.8
  - Burnett's (milk-alkali) 275.42
  - Burnier's (hypophyseal dwarfism) 253.3
  - burning feet 266.2
  - Bywaters' 958.5
  - Caffey's (infantile cortical hyperostosis) 756.59
  - Calvé-Legg-Perthes (osteochrondrosis, femoral capital) 732.1
  - Caplan (-Colinet) syndrome 714.81
  - capsular thrombosis (*see also* Thrombosis, brain) 434.0 5th
  - carbohydrate-deficient glycoprotein (CDGS) 271.8
  - carcinogenic thrombophlebitis 453.1
  - carcinoid 259.2
  - cardiac asthma (*see also* Failure, ventricular, left) 428.1
  - cardiacos negros 416.0
  - cardiofaciocutaneous 759.89 ●
  - cardiopulmonary obesity 278.8
  - cardiorenal (*see also* Hypertension, cardiorenal) 404.90
  - cardiorespiratory distress (idiopathic), newborn 769
  - cardiovascular renal (*see also* Hypertension, cardiorenal) 404.90
  - cardiovasorenal 272.7
  - Carini's (ichthyosis congenita) 757.1
  - carotid
    - artery (internal) 435.8
    - body or sinus 337.01
  - carpal tunnel 354.0
  - Carpenter's 759.89
  - Cassidy (-Scholte) (malignant carcinoid) 259.2
  - cat-cry 758.31
  - cauda equina 344.60
  - causalgia 355.9
    - lower limb 355.71
    - upper limb 354.4
  - cavernous sinus 437.6
  - celiac 579.0
    - artery compression 447.4
    - axis 447.4
  - central pain 338.0
  - cerebellomedullary malformation (*see also* Spina bifida) 741.0 5th
  - cerebral gigantism 253.0
  - cerebrohepatorenal 759.89
  - cervical (root) (spine) NEC 723.8
    - disc 722.71
    - posterior, sympathetic 723.2
    - rib 353.0
    - sympathetic paralysis 337.09
    - traumatic (acute) NEC 847.0
  - cervicobrachial (diffuse) 723.3
  - cervicocranial 723.2
  - cervicodorsal outlet 353.2
  - Céstan's 344.89
  - Céstan (-Raymond) 433.8 5th
  - Céstan-Chenais 344.89
  - chancriform 114.1
  - Charcôt's (intermittent claudication) 443.9
    - angina cruris 443.9
    - due to atherosclerosis 440.21
  - Charcôt-Marie-Tooth 356.1
  - Charcôt-Weiss-Baker 337.01
  - CHARGE association 759.89
  - Cheadle (-Möller) (-Barlow) (infantile scurvy) 267
  - Chédiak-Higashi (-Steinbrinck) (congenital gigantism of peroxidase granules) 288.2
  - chest wall 786.52
  - Chiari's (hepatic vein thrombosis) 453.0
  - Chiari-Frommel 676.6 5th
  - chiasmatic 368.41
  - Chilaiditi's (subphrenic displacement, colon) 751.4
  - chondroectodermal dysplasia 756.55
  - chorea-athetosis-agitans 275.1
  - Christian's (chronic histiocytosis X) 277.89
  - chromosome 4 short arm deletion 758.39
  - chronic pain 338.4
  - Churg-Strauss 446.4
  - Clarke-Hadfield (pancreatic infantilism) 577.8
  - Claude's 352.6
  - Claude Bernard-Horner (*see also* Neuropathy, peripheral, autonomic) 337.9
  - Clérambault's
    - automatism 348.8<u>9</u> ▲
    - erotomania 297.8
  - Clifford's (postmaturity) 766.22
  - climacteric 627.2
  - Clouston's (hidrotic ectodermal dysplasia) 757.31
  - clumsiness 315.4
  - Cockayne's (microencephaly and dwarfism) 759.89
  - Cockayne-Weber (epidermolysis bullosa) 757.39
  - Coffin-Lowry 759.89
  - Cogan's (nonsyphilitic interstitial keratitis) 370.52
  - cold injury (newborn) 778.2
  - Collet (-Sicard) 352.6
  - combined immunity deficiency 279.2
  - compartment(al) (anterior) (deep) (posterior) 958.8
    - nontraumatic
      - abdomen 729.73
      - arm 729.71
      - buttock 729.72
      - fingers 729.71
      - foot 729.72
      - forearm 729.71
      - hand 729.71
      - hip 729.72
      - leg 729.72
      - lower extremity 729.72
      - shoulder 729.71
      - specified site NEC 729.79
      - thigh 729.72
      - toes 729.72
      - upper extremity 729.71
      - wrist 729.71
    - post-surgical (*see also* Syndrome, compartment, non-traumatic) 998.89
    - traumatic 958.90
      - abdomen 958.93
      - arm 958.91
      - buttock 958.92
      - fingers 958.91
      - foot 958.92
      - forearm 958.91
      - hand 958.91
      - hip 958.92
      - leg 958.92
      - lower extremity 958.92
      - shoulder 958.91
      - specified site NEC 958.99
      - thigh 958.92
      - tibial 958.92
      - toes 958.92
      - upper extremity 958.91
      - wrist 958.91
  - complex regional pain - *see also* Dystrophy, sympathetic
    - type I - *see* Dystrophy, sympathetic (posttraumatic) (reflex)
    - type II - *see* Causalgia
  - compression 958.5
    - cauda equina 344.60
      - with neurogenic bladder 344.61
  - concussion 310.2
  - congenital
    - affecting more than one system 759.7
      - specified type NEC 759.89
    - congenital central alveolar hypoventilation 327.25
    - facial diplegia 352.6
    - muscular hypertrophy-cerebral 759.89
  - congestion-fibrosis (pelvic) 625.5
  - conjunctivourethrosynovial 099.3
  - Conn (-Louis) (primary aldosteronism) 255.12
  - Conradi (-Hünermann) (chondrodysplasia calcificans congenita) 756.59
  - conus medullaris 336.8
  - Cooke-Apert-Gallais (adrenogenital) 255.2
  - Cornelia de Lange's (Amsterdam dwarf, mental retardation, and brachycephaly) 759.8 5th
  - coronary insufficiency or intermediate 411.1
  - cor pulmonale 416.9

Syndrome

Syndrome – *continued*
- Launois-Cléret (adiposogenital dystrophy) 253.8
- Laurence-Moon (-Bardet)-Biedl (obesity, polydactyly, and mental retardation) 759.89
- Lawford's (encephalocutaneous angiomatosis) 759.6
- lazy
  - leukocyte 288.09
  - posture 728.3
- Lederer-Brill (acquired infectious hemolytic anemia) 283.19
- Legg-Calvé-Perthes (osteochondrosis capital femoral) 732.1
- Lemiere 451.89
- Lennox-Gastaut syndrome 345.0 5th
  - with tonic seizures 345.1 5th
- Lennox's (*see also* Epilepsy) 345.0 5th
- lenticular 275.1
- Léopold-Lévi's (paroxysmal thyroid instability) 242.9 5th
- Lepore hemoglobin 282.49
- Léri-Weill 756.59
- Leriche's (aortic bifurcation occlusion) 444.0
- Lermoyez's (*see also* Disease, Ménière's) 386.00
- Lesch-Nyhan (hypoxanthine-guanine-phosphroibosyltransferase deficiency) 277.2
- leukoencephalopathy, reversible, posterior 348.5 5th
- Lev's (acquired complete heart block) 426.0
- Levi's (pituitary dwarfism) 253.3
- Lévy-Roussy 334.3
- Lichtheim's (subacute combined sclerosis with pernicious anemia) 281.0 *[336.2]*
- Li-Fraumeni V84.01
- Lightwood's (renal tubular acidosis) 588.89
- Lignac (-de Toni) (-Fanconi) (-Debré) (cystinosis) 270.0
- Likoff's (angina in menopausal women) 413.9
- liver-kidney 572.4
- Lloyd's 258.1
- lobotomy 310.0
- Löffler's (eosinophilic pneumonitis) 518.3
- Löfgren's (sarcoidosis) 135
- long arm 18 or 21 deletion 758.39
- Looser (-Debray)-Milkman (osteomalacia with pseudofractures) 268.2
- Lorain-Levi (pituitary dwarfism) 253.3
- Louis-Bar (ataxia-telangiectasia) 334.8
- low
  - atmospheric pressure 993.2
  - back 724.2
    - psychogenic 306.0
  - output (cardiac) (*see also* Failure, heart) 428.9
- Lowe's (oculocerebrorenal dystrophy) 270.8
- Lowe-Terrey-MacLachlan (oculocerebrorenal dystrophy) 270.8
- lower radicular, newborn 767.4
- Lown (-Ganong)-Levine (short P-R internal, normal QRS complex, and supraventricular tachycardia) 426.81
- Lucey-Driscoll (jaundice due to delayed conjugation) 774.30
- Luetscher's (dehydration) 276.51
- lumbar vertebral 724.4
- Lutembacher's (atrial septal defect with mitral stenosis) 745.5
- Lyell's (toxic epidermal necrolysis) 695.15
  - due to drug
    - correct substance properly administered 695.15

Syndrome – *continued*
- Lyell's – *continued*
  - due to drug – *continued*
    - overdose or wrong substance given or taken 977.9
      - specified drug - *see* Table of Drugs and Chemicals
- MacLeod's 492.8
- macrogenitosomia praecox 259.8
- macroglobulinemia 273.3
- macrophage activation 288.4
- Maffucci's (dyschondroplasia with hemangiomas) 756.4
- Magenblase 306.4
- magnesium-deficiency 781.7
- malabsorption 579.9
  - postsurgical 579.3
  - spinal fluid 331.3
- Mal de Debarquement 780.4
- malignant carcinoid 259.2
- Mallory-Weiss 530.7
- mandibulofacial dysostosis 756.0
- manic-depressive (*see also* Psychosis, affective) 296.80
- Mankowsky's (familial dysplastic osteopathy) 731.2
- maple syrup (urine) 270.3
- Marable's (celiac artery compression) 447.4
- Marchesani (-Weill) (brachymorphism and ectopia lentis) 759.89
- Marchiafava-Bignami 341.8
- Marchiafava-Micheli (paroxysmal nocturnal hemoglobinuria) 283.2
- Marcus Gunn's (jaw-winking syndrome) 742.8
- Marfan's (arachnodactyly) 759.82
  - meaning congenital syphilis 090.49
    - with luxation of lens 090.49 *[379.32]*
- Marie's (acromegaly) 253.0
  - primary or idiopathic (acropachyderma) 757.39
  - secondary (hypertrophic pulmonary osteoarthropathy) 731.2
- Markus-Adie 379.46
- Maroteaux-Lamy (mucopolysaccharidosis VI) 277.5
- Martin's 715.27
- Martin-Albright (pseudohypoparathyroidism) 275.49
- Martorell-Fabré (pulseless disease) 446.7
- massive aspiration of newborn 770.18
- Masters-Allen 620.6
- mastocytosis 757.33
- maternal hypotension 669.2 5th
- maternal obesity 646.1 5th
- May (-Hegglin) 288.2
- McArdle (-Schmid) (-Pearson) (glycogenosis V) 271.0
- McCune-Albright (osteitis fibrosa disseminata) 756.59
- McQuarrie's (idiopathic familial hypoglycemia) 251.2
- meconium
  - aspiration 770.12
  - plug (newborn) NEC 777.1
- median arcuate ligament 447.4
- mediastinal fibrosis 519.3
- Meekeren-Ehlers-Danlos 756.83
- Meige (blepharospasm-oromandibular dystonia) 333.82
  - -Milroy (chronic hereditary edema) 757.0
- MELAS (mitochondrial encephalopathy, lactic acidosis and stroke-like episodes) 277.87
- Melkersson (-Rosenthal) 351.8
- MEN (multiple endocrine neoplasia)
  - type I 258.01
  - type IIA 258.02
  - type IIB 258.03
- Mende's (ptosis-epicanthus) 270.2

Syndrome – *continued*
- Mendelson's (resulting from a procedure) 997.39
  - during labor 668.0 5th
  - obstetric 668.0 5th
- Ménétrier's (hypertrophic gastritis) 535.2 5th
- Ménière's (*see also* Disease, Ménière's) 386.00
- meningo-eruptive 047.1
- Menkes' 759.89
  - glutamic acid 759.89
  - maple syrup (urine) disease 270.3
- menopause 627.2
  - postartificial 627.4
- menstruation 625.4
- MERRF (myoclonus with epilepsy and with ragged red fibers) 277.87
- mesenteric
  - artery, superior 557.1
  - vascular insufficiency (with gangrene) 557.1
- metabolic 277.7
- metastatic carcinoid 259.2
- Meyenburg-Altherr-Uehlinger 733.99
- Meyer-Schwickerath and Weyers (dysplasia oculodentodigitalis) 759.89
- Micheli-Rietti (thalassemia minor) 282.49
- Michotte's 721.5
- micrognathia-glossoptosis 756.0
- microphthalmos (congenital) 759.89
- midbrain 348.89 ▲
- middle
  - lobe (lung) (right) 518.0
  - radicular 353.0
- Miescher's
  - familial acanthosis nigricans 701.2
  - granulomatosis disciformis 709.3
- Mieten's 759.89
- migraine 346.0 5th
- Mikity-Wilson (pulmonary dysmaturity) 770.7
- Mikulicz's (dryness of mouth, absent or decreased lacrimation) 527.1
- milk alkali (milk drinkers') 275.42
- Milkman (-Looser) (osteomalacia with pseudofractures) 268.2
- Millard-Gubler 344.89
- Miller-Dieker 758.33
- Miller Fisher's 357.0
- Milles' (encephalocutaneous angiomatosis) 759.6
- Minkowski-Chauffard (*see also* Spherocytosis) 282.0
- Mirizzi's (hepatic duct stenosis) 576.2
  - with calculus, cholelithiasis, or stones - *see* Choledocholithiasis
- mitochondrial neurogastrointestinal encephalopathy (MNGIE) 277.87
- mitral
  - click (-murmur) 785.2
  - valve prolapse 424.0
- MNGIE (mitochondrial neurogastrointestinal encephalopathy) 277.87
- Möbius'
  - congenital oculofacial paralysis 352.6
  - ophthalmoplegic migraine 346.2 5th
- Mohr's (types I and II) 759.89
- monofixation 378.34
- Moore's (*see also* Epilepsy) 345.5 5th
- Morel-Moore (hyperostosis frontalis interna) 733.3
- Morel-Morgagni (hyperostosis frontalis interna) 733.3
- Morgagni (-Stewart-Morel) (hyperostosis frontalis interna) 733.3
- Morgagni-Adams-Stokes (syncope with heart block) 426.9
- Morquio (-Brailsford) (-Ullrich) (mucopolysaccharidosis IV) 277.5
- Morris (testicular feminization) 259.51

Syndrome – *continued*
- Morton's (foot) (metatarsalgia) (metatarsal neuralgia) (neuralgia) (neuroma) (toe) 355.6
- Moschcowitz (-Singer-Symmers) (thrombotic thrombocytopenic purpura) 446.6
- Mounier-Kuhn 748.3
  - with
    - acute exacerbation 494.1
    - bronchiectasis 494.0
      - with (acute) exacerbation 494.1
  - acquired 519.19
    - with bronchiectasis 494.0
      - with (acute) exacerbation 494.1
- Mucha-Haberman (acute parapsoriasis varioliformis) 696.2
- mucocutaneous lymph node (acute) (febrile) (infantile) (MCLS) 446.1
- multiple
  - deficiency 260
  - endocrine neoplasia (MEN)
    - type I 258.01
    - type IIA 258.02
    - type IIB 258.03
  - operations 301.51
- Munchausen's 301.51
- Munchmeyer's (exostosis luxurians) 728.11
- Murchison-Sanderson - *see* Disease, Hodgkin's
- myasthenic - *see* Myasthenia, syndrome
- myelodysplastic 238.75
  - with 5q deletion 238.74
  - high grade with 5q deletion 238.73
  - therapy-related 289.83
- myeloproliferative (chronic) (M9960/1) 238.79
- myofascial pain NEC 729.1
- Naffziger's 353.0
- Nager-de Reynier (dysostosis mandibularis) 756.0
- nail-patella (hereditary osteo-onychodysplasia) 756.89
- NARP (neuropathy, ataxia and retinitis pigmentosa) 277.87
- Nebécourt's 253.3
- Neill Dingwall (microencephaly and dwarfism) 759.89
- nephrotic (*see also* Nephrosis) 581.9
  - diabetic 250.4 5th *[581.81]*
    - due to secondary diabetes 249.4 5th *[581.81]*
- Netherton's (ichthyosiform erythroderma) 757.1
- neurocutaneous 759.6
- neuroleptic malignant 333.92
- Nezelof's (pure alymphocytosis) 279.13
- Niemann-Pick (lipid histiocytosis) 272.7
- Nonne-Milroy-Meige (chronic hereditary edema) 757.0
- nonsense 300.16
- Noonan's 759.89
- Nothnagel's
  - ophthalmoplegia-cerebellar ataxia 378.52
  - vasomotor acroparesthesia 443.89
- nucleus ambiguous-hypoglossal 352.6
- OAV (oculoauriculovertebral dysplasia) 756.0
- obsessional 300.3
- oculocutaneous 364.24
- oculomotor 378.81
- oculourethroarticular 099.3
- Ogilvie's (sympathicotonic colon obstruction) 560.89
- ophthalmoplegia-cerebellar ataxia 378.52
- Oppenheim-Urbach (necrobiosis lipoidica diabeticorum) 250.8 5th *[709.3]*
  - due to secondary diabetes 249.8 5th *[709.3]*
- oral-facial-digital 759.89

Syndrome

Syndrome - *continued*
- organic
  - affective NEC 293.83
    - drug-induced 292.84
  - anxiety 293.84
  - delusional 293.81
    - alcohol-induced 291.5
    - drug-induced 292.11
    - due to or associated with
      - arteriosclerosis 290.42
      - presenile brain disease 290.12
      - senility 290.20
  - depressive 293.83
    - drug-induced 292.84
    - due to or associated with
      - arteriosclerosis 290.43
      - presenile brain disease 290.13
      - senile brain disease 290.21
  - hallucinosis 293.82
    - drug-induced 292.84
- organic affective 293.83
  - induced by drug 292.84
- organic personality 310.1
  - induced by drug 292.89
- Ormond's 593.4
- ordigitofacial 759.89
- orthostatic hypotensive-dysautonomic-dyskinetic 333.0
- Osler-Weber-Rendu (familial hemmorrhagic telangiectasia) 448.0
- osteodermopathic hyperostosis 757.39
- osteoporosis-osteomalacia 268.2
- Österreicher-Turner (hereditary osteo-onychodysplasia) 756.89
- os trigonum 755.69
- Ostrum-Furst 756.59
- otolith 386.19
- otopalatodigital 759.89
- outlet (thoracic) 353.0
- ovarian remnant 620.8
- Owren's (*see also* Defect, coagulation) 286.3
- OX 758.6
- pacemaker 429.4
- Paget-Schroetter (intermittent venous claudication) 453.89 ▲
- pain - *see also* Pain
  - central 338.0
  - chronic 338.4
  - complex regional 355.9
    - type I 337.20
      - lower limb 337.22
      - specified site NEC 337.29
      - upper limb 337.21
    - type II
      - lower limb 355.71
      - upper limb 354.4
  - myelopathic 338.0
  - thalamic (hyperesthetic) 338.0
- painful
  - apicocostal vertebral (M8010/3) 162.3
  - arc 726.19
  - bruising 287.2
  - feet 266.2
- Pancoast's (carcinoma, pulmonary apex) (M8010/3) 162.3
- panhypopituitary (postpartum) 253.2
- papillary muscle 429.81
  - with myocardial infarction 410.8 5th
- Papillon-Léage and Psaume (orodigitofacial dysostosis) 759.89
- parabiotic (transfusion)
  - donor (twin) 772.0
  - recipient (twin) 776.4
- paralysis agitans 332.0
- paralytic 344.9
  - specified type NEC 344.89
- paraneoplastic- *see* condition
- Parinaud's (paralysis of conjugate upward gaze) 378.81
  - oculoglandular 372.02

Syndrome - *continued*
- Parkes Weber and Dimitri (encephalocutaneous angiomatosis) 759.6
- Parkinson's (*see also* Parkinsonism) 332.0
- parkinsonian (*see also* Parkinsonism) 332.0
- Parry's (exophthalmic goiter) 242.0 5th
- Parry-Romberg 349.89
- Parsonage-Aldren-Turner 353.5
- Parsonage-Turner 353.5
- Patau's (trisomy D_1) 758.1
- patella clunk 719.66
- patellofemoral 719.46
- Paterson (-Brown) (-Kelly) (sideropenic dysphagia) 280.8
- Payr's (splenic flexure syndrome) 569.89
- pectoral girdle 447.8
- pectoralis minor 447.8
- Pelger-Huët (hereditary hyposegmentation) 288.2
- pellagra-cerebellar ataxia-renal aminoaciduria 270.0
- Pellegrini-Stieda 726.62
- pellagroid 265.2
- Pellizzi's (pineal) 259.8
- pelvic congestion (-fibrosis) 625.5
- Pendred's (familial goiter with deaf-mutism) 243
- Penfield's (*see also* Epilepsy) 345.5 5th
- Penta X 758.81
- peptic ulcer - *see* Ulcer, peptic 533.9 5th
- perabduction 447.8
- periodic 277.31
- periurethral fibrosis 593.4
- persistent fetal circulation 747.83
- Petges-Cléjat (poikilodermatomyositis) 710.3
- Peutz-Jeghers 759.6
- Pfeiffer (acrocephalosyndactyly) 755.55
- phantom limb 353.6
- pharyngeal pouch 279.11
- Pick's (pericardial pseudocirrhosis of liver) 423.2
  - heart 423.2
  - liver 423.2
- Pick-Herxheimer (diffuse idiopathic cutaneous atrophy) 701.8
- Pickwickian (cardiopulmonary obesity) 278.8
- PIE (pulmonary infiltration with eosinophilia 518.3
- Pierre Marie-Bamberger (hypertrophic pulmonary osteoarthropathy) 731.2
- Pierre Mauriac's (diabetes-dwarfism-obesity) 258.1
- Pierre Robin 756.0
- pigment dispersion, iris 364.53
- pineal 259.8
- pink puffer 492.8
- pituitary 253.0
- placental
  - dysfunction 762.2
  - insufficiency 762.2
  - transfusion 762.3
- plantar fascia 728.71
- plateau iris 364.82
- plica knee 727.83
- Plummer-Vinson (sideropenic dysphagia) 280.8
- pluricarential of infancy 260
- plurideficiency of infancy 260
- pluriglandular (compensatory) 258.8
- polycarential of infancy 260
- polyglandular 258.8
- polysplenia 759.0
- pontine 433.8 5th
- popliteal
  - artery entrapment 447.8
  - web 756.89
- postartificial menopause 627.4
- postcardiac injury
  - postcardiotomy 429.4
  - postmyocardial infarction 411.0

Syndrome - *continued*
- postcardiotomy 429.4
- postcholecystectomy 576.0
- postcommissurotomy 429.4
- postconcussional 310.2
- postcontusional 310.2
- postencephalitic 310.8
- posterior
  - cervical sympathetic 723.2
  - fossa compression 348.4
  - inferior cerebellar artery (*see also* Disease, cerebrovascular, acute) 436
  - reversible encephalopathy (PRES) 348.39
- postgastrectomy (dumping) 564.2
- post-gastric surgery 564.2
- posthepatitis 780.79
- postherpetic (neuralgia) (zoster) 053.19
  - geniculate ganglion 053.11
  - ophthalmica 053.19
- postimmunization - *see* Complications, vaccination
- postinfarction 411.0
- postinfluenza (asthenia) 780.79
- postirradiation 990
- postlaminectomy 722.80
  - cervical, cervicothoracic 722.81
  - lumbar, lumbosacral 722.83
  - thoracic, thoracolumbar 722.82
- postleukotomy 310.0
- postlobotomy 310.0
- postmastectomy lymphedema 457.0
- postmature (of newborn) 766.22
- postmyocardial infarction 411.0
- postoperative NEC 998.9
  - blind loop 579.2
- postpartum panhypopituitary 253.2
- postperfusion NEC 999.89
  - bone marrow 996.85
- postpericardiotomy 429.4
- postphlebitic (asymptomatic) 459.10
  - with
    - complications NEC 459.19
    - inflammation 459.12
      - and ulcer 459.13
    - stasis dermatitis 459.12
      - with ulcer 459.13
    - ulcer 459.11
      - with inflammation 459.13
- postpolio (myelitis) 138
- postvagotomy 564.2
- postvalvulotomy 429.4
- postviral (asthenia) NEC 780.79
- Potain's (gastrectasis with dyspepsia) 536.1
- potassium intoxication 276.7
- Potter's 753.0
- Prader (-Labhart)-Willi (-Fanconi) 759.81
- preinfarction 411.1
- preleukemic 238.75
- premature senility 259.8
- premenstrual 625.4
- premenstrual tension 625.4
- pre ulcer 536.9
- Prinzmetal-Massumi (anterior chest wall syndrome) 786.52
- Profichet's 729.90
- progeria 259.8
- progressive pallidal degeneration 333.0
- prolonged gestation 766.22
- Proteus (dermal hypoplasia) 757.39
- prune belly 756.71
- prurigo-asthma 691.8
- pseudocarpal tunnel (sublimis) 354.0
- pseudohermaphroditism-virilism-hirsutism 255.2
- pseudoparalytica 358.00
- pseudo-Turner's 759.89
- psycho-organic 293.9
  - acute 293.0
  - anxiety type 293.84
  - depressive type 293.83
  - hallucinatory type 293.82

Syndrome - *continued*
- psycho-organic - *continued*
  - nonpsychotic severity 310.1
    - specified focal (partial) NEC 310.8
  - paranoid type 293.81
  - specified type NEC 293.89
  - subacute 293.1
- pterygolymphangiectasia 758.6
- ptosis-epicanthus 270.2
- pulmonary
  - arteriosclerosis 416.0
  - hypoperfusion (idiopathic) 769
  - renal (hemorrhagic) 446.21
- pulseless 446.7
- Putnam-Dana (subacute combined sclerosis with pernicious anemia) 281.0 *[336.2]*
- pyloroduodenal 537.89
- pyramidopallidonigral 332.0
- pyriformis 355.0
- QT interval prolongation 426.82
- radicular NEC 729.2
  - lower limbs 724.4
  - upper limbs 723.4
    - newborn 767.4
- Raeder-Harbitz (pulseless disease) 446.7
- Ramsay Hunt's
  - dyssynergia cerebellaris myoclonica 334.2
  - herpetic geniculate ganglionitis 053.11
- rapid time-zone change 327.35
- Raymond (-Céstan) 433.8 5th
- Raynaud's (paroxysmal digital cyanosis) 443.0
- RDS (respiratory distress syndrome, newborn) 769
- Refsum's (heredopathia atactica polyneuritiformis) 356.3
- Reichmann's (gastrosuccorrhea) 536.8
- Reifenstein's (hereditary familial hypogonadism, male) 259.52
- Reilly's (*see also* Neuropathy, peripheral, autonomic 337.9
- Reiter's 099.3
- renal glomerulohyalinosis-diabetic 250.4 5th *[581.81]*
  - due to secondary diabetes 249.4 5th *[581.81]*
- Rendu-Osler-Weber (familial hemorrhagic telangiectasia) 448.0
- renofacial (congenital biliary fibroangiomatosis) 753.0
- Rénon-Delille 253.8
- respiratory distress (idiopathic) (newborn) 769
  - adult (following shock, surgery, or trauma) 518.5
    - specified NEC 518.82
  - type II 770.6
- restless legs (RLS) 333.94
- retinoblastoma (familial) 190.5
- retraction (Duane's) 378.71
- retroperitoneal fibrosis 593.4
- retroviral seroconversion (acute) V08
- Rett's 330.8
- Reye's 331.81
- Reye-Sheehan (postpartum pituitary necrosis) 253.2
- Riddoch's (visual disorientation) 368.16
- Ridley's (*see also* Failure, ventricular, left) 428.1
- Rieger's (mesodermal dysgenesis, anterior ocular segment) 743.44
- Rietti-Greppi-Micheli (thalassemia minor) 282.49
- right ventricular obstruction - *see* Failure heart
- Riley-Day (familial dysautonomia) 742.8
- Robin's 756.0
- Rokitansky-Kuster-Hauser (congenital absence, vagina) 752.49
- Romano-Ward (prolonged QT interval syndrome) 426.82
- Romberg's 349.89

- **Syndrome** – *continued*
  - trisomy – *continued*
    - 20 758.5
    - 21 or G (mongolism) 758.0
    - 22 or G (mongolism) 758.0
    - G 758.0
  - Troisier-Hanot-Chauffard (bronze diabetes) 275.0
  - tropical wet feet 991.4
  - Trousseau's (thrombophlebitis migrans visceral cancer) 453.1
  - Türk's (ocular retraction syndrome) 378.71
  - Turner's 758.6
  - Turner-Varny 758.6
  - tumor lysis (following antineoplastic drug therapy) (spontaneous) 277.88 ●
  - Twiddler's (due to)
    - automatic implantable defibrillator 996.04
    - pacemaker 996.01
  - twin-to-twin transfusion 762.3
    - recipient twin 776.4
  - Uehlinger's (acropachyderma) 757.39
  - Ullrich (-Bonnevie) (-Turner) 758.6
  - Ullrich-Feichtiger 759.89
  - underwater blast injury (abdominal) (*see also* Injury, internal, abdomen) 868.00
  - universal joint, cervix 620.6
  - Unverricht (-Lundborg) 345.1 ▲
  - Unverricht-Wagner (dermatomyositis) 710.3
  - upward gaze 378.81
  - Urbach-Oppenheim (necrobiosis lipoidica diabeticorum) 250.8 [5th] *[709.3]*
    - due to secondary diabetes 249.8 [5th] *[709.3]*
  - Urbach-Wiethe (lipoid proteinosis) 272.8
  - uremia, chronic 585.9
  - urethral 597.81
  - urethro-oculoarticular 099.3
  - urethro-oculosynovial 099.3
  - urohepatic 572.4
  - uveocutaneous 364.24
  - uveomeningeal, uveomeningitis 363.22
  - vagohypoglossal 352.6
  - vagovagal 780.2
  - van Buchem's (hyperostosis corticalis) 733.3
  - van der Hoeve's (brittle bones and blue sclera, deafness) 756.51
  - van der Hoeve-Halbertsma-Waardenburg (ptosis-epicanthus) 270.2
  - van der Hoeve-Waarderburg-Gualdi (ptosis-epicanthus) 270.2
  - vanishing twin 651.33
  - van Neck-Odelberg (juvenile osteochondrosis) 732.1
  - vascular splanchnic 557.0
  - vasomotor 443.9
  - vasovagal 780.2
  - VATER 759.89
  - Velo-cardio-facial 758.32
  - vena cava (inferior) (superior) (obstruction) 459.2
  - Verbiest's (claudicatio intermittens spinalis) 435.1
  - Vernet's 352.6
  - vertebral
    - artery 435.1
      - compression 721.1
    - lumbar 724.4
    - steal 435.1
  - vertebrogenic (pain) 724.5
  - vertiginous NEC 386.9
  - video display tube 723.8
  - Villaret's 352.6
  - Vinson-Plummer (sideropenic dysphagia) 280.8
  - virilizing adrenocortical hyperplasia, congenital 255.2
  - virus, viral 079.99
  - visceral larval migrans 128.0
  - visual disorientation 368.16
  - vitamin B_6 deficiency 266.1
  - vitreous touch 997.99
  - Vogt's (corpus striatum) 333.71
  - Vogt-Koyanagi 364.24
  - Volkmann's 958.6
  - von Bechterew-Stumpell (ankylosing spondylitis) 720.0
  - von Graefe's 378.72
  - von Hippel-Lindau (angiomatosis retinocerebellosa) 759.6
  - von Schroetter's (intermittent venous claudication) 453.89 ▲
  - von Willebrand (-Jürgens) (angiohemophilia) 286.4
  - Waardenburg-Klein (ptosis epicanthus) 270.2
  - Wagner (-Unverricht) (dermatomyositis) 710.3
  - Waldenström's (macroglobulinemia) 273.3
  - Waldenström-Kjellberg (sideropenic dysphagia) 280.8
  - Wallenberg's (posterior inferior cerebellar artery) (*see also* Disease, cerebrovascular, acute) 436
  - Waterhouse (-Friderichsen) 036.3
  - water retention 276.6
  - Weber's 344.89
  - Weber-Christian (nodular nonsuppurative panniculitis) 729.30
  - Weber-Cockayne (epidermolysis bullosa) 757.39
  - Weber-Dimitri (encephalocutaneous angiomatosis) 759.6
  - Weber-Gubler 344.89
  - Weber-Leyden 344.89
  - Weber-Osler (familial hemorrhagic telangiectasia) 448.0
  - Wegener's (necrotizing respiratory granulomatosis) 446.4
  - Weill-Marchesani (brachymorphism and ectopia lentis) 759.89
  - Weingarten's (tropical eosinophilia) 518.3
  - Weiss-Baker (carotid sinus syncope) 337.01
  - Weissenbach-Thibierge (cutaneous systemic sclerosis) 710.1
  - Werdnig-Hoffmann 335.0
  - Werlhof-Wichmann (*see also* Purpura, thrombocytopenic) 287.39
  - Wermer's (polyendocrine adenomatosis) 258.01
  - Werner's (progeria adultorum) 259.8
  - Wernicke's (nonalcoholic) (superior hemorrhagic polioencephalitis) 265.1
  - Wernicke-Korsakoff (nonalcoholic) 294.0
    - alcoholic 291.1
  - Westphal-Strümpell (hepatolenticular degeneration) 275.1
  - wet
    - brain (alcoholic) 303.9 [5th]
    - feet (maceration) (tropical) 991.4
    - lung
      - adult 518.5
      - newborn 770.6
  - whiplash 847.0
  - Whipple's (intestinal lipodystrophy) 040.2
  - "whistling face" (craniocarpotarsal dystrophy) 759.89
  - Widal (-Abrami) (acquired hemolytic jaundice) 283.9
  - Wilkie's 557.1
  - Wilkinson-Sneddon (subcorneal pustular dermatosis) 694.1
  - Willan-Plumbe (psoriasis) 696.1
  - Willebrand (-Jürgens) (angiohemophilia) 286.4
  - Willi-Prader (hypogenital dystrophy with diabetic tendency) 759.81
  - Wilson's (hepatolenticular degeneration) 275.1
  - Wilson-Mikity 770.7
  - Wiskott-Aldrich (eczema-thrombocytopenia) 279.12
  - withdrawal
    - alcohol 291.81
    - drug 292.0
      - infant of dependent mother 779.5
  - Woakes' (ethmoiditis) 471.1
  - Wolff-Parkinson-White (anomalous atrioventricular excitation) 426.7
  - Wright's (hyperabduction) 447.8
  - X
    - cardiac 413.9
    - dysmetabolic 277.7
  - xiphoidalgia 733.99
  - XO 758.6
  - XXX 758.81
  - XXXXY 758.81
  - XXY 758.7
  - yellow vernix (placental dysfunction) 762.2
  - Zahorsky's 074.0
  - Zellweger 277.86
  - Zieve's (jaundice, hyperlipemia and hemolytic anemia) 571.1
  - Zollinger-Ellison (gastric hypersecretion with pancreatic islet cell tumor) 251.5
  - Zuelzer-Ogden (nutritional megaloblastic anemia) 281.2
- **Synechia** (iris) (pupil) 364.70
  - anterior 364.72
    - peripheral 364.73
  - intrauterine (traumatic) 621.5
  - posterior 364.71
  - vulvae, congenital 752.49
- **Synesthesia** (*see also* Disturbance, sensation) 782.0
- **Synodontia** 520.2
- **Synophthalmus** 759.89
- **Synorchidism** 752.89
- **Synorchism** 752.89
- **Synostosis** (congenital) 756.59
  - astragaloscaphoid 755.67
  - radioulnar 755.53
  - talonavicular (bar) 755.67
  - tarsal 755.67
- **Synovial** - *see* condition
- **Synovioma** (M9040/3) - *see also* Neoplasm, connective tissue, malignant
  - benign (M9040/0) - *see* Neoplasm, connective tissue, benign
- **Synoviosarcoma** (M9040/3) - *see* Neoplasm, connective tissue, malignant
- **Synovitis** (see also Tenosynovitis) 727.00
  - chronic crepitant, wrist 727.2
  - due to crystals - *see* Arthritis, due to crystals
  - gonococcal 098.51
  - gouty 274.00 ▲
  - specified NEC 727.09
  - syphilitic 095.7
    - congenital 090.0
  - traumatic, current - *see* Sprain, by site
  - tuberculous - *see* Tuberculosis, synovitis
  - villonodular 719.20
    - ankle 719.27
    - elbow 719.22
    - foot 719.27
    - hand 719.24
    - hip 719.25
    - knee 719.26
    - multiple sites 719.29
    - pelvic region 719.25
    - shoulder (region) 719.21
    - specified site NEC 719.28
    - wrist 719.23
- **Syphilide** 091.3
  - congenital 090.0
  - newborn 090.0
  - tubercular 095.8
    - congenital 090.0
- **Syphilis, syphilitic** (acquired) 097.9
  - with lung involvement 095.1
- **Syphilis, syphilitic** – *continued*
  - abdomen (late) 095.2
  - acoustic nerve 094.86
  - adenopathy (secondary) 091.4
  - adrenal (gland) 095.8
    - with cortical hypofunction 095.8
  - age under 2 years NEC (*see also* Syphilis, congenital) 090.9
    - acquired 097.9
  - alopecia (secondary) 091.82
  - anemia 095.8
  - aneurysm (artery) (ruptured) 093.89
    - aorta 093.0
    - central nervous system 094.89
    - congenital 090.5
  - anus 095.8
    - primary 091.1
    - secondary 091.3
  - aorta, aortic (arch) (abdominal) (insufficiency) (pulmonary) (regurgitation) (stenosis) (thoracic) 093.89
    - aneurysm 093.0
  - arachnoid (adhesive) 094.2
  - artery 093.89
    - cerebral 094.89
    - spinal 094.89
  - arthropathy (neurogenic) (tabetic) 094.0 *[713.5]*
  - asymptomatic - *see* Syphilis, latent
  - ataxia, locomotor (progressive) 094.0
  - atrophoderma maculatum 091.3
  - auricular fibrillation 093.89
  - Bell's palsy 094.89
  - bladder 095.8
  - bone 095.5
    - secondary 091.61
  - brain 094.89
  - breast 095.8
  - bronchus 095.8
  - bubo 091.0
  - bulbar palsy 094.89
  - bursa (late) 095.7
  - cardiac decompensation 093.89
  - cardiovascular (early) (late) (primary) (secondary) (tertiary) 093.9
    - specified type and site NEC 093.89
  - causing death under 2 years of age (*see also* Syphilis, congenital) 090.9
    - stated to be acquired NEC 097.9
  - central nervous system (any site) (early) (late) (latent) (primary) (recurrent) (relapse) (secondary) (tertiary) 094.9
    - with
      - ataxia 094.0
      - paralysis, general 094.1
        - juvenile 090.40
      - paresis (general) 094.1
        - juvenile 090.40
      - tabes (dorsalis) 094.0
        - juvenile 090.40
      - taboparesis 094.1
        - juvenile 090.40
    - aneurysm (ruptured) 094.87
    - congenital 090.40
    - juvenile 090.40
    - remission in (sustained) 094.9
    - serology doubtful, negative, or positive 094.9
    - specified nature or site NEC 094.89
    - vascular 094.89
  - cerebral 094.89
    - meningovascular 094.2
    - nerves 094.89
    - sclerosis 094.89
    - thrombosis 094.89
  - cerebrospinal 094.89
    - tabetic 094.0
  - cerebrovascular 094.89
  - cervix 095.8
  - chancre (multiple) 091.0
    - extragenital 091.2
    - Rollet's 091.2

Syphilis, syphilitic

Syphilis, syphilitic – *continued*
primary – *continued*
genital 091.0
lip 091.2
specified site NEC 091.2
tonsils 091.2
prostate 095.8
psychosis (intracranial gumma) 094.89
ptosis (eyelid) 094.89
pulmonary (late) 095.1
artery 093.89
pulmonum 095.1
pyelonephritis 095.4
recently acquired, symptomatic NEC 091.89
rectum 095.8
respiratory tract 095.8
retina
late 094.83
neurorecidive 094.83
retrobulbar neuritis 094.85
salpingitis 095.8
sclera (late) 095.0
sclerosis
cerebral 094.89
coronary 093.89
multiple 094.89
subacute 094.89
scotoma (central) 095.8
scrotum 095.8
secondary (and primary) 091.9
adenopathy 091.4
anus 091.3
bone 091.61
cardiovascular 093.9
central nervous system 094.9
chorioretinitis, choroiditis 091.51
hepatitis 091.62
liver 091.62
lymphadenitis 091.4
meningitis, acute 091.81
mouth 091.3
mucous membranes 091.3
periosteum 091.61
periostitis 091.61
pharynx 091.3
relapse (treated) (untreated) 091.7
skin 091.3
specified form NEC 091.89
tonsil 091.3
ulcer 091.3
viscera 091.69
vulva 091.3
seminal vesicle (late) 095.8
seronegative
with signs or symptoms - *see* Syphilis, by site and stage
seropositive
with signs or symptoms - *see* Syphilis, by site or stage
follow-up of latent syphilis - *see* Syphilis, latent
only finding - *see* Syphilis, latent
seventh nerve (paralysis) 094.89
sinus 095.8
sinusitis 095.8
skeletal system 095.5
skin (early) (secondary) (with ulceration) 091.3
late or tertiary 095.8
small intestine 095.8
spastic spinal paralysis 094.0
spermatic cord (late) 095.8
spinal (cord) 094.89
with
paresis 094.1
tabes 094.0
spleen 095.8
splenomegaly 095.8
spondylitis 095.5
staphyloma 095.8
stigmata (congenital) 090.5
stomach 095.8
synovium (late) 095.7

Syphilis, syphilitic – *continued*
tabes dorsalis (early) (late) 094.0
juvenile 090.40
tabetic type 094.0
juvenile 090.40
taboparesis 094.1
juvenile 090.40
tachycardia 093.89
tendon (late) 095.7
tertiary 097.0
with symptoms 095.8
cardiovascular 093.9
central nervous system 094.9
multiple NEC 095.8
specified site NEC 095.8
testis 095.8
thorax 095.8
throat 095.8
thymus (gland) 095.8
thyroid (late) 095.8
tongue 095.8
tonsil (lingual) 095.8
primary 091.2
secondary 091.3
trachea 095.8
tricuspid valve 093.23
tumor, brain 094.89
tunica vaginalis (late) 095.8
ulcer (any site) (early) (secondary) 091.3
late 095.9
perforating 095.9
foot 094.0
urethra (stricture) 095.8
urogenital 095.8
uterus 095.8
uveal tract (secondary) 091.50
late 095.8 *[363.13]*
uveitis (secondary) 091.50
late 095.8 *[363.13]*
uvula (late) 095.8
perforated 095.8
vagina 091.0
late 095.8
valvulitis NEC 093.20
vascular 093.89
brain or cerebral 094.89
vein 093.89
cerebral 094.89
ventriculi 095.8
vesicae urinariae 095.8
viscera (abdominal) 095.2
secondary 091.69
vitreous (hemorrhage) (opacities) 095.8
vulva 091.0
late 095.8
secondary 091.3
Syphiloma 095.9
cardiovascular system 093.9
central nervous system 094.9
circulatory system 093.9
congenital 090.5
Syphilophobia 300.29
Syringadenoma (M8400/0) - *see also* Neoplasm, skin, benign
papillary (M8406/0) - *see* Neoplasm, skin, benign
Syringobulbia 336.0
Syringocarcinoma (M8400/3) - *see* Neoplasm, skin, malignant
Syringocystadenoma (M8400/0) - *see also* Neoplasm, skin, benign
papillary (M8406/0) - *see* Neoplasm, skin, benign
Syringocystoma (M8407/0) - *see* Neoplasm, skin, benign
Syringoma (M8407/0) - *see also* Neoplasm, skin, benign
chondroid (M8940/0) - *see* Neoplasm, by site, benign
Syringomyelia 336.0
Syringomyelitis 323.9
late effect - *see* category 326
Syringomyelocele (*see also* Spina bifida) 741.9 5th

Syringopontia 336.0
System, systemic - *see also* condition
disease, combined - *see* Degeneration, combined
fibrosclerosing syndrome 710.8
inflammatory response syndrome (SIRS) 995.90
due to
infectious process 995.91
with acute organ dysfunction 995.92
non-infectious process 995.93
with acute organ dysfunction 995.94
lupus erythematosus 710.0
inhibitor 286.5

T

Tab - *see* Tag
Tabacism 989.84
Tabacosis 989.84
Tabardillo 080
flea-borne 081.0
louse-borne 080
Tabes, tabetic
with
central nervous system syphilis 094.0
Charcôt's joint 094.0 *[713.5]*
cord bladder 094.0
crisis, viscera (any) 094.0
paralysis, general 094.1
paresis (general) 094.1
perforating ulcer 094.0
arthropathy 094.0 *[713.5]*
bladder 094.0
bone 094.0
cerebrospinal 094.0
congenital 090.40
conjugal 094.0
dorsalis 094.0
neurosyphilis 094.0
early 094.0
juvenile 090.40
latent 094.0
mesenterica (*see also* Tuberculosis) 014.8 5th
paralysis insane, general 094.1
peripheral (nonsyphilitic) 799.89
spasmodic 094.0
not dorsal or dorsalis 343.9
syphilis (cerebrospinal) 094.0
Taboparalysis 094.1
Taboparesis (remission) 094.1
with
Charcôt's joint 094.1 *[713.5]*
cord bladder 094.1
perforating ulcer 094.1
juvenile 090.40
Tache noir 923.20
Tachyalimentation 579.3
Tachyarrhythmia, tachyrhythmia - *see also* Tachycardia
paroxysmal with sinus bradycardia 427.81
Tachycardia 785.0
atrial 427.89
auricular 427.89
AV nodal re-entry (re-entrant) 427.89
junctional ectopic 427.0
newborn 779.82
nodal 427.89
nonparoxysmal atrioventricular 426.89
nonparoxysmal atrioventricular (nodal) 426.89
nonsustained 427.2
paroxysmal 427.2
with sinus bradycardia 427.81
atrial (PAT) 427.0
psychogenic 316 *[427.0]*
atrioventricular (AV) 427.0
psychogenic 316 *[427.0]*
essential 427.2

Tachycardia – *continued*
paroxysmal – *continued*
junctional 427.0
nodal 427.0
psychogenic 316 *[427.2]*
atrial 316 *[427.0]*
supraventricular 316 *[427.0]*
ventricular 316 *[427.1]*
supraventricular 427.0
psychogenic 316 *[427.0]*
ventricular 427.1
psychogenic 316 *[427.1]*
postoperative 997.1
psychogenic 306.2
sick sinus 427.81
sinoauricular 427.89
sinus 427.89
supraventricular 427.89
sustained 427.2
supraventricular 427.0
ventricular 427.1
ventricular (paroxysmal) 427.1
psychogenic 316 *[427.1]*
Tachygastria 536.8
Tachypnea 786.06
hysterical 300.11
newborn (idiopathic) (transitory) 770.6
psychogenic 306.1
transitory, of newborn 770.6
Taenia (infection) (infestation) (*see also* Infestation, taenia) 123.3
diminuta 123.6
echinococcal infestation (*see also* Echinococcus) 122.9
nana 123.6
saginata infestation 123.2
solium (intestinal form) 123.0
larval form 123.1
Taeniasis (intestine) (*see also* Infestation, taenia) 123.3
saginata 123.2
solium 123.0
Taenzer's disease 757.4
Tag (hypertrophied skin) (infected) 701.9
adenoid 474.8
anus 455.9
endocardial (*see also* Endocarditis) 424.90
hemorrhoidal 455.9
hymen 623.8
perineal 624.8
preauricular 744.1
rectum 455.9
sentinel 455.9
skin 701.9
accessory 757.39
anus 455.9
congenital 757.39
preauricular 744.1
rectum 455.9
tonsil 474.8
urethra, urethral 599.84
vulva 624.8
Tahyna fever 062.5
Takayasu (-Onishi) **disease or syndrome** (pulseless disease) 446.7
Takotsubo syndrome 429.83
Talc granuloma 728.82
in operation wound 998.7
Talcosis 502
Talipes (congenital) 754.70
acquired NEC 736.79
planus 734
asymmetric 754.79
acquired 736.79
calcaneovalgus 754.62
acquired 736.76
calcaneovarus 754.59
acquired 736.76
calcaneus 754.79
acquired 736.76
cavovarus 754.59
acquired 736.75
cavus 754.71
acquired 736.73

Syphilis, syphilitic – Talipes

- **Talipes** – *continued*
  - equinovalgus 754.69
    - acquired 736.72
  - equinovarus 754.51
    - acquired 736.71
  - equinus 754.79
    - acquired, NEC 736.72
  - percavus 754.71
    - acquired 736.73
  - planovalgus 754.69
    - acquired 736.79
  - planus (acquired) (any degree) 734
    - congenital 754.61
    - due to rickets 268.1
  - valgus 754.60
    - acquired 736.79
  - varus 754.50
    - acquired 736.79
- **Talma's disease** 728.85
- **Talon noir** 924.20
  - hand 923.20
  - heel 924.20
  - toe 924.3
- **Tamponade heart** (Rose's) (*see also* Pericarditis) 423.3
- **Tanapox** 059.21
- **Tangier disease** (familial high-density lipoprotein deficiency) 272.5
- **Tank ear** 380.12
- **Tantrum** (childhood) (*see also* Disturbance, conduct) 312.1 5th
- **Tapeworm** (infection) (infestation) (*see also* Infestation, tapeworm) 123.9
- **Tapia's syndrome** 352.6
- **Tarantism** 297.8
- **Target-oval cell anemia** 282.49
- **Tarlov's cyst** 355.9
- **Tarral-Besnier disease** (pityriasis rubra pilaris) 696.4
- **Tarsalgia** 729.2
- **Tarsal tunnel syndrome** 355.5
- **Tarsitis** (eyelid) 373.00
  - syphilitic 095.8 *[373.00]*
  - tuberculous (*see also* Tuberculosis) 017.0 5th *[373.4]*
- **Tartar** (teeth) 523.6
- **Tattoo** (mark) 709.09
- **Taurodontism** 520.2
- **Taussig-Bing defect, heart, or syndrome** (transposition, aorta and overriding pulmonary artery) 745.11
- **Tay's choroiditis** 363.41
- **Tay-Sachs**
  - amaurotic familial idiocy 330.1
  - disease 330.1
- **Taybi's syndrome** (otopalatodigital) 759.89
- **Taylor's**
  - disease (diffuse idiopathic cutaneous atrophy) 701.8
  - syndrome 625.5
- **TBI** (traumatic brain injury) (*see also* Injury, intracranial) 854.0 5th ●
  - with skull fracture - *see* Fracture, skull, by site ●
- **Tear, torn** (traumatic) - *see also* Wound, open, by site
  - anus, anal (sphincter) 863.89
    - with open wound in cavity 863.99
    - complicating delivery (healed) (old) 654.8 5th
      - with mucosa 664.3 5th
      - not associated with third-degree perineal laceration 664.6 5th
    - nontraumatic, nonpuerperal (healed) (old) 569.43
  - articular cartilage, old (*see also* Disorder, cartilage, articular) 718.0 5th
  - bladder
    - with
      - abortion - *see* Abortion, by type, with damage to pelvic organs
      - ectopic pregnancy (*see also* categories 633.0-633.9) 639.2

- **Tear, torn** – *continued*
  - bladder – *continued*
    - with – *continued*
      - molar pregnancy (*see also* categories 630-632) 639.2
    - following
      - abortion 639.2
      - ectopic or molar pregnancy 639.2
    - obstetrical trauma 665.5 5th
  - bowel
    - with
      - abortion - *see* Abortion, by type, with damage to pelvic organs
      - ectopic pregnancy (*see also* categories 633.0-633.9) 639.2
      - molar pregnancy (*see also* categories 630-632) 639.2
    - following
      - abortion 639.2
      - ectopic or molar pregnancy 639.2
    - obstetrical trauma 665.5 5th
  - broad ligament
    - with
      - abortion - *see* Abortion, by type, with damage to pelvic organs
      - ectopic pregnancy (*see also* categories 633.0-633.9) 639.2
      - molar pregnancy (*see also* categories 630-632) 639.2
    - following
      - abortion 639.2
      - ectopic or molar pregnancy 639.2
    - obstetrical trauma 665.6 5th
  - bucket handle (knee) (meniscus) - *see* Tear, meniscus
  - capsule
    - joint - *see* Sprain, by site
    - spleen - *see* Laceration, spleen, capsule
  - cartilage - *see also* Sprain, by site
    - articular, old (*see also* Disorder, cartilage, articular) 718.0 5th
    - knee - *see* Tear, meniscus
    - semilunar (knee) (current injury) - *see* Tear, meniscus
  - cervix
    - with
      - abortion - *see* Abortion, by type, with damage to pelvic organs
      - ectopic pregnancy (*see also* categories 633.0-633.9) 639.2
      - molar pregnancy (*see also* categories 630-632) 639.2
    - following
      - abortion 639.2
      - ectopic or molar pregnancy 639.2
    - obstetrical trauma (current) 665.3 5th
    - old 622.3
  - dural 349.31
    - accidental puncture or laceration during a procedure 349.31
    - incidental (inadvertent) 349.31
    - nontraumatic NEC 349.39
  - internal organ (abdomen, chest, or pelvis) - *see* Injury, internal, by site
  - ligament - *see also* Sprain, by site
    - with open wound - *see* Wound, open by site
  - meniscus (knee) (current injury) 836.2
    - bucket handle 836.0
      - old 717.0
    - lateral 836.1
      - anterior horn 836.1
        - old 717.42
      - bucket handle 836.1
        - old 717.41
      - old 717.40
      - posterior horn 836.1
        - old 717.43
      - specified site NEC 836.1
        - old 717.49
    - medial 836.0
      - anterior horn 836.0
        - old 717.1

- **Tear, torn** – *continued*
  - meniscus – *continued*
    - medial – *continued*
      - bucket handle 836.0
        - old 717.0
      - old 717.3
      - posterior horn 836.0
        - old 717.2
    - old NEC 717.5
    - site other than knee - *see* Sprain, by site
  - muscle - *see also* Sprain, by site
    - with open wound - *see* Wound, open by site
  - pelvic
    - floor, complicating delivery 664.1 5th
    - organ NEC
      - with
        - abortion - *see* Abortion, by type, with damage to pelvic organs
        - ectopic pregnancy (*see also* categories 633.0-633.9) 639.2
        - molar pregnancy (*see also* categories 630-632) 639.2
      - following
        - abortion 639.2
        - ectopic or molar pregnancy 639.2
      - obstetrical trauma 665.5 5th
  - perineum - *see also* Laceration, perineum
    - obstetrical trauma 665.5 5th
  - periurethral tissue
    - with
      - abortion - *see* Abortion, by type, with damage to pelvic organs
      - ectopic pregnancy (*see also* categories 633.0-633.9) 639.2
      - molar pregnancy (*see also* categories 630-632) 639.2
    - following
      - abortion 639.2
      - ectopic or molar pregnancy 639.2
    - obstetrical trauma 665.5 5th
  - rectovaginal septum - *see* Laceration, rectovaginal septum
  - retina, retinal (recent) (with detachment) 361.00
    - without detachment 361.30
    - dialysis (juvenile) (with detachment) 361.04
    - giant (with detachment) 361.03
    - horseshoe (without detachment) 361.32
    - multiple (with detachment) 361.02
      - without detachment 361.33
    - old
      - delimited (partial) 361.06
      - partial 361.06
      - total or subtotal 361.07
    - partial (without detachment)
      - giant 361.03
      - multiple defects 361.02
      - old (delimited) 361.06
      - single defect 361.01
    - round hole (without detachment) 361.31
    - single defect (with detachment) 361.01
    - total or subtotal (recent) 361.05
      - old 361.07
  - rotator cuff (traumatic) 840.4
    - current injury 840.4
    - degenerative 726.10
    - nontraumatic 727.61
  - semilunar cartilage, knee (*see also* Tear, meniscus) 836.2
    - old 717.5
  - tendon - *see also* Sprain, by site
    - with open wound - *see* Wound, open by site
  - tentorial, at birth 767.0
  - umbilical cord
    - affecting fetus or newborn 772.0
    - complicating delivery 663.8 5th

- **Tear, torn** (traumatic) – *continued*
  - urethra
    - with
      - abortion - *see* Abortion, by type, with damage to pelvic organs
      - ectopic pregnancy (*see also* categories 633.0-633.9) 639.2
      - molar pregnancy (*see also* categories 630-632) 639.2
    - following
      - abortion 639.2
      - ectopic or molar pregnancy 639.2
    - obstetrical trauma 665.5 5th
  - uterus - *see* Injury, internal, uterus
  - vagina - *see* Laceration, vagina
  - vessel, from catheter 998.2
  - vulva, complicating delivery 664.0 5th
- **Tear stone** 375.57
- **Teeth, tooth** - *see also* condition
  - grinding 306.8
  - prenatal 520.6
- **Teething** 520.7
  - syndrome 520.7
- **Tegmental syndrome** 344.89
- **Telangiectasia, telangiectasis** (verrucous) 448.9
  - ataxic (cerebellar) 334.8
  - familial 448.0
  - hemorrhagic, hereditary (congenital) (senile) 448.0
  - hereditary hemorrhagic 448.0
  - retina 362.15
  - spider 448.1
- **Telecanthus** (congenital) 743.63
- **Telescoped bowel or intestine** (*see also* Intussusception) 560.0
- **Teletherapy, adverse effect NEC** 990
- **Telogen effluvium** 704.02
- **Temperature**
  - body, high (of unknown origin) (*see also* Pyrexia) 780.60
  - cold, trauma from 991.9
    - newborn 778.2
    - specified effect NEC 991.8
  - high
    - body (of unknown origin) (*see also* Pyrexia) 780.60
    - trauma from - *see* Heat
- **Temper tantrum** (childhood) (*see also* Disturbance, conduct) 312.1 5th
- **Temple** - *see* condition
- **Temporal** - *see also* condition
  - lobe syndrome 310.0
- **Temporomandibular joint-pain-dysfunction syndrome** 524.60
- **Temporosphenoidal** - *see* condition
- **Tendency**
  - bleeding (*see also* Defect, coagulation) 286.9
  - homosexual, ego-dystonic 302.0
  - paranoid 301.0
  - suicide 300.9
- **Tenderness**
  - abdominal (generalized) (localized) 789.6 5th
  - rebound 789.6 5th
  - skin 782.0
- **Tendinitis, tendonitis** (*see also* Tenosynovitis) 726.90
  - Achilles 726.71
  - adhesive 726.90
    - shoulder 726.0
  - calcific 727.82
    - shoulder 726.11
  - gluteal 726.5
  - patellar 726.64
  - peroneal 726.79
  - pes anserinus 726.61
  - psoas 726.5
  - tibialis (anterior) (posterior) 726.72
  - trochanteric 726.5
- **Tendon** - *see* condition
- **Tendosynovitis** - *see* Tenosynovitis
- **Tendovaginitis** - *see* Tenosynovitis

Tenesmus 787.99
- rectal 787.99
- vesical 788.99

Tenia - *see* Taenia
Teniasis - *see* Taeniasis
Tennis elbow 726.32
Tenonitis - *see also* Tenosynovitis
- eye (capsule) 376.04

Tenontosynovitis - *see* Tenosynovitis
Tenontothecitis - *see* Tenosynovitis
Tenophyte 727.9
Tenosynovitis (*see also* Synovitis) 727.00
- adhesive 726.90
  - shoulder 726.0
- ankle 727.06
- bicipital (calcifying) 726.12
- buttock 727.09
- due to crystals - *see* Arthritis, due to crystals
- elbow 727.09
- finger 727.05
- foot 727.06
- gonococcal 098.51
- hand 727.05
- hip 727.09
- knee 727.09
- radial styloid 727.04
- shoulder 726.10
  - adhesive 726.0
- specified NEC 727.09
- spine 720.1
- supraspinatus 726.10
- toe 727.06
- tuberculous - *see* Tuberculosis, tenosynovitis
- wrist 727.05

Tenovaginitis - *see* Tenosynovitis
Tension
- arterial, high (*see also* Hypertension) 401.9
  - without diagnosis of hypertension 796.2
- headache 307.81
- intraocular (elevated) 365.00
- nervous 799.21 ▲
- ocular (elevated) 365.00
- pneumothorax 512.0
- iatrogenic 512.1
  - postoperative 512.1
  - spontaneous 512.0
- premenstrual 625.4
- state 300.9

Tentorium - *see* condition
Teratencephalus 759.89
Teratism 759.7
Teratoblastoma (malignant) (M9080/3) - *see* Neoplasm, by site, malignant
Teratocarcinoma (M9081/3) - *see also* Neoplasm, by site, malignant
- liver 155.0

Teratoma (solid) (M9080/1) - *see also* Neoplasm, by site, uncertain behavior
- adult (cystic) (M9080/0) - *see* Neoplasm, by site, benign
- and embryonal carcinoma, mixed (M9081/3) - *see* Neoplasm, by site, malignant
- benign (M9080/0) - *see* Neoplasm, by site, benign
- combined with choriocarcinoma (M9101/3) - *see* Neoplasm, by site, malignant
- cystic (adult) (M9080/0) - *see* Neoplasm, by site, benign
- differentiated type (M9080/0) - *see* Neoplasm, by site, benign
- embryonal (M9080/3) - *see also* Neoplasm, by site, malignant
  - liver 155.0
- fetal
  - sacral, causing fetopelvic disproportion 653.7 [5th]
- immature (M9080/3) - *see* Neoplasm, by site, malignant

Teratoma – *continued*
- liver (M9080/3) 155.0
  - adult, benign, cystic, differentiated type, or mature (M9080/0) 211.5
- malignant (M9080/3) - *see also* Neoplasm, by site, malignant
  - anaplastic type (M9082/3) - *see* Neoplasm, by site, malignant
  - intermediate type (M9083/3) - *see* Neoplasm, by site, malignant
  - liver (M9080/3) 155.0
  - trophoblastic (M9102/3)
    - specified site - *see* Neoplasm, by site, malignant
    - unspecified site 186.9
  - undifferentiated type (M9082/3) - *see* Neoplasm, by site, malignant
- mature (M9080/0) - *see* Neoplasm, by site, benign
  - malignant (M9080/3) - *see* Neoplasm, by site, malignant
- ovary (M9080/0) 220
  - embryonal, immature, or malignant (M9080/3) 183.0
- suprasellar (M9080/3) - *see* Neoplasm, by site, malignant
- testis (M9080/3) 186.9
  - adult, benign, cystic, differentiated type or mature (M9080/0) 222.0
  - undescended 186.0

Terminal care V66.7
Termination
- anomalous - *see also* Malposition, congenital
  - portal vein 747.49
  - right pulmonary vein 747.42
- pregnancy (legal) (therapeutic) (*see* Abortion, legal) 635.9 [5th]
  - fetus NEC 779.6
  - illegal (*see also* Abortion, illegal) 636.9 [5th]

Ternidens diminutus infestation 127.7
Terrors, night (child) 307.46
Terry's syndrome (*see also* Retinopathy of prematurity) 362.21
Tertiary - *see* condition
Tessellated fundus, retina (tigroid) 362.89
Test(s)
- adequacy
  - hemodialysis V56.31
  - peritoneal dialysis V56.32
- AIDS virus V72.69 ▲
- allergen V72.7
- bacterial disease NEC (*see also* Screening, by name of disease) V74.9
- basal metabolic rate V72.69 ▲
- blood~~-alcohol V70.4~~ ▲
  - alcohol V70.4 ●
  - drug V70.4 ●
    - for therapeutic drug monitoring V58.83 ●
  - for routine general physical examination V72.62 ●
  - prior to treatment or procedure V72.63 ●
  - typing V72.86 ●
    - Rh typing V72.86 ●
- ~~blood-drug V70.4~~
  - ~~for therapeutic drug monitoring V58.83~~
- ~~blood typing V72.86~~
  - ~~Rh typing V72.86~~
- developmental, infant or child V20.2
- Dick V74.8
- fertility V26.21
- genetic
  - female V26.32
  - for genetic disease carrier status
    - female V26.31
    - male V26.34
  - male V26.39
- hearing V72.19
  - following failed hearing screening V72.11

Test(s) – *continued*
- hearing – *continued*
  - routine, for infant and child V20.2 ●
- HIV V72.69 ▲
- human immunodeficiency virus V72.69 ▲
- immunity status V72.61 ●
- Kveim V82.89
- laboratory V72.60 ▲
  - for medicolegal reason V70.4
  - ordered as part of a routine general medical examination V72.62 ●
  - pre-operative V72.63 ●
  - pre-procedural V72.63 ●
  - specified NEC V72.69 ●
- male partner of habitual aborter V26.35
- Mantoux (for tuberculosis) V74.1
- mycotic organism V75.4
- nuchal translucency V28.89
- parasitic agent NEC V75.8
- paternity V70.4
- peritoneal equilibration V56.32
- pregnancy
  - negative result V72.41
  - positive result V72.42
    - first pregnancy V72.42
  - unconfirmed V72.40
- preoperative V72.84
  - cardiovascular V72.81
  - respiratory V72.82
  - specified NEC V72.83
- procreative management NEC V26.29
  - genetic disease carrier status
    - female V26.31
    - male V26.34
- Rh typing V72.86
- sarcoidosis V82.89
- Schick V74.3
- Schultz-Charlton V74.8
- skin, diagnostic
  - allergy V72.7
  - bacterial agent NEC (*see also* Screening, by name of disease) V74.9
  - Dick V74.8
  - hypersensitivity V72.7
  - Kveim V82.89
  - Mantoux V74.1
  - mycotic organism V75.4
  - parasitic agent NEC V75.8
  - sarcoidosis V82.89
  - Schick V74.3
  - Schultz-Charlton V74.8
  - tuberculin V74.1
- specified type NEC V72.85
- tuberculin V74.1
- vision V72.0
  - routine, for infant and child V20.2 ●
- Wassermann
  - positive (*see also* Serology for syphilis, positive) 097.1
    - false 795.6

Testicle, testicular, testis - *see also* condition
- feminization (syndrome) 259.51

Tetanus, tetanic (cephalic) (convulsions) 037
- with
  - abortion - *see* Abortion, by type, with sepsis
  - ectopic pregnancy (*see also* categories 633.0-633.9) 639.0
  - molar pregnancy (*see* categories 630-632) 639.0
- following
  - abortion 639.0
  - ectopic or molar pregnancy 639.0
- inoculation V03.7
  - reaction (due to serum) - *see* Complications, vaccination
- neonatorum 771.3
- puerperal, postpartum, childbirth 670.8 [5th] ▲

Tetany, tetanic 781.7
- alkalosis 276.3
- associated with rickets 268.0

Tetany, tetanic – *continued*
- convulsions 781.7
  - hysterical 300.11
- functional (hysterical) 300.11
- hyperkinetic 781.7
  - hysterical 300.11
- hyperpnea 786.01
  - hysterical 300.11
  - psychogenic 306.1
- hyperventilation 786.01
  - hysterical 300.11
  - psychogenic 306.1
- hypocalcemic, neonatal 775.4
- hysterical 300.11
- neonatal 775.4
- parathyroid (gland) 252.1
- parathyroprival 252.1
- postoperative 252.1
- postthyroidectomy 252.1
- pseudotetany 781.7
  - hysterical 300.11
- psychogenic 306.1
  - specified as conversion reaction 300.11

Tetralogy of Fallot 745.2
Tetraplegia - *see* **Quadriplegia**
Thailand hemorrhagic fever 065.4
Thalassanemia 282.49
Thalassemia (alpha) (beta) (disease) (Hb-C) (Hb-D) (Hb-E) (Hb-H) (Hb-I) (high fetal gene) (high fetal hemoglobin) (intermedia) (major) (minima) (minor) (mixed) (trait) (with other hemoglobinopathy) 282.49
- Hb-S (without crisis) 282.41
  - with
    - crisis 282.42
    - vaso-occlusive pain 282.42
- sickle-cell (without crisis) 282.41
  - with
    - crisis 282.42
    - vaso-occlusive pain 282.42

Thalassemic variants 282.49
Thaysen-Gee disease (nontropical sprue) 579.0
Thecoma (M8600/0) 220
- malignant (M8600/3) 183.0

Thelarche, precocious 259.1
Thelitis 611.0
- puerperal, postpartum 675.0 [5th]

Therapeutic - *see* condition
Therapy V57.9
- blood transfusion, without reported diagnosis V58.2
- breathing V57.0
- chemotherapy, antineoplastic V58.11
  - fluoride V07.31
  - prophylactic NEC V07.39
- dialysis (intermittent) (treatment)
  - extracorporeal V56.0
  - peritoneal V56.8
  - renal V56.0
  - specified type NEC V56.8
- exercise NEC V57.1
  - breathing V57.0
- extracorporeal dialysis (renal) V56.0
- fluoride prophylaxis V07.31
- hemodialysis V56.0
- hormone replacement (postmenopausal) V07.4
- immunotherapy antineoplastic V58.12
- long term oxygen therapy V46.2
- occupational V57.21
- orthoptic V57.4
- orthotic V57.81
- peritoneal dialysis V56.8
- physical NEC V57.1
- postmenopausal hormone replacement V07.4
- radiation V58.0
- speech(-language) V57.3 ▲
- vocational V57.22

Thermalgesia 782.0
Thermalgia 782.0
Thermanalgesia 782.0

- **Thermanesthesia** 782.0
- **Thermic** - *see* condition
- **Thermography** (abnormal) 793.99
  - breast 793.89
- **Thermoplegia** 992.0
- **Thesaurismosis**
  - amyloid 277.39
  - bilirubin 277.4
  - calcium 275.40
  - cystine 270.0
  - glycogen (*see also* Disease, glycogen storage) 271.0
  - kerasin 272.7
  - lipoid 272.7
  - melanin 255.41
  - phosphatide 272.7
  - urate 274.9
- **Thiaminic deficiency** 265.1
  - with beriberi 265.0
- **Thibierge-Weissenbach syndrome** (cutaneous systemic sclerosis) 710.1
- **Thickened endometrium** 793.5
- **Thickening**
  - bone 733.99
    - extremity 733.99
  - breast 611.79
  - hymen 623.3
  - larynx 478.79
  - nail 703.8
    - congenital 757.5
  - periosteal 733.99
  - pleura (*see also* Pleurisy) 511.0
  - skin 782.8
  - subepiglottic 478.79
  - tongue 529.8
  - valve, heart - *see* Endocarditis
- **Thiele syndrome** 724.6
- **Thigh** - *see* condition
- **Thinning vertebra** (*see also* Osteoporosis) 733.00
- **Thirst, excessive** 783.5
  - due to deprivation of water 994.3
- **Thomsen's disease** 359.22
- **Thomson's disease** (congenital poikiloderma) 757.33
- **Thoracic** - *see also* condition
  - kidney 753.3
  - outlet syndrome 353.0
  - stomach - *see* Hernia, diaphragm
- **Thoracogastroschisis** (congenital) 759.89
- **Thoracopagus** 759.4
- **Thoracoschisis** 756.3
- **Thoracoscopic surgical procedure converted to open procedure** V64.42
- **Thorax** - *see* condition
- **Thorn's syndrome** (*see also* Disease, renal) 593.9
- **Thornwaldt's, Tornwaldt's**
  - bursitis (pharyngeal) 478.29
  - cyst 478.26
  - disease (pharyngeal bursitis) 478.29
- **Thorson-Biörck syndrome** (malignant carcinoid) 259.2
- **Threadworm** (infection) (infestation) 127.4
- **Threatened**
  - abortion or miscarriage 640.0 [5th]
    - with subsequent abortion (*see also* Abortion, spontaneous) 634.9 [5th]
    - affecting fetus 762.1
  - labor 644.1 [5th]
    - affecting fetus or newborn 761.8
    - premature 644.0 [5th]
  - miscarriage 640.0 [5th]
    - affecting fetus 762.1
  - premature
    - delivery 644.2 [5th]
      - affecting fetus or newborn 761.8
    - labor 644.0 [5th]
      - before 22 completed weeks gestation 640.0 [5th]
- **Three-day fever** 066.0
- **Threshers' lung** 495.0
- **Thrix annulata** (congenital) 757.4
- **Throat** - *see* condition
- **Thrombasthenia** (Glanzmann's) (hemorrhagic) (hereditary) 287.1
- **Thromboangiitis** 443.1
  - obliterans (general) 443.1
    - cerebral 437.1
    - vessels
      - brain 437.1
      - spinal cord 437.1
- **Thromboarteritis** - *see* Arteritis
- **Thromboasthenia** (Glanzmann's) (hemorrhagic) (hereditary) 287.1
- **Thrombocytasthenia** (Glanzmann's) 287.1
- **Thrombocythemia** (primary) (M9962/1) 238.71
  - essential 238.71
  - hemorrhagic 238.71
  - idiopathic (hemorrhagic) (M9962/1) 238.71
- **Thrombocytopathy** (dystrophic) (granulopenic) 287.1
- **Thrombocytopenia, thrombocytopenic** 287.5
  - with
    - absent radii (TAR) syndrome 287.33
    - giant hemangioma 287.39
  - amegakaryocytic, congenital 287.33
  - congenital 287.33
  - cyclic 287.39
  - dilutional 287.4
  - due to
    - drugs 287.4
    - extracorporeal circulation of blood 287.4
    - massive blood transfusion 287.4
    - platelet alloimmunization 287.4
  - essential 287.30
  - fetal 678.0 [5th]
  - heparin-induced (HIT) 289.84
  - hereditary 287.33
  - Kasabach-Merritt 287.39
  - neonatal, transitory 776.1
    - due to
      - exchange transfusion 776.1
      - idiopathic maternal thrombocytopenia 776.1
      - isoimmunization 776.1
  - primary 287.30
  - puerperal, postpartum 666.3 [5th]
  - purpura (*see also* Purpura, thrombocytopenic) 287.30
    - thrombotic 446.6
  - secondary 287.4
  - sex-linked 287.39
- **Thrombocytosis** 238.71
  - essential 238.71
  - primary 238.71
- **Thromboembolism** - *see* Embolism
- **Thrombopathy** (Bernard-Soulier) 287.1
  - constitutional 286.4
  - Willebrand-Jürgens (angiohemophilia) 286.4
- **Thrombopenia** (*see also* Thrombocytopenia) 287.5
- **Thrombophlebitis** 451.9
  - antecubital vein 451.82
  - antepartum (superficial) 671.2 [5th]
    - affecting fetus or newborn 760.3
    - deep 671.3 [5th]
  - arm 451.89
    - deep 451.83
    - superficial 451.82
  - breast, superficial 451.89
  - cavernous (venous) sinus - *see* Thrombophlebitis, intracranial venous sinus
  - cephalic vein 451.82
  - cerebral (sinus) (vein) 325
    - late effect - *see* category 326
    - nonpyogenic 437.6
      - in pregnancy or puerperium 671.5 [5th]
      - late effect - *see* Late effect(s) (of) cerebrovascular disease

Thrombophlebitis – *continued*

  - due to implanted device - *see* Complications, due to (presence of) any device, implant, or graft classified to 996.0-996.5 NEC
  - during or resulting from a procedure NEC 997.2
  - femoral 451.11
  - femoropopliteal 451.19
  - following infusion, perfusion, or transfusion 999.2
  - hepatic (vein) 451.89
  - idiopathic, recurrent 453.1
  - iliac vein 451.81
  - iliofemoral 451.11
  - intracranial venous sinus (any) 325
    - late effect - *see* category 326
    - nonpyogenic 437.6
      - in pregnancy or puerperium 671.5 [5th]
      - late effect - *see* Late effect(s) (of) cerebrovascular disease
  - jugular vein 451.89
  - lateral (venous) sinus - *see* Thrombophlebitis, intracranial venous sinus
  - leg 451.2
    - deep (vessels) 451.19
      - femoral vein 451.11
      - specified vessel NEC 451.19
    - superficial (vessels) 451.0
      - femoral vein 451.11
  - longitudinal (venous) sinus - *see* Thrombophlebitis, intracranial venous sinus
  - lower extremity 451.2
    - deep (vessels) 451.19
      - femoral vein 451.11
      - specified vessel NEC 451.19
    - superficial (vessels) 451.0
  - migrans, migrating 453.1
  - pelvic
    - with
      - abortion - *see* Abortion, by type, with sepsis
      - ectopic pregnancy (*see also* categories 633.0-633.9) 639.0
      - molar pregnancy (*see also* categories 630-632) 639.0
    - following
      - abortion 639.0
      - ectopic or molar pregnancy 639.0
    - puerperal 671.4 [5th]
  - popliteal vein 451.19
  - portal (vein) 572.1
  - postoperative 997.2
  - pregnancy (superficial) 671.2 [5th]
    - affecting fetus or newborn 760.3
    - deep 671.3 [5th]
  - puerperal, postpartum, childbirth (extremities) (superficial) 671.2 [5th]
    - deep 671.4 [5th]
    - pelvic 671.4 [5th]
    - septic 670.3 [5th] ●
    - specified site NEC 671.5 [5th]
  - radial vein 451.82
  - saphenous (greater) (lesser) 451.0
  - sinus (intracranial) - *see* Thrombophlebitis, intracranial venous sinus
  - specified site NEC 451.89
  - tibial vein 451.19
- **Thrombosis, thrombotic** (marantic) (multiple) (progressive) (vein) (vessel) 453.9
  - with childbirth or during the puerperium - *see* Thrombosis, puerperal, postpartum
  - antepartum - *see* Thrombosis, pregnancy
  - aorta, aortic 444.1
    - abdominal 444.0
    - bifurcation 444.0
    - saddle 444.0
    - terminal 444.0

Thrombosis, thrombotic – *continued*

  - aorta, aortic – *continued*
    - thoracic 444.1
    - valve - *see* Endocarditis, aortic
  - apoplexy (*see also* Thrombosis, brain) 434.0 [5th]
    - late effect - *see* Late effect(s) (of) cerebrovascular disease
  - appendix, septic - *see* Appendicitis, acute
  - arteriolar-capillary platelet, disseminated 446.6
  - artery, arteries (postinfectional) 444.9
    - auditory, internal 433.8
    - basilar (*see also* Occlusion, artery, basilar) 433.0 [5th]
    - carotid (common) (internal) (*see also* Occlusion, artery, carotid) 433.1 [5th]
      - with other precerebral artery 433.3 [5th]
    - cerebellar (anterior inferior) (posterior inferior) (superior) 433.8 [5th]
    - cerebral (*see also* Thrombosis, brain) 434.0 [5th]
    - choroidal (anterior) 433.8 [5th]
    - communicating posterior 433.8 [5th]
    - coronary (*see also* Infarct, myocardium) 410.9 [5th]
      - without myocardial infarction 411.81
      - due to syphilis 093.89
      - healed or specified as old 412
    - extremities 444.22
      - lower 444.22
      - upper 444.21
    - femoral 444.22
    - hepatic 444.89
    - hypophyseal 433.8 [5th]
    - meningeal, anterior or posterior 433.8 [5th]
    - mesenteric (with gangrene) 557.0
    - ophthalmic (*see also* Occlusion, retina) 362.30
    - pontine 433.8 [5th]
    - popliteal 444.22
    - precerebral - *see* Occlusion, artery, precerebral NEC
    - pulmonary 415.19
      - iatrogenic 415.11
      - personal history of V12.51 ●
      - postoperative 415.11
      - septic 415.12
    - renal 593.81
    - retinal (*see also* Occlusion, retina) 362.30
    - specified site NEC 444.89
    - spinal, anterior or posterior 433.8 [5th]
    - traumatic (complication) (early) (*see also* Injury, blood vessel, by site) 904.9
    - vertebral (*see also* Occlusion, artery, vertebral) 433.2 [5th]
      - with other precerebral artery 433.3 [5th]
  - atrial (endocardial) 424.90
    - without endocarditis 429.89
    - due to syphilis 093.89
  - auricular (*see also* Infarct, myocardium) 410.9 [5th]
  - axillary (acute) (vein) 453.84 ▲
    - chronic 453.74 ●
    - personal history of V12.51 ●
  - basilar (artery) (*see also* Occlusion, artery, basilar) 433.0 [5th]
  - bland NEC 453.9
  - brain (artery) (stem) 434.0 [5th]
    - due to syphilis 094.89
    - iatrogenic 997.02
    - late effect - *see* Late effect(s) (of) cerebrovascular disease
    - postoperative 997.02
    - puerperal, postpartum, childbirth 674.0 [5th]

Thrombosis, thrombotic – Thyroid

Thyroiditis 245.9
- acute (pyogenic) (suppurative) 245.0
  - nonsuppurative 245.0
- autoimmune 245.2
- chronic (nonspecific) (sclerosing) 245.8
  - fibrous 245.3
  - lymphadenoid 245.2
  - lymphocytic 245.2
  - lymphoid 245.2
- complicating pregnancy, childbirth, or puerperium 648.1 [5th]
- de Quervain's (subacute granulomatous) 245.1
- fibrous (chronic) 245.3
- giant (cell) (follicular) 245.1
- granulomatous (de Quervain's) (subacute) 245.1
- Hashimoto's (struma lymphomatosa) 245.2
- iatrogenic 245.4
- invasive (fibrous) 245.3
- ligneous 245.3
- lymphocytic (chronic) 245.2
- lymphoid 245.2
- lymphomatous 245.2
- pseudotuberculous 245.1
- pyogenic 245.0
- radiation 245.4
- Riedel's (ligneous) 245.3
- subacute 245.1
- suppurative 245.0
- tuberculous (*see also* Tuberculosis) 017.5 [5th]
- viral 245.1
- woody 245.3

Thyrolingual duct, persistent 759.2

Thyromegaly 240.9

Thyrotoxic
- crisis or storm (*see also* Thyrotoxicosis) 242.9 [5th]
- heart failure (*see also* Thyrotoxicosis) 242.9 [5th] *[425.7]*

Thyrotoxicosis 242.9 [5th]

Note *Use the following fifth-digit subclassification with category 242:*

0 without mention of thyrotoxic crisis or storm

1 with mention of thyrotoxic crisis or storm

- with
  - goiter (diffuse) 242.0 [5th]
    - adenomatous 242.3 [5th]
      - multinodular 242.2 [5th]
      - uninodular 242.1 [5th]
    - nodular 242.3 [5th]
      - multinodular 242.2 [5th]
      - uninodular 242.1 [5th]
  - infiltrative
    - dermopathy 242.0 [5th]
    - ophthalmopathy 242.0 [5th]
  - thyroid acropachy 242.0 [5th]
- complicating pregnancy, childbirth, or puerperium 648.1 [5th]
- due to
  - ectopic thyroid nodule 242.4 [5th]
  - ingestion of (excessive) thyroid material 242.8 [5th]
  - specified cause NEC 242.8 [5th]
- factitia 242.8 [5th]
- heart 242.9 [5th] *[425.7]*
- neonatal (transient) 775.3

TIA (transient ischemic attack) 435.9
- with transient neurologic deficit 435.9
- late effect - *see* Late effect(s) (of) cerebrovascular disease

Tibia vara 732.4

Tic 307.20
- breathing 307.20
- child problem 307.21
- compulsive 307.22
- convulsive 307.20

Tic – *continued*
- degenerative (generalized) (localized) 333.3
  - facial 351.8
- douloureux (*see also* Neuralgia, trigeminal) 350.1
  - atypical 350.2
- habit 307.20
  - chronic (motor or vocal) 307.22
  - transient (of childhood) 307.21
- lid 307.20
  - transient (of childhood) 307.21
- motor-verbal 307.23
- occupational 300.89
- orbicularis 307.20
  - transient (of childhood) 307.21
- organic origin 333.3
- postchoreic - *see* Chorea
- psychogenic 307.20
  - compulsive 307.22
- salaam 781.0
- spasm 307.20
  - chronic (motor or vocal) 307.22
  - transient (of childhood) 307.21

Tick (-borne) fever NEC 066.1
- American mountain 066.1
- Colorado 066.1
- hemorrhagic NEC 065.3
  - Crimean 065.0
  - Kyasanur Forest 065.2
  - Omsk 065.1
- mountain 066.1
- nonexanthematous 066.1

Tick-bite fever NEC 066.1
- African 087.1
- Colorado (virus) 066.1
- Rocky Mountain 082.0

Tick paralysis 989.5

Tics and spasms, compulsive 307.22

Tietze's disease or syndrome 733.6

Tight, tightness
- anus 564.89
- chest 786.59
- fascia (lata) 728.9
- foreskin (congenital) 605
- hymen 623.3
- introitus (acquired) (congenital) 623.3
- rectal sphincter 564.89
- tendon 727.81
  - Achilles (heel) 727.81
- urethral sphincter 598.9

Tilting vertebra 737.9

Timidity, child 313.21

Tinea (intersecta) (tarsi) 110.9
- amiantacea 110.0
- asbestina 110.0
- barbae 110.0
- beard 110.0
- black dot 110.0
- blanca 111.2
- capitis 110.0
- corporis 110.5
- cruris 110.3
- decalvans 704.09
- flava 111.0
- foot 110.4
- furfuracea 111.0
- imbricata (Tokelau) 110.5
- lepothrix 039.0
- manuum 110.2
- microsporic (*see also* Dermatophytosis) 110.9
- nigra 111.1
- nodosa 111.2
- pedis 110.4
- scalp 110.0
- specified site NEC 110.8
- sycosis 110.0
- tonsurans 110.0
- trichophytic (*see also* Dermatophytosis) 110.9
- unguium 110.1
- versicolor 111.0

Tingling sensation (*see also* Disturbance, sensation) 782.0

Tin-miners' lung 503

Tinnitus (aurium) 388.30
- audible 388.32
- objective 388.32
- subjective 388.31

Tipped, teeth 524.33

Tipping
- pelvis 738.6
  - with disproportion (fetopelvic) 653.0 [5th]
    - affecting fetus or newborn 763.1
    - causing obstructed labor 660.1 [5th]
      - affecting fetus or newborn 763.1
- teeth 524.33

Tiredness 780.79

Tissue - *see* condition

Tobacco
- abuse (affecting health) NEC (*see also* Abuse, drugs, nondependent) 305.1
- heart 989.84
- use disorder complicating pregnancy, childbirth, or the puerperium 649.0 [5th]

Tobias' syndrome (carcinoma, pulmonary apex) (M8010/3) 162.3

Tocopherol deficiency 269.1

Todd's
- cirrhosis - *see* Cirrhosis, biliary
- paralysis (postepileptic transitory paralysis) 344.89

Toe - *see* condition

Toilet, artificial opening (*see also* Attention to, artificial, opening) V55.9

Tokelau ringworm 110.5

Tollwut 071

Tolosa-Hunt syndrome 378.55

Tommaselli's disease
- correct substance properly administered 599.70
- overdose or wrong substance given or taken 961.4

Tongue - *see also* condition
- worms 134.1

Tongue tie 750.0

Toni-Fanconi syndrome (cystinosis) 270.0

Tonic pupil 379.46

Tonsil - *see* condition

Tonsillitis (acute) (catarrhal) (croupous) (follicular) (gangrenous) (infective) (lacunar) (lingual) (malignant) (membranous) (phlegmonous) (pneumococcal) (pseudomembranous) (purulent) (septic) (staphylococcal) (subacute) (suppurative) (toxic) (ulcerative) (vesicular) (viral) 463
- with influenza, flu, or grippe 487.1
- chronic 474.00
- diphtheritic (membranous) 032.0
- hypertrophic 474.00
- influenzal 487.1
- parenchymatous 475
- streptococcal 034.0
- tuberculous (*see also* Tuberculosis) 012.8 [5th]
- Vincent's 101

Tonsillopharyngitis 465.8

Tooth, teeth - *see* condition

Toothache 525.9

Topagnosis 782.0

Tophi (gouty) 274.00 ▲
- ear 274.81
- heart 274.82
- specified site NEC 274.82

TORCH infection - (*see also* Infection, congenital) 760.2

Torn - *see* Tear, torn

Tornwaldt's bursitis (disease) (pharyngeal bursitis) 478.29
- cyst 478.26

Torpid liver 573.9

Torsion
- accessory tube 620.5

Torsion – *continued*
- adnexa (female) 620.5
- aorta (congenital) 747.29
  - acquired 447.1
- appendix
  - epididymis 608.24
  - testis 608.23
- bile duct 576.8
  - with calculus, choledocholithiasis or stones - *see* Choledocholithiasis
  - congenital 751.69
- bowel, colon, or intestine 560.2
- cervix *see* - Malposition, uterus
- duodenum 537.3
- dystonia - *see* Dystonia, torsion
- epididymis 608.24
  - appendix 608.24
- fallopian tube 620.5
- gallbladder (*see also* Disease, gallbladder) 575.8
  - congenital 751.69
- gastric 537.89
- hydatid of Morgagni (female) 620.5
- kidney (pedicle) 593.89
- Meckel's diverticulum (congenital) 751.0
- mesentery 560.2
- omentum 560.2
- organ or site, congenital NEC - *see* Anomaly, specified type NEC
- ovary (pedicle) 620.5
  - congenital 752.0
- oviduct 620.5
- penis 607.89
  - congenital 752.69
- renal 593.89
- spasm - *see* Dystonia, torsion
- spermatic cord 608.22
  - extravaginal 608.21
  - intravaginal 608.22
- spleen 289.59
- testicle, testis 608.20
  - appendix 608.23
- tibia 736.89
- umbilical cord - *see* Compression, umbilical cord
- uterus (*see also* Malposition, uterus) 621.6

Torticollis (intermittent) (spastic) 723.5
- congenital 754.1
  - sternomastoid 754.1
- due to birth injury 767.8
- hysterical 300.11
- ocular 781.93
- psychogenic 306.0
  - specified as conversion reaction 300.11
- rheumatic 723.5
- rheumatoid 714.0
- spasmodic 333.83
- traumatic, current NEC 847.0

Tortuous
- artery 447.1
- fallopian tube 752.19
- organ or site, congenital NEC - *see* Distortion
- renal vessel (congenital) 747.62
- retina vessel (congenital) 743.58
  - acquired 362.17
- ureter 593.4
- urethra 599.84
- vein - *see* Varicose, vein

Torula, torular (infection) 117.5
- histolytica 117.5
- lung 117.5

Torulosis 117.5

Torus
- fracture
  - fibula 823.41
    - with tibia 823.42
  - humerus 812.49 ●
  - radius 813.45
  - tibia (alone) 823.40 ▲
    - with fibula 823.42
    - with ulna 813.47 ●
  - ulna (alone) 813.46 ●
    - with radius 813.47 ●

Thyroiditis – Torus

- **Torus** – *continued*
  - mandibularis 526.81
  - palatinus 526.81
- **Touch, vitreous** 997.99
- **Touraine's syndrome** (hereditary osteo-onychodysplasia) 756.89
- **Touraine-Solente-Golé syndrome** (acropachyderma) 757.39
- **Tourette's disease** (motor-verbal tic) 307.23
- **Tower skull** 756.0
  - with exophthalmos 756.0
- **Toxemia** 799.89
  - with
    - abortion - *see* Abortion, by type, with toxemia
  - bacterial - *see* Septicemia
  - biliary (*see also* Disease, biliary) 576.8
  - burn - *see* Burn, by site
  - congenital NEC 779.89
  - eclamptic 642.6 [5th]
    - with pre-existing hypertension 642.7 [5th]
  - erysipelatous (*see also* Erysipelas) 035
  - fatigue 799.89
  - fetus or newborn NEC 779.89
  - food (*see also* Poisoning, food) 005.9
  - gastric 537.89
  - gastrointestinal 558.2
  - intestinal 558.2
  - kidney (*see also* Disease, renal) 593.9
  - lung 518.89
  - malarial NEC (*see also* Malaria) 084.6
  - maternal (of pregnancy), affecting fetus or newborn 760.0
  - myocardial - *see* Myocarditis, toxic
  - of pregnancy (mild) (pre-eclamptic) 642.4 [5th]
    - with
      - convulsions 642.6 [5th]
      - pre-existing hypertension 642.7 [5th]
    - affecting fetus or newborn 760.0
    - severe 642.5 [5th]
  - pre-eclamptic - *see* Toxemia, of pregnancy
  - puerperal, postpartum - *see* Toxemia, of pregnancy
  - pulmonary 518.89
  - renal (*see also* Disease, renal) 593.9
  - septic (*see also* Septicemia) 038.9
  - small intestine 558.2
  - staphylococcal 038.10
    - aureus 038.11
    - due to food 005.0
    - specified organism NEC 038.19
  - stasis 799.89
  - stomach 537.89
  - uremic (*see also* Uremia) 586
  - urinary 586
- **Toxemica cerebropathia psychica** (nonalcoholic) 294.0
  - alcoholic 291.1
- **Toxic** (poisoning) - *see also* condition
  - from drug or poison - *see* Table of Drugs and Chemicals
  - oil syndrome 710.5
  - shock syndrome 040.82
  - thyroid (gland) (*see also* Thyrotoxicosis) 242.9 [5th]
- **Toxicemia** - *see* Toxemia
- **Toxicity**
  - dilantin
    - asymptomatic 796.0
    - symptomatic -*see* Table of Drugs and Chemicals
  - drug
    - asymptomatic 796.0
    - symptomatic- *see* Table of Drugs and Chemicals
  - fava bean 282.2
  - from drug or poison
    - asymptomatic 796.0
    - symptomatic- *see* Table of Drugs and Chemicals
- **Toxicosis** (*see also* Toxemia) 799.89
  - capillary, hemorrhagic 287.0
- **Toxinfection** 799.89
  - gastrointestinal 558.2
- **Toxocariasis** 128.0
- **Toxoplasma infection, generalized** 130.9
- **Toxoplasmosis** (acquired) 130.9
  - with pneumonia 130.4
  - congenital, active 771.2
  - disseminated (multisystemic) 130.8
  - maternal
    - with suspected damage to fetus affecting management of pregnancy 655.4 [5th]
    - affecting fetus or newborn 760.2
      - manifest toxoplasmosis in fetus or newborn 771.2
  - multiple sites 130.8
  - multisystemic disseminated 130.8
  - specified site NEC 130.7
- **Trabeculation, bladder** 596.8
- **Trachea** - *see* condition
- **Tracheitis** (acute) (catarrhal) (infantile) (membranous) (plastic) (pneumococcal) (septic) (suppurative) (viral) 464.10
  - with
    - bronchitis 490
      - acute or subacute 466.0
      - chronic 491.8
      - tuberculosis - *see* Tuberculosis, pulmonary
    - laryngitis (acute) 464.20
      - with obstruction 464.21
      - chronic 476.1
      - tuberculous (*see also* Tuberculosis, larynx) 012.3 [5th]
    - obstruction 464.11
  - chronic 491.8
    - with
      - bronchitis (chronic) 491.8
      - laryngitis (chronic) 476.1
    - due to external agent - *see* Condition, respiratory, chronic, due to
  - diphtheritic (membranous) 032.3
    - due to external agent - *see* Inflammation, respiratory, upper, due to
  - edematous 464.11
  - influenzal 487.1
  - streptococcal 034.0
  - syphilitic 095.8
  - tuberculous (*see also* Tuberculosis) 012.8 [5th]
- **Trachelitis** (nonvenereal) (*see also* Cervicitis) 616.0
  - trichomonal 131.09
- **Tracheobronchial** - *see* condition
- **Tracheobronchitis** (*see also* Bronchitis) 490
  - acute or subacute 466.0
    - with bronchospasm or obstruction 466.0
  - chronic 491.8
  - influenzal 487.1
  - senile 491.8
- **Tracheobronchomegaly** (congenital) 748.3
  - with bronchiectasis 494.0
    - with (acute) exacerbation 494.1
  - acquired 519.19
    - with bronchiectasis 494.0
      - with (acute) exacerbation 494.1
- **Tracheobronchopneumonitis** - *see* Pneumonia, broncho
- **Tracheocele** (external) (internal) 519.19
  - congenital 748.3
- **Tracheomalacia** 519.19
  - congenital 748.3
- **Tracheopharyngitis** (acute) 465.8
  - chronic 478.9
    - due to external agent - *see* Condition, respiratory, chronic, due to
  - due to external agent - *see* Inflammation, respiratory, upper, due to
- **Tracheostenosis** 519.19
  - congenital 748.3
- **Tracheostomy**
  - attention to V55.0
  - complication 519.00
  - granuloma 519.09
  - hemorrhage 519.09
  - infection 519.01
  - malfunctioning 519.02
  - obstruction 519.09
  - sepsis 519.01
  - status V44.0
  - stenosis 519.02
- **Trachoma, trachomatous** 076.9
  - active (stage) 076.1
  - contraction of conjunctiva 076.1
  - dubium 076.0
  - healed or late effect 139.1
  - initial (stage) 076.0
  - Türck's (chronic catarrhal laryngitis) 476.0
- **Trachyphonia** 784.49
- **Training**
  - insulin pump V65.46
  - orthoptic V57.4
  - orthotic V57.81
- **Train sickness** 994.6
- **Trait**
  - hemoglobin
    - abnormal NEC 282.7
      - with thalassemia 282.49
    - C (*see also* Disease, hemoglobin, C) 282.7
      - with elliptocytosis 282.7
    - S (Hb-S) 282.5
  - Lepore 282.49
    - with other abnormal hemoglobin NEC 282.49
  - paranoid 301.0
  - sickle-cell 282.5
    - with
      - elliptocytosis 282.5
      - spherocytosis 282.5
- **Traits, paranoid** 301.0
- **Tramp** V60.0
- **Trance** 780.09
  - hysterical 300.13
- **Transaminasemia** 790.4
- **Transfusion, blood**
  - donor V59.01
    - stem cells V59.02
  - fetal twin to twin 678.0 [5th]
  - incompatible ~~999.6~~ ▲
    - ABO 999.6 ●
    - minor blood group 999.89 ●
  - reaction or complication - *see* Complications, transfusion
  - related acute lung injury (TRALI) 518.7
  - syndrome
    - fetomaternal 772.0
    - twin-to-twin
      - blood loss (donor twin) 772.0
      - recipient twin 776.4
  - twin to twin fetal 678.0 [5th]
  - without reported diagnosis V58.2
- **Transient** - *see also* condition
  - alteration of awareness 780.02
  - blindness 368.12
  - deafness (ischemic) 388.02
  - global amnesia 437.7
  - hyperglycemia (post-procedural) 790.29 ●
  - hypoglycemia (post-procedural) 251.2 ●
  - person (homeless) NEC V60.0
- **Transitional, lumbosacral joint of vertebra** 756.19
- **Translocation**
  - autosomes NEC 758.5
    - 13-15 758.1
    - 16-18 758.2
    - 21 or 22 758.0
    - balanced in normal individual 758.4
    - D_1 758.1
    - E_3 758.2
    - G 758.0
  - balanced autosomal in normal individual 758.4
- **Translocation** – *continued*
  - chromosomes NEC 758.89
  - Down's syndrome 758.0
- **Translucency, iris** 364.53
- **Transmission of chemical substances through the placenta** (affecting fetus or newborn) 760.70
  - alcohol 760.71
  - anticonvulsants 760.77
  - antifungals 760.74
- **Transmission of chemical substances through the placenta** (affecting fetus or newborn) – *continued*
  - anti-infective agents 760.74
  - antimetabolics 760.78
  - cocaine 760.75
  - "crack" 760.75
  - diethylstilbestrol [DES] 760.76
  - hallucinogenic agents 760.73
  - medicinal agents NEC 760.79
  - narcotics 760.72
  - obstetric anesthetic or analgesic drug 763.5
  - specified agent NEC 760.79
  - suspected, affecting management of pregnancy 655.5 [5th]
- **Transplant**(ed)
  - bone V42.4
    - marrow V42.81
  - complication - *see also* Complications, due to (presence of) any device, implant, or graft classified to 996.0-996.5 NEC
    - bone marrow 996.85
    - corneal graft NEC 996.79
      - infection or inflammation 996.69
      - reaction 996.51
      - rejection 996.51
    - organ (failure) (immune or nonimmune cause) (infection) (rejection) 996.80
      - bone marrow 996.85
      - heart 996.83
      - intestines 996.87
      - kidney 996.81
      - liver 996.82
      - lung 996.84
      - pancreas 996.86
      - specified NEC 996.89
    - previously removed due to complication, failure, rejection or infection V45.87
    - removal status V45.87
    - skin NEC 996.79
      - infection or inflammation 996.69
      - rejection 996.52
        - artificial 996.55
        - decellularized allodermis 996.55
  - cornea V42.5
  - hair V50.0
  - heart V42.1
    - valve V42.2
  - intestine V42.84
  - kidney V42.0
  - liver V42.7
  - lung V42.6
  - organ V42.9
    - specified NEC V42.89
  - pancreas V42.83
  - peripheral stem cells V42.82
  - skin V42.3
  - stem cells, peripheral V42.82
  - tissue V42.9
    - specified NEC V42.89
- **Transplants, ovarian, endometrial** 617.1
- **Transposed** - *see* Transposition
- **Transposition** (congenital) - *see also* Malposition, congenital
  - abdominal viscera 759.3
  - aorta (dextra) 745.11
  - appendix 751.5
  - arterial trunk 745.10
  - colon 751.5

Tuberculosis, tubercular, tuberculous (calcification) (calcified) (caseous) (chromogenic acid-fast bacilli) (congenital) (degeneration) (disease) (fibrocaseous) (fistula) (gangrene) (interstitial) (isolated circumscribed lesions) (necrosis) (parenchymatous) (ulcerative) 011.9 5th

Note *Use the following fifth-digit subclassification with categories 010-018:*

- 0 unspecified
- 1 bacteriological or histological examination not done
- 2 bacteriological or histological examination unknown (at present)
- 3 tubercle bacilli found (in sputum) by microscopy
- 4 tubercle bacilli not found (in sputum) by microscopy, but found by bacterial culture
- 5 tubercle bacilli not found by bacteriological examination, but tuberculosis confirmed histologically
- 6 tubercle bacilli not found by bacteriological or histological examination, but tuberculosis confirmed by other methods [inoculation of animals]

For tuberculous conditions specified as late effects or sequelae, see category 137.

- abdomen 014.8 5th
  - lymph gland 014.8 5th
- abscess 011.9 5th
  - arm 017.9 5th
  - bone (*see also* Osteomyelitis, due to, tuberculosis) 015.9 5th *[730.8]*
    - hip 015.1 5th *[730.85]*
    - knee 015.2 5th *[730.86]*
    - sacrum 015.0 5th *[730.88]*
    - specified site NEC 015.7 5th *[730.88]*
    - spinal 015.0 5th *[730.88]*
    - vertebra 015.0 5th *[730.88]*
  - brain 013.3 5th
  - breast 017.9 5th
  - Cowper's gland 016.5 5th
  - dura (mater) 013.8 5th
    - brain 013.3 5th
    - spinal cord 013.5 5th
  - epidural 013.8 5th
    - brain 013.3 5th
    - spinal cord 013.5 5th
  - frontal sinus - *see* Tuberculosis, sinus
  - genital organs NEC 016.9 5th
    - female 016.7 5th
    - male 016.5 5th
  - genitourinary NEC 016.9 5th
  - gland (lymphatic) - *see* Tuberculosis, lymph gland
  - hip 015.1 5th
  - iliopsoas 015.0 5th *[730.88]*
  - intestine 014.8 5th
  - ischiorectal 014.8 5th
  - joint 015.9 5th
    - hip 015.1 5th
    - knee 015.2 5th
    - specified joint NEC 015.8 5th
    - vertebral 015.0 5th *[730.88]*
  - kidney 016.0 5th *[590.81]*
  - knee 015.2 5th
  - lumbar 015.0 5th *[730.88]*
  - lung 011.2 5th
    - primary, progressive 010.8 5th
  - meninges (cerebral) (spinal) 013.0 5th
  - pelvic 016.9 5th
    - female 016.7 5th
    - male 016.5 5th
  - perianal 014.8 5th
    - fistula 014.8 5th
  - perinephritic 016.0 5th *[590.81]*

Tuberculosis, tubercular, tuberculous *– continued*

- abscess *– continued*
  - perineum 017.9 5th
  - perirectal 014.8 5th
  - psoas 015.0 5th *[730.88]*
  - rectum 014.8 5th
  - retropharyngeal 012.8 5th
  - sacrum 015.0 5th *[730.88]*
  - scrofulous 017.2 5th
  - scrotum 016.5 5th
  - skin 017.0 5th
    - primary 017.0 5th
  - spinal cord 013.5 5th
  - spine or vertebra (column) 015.0 5th *[730.88]*
  - strumous 017.2 5th
  - subdiaphragmatic 014.8 5th
  - testis 016.5 5th
  - thigh 017.9 5th
  - urinary 016.3 5th
    - kidney 016.0 5th *[590.81]*
  - uterus 016.7 5th
- accessory sinus - *see* Tuberculosis, sinus
- Addison's disease 017.6 5th
- adenitis (*see also* Tuberculosis, lymph gland) 017.2 5th
- adenoids 012.8 5th
- adenopathy (*see also* Tuberculosis, lymph gland) 017.2 5th
  - tracheobronchial 012.1 5th
    - primary progressive 010.8 5th
- adherent pericardium 017.9 5th *[420.0]*
- adnexa (uteri) 016.7 5th
- adrenal (capsule) (gland) 017.6 5th
- air passage NEC 012.8 5th
- alimentary canal 014.8 5th
- anemia 017.9 5th
- ankle (joint) 015.8 5th
  - bone 015.5 5th *[730.87]*
- anus 014.8 5th
- apex (*see also* Tuberculosis, pulmonary) 011.9 5th
- apical (*see also* Tuberculosis, pulmonary) 011.9 5th
- appendicitis 014.8 5th
- appendix 014.8 5th
- arachnoid 013.0 5th
- artery 017.9 5th
- arthritis (chronic) (synovial) 015.9 5th *[711.40]*
  - ankle 015.8 5th *[730.87]*
  - hip 015.1 5th *[711.45]*
  - knee 015.2 5th *[711.46]*
  - specified site NEC 015.8 5th *[711.48]*
  - spine or vertebra (column) 015.0 5th *[720.81]*
  - wrist 015.8 5th *[730.83]*
- articular - *see* Tuberculosis, joint
- ascites 014.0 5th
- asthma (*see also* Tuberculosis, pulmonary) 011.9 5th
- axilla, axillary 017.2 5th
  - gland 017.2 5th
- bilateral (*see also* Tuberculosis, pulmonary) 011.9 5th
- bladder 016.1 5th
- bone (*see also* Osteomyelitis, due to, tuberculosis) 015.9 5th *[730.8]*
  - hip 015.1 5th *[730.85]*
  - knee 015.2 5th *[730.86]*
  - limb NEC 015.5 5th *[730.88]*
  - sacrum 015.0 5th *[730.88]*
  - specified site NEC 015.7 5th *[730.88]*
  - spinal or vertebral column 015.0 5th *[730.88]*
- bowel 014.8 5th
  - miliary 018.9 5th
- brain 013.2 5th
- breast 017.9 5th
- broad ligament 016.7 5th
- bronchi, bronchial, bronchus 011.3 5th
  - ectasia, ectasis 011.5 5th

Tuberculosis, tubercular, tuberculous *– continued*

- bronchi, bronchial, bronchus *– continued*
  - fistula 011.3 5th
    - primary, progressive 010.8 5th
  - gland 012.1 5th
    - primary, progressive 010.8 5th
  - isolated 012.2 5th
  - lymph gland or node 012.1 5th
    - primary, progressive 010.8 5th
- bronchiectasis 011.5 5th
- bronchitis 011.3 5th
- bronchopleural 012.0 5th
- bronchopneumonia, bronchopneumonic 011.6 5th
- bronchorrhagia 011.3 5th
- bronchotracheal 011.3 5th
  - isolated 012.2 5th
- bronchus - *see* Tuberculosis, bronchi
- bronze disease (Addison's) 017.6 5th
- buccal cavity 017.9 5th
- bulbourethral gland 016.5 5th
- bursa (*see also* Tuberculosis, joint) 015.9 5th
- cachexia NEC (*see also* Tuberculosis, pulmonary) 011.9 5th
- cardiomyopathy 017.9 5th *[425.8]*
- caries (*see also* Tuberculosis, bone) 015.9 5th *[730.8]*
- cartilage (*see also* Tuberculosis, bone) 015.9 5th *[730.8]*
  - intervertebral 015.0 5th *[730.88]*
- catarrhal (*see also* Tuberculosis, pulmonary) 011.9 5th
- cecum 014.8 5th
- cellular tissue (primary) 017.0 5th
- cellulitis (primary) 017.0 5th
- central nervous system 013.9 5th
  - specified site NEC 013.8 5th
- cerebellum (current) 013.2 5th
- cerebral (current) 013.2 5th
  - meninges 013.0 5th
- cerebrospinal 013.6 5th
  - meninges 013.0 5th
- cerebrum (current) 013.2 5th
- cervical 017.2 5th
  - gland 017.2 5th
  - lymph nodes 017.2 5th
- cervicitis (uteri) 016.7 5th
- cervix 016.7 5th
- chest (*see also* Tuberculosis, pulmonary) 011.9 5th
- childhood type or first infection 010.0 5th
- choroid 017.3 5th *[363.13]*
- choroiditis 017.3 5th *[363.13]*
- ciliary body 017.3 5th *[364.11]*
- colitis 014.8 5th
- colliers' 011.4 5th
- colliquativa (primary) 017.0 5th
- colon 014.8 5th
  - ulceration 014.8 5th
- complex, primary 010.0 5th
- complicating pregnancy, childbirth, or puerperium 647.3 5th
  - affecting fetus or newborn 760.2
- congenital 771.2
- conjunctiva 017.3 5th *[370.31]*
- connective tissue 017.9 5th
  - bone - *see* Tuberculosis, bone
- contact V01.1
- converter (tuberculin skin test) (without disease) 795.5
- cornea (ulcer) 017.3 5th *[370.31]*
- Cowper's gland 016.5 5th
- coxae 015.1 5th *[730.85]*
- coxalgia 015.1 5th *[730.85]*
- cul-de-sac of Douglas 014.8 5th
- curvature, spine 015.0 5th *[737.40]*
- cutis (colliquativa) (primary) 017.0 5th
- cyst, ovary 016.6 5th
- cystitis 016.1 5th
- dacryocystitis 017.3 5th *[375.32]*
- dactylitis 015.5 5th
- diarrhea 014.8 5th

Tuberculosis, tubercular, tuberculous *– continued*

- diffuse (*see also* Tuberculosis, miliary) 018.9 5th
  - lung - *see* Tuberculosis, pulmonary
  - meninges 013.0 5th
- digestive tract 014.8 5th
- disseminated (*see also* Tuberculosis, miliary) 018.9 5th
  - meninges 013.0 5th
- duodenum 014.8 5th
- dura (mater) 013.9 5th
  - abscess 013.8 5th
    - cerebral 013.3 5th
    - spinal 013.5 5th
- dysentery 014.8 5th
- ear (inner) (middle) 017.4 5th
  - bone 015.6 5th
  - external (primary) 017.0 5th
  - skin (primary) 017.0 5th
- elbow 015.8 5th
- emphysema - *see* Tuberculosis, pulmonary
- empyema 012.0 5th
- encephalitis 013.6 5th
- endarteritis 017.9 5th
- endocarditis (any valve) 017.9 5th *[424.91]*
- endocardium (any valve) 017.9 5th *[424.91]*
- endocrine glands NEC 017.9 5th
- endometrium 016.7 5th
- enteric, enterica 014.8 5th
- enteritis 014.8 5th
- enterocolitis 014.8 5th
- epididymis 016.4 5th
- epididymitis 016.4 5th
- epidural abscess 013.8 5th
  - brain 013.3 5th
  - spinal cord 013.5 5th
- epiglottis 012.3 5th
- episcleritis 017.3 5th *[379.00]*
- erythema (induratum) (nodosum) (primary) 017.1 5th
- esophagus 017.8 5th
- Eustachian tube 017.4 5th
- exposure to V01.1
- exudative 012.0 5th
  - primary, progressive 010.1 5th
- eye 017.3 5th
- eyelid (primary) 017.0 5th
  - lupus 017.0 5th *[373.4]*
- fallopian tube 016.6 5th
- fascia 017.9 5th
- fauces 012.8 5th
- finger 017.9 5th
- first infection 010.0 5th
- fistula, perirectal 014.8 5th
- Florida 011.6 5th
- foot 017.9 5th
- funnel pelvis 137.3
- gallbladder 017.9 5th
- galloping (*see also* Tuberculosis, pulmonary) 011.9 5th
- ganglionic 015.9 5th
- gastritis 017.9 5th
- gastrocolic fistula 014.8 5th
- gastroenteritis 014.8 5th
- gastrointestinal tract 014.8 5th
- general, generalized 018.9 5th
  - acute 018.0 5th
  - chronic 018.8 5th
- genital organs NEC 016.9 5th
  - female 016.7 5th
  - male 016.5 5th
- genitourinary NEC 016.9 5th
- genu 015.2 5th
- glandulae suprarenalis 017.6 5th
- glandular, general 017.2 5th
- glottis 012.3 5th
- grinders' 011.4 5th
- groin 017.2 5th
- gum 017.9 5th
- hand 017.9 5th
- heart 017.9 5th *[425.8]*
- hematogenous - *see* Tuberculosis, miliary

Tuberculosis, tubercular, tuberculous *- continued*
- hemoptysis (*see also* Tuberculosis, pulmonary) 011.9 5th
- hemorrhage NEC (*see also* Tuberculosis, pulmonary) 011.9 5th
- hemothorax 012.0 5th
- hepatitis 017.9 5th
- hilar lymph nodes 012.1 5th
  - primary, progressive 010.8 5th
- hip (disease) (joint) 015.1 5th
  - bone 015.1 5th *[730.85]*
- hydrocephalus 013.8 5th
- hydropneumothorax 012.0 5th
- hydrothorax 012.0 5th
- hypoadrenalism 017.6 5th
- hypopharynx 012.8 5th
- ileocecal (hyperplastic) 014.8 5th
- ileocolitis 014.8 5th
- ileum 014.8 5th
- iliac spine (superior) 015.0 5th *[730.88]*
- incipient NEC (*see also* Tuberculosis, pulmonary) 011.9 5th
- indurativa (primary) 017.1 5th
- infantile 010.0 5th
- infection NEC 011.9 5th
  - without clinical manifestation 010.0 5th
- infraclavicular gland 017.2 5th
- inguinal gland 017.2 5th
- inguinalis 017.2 5th
- intestine (any part) 014.8 5th
- iris 017.3 5th *[364.11]*
- iritis 017.3 5th *[364.11]*
- ischiorectal 014.8 5th
- jaw 015.7 5th *[730.88]*
- jejunum 014.8 5th
- joint 015.9 5th
  - hip 015.1 5th
  - knee 015.2 5th
  - specified site NEC 015.8 5th
  - vertebral 015.0 5th *[730.88]*
- keratitis 017.3 5th *[370.31]*
  - interstitial 017.3 5th *[370.59]*
- keratoconjunctivitis 017.3 5th *[370.31]*
- kidney 016.0 5th
- knee (joint) 015.2 5th
- kyphoscoliosis 015.0 5th *[737.43]*
- kyphosis 015.0 5th *[737.41]*
- lacrimal apparatus, gland 017.3 5th
- laryngitis 012.3 5th
- larynx 012.3 5th
- leptomeninges, leptomeningitis (cerebral) (spinal) 013.0 5th
- lichenoides (primary) 017.0 5th
- linguae 017.9 5th
- lip 017.9 5th
- liver 017.9 5th
- lordosis 015.0 5th *[737.42]*
- lung - *see* Tuberculosis, pulmonary
- luposa 017.0 5th
  - eyelid 017.0 5th *[373.4]*
- lymphadenitis - *see* Tuberculosis, lymph gland
- lymphangitis - *see* Tuberculosis, lymph gland
- lymphatic (gland) (vessel) - *see* Tuberculosis, lymph gland
- lymph gland or node (peripheral) 017.2 5th
  - abdomen 014.8 5th
  - bronchial 012.1 5th
    - primary, progressive 010.8 5th
  - cervical 017.2 5th
  - hilar 012.1 5th
    - primary, progressive 010.8 5th
  - intrathoracic 012.1 5th
    - primary, progressive 010.8 5th
  - mediastinal 012.1 5th
    - primary, progressive 010.8 5th
  - mesenteric 014.8 5th
  - peripheral 017.2 5th
  - retroperitoneal 014.8 5th
  - tracheobronchial 012.1 5th
    - primary, progressive 010.8 5th

Tuberculosis, tubercular, tuberculous *- continued*
- malignant NEC (*see also* Tuberculosis, pulmonary) 011.9 5th
- mammary gland 017.9 5th
- marasmus NEC (*see also* Tuberculosis, pulmonary) 011.9 5th
- mastoiditis 015.6 5th
- maternal, affecting fetus or newborn 760.2
- mediastinal (lymph) gland or node 012.1 5th
  - primary, progressive 010.8 5th
- mediastinitis 012.8 5th
  - primary, progressive 010.8 5th
- mediastinopericarditis 017.9 5th *[420.0]*
- mediastinum 012.8 5th
  - primary, progressive 010.8 5th
- medulla 013.9 5th
  - brain 013.2 5th
  - spinal cord 013.4 5th
- melanosis, Addisonian 017.6 5th
- membrane, brain 013.0 5th
- meninges (cerebral) (spinal) 013.0 5th
- meningitis (basilar) (brain) (cerebral) (cerebrospinal) (spinal) 013.0 5th
- meningoencephalitis 013.0 5th
- mesentery, mesenteric 014.8 5th
  - lymph gland or node 014.8 5th
- miliary (any site) 018.9 5th
  - acute 018.0 5th
  - chronic 018.8 5th
  - specified type NEC 018.8 5th
- millstone makers' 011.4 5th
- miners' 011.4 5th
- moulders' 011.4 5th
- mouth 017.9 5th
- multiple 018.9 5th
  - acute 018.0 5th
  - chronic 018.8 5th
- muscle 017.9 5th
- myelitis 013.6 5th
- myocarditis 017.9 5th *[422.0]*
- myocardium 017.9 5th *[422.0]*
- nasal (passage) (sinus) 012.8 5th
- nasopharynx 012.8 5th
- neck gland 017.2 5th
- nephritis 016.0 5th *[583.81]*
- nerve 017.9 5th
- nose (septum) 012.8 5th
- ocular 017.3 5th
- old NEC 137.0
  - without residuals V12.01
- omentum 014.8 5th
- oophoritis (acute) (chronic) 016.6 5th
- optic 017.3 5th *[377.39]*
  - nerve trunk 017.3 5th *[377.39]*
  - papilla, papillae 017.3 5th *[377.39]*
- orbit 017.3 5th
- orchitis 016.5 5th *[608.81]*
- organ, specified NEC 017.9 5th
- orificialis (primary) 017.0 5th
- osseous (*see also* Tuberculosis, bone) 015.9 5th *[730.8]* 5th
- osteitis (*see also* Tuberculosis, bone) 015.9 5th *[730.8]* 5th
- osteomyelitis (*see also* Tuberculosis, bone) 015.9 5th *[730.8]* 5th
- otitis (media) 017.4 5th
- ovaritis (acute) (chronic) 016.6 5th
- ovary (acute) (chronic) 016.6 5th
- oviducts (acute) (chronic) 016.6 5th
- pachymeningitis 013.0 5th
- palate (soft) 017.9 5th
- pancreas 017.9 5th
- papulonecrotic (primary) 017.0 5th
- parathyroid glands 017.9 5th
- paronychia (primary) 017.0 5th
- parotid gland or region 017.9 5th
- pelvic organ NEC 016.9 5th
  - female 016.7 5th
  - male 016.5 5th
- pelvis (bony) 015.7 5th *[730.85]*
- penis 016.5 5th
- peribronchitis 011.3 5th

Tuberculosis, tubercular, tuberculous *- continued*
- pericarditis 017.9 5th *[420.0]*
- pericardium 017.9 5th *[420.0]*
- perichondritis, larynx 012.3 5th
- perineum 017.9 5th
- periostitis (*see also* Tuberculosis, bone) 015.9 5th *[730.8]* 5th
- periphlebitis 017.9 5th
  - eye vessel 017.3 5th *[362.18]*
  - retina 017.3 5th *[362.18]*
- perirectal fistula 014.8 5th
- peritoneal gland 014.8 5th
- peritoneum 014.0 5th
- peritonitis 014.0 5th
- pernicious NEC (*see also* Tuberculosis, pulmonary) 011.9 5th
- pharyngitis 012.8 5th
- pharynx 012.8 5th
- phlyctenulosis (conjunctiva) 017.3 5th *[370.31]*
- phthisis NEC (*see also* Tuberculosis, pulmonary) 011.9 5th
- pituitary gland 017.9 5th
- placenta 016.7 5th
- pleura, pleural, pleurisy, pleuritis (fibrinous) (obliterative) (purulent) (simple plastic) (with effusion) 012.0 5th
  - primary, progressive 010.1 5th
- pneumonia, pneumonic 011.6 5th
- pneumothorax 011.7 5th
- polyserositis 018.9 5th
  - acute 018.0 5th
  - chronic 018.8 5th
- potters' 011.4 5th
- prepuce 016.5 5th
- primary 010.9 5th
  - complex 010.0 5th
  - complicated 010.8 5th
    - with pleurisy or effusion 010.1 5th
  - progressive 010.8 5th
    - with pleurisy or effusion 010.1 5th
  - skin 017.0 5th
- proctitis 014.8 5th
- prostate 016.5 5th *[601.4]*
- prostatitis 016.5 5th *[601.4]*
- pulmonaris (*see also* Tuberculosis, pulmonary) 011.9 5th
- pulmonary (artery) (incipient) (malignant) (multiple round foci) (pernicious) (reinfection stage) 011.9 5th
  - cavitated or with cavitation 011.2 5th
    - primary, progressive 010.8 5th
  - childhood type or first infection 010.0 5th
  - chromogenic acid-fast bacilli 795.39
  - fibrosis or fibrotic 011.4 5th
  - infiltrative 011.0 5th
    - primary, progressive 010.9 5th
  - nodular 011.1 5th
  - specified NEC 011.8 5th
  - sputum positive only 795.39
  - status following surgical collapse of lung NEC 011.9 5th
- pyelitis 016.0 5th *[590.81]*
- pyelonephritis 016.0 5th *[590.81]*
- pyemia - *see* Tuberculosis, miliary
- pyonephrosis 016.0 5th
- pyopneumothorax 012.0 5th
- pyothorax 012.0 5th
- rectum (with abscess) 014.8 5th
  - fistula 014.8 5th
- reinfection stage (*see also* Tuberculosis, pulmonary) 011.9 5th
- renal 016.0 5th
- renis 016.0 5th
- reproductive organ 016.7 5th
- respiratory NEC (*see also* Tuberculosis, pulmonary) 011.9 5th
  - specified site NEC 012.8 5th
- retina 017.3 5th *[363.13]*

Tuberculosis, tubercular, tuberculous *- continued*
- retroperitoneal (lymph gland or node) 014.8 5th
  - gland 014.8 5th
- retropharyngeal abscess 012.8 5th
- rheumatism 015.9 5th
- rhinitis 012.8 5th
- sacroiliac (joint) 015.8 5th
- sacrum 015.0 5th *[730.88]*
- salivary gland 017.9 5th
- salpingitis (acute) (chronic) 016.6 5th
- sandblasters' 011.4 5th
- sclera 017.3 5th *[379.09]*
- scoliosis 015.0 5th *[737.43]*
- scrofulous 017.2 5th
- scrotum 016.5 5th
- seminal tract or vesicle 016.5 5th *[608.81]*
- senile NEC (*see also* Tuberculosis, pulmonary) 011.9 5th
- septic NEC (*see also* Tuberculosis, miliary) 018.9 5th
- shoulder 015.8 5th
  - blade 015.7 5th *[730.8]*
- sigmoid 014.8 5th
- sinus (accessory) (nasal) 012.8 5th
  - bone 015.7 5th *[730.88]*
  - epididymis 016.4 5th
- skeletal NEC (*see also* Osteomyelitis, due to tuberculosis) 015.9 5th *[730.8]*
- skin (any site) (primary) 017.0 5th
- small intestine 014.8 5th
- soft palate 017.9 5th
- spermatic cord 016.5 5th
- spinal
  - column 015.0 5th *[730.88]*
  - cord 013.4 5th
  - disease 015.0 5th *[730.88]*
  - medulla 013.4 5th
  - membrane 013.0 5th
  - meninges 013.0 5th
- spine 015.0 5th *[730.88]*
- spleen 017.7 5th
- splenitis 017.7 5th
- spondylitis 015.0 5th *[720.81]*
- spontaneous pneumothorax - *see* Tuberculosis, pulmonary
- sternoclavicular joint 015.8 5th
- stomach 017.9 5th
- stonemasons' 011.4 5th
- struma 017.2 5th
- subcutaneous tissue (cellular) (primary) 017.0 5th
- subcutis (primary) 017.0 5th
- subdeltoid bursa 017.9 5th
- submaxillary 017.9 5th
  - region 017.9 5th
- supraclavicular gland 017.2 5th
- suprarenal (capsule) (gland) 017.6 5th
- swelling, joint (*see also* Tuberculosis, joint) 015.9 5th
- symphysis pubis 015.7 5th *[730.88]*
- synovitis 015.9 5th *[727.01]*
  - hip 015.1 5th *[727.01]*
  - knee 015.2 5th *[727.01]*
  - specified site NEC 015.8 5th *[727.01]*
  - spine or vertebra 015.0 5th *[727.01]*
- systemic - *see* Tuberculosis, miliary
- tarsitis (eyelid) 017.0 5th *[373.4]*
  - ankle (bone) 015.5 5th *[730.87]*
- tendon (sheath) - *see* Tuberculosis, tenosynovitis
- tenosynovitis 015.9 5th *[727.01]*
  - hip 015.1 5th *[727.01]*
  - knee 015.2 5th *[727.01]*
  - specified site NEC 015.8 5th *[727.01]*
  - spine or vertebra 015.0 5th *[727.01]*
- testis 016.5 5th *[608.81]*
- throat 012.8 5th
- thymus gland 017.9 5th
- thyroid gland 017.5 5th
- toe 017.9 5th
- tongue 017.9 5th
- tonsil (lingual) 012.8 5th

Tuberculosis, tubercular, tuberculous – *continued*
- tonsillitis 012.8 5th
- trachea, tracheal 012.8 5th
  - gland 012.1 5th
    - primary, progressive 010.8 5th
  - isolated 012.2 5th
- tracheobronchial 011.3 5th
  - glandular 012.1 5th
    - primary, progressive 010.8 5th
  - isolated 012.2 5th
  - lymph gland or node 012.1 5th
    - primary, progressive 010.8 5th
- tubal 016.6 5th
- tunica vaginalis 016.5 5th
- typhlitis 014.8 5th
- ulcer (primary) (skin) 017.0 5th
  - bowel or intestine 014.8 5th
  - specified site NEC - *see* Tuberculosis, by site
- unspecified site - *see* Tuberculosis, pulmonary
- ureter 016.2 5th
- urethra, urethral 016.3 5th
- urinary organ or tract 016.3 5th
  - kidney 016.0 5th
- uterus 016.7 5th
- uveal tract 017.3 5th *[363.13]*
- uvula 017.9 5th
- vaccination, prophylactic (against) V03.2
- vagina 016.7 5th
- vas deferens 016.5 5th
- vein 017.9 5th
- verruca (primary) 017.0 5th
- verrucosa (cutis) (primary) 017.0 5th
- vertebra (column) 015.0 5th *[730.88]*
- vesiculitis 016.5 5th *[608.81]*
- viscera NEC 014.8 5th
- vulva 016.7 5th *[616.51]*
- wrist (joint) 015.8 5th
  - bone 015.5 5th *[730.83]*

Tuberculum
- auriculae 744.29
- occlusal 520.2
- paramolare 520.2

Tuberosity
- jaw, excessive 524.07
- maxillary, entire 524.07

Tuberous sclerosis (brain) 759.5

Tubo-ovarian - *see* condition

Tuboplasty, after previous sterilization V26.0

Tubotympanitis 381.10

Tularemia 021.9
- with
  - conjunctivitis 021.3
  - pneumonia 021.2
- bronchopneumonic 021.2
- conjunctivitis 021.3
- cryptogenic 021.1
- disseminated 021.8
- enteric 021.1
- generalized 021.8
- glandular 021.8
- intestinal 021.1
- oculoglandular 021.3
- ophthalmic 021.3
- pneumonia 021.2
- pulmonary 021.2
- specified NEC 021.8
- typhoidal 021.1
- ulceroglandular 021.0
- vaccination, prophylactic (against) V03.4

Tularensis conjunctivitis 021.3

Tumefaction - *see also* Swelling
- liver (*see also* Hypertrophy, liver) 789.1

Tumor (M8000/1) - *see also* Neoplasm, by site, unspecified nature
- Abrikossov's (M9580/0) - *see also* Neoplasm, connective tissue, benign
  - malignant (M9580/3) - *see* Neoplasm, connective tissue, malignant
- acinar cell (M8550/1) - *see* Neoplasm, by site, uncertain behavior
- acinic cell (M8550/1) - *see* Neoplasm, by site, uncertain behavior
- adenomatoid (M9054/0) - *see also* Neoplasm, by site, benign
  - odontogenic (M9300/0) 213.1
    - upper jaw (bone) 213.0
- adnexal (skin) (M8390/0) - *see* Neoplasm, skin, benign
- adrenal
  - cortical (benign) (M8370/0) 227.0
    - malignant (M8370/3) 194.0
  - rest (M8671/0) - *see* Neoplasm, by site, benign
- alpha cell (M8152/0)
  - malignant (M8152/3)
    - pancreas 157.4
    - specified site NEC - *see* Neoplasm, by site, malignant
    - unspecified site 157.4
  - pancreas 211.7
  - specified site NEC - *see* Neoplasm, by site, benign
  - unspecified site 211.7
- aneurysmal (*see also* Aneurysm) 442.9
- aortic body (M8691/1) 237.3
  - malignant (M8691/3) 194.6
- argentaffin (M8241/1) - *see* Neoplasm, by site, uncertain behavior
- basal cell (M8090/1) - *see also* Neoplasm, skin, uncertain behavior
- benign (M8000/0) - *see* Neoplasm, by site, benign
- beta cell (M8151/0)
  - malignant (M8151/3)
    - pancreas 157.4
    - specified site - *see* Neoplasm, by site, malignant
    - unspecified site 157.4
  - pancreas 211.7
  - specified site NEC - *see* Neoplasm, by site, benign
  - unspecified site 211.7
- blood - *see* Hematoma
- brenner (M9000/0) 220
  - borderline malignancy (M9000/1) 236.2
  - malignant (M9000/3) 183.0
  - proliferating (M9000/1) 236.2
- Brooke's (M8100/0) - *see* Neoplasm, skin, benign
- brown fat (M8880/0) - *see* Lipoma, by site
- Burkitt's (M9750/3) 200.2 5th
- calcifying epithelial odontogenic (M9340/0) 213.1
  - upper jaw (bone) 213.0
- carcinoid (M8240/1) 209.60
  - benign 209.60
    - appendix 209.51
    - ascending colon 209.53
    - bronchus 209.61
    - cecum 209.52
    - colon 209.50
    - descending colon 209.55
    - duodenum 209.41
    - foregut 209.65
    - hindgut 209.67
    - ileum 209.43
    - jejunum 209.42
    - kidney 209.64
    - large intestine 209.50
    - lung 209.61
    - midgut 209.66
    - rectum 209.57
    - sigmoid colon 209.56
    - small intestine 209.40
    - specified NEC 209.69
    - stomach 209.63
    - thymus 209.62
    - transverse colon 209.54
  - malignant (of) 209.20
    - appendix 209.11

Tumor – *continued*
- carcinoid – *continued*
  - malignant (of) – *continued*
    - ascending colon 209.13
    - bronchus 209.21
    - cecum 209.12
    - colon 209.10
    - descending colon 209.15
    - duodenum 209.01
    - foregut 209.25
    - hindgut 209.27
    - ileum 209.03
    - jejunum 209.02
    - kidney 209.24
    - large intestine 209.10
    - lung 209.21
    - midgut 209.26
    - rectum 209.17
    - sigmoid colon 209.16
    - small intestine 209.00
    - specified NEC 209.29
    - stomach 209.23
    - thymus 209.22
    - transverse colon 209.14
  - ~~neuroendocrine 209.60~~
    - ~~malignant poorly differentiated 209.30~~
  - secondary - *see* Tumor, neuroendocrine, secondary ●
- carotid body (M8692/1) 237.3
  - malignant (M8692/3) 194.5
- Castleman's (mediastinal lymph node hyperplasia) 785.6
- cells (M8001/1) - *see also* Neoplasm, by site, unspecified nature
  - benign (M8001/0) - *see* Neoplasm, by site, benign
  - malignant (M8001/3) - *see* Neoplasm, by site, malignant
  - uncertain whether benign or malignant (M8001/1) - *see* Neoplasm, by site, uncertain nature
- cervix
  - in pregnancy or childbirth 654.6 5th
    - affecting fetus or newborn 763.89
    - causing obstructed labor 660.2 5th
      - affecting fetus or newborn 763.1
- chondromatous giant cell (M9230/0) - *see* Neoplasm, bone, benign
- chromaffin (M8700/0) - *see also* Neoplasm, by site, benign
  - malignant (M8700/3) - *see* Neoplasm, by site, malignant
- Cock's peculiar 706.2
- Codman's (benign chondroblastoma) (M9230/0) - *see* Neoplasm, bone, benign
- dentigerous, mixed (M9282/0) 213.1
  - upper jaw (bone) 213.0
- dermoid (M9084/0) - *see* Neoplasm, by site, benign
  - with malignant transformation (M9084/3) 183.0
- desmoid (extra-abdominal) (M8821/1) - *see also* Neoplasm, connective tissue, uncertain behavior
  - abdominal (M8822/1) - *see* Neoplasm, connective tissue, uncertain behavior
- embryonal (mixed) (M9080/1) - *see also* Neoplasm, by site, uncertain behavior
  - liver (M9080/3) 155.0
- endodermal sinus (M9071/3)
  - specified site - *see* Neoplasm, by site, malignant
  - unspecified site
    - female 183.0
    - male 186.9
- epithelial
  - benign (M8010/0) - *see* Neoplasm, by site, benign

Tumor – *continued*
- epithelial – *continued*
  - malignant (M8010/3) - *see* Neoplasm, by site, malignant
- Ewing's (M9260/3) - *see* Neoplasm, bone, malignant
- fatty - *see* Lipoma
- fetal, causing disproportion 653.7 5th
  - causing obstructed labor 660.1 5th
- fibroid (M8890/0) - *see* Leiomyoma
- G cell (M8153/1)
  - malignant (M8153/3)
    - pancreas 157.4
    - specified site NEC - *see* Neoplasm, by site, malignant
    - unspecified site 157.4
  - specified site - *see* Neoplasm, by site, uncertain behavior
  - unspecified site 235.5
- giant cell (type) (M8003/1) - *see also* Neoplasm, by site, unspecified nature
  - bone (M9250/1) 238.0
    - malignant (M9250/3) - *see* Neoplasm, bone, malignant
  - chondromatous (M9230/0) - *see* Neoplasm, bone, benign
  - malignant (M8003/3) - *see* Neoplasm, by site, malignant
  - peripheral (gingiva) 523.8
  - soft parts (M9251/1) - *see also* Neoplasm, connective tissue, uncertain behavior
    - malignant (M9251/3) - *see* Neoplasm, connective tissue, malignant
  - tendon sheath 727.02
- glomus (M8711/0) - *see also* Hemangioma, by site
  - jugulare (M8690/1) 237.3
    - malignant (M8690/3) 194.6
- gonadal stromal (M8590/1) - *see* Neoplasm, by site, uncertain behavior
- granular cell (M9580/0) - *see also* Neoplasm, connective tissue, benign
  - malignant (M9580/3) - *see* Neoplasm, connective tissue, malignant
- granulosa cell (M8620/1) 236.2
  - malignant (M8620/3) 183.0
- granulosa cell-theca cell (M8621/1) 236.2
  - malignant (M8621/3) 183.0
- Grawitz's (hypernephroma) (M8312/3) 189.0
- hazard-crile (M8350/3) 193
- hemorrhoidal - *see* Hemorrhoids
- hilar cell (M8660/0) 220
- Hürthle cell (benign) (M8290/0) 226
  - malignant (M8290/3) 193
- hydatid (*see also* Echinococcus) 122.9
- hypernephroid (M8311/1) - *see also* Neoplasm, by site, uncertain behavior
- interstitial cell (M8650/1) - *see also* Neoplasm, by site, uncertain behavior
  - benign (M8650/0) - *see* Neoplasm, by site, benign
  - malignant (M8650/3) - *see* Neoplasm, by site, malignant
- islet cell (M8150/0)
  - malignant (M8150/3)
    - pancreas 157.4
    - specified site - *see* Neoplasm, by site, malignant
    - unspecified site 157.4
  - pancreas 211.7
  - specified site NEC - *see* Neoplasm, by site, benign
  - unspecified site 211.7
- juxtaglomerular (M8361/1) 236.91
- Krukenberg's (M8490/6) 198.6
- Leydig cell (M8650/1)

Typhoid – *continued*
- carrier (suspected) of V02.1
- cholecystitis (current) 002.0
- clinical (Widal and blood test negative) 002.0
- endocarditis 002.0 *[421.1]*
- inoculation reaction - *see* Complications, vaccination
- meningitis 002.0 *[320.7]*
- mesenteric lymph nodes 002.0
- myocarditis 002.0 *[422.0]*
- osteomyelitis (*see also* Osteomyelitis, due to, typhoid) 002.0 *[730.8]* [5th]
- perichondritis, larynx 002.0 *[478.71]*
- pneumonia 002.0 *[484.8]*
- spine 002.0 *[720.81]*
- ulcer (perforating) 002.0
- vaccination, prophylactic (against) V03.1
- Widal negative 002.0

Typhomalaria (fever) (*see also* Malaria) 084.6

Typhomania 002.0

Typhoperitonitis 002.0

Typhus (fever) 081.9
- abdominal, abdominalis 002.0
- African tick 082.1
- amarillic (*see also* Fever, Yellow) 060.9
- brain 081.9
- cerebral 081.9
- classical 080
- endemic (flea-borne) 081.0
- epidemic (louse-borne) 080
- exanthematic NEC 080
- exanthematicus SAI 080
  - brillii SAI 081.1
  - Mexicanus SAI 081.0
  - pediculo vestimenti causa 080
  - typhus murinus 081.0
- flea-borne 081.0
- Indian tick 082.1
- Kenya tick 082.1
- louse-borne 080
- Mexican 081.0
  - flea-borne 081.0
  - louse-borne 080
  - tabardillo 080
- mite-borne 081.2
- murine 081.0
- North Asian tick-borne 082.2
- petechial 081.9
- Queensland tick 082.3
- rat 081.0
- recrudescent 081.1
- recurrent (*see also* Fever, relapsing) 087.9
- S€o Paulo 082.0
- scrub (China) (India) (Malaya) (New Guinea) 081.2
- shop (of Malaya) 081.0
- Siberian tick 082.2
- tick-borne NEC 082.9
- tropical 081.2
- vaccination, prophylactic (against) V05.8

Tyrosinemia 270.2
- neonatal 775.89

Tyrosinosis (Medes) (Sakai) 270.2

Tyrosinuria 270.2

Tyrosyluria 270.2

Uehlinger's syndrome (acropachyderma) 757.39

Uhl's anomaly or disease (hypoplasia of myocardium, right ventricle) 746.84

Ulcer, ulcerated, ulcerating, ulceration, ulcerative 707.9
- with gangrene 707.9 *[785.4]*
- abdomen (wall) (*see also* Ulcer, skin) 707.8
- ala, nose 478.19
- alveolar process 526.5
- amebic (intestine) 006.9
  - skin 006.6

Ulcer, ulcerated, ulcerating, ulceration, ulcerative – *continued*
- anastomotic - *see* Ulcer, gastrojejunal
- anorectal 569.41
- antral - *see* Ulcer, stomach
- anus (sphincter) (solitary) 569.41
  - varicose - *see* Varicose, ulcer, anus
- aorta - *see* Aneurysm
- aphthous (oral) (recurrent) 528.2
  - genital organ(s)
    - female 616.50
    - male 608.89
  - mouth 528.2
- arm (*see also* Ulcer, skin) 707.8
- arteriosclerotic plaque - *see* Arteriosclerosis, by site
- artery NEC 447.2
  - without rupture 447.8
- atrophic NEC - *see* Ulcer, skin
- Barrett's (chronic peptic ulcer of esophagus) 530.85
- bile duct 576.8
- bladder (solitary) (sphincter) 596.8
  - bilharzial (*see also* Schistosomiasis) 120.9 *[595.4]*
  - submucosal (*see also* Cystitis) 595.1
  - tuberculous (*see also* Tuberculosis) 016.1 [5th]
- bleeding NEC - *see* Ulcer, peptic, with hemorrhage
- bone 730.9 [5th]
- bowel (*see also* Ulcer, intestine) 569.82
- breast 611.0
- bronchitis 491.8
- bronchus 519.19
- buccal (cavity) (traumatic) 528.9
- burn (acute) - *see* Ulcer, duodenum
- Buruli 031.1
- buttock (*see also* Ulcer, skin) 707.8
  - decubitus (*see also* Ulcer, pressure) 707.00
- cancerous (M8000/3) - *see* Neoplasm, by site, malignant
- cardia - *see* Ulcer, stomach
- cardio-esophageal (peptic) 530.20
  - with bleeding 530.21
- cecum (*see also* Ulcer, intestine) 569.82
- cervix (uteri) (trophic) 622.0
  - with mention of cervicitis 616.0
- chancroidal 099.0
- chest (wall) (*see also* Ulcer, skin) 707.8
- Chiclero 085.4
- chin (pyogenic) (*see also* Ulcer, skin) 707.8
- chronic (cause unknown) - *see also* Ulcer, skin
  - penis 607.89
- Cochin-China 085.1
- colitis - *see* Colitis, ulcerative
- colon (*see also* Ulcer, intestine) 569.82
- conjunctiva (acute) (postinfectional) 372.00
- cornea (infectional) 370.00
  - with perforation 370.06
  - annular 370.02
  - catarrhal 370.01
  - central 370.03
  - dendritic 054.42
  - marginal 370.01
  - mycotic 370.05
  - phlyctenular, tuberculous (*see also* Tuberculosis) 017.3 [5th] *[370.31]*
  - ring 370.02
  - rodent 370.07
  - serpent, serpiginous 370.04
  - superficial marginal 370.01
  - tuberculous (*see also* Tuberculosis) 017.3 [5th] *[370.31]*
- corpus cavernosum (chronic) 607.89
- crural - *see* Ulcer, lower extremity
- Curling's - *see* Ulcer, duodenum
- Cushing's - *see* Ulcer, peptic
- cystitis (interstitial) 595.1

Ulcer, ulcerated, ulcerating, ulceration, ulcerative – *continued*
- decubitus (unspecified site) (*see also* Ulcer, pressure) 707.00
  - with gangrene 707.00 *[785.4]*
  - ankle 707.06
  - back
    - lower 707.03
    - upper 707.02
  - buttock 707.05
  - coccyx 707.03 ●
  - elbow 707.01
  - head 707.09
  - heel 707.07
  - hip 707.04
  - other site 707.09
  - sacrum 707.03
  - shoulder blades 707.02
- dendritic 054.42
- diabetes, diabetic (mellitus) 250.8 [5th] *[707.9]*
  - due to secondary diabetes 249.8 [5th] *[707.9]*
  - lower limb 250.8 [5th] *[707.10]*
    - ankle 250.8 [5th] *[707.13]*
      - due to secondary diabetes 249.8 [5th] *[707.13]*
    - calf 250.8 [5th] *[707.12]*
      - due to secondary diabetes 249.8 [5th] *[707.12]*
    - due to secondary diabetes 249.8 [5th] *[707.10]*
    - foot 250.8 [5th] *[707.15]*
      - due to secondary diabetes 249.8 [5th] *[707.15]*
    - heel 250.8 [5th] *[707.14]*
      - due to secondary diabetes 249.8 [5th] *[707.14]*
    - knee 250.8 [5th] *[707.19]*
      - due to secondary diabetes 249.8 [5th] *[707.19]*
    - specified site NEC 250.8 [5th] *[707.19]*
      - due to secondary diabetes 249.8 [5th] *[707.19]*
    - thigh 250.8 [5th] *[707.11]*
      - due to secondary diabetes 249.8 [5th] *[707.11]*
    - toes 250.8 [5th] *[707.15]*
      - due to secondary diabetes 249.8 [5th] *[707.15]*
  - specified site NEC 250.8 [5th] *[707.8]*
    - due to secondary diabetes 249.8 [5th] *[707.8]*
- Dieulafoy - *see* Lesion, Dieulafoy
- due to
  - infection NEC - *see* Ulcer, skin
  - radiation, radium - *see* Ulcer, by site
  - trophic disturbance (any region) - *see* Ulcer, skin
  - x-ray - *see* Ulcer, by site
- duodenum, duodenal (eroded) (peptic) 532.9 [5th]

Note *Use the following fifth-digit subclassification with categories 531-534:*

0	without mention of obstruction
1	with obstruction

  - with
    - hemorrhage (chronic) 532.4 [5th]
      - and perforation 532.6 [5th]
    - perforation (chronic) 532.5 [5th]
      - and hemorrhage 532.6 [5th]
  - acute 532.3 [5th]
    - with
      - hemorrhage 532.0 [5th]
        - and perforation 532.2 [5th]
      - perforation 532.1 [5th]
        - and hemorrhage 532.2 [5th]
  - bleeding (recurrent) - *see* Ulcer, duodenum, with hemorrhage

Ulcer, ulcerated, ulcerating, ulceration, ulcerative – *continued*
- duodenum, duodenal – *continued*
  - chronic 532.7 [5th]
    - with
      - hemorrhage 532.4 [5th]
        - and perforation 532.6 [5th]
      - perforation 532.5 [5th]
        - and hemorrhage 532.6 [5th]
  - penetrating - *see* Ulcer, duodenum, with perforation
  - perforating - *see* Ulcer, duodenum, with perforation
- dysenteric NEC 009.0
- elusive 595.1
- endocarditis (any valve) (acute) (chronic) (subacute) 421.0
- enteritis - *see* Colitis, ulcerative
- enterocolitis 556.0
- epiglottis 478.79
- esophagus (peptic) 530.20
  - with bleeding 530.21
  - due to ingestion
    - aspirin 530.20
    - chemicals 530.20
    - medicinal agents 530.20
  - fungal 530.20
  - infectional 530.20
  - varicose (*see also* Varix, esophagus) 456.1
    - bleeding (*see also* Varix, esophagus, bleeding) 456.0
- eye NEC 360.00
  - dendritic 054.42
- eyelid (region) 373.01
- face (*see also* Ulcer, skin) 707.8
- fauces 478.29
- Fenwick (-Hunner) (solitary) (*see also* Cystitis) 595.1
- fistulous NEC - *see* Ulcer, skin
- foot (indolent) (*see also* Ulcer, lower extremity) 707.15
  - perforating 707.15
    - leprous 030.1
    - syphilitic 094.0
  - trophic 707.15
  - varicose 454.0
    - inflamed or infected 454.2
- frambesial, initial or primary 102.0
- gallbladder or duct 575.8
- gall duct 576.8
- gangrenous (*see also* Gangrene) 785.4
- gastric - *see* Ulcer, stomach
- gastrocolic - *see* Ulcer, gastrojejunal
- gastroduodenal - *see* Ulcer, peptic
- gastroesophageal - *see* Ulcer, stomach
- gastrohepatic - *see* Ulcer, stomach
- gastrointestinal - *see* Ulcer, gastrojejunal
- gastrojejunal (eroded) (peptic) 534.9 [5th]

Note *Use the following fifth-digit subclassification with categories 531-534:*

0	without mention of obstruction
1	with obstruction

  - with
    - hemorrhage (chronic) 534.4 [5th]
      - and perforation 534.6 [5th]
    - perforation 534.5 [5th]
      - and hemorrhage 534.6 [5th]
  - acute 534.3 [5th]
    - with
      - hemorrhage 534.0 [5th]
        - and perforation 534.2 [5th]
      - perforation 534.1 [5th]
        - and hemorrhage 534.2 [5th]
  - bleeding (recurrent) - *see* Ulcer, gastrojejunal, with hemorrhage
  - chronic 534.7 [5th]
    - with
      - hemorrhage 534.4 [5th]
        - and perforation 534.6 [5th]
      - perforation 534.5 [5th]
        - and hemorrhage 534.6 [5th]

Typhoid – Ulcer, ulcerated, ulcerating, ulceration, ulcerative

Ulcer, ulcerated, ulcerating, ulceration, ulcerative – *continued*
- gastrojejunal – *continued*
  - penetrating - *see* Ulcer, gastrojejunal, with perforation
  - perforating - *see* Ulcer, gastrojejunal, with perforation
- gastrojejunocolic - *see* Ulcer, gastrojejunal
- genital organ
  - female 629.89
  - male 608.89
- gingiva 523.8
- gingivitis 523.10
- glottis 478.79
- granuloma of pudenda 099.2
- groin (*see also* Ulcer, skin) 707.8
- gum 523.8
- gumma, due to yaws 102.4
- hand (*see also* Ulcer, skin) 707.8
- hard palate 528.9
- heel (*see also* Ulcer, lower extremity) 707.14
  - decubitus (*see also* Ulcer, pressure) 707.07
- hemorrhoids 455.8
  - external 455.5
  - internal 455.2
- hip (*see also* Ulcer, skin) 707.8
  - decubitus (*see also* Ulcer, pressure) 707.04
- Hunner's 595.1
- hypopharynx 478.29
- hypopyon (chronic) (subacute) 370.04
- hypostaticum - *see* Ulcer, varicose
- ileocolitis 556.1
- ileum (*see also* Ulcer, intestine) 569.82
- intestine, intestinal 569.82
  - with perforation 569.83
  - amebic 006.9
  - duodenal - *see* Ulcer, duodenum
  - granulocytopenic (with hemorrhage) 288.09
  - marginal 569.82
  - perforating 569.83
  - small, primary 569.82
  - stercoraceous 569.82
  - stercoral 569.82
  - tuberculous (*see also* Tuberculosis) 014.8 [5th]
  - typhoid (fever) 002.0
  - varicose 456.8
- ischemic 707.9
  - lower extremity (*see also* Ulcer, lower extremity) 707.10
    - ankle 707.13
    - calf 707.12
    - foot 707.15
    - heel 707.14
    - knee 707.19
    - specified site NEC 707.19
    - thigh 707.11
    - toes 707.15
- jejunum, jejunal - *see* Ulcer, gastrojejunal
- keratitis (*see also* Ulcer, cornea) 370.00
- knee - *see* Ulcer, lower extremity
- labium (majus) (minus) 616.50
- laryngitis (*see also* Laryngitis) 464.00
  - with obstruction 464.01
- larynx (aphthous) (contact) 478.79
  - diphtheritic 032.3
- leg - *see* Ulcer, lower extremity
- lip 528.5
- Lipschütz's 616.50
- lower extremity (atrophic) (chronic) (neurogenic) (perforating) (pyogenic) (trophic) (tropical) 707.10
  - with gangrene (*see also* Ulcer, lower extremity) 707.10 *[785.4]*
    - arteriosclerotic 440.24
  - ankle 707.13
  - arteriosclerotic 440.23
    - with gangrene 440.24
  - calf 707.12
  - decubitus (*see also* Ulcer, pressure) 707.00
    - with gangrene 707.00 *[785.4]*
    - ankle 707.06
    - buttock 707.05
    - heel 707.07
    - hip 707.04
  - foot 707.15
  - heel 707.14
  - knee 707.19
  - specified site NEC 707.19
  - thigh 707.11
  - toes 707.15
  - varicose 454.0
    - inflamed or infected 454.2
- luetic - *see* Ulcer, syphilitic
- lung 518.89
  - tuberculous (*see also* Tuberculosis) 011.2 [5th]
- malignant (M8000/3) - *see* Neoplasm, by site, malignant
- marginal NEC - *see* Ulcer, gastrojejunal
- meatus (urinarius) 597.89
- Meckel's diverticulum 751.0
- Meleney's (chronic undermining) 686.09
- Mooren's (cornea) 370.07
- mouth (traumatic) 528.9
- mycobacterial (skin) 031.1
- nasopharynx 478.29
- navel cord (newborn) 771.4
- neck (*see also* Ulcer, skin) 707.8
  - uterus 622.0
- neurogenic NEC - *see* Ulcer, skin
- nose, nasal (infectional) (passage) 478.19
  - septum 478.19
    - varicose 456.8
  - skin - *see* Ulcer, skin
  - spirochetal NEC 104.8
- oral mucosa (traumatic) 528.9
- palate (soft) 528.9
- penetrating NEC - *see* Ulcer, peptic, with perforation
- penis (chronic) 607.89
- peptic (site unspecified) 533.9 [5th]

Note *Use the following fifth-digit subclassification with categories 531-534:*

0	without mention of obstruction
1	with obstruction

  - with
    - hemorrhage 533.4 [5th]
      - and perforation 533.6 [5th]
    - perforation (chronic) 533.5 [5th]
      - and hemorrhage 533.6 [5th]
  - acute 533.3 [5th]
    - with
      - hemorrhage 533.0 [5th]
        - and perforation 533.2 [5th]
      - perforation 533.1 [5th]
        - and hemorrhage 533.2 [5th]
  - bleeding (recurrent) - *see* Ulcer, peptic, with hemorrhage
  - chronic 533.7 [5th]
    - with
      - hemorrhage 533.4 [5th]
        - and perforation 533.6 [5th]
      - perforation 533.5 [5th]
        - and hemorrhage 533.6 [5th]
  - penetrating - *see* Ulcer, peptic, with perforation
- perforating NEC (*see also* Ulcer, peptic, with perforation) 533.5 [5th]
  - skin 707.9
- perineum (*see also* Ulcer, skin) 707.8
- peritonsillar 474.8
- phagedenic (tropical) NEC - *see* Ulcer, skin
- pharynx 478.29
- phlebitis - *see* Phlebitis
- plaster (*see also* Ulcer, pressure) 707.00
- popliteal space - *see* Ulcer, lower extremity
- postpyloric - *see* Ulcer, duodenum
- prepuce 607.89
- prepyloric - *see* Ulcer, stomach
- pressure 707.00
  - with
    - abrasion, blister, partial thickness skin loss involving epidermis and/or dermis 707.22
    - full thickness skin loss involving damage or necrosis of subcutaneous tissue 707.23
    - gangrene 707.00 *[785.4]*
    - necrosis of soft tissues through to underlying muscle, tendon, or bone 707.24
  - ankle 707.06
  - back
    - lower 707.03
    - upper 707.02
  - buttock 707.05
  - coccyx 707.03 ●
  - elbow 707.01
  - head 707.09
  - healed - omit code
  - healing - code to Ulcer, pressure, by stage
  - heel 707.07
  - hip 707.04
  - other site 707.09
  - sacrum 707.03
  - shoulder blades 707.02
  - stage
    - I (healing) 707.21
    - II (healing) 707.22
    - III (healing) 707.23
    - IV (healing) 707.24
    - unspecified (healing) 707.20
  - unstageable 707.25
- primary of intestine 569.82
  - with perforation 569.83
- proctitis 556.2
  - with ulcerative sigmoiditis 556.3
- prostate 601.8
- pseudopeptic - *see* Ulcer, peptic
- pyloric - *see* Ulcer, stomach
- rectosigmoid 569.82
  - with perforation 569.83
- rectum (sphincter) (solitary) 569.41
  - stercoraceous, stercoral 569.41
  - varicose - *see* Varicose, ulcer, anus
- retina (*see also* Chorioretinitis) 363.20
- rodent (M8090/3) - *see also* Neoplasm, skin, malignant
  - cornea 370.07
- round - *see* Ulcer, stomach
- sacrum (region) (*see also* Ulcer, skin) 707.8
- Saemisch's 370.04
- scalp (*see also* Ulcer, skin) 707.8
- sclera 379.09
- scrofulous (*see also* Tuberculosis) 017.2 [5th]
- scrotum 608.89
  - tuberculous (*see also* Tuberculosis) 016.5 [5th]
  - varicose 456.4
- seminal vesicle 608.89
- sigmoid 569.82
  - with perforation 569.83
- skin (atrophic) (chronic) (neurogenic) (non-healing) (perforating) (pyogenic) (trophic) 707.9
  - with gangrene 707.9 *[785.4]*
  - amebic 006.6
  - decubitus (*see also* Ulcer, pressure) 707.00
    - with gangrene 707.00 *[785.4]*
  - in granulocytopenia 288.09
  - lower extremity (*see also* Ulcer, lower extremity) 707.10
    - with gangrene 707.10 *[785.4]*
      - arteriosclerotic 440.24
    - ankle 707.13
    - arteriosclerotic 440.23
      - with gangrene 440.24
    - calf 707.12
    - foot 707.15
    - heel 707.14
    - knee 707.19
    - specified site NEC 707.19
    - thigh 707.11
    - toes 707.15
  - mycobacterial 031.1
  - syphilitic (early) (secondary) 091.3
  - tuberculous (primary) (*see also* Tuberculosis) 017.0 [5th]
  - varicose - *see* Ulcer, varicose
- sloughing NEC - *see* Ulcer, skin
- soft palate 528.9
- solitary, anus or rectum (sphincter) 569.41
- sore throat 462
  - streptococcal 034.0
- spermatic cord 608.89
- spine (tuberculous) 015.0 [5th] *[730.88]*
- stasis (leg) (venous) 454.0
  - with varicose veins 454.0
  - without varicose veins 459.81
  - inflamed or infected 454.2
- stercoral, stercoraceous 569.82
  - with perforation 569.83
  - anus or rectum 569.41
- stoma, stomal - *see* Ulcer, gastrojejunal
- stomach (eroded) (peptic) (round) 531.9 [5th]

Note *Use the following fifth-digit subclassification with categories 531-534:*

0	without mention of obstruction
1	with obstruction

  - with
    - hemorrhage 531.4 [5th]
      - and perforation 531.6 [5th]
    - perforation (chronic) 531.5 [5th]
      - and hemorrhage 531.6 [5th]
  - acute 531.3 [5th]
    - with
      - hemorrhage 531.0 [5th]
        - and perforation 531.2 [5th]
      - perforation 531.1 [5th]
        - and hemorrhage 531.2 [5th]
  - bleeding (recurrent) - *see* Ulcer, stomach, with hemorrhage
  - chronic 531.7 [5th]
    - with
      - hemorrhage 531.4 [5th]
        - and perforation 531.6 [5th]
      - perforation 531.5 [5th]
        - and hemorrhage 531.6 [5th]
  - penetrating - *see* Ulcer, stomach, with perforation
  - perforating - *see* Ulcer, stomach, with perforation
- stomatitis 528.00
- stress - *see* Ulcer, peptic
- strumous (tuberculous) (*see also* Tuberculosis) 017.2 [5th]
- submental (*see also* Ulcer, skin) 707.8
- submucosal, bladder 595.1
- syphilitic (any site) (early) (secondary) 091.3
  - late 095.9
  - perforating 095.9
    - foot 094.0
- testis 608.89
- thigh - *see* Ulcer, lower extremity
- throat 478.29
  - diphtheritic 032.0
- toe - *see* Ulcer, lower extremity
- tongue (traumatic) 529.0
- tonsil 474.8
  - diphtheritic 032.0
- trachea 519.19

Ulcer, ulcerated, ulcerating, ulceration, ulcerative – *continued*
trophic - *see* Ulcer, skin
tropical NEC (*see also* Ulcer, skin) 707.9
tuberculous - *see* Tuberculosis, ulcer
tunica vaginalis 608.89
turbinate 730.9 5th
typhoid (fever) 002.0
perforating 002.0
umbilicus (newborn) 771.4
unspecified site NEC - *see* Ulcer, skin
urethra (meatus) (*see also* Urethritis) 597.89
uterus 621.8
cervix 622.0
with mention of cervicitis 616.0
neck 622.0
with mention of cervicitis 616.0
vagina 616.89
valve, heart 421.0
varicose (lower extremity, any part) 454.0
anus - *see* Varicose, ulcer, anus
broad ligament 456.5
varicose (lower extremity, any part) – *continued*
esophagus (*see also* Varix, esophagus) 456.1
bleeding (*see also* Varix, esophagus, bleeding) 456.0
inflamed or infected 454.2
nasal septum 456.8
perineum 456.6
rectum - *see* Varicose, ulcer, anus
scrotum 456.4
specified site NEC 456.8
sublingual 456.3
vulva 456.6
vas deferens 608.89
vesical (*see also* Ulcer, bladder) 596.8
vulva (acute) (infectional) 616.50
Behçet's syndrome 136.1 *[616.51]*
herpetic 054.12
tuberculous 016.7 5th *[616.51]*
vulvobuccal, recurring 616.50
x-ray - *see* Ulcer, by site
yaws 102.4
Ulcerosa scarlatina 034.1
Ulcus - *see also* Ulcer
cutis tuberculosum (*see also* Tuberculosis) 017.0 5th
duodeni - *see* Ulcer, duodenum
durum 091.0
extragenital 091.2
gastrojejunale - *see* Ulcer, gastrojejunal
hypostaticum - *see* Ulcer, varicose
molle (cutis) (skin) 099.0
serpens corneae (pneumococcal) 370.04
ventriculi - *see* Ulcer, stomach
Ulegyria 742.4
Ulerythema
acneiforma 701.8
centrifugum 695.4
ophryogenes 757.4
Ullrich (-Bonnevie) (-Turner) syndrome 758.6
Ullrich-Feichtiger syndrome 759.89
Ulnar - *see* condition
Ulorrhagia 523.8
Ulorrhea 523.8
Umbilicus, umbilical - *see also* condition
cord necrosis, affecting fetus or newborn 762.6
Unacceptable
existing dental restoration
contours 525.65
morphology 525.65
Unavailability of medical facilities (at) V63.9
due to
investigation by social service agency V63.8
lack of services at home V63.1
remoteness from facility V63.0
waiting list V63.2
Unavailability of medical facilities (at) – *continued*
home V63.1
outpatient clinic V63.0
specified reason NEC V63.8
Uncinaria americana infestation 126.1
Uncinariasis (*see also* Ancylostomiasis) 126.9
Unconscious, unconsciousness 780.09
Underdevelopment - *see also* Undeveloped
sexual 259.0
Underfill, endodontic 526.63
Undernourishment 269.9
Undernutrition 269.9
Under observation - *see* Observation
Underweight 783.22
for gestational age - *see* Light-for-dates
Underwood's disease (sclerema neonatorum) 778.1
Undescended - *see also* Malposition, congenital
cecum 751.4
colon 751.4
testis 752.51
Undetermined diagnosis or cause 799.9
Undeveloped, undevelopment - *see also* Hypoplasia
brain (congenital) 742.1
cerebral (congenital) 742.1
fetus or newborn 764.9 5th
heart 746.89
lung 748.5
testis 257.2
uterus 259.0
Undiagnosed (disease) 799.9
Undulant fever (*see also* Brucellosis) 023.9
Unemployment, anxiety concerning V62.0
Unequal leg (acquired) (length) 736.81
congenital 755.30
Unerupted teeth, tooth 520.6
Unextracted dental root 525.3
Unguis incarnatus 703.0
Unicornis uterus 752.3
Unicorporeus uterus 752.3
Uniformis uterus 752.3
Unilateral - *see also* condition
development, breast 611.89
organ or site, congenital NEC - *see* Agenesis
vagina 752.49
Unilateralis uterus 752.3
Unilocular heart 745.8
Uninhibited bladder 596.54
with cauda equina syndrome 344.61
neurogenic (*see also* Neurogenic, bladder) 596.54
Union, abnormal - *see also* Fusion
divided tendon 727.89
larynx and trachea 748.3
Universal
joint, cervix 620.6
mesentery 751.4
Unknown
cause of death 799.9
diagnosis 799.9
Unna's disease (seborrheic dermatitis) 690.10
Unresponsiveness, adrenocorticotropin (ACTH) 255.41
Unsatisfactory
restoration, tooth (existing) 525.60
specified NEC 525.69
cytology smear
anal 796.78
cervical 795.08
vaginal 795.18
Unsoundness of mind (*see also* Psychosis) 298.9
Unspecified cause of death 799.9
Unstable
back NEC 724.9
colon 569.89
joint - *see* Instability, joint
Unstable – *continued*
lie 652.0 5th
affecting fetus or newborn (before labor) 761.7
causing obstructed labor 660.0 5th
affecting fetus or newborn 763.1
lumbosacral joint (congenital) 756.19
acquired 724.6
sacroiliac 724.6
spine NEC 724.9
Untruthfulness, child problem (*see also* Disturbance, conduct) 312.0 5th
Unverricht (-Lundborg) disease, syndrome, or epilepsy 345.1 ▲
Unverricht-Wagner syndrome (dermatomyositis) 710.3
Upper respiratory - *see* condition
Upset
gastric 536.8
psychogenic 306.4
gastrointestinal 536.8
psychogenic 306.4
virus (*see also* Enteritis, viral) 008.8
intestinal (large) (small) 564.9
psychogenic 306.4
menstruation 626.9
Upset – *continued*
mental 300.9
stomach 536.8
psychogenic 306.4
Urachus - *see also* condition
patent 753.7
persistent 753.7
Uratic arthritis 274.00 ▲
Urbach's lipoid proteinosis 272.8
Urbach-Oppenheim disease or syndrome (necrobiosis lipoidica diabeticorum) 250.8 5th *[709.3]*
due to secondary diabetes 249.8 5th *[709.3]*
Urbach-Wiethe disease or syndrome (lipoid proteinosis) 272.8
Urban yellow fever 060.1
Urea, blood, high - *see* Uremia
Uremia, uremic (absorption) (amaurosis) (amblyopia) (aphasia) (apoplexy) (coma) (delirium) (dementia) (dropsy) (dyspnea) (fever) (intoxication) (mania) (paralysis) (poisoning) (toxemia) (vomiting) 586
with
abortion - *see* Abortion, by type, with renal failure
ectopic pregnancy (*see also* categories 633.0-633.9) 639.3
hypertension (*see also* Hypertension, kidney) 403.91
molar pregnancy (*see also* categories 630-632) 639.3
chronic 585.9
complicating
abortion 639.3
ectopic or molar pregnancy 639.3
hypertension (*see also* Hypertension, kidney) 403.91
labor and delivery 669.3 5th
congenital 779.89
extrarenal 788.99
hypertensive (chronic) (*see also* Hypertension, kidney) 403.91
maternal NEC, affecting fetus or newborn 760.1
neuropathy 585.9 *[357.4]*
pericarditis 585.9 *[420.0]*
prerenal 788.99
pyelitic (*see also* Pyelitis) 590.80
Ureter, ureteral - *see* condition
Ureteralgia 788.0
Ureterectasis 593.89
Ureteritis 593.89
cystica 590.3
due to calculus 592.1
Ureteritis – *continued*
gonococcal (acute) 098.19
chronic or duration of 2 months or over 098.39
nonspecific 593.89
Ureterocele (acquired) 593.89
congenital 753.23
Ureterolith 592.1
Ureterolithiasis 592.1
Ureterostomy status V44.6
with complication 997.5
Urethra, urethral - *see* condition
Urethralgia 788.99
Urethritis (abacterial) (acute) (allergic) (anterior) (chronic) (nonvenereal) (posterior) (recurrent) (simple) (subacute) (ulcerative) (undifferentiated) 597.80
diplococcal (acute) 098.0
chronic or duration of 2 months or over 098.2
due to Trichomonas (vaginalis) 131.02
gonococcal (acute) 098.0
chronic or duration of 2 months or over 098.2
nongonococcal (sexually transmitted) 099.40
Chlamydia trachomatis 099.41
Reiter's 099.3
specified organism NEC 099.49
nonspecific (sexually transmitted) (*see also* Urethritis, nongonococcal) 099.40
not sexually transmitted 597.80
Reiter's 099.3
trichomonal or due to Trichomonas (vaginalis) 131.02
tuberculous (*see also* Tuberculosis) 016.3 5th
venereal NEC (*see also* Urethritis, nongonococcal) 099.40
Urethrocele
female 618.03
with uterine prolapse 618.4
complete 618.3
incomplete 618.2
male 599.5
Urethrolithiasis 594.2
Urethro-oculoarticular syndrome 099.3
Urethro-oculosynovial syndrome 099.3
Urethrorectal - *see* condition
Urethrorrhagia 599.84
Urethrorrhea 788.7
Urethrostomy status V44.6
with complication 997.5
Urethrotrigonitis 595.3
Urethrovaginal - *see* condition
Urhidrosis, uridrosis 705.89
Uric acid
diathesis 274.9
in blood 790.6
Uricacidemia 790.6
Uricemia 790.6
Uricosuria 791.9
Urination
frequent 788.41
painful 788.1
urgency 788.63
Urine, urinary - *see also* condition
abnormality NEC 788.69
blood in (*see also* Hematuria) 599.70
discharge, excessive 788.42
enuresis 788.30
nonorganic origin 307.6
extravasation 788.8
frequency 788.41
hesitancy 788.64
incontinence 788.30
active 788.30
female 788.30
stress 625.6
and urge 788.33

Urine, urinary – *continued*
- incontinence – *continued*
  - male 788.30
    - stress 788.32
      - and urge 788.33
    - mixed (stress and urge) 788.33
    - neurogenic 788.39
    - nonorganic origin 307.6
    - overflow 788.38
    - stress (female) 625.6
      - male NEC 788.32
- intermittent stream 788.61
- pus in 791.9
- retention or stasis NEC 788.20
  - bladder, incomplete emptying 788.21
  - psychogenic 306.53
  - specified NEC 788.29
- secretion
  - deficient 788.5
  - excessive 788.42
  - frequency 788.41
- strain 788.65
- stream
  - intermittent 788.61
  - slowing 788.62
  - splitting 788.61
  - weak 788.62
- urgency 788.63

Urinemia - *see* Uremia

Urinoma NEC 599.9
- bladder 596.8
- kidney 593.89
- renal 593.89
- ureter 593.89
- urethra 599.84

Uroarthritis, infectious 099.3

Urodialysis 788.5

Urolithiasis 592.9

Uronephrosis 593.89

Uropathy 599.9
- obstructive 599.60

Urosepsis 599.0
- meaning sepsis 995.91
- meaning urinary tract infection 599.0

Urticaria 708.9
- with angioneurotic edema 995.1
  - hereditary 277.6
- allergic 708.0
- cholinergic 708.5
- chronic 708.8
- cold, familial 708.2
- dermatographic 708.3
- due to
  - cold or heat 708.2
  - drugs 708.0
  - food 708.0
  - inhalants 708.0
  - plants 708.8
  - serum 999.5
- factitial 708.3
- giant 995.1
  - hereditary 277.6
- gigantea 995.1
  - hereditary 277.6
- idiopathic 708.1
- larynx 995.1
  - hereditary 277.6
- neonatorum 778.8
- nonallergic 708.1
- papulosa (Hebra) 698.2
- perstans hemorrhagica 757.39
- pigmentosa 757.33
- recurrent periodic 708.8
- serum 999.5
- solare 692.72
- specified type NEC 708.8
- thermal (cold) (heat) 708.2
- vibratory 708.4

Urticarioides acarodermatitis 133.9

Use of
- methadone 304.00
- nonprescribed drugs (*see also* Abuse, drugs, nondependent) 305.9 5th
- patent medicines (*see also* Abuse, drugs, nondependent) 305.9 5th

Usher-Senear disease (pemphigus erythematosus) 694.4

Uta 085.5

Uterine size-date discrepancy 649.6 5th

Uteromegaly 621.2

Uterovaginal - *see* condition

Uterovesical - *see* condition

Uterus - *see* condition

Utriculitis (utriculus prostaticus) 597.89

Uveal - *see* condition

Uveitis (anterior) (*see also* Iridocyclitis) 364.3
- acute or subacute 364.00
  - due to or associated with
    - gonococcal infection 098.41
    - herpes (simplex) 054.44
    - zoster 053.22
  - primary 364.01
  - recurrent 364.02
  - secondary (noninfectious) 364.04
    - infectious 364.03
- allergic 360.11
- chronic 364.10
  - due to or associated with
    - sarcoidosis 135 *[364.11]*
    - tuberculosis (*see also* Tuberculosis) 017.3 5th *[364.11]*
- due to
  - operation 360.11
  - toxoplasmosis (acquired) 130.2
    - congenital (active) 771.2
- granulomatous 364.10
- heterochromic 364.21
- lens-induced 364.23
- nongranulomatous 364.00
- posterior 363.20
  - disseminated - *see* Chorioretinitis, disseminated
  - focal - *see* Chorioretinitis, focal
- recurrent 364.02
- sympathetic 360.11
- syphilitic (secondary) 091.50
  - congenital 090.0 *[363.13]*
  - late 095.8 *[363.13]*
- tuberculous (*see also* Tuberculosis) 017.3 5th *[364.11]*

Uveoencephalitis 363.22

Uveokeratitis (*see also* Iridocyclitis) 364.3

Uveoparotid fever 135

Uveoparotitis 135

Uvula - *see* condition

Uvulitis (acute) (catarrhal) (chronic) (gangrenous) (membranous) (suppurative) (ulcerative) 528.3

V

Vaccination
- complication or reaction - *see* Complications, vaccination
- delayed V64.00
- not carried out V64.00
  - because of
    - acute illness V64.01
    - allergy to vaccine or component V64.04
    - caregiver refusal V64.05
    - chronic illness V64.02
    - guardian refusal V64.05
    - immune compromised state V64.03
    - parent refusal V64.05
    - patient had disease being vaccinated against V64.08
    - patient refusal V64.06
    - reason NEC V64.09
    - religious reasons V64.07
- prophylactic (against) V05.9
  - arthropod-borne viral
    - disease NEC V05.1
    - encephalitis V05.0
  - chicken pox V05.4
  - cholera (alone) V03.0
    - with typhoid-paratyphoid (cholera + TAB) V06.0
  - common cold V04.7
  - diphtheria (alone) V03.5
    - with
      - poliomyelitis (DTP + polio) V06.3
      - tetanus V06.5
        - pertussis combined [DTP] (DTaP) V06.1
      - typhoid-paratyphoid (DTP + TAB) V06.2
  - disease (single) NEC V05.9
    - bacterial NEC V03.9
      - specified type NEC V03.89
    - combination NEC V06.9
      - specified type NEC V06.8
    - specified type NEC V05.8
  - encephalitis, viral, arthropod-borne V05.0
  - Hemophilus influenzae, type B [Hib] V03.81
  - hepatitis, viral V05.3
  - influenza V04.81
    - with
      - Streptococcus pneumoniae [pneumococcus] V06.6
  - leishmaniasis V05.2
  - measles (alone) V04.2
    - with mumps-rubella (MMR) V06.4
  - mumps (alone) V04.6
    - with measles and rubella (MMR) V06.4
  - pertussis alone V03.6
  - plague V03.3
  - poliomyelitis V04.0
    - with diphtheria-tetanus-pertussis (DTP polio) V06.3
  - rabies V04.5
  - respiratory syncytial virus (RSV) V04.82
  - rubella (alone) V04.3
    - with measles and mumps (MMR) V06.4
  - smallpox V04.1
  - Streptococcus pneumoniae [pneumococcus] V03.82
    - with
      - influenza V06.6
  - tetanus toxoid (alone) V03.7
    - with diphtheria [Td] [DT] V06.5
      - with
        - pertussis (DTP) (DTaP) V06.1
          - with poliomyelitis (DTP + polio) V06.3
  - tuberculosis (BCG) V03.2
  - tularemia V03.4
  - typhoid-paratyphoid (TAB) (alone) V03.1
    - with diphtheria-tetanus-pertussis (TAB + DTP) V06.2
  - varicella V05.4
  - viral
    - disease NEC V04.89
    - encephalitis, arthropod-borne V05.0
    - hepatitis V05.3
  - yellow fever V04.4

Vaccinia (generalized) 999.0
- congenital 771.2
- conjunctiva 999.39
- eyelids 999.0 *[373.5]*
- localized 999.39
- nose 999.39
- not from vaccination 051.02
  - eyelid 051.02 *[373.5]*
- sine vaccinatione 051.02
- without vaccination 051.02

Vacuum
- extraction of fetus or newborn 763.3
- in sinus (accessory) (nasal) (*see also* Sinusitis) 473.9

Vagabond V60.0

Vagabondage V60.0

Vagabonds' disease 132.1

Vagina, vaginal - *see also* condition
- high risk human papillomavirus (HPV) DNA test positive 795.15
- low risk human papillomavirus (HPV) DNA test positive 795.19

Vaginalitis (tunica) 608.4

Vaginismus (reflex) 625.1
- functional 306.51
- hysterical 300.11
- psychogenic 306.51

Vaginitis (acute) (chronic) (circumscribed) (diffuse) (emphysematous) (Hemophilus vaginalis) (nonspecific) (nonvenereal) (ulcerative) 616.10
- with
  - abortion - *see* Abortion, by type, with sepsis
  - ectopic pregnancy (*see also* categories 633.0-633.9) 639.0
  - molar pregnancy (*see also* categories 630-632) 639.0
- adhesive, congenital 752.49
- atrophic, postmenopausal 627.3
- bacterial 616.10
- blennorrhagic (acute) 098.0
  - chronic or duration of 2 months or over 098.2
- candidal 112.1
- chlamydial 099.53
- complicating pregnancy or puerperium 646.6 5th
  - affecting fetus or newborn 760.8
- congenital (adhesive) 752.49
- due to
  - C. albicans 112.1
  - Trichomonas (vaginalis) 131.01
- following
  - abortion 639.0
  - ectopic or molar pregnancy 639.0
- gonococcal (acute) 098.0
  - chronic or duration of 2 months or over 098.2
- granuloma 099.2
- Monilia 112.1
- mycotic 112.1
- pinworm 127.4 *[616.11]*
- postirradiation 616.10
- postmenopausal atrophic 627.3
- senile (atrophic) 627.3
- syphilitic (early) 091.0
  - late 095.8
- trichomonal 131.01
- tuberculous (*see also* Tuberculosis) 016.7 5th
- venereal NEC 099.8

Vaginosis - *see* Vaginitis

Vagotonia 352.3

Vagrancy V60.0

VAIN I (vaginal intraepithelial neoplasia I) 623.0

VAIN II (vaginal intraepithelial neoplasia II) 623.0

VAIN III (vaginal intraepithelial neoplasia III) 233.31

Vallecula - *see* condition

Valley fever 114.0

Valsuani's disease (progressive pernicious anemia, puerperal) 648.2 5th

Valve, valvular (formation) - *see also* condition
- cerebral ventricle (communicating) in situ V45.2
- cervix, internal os 752.49
- colon 751.5
- congenital NEC - *see* Atresia
- formation congenital NEC - *see* Atresia
- heart defect - *see* Anomaly, heart, valve

Urine, urinary – Valve, valvular

Valve, valvular – *continued*
  ureter 753.29
    pelvic junction 753.21
    vesical orifice 753.22
  urethra 753.6
Valvulitis (chronic) (*see also* Endocarditis) 424.90
  rheumatic (chronic) (inactive) (with chorea) 397.9
    active or acute (aortic) (mitral) (pulmonary) (tricuspid) 391.1
  syphilitic NEC 093.20
    aortic 093.22
    mitral 093.21
    pulmonary 093.24
    tricuspid 093.23
Valvulopathy - *see* Endocarditis
van Bogaert's leukoencephalitis (sclerosing) (subacute) 046.2
van Bogaert-Nijssen (-Peiffer) disease 330.0
van Buchem's syndrome (hyperostosis corticalis) 733.3
van Creveld-von Gierke disease (glycogenosis I) 271.0
van den Bergh's disease (enterogenous cyanosis) 289.7
van der Hoeve's syndrome (brittle bones and blue sclera, deafness) 756.51
van der Hoeve-Halbertsma-Waardenburg syndrome (ptosis-epicanthus) 270.2
van der Hoeve-Waardenburg-Gualdi syndrome (ptosis-epicanthus) 270.2
Vancomycin (glycopeptide)
  intermediate staphylococcus aureus (VISA/GISA) V09.8 [5th]
  resistant
    enterococcus (VRE) V09.8 [5th]
    staphylococcus aureus (VRSA/GRSA) V09.8 [5th]
Vanillism 692.89
Vanishing lung 492.0
Vanishing twin 651.33
van Neck (-Odelberg) disease or syndrome (juvenile osteochondrosis) 732.1
Vapor asphyxia or suffocation NEC 987.9
  specified agent - *see* Table of Drugs and Chemicals
Vaquez's disease (M9950/1) 238.4
Vaquez-Osler disease (polycythemia vera) (M9950/1) 238.4
Variance, lethal ball, prosthetic heart valve 996.02
Variants, thalassemic 282.49
Variations in hair color 704.3
Varicella 052.9
  with
    complication 052.8
      specified NEC 052.7
    pneumonia 052.1
  exposure to V01.71
  vaccination and inoculation (against) (prophylactic) V05.4
Varices - *see* Varix
Varicocele (scrotum) (thrombosed) 456.4
  ovary 456.5
  perineum 456.6
  spermatic cord (ulcerated) 456.4
Varicose
  aneurysm (ruptured) (*see also* Aneurysm) 442.9
  dermatitis (lower extremity) - *see* Varicose, vein, inflamed or infected
  eczema - *see* Varicose, vein
  phlebitis - *see* Varicose, vein, inflamed or infected
  placental vessel - *see* Placenta, abnormal
  tumor - *see* Varicose, vein
  ulcer (lower extremity, any part) 454.0
    anus 455.8
      external 455.5
      internal 455.2

Varicose – *continued*
  ulcer – *continued*
    esophagus (*see also* Varix, esophagus) 456.1
      bleeding (*see also* Varix, esophagus, bleeding) 456.0
    inflamed or infected 454.2
    nasal septum 456.8
    perineum 456.6
    rectum - *see* Varicose, ulcer, anus
    scrotum 456.4
    specified site NEC 456.8
  vein (lower extremity) (ruptured) (*see also* Varix) 454.9
    with
      complications NEC 454.8
      edema 454.8
      inflammation or infection 454.1
        ulcerated 454.2
      pain 454.8
      stasis dermatitis 454.1
        with ulcer 454.2
      swelling 454.8
      ulcer 454.0
        inflamed or infected 454.2
    anus - *see* Hemorrhoids
    broad ligament 456.5
    congenital (peripheral) 747.60
      gastrointestinal 747.61
      lower limb 747.64
      renal 747.62
      specified NEC 747.69
      upper limb 747.63
    esophagus (ulcerated (*see also* Varix, esophagus) 456.1
      bleeding (*see also* Varix, esophagus, bleeding) 456.0
    inflamed or infected 454.1
      with ulcer 454.2
    in pregnancy or puerperium 671.0 [5th]
      vulva or perineum 671.1 [5th]
    nasal septum (with ulcer) 456.8
    pelvis 456.5
    perineum 456.6
      in pregnancy, childbirth, or puerperium 671.1 [5th]
    rectum - *see* Hemorrhoids
    scrotum (ulcerated) 456.4
    specified site NEC 456.8
    sublingual 456.3
    ulcerated 454.0
      inflamed or infected 454.2
    umbilical cord, affecting fetus or newborn 762.6
    urethra 456.8
    vulva 456.6
      in pregnancy, childbirth, or puerperium 671.1 [5th]
  vessel - *see also* Varix
    placenta - *see* Placenta, abnormal
Varicosis, varicosities, varicosity (*see also* Varix) 454.9
Variola 050.9
  hemorrhagic (pustular) 050.0
  major 050.0
  minor 050.1
  modified 050.2
Varioloid 050.2
Variolosa, purpura 050.0
Varix (lower extremity) (ruptured) 454.9
  with
    complications NEC 454.8
    edema 454.8
    inflammation or infection 454.1
      with ulcer 454.2
    pain 454.8
    stasis dermatitis 454.1
      with ulcer 454.2
    swelling 454.8
    ulcer 454.0
      with inflammation or infection 454.2
  aneurysmal (*see also* Aneurysm) 442.9
  anus - *see* Hemorrhoids

Varix – *continued*
  arteriovenous (congenital) (peripheral) NEC 747.60
    gastrointestinal 747.61
    lower limb 747.64
    renal 747.62
    specified NEC 747.69
    spinal 747.82
    upper limb 747.63
  bladder 456.5
  broad ligament 456.5
  congenital (peripheral) 747.60
  esophagus (ulcerated) 456.1
    bleeding 456.0
      in
        cirrhosis of liver 571.5 *[456.20]*
        portal hypertension 572.3 *[456.20]*
    congenital 747.69
    in
      cirrhosis of liver 571.5 *[456.21]*
        with bleeding 571.5 *[456.20]*
      portal hypertension 572.3 *[456.21]*
        with bleeding 572.3 *[456.20]*
  gastric 456.8
  inflamed or infected 454.1
    ulcerated 454.2
  in pregnancy or puerperium 671.0 [5th]
    perineum 671.1 [5th]
    vulva 671.1 [5th]
  labia (majora) 456.6
  orbit 456.8
    congenital 747.69
  ovary 456.5
  papillary 448.1
  pelvis 456.5
  perineum 456.6
    in pregnancy or puerperium 671.1 [5th]
  pharynx 456.8
  placenta - *see* Placenta, abnormal
  prostate 456.8
  rectum - *see* Hemorrhoids
  renal papilla 456.8
  retina 362.17
  scrotum (ulcerated) 456.4
  sigmoid colon 456.8
  specified site NEC 456.8
  spinal (cord) (vessels) 456.8
  spleen, splenic (vein) (with phlebolith) 456.8
  sublingual 456.3
  ulcerated 454.0
    inflamed or infected 454.2
  umbilical cord, affecting fetus or newborn 762.6
  uterine ligament 456.5
  vocal cord 456.8
  vulva 456.6
    in pregnancy, childbirth, or puerperium 671.1 [5th]
Vasa previa 663.5 [5th]
  affecting fetus or newborn 762.6
  hemorrhage from, affecting fetus or newborn 772.0
Vascular - *see also* condition
  loop on papilla (optic) 743.57
  sheathing, retina 362.13
  spasm 443.9
  spider 448.1
Vascularity, pulmonary, congenital 747.3
Vascularization
  choroid 362.16
  cornea 370.60
    deep 370.63
    localized 370.61
  retina 362.16
  subretinal 362.16
Vasculitis 447.6
  allergic 287.0
  cryoglobulinemic 273.2
  disseminated 447.6
  kidney 447.8
  leukocytoclastic 446.29
  nodular 695.2

Vasculitis – *continued*
  retinal 362.18
  rheumatic - *see* Fever, rheumatic
Vasculopathy
  cardiac allograft 996.83
Vas deferens - *see* condition
Vas deferentitis 608.4
Vasectomy, admission for V25.2
Vasitis 608.4
  nodosa 608.4
  scrotum 608.4
  spermatic cord 608.4
  testis 608.4
  tuberculous (*see also* Tuberculosis) 016.5 [5th]
  tunica vaginalis 608.4
  vas deferens 608.4
Vasodilation 443.9
Vasomotor - *see* condition
Vasoplasty, after previous sterilization V26.0
Vasoplegia, splanchnic (*see also* Neuropathy, peripheral, autonomic) 337.9
Vasospasm 443.9
  cerebral (artery) 435.9
    with transient neurologic deficit 435.9
  coronary 413.1
  nerve
    arm NEC 354.9
    autonomic 337.9
    brachial plexus 353.0
    cervical plexus 353.2
    leg NEC 355.8
    lower extremity NEC 355.8
    peripheral NEC 335.9
    spinal NEC 355.9
    sympathetic 337.9
    upper extremity NEC 354.9
  peripheral NEC 443.9
  retina (artery) (*see also* Occlusion, retinal, artery) 362.30
Vasospastic - *see* condition
Vasovagal attack (paroxysmal) 780.2
  psychogenic 306.2
Vater's ampulla - *see* condition
VATER syndrome 759.89
vCJD (variant Creutzfeldt-Jakob disease) 046.11
Vegetation, vegetative
  adenoid (nasal fossa) 474.2
  consciousness (persistent) 780.03
  endocarditis (acute) (any valve) (chronic) (subacute) 421.0
  heart (mycotic) (valve) 421.0
  state (persistent) 780.03
Veil
  Jackson's 751.4
  over face (causing asphyxia) 768.9
Vein, venous - *see* condition
Veldt sore (*see also* Ulcer, skin) 707.9
Velo-cardio-facial syndrome 758.32
Velpeau's hernia - *see* Hernia, femoral
Venereal
  balanitis NEC 099.8
  bubo 099.1
  disease 099.9
    specified nature or type NEC 099.8
  granuloma inguinale 099.2
  lymphogranuloma (Durand-Nicolas-Favre), any site 099.1
  salpingitis 098.37
  urethritis (*see also* Urethritis, nongonococcal) 099.40
  vaginitis NEC 099.8
  warts 078.11
Vengefulness, in child (*see also* Disturbance, conduct) 312.0 [5th]
Venofibrosis 459.89
Venom, venomous
  bite or sting (animal or insect) 989.5
  poisoning 989.5
Venous - *see* condition
Ventouse delivery NEC 669.5 [5th]
  affecting fetus or newborn 763.3

Valve, valvular – Ventouse delivery

Ventral - *see* condition
Ventricle, ventricular - *see also* condition
- escape 427.69
- standstill (*see also* Arrest, cardiac) 427.5

Ventriculitis, cerebral (*see also* Meningitis) 322.9
Ventriculostomy status V45.2
Verbiest's syndrome (claudicatio intermittens spinalis) 435.1
Vernet's syndrome 352.6
Verneuil's disease (syphilitic bursitis) 095.7
Verruca (filiformis) 078.10
- acuminata (any site) 078.11
- necrogenica (primary) (*see also* Tuberculosis) 017.0 5th
- peruana 088.0
- peruviana 088.0
- plana (juvenilis) 078.19
- plantaris 078.12
- seborrheica 702.19
  - inflamed 702.11
- senilis 702.0
- tuberculosa (primary) (*see also* Tuberculosis) 017.0 5th
- venereal 078.11
- viral 078.10
  - specified NEC 078.19
- vulgaris 078.10

Verrucosities (*see also* Verruca) 078.10
Verrucous endocarditis (acute) (any valve) (chronic) (subacute) 710.0 *[424.91]*
- nonbacterial 710.0 *[424.91]*

Verruga
- peruana 088.0
- peruviana 088.0

Verse's disease (calcinosis intervertebralis) 275.49 *[722.90]*
Version
- before labor, affecting fetus or newborn 761.7
- cephalic (correcting previous malposition) 652.1 5th
  - affecting fetus or newborn 763.1
- cervix- *see* Version, uterus
- uterus (postinfectional) (postpartal, old) (*see also* Malposition, uterus) 621.6
  - forward - *see* Anteversion, uterus
  - lateral - *see* Lateroversion, uterus

Vertebra, vertebral - *see* condition
Vertigo 780.4
- auditory 386.19
- aural 386.19
- benign paroxysmal positional 386.11
- central origin 386.2
- cerebral 386.2
- Dix and Hallpike (epidemic) 386.12
- endemic paralytic 078.81
- epidemic 078.81
  - Dix and Hallpike 386.12
  - Gerlier's 078.81
  - Pedersen's 386.12
  - vestibular neuronitis 386.12
- epileptic - *see* Epilepsy
- Gerlier's (epidemic) 078.81
- hysterical 300.11
- labyrinthine 386.10
- laryngeal 786.2
- malignant positional 386.2
- Ménière's (*see also* Disease, Ménière's) 386.00
- menopausal 627.2
- otogenic 386.19
- paralytic 078.81
- paroxysmal positional, benign 386.11
- Pedersen's (epidemic) 386.12
- peripheral 386.10
  - specified type NEC 386.19
- positional
  - benign paroxysmal 386.11
  - malignant 386.2

Verumontanitis (chronic) (*see also* Urethritis) 597.89
Vesania (*see also* Psychosis) 298.9
Vesical - *see* condition
Vesicle
- cutaneous 709.8
- seminal - *see* condition
- skin 709.8

Vesicocolic - *see* condition
Vesicoperineal - *see* condition
Vesicorectal - *see* condition
Vesicourethrorectal - *see* condition
Vesicovaginal - *see* condition
Vesicular - *see* condition
Vesiculitis (seminal) 608.0
- amebic 006.8
- gonorrheal (acute) 098.14
  - chronic or duration of 2 months or over 098.34
- trichomonal 131.09
- tuberculous (*see also* Tuberculosis) 016.5 5th *[608.81]*

Vestibulitis (ear) (*see also* Labyrinthitis) 386.30
- nose (external) 478.19
- vulvar 625.71

Vestibulopathy, acute peripheral (recurrent) 386.12
Vestige, vestigial - *see also* Persistence
- branchial 744.41
- structures in vitreous 743.51

Vibriosis NEC 027.9
Vidal's disease (lichen simplex chronicus) 698.3
Video display tube syndrome 723.8
Vienna-type encephalitis 049.8
Villaret's syndrome 352.6
Villous - *see* condition
VIN I (vulvar intraepithelial neoplasia I) 624.01
VIN II (vulvar intraepithelial neoplasia II) 624.02
VIN III (vulvar intraepithelial neoplasia III) 233.32
Vincent's
- angina 101
- bronchitis 101
- disease 101
- gingivitis 101
- infection (any site) 101
- laryngitis 101
- stomatitis 101
- tonsillitis 101

Vinson-Plummer syndrome (sideropenic dysphagia) 280.8
Viosterol deficiency (*see also* Deficiency, calciferol) 268.9
Virchow's disease 733.99
Viremia 790.8
Virilism (adrenal) (female) NEC 255.2
- with
  - 3-beta-hydroxysteroid dehydrogenase defect 255.2
  - 11-hydroxylase defect 255.2
  - 21-hydroxylase defect 255.2
  - adrenal
    - hyperplasia 255.2
    - insufficiency (congenital) 255.2
  - cortical hyperfunction 255.2

Virilization (female) (suprarenal) (*see also* Virilism) 255.2
- isosexual 256.4

Virulent bubo 099.0
Virus, viral - *see also* condition
- infection NEC (*see also* Infection, viral) 079.99
- septicemia 079.99
- yaba monkey tumor 059.22

VISA (vancomycin intermediate staphylococcus aureus) V09.8 5th
Viscera, visceral - *see* condition
Visceroptosis 569.89
Visible peristalsis 787.4
Vision, visual
- binocular, suppression 368.31
- blurred, blurring 368.8
  - hysterical 300.11

Vision, visual – *continued*
- defect, defective (*see also* Impaired, vision) 369.9
- disorientation (syndrome) 368.16
- disturbance NEC (*see also* Disturbance, vision) 368.9
  - hysterical 300.11
- examination V72.0
- field, limitation 368.40
- fusion, with defective steropsis 368.33
- hallucinations 368.16
- halos 368.16
- loss 369.9
  - both eyes (*see also* Blindness, both eyes) 369.3
  - complete (*see also* Blindness, both eyes) 369.00
  - one eye 369.8
  - sudden 368.16
- low (both eyes) 369.20
  - one eye (other eye normal) (*see also* Impaired, vision) 369.70
    - blindness, other eye 369.10
- perception, simultaneous without fusion 368.32
- tunnel 368.45

Vitality, lack or want of 780.79
- newborn 779.89

Vitamin deficiency NEC (*see also* Deficiency, vitamin) 269.2
Vitelline duct, persistent 751.0
Vitiligo 709.01
- due to pinta (carate) 103.2
- eyelid 374.53
- vulva 624.8

Vitium cordis - *see* Disease, heart
Vitreous - *see also* condition
- touch syndrome 997.99

VLCAD (long chain/very long chain acyl CoA dehydrogenase deficiency, LCAD) 277.85
Vocal cord - *see* condition
Vocational rehabilitation V57.22
Vogt's (Cecile) disease or syndrome 333.7 5th
Vogt-Koyanagi syndrome 364.24
Vogt-Spielmeyer disease (amaurotic familial idiocy) 330.1
Voice
- change (*see also* Dysphonia) 784.49
- loss (*see also* Aphonia) 784.41

Volhard-Fahr disease (malignant nephrosclerosis) 403.00
Volhynian fever 083.1
Volkmann's ischemic contracture or paralysis (complicating trauma) 958.6
Voluntary starvation 307.1
Volvulus (bowel) (colon) (intestine) 560.2
- with
  - hernia - *see also* Hernia, by site, with obstruction
    - gangrenous - *see* Hernia, by site, with gangrene
  - perforation 560.2
- congenital 751.5
- duodenum 537.3
- fallopian tube 620.5
- oviduct 620.5
- stomach (due to absence of gastrocolic ligament) 537.89

Vomiting 787.03
- with nausea 787.01
- allergic 535.4 5th
- asphyxia 933.1
- bilious (cause unknown) 787.04 ▲
  - following gastrointestinal surgery 564.3
  - newborn 779.32 ●
- blood (*see also* Hematemesis) 578.0
- causing asphyxia, choking, or suffocation (*see also* Asphyxia, food) 933.1
- cyclical 536.2
  - associated with migraine 346.2 5th
  - psychogenic 306.4

Vomiting – *continued*
- epidemic 078.82
- fecal matter 569.87 ▲
- following gastrointestinal surgery 564.3
- functional 536.8
  - psychogenic 306.4
- habit 536.2
- hysterical 300.11
- nervous 306.4
- neurotic 306.4
- newborn 779.33 ▲
  - bilous 779.32 ●
- of or complicating pregnancy 643.9 5th
  - due to
    - organic disease 643.8 5th
    - specific cause NEC 643.8 5th
  - early - *see* Hyperemesis, gravidarum
  - late (after 22 completed weeks of gestation) 643.2 5th
- pernicious or persistent 536.2
  - complicating pregnancy - *see* Hyperemesis, gravidarum
  - psychogenic 306.4
- physiological 787.03 ▲
  - bilious 787.04 ●
- psychic 306.4
- psychogenic 307.54
- stercoral 569.89
- uncontrollable 536.2
  - psychogenic 306.4
- uremic - *see* Uremia
- winter 078.82

von Bechterew (-Strümpell) disease or syndrome (ankylosing spondylitis) 720.0
von Bezold's abscess 383.01
von Economo's disease (encephalitis lethargica) 049.8
von Eulenburg's disease (congenital paramyotonia) 359.29
von Gierke's disease (glycogenosis I) 271.0
von Gies' joint 095.8
von Graefe's disease or syndrome 378.72
von Hippel (-Lindau) disease or syndrome (retinocerebral angiomatosis) 759.6
von Jaksch's anemia or disease (pseudoleukemia infantum) 285.8
von Recklinghausen's
- disease or syndrome (nerves) (skin) (M9540/1) 237.71
  - bones (osteitis fibrosa cystica) 252.01
- tumor (M9540/1) 237.71

von Recklinghausen-Applebaum disease (hemochromatosis) 275.0
von Schroetter's syndrome (intermittent venous claudication) 453.89 ▲
von Willebrand (-Jürgens) (-Minot) disease or syndrome (angiohemophilia) 286.4
von Zambusch's disease (lichen sclerosus et atrophicus) 701.0
Voorhoeve's disease or dyschondroplasia 756.4
Vossius' ring 921.3
- late effect 366.21

Voyeurism 302.82
VRE (vancomycin resistant enterococcus) V09.8 5th
Vrolik's disease (osteogenesis imperfecta) 756.51
VRSA (vancomycin resistant staphylococcus aureus) V09.8 5th
Vulva - *see* condition
Vulvismus 625.1
Vulvitis (acute) (allergic) (chronic) (gangrenous) (hypertrophic) (intertriginous) 616.10
- with
  - abortion - *see* Abortion, by type, with sepsis
  - ectopic pregnancy (*see also* categories 633.0-633.9) 639.0
  - molar pregnancy (*see also* categories 630-632) 639.0
- adhesive, congenital 752.49

Ventral – Vulvitis

Vulvitis – *continued*
- blennorrhagic (acute) 098.0
  - chronic or duration of 2 months or over 098.2
- chlamydial 099.53
- complicating pregnancy or puerperium 646.6 5th
- due to Ducrey's bacillus 099.0
- following
  - abortion 639.0
  - ectopic or molar pregnancy 639.0
- gonococcal (acute) 098.0
  - chronic or duration of 2 months or over 098.2
- herpetic 054.11
- leukoplakic 624.09
- monilial 112.1
- puerperal, postpartum, childbirth 646.6 5th
- syphilitic (early) 091.0
  - late 095.8
- trichomonal 131.01

Vulvodynia 625.70
- specified NEC 625.79

Vulvorectal - *see* condition

Vulvovaginitis (*see also* Vulvitis) 616.10
- amebic 006.8
- chlamydial 099.53
- gonococcal (acute) 098.0
  - chronic or duration of 2 months or over 098.2
- herpetic 054.11
- monilial 112.1
- trichomonal (Trichomonas vaginalis) 131.01

W

Waardenburg's syndrome 756.89
- meaning ptosis-epicanthus 270.2

Waardenburg-Klein syndrome (ptosis-epicanthus) 270.2

Wagner's disease (colloid milium) 709.3

Wagner (-Unverricht) syndrome (dermatomyositis) 710.3

Waiting list, person on V63.2
- undergoing social agency investigation V63.8

Wakefulness disorder (*see also* Hypersomnia) 780.54
- nonorganic origin 307.43

Waldenström's
- disease (osteochondrosis, capital femoral) 732.1
- hepatitis (lupoid hepatitis) 571.49
- hypergammaglobulinemia 273.0
- macroglobulinemia 273.3
- purpura, hypergammaglobulinemic 273.0
- syndrome (macroglobulinemia) 273.3

Waldenström-Kjellberg syndrome (sideropenic dysphagia) 280.8

Walking
- difficulty 719.7
  - psychogenic 307.9
- sleep 307.46
  - hysterical 300.13

Wall, abdominal - *see* condition

Wallenberg's syndrome (posterior inferior cerebellar artery) (*see also* Disease, cerebrovascular, acute) 436

Wallgren's
- disease (obstruction of splenic vein with collateral circulation) 459.89
- meningitis (*see also* Meningitis, aseptic) 047.9

Wandering
- acetabulum 736.39
- gallbladder 751.69
- kidney, congenital 753.3
- organ or site, congenital NEC - *see* Malposition, congenital
- pacemaker (atrial) (heart) 427.89

Wandering – *continued*
- spleen 289.59

Wardrop's disease (with lymphangitis) 681.9
- finger 681.02
- toe 681.11

War neurosis 300.16

Wart (digitate) (filiform) (infectious) (viral) 078.10
- common 078.19
- external genital organs (venereal) 078.11
- fig 078.19
- flat 078.19
- genital 078.11
- Hassall-Henle's (of cornea) 371.41
- Henle's (of cornea) 371.41
- juvenile 078.19
- moist 078.10
- Peruvian 088.0
- plantar 078.12
- prosector (*see also* Tuberculosis) 017.0 5th
- seborrheic 702.19
  - inflamed 702.11
- senile 702.0
- specified NEC 078.19
- syphilitic 091.3
- tuberculous (*see also* Tuberculosis) 017.0 5th
- venereal (female) (male) 078.11

Warthin's tumor (salivary gland) (M8561/0) 210.2

Washerwoman's itch 692.4

Wassilieff's disease (leptospiral jaundice) 100.0

Wasting
- disease 799.4
  - due to malnutrition 261
- extreme (due to malnutrition) 261
- muscular NEC 728.2
- palsy, paralysis 335.21
- pelvic muscle 618.83

Water
- clefts 366.12
- deprivation of 994.3
- in joint (*see also* Effusion, joint) 719.0 5th
- intoxication 276.6
- itch 120.3
- lack of 994.3
- loading 276.6
- on
  - brain - *see* Hydrocephalus
  - chest 511.89
- poisoning 276.6

Waterbrash 787.1

Water-hammer pulse (*see also* Insufficiency, aortic) 424.1

Waterhouse (-Friderichsen) disease or syndrome 036.3

Water-losing nephritis 588.89

Watermelon stomach 537.82
- with hemorrhage 537.83
- without hemorrhage 537.82

Wax in ear 380.4

Waxy
- degeneration, any site 277.39
- disease 277.39
- kidney 277.39 *[583.81]*
- liver (large) 277.39
- spleen 277.39

Weak, weakness (generalized) 780.79
- arches (acquired) 734
  - congenital 754.61
- bladder sphincter 596.59
- congenital 779.89
- eye muscle - *see* Strabismus
- facial 781.94
- foot (double) - *see* Weak, arches
- heart, cardiac (*see also* Failure, heart) 428.9
  - congenital 746.9
- mind 317
- muscle (generalized) 728.87
- myocardium (*see also* Failure, heart) 428.9
- newborn 779.89

Weak, weakness – *continued*
- pelvic fundus
  - pubocervical tissue 618.81
  - rectovaginal tissue 618.82
- pulse 785.9
- senile 797
- urinary stream 788.62
- valvular - *see* Endocarditis

Wear, worn, tooth, teeth (approximal) (hard tissues) (interproximal) (occlusal) - *see also* Attrition, teeth 521.10

Weather, weathered
- effects of
  - cold NEC 991.9
    - specified effect NEC 991.8
  - hot (*see also* Heat) 992.9
- skin 692.74

Web, webbed (congenital) - *see also* Anomaly, specified type NEC
- canthus 743.63
- digits (*see also* Syndactylism) 755.10
- duodenal 751.5
- esophagus 750.3
- fingers (*see also* Syndactylism, fingers) 755.11
- larynx (glottic) (subglottic) 748.2
- neck (pterygium colli) 744.5
- Paterson-Kelly (sideropenic dysphagia) 280.8
- popliteal syndrome 756.89
- toes (*see also* Syndactylism, toes) 755.13

Weber's paralysis or syndrome 344.89

Weber-Christian disease or syndrome (nodular nonsuppurative panniculitis) 729.30

Weber-Cockayne syndrome (epidermolysis bullosa) 757.39

Weber-Dimitri syndrome 759.6

Weber-Gubler syndrome 344.89

Weber-Leyden syndrome 344.89

Weber-Osler syndrome (familial hemorrhagic telangiectasia) 448.0

Wedge-shaped or wedging vertebra (*see also* Osteoporosis) 733.00

Wegener's granulomatosis or syndrome 446.4

Wegner's disease (syphilitic osteochondritis) 090.0

Weight
- gain (abnormal) (excessive) 783.1
  - during pregnancy 646.1 5th
    - insufficient 646.8 5th
- less than 1000 grams at birth 765.0 5th
- loss (cause unknown) 783.21

Weightlessness 994.9

Weil's disease (leptospiral jaundice) 100.0

Weill-Marchesani syndrome (brachymorphism and ectopia lentis) 759.89

Weingarten's syndrome (tropical eosinophilia) 518.3

Weir Mitchell's disease (erythromelalgia) 443.82

Weiss-Baker syndrome (carotid sinus syncope) 337.01

Weissenbach-Thibierge syndrome (cutaneous systemic sclerosis) 710.1

Wen (*see also* Cyst, sebaceous) 706.2

Wenckebach's phenomenon, heart block (second degree) 426.13

Werdnig-Hoffmann syndrome (muscular atrophy) 335.0

Werlhof's disease (*see also* Purpura, thrombocytopenic) 287.39

Werlhof-Wichmann syndrome (*see also* Purpura, thrombocytopenic) 287.39

Wermer's syndrome or disease (polyendocrine adenomatosis) 258.01

Werner's disease or syndrome (progeria adultorum) 259.8

Werner-His disease (trench fever) 083.1

Werner-Schultz disease (agranulocytosis) 288.09

Wernicke's encephalopathy, disease, or syndrome (superior hemorrhagic polioencephalitis) 265.1

Wernicke-Korsakoff syndrome or psychosis (nonalcoholic) 294.0
- alcoholic 291.1

Wernicke-Posadas disease (*see also* Coccidioidomycosis) 114.9

Wesselsbron fever 066.3

West African fever 084.8

West Nile
- encephalitis 066.41
- encephalomyelitis 066.41
- fever 066.40
  - with
    - cranial nerve disorders 066.42
    - encephalitis 066.41
    - optic neuritis 066.42
    - other complications 066.49
    - other neurologic manifestations 066.42
    - polyradiculitis 066.42
- virus 066.40

Westphal-Strümpell syndrome (hepatolenticular degeneration) 275.1

Wet
- brain (alcoholic) (*see also* Alcoholism) 303.9 5th
- feet, tropical (syndrome) (maceration) 991.4
- lung (syndrome)
  - adult 518.5
  - newborn 770.6

Wharton's duct - *see* condition

Wheal 709.8

Wheelchair confinement status V46.3

Wheezing 786.07

Whiplash injury or syndrome 847.0

Whipple's disease or syndrome (intestinal lipodystrophy) 040.2

Whipworm 127.3

"Whistling face" syndrome (craniocarpotarsal dystrophy) 759.89

White - *see also* condition
- kidney
  - large - *see* Nephrosis
  - small 582.9
- leg, puerperal, postpartum, childbirth 671.4 5th
  - nonpuerperal 451.19
- mouth 112.0
- patches of mouth 528.6
- sponge nevus of oral mucosa 750.26
- spot lesions, teeth 521.01

White's disease (congenital) (keratosis follicularis) 757.39

Whitehead 706.2

Whitlow (with lymphangitis) 681.01
- herpetic 054.6

Whitmore's disease or fever (melioidosis) 025

Whooping cough 033.9
- with pneumonia 033.9 *[484.3]*
- due to
  - Bordetella
    - bronchoseptica 033.8
      - with pneumonia 033.8 *[484.3]*
    - parapertussis 033.1
      - with pneumonia 033.1 *[484.3]*
    - pertussis 033.0
      - with pneumonia 033.0 *[484.3]*
  - specified organism NEC 033.8
    - with pneumonia 033.8 *[484.3]*
- vaccination, prophylactic (against) V03.6

Wichmann's asthma (laryngismus stridulus) 478.75

Widal (-Abrami) syndrome (acquired hemolytic jaundice) 283.9

Widening aorta (*see also* Aneurysm, aorta) 441.9
- ruptured 441.5

Wilkie's disease or syndrome 557.1

Wilkinson-Sneddon disease or syndrome (subcorneal pustular dermatosis) 694.1

Note *For fracture with open wound, see Fracture.*

For laceration, traumatic rupture, tear, or penetrating wound of internal organs, such as heart, lung, liver, kidney, pelvic organs, etc., whether or not accompanied by open wound or fracture in the same region, see Injury, internal.

For contused wound, see Contusion. For crush injury, see Crush. For abrasion, insect bite (nonvenomous), blister, or scratch, see Injury, superficial.

Complicated includes wounds with:

delayed healing
delayed treatment
foreign body
primary infection

For late effect of open wound, see Late, effect, wound, open, by site.

Willan's lepra – Wound, open

- **Wound, open** – *continued*
  - inguinal region 879.4
    - complicated 879.5
  - instep 892.0
    - with tendon involvement 892.2
    - complicated 892.1
  - interscapular region 876.0
    - complicated 876.1
  - intracranial - *see* Injury, intracranial, with open intracranial wound
  - intraocular 871.9
    - with
      - partial loss (of intraocular tissue) 871.2
      - prolapse or exposure (of intraocular tissue) 871.1
    - laceration (*see also* Laceration, eyeball) 871.4
    - penetrating 871.7
      - with foreign body (nonmagnetic) 871.6
        - magnetic 871.5
    - without prolapse (of intraocular tissue) 871.0
  - iris (*see also* Wound, open, eyeball) 871.9
  - jaw (fracture not involved) 873.44
    - with fracture - *see* Fracture, jaw
    - complicated 873.54
  - knee 891.0
    - with tendon involvement 891.2
    - complicated 891.1
  - labium (majus) (minus) 878.4
    - complicated 878.5
  - lacrimal apparatus, gland, or sac 870.8
    - with laceration of eyelid 870.2
  - larynx 874.01
    - with trachea 874.00
      - complicated 874.10
    - complicated 874.11
  - leg (multiple) 891.0
    - with tendon involvement 891.2
    - complicated 891.1
    - lower 891.0
      - with tendon involvement 891.2
      - complicated 891.1
    - thigh 890.0
      - with tendon involvement 890.2
      - complicated 890.1
    - upper 890.0
      - with tendon involvement 890.2
      - complicated 890.1
  - lens (eye) (alone) (*see also* Cataract, traumatic) 366.20
    - with involvement of other eye structures - *see* Wound, open, eyeball
  - limb
    - lower (multiple) NEC 894.0
      - with tendon involvement 894.2
      - complicated 894.1
    - upper (multiple) NEC 884.0
      - with tendon involvement 884.2
      - complicated 884.1
  - lip 873.43
    - complicated 873.53
  - loin 876.0
    - complicated 876.1
  - lumbar region 876.0
    - complicated 876.1
  - malar region 873.41
    - complicated 873.51
  - mastoid region 873.49
    - complicated 873.59
  - mediastinum - *see* Injury, internal, mediastinum
  - midthoracic region 875.0
    - complicated 875.1
  - mouth 873.60
    - complicated 873.70
    - floor 873.64
      - complicated 873.74
    - multiple sites 873.69
      - complicated 873.79

- **Wound, open** – *continued*
  - mouth – *continued*
    - specified site NEC 873.69
      - complicated 873.79
  - multiple, unspecified site(s) 879.8

Note *Multiple open wounds of sites classifiable to the same four-digit category should be classified to that category unless they are in different limbs.*

Multiple open wounds of sites classifiable to different four-digit categories, or to different limbs, should be coded separately.

-
  -
    - complicated 879.9
    - lower limb(s) (one or both) (sites classifiable to more than one three-digit category in 890-893) 894.0
      - with tendon involvement 894.2
      - complicated 894.1
    - upper limb(s) (one or both) (sites classifiable to more than one three-digit category in 880-883) 884.0
      - with tendon involvement 884.2
      - complicated 884.1
  - muscle - *see* Sprain, by site
  - nail
    - finger(s) 883.0
      - complicated 883.1
    - thumb 883.0
      - complicated 883.1
    - toe(s) 893.0
      - complicated 893.1
  - nape (neck) 874.8
    - complicated 874.9
    - specified part NEC 874.8
      - complicated 874.9
  - nasal - *see also* Wound, open, nose
    - cavity 873.22
      - complicated 873.32
    - septum 873.21
      - complicated 873.31
    - sinuses 873.23
      - complicated 873.33
  - nasopharynx 873.22
    - complicated 873.32
  - neck 874.8
    - complicated 874.9
    - nape 874.8
      - complicated 874.9
    - specified part NEC 874.8
      - complicated 874.9
  - nerve - *see* Injury, nerve, by site
  - non-healing surgical 998.83
  - nose 873.20
    - complicated 873.30
    - multiple sites 873.29
      - complicated 873.39
    - septum 873.21
      - complicated 873.31
    - sinuses 873.23
      - complicated 873.33
  - occipital region - *see* Wound, open, scalp
  - ocular NEC 871.9
    - adnexa 870.9
      - specified region NEC 870.8
    - laceration (*see also* Laceration, ocular) 871.4
    - muscle (extraocular) 870.3
      - with foreign body 870.4
      - eyelid 870.1
      - intraocular - *see* Wound, open, eyeball
    - penetrating (*see also* Penetrating wound, ocular) 871.7
  - orbit 870.8
    - penetrating 870.3
      - with foreign body 870.4
  - orbital region 870.9
  - ovary - *see* Injury, internal, pelvic organs

- **Wound, open** – *continued*
  - palate 873.65
    - complicated 873.75
  - palm 882.0
    - with tendon involvement 882.2
    - complicated 882.1
  - parathyroid (gland) 874.2
    - complicated 874.3
  - parietal region - *see* Wound, open, scalp
  - pelvic floor or region 879.6
    - complicated 879.7
  - penis 878.0
    - complicated 878.1
  - perineum 879.6
    - complicated 879.7
  - periocular area 870.8
    - laceration of skin 870.0
  - pharynx 874.4
    - complicated 874.5
  - pinna 872.01
    - complicated 872.11
  - popliteal space 891.0
    - with tendon involvement 891.2
    - complicated 891.1
  - prepuce 878.0
    - complicated 878.1
  - pubic region 879.2
    - complicated 879.3
  - pudenda 878.8
    - complicated 878.9
  - rectovaginal septum 878.8
    - complicated 878.9
  - sacral region 877.0
    - complicated 877.1
  - sacroiliac region 877.0
    - complicated 877.1
  - salivary (ducts) (glands) 873.69
    - complicated 873.79
  - scalp 873.0
    - complicated 873.1
  - scalpel, fetus or newborn 767.8
  - scapular region 880.01
    - with tendon involvement 880.21
    - complicated 880.11
    - involving other sites of upper arm 880.09
      - with tendon involvement 880.29
      - complicated 880.19
  - sclera (*see also* Wound, open, intraocular) 871.9
  - scrotum 878.2
    - complicated 878.3
  - seminal vesicle - *see* Injury, internal, pelvic organs
  - shin 891.0
    - with tendon involvement 891.2
    - complicated 891.1
  - shoulder 880.00
    - with tendon involvement 880.20
    - complicated 880.10
    - involving other sites of upper arm 880.09
      - with tendon involvement 880.29
      - complicated 880.19
  - skin NEC 879.8
    - complicated 879.9
  - skull - *see also* Injury, intracranial, with open intracranial wound
    - with skull fracture - *see* Fracture, skull
  - spermatic cord (scrotal) 878.2
    - complicated 878.3
    - pelvic region - *see* Injury, internal, spermatic cord
  - spinal cord - *see* Injury, spinal
  - sternal region 875.0
    - complicated 875.1
  - subconjunctival - *see* Wound, open, intraocular
  - subcutaneous NEC 879.8
    - complicated 879.9
  - submaxillary region 873.44
    - complicated 873.54
  - submental region 873.44
    - complicated 873.54

- **Wound, open** – *continued*
  - subungual
    - finger(s) (thumb) - *see* Wound, open, finger
    - toe(s) - *see* Wound, open, toe
  - supraclavicular region 874.8
    - complicated 874.9
  - supraorbital 873.42
    - complicated 873.52
  - surgical, non-healing 998.83
  - temple 873.49
    - complicated 873.59
  - temporal region 873.49
    - complicated 873.59
  - testis 878.2
    - complicated 878.3
  - thigh 890.0
    - with tendon involvement 890.2
    - complicated 890.1
  - thorax, thoracic (external) 875.0
    - complicated 875.1
  - throat 874.8
    - complicated 874.9
  - thumb (nail) (subungual) 883.0
    - with tendon involvement 883.2
    - complicated 883.1
  - thyroid (gland) 874.2
    - complicated 874.3
  - toe(s) (nail) (subungual) 893.0
    - with tendon involvement 893.2
    - complicated 893.1
  - tongue 873.64
    - complicated 873.74
  - tonsil - *see* Wound, open, neck
  - trachea (cervical region) 874.02
    - with larynx 874.00
      - complicated 874.10
    - complicated 874.12
    - intrathoracic - *see* Injury, internal, trachea
  - trunk (multiple) NEC 879.6
    - complicated 879.7
    - specified site NEC 879.6
      - complicated 879.7
  - tunica vaginalis 878.2
    - complicated 878.3
  - tympanic membrane 872.61
    - complicated 872.71
  - tympanum 872.61
    - complicated 872.71
  - umbilical region 879.2
    - complicated 879.3
  - ureter - *see* Injury, internal, ureter
  - urethra - *see* Injury, internal, urethra
  - uterus - *see* Injury, internal, uterus
  - uvula 873.69
    - complicated 873.79
  - vagina 878.6
    - complicated 878.7
  - vas deferens - *see* Injury, internal, vas deferens
  - vitreous (humor) 871.2
  - vulva 878.4
    - complicated 878.5
  - wrist 881.02
    - with tendon involvement 881.22
    - complicated 881.12
- **Wright's syndrome** (hyperabduction) 447.8
  - pneumonia 390 *[517.1]*
- **Wringer injury** - *see* Crush injury, by site
- **Wrinkling of skin** 701.8
- **Wrist** - *see also* condition
  - drop (acquired) 736.05
- **Wrong drug** (given in error) NEC 977.9
  - specified drug or substance - *see* Table of Drugs and Chemicals
- **Wry neck** - *see also* Torticollis
  - congenital 754.1
- **Wuchereria infestation** 125.0
  - bancrofti 125.0
  - Brugia malayi 125.1
  - malayi 125.1
- **Wuchereriasis** 125.0
- **Wuchereriosis** 125.0

Wuchernde struma langhans (M8332/3) 193

Xanthelasma 272.2
- eyelid 272.2 *[374.51]*
- palpebrarum 272.2 *[374.51]*

Xanthelasmatosis (essential) 272.2
Xanthelasmoidea 757.33
Xanthine stones 277.2
Xanthinuria 277.2
Xanthofibroma (M8831/0) - *see* Neoplasm, connective tissue, benign
Xanthoma(s), xanthomatosis 272.2
- with
  - hyperlipoproteinemia
    - type I 272.3
    - type III 272.2
    - type IV 272.1
    - type V 272.3
- bone 272.7
- craniohypophyseal 277.89
- cutaneotendinous 272.7
- diabeticorum 250.8 5th *[272.2]*
  - due to secondary diabetes 249.8 5th *[272.2]*
- disseminatum 272.7
- eruptive 272.2
- eyelid 272.2 *[374.51]*
- familial 272.7
- hereditary 272.7
- hypercholesterinemic 272.0
- hypercholesterolemic 272.0
- hyperlipemic 272.4
- hyperlipidemic 272.4
- infantile 272.7
- joint 272.7
- juvenile 272.7
- multiple 272.7
- multiplex 272.7
- primary familial 272.7
- tendon (sheath) 272.7
- tuberosum 272.2

Xanthoma(s), xanthomatosis – *continued*
- tuberous 272.2
- tubo-eruptive 272.2

Xanthosis 709.09
- surgical 998.81

Xenophobia 300.29
Xeroderma (congenital) 757.39
- acquired 701.1
  - eyelid 373.33
- eyelid 373.33
- pigmentosum 757.33
- vitamin A deficiency 264.8

Xerophthalmia 372.53
- vitamin A deficiency 264.7

Xerosis
- conjunctiva 372.53
  - with Bitôt's spot 372.53
    - vitamin A deficiency 264.1
  - vitamin A deficiency 264.0
- cornea 371.40
  - with corneal ulceration 370.00
    - vitamin A deficiency 264.3
  - vitamin A deficiency 264.2
- cutis 706.8
- skin 706.8

Xerostomia 527.7
Xiphodynia 733.90
Xiphoidalgia 733.90
Xiphoiditis 733.99
Xiphopagus 759.4
XO syndrome 758.6
X-ray
- effects, adverse, NEC 990
- of chest
  - for suspected tuberculosis V71.2
  - routine V72.5

XXX syndrome 758.81
XXXXY syndrome 758.81
XXY syndrome 758.7
Xyloketosuria 271.8
Xylosuria 271.8
Xylulosuria 271.8
XYY syndrome 758.81

Y

Yaba monkey tumor virus 059.22
Yawning 786.09
- psychogenic 306.1

Yaws 102.9
- bone or joint lesions 102.6
- butter 102.1
- chancre 102.0
- cutaneous, less than five years after infection 102.2
- early (cutaneous) (macular) (maculopapular) (micropapular) (papular) 102.2
  - frambeside 102.2
  - skin lesions NEC 102.2
- eyelid 102.9 *[373.4]*
- ganglion 102.6
- gangosis, gangosa 102.5
- gumma, gummata 102.4
  - bone 102.6
- gummatous
  - frambeside 102.4
  - osteitis 102.6
  - periostitis 102.6
- hydrarthrosis 102.6
- hyperkeratosis (early) (late) (palmar) (plantar) 102.3
- initial lesions 102.0
- joint lesions 102.6
- juxta-articular nodules 102.7
- late nodular (ulcerated) 102.4
- latent (without clinical manifestations) (with positive serology) 102.8
- mother 102.0
- mucosal 102.7
- multiple papillomata 102.1
- nodular, late (ulcerated) 102.4
- osteitis 102.6
- papilloma, papillomata (palmar) (plantar) 102.1
- periostitis (hypertrophic) 102.6
- ulcers 102.4

Yaws – *continued*
- wet crab 102.1

Yeast infection (*see also* Candidiasis) 112.9
Yellow
- atrophy (liver) 570
  - chronic 571.8
  - resulting from administration of blood, plasma, serum, or other biological substance (within 8 months of administration) - *see* Hepatitis, viral
- fever - *see* Fever, yellow
- jack (*see also* Fever, yellow) 060.9
- jaundice (*see also* Jaundice) 782.4

Yersinia septica 027.8

Zagari's disease (xerostomia) 527.7
Zahorsky's disease (exanthema subitum) (*see also* Exanthem subitum) 058.10
- syndrome (herpangina) 074.0

Zellweger syndrome 277.86
Zenker's diverticulum (esophagus) 530.6
Ziehen-Oppenheim disease 333.6
Zieve's syndrome (jaundice, hyperlipemia, and hemolytic anemia) 571.1
Zika fever 066.3
Zollinger-Ellison syndrome (gastric hypersecretion with pancreatic islet cell tumor) 251.5
Zona (*see also* Herpes, zoster) 053.9
Zoophilia (erotica) 302.1
Zoophobia 300.29
Zoster (herpes) (*see also* Herpes, zoster) 053.9
Zuelzer (-Ogden) anemia or syndrome (nutritional megaloblastic anemia) 281.2
Zygodactyly (*see also* Syndactylism) 755.10
Zygomycosis 117.7
Zymotic - *see* condition

Wuchernde struma langhans – Zymotic

Table of Drugs and Chemicals

INDEX TO POISONING AND EXTERNAL CAUSES OF ADVERSE EFFECTS OF DRUGS AND OTHER CHEMICAL SUBSTANCES

This table contains a classification of drugs and other chemical substances to identify poisoning states and external causes of adverse effects.

Each of the listed substances in the table is assigned a code according to the poisoning classification (960-989). These codes are used when there is a statement of poisoning, overdose, wrong substance given or taken, or intoxication.

The table also contains a listing of external causes of adverse effects. An adverse effect is a pathologic manifestation due to ingestion or exposure to drugs or other chemical substances (e.g., dermatitis, hypersensitivity reaction, aspirin gastritis). The adverse effect is to be identified by the appropriate code found in Section 1, Index to Diseases and Injuries. An external cause code can then be used to identify the circumstances involved. The table headings pertaining to external causes are defined below:

Accidental poisoning (E850-E869) – accidental overdose of drug, wrong substance given or taken, drug taken inadvertently, accidents in the usage of drugs and biologicals in medical and surgical procedures, and to show external causes of poisonings classifiable to 980-989.

Therapeutic use (E930-E949) – a correct substance properly administered in therapeutic or prophylactic dosage as the external cause of adverse effects.

Suicide attempt (E950-E952) – instances in which self-inflicted injuries or poisonings are involved.

Assault (E961-E962) – injury or poisoning inflicted by another person with the intent to injure or kill.

Undetermined (E980-E982)–to be used when the intent of the poisoning or injury cannot be determined whether it was intentional or accidental.

The American Hospital Formulary Service (AHFS) list numbers are included in the table to help classify new drugs not identified in the table by name. The AHFS list numbers are keyed to the continually revised AHFS (American Hospital Formulary Service, 2 vol. Washington, D.C.: American Society of Hospital Pharmacists, 1959-). These listings are found in the table under the main term **Drug**.

Excluded from the table are radium and other radioactive substances. The classification of adverse effects and complications pertaining to these substances will be found in Index to Diseases and Injuries, and Index to External Causes of Injuries.

Although certain substances are indexed with one or more subentries, the majority are listed according to one use or state. It is recognized that many substances may be used in various ways, in medicine and in industry, and may cause adverse effects whatever the state of the agent (solid, liquid, or fumes arising from a liquid). In cases in which the reported data indicate a use or state not in the table, or which is clearly different from the one listed, an attempt should be made to classify the substance in the form which most nearly expresses the reported facts.

ICD-9-CM Official Guidelines (Chapter 19):

Introduction: *These guidelines are provided for those who are currently collecting E codes in order that there will be standardization in the process. If your institution plans to begin collecting E codes, these guidelines are to be applied. The use of E codes is supplemental to the application of ICD-9-CM diagnosis codes. E codes are never to be recorded as principal diagnoses (first-listed in non-inpatient setting) and are not required for reporting to CMS.*

External causes of injury and poisoning codes (E codes) are intended to provide data for injury research and evaluation of injury prevention strategies. E codes capture how the injury or poisoning happened (cause), the intent (unintentional or accidental; or intentional, such as suicide or assault), and the place where the event occurred.

c. ***Adverse Effects of Drugs, Medicinal and Biological Substances Guidelines***

1) *Do not code directly from the Table of Drugs and Chemicals. Always refer back to the Tabular List.*
2) *Use as many codes as necessary to describe completely all drugs, medicinal or biological substances.*
3) *If the same E code would describe the causative agent for more than one adverse reaction, assign the code only once.*
4) *If two or more drugs, medicinal or biological substances are reported, code each individually unless the combination code is listed in the Table of Drugs and Chemicals. In that case, assign the E code for the combination.*
5) *When a reaction results from the interaction of a drug(s) and alcohol, use poisoning codes and E codes for both.*
6) *If the reporting format limits the number of E codes that can be used in reporting clinical data, code the one most related to the principal diagnosis. Include at least one from each category (cause, intent, place) if possible.*

   If there are different fourth digit codes in the same three digit category, use the code for "Other specified" of that category. If there is no "Other specified" code in that category, use the appropriate "Unspecified" code in that category.

   If the codes are in different three digit categories, assign the appropriate E code for other multiple drugs and medicinal substances.
7) *Codes from the E930-E949 series must be used to identify the causative substance for an adverse effect of drug, medicinal and biological substances, correctly prescribed and properly administered. The effect, such as tachycardia, delirium, gastrointestinal hemorrhaging, vomiting, hypokalemia, hepatitis, renal failure, or respiratory failure, is coded and followed by the appropriate code from the E930-E949 series.*

Drug, chemical	Poisoning	External Cause (E Code): Accident	Therapeutic Use	Suicide Attempt	Assault	Undetermined
1-propanol	980.3	E860.4	–	E950.9	E962.1	E980.9
2-propanol	980.2	E860.3	–	E950.9	E962.1	E980.9
2,4-D (dichlorophenoxyacetic acid)	989.4	E863.5	–	E950.6	E962.1	E980.7
2,4-toluene diisocyanate	983.0	E864.0	–	E950.7	E962.1	E980.6
2,4,5-T (trichlorophenoxyacetic acid)	989.2	E863.5	–	E950.6	E962.1	E980.7
14-hydroxydihydromorphinone	965.09	E850.2	E935.2	E950.0	E962.0	E980.0
ABOB	961.7	E857	E931.7	E950.4	E962.0	E980.4
Abrus (seed)	988.2	E865.3	–	E950.9	E962.1	E980.9
Absinthe	980.0	E860.1	–	E950.9	E962.1	E980.9
beverage	980.0	E860.0	–	E950.9	E962.1	E980.9
Acenocoumarin, acenocoumarol	964.2	E858.2	E934.2	E950.4	E962.0	E980.4
Acepromazine	969.1	E853.0	E939.1	E950.3	E962.0	E980.3
Acetal	982.8	E862.4	–	E950.9	E962.1	E980.9
Acetaldehyde (vapor)	987.8	E869.8	–	E952.8	E962.2	E982.8
liquid	989.89	E866.8	–	E950.9	E962.1	E980.9
Acetaminophen	965.4	E850.4	E935.4	E950.0	E962.0	E980.0
Acetaminosalol	965.1	E850.3	E935.3	E950.0	E962.0	E980.0
Acetanilid(e)	965.4	E850.4	E935.4	E950.0	E962.0	E980.0
Acetarsol, acetarsone	961.1	E857	E931.1	E950.4	E962.0	E980.4
Acetazolamide	974.2	E858.5	E944.2	E950.4	E962.0	E980.4
Acetic						
acid	983.1	E864.1	–	E950.7	E962.1	E980.6
with sodium acetate (ointment)	976.3	E858.7	E946.3	E950.4	E962.0	E980.4
irrigating solution	974.5	E858.5	E944.5	E950.4	E962.0	E980.4
lotion	976.2	E858.7	E946.2	E950.4	E962.0	E980.4
anhydride	983.1	E864.1	–	E950.7	E962.1	E980.6
ether (vapor)	982.8	E862.4	–	E950.9	E962.1	E980.9
Acetohexamide	962.3	E858.0	E932.3	E950.4	E962.0	E980.4
Acetomenaphihone	964.3	E858.2	E934.3	E950.4	E962.0	E980.4
Acetomorphine	965.01	E850.0	E935.0	E950.0	E962.0	E980.0
Acetone (oils) (vapor)	982.8	E862.4	–	E950.9	E962.1	E980.9
Acetophenazine (maleate)	969.1	E853.0	E939.1	E950.3	E962.0	E980.3
Acetophenetidin	965.4	E850.4	E935.4	E950.0	E962.0	E980.0
Acetophenone	982.0	E862.4	–	E950.9	E962.1	E980.9
Acetorphine	965.09	E850.2	E935.2	E950.0	E962.0	E980.0
Acetosulfone (sodium)	961.8	E857	E931.8	E950.4	E962.0	E980.4
Acetrizoate (sodium)	977.8	E858.8	E947.8	E950.4	E962.0	E980.4
Acetylcarbromal	967.3	E852.2	E937.3	E950.2	E962.0	E980.2
Acetylcholine (chloride)	971.0	E855.3	E941.0	E950.4	E962.0	E980.4
Acetylcysteine	975.5	E858.6	E945.5	E950.4	E962.0	E980.4
Acetyldigitoxin	972.1	E858.3	E942.1	E950.4	E962.0	E980.4
Acetyldihydrocodeine	965.09	E850.2	E935.2	E950.0	E962.0	E980.0
Acetyldihydrocodeinone	965.09	E850.2	E935.2	E950.0	E962.0	E980.0
Acetylene (gas) (industrial)	987.1	E868.1	–	E951.8	E962.2	E981.8
incomplete combustion of – *see* Carbon monoxide, fuel, utility						
tetrachloride (vapor)	982.3	E862.4	–	E950.9	E962.1	E980.9
Acetyliodosalicylic acid	965.1	E850.3	E935.3	E950.0	E962.0	E980.0
Acetylphenylhydrazine	965.8	E850.8	E935.8	E950.0	E962.0	E980.0
Acetylsalicylic acid	965.1	E850.3	E935.3	E950.0	E962.0	E980.0
Achromycin	960.4	E856	E930.4	E950.4	E962.0	E980.4
ophthalmic preparation	976.5	E858.7	E946.5	E950.4	E962.0	E980.4
topical NEC	976.0	E858.7	E946.0	E950.4	E962.0	E980.4
Acidifying agents	963.2	E858.1	E933.2	E950.4	E962.0	E980.4
Acids (corrosive) NEC	983.1	E864.1	–	E950.7	E962.1	E980.6
Aconite (wild)	988.2	E865.4	–	E950.9	E962.1	E980.9
Aconitine (liniment)	976.8	E858.7	E946.8	E950.4	E962.0	E980.4
Aconitum ferox	988.2	E865.4	–	E950.9	E962.1	E980.9
Acridine	983.0	E864.0	–	E950.7	E962.1	E980.6
vapor	987.8	E869.8	–	E952.8	E962.2	E982.8
Acriflavine	961.9	E857	E931.9	E950.4	E962.0	E980.4
Acrisorcin	976.0	E858.7	E946.0	E950.4	E962.0	E980.4
Acrolein (gas)	987.8	E869.8	–	E952.8	E962.2	E982.8
liquid	989.89	E866.8	–	E950.9	E962.1	E980.9
Actaea spicata	988.2	E865.4	–	E950.9	E962.1	E980.9
Acterol	961.5	E857	E931.5	E950.4	E962.0	E980.4
ACTH	962.4	E858.0	E932.4	E950.4	E962.0	E980.4
Acthar	962.4	E858.0	E932.4	E950.4	E962.0	E980.4
Actinomycin (C) (D)	960.7	E856	E930.7	E950.4	E962.0	E980.4
Adalin (acetyl)	967.3	E852.2	E937.3	E950.2	E962.0	E980.2
Adenosine (phosphate)	977.8	E858.8	E947.8	E950.4	E962.0	E980.4
Adhesives	989.89	E866.6	–	E950.9	E962.1	E980.9
ADH	962.5	E858.0	E932.5	E950.4	E962.0	E980.4
Adicillin	960.0	E856	E930.0	E950.4	E962.0	E980.4
Adiphenine	975.1	E855.6	E945.1	E950.4	E962.0	E980.4
Adjunct, pharmaceutical	977.4	E858.8	E947.4	E950.4	E962.0	E980.4
Adrenal (extract, cortex or medulla) (glucocorticoids) (hormones) (mineralocorticoids)	962.0	E858.0	E932.0	E950.4	E962.0	E980.4
ENT agent	976.6	E858.7	E946.6	E950.4	E962.0	E980.4
ophthalmic preparation	976.5	E858.7	E946.5	E950.4	E962.0	E980.4

Drug, chemical	Poisoning	External Cause (E Code): Accident	Therapeutic Use	Suicide Attempt	Assault	Undetermined
Adrenal – *continued*						
topical NEC	976.0	E858.7	E946.0	E950.4	E962.0	E980.4
Adrenalin	971.2	E855.5	E941.2	E950.4	E962.0	E980.4
Adrenergic blocking agents	971.3	E855.6	E941.3	E950.4	E962.0	E980.4
Adrenergics	971.2	E855.5	E941.2	E950.4	E962.0	E980.4
Adrenochrome (derivatives)	972.8	E858.3	E942.8	E950.4	E962.0	E980.4
Adrenocorticotropic hormone	962.4	E858.0	E932.4	E950.4	E962.0	E980.4
Adrenocorticotropin	962.4	E858.0	E932.4	E950.4	E962.0	E980.4
Adriamycin	960.7	E856	E930.7	E950.4	E962.0	E980.4
Aerosol spray – *see* Sprays						
Aerosporin	960.8	E856	E930.8	E950.4	E962.0	E980.4
ENT agent	976.6	E858.7	E946.6	E950.4	E962.0	E980.4
ophthalmic preparation	976.5	E858.7	E946.5	E950.4	E962.0	E980.4
topical NEC	976.0	E858.7	E946.0	E950.4	E962.0	E980.4
Aethusa cynapium	988.2	E865.4	–	E950.9	E962.1	E980.9
Afghanistan black	969.6	E854.1	E939.6	E950.3	E962.0	E980.3
Aflatoxin	989.7	E865.9	–	E950.9	E962.1	E980.9
African boxwood	988.2	E865.4	–	E950.9	E962.1	E980.9
Agar (-agar)	973.3	E858.4	E943.3	E950.4	E962.0	E980.4
Agricultural agent NEC	989.89	E863.9	–	E950.6	E962.1	E980.7
Agrypnal	967.0	E851	E937.0	E950.1	E962.0	E980.1
Air contaminant(s), source or type not specified	987.9	E869.9	–	E952.9	E962.2	E982.9
specified type – *see* specific substance						
Akee	988.2	E865.4	–	E950.9	E962.1	E980.9
Akrinol	976.0	E858.7	E946.0	E950.4	E962.0	E980.4
Alantolactone	961.6	E857	E931.6	E950.4	E962.0	E980.4
Albamycin	960.8	E856	E930.8	E950.4	E962.0	E980.4
Albumin (normal human serum)	964.7	E858.2	E934.7	E950.4	E962.0	E980.4
Albuterol	975.7	E858.6	E945.7	E950.4	E962.0	E980.4
Alcohol	980.9	E860.9	–	E950.9	E962.1	E980.9
absolute	980.0	E860.1	–	E950.9	E962.1	E980.9
beverage	980.0	E860.0	E947.8	E950.9	E962.1	E980.9
amyl	980.3	E860.4	–	E950.9	E962.1	E980.9
antifreeze	980.1	E860.2	–	E950.9	E962.1	E980.9
butyl	980.3	E860.4	–	E950.9	E962.1	E980.9
dehydrated	980.0	E860.1	–	E950.9	E862.1	E980.9
beverage	980.0	E860.0	E947.8	E950.9	E962.1	E980.9
denatured	980.0	E860.1	–	E950.9	E962.1	E980.9
deterrents	977.3	E858.8	E947.3	E950.4	E962.0	E980.4
diagnostic (gastric function)	977.8	E858.8	E947.8	E950.4	E962.0	E980.4
ethyl	980.0	E860.1	–	E950.9	E962.1	E980.9
beverage	980.0	E860.0	E947.8	E950.9	E962.1	E980.9
grain	980.0	E860.1	–	E950.9	E962.1	E980.9
beverage	980.0	E860.0	E947.8	E950.9	E962.1	E980.9
industrial	980.9	E860.9	–	E950.9	E962.1	E980.9
isopropyl	980.2	E860.3	–	E950.9	E962.1	E980.9
methyl	980.1	E860.2	–	E950.9	E962.1	E980.9
preparation for consumption	980.0	E860.0	E947.8	E950.9	E962.1	E980.9
propyl	980.3	E860.4	–	E950.9	E962.1	E980.9
secondary	980.2	E860.3	–	E950.9	E962.1	E980.9
radiator	980.1	E860.2	–	E950.9	E962.1	E980.9
rubbing	980.2	E860.3	–	E950.9	E962.1	E980.9
specified type NEC	980.8	E860.8	–	E950.9	E962.1	E980.9
surgical	980.9	E860.9	–	E950.9	E962.1	E980.9
vapor (from any type of alcohol)	987.8	E869.8	–	E952.8	E962.2	E982.8
wood	980.1	E860.2	–	E950.9	E962.1	E980.9
Alcuronium chloride	975.2	E858.6	E945.2	E950.4	E962.0	E980.4
Aldacione	974.4	E858.5	E944.4	E950.4	E962.0	E980.4
Aldicarb	989.3	E863.2	–	E950.6	E962.1	E980.7
Aldomet	972.6	E858.3	E942.6	E950.4	E962.0	E980.4
Aldosterone	962.0	E858.0	E932.0	E950.4	E962.0	E980.4
Aldrin (dust)	989.2	E863.0	–	E950.6	E962.1	E980.7
Algeldrate	973.0	E858.4	E943.0	E950.4	E962.0	E980.4
Alidase	963.4	E858.1	E933.4	E950.4	E962.0	E980.4
Aliphatic thiocyanates	989.0	E866.8	–	E950.9	E962.1	E980.9
Alkaline antiseptic solution (aromatic)	976.6	E858.7	E946.6	E950.4	E962.0	E980.4
Alkalinizing agents (medicinal)	963.3	E858.1	E933.3	E950.4	E962.0	E980.4
Alkalis, caustic	983.2	E864.2	–	E950.7	E962.1	E980.6
Alkalizing agents (medicinal)	963.3	E858.1	E933.3	E950.4	E962.0	E980.4
Alka-seltzer	965.1	E850.3	E935.3	E950.0	E962.0	E980.0
Alkavervir	972.6	E858.3	E942.6	E950.4	E962.0	E980.4
Allegron ▲	969.05	E854.0	E939.0	E950.3	E962.0	E980.3
Alleve - *see* Naproxen						
Allobarbital, allobarbitone	967.0	E851	E937.0	E950.1	E962.0	E980.1
Allopurinol	974.7	E858.5	E944.7	E950.4	E962.0	E980.4
Allylestrenol	962.2	E858.0	E932.2	E950.4	E962.0	E980.4
Allylisopropylacetylurea	967.8	E852.8	E937.8	E950.2	E962.0	E980.2
Allylisopropylmalonylurea	967.0	E851	E937.0	E950.1	E962.0	E980.1
Allyltribromide	967.3	E852.2	E937.3	E950.2	E962.0	E980.2

Drug, chemical	Poisoning	External Cause (E Code)				
		Accident	Therapeutic Use	Suicide Attempt	Assault	Undetermined
Aloe, aloes, aloin	973.1	E858.4	E943.1	E950.4	E962.0	E980.4
Alosetron	973.8	E858.4	E943.8	E950.4	E962.0	E980.4
Aloxidone	966.0	E855.0	E936.0	E950.4	E962.0	E980.4
Aloxiprin	965.1	E850.3	E935.3	E950.0	E962.0	E980.0
Alpha-1 blockers	971.3	E855.6	E941.3	E950.4	E962.0	E980.4
Alpha amylase	963.4	E858.1	E933.4	E950.4	E962.0	E980.4
Alphaprodine (hydrochloride)	965.09	E850.2	E935.2	E950.0	E962.0	E980.0
Alpha tocopherol	963.5	E858.1	E933.5	E950.4	E962.0	E980.4
Alseroxylon	972.6	E858.3	E942.6	E950.4	E962.0	E980.4
Alum (ammonium) (potassium)	983.2	E864.2	–	E950.7	E962.1	E980.6
medicinal (astringent) NEC	976.2	E858.7	E946.2	E950.4	E962.0	E980.4
Aluminium, aluminum (gel) (hydroxide)	973.0	E858.4	E943.0	E950.4	E962.0	E980.4
acetate solution	976.2	E858.7	E946.2	E950.4	E962.0	E980.4
aspirin	965.1	E850.3	E935.3	E950.0	E962.0	E980.0
carbonate	973.0	E858.4	E943.0	E950.4	E962.0	E980.4
glycinate	973.0	E858.4	E943.0	E950.4	E962.0	E980.4
nicotinate	972.2	E858.3	E942.2	E950.4	E962.0	E980.4
ointment (surgical) (topical)	976.3	E858.7	E946.3	E950.4	E962.0	E980.4
phosphate	973.0	E858.4	E943.0	E950.4	E962.0	E980.4
subacetate	976.2	E858.7	E946.2	E950.4	E962.0	E980.4
topical NEC	976.3	E858.7	E946.3	E950.4	E962.0	E980.4
Alurate	967.0	E851	E937.0	E950.1	E962.0	E980.1
Alverine (citrate)	975.1	E858.6	E945.1	E950.4	E962.0	E980.4
Alvodine	965.09	E850.2	E935.2	E950.0	E962.0	E980.0
Amanita phalloides	988.1	E865.5	–	E950.9	E962.1	E980.9
Amantadine (hydrochloride)	966.4	E855.0	E936.4	E950.4	E962.0	E980.4
Ambazone	961.9	E857	E931.9	E950.4	E962.0	E980.4
Ambenonium	971.0	E855.3	E941.0	E950.4	E962.0	E980.4
Ambutonium bromide	971.1	E855.4	E941.1	E950.4	E962.0	E980.4
Ametazole	977.8	E858.8	E947.8	E950.4	E962.0	E980.4
Amethocaine (infiltration) (topical)	968.5	E855.2	E938.5	E950.4	E962.0	E980.4
nerve block (peripheral) (plexus)	968.6	E855.2	E938.6	E950.4	E962.0	E980.4
spinal	968.7	E855.2	E938.7	E950.4	E962.0	E980.4
Amethopterin	963.1	E858.1	E933.1	E950.4	E962.0	E980.4
Amfepramone	977.0	E858.8	E947.0	E950.4	E962.0	E980.4
Amidon	965.02	E850.1	E935.1	E950.0	E962.0	E980.0
Amidopyrine	965.5	E850.5	E935.5	E950.0	E962.0	E980.0
Aminacrine	976.0	E858.7	E946.0	E950.4	E962.0	E980.4
Aminitrozole	961.5	E857	E931.5	E950.4	E962.0	E980.4
Aminoacetic acid	974.5	E858.5	E944.5	E950.4	E962.0	E980.4
Amino acids	974.5	E858.5	E944.5	E950.4	E962.0	E980.4
Aminocaproic acid	964.4	E858.2	E934.4	E950.4	E962.0	E980.4
Aminoethylisothiourium	963.8	E858.1	E933.8	E950.4	E962.0	E980.4
Aminoglutethimide	966.3	E855.0	E936.3	E950.4	E962.0	E980.4
Aminometradine	974.3	E858.5	E944.3	E950.4	E962.0	E980.4
Aminopentamide	971.1	E855.4	E941.1	E950.4	E962.0	E980.4
Aminophenazone	965.5	E850.5	E935.5	E950.0	E962.0	E980.0
Aminophenol	983.0	E864.0	–	E950.7	E962.1	E980.6
Aminophenylpyridone	969.5	E853.8	E939.5	E950.3	E962.0	E980.3
Aminophyllin	975.7	E858.6	E945.7	E950.4	E962.0	E980.4
Aminopterin	963.1	E858.1	E933.1	E950.4	E962.0	E980.4
Aminopyrine	965.5	E850.5	E935.5	E950.0	E962.0	E980.0
Aminosalicylic acid	961.8	E857	E931.8	E950.4	E962.0	E980.4
Amiphenazole	970.1	E854.3	E940.1	E950.4	E962.0	E980.4
Amiquinsin	972.6	E858.3	E942.6	E950.4	E962.0	E980.4
Amisometradine	974.3	E858.5	E944.3	E950.4	E962.0	E980.4
Amitriptyline ▲	969.05	E854.0	E939.0	E950.3	E962.0	E980.3
Ammonia (fumes) (gas) (vapor)	987.8	E869.8	–	E952.8	E962.2	E982.8
liquid (household) NEC	983.2	E861.4	–	E950.7	E962.1	E980.6
spirit, aromatic	970.8	E854.3	E940.8	E950.4	E962.0	E980.4
Ammoniated mercury	976.0	E858.7	E946.0	E950.4	E962.0	E980.4
Ammonium						
carbonate	983.2	E864.2	–	E950.7	E962.1	E980.6
chloride (acidifying agent)	963.2	E858.1	E933.2	E950.4	E962.0	E980.4
expectorant	975.5	E858.6	E945.5	E950.4	E962.0	E980.4
compounds (household) NEC	983.2	E861.4	–	E950.7	E962.1	E980.6
fumes (any usage)	987.8	E869.8	–	E952.8	E962.2	E982.8
industrial	983.2	E864.2	–	E950.7	E962.1	E980.6
ichthyosulronate	976.4	E858.7	E946.4	E950.4	E962.0	E980.4
mandelate	961.9	E857	E931.9	E950.4	E962.0	E980.4
Amobarbital	967.0	E851	E937.0	E950.1	E962.0	E980.1
Amodiaquin(e)	961.4	E857	E931.4	E950.4	E962.0	E980.4
Amopyroquin(e)	961.4	E857	E931.4	E950.4	E962.0	E980.4
Amphenidone	969.5	E853.8	E939.5	E950.3	E962.0	E980.3
Amphetamine ▲	969.72	E854.2	E939.7	E950.3	E962.0	E980.3
Amphomycin	960.8	E856	E930.8	E950.4	E962.0	E980.4
Amphotericin B	960.1	E856	E930.1	E950.4	E962.0	E980.4
topical	976.0	E858.7	E946.0	E950.4	E962.0	E980.4
Ampicillin	960.0	E856	E930.0	E950.4	E962.0	E980.4
Amprotropine	971.1	E855.4	E941.1	E950.4	E962.0	E980.4
Amygdalin	977.8	E858.8	E947.8	E950.4	E962.0	E980.4
Amyl						
acetate (vapor)	982.8	E862.4	–	E950.9	E962.1	E980.9
alcohol	980.3	E860.4	–	E950.9	E962.1	E980.9
nitrite (medicinal)	972.4	E858.3	E942.4	E950.4	E962.0	E980.4
Amylase (alpha)	963.4	E858.1	E933.4	E950.4	E962.0	E980.4
Amylene hydrate	980.8	E860.8	–	E950.9	E962.1	E980.9
Amylobarbitone	967.0	E851	E937.0	E950.1	E962.0	E980.1
Amylocaine	968.9	E855.2	E938.9	E950.4	E962.0	E980.4
infiltration (subcutaneous)	968.5	E855.2	E938.5	E950.4	E962.0	E980.4
nerve block (peripheral) (plexus)	968.6	E855.2	E938.6	E950.4	E962.0	E980.4
spinal	968.7	E855.2	E938.7	E950.4	E962.0	E980.4
topical (surface)	968.5	E855.2	E938.5	E950.4	E962.0	E980.4
Amytal (sodium)	967.0	E851	E937.0	E950.1	E962.0	E980.1
Analeptics	970.0	E854.3	E940.0	E950.4	E962.0	E980.4
Analgesics	965.9	E850.9	E935.9	E950.0	E962.0	E980.0
aromatic NEC	965.4	E850.4	E935.4	E950.0	E962.0	E980.0
non-narcotic NEC	965.7	E850.7	E935.7	E950.0	E962.0	E980.0
specified NEC	965.8	E850.8	E935.8	E950.0	E962.0	E980.0
Anamirta cocculus	988.2	E865.3	–	E950.9	E962.1	E980.9
Ancillin	960.0	E856	E930.0	E950.4	E962.0	E980.4
Androgens (anabolic congeners)	962.1	E858.0	E932.1	E950.4	E962.0	E980.4
Androstalone	962.1	E858.0	E932.1	E950.4	E962.0	E980.4
Androsterone	962.1	E858.0	E932.1	E950.4	E962.0	E980.4
Anemone pulsatilla	988.2	E865.4	–	E950.9	E962.1	E980.9
Anesthesia, anesthetic (general) NEC	968.4	E855.1	E938.4	E950.4	E962.0	E980.4
block (nerve) (plexus)	968.6	E855.2	E938.6	E950.4	E962.0	E980.4
gaseous NEC	968.2	E855.1	E938.2	E950.4	E962.0	E980.4
halogenated hydrocarbon derivatives NEC	968.2	E855.1	E938.2	E950.4	E962.0	E980.4
infiltration (intradermal) (subcutaneous) (submucosal)	968.5	E855.2	E938.5	E950.4	E962.0	E980.4
intravenous	968.3	E855.1	E938.3	E950.4	E962.0	E980.4
local NEC	968.9	E855.2	E938.9	E950.4	E962.0	E980.4
nerve blocking (peripheral) (plexus)	968.6	E855.2	E938.6	E950.4	E962.0	E980.4
rectal NEC	968.3	E855.1	E938.3	E950.4	E962.0	E980.4
spinal	968.7	E855.2	E938.7	E950.4	E962.0	E980.4
surface	968.5	E855.2	E938.5	E950.4	E962.0	E980.4
topical	968.5	E855.2	E938.5	E950.4	E962.0	E980.4
Aneurine	963.5	E858.1	E933.5	E950.4	E962.0	E980.4
Anginine - *see* Glyceryl trinitrate	971.2	E855.5	E941.2	E950.4	E962.0	E980.4
Angio-Conray	977.8	E858.8	E947.8	E950.4	E962.0	E980.4
Angiotensin	971.2	E855.5	E941.2	E950.4	E962.0	E980.4
Anhydrohydroxyprogesterone	962.2	E858.0	E932.2	E950.4	E962.0	E980.4
Anhydron	974.3	E858.5	E944.3	E950.4	E962.0	E980.4
Anileridine	965.09	E850.2	E935.2	E950.0	E962.0	E980.0
Aniline (dye) (liquid)	983.0	E864.0	–	E950.7	E962.1	E980.6
analgesic	965.4	E850.4	E935.4	E950.0	E962.0	E980.0
derivatives, therapeutic NEC	965.4	E850.4	E935.4	E950.0	E962.0	E980.0
vapor	987.8	E869.8	–	E952.8	E962.2	E982.8
Anisindione	964.2	E858.2	E934.2	E950.4	E962.0	E980.4
Aniscoropine	971.1	E855.4	E941.1	E950.4	E962.0	E980.4
Anorexic agents	977.0	E858.8	E947.0	E950.4	E962.0	E980.4
Ant (bite) (sting)	989.5	E905.5	–	E950.9	E962.1	E980.9
Antabuse	977.3	E858.8	E947.3	E950.4	E962.0	E980.4
Antacids	973.0	E858.4	E943.0	E950.4	E962.0	E980.4
Antazoline	963.0	E858.1	E933.0	E950.4	E962.0	E980.4
Anthelmintics	961.6	E857	E931.6	E950.4	E962.0	E980.4
Anthralin	976.4	E858.7	E946.4	E950.4	E962.0	E980.4
Anthramycin	960.7	E856	E930.7	E950.4	E962.0	E980.4
Antiadrenergics	971.3	E855.6	E941.3	E950.4	E962.0	E980.4
Antiallergic agents	963.0	E858.1	E933.0	E950.4	E962.0	E980.4
Antianemic agents NEC	964.1	E858.2	E934.1	E950.4	E962.0	E980.4
Antiaris toxicaria	988.2	E865.4	–	E950.9	E962.1	E980.9
Antiarteriesclerotic agents	972.2	E858.3	E942.2	E950.4	E962.0	E980.4
Antiasthmatics	975.7	E858.6	E945.7	E950.4	E962.0	E980.4
Antibiotics	960.9	E856	E930.9	E950.4	E962.0	E980.4
antifungal	960.1	E856	E930.1	E950.4	E962.0	E980.4
antimycobacterial	960.6	E856	E930.6	E950.4	E962.0	E980.4
antineoplastic	960.7	E856	E930.7	E950.4	E962.0	E980.4
cephalosporin (group)	960.5	E856	E930.5	E950.4	E962.0	E980.4
chloramphenicol (group)	960.2	E856	E930.2	E950.4	E962.0	E980.4
macrolides	960.3	E856	E930.3	E950.4	E962.0	E980.4
specified NEC	960.8	E856	E930.8	E950.4	E962.0	E980.4
tetracycline (group)	960.4	E856	E930.4	E950.4	E962.0	E980.4
Anticancer agents NEC	963.1	E858.1	E933.1	E950.4	E962.0	E980.4
antibiotics	960.7	E856	E930.7	E950.4	E962.0	E980.4
Anticholinergics	971.1	E855.4	E941.1	E950.4	E962.0	E980.4
Anticholinesterase (organo-phosphorus) (reversible)	971.0	E855.3	E941.0	E950.4	E962.0	E980.4

Drug, chemical	Poisoning	External Cause (E Code)				
		Accident	Therapeutic Use	Suicide Attempt	Assault	Undetermined
Anticoagulants	964.2	E858.2	E934.2	E950.4	E962.0	E980.4
antagonists	964.5	E858.2	E934.5	E950.4	E962.0	E980.4
Anti-common cold agents NEC	975.6	E858.6	E945.6	E950.4	E962.0	E980.4
Anticonvulsants NEC	966.3	E855.0	E936.3	E950.4	E962.0	E980.4
Antidepressants ▲	969.00	E854.0	E939.0	E950.3	E962.0	E980.3
monoamine oxidase inhibitors (MAOI) ●	969.01	E854.0	E939.0	E950.3	E962.0	E980.3
specified type NEC ●	969.09	E854.0	E939.0	E950.3	E962.0	E980.3
SSNRI (selective serotonin and norepinephrine reuptake inhibitors) ●	969.02	E854.0	E939.0	E950.3	E962.0	E980.3
SSRI (selective serotonin reuptake inhibitors) ●	969.03	E854.0	E939.0	E950.3	E962.0	E980.3
tetracyclic ●	969.04	E854.0	E939.0	E950.3	E962.0	E980.3
tricyclic ●	969.05	E854.0	E939.0	E950.3	E962.0	E980.3
Antidiabetic agents	962.3	E858.0	E932.3	E950.4	E962.0	E980.4
Antidiarrheal agents	973.5	E858.4	E943.5	E950.4	E962.0	E980.4
Antidiuretic hormone	962.5	E858.0	E932.5	E950.4	E962.0	E980.4
Antidotes NEC	977.2	E858.8	E947.2	E950.4	E962.0	E980.4
Antiemetic agents	963.0	E858.1	E933.0	E950.4	E962.0	E980.4
Antiepilepsy agent NEC	966.3	E855.0	E936.3	E950.4	E962.0	E980.4
Antifertility pills	962.2	E858.0	E932.2	E950.4	E962.0	E980.4
Antiflatulents	973.8	E858.4	E943.8	E950.4	E962.0	E980.4
Antifreeze	989.89	E866.8	–	E950.9	E962.1	E980.9
alcohol	980.1	E860.2	–	E950.9	E962.1	E980.9
ethylene glycol	982.8	E862.4	–	E950.9	E962.1	E980.9
Antifungals (nonmedicinal) (sprays)	989.4	E863.6	–	E950.6	E962.1	E980.7
medicinal NEC	961.9	E857	E931.9	E950.4	E962.0	E980.4
antibiotic	960.1	E856	E930.1	E950.4	E962.0	E980.4
topical	976.0	E858.7	E946.0	E950.4	E962.0	E980.4
Antigastric secretion agents	973.0	E858.4	E943.0	E950.4	E962.0	E980.4
Antihelmintics	961.6	E857	E931.6	E950.4	E962.0	E980.4
Antihemophilic factor (human)	964.7	E858.2	E934.7	E950.4	E962.0	E980.4
Antihistamine	963.0	E858.1	E933.0	E950.4	E962.0	E980.4
Antihypertensive agents NEC	972.6	E858.3	E942.6	E950.4	E962.0	E980.4
Anti-infectives NEC	961.9	E857	E931.9	E950.4	E962.0	E980.4
antibiotics	960.9	E856	E930.9	E950.4	E962.0	E980.4
specified NEC	960.8	E856	E930.8	E950.4	E962.0	E980.4
anthelmintic	961.6	E857	E931.6	E950.4	E962.0	E980.4
antimalarial	961.4	E857	E931.4	E950.4	E962.0	E980.4
antimycobacterial NEC	961.8	E857	E931.8	E950.4	E962.0	E980.4
antibiotics	960.6	E856	E930.6	E950.4	E962.0	E980.4
antiprotozoal NEC	961.5	E857	E931.5	E950.4	E962.0	E980.4
blood	961.4	E857	E931.4	E950.4	E962.0	E980.4
antiviral	961.7	E857	E931.7	E950.4	E962.0	E980.4
arsenical	961.1	E857	E931.1	E950.4	E962.0	E980.4
ENT agents	976.6	E858.7	E946.6	E950.4	E962.0	E980.4
heavy metals NEC	961.2	E857	E931.2	E950.4	E962.0	E980.4
local	976.0	E858.7	E946.0	E950.4	E962.0	E980.4
ophthalmic preparation	976.5	E858.7	E946.5	E950.4	E962.0	E980.4
topical NEC	976.0	E858.7	E946.0	E950.4	E962.0	E980.4
Anti-inflammatory agents (topical)	976.0	E858.7	E946.0	E950.4	E962.0	E980.4
Antiknock (tetraethyl lead)	984.1	E862.1	–	E950.9	E962.1	E980.9
Antilipemics	972.2	E858.3	E942.2	E950.4	E962.0	E980.4
Antimalarials	961.4	E857	E931.4	E950.4	E962.0	E980.4
Antimony (compounds) (vapor) NEC	985.4	E866.2	–	E950.9	E962.1	E980.9
anti-infectives	961.2	E857	E931.2	E950.4	E962.0	E980.4
pesticides (vapor)	985.4	E863.4	–	E950.6	E962.2	E980.7
potassium tartrate	961.2	E857	E931.2	E950.4	E962.0	E980.4
tartrated	961.2	E857	E931.2	E950.4	E962.0	E980.4
Antimuscarinic agents	971.1	E855.4	E941.1	E950.4	E962.0	E980.4
Antimycobacterials NEC	961.8	E857	E931.8	E950.4	E962.0	E980.4
antibiotics	960.6	E856	E930.6	E950.4	E962.0	E980.4
Antineoplastic agents	963.1	E858.1	E933.1	E950.4	E962.0	E980.4
antibiotics	960.7	E856	E930.7	E950.4	E962.0	E980.4
Anti-Parkinsonism agents	966.4	E855.0	E936.4	E950.4	E962.0	E980.4
Antiphlogistics	965.69	E850.6	E935.6	E950.0	E962.0	E980.0
Antiprotozoals NEC	961.5	E857	E931.5	E950.4	E962.0	E980.4
blood	961.4	E857	E931.4	E950.4	E962.0	E980.4
Antipruritics (local)	976.1	E858.7	E946.1	E950.4	E962.0	E980.4
Antipsychotic agents NEC	969.3	E853.8	E939.3	E950.3	E962.0	E980.3
Antipyretics	965.9	E850.9	E935.9	E950.0	E962.0	E980.0
specified NEC	965.8	E850.8	E935.8	E950.0	E962.0	E980.0
Antipyrine	965.5	E850.5	E935.5	E950.0	E962.0	E980.0
Antirabies serum (equine)	979.9	E858.8	E949.9	E950.4	E962.0	E980.4
Antirheumatics	965.69	E850.6	E935.6	E950.0	E962.0	E980.0
Antiseborrheics	976.4	E858.7	E946.4	E950.4	E962.0	E980.4
Antiseptics (external) (medicinal)	976.0	E858.7	E946.0	E950.4	E962.0	E980.4
Antistine	963.0	E858.1	E933.0	E950.4	E962.0	E980.4
Antithyroid agents	962.8	E858.0	E932.8	E950.4	E962.0	E980.4
Antitoxin, any	979.9	E858.8	E949.9	E950.4	E962.0	E980.4

Drug, chemical	Poisoning	External Cause (E Code)				
		Accident	Therapeutic Use	Suicide Attempt	Assault	Undetermined
Antituberculars	961.8	E857	E931.8	E950.4	E962.0	E980.4
antibiotics	960.6	E856	E930.6	E950.4	E962.0	E980.4
Antitussives	975.4	E858.6	E945.4	E950.4	E962.0	E980.4
Antivaricose agents (sclerosing)	972.7	E858.3	E942.7	E950.4	E962.0	E980.4
Antivenin (crotaline) (spider-bite)	979.9	E858.8	E949.9	E950.4	E962.0	E980.4
Antivert	963.0	E858.1	E933.0	E950.4	E962.0	E980.4
Antivirals NEC	961.7	E857	E931.7	E950.4	E962.0	E980.4
Ant poisons – *see* Pesticides						
Antrol	989.4	E863.4	–	E950.6	E962.1	E980.7
fungicide	989.4	E863.6	–	E950.6	E962.1	E980.7
Apomorphine hydrochloride (emetic)	973.6	E858.4	E943.6	E950.4	E962.0	E980.4
Appetite depressants, central	977.0	E858.8	E947.0	E950.4	E962.0	E980.4
Apresoline	972.6	E858.3	E942.6	E950.4	E962.0	E980.4
Aprobarbital, aprobarbitone	967.0	E851	E937.0	E950.1	E962.0	E980.1
Apronalide	967.8	E852.8	E937.8	E950.2	E962.0	E980.2
Aqua fortis	983.1	E864.1	–	E950.7	E962.1	E980.6
Arachis oil (topical)	976.3	E858.7	E946.3	E950.4	E962.0	E980.4
cathartic	973.2	E858.4	E943.2	E950.4	E962.0	E980.4
Aralen	961.4	E857	E931.4	E950.4	E962.0	E980.4
Arginine salts	974.5	E858.5	E944.5	E950.4	E962.0	E980.4
Argyrol	976.0	E858.7	E946.0	E950.4	E962.0	E980.4
ENT agent	976.6	E858.7	E946.6	E950.4	E962.0	E980.4
ophthalmic preparation	976.5	E858.7	E946.5	E950.4	E962.0	E980.4
Aristocort	962.0	E858.0	E932.0	E950.4	E962.0	E980.4
ENT agent	976.6	E858.7	E946.6	E950.4	E962.0	E980.4
ophthalmic preparation	976.5	E858.7	E946.5	E950.4	E962.0	E980.4
topical NEC	976.0	E858.7	E946.0	E950.4	E962.0	E980.4
Aromatics, corrosive	983.0	E864.0	–	E950.7	E962.1	E980.6
disinfectants	983.0	E861.4	–	E950.7	E962.1	E980.6
Arsenate of lead (insecticide)	985.1	E863.4	–	E950.8	E962.1	E980.8
herbicide	985.1	E863.5	–	E950.8	E962.1	E980.8
Arsenic, arsenicals (compounds) (dust) (fumes) (vapor) NEC	985.1	E866.3	–	E950.8	E962.1	E980.8
anti-infectives	961.1	E857	E931.1	E950.4	E962.0	E980.4
pesticide (dust) (fumes)	985.1	E863.4	–	E950.8	E962.1	E980.8
Arsine (gas)	985.1	E866.3	–	E950.8	E962.1	E980.8
Arsphenamine (silver)	961.1	E857	E931.1	E950.4	E962.0	E980.4
Arsthinol	961.1	E857	E931.1	E950.4	E962.0	E980.4
Artane	971.1	E855.4	E941.1	E950.4	E962.0	E980.4
Arthropod (venomous) NEC	989.5	E905.5	–	E950.9	E962.1	E980.9
Asbestos	989.81	E866.8	–	E950.9	E962.1	E980.9
Ascaridole	961.6	E857	E931.6	E950.4	E962.0	E980.4
Ascorbic acid	963.5	E858.1	E933.5	E950.4	E962.0	E980.4
Asiaticoside	976.0	E858.7	E946.0	E950.4	E962.0	E980.4
Aspidium (oleoresin)	961.6	E857	E931.6	E950.4	E962.0	E980.4
Aspirin	965.1	E850.3	E935.3	E950.0	E962.0	E980.0
Astringents (local)	976.2	E858.7	E946.2	E950.4	E962.0	E980.4
Atabrine	961.3	E857	E931.3	E950.4	E962.0	E980.4
Ataractics	969.5	E853.8	E939.5	E950.3	E962.0	E980.3
Atonia drug, intestinal	973.3	E858.4	E943.3	E950.4	E962.0	E980.4
Atophan	974.7	E858.5	E944.7	E950.4	E962.0	E980.4
Atropine	971.1	E855.4	E941.1	E950.4	E962.0	E980.4
Attapulgite	973.5	E858.4	E943.5	E950.4	E962.0	E980.4
Attenuvaxe	979.4	E858.8	E949.4	E950.4	E962.0	E980.4
Aureomycin	960.4	E856	E930.4	E950.4	E962.0	E980.4
ophthalmic preparation	976.5	E858.7	E946.5	E950.4	E962.0	E980.4
topical NEC	976.0	E858.7	E946.0	E950.4	E962.0	E980.4
Aurothioglucose	965.69	E850.6	E935.6	E950.0	E962.0	E980.0
Aurothioglycanide	965.69	E850.6	E935.6	E950.0	E962.0	E980.0
Aurothiomalate	965.69	E850.6	E935.6	E950.0	E962.0	E980.0
Automobile fuel	981	E862.1	–	E950.9	E962.1	E980.9
Autonomic nervous system agents NEC	971.9	E855.9	E941.9	E950.4	E962.0	E980.4
Avlosulfon	961.8	E857	E931.8	E950.4	E962.0	E980.4
Avomine	967.8	E852.8	E937.8	E950.2	E962.0	E980.2
Azacyclonol	969.5	E853.8	E939.5	E950.3	E962.0	E980.3
Azapetine	971.3	E855.6	E941.3	E950.4	E962.0	E980.4
Azaribine	963.1	E858.1	E933.1	E950.4	E962.0	E980.4
Azaserine	960.7	E856	E930.7	E950.4	E962.0	E980.4
Azathioprine	963.1	E858.1	E933.1	E950.4	E962.0	E980.4
Azosulfamide	961.0	E857	E931.0	E950.4	E962.0	E980.4
Azulfidine	961.0	E857	E931.0	E950.4	E962.0	E980.4
Azuresin	977.8	E858.8	E947.8	E950.4	E962.0	E980.4
Bacimycin	976.0	E858.7	E946.0	E950.4	E962.0	E980.4
ophthalmic preparation	976.5	E858.7	E946.5	E950.4	E962.0	E980.4
Bacitracin	960.8	E856	E930.8	E950.4	E962.0	E980.4
ENT agent	976.6	E858.7	E946.6	E950.4	E962.0	E980.4
ophthalmic preparation	976.5	E858.7	E946.5	E950.4	E962.0	E980.4
topical NEC	976.0	E858.7	E946.0	E950.4	E962.0	E980.4
Baking soda	963.3	E858.1	E933.3	E950.4	E962.0	E980.4
BAL	963.8	E858.1	E933.8	E950.4	E962.0	E980.4

4th Fourth Digit Required 5th Fifth Digit Required | *[code]* Manifestation Code | ● New Line ▲ Revised Line text New Text ~~text~~ Deleted text

Drug, chemical	Poisoning	External Cause (E Code) Accident	Therapeutic Use	Suicide Attempt	Assault	Undetermined
Bamethan (sulfate)	972.5	E858.3	E942.5	E950.4	E962.0	E980.4
Bamipine	963.0	E858.1	E933.0	E950.4	E962.0	E980.4
Baneberry	988.2	E865.4	–	E950.9	E962.1	E980.9
Banewort	988.2	E865.4	–	E950.9	E962.1	E980.9
Barbenyl	967.0	E851	E937.0	E950.1	E962.0	E980.1
Barbital, barbitone	967.0	E851	E937.0	E950.1	E962.0	E980.1
Barbiturates, barbituric acid	967.0	E851	E937.0	E950.1	E962.0	E980.1
anesthetic (intravenous)	968.3	E855.1	E938.3	E950.4	E962.0	E980.4
Barium (carbonate) (chloride) (sulfate)	985.8	E866.4	–	E950.9	E962.1	E980.9
diagnostic agent	977.8	E858.8	E947.8	E950.4	E962.0	E980.4
pesticide	985.8	E863.4	–	E950.6	E962.1	E980.7
rodenticide	985.8	E863.7	–	E950.6	E962.1	E980.7
Barrier cream	976.3	E858.7	E946.3	E950.4	E962.0	E980.4
Battery acid or fluid	983.1	E864.1	–	E950.7	E962.1	E980.6
Bay rum	980.8	E860.8	–	E950.9	E962.1	E980.9
BCG vaccine	978.0	E858.8	E948.0	E950.4	E962.0	E980.4
Bearsfoot	988.2	E865.4	–	E950.9	E962.1	E980.9
Beclamide	966.3	E855.0	E936.3	E950.4	E962.0	E980.4
Bee (sting) (venom)	989.5	E905.3	–	E950.9	E962.1	E980.9
Belladonna (alkaloids)	971.1	E855.4	E941.1	E950.4	E962.0	E980.4
Bemegride	970.0	E854.3	E940.0	E950.4	E962.0	E980.4
Benactyzine	969.8	E855.8	E939.8	E950.3	E962.0	E980.3
Benadryl	963.0	E858.1	E933.0	E950.4	E962.0	E980.4
Bendrofluazide	974.3	E858.5	E944.3	E950.4	E962.0	E980.4
Bendroflumethiazide	974.3	E858.5	E944.3	E950.4	E962.0	E980.4
Benemid	974.7	E858.5	E944.7	E950.4	E962.0	E980.4
Benethamine penicillin G	960.0	E856	E930.0	E950.4	E962.0	E980.4
Benisone	976.0	E858.7	E946.0	E950.4	E962.0	E980.4
Benoquin	976.8	E858.7	E946.8	E950.4	E962.0	E980.4
Benoxinate	968.5	E855.2	E938.5	E950.4	E962.0	E980.4
Bentonite	976.3	E858.7	E946.3	E950.4	E962.0	E980.4
Benzalkonium (chloride)	976.0	E858.7	E946.0	E950.4	E962.0	E980.4
ophthalmic preparation	976.5	E858.7	E946.5	E950.4	E962.0	E980.4
Benzamidosalicylate (calcium)	961.8	E857	E931.8	E950.4	E962.0	E980.4
Benzathine penicillin	960.0	E856	E930.0	E950.4	E962.0	E980.4
Benzcarbimine	963.1	E858.1	E933.1	E950.4	E962.0	E980.4
Benzedrex	971.2	E855.5	E941.2	E950.4	E962.0	E980.4
Benzedrine (amphetamine) ▲	969.72	E854.2	E939.7	E950.3	E962.0	E980.3
Benzene (acetyl) (dimethyl) (methyl) (solvent) (vapor)	982.0	E862.4	–	E950.9	E962.1	E980.9
hexachloride (gamma) (insecticide) (vapor)	989.2	E863.0	–	E950.6	E962.1	E980.7
Benzethonium	976.0	E858.7	E946.0	E950.4	E962.0	E980.4
Benzhexol (chloride)	966.4	E855.0	E936.4	E950.4	E962.0	E980.4
Benzilonium	971.1	E855.4	E941.1	E950.4	E962.0	E980.4
Benzin(e) – *see* Ligroin						
Benziodarone	972.4	E858.3	E942.4	E950.4	E962.0	E980.4
Benzocaine	968.5	E855.2	E938.5	E950.4	E962.0	E980.4
Benzodiapin	969.4	E853.2	E939.4	E950.3	E962.0	E980.3
Benzodiazepines (tranquilizers) NEC	969.4	E853.2	E939.4	E950.3	E962.0	E980.3
Benzoic acid (with salicylic acid) (anti-infective)	976.0	E858.7	E946.0	E950.4	E962.0	E980.4
Benzoin	976.3	E858.7	E946.3	E950.4	E962.0	E980.4
Benzol (vapor)	982.0	E862.4	–	E950.9	E962.1	E980.9
Benzomorphan	965.09	E850.2	E935.2	E950.0	E962.0	E980.0
Benzonatate	975.4	E858.6	E945.4	E950.4	E962.0	E980.4
Benzothiadiazides	974.3	E858.5	E944.3	E950.4	E962.0	E980.4
Benzoylpas	961.8	E857	E931.8	E950.4	E962.0	E980.4
Benzperidol	969.5	E853.8	E939.5	E950.3	E962.0	E980.3
Benzphetamine	977.0	E858.8	E947.0	E950.4	E962.0	E980.4
Benzpyrinium	971.0	E855.3	E941.0	E950.4	E962.0	E980.4
Benzquinamide	963.0	E858.1	E933.0	E950.4	E962.0	E980.4
Benzthiazide	974.3	E858.5	E944.3	E950.4	E962.0	E980.4
Benztropine	971.1	E855.4	E941.1	E950.4	E962.0	E980.4
Benzyl						
acetate	982.8	E862.4	–	E950.9	E962.1	E980.9
benzoate (anti-infective)	976.0	E858.7	E946.0	E950.4	E962.0	E980.4
morphine	965.09	E850.2	E935.2	E950.0	E962.0	E980.0
penicillin	960.0	E856	E930.0	E950.4	E962.0	E980.4
Bephenium hydroxynapthoate	961.6	E857	E931.6	E950.4	E962.0	E980.4
Bergamot oil	989.89	E866.8	–	E950.9	E962.1	E980.9
Berries, poisonous	988.2	E865.3	–	E950.9	E962.1	E980.9
Beryllium (compounds) (fumes)	985.3	E866.4	–	E950.9	E962.1	E980.9
Beta-carotene	976.3	E858.7	E946.3	E950.4	E962.0	E980.4
Beta-Chlor	967.1	E852.0	E937.1	E950.2	E962.0	E980.2
Betamethasone	962.0	E858.0	E932.0	E950.4	E962.0	E980.4
topical	976.0	E858.7	E946.0	E950.4	E962.0	E980.4
Betazole	977.8	E858.8	E947.8	E950.4	E962.0	E980.4
Bethanechol	971.0	E855.3	E941.0	E950.4	E962.0	E980.4

Drug, chemical	Poisoning	External Cause (E Code) Accident	Therapeutic Use	Suicide Attempt	Assault	Undetermined
Bethanidine	972.6	E858.3	E942.6	E950.4	E962.0	E980.4
Betula oil	976.3	E858.7	E946.3	E950.4	E962.0	E980.4
Bhang	969.6	E854.1	E939.6	E950.3	E962.0	E980.3
Bialamicol	961.5	E857	E931.5	E950.4	E962.0	E980.4
Bichloride of mercury – *see* Mercury, chloride						
Bichromates (calcium) (crystals) (potassium) (sodium)	983.9	E864.3	–	E950.7	E962.1	E980.6
fumes	987.8	E869.8	–	E952.8	E962.2	E982.8
Biguanide derivatives, oral	962.3	E858.0	E932.3	E950.4	E962.0	E980.4
Biligrafin	977.8	E858.8	E947.8	E950.4	E962.0	E980.4
Bilopaque	977.8	E858.8	E947.8	E950.4	E962.0	E980.4
Bioflavonoids	972.8	E858.3	E942.8	E950.4	E962.0	E980.4
Biological substance NEC	979.9	E858.8	E949.9	E950.4	E962.0	E980.4
Biperiden	966.4	E855.0	E936.4	E950.4	E962.0	E980.4
Bisacodyl	973.1	E858.4	E943.1	E950.4	E962.0	E980.4
Bishydroxycoumarin	964.2	E858.2	E934.2	E950.4	E962.0	E980.4
Bismarsen	961.1	E857	E931.1	E950.4	E962.0	E980.4
Bismuth (compounds) NEC	985.8	E866.4	–	E950.9	E962.1	E980.9
anti-infectives	961.2	E857	E931.2	E950.4	E962.0	E980.4
subcarbonate	973.5	E858.4	E943.5	E950.4	E962.0	E980.4
sulfarsphenamine	961.1	E857	E931.1	E950.4	E962.0	E980.4
Bisphosphonates						
intravenous	963.1	E858.1	E933.7	E950.4	E962.0	E980.4
oral	963.1	E858.1	E933.6	E950.4	E962.0	E980.4
Bithionol	961.6	E857	E931.6	E950.4	E962.0	E980.4
Bitter almond oil	989.0	E866.8	–	E950.9	E962.1	E980.9
Bittersweet	988.2	E865.4	–	E950.9	E962.1	E930.9
Black						
flag	989.4	E863.4	–	E950.6	E962.1	E980.7
henbane	988.2	E865.4	–	E950.9	E962.1	E980.9
leaf (40)	989.4	E863.4	–	E950.6	E962.1	E980.7
widow spider (bite)	989.5	E905.1	–	E950.9	E962.1	E980.9
antivenin	979.9	E858.8	E949.9	E950.4	E962.0	E980.4
Blast furnace gas (carbon monoxide from)	986	E868.8	–	E952.1	E962.2	E982.1
Bleach NEC	983.9	E864.3	–	E950.7	E962.1	E980.6
Bleaching solutions	983.9	E864.3	–	E950.7	E962.1	E980.6
Bleomycin (sulfate)	960.7	E856	E930.7	E950.4	E962.0	E980.4
Blockain	968.9	E855.2	E938.9	E950.4	E962.0	E980.4
infiltration (subcutaneous)	968.5	E855.2	E938.5	E950.4	E962.0	E980.4
nerve block (peripheral) (plexus)	968.6	E855.2	E938.6	E950.4	E962.0	E980.4
topical (surface)	968.5	E855.2	E938.5	E950.4	E962.0	E980.4
Blood (derivatives) (natural) (plasma) (whole)	964.7	E858.2	E934.7	E950.4	E962.0	E980.4
affecting agent	964.9	E858.2	E934.9	E950.4	E962.0	E980.4
specified NEC	964.8	E858.2	E934.8	E950.4	E962.0	E980.4
substitute (macromolecular)	964.8	E858.2	E934.8	E950.4	E962.0	E980.4
Blue velvet	965.09	E850.2	E935.2	E950.0	E962.0	E980.0
Bone meal	989.89	E866.5	–	E950.9	E962.1	E980.9
Bonine	963.0	E858.1	E933.0	E950.4	E962.0	E980.4
Boracic acid	976.0	E858.7	E946.0	E950.4	E962.0	E980.4
ENT agent	976.6	E858.7	E946.6	E950.4	E962.0	E980.4
ophthalmic preparation	976.5	E858.7	E946.5	E950.4	E962.0	E980.4
Borate (cleanser) (sodium)	989.6	E861.3	–	E950.9	E962.1	E980.9
Borax (cleanser)	989.6	E861.3	–	E950.9	E962.1	E980.9
Boric acid	976.0	E858.7	E946.0	E950.4	E962.0	E980.4
ENT agent	976.6	E858.7	E946.6	E950.4	E962.0	E980.4
ophthalmic preparation	976.5	E858.7	E946.5	E950.4	E962.0	E980.4
Boron hydride NEC	989.89	E866.8	–	E950.9	E962.1	E980.9
fumes or gas	987.8	E869.8	–	E952.8	E962.2	E982.8
Botox	975.3	E858.6	E945.3	E950.4	E962.0	E980.4
Brake fluid vapor	987.8	E869.8	–	E952.8	E962.2	E982.8
Brass (compounds) (fumes)	985.8	E866.4	–	E950.9	E962.1	E980.9
Brasso	981	E861.3	–	E950.9	E962.1	E980.9
Bretylium (tosylate)	972.6	E858.3	E942.6	E950.4	E962.0	E980.4
Brevital (sodium)	968.3	E855.1	E938.3	E950.4	E962.0	E980.4
British antilewisite	963.8	E858.1	E933.8	E950.4	E962.0	E980.4
Bromal (hydrate)	967.3	E852.2	E937.3	E950.2	E962.0	E980.2
Bromelains	963.4	E858.1	E933.4	E950.4	E962.0	E980.4
Bromides NEC	967.3	E852.2	E937.3	E950.2	E962.0	E980.2
Bromine (vapor)	987.8	E869.8	–	E952.8	E962.2	E982.8
compounds (medicinal)	967.3	E852.2	E937.3	E950.2	E962.0	E980.2
Bromisovalum	967.3	E852.2	E937.3	E950.2	E962.0	E980.2
Bromobenzyl cyanide	987.5	E869.3	–	E952.8	E962.2	E982.8
Bromodiphenhydramine	963.0	E858.1	E933.0	E950.4	E962.0	E980.4
Bromoform	967.3	E852.2	E937.3	E950.2	E962.0	E980.2
Bromophenol blue reagent	977.8	E858.8	E947.8	E950.4	E962.0	E980.4
Bromosalicylhydroxamic acid	961.8	E857	E931.8	E950.4	E962.0	E980.4
Bromo-seltzer	965.4	E850.4	E935.4	E950.0	E962.0	E980.0
Brompheniramine	963.0	E858.1	E933.0	E950.4	E962.0	E980.4
Bromural	967.3	E852.2	E937.3	E950.2	E962.0	E980.2

Drug, chemical	Poisoning	External Cause (E Code)				
		Accident	Therapeutic Use	Suicide Attempt	Assault	Undetermined
Brown spider (bite) (venom)	989.5	E905.1	–	E950.9	E962.1	E980.9
Brucia	988.2	E865.3	–	E950.9	E962.1	E980.9
Brucine	989.1	E863.7	–	E950.6	E962.1	E980.7
Brunswick green – *see* Copper						
Bruten – *see* Ibuprofen						
Bryonia (alba) (dioica)	988.2	E865.4	–	E950.9	E962.1	E980.9
Buclizine	969.5	E853.8	E939.5	E950.3	E962.0	E980.3
Bufferin	965.1	E850.3	E935.3	E950.0	E962.0	E980.0
Bufotenine	969.6	E854.1	E939.6	E950.3	E962.0	E980.3
Buphenine	971.2	E855.5	E941.2	E950.4	E962.0	E980.4
Bupivacaine	968.9	E855.2	E938.9	E950.4	E962.0	E980.4
infiltration (subcutaneous)	968.5	E855.2	E938.5	E950.4	E962.0	E980.4
nerve block (peripheral) (plexus)	968.6	E855.2	E938.6	E950.4	E962.0	E980.4
Busulfan	963.1	E858.1	E933.1	E950.4	E962.0	E980.4
Butabarbital (sodium)	967.0	E851	E937.0	E950.1	E962.0	E980.1
Butabarbitone	967.0	E851	E937.0	E950.1	E962.0	E980.1
Butabarpal	967.0	E851	E937.0	E950.1	E962.0	E980.1
Butacaine	968.5	E855.2	E938.5	E950.4	E962.0	E980.4
Butallylonal	967.0	E851	E937.0	E950.1	E962.0	E980.1
Butane (distributed in mobile container)	987.0	E868.0	–	E951.1	E962.2	E981.1
distributed through pipes	987.0	E867	–	E951.0	E962.2	E981.0
incomplete combustion of – *see* Carbon monoxide, butane						
Butanol	980.3	E860.4	–	E950.9	E962.1	E980.9
Butanone	982.8	E862.4	–	E950.9	E962.1	E980.9
Butaperazine	969.1	E853.0	E939.1	E950.3	E962.0	E980.3
Butazolidin	965.5	E850.5	E935.5	E950.0	E962.0	E980.0
Butethal	967.0	E851	E937.0	E950.1	E962.0	E980.1
Butethamate	971.1	E855.4	E941.1	E950.4	E962.0	E980.4
Buthalitone (sodium)	968.3	E855.1	E938.3	E950.4	E962.0	E980.4
Butisol (sodium)	967.0	E851	E937.0	E950.1	E962.0	E980.1
Butobarbital, butobarbitone	967.0	E851	E937.0	E950.1	E962.0	E980.1
Butriptyline ▲	969.05	E854.0	E939.0	E950.3	E962.0	E980.3
Buttercups	988.2	E865.4	–	E950.9	E962.1	E980.9
Butter of antimony – *see* Antimony						
Butyl						
acetate (secondary)	982.8	E862.4	–	E950.9	E962.1	E980.9
alcohol	980.3	E860.4	–	E950.9	E962.1	E980.9
carbinol	980.8	E860.8	–	E950.9	E962.1	E980.9
carbitol	982.8	E862.4	–	E950.9	E962.1	E980.9
cellosolve	982.8	E862.4	–	E950.9	E962.1	E980.9
chloral (hydrate)	967.1	E852.0	E937.1	E950.2	E962.0	E980.2
formate	982.8	E862.4	–	E950.9	E962.1	E980.9
scopolammonium bromide	971.1	E855.4	E941.1	E950.4	E962.0	E980.4
Butyn	968.5	E855.2	E938.5	E950.4	E962.0	E980.4
Butyrophenone (-based tranquilizers)	969.2	E853.1	E939.2	E950.3	E962.0	E980.3
Cacodyl, cacodylic acid – *see* Arsenic						
Cactinomycin	960.7	E856	E930.7	E950.4	E962.0	E980.4
Cade oil	976.4	E858.7	E946.4	E950.4	E962.0	E980.4
Cadmium (chloride) (compounds) (dust) (fumes) (oxide)	985.5	E866.4	–	E950.9	E962.1	E980.9
sulfide (medicinal) NEC	976.4	E858.7	E946.4	E950.4	E962.0	E980.4
Caffeine ▲	969.71	E854.2	E939.7	E950.3	E962.0	E980.3
Calabar bean	988.2	E865.4	–	E950.9	E962.1	E980.9
Caladium seguinium	988.2	E865.4	–	E950.9	E962.1	E980.9
Calamine (liniment) (lotion)	976.3	E858.7	E946.3	E950.4	E962.0	E980.4
Calciferol	963.5	E858.1	E933.5	E950.4	E962.0	E980.4
Calcium (salts) NEC	974.5	E858.5	E944.5	E950.4	E962.0	E980.4
acetylsalicylate	965.1	E850.3	E935.3	E950.0	E962.0	E980.0
benzamidosalicylate	961.8	E857	E931.8	E950.4	E962.0	E980.4
carbaspirin	965.1	E850.3	E935.3	E950.0	E962.0	E980.0
carbimide (citrated)	977.3	E858.8	E947.3	E950.4	E962.0	E980.4
carbonate (antacid)	973.0	E858.4	E943.0	E950.4	E962.0	E980.4
cyanide (citrated)	977.3	E858.8	E947.3	E950.4	E962.0	E980.4
dioctyl sulfosuccinate	973.2	E858.4	E943.2	E950.4	E962.0	E980.4
disodium edathamil	963.8	E858.1	E933.8	E950.4	E962.0	E980.4
disodium edetate	963.8	E858.1	E933.8	E950.4	E962.0	E980.4
EDTA	963.8	E858.1	E933.8	E950.4	E962.0	E980.4
hydrate, hydroxide	983.2	E864.2	–	E950.7	E962.1	E980.6
mandelate	961.9	E857	E931.9	E950.4	E962.0	E980.4
oxide	983.2	E864.2	–	E950.7	E962.1	E980.6
Calomel – *see* Mercury, chloride						
Caloric agents NEC	974.5	E858.5	E944.5	E950.4	E962.0	E980.4
Calusterone	963.1	E858.1	E933.1	E950.4	E962.0	E980.4
Camoquin	961.4	E857	E931.4	E950.4	E962.0	E980.4
Camphor (oil)	976.1	E858.7	E946.1	E950.4	E962.0	E980.4
Candeptin	976.0	E858.7	E946.0	E950.4	E962.0	E980.4
Candicidin	976.0	E858.7	E946.0	E950.4	E962.0	E980.4
Cannabinols	969.6	E854.1	E939.6	E950.3	E962.0	E980.3
Cannabis (derivatives) (indica) (sativa)	969.6	E854.1	E939.6	E950.3	E962.0	E980.3
Canned heat	980.1	E860.2	–	E950.9	E962.1	E980.9
Cantharides, cantharidin, cantharis	976.8	E858.7	E946.8	E950.4	E962.0	E980.4
Capillary agents	972.8	E858.3	E942.8	E950.4	E962.0	E980.4
Capreomycin	960.6	E856	E930.6	E950.4	E962.0	E980.4
Captodiame, captodiamine	969.5	E853.8	E939.5	E950.3	E962.0	E980.3
Caramiphen (hydrochloride)	971.1	E855.4	E941.1	E950.4	E962.0	E980.4
Carbachol	971.0	E855.3	E941.0	E950.4	E962.0	E980.4
Carbacrylamine resins	974.5	E858.5	E944.5	E950.4	E962.0	E980.4
Carbamate (sedative)	967.8	E852.8	E937.8	E950.2	E962.0	E980.2
herbicide	989.3	E863.5	–	E950.6	E962.1	E980.7
insecticide	989.3	E863.2	–	E950.6	E962.1	E980.7
Carbamazepine	966.3	E855.0	E936.3	E950.4	E962.0	E980.4
Carbamic esters	967.8	E852.8	E937.8	E950.2	E962.0	E980.2
Carbamide	974.4	E858.5	E944.4	E950.4	E962.0	E980.4
topical	976.8	E858.7	E946.8	E950.4	E962.0	E980.4
Carbamylcholine chloride	971.0	E855.3	E941.0	E950.4	E962.0	E980.4
Carbarsone	961.1	E857	E931.1	E950.4	E962.0	E980.4
Carbaryl	989.3	E863.2	–	E950.6	E962.1	E980.7
Carbaspirin	965.1	E850.3	E935.3	E950.0	E962.0	E980.0
Carbazochrome	972.8	E858.3	E942.8	E950.4	E962.0	E980.4
Carbenicillin	960.0	E856	E930.0	E950.4	E962.0	E980.4
Carbenoxolone	973.8	E858.4	E943.8	E950.4	E962.0	E980.4
Carbetapentane	975.4	E858.6	E945.4	E950.4	E962.0	E980.4
Carbimazole	962.8	E858.0	E932.8	E950.4	E962.0	E980.4
Carbinol	980.1	E860.2	–	E950.9	E962.1	E980.9
Carbinoxamine	963.0	E858.1	E933.0	E950.4	E962.0	E980.4
Carbitol	982.8	E862.4	–	E950.9	E962.1	E980.9
Carbocaine	968.9	E855.2	E938.9	E950.4	E962.0	E980.4
infiltration (subcutaneous)	968.5	E855.2	E938.5	E950.4	E962.0	E980.4
nerve block (peripheral) (plexus)	968.6	E855.2	E938.6	E950.4	E962.0	E980.4
topical (surface)	968.5	E855.2	E938.5	E950.4	E962.0	E980.4
Carbol-fuchsin solution	976.0	E858.7	E946.0	E950.4	E962.0	E980.4
Carbolic acid (*see also* Phenol)	983.0	E864.0	–	E950.7	E962.1	E980.6
Carbomycin	960.8	E856	E930.8	E950.4	E962.0	E980.4
Carbon						
bisulfide (liquid) (vapor)	982.2	E862.4	–	E950.9	E962.1	E980.9
dioxide (gas)	987.8	E869.8	–	E952.8	E962.2	E982.8
disulfide (liquid) (vapor)	982.2	E862.4	–	E950.9	E962.1	E980.9
monoxide (from incomplete combustion of) (in) NEC	986	E868.9	–	E952.1	E962.2	E982.1
blast furnace gas	986	E868.8	–	E952.1	E962.2	E982.1
butane (distributed in mobile container)	986	E868.0	–	E951.1	E962.2	E981.1
distributed through pipes	986	E867	–	E951.0	E962.2	E981.0
charcoal fumes	986	E868.3	–	E952.1	E962.2	E982.1
coal gas (piped)	986	E867	–	E951.0	E962.2	E981.0
solid (in domestic stoves, fireplaces)	986	E868.3	–	E952.1	E962.2	E982.1
coke (in domestic stoves, fireplaces)	986	E868.3	–	E952.1	E962.2	E982.1
exhaust gas (motor) not in transit	986	E868.2	–	E952.0	E962.2	E982.0
combustion engine, any not in watercraft	986	E868.2	–	E952.0	E962.2	E982.0
farm tractor, not in transit	986	E868.2	–	E952.0	E962.2	E982.0
gas engine	986	E868.2	–	E952.0	E962.2	E982.0
motor pump	986	E868.2	–	E952.0	E962.2	E982.0
motor vehicle, not in transit	986	E868.2	–	E952.0	E962.2	E982.0
fuel (in domestic use)	986	E868.3	–	E952.1	E962.2	E982.1
gas (piped)	986	E867	–	E951.0	E962.2	E981.0
in mobile container	986	E868.0	–	E951.1	E962.2	E981.1
utility	986	E868.1	–	E951.8	E962.2	E981.1
in mobile container	986	E868.0	–	E951.1	E962.2	E981.1
piped (natural)	986	E867	–	E951.0	E962.2	E981.0
illuminating gas	986	E868.1	–	E951.8	E962.2	E981.8
industrial fuels or gases, any	986	E868.8	–	E952.1	E962.2	E982.1
kerosene (in domestic stoves, fireplaces)	986	E868.3	–	E952.1	E962.2	E982.1
kiln gas or vapor	986	E868.8	–	E952.1	E962.2	E982.1
motor exhaust gas, not in transit	986	E868.2	–	E952.0	E962.2	E982.0
piped gas (manufactured) (natural)	986	E867	–	E951.0	E962.2	E981.0
producer gas	986	E868.8	–	E952.1	E962.2	E982.1
propane (distributed in mobile container)	986	E868.0	–	E951.1	E962.2	E981.1
distributed through pipes	986	E867	–	E951.0	E962.2	E981.0
specified source NEC	986	E868.8	–	E952.1	E962.2	E982.1
stove gas	986	E868.1	–	E951.8	E962.2	E981.8
piped	986	E867	–	E951.0	E962.2	E981.0

Drug, chemical	Poisoning	External Cause (E Code)				
		Accident	Therapeutic Use	Suicide Attempt	Assault	Undetermined
Carbon – *continued*						
monoxide – *continued*						
utility gas	986	E868.1	–	E951.8	E962.2	E981.8
piped	986	E867	–	E951.0	E962.2	E981.0
water gas	986	E868.1	–	E951.8	E962.2	E981.8
wood (in domestic stoves, fireplaces)	986	E868.3	–	E952.1	E962.2	E982.1
tetrachloride (vapor) NEC	987.8	E869.8	–	E952.8	E962.2	E982.8
liquid (cleansing agent) NEC	982.1	E861.3	–	E950.9	E962.1	E980.9
solvent	982.1	E862.4	–	E950.9	E962.1	E980.9
Carbonic acid (gas)	987.8	E869.8	–	E952.8	E962.2	E982.8
anhydrase inhibitors	974.2	E858.5	E944.2	E950.4	E962.0	E980.4
Carbowax	976.3	E858.7	E946.3	E950.4	E962.0	E980.4
Carbrital	967.0	E851	E937.0	E950.1	E962.0	E980.1
Carbromal (derivatives)	967.3	E852.2	E937.3	E950.2	E962.0	E980.2
Cardiac						
depressants	972.0	E858.3	E942.0	E950.4	E962.0	E980.4
rhythm regulators	972.0	E858.3	E942.0	E950.4	E962.0	E980.4
Cardiografin	977.8	E858.8	E947.8	E950.4	E962.0	E980.4
Cardio-green	977.8	E858.8	E947.8	E950.4	E962.0	E980.4
Cardiotonic glycosides	972.1	E858.3	E942.1	E950.4	E962.0	E980.4
Cardiovascular agents NEC	972.9	E858.3	E942.9	E950.4	E962.0	E980.4
Cardrase	974.2	E858.5	E944.2	E950.4	E962.0	E980.4
Carfusin	976.0	E858.7	E946.0	E950.4	E962.0	E980.4
Carisoprodol	968.0	E855.1	E938.0	E950.4	E962.0	E980.4
Carmustine	963.1	E858.1	E933.1	E950.4	E962.0	E980.4
Carotene	963.5	E858.1	E933.5	E950.4	E962.0	E980.4
Carphenazine (maleate)	969.1	E853.0	E939.1	E950.3	E962.0	E980.3
Carter's Little Pills	973.1	E858.4	E943.1	E950.4	E962.0	E980.4
Cascara (sagrada)	973.1	E858.4	E943.1	E950.4	E962.0	E980.4
Cassava	988.2	E865.4	–	E950.9	E962.1	E980.9
Castellani's paint	976.0	E858.7	E946.0	E950.4	E962.0	E980.4
Castor						
bean	988.2	E865.3	–	E950.9	E962.1	E980.9
oil	973.1	E858.4	E943.1	E950.4	E962.0	E980.4
Caterpillar (sting)	989.5	E905.5	–	E950.9	E962.1	E980.9
Catha (edulis)	970.8	E854.3	E940.8	E950.4	E962.0	E980.4
Cathartics NEC	973.3	E858.4	E943.3	E950.4	E962.0	E980.4
contact	973.1	E858.4	E943.1	E950.4	E962.0	E980.4
emollient	973.2	E858.4	E943.2	E950.4	E962.0	E980.4
intestinal irritants	973.1	E858.4	E943.1	E950.4	E962.0	E980.4
saline	973.3	E858.4	E943.3	E950.4	E962.0	E980.4
Cathomycin	960.8	E856	E930.8	E950.4	E962.0	E980.4
Caustic(s)	983.9	E864.4	–	E950.7	E962.1	E980.6
alkali	983.2	E864.2	–	E950.7	E962.1	E980.6
hydroxide	983.2	E864.2	–	E950.7	E962.1	E980.6
potash	983.2	E864.2	–	E950.7	E962.1	E980.6
soda	983.2	E864.2	–	E950.7	E962.1	E980.6
specified NEC	983.9	E864.3	–	E950.7	E962.1	E980.6
Ceepryn	976.0	E858.7	E946.0	E950.4	E962.0	E980.4
ENT agent	976.6	E858.7	E946.6	E950.4	E962.0	E980.4
lozenges	976.6	E858.7	E946.6	E950.4	E962.0	E980.4
Celestone	962.0	E858.0	E932.0	E950.4	E962.0	E980.4
topical	976.0	E858.7	E946.0	E950.4	E962.0	E980.4
Cellosolve	982.8	E862.4	–	E950.9	E962.1	E980.9
Cell stimulants and proliferants	976.8	E858.7	E946.8	E950.4	E962.0	E980.4
Cellulose derivatives, cathartic	973.3	E858.4	E943.3	E950.4	E962.0	E980.4
nitrates (topical)	976.3	E858.7	E946.3	E950.4	E962.0	E980.4
Centipede (bite)	989.5	E905.4	–	E950.9	E962.1	E980.9
Central nervous system						
depressants	968.4	E855.1	E938.4	E950.4	E962.0	E980.4
anesthetic (general) NEC	968.4	E855.1	E938.4	E950.4	E962.0	E980.4
gases NEC	968.2	E855.1	E938.2	E950.4	E962.0	E980.4
intravenous	968.3	E855.1	E938.3	E950.4	E962.0	E980.4
barbiturates	967.0	E851	E937.0	E950.1	E962.0	E980.1
bromides	967.3	E852.2	E937.3	E950.2	E962.0	E980.2
cannabis sativa	969.6	E854.1	E939.6	E950.3	E962.0	E980.3
chloral hydrate	967.1	E852.0	E937.1	E950.2	E962.0	E980.2
hallucinogenics	969.6	E854.1	E939.6	E950.3	E962.0	E980.3
hypnotics	967.9	E852.9	E937.9	E950.2	E962.0	E980.2
specified NEC	967.8	E852.8	E937.8	E950.2	E962.0	E980.2
muscle relaxants	968.0	E855.1	E938.0	E950.4	E962.0	E980.4
paraldehyde	967.2	E852.1	E937.2	E950.2	E962.0	E980.2
sedatives	967.9	E852.9	E937.9	E950.2	E962.0	E980.2
mixed NEC	967.6	E852.5	E937.6	E950.2	E962.0	E980.2
specified NEC	967.8	E852.8	E937.8	E950.2	E962.0	E980.2
muscle-tone depressants	968.0	E855.1	E938.0	E950.4	E962.0	E980.4
stimulants	970.9	E854.3	E940.9	E950.4	E962.0	E980.4
amphetamines ▲	969.72	E854.2	E939.7	E950.3	E962.0	E980.3
analeptics	970.0	E854.3	E940.0	E950.4	E962.0	E980.4
antidepressants ▲	969.00	E854.0	E939.0	E950.3	E962.0	E980.3
opiate antagonists	970.1	E854.3	E940.1	E950.4	E962.0	E980.4
specified NEC	970.8	E854.3	E940.8	E950.4	E962.0	E980.4
Cephalexin	960.5	E856	E930.5	E950.4	E962.0	E980.4
Cephaloglycin	960.5	E856	E930.5	E950.4	E962.0	E980.4
Cephaloridine	960.5	E856	E930.5	E950.4	E962.0	E980.4
Cephalosporins NEC	960.5	E856	E930.5	E950.4	E962.0	E980.4
N (adicillin)	960.0	E856	E930.0	E950.4	E962.0	E980.4
Cephalothin (sodium)	960.5	E856	E930.5	E950.4	E962.0	E980.4
Cerbera (odallam)	988.2	E865.4	–	E950.9	E962.1	E980.9
Cerberin	972.1	E858.3	E942.1	E950.4	E962.0	E980.4
Cerebral stimulants	970.9	E854.3	E940.9	E950.4	E962.0	E980.4
psychotherapeutic ▲	969.79	E854.2	E939.7	E950.3	E962.0	E980.3
specified NEC	970.8	E854.3	E940.8	E950.4	E962.0	E980.4
Cetalkonium (chloride)	976.0	E858.7	E946.0	E950.4	E962.0	E980.4
Cetoxime	963.0	E858.1	E933.0	E950.4	E962.0	E980.4
Cetrimide	976.2	E858.7	E946.2	E950.4	E962.0	E980.4
Cetylpyridinium	976.0	E858.7	E946.0	E950.4	E962.0	E980.4
ENT agent	976.6	E858.7	E946.6	E950.4	E962.0	E980.4
lozenges	976.6	E858.7	E946.6	E950.4	E962.0	E980.4
Cevadilla – *see* Sabadilla						
Cevitamic acid	963.5	E858.1	E933.5	E950.4	E962.0	E980.4
Chalk, precipitated	973.0	E858.4	E943.0	E950.4	E962.0	E980.4
Charcoal						
fumes (carbon monoxide)	986	E868.3	–	E952.1	E962.2	E982.1
industrial	986	E868.8	–	E952.1	E962.2	E982.1
medicinal (activated)	973.0	E858.4	E943.0	E950.4	E962.0	E980.4
Chelating agents NEC	977.2	E858.8	E947.2	E950.4	E962.0	E980.4
Chelidonium majus	988.2	E865.4	–	E950.9	E962.1	E980.9
Chemical substance	989.9	E866.9	–	E950.9	E962.1	E980.9
specified NEC	989.89	E866.8	–	E950.9	E962.1	E980.9
Chemotherapy, antineoplastic	963.1	E858.1	E933.1	E950.4	E962.0	E980.4
Chenopodium (oil)	961.6	E857	E931.6	E950.4	E962.0	E980.4
Cherry laurel	988.2	E865.4	–	E950.9	E962.1	E980.9
Chiniofon	961.3	E857	E931.3	E950.4	E962.0	E980.4
Chlophedianol	975.4	E858.6	E945.4	E950.4	E962.0	E980.4
Chloral (betaine) (formamide) (hydrate)	967.1	E852.0	E937.1	E950.2	E962.0	E980.2
Chloralamide	967.1	E852.0	E937.1	E950.2	E962.0	E980.2
Chlorambucil	963.1	E858.1	E933.1	E950.4	E962.0	E980.4
Chloramphenicol	960.2	E856	E930.2	E950.4	E962.0	E980.4
ENT agent	976.6	E858.7	E946.6	E950.4	E962.0	E980.4
ophthalmic preparation	976.5	E858.7	E946.5	E950.4	E962.0	E980.4
topical NEC	976.0	E858.7	E946.0	E950.4	E962.0	E980.4
Chlorate(s) (potassium) (sodium) NEC	983.9	E864.3	–	E950.7	E962.1	E980.6
herbicides	989.4	E863.5	–	E950.6	E962.1	E980.7
Chlorcylizine	963.0	E858.1	E933.0	E950.4	E962.0	E980.4
Chlordan(e) (dust)	989.2	E863.0	–	E950.6	E962.1	E980.7
Chlordantoin	976.0	E858.7	E946.0	E950.4	E962.0	E980.4
Chlordiazepoxide	969.4	E853.2	E939.4	E950.3	E962.0	E980.3
Chloresium	976.8	E858.7	E946.8	E950.4	E962.0	E980.4
Chlorethiazol	967.1	E852.0	E937.1	E950.2	E962.0	E980.2
Chlorethyl – *see* Ethyl, chloride						
Chloretone	967.1	E852.0	E937.1	E950.2	E962.0	E980.2
Chlorex	982.3	E862.4	–	E950.9	E962.1	E980.9
Chlorhexadol	967.1	E852.0	E937.1	E950.2	E962.0	E980.2
Chlorhexidine (hydrochloride)	976.0	E858.7	E946.0	E950.4	E962.0	E980.4
Chlorhydroxyquinolin	976.0	E858.7	E946.0	E950.4	E962.0	E980.4
Chloride of lime (bleach)	983.9	E864.3	–	E950.7	E962.1	E980.6
Chlorinated						
camphene	989.2	E863.0	–	E950.6	E962.1	E980.7
diphenyl	989.89	E866.8	–	E950.9	E962.1	E980.9
hydrocarbons NEC	989.2	E863.0	–	E950.6	E962.1	E980.7
solvent	982.3	E862.4	–	E950.9	E962.1	E980.9
lime (bleach)	983.9	E864.3	–	E950.7	E962.1	E980.6
naphthalene – *see* Naphthalene						
pesticides NEC	989.2	E863.0	–	E950.6	E962.1	E980.7
soda – *see* Sodium, hypochlorite						
Chlorine (fumes) (gas)	987.6	E869.8	–	E952.8	E962.2	E982.8
bleach	983.9	E864.3	–	E950.7	E962.1	E980.6
compounds NEC	983.9	E864.3	–	E950.7	E962.1	E980.6
disinfectant	983.9	E861.4	–	E950.7	E962.1	E980.6
releasing agents NEC	983.9	E864.3	–	E950.7	E962.1	E980.6
Chlorisondamine	972.3	E858.3	E942.3	E950.4	E962.0	E980.4
Chlormadinone	962.2	E858.0	E932.2	E950.4	E962.0	E980.4
Chlormerodrin	974.0	E858.5	E944.0	E950.4	E962.0	E980.4
Chlormethiazole	967.1	E852.0	E937.1	E950.2	E962.0	E980.2
Chlormethylenecycline	960.4	E856	E930.4	E950.4	E962.0	E980.4
Chlormezanone	969.5	E853.8	E939.5	E950.3	E962.0	E980.3
Chloroacetophenone	987.5	E869.3	–	E952.8	E962.2	E982.8
Chloroaniline	983.0	E864.0	–	E950.7	E962.1	E980.6
Chlorobenzene, chlorobenzol	982.0	E862.4	–	E950.9	E962.1	E980.9
Chlorobutanol	967.1	E852.0	E937.1	E950.2	E962.0	E980.2
Chlorodinitrobenzene	983.0	E864.0	–	E950.7	E962.1	E980.6
dust or vapor	987.8	E869.8	–	E952.8	E962.2	E982.8

Drug, chemical	Poisoning	External Cause (E Code) Accident	Therapeutic Use	Suicide Attempt	Assault	Undetermined
Chloroethane – *see* Ethyl, chloride						
Chloroform (fumes) (vapor)	987.8	E869.8	–	E952.8	E962.2	E932.8
anesthetic (gas)	968.2	E855.1	E938.2	E950.4	E962.0	E980.4
liquid NEC	968.4	E855.1	E938.4	E950.4	E962.0	E980.4
solvent	982.3	E862.4	–	E950.9	E962.1	E980.9
Chloroguanide	961.4	E857	E931.4	E950.4	E962.0	E980.4
Chloromycetin	960.2	E856	E930.2	E950.4	E962.0	E980.4
ENT agent	976.6	E858.7	E946.6	E950.4	E962.0	E980.4
ophthalmic preparation	976.5	E858.7	E946.5	E950.4	E962.0	E980.4
otic solution	976.6	E858.7	E946.6	E950.4	E962.0	E980.4
topical NEC	976.0	E858.7	E946.0	E950.4	E962.0	E980.4
Chloronitrobenzene	983.0	E864.0	–	E950.7	E962.1	E980.6
dust or vapor	987.8	E869.8	–	E952.8	E962.2	E982.8
Chlorophenol	983.0	E864.0	–	E950.7	E962.1	E980.6
Chlorophenothane	989.2	E863.0	–	E950.6	E962.1	E980.7
Chlorophyll (derivatives)	976.8	E858.7	E946.8	E950.4	E962.0	E980.4
Chloropicrin (fumes)	987.8	E869.8	–	E952.8	E962.2	E982.8
fumigant	989.4	E863.8	–	E950.6	E962.1	E980.7
fungicide	989.4	E863.6	–	E950.6	E962.1	E980.7
pesticide (fumes)	989.4	E863.4	–	E950.6	E962.1	E980.7
Chloroprocaine	968.9	E855.2	E938.9	E950.4	E962.0	E980.4
infiltration (subcutaneous)	968.5	E855.2	E938.5	E950.4	E962.0	E980.4
nerve block (peripheral) (plexus)	968.6	E855.2	E938.6	E950.4	E962.0	E980.4
Chloroptic	976.5	E858.7	E946.5	E950.4	E962.0	E980.4
Chloropurine	963.1	E858.1	E933.1	E950.4	E962.0	E980.4
Chloroquine (hydrochloride) (phosphate)	961.4	E857	E931.4	E950.4	E962.0	E980.4
Chlorothen	963.0	E858.1	E933.0	E950.4	E962.0	E980.4
Chlorothiazide	974.3	E858.5	E944.3	E950.4	E962.0	E980.4
Chlorotrianisene	962.2	E858.0	E932.2	E950.4	E962.0	E980.4
Chlorovinyldichloroarsine	985.1	E866.3	–	E950.8	E962.1	E980.8
Chloroxylenol	976.0	E858.7	E946.0	E950.4	E962.0	E980.4
Chlorphenesin (carbamate)	968.0	E855.1	E938.0	E950.4	E962.0	E980.4
topical (antifungal)	976.0	E858.7	E946.0	E950.4	E962.0	E980.4
Chlorpheniramine	963.0	E858.1	E933.0	E950.4	E962.0	E980.4
Chlorphenoxamine	966.4	E855.0	E936.4	E950.4	E962.0	E980.4
Chlorphentermine	977.0	E858.8	E947.0	E950.4	E962.0	E980.4
Chlorproguanil	961.4	E857	E931.4	E950.4	E962.0	E980.4
Chlorpromazine	969.1	E853.0	E939.1	E950.3	E962.0	E980.3
Chlorpropamide	962.3	E858.0	E932.3	E950.4	E962.0	E980.4
Chlorprothixene	969.3	E853.8	E939.3	E950.3	E962.0	E980.3
Chlorquinaldol	976.0	E858.7	E946.0	E950.4	E962.0	E980.4
Chlortetracycline	960.4	E856	E930.4	E950.4	E962.0	E980.4
Chlorthalidone	974.4	E858.5	E944.4	E950.4	E962.0	E980.4
Chlortrianisene	962.2	E858.0	E932.2	E950.4	E962.0	E980.4
Chlor-Trimeton	963.0	E858.1	E933.0	E950.4	E962.0	E980.4
Chlorzoxazone	968.0	E855.1	E938.0	E950.4	E962.0	E980.4
Choke damp	987.8	E869.8	–	E952.8	E962.2	E982.8
Cholebrine	977.8	E858.8	E947.8	E950.4	E962.0	E980.4
Cholera vaccine	978.2	E858.8	E948.2	E950.4	E962.0	E980.4
Cholesterol-lowering agents	972.2	E858.3	E942.2	E950.4	E962.0	E980.4
Cholestyramine (resin)	972.2	E858.3	E942.2	E950.4	E962.0	E980.4
Cholic acid	973.4	E858.4	E943.4	E950.4	E962.0	E980.4
Choline						
dihydrogen citrate	977.1	E858.8	E947.1	E950.4	E962.0	E980.4
salicylate	965.1	E850.3	E935.3	E950.0	E962.0	E980.0
theophyllinate	974.1	E858.5	E944.1	E950.4	E962.0	E980.4
Cholinergics	971.0	E855.3	E941.0	E950.4	E962.0	E980.4
Cholograrin	977.8	E858.8	E947.8	E950.4	E962.0	E980.4
Chorionic gonadoiropin	962.4	E858.0	E932.4	E950.4	E962.0	E980.4
Chromates	983.9	E864.3	–	E950.7	E962.1	E980.6
dust or mist	987.8	E869.8	–	E952.8	E962.2	E982.8
lead	984.0	E866.0	–	E950.9	E962.1	E980.9
paint	984.0	E861.5	–	E950.9	E962.1	E980.9
Chromic acid	983.9	E864.3	–	E950.7	E962.1	E980.6
dust or mist	987.8	E869.8	–	E952.8	E962.2	E982.8
Chromium	985.6	E866.4	–	E950.9	E962.1	E980.9
compounds – *see* Chromates						
Chromonar	972.4	E858.3	E942.4	E950.4	E962.0	E980.4
Chromyl chloride	983.9	E864.3	–	E950.7	E962.1	E980.6
Chrysarobin (ointment)	976.4	E858.7	E946.4	E950.4	E962.0	E980.4
Chrysazin	973.1	E858.4	E943.1	E950.4	E962.0	E980.4
Chymar	963.4	E858.1	E933.4	E950.4	E962.0	E980.4
ophthalmic preparation	976.5	E858.7	E946.5	E950.4	E962.0	E980.4
Chymotrypsin	963.4	E858.1	E933.4	E950.4	E962.0	E980.4
ophthalmic preparation	976.5	E858.7	E946.5	E950.4	E962.0	E980.4
Cicuta maculata or virosa	988.2	E865.4	–	E950.9	E962.1	E980.9
Cigarette lighter fluid	981	E862.1	–	E950.9	E962.1	E980.9
Cinchocaine (spinal)	968.7	E855.2	E938.7	E950.4	E962.0	E980.4
topical (surface)	968.5	E855.2	E938.5	E950.4	E962.0	E980.4
Cinchona	961.4	E857	E931.4	E950.4	E962.0	E980.4
Cinchonine alkaloids	961.4	E857	E931.4	E950.4	E962.0	E980.4
Cinchophen	974.7	E858.5	E944.7	E950.4	E962.0	E980.4
Cinnarizine	963.0	E858.1	E933.0	E950.4	E962.0	E980.4
Citanest	968.9	E855.2	E938.9	E950.4	E962.0	E980.4
infiltration (subcutaneous)	968.5	E855.2	E938.5	E950.4	E962.0	E980.4
nerve block (peripheral) (plexus)	968.6	E855.2	E938.6	E950.4	E962.0	E980.4
Citric acid	989.89	E866.8	–	E950.9	E962.1	E980.9
Citrovorum factor	964.1	E858.2	E934.1	E950.4	E962.0	E980.4
Claviceps purpurea	988.2	E865.4	–	E950.9	E962.1	E980.9
Cleaner, cleansing agent NEC	989.89	E861.3	–	E950.9	E962.1	E980.9
of paint or varnish	982.8	E862.9	–	E950.9	E962.1	E980.9
Clematis vitalba	988.2	E865.4	–	E950.9	E962.1	E980.9
Clemizole	963.0	E858.1	E933.0	E950.4	E962.0	E980.4
penicillin	960.0	E856	E930.0	E950.4	E962.0	E980.4
Clidinium	971.1	E855.4	E941.1	E950.4	E962.0	E980.4
Clindamycin	960.8	E856	E930.8	E950.4	E962.0	E980.4
Cliradon	965.09	E850.2	E935.2	E950.0	E962.0	E980.0
Clocortolone	962.0	E858.0	E932.0	E950.4	E962.0	E980.4
Clofedanol	975.4	E858.6	E945.4	E950.4	E962.0	E980.4
Clofibrate	972.2	E858.3	E942.2	E950.4	E962.0	E980.4
Clomethiazole	967.1	E852.0	E937.1	E950.2	E962.0	E980.2
Clomiphene	977.8	E858.8	E947.8	E950.4	E962.0	E980.4
Clonazepam	969.4	E853.2	E939.4	E950.3	E962.0	E980.3
Clonidine	972.6	E858.3	E942.6	E950.4	E962.0	E980.4
Clopamide	974.3	E858.5	E944.3	E950.4	E962.0	E980.4
Clorazepate	969.4	E853.2	E939.4	E950.3	E962.0	E980.3
Clorexolone	974.4	E858.5	E944.4	E950.4	E962.0	E980.4
Clorox (bleach)	983.9	E864.3	–	E950.7	E962.1	E980.6
Clortermine	977.0	E858.8	E947.0	E950.4	E962.0	E980.4
Clotrimazole	976.0	E858.7	E946.0	E950.4	E962.0	E980.4
Cloxacillin	960.0	E856	E930.0	E950.4	E962.0	E980.4
Coagulants NEC	964.5	E858.2	E934.5	E950.4	E962.0	E980.4
Coal (carbon monoxide from) – *see also* Carbon, monoxide, coal						
oil – *see* Kerosene						
tar NEC	983.0	E864.0	–	E950.7	E962.1	E980.6
fumes	987.8	E869.8	–	E952.8	E962.2	E982.8
medicinal (ointment)	976.4	E858.7	E946.4	E950.4	E962.0	E980.4
analgesics NEC	965.5	E850.5	E935.5	E950.0	E962.0	E980.0
naphtha (solvent)	981	E862.0	–	E950.9	E962.1	E980.9
Cobalt (fumes) (industrial)	985.8	E866.4	–	E950.9	E962.1	E980.9
Cobra (venom)	989.5	E905.0	–	E950.9	E962.1	E980.9
Coca (leaf)	970.8	E854.3	E940.8	E950.4	E962.0	E980.4
Cocaine (hydrochloride) (salt)	970.8	E854.3	E940.8	E950.4	E962.0	E980.4
topical anesthetic	968.5	E855.2	E938.5	E950.4	E962.0	E980.4
Coccidioidin	977.8	E858.8	E947.8	E950.4	E962.0	E980.4
Cocculus indicus	988.2	E865.3	–	E950.9	E962.1	E980.9
Cochineal	989.89	E866.8	–	E950.9	E962.1	E980.9
medicinal products	977.4	E858.8	E947.4	E950.4	E962.0	E980.4
Codeine	965.09	E850.2	E935.2	E950.0	E962.0	E980.0
Coffee	989.89	E866.8	–	E950.9	E962.1	E980.9
Cogentin	971.1	E855.4	E941.1	E950.4	E962.0	E980.4
Coke fumes or gas (carbon monoxide)	986	E868.3	–	E952.1	E962.2	E982.1
industrial use	986	E868.8	–	E952.1	E962.2	E982.1
Colace	973.2	E858.4	E943.2	E950.4	E962.0	E980.4
Coichicine	974.7	E858.5	E944.7	E950.4	E962.0	E980.4
Coichicum	988.2	E865.3	–	E950.9	E962.1	E980.9
Cold cream	976.3	E858.7	E946.3	E950.4	E962.0	E980.4
Colestipol	972.2	E858.3	E942.2	E950.4	E962.0	E980.4
Colistimethate	960.8	E856	E930.8	E950.4	E962.0	E980.4
Colistin	960.8	E856	E930.8	E950.4	E962.0	E980.4
Coliagenase	976.8	E858.7	E946.8	E950.4	E962.0	E980.4
Collagen	977.8	E866.8	E947.8	E950.9	E962.1	E980.9
Collodion (flexible)	976.3	E858.7	E946.3	E950.4	E962.0	E980.4
Colocynth	973.1	E858.4	E943.1	E950.4	E962.0	E980.4
Coloring matter – *see* Dye(s)						
Combustion gas – *see* Carbon, monoxide						
Compazine	969.1	E853.0	E939.1	E950.3	E962.0	E980.3
Compound						
42 (warfarin)	989.4	E863.7	–	E950.6	E962.1	E980.7
269 (endrin)	989.2	E863.0	–	E950.6	E962.1	E980.7
497 (dieldrin)	989.2	E863.0	–	E950.6	E962.1	E980.7
1080 (sodium fluoroacetate)	989.4	E863.7	–	E950.6	E962.1	E980.7
3422 (parathion)	989.3	E863.1	–	E950.6	E962.1	E980.7
3911 (phorate)	989.3	E863.1	–	E950.6	E962.1	E980.7
3956 (toxaphene)	989.2	E863.0	–	E950.6	E962.1	E980.7
4049 (malathion)	989.3	E863.1	–	E950.6	E962.1	E980.7
4124 (dicapthon)	989.4	E863.4	–	E950.6	E962.1	E980.7
E (cortisone)	962.0	E858.0	E932.0	E950.4	E962.0	E980.4
F (hydrocortisone)	962.0	E858.0	E932.0	E950.4	E962.0	E980.4
Congo red	977.8	E858.8	E947.8	E950.4	E962.0	E980.4

Drug, chemical	Poisoning	External Cause (E Code)				
		Accident	Therapeutic Use	Suicide Attempt	Assault	Undetermined
Coniine, conine	965.7	E850.7	E935.7	E950.0	E962.0	E980.0
Conium (maculatum)	988.2	E865.4	–	E950.9	E962.1	E980.9
Conjugated estrogens (equine)	962.2	E858.0	E932.2	E950.4	E962.0	E980.4
Contac	975.6	E858.6	E945.6	E950.4	E962.0	E980.4
Contact lens solution	976.5	E858.7	E946.5	E950.4	E962.0	E980.4
Contraceptives (oral)	962.2	E858.0	E932.2	E950.4	E962.0	E980.4
vaginal	976.8	E858.7	E946.8	E950.4	E962.0	E980.4
Contrast media (roentgenographic)	977.8	E858.8	E947.8	E950.4	E962.0	E980.4
Convallaria majalis	988.2	E865.4	–	E950.9	E962.1	E980.9
Copper (dust) (fumes) (salts) NEC	985.8	E866.4	–	E950.9	E962.1	E980.9
arsenate, arsenite	985.1	E866.3	–	E950.8	E962.1	E980.8
insecticide	985.1	E863.4	–	E950.8	E962.1	E980.8
emetic	973.6	E858.4	E943.6	E950.4	E962.0	E980.4
fungicide	985.8	E863.6	–	E950.6	E962.1	E980.7
insecticide	985.8	E863.4	–	E950.6	E962.1	E980.7
oleate	976.0	E858.7	E946.0	E950.4	E962.0	E980.4
sulfate	983.9	E864.3	–	E950.7	E962.1	E980.6
fungicide	983.9	E863.6	–	E950.7	E962.1	E980.6
cupric	973.6	E858.4	E943.6	E950.4	E962.0	E980.4
cuprous	983.9	E864.3	–	E950.7	E962.1	E980.6
Copperhead snake (bite) (venom)	989.5	E905.0	–	E950.9	E962.1	E980.9
Coral (sting)	989.5	E905.6	–	E950.9	E962.1	E980.9
snake (bite) (venom)	989.5	E905.0	–	E950.9	E962.1	E980.9
Cordran	976.0	E858.7	E946.0	E950.4	E962.0	E980.4
Corn cures	976.4	E858.7	E946.4	E950.4	E962.0	E980.4
Cornhusker's lotion	976.3	E858.7	E946.3	E950.4	E962.0	E980.4
Corn starch	976.3	E858.7	E946.3	E950.4	E962.0	E980.4
Corrosive	983.9	E864.4	–	E950.7	E962.1	E980.6
acids NEC	983.1	E864.1	–	E950.7	E962.1	E980.6
aromatics	983.0	E864.0	–	E950.7	E962.1	E980.6
disinfectant	983.0	E861.4	–	E950.7	E962.1	E980.6
fumes NEC	987.9	E869.9	–	E952.9	E962.2	E982.9
specified NEC	983.9	E864.3	–	E950.7	E962.1	E980.6
sublimate – *see* Mercury, chloride						
Cortate	962.0	E858.0	E932.0	E950.4	E962.0	E980.4
Cort-Dome	962.0	E858.0	E932.0	E950.4	E962.0	E980.4
ENT agent	976.6	E858.7	E946.6	E950.4	E962.0	E980.4
ophthalmic preparation	976.5	E858.7	E946.5	E950.4	E962.0	E980.4
topical NEC	976.0	E858.7	E946.0	E950.4	E962.0	E980.4
Cortef	962.0	E858.0	E932.0	E950.4	E962.0	E980.4
ENT agent	976.6	E858.7	E946.6	E950.4	E962.0	E980.4
ophthalmic preparation	976.5	E858.7	E946.5	E950.4	E962.0	E980.4
topical NEC	976.0	E858.7	E946.0	E950.4	E962.0	E980.4
Corticosteroids (fluorinated)	962.0	E858.0	E932.0	E950.4	E962.0	E980.4
ENT agent	976.6	E858.7	E946.6	E950.4	E962.0	E980.4
ophthalmic preparation	976.5	E858.7	E946.5	E950.4	E962.0	E980.4
topical NEC	976.0	E858.7	E946.0	E950.4	E962.0	E980.4
Corticotropin	962.4	E858.0	E932.4	E950.4	E962.0	E980.4
Cortisol	962.0	E858.0	E932.0	E950.4	E962.0	E980.4
ENT agent	976.6	E858.7	E946.6	E950.4	E962.0	E980.4
ophthalmic preparation	976.5	E858.7	E946.5	E950.4	E962.0	E980.4
topical NEC	976.0	E858.7	E946.0	E950.4	E962.0	E980.4
Cortisone derivatives (acetate)	962.0	E858.0	E932.0	E950.4	E962.0	E980.4
ENT agent	976.6	E858.7	E946.6	E950.4	E962.0	E980.4
ophthalmic preparation	976.5	E858.7	E946.5	E950.4	E962.0	E980.4
topical NEC	976.0	E858.7	E946.0	E950.4	E962.0	E980.4
Cortogen	962.0	E858.0	E932.0	E950.4	E962.0	E980.4
ENT agent	976.6	E858.7	E946.6	E950.4	E962.0	E980.4
ophthalmic preparation	976.5	E858.7	E946.5	E950.4	E962.0	E980.4
Cortone	962.0	E858.0	E932.0	E950.4	E962.0	E980.4
ENT agent	976.6	E858.7	E946.6	E950.4	E962.0	E980.4
ophthalmic preparation	976.5	E858.7	E946.5	E950.4	E962.0	E980.4
Cortril	962.0	E858.0	E932.0	E950.4	E962.0	E980.4
ENT agent	976.6	E858.7	E946.6	E950.4	E962.0	E980.4
ophthalmic preparation	976.5	E858.7	E946.5	E950.4	E962.0	E980.4
topical NEC	976.0	E858.7	E946.0	E950.4	E962.0	E980.4
Cosmetics	989.89	E866.7	–	E950.9	E962.1	E980.9
Cosyntropin	977.8	E858.8	E947.8	E950.4	E962.0	E980.4
Cotarnine	964.5	E858.2	E934.5	E950.4	E962.0	E980.4
Cottonseed oil	976.3	E858.7	E946.3	E950.4	E962.0	E980.4
Cough mixtures (antitussives)	975.4	E858.6	E945.4	E950.4	E962.0	E980.4
containing opiates	965.09	E850.2	E935.2	E950.0	E962.0	E980.0
expectorants	975.5	E858.6	E945.5	E950.4	E962.0	E980.4
Coumadin	964.2	E858.2	E934.2	E950.4	E962.0	E980.4
rodenticide	989.4	E863.7	–	E950.6	E962.1	E980.7
Coumarin	964.2	E858.2	E934.2	E950.4	E962.0	E980.4
Coumetarol	964.2	E858.2	E934.2	E950.4	E962.0	E980.4
Cowbane	988.2	E865.4	–	E950.9	E962.1	E980.9
Cozyme	963.5	E858.1	E933.5	E950.4	E962.0	E980.4
Crack	970.8	E854.3	E940.8	E950.4	E962.0	E980.4
Creolin	983.0	E864.0	–	E950.7	E962.1	E980.6
disinfectant	983.0	E861.4	–	E950.7	E962.1	E980.6
Creosol (compound)	983.0	E864.0	–	E950.7	E962.1	E980.6
Creosote (beechwood) (coal tar)	983.0	E864.0	–	E950.7	E962.1	E980.6
medicinal (expectorant)	975.5	E858.6	E945.5	E950.4	E962.0	E980.4
syrup	975.5	E858.6	E945.5	E950.4	E962.0	E980.4
Cresol	983.0	E864.0	–	E950.7	E962.1	E980.6
disinfectant	983.0	E861.4	–	E950.7	E962.1	E980.6
Cresylic acid	983.0	E864.0	–	E950.7	E962.1	E980.6
Cropropamide	965.7	E850.7	E935.7	E950.0	E962.0	E980.0
with crotethamide	970.0	E854.3	E940.0	E950.4	E962.0	E980.4
Crotamiton	976.0	E858.7	E946.0	E950.4	E962.0	E980.4
Crotethamide	965.7	E850.7	E935.7	E950.0	E962.0	E980.0
with cropropamide	970.0	E854.3	E940.0	E950.4	E962.0	E980.4
Croton (oil)	973.1	E858.4	E943.1	E950.4	E962.0	E980.4
chloral	967.1	E852.0	E937.1	E950.2	E962.0	E980.2
Crude oil	981	E862.1	–	E950.9	E962.1	E980.9
Cryogenine	965.8	E850.8	E935.8	E950.0	E962.0	E980.0
Cryolite (pesticide)	989.4	E863.4	–	E950.6	E962.1	E980.7
Cryptenamine	972.6	E858.3	E942.6	E950.4	E962.0	E980.4
Crystal violet	976.0	E858.7	E946.0	E950.4	E962.0	E980.4
Cuckoopint	988.2	E865.4	–	E950.9	E962.1	E980.9
Cumetharol	964.2	E858.2	E934.2	E950.4	E962.0	E980.4
Cupric sulfate	973.6	E858.4	E943.6	E950.4	E962.0	E980.4
Cuprous sulfate	983.9	E864.3	–	E950.7	E962.1	E980.6
Curare, curarine	975.2	E858.6	E945.2	E950.4	E962.0	E980.4
Cyanic acid – *see* Cyanide(s)						
Cyanide(s) (compounds) (hydrogen) (potassium) (sodium) NEC	989.0	E866.8	–	E950.9	E962.1	E980.9
dust or gas (inhalation) NEC	987.7	E869.8	–	E952.8	E962.2	E982.8
fumigant	989.0	E863.8	–	E950.6	E962.1	E980.7
mercuric – *see* Mercury						
pesticide (dust) (fumes)	989.0	E863.4	–	E950.6	E962.1	E980.7
Cyanocobalamin	964.1	E858.2	E934.1	E950.4	E962.0	E980.4
Cyanogen (chloride) (gas) NEC	987.8	E869.8	–	E952.8	E962.2	E982.8
Cyclaine	968.5	E855.2	E938.5	E950.4	E962.0	E980.4
Cyclamen europaeum	988.2	E865.4	–	E950.9	E962.1	E980.9
Cyclandelate	972.5	E858.3	E942.5	E950.4	E962.0	E980.4
Cyclazocine	965.09	E850.2	E935.2	E950.0	E962.0	E980.0
Cyclizine	963.0	E858.1	E933.0	E950.4	E962.0	E980.4
Cyclobarbital, cyclobarbitone	967.0	E851	E937.0	E950.1	E962.0	E980.1
Cycloguanil	961.4	E857	E931.4	E950.4	E962.0	E980.4
Cyclohexane	982.0	E862.4	–	E950.9	E962.1	E980.9
Cyclohexanol	980.8	E860.8	–	E950.9	E962.1	E980.9
Cyclohexanone	982.8	E862.4	–	E950.9	E962.1	E980.9
Cyclomethycaine	968.5	E855.2	E938.5	E950.4	E962.0	E980.4
Cyclopentamine	971.2	E855.5	E941.2	E950.4	E962.0	E980.4
Cyclopenthiazide	974.3	E858.5	E944.3	E950.4	E962.0	E980.4
Cyclopentolate	971.1	E855.4	E941.1	E950.4	E962.0	E980.4
Cyclophosphamide	963.1	E858.1	E933.1	E950.4	E962.0	E980.4
Cyclopropane	968.2	E855.1	E938.2	E950.4	E962.0	E980.4
Cycloserine	960.6	E856	E930.6	E950.4	E962.0	E980.4
Cyclothiazide	974.3	E858.5	E944.3	E950.4	E962.0	E980.4
Cycrimine	966.4	E855.0	E936.4	E950.4	E962.0	E980.4
Cymarin	972.1	E858.3	E942.1	E950.4	E962.0	E980.4
Cyproheptadine	963.0	E858.1	E933.0	E950.4	E962.0	E980.4
Cyprolidol ▲	969.09	E854.0	E939.0	E950.3	E962.0	E980.3
Cytarabine	963.1	E858.1	E933.1	E950.4	E962.0	E980.4
Cytisus						
laburnum	988.2	E865.4	–	E950.9	E962.1	E980.9
scoparius	988.2	E865.4	–	E950.9	E962.1	E980.9
Cytomel	962.7	E858.0	E932.7	E950.4	E962.0	E980.4
Cytosine (antineoplastic)	963.1	E858.1	E933.1	E950.4	E962.0	E980.4
Cytoxan	963.1	E858.1	E933.1	E950.4	E962.0	E980.4
Dacarbazine	963.1	E858.1	E933.1	E950.4	E962.0	E980.4
Dactinomycin	960.7	E856	E930.7	E950.4	E962.0	E980.4
DADPS	961.8	E857	E931.8	E950.4	E962.0	E980.4
Dakin's solution (external)	976.0	E858.7	E946.0	E950.4	E962.0	E980.4
Dalmane	969.4	E853.2	E939.4	E950.3	E962.0	E980.3
DAM	977.2	E858.8	E947.2	E950.4	E962.0	E980.4
Danilone	964.2	E858.2	E934.2	E950.4	E962.0	E980.4
Danthron	973.1	E858.4	E943.1	E950.4	E962.0	E980.4
Dantrolene	975.2	E858.6	E945.2	E950.4	E962.0	E980.4
Daphne (gnidium) (mezereum)	988.2	E865.4	–	E950.9	E962.1	E980.9
berry	988.2	E865.3	–	E950.9	E962.1	E980.9
Dapsone	961.8	E857	E931.8	E950.4	E962.0	E980.4
Daraprim	961.4	E857	E931.4	E950.4	E962.0	E980.4
Darnel	988.2	E865.3	–	E950.9	E962.1	E980.9
Darvon	965.8	E850.8	E935.8	E950.0	E962.0	E980.0
Daunorubicin	960.7	E856	E930.7	E950.4	E962.0	E980.4
DBI	962.3	E858.0	E932.3	E950.4	E962.0	E980.4
D-Con (rodenticide)	989.4	E863.7	–	E950.6	E962.1	E980.7
DDS	961.8	E857	E931.8	E950.4	E962.0	E980.4
DDT	989.2	E863.0	–	E950.6	E962.1	E980.7

Drug, chemical	Poisoning	External Cause (E Code)				
		Accident	Therapeutic Use	Suicide Attempt	Assault	Undetermined
Deadly nightshade	988.2	E865.4	–	E950.9	E962.1	E980.9
berry	988.2	E865.3	–	E950.9	E962.1	E980.9
Deanol ▲	969.79	E854.2	E939.7	E950.3	E962.0	E980.3
Debrisoquine	972.6	E858.3	E942.6	E950.4	E962.0	E980.4
Decaborane	989.89	E866.8	–	E950.9	E962.1	E980.9
fumes	987.8	E869.8	–	E952.8	E962.2	E982.8
Decadron	962.0	E858.0	E932.0	E950.4	E962.0	E980.4
ENT agent	976.6	E858.7	E946.6	E950.4	E962.0	E980.4
ophthalmic preparation	976.5	E858.7	E946.5	E950.4	E962.0	E980.4
topical NEC	976.0	E858.7	E946.0	E950.4	E962.0	E980.4
Decahydronaphthalene	982.0	E862.4	–	E950.9	E962.1	E980.9
Decalin	982.0	E862.4	–	E950.9	E962.1	E980.9
Decamethonium	975.2	E858.6	E945.2	E950.4	E962.0	E980.4
Decholin	973.4	E858.4	E943.4	E950.4	E962.0	E980.4
sodium (diagnostic)	977.8	E858.8	E947.8	E950.4	E962.0	E980.4
Declomycin	960.4	E856	E930.4	E950.4	E962.0	E980.4
Deferoxamine	963.8	E858.1	E933.8	E950.4	E962.0	E980.4
Dehydrocholic acid	973.4	E858.4	E943.4	E950.4	E962.0	E980.4
DeKalin	982.0	E862.4	–	E950.9	E962.1	E980.9
Delalutin	962.2	E858.0	E932.2	E950.4	E962.0	E980.4
Delphinium	988.2	E865.3	–	E950.9	E962.1	E980.9
Deltasone	962.0	E858.0	E932.0	E950.4	E962.0	E980.4
Deltra	962.0	E858.0	E932.0	E950.4	E962.0	E980.4
Delvinal	967.0	E851	E937.0	E950.1	E962.0	E980.1
Demecarium (bromide)	971.0	E855.3	E941.0	E950.4	E962.0	E980.4
Demeclocycline	960.4	E856	E930.4	E950.4	E962.0	E980.4
Demecolcine	963.1	E858.1	E933.1	E950.4	E962.0	E980.4
Demelanizing agents	976.8	E858.7	E946.8	E950.4	E962.0	E980.4
Demerol	965.09	E850.2	E935.2	E950.0	E962.0	E980.0
Demethylchlortetracycline	960.4	E856	E930.4	E950.4	E962.0	E980.4
Demethyltetracycline	960.4	E856	E930.4	E950.4	E962.0	E980.4
Demeton	989.3	E863.1	–	E950.6	E962.1	E980.7
Demulcents	976.3	E858.7	E946.3	E950.4	E962.0	E980.4
Demulen	962.2	E858.0	E932.2	E950.4	E962.0	E980.4
Denatured alcohol	980.0	E860.1	–	E950.9	E962.1	E980.9
Dendrid	976.5	E858.7	E946.5	E950.4	E962.0	E980.4
Dental agents, topical	976.7	E858.7	E946.7	E950.4	E962.0	E980.4
Deodorant spray (feminine hygiene)	976.8	E858.7	E946.8	E950.4	E962.0	E980.4
Deoxyribonuclease	963.4	E858.1	E933.4	E950.4	E962.0	E980.4
Depressants						
appetite, central	977.0	E858.8	E947.0	E950.4	E962.0	E980.4
cardiac	972.0	E858.3	E942.0	E950.4	E962.0	E980.4
central nervous system (anesthetic)	968.4	E855.1	E938.4	E950.4	E962.0	E980.4
psychotherapeutic	969.5	E853.9	E939.5	E950.3	E962.0	E980.3
Dequalinium	976.0	E858.7	E946.0	E950.4	E962.0	E980.4
Dermolate	976.2	E858.7	E946.2	E950.4	E962.0	E980.4
DES	962.2	E858.0	E932.2	E950.4	E962.0	E980.4
Desenex	976.0	E858.7	E946.0	E950.4	E962.0	E980.4
Deserpidine	972.6	E858.3	E942.6	E950.4	E962.0	E980.4
Desianoside	972.1	E858.3	E942.1	E950.4	E962.0	E980.4
Desipramine ▲	969.05	E854.0	E939.0	E950.3	E962.0	E980.3
Desocodeine	965.09	E850.2	E935.2	E950.0	E962.0	E980.0
Desomorphine	965.09	E850.2	E935.2	E950.0	E962.0	E980.0
Desonide	976.0	E858.7	E946.0	E950.4	E962.0	E980.4
Desoxycorticosterone derivatives	962.0	E858.0	E932.0	E950.4	E962.0	E980.4
Desoxyephedrine ▲	969.72	E854.2	E939.7	E950.3	E962.0	E980.3
DET	969.6	E854.1	E939.6	E950.3	E962.0	E980.3
Detergents (ingested) (synthetic)	989.6	E861.0	–	E950.9	E962.1	E980.9
external medication	976.2	E858.7	E946.2	E950.4	E962.0	E980.4
Deterrent, alcohol	977.3	E858.8	E947.3	E950.4	E962.0	E980.4
Detrothyronine	962.7	E858.0	E932.7	E950.4	E962.0	E980.4
Dettol (external medication)	976.0	E858.7	E946.0	E950.4	E962.0	E980.4
Dexamethasone	962.0	E858.0	E932.0	E950.4	E962.0	E980.4
ENT agent	976.6	E858.7	E946.6	E950.4	E962.0	E980.4
ophthalmic preparation	976.5	E858.7	E946.5	E950.4	E962.0	E980.4
topical NEC	976.0	E858.7	E946.0	E950.4	E962.0	E980.4
Dexamphetamine ▲	969.72	E854.2	E939.7	E950.3	E962.0	E980.3
Dexedrine ▲	969.72	E854.2	E939.7	E950.3	E962.0	E980.3
Dexpanthenol	963.5	E858.1	E933.5	E950.4	E962.0	E980.4
Dextran	964.8	E858.2	E934.8	E950.4	E962.0	E980.4
Dextriferron	964.0	E858.2	E934.0	E950.4	E962.0	E980.4
Dextroamphetamine ▲	969.72	E854.2	E939.7	E950.3	E962.0	E980.3
Dextro calcium pantothenate	963.5	E858.1	E933.5	E950.4	E962.0	E980.4
Dextromethorphan	975.4	E858.6	E945.4	E950.4	E962.0	E980.4
Dextromoramide	965.09	E850.2	E935.2	E950.0	E962.0	E980.0
Dextro pantothenyl alcohol	963.5	E858.1	E933.5	E950.4	E962.0	E980.4
topical	976.8	E858.7	E946.8	E950.4	E962.0	E980.4
Dextropropoxyphene (hydrochloride)	965.8	E850.8	E935.8	E950.0	E962.0	E980.0
Dextrorphan	965.09	E850.2	E935.2	E950.0	E962.0	E980.0
Dextrose NEC	974.5	E858.5	E944.5	E950.4	E962.0	E980.4
Dextrothyroxin	962.7	E858.0	E932.7	E950.4	E962.0	E980.4
DFP	971.0	E855.3	E941.0	E950.4	E962.0	E980.4
DHE-45	972.9	E858.3	E942.9	E950.4	E962.0	E980.4
Diabinese	962.3	E858.0	E932.3	E950.4	E962.0	E980.4
Diacetyl monoxime	977.2	E858.8	E947.2	E950.4	E962.0	E980.4
Diacetylmorphine	965.01	E850.0	E935.0	E950.0	E962.0	E980.0
Diagnostic agents	977.8	E858.8	E947.8	E950.4	E962.0	E980.4
Dial (soap)	976.2	E858.7	E946.2	E950.4	E962.0	E980.4
sedative	967.0	E851	E937.0	E950.1	E962.0	E980.1
Diallylbarbituric acid	967.0	E851	E937.0	E950.1	E962.0	E980.1
Diaminodiphenylsulfone	961.8	E857	E931.8	E950.4	E962.0	E980.4
Diamorphine	965.01	E850.0	E935.0	E950.0	E962.0	E980.0
Diamox	974.2	E858.5	E944.2	E950.4	E962.0	E980.4
Diamthazole	976.0	E858.7	E946.0	E950.4	E962.0	E980.4
Diaphenylsulfone	961.8	E857	E931.8	E950.4	E962.0	E980.4
Diasone (sodium)	961.8	E857	E931.8	E950.4	E962.0	E980.4
Diazepam	969.4	E853.2	E939.4	E950.3	E962.0	E980.3
Diazinon	989.3	E863.1	–	E950.6	E962.1	E980.7
Diazomethane (gas)	987.8	E869.8	–	E952.8	E962.2	E982.8
Diazoxide	972.5	E858.3	E942.5	E950.4	E962.0	E980.4
Dibenamine	971.3	E855.6	E941.3	E950.4	E962.0	E980.4
Dibenzheptropine	963.0	E858.1	E933.0	E950.4	E962.0	E980.4
Dibenzyline	971.3	E855.6	E941.3	E950.4	E962.0	E980.4
Diborane (gas)	987.8	E869.8	–	E952.8	E962.2	E982.8
Dibromomannitol	963.1	E858.1	E933.1	E950.4	E962.0	E980.4
Dibucaine (spinal)	968.7	E855.2	E938.7	E950.4	E962.0	E980.4
topical (surface)	968.5	E855.2	E938.5	E950.4	E962.0	E980.4
Dibunate sodium	975.4	E858.6	E945.4	E950.4	E962.0	E980.4
Dibutoline	971.1	E855.4	E941.1	E950.4	E962.0	E980.4
Dicapthon	989.4	E863.4	–	E950.6	E962.1	E980.7
Dichloralphenazone	967.1	E852.0	E937.1	E950.2	E962.0	E980.2
Dichlorodifluoromethane	987.4	E869.2	–	E952.8	E962.2	E982.8
Dichloroethane	982.3	E862.4	–	E950.9	E962.1	E980.9
Dichloroethylene	982.3	E862.4	–	E950.9	E962.1	E980.9
Dichloroethyl sulfide	987.8	E869.8	–	E952.8	E962.2	E982.8
Dichlorohydrin	982.3	E862.4	–	E950.9	E962.1	E980.9
Dichloromethane (solvent) (vapor)	982.3	E862.4	–	E950.9	E962.1	E980.9
Dichlorophen(e)	961.6	E857	E931.6	E950.4	E962.0	E980.4
Dichlorphenamide	974.2	E858.5	E944.2	E950.4	E962.0	E980.4
Dichlorvos	989.3	E863.1	–	E950.6	E962.1	E980.7
Diclofenac sodium	965.69	E850.6	E935.6	E950.0	E962.0	E980.0
Dicoumarin, dicumarol	964.2	E858.2	E934.2	E950.4	E962.0	E980.4
Dicyanogen (gas)	987.8	E869.8	–	E952.8	E962.2	E982.8
Dicyclomine	971.1	E855.4	E941.1	E950.4	E962.0	E980.4
Dieldrin (vapor)	989.2	E863.0	–	E950.6	E962.1	E980.7
Dienestrol	962.2	E858.0	E932.2	E950.4	E962.0	E980.4
Dietetics	977.0	E858.8	E947.0	E950.4	E962.0	E980.4
Diethazine	966.4	E855.0	E936.4	E950.4	E962.0	E980.4
Diethyl						
barbituric acid	967.0	E851	E937.0	E950.1	E962.0	E980.1
carbamazine	961.6	E857	E931.6	E950.4	E962.0	E980.4
carbinol	980.8	E860.8	–	E950.9	E962.1	E980.9
carbonate	982.8	E862.4	–	E950.9	E962.1	E980.9
ether (vapor) – *see* Ether(s)						
propion	977.0	E858.8	E947.0	E950.4	E962.0	E980.4
stilbestrol	962.2	E858.0	E932.2	E950.4	E962.0	E980.4
Diethylene						
dioxide	982.8	E862.4	–	E950.9	E962.1	E980.9
glycol (monoacetate) (monoethyl ether)	982.8	E862.4	–	E950.9	E962.1	E980.9
Diethylsulfone-diethylmethane	967.8	E852.8	E937.8	E950.2	E962.0	E980.2
Difencloxazine	965.09	E850.2	E935.2	E950.0	E962.0	E980.0
Diffusin	963.4	E858.1	E933.4	E950.4	E962.0	E980.4
Diflos	971.0	E855.3	E941.0	E950.4	E962.0	E980.4
Digestants	973.4	E858.4	E943.4	E950.4	E962.0	E980.4
Digitalin(e)	972.1	E858.3	E942.1	E950.4	E962.0	E980.4
Digitalis glycosides	972.1	E858.3	E942.1	E950.4	E962.0	E980.4
Digitoxin	972.1	E858.3	E942.1	E950.4	E962.0	E980.4
Digoxin	972.1	E858.3	E942.1	E950.4	E962.0	E980.4
Dihydrocodeine	965.09	E850.2	E935.2	E950.0	E962.0	E980.0
Dihydrocodeinone	965.09	E850.2	E935.2	E950.0	E962.0	E980.0
Dihydroergocristine	972.9	E858.3	E942.9	E950.4	E962.0	E980.4
Dihydroergotamine	972.9	E858.3	E942.9	E950.4	E962.0	E980.4
Dihydroergotoxine	972.9	E858.3	E942.9	E950.4	E962.0	E980.4
Dihydrohydroxycodeinone	965.09	E850.2	E935.2	E950.0	E962.0	E980.0
Dihydrohydroxymorphinone	965.09	E850.2	E935.2	E950.0	E962.0	E980.0
Dihydroisocodeine	965.09	E850.2	E935.2	E950.0	E962.0	E980.0
Dihydromorphine	965.09	E850.2	E935.2	E950.0	E962.0	E980.0
Dihydromorphinone	965.09	E850.2	E935.2	E950.0	E962.0	E980.0
Dihydrostreptomycin	960.6	E856	E930.6	E950.4	E962.0	E980.4
Dihydrotachysterol	962.6	E858.0	E932.6	E950.4	E962.0	E980.4
Dihydroxyanthraquinone	973.1	E858.4	E943.1	E950.4	E962.0	E980.4
Dihydroxycodeinone	965.09	E850.2	E935.2	E950.0	E962.0	E980.0

Drug, chemical	Poisoning	External Cause (E Code)				
		Accident	Therapeutic Use	Suicide Attempt	Assault	Undetermined
Diiodohydroxyquin	961.3	E857	E931.3	E950.4	E962.0	E980.4
topical	976.0	E858.7	E946.0	E950.4	E962.0	E980.4
Diiodohydroxyquinoline	961.3	E857	E931.3	E950.4	E962.0	E980.4
Dilantin	966.1	E855.0	E936.1	E950.4	E962.0	E980.4
Dilaudid	965.09	E850.2	E935.2	E950.0	E962.0	E980.0
Diloxanide	961.5	E857	E931.5	E950.4	E962.0	E980.4
Dimefline	970.0	E854.3	E940.0	E950.4	E962.0	E980.4
Dimenhydrinate	963.0	E858.1	E933.0	E950.4	E962.0	E980.4
Dimercaprol	963.8	E858.1	E933.8	E950.4	E962.0	E980.4
Dimercaptopropanol	963.8	E858.1	E933.8	E950.4	E962.0	E980.4
Dimetane	963.0	E858.1	E933.0	E950.4	E962.0	E980.4
Dimethicone	976.3	E858.7	E946.3	E950.4	E962.0	E980.4
Dimethindene	963.0	E858.1	E933.0	E950.4	E962.0	E980.4
Dimethisoquin	968.5	E855.2	E938.5	E950.4	E962.0	E980.4
Dimethisterone	962.2	E858.0	E932.2	E950.4	E962.0	E980.4
Dimethoxanate	975.4	E858.6	E945.4	E950.4	E962.0	E980.4
Dimethyl						
arsine, arsinic acid – *see* Arsenic						
carbinol	980.2	E860.3	–	E950.9	E962.1	E980.9
diguanide	962.3	E858.0	E932.3	E950.4	E962.0	E980.4
ketone	982.8	E862.4	–	E950.9	E962.1	E980.9
vapor	987.8	E869.8	–	E952.8	E962.2	E982.8
meperidine	965.09	E850.2	E935.2	E950.0	E962.0	E980.0
parathion	989.3	E863.1	–	E950.6	E962.1	E980.7
polysiloxane	973.8	E858.4	E943.8	E950.4	E962.0	E980.4
sulfate (fumes)	987.8	E869.8	–	E952.8	E962.2	E982.8
liquid	983.9	E864.3	–	E950.7	E962.1	E980.6
sulfoxide NEC	982.8	E862.4	–	E950.9	E962.1	E980.9
medicinal	976.4	E858.7	E946.4	E950.4	E962.0	E980.4
triptamine	969.6	E854.1	E939.6	E950.3	E962.0	E980.3
tubocurarine	975.2	E858.6	E945.2	E950.4	E962.0	E980.4
Dindevan	964.2	E858.2	E934.2	E950.4	E962.0	E980.4
Dinitro (-ortho-) **cresol** (herbicide) (spray)	989.4	E863.5	–	E950.6	E962.1	E980.7
insecticide	989.4	E863.4	–	E950.6	E962.1	E980.7
Dinitrobenzene	983.0	E864.0	–	E950.7	E962.1	E980.6
vapor	987.8	E869.8	–	E952.8	E962.2	E982.8
Dinitro-orthocresol (herbicide)	989.4	E863.5	–	E950.6	E962.1	E980.7
insecticide	989.4	E863.4	–	E950.6	E962.1	E980.7
Dinitrophenol (herbicide) (spray)	989.4	E863.5	–	E950.6	E962.1	E980.7
insecticide	989.4	E863.4	–	E950.6	E962.1	E980.7
Dinoprost	975.0	E858.6	E945.0	E950.4	E962.0	E980.4
Dioctyl sulfosuccinate (calcium) (sodium)	973.2	E858.4	E943.2	E950.4	E962.0	E980.4
Diodoquin	961.3	E857	E931.3	E950.4	E962.0	E980.4
Dione derivatives NEC	966.3	E855.0	E936.3	E950.4	E962.0	E980.4
Dionin	965.09	E850.2	E935.2	E950.0	E962.0	E980.0
Dioxane	982.8	E862.4	–	E950.9	E962.1	E980.9
Dioxin – *see* herbicide						
Dioxyline	972.5	E858.3	E942.5	E950.4	E962.0	E980.4
Dipentene	982.8	E862.4	–	E950.9	E962.1	E980.9
Diphemanil	971.1	E855.4	E941.1	E950.4	E962.0	E980.4
Diphenadione	964.2	E858.2	E934.2	E950.4	E962.0	E980.4
Diphenhydramine	963.0	E858.1	E933.0	E950.4	E962.0	E980.4
Diphenidol	963.0	E858.1	E933.0	E950.4	E962.0	E980.4
Diphenoxylate	973.5	E858.4	E943.5	E950.4	E962.0	E980.4
Diphenylchloroarsine	985.1	E866.3	–	E950.8	E962.1	E980.8
Diphenylhydantoin (sodium)	966.1	E855.0	E936.1	E950.4	E962.0	E980.4
Diphenylpyraline	963.0	E858.1	E933.0	E950.4	E962.0	E980.4
Diphtheria antitoxin	979.9	E858.8	E949.9	E950.4	E962.0	E980.4
toxoid	978.5	E858.8	E948.5	E950.4	E962.0	E980.4
with tetanus toxoid	978.9	E858.8	E948.9	E950.4	E962.0	E980.4
with pertussis component	978.6	E858.8	E948.6	E950.4	E962.0	E980.4
vaccine	978.5	E858.8	E948.5	E950.4	E962.0	E980.4
Dipipanone	965.09	E850.2	E935.2	E950.0	E962.0	E980.0
Diplovax	979.5	E858.8	E949.5	E950.4	E962.0	E980.4
Diprophylline	975.1	E858.6	E945.1	E950.4	E962.0	E980.4
Dipyridamole	972.4	E858.3	E942.4	E950.4	E962.0	E980.4
Dipyrone	965.5	E850.5	E935.5	E950.0	E962.0	E980.0
Diquat	989.4	E863.5	–	E950.6	E962.1	E980.7
Disinfectant NEC	983.9	E861.4	–	E950.7	E962.1	E980.6
alkaline	983.2	E861.4	–	E950.7	E962.1	E980.6
aromatic	983.0	E861.4	–	E950.7	E962.1	E980.6
Disipal	966.4	E855.0	E936.4	E950.4	E962.0	E980.4
Disodium edetate	963.8	E858.1	E933.8	E950.4	E962.0	E980.4
Disulfamide	974.4	E858.5	E944.4	E950.4	E962.0	E980.4
Disulfanilamide	961.0	E857	E931.0	E950.4	E962.0	E980.4
Disulfiram	977.3	E858.8	E947.3	E950.4	E962.0	E980.4
Dithiazanine	961.6	E857	E931.6	E950.4	E962.0	E980.4
Dithioglycerol	963.8	E858.1	E933.8	E950.4	E962.0	E980.4
Dithranol	976.4	E858.7	E946.4	E950.4	E962.0	E980.4
Diucardin	974.3	E858.5	E944.3	E950.4	E962.0	E980.4

Drug, chemical	Poisoning	External Cause (E Code)				
		Accident	Therapeutic Use	Suicide Attempt	Assault	Undetermined
Diupres	974.3	E858.5	E944.3	E950.4	E962.0	E980.4
Diuretics NEC	974.4	E858.5	E944.4	E950.4	E962.0	E980.4
carbonic acid anhydrase inhibitors	974.2	E858.5	E944.2	E950.4	E962.0	E980.4
mercurial	974.0	E858.5	E944.0	E950.4	E962.0	E980.4
osmotic	974.4	E858.5	E944.4	E950.4	E962.0	E980.4
purine derivatives	974.1	E858.5	E944.1	E950.4	E962.0	E980.4
saluretic	974.3	E858.5	E944.3	E950.4	E962.0	E980.4
Diuril	974.3	E858.5	E944.3	E950.4	E962.0	E980.4
Divinyl ether	968.2	E855.1	E938.2	E950.4	E962.0	E980.4
D-lysergic acid diethylamide	969.6	E854.1	E939.6	E950.3	E962.0	E980.3
DMCT	960.4	E856	E930.4	E950.4	E962.0	E980.4
DMSO	982.8	E862.4	–	E950.9	E962.1	E980.9
DMT	969.6	E854.1	E939.6	E950.3	E962.0	E980.3
DNOC	989.4	E863.5	–	E950.6	E962.1	E980.7
DOCA	962.0	E858.0	E932.0	E950.4	E962.0	E980.4
Dolophine	965.02	E850.1	E935.1	E950.0	E962.0	E980.0
Doloxene	965.8	E850.8	E935.8	E950.0	E962.0	E980.0
DOM	969.6	E854.1	E939.6	E950.3	E962.0	E980.3
Domestic gas – *see* Gas, utility						
Domiphen (bromide) (lozenges)	976.6	E858.7	E946.6	E950.4	E962.0	E980.4
Dopa (levo)	966.4	E855.0	E936.4	E950.4	E962.0	E980.4
Dopamine	971.2	E855.5	E941.2	E950.4	E962.0	E980.4
Doriden	967.5	E852.4	E937.5	E950.2	E962.0	E980.2
Dormiral	967.0	E851	E937.0	E950.1	E962.0	E980.1
Dormison	967.8	E852.8	E937.8	E950.2	E962.0	E980.2
Dornase	963.4	E858.1	E933.4	E950.4	E962.0	E980.4
Dorsacaine	968.5	E855.2	E938.5	E950.4	E962.0	E980.4
Dothiepin hydrochloride ▲	969.05	E854.0	E939.0	E950.3	E962.0	E980.3
Doxapram	970.0	E854.3	E940.0	E950.4	E962.0	E980.4
Doxepin ▲	969.05	E854.0	E939.0	E950.3	E962.0	E980.3
Doxorubicin	960.7	E856	E930.7	E950.4	E962.0	E980.4
Doxycycline	960.4	E856	E930.4	E950.4	E962.0	E980.4
Doxylamine	963.0	E858.1	E933.0	E950.4	E962.0	E980.4
Dramamine	963.0	E858.1	E933.0	E950.4	E962.0	E980.4
Drano (drain cleaner)	983.2	E864.2	–	E950.7	E962.1	E980.6
Dromoran	965.09	E850.2	E935.2	E950.0	E962.0	E980.0
Dromostanolone	962.1	E858.0	E932.1	E950.4	E962.0	E980.4
Droperidol	969.2	E853.1	E939.2	E950.3	E962.0	E980.3
Drotrecogin alfa	964.2	E858.2	E934.2	E950.4	E962.0	E980.4
Drug	977.9	E858.9	E947.9	E950.5	E962.0	E980.5
specified NEC	977.8	E858.8	E947.8	E950.4	E962.0	E980.4
AHFS List						
4:00 antihistamine drugs	963.0	E858.1	E933.0	E950.4	E962.0	E980.4
8:04 amebacides	961.5	E857	E931.5	E950.4	E962.0	E980.4
arsenical anti-infectives	961.1	E857	E931.1	E950.4	E962.0	E980.4
quinoline derivatives	961.3	E857	E931.3	E950.4	E962.0	E980.4
8:08 anthelmintics	961.6	E857	E931.6	E950.4	E962.0	E980.4
quinoline derivatives	961.3	E857	E931.3	E950.4	E962.0	E980.4
8:12.04 antifungal antibiotics	960.1	E856	E930.1	E950.4	E962.0	E980.4
8:12.06 cephalosporins	960.5	E856	E930.5	E950.4	E962.0	E980.4
8:12.08 chloramphenicol	960.2	E856	E930.2	E950.4	E962.0	E980.4
8:12.12 erythromycins	960.3	E856	E930.3	E950.4	E962.0	E980.4
8:12.16 penicillins	960.0	E856	E930.0	E950.4	E962.0	E980.4
8:12.20 streptomycins	960.6	E856	E930.6	E950.4	E962.0	E980.4
8:12.24 tetracyclines	960.4	E856	E930.4	E950.4	E962.0	E980.4
8:12.28 other antibiotics	960.8	E856	E930.8	E950.4	E962.0	E980.4
antimycobacterial	960.6	E856	E930.6	E950.4	E962.0	E980.4
macrolides	960.3	E856	E930.3	E950.4	E962.0	E980.4
8:16 antituberculars	961.8	E857	E931.8	E950.4	E962.0	E980.4
antibiotics	960.6	E856	E930.6	E950.4	E962.0	E980.4
8:18 antivirals	961.7	E857	E931.7	E950.4	E962.0	E980.4
8:20 plasmodicides (antimalarials)	961.4	E857	E931.4	E950.4	E962.0	E980.4
8:24 sulfonamides	961.0	E857	E931.0	E950.4	E962.0	E980.4
8:26 sulfones	961.8	E857	E931.8	E950.4	E962.0	E980.4
8:28 treponemicides	961.2	E857	E931.2	E950.4	E962.0	E980.4
8:32 trichomonacides	961.5	E857	E931.5	E950.4	E962.0	E980.4
quinoline derivatives	961.3	E857	E931.3	E950.4	E962.0	E980.4
nitrofuran derivatives	961.9	E857	E931.9	E950.4	E962.0	E980.4
8:36 urinary germicides	961.9	E857	E931.9	E950.4	E962.0	E980.4
quinoline derivatives	961.3	E857	E931.3	E950.4	E962.0	E980.4
8:40 other anti-infectives	961.9	E857	E931.9	E950.4	E962.0	E980.4
10:00 antineoplastic agents	963.1	E858.1	E933.1	E950.4	E962.0	E980.4
antibiotics	960.7	E856	E930.7	E950.4	E962.0	E980.4
progestogens	962.2	E858.0	E932.2	E950.4	E962.0	E980.4
12:04 parasympatho-mimetic (cholinergic) agents	971.0	E855.3	E941.0	E950.4	E962.0	E980.4
12:08 parasympatholytic (cholinergic-blocking) agents	971.1	E855.4	E941.1	E950.4	E962.0	E980.4
12:12 Sympathomimetic (adrenergic) agents	971.2	E855.5	E941.2	E950.4	E962.0	E980.4
12:16 sympatholytic (adrenergic-blocking) agents	971.3	E855.6	E941.3	E950.4	E962.0	E980.4

Drug, chemical	Poisoning	External Cause (E Code)				
		Accident	Therapeutic Use	Suicide Attempt	Assault	Undetermined
Drug – continued						
AHFS List – *continued*						
12:20 skeletal muscle relaxants						
central nervous system muscle-tone depressants	968.0	E855.1	E938.0	E950.4	E962.0	E980.4
myoneural blocking agents	975.2	E858.6	E945.2	E950.4	E962.0	E980.4
16:00 blood derivatives	964.7	E858.2	E934.7	E950.4	E962.0	E980.4
20:04 antianemia drugs	964.1	E858.2	E934.1	E950.4	E962.0	E980.4
20:04.04 iron preparations	964.0	E858.2	E934.0	E950.4	E962.0	E980.4
20:04.08 liver and stomach preparations	964.1	E858.2	E934.1	E950.4	E962.0	E980.4
20:12.04 anticoagulants	964.2	E858.2	E934.2	E950.4	E962.0	E980.4
20:12.08 antiheparin agents	964.5	E858.2	E934.5	E950.4	E962.0	E980.4
20:12.12 coagulants	964.5	E858.2	E934.5	E950.4	E962.0	E980.4
20:12.16 hemostatics NEC	964.5	E858.2	E934.5	E950.4	E962.0	E980.4
capillary active drugs	972.8	E858.3	E942.8	E950.4	E962.0	E980.4
24:04 cardiac drugs	972.9	E858.3	E942.9	E950.4	E962.0	E980.4
cardiotonic agents	972.1	E858.3	E942.1	E950.4	E962.0	E980.4
rhythm regulators	972.0	E858.3	E942.0	E950.4	E962.0	E980.4
24:06 antilipemic agents	972.2	E858.3	E942.2	E950.4	E962.0	E980.4
thyroid derivatives	962.7	E858.0	E932.7	E950.4	E962.0	E980.4
24:08 hypotensive agents	972.6	E858.3	E942.6	E950.4	E962.0	E980.4
adrenergic blocking agents	971.3	E855.6	E941.3	E950.4	E962.0	E980.4
ganglion blocking agents	972.3	E858.3	E942.3	E950.4	E962.0	E980.4
vasodilators	972.5	E858.3	E942.5	E950.4	E962.0	E980.4
24:12 vasodilating agents NEC	972.5	E858.3	E942.5	E950.4	E962.0	E980.4
coronary	972.4	E858.3	E942.4	E950.4	E962.0	E980.4
nicotinic acid derivatives	972.2	E858.3	E942.2	E950.4	E962.0	E980.4
24:16 sclerosing agents	972.7	E858.3	E942.7	E950.4	E962.0	E980.4
28:04 general anesthetics	968.4	E855.1	E938.4	E950.4	E962.0	E980.4
gaseous anesthetics	968.2	E855.1	E938.2	E950.4	E962.0	E980.4
halothane	968.1	E855.1	E938.1	E950.4	E962.0	E980.4
intravenous anesthetics	968.3	E855.1	E938.3	E950.4	E962.0	E980.4
28:08 analgesics and antipyretics	965.9	E850.9	E935.9	E950.0	E962.0	E980.0
antirheumatics	965.69	E850.6	E935.6	E950.0	E962.0	E980.0
aromatic analgesics	965.4	E850.4	E935.4	E950.0	E962.0	E980.0
non-narcotic NEC	965.7	E850.7	E935.7	E950.0	E962.0	E980.0
opium alkaloids	965.00	E850.2	E935.2	E950.0	E962.0	E980.0
heroin	965.01	E850.0	E935.0	E950.0	E962.0	E980.0
methadone	965.02	E850.1	E935.1	E950.0	E962.0	E980.0
specified type NEC	965.09	E850.2	E935.2	E950.0	E962.0	E980.0
pyrazole derivatives	965.5	E850.5	E935.5	E950.0	E962.0	E980.0
salicylates	965.1	E850.3	E935.3	E950.0	E962.0	E980.0
specified NEC	965.8	E850.8	E935.8	E950.0	E962.0	E980.0
28:10 narcotic antagonists	970.1	E854.3	E940.1	E950.4	E962.0	E980.4
28:12 anticonvulsants	966.3	E855.0	E936.3	E950.4	E962.0	E980.4
barbiturates	967.0	E851	E937.0	E950.1	E962.0	E980.1
benzodiazepine-based tranquilizers	969.4	E853.2	E939.4	E950.3	E962.0	E980.3
bromides	967.3	E852.2	E937.3	E950.2	E962.0	E980.2
hydantoinderivatives	966.1	E855.0	E936.1	E950.4	E962.0	E980.4
oxazolidine (derivatives)	966.0	E855.0	E936.0	E950.4	E962.0	E980.4
succinimides	966.2	E855.0	E936.2	E950.4	E962.0	E980.4
28:16.04 anti-depressants ▲	969.00	E854.0	E939.0	E950.3	E962.0	E980.3
28:16.08 tranquilizers	969.5	E853.9	E939.5	E950.3	E962.0	E980.3
benzodiazepine-based	969.4	E853.2	E939.4	E950.3	E962.0	E980.3
butyrophenone-based	969.2	E853.1	E939.2	E950.3	E962.0	E980.3
major NEC	969.3	E853.8	E939.3	E950.3	E962.0	E980.3
phenothiazine-based	969.1	E853.0	E939.1	E950.3	E962.0	E980.3
28:16.12 other psychotherapeutic agents	969.8	E855.8	E939.8	E950.3	E962.0	E980.3
28:20 respiratory and cerebral stimulants	970.9	E854.3	E940.9	E950.4	E962.0	E980.4
analeplics	970.0	E854.3	E940.0	E950.4	E962.0	E980.4
anorexigenic agents	977.0	E858.8	E947.0	E950.4	E962.0	E980.4
psychostimulants ▲	969.70	E854.2	E939.7	E950.3	E962.0	E980.3
specified NEC	970.8	E854.3	E940.8	E950.4	E962.0	E980.4
28:24 sedatives and hypnotics	967.9	E852.9	E937.9	E950.2	E962.0	E980.2
barbiturates	967.0	E851	E937.0	E950.1	E962.0	E980.1
benzodiazepine-based tranquilizers	969.4	E853.2	E939.4	E950.3	E962.0	E980.3
chloral hydrate (group)	967.1	E852.0	E937.1	E950.2	E962.0	E980.2
glutethamide group	967.5	E852.4	E937.5	E950.2	E962.0	E980.2
intravenous anesthetics	968.3	E855.1	E938.3	E950.4	E962.0	E980.4
methaqualone (compounds)	967.4	E852.3	E937.4	E950.2	E962.0	E980.2
paraldehyde	967.2	E852.1	E937.2	E950.2	E962.0	E980.2
phenothiazine-based tranquilizers	969.1	E853.0	E939.1	E950.3	E962.0	E980.3
specified NEC	967.8	E852.8	E937.8	E950.2	E962.0	E980.2
thiobarbiturates	968.3	E855.1	E938.3	E950.4	E962.0	E980.4
tranquilizer NEC	969.5	E853.9	E939.5	E950.3	E962.0	E980.3
36:04 to 36:88 diagnostic agents	977.8	E858.8	E947.8	E950.4	E962.0	E980.4

Drug, chemical	Poisoning	External Cause (E Code)				
		Accident	Therapeutic Use	Suicide Attempt	Assault	Undetermined
Drug – continued						
AHFS List – *continued*						
40:00 electrolyte, caloric, and water balance agents NEC	974.5	E858.5	E944.5	E950.4	E962.0	E980.4
40:04 acidifying agents	963.2	E858.1	E933.2	E950.4	E962.0	E980.4
40:08 alkalinizing agents	963.3	E858.1	E933.3	E950.4	E962.0	E980.4
40:10 ammonia detoxicants	974.5	E858.5	E944.5	E950.4	E962.0	E980.4
40:12 replacement solutions	974.5	E858.5	E944.5	E950.4	E962.0	E980.4
plasma expanders	964.8	E858.2	E934.8	E950.4	E962.0	E980.4
40:16 sodium-removing resins	974.5	E858.5	E944.5	E950.4	E962.0	E980.4
40:18 potassium-removing resins	974.5	E858.5	E944.5	E950.4	E962.0	E980.4
40:20 caloric agents	974.5	E858.5	E944.5	E950.4	E962.0	E980.4
40:24 salt and sugar substitutes	974.5	E858.5	E944.5	E950.4	E962.0	E980.4
40:28 diuretics NEC	974.4	E858.5	E944.4	E950.4	E962.0	E980.4
carbonic acid anhydrase inhibitors	974.2	E858.5	E944.2	E950.4	E962.0	E980.4
mercurials	974.0	E858.5	E944.0	E950.4	E962.0	E980.4
purine derivatives	974.1	E858.5	E944.1	E950.4	E962.0	E980.4
saluretics	974.3	E858.5	E944.3	E950.4	E962.0	E980.4
thiazides	974.3	E858.5	E944.3	E950.4	E962.1	E980.4
40:36 irrigating solutions	974.5	E858.5	E944.5	E950.4	E962.0	E980.4
40:40 uricosuric agents	974.7	E858.5	E944.7	E950.4	E962.0	E980.4
44:00 enzymes	963.4	E858.1	E933.4	E950.4	E962.0	E980.4
fibrinolysis-affecting agents	964.4	E858.2	E934.4	E950.4	E962.0	E980.4
gastric agents	973.4	E858.4	E943.4	E950.4	E962.0	E980.4
48:00 expectorants and cough preparations						
antihistamine agents	963.0	E858.1	E933.0	E950.4	E962.0	E980.4
antitussives	975.4	E858.6	E945.4	E950.4	E962.0	E980.4
codeine derivatives	965.09	E850.2	E935.2	E950.0	E962.0	E980.0
expectorants	975.5	E858.6	E945.5	E950.4	E962.0	E980.4
narcotic agents NEC	965.09	E850.2	E935.2	E950.0	E962.0	E980.0
52:04 anti-infectives (EENT)						
ENT agent	976.6	E858.7	E946.6	E950.4	E962.0	E980.4
ophthalmic preparation	976.5	E858.7	E946.5	E950.4	E962.0	E980.4
52:04.04 antibiotics (EENT)						
ENT agent	976.6	E858.7	E946.6	E950.4	E962.0	E980.4
ophthalmic preparation	976.5	E858.7	E946.5	E950.4	E962.0	E980.4
52:04.06 antivirals (EENT)						
ENT agent	976.6	E858.7	E946.6	E950.4	E962.0	E980.4
ophthalmic preparation	976.5	E858.7	E946.5	E950.4	E962.0	E980.4
52:04.08 sulfonamides (EENT)						
ENT agent	976.6	E858.7	E946.6	E950.4	E962.0	E980.4
ophthalmic preparation	976.5	E858.7	E946.5	E950.4	E962.0	E980.4
52:04.12 miscellaneous anti-infectives (EENT)						
ENT agent	976.6	E858.7	E946.6	E950.4	E962.0	E980.4
ophthalmic preparation	976.5	E858.7	E946.5	E950.4	E962.0	E980.4
52:08 anti-inflammatory agents (EENT)						
ENT agent	976.6	E858.7	E946.6	E950.4	E962.0	E980.4
ophthalmic preparation	976.5	E858.7	E946.5	E950.4	E962.0	E980.4
52:10 carbonic anhydrase inhibitors	974.2	E858.5	E944.2	E950.4	E962.0	E980.4
52:12 contact lens solutions	976.5	E858.7	E946.5	E950.4	E962.0	E980.4
52:16 local anesthetics (EENT)	968.5	E855.2	E938.5	E950.4	E962.0	E980.4
52:20 miotics	971.0	E855.3	E941.0	E950.4	E962.0	E980.4
52:24 mydriatics						
adrenergics	971.2	E855.5	E941.2	E950.4	E962.0	E980.4
anticholinergics	971.1	E855.4	E941.1	E950.4	E962.0	E980.4
antimuscarinics	971.1	E855.4	E941.1	E950.4	E962.0	E980.4
parasympatholytics	971.1	E855.4	E941.1	E950.4	E962.0	E980.4
spasmolytics	971.1	E855.4	E941.1	E950.4	E962.0	E980.4
sympathomimetics	971.2	E855.5	E941.2	E950.4	E962.0	E980.4
52:28 mouth washes and gargles	976.6	E858.7	E946.6	E950.4	E962.0	E980.4
52:32 vasoconstrictors (EENT)	971.2	E855.5	E941.2	E950.4	E962.0	E980.4
52:36 unclassified agents (EENT)						
ENT agent	976.6	E858.7	E946.6	E950.4	E962.0	E980.4
ophthalmic preparation	976.5	E858.7	E946.5	E950.4	E962.0	E980.4
56:04 antacids and adsorbents	973.0	E858.4	E943.0	E950.4	E962.0	E980.4
56:08 antidiarrhea agents	973.5	E858.4	E943.5	E950.4	E962.0	E980.4
56:10 antiflatulents	973.8	E858.4	E943.8	E950.4	E962.0	E980.4
56:12 cathartics NEC	973.3	E858.4	E943.3	E950.4	E962.0	E980.4
emollients	973.2	E858.4	E943.2	E950.4	E962.0	E980.4
irritants	973.1	E858.4	E943.1	E950.4	E962.0	E980.4
56:16 digestants	973.4	E858.4	E943.4	E950.4	E962.0	E980.4
56:20 emetics and antiemetics						
antiemetics	963.0	E858.1	E933.0	E950.4	E962.0	E980.4
emetics	973.6	E858.4	E943.6	E950.4	E962.0	E980.4
56:24 lipotropic agents	977.1	E858.8	E947.1	E950.4	E962.0	E980.4
56:40 miscellaneous G.I. drugs	973.8	E858.4	E943.8	E950.4	E962.0	E980.4
60:00 gold compounds	965.69	E850.6	E935.6	E950.0	E962.0	E980.0

Drug, chemical	Poisoning	External Cause (E Code) Accident	Therapeutic Use	Suicide Attempt	Assault	Undetermined
Drug – *continued*						
AHFS List – *continued*						
64:00 heavy metal antagonists	963.8	E858.1	E933.8	E950.4	E962.0	E980.4
68:04 adrenals	962.0	E858.0	E932.0	E950.4	E962.0	E980.4
68:08 androgens	962.1	E858.0	E932.1	E950.4	E962.0	E980.4
68:12 contraceptives, oral	962.2	E858.0	E932.2	E950.4	E962.0	E980.4
68:16 estrogens	962.2	E858.0	E932.2	E950.4	E962.0	E980.4
68:18 gonadotropins	962.4	E858.0	E932.4	E950.4	E962.0	E980.4
68:20 insulins and antidiabetic agents	962.3	E858.0	E932.3	E950.4	E962.0	E980.4
68:20.08 insulins	962.3	E858.0	E932.3	E950.4	E962.0	E980.4
68:24 parathyroid	962.6	E858.0	E932.6	E950.4	E962.0	E980.4
68:28 pituitary (posterior)	962.5	E858.0	E932.5	E950.4	E962.0	E980.4
anterior	962.4	E858.0	E932.4	E950.4	E962.0	E980.4
68:32 progestogens	962.2	E858.0	E932.2	E950.4	E962.0	E980.4
68:34 other corpus luteum hormones NEC	962.2	E858.0	E932.2	E950.4	E962.0	E980.4
68:36 thyroid and antithyroid						
antithyroid	962.8	E858.0	E932.8	E950.4	E962.0	E980.4
thyroid (derivatives)	962.7	E858.0	E932.7	E950.4	E962.0	E980.4
72:00 local anesthetics NEC	968.9	E855.2	E938.9	E950.4	E962.0	E980.4
topical (surface)	968.5	E855.2	E938.5	E950.4	E962.0	E980.4
infiltration (intradermal) (subcutaneous) (submucosal)	968.5	E855.2	E938.5	E950.4	E962.0	E980.4
nerve blocking (peripheral) (plexus) (regional)	968.6	E855.2	E938.6	E950.4	E962.0	E980.4
spinal	968.7	E855.2	E938.7	E950.4	E962.0	E980.4
76:00 oxytocics	975.0	E858.6	E945.0	E950.4	E962.0	E980.4
78:00 radioactive agents	990	–	–	–	–	–
80:04 serums NEC	979.9	E858.8	E949.9	E950.4	E962.0	E980.4
immune gamma globulin (human)	964.6	E858.2	E934.6	E950.4	E962.0	E980.4
80:08 toxoids NEC	978.8	E858.8	E948.8	E950.4	E962.0	E980.4
diphtheria	978.5	E858.8	E948.5	E950.4	E962.0	E980.4
and tetanus	978.9	E858.8	E948.9	E950.4	E962.0	E980.4
with pertussis component	978.6	E858.8	E948.6	E950.4	E962.0	E980.4
tetanus	978.4	E858.8	E948.4	E950.4	E962.0	E980.4
and diphtheria	978.9	E858.8	E948.9	E950.4	E962.0	E980.4
with pertussis component	978.6	E858.8	E948.6	E950.4	E962.0	E980.4
80:12 vaccines	979.9	E858.8	E949.9	E950.4	E962.0	E980.4
bacterial NEC	978.8	E858.8	E948.8	E950.4	E962.0	E980.4
with						
other bacterial components	978.9	E858.8	E948.9	E950.4	E962.0	E980.4
pertussis component	978.6	E858.8	E948.6	E950.4	E962.0	E980.4
viral and rickettsial components	979.7	E858.8	E949.7	E950.4	E962.0	E980.4
rickettsial NEC	979.6	E858.8	E949.6	E950.4	E962.0	E980.4
with						
bacterial component	979.7	E858.8	E949.7	E950.4	E962.0	E980.4
pertussis component	978.6	E858.8	E948.6	E950.4	E962.0	E980.4
viral component	979.7	E858.8	E949.7	E950.4	E962.0	E980.4
viral NEC	979.6	E858.8	E949.6	E950.4	E962.0	E980.4
with						
bacterial component	979.7	E858.8	E949.7	E950.4	E962.0	E980.4
pertussis component	978.6	E858.8	E948.6	E950.4	E962.0	E980.4
rickettsial component	979.7	E858.8	E949.7	E950.4	E962.0	E980.4
84:04.04 antibiotics (skin and mucous membrane)	976.0	E858.7	E946.0	E950.4	E962.0	E980.4
84:04.08 fungicides (skin and mucous membrane)	976.0	E858.7	E946.0	E950.4	E962.0	E980.4
84:04.12 scabicides and pediculicides (skin and mucous membrane)	976.0	E858.7	E946.0	E950.4	E962.0	E980.4
84:04.16 miscellaneous local anti-infectives (skin and mucous membrane)	976.0	E858.7	E946.0	E950.4	E962.0	E980.4
84:06 anti-inflammatory agents (skin and mucous membrane)	976.0	E858.7	E946.0	E950.4	E962.0	E980.4
84:08 antipruritics and local anesthetics						
antipruritics	976.1	E858.7	E946.1	E950.4	E962.0	E980.4
local anesthetics	968.5	E855.2	E938.5	E950.4	E962.0	E980.4
84:12 astringents	976.2	E858.7	E946.2	E950.4	E962.0	E980.4
84:16 cell stimulants and proliferants	976.8	E858.7	E946.8	E950.4	E962.0	E980.4
84:20 detergents	976.2	E858.7	E946.2	E950.4	E962.0	E980.4
84:24 emollients, demulcents, and protectants	976.3	E858.7	E946.3	E950.4	E962.0	E980.4
84:28 keratolytic agents	976.4	E858.7	E946.4	E950.4	E962.0	E980.4
84:32 keratoplastic agents	976.4	E858.7	E946.4	E950.4	E962.0	E980.4
84:36 miscellaneous agents (skin and mucous membrane)	976.8	E858.7	E946.8	E950.4	E962.0	E980.4

Drug, chemical	Poisoning	External Cause (E Code) Accident	Therapeutic Use	Suicide Attempt	Assault	Undetermined
Drug – *continued*						
AHFS List – *continued*						
86:00 spasmolytic agents	975.1	E858.6	E945.1	E950.4	E962.0	E980.4
antiasthmatics	975.7	E858.6	E945.7	E950.4	E962.0	E980.4
papaverine	972.5	E858.3	E942.5	E950.4	E962.0	E980.4
theophylline	974.1	E858.5	E944.1	E950.4	E962.0	E980.4
88:04 vitamin A	963.5	E858.1	E933.5	E950.4	E962.0	E980.4
88:08 vitamin B complex	963.5	E858.1	E933.5	E950.4	E962.0	E980.4
hematopoietic vitamin	964.1	E858.2	E934.1	E950.4	E962.0	E980.4
nicotinic acid derivatives	972.2	E858.3	E942.2	E950.4	E962.0	E980.4
88:12 vitamin C	963.5	E858.1	E933.5	E950.4	E962.0	E980.4
88:16 vitamin D	963.5	E858.1	E933.5	E950.4	E962.0	E980.4
88:20 vitamin E	963.5	E858.1	E933.5	E950.4	E962.0	E980.4
88:24 vitamin K activity	964.3	E858.2	E934.3	E950.4	E962.0	E980.4
88:28 multivitamin preparations	963.5	E858.1	E933.5	E950.4	E962.0	E980.4
92:00 unclassified therapeutic agents	977.8	E858.8	E947.8	E950.4	E962.0	E980.4
Duboisine	971.1	E855.4	E941.1	E950.4	E962.0	E980.4
Dulcolax	973.1	E858.4	E943.1	E950.4	E962.0	E980.4
Duponol (C) (EP)	976.2	E858.7	E946.2	E950.4	E962.0	E980.4
Durabolin	962.1	E858.0	E932.1	E950.4	E962.0	E980.4
Dyclone	968.5	E855.2	E938.5	E950.4	E962.0	E980.4
Dyclonine	968.5	E855.2	E938.5	E950.4	E962.0	E980.4
Dydrogesterone	962.2	E858.0	E932.2	E950.4	E962.0	E980.4
Dyes NEC	989.89	E866.8	–	E950.9	E962.1	E980.9
diagnostic agents	977.8	E858.8	E947.8	E950.4	E962.0	E980.4
pharmaceutical NEC	977.4	E858.8	E947.4	E950.4	E962.0	E980.4
Dyfols	971.0	E855.3	E941.0	E950.4	E962.0	E980.4
Dymelor	962.3	E858.0	E932.3	E950.4	E962.0	E980.4
Dynamite	989.89	E866.8	–	E950.9	E962.1	E980.9
fumes	987.8	E869.8	–	E952.8	E962.2	E982.8
Dyphylline	975.1	E858.6	E945.1	E950.4	E962.0	E980.4
Ear preparations	976.6	E858.7	E946.6	E950.4	E962.0	E980.4
Echothiopate, ecothiopate	971.0	E855.3	E941.0	E950.4	E962.0	E980.4
Ecstasy ▲	969.72	E854.2	E939.7	E950.3	E962.0	E980.3
Ectylurea	967.8	E852.8	E937.8	E950.2	E962.0	E980.2
Edathamil disodium	963.8	E858.1	E933.8	E950.4	E962.0	E980.4
Edecrin	974.4	E858.5	E944.4	E950.4	E962.0	E980.4
Edetate, disodium (calcium)	963.8	E858.1	E933.8	E950.4	E962.0	E980.4
Edrophonium	971.0	E855.3	E941.0	E950.4	E962.0	E980.4
Elase	976.8	E858.7	E946.8	E950.4	E962.0	E980.4
Elaterium	973.1	E858.4	E943.1	E950.4	E962.0	E980.4
Elder	988.2	E865.4	–	E950.9	E962.1	E980.9
berry, (unripe)	988.2	E865.3	–	E950.9	E962.1	E980.9
Electrolytes NEC	974.5	E858.5	E944.5	E950.4	E962.0	E980.4
Electrolytic agent NEC	974.5	E858.5	E944.5	E950.4	E962.0	E980.4
Embramine	963.0	E858.1	E933.0	E950.4	E962.0	E980.4
Emetics	973.6	E858.4	E943.6	E950.4	E962.0	E980.4
Emetine (hydrochloride)	961.5	E857	E931.5	E950.4	E962.0	E980.4
Emollients	976.3	E858.7	E946.3	E950.4	E962.0	E980.4
Emylcamate	969.5	E853.8	E939.5	E950.3	E962.0	E980.3
Encyprate ▲	969.09	E854.0	E939.0	E950.3	E962.0	E980.3
Endocaine	968.5	E855.2	E938.5	E950.4	E962.0	E980.4
Endrin	989.2	E863.0	–	E950.6	E962.1	E980.7
Enflurane	968.2	E855.1	E938.2	E950.4	E962.0	E980.4
Enovid	962.2	E858.0	E932.2	E950.4	E962.0	E980.4
ENT preparations (anti-infectives)	976.6	E858.7	E946.6	E950.4	E962.0	E980.4
Enzodase	963.4	E858.1	E933.4	E950.4	E962.0	E980.4
Enzymes NEC	963.4	E858.1	E933.4	E950.4	E962.0	E980.4
Epanutin	966.1	E855.0	E936.1	E950.4	E962.0	E980.4
Ephedra (tincture)	971.2	E855.5	E941.2	E950.4	E962.0	E980.4
Ephedrine	971.2	E855.5	E941.2	E950.4	E962.0	E980.4
Epiestriol	962.2	E858.0	E932.2	E950.4	E962.0	E980.4
Epilim – *see* Sodium valproate						
Epinephrine	971.2	E855.5	E941.2	E950.4	E962.0	E980.4
Epsom salt	973.3	E858.4	E943.3	E950.4	E962.0	E980.4
Equanil	969.5	E853.8	E939.5	E950.3	E962.0	E980.3
Equisetum (diuretic)	974.4	E858.5	E944.4	E950.4	E962.0	E980.4
Ergometrine	975.0	E858.6	E945.0	E950.4	E962.0	E980.4
Ergonovine	975.0	E858.6	E945.0	E950.4	E962.0	E980.4
Ergot NEC	988.2	E865.4	–	E950.9	E962.1	E980.9
medicinal (alkaloids)	975.0	E858.6	E945.0	E950.4	E962.0	E980.4
Ergotamine (tartrate) (for migraine) NEC	972.9	E858.3	E942.9	E950.4	E962.0	E980.4
Ergotrate	975.0	E858.6	E945.0	E950.4	E962.0	E980.4
Erythrityl tetranitrate	972.4	E858.3	E942.4	E950.4	E962.0	E980.4
Erythrol tetranitrate	972.4	E858.3	E942.4	E950.4	E962.0	E980.4
Erythromycin	960.3	E856	E930.3	E950.4	E962.0	E980.4
ophthalmic preparation	976.5	E858.7	E946.5	E950.4	E962.0	E980.4
topical NEC	976.0	E858.7	E946.0	E950.4	E962.0	E980.4
Eserine	971.0	E855.3	E941.0	E950.4	E962.0	E980.4
Eskabarb	967.0	E851	E937.0	E950.1	E962.0	E980.1

Drug, chemical	Poisoning	External Cause (E Code)				
		Accident	Therapeutic Use	Suicide Attempt	Assault	Undetermined
Eskalith	969.8	E855.8	E939.8	E950.3	E962.0	E980.3
Estradiol (cypionate) (dipropionate) (valerate)	962.2	E858.0	E932.2	E950.4	E962.0	E980.4
Estriol	962.2	E858.0	E932.2	E950.4	E962.0	E980.4
Estrogens (with progestogens)	962.2	E858.0	E932.2	E950.4	E962.0	E980.4
Estrone	962.2	E858.0	E932.2	E950.4	E962.0	E980.4
Etafedrine	971.2	E855.5	E941.2	E950.4	E962.0	E980.4
Ethacrynate sodium	974.4	E858.5	E944.4	E950.4	E962.0	E980.4
Ethacrynic acid	974.4	E858.5	E944.4	E950.4	E962.0	E980.4
Ethambutol	961.8	E857	E931.8	E950.4	E962.0	E980.4
Ethamide	974.2	E858.5	E944.2	E950.4	E962.0	E980.4
Ethamivan	970.0	E854.3	E940.0	E950.4	E962.0	E980.4
Ethamsylate	964.5	E858.2	E934.5	E950.4	E962.0	E980.4
Ethanol	980.0	E860.1	–	E950.9	E962.1	E980.9
beverage	980.0	E860.0	–	E950.9	E962.1	E980.9
Ethchlorvynol	967.8	E852.8	E937.8	E950.2	E962.0	E980.2
Ethebenecid	974.7	E858.5	E944.7	E950.4	E962.0	E980.4
Ether(s) (diethyl) (ethyl) (vapor)	987.8	E869.8	–	E952.8	E962.2	E982.8
anesthetic	968.2	E855.1	E938.2	E950.4	E962.0	E980.4
petroleum – *see* Ligroin solvent	982.8	E862.4	–	E950.9	E962.1	E980.9
Ethidine chloride (vapor)	987.8	E869.8	–	E952.8	E962.2	E982.8
liquid (solvent)	982.3	E862.4	–	E950.9	E962.1	E980.9
Ethinamate	967.8	E852.8	E937.8	E950.2	E962.0	E980.2
Ethinylestradiol	962.2	E858.0	E932.2	E950.4	E962.0	E980.4
Ethionamide	961.8	E857	E931.8	E950.4	E962.0	E980.4
Ethisterone	962.2	E858.0	E932.2	E950.4	E962.0	E980.4
Ethobral	967.0	E851	E937.0	E950.1	E962.0	E980.1
Ethocaine (infiltration) (topical)	968.5	E855.2	E938.5	E950.4	E962.0	E980.4
nerve block (peripheral) (plexus)	968.6	E855.2	E938.6	E950.4	E962.0	E980.4
spinal	968.7	E855.2	E938.7	E950.4	E962.0	E980.4
Ethoheptazine (citrate)	965.7	E850.7	E935.7	E950.0	E962.0	E980.0
Ethopropazine	966.4	E855.0	E936.4	E950.4	E962.0	E980.4
Ethosuximide	966.2	E855.0	E936.2	E950.4	E962.0	E980.4
Ethotoin	966.1	E855.0	E936.1	E950.4	E962.0	E980.4
Ethoxazene	961.9	E857	E931.9	E950.4	E962.0	E980.4
Ethoxzolamide	974.2	E858.5	E944.2	E950.4	E962.0	E980.4
Ethyl						
acetate (vapor)	982.8	E862.4	–	E950.9	E962.1	E980.9
alcohol	980.0	E860.1	–	E950.9	E962.1	E980.9
beverage	980.0	E860.0	–	E950.9	E962.1	E980.9
aldehyde (vapor)	987.8	E869.8	–	E952.8	E962.2	E982.8
liquid	989.89	E866.8	–	E950.9	E962.1	E980.9
aminobenzoate	968.5	E855.2	E938.5	E950.4	E962.0	E980.4
biscoumacetate	964.2	E858.2	E934.2	E950.4	E962.0	E980.4
bromide (anesthetic)	968.2	E855.1	E938.2	E950.4	E962.0	E980.4
carbamate (antineoplastic)	963.1	E858.1	E933.1	E950.4	E962.0	E980.4
carbinol	980.3	E860.4	–	E950.9	E962.1	E980.9
chaulmoograte	961.8	E857	E931.8	E950.4	E962.0	E980.4
chloride (vapor)	987.8	E869.8	–	E952.8	E962.2	E982.8
anesthetic (local)	968.5	E855.2	E938.5	E950.4	E962.0	E980.4
inhaled	968.2	E855.1	E938.2	E950.4	E962.0	E980.4
solvent	982.3	E862.4	–	E950.9	E962.1	E980.9
estranol	962.1	E858.0	E932.1	E950.4	E962.0	E980.4
ether – *see* Ether(s)						
formate (solvent) NEC	982.8	E862.4	–	E950.9	E962.1	E980.9
iodoacetate	987.5	E869.3	–	E952.8	E962.2	E982.8
lactate (solvent) NEC	982.8	E862.4	–	E950.9	E962.1	E980.9
methylcarbinol	980.8	E860.8	–	E950.9	E962.1	E980.9
morphine	965.09	E850.2	E935.2	E950.0	E962.0	E980.0
Ethylene (gas)	987.1	E869.8	–	E952.8	E962.2	E982.8
anesthetic (general)	968.2	E855.1	E938.2	E950.4	E962.0	E980.4
chlorohydrin (vapor)	982.3	E862.4	–	E950.9	E962.1	E980.9
dichloride (vapor)	982.3	E862.4	–	E950.9	E962.1	E980.9
glycol(s) (any) (vapor)	982.8	E862.4	–	E950.9	E962.1	E980.9
Ethylidene						
chloride NEC	982.3	E862.4	–	E950.9	E962.1	E980.9
diethyl ether	982.8	–	E862.4	E950.9	E962.1	E980.9
Ethynodiol	962.2	E858.0	E932.2	E950.4	E962.0	E980.4
Etidocaine	968.9	E855.2	E938.9	E950.4	E962.0	E980.4
infiltration (subcutaneous)	968.5	E855.2	E938.5	E950.4	E962.0	E980.4
nerve (peripheral) (plexus)	968.6	E855.2	E938.6	E950.4	E962.0	E980.4
Etilfen	967.0	E851	E937.0	E950.1	E962.0	E980.1
Etomide	965.7	E850.7	E935.7	E950.0	E962.0	E980.0
Etorphine	965.09	E850.2	E935.2	E950.0	E962.0	E980.0
Etoval	967.0	E851	E937.0	E950.1	E962.0	E980.1
Etryptamine ▲	969.01	E854.0	E939.0	E950.3	E962.0	E980.3
Eucaine	968.5	E855.2	E938.5	E950.4	E962.0	E980.4
Eucalyptus (oil) NEC	975.5	E858.6	E945.5	E950.4	E962.0	E980.4
Eucatropine	971.1	E855.4	E941.1	E950.4	E962.0	E980.4
Eucodal	965.09	E850.2	E935.2	E950.0	E962.0	E980.0
Euneryl	967.0	E851	E937.0	E950.1	E962.0	E980.1
Euphthalmine	971.1	E855.4	E941.1	E950.4	E962.0	E980.4

Drug, chemical	Poisoning	External Cause (E Code)				
		Accident	Therapeutic Use	Suicide Attempt	Assault	Undetermined
Eurax	976.0	E858.7	E946.0	E950.4	E962.0	E980.4
Euresol	976.4	E858.7	E946.4	E950.4	E962.0	E980.4
Euthroid	962.7	E858.0	E932.7	E950.4	E962.0	E980.4
Evans blue	977.8	E858.8	E947.8	E950.4	E962.0	E980.4
Evipal	967.0	E851	E937.0	E950.1	E962.0	E980.1
sodium	968.3	E855.1	E938.3	E950.4	E962.0	E980.4
Evipan	967.0	E851	E937.0	E950.1	E962.0	E980.1
sodium	968.3	E855.1	E938.3	E950.4	E962.0	E980.4
Exalgin	965.4	E850.4	E935.4	E950.0	E962.0	E980.0
Excipients, pharmaceutical	977.4	E858.8	E947.4	E950.4	E962.0	E980.4
Exhaust gas – *see* Carbon, monoxide						
Ex-Lax (phenolphthalein)	973.1	E858.4	E943.1	E950.4	E962.0	E980.4
Expectorants	975.5	E858.6	E945.5	E950.4	E962.0	E980.4
External medications (skin) (mucous membrane)	976.9	E858.7	E946.9	E950.4	E962.0	E980.4
dental agent	976.7	E858.7	E946.7	E950.4	E962.0	E980.4
ENT agent	976.6	E858.7	E946.6	E950.4	E962.0	E980.4
ophthalmic preparation	976.5	E858.7	E946.5	E950.4	E962.0	E980.4
specified NEC	976.8	E858.7	E946.8	E950.4	E962.0	E980.4
Eye agents (anti-infective)	976.5	E858.7	E946.5	E950.4	E962.0	E980.4
Factor IX complex (human)	964.5	E858.2	E934.5	E950.4	E962.0	E980.4
Fecal softeners	973.2	E858.4	E943.2	E950.4	E962.0	E980.4
Fenbutrazate	977.0	E858.8	E947.0	E950.4	E962.0	E980.4
Fencamfamin	970.8	E854.3	E940.8	E950.4	E962.0	E980.4
Fenfluramine	977.0	E858.8	E947.0	E950.4	E962.0	E980.4
Fenoprofen	965.61	E850.6	E935.6	E950.0	E962.0	E980.0
Fentanyl	965.09	E850.2	E935.2	E950.0	E962.0	E980.0
Fentazin	969.1	E853.0	E939.1	E930.3	E962.0	E980.3
Fenticlor, fentichlor	976.0	E858.7	E946.0	E950.4	E962.0	E980.4
Fer de lance (bite) (venom)	989.5	E905.0	–	E950.9	E962.1	E980.9
Ferric – *see* Iron						
Ferrocholinate	964.0	E858.2	E934.0	E950.4	E962.0	E980.4
Ferrous fumerate, gluconate, lactate, salt NEC, sulfate (medicinal)	964.0	E858.2	E934.0	E950.4	E962.0	E980.4
Ferrum – *see* Iron						
Fertilizers NEC	989.89	E866.5	–	E950.9	E962.1	E980.4
with herbicide mixture	989.4	E863.5	–	E950.6	E962.1	E980.7
Fibrinogen (human)	964.7	E858.2	E934.7	E950.4	E962.0	E980.4
Fibrinolysin	964.4	E858.2	E934.4	E950.4	E962.0	E980.4
Fibrinolysis-affecting agents	964.4	E858.2	E934.4	E950.4	E962.0	E980.4
Filix mas	961.6	E857	E931.6	E950.4	E962.0	E980.4
Fiorinal	965.1	E850.3	E935.3	E950.0	E962.0	E980.0
Fire damp	987.1	E869.8	–	E952.8	E962.2	E982.8
Fish, nonbacterial or noxious	988.0	E865.2	–	E950.9	E962.1	E980.9
shell	988.0	E865.1	–	E950.9	E962.1	E980.9
Flagyl	961.5	E857	E931.5	E950.4	E962.0	E980.4
Flavoxate	975.1	E858.6	E945.1	E950.4	E962.0	E980.4
Flaxedil	975.2	E858.6	E945.2	E950.4	E962.0	E980.4
Flaxseed (medicinal)	976.3	E858.7	E946.3	E950.4	E962.0	E980.4
Florantyrone	973.4	E858.4	E943.4	E950.4	E962.0	E980.4
Floraquin	961.3	E857	E931.3	E950.4	E962.0	E980.4
Florinef	962.0	E858.0	E932.0	E950.4	E962.0	E980.4
ENT agent	976.6	E858.7	E946.6	E950.4	E962.0	E980.4
ophthalmic preparation	976.5	E858.7	E946.5	E950.4	E962.0	E980.4
topical NEC	976.0	E858.7	E946.0	E950.4	E962.0	E980.4
Flowers of sulfur	976.4	E858.7	E946.4	E950.4	E962.0	E980.4
Flomax	971.3	E855.6	E941.3	E950.4	E962.0	E980.4
Floxuridine	963.1	E858.1	E933.1	E950.4	E962.0	E980.4
Flucytosine	961.9	E857	E931.9	E950.4	E962.0	E980.4
Fludrocortisone	962.0	E858.0	E932.0	E950.4	E962.0	E980.4
ENT agent	976.6	E858.7	E946.6	E950.4	E962.0	E980.4
ophthalmic preparation	976.5	E858.7	E946.5	E950.4	E962.0	E980.4
topical NEC	976.0	E858.7	E946.0	E950.4	E962.0	E980.4
Flumethasone	976.0	E858.7	E946.0	E950.4	E962.0	E980.4
Flumethiazide	974.3	E858.5	E944.3	E950.4	E962.0	E980.4
Flumidin	961.7	E857	E931.7	E950.4	E962.0	E980.4
Flunitrazepam	969.4	E853.2	E939.4	E950.3	E962.0	E980.3
Fluocinolone	976.0	E858.7	E946.0	E950.4	E962.0	E980.4
Fluocortolone	962.0	E858.0	E932.0	E950.4	E962.0	E980.4
Fluohydrocortisone	962.0	E858.0	E932.0	E950.4	E962.0	E980.4
ENT agent	976.6	E858.7	E946.6	E950.4	E962.0	E980.4
ophthalmic preparation	976.5	E858.7	E946.5	E950.4	E962.0	E980.4
topical NEC	976.0	E858.7	E946.0	E950.4	E962.0	E980.4
Fluonid	976.0	E858.7	E946.0	E950.4	E962.0	E980.4
Fluopromazine	969.1	E853.0	E939.1	E950.3	E962.0	E980.3
Fluoracetate	989.4	E863.7	–	E950.6	E962.1	E980.7
Fluorescein (sodium)	977.8	E858.8	E947.8	E950.4	E962.0	E980.4
Fluoride(s) (pesticides) (sodium) NEC	989.4	E863.4	–	E950.6	E962.1	E980.7
hydrogen – *see* Hydrofluoric acid						
medicinal	976.7	E858.7	E946.7	E950.4	E962.0	E980.4

Drug, chemical	Poisoning	External Cause (E Code) Accident	Therapeutic Use	Suicide Attempt	Assault	Undetermined
Fluoride(s) – *continued*						
not pesticide NEC	983.9	E864.4	–	E950.7	E962.1	E980.6
stannous	976.7	E858.7	E946.7	E950.4	E962.0	E980.4
Fluorinated corticosteroids	962.0	E858.0	E932.0	E950.4	E962.0	E980.4
Fluorine (compounds) (gas)	987.8	E869.8	–	E952.8	E962.2	E982.8
salt – *see* Fluoride(s)						
Fluoristan	976.7	E858.7	E946.7	E950.4	E962.0	E980.4
Fluoroacetate	989.4	E863.7	–	E950.6	E962.1	E980.7
Fluorodeoxyuridine	963.1	E858.1	E933.1	E950.4	E962.0	E980.4
Fluorometholone (topical) NEC	976.0	E858.7	E946.0	E950.4	E962.0	E980.4
ophthalmic preparation	976.5	E858.7	E946.5	E950.4	E962.0	E980.4
Fluorouracil	963.1	E858.1	E933.1	E950.4	E962.0	E980.4
Fluothane	968.1	E855.1	E938.1	E950.4	E962.0	E980.4
Fluoxetine hydrochloride ▲	969.03	E854.0	E939.0	E950.3	E962.0	E980.3
Fluoxymesterone	962.1	E858.0	E932.1	E950.4	E962.0	E980.4
Fluphenazine	969.1	E853.0	E939.1	E950.3	E962.0	E980.3
Fluprednisolone	962.0	E858.0	E932.0	E950.4	E962.0	E980.4
Flurandrenolide	976.0	E858.7	E946.0	E950.4	E962.0	E980.4
Flurazepam (hydrochloride)	969.4	E853.2	E939.4	E950.3	E962.0	E980.3
Flurbiprofen	965.61	E850.6	E935.6	E950.0	E962.0	E980.0
Flurobate	976.0	E858.7	E946.0	E950.4	E962.0	E980.4
Flurothyl	969.8	E855.8	E939.8	E950.3	E962.0	E980.3
Fluroxene	968.2	E855.1	E938.2	E950.4	E962.0	E980.4
Folacin	964.1	E858.2	E934.1	E950.4	E962.0	E980.4
Folic acid	964.1	E858.2	E934.1	E950.4	E962.0	E980.4
Follicle stimulating hormone	962.4	E858.0	E932.4	E950.4	E962.0	E980.4
Food, foodstuffs, nonbacterial or noxious	988.9	E865.9	–	E950.9	E962.1	E980.9
berries, seeds	988.2	E865.3	–	E950.9	E962.1	E980.9
fish	988.0	E865.2	–	E950.9	E962.1	E980.9
mushrooms	988.1	E865.5	–	E950.9	E962.1	E980.9
plants	988.2	E865.9	–	E950.9	E962.1	E980.9
specified type NEC	988.2	E865.4	–	E950.9	E962.1	E980.9
shellfish	988.0	E865.1	–	E950.9	E962.1	E980.9
specified NEC	988.8	E865.8	–	E950.9	E962.1	E980.9
Fool's parsley	988.2	E865.4	–	E950.9	E962.1	E980.9
Formaldehyde (solution)	989.89	E861.4	–	E950.9	E962.1	E980.9
fungicide	989.4	E863.6	–	E950.6	E962.1	E980.7
gas or vapor	987.8	E869.8	–	E952.8	E962.2	E982.8
Formalin	989.89	E861.4	–	E950.9	E962.1	E980.9
fungicide	989.4	E863.6	–	E950.6	E962.1	E980.7
vapor	987.8	E869.8	–	E952.8	E962.2	E982.8
Formic acid	983.1	E864.1	–	E950.7	E962.1	E980.6
vapor	987.8	E869.8	–	E952.8	E962.2	E982.8
Fowler's solution	985.1	E866.3	–	E950.8	E962.1	E980.8
Foxglove	988.2	E865.4	–	E950.9	E962.1	E980.9
Fox green	977.8	E858.8	E947.8	E950.4	E962.0	E980.4
Framycetin	960.8	E856	E930.8	E950.4	E962.0	E980.4
Frangula (extract)	973.1	E858.4	E943.1	E950.4	E962.0	E980.4
Frei antigen	977.8	E858.8	E947.8	E950.4	E962.0	E980.4
Freons	987.4	E869.2	–	E952.8	E962.2	E982.8
Fructose	974.5	E858.5	E944.5	E950.4	E962.0	E980.4
Frusemide	974.4	E858.5	E944.4	E950.4	E962.0	E980.4
FSH	962.4	E858.0	E932.4	E950.4	E962.0	E980.4
Fuel						
automobile	981	E862.1	–	E950.9	E962.1	E980.9
exhaust gas, not in transit	986	E868.2	–	E952.0	E962.2	E982.0
vapor NEC	987.1	E869.8	–	E952.8	E962.2	E982.8
gas (domestic use) – *see also* Carbon, monoxide, fuel utility	987.1	E868.1	–	E951.8	E962.2	E981.8
incomplete combustion of – *see* Carbon, monoxide, fuel, utility						
in mobile container	987.0	E868.0	–	E951.1	E962.2	E981.1
piped (natural)	987.1	E867	–	E951.0	E962.2	E981.0
industrial, incomplete combustion	986	E868.3	–	E952.1	E962.2	E982.1
Fugillin	960.8	E856	E930.8	E950.4	E962.0	E980.4
Fulminate of mercury	985.0	E866.1	–	E950.9	E962.1	E980.9
Fulvicin	960.1	E856	E930.1	E950.4	E962.0	E980.4
Fumadil	960.8	E856	E930.8	E950.4	E962.0	E980.4
Fumagillin	960.8	E856	E930.8	E950.4	E962.0	E980.4
Fumes (from)	987.9	E869.9	–	E952.9	E962.2	E982.9
carbon monoxide – *see* Carbon, monoxide						
charcoal (domestic use)	986	E868.3	–	E952.1	E962.2	E982.1
chloroform – *see* Chloroform						
coke (in domestic stoves, fireplaces)	986	E868.3	–	E952.1	E962.2	E982.1
corrosive NEC	987.8	E869.8	–	E952.8	E962.2	E982.8
ether – *see* Ether(s)						
freons	987.4	E869.2	–	E952.8	E962.2	E982.8

Drug, chemical	Poisoning	External Cause (E Code) Accident	Therapeutic Use	Suicide Attempt	Assault	Undetermined
Fumes – *continued*						
hydrocarbons	987.1	E869.8	–	E952.8	E962.2	E982.8
petroleum (liquefied)	987.0	E868.0	–	E951.1	E962.2	E981.1
distributed through pipes (pure or mixed with air)	987.0	E867	–	E951.0	E962.2	E981.0
lead – *see* Lead						
metals – *see* specified metal						
nitrogen dioxide	987.2	E869.0	–	E952.8	E962.2	E982.8
pesticides – *see* Pesticides						
petroleum (liquefied)	987.0	E868.0	–	E951.1	E962.2	E981.1
distributed through pipes (pure or mixed with air)	987.0	E867	–	E951.0	E962.2	E981.0
polyester	987.8	E869.8	–	E952.8	E962.2	E982.8
specified source, other (*see* also substance specified)	987.8	E869.8	–	E952.8	E962.2	E982.8
sulfur dioxide	987.3	E869.1	–	E952.8	E962.2	E982.8
Fumigants	989.4	E863.8	–	E950.6	E962.1	E980.7
Fungi, noxious, used as food	988.1	E865.5	–	E950.9	E962.1	E980.9
Fungicides (*see also* Antifungals)	989.4	E863.6	–	E950.6	E962.1	E980.7
Fungizone	960.1	E856	E930.1	E950.4	E962.0	E980.4
topical	976.0	E858.7	E946.0	E950.4	E962.0	E980.4
Furacin	976.0	E858.7	E946.0	E950.4	E962.0	E980.4
Furadantin	961.9	E857	E931.9	E950.4	E962.0	E980.4
Furazolidone	961.9	E857	E931.9	E950.4	E962.0	E980.4
Furnace (coal burning) (domestic), **gas from**	986	E868.3	–	E952.1	E962.2	E982.1
industrial	986	E868.8	–	E952.1	E962.2	E982.1
Furniture polish	989.89	E861.2	–	E950.9	E962.1	E980.9
Furosemide	974.4	E858.5	E944.4	E950.4	E962.0	E980.4
Furoxone	961.9	E857	E931.9	E950.4	E962.0	E980.4
Fusel oil (amyl) (butyl) (propyl)	980.3	E860.4	–	E950.9	E962.1	E980.9
Fusidic acid	960.8	E856	E930.8	E950.4	E962.0	E980.4
Gallamine	975.2	E858.6	E945.2	E950.4	E962.0	E980.4
Gallotannic acid	976.2	E858.7	E946.2	E950.4	E962.0	E980.4
Gamboge	973.1	E858.4	E943.1	E950.4	E962.0	E980.4
Gamimune	964.6	E858.2	E934.6	E950.4	E962.0	E980.4
Gamma-benzene hexachloride (vapor)	989.2	E863.0	–	E950.6	E962.1	E980.7
Gamma globulin	964.6	E858.2	E934.6	E950.4	E962.0	E980.4
Gamma Hydroxy Butyrate (GHB)	968.4	E855.1	E938.4	E950.4	E962.0	E980.4
Gamulin	964.6	E858.2	E934.6	E950.4	E962.0	E980.4
Ganglionic blocking agents	972.3	E858.3	E942.3	E950.4	E962.0	E980.4
Ganja	969.6	E854.1	E939.6	E950.3	E962.0	E980.3
Garamycin	960.8	E856	E930.8	E950.4	E962.0	E980.4
ophthalmic preparation	976.5	E858.7	E946.5	E950.4	E962.0	E980.4
topical NEC	976.0	E858.7	E946.0	E950.4	E962.0	E980.4
Gardenal	967.0	E851	E937.0	E950.1	E962.0	E980.1
Gardepanyl	967.0	E851	E937.0	E950.1	E962.0	E980.1
Gas	987.9	E869.9	–	E952.9	E962.2	E982.9
acetylene	987.1	E868.1	–	E951.8	E962.2	E981.8
incomplete combustion of – *see* Carbon, monoxide, fuel, utility						
air contaminants, source or type not specified	987.9	E869.9	–	E952.9	E962.2	E982.9
anesthetic (general) NEC	968.2	E855.1	E938.2	E950.4	E962.0	E980.4
blast furnace	986	E868.8	–	E952.1	E962.2	E982.1
butane – *see* Butane						
carbon monoxide – *see* Carbon, monoxide						
chlorine	987.6	E869.8	–	E952.8	E962.2	E982.8
coal – *see* Carbon,monoxide, coal						
cyanide	987.7	E869.8	–	E952.8	E962.2	E982.8
dicyanogen	987.8	E869.8	–	E952.8	E962.2	E982.8
domestic – *see* Gas, utility						
exhaust – *see* Carbon, monoxide, exhaust gas						
from wood- or coal-burning stove or fireplace	986	E868.3	–	E952.1	E962.2	E982.1
fuel (domestic use) – *see also* Carbon, monoxide, fuel						
industrial use	986	E868.8	–	E952.1	E962.2	E982.1
utility	987.1	E868.1	–	E951.8	E962.2	E981.8
incomplete combustion of – *see* Carbon, monoxide, fuel, utility						
in mobile container	987.0	E868.0	–	E951.1	E962.2	E981.1
piped (natural)	987.1	E867	–	E951.0	E962.2	E981.0
garage	986	E868.2	–	E952.0	E962.2	E982.0

Drug, chemical	Poisoning	External Cause (E Code): Accident	Therapeutic Use	Suicide Attempt	Assault	Undetermined
Gas – *continued*						
hydrocarbon NEC	987.1	E869.8	–	E952.8	E962.2	E982.8
incomplete combustion of – *see* Carbon, monoxide, fuel, utility						
liquefied (mobile container)	987.0	E868.0	–	E951.1	E962.2	E981.1
piped	987.0	E867	–	E951.0	E962.2	E981.0
hydrocyanic acid	987.7	E869.8	–	E952.8	E962.2	E982.8
illuminating – *see* Gas,utility						
incomplete combustion, any – *see* Carbon,monoxide						
kiln	986	E868.8	–	E952.1	E962.2	E982.1
lacrimogenic	987.5	E869.3	–	E952.8	E962.2	E982.8
marsh	987.1	E869.8	–	E952.8	E962.2	E982.8
motor exhaust, not in transit	986	E868.8	–	E952.1	E962.2	E982.1
mustard – *see* Mustard, gas natural	987.1	E867	–	E951.0	E962.2	E981.0
nerve (war)	987.9	E869.9	–	E952.9	E962.2	E982.
oils	981	E862.1	–	E950.9	E962.1	E980.9
petroleum (liquefied) (distributed in mobile containers)	987.0	E868.0	–	E951.1	E962.2	E981.1
piped (pure or mixed with air)	987.0	E867	–	E951.1	E962.2	E981.1
piped (manufactured) (natural) NEC	987.1	E867	–	E951.0	E962.2	E981.0
producer	986	E868.8	–	E952.1	E962.2	E982.1
propane – *see* Propane						
refrigerant (freon)	987.4	E869.2	–	E952.8	E962.2	E982.8
not freon	987.9	E869.9	–	E952.9	E962.2	E982.9
sewer	987.8	E869.8	–	E952.8	E962.2	E982.8
specified source NEC (*see also* substance specified)	987.8	E869.8	–	E952.8	E962.2	E982.8
stove – *see* Gas, utility						
tear	987.5	E869.3	–	E952.8	E962.2	E982.8
utility (for cooking, heating, or lighting) (piped) NEC	987.1	E868.1	–	E951.8	E962.2	E981.8
incomplete combustion of – *see* Carbon, monoxide, fuel, utilty						
in mobile container	987.0	E868.0	–	E951.1	E962.2	E981.1
piped (natural)	987.1	E867	–	E951.0	E962.2	E981.0
water	987.1	E868.1	–	E951.8	E962.2	E981.8
incomplete combustion of – *see* Carbon, monoxide, fuel, utility						
Gaseous substance – *see* Gas						
Gasoline, gasolene	981	E862.1	–	E950.9	E962.1	E980.9
vapor	987.1	E869.8	–	E952.8	E962.2	E982.8
Gastric enzymes	973.4	E858.4	E943.4	E950.4	E962.0	E980.4
Gastrografin	977.8	E858.8	E947.8	E950.4	E962.0	E980.4
Gastrointestinal agents	973.9	E858.4	E943.9	E950.4	E962.0	E980.4
specified NEC	973.8	E858.4	E943.8	E950.4	E962.0	E980.4
Gaultheria procumbens	988.2	E865.4	–	E950.9	E962.1	E980.9
Gelatin (intravenous)	964.8	E858.2	E934.8	E950.4	E962.0	E980.4
absorbable (sponge)	964.5	E858.2	E934.5	E950.4	E962.0	E980.4
Gelfilm	976.8	E858.7	E946.8	E950.4	E962.0	E980.4
Gelfoam	964.5	E858.2	E934.5	E950.4	E962.0	E980.4
Gelsemine	970.8	E854.3	E940.8	E950.4	E962.0	E980.4
Gelsemium (sempervirens)	988.2	E865.4	–	E950.9	E962.1	E980.9
Gemonil	967.0	E851	E937.0	E950.1	E962.0	E980.1
Gentamicin	960.8	E856	E930.8	E950.4	E962.0	E980.4
ophthalmic preparation	976.5	E858.7	E946.5	E950.4	E962.0	E980.4
topical NEC	976.0	E858.7	E946.0	E950.4	E962.0	E980.4
Gentian violet	976.0	E858.7	E946.0	E950.4	E962.0	E980.4
Gexane	976.0	E858.7	E946.0	E950.4	E962.0	E980.4
Gila monster (venom)	989.5	E905.0	–	E950.9	E962.1	E980.9
Ginger, Jamaica	989.89	E866.8	–	E950.9	E962.1	E980.9
Gitalin	972.1	E858.3	E942.1	E950.4	E962.0	E980.4
Gitoxin	972.1	E858.3	E942.1	E950.4	E962.0	E980.4
Glandular extract (medicinal) NEC	977.9	E858.9	E947.9	E950.5	E962.0	E980.5
Glaucarubin	961.5	E857	E931.5	E950.4	E962.0	E980.4
Globin zinc insulin	962.3	E858.0	E932.3	E950.4	E962.0	E980.4
Glucagon	962.3	E858.0	E932.3	E950.4	E962.0	E980.4
Glucochloral	967.1	E852.0	E937.1	E950.2	E962.0	E980.2
Glucocorticoids	962.0	E858.0	E932.0	E950.4	E962.0	E980.4
Glucose	974.5	E858.5	E944.5	E950.4	E962.0	E980.4
oxidase reagent	977.8	E858.8	E947.8	E950.4	E962.0	E980.4
Glucosulfone sodium	961.8	E857	E931.8	E950.4	E962.0	E980.4
Glue(s)	989.89	E866.6	–	E950.9	E962.1	E980.9
Glutamic acid (hydrochloride)	973.4	E858.4	E943.4	E950.4	E962.0	E980.4
Glutalhione	963.8	E858.1	E933.8	E950.4	E962.0	E980.4
Glutaraldehyde	989.89	E861.4	–	E950.9	E962.1	E980.9
Glutethimide (group)	967.5	E852.4	E937.5	E950.2	E962.0	E980.2
Glycerin (lotion)	976.3	E858.7	E946.3	E950.4	E962.0	E980.4
Glycerol (topical)	976.3	E858.7	E946.3	E950.4	E962.0	E980.4

Drug, chemical	Poisoning	External Cause (E Code): Accident	Therapeutic Use	Suicide Attempt	Assault	Undetermined
Glyceryl						
gualacolate	975.5	E858.6	E945.5	E950.4	E962.0	E980.4
triacetate (topical)	976.0	E858.7	E946.0	E950.4	E962.0	E980.4
trinitrate	972.4	E858.3	E942.4	E950.4	E962.0	E980.4
Glycine	974.5	E858.5	E944.5	E950.4	E962.0	E980.4
Glycobiarsol	961.1	E857	E931.1	E950.4	E962.0	E980.4
Glycols (ether)	982.8	E862.4	–	E950.9	E962.1	E980.9
Glycopyrrolate	971.1	E855.4	E941.1	E950.4	E962.0	E980.4
Glymidine	962.3	E858.0	E932.3	E950.4	E962.0	E980.4
Gold (compounds) (salts)	965.69	E850.6	E935.6	E950.0	E962.0	E980.0
Golden sulfide of antimony	985.4	E866.2	–	E950.9	E962.1	E980.9
Goldylocks	988.2	E865.4	–	E950.9	E962.1	E980.9
Gonadal tissue extract	962.9	E858.0	E932.9	E950.4	E962.0	E980.4
female	962.2	E858.0	E932.2	E950.4	E962.0	E980.4
male	962.1	E858.0	E932.1	E950.4	E962.0	E980.4
Gonadotropin	962.4	E858.0	E932.4	E950.4	E962.0	E980.4
Grain alcohol	980.0	E860.1	–	E950.9	E962.1	E980.9
beverage	980.0	E860.0	–	E950.9	E962.1	E980.9
Gramicidin	960.8	E856	E930.8	E950.4	E962.0	E980.4
Gratiola officinalis	988.2	E865.4	–	E950.9	E962.1	E980.9
Grease	989.89	E866.8	–	E950.9	E962.1	E980.9
Green hellebore	988.2	E865.4	–	E950.9	E962.1	E980.9
Green soap	976.2	E858.7	E946.2	E950.4	E962.0	E980.4
Grifulvin	960.1	E856	E930.1	E950.4	E962.0	E980.4
Griseofulvin	960.1	E856	E930.1	E950.4	E962.0	E980.4
Growth hormone	962.4	E858.0	E932.4	E950.4	E962.0	E980.4
Guaiacol	975.5	E858.6	E945.5	E950.4	E962.0	E980.4
Giuaiac reagent	977.8	E858.8	E947.8	E950.4	E962.0	E980.4
Guaifenesin	975.5	E858.6	E945.5	E950.4	E962.0	E980.4
Guaiphenesin	975.5	E858.6	E945.5	E950.4	E962.0	E980.4
Guanatol	961.4	E857	E931.4	E950.4	E962.0	E980.4
Guanethidine	972.6	E858.3	E942.6	E950.4	E962.0	E980.4
Guano	989.89	E866.5	–	E950.9	E962.1	E980.9
Guanochlor	972.6	E858.3	E942.6	E950.4	E962.0	E980.4
Guanoctine	972.6	E858.3	E942.6	E950.4	E962.0	E980.4
Guanoxan	972.6	E858.3	E942.6	E950.4	E962.0	E980.4
Hair treatment agent NEC	976.4	E858.7	E946.4	E950.4	E962.0	E980.4
Halcinonide	976.0	E858.7	E946.0	E950.4	E962.0	E980.4
Halethazole	976.0	E858.7	E946.0	E950.4	E962.0	E980.4
Hallucinogens	969.6	E854.1	E939.6	E950.3	E962.0	E980.3
Haloperidol	969.2	E853.1	E939.2	E950.3	E962.0	E980.3
Haloprogin	976.0	E858.7	E946.0	E950.4	E962.0	E980.4
Halotex	976.0	E858.7	E946.0	E950.4	E962.0	E980.4
Halothane	968.1	E855.1	E938.1	E950.4	E962.0	E980.4
Halquinols	976.0	E858.7	E946.0	E950.4	E962.0	E980.4
Hand sanitizer	976.0	E858.7	E946.0	E950.4	E962.0	E980.4
Harmonyl	972.6	E858.3	E942.6	E950.4	E962.0	E980.4
Hartmann's solution	974.5	E858.5	E944.5	E950.4	E962.0	E980.4
Hashish	969.6	E854.1	E939.6	E950.3	E962.0	E980.3
Hawaiian wood rose seeds	969.6	E854.1	E939.6	E950.3	E962.0	E980.3
Headache cures, drugs, powders NEC	977.9	E858.9	E947.9	E950.5	E962.0	E980.9
Heavenly Blue (morning glory)	969.6	E854.1	E939.6	E950.3	E962.0	E980.3
Heavy metal						
antagonists	963.8	E858.1	E933.8	E950.4	E962.0	E980.4
anti-infectives	961.2	E857	E931.2	E950.4	E962.0	E980.4
Hedaquinium	976.0	E858.7	E946.0	E950.4	E962.0	E980.4
Hedge hyssop	988.2	E865.4	–	E950.9	E962.1	E980.9
Heet	976.8	E858.7	E946.8	E950.4	E962.0	E980.4
Helenin	961.6	E857	E931.6	E950.4	E962.0	E980.4
Hellebore (black) (green) (white)	988.2	E865.4	–	E950.9	E962.1	E980.9
Hemlock	988.2	E865.4	–	E950.9	E962.1	E980.9
Hemostatics	964.5	E858.2	E934.5	E950.4	E962.0	E980.4
capillary active drugs	972.8	E858.3	E942.8	E950.4	E962.0	E980.4
Henbane	988.2	E865.4	–	E950.9	E962.1	E980.9
Heparin (sodium)	964.2	E858.2	E934.2	E950.4	E962.0	E980.4
Heptabarbital, heptabarbitone	967.0	E851	E937.0	E950.1	E962.0	E980.1
Heptachlor	989.2	E863.0	–	E950.6	E962.1	E980.7
Heptalgin	965.09	E850.2	E935.2	E950.0	E962.0	E980.0
Herbicides	989.4	E863.5	–	E950.6	E962.1	E980.7
Heroin	965.01	E850.0	E935.0	E950.0	E962.0	E980.0
Herplex	976.5	E858.7	E946.5	E950.4	E962.0	E980.4
HES	964.8	E858.2	E934.8	E950.4	E962.0	E980.4
Hetastarch	964.8	E858.2	E934.8	E950.4	E962.0	E980.4
Hexachlorocyclohexane	989.2	E863.0	–	E950.6	E962.1	E980.7
Hexachlorophene	976.2	E858.7	E946.2	E950.4	E962.0	E980.4
Hexadimethrine (bromide)	964.5	E858.2	E934.5	E950.4	E962.0	E980.4
Hexanuorenium	975.2	E858.6	E945.2	E950.4	E962.0	E980.4
Hexa-germ	976.2	E858.7	E946.2	E950.4	E962.0	E980.4
Hexahydrophenol	980.8	E860.8	–	E950.9	E962.1	E980.9
Hexalin	980.8	E860.8	–	E950.9	E962.1	E980.9
Hexamethonium	972.3	E858.3	E942.3	E950.4	E962.0	E980.4

4th Fourth Digit Required | 5th Fifth Digit Required | *[code]* Manifestation Code | ● New Line | ▲ Revised Line | <u>text</u> New Text | ~~text~~ Deleted text

Drug, chemical	Poisoning	External Cause (E Code) Accident	Therapeutic Use	Suicide Attempt	Assault	Undetermined
Hexamethyleneamine	961.9	E857	E931.9	E950.4	E962.0	E980.4
Hexamine	961.9	E857	E931.9	E950.4	E962.0	E980.4
Hexanone	982.8	E862.4	–	E950.9	E962.1	E980.9
Hexapropymate	967.8	E852.8	E937.8	E950.2	E962.0	E980.2
Hexestrol	962.2	E858.0	E932.2	E950.4	E962.0	E980.4
Hexethal (sodium)	967.0	E851	E937.0	E950.1	E962.0	E980.1
Hexetidine	976.0	E858.7	E946.0	E950.4	E962.0	E980.4
Hexobarbital, hexobarbitone	967.0	E851	E937.0	E950.1	E962.0	E980.1
sodium (anesthetic)	968.3	E855.1	E938.3	E950.4	E962.0	E980.4
soluble	968.3	E855.1	E938.3	E950.4	E962.0	E980.4
Hexocyclium	971.1	E855.4	E941.1	E950.4	E962.0	E980.4
Hexoestrol	962.2	E858.0	E932.2	E950.4	E962.0	E980.4
Hexone	982.8	E862.4	–	E950.9	E962.1	E980.9
Hexylcaine	968.5	E855.2	E938.5	E950.4	E962.0	E980.4
Hexylresorcinol	961.6	E857	E931.6	E950.4	E962.0	E980.4
Hinkle's pills	973.1	E858.4	E943.1	E950.4	E962.0	E980.4
Histalog	977.8	E858.8	E947.8	E950.4	E962.0	E980.4
Histamine (phosphate)	972.5	E858.3	E942.5	E950.4	E962.0	E980.4
Histoplasmin	977.8	E858.8	E947.8	E950.4	E962.0	E980.4
Holly berries	988.2	E865.3	–	E950.9	E962.1	E980.9
Homatropine	971.1	E855.4	E941.1	E950.4	E962.0	E980.4
Homo-tet	964.6	E858.2	E934.6	E950.4	E962.0	E980.4
Hormones (synthetic substitute)						
NEC	962.9	E858.0	E932.9	E950.4	E962.0	E980.4
adrenal cortical steroids	962.0	E858.0	E932.0	E950.4	E962.0	E980.4
antidiabetic agents	962.3	E858.0	E932.3	E950.4	E962.0	E980.4
follicle stimulating	962.4	E858.0	E932.4	E950.4	E962.0	E980.4
gonadotropic	962.4	E858.0	E932.4	E950.4	E962.0	E980.4
growth	962.4	E858.0	E932.4	E950.4	E962.0	E980.4
ovarian (substitutes)	962.2	E858.0	E932.2	E950.4	E962.0	E980.4
parathyroid (derivatives)	962.6	E858.0	E932.6	E950.4	E962.0	E980.4
pituitary (posterior)	962.5	E858.0	E932.5	E950.4	E962.0	E980.4
anterior	962.4	E858.0	E932.4	E950.4	E962.0	E980.4
thyroid (derivative)	962.7	E858.0	E932.7	E950.4	E962.0	E980.4
Hornet (sting)	989.5	E905.3	–	E950.9	E962.1	E980.9
Horticulture agent NEC	989.4	E863.9	–	E950.6	E962.1	E980.7
Hyaluronidase	963.4	E858.1	E933.4	E950.4	E962.0	E980.4
Hyazyme	963.4	E858.1	E933.4	E950.4	E962.0	E980.4
Hycodan	965.09	E850.2	E935.2	E950.0	E962.0	E980.0
Hydantoin derivatives	966.1	E855.0	E936.1	E950.4	E962.0	E980.4
Hydeltra	962.0	E858.0	E932.0	E950.4	E962.0	E980.4
Hydergine	971.3	E855.6	E941.3	E950.4	E962.0	E980.4
Hydrabamine penicillin	960.0	E856	E930.0	E950.4	E962.0	E980.4
Hydralazine, hydrallazine	972.6	E858.3	E942.6	E950.4	E962.0	E980.4
Hydrargaphen	976.0	E858.7	E946.0	E950.4	E962.0	E980.4
Hydrazine	983.9	E864.3	–	E950.7	E962.1	E980.6
Hydriodic acid	975.5	E858.6	E945.5	E950.4	E962.0	E980.4
Hydrocarbon gas	987.1	E869.8	–	E952.8	E962.2	E982.8
incomplete combustion of – *see* Carbon, monoxide, fuel, utility						
liquefied (mobile container)	987.0	E868.0	–	E951.1	E962.2	E981.1
piped (natural)	987.0	E867	–	E951.0	E962.2	E981.0
Hydrochloric acid (liquid)	983.1	E864.1	–	E950.7	E962.1	E980.6
medicinal	973.4	E858.4	E943.4	E950.4	E962.0	E980.4
vapor	987.8	E869.8	–	E952.8	E962.2	E982.8
Hydrochlorothiazide	974.3	E858.5	E944.3	E950.4	E962.0	E980.4
Hydrocodone	965.09	E850.2	E935.2	E950.0	E962.0	E980.0
Hydrocortisone	962.0	E858.0	E932.0	E950.4	E962.0	E980.4
ENT agent	976.6	E858.7	E946.6	E950.4	E962.0	E980.4
ophthalmic preparation	976.5	E858.7	E946.5	E950.4	E962.0	E980.4
topical NEC	976.0	E858.7	E946.0	E950.4	E962.0	E980.4
Hydrocortone	962.0	E858.0	E932.0	E950.4	E962.0	E980.4
ENT agent	976.6	E858.7	E946.6	E950.4	E962.0	E980.4
ophthalmic preparation	976.5	E858.7	E946.5	E950.4	E962.0	E980.4
topical NEC	976.0	E858.7	E946.0	E950.4	E962.0	E980.4
Hydrocyanic acid – *see* Cyanide(s)						
Hydroflumethiazide	974.3	E858.5	E944.3	E950.4	E962.0	E980.4
Hydrofluoric acid (liquid)	983.1	E864.1	–	E950.7	E962.1	E980.6
vapor	987.8	E869.8	–	E952.8	E962.2	E982.8
Hydrogen	987.8	E869.8	–	E952.8	E962.2	E982.8
arsenide	985.1	E866.3	–	E950.8	E962.1	E980.8
arseniureted	985.1	E866.3	–	E950.8	E962.1	E980.8
cyanide (salts)	989.0	E866.8	–	E950.9	E962.1	E980.9
gas	987.7	E869.8	–	E952.8	E962.2	E982.8
fluoride (liquid)	983.1	E864.1	–	E950.7	E962.1	E980.6
vapor	987.8	E869.8	–	E952.8	E962.2	E982.8
peroxide (solution)	976.6	E858.7	E946.6	E950.4	E962.0	E980.4
phosphureted	987.8	E869.8	–	E952.8	E962.2	E982.8
sulfide (gas)	987.8	E869.8	–	E952.8	E962.2	E982.8
arseniureted	985.1	E866.3	–	E950.8	E962.1	E980.8
sulfureted	987.8	E869.8	–	E952.8	E962.2	E982.8
Hydromorphinol	965.09	E850.2	E935.2	E950.0	E962.0	E980.0
Hydromorphinone	965.09	E850.2	E935.2	E950.0	E962.0	E980.0
Hydromorphone	965.09	E850.2	E935.2	E950.0	E962.0	E980.0
Hydromox	974.3	E858.5	E944.3	E950.4	E962.0	E980.4
Hydrophilic lotion	976.3	E858.7	E946.3	E950.4	E962.0	E980.4
Hydroquinone	983.0	E864.0	–	E950.7	E962.1	E980.6
vapor	987.8	E869.8	–	E952.8	E962.2	E982.8
Hydrosulfuric acid (gas)	987.8	E869.8	–	E952.8	E962.2	E982.8
Hydrous wool fat (lotion)	976.3	E858.7	E946.3	E950.4	E962.0	E980.4
Hydroxide, caustic	983.2	E864.2	–	E950.7	E962.1	E980.6
Hydroxocobalamin	964.1	E858.2	E934.1	E950.4	E962.0	E980.4
Hydroxyamphetamine	971.2	E858.5	E941.2	E950.4	E962.0	E980.4
Hydroxychloroquine	961.4	E857	E931.4	E950.4	E962.0	E980.4
Hydroxydihydrocodeinone	965.09	E850.2	E935.2	E950.0	E962.0	E980.0
Hydroxyethyl starch	964.8	E858.2	E934.8	E950.4	E962.0	E980.4
Hydroxyphenamate	969.5	E853.8	E939.5	E950.3	E962.0	E980.3
Hydroxyphenylbutazone	965.5	E850.5	E935.5	E950.0	E962.0	E980.0
Hydroxyprogesterone	962.2	E858.0	E932.2	E950.4	E962.0	E980.4
Hydroxyquinoline derivatives	961.3	E857	E931.3	E950.4	E962.0	E980.4
Hydroxystilbamidine	961.5	E857	E931.5	E950.4	E962.0	E980.4
Hydroxyurea	963.1	E858.1	E933.1	E950.4	E962.0	E980.4
Hydroxyzine	969.5	E853.8	E939.5	E950.3	E962.0	E980.3
Hyoscine (hydrobromide)	971.1	E855.4	E941.1	E950.4	E962.0	E980.4
Hyoscyamine	971.1	E855.4	E941.1	E950.4	E962.0	E980.4
Hyoscyamus (albus) (niger)	988.2	E865.4	–	E950.9	E962.1	E980.9
Hypaque	977.8	E858.8	E947.8	E950.4	E962.0	E980.4
Hypertussis	964.6	E858.2	E934.6	E950.4	E962.0	E980.4
Hypnotics NEC	967.9	E852.9	E937.9	E950.2	E962.0	E980.2
Hypochlorites – *see* Sodium, hypochlorite						
Hypotensive agents NEC	972.6	E858.3	E942.6	E950.4	E962.0	E980.4
Ibufenac	965.69	E850.6	E935.6	E950.0	E962.0	E980.0
Ibuprofen	965.61	E850.6	E935.6	E950.0	E962.0	E980.0
ICG	977.8	E858.8	E947.8	E950.4	E962.0	E980.4
Ichthammol	976.4	E858.7	E946.4	E950.4	E962.0	E980.4
Ichthyol	976.4	E858.7	E946.4	E950.4	E962.0	E980.4
Idoxuridine	976.5	E858.7	E946.5	E950.4	E962.0	E980.4
IDU	976.5	E858.7	E946.5	E950.4	E962.0	E980.4
Iletin	962.3	E858.0	E932.3	E950.4	E962.0	E980.4
Ilex	988.2	E865.4	–	E950.9	E962.1	E980.9
Illuminating gas – *see* Gas, utility						
Ilopan	963.5	E858.1	E933.5	E950.4	E962.0	E980.4
Ilotycin	960.3	E856	E930.3	E950.4	E962.0	E980.4
ophthalmic preparation	976.5	E858.7	E946.5	E950.4	E962.0	E980.4
topical NEC	976.0	E858.7	E946.0	E950.4	E962.0	E980.4
Imipramine ▲	969.05	E854.0	E939.0	E950.3	E962.0	E980.3
Immu-G	964.6	E858.2	E934.6	E950.4	E962.0	E980.4
Immuglobin	964.6	E858.2	E934.6	E950.4	E962.0	E980.4
Immune serum globulin	964.6	E858.2	E934.6	E950.4	E962.0	E980.4
Immunosuppressive agents	963.1	E858.1	E933.1	E950.4	E962.0	E980.4
Immu-tetanus	964.6	E858.2	E934.6	E950.4	E962.0	E980.4
Indandione (derivatives)	964.2	E858.2	E934.2	E950.4	E962.0	E980.4
Inderal	972.0	E858.3	E942.0	E950.4	E962.0	E980.4
Indian						
hemp	969.6	E854.1	E939.6	E950.3	E962.0	E980.3
tobacco	988.2	E865.4	–	E950.9	E962.1	E980.9
Indigo carmine	977.8	E858.8	E947.8	E950.4	E962.0	E980.4
Indocin	965.69	E850.6	E935.6	E950.0	E962.0	E980.0
Indocyanine green	977.8	E858.8	E947.8	E950.4	E962.0	E980.4
Indomethacin	965.69	E850.6	E935.6	E950.0	E962.0	E980.0
Industrial						
alcohol	980.9	E860.9	–	E950.9	E962.1	E980.9
fumes	987.8	E869.8	–	E952.8	E962.2	E982.8
solvents (fumes) (vapors)	982.8	E862.9	–	E950.9	E962.1	E980.9
Influenza vaccine	979.6	E858.8	E949.6	E950.4	E962.0	E982.8
Ingested substances NEC	989.9	E866.9	–	E950.9	E962.1	E980.9
INH (isoniazid)	961.8	E857	E931.8	E950.4	E962.0	E980.4
Inhalation, gas (noxious) – *see* Gas						
Ink	989.89	E866.8	–	E950.9	E962.1	E980.9
Innovar	967.6	E852.5	E937.6	E950.2	E962.0	E980.2
Inositol niacinate	972.2	E858.3	E942.2	E950.4	E962.0	E980.4
Inproquone	963.1	E858.1	E933.1	E950.4	E962.0	E980.4
Insect (sting), venomous	989.5	E905.5	–	E950.9	E962.1	E980.9
Insecticides (*see also* Pesticides)	989.4	E863.4	–	E950.6	E962.1	E980.7
chlorinated	989.2	E863.0	–	E950.6	E962.1	E980.7
mixtures	989.4	E863.3	–	E950.6	E962.1	E980.7
organochlorine (compounds)	989.2	E863.0	–	E950.6	E962.1	E980.7
organophosphorus (compounds)	989.3	E863.1	–	E950.6	E962.1	E980.7
Insular tissue extract	962.3	E858.0	E932.3	E950.4	E962.0	E980.4
Insulin (amorphous) (globin) (isophane) (Lente) (NPH) (prolamine)(Semilente) (Ultralente) (zinc)	962.3	E858.0	E932.3	E950.4	E962.0	E980.4

Drug, chemical	Poisoning	External Cause (E Code)				
		Accident	Therapeutic Use	Suicide Attempt	Assault	Undetermined
Intranarcon	968.3	E855.1	E938.3	E950.4	E962.0	E980.4
Inulin	977.8	E858.8	E947.8	E950.4	E962.0	E980.4
Invert sugar	974.5	E858.5	E944.5	E950.4	E962.0	E980.4
Inza – *see* Naproxen						
Iodide NEC (*see also* Iodine)	976.0	E858.7	E946.0	E950.4	E962.0	E980.4
mercury (ointment)	976.0	E858.7	E946.0	E950.4	E962.0	E980.4
methylate	976.0	E858.7	E946.0	E950.4	E962.0	E980.4
potassium (expectorant) NEC	975.5	E858.6	E945.5	E950.4	E962.0	E980.4
Iodinated glycerol	975.5	E858.6	E945.5	E950.4	E962.0	E980.4
Iodine (antiseptic, external) (tincture) NEC	976.0	E858.7	E946.0	E950.4	E962.0	E980.4
diagnostic	977.8	E858.8	E947.8	E950.4	E962.0	E980.4
for thyroid conditions (antithyroid)	962.8	E858.0	E932.8	E950.4	E962.0	E980.4
vapor	987.8	E869.8	–	E952.8	E962.2	E982.8
Iodized oil	977.8	E858.8	E947.8	E950.4	E962.0	E980.4
Iodobismitol	961.2	E857	E931.2	E950.4	E962.0	E980.4
Iodochlorhydroxyquin	961.3	E857	E931.3	E950.4	E962.0	E980.4
topical	976.0	E858.7	E946.0	E950.4	E962.0	E980.4
Iodoform	976.0	E858.7	E946.0	E950.4	E962.0	E980.4
Iodopanoic acid	977.8	E858.8	E947.8	E950.4	E962.0	E980.4
Iodophthalein	977.8	E858.8	E947.8	E950.4	E962.0	E980.4
Ion exchange resins	974.5	E858.5	E944.5	E950.4	E962.0	E980.4
Iopanoic acid	977.8	E858.8	E947.8	E950.4	E962.0	E980.4
Iophendylate	977.8	E858.8	E947.8	E950.4	E962.0	E980.4
Iothiouracil	962.8	E858.0	E932.8	E950.4	E962.0	E980.4
Ipecac	973.6	E858.4	E943.6	E950.4	E962.0	E980.4
Ipecacuanha	973.6	E858.4	E943.6	E950.4	E962.0	E980.4
Ipodate	977.8	E858.8	E947.8	E950.4	E962.0	E980.4
Ipral	967.0	E851	E937.0	E950.1	E962.0	E980.1
Ipratropium	975.1	E858.6	E945.1	E950.4	E962.0	E980.4
Iproniazid ▲	969.01	E854.0	E939.0	E950.3	E962.0	E980.3
Iron (compounds) (medicinal) (preparations)	964.0	E858.2	E934.0	E950.4	E962.0	E980.4
dextran	964.0	E858.2	E934.0	E950.4	E962.0	E980.4
nonmedicinal (dust) (fumes) NEC	985.8	E866.4	–	E950.9	E962.1	E980.9
Irritant drug	977.9	E858.9	E947.9	E950.5	E962.0	E980.5
Ismelin	972.6	E858.3	E942.6	E950.4	E962.0	E980.4
Isoamyl nitrite	972.4	E858.3	E942.4	E950.4	E962.0	E980.4
Isobutyl acetate	982.8	E862.4	–	E950.9	E962.1	E980.9
Isocarboxazid ▲	969.01	E854.0	E939.0	E950.3	E962.0	E980.3
Isoephedrine	971.2	E855.5	E941.2	E950.4	E962.0	E980.4
Isoetharine	971.2	E855.5	E941.2	E950.4	E962.0	E980.4
Isofluorophate	971.0	E855.3	E941.0	E950.4	E962.0	E980.4
Isoniazid (INH)	961.8	E857	E931.8	E950.4	E962.0	E980.4
Isopentaquine	961.4	E857	E931.4	E950.4	E962.0	E980.4
Isophane insulin	962.3	E858.0	E932.3	E950.4	E962.0	E980.4
Isopregnenone	962.2	E858.0	E932.2	E950.4	E962.0	E980.4
Isoprenaline	971.2	E855.5	E941.2	E950.4	E962.0	E980.4
Isopropamide	971.1	E855.4	E941.1	E950.4	E962.0	E980.4
Isopropanol	980.2	E860.3	–	E950.9	E962.1	E980.9
topical (germicide)	976.0	E858.7	E946.0	E950.4	E962.0	E980.4
Isopropyl						
acetate	982.8	E862.4	–	E950.9	E962.1	E980.9
alcohol	980.2	E860.3	–	E950.9	E962.1	E980.9
topical (germicide)	976.0	E858.7	E946.0	E950.4	E962.0	E980.4
ether	982.8	E862.4	–	E950.9	E962.1	E980.9
Isoproterenol	971.2	E855.5	E941.2	E950.4	E962.0	E980.4
Isosorbide dinitrate	972.4	E858.3	E942.4	E950.4	E962.0	E980.4
Isothipendyl	963.0	E858.1	E933.0	E950.4	E962.0	E980.4
Isoxazolyl penicillin	960.0	E856	E930.0	E950.4	E962.0	E980.4
Isoxsuprine hydrochloride	972.5	E858.3	E942.5	E950.4	E962.0	E980.4
I-thyroxine sodium	962.7	E858.0	E932.7	E950.4	E962.0	E980.4
Jaborandi (pilocarpus) (extract)	971.0	E855.3	E941.0	E950.4	E962.0	E980.4
Jalap	973.1	E858.4	E943.1	E950.4	E962.0	E980.4
Jamaica						
dogwood (bark)	965.7	E850.7	E935.7	E950.0	E962.0	E980.0
ginger	989.89	E866.8	–	E950.9	E962.1	E980.9
Jatropha	988.2	E865.4	–	E950.9	E962.1	E980.9
curcas	988.2	E865.3	–	E950.9	E962.1	E980.9
Jectofer	964.0	E858.2	E934.0	E950.4	E962.0	E980.4
Jellyfish (sting)	989.5	E905.6	–	E950.9	E962.1	E980.9
Jequirity (bean)	988.2	E865.3	–	E950.9	E962.1	E980.9
Jimson weed	988.2	E865.4	–	E950.9	E962.1	E980.9
seeds	988.2	E865.3	–	E950.9	E962.1	E980.9
Juniper tar (oil) (ointment)	976.4	E858.7	E946.4	E950.4	E962.0	E980.4
Kallikrein	972.5	E858.3	E942.5	E950.4	E962.0	E980.4
Kanamycin	960.6	E856	E930.6	E950.4	E962.0	E980.4
Kantrex	960.6	E856	E930.6	E950.4	E962.0	E980.4
Kaolin	973.5	E858.4	E943.5	E950.4	E962.0	E980.4
Karaya (gum)	973.3	E858.4	E943.3	E950.4	E962.0	E980.4
Kemithal	968.3	E855.1	E938.3	E950.4	E962.0	E980.4
Kenacort	962.0	E858.0	E932.0	E950.4	E962.0	E980.4

Drug, chemical	Poisoning	External Cause (E Code)				
		Accident	Therapeutic Use	Suicide Attempt	Assault	Undetermined
Keratolytics	976.4	E858.7	E946.4	E950.4	E962.0	E980.4
Keratoplastics	976.4	E858.7	E946.4	E950.4	E962.0	E980.4
Kerosene, kerosine (fuel) (solvent) NEC	981	E862.1	–	E950.9	E962.1	E980.9
insecticide	981	E863.4	–	E950.6	E962.1	E980.7
vapor	987.1	E869.8	–	E952.8	E962.2	E982.8
Ketamine	968.3	E855.1	E938.3	E950.4	E962.0	E980.4
Ketobemidone	965.09	E850.2	E935.2	E950.0	E962.0	E980.0
Ketols	982.8	E862.4	–	E950.9	E962.1	E980.9
Ketone oils	982.8	E862.4	–	E950.9	E962.1	E980.9
Ketoprofen	965.61	E850.6	E935.6	E950.0	E962.0	E980.0
Kiln gas or vapor (carbon monoxide)	986	E868.8	–	E952.1	E962.2	E982.1
Konsyl	973.3	E858.4	E943.3	E950.4	E962.0	E980.4
Kosam seed	988.2	E865.3	–	E950.9	E962.1	E980.9
Krait (venom)	989.5	E905.0	–	E950.9	E962.1	E980.9
Kwell (insecticide)	989.2	E863.0	–	E950.6	E962.1	E980.7
anti-infective (topical)	976.0	E858.7	E946.0	E950.4	E962.0	E980.4
Laburnum (flowers) (seeds)	988.2	E865.3	–	E950.9	E962.1	E980.9
leaves	988.2	E865.4	–	E950.9	E962.1	E980.9
Lacquers	989.89	E861.6	–	E950.9	E962.1	E980.9
Lacrimogenic gas	987.5	E869.3	–	E952.8	E962.2	E982.8
Lactic acid	983.1	E864.1	–	E950.7	E962.1	E980.6
Lactobacillus acidophilus	973.5	E858.4	E943.5	E950.4	E962.0	E980.4
Lactoflavin	963.5	E858.1	E933.5	E950.4	E962.0	E980.4
Lactuca (virosa) (extract)	967.8	E852.8	E937.8	E950.2	E962.0	E980.2
Lactucarium	967.8	E852.8	E937.8	E950.2	E962.0	E980.2
Laevulose	974.5	E858.5	E944.5	E950.4	E962.0	E980.4
Lanatoside (C)	972.1	E858.3	E942.1	E950.4	E962.0	E980.4
Lanolin (lotion)	976.3	E858.7	E946.3	E950.4	E962.0	E980.4
Largactil	969.1	E853.0	E939.1	E950.3	E962.0	E980.3
Larkspur	988.2	E865.3	–	E950.9	E962.1	E980.9
Laroxyl ▲	969.05	E854.0	E939.0	E950.3	E962.0	E980.3
Lasix	974.4	E858.5	E944.4	E950.4	E962.0	E980.4
Latex	989.82	E866.8	–	E950.9	E962.1	E980.9
Lathyrus (seed)	988.2	E865.3	–	E950.9	E962.1	E980.9
Laudanum	965.09	E850.2	E935.2	E950.0	E962.0	E980.0
Laudexium	975.2	E858.6	E945.2	E950.4	E962.0	E980.4
Laurel, black or cherry	988.2	E865.4	–	E950.9	E962.1	E980.9
Laurolinium	976.0	E858.7	E946.0	E950.4	E962.0	E980.4
Lauryl sulfoacetate	976.2	E858.7	E946.2	E950.4	E962.0	E980.4
Laxatives NEC	973.3	E858.4	E943.3	E950.4	E962.0	E980.4
emollient	973.2	E858.4	E943.2	E950.4	E962.0	E980.4
L-dopa	966.4	E855.0	E936.4	E950.4	E962.0	E980.4
L-Tryptophan – *see* amino acid						
Lead (dust) (fumes) (vapor) NEC	984.9	E866.0	–	E950.9	E962.1	E980.9
acetate (dust)	984.1	E866.0	–	E950.9	E962.1	E980.9
anti-infectives	961.2	E857	E931.2	E950.4	E962.0	E980.4
antiknock compound (tetraethyl)	984.1	E862.1	–	E950.9	E962.1	E980.9
arsenate, arsenite (dust) (insecticide) (vapor)	985.1	E863.4	–	E950.8	E962.1	E980.8
herbicide	985.1	E863.5	–	E950.8	E962.1	E980.8
carbonate	984.0	E866.0	–	E950.9	E962.1	E980.9
paint	984.0	E861.5	–	E950.9	E962.1	E980.9
chromate	984.0	E866.0	–	E950.9	E962.1	E980.9
paint	984.0	E861.5	–	E950.9	E962.1	E980.9
dioxide	984.0	E866.0	–	E950.9	E962.1	E980.9
inorganic (compound)	984.0	E866.0	–	E950.9	E962.1	E980.9
paint	984.0	E861.5	–	E950.9	E962.1	E980.9
iodide	984.0	E866.0	–	E950.9	E962.1	E980.9
pigment (paint)	984.0	E861.5	–	E950.9	E962.1	E980.9
monoxide (dust)	984.0	E866.0	–	E950.9	E962.1	E980.9
paint	984.0	E861.5	–	E950.9	E962.1	E980.9
organic	984.1	E866.0	–	E950.9	E962.1	E980.9
oxide	984.0	E866.0	–	E950.9	E962.1	E980.9
paint	984.0	E861.5	–	E950.9	E962.1	E980.9
paint	984.0	E861.5	–	E950.9	E962.1	E980.9
salts	984.0	E866.0	–	E950.9	E962.1	E980.9
specified compound NEC	984.8	E866.0	–	E950.9	E962.1	E980.9
tetra-ethyl	984.1	E862.1	–	E950.9	E962.1	E980.9
Lebanese red	969.6	E854.1	E939.6	E950.3	E962.0	E980.3
Lente lietin (insulin)	962.3	E858.0	E932.3	E950.4	E962.0	E980.4
Leptazol	970.0	E854.3	E940.0	E950.4	E962.0	E980.4
Leritine	965.09	E850.2	E935.2	E950.0	E962.0	E980.0
Letter	962.7	E858.0	E932.7	E950.4	E962.0	E980.4
Lettuce opium	967.8	E852.8	E937.8	E950.2	E962.0	E980.2
Leucovorin (factor)	964.1	E858.2	E934.1	E950.4	E962.0	E980.4
Leukeran	963.1	E858.1	E933.1	E950.4	E962.0	E980.4
Levalbuterol	975.7	E858.6	E945.7	E950.4	E962.0	E980.4
Levallorphan	970.1	E854.3	E940.1	E950.4	E962.0	E980.4
Levanil	967.8	E852.8	E937.8	E950.2	E962.0	E980.2
Levarterenol	971.2	E855.5	E941.2	E950.4	E962.0	E980.4

Drug, chemical	Poisoning	External Cause (E Code)				
		Accident	Therapeutic Use	Suicide Attempt	Assault	Undetermined
Levodopa	966.4	E855.0	E936.4	E950.4	E962.0	E980.4
Levo-dromoran	965.09	E850.2	E935.2	E950.0	E962.0	E980.0
Levoid	962.7	E858.0	E932.7	E950.4	E962.0	E980.4
Levo-iso-methadone	965.02	E850.1	E935.1	E950.0	E962.0	E980.0
Levomepromazine	967.8	E852.8	E937.8	E950.2	E962.0	E980.2
Levoprome	967.8	E852.8	E937.8	E950.2	E962.0	E980.2
Levopropoxyphene	975.4	E858.6	E945.4	E950.4	E962.0	E980.4
Levorphan, levophanol	965.09	E850.2	E935.2	E950.0	E962.0	E980.0
Levothyroxine (sodium)	962.7	E858.0	E932.7	E950.4	E962.0	E980.4
Levsin	971.1	E855.4	E941.1	E950.4	E962.0	E980.4
Levulose	974.5	E858.5	E944.5	E950.4	E962.0	E980.4
Lewisite (gas)	985.1	E866.3	–	E950.8	E962.1	E980.8
Librium	969.4	E853.2	E939.4	E950.3	E962.0	E980.3
Lidex	976.0	E858.7	E946.0	E950.4	E962.0	E980.4
Lidocaine (infiltration) (topical)	968.5	E855.2	E938.5	E950.4	E962.0	E980.4
nerve block (peripheral) (plexus)	968.6	E855.2	E938.6	E950.4	E962.0	E980.4
spinal	968.7	E855.2	E938.7	E950.4	E962.0	E980.4
Lighter fluid	981	E862.1	–	E950.9	E962.1	E980.9
Lignocaine (infiltration) (topical)	968.5	E855.2	E938.5	E950.4	E962.0	E980.4
nerve block (peripheral) (plexus)	968.6	E855.2	E938.6	E950.4	E962.0	E980.4
spinal	968.7	E855.2	E938.7	E950.4	E962.0	E980.4
Ligroin(e) (solvent)	981	E862.0	–	E950.9	E962.1	E980.9
vapor	987.1	E869.8	–	E952.8	E962.2	E982.8
Ligustrum vulgare	988.2	E865.3	–	E950.9	E962.1	E980.9
Lily of the valley	988.2	E865.4	–	E950.9	E962.1	E980.9
Lime (chloride)	983.2	E864.2	–	E950.7	E962.1	E980.6
solution, sulferated	976.4	E858.7	E946.4	E950.4	E962.0	E980.4
Limonene	982.8	E862.4	–	E950.9	E962.1	E980.9
Lincomycin	960.8	E856	E930.8	E950.4	E962.0	E980.4
Lindane (insecticide) (vapor)	989.2	E863.0	–	E950.6	E962.1	E980.7
anti-infective (topical)	976.0	E858.7	E946.0	E950.4	E962.0	E980.4
Liniments NEC	976.9	E858.7	E946.9	E950.4	E962.0	E980.4
Linoleic acid	972.2	E858.3	E942.2	E950.4	E962.0	E980.4
Liothyronine	962.7	E858.0	E932.7	E950.4	E962.0	E980.4
Liotrix	962.7	E858.0	E932.7	E950.4	E962.0	E980.4
Lipancreatin	973.4	E858.4	E943.4	E950.4	E962.0	E980.4
Lipo-Lutin	962.2	E858.0	E932.2	E950.4	E962.0	E980.4
Lipotropic agents	977.1	E858.8	E947.1	E950.4	E962.0	E980.4
Liquefied petroleum gases	987.0	E868.0	–	E951.1	E962.2	E981.1
piped (pure or mixed with air)	987.0	E867	–	E951.0	E962.2	E981.0
Liquid petrolatum	973.2	E858.4	E943.2	E950.4	E962.0	E980.4
substance	989.9	E866.9	–	E950.9	E962.1	E980.9
specified NEC	989.89	E866.8	–	E950.9	E962.1	E980.9
Lirugen	979.4	E858.8	E949.4	E950.4	E962.0	E980.4
Lithane	969.8	E855.8	E939.8	E950.3	E962.0	E980.3
Lithium	985.8	E866.4	–	E950.9	E962.1	E980.9
carbonate	969.8	E855.8	E939.8	E950.3	E962.0	E980.3
Lithonate	969.8	E855.8	E939.8	E950.3	E962.0	E980.3
Liver (extract) (injection) (preparations)	964.1	E858.2	E934.1	E950.4	E962.0	E980.4
Lizard (bite) (venom)	989.5	E905.0	–	E950.9	E962.1	E980.9
LMD	964.8	E858.2	E934.8	E950.4	E962.0	E980.4
Lobelia	988.2	E865.4	–	E950.9	E962.1	E980.9
Lobeline	970.0	E854.3	E940.0	E950.4	E962.0	E980.4
Locorten	976.0	E858.7	E946.0	E950.4	E962.0	E980.4
Lolium temulentum	988.2	E865.3	–	E950.9	E962.1	E980.9
Lomotil	973.5	E858.4	E943.5	E950.4	E962.0	E980.4
Lomustine	963.1	E858.1	E933.1	E950.4	E962.0	E980.4
Lophophora williamsii	969.6	E854.1	E939.6	E950.3	E962.0	E980.3
Lorazepam	969.4	E853.2	E939.4	E950.3	E962.0	E980.3
Lotions NEC	976.9	E858.7	E946.9	E950.4	E962.0	E980.4
Lotronex	973.8	E858.4	E943.8	E950.4	E962.0	E980.4
Lotusate	967.0	E851	E937.0	E950.1	E962.0	E980.1
Lowila	976.2	E858.7	E946.2	E950.4	E962.0	E980.4
Loxapine	969.3	E853.8	E939.3	E950.3	E962.0	E980.3
Lozenges (throat)	976.6	E858.7	E946.6	E950.4	E962.0	E980.4
LSD (25)	969.6	E854.1	E939.6	E950.3	E962.0	E980.3
Lubricating oil NEC	981	E862.2	–	E950.9	E962.1	E980.9
Lucanthone	961.6	E857	E931.6	E950.4	E962.0	E980.4
Luminal	967.0	E851	E937.0	E950.1	E962.0	E980.1
Lung irritant (gas) NEC	987.9	E869.9	–	E952.9	E962.2	E982.9
Lutocylol	962.2	E858.0	E932.2	E950.4	E962.0	E980.4
Lutromone	962.2	E858.0	E932.2	E950.4	E962.0	E980.4
Lututrin	975.0	E858.6	E945.0	E950.4	E962.0	E980.4
Lye (concentrated)	983.2	E864.2	–	E950.7	E962.1	E980.6
Lygranum (skin test)	977.8	E858.8	E947.8	E950.4	E962.0	E980.4
Lymecycline	960.4	E856	E930.4	E950.4	E962.0	E980.4
Lymphogranuloma venereum antigen	977.8	E858.8	E947.8	E950.4	E962.0	E980.4
Lynestrenol	962.2	E858.0	E932.2	E950.4	E962.0	E980.4
Lyovac Sodium Edecrin	974.4	E858.5	E944.4	E950.4	E962.0	E980.4
Lypressin	962.5	E858.0	E932.5	E950.4	E962.0	E980.4

Drug, chemical	Poisoning	External Cause (E Code)				
		Accident	Therapeutic Use	Suicide Attempt	Assault	Undetermined
Lysergic acid (amide) (diethylamide)	969.6	E854.1	E939.6	E950.3	E962.0	E980.3
Lysergide	969.6	E854.1	E939.6	E950.3	E962.0	E980.3
Lysine vasopressin	962.5	E858.0	E932.5	E950.4	E962.0	E980.4
Lysol	983.0	E864.0	–	E950.7	E962.1	E980.6
Lytta (vitatta)	976.8	E858.7	E946.8	E950.4	E962.0	E980.4
Mace	987.5	E869.3	–	E952.8	E962.2	E982.8
Macrolides (antibiotics)	960.3	E856	E930.3	E950.4	E962.0	E980.4
Mafenide	976.0	E858.7	E946.0	E950.4	E962.0	E980.4
Magaldrate	973.0	E858.4	E943.0	E950.4	E962.0	E980.4
Magic mushroom	969.6	E854.1	E939.6	E950.3	E962.0	E980.3
Magnamycin	960.8	E856	E930.8	E950.4	E962.0	E980.4
Magnesia magma	973.0	E858.4	E943.0	E950.4	E962.0	E980.4
Magnesium (compounds) (fumes) NEC	985.8	E866.4	–	E950.9	E962.1	E980.9
antacid	973.0	E858.4	E943.0	E950.4	E962.0	E980.4
carbonate	973.0	E858.4	E943.0	E950.4	E962.0	E980.4
cathartic	973.3	E858.4	E943.3	E950.4	E962.0	E980.4
citrate	973.3	E858.4	E943.3	E950.4	E962.0	E980.4
hydroxide	973.0	E858.4	E943.0	E950.4	E962.0	E980.4
oxide	973.0	E858.4	E943.0	E950.4	E962.0	E980.4
sulfate (oral)	973.3	E858.4	E943.3	E950.4	E962.0	E980.4
intravenous	966.3	E855.0	E936.3	E950.4	E962.0	E980.4
trisilicate	973.0	E858.4	E943.0	E950.4	E962.0	E980.4
Malathion (insecticide)	989.3	E863.1	–	E950.6	E962.1	E980.7
Male fern (oleoresin)	961.6	E857	E931.6	E950.4	E962.0	E980.4
Mandelic acid	961.9	E857	E931.9	E950.4	E962.0	E980.4
Manganese compounds (fumes) NEC	985.2	E866.4	–	E950.9	E962.1	E980.9
Mannitol (diuretic) (medicinal) NEC	974.4	E858.5	E944.4	E950.4	E962.0	E980.4
hexanitrate	972.4	E858.3	E942.4	E950.4	E962.0	E980.4
mustard	963.1	E858.1	E933.1	E950.4	E962.0	E980.4
Mannomustine	963.1	E858.1	E933.1	E950.4	E962.0	E980.4
MAO inhibitors ▲	969.01	E854.0	E939.0	E950.3	E962.0	E980.3
Mapharsen	961.1	E857	E931.1	E950.4	E962.0	E980.4
Marcaine	968.9	E855.2	E938.9	E950.4	E962.0	E980.4
infiltration (subcutaneous)	968.5	E855.2	E938.5	E950.4	E962.0	E980.4
nerve block (peripheral) (plexus)	968.6	E855.2	E938.6	E950.4	E962.0	E980.4
Marezine	963.0	E858.1	E933.0	E950.4	E962.0	E980.4
Marihuana, marijuana (derivatives)	969.6	E854.1	E939.6	E950.3	E962.0	E980.3
Marine animals or plants (sting)	989.5	E905.6	–	E950.9	E962.1	E980.9
Marplan ▲	969.01	E854.0	E939.0	E950.3	E962.0	E980.3
Marsh gas	987.1	E869.8	–	E952.8	E962.2	E982.8
Marsilid ▲	969.01	E854.0	E939.0	E950.3	E962.0	E980.3
Matulane	963.1	E858.1	E933.1	E950.4	E962.0	E980.4
Mazindol	977.0	E858.8	E947.0	E950.4	E962.0	E980.4
MDMA ▲	969.72	E854.2	E939.7	E950.3	E962.0	E980.3
Meadow saffron	988.2	E865.3	–	E950.9	E962.1	E980.9
Measles vaccine	979.4	E858.8	E949.4	E950.4	E962.0	E980.4
Meat, noxious or nonbacterial	988.8	E865.0	–	E950.9	E962.1	E980.9
Mebanazine ▲	969.01	E854.0	E939.0	E950.3	E962.0	E980.3
Mebaral	967.0	E851	E937.0	E950.1	E962.0	E980.1
Mebendazole	961.6	E857	E931.6	E950.4	E962.0	E980.4
Mebeverine	975.1	E858.6	E945.1	E950.4	E962.0	E980.4
Mebhydroline	963.0	E858.1	E933.0	E950.4	E962.0	E980.4
Mebrophenhydramine	963.0	E858.1	E933.0	E950.4	E962.0	E980.4
Mebutamate	969.5	E853.8	E939.5	E950.3	E962.0	E980.3
Mecamylamine (chloride)	972.3	E858.3	E942.3	E950.4	E962.0	E980.4
Mechlorethamine hydrochloride	963.1	E858.1	E933.1	E950.4	E962.0	E980.4
Meclizene (hydrochloride)	963.0	E858.1	E933.0	E950.4	E962.0	E980.4
Meclofenoxate	970.0	E854.3	E940.0	E950.4	E962.0	E980.4
Meclozine (hydrochloride)	963.0	E858.1	E933.0	E950.4	E962.0	E980.4
Medazepam	969.4	E853.2	E939.4	E950.3	E962.0	E980.3
Medicine, medicinal substance	977.9	E858.9	E947.9	E950.5	E962.0	E980.5
specified NEC	977.8	E858.8	E947.8	E950.4	E962.0	E980.4
Medinal	967.0	E851	E937.0	E950.1	E962.0	E980.1
Medomin	967.0	E851	E937.0	E950.1	E962.0	E980.1
Medroxyprogesterone	962.2	E858.0	E932.2	E950.4	E962.0	E980.4
Medrysone	976.5	E858.7	E946.5	E950.4	E962.0	E980.4
Mefenamic acid	965.7	E850.7	E935.7	E950.0	E962.0	E980.0
Megahallucinogen	969.6	E854.1	E939.6	E950.3	E962.0	E980.3
Megestrol	962.2	E858.0	E932.2	E950.4	E962.0	E980.4
Meglumine	977.8	E858.8	E947.8	E950.4	E962.0	E980.4
Meladinin	976.3	E858.7	E946.3	E950.4	E962.0	E980.4
Melanizing agents	976.3	E858.7	E946.3	E950.4	E962.0	E980.4
Melarsoprol	961.1	E857	E931.1	E950.4	E962.0	E980.4
Melia azedarach	988.2	E865.3	–	E950.9	E962.1	E980.9
Mellaril	969.1	E853.0	E939.1	E950.3	E962.0	E980.3
Meloxine	976.3	E858.7	E946.3	E950.4	E962.0	E980.4
Melphalan	963.1	E858.1	E933.1	E950.4	E962.0	E980.4
Memantine hydrochloride	969.8	E854.8	E939.8	E950.3	E962.0	E980.3
Menadiol sodium diphosphate	964.3	E858.2	E934.3	E950.4	E962.0	E980.4
Menadione (sodium bisulfite)	964.3	E858.2	E934.3	E950.4	E962.0	E980.4

Drug, chemical	Poisoning	External Cause (E Code) Accident	Therapeutic Use	Suicide Attempt	Assault	Undetermined
Menaphthone	964.3	E858.2	E934.3	E950.4	E962.0	E980.4
Meningococcal vaccine	978.8	E858.8	E948.8	E950.4	E962.0	E980.4
Menningovax-C	978.8	E858.8	E948.8	E950.4	E962.0	E980.4
Menotropins	962.4	E858.0	E932.4	E950.4	E962.0	E980.4
Menthol NEC	976.1	E858.7	E946.1	E950.4	E962.0	E980.4
Mepacrine	961.3	E857	E931.3	E950.4	E962.0	E980.4
Meparfynol	967.8	E852.8	E937.8	E950.2	E962.0	E980.2
Mepazine	969.1	E853.0	E939.1	E950.3	E962.0	E980.3
Mepenzolate	971.1	E855.4	E941.1	E950.4	E962.0	E980.4
Meperidine	965.09	E850.2	E935.2	E950.0	E962.0	E980.0
Mephenamin(e)	966.4	E855.0	E936.4	E950.4	E962.0	E980.4
Mephenesin (carbamate)	968.0	E855.1	E938.0	E950.4	E962.0	E980.4
Mephenoxalone	969.5	E853.8	E939.5	E950.3	E962.0	E980.3
Mephentermine	971.2	E855.5	E941.2	E950.4	E962.0	E980.4
Mephenytoin	966.1	E855.0	E936.1	E950.4	E962.0	E980.4
Mephobarbital	967.0	E851	E937.0	E950.1	E962.0	E980.1
Mepiperphenidol	971.1	E855.4	E941.1	E950.4	E962.0	E980.4
Mepivacaine	968.9	E855.2	E938.9	E950.4	E962.0	E980.4
infiltration(subcutaneous)	968.5	E855.2	E938.5	E950.4	E962.0	E980.4
nerve block (peripheral) (plexus)	968.6	E855.2	E938.6	E950.4	E962.0	E980.4
topical (surface)	968.5	E855.2	E938.5	E950.4	E962.0	E980.4
Meprednisone	962.0	E858.0	E932.0	E950.4	E962.0	E980.4
Meprobam	969.5	E853.8	E939.5	E950.3	E962.0	E980.3
Meprobamate	969.5	E853.8	E939.5	E950.3	E962.0	E980.3
Mepyramine (maleate)	963.0	E858.1	E933.0	E950.4	E962.0	E980.4
Meralluride	974.0	E858.5	E944.0	E950.4	E962.0	E980.4
Merbaphen	974.0	E858.5	E944.0	E950.4	E962.0	E980.4
Merbromin	976.0	E858.7	E946.0	E950.4	E962.0	E980.4
Mercaplomerin	974.0	E858.5	E944.0	E950.4	E962.0	E980.4
Mercaptopurine	963.1	E858.1	E933.1	E950.4	E962.0	E980.4
Mercumatilin	974.0	E858.5	E944.0	E950.4	E962.0	E980.4
Mercuramide	974.0	E858.5	E944.0	E950.4	E962.0	E980.4
Mercuranin	976.0	E858.7	E946.0	E950.4	E962.0	E980.4
Mercurochrome	976.0	E858.7	E946.0	E950.4	E962.0	E980.4
Mercury, mercuric, mercurous (compounds) (cyanide) (fumes) (nonmedicinal) (vapor) NEC	985.0	E866.1	–	E950.9	E962.1	E980.9
ammoniated	976.0	E858.7	E946.0	E950.4	E962.0	E980.4
anti-infective	961.2	E857	E931.2	E950.4	E962.0	E980.4
topical	976.0	E858.7	E946.0	E950.4	E962.0	E980.4
chloride (antiseptic) NEC	976.0	E858.7	E946.0	E950.4	E962.0	E980.4
fungicide	985.0	E863.6	–	E950.6	E962.1	E980.7
diuretic compounds	974.0	E858.5	E944.0	E950.4	E962.0	E980.4
fungicide	985.0	E863.6	–	E950.6	E962.1	E980.7
organic (fungicide)	985.0	E863.6	–	E950.6	E962.1	E980.7
Merethoxylline	974.0	E858.5	E944.0	E950.4	E962.0	E980.4
Mersalyl	974.0	E858.5	E944.0	E950.4	E962.0	E980.4
Merthiolate (topical)	976.0	E858.7	E946.0	E950.4	E962.0	E980.4
ophthalmic preparation	976.5	E858.7	E946.5	E950.4	E962.0	E980.4
Meruvax	979.4	E858.8	E949.4	E950.4	E962.0	E980.4
Mescal buttons	969.6	E854.1	E939.6	E950.3	E962.0	E980.3
Mescaline (salts)	969.6	E854.1	E939.6	E950.3	E962.0	E980.3
Mesoridazine besylate	969.1	E853.0	E939.1	E950.3	E962.0	E980.3
Mestanolone	962.1	E858.0	E932.1	E950.4	E962.0	E980.4
Mestranol	962.2	E858.0	E932.2	E950.4	E962.0	E980.4
Metactesylacetate	976.0	E858.7	E946.0	E950.4	E962.0	E980.4
Metaldehyde (snail killer) **NEC**	989.4	E863.4	–	E950.6	E962.1	E980.7
Metals (heavy) (nonmedicinal) NEC	985.9	E866.4	–	E950.9	E962.1	E980.9
dust, fumes, or vapor NEC	985.9	E866.4	–	E950.9	E962.1	E980.9
light NEC	985.9	E866.4	–	E950.9	E962.1	E980.9
dust, fumes, or vapor NEC	985.9	E866.4	–	E950.9	E962.1	E980.9
pesticides (dust) (vapor)	985.9	E863.4	–	E950.6	E962.1	E980.7
Metamucil	973.3	E858.4	E943.3	E950.4	E962.0	E980.4
Metaphen	976.0	E858.7	E946.0	E950.4	E962.0	E980.4
Metaproterenol	975.1	E858.6	E945.1	E950.4	E962.0	E980.4
Metaraminol	972.8	E858.3	E942.8	E950.4	E962.0	E980.4
Metaxalone	968.0	E855.1	E938.0	E950.4	E962.0	E980.4
Metformin	962.3	E858.0	E932.3	E950.4	E962.0	E980.4
Methacycline	960.4	E856	E930.4	E950.4	E962.0	E980.4
Methadone	965.02	E850.1	E935.1	E950.0	E962.0	E980.0
Methallenestril	962.2	E858.0	E932.2	E950.4	E962.0	E980.4
Methamphetamine ▲	969.72	E854.2	E939.7	E950.3	E962.0	E980.3
Methandienone	962.1	E858.0	E932.1	E950.4	E962.0	E980.4
Methandriol	962.1	E858.0	E932.1	E950.4	E962.0	E980.4
Methandrostenolone	962.1	E858.0	E932.1	E950.4	E962.0	E980.4
Methane gas	987.1	E869.8	–	E952.8	E962.2	E982.8
Methanol	980.1	E860.2	–	E950.9	E962.1	E980.9
vapor	987.8	E869.8	–	E952.8	E962.2	E982.8
Methantheline	971.1	E855.4	E941.1	E950.4	E962.0	E980.4
Methaphenilene	963.0	E858.1	E933.0	E950.4	E962.0	E980.4
Methapyrilene	963.0	E858.1	E933.0	E950.4	E962.0	E980.4
Methaqualone (compounds)	967.4	E852.3	E937.4	E950.2	E962.0	E980.2

Drug, chemical	Poisoning	External Cause (E Code) Accident	Therapeutic Use	Suicide Attempt	Assault	Undetermined
Metharbital, metharbitone	967.0	E851	E937.0	E950.1	E962.0	E980.1
Methazolamide	974.2	E858.5	E944.2	E950.4	E962.0	E980.4
Methdilazine	963.0	E858.1	E933.0	E950.4	E962.0	E980.4
Methedrine ▲	969.72	E854.2	E939.7	E950.3	E962.0	E980.3
Methenamine (mandelate)	961.9	E857	E931.9	E950.4	E962.0	E980.4
Methenolone	962.1	E858.0	E932.1	E950.4	E962.0	E980.4
Methergine	975.0	E858.6	E945.0	E950.4	E962.0	E980.4
Methiacil	962.8	E858.0	E932.8	E950.4	E962.0	E980.4
Methicillin (sodium)	960.0	E856	E930.0	E950.4	E962.0	E980.4
Methimazole	962.8	E858.0	E932.8	E950.4	E962.0	E980.4
Methionine	977.1	E858.8	E947.1	E950.4	E962.0	E980.4
Methisazone	961.7	E857	E931.7	E950.4	E962.0	E980.4
Methitural	967.0	E851	E937.0	E950.1	E962.0	E980.1
Methixene	971.1	E855.4	E941.1	E950.4	E962.0	E980.4
Methobarbital, methobarbitone	967.0	E851	E937.0	E950.1	E962.0	E980.1
Methocarbamol	968.0	E855.1	E938.0	E950.4	E962.0	E980.4
Methohexital, methohexitone (sodium)	968.3	E855.1	E938.3	E950.4	E962.0	E980.4
Methoin	966.1	E855.0	E936.1	E950.4	E962.0	E980.4
Methopholine	965.7	E850.7	E935.7	E950.0	E962.0	E980.0
Methorate	975.4	E858.6	E945.4	E950.4	E962.0	E980.4
Methoserpidine	972.6	E858.3	E942.6	E950.4	E962.0	E980.4
Methotrexate	963.1	E858.1	E933.1	E950.4	E962.0	E980.4
Methotrimeprazine	967.8	E852.8	E937.8	E950.2	E962.0	E980.2
Methoxa-Dome	976.3	E858.7	E946.3	E950.4	E962.0	E980.4
Methoxamine	971.2	E855.5	E941.2	E950.4	E962.0	E980.4
Methoxsalen	976.3	E858.7	E946.3	E950.4	E962.0	E980.4
Methoxybenzyl penicillin	960.0	E856	E930.0	E950.4	E962.0	E980.4
Methoxychlor	989.2	E863.0	–	E950.6	E962.1	E980.7
Methoxyflurane	968.2	E855.1	E938.2	E950.4	E962.0	E980.4
Methoxyphenamine	971.2	E855.5	E941.2	E950.4	E962.0	E980.4
Methoxypromazine	969.1	E853.0	E939.1	E950.3	E962.0	E980.3
Methoxypsoralen	976.3	E858.7	E946.3	E950.4	E962.0	E980.4
Methscopolamine (bromide)	971.1	E855.4	E941.1	E950.4	E962.0	E980.4
Methsuximide	966.2	E855.0	E936.2	E950.4	E962.0	E980.4
Methyclothiazide	974.3	E858.5	E944.3	E950.4	E962.0	E980.4
Methyl						
acetate	982.8	E862.4	–	E950.9	E962.1	E980.9
acetone II	982.8	E862.4	–	E950.9	E962.1	E980.9
alcohol	980.1	E860.2	–	E950.9	E962.1	E980.9
amphetamine ▲	969.72	E854.2	E939.7	E950.3	E962.0	E980.3
androstanolone	962.1	E858.0	E932.1	E950.4	E962.0	E980.4
atropine	971.1	E855.4	E941.1	E950.4	E962.0	E980.4
benzene	982.0	E862.4	–	E950.9	E962.1	E980.9
bromide (gas)	987.8	E869.8	–	E952.8	E962.2	E982.8
fumigant	987.8	E863.8	–	E950.6	E962.2	E980.7
butanol	980.8	E860.8	–	E950.9	E962.1	E980.9
carbinol	980.1	E860.2	–	E950.9	E962.1	E980.9
cellosolve	982.8	E862.4	–	E950.9	E962.1	E980.9
cellulose	973.3	E858.4	E943.3	E950.4	E962.0	E980.4
chloride (gas)	987.8	E869.8	–	E952.8	E962.2	E982.8
cyclohexane	982.8	E862.4	–	E950.9	E962.1	E980.9
cyclohexanone	982.8	E862.4	–	E950.9	E962.1	E980.9
dihydromorphinone	965.09	E850.2	E935.2	E950.0	E962.0	E980.0
ergometrine	975.0	E858.6	E945.0	E950.4	E962.0	E980.4
ergonovine	975.0	E858.6	E945.0	E950.4	E962.0	E980.4
ethyl ketone	982.8	E862.4	–	E950.9	E962.1	E980.9
hydrazine	983.9	E864.3	–	E950.7	E962.1	E980.6
isobutyl ketone	982.8	E862.4	–	E950.9	E962.1	E980.9
morphine NEC	965.09	E850.2	E935.2	E950.0	E962.0	E980.0
parafynol	967.8	E852.8	E937.8	E950.2	E962.0	E980.2
parathion	989.3	E863.1	–	E950.6	E962.1	E980.7
pentynol NEC	967.8	E852.8	E937.8	E950.2	E962.0	E980.2
peridol	969.2	E853.1	E939.2	E950.3	E962.0	E980.3
phenidate ▲	969.73	E854.2	E939.7	E950.3	E962.0	E980.3
prednisolone	962.0	E858.0	E932.0	E950.4	E962.0	E980.4
ENT agent	976.6	E858.7	E946.6	E950.4	E962.0	E980
ophthalmic preparation	976.5	E858.7	E946.5	E950.4	E962.0	E980.4
topical NEC	976.0	E858.7	E946.0	E950.4	E962.0	E980.4
propylcarbinol	980.8	E860.8	–	E950.9	E962.1	E980.9
rosaniline NEC	976.0	E858.7	E946.0	E950.4	E962.0	E980.4
salicylate NEC	976.3	E858.7	E946.3	E950.4	E962.0	E980.4
sulfate (fumes)	987.8	E869.8	–	E952.8	E962.2	E982.8
liquid	983.9	E864.3	–	E950.7	E962.1	E980.6
sulfonal	967.8	E852.8	E937.8	E950.2	E962.0	E980.2
testosterone	962.1	E858.0	E932.1	E950.4	E962.0	E980.4
thiouracil	962.8	E858.0	E932.8	E950.4	E962.0	E980.4
Methylated spirit	980.0	E860.1	–	E950.9	E962.1	E980.9
Methyldopa	972.6	E858.3	E942.6	E950.4	E962.0	E980.4
Methylene						
blue	961.9	E857	E931.9	E950.4	E962.0	E980.4

Drug, chemical	Poisoning	External Cause (E Code) Accident	Therapeutic Use	Suicide Attempt	Assault	Undetermined
Methylene – *continued*						
chloride or dichloride (solvent) NEC	982.3	E862.4	–	E950.9	E962.1	E980.9
Methylhexabital	967.0	E851	E937.0	E950.1	E962.0	E980.1
Methylparaben (ophthalmic)	976.5	E858.7	E946.5	E950.4	E962.0	E980.4
Methyprylon	967.5	E852.4	E937.5	E950.2	E962.0	E980.2
Methysergide	971.3	E855.6	E941.3	E950.4	E962.0	E980.4
Metoclopramide	963.0	E858.1	E933.0	E950.4	E962.0	E980.4
Metofoline	965.7	E850.7	E935.7	E950.0	E962.0	E980.0
Metopon	965.09	E850.2	E935.2	E950.0	E962.0	E980.0
Metronidazole	961.5	E857	E931.5	E950.4	E962.0	E980.4
Metycaine	968.9	E855.2	E938.9	E950.4	E962.0	E980.4
infiltration (subcutaneous)	968.5	E855.2	E938.5	E950.4	E962.0	E980.4
nerve block (peripheral) (plexus)	968.6	E855.2	E938.6	E950.4	E962.0	E980.4
topical (surface)	968.5	E855.2	E938.5	E950.4	E962.0	E980.4
Metyrapone	977.8	E858.8	E947.8	E950.4	E962.0	E980.4
Mevinphos	989.3	E863.1	–	E950.6	E962.1	E980.7
Mezereon (berries)	988.2	E865.3	–	E950.9	E962.1	E980.9
Micatin	976.0	E858.7	E946.0	E950.4	E962.0	E980.4
Miconazole	976.0	E858.7	E946.0	E950.4	E962.0	E980.4
Mifepristone	962.9	E858.0	E932.9	E950.4	E962.0	E980.4
Midol	965.1	E850.3	E935.3	E950.0	E962.0	E980.0
Milk of magnesia	973.0	E858.4	E943.0	E950.4	E962.0	E980.4
Millipede (tropical) (venomous)	989.5	E905.4	–	E950.9	E962.1	E980.9
Miltown	969.5	E853.8	E939.5	E950.3	E962.0	E980.3
Mineral						
oil (medicinal)	973.2	E858.4	E943.2	E950.4	E962.0	E980.4
nonmedicinal	981	E862.1	–	E950.9	E962.1	E980.9
topical	976.3	E858.7	E946.3	E950.4	E962.0	E980.4
salts NEC	974.6	E858.5	E944.6	E950.4	E962.0	E980.4
spirits	981	E862.0	–	E950.9	E962.1	E980.9
Minocycline	960.4	E856	E930.4	E950.4	E962.0	E980.4
Mithramycin (antineoplastic)	960.7	E856	E930.7	E950.4	E962.0	E980.4
Mitobronitol	963.1	E858.1	E933.1	E950.4	E962.0	E980.4
Mitomycin (antineoplastic)	960.7	E856	E930.7	E950.4	E962.0	E980.4
Mitotane	963.1	E858.1	E933.1	E950.4	E962.0	E980.4
Moderil	972.6	E858.3	E942.6	E950.4	E962.0	E980.4
Mogadon – *see* Nitrazepam						
Molindone	969.3	E853.8	E939.3	E950.3	E962.0	E980.3
Monistat	976.0	E858.7	E946.0	E950.4	E962.0	E980.4
Monkshood	988.2	E865.4	–	E950.9	E962.1	E980.9
Monoamine oxidase inhibitors ▲	969.01	E854.0	E939.0	E950.3	E962.0	E980.3
Monochlorobenzene	982.0	E862.4	–	E950.9	E962.1	E980.9
Monosodium glutamate	989.89	E866.8	–	E950.9	E962.1	E980.9
Monoxide, carbon – *see* Carbon, monoxide						
Moperone	969.2	E853.1	E939.2	E950.3	E962.0	E980.3
Morning glory seeds	969.6	E854.1	E939.6	E950.3	E962.0	E980.3
Moroxydine (hydrochloride)	961.7	E857	E931.7	E950.4	E962.0	E980.4
Morphazinamide	961.8	E857	E931.8	E950.4	E962.0	E980.4
Morphinans	965.09	E850.2	E935.2	E950.0	E962.0	E980.0
Morphine NEC	965.09	E850.2	E935.2	E950.0	E962.0	E980.0
antagonists	970.1	E854.3	E940.1	E950.4	E962.0	E980.4
Morpholinylethylmorphine	965.09	E850.2	E935.2	E950.0	E962.0	E980.0
Morrhuate sodium	972.7	E858.3	E942.7	E950.4	E962.0	E980.4
Moth balls (*see also* Pesticides)	989.4	E863.4	–	E950.6	E962.1	E980.7
naphthalene	983.0	E863.4	–	E950.7	E962.1	E980.6
Motor exhaust gas – *see* Carbon, monoxide, exhaust gas						
Mouth wash	976.6	E858.7	E946.6	E950.4	E962.0	E980.4
Mucolytic agent	975.5	E858.6	E945.5	E950.4	E962.0	E980.4
Mucomyst	975.5	E858.6	E945.5	E950.4	E962.0	E980.4
Mucous membrane agents (external)	976.9	E858.7	E946.9	E950.4	E962.0	E980.4
specified NEC	976.8	E858.7	E946.8	E950.4	E962.0	E980.4
Mumps						
immune globulin (human)	964.6	E858.2	E934.6	E950.4	E962.0	E980.4
skin test antigen	977.8	E858.8	E947.8	E950.4	E962.0	E980.4
vaccine	979.6	E858.8	E949.6	E950.4	E962.0	E980.4
Mumpsvax	979.6	E858.8	E949.6	E950.4	E962.0	E980.4
Muriatic acid – *see* Hydrochloric acid						
Muscarine	971.0	E855.3	E941.0	E950.4	E962.0	E980.4
Muscle affecting agents NEC	975.3	E858.6	E945.3	E950.4	E962.0	E980.4
oxytocic	975.0	E858.6	E945.0	E950.4	E962.0	E980.4
relaxants	975.3	E858.6	E945.3	E950.4	E962.0	E980.4
central nervous system	968.0	E855.1	E938.0	E950.4	E962.0	E980.4
skeletal	975.2	E858.6	E945.2	E950.4	E962.0	E980.4
smooth	975.1	E858.6	E945.1	E950.4	E962.0	E980.4
Mushrooms, noxious	988.1	E865.5	–	E950.9	E962.1	E980.9
Mussel, noxious	988.0	E865.1	–	E950.9	E962.1	E980.9
Mustard (emetic)	973.6	E858.4	E943.6	E950.4	E962.0	E980.4
gas	987.8	E869.8	–	E952.8	E962.2	E982.8
nitrogen	963.1	E858.1	E933.1	E950.4	E962.0	E980.4
Mustine	963.1	E858.1	E933.1	E950.4	E962.0	E980.4
M-vac	979.4	E858.8	E949.4	E950.4	E962.0	E980.4
Mycifradin	960.8	E856	E930.8	E950.4	E962.0	E980.4
topical	976.0	E858.7	E946.0	E950.4	E962.0	E980.4
Mycitracin	960.8	E856	E930.8	E950.4	E962.0	E980.4
ophthalmic preparation	976.5	E858.7	E946.5	E950.4	E962.0	E980.4
Mycostatin	960.1	E856	E930.1	E950.4	E962.0	E980.4
topical	976.0	E858.7	E946.0	E950.4	E962.0	E980.4
Mydriacyl	971.1	E855.4	E941.1	E950.4	E962.0	E980.4
Myelobromal	963.1	E858.1	E933.1	E950.4	E962.0	E980.4
Myleran	963.1	E858.1	E933.1	E950.4	E962.0	E980.4
Myochrysin(e)	965.69	E850.6	E935.6	E950.0	E962.0	E980.0
Myoneural blocking agents	975.2	E858.6	E945.2	E950.4	E962.0	E980.4
Myristica fragrans	988.2	E865.3	–	E950.9	E962.1	E980.9
Myristicin	988.2	E865.3	–	E950.9	E962.1	E980.9
Mysoline	966.3	E855.0	E936.3	E950.4	E962.0	E980.4
Nafcillin (sodium)	960.0	E856	E930.0	E950.4	E962.0	E980.4
Nail polish remover	982.8	E862.4	–	E950.9	E962.1	E908.9
Nalidixic acid	961.9	E857	E931.9	E950.4	E962.0	E980.4
Nalorphine	970.1	E854.3	E940.1	E950.4	E962.0	E980.4
Naloxone	970.1	E854.3	E940.1	E950.4	E962.0	E980.4
Namenda	969.8	E854.8	E939.8	E950.3	E962.0	E980.3
Nandrolone (decanoate) (phenproprioate)	962.1	E858.0	E932.1	E950.4	E962.0	E980.4
Naphazoline	971.2	E855.5	E941.2	E950.4	E962.0	E980.4
Naphtha (painter's) (petroleum)	981	E862.0	–	E950.9	E962.1	E980.9
solvent	981	E862.0	–	E950.9	E962.1	E980.9
vapor	987.1	E869.8	–	E952.8	E962.2	E982.8
Naphthalene (chlorinated)	983.0	E864.0	–	E950.7	E962.1	E980.6
insecticide or moth repellent	983.0	E863.4	–	E950.7	E962.1	E980.6
vapor	987.8	E869.8	–	E952.8	E962.2	E982.8
Naphthol	983.0	E864.0	–	E950.7	E962.1	E980.6
Naphthylamine	983.0	E864.0	–	E950.7	E962.1	E980.6
Naprosyn – *see* Naproxen						
Naproxen	965.61	E850.6	E935.6	E950.0	E962.0	E980.0
Narcotic (drug)	967.9	E852.9	E937.9	E950.2	E962.0	E980.2
analgesic NEC	965.8	E850.8	E935.8	E950.0	E962.0	E980.0
antagonist	970.1	E854.3	E940.1	E950.4	E962.0	E980.4
specified NEC	967.8	E852.8	E937.8	E950.2	E962.0	E980.2
Narcotine	975.4	E858.6	E945.4	E950.4	E962.0	E980.4
Nardil ▲	969.01	E854.0	E939.0	E950.3	E962.0	E980.3
Natrium cyanide – *see* Cyanide(s)						
Natural						
blood (product)	964.7	E858.2	E934.7	E950.4	E962.0	E980.4
gas (piped)	987.1	E867	–	E951.0	E962.2	E981.0
incomplete combustion	986	E867	–	E951.0	E962.2	E981.0
Nealbarbital, nealbarbitone	967.0	E851	E937.0	E950.1	E962.0	E980.1
Nectadon	975.4	E858.6	E945.4	E950.4	E962.0	E980.4
Nematocyst (sting)	989.5	E905.6	–	E950.9	E962.1	E980.9
Nembutal	967.0	E851	E937.0	E950.1	E962.0	E980.1
Neoarsphenamine	961.1	E857	E931.1	E950.4	E962.0	E980.4
Neocinchophen	974.7	E858.5	E944.7	E950.4	E962.0	E980.4
Neomycin	960.8	E856	E930.8	E950.4	E962.0	E980.4
ENT agent	976.6	E858.7	E946.6	E950.4	E962.0	E980.4
ophthalmic preparation	976.5	E858.7	E946.5	E950.4	E962.0	E980.4
topical NEC	976.0	E858.7	E946.0	E950.4	E962.0	E980.4
Neonal	967.0	E851	E937.0	E950.1	E962.0	E980.1
Neoprontosil	961.0	E857	E931.0	E950.4	E962.0	E980.4
Neosalvarsan	961.1	E857	E931.1	E950.4	E962.0	E980.4
Neosilversalvarsan	961.1	E857	E931.1	E950.4	E962.0	E980.4
Neosporin	960.8	E856	E930.8	E950.4	E962.0	E980.4
ENT agent	976.6	E858.7	E946.6	E950.4	E962.0	E980.4
opthalmic preparation	976.5	E858.7	E946.5	E950.4	E962.0	E980.4
topical NEC	976.0	E858.7	E946.0	E950.4	E962.0	E980.4
Neostigmine	971.0	E855.3	E941.0	E950.4	E962.0	E980.4
Neraval	967.0	E851	E937.0	E950.1	E962.0	E980.1
Neravan	967.0	E851	E937.0	E950.1	E962.0	E980.1
Nerium oleander	988.2	E865.4	–	E950.9	E962.1	E980.9
Nerve gases (war)	987.9	E869.9	–	E952.9	E962.2	E982.9
Nesacaine	968.9	E855.2	E938.9	E950.4	E962.0	E980.4
infiltration(subcutaneous)	968.5	E855.2	E938.5	E950.4	E962.0	E980.4
nerve block (peripheral) (plexus)	968.6	E855.2	E938.6	E950.4	E962.0	E980.4
Neurobarb	967.0	E851	E937.0	E950.1	E962.0	E980.1
Neuroleptics NEC	969.3	E853.8	E939.3	E950.3	E962.0	E980.3
Neuroprotective agent	977.8	E858.8	E947.8	E950.4	E962.0	E980.4
Neutral spirits	980.0	E860.1	–	E950.9	E962.1	E980.9
beverage	980.0	E860.0	–	E950.9	E962.1	E980.9
Niacin, niacinamide	972.2	E858.3	E942.2	E950.4	E962.0	E980.4
Nialamide ▲	969.01	E854.0	E939.0	E950.3	E962.0	E980.3

Drug, chemical	Poisoning	External Cause (E Code)				
		Accident	Therapeutic Use	Suicide Attempt	Assault	Undetermined
Nickle (carbonyl) (compounds) (fumes) (tetracarbonyl) (vapor)	985.8	E866.4	–	E950.9	E962.1	E980.9
Niclosamide	961.6	E857	E931.6	E950.4	E962.0	E980.4
Nicomorphine	965.09	E850.2	E935.2	E950.0	E962.0	E980.0
Nicotinamide	972.2	E858.3	E942.2	E950.4	E962.0	E980.4
Nicotine (insecticide) (spray) (sulfate) NEC	989.4	E863.4	–	E950.6	E962.1	E980.7
not insecticide	989.89	E866.8	–	E950.9	E962.1	E980.9
Nicotinic acid (derivatives)	972.2	E858.3	E942.2	E950.4	E962.0	E980.4
Nicotinyl alcohol	972.2	E858.3	E942.2	E950.4	E962.0	E980.4
Nicoumalone	964.2	E858.2	E934.2	E950.4	E962.0	E980.4
Nifenazone	965.5	E850.5	E935.5	E950.0	E962.0	E980.0
Nifuraldezone	961.9	E857	E931.9	E950.4	E962.0	E980.4
Nightshade (deadly)	988.2	E865.4	–	E950.9	E962.1	E980.9
Nikethamide	970.0	E854.3	E940.0	E950.4	E962.0	E980.4
Nilstat	960.1	E856	E930.1	E950.4	E962.0	E980.4
topical	976.0	E858.7	E946.0	E950.4	E962.0	E980.4
Nimodipine	977.8	E858.8	E947.8	E950.4	E962.0	E980.4
Niridazole	961.6	E857	E931.6	E950.4	E962.0	E980.4
Nisentil	965.09	E850.2	E935.2	E950.0	E962.0	E980.0
Nitrates	972.4	E858.3	E942.4	E950.4	E962.0	E980.4
Nitrazepam	969.4	E853.2	E939.4	E950.3	E962.0	E980.3
Nitric						
acid (liquid)	983.1	E864.1	–	E950.7	E962.1	E980.6
vapor	987.8	E869.8	–	E952.8	E962.2	E982.8
oxide (gas)	987.2	E869.0	–	E952.8	E962.2	E982.8
Nitrite, amyl (medicinal) (vapor)	972.4	E858.3	E942.4	E950.4	E962.0	E980.4
Nitroaniline	983.0	E864.0	–	E950.7	E962.1	E980.6
vapor	987.8	E869.8	–	E952.8	E962.2	E982.8
Nitrobenzene, nitrobenzol	983.0	E864.0	–	E950.7	E962.1	E980.6
vapor	987.8	E869.8	–	E952.8	E962.2	E982.8
Nitrocellulose	976.3	E858.7	E946.3	E950.4	E962.0	E980.4
Nitrofuran derivatives	961.9	E857	E931.9	E950.4	E962.0	E980.4
Nitrofurantoin	961.9	E857	E931.9	E950.4	E962.0	E980.4
Nitrofurazone	976.0	E858.7	E946.0	E950.4	E962.0	E980.4
Nitrogen (dioxide) (gas) (oxide)	987.2	E869.0	–	E952.8	E962.2	E982.8
mustard (antineoplastic)	963.1	E858.1	E933.1	E950.4	E962.0	E980.4
Nitroglycerin, nitroglycerol (medicinal)	972.4	E858.3	E942.4	E950.4	E962.0	E980.4
nonmedicinal	989.89	E866.8	–	E950.9	E962.1	E980.9
fumes	987.8	E869.8	–	E952.8	E962.2	E982.8
Nitrohydrochloric acid	983.1	E864.1	–	E950.7	E962.1	E980.6
Nitromersol	976.0	E858.7	E946.0	E950.4	E962.0	E980.4
Nitronaphthalene	983.0	E864.0	–	E950.7	E962.2	E980.6
Nitrophenol	983.0	E864.0	–	E950.7	E962.2	E980.6
Nitrothiazol	961.6	E857	E931.6	E950.4	E962.0	E980.4
Nitrotoluene, nitrotoluol	983.0	E864.0	–	E950.7	E962.1	E980.6
vapor	987.8	E869.8	–	E952.8	E962.2	E982.8
Nitrous	968.2	E855.1	E938.2	E950.4	E962.0	E980.4
acid (liquid)	983.1	E864.1	–	E950.7	E962.1	E980.6
fumes	987.2	E869.0	–	E952.8	E962.2	E982.8
oxide (anesthetic) NEC	968.2	E855.1	E938.2	E950.4	E962.0	E980.4
Nitrozone	976.0	E858.7	E946.0	E950.4	E962.0	E980.4
Noctec	967.1	E852.0	E937.1	E950.2	E962.0	E980.2
Noludar	967.5	E852.4	E937.5	E950.2	E962.0	E980.2
Noptil	967.0	E851	E937.0	E950.1	E962.0	E980.1
Noradrenalin	971.2	E855.5	E941.2	E950.4	E962.0	E980.4
Noramidopyrine	965.5	E850.5	E935.5	E950.0	E962.0	E980.0
Norepinephrine	971.2	E855.5	E941.2	E950.4	E962.0	E980.4
Norethandrolone	962.1	E858.0	E932.1	E950.4	E962.0	E980.4
Norethindrone	962.2	E858.0	E932.2	E950.4	E962.0	E980.4
Norethisterone	962.2	E858.0	E932.2	E950.4	E962.0	E980.4
Norethynodrel	962.2	E858.0	E932.2	E950.4	E962.0	E980.4
Norlestrin	962.2	E858.0	E932.2	E950.4	E962.0	E980.4
Norlutin	962.2	E858.0	E932.2	E950.4	E962.0	E980.4
Normison – *see* Benzodiazepines						
Normorphine	965.09	E850.2	E935.2	E950.0	E962.0	E980.0
Nortriptyline ▲	969.0<u>5</u>	E854.0	E939.0	E950.3	E962.0	E980.3
Noscapine	975.4	E858.6	E945.4	E950.4	E962.0	E980.4
Nose preparations	976.6	E858.7	E946.6	E950.4	E962.0	E980.4
Novobiocin	960.8	E856	E930.8	E950.4	E962.0	E980.4
Novocain (infiltration) (topical)	968.5	E855.2	E938.5	E950.4	E962.0	E980.4
nerve block (peripheral) (plexus)	968.6	E855.2	E938.6	E950.4	E962.0	E980.4
spinal	968.7	E855.2	E938.7	E950.4	E962.0	E980.4
Noxythiolin	961.9	E857	E931.9	E950.4	E962.0	E980.4
NPH Iletin (insulin)	962.3	E858.0	E932.3	E950.4	E962.0	E980.4
Numorphan	965.09	E850.2	E935.2	E950.0	E962.0	E980.0
Nunol	967.0	E851	E937.0	E950.1	E962.0	E980.1
Nupercaine (spinal anesthetic)	968.7	E855.2	E938.7	E950.4	E962.0	E980.4
topical (surface)	968.5	E855.2	E938.5	E950.4	E962.0	E980.4
Nutmeg oil (liniment)	976.3	E858.7	E946.3	E950.4	E962.0	E980.4
Nux vomica	989.1	E863.7	–	E950.6	E962.1	E980.7
Nydrazid	961.8	E857	E931.8	E950.4	E962.0	E980.4
Nylidrin	971.2	E855.5	E941.2	E950.4	E962.0	E980.4
Nystatin	960.1	E856	E930.1	E950.4	E962.0	E980.4
topical	976.0	E858.7	E946.0	E950.4	E962.0	E980.4
Nytol	963.0	E858.1	E933.0	E950.4	E962.0	E980.4
Oblivion	967.8	E852.8	E937.8	E950.2	E962.0	E980.2
Octyl nitrite	972.4	E858.3	E942.4	E950.4	E962.0	E980.4
Oestradiol (cypionate) (dipropionate) (valerate)	962.2	E858.0	E932.2	E950.4	E962.0	E980.4
Oestriol	962.2	E858.0	E932.2	E950.4	E962.0	E980.4
Oestrone	962.2	E858.0	E932.2	E950.4	E962.0	E980.4
Oil (of) NEC	989.89	E866.8	–	E950.9	E962.1	E980.9
bitter almond	989.0	E866.8	–	E950.9	E962.1	E980.9
camphor	976.1	E858.7	E946.1	E950.4	E962.0	E980.4
colors	989.89	E861.6	–	E950.9	E962.1	E980.9
fumes	987.8	E869.8	–	E952.8	E962.2	E982.8
lubricating	981	E862.2	–	E950.9	E962.1	E980.9
specified source, other – *see* substance specified						
vitriol (liquid)	983.1	E864.1	–	E950.7	E962.1	E980.6
fumes	987.8	E869.8	–	E952.8	E962.2	E982.8
wintergreen (bitter) NEC	976.3	E858.7	E946.3	E950.4	E962.0	E980.4
Ointments NEC	976.9	E858.7	E946.9	E950.4	E962.0	E980.4
Oleander	988.2	E865.4	–	E950.9	E962.1	E980.9
Oleandomycin	960.3	E856	E930.3	E950.4	E962.0	E980.4
Oleovitamin A	963.5	E858.1	E933.5	E950.4	E962.0	E980.4
Oleum ricini	973.1	E858.4	E943.1	E950.4	E962.0	E980.4
Olive oil (medicinal) **NEC**	973.2	E858.4	E943.2	E950.4	E962.0	E980.4
OMPA	989.3	E863.1	–	E950.6	E962.1	E980.7
Oncovin	963.1	E858.1	E933.1	E950.4	E962.0	E980.4
Ophthaine	968.5	E855.2	E938.5	E950.4	E962.0	E980.4
Ophthetic	968.5	E855.2	E938.5	E950.4	E962.0	E980.4
Opiates, opioids, opium NEC	965.00	E850.2	E935.2	E950.0	E962.0	E980.0
antagonists	970.1	E854.3	E940.1	E950.4	E962.0	E980.4
Oracon	962.2	E858.0	E932.2	E950.4	E962.0	E980.4
Oragrafin	977.8	E858.8	E947.8	E950.4	E962.0	E980.4
Oral contraceptives	962.2	E858.0	E932.2	E950.4	E962.0	E980.4
Orciprenaline	975.1	E858.6	E945.1	E950.4	E962.0	E980.4
Organidin	975.5	E858.6	E945.5	E950.4	E962.0	E980.4
Organophosphates	989.3	E863.1	–	E950.6	E962.1	E980.7
Orimune	979.5	E858.8	E949.5	E950.4	E962.0	E980.4
Orinase	962.3	E858.0	E932.3	E950.4	E962.0	E980.4
Orphenadrine	966.4	E855.0	E936.4	E950.4	E962.0	E980.4
Ortal (sodium)	967.0	E851	E937.0	E950.1	E962.0	E980.1
Orthoboric acid	976.0	E858.7	E946.0	E950.4	E962.0	E980.4
ENT agent	976.6	E858.7	E946.6	E950.4	E962.0	E980.4
ophthalmic preparation	976.5	E858.7	E946.5	E950.4	E962.0	E980.4
Orthocaine	968.5	E855.2	E938.5	E950.4	E962.0	E980.4
Ortho-Novum	962.2	E858.0	E932.2	E950.4	E962.0	E980.4
Orthotolidine (reagent)	977.8	E858.8	E947.8	E950.4	E962.0	E980.4
Osmic acid (liquid)	983.1	E864.1	–	E950.7	E962.1	E980.6
fumes	987.8	E869.8	–	E952.8	E962.2	E982.8
Osmotic diuretics	974.4	E858.5	E944.4	E950.4	E962.0	E980.4
Ouabain	972.1	E858.3	E942.1	E950.4	E962.0	E980.4
Ovarian hormones (synthetic substitutes)	962.2	E858.0	E932.2	E950.4	E962.0	E980.4
Ovral	962.2	E858.0	E932.2	E950.4	E962.0	E980.4
Ovulation suppressants	962.2	E858.0	E932.2	E950.4	E962.0	E980.4
Ovulen	962.2	E858.0	E932.2	E950.4	E962.0	E980.4
Oxacillin (sodium)	960.0	E856	E930.0	E950.4	E962.0	E980.4
Oxalic acid	983.1	E864.1	–	E950.7	E962.1	E980.6
Oxanamide	969.5	E853.8	E939.5	E950.3	E962.0	E980.3
Oxandrolone	962.1	E858.0	E932.1	E950.4	E962.0	E980.4
Oxaprozin	965.61	E850.6	E935.6	E950.0	E962.0	E980.0
Oxazepam	969.4	E853.2	E939.4	E950.3	E962.0	E980.3
Oxazolidine derivatives	966.0	E855.0	E936.0	E950.4	E962.0	E980.4
Ox bile extract	973.4	E858.4	E943.4	E950.4	E962.0	E980.4
Oxedrine	971.2	E855.5	E941.2	E950.4	E962.0	E980.4
Oxeladin	975.4	E858.6	E945.4	E950.4	E962.0	E980.4
Oxethazaine NEC	968.5	E855.2	E938.5	E950.4	E962.0	E980.4
Oxidizing agents NEC	983.9	E864.3	–	E950.7	E962.1	E980.6
Oxolinic acid	961.3	E857	E931.3	E950.4	E962.0	E980.4
Oxophenarsine	961.1	E857	E931.1	E950.4	E962.0	E980.4
Oxsoralen	976.3	E858.7	E946.3	E950.4	E962.0	E980.4
Oxtriphylline	976.7	E858.6	E945.7	E950.4	E962.0	E980.4
Oxybuprocaine	968.5	E855.2	E938.5	E950.4	E962.0	E980.4
Oxybutynin	975.1	E858.6	E945.1	E950.4	E962.0	E980.4
Oxycodone	965.09	E850.2	E935.2	E950.0	E962.0	E980.0
Oxygen	987.8	E869.8	–	E952.8	E962.2	E982.8
Oxylone	976.0	E858.7	E946.0	E950.4	E962.0	E980.4
ophthalmic preparation	976.5	E858.7	E946.5	E950.4	E962.0	E980.4
Oxymesterone	962.1	E858.0	E932.1	E950.4	E962.0	E980.4

Drug, chemical	Poisoning	External Cause (E Code) Accident	Therapeutic Use	Suicide Attempt	Assault	Undetermined
Oxymetazoline	971.2	E855.5	E941.2	E950.4	E962.0	E980.4
Oxymetholone	962.1	E858.0	E932.1	E950.4	E962.0	E980.4
Oxymorphone	965.09	E850.2	E935.2	E950.0	E962.0	E980.0
Oxypertine ▲	969.09	E854.0	E939.0	E950.3	E962.0	E980.3
Oxyphenbutazone	965.5	E850.5	E935.5	E950.0	E962.0	E980.0
Oxyphencyclimine	971.1	E855.4	E941.1	E950.4	E962.0	E980.4
Oxyphenisatin	973.1	E858.4	E943.1	E950.4	E962.0	E980.4
Oxyphenonium	971.1	E855.4	E941.1	E950.4	E962.0	E980.4
Oxyquinoline	961.3	E857	E931.3	E950.4	E962.0	E980.4
Oxytetracycline	960.4	E856	E930.4	E950.4	E962.0	E980.4
Oxytocics	975.0	E858.6	E945.0	E950.4	E962.0	E980.4
Oxytocin	975.0	E858.6	E945.0	E950.4	E962.0	E980.4
Ozone	987.8	E869.8	–	E952.8	E962.2	E982.8
PABA	976.3	E858.7	E946.3	E950.4	E962.0	E980.4
Packed red cells	964.7	E858.2	E934.7	E950.4	E962.0	E980.4
Paint NEC	989.89	E861.6	–	E950.9	E962.1	E980.9
cleaner	982.8	E862.9	–	E950.9	E962.1	E980.9
fumes NEC	987.8	E869.8	–	E952.8	E962.1	E982.8
lead (fumes)	984.0	E861.5	–	E950.9	E962.1	E980.9
solvent NEC	982.8	E862.9	–	E950.9	E962.1	E980.9
stripper	982.8	E862.9	–	E950.9	E962.1	E980.9
Palfium	965.09	E850.2	E935.2	E950.0	E962.0	E980.0
Palivizumab	979.9	E858.8	E949.6	E950.4	E962.0	E980.4
Paludrine	961.4	E857	E931.4	E950.4	E962.0	E980.4
PAM	977.2	E855.8	E947.2	E950.4	E962.0	E980.4
Pamaquine (naphthoute)	961.4	E857	E931.4	E950.4	E962.0	E980.4
Pamprin	965.1	E850.3	E935.3	E950.0	E962.0	E980.0
Panadol	965.4	E850.4	E935.4	E950.0	E962.0	E980.0
Pancreatic dornase (mucolytic)	963.4	E858.1	E933.4	E950.4	E962.0	E980.4
Pancreatin	973.4	E858.4	E943.4	E950.4	E962.0	E980.4
Pancrelipase	973.4	E858.4	E943.4	E950.4	E962.0	E980.4
Pangamic acid	963.5	E858.1	E933.5	E950.4	E962.0	E980.4
Panthenol	963.5	E858.1	E933.5	E950.4	E962.0	E980.4
topical	976.8	E858.7	E946.8	E950.4	E962.0	E980.4
Pantopaque	977.8	E858.8	E947.8	E950.4	E962.0	E980.4
Pantopon	965.00	E850.2	E935.2	E950.0	E962.0	E980.0
Pantothenic acid	963.5	E858.1	E933.5	E950.4	E962.0	E980.4
Panwarfin	964.2	E858.2	E934.2	E950.4	E962.0	E980.4
Papain	973.4	E858.4	E943.4	E950.4	E962.0	E980.4
Papaverine	972.5	E858.3	E942.5	E950.4	E962.0	E980.4
Para-aminobenzoic acid	976.3	E858.7	E946.3	E950.4	E962.0	E980.4
Para-aminophenol derivatives	965.4	E850.4	E935.4	E950.0	E962.0	E980.0
Para-aminosalicylic acid (derivatives)	961.8	E857	E931.8	E950.4	E962.0	E980.4
Paracetaldehyde (medicinal)	967.2	E852.1	E937.2	E950.2	E962.0	E980.2
Paracetamol	965.4	E850.4	E935.4	E950.0	E962.0	E980.0
Paracodin	965.09	E850.2	E935.2	E950.0	E962.0	E980.0
Paradione	966.0	E855.0	E936.0	E950.4	E962.0	E980.4
Paraffin(s) (wax)	981	E862.3	–	E950.9	E962.1	E980.9
liquid (medicinal)	973.2	E858.4	E943.2	E950.4	E962.0	E980.4
nonmedicinal (oil)	981	E962.1	–	E950.9	E962.1	E980.9
Paraldehyde (medicinal)	967.2	E852.1	E937.2	E950.2	E962.0	E980.2
Paramethadione	966.0	E855.0	E936.0	E950.4	E962.0	E980.4
Paramethasone	962.0	E858.0	E932.0	E950.4	E962.0	E980.4
Paraquat	989.4	E863.5	–	E950.6	E962.1	E980.7
Parasympatholytics	971.1	E855.4	E941.1	E950.4	E962.0	E980.4
Parasympathomimetics	971.0	E855.3	E941.0	E950.4	E962.0	E980.4
Parathion	989.3	E863.1	–	E950.6	E962.1	E980.7
Parathormone	962.6	E858.0	E932.6	E950.4	E962.0	E980.4
Parathyroid (derivatives)	962.6	E858.0	E932.6	E950.4	E962.0	E980.4
Paratyphoid vaccine	978.1	E858.8	E948.1	E950.4	E962.0	E980.4
Paredrine	971.2	E855.5	E941.2	E950.4	E962.0	E980.4
Paregoric	965.00	E850.2	E935.2	E950.0	E962.0	E980.0
Pargyline	972.3	E858.3	E942.3	E950.4	E962.0	E980.4
Paris green	985.1	E866.3	–	E950.8	E962.1	E980.8
insecticide	985.1	E863.4	–	E950.8	E962.1	E980.8
Parnate ▲	969.01	E854.0	E939.0	E950.3	E962.0	E980.3
Paromomycin	960.8	E856	E930.8	E950.4	E962.0	E980.4
Paroxypropione	963.1	E858.1	E933.1	E950.4	E962.0	E980.4
Parzone	965.09	E850.2	E935.2	E950.0	E962.0	E980.0
PAS	961.8	E857	E931.8	E950.4	E962.0	E980.4
PCBs	981	E862.3	–	E950.9	E962.1	E980.9
PCP (pentachlorophenol)	989.4	E863.6	–	E950.6	E962.1	E980.7
herbicide	989.4	E863.5	–	E950.6	E962.1	E980.7
insecticide	989.4	E863.4	–	E950.6	E962.1	E980.7
phencyclidine	968.3	E855.1	E938.3	E950.4	E962.0	E980.4
Peach kernel oil (emulsion)	973.2	E858.4	E943.2	E950.4	E962.0	E980.4
Peanut oil (emulsion) NEC	973.2	E858.4	E943.2	E950.4	E962.0	E980.4
topical	976.3	E858.7	E946.3	E950.4	E962.0	E980.4
Pearly Gates (morning glory seeds)	969.6	E854.1	E939.6	E950.3	E962.0	E980.3
Pecazine	969.1	E853.0	E939.1	E950.3	E962.0	E980.3
Pecilocin	960.1	E856	E930.1	E950.4	E962.0	E980.4

Drug, chemical	Poisoning	External Cause (E Code) Accident	Therapeutic Use	Suicide Attempt	Assault	Undetermined
Pectin (with kaolin) NEC	973.5	E858.4	E943.5	E950.4	E962.0	E980.4
Pelletierine tannate	961.6	E857	E931.6	E950.4	E962.0	E980.4
Pemoline ▲	969.79	E854.2	E939.7	E950.3	E962.0	E980.3
Pempidine	972.3	E858.3	E942.3	E950.4	E962.0	E980.4
Penamecillin	960.0	E856	E930.0	E950.4	E962.0	E980.4
Penethamate hydriodide	960.0	E856	E930.0	E950.4	E962.0	E980.4
Penicillamine	963.8	E858.1	E933.8	E950.4	E962.0	E980.4
Penicillin (any type)	960.0	E856	E930.0	E950.4	E962.0	E980.4
Penicillinase	963.4	E858.1	E933.4	E950.4	E962.0	E980.4
Pentachlorophenol (fungicide)	989.4	E863.6	–	E950.6	E962.1	E980.7
herbicide	989.4	E863.5	–	E950.6	E962.1	E980.7
insecticide	989.4	E863.4	–	E950.6	E962.1	E980.7
Pentaerythritol	972.4	E858.3	E942.4	E950.4	E962.0	E980.4
chloral	967.1	E852.0	E937.1	E950.2	E962.0	E980.2
tetranitrate NEC	972.4	E858.3	E942.4	E950.4	E962.0	E980.4
Pentagastrin	977.8	E858.8	E947.8	E950.4	E962.0	E980.4
Pentalin	982.3	E862.4	–	E950.9	E962.1	E980.9
Pentamethonium (bromide)	972.3	E858.3	E942.3	E950.4	E962.0	E980.4
Pentamidine	961.5	E857	E931.5	E950.4	E962.0	E980.4
Pentanol	980.8	E860.8	–	E950.9	E962.1	E980.9
Pentaquine	961.4	E857	E931.4	E950.4	E962.0	E980.4
Peniazocine	965.8	E850.8	E935.8	E950.0	E962.0	E980.0
Penthienate	971.1	E855.4	E941.1	E950.4	E962.0	E980.4
Pentobarbital, pentobarbitone (sodium)	967.0	E851	E937.0	E950.1	E962.0	E980.1
Pentolinium (tartrate)	972.3	E858.3	E942.3	E950.4	E962.0	E980.4
Pentothal	968.3	E855.1	E938.3	E950.4	E962.0	E980.4
Pentyleneteirazol	970.0	E854.3	E940.0	E950.4	E962.0	E980.4
Pentylsalicylamide	961.8	E857	E931.8	E950.4	E962.0	E980.4
Pepsin	973.4	E858.4	E943.4	E950.4	E962.0	E980.4
Peptavlon	977.8	E858.8	E947.8	E950.4	E962.0	E980.4
Percaine (spinal)	968.7	E855.2	E938.7	E950.4	E962.0	E980.4
topical (surface)	968.5	E855.2	E938.5	E950.4	E962.0	E980.4
Perchloroethylene (vapor)	982.3	E862.4	–	E950.9	E962.1	E980.9
medicinal	961.6	E857	E931.6	E950.4	E962.0	E980.4
Percodan	965.09	E850.2	E935.2	E950.0	E962.0	E980.0
Percogesic	965.09	E850.2	E935.2	E950.0	E962.0	E980.0
Percorten	962.0	E858.0	E932.0	E950.4	E962.0	E980.4
Pergonal	962.4	E858.0	E932.4	E950.4	E962.0	E980.4
Perhexiline	972.4	E858.3	E942.4	E950.4	E962.0	E980.4
Periactin	963.0	E858.1	E933.0	E950.4	E962.0	E980.4
Periclor	967.1	E852.0	E937.1	E950.2	E962.0	E980.2
Pericyazine	969.1	E853.0	E939.1	E950.3	E962.0	E980.3
Peritrate	972.4	E858.3	E942.4	E950.4	E962.0	E980.4
Permanganates NEC	983.9	E864.3	–	E950.7	E962.1	E980.6
potassium (topical)	976.0	E858.7	E946.0	E950.4	E962.0	E980.4
Pernocton	967.0	E851	E937.0	E950.1	E962.0	E980.1
Pernoston	967.0	E851	E937.0	E950.1	E962.0	E980.1
Peronin(e)	965.09	E850.2	E935.2	E950.0	E962.0	E980.0
Perphenazine	969.1	E853.0	E939.1	E950.3	E962.0	E980.3
Pertofrane ▲	969.05	E854	E939.0	E950.3	E962.0	E980.3
Pertussis						
immune serum (human)	964.6	E858.2	E934.6	E950.4	E962.0	E980.4
vaccine (with diphtheria toxoid) (with tetanus toxoid)	978.6	E858.8	E948.6	E950.4	E962.0	E980.4
Peruvian balsam	976.8	E858.7	E946.8	E950.4	E962.0	E980.4
Pesticides (dust) (fumes) (vapor)	989.4	E863.4	–	E950.6	E962.1	E980.7
arsenic	985.1	E863.4	–	E950.8	E962.1	E980.8
chlorinated	989.2	E863.0	–	E950.6	E962.1	E980.7
cyanide	989.0	E863.4	–	E950.6	E962.1	E980.7
kerosene	981	E863.4	–	E950.6	E962.1	E980.7
mixture (of compounds)	989.4	E863.3	–	E950.6	E962.1	E980.7
naphthalene	983.0	E863.4	–	E950.7	E962.1	E980.6
organochlorine (compounds)	989.2	E863.0	–	E950.6	E962.1	E980.7
petroleum (distillate) (products) NEC	981	E863.4	–	E950.6	E962.1	E980.7
specified ingredient NEC	989.4	E863.4	–	E950.6	E962.1	E980.7
strychnine	989.1	E863.4	–	E950.6	E962.1	E980.7
thallium	985.8	E863.7	–	E950.6	E962.1	E980.7
Pethidine (hydrochloride)	965.09	E850.2	E935.2	E950.0	E962.0	E980.0
Petrichloral	967.1	E852.0	E937.1	E950.2	E962.0	E980.2
Petrol	981	E862.1	–	E950.9	E962.1	E980.9
vapor	987.1	E869.8	–	E952.8	E962.2	E982.8
Petrolatum (jelly) (ointment)	976.3	E858.7	E946.3	E950.4	E962.0	E980.4
hydrophilic	976.3	E858.7	E946.3	E950.4	E962.0	E980.4
liquid	973.2	E858.4	E943.2	E950.4	E962.0	E980.4
topical	976.3	E858.7	E946.3	E950.4	E962.0	E980.4
nonmedicinal	981	E862.1	–	E950.9	E962.1	E980.9
Petroleum (cleaners) (fuels) (products) NEC	981	E862.1	–	E950.9	E962.1	E980.9
benzin(e) – *see* Ligroin						
ether – *see* Ligroin						

Drug, chemical	Poisoning	External Cause (E Code) Accident	Therapeutic Use	Suicide Attempt	Assault	Undetermined
Petroleum – *continued*						
jelly – *see* Petrolatum						
naphtha – *see* Ligroin						
pesticide	981	E863.4	–	E950.6	E962.1	E980.7
solids	981	E862.3	–	E950.9	E962.1	E980.9
solvents	981	E862.0	–	E950.9	E962.1	E980.9
vapor	987.1	E869.8	–	E952.8	E962.2	E982.8
Peyote	969.6	E854.1	E939.6	E950.3	E962.0	E980.3
Phanodorm, phanodorn	967.0	E851	E937.0	E950.1	E962.0	E980.1
Phanquinone, phanquone	961.5	E857	E931.5	E950.4	E962.0	E980.4
Pharmaceutical excipient or adjunct	977.4	E858.8	E947.4	E950.4	E962.0	E980.4
Phenacemide	966.3	E855.0	E936.3	E950.4	E962.0	E980.4
Phenacetin	965.4	E850.4	E935.4	E950.0	E962.0	E980.0
Phenadoxone	965.09	E850.2	E935.2	E950.0	E962.0	E980.0
Phenaglycodol	969.5	E853.8	E939.5	E950.3	E962.0	E980.3
Phenantoin	966.1	E855.0	E936.1	E950.4	E962.0	E980.4
Phenaphthazine reagent	977.8	E858.8	E947.8	E950.4	E962.0	E980.4
Phenazocine	965.09	E850.2	E935.2	E950.0	E962.0	E980.0
Phenazone	965.5	E850.5	E935.5	E950.0	E962.0	E980.0
Phenazopyridine	976.1	E858.7	E946.1	E950.4	E962.0	E980.4
Phenbenicillin	960.0	E856	E930.0	E950.4	E962.0	E980.4
Phenbutrazate	977.0	E858.8	E947.0	E950.4	E962.0	E980.4
Phencyclidine	968.3	E855.1	E938.3	E950.4	E962.0	E980.4
Phendimetrazine	977.0	E858.8	E947.0	E950.4	E962.0	E980.4
Phenelzine ▲	969.01	E854.0	E939.0	E950.3	E962.0	E980.3
Phenergan	967.8	E852.8	E937.8	E950.2	E962.0	E980.2
Phenethicillin (potassium)	960.0	E856	E930.0	E950.4	E962.0	E980.4
Phenetsal	965.1	E850.3	E935.3	E950.0	E962.0	E980.0
Pheneturide	966.3	E855.0	E936.3	E950.4	E962.0	E980.4
Phenformin	962.3	E858.0	E932.3	E950.4	E962.0	E980.4
Phenglutarimide	971.1	E855.4	E941.1	E950.4	E962.0	E980.4
Phenicarbazide	965.8	E850.8	E935.8	E950.0	E962.0	E980.0
Phenindamine (tartrate)	963.0	E858.1	E933.0	E950.4	E962.0	E980.4
Phenindione	964.2	E858.2	E934.2	E950.4	E962.0	E980.4
Phenprazine ▲	969.01	E854.0	E939.0	E950.3	E962.0	E980.3
Pheniramine (maleate)	963.0	E858.1	E933.0	E950.4	E962.0	E980.4
Phenmetrazine	977.0	E858.8	E947.0	E950.4	E962.0	E980.4
Phenobal	967.0	E851	E937.0	E950.1	E962.0	E980.1
Phenobarbital	967.0	E851	E937.0	E950.1	E962.0	E980.1
Phenobarbitone	967.0	E851	E937.0	E950.1	E962.0	E980.1
Phenoctide	976.0	E858.7	E946.0	E950.4	E962.0	E980.4
Phenol (derivatives) NEC	983.0	E864.0	–	E950.7	E962.1	E980.6
disinfectant	983.0	E864.0	–	E950.7	E962.1	E980.6
pesticide	989.4	E863.4	–	E950.6	E962.1	E980.7
red	977.8	E858.8	E947.8	E950.4	E962.0	E980.4
Phenolphthalein	973.1	E858.4	E943.1	E950.4	E962.0	E980.4
Phenolsulfonphthalein	977.8	E858.8	E947.8	E950.4	E962.0	E980.4
Phenomorphan	965.09	E850.2	E935.2	E950.0	E962.0	E980.0
Phenonyl	967.0	E851	E937.0	E950.1	E962.0	E980.1
Phenoperidine	965.09	E850.2	E935.2	E950.0	E962.0	E980.0
Phenoquin	974.7	E858.5	E944.7	E950.4	E962.0	E980.4
Phenothiazines (tranquilizers) NEC	969.1	E853.0	E939.1	E950.3	E962.0	E980.3
insecticide	989.3	E863.4	–	E950.6	E962.1	E980.7
Phenoxybenzamine	971.3	E855.6	E941.3	E950.4	E962.0	E980.4
Phenoxymethyl penicillin	960.0	E856	E930.0	E950.4	E962.0	E980.4
Phenprocoumon	964.2	E858.2	E934.2	E950.4	E962.0	E980.4
Phensuximide	966.2	E855.0	E936.2	E950.4	E962.0	E980.4
Phentermine	977.0	E858.8	E947.0	E950.4	E962.0	E980.4
Phentolamine	971.3	E855.6	E941.3	E950.4	E962.0	E980.4
Phenyl						
butazone	965.5	E850.5	E935.5	E950.0	E962.0	E980.0
enediamine	983.0	E864.0	–	E950.7	E962.1	E980.6
hydrazine	983.0	E864.0	–	E950.7	E962.1	E980.6
antineoplastic	963.1	E858.1	E933.1	E950.4	E962.0	E980.4
mercuric compounds – *see* Mercury						
salicylate	976.3	E858.7	E946.3	E950.4	E962.0	E980.4
Phenylephrin	971.2	E855.5	E941.2	E950.4	E962.0	E980.4
Phenylethylbiguanide	962.3	E858.0	E932.3	E950.4	E962.0	E980.4
Phenylpropanolamine	971.2	E855.5	E941.2	E950.4	E962.0	E980.4
Phenylsulfthion	989.3	E863.1	–	E950.6	E962.1	E980.7
Phenyramidol, phenyramidon	965.7	E850.7	E935.7	E950.0	E962.0	E980.0
Phenytoin	966.1	E855.0	E936.1	E950.4	E962.0	E980.4
pHisoHex	976.2	E858.7	E946.2	E950.4	E962.0	E980.4
Pholcodine	965.09	E850.2	E935.2	E950.0	E962.0	E980.0
Phorate	989.3	E863.1	–	E950.6	E962.1	E980.7
Phosdrin	989.3	E863.1	–	E950.6	E962.1	E980.7
Phosgene (gas)	987.8	E869.8	–	E952.8	E962.2	E982.8
Phosphate (tricresyl)	989.89	E866.8	–	E950.9	E962.1	E980.9
organic	989.3	E863.1	–	E950.6	E962.1	E980.7
solvent	982.8	E862.4	–	E950.9	E926.1	E980.9

Drug, chemical	Poisoning	External Cause (E Code) Accident	Therapeutic Use	Suicide Attempt	Assault	Undetermined
Phosphine	987.8	E869.8	–	E952.8	E962.2	E982.8
fumigant	987.8	E863.8	–	E950.6	E962.2	E980.7
Phospholine	971.0	E855.3	E941.0	E950.4	E962.0	E980.4
Phosphoric acid	983.1	E864.1	–	E950.7	E962.1	E980.6
Phosphorus (compounds) NEC	983.9	E864.3	–	E950.7	E962.1	E980.6
rodenticide	983.9	E863.7	–	E950.7	E962.1	E980.6
Phthalimidoglutarimide	967.8	E852.8	E937.8	E950.2	E962.0	E980.2
Phthalylsulfathiazole	961.0	E857	E931.0	E950.4	E962.0	E980.4
Phylloquinone	964.3	E858.2	E934.3	E950.4	E962.0	E980.4
Physeptone	965.02	E850.1	E935.1	E950.0	E962.0	E980.0
Physostigma venenosum	988.2	E865.4	–	E950.9	E962.1	E980.9
Physostigmine	971.0	E855.3	E941.0	E950.4	E962.0	E980.4
Phytolacca decandra	988.2	E865.4	–	E950.9	E962.1	E980.9
Phytomenadione	964.3	E858.2	E934.3	E950.4	E962.0	E980.4
Phytonadione	964.3	E858.2	E934.3	E950.4	E962.0	E980.4
Picric (acid)	983.0	E864.0	–	E950.7	E962.1	E980.6
Picrotoxin	970.0	E854.3	E940.0	E950.4	E962.0	E980.4
Pilocarpine	971.0	E855.3	E941.0	E950.4	E962.0	E980.4
Pilocarpus (jaborandi) **extract**	971.0	E855.3	E941.0	E950.4	E962.0	E980.4
Pimaricin	960.1	E856	E930.1	E950.4	E962.0	E980.4
Piminodine	965.09	E850.2	E935.2	E950.0	E962.0	E980.0
Pine oil, pinesol (disinfectant)	983.9	E861.4	–	E950.7	E962.1	E980.6
Pinkroot	961.6	E857	E931.6	E950.4	E962.0	E980.4
Pipadone	965.09	E850.2	E935.2	E950.0	E962.0	E980.0
Pipamazine	963.0	E858.1	E933.0	E950.4	E962.0	E980.4
Pipazethate	975.4	E858.6	E945.4	E950.4	E962.0	E980.4
Pipenzolate	971.1	E855.4	E941.1	E950.4	E962.0	E980.4
Piperacetazine	969.1	E853.0	E939.1	E950.3	E962.0	E980.3
Piperazine NEC	961.6	E857	E931.6	E950.4	E962.0	E980.4
estrone sulfate	962.2	E858.0	E932.2	E950.4	E962.0	E980.4
Piper cubeba	988.2	E865.4	–	E950.9	E962.1	E980.9
Piperidione	975.4	E858.6	E945.4	E950.4	E962.0	E980.4
Piperidolate	971.1	E855.4	E941.1	E950.4	E962.0	E980.4
Piperocaine	968.9	E855.2	E938.9	E950.4	E962.0	E980.4
infiltration (subcutaneous)	968.5	E855.2	E938.5	E950.4	E962.0	E980.4
nerve block (peripheral) (plexus)	968.6	E855.2	E938.6	E950.4	E962.0	E980.4
topical (surface)	968.5	E855.2	E938.5	E950.4	E962.0	E980.4
Pipobroman	963.1	E858.1	E933.1	E950.4	E962.0	E980.4
Pipradrol	970.8	E854.3	E940.8	E950.4	E962.0	E980.4
Piscidia (bark) (erythrina)	965.7	E850.7	E935.7	E950.0	E962.0	E980.0
Pitch	983.0	E864.0	–	E950.7	E962.1	E980.6
Pitkin's solution	968.7	E855.2	E938.7	E950.4	E962.0	E980.4
Pitocin	975.0	E858.6	E945.0	E950.4	E962.0	E980.4
Pitressin (tannate)	962.5	E858.0	E932.5	E950.4	E962.0	E980.4
Pituitary extracts (posterior)	962.5	E858.0	E932.5	E950.4	E962.0	E980.4
anterior	962.4	E858.0	E932.4	E950.4	E962.0	E980.4
Pituitrin	962.5	E858.0	E932.5	E950.4	E962.0	E980.4
Placental extract	962.9	E858.0	E932.9	E950.4	E962.0	E980.4
Placidyl	967.8	E852.8	E937.8	E950.2	E962.0	E980.2
Plague vaccine	978.3	E858.8	E948.3	E950.4	E962.0	E980.4
Plant foods or fertilizers NEC	989.89	E866.5	–	E950.9	E962.1	E980.9
mixed with herbicides	989.4	E863.5	–	E950.6	E962.1	E930.7
Plants, noxious, used as food	988.2	E865.9	–	E950.9	E962.1	E980.9
berries and seeds	988.2	E865.3	–	E950.9	E962.1	E980.9
specified type NEC	988.2	E865.4	–	E950.9	E962.1	E980.9
Plasma (blood)	964.7	E858.2	E934.7	E950.4	E962.0	E980.4
expanders	964.8	E858.2	E934.8	E950.4	E962.0	E980.4
Plasmanate	964.7	E858.2	E934.7	E950.4	E962.0	E980.4
Plegicil	969.1	E853.0	E939.1	E950.3	E962.0	E980.3
Podophyllin	976.4	E858.7	E946.4	E950.4	E962.0	E980.4
Podophyllum resin	976.4	E858.7	E946.4	E950.4	E962.0	E980.4
Poison NEC	989.9	E866.9	–	E950.9	E962.1	E980.9
Poisonous berries	988.2	E865.3	–	E950.9	E962.1	E980.9
Pokeweed (any part)	988.2	E865.4	–	E950.9	E962.1	E980.9
Poldine	971.1	E855.4	E941.1	E950.4	E962.0	E980.4
Poliomyelitis vaccine	979.5	E858.8	E949.5	E950.4	E962.0	E980.4
Poliovirus vaccine	979.5	E858.8	E949.5	E950.4	E962.0	E980.4
Polish (car) (floor) (furniture) (metal) (silver)	989.89	E861.2	–	E950.9	E962.1	E980.9
abrasive	989.89	E861.3	–	E950.9	E962.1	E980.9
porcelain	989.89	E861.3	–	E950.9	E962.1	E980.9
Poloxalkol	973.2	E858.4	E943.2	E950.4	E962.0	E980.4
Polyaminostyrene resins	974.5	E858.5	E944.5	E950.4	E962.0	E980.4
Polychlorinated biphenyl – *see* PCBs						
Polycycline	960.4	E856	E930.4	E950.4	E962.0	E980.4
Polyester resin hardener	982.8	E862.4	–	E950.9	E962.1	E980.9
fumes	987.8	E869.8	–	E952.8	E962.2	E982.8
Polyestradiol (phosphate)	962.2	E858.0	E932.2	E950.4	E962.0	E980.4
Polyethanolamine alkyl sulfate	976.2	E858.7	E946.2	E950.4	E962.0	E980.4
Polyethylene glycol	976.3	E858.7	E946.3	E950.4	E962.0	E980.4
Polyferose	964.0	E858.2	E934.0	E950.4	E962.0	E980.4

Drug, chemical	Poisoning	External Cause (E Code) Accident	Therapeutic Use	Suicide Attempt	Assault	Undetermined
Polymyxin B	960.8	E856	E930.8	E950.4	E962.0	E980.4
ENT agent	976.6	E858.7	E946.6	E950.4	E962.0	E980.4
ophthalmic preparation	976.5	E858.7	E946.5	E950.4	E962.0	E980.4
topical NEC	976.0	E858.7	E946.0	E950.4	E962.0	E980.4
Polynoxylin(e)	976.0	E858.7	E946.0	E950.4	E962.0	E980.4
Polyoxymethyleneurea	976.0	E858.7	E946.0	E950.4	E962.0	E980.4
Polytetrafluoroethylene (inhaled)	987.8	E869.8	–	E952.8	E962.2	E982.8
Polythiazide	974.3	E858.5	E944.3	E950.4	E962.0	E980.4
Polyvinylpyrrolidone	964.8	E858.2	E934.8	E950.4	E962.0	E980.4
Pontocaine (hydrochloride) (infiltration) (topical)	968.5	E855.2	E938.5	E950.4	E962.0	E980.4
nerve block (peripheral) (plexus)	968.6	E855.2	E938.6	E950.4	E962.0	E980.4
spinal	968.7	E855.2	E938.7	E950.4	E962.0	E980.4
Pot	969.6	E854.1	E939.6	E950.3	E962.0	E980.3
Potash (caustic)	983.2	E864.2	–	E950.7	E962.1	E980.6
Potassic saline injection (lactated)	974.5	E858.5	E944.5	E950.4	E962.0	E980.4
Potassium (salts) NEC	974.5	E858.5	E944.5	E950.4	E962.0	E980.4
aminosalicylate	961.8	E857	E931.8	E950.4	E962.0	E980.4
arsenite (solution)	985.1	E866.3	–	E950.8	E962.1	E980.8
bichromate	983.9	E864.3	–	E950.7	E962.1	E980.6
bisulfate	983.9	E864.3	–	E950.7	E962.1	E980.6
bromide (medicinal) NEC	967.3	E852.2	E937.3	E950.2	E962.0	E980.2
carbonate	983.2	E864.2	–	E950.7	E962.1	E980.6
chlorate NEC	983.9	E864.3	–	E950.7	E962.1	E980.6
cyanide – *see*, Cyanide						
hydroxide	983.2	E864.2	–	E950.7	E962.1	E980.6
iodide (expectorant) NEC	975.5	E858.6	E945.5	E950.4	E962.0	E980.4
nitrate	989.89	E866.8	–	E950.9	E962.1	E980.9
oxalate	983.9	E864.3	–	E950.7	E962.1	E980.6
perchlorate NEC	977.8	E858.8	E947.8	E950.4	E962.0	E980.4
antithyroid	962.8	E858.0	E932.8	E950.4	E962.0	E980.4
permanganate	976.0	E858.7	E946.0	E950.4	E962.0	E980.4
nonmedicinal	983.9	E864.3	–	E950.7	E962.1	E980.6
Povidone-iodine (anti-infective) NEC	976.0	E858.7	E946.0	E950.4	E962.0	E980.4
Practolol	972.0	E858.3	E942.0	E950.4	E962.0	E980.4
Pralidoxime (chloride)	977.2	E858.8	E947.2	E950.4	E962.0	E980.4
Pramoxine	968.5	E855.2	E938.5	E950.4	E962.0	E980.4
Prazosin	972.6	E858.3	E942.6	E950.4	E962.0	E980.4
Prednisolone	962.0	E858.0	E932.0	E950.4	E962.0	E980.4
ENT agent	976.6	E858.7	E946.6	E950.4	E962.0	E980.4
ophthalmic preparation	976.5	E858.7	E946.5	E950.4	E962.0	E980.4
topical NEC	976.0	E858.7	E946.0	E950.4	E962.0	E980.4
Prednisone	962.0	E858.0	E932.0	E950.4	E962.0	E980.4
Pregnanediol	962.2	E858.0	E932.2	E950.4	E962.0	E980.4
Pregneninolone	962.2	E858.0	E932.2	E950.4	E962.0	E980.4
Preludin	977.0	E858.8	E947.0	E950.4	E962.0	E980.4
Premarin	962.2	E858.0	E932.2	E950.4	E962.0	E980.4
Prenylamine	972.4	E858.3	E942.4	E950.4	E962.0	E980.4
Preparation H	976.8	E858.7	E946.8	E950.4	E962.0	E980.4
Preservatives	989.89	E866.8	–	E950.9	E962.1	E980.9
Pride of China	988.2	E865.3	–	E950.9	E962.1	E980.9
Prilocaine	968.9	E855.2	E938.9	E950.4	E962.0	E980.4
infiltration (subcutaneous)	968.5	E855.2	E938.5	E950.4	E962.0	E980.4
nerve block (peripheral) (plexus)	968.6	E855.2	E938.6	E950.4	E962.0	E980.4
Primaquine	961.4	E857	E931.4	E950.4	E962.0	E980.4
Primidone	966.3	E855.0	E936.3	E950.4	E962.0	E980.4
Primula (veris)	988.2	E865.4	–	E950.9	E962.1	E980.9
Prinadol	965.09	E850.2	E935.2	E950.0	E962.0	E980.0
Priscol, Priscoline	971.3	E855.6	E941.3	E950.4	E962.0	E980.4
Privet	988.2	E865.4	–	E950.9	E962.1	E980.9
Privine	971.2	E855.5	E941.2	E950.4	E962.0	E980.4
Pro-Banthine	971.1	E855.4	E941.1	E950.4	E962.0	E980.4
Probarbital	967.0	E851	E937.0	E950.1	E962.0	E980.1
Probenecid	974.7	E858.5	E944.7	E950.4	E962.0	E980.4
Procainamide (hydrochloride)	972.0	E858.3	E942.0	E950.4	E962.0	E980.4
Procaine (hydrochloride) (infiltration) (topical)	968.5	E855.2	E938.5	E950.4	E962.0	E980.4
nerve block (periphreal) (plexus)	968.6	E855.2	E938.6	E950.4	E962.0	E980.4
penicillin G	960.0	E856	E930.0	E950.4	E962.0	E980.4
spinal	968.7	E855.2	E938.7	E950.4	E962.0	E980.4
Procalmidol	969.5	E853.8	E939.5	E950.3	E962.0	E980.3
Procarbazine	963.1	E858.1	E933.1	E950.4	E962.0	E980.4
Prochlorperazine	969.1	E853.0	E939.1	E950.3	E962.0	E980.3
Procyclidine	966.4	E855.0	E936.4	E950.4	E962.0	E980.4
Producer gas	986	E868.8	–	E952.1	E962.2	E982.1
Profenamine	966.4	E855.0	E936.4	E950.4	E962.0	E980.4
Profenil	975.1	E858.6	E945.1	E950.4	E962.0	E980.4
Progesterones	962.2	E858.0	E932.2	E950.4	E962.0	E980.4
Progestin	962.2	E858.0	E932.2	E950.4	E962.0	E980.4
Progestogens (with estrogens)	962.2	E858.0	E932.2	E950.4	E962.0	E980.4
Progestone	962.2	E858.0	E932.2	E950.4	E962.0	E980.4
Proguanil	961.4	E857	E931.4	E950.4	E962.0	E980.4
Prolactin	962.4	E858.0	E932.4	E950.4	E962.0	E980.4
Proloid	962.7	E858.0	E932.7	E950.4	E962.0	E980.4
Proluton	962.2	E858.0	E932.2	E950.4	E962.0	E980.4
Promacetin	961.8	E857	E931.8	E950.4	E962.0	E980.4
Promazine	969.1	E853.0	E939.1	E950.3	E962.0	E980.3
Promedol	965.09	E850.2	E935.2	E950.0	E962.0	E980.0
Promethazine	967.8	E852.8	E937.8	E950.2	E962.0	E980.2
Promin	961.8	E857	E931.8	E950.4	E962.0	E980.4
Pronestyl (hydrochloride)	972.0	E858.3	E942.0	E950.4	E962.0	E980.4
Pronetalol, pronethalol	972.0	E858.3	E942.0	E950.4	E962.0	E980.4
Prontosil	961.0	E857	E931.0	E950.4	E962.0	E980.4
Propamidine isethionate	961.5	E857	E931.5	E950.4	E962.0	E980.4
Propanal (medicinal)	967.8	E852.8	E937.8	E950.2	E962.0	E980.2
Propane (gas) (distributed in mobile container)	987.0	E868.0	–	E951.1	E962.2	E981.1
distributed through pipes	987.0	E867	–	E951.0	E962.2	E981.0
incomplete combustion of – *see* Carbon monoxide, Propane						
Propanidid	968.3	E855.1	E938.3	E950.4	E962.0	E980.4
Propanol	980.3	E860.4	–	E950.9	E962.1	E980.9
Propantheline	971.1	E855.4	E941.1	E950.4	E962.0	E980.4
Proparacaine	968.5	E855.2	E938.5	E950.4	E962.0	E980.4
Propatyl nitrate	972.4	E858.3	E942.4	E950.4	E962.0	E980.4
Propicillin	960.0	E856	E930.0	E950.4	E962.0	E980.4
Propiolactone (vapor)	987.8	E869.8	–	E952.8	E962.2	E982.8
Propiomazine	967.8	E852.8	E937.8	E950.2	E962.0	E980.2
Propionaidehyde (medicinal)	967.8	E852.8	E937.8	E950.2	E962.0	E980.2
Propionate compound	976.0	E858.7	E946.0	E950.4	E962.0	E980.4
Propion gel	976.0	E858.7	E946.0	E950.4	E962.0	E980.4
Propitocaine	968.9	E855.2	E938.9	E950.4	E962.0	E980.4
infiltration (subcutaneous)	968.5	E855.2	E938.5	E950.4	E962.0	E980.4
nerve block (peripheral) (plexus)	968.6	E855.2	E938.6	E950.4	E962.0	E980.4
Propoxur	989.3	E863.2	–	E950.6	E962.1	E980.7
Propoxycaine	968.9	E855.2	E938.9	E950.4	E962.0	E980.4
infiltration (subcutaneous)	968.5	E855.2	E938.5	E950.4	E962.0	E980.4
nerve block (peripheral) (plexus)	968.6	E855.2	E938.6	E950.4	E962.0	E980.4
topical (surface)	968.5	E855.2	E938.5	E950.4	E962.0	E980.4
Propoxyphene (hydrochloride)	965.8	E850.8	E935.8	E950.0	E962.0	E980.0
Propranolol	972.0	E858.3	E942.0	E950.4	E962.0	E980.4
Propyl						
alcohol	980.3	E860.4	–	E950.9	E962.1	E980.9
carbinol	980.3	E860.4	–	E950.9	E962.1	E980.9
hexadrine	971.2	E855.5	E941.2	E950.4	E962.0	E980.4
iodone	977.8	E858.8	E947.8	E950.4	E962.0	E980.4
thiouracil	962.8	E858.0	E932.8	E950.4	E962.0	E980.4
Propylene	987.1	E869.8	–	E952.8	E962.2	E982.8
Propylparaben (ophthalmic)	976.5	E858.7	E946.5	E950.4	E962.0	E980.4
Proscillaridin	972.1	E858.3	E942.1	E950.4	E962.0	E980.4
Prostaglandins	975.0	E858.6	E945.0	E950.4	E962.0	E980.4
Prostigmin	971.0	E855.3	E941.0	E950.4	E962.0	E980.4
Protamine (sulfate)	964.5	E858.2	E934.5	E950.4	E962.0	E980.4
zinc insulin	962.3	E858.0	E932.3	E950.4	E962.0	E980.4
Protectants (topical)	976.3	E858.7	E946.3	E950.4	E962.0	E980.4
Protein hydrolysate	974.5	E858.5	E944.5	E950.4	E962.0	E980.4
Prothiaden – *see* Dothiepin hydrochloride						
Prothionamide	961.8	E857	E931.8	E950.4	E962.0	E980.4
Prothipendyl	969.5	E853.8	E939.5	E950.3	E962.0	E980.3
Protokylol	971.2	E855.5	E941.2	E950.4	E962.0	E980.4
Protopam	977.2	E858.8	E947.2	E950.4	E962.0	E980.4
Protoveratrine(s) (A) (B)	972.6	E858.3	E942.6	E950.4	E962.0	E980.4
Protriptyline ▲	969.05	E854.0	E939.0	E950.3	E962.0	E980.3
Provera	962.2	E858.0	E932.2	E950.4	E962.0	E980.4
Provitamin A	963.5	E858.1	E933.5	E950.4	E962.0	E980.4
Proxymetacaine	968.5	E855.2	E938.5	E950.4	E962.0	E980.4
Proxyphylline	975.1	E858.6	E945.1	E950.4	E962.0	E980.4
Prozac – *see* Fluoxetine hydrochloride						
Prunus						
laurocerasus	988.2	E865.4	–	E950.9	E962.1	E980.9
virginiana	988.2	E865.4	–	E950.9	E962.1	E980.9
Prussic acid	989.0	E866.8	–	E950.9	E962.1	E980.9
vapor	987.7	E869.8	–	E952.8	E962.2	E982.8
Pseudoephedrine	971.2	E855.5	E941.2	E950.4	E962.0	E980.4
Psilocin	969.6	E854.1	E939.6	E950.3	E962.0	E980.3
Psilocybin	969.6	E854.1	E939.6	E950.3	E962.0	E980.3
PSP	977.8	E858.8	E947.8	E950.4	E962.0	E980.4
Psychedelic agents	969.6	E854.1	E939.6	E950.3	E962.0	E980.3
Psychodysleptics	969.6	E854.1	E939.6	E950.3	E962.0	E980.3
Psychostimulants ▲	969.70	E854.2	E939.7	E950.3	E962.0	E980.3

Drug, chemical	Poisoning	External Cause (E Code)				
		Accident	Therapeutic Use	Suicide Attempt	Assault	Undetermined
Psychotherapeutic agents	969.9	E855.9	E939.9	E950.3	E962.0	E980.3
antidepressants ▲	969.00	E854.0	E939.0	E950.3	E962.0	E980.3
specified NEC	969.8	E855.8	E939.8	E950.3	E962.0	E980.3
tranquilizers NEC	969.5	E853.9	E939.5	E950.3	E962.0	E980.3
Psychotomimetic agents	969.6	E854.1	E939.6	E950.3	E962.0	E980.3
Psychotropic agents	969.9	E854.8	E939.9	E950.3	E962.0	E980.3
specified NEC	969.8	E854.8	E939.8	E950.3	E962.0	E980.3
Psyllium	973.3	E858.4	E943.3	E950.4	E962.0	E980.4
Pteroylglutamic acid	964.1	E858.2	E934.1	E950.4	E962.0	E980.4
Pteroyltriglutamate	963.1	E858.1	E933.1	E950.4	E962.0	E980.4
PTFE	987.8	E869.8	–	E952.8	E962.2	E982.8
Pulsatilla	988.2	E865.4	–	E950.9	E962.1	E980.9
Purex (bleach)	983.9	E864.3	–	E950.7	E962.1	E980.6
Purine diuretics	974.1	E858.5	E944.1	E950.4	E962.0	E980.4
Purinethol	963.1	E858.1	E933.1	E950.4	E962.0	E980.4
PVP	964.8	E858.2	E934.8	E950.4	E962.0	E980.4
Pyrabital	965.7	E850.7	E935.7	E950.0	E962.0	E980.0
Pyramidon	965.5	E850.5	E935.5	E950.0	E962.0	E980.0
Pyrantel (pamoate)	961.6	E857	E931.6	E950.4	E962.0	E980.4
Pyrathiazine	963.0	E858.1	E933.0	E950.4	E962.0	E980.4
Pyrazinamide	961.8	E857	E931.8	E950.4	E962.0	E980.4
Pyrazinoic acid (amide)	961.8	E857	E931.8	E950.4	E962.0	E980.4
Pyrazole (derivatives)	965.5	E850.5	E935.5	E950.0	E962.0	E980.0
Pyrazolone (analgesics)	965.5	E850.5	E935.5	E950.0	E962.0	E980.0
Pyrethrins, pyrethrum	989.4	E863.4	–	E950.6	E962.1	E980.7
Pyribenzamine	963.0	E858.1	E933.0	E950.4	E962.0	E980.4
Pyridine (liquid) (vapor)	982.0	E862.4	–	E950.9	E962.1	E980.9
aldoxime chloride	977.2	E858.8	E947.2	E950.4	E962.0	E980.4
Pyridium	976.1	E858.7	E946.1	E950.4	E962.0	E980.4
Pyridostigmine	971.0	E855.3	E941.0	E950.4	E962.0	E980.4
Pyridoxine	963.5	E858.1	E933.5	E950.4	E962.0	E980.4
Pyrilamine	963.0	E858.1	E933.0	E950.4	E962.0	E980.4
Pyrimethamine	961.4	E857	E931.4	E950.4	E962.0	E980.4
Pyrogallic acid	983.0	E864.0	–	E950.7	E962.1	E980.6
Pyroxylin	976.3	E858.7	E946.3	E950.4	E962.0	E980.4
Pyrrobutamine	963.0	E858.1	E933.0	E950.4	E962.0	E980.4
Pyrrocitine	968.5	E855.2	E938.5	E950.4	E962.0	E980.4
Pyrvinium (pamoate)	961.6	E857	E931.6	E950.4	E962.0	E980.4
PZI	962.3	E858.0	E932.3	E950.4	E962.0	E980.4
Quaalude	967.4	E852.3	E937.4	E950.2	E962.0	E980.2
Quaternary ammonium derivatives	971.1	E855.4	E941.1	E950.4	E962.0	E980.4
Quicklime	983.2	E864.2	–	E950.7	E962.1	E980.6
Quinacrine	961.3	E857	E931.3	E950.4	E962.0	E980.4
Quinaglute	972.0	E858.3	E942.0	E950.4	E962.0	E980.4
Quinalbarbitone	967.0	E851	E937.0	E950.1	E962.0	E980.1
Quinestradiol	962.2	E858.0	E932.2	E950.4	E962.0	E980.4
Quinethazone	974.3	E858.5	E944.3	E950.4	E962.0	E980.4
Quinidine (gluconate) (polygalacturonate) (salts) (sulfate)	972.0	E858.3	E942.0	E950.4	E962.0	E980.4
Quinine	961.4	E857	E931.4	E950.4	E962.0	E980.4
Quiniobine	961.3	E857	E931.3	E950.4	E962.0	E980.4
Quinolines	961.3	E857	E931.3	E950.4	E962.0	E980.4
Quotane	968.5	E855.2	E938.5	E950.4	E962.0	E980.4
Rabies						
immune globulin (human)	964.6	E858.2	E934.6	E950.4	E962.0	E980.4
vaccine	979.1	E858.8	E949.1	E950.4	E962.0	E980.4
Racemoramide	965.09	E850.2	E935.2	E950.0	E962.0	E980.0
Racemorphan	965.09	E850.2	E935.2	E950.0	E962.0	E980.0
Radiator alcohol	980.1	E860.2	–	E950.9	E962.1	E980.9
Radio-opaque (drugs) (materials)	977.8	E858.8	E947.8	E950.4	E962.0	E980.4
Ranunculus	988.2	E865.4	–	E950.9	E962.1	E980.9
Rat poison	989.4	E863.7	–	E950.6	E962.1	E980.7
Rattlesnake (venom)	989.5	E905.0	–	E950.9	E962.1	E980.9
Raudixin	972.6	E858.3	E942.6	E950.4	E962.0	E980.4
Rautensin	972.6	E858.3	E942.6	E950.4	E962.0	E980.4
Rautina	972.6	E858.3	E942.6	E950.4	E962.0	E980.4
Rautotal	972.6	E858.3	E942.6	E950.4	E962.0	E980.4
Rauwiloid	972.6	E858.3	E942.6	E950.4	E962.0	E980.4
Rauwoldin	972.6	E858.3	E942.6	E950.4	E962.0	E980.4
Rauwolfia (alkaloids)	972.6	E858.3	E942.6	E950.4	E962.0	E980.4
Realgar	985.1	E866.3	–	E950.8	E962.1	E980.8
Red cells, packed	964.7	E858.2	E934.7	E950.4	E962.0	E980.4
Reducing agents, industrial NEC	983.9	E864.3	–	E950.7	E962.1	E980.6
Refrigerant gas (freon)	987.4	E869.2	–	E952.8	E962.2	E982.8
not freon	987.9	E869.9	–	E952.9	E962.2	E982.9
Regroton	974.4	E858.5	E944.4	E950.4	E962.0	E980.4
Rela	968.0	E855.1	E938.0	E950.4	E962.0	E980.4
Relaxants, skeletal muscle (autonomic)	975.2	E858.6	E945.2	E950.4	E962.0	E980.4
central nervous system	968.0	E855.1	E938.0	E950.4	E962.0	E980.4
Renese	974.3	E858.5	E944.3	E950.4	E962.0	E980.4

Drug, chemical	Poisoning	External Cause (E Code)				
		Accident	Therapeutic Use	Suicide Attempt	Assault	Undetermined
Renografin	977.8	E858.8	E947.8	E950.4	E962.0	E980.4
Replacement solutions	974.5	E858.5	E944.5	E950.4	E962.0	E980.4
Rescinnamine	972.6	E858.3	E942.6	E950.4	E962.0	E980.4
Reserpine	972.6	E858.3	E942.6	E950.4	E962.0	E980.4
Resorcin, resorcinol	976.4	E858.7	E946.4	E950.4	E962.0	E980.4
Respaire	975.5	E858.6	E945.5	E950.4	E962.0	E980.4
Respiratory agents NEC	975.8	E858.6	E945.8	E950.4	E962.0	E980.4
Retinoic acid	976.8	E858.7	E946.8	E950.4	E962.0	E980.4
Retinol	963.5	E858.1	E933.5	E950.4	E962.0	E980.4
Rh (D) immune globulin (human)	964.6	E858.2	E934.6	E950.4	E962.0	E980.4
Rhodine	965.1	E850.3	E935.3	E950.0	E962.0	E980.0
RhoGAM	964.6	E858.2	E934.6	E950.4	E962.0	E980.4
Riboflavin	963.5	E858.1	E933.5	E950.4	E962.0	E980.4
Ricin	989.8	E866.8	–	E950.9	E962.1	E980.9
Ricinus communis	988.2	E865.3	–	E950.9	E962.1	E980.9
Rickettsial vaccine NEC	979.6	E858.8	E949.6	E950.4	E962.0	E980.4
with viral and bacterial vaccine	979.7	E858.8	E949.7	E950.4	E962.0	E980.4
Rifampin	960.6	E856	E930.6	E950.4	E962.0	E980.4
Rimifon	961.8	E857	E931.8	E950.4	E962.0	E980.4
Ringer's injection (lactated)	974.5	E858.5	E944.5	E950.4	E962.0	E980.4
Ristocetin	960.8	E856	E930.8	E950.4	E962.0	E980.4
Ritalin ▲	969.73	E854.2	E939.7	E950.3	E962.0	E980.3
Roach killers – *see* Pesticides						
Rocky Mountain spotted fever vaccine	979.6	E858.8	E949.6	E950.4	E962.0	E980.4
Rodenticides	989.4	E863.7	–	E950.6	E962.1	E980.7
Rohypnol	969.4	E853.2	E939.4	E950.3	E962.0	E980.3
Rolaids	973.0	E858.4	E943.0	E950.4	E962.0	E980.4
Rolitetracycline	960.4	E856	E930.4	E950.4	E962.0	E980.4
Romilar	975.4	E858.6	E945.4	E950.4	E962.0	E980.4
Rose water ointment	976.3	E858.7	E946.3	E950.4	E962.0	E980.4
Rotenone	989.4	E863.7	–	E950.6	E962.1	E980.7
Rotoxamine	963.0	E858.1	E933.0	E950.4	E962.0	E980.4
Rough-on-rats	989.4	E863.7	–	E950.6	E962.1	E980.7
RU486	962.9	E858.0	E932.9	E950.4	E962.0	E980.4
Rubbing alcohol	980.2	E860.3	–	E950.9	E962.1	E980.9
Rubella virus vaccine	979.4	E858.8	E949.4	E950.4	E962.0	E980.4
Rubelogen	979.4	E858.8	E949.4	E950.4	E962.0	E980.4
Rubeovax	979.4	E858.8	E949.4	E950.4	E962.0	E980.4
Rubidomycin	960.7	E856	E930.7	E950.4	E962.0	E980.4
Rue	988.2	E865.4	–	E950.9	E962.1	E980.9
Ruta	988.2	E865.4	–	E950.9	E962.1	E980.9
Sabadilla (medicinal)	976.0	E858.7	E946.0	E950.4	E962.0	E980.4
pesticide	989.4	E863.4	–	E950.6	E962.1	E980.7
Sabin oral vaccine	979.5	E858.8	E949.5	E950.4	E962.0	E980.4
Saccharated iron oxide	964.0	E858.2	E934.0	E950.4	E962.0	E980.4
Saccharin	974.5	E858.5	E944.5	E950.4	E962.0	E980.4
Safflower oil	972.2	E858.3	E942.2	E950.4	E962.0	E980.4
Salbutamol sulfate	975.7	E858.6	E945.7	E950.4	E962.0	E980.4
Salicylamide	965.1	E850.3	E935.3	E950.0	E962.0	E980.0
Salicylate(s)	965.1	E850.3	E935.3	E950.0	E962.0	E980.0
methyl	976.3	E858.7	E946.3	E950.4	E962.0	E980.4
theobromine calcium	974.1	E858.5	E944.1	E950.4	E962.0	E980.4
Salicylazosulfapyridine	961.0	E857	E931.0	E950.4	E962.0	E980.4
Salicylhydroxamic acid	976.0	E858.7	E946.0	E950.4	E962.0	E980.4
Salicylic acid (keratolytic) NEC	976.4	E858.7	E946.4	E950.4	E962.0	E980.4
congeners	965.1	E850.3	E935.3	E950.0	E962.0	E980.0
salts	965.1	E850.3	E935.3	E950.0	E962.0	E980.0
Saliniazid	961.8	E857	E931.8	E950.4	E962.0	E980.4
Salol	976.3	E858.7	E946.3	E950.4	E962.0	E980.4
Salt (substitute) **NEC**	974.5	E858.5	E944.5	E950.4	E962.0	E980.4
Saluretics	974.3	E858.5	E944.3	E950.4	E962.0	E980.4
Saluron	974.3	E858.5	E944.3	E950.4	E962.0	E980.4
Salvarsan 606 (neosilver) (silver)	961.1	E857	E931.1	E950.4	E962.0	E980.4
Sambucus canadensis	988.2	E865.4	–	E950.9	E962.1	E980.9
berry	988.2	E865.3	–	E950.9	E962.1	E980.9
Sandril	972.6	E858.3	E942.6	E950.4	E962.0	E980.4
Sanguinaria canadensis	988.2	E865.4	–	E950.9	E962.1	E980.9
Saniflush (cleaner)	983.9	E861.3	–	E950.7	E962.1	E980.6
Santonin	961.6	E857	E931.6	E950.4	E962.0	E980.4
Santyl	976.8	E858.7	E946.8	E950.4	E962.0	E980.4
Sarkomycin	960.7	E856	E930.7	E950.4	E962.0	E980.4
Saroten ▲	969.05	E854.0	E939.0	E950.3	E962.0	E980.3
Saturnine – *see* Lead						
Savin (oil)	976.4	E858.7	E946.4	E950.4	E962.0	E980.4
Scammony	973.1	E858.4	E943.1	E950.4	E962.0	E980.4
Scarlet red	976.8	E858.7	E946.8	E950.4	E962.0	E980.4
Scheele's green	985.1	E866.3	–	E950.8	E962.1	E980.8
insecticide	985.1	E863.4	–	E950.8	E962.1	E980.8
Schradan	989.3	E863.1	–	E950.6	E962.1	E980.7
Schweinfurt(h) green	985.1	E866.3	–	E950.8	E962.1	E980.8
insecticide	985.1	E863.4	–	E950.8	E962.1	E980.8

4th Fourth Digit Required | 5th Fifth Digit Required | *[code]* Manifestation Code | ● New Line | ▲ Revised Line | text New Text | ~~text~~ Deleted text

Drug, chemical	Poisoning	External Cause (E Code): Accident	Therapeutic Use	Suicide Attempt	Assault	Undetermined
Scilla – *see* Squill						
Sclerosing agents	972.7	E858.3	E942.7	E950.4	E962.0	E980.4
Scopolamine	971.1	E855.4	E941.1	E950.4	E962.0	E980.4
Scouring powder	989.89	E861.3	–	E950.9	E962.1	E980.9
Sea						
anemone (sting)	989.5	E905.6	–	E950.9	E962.1	E980.9
cucumber (sting)	989.5	E905.6	–	E950.9	E962.1	E980.9
snake (bite) (venom)	989.5	E905.0	–	E950.9	E962.1	E980.9
urchin spine (puncture)	989.5	E905.6	–	E950.9	E962.1	E980.9
Secbutabarbital	967.0	E851	E937.0	E950.1	E962.0	E980.1
Secbutabarbitone	967.0	E851	E937.0	E950.1	E962.0	E980.1
Secobarbital	967.0	E851	E937.0	E950.1	E962.0	E980.1
Seconal	967.0	E851	E937.0	E950.1	E962.0	E980.1
Secretin	977.8	E858.8	E947.8	E950.4	E962.0	E980.4
Sedatives, nonbarbiturate	967.9	E852.9	E937.9	E950.2	E962.0	E980.2
specified NEC	967.8	E852.8	E937.8	E950.2	E962.0	E980.2
Sedormid	967.8	E852.8	E937.8	E950.2	E962.0	E980.2
Seed (plant)	988.2	E865.3	–	E950.9	E962.1	E980.9
disinfectant or dressing	989.89	E866.5	–	E950.9	E962.1	E980.9
Selective serotonin and norepinephrine reuptake inhibitors (SSNRI) ●	969.02	E854.0	E939.0	E950.3	E962.0	E980.3
Selective serotonin reuptake inhibitors (SSRI) ●	969.03	E854.0	E939.0	E950.3	E962.0	E980.3
Selenium (fumes) NEC	985.8	E866.4	–	E950.9	E962.1	E980.9
disulfide or sulfide	976.4	E858.7	E946.4	E950.4	E962.0	E980.4
Selsun	976.4	E858.7	E946.4	E950.4	E962.0	E980.4
Senna	973.1	E858.4	E943.1	E950.4	E962.0	E980.4
Septisol	976.2	E858.7	E946.2	E950.4	E962.0	E980.4
Serax	969.4	E853.2	E939.4	E950.3	E962.0	E980.3
Serenesil	967.8	E852.8	E937.8	E950.2	E962.0	E980.2
Serenium (hydrochloride)	961.9	E857	E931.9	E950.4	E962.0	E980.4
Serepax – *see* Oxazepam						
Sernyl	968.3	E855.1	E938.3	E950.4	E962.0	E980.4
Serotonin	977.8	E858.8	E947.8	E950.4	E962.0	E980.4
Serpasil	972.6	E858.3	E942.6	E950.4	E962.0	E980.4
Sewer gas	987.8	E869.8	–	E952.8	E962.2	E982.8
Shampoo	989.6	E861.0	–	E950.9	E962.1	E980.9
Shellfish, nonbacterial or noxious	988.0	E865.1	–	E950.9	E962.1	E980.9
Silicones NEC	989.83	E866.8	E947.8	E950.9	E962.1	E980.9
Silvadene	976.0	E858.7	E946.0	E950.4	E962.0	E980.4
Silver (compound) (medicinal) NEC	976.0	E858.7	E946.0	E950.4	E962.0	E980.4
anti-infectives	976.0	E858.7	E946.0	E950.4	E962.0	E980.4
arsphenamine	961.1	E857	E931.1	E950.4	E962.0	E980.4
nitrate	976.0	E858.7	E946.0	E950.4	E962.0	E980.4
ophthalmic preparation	976.5	E858.7	E946.5	E950.4	E962.0	E980.4
toughened (keratolytic)	976.4	E858.7	E946.4	E950.4	E962.0	E980.4
nonmedicinal (dust)	985.8	E866.4	–	E950.9	E962.1	E980.9
protein (mild) (strong)	976.0	E858.7	E946.0	E950.4	E962.0	E980.4
salvarsan	961.1	E857	E931.1	E950.4	E962.0	E980.4
Simethicone	973.8	E858.4	E943.8	E950.4	E962.0	E980.4
Sinequan ▲	969.05	E854.0	E939.0	E950.3	E962.0	E980.3
Singoserp	972.6	E858.3	E942.6	E950.4	E962.0	E980.4
Sintrom	964.2	E858.2	E934.2	E950.4	E962.0	E980.4
Sitosterols	972.2	E858.3	E942.2	E950.4	E962.0	E980.4
Skeletal muscle relaxants	975.2	E858.6	E945.2	E950.4	E962.0	E980.4
Skin agents (external)	976.9	E858.7	E946.9	E950.4	E962.0	E980.4
specified NEC	976.8	E858.7	E946.8	E950.4	E962.0	E980.4
test antigen	977.8	E858.8	E947.8	E950.4	E962.0	E980.4
Sleep-eze	963.0	E858.1	E933.0	E950.4	E962.0	E980.4
Sleeping draught (drug) (pill) (tablet)	967.9	E852.9	E937.9	E950.2	E962.0	E980.2
Smallpox vaccine	979.0	E858.8	E949.0	E950.4	E962.0	E980.4
Smelter fumes NEC	985.9	E866.4	–	E950.9	E962.1	E980.9
Smog	987.3	E869.1	–	E952.8	E962.2	E982.8
Smoke NEC	987.9	E869.9	–	E952.9	E962.2	E982.9
Smooth muscle relaxant	975.1	E858.6	E945.1	E950.4	E962.0	E980.4
Snail killer	989.4	E863.4	–	E950.6	E962.1	E980.7
Snake (bite) (venom)	989.5	E905.0	–	E950.9	E962.1	E980.9
Snuff	989.89	E866.8	–	E950.9	E962.1	E980.9
Soap (powder) (product)	989.6	E861.1	–	E950.9	E962.1	E980.9
medicinal, soft	976.2	E858.7	E946.2	E950.4	E962.0	E980.4
Soda (caustic)	983.2	E864.2	–	E950.7	E962.1	E980.6
bicarb	963.3	E858.1	E933.3	E950.4	E962.0	E980.4
chlorinated – *see* Sodium, hypochlorite						
Sodium						
acetosulfone	961.8	E857	E931.8	E950.4	E962.0	E980.4
acetrizoate	977.8	E858.8	E947.8	E950.4	E962.0	E980.4
amytal	967.0	E851	E937.0	E950.1	E962.0	E980.1
arsenate – *see* Arsenic						
bicarbonate	963.3	E858.1	E933.3	E950.4	E962.0	E980.4
Sodium – *continued*						
bichromate	983.9	E864.3	–	E950.7	E962.1	E980.6
biphosphate	963.2	E858.1	E933.2	E950.4	E962.0	E980.4
bisulfate	983.9	E864.3	–	E950.7	E962.1	E980.6
borate (cleanser)	989.6	E861.3	–	E950.9	E962.1	E980.9
bromide NEC	967.3	E852.2	E937.3	E950.2	E962.0	E980.2
cacodylate (nonmedicinal) NEC	978.8	E858.8	E948.8	E950.4	E962.0	E980.4
anti-infective	961.1	E857	E931.1	E950.4	E962.0	E980.4
herbicide	989.4	E863.5	–	E950.6	E962.1	E980.7
calcium edetate	963.8	E858.1	E933.8	E950.4	E962.0	E980.4
carbonate NEC	983.2	E864.2	–	E950.7	E962.1	E980.6
chlorate NEC	983.9	E864.3	–	E950.7	E962.1	E980.6
herbicide	983.9	E863.5	–	E950.7	E962.1	E980.6
chloride NEC	974.5	E858.5	E944.5	E950.4	E962.0	E980.4
chromate	983.9	E864.3	–	E950.7	E962.1	E980.6
citrate	963.3	E858.1	E933.3	E950.4	E962.0	E980.4
cyanide – *see* Cyanide(s)						
cyclamate	974.5	E858.5	E944.5	E950.4	E962.0	E980.4
diatrizoate	977.8	E858.8	E947.8	E950.4	E962.0	E980.4
dibunate	975.4	E858.6	E945.4	E950.4	E962.0	E980.4
dioctyl sulfosuccinate	973.2	E858.4	E943.2	E950.4	E962.0	E980.4
edetate	963.8	E858.1	E933.8	E950.4	E962.0	E980.4
ethacrynate	974.4	E858.5	E944.4	E950.4	E962.0	E980.4
fluoracetate (dust) (rodenticide)	989.4	E863.7	–	E950.6	E962.1	E980.7
fluoride – *see* Fluoride(s)						
free salt	974.5	E858.5	E944.5	E950.4	E962.0	E980.4
glucosulfone	961.8	E857	E931.8	E950.4	E962.0	E980.4
hydroxide	983.2	E864.2	–	E950.7	E962.1	E980.6
hypochlorite (bleach) NEC	983.9	E864.3	–	E950.7	E962.1	E980.6
disinfectant	983.9	E861.4	–	E950.7	E962.1	E980.6
medicinal (anti-infective) (external)	976.0	E858.7	E946.0	E950.4	E962.0	E980.4
vapor	987.8	E869.8	–	E952.8	E962.2	E982.8
hyposulfite	976.0	E858.7	E946.0	E950.4	E962.0	E980.4
indigotindisulfonate	977.8	E858.8	E947.8	E950.4	E962.0	E980.4
iodide	977.8	E858.8	E947.8	E950.4	E962.0	E980.4
iothalamate	977.8	E858.8	E947.8	E950.4	E962.0	E980.4
iron edetate	964.0	E858.2	E934.0	E950.4	E962.0	E980.4
lactate	963.3	E858.1	E933.3	E950.4	E962.0	E980.4
lauryl sulfate	976.2	E858.7	E946.2	E950.4	E962.0	E980.4
L-triiodothyronine	962.7	E858.0	E932.7	E950.4	E962.0	E980.4
metrizoate	977.8	E858.8	E947.8	E950.4	E962.0	E980.4
monofluoracetate (dust) (rodenticide)	989.4	E863.7	–	E950.6	E962.1	E980.7
morrhuate	972.7	E858.3	E942.7	E950.4	E962.0	E980.4
nafcillin	960.0	E856	E930.0	E950.4	E962.0	E980.4
nitrate (oxidizing agent)	983.9	E864.3	–	E950.7	E962.1	E980.6
nitrite (medicinal)	972.4	E858.3	E942.4	E950.4	E962.0	E980.4
nitroferricyanide	972.6	E858.3	E942.6	E950.4	E962.0	E980.4
nitroprusside	972.6	E858.3	E942.6	E950.4	E962.0	E980.4
para-aminohippurate	977.8	E858.8	E947.8	E950.4	E962.0	E980.4
perborate (non-medicinal) NEC	989.89	E866.8	–	E950.9	E962.1	E980.9
medicinal	976.6	E858.7	E946.6	E950.4	E962.0	E980.4
soap	989.6	E861.1	–	E950.9	E962.1	E980.9
percarbonate – *see* Sodium, perborate						
phosphate	973.3	E858.4	E943.3	E950.4	E962.0	E980.4
polystyrene sulfonate	974.5	E858.5	E944.5	E950.4	E962.0	E980.4
propionate	976.0	E858.7	E946.0	E950.4	E962.0	E980.4
psylliate	972.7	E858.3	E942.7	E950.4	E962.0	E980.4
removing resins	974.5	E858.5	E944.5	E950.4	E962.0	E980.4
salicylate	965.1	E850.3	E935.3	E950.0	E962.0	E980.0
sulfate	973.3	E858.4	E943.3	E950.4	E962.0	E980.4
sulfoxone	961.8	E857	E931.8	E950.4	E962.0	E980.4
tetradecyl sulfate	972.7	E858.3	E942.7	E950.4	E962.0	E980.4
thiopental	968.3	E855.1	E938.3	E950.4	E962.0	E980.4
thiosalicylate	965.1	E850.3	E935.3	E950.0	E962.0	E980.0
thiosulfate	976.0	E858.7	E946.0	E950.4	E962.0	E980.4
tolbutdmide	977.8	E858.8	E947.8	E950.4	E962.0	E980.4
tyropanoate	977.8	E858.8	E947.8	E950.4	E962.0	E980.4
valproate	966.3	E855.0	E936.3	E950.4	E962.0	E980.4
Solanine	977.8	E858.8	E947.8	E950.4	E962.0	E980.4
Solanum dulcamara	988.2	E865.4	–	E950.9	E962.1	E980.9
Solapsone	961.8	E857	E931.8	E950.4	E962.0	E980.4
Solasulfone	961.8	E857	E931.8	E950.4	E962.0	E980.4
Soldering fluid	983.1	E864.1	–	E950.7	E962.1	E980.6
Solid substance	989.9	E866.9	–	E950.9	E962.1	E980.9
specified NEC	989.9	E866.8	–	E950.9	E962.1	E980.9
Solvents, industrial	982.8	E862.9	–	E950.9	E962.1	E980.9
naphtha	981	E862.0	–	E950.9	E962.1	E980.9
petroleum	981	E862.0	–	E950.9	E962.1	E980.9
specified NEC	982.8	E862.4	–	E950.9	E962.1	E980.9

Drug, chemical	Poisoning	External Cause (E Code)				
		Accident	Therapeutic Use	Suicide Attempt	Assault	Undetermined
Soma	968.0	E855.1	E938.0	E950.4	E962.0	E980.4
Somatotropin	962.4	E858.0	E932.4	E950.4	E962.0	E980.4
Sominex	963.0	E858.1	E933.0	E950.4	E962.0	E980.4
Somnos	967.1	E852.0	E937.1	E950.2	E962.0	E980.2
Somonal	967.0	E851	E937.0	E950.1	E962.0	E980.1
Soneryl	967.0	E851	E937.0	E950.1	E962.0	E980.1
Soothing syrup	977.9	E858.9	E947.9	E950.5	E962.0	E980.5
Sopor	967.4	E852.3	E937.4	E950.2	E962.0	E980.2
Soporific drug	967.9	E852.9	E937.9	E950.2	E962.0	E980.2
specified type NEC	967.8	E852.8	E937.8	E950.2	E962.0	E980.2
Sorbitol NEC	977.4	E858.8	E947.4	E950.4	E962.0	E980.4
Sotradecol	972.7	E858.3	E942.7	E950.4	E962.0	E980.4
Spacoline	975.1	E858.6	E945.1	E950.4	E962.0	E980.4
Spanish fly	976.8	E858.7	E946.8	E950.4	E962.0	E980.4
Sparine	969.1	E853.0	E939.1	E950.3	E962.0	E980.3
Sparteine	975.0	E858.6	E945.0	E950.4	E962.0	E980.4
Spasmolytics	975.1	E858.6	E945.1	E950.4	E962.0	E980.4
anticholinergics	971.1	E855.4	E941.1	E950.4	E962.0	E980.4
Spectinomycin	960.8	E856	E930.8	E950.4	E962.0	E980.4
Speed ▲	969.72	E854.2	E939.7	E950.3	E962.0	E980.3
Spermicides	976.8	E858.7	E946.8	E950.4	E962.0	E980.4
Spider (bite) (venom)	989.5	E905.1	–	E950.9	E962.1	E980.9
antivenin	979.9	E858.8	E949.9	E950.4	E962.0	E980.4
Spigelia (root)	961.6	E857	E931.6	E950.4	E962.0	E980.4
Spiperone	969.2	E853.1	E939.2	E950.3	E962.0	E980.3
Spiramycin	960.3	E856	E930.3	E950.4	E962.0	E980.4
Spirilene	969.5	E853.8	E939.5	E950.3	E962.0	E980.3
Spirit(s) (neutral) NEC	980.0	E860.1	–	E950.9	E962.1	E980.9
beverage	980.0	E860.0	–	E950.9	E962.1	E980.9
industrial	980.9	E860.9	–	E950.9	E962.1	E980.9
mineral	981	E862.0	–	E950.9	E962.1	E980.9
of salt – *see* Hydrochloric acid						
surgical	980.9	E860.9	–	E950.9	E962.1	E980.9
Spironolactone	974.4	E858.5	E944.4	E950.4	E962.0	E980.4
Sponge, absorbable (gelatin)	964.5	E858.2	E934.5	E950.4	E962.0	E980.4
Sporostacin	976.0	E858.7	E946.0	E950.4	E962.0	E980.4
Sprays (aerosol)	989.89	E866.8	–	E950.9	E962.1	E980.9
cosmetic	989.89	E866.7	–	E950.9	E962.1	E980.9
medicinal NEC	977.9	E858.9	E947.9	E950.5	E962.0	E980.5
pesticides – *see* Pesticides						
specified content – *see* substance specified						
Spurge flax	988.2	E865.4	–	E950.9	E962.1	E980.9
Spurges	988.2	E865.4	–	E950.9	E962.1	E980.9
Squill (expectorant) NEC	975.5	E858.6	E945.5	E950.4	E962.0	E980.4
rat poison	989.4	E863.7	–	E950.6	E962.1	E980.7
Squirting cucumber (cathartic)	973.1	E858.4	E943.1	E950.4	E962.0	E980.4
SSNRI (selective serotonin and norepinephrine reuptake inhibitors) ●	969.02	E854.0	E939.0	E950.3	E962.0	E980.3
SSRI (selective serotonin reuptake inhibitors) ●	969.03	E854.0	E939.0	E950.3	E962.0	E980.3
Stains	989.89	E866.8	–	E950.9	E962.1	E980.9
Stannous – *see also* Tin						
fluoride	976.7	E858.7	E946.7	E950.4	E962.0	E980.4
Stanolone	962.1	E858.0	E932.1	E950.4	E962.0	E980.4
Stanozolol	962.1	E858.0	E932.1	E950.4	E962.0	E980.4
Staphisagria or stavesacre (pediculicide)	976.0	E858.7	E946.0	E950.4	E962.0	E980.4
Stelazine	969.1	E853.0	E939.1	E950.3	E962.0	E980.3
Stemetil	969.1	E853.0	E939.1	E950.3	E962.0	E980.3
Sterculia (cathartic) (gum)	973.3	E858.4	E943.3	E950.4	E962.0	E980.4
Sternutator gas	987.8	E869.8	–	E952.8	E962.2	E982.8
Steroids NEC	962.0	E858.0	E932.0	E950.4	E962.0	E980.4
ENT agent	976.6	E858.7	E946.6	E950.4	E962.0	E980.4
ophthalmic preparation	976.5	E858.7	E946.5	E950.4	E962.0	E980.4
topical NEC	976.0	E858.7	E946.0	E950.4	E962.0	E980.4
Stibine	985.8	E866.4	–	E950.9	E962.1	E980.9
Stibophen	961.2	E857	E931.2	E950.4	E962.0	E980.4
Stilbamide, stilbamidine	961.5	E857	E931.5	E950.4	E962.0	E980.4
Stilbestrol	962.2	E858.0	E932.2	E950.4	E962.0	E980.4
Stimulants (central nervous system)	970.9	E854.3	E940.9	E950.4	E962.0	E980.4
analeptics	970.0	E854.3	E940.0	E950.4	E962.0	E980.4
opiate antagonist	970.1	E854.3	E940.1	E950.4	E962.0	E980.4
psychotherapeutic NEC ▲	969.09	E854.0	E939.0	E950.3	E962.0	E980.3
specified NEC	970.8	E854.3	E940.8	E950.4	E962.0	E980.4
Storage batteries (acid) (cells)	983.1	E864.1	–	E950.7	E962.1	E980.6
Stovaine	968.9	E855.2	E938.9	E950.4	E962.0	E980.4
infiltration (subcutaneous)	968.5	E855.2	E938.5	E950.4	E962.0	E980.4
nerve block (peripheral) (plexus)	968.6	E855.2	E938.6	E950.4	E962.0	E980.4
spinal	968.7	E855.2	E938.7	E950.4	E962.0	E980.4
topical (surface)	968.5	E855.2	E938.5	E950.4	E962.0	E980.4

Drug, chemical	Poisoning	External Cause (E Code)				
		Accident	Therapeutic Use	Suicide Attempt	Assault	Undetermined
Stovarsal	961.1	E857	E931.1	E950.4	E962.0	E980.4
Stove gas – *see* Gas, utility						
Stoxil	976.5	E858.7	E946.5	E950.4	E962.0	E980.4
STP	969.6	E854.1	E939.6	E950.3	E962.0	E980.3
Stramonium (medicinal) NEC	971.1	E855.4	E941.1	E950.4	E962.0	E980.4
natural state	988.2	E865.4	–	E950.9	E962.1	E980.9
Streptodornase	964.4	E858.2	E934.4	E950.4	E962.0	E980.4
Streptoduocin	960.6	E856	E930.6	E950.4	E962.0	E980.4
Streptokinase	964.4	E858.2	E934.4	E950.4	E962.0	E980.4
Streptomycin	960.6	E856	E930.6	E950.4	E962.0	E980.4
Streptozocin	960.7	E856	E930.7	E950.4	E962.0	E980.4
Stripper (paint) (solvent)	982.8	E862.9	–	E950.9	E962.1	E980.9
Strobane	989.2	E863.0	–	E950.6	E962.1	E980.7
Strophanthin	972.1	E858.3	E942.1	E950.4	E962.0	E980.4
Strophanthus hispidus or kombe	988.2	E865.4	–	E950.9	E962.1	E980.9
Strychnine (rodenticide) (salts)	989.1	E863.7	–	E950.6	E962.1	E980.7
medicinal NEC	970.8	E854.3	E940.8	E950.4	E962.0	E980.4
Strychnos (ignatii) – *see* Strychnine						
Styramate	968.0	E855.1	E938.0	E950.4	E962.0	E980.4
Styrene	983.0	E864.0	–	E950.7	E962.1	E980.6
Succinimide (anticonvulsant)	966.2	E855.0	E936.2	E950.4	E962.0	E980.4
mercuric – *see* Mercury						
Succinylcholine	975.2	E858.6	E945.2	E950.4	E962.0	E980.4
Succinylsulfathiazole	961.0	E857	E931.0	E950.4	E962.0	E980.4
Sucrose	974.5	E858.5	E944.5	E950.4	E962.0	E980.4
Sulfacetamide	961.0	E857	E931.0	E950.4	E962.0	E980.4
ophthalmic preparation	976.5	E858.7	E946.5	E950.4	E962.0	E980.4
Sulfachlorpyridazine	961.0	E857	E931.0	E950.4	E962.0	E980.4
Sulfacytine	961.0	E857	E931.0	E950.4	E962.0	E980.4
Sulfadiazine	961.0	E857	E931.0	E950.4	E962.0	E980.4
silver (topical)	976.0	E858.7	E946.0	E950.4	E962.0	E980.4
Sulfadimethoxine	961.0	E857	E931.0	E950.4	E962.0	E980.4
Sulfadimidine	961.0	E857	E931.0	E950.4	E962.0	E980.4
Sulfaethidole	961.0	E857	E931.0	E950.4	E962.0	E980.4
Sulfafurazole	961.0	E857	E931.0	E950.4	E962.0	E980.4
Sulfaguanidine	961.0	E857	E931.0	E950.4	E962.0	E980.4
Sulfamerazine	961.0	E857	E931.0	E950.4	E962.0	E980.4
Sulfameter	961.0	E857	E931.0	E950.4	E962.0	E980.4
Sulfamethizole	961.0	E857	E931.0	E950.4	E962.0	E980.4
Sulfamethoxazole	961.0	E857	E931.0	E950.4	E962.0	E980.4
Sulfamethoxydiazine	961.0	E857	E931.0	E950.4	E962.0	E980.4
Sulfamethoxypyridazine	961.0	E857	E931.0	E950.4	E962.0	E980.4
Sulfamethylthiazole	961.0	E857	E931.0	E950.4	E962.0	E980.4
Sulfamylon	976.0	E858.7	E946.0	E950.4	E962.0	E980.4
Sulfan blue (diagnostic dye)	977.8	E858.8	E947.8	E950.4	E962.0	E980.4
Sulfanilamide	961.0	E857	E931.0	E950.4	E962.0	E980.4
Sulfanilylguanidine	961.0	E857	E931.0	E950.4	E962.0	E980.4
Sulfaphenazole	961.0	E857	E931.0	E950.4	E962.0	E980.4
Sulfaphenylthiazole	961.0	E857	E931.0	E950.4	E962.0	E980.4
Sulfaproxyline	961.0	E857	E931.0	E950.4	E962.0	E980.4
Sulfapyridine	961.0	E857	E931.0	E950.4	E962.0	E980.4
Sulfapyrimidine	961.0	E857	E931.0	E950.4	E962.0	E980.4
Sulfarsphenamine	961.1	E857	E931.1	E950.4	E962.0	E980.4
Sulfasalazine	961.0	E857	E931.0	E950.4	E962.0	E980.4
Sulfasomizole	961.0	E857	E931.0	E950.4	E962.0	E980.4
Sulfasuxidine	961.0	E857	E931.0	E950.4	E962.0	E980.4
Sulfinpyrazone	974.7	E858.5	E944.7	E950.4	E962.0	E980.4
Sulfisoxazole	961.0	E857	E931.0	E950.4	E962.0	E980.4
ophthalmic preparation	976.5	E858.7	E946.5	E950.4	E962.0	E980.4
Sulfomyxin	960.8	E856	E930.8	E950.4	E962.0	E980.4
Sulfonal	967.8	E852.8	E937.8	E950.2	E962.0	E980.2
Sulfonamides (mixtures)	961.0	E857	E931.0	E950.4	E962.0	E980.4
Sulfones	961.8	E857	E931.8	E950.4	E962.0	E980.4
Sulfonethylmethane	967.8	E852.8	E937.8	E950.2	E962.0	E980.2
Sulfonmethane	967.8	E852.8	E937.8	E950.2	E962.0	E980.2
Sulfonphthal, sulfonphthol	977.8	E858.8	E947.8	E950.4	E962.0	E980.4
Sulfonylurea derivatives, oral	962.3	E858.0	E932.3	E950.4	E962.0	E980.4
Sulfoxone	961.8	E857	E931.8	E950.4	E962.0	E980.4
Sulfur, sulfureted, sulfuric, sulfurous, sulfuryl (compounds) NEC	989.89	E866.8	–	E950.9	E962.1	E980.9
acid	983.1	E864.1	–	E950.7	E962.1	E980.6
dioxide	987.3	E869.1	–	E952.8	E962.2	E982.8
ether – *see* Ether(s)						
hydrogen	987.8	E869.8	–	E952.8	E962.2	E982.8
medicinal (keratolytic) (ointment) NEC	976.4	E858.7	E946.4	E950.4	E962.0	E980.4
pesticide (vapor)	989.4	E863.4	–	E950.6	E962.1	E980.7
vapor NEC	987.8	E869.8	–	E952.8	E962.2	E982.8
Sulkowitch's reagent	977.8	E858.8	E947.8	E950.4	E962.0	E980.4
Sulph – *see also* Sulf-						
Sulphadione	961.8	E857	E931.8	E950.4	E962.0	E980.4

Drug, chemical	Poisoning	External Cause (E Code) Accident	Therapeutic Use	Suicide Attempt	Assault	Undetermined
Sulthiame, sultiame	966.3	E855.0	E936.3	E950.4	E962.0	E980.4
Superinone	975.5	E858.6	E945.5	E950.4	E962.0	E980.4
Suramin	961.5	E857	E931.5	E950.4	E962.0	E980.4
Surfacaine	968.5	E855.2	E938.5	E950.4	E962.0	E980.4
Surital	968.3	E855.1	E938.3	E950.4	E962.0	E980.4
Sutilains	976.8	E858.7	E946.8	E950.4	E962.0	E980.4
Suxamethonium (bromide) (chloride) (iodide)	975.2	E858.6	E945.2	E950.4	E962.0	E980.4
Suxethonium (bromide)	975.2	E858.6	E945.2	E950.4	E962.0	E980.4
Sweet oil (birch)	976.3	E858.7	E946.3	E950.4	E962.0	E980.4
Sym-dichloroethyl ether	982.3	E862.4	–	E950.9	E962.1	E980.9
Sympatholytics	971.3	E855.6	E941.3	E950.4	E962.0	E980.4
Sympathomimetics	971.2	E855.5	E941.2	E950.4	E962.0	E980.4
Synagis	979.6	E858.8	E949.6	E950.4	E962.0	E980.4
Synalar	976.0	E858.7	E946.0	E950.4	E962.0	E980.4
Synthroid	962.7	E858.0	E932.7	E950.4	E962.0	E980.4
Syntocinon	975.0	E858.6	E945.0	E950.4	E962.0	E950.4
Syrosingopine	972.6	E858.3	E942.6	E950.4	E962.0	E980.4
Systemic agents (primarily)	963.9	E858.1	E933.9	E950.4	E962.0	E980.4
specified NEC	963.8	E858.1	E933.8	E950.4	E962.0	E980.4
Tablets (*see also* specified substance)	977.9	E858.9	E947.9	E950.5	E962.0	E980.5
Tace	962.2	E858.0	E932.2	E950.4	E962.0	E980.4
Tacrine	971.0	E855.3	E941.0	E950.4	E962.0	E980.4
Talbutal	967.0	E851	E937.0	E950.1	E962.0	E980.1
Talc	976.3	E858.7	E946.3	E950.4	E962.0	E980.4
Talcum	976.3	E858.7	E946.3	E950.4	E962.0	E980.4
Tamsulosin	971.3	E855.6	E941.3	E950.4	E962.0	E980.4
Tandearil, tanderil	965.5	E850.5	E935.5	E950.0	E962.0	E980.0
Tannic acid	983.1	E864.1	–	E950.7	E962.1	E980.6
medicinal (astringent)	976.2	E858.7	E946.2	E950.4	E962.0	E980.4
Tannin – *see* Tannic acid						
Tansy	988.2	E865.4	–	E950.9	E962.1	E980.9
TAO	960.3	E856	E930.3	E950.4	E962.0	E980.4
Tapazole	962.8	E858.0	E932.8	E950.4	E962.0	E980.4
Tar NEC	983.0	E864.0	–	E950.7	E962.1	E980.6
camphor – *see* Naphthalene						
fumes	987.8	E869.8	–	E952.8	E962.2	E982.8
Taractan	969.3	E853.8	E939.3	E950.3	E962.0	E980.3
Tarantula (venomous)	989.5	E905.1	–	E950.9	E962.1	E980.9
Tartar emetic (anti-infective)	961.2	E857	E931.2	E950.4	E962.0	E980.4
Tartaric acid	983.1	E864.1	–	E950.7	E962.1	E980.6
Tartrated antimony (anti-infective)	961.2	E857	E931.2	E950.4	E962.0	E980.4
TCA – *see* Trichloroacetic acid						
TDI	983.0	E864.0	–	E950.7	E962.1	E980.6
vapor	987.8	E869.8	–	E952.8	E962.2	E982.8
Tear gas	987.5	E869.3	–	E952.8	E962.2	E982.8
Teclothiazide	974.3	E858.5	E944.3	E950.4	E962.0	E980.4
Tegretol	966.3	E855.0	E936.3	E950.4	E962.0	E980.4
Telepaque	977.8	E858.8	E947.8	E950.4	E962.0	E980.4
Tellurium	985.8	E866.4	–	E950.9	E962.1	E980.9
fumes	985.8	E866.4	–	E950.9	E962.1	E980.9
TEM	963.1	E858.1	E933.1	E950.4	E962.0	E980.4
Temazepan – *see* Benzodiazepines						
TEPA	963.1	E858.1	E933.1	E950.4	E962.0	E980.4
TEPP	989.3	E863.1	–	E950.6	E962.1	E980.7
Terbutaline	971.2	E855.5	E941.2	E950.4	E962.0	E980.4
Teroxalene	961.6	E857	E931.6	E950.4	E962.0	E980.4
Terpin hydrate	975.5	E858.6	E945.5	E950.4	E962.0	E980.4
Terramycin	960.4	E856	E930.4	E950.4	E962.0	E980.4
Tessalon	975.4	E858.6	E945.4	E950.4	E962.0	E980.4
Testosterone	962.1	E858.0	E932.1	E950.4	E962.0	E980.4
Tetanus (vaccine)	978.4	E858.8	E948.4	E950.4	E962.0	E980.4
antitoxin	979.9	E858.8	E949.9	E950.4	E962.0	E980.4
immune globulin (human)	964.6	E858.2	E934.6	E950.4	E962.0	E980.4
toxoid	978.4	E858.8	E948.4	E950.4	E962.0	E980.4
with diphtheria toxoid	978.9	E858.8	E948.9	E950.4	E962.0	E980.4
with pertussis	978.6	E858.8	E948.6	E950.4	E962.0	E980.4
Tetrabenazine	969.5	E853.8	E939.5	E950.3	E962.0	E980.3
Tetracaine (infiltration) (topical)	968.5	E855.2	E938.5	E950.4	E962.0	E980.4
nerve block (peripheral) (plexus)	968.6	E855.2	E938.6	E950.4	E962.0	E980.4
spinal	968.7	E855.2	E938.7	E950.4	E962.0	E980.4
Tetrachlorethylene – *see* Tetrachloroethylene						
Tetrachlormethiazide	974.3	E858.5	E944.3	E950.4	E962.0	E980.4
Tetrachloroethane (liquid) (vapor)	982.3	E862.4	–	E950.9	E962.1	E980.9
paint or varnish	982.3	E861.6	–	E950.9	E962.1	E980.9
Tetrachloroethylene (liquid) (vapor)	982.3	E862.4	–	E950.9	E962.1	E980.9
medicinal	961.6	E857	E931.6	E950.4	E962.0	E980.4
Tetrachloromethane – *see* Carbon, tetrachloride						
Tetracycline	960.4	E856	E930.4	E950.4	E962.0	E980.4
ophthalmic preparation	976.5	E858.7	E946.5	E950.4	E962.0	E980.4
Tetracycline – *continued*						
topical NEC	976.0	E858.7	E946.0	E950.4	E962.0	E980.4
Tetraethylammonium chloride	972.3	E858.3	E942.3	E950.4	E962.0	E980.4
Tetraethyl lead (antiknock compound)	984.1	E862.1	–	E950.9	E962.1	E980.9
Tetraethyl pyrophosphate	989.3	E863.1	–	E950.6	E962.1	E980.7
Tetraethylthiuram disulfide	977.3	E858.8	E947.3	E950.4	E962.0	E980.4
Tetrahydroaminoacridine	971.0	E855.3	E941.0	E950.4	E962.0	E980.4
Tetrahydrocannabinol	969.6	E854.1	E939.6	E950.3	E962.0	E980.3
Tetrahydronaphthalene	982.0	E862.4	–	E950.9	E962.1	E980.9
Tetrahydrozoline	971.2	E855.5	E941.2	E950.4	E962.0	E980.4
Tetralin	982.0	E862.4	–	E950.9	E962.1	E980.9
Tetramethylthiuram (disulfide) NEC	989.4	E863.6	–	E950.6	E962.1	E980.7
medicinal	976.2	E858.7	E946.2	E950.4	E962.0	E980.4
Tetronal	967.8	E852.8	E937.8	E950.2	E962.0	E980.2
Tetryl	983.0	E864.0	–	E950.7	E962.1	E980.6
Thalidomide	967.8	E852.8	E937.8	E950.2	E962.0	E980.2
Thallium (compounds) (dust) NEC	985.8	E866.4	–	E950.9	E962.1	E980.9
pesticide (rodenticide)	985.8	E863.7	–	E950.6	E962.1	E980.7
THC	969.6	E854.1	E939.6	E950.3	E962.0	E980.3
Thebacon	965.09	E850.2	E935.2	E950.0	E962.0	E980.0
Thebaine	965.09	E850.2	E935.2	E950.0	E962.0	E980.0
Theobromine (calcium salicylate)	974.1	E858.5	E944.1	E950.4	E962.0	E980.4
Theophylline (diuretic)	974.1	E858.5	E944.1	E950.4	E962.0	E980.4
ethylenediamine	975.7	E858.6	E945.7	E950.4	E962.0	E980.4
Thiabendazole	961.6	E857	E931.6	E950.4	E962.0	E980.4
Thialbarbital, thialbarbitone	968.3	E855.1	E938.3	E950.4	E962.0	E980.4
Thiamine	963.5	E858.1	E933.5	E950.4	E962.0	E980.4
Thiamylal (sodium)	968.3	E855.1	E938.3	E950.4	E962.0	E980.4
Thiazesim ▲	969.09	E854.0	E939.0	E950.3	E962.0	E980.3
Thiazides (diuretics)	974.3	E858.5	E944.3	E950.4	E962.0	E980.4
Thiethylperazine	963.0	E858.1	E933.0	E950.4	E962.0	E980.4
Thimerosal (topical)	976.0	E858.7	E946.0	E950.4	E962.0	E980.4
ophthalmic preparation	976.5	E858.7	E946.5	E950.4	E962.0	E980.4
Thioacetazone	961.8	E857	E931.8	E950.4	E962.0	E980.4
Thiobarbiturates	968.3	E855.1	E938.3	E950.4	E962.0	E980.4
Thiobismol	961.2	E857	E931.2	E950.4	E962.0	E980.4
Thiocarbamide	962.8	E858.0	E932.8	E950.4	E962.0	E980.4
Thiocarbarsone	961.1	E857	E931.1	E950.4	E962.0	E980.4
Thiocarlide	961.8	E857	E931.8	E950.4	E962.0	E980.4
Thioguanine	963.1	E858.1	E933.1	E950.4	E962.0	E980.4
Thiomercaptomerin	974.0	E858.5	E944.0	E950.4	E962.0	E980.4
Thiomerin	974.0	E858.5	E944.0	E950.4	E962.0	E980.4
Thiopental, thiopentone (sodium)	968.3	E855.1	E938.3	E950.4	E962.0	E980.4
Thiopropazate	969.1	E853.0	E939.1	E950.3	E962.0	E980.3
Thioproperazine	969.1	E853.0	E939.1	E950.3	E962.0	E980.3
Thioridazine	969.1	E853.0	E939.1	E950.3	E962.0	E980.3
Thio-TEPA, thiotepa	963.1	E858.1	E933.1	E950.4	E962.0	E980.4
Thiothixene	969.3	E853.8	E939.3	E950.3	E962.0	E980.3
Thiouracil	962.8	E858.0	E932.8	E950.4	E962.0	E980.4
Thiourea	962.8	E858.0	E932.8	E950.4	E962.0	E980.4
Thiphenamil	971.1	E855.4	E941.1	E950.4	E962.0	E980.4
Thiram NEC	989.4	E863.6	–	E950.6	E962.1	E980.7
medicinal	976.2	E858.7	E946.2	E950.4	E962.0	E980.4
Thonzylamine	963.0	E858.1	E933.0	E950.4	E962.0	E980.4
Thorazine	969.1	E853.0	E939.1	E950.3	E962.0	E980.3
Thornapple	988.2	E865.4	–	E950.9	E962.1	E980.9
Throat preparation (lozenges) **NEC**	976.6	E858.7	E946.6	E950.4	E962.0	E980.4
Thrombin	964.5	E858.2	E934.5	E950.4	E962.0	E980.4
Thrombolysin	964.4	E858.2	E934.4	E950.4	E962.0	E980.4
Thymol	983.0	E864.0	–	E950.7	E962.1	E980.6
Thymus extract	962.9	E858.0	E932.9	E950.4	E962.0	E980.4
Thyroglobulin	962.7	E858.0	E932.7	E950.4	E962.0	E980.4
Thyroid (derivatives) (extract)	962.7	E858.0	E932.7	E950.4	E962.0	E980.4
Thyrolar	962.7	E858.0	E932.7	E950.4	E962.0	E980.4
Thyrothrophin, thyrotropin	977.8	E858.8	E947.8	E950.4	E962.0	E980.4
Thyroxin(e)	962.7	E858.0	E932.7	E950.4	E962.0	E980.4
Tigan	963.0	E858.1	E933.0	E950.4	E962.0	E980.4
Tigloidine	968.0	E855.1	E938.0	E950.4	E962.0	E980.4
Tin (chloride) (dust) (oxide) NEC	985.8	E866.4	–	E950.9	E962.1	E980.9
anti-infectives	961.2	E857	E931.2	E950.4	E962.0	E980.4
Tinactin	976.0	E858.7	E946.0	E950.4	E962.0	E980.4
Tincture, iodine – *see* Iodine						
Tindal	969.1	E853.0	E939.1	E950.3	E962.0	E980.3
Titanium (compounds) (vapor)	985.8	E866.4	–	E950.9	E962.1	E980.9
ointment	976.3	E858.7	E946.3	E950.4	E962.0	E980.4
Titroid	962.7	E858.0	E932.7	E950.4	E962.0	E980.4
TMTD – *see* Tetramethylthiuram disulfide						
TNT	989.89	E866.8	–	E950.9	E962.1	E980.9
fumes	987.8	E869.8	–	E952.8	E962.2	E982.8

Drug, chemical	Poisoning	External Cause (E Code)				
		Accident	Therapeutic Use	Suicide Attempt	Assault	Undetermined
Toadstool	988.1	E865.5	–	E950.9	E962.1	E980.9
Tobacco NEC	989.84	E866.8	–	E950.9	E962.1	E980.9
Indian	988.2	E865.4	–	E950.9	E962.1	E980.9
smoke, second-hand	987.8	E869.4	–	–	–	–
Tocopherol	963.5	E858.1	E933.5	E950.4	E962.0	E980.4
Tocosamine	975.0	E858.6	E945.0	E950.4	E962.0	E980.4
Tofranil ▲	969.05	E854.0	E939.0	E950.3	E962.0	E980.3
Toilet deodorizer	989.89	E866.8	–	E950.9	E962.1	E980.9
Tolazamide	962.3	E858.0	E932.3	E950.4	E962.0	E980.4
Tolazoline	971.3	E855.6	E941.3	E950.4	E962.0	E980.4
Tolbutamide	962.3	E858.0	E932.3	E950.4	E962.0	E980.4
sodium	977.8	E858.8	E947.8	E950.4	E962.0	E980.4
Tolmetin	965.69	E850.6	E935.6	E950.0	E962.0	E980.0
Tolnaftate	976.0	E858.7	E946.0	E950.4	E962.0	E980.4
Tolpropamine	976.1	E858.7	E946.1	E950.4	E962.0	E980.4
Tolserol	968.0	E855.1	E938.0	E950.4	E962.0	E980.4
Toluene (liquid) (vapor)	982.0	E862.4	–	E950.9	E962.1	E980.9
diisocyanate	983.0	E864.0	–	E950.7	E962.1	E980.6
Toluidine	983.0	E864.0	–	E950.7	E962.1	E980.6
vapor	987.8	E869.8	–	E952.8	E962.2	E982.8
Toluol (liquid) (vapor)	982.0	E862.4	–	E950.9	E962.1	E980.9
Tolylene-2,4-diisocyanate	983.0	E864.0	–	E950.7	E962.1	E980.6
Tonics, cardiac	972.1	E858.3	E942.1	E950.4	E962.0	E980.4
Toxaphene (dust) (spray)	989.2	E863.0	–	E950.6	E962.1	E980.7
Toxoids NEC	978.8	E858.8	E948.8	E950.4	E962.0	E980.4
Tractor fuel NEC	981	E862.1	–	E950.9	E962.1	E980.9
Tragacanth	973.3	E858.4	E943.3	E950.4	E962.0	E980.4
Traniazoline	971.2	E855.5	E941.2	E950.4	E962.0	E980.4
Tranquilizers	969.5	E853.9	E939.5	E950.3	E962.0	E980.3
benzodiazepine-based	969.4	E853.2	E939.4	E950.3	E962.0	E980.3
butyropherione-based	969.2	E853.1	E939.2	E950.3	E962.0	E980.3
major NEC	969.3	E853.8	E939.3	E950.3	E962.0	E980.3
phenothiazine-based	969.1	E853.0	E939.1	E950.3	E962.0	E980.3
specified NEC	969.5	E853.8	E939.5	E950.3	E962.0	E980.3
Trantoin	961.9	E857	E931.9	E950.4	E962.0	E980.4
Tranxene	969.4	E853.2	E939.4	E950.3	E962.0	E980.3
Tranylcypromine (sulfate) ▲	969.01	E854.0	E939.0	E950.3	E962.0	E980.3
Trasentine	975.1	E858.6	E945.1	E950.4	E962.0	E980.4
Travert	974.5	E858.5	E944.5	E950.4	E962.0	E980.4
Trecator	961.8	E857	E931.8	E950.4	E962.0	E980.4
Tretinoin	976.8	E858.7	E946.8	E950.4	E962.0	E980.4
Triacetin	976.0	E858.7	E946.0	E950.4	E962.0	E980.4
Triacetyloleandomycin	960.3	E856	E930.3	E950.4	E962.0	E980.4
Triamcinolone	962.0	E858.0	E932.0	E950.4	E962.0	E980.4
ENT agent	976.6	E858.7	E946.6	E950.4	E962.0	E980.4
ophthalmic preparation	976.5	E858.7	E946.5	E950.4	E962.0	E980.4
topical NEC	976.0	E858.7	E946.0	E950.4	E962.0	E980.4
Triamterene	974.4	E858.5	E944.4	E950.4	E962.0	E980.4
Triaziquone	963.1	E858.1	E933.1	E950.4	E962.0	E980.4
Tribromacetaldehyde	967.3	E852.2	E937.3	E950.2	E962.0	E980.2
Tribromoethanol	968.2	E855.1	E938.2	E950.4	E962.0	E980.4
Tribromomethane	967.3	E852.2	E937.3	E950.2	E962.0	E980.2
Trichlorethane	982.3	E862.4	–	E950.9	E962.1	E980.9
Trichlormethiazide	974.3	E858.5	E944.3	E950.4	E962.0	E980.4
Trichloroacetic acid	983.1	E864.1	–	E950.7	E962.1	E980.6
medicinal (keratolytic)	976.4	E858.7	E946.4	E950.4	E962.0	E980.4
Trichloroethanol	967.1	E852.0	E937.1	E950.2	E962.0	E980.2
Trichloroethylene (liquid) (vapor)	982.3	E862.4	–	E950.9	E962.1	E980.9
anesthetic (gas)	968.2	E855.1	E938.2	E950.4	E962.0	E980.4
Trichloroethyl phosphate	967.1	E852.0	E937.1	E950.2	E962.0	E980.2
Trichlorofluoromethane NEC	987.4	E869.2	–	E952.8	E962.2	E982.8
Trichlorotriethylamine	963.1	E858.1	E933.1	E950.4	E962.0	E980.4
Trichomonacides NEC	961.5	E857	E931.5	E950.4	E962.0	E980.4
Trichomycin	960.1	E856	E930.1	E950.4	E962.0	E980.4
Triclofos	967.1	E852.0	E937.1	E950.2	E962.0	E980.2
Tricresyl phosphate	989.89	E866.8	–	E950.9	E962.1	E980.9
solvent	982.8	E862.4	–	E950.9	E962.1	E980.9
Tricyclamol	966.4	E855.0	E936.4	E950.4	E962.0	E980.4
Tridesilon	976.0	E858.7	E946.0	E950.4	E962.0	E980.4
Tridihexethyl	971.1	E855.4	E941.1	E950.4	E962.0	E980.4
Tridione	966.0	E855.0	E936.0	E950.4	E962.0	E980.4
Triethanolamine NEC	983.2	E864.2	–	E950.7	E962.1	E980.6
detergent	983.2	E861.0	–	E950.7	E962.1	E980.6
trinitrate	972.4	E858.3	E942.4	E950.4	E962.0	E980.4
Triethanomelamine	963.1	E858.1	E933.1	E950.4	E962.0	E980.4
Triethylene melamine	963.1	E858.1	E933.1	E950.4	E962.0	E980.4
Triethylenephosphoramide	963.1	E858.1	E933.1	E950.4	E962.0	E980.4
Triethylenethiophos-phoramide	963.1	E858.1	E933.1	E950.4	E962.0	E980.4
Trifluoperazine	969.1	E853.0	E939.1	E950.3	E962.0	E980.3
Trifluperidol	969.2	E853.1	E939.2	E950.3	E962.0	E980.3
Triflupromazine	969.1	E853.0	E939.1	E950.3	E962.0	E980.3
Trihexyphenidyl	971.1	E855.4	E941.1	E950.4	E962.0	E980.4

Drug, chemical	Poisoning	External Cause (E Code)				
		Accident	Therapeutic Use	Suicide Attempt	Assault	Undetermined
Triiodothyronine	962.7	E858.0	E932.7	E950.4	E962.0	E980.4
Trilene	968.2	E855.1	E938.2	E950.4	E962.0	E980.4
Trimeprazine	963.0	E858.1	E933.0	E950.4	E962.0	E980.4
Trimetazidine	972.4	E858.3	E942.4	E950.4	E962.0	E980.4
Trimethadione	966.0	E855.0	E936.0	E950.4	E962.0	E980.4
Trimethaphan	972.3	E858.3	E942.3	E950.4	E962.0	E980.4
Trimethidinium	972.3	E858.3	E942.3	E950.4	E962.0	E980.4
Trimethobenzamide	963.0	E858.1	E933.0	E950.4	E962.0	E980.4
Trimethylcarbinol	980.8	E860.8	–	E950.9	E962.1	E980.9
Trimethylpsoralen	976.3	E858.7	E946.3	E950.4	E962.0	E980.4
Trimeton	963.0	E858.1	E933.0	E950.4	E962.0	E980.4
Trimipramine ▲	969.05	E854.0	E939.0	E950.3	E962.0	E980.3
Trimustine	963.1	E858.1	E933.1	E950.4	E962.0	E980.4
Trinitrin	972.4	E858.3	E942.4	E950.4	E962.0	E980.4
Trinitrophenol	983.0	E864.0	–	E950.7	E962.1	E980.6
Trinitrotoluene	989.89	E866.8	–	E950.9	E962.1	E980.9
fumes	987.8	E869.8	–	E952.8	E962.2	E982.8
Trional	967.8	E852.8	E937.8	E950.2	E962.0	E980.2
Trioxide of arsenic – *see* Arsenic						
Trioxsalen	976.3	E858.7	E946.3	E950.4	E962.0	E980.4
Tripelennamine	963.0	E858.1	E933.0	E950.4	E962.0	E980.4
Triperidol	969.2	E853.1	E939.2	E950.3	E962.0	E980.3
Triprolidine	963.0	E858.1	E933.0	E950.4	E962.0	E980.4
Trisoralen	976.3	E858.7	E946.3	E950.4	E962.0	E980.4
Troleandomycin	960.3	E856	E930.3	E950.4	E962.0	E980.4
Trolnitrate (phosphate)	972.4	E858.3	E942.4	E950.4	E962.0	E980.4
Trometamol	963.3	E858.1	E933.3	E950.4	E962.0	E980.4
Tromethamine	963.3	E858.1	E933.3	E950.4	E962.0	E980.4
Tronothane	968.5	E855.2	E938.5	E950.4	E962.0	E980.4
Tropicamide	971.1	E855.4	E941.1	E950.4	E962.0	E980.4
Troxidone	966.0	E855.0	E936.0	E950.4	E962.0	E980.4
Tryparsamide	961.1	E857	E931.1	E950.4	E962.0	E980.4
Trypsin	963.4	E858.1	E933.4	E950.4	E962.0	E980.4
Tryptizol ▲	969.05	E854.0	E939.0	E950.3	E962.0	E980.3
Tuaminoheptane	971.2	E855.5	E941.2	E950.4	E962.0	E980.4
Tuberculin (old)	977.8	E858.8	E947.8	E950.4	E962.0	E980.4
Tubocurare	975.2	E858.6	E945.2	E950.4	E962.0	E980.4
Tubocurarine	975.2	E858.6	E945.2	E950.4	E962.0	E980.4
Turkish green	969.6	E854.1	E939.6	E950.3	E962.0	E980.3
Turpentine (spirits of) (liquid) (vapor)	982.8	E862.4	–	E950.9	E962.1	E980.9
Tybamate	969.5	E853.8	E939.5	E950.3	E962.0	E980.3
Tyloxapol	975.5	E858.6	E945.5	E950.4	E962.0	E980.4
Tymazoline	971.2	E855.5	E941.2	E950.4	E962.0	E980.4
Typhoid vaccine	978.1	E858.8	E948.1	E950.4	E962.0	E980.4
Typhus vaccine	979.2	E858.8	E949.2	E950.4	E962.0	E980.4
Tyrothricin	976.0	E858.7	E946.0	E950.4	E962.0	E980.4
ENT agent	976.6	E858.7	E946.6	E950.4	E962.0	E980.4
ophthalmic preparation	976.5	E858.7	E946.5	E950.4	E962.0	E980.4
Undecenoic acid	976.0	E858.7	E946.0	E950.4	E962.0	E980.4
Undecylenic acid	976.0	E858.7	E946.0	E950.4	E962.0	E980.4
Unna's boot	976.3	E858.7	E946.3	E950.4	E962.0	E980.4
Uracil mustard	963.1	E858.1	E933.1	E950.4	E962.0	E980.4
Uramustine	963.1	E858.1	E933.1	E950.4	E962.0	E980.4
Urari	975.2	E858.6	E945.2	E950.4	E962.0	E980.4
Urea	974.4	E858.5	E944.4	E950.4	E962.0	E980.4
topical	976.8	E858.7	E946.8	E950.4	E962.0	E980.4
Urethan(e) (antineoplastic)	963.1	E858.1	E933.1	E950.4	E962.0	E980.4
Urginea (maritima) (scilla) – *see* Squill						
Uric acid metabolism agents NEC	974.7	E858.5	E944.7	E950.4	E962.0	E980.4
Urokinase	964.4	E858.2	E934.4	E950.4	E962.0	E980.4
Urokon	977.8	E858.8	E947.8	E950.4	E962.0	E980.4
Urotropin	961.9	E857	E931.9	E950.4	E962.0	E980.4
Urtica	988.2	E865.4	–	E950.9	E962.1	E980.9
Utility gas – *see* Gas, utility						
Vaccine NEC	979.9	E858.8	E949.9	E950.4	E962.0	E980.4
bacterial NEC	978.8	E858.8	E948.8	E950.4	E962.0	E980.4
with						
other bacterial component	978.9	E858.8	E948.9	E950.4	E962.0	E980.
pertussis component	978.6	E858.8	E948.6	E950.4	E962.0	E980.4
viral-rickettsial component	979.7	E858.8	E949.7	E950.4	E962.0	E980.4
mixed NEC	978.9	E858.8	E948.9	E950.4	E962.0	E980.4
BCG	978.0	E858.8	E948.0	E950.4	E962.0	E980.4
cholera	978.2	E858.8	E948.2	E950.4	E962.0	E980.4
diphtheria	978.5	E858.8	E948.5	E950.4	E962.0	E980.4
influenza	979.6	E858.8	E949.6	E950.4	E962.0	E980.4
measles	979.4	E858.8	E949.4	E950.4	E962.0	E980.4
meningococcal	978.8	E858.8	E948.8	E950.4	E962.0	E980.4
mumps	979.6	E858.8	E949.6	E950.4	E962.0	E980.4
paratyphoid	978.1	E858.8	E948.1	E950.4	E962.0	E980.4

Drug, chemical	Poisoning	External Cause (E Code)				
		Accident	Therapeutic Use	Suicide Attempt	Assault	Undetermined
Vaccine – *continued*						
pertussis (with diphtheria toxoid) (with tetanus toxoid)	978.6	E858.8	E948.6	E950.4	E962.0	E980.4
plague	978.3	E858.8	E948.3	E950.4	E962.0	E980.4
poliomyelitis	979.5	E858.8	E949.5	E950.4	E962.0	E980.4
poliovirus	979.5	E858.8	E949.5	E950.4	E962.0	E980.4
rabies	979.1	E858.8	E949.1	E950.4	E962.0	E980.4
respiratory syncytial virus	979.6	E858.8	E949.6	E950.4	E962.0	E980.4
rickettsial NEC	979.6	E858.8	E949.6	E950.4	E962.0	E980.4
with bacterial component	979.7	E858.8	E949.7	E950.4	E962.0	E980.4
pertussis component	978.6	E858.8	E948.6	E950.4	E962.0	E980.4
viral component	979.7	E858.8	E949.7	E950.4	E962.0	E980.4
Rocky mountain spotted fever	979.6	E858.8	E949.6	E950.4	E962.0	E980.4
rotavirus	979.6	E858.8	E949.6	E950.4	E962.0	E980.4
rubella virus	979.4	E858.8	E949.4	E950.4	E962.0	E980.4
sabin oral	979.5	E858.8	E949.5	E950.4	E962.0	E980.4
smallpox	979.0	E858.8	E949.0	E950.4	E962.0	E980.4
tetanus	978.4	E858.8	E948.4	E950.4	E962.0	E980.4
typhoid	978.1	E858.8	E948.1	E950.4	E962.0	E980.4
typhus	979.2	E858.8	E949.2	E950.4	E962.0	E980.4
viral NEC	979.6	E858.8	E949.6	E950.4	E962.0	E980.4
with						
bacterial component	979.7	E858.8	E949.7	E950.4	E962.0	E980.4
pertussis component	978.6	E858.8	E948.6	E950.4	E962.0	E980.4
rickettsial component	979.7	E858.8	E949.7	E950.4	E962.0	E980.4
yellow fever	979.3	E858.8	E949.3	E950.4	E962.0	E980.4
Vaccinia immune globulin (human)	964.6	E858.2	E934.6	E950.4	E962.0	E980.4
Vaginal contraceptives	976.8	E858.7	E946.8	E950.4	E962.0	E980.4
Valethamate	971.1	E855.4	E941.1	E950.4	E962.0	E980.4
Valisone	976.0	E858.7	E946.0	E950.4	E962.0	E980.4
Valium	969.4	E853.2	E939.4	E950.3	E962.0	E980.3
Valmid	967.8	E852.8	E937.8	E950.2	E962.0	E980.2
Vanadium	985.8	E866.4	–	E950.9	E962.1	E980.9
Vancomycin	960.8	E856	E930.8	E950.4	E962.0	E980.4
Vapor (*see also* Gas)	987.9	E869.9	–	E952.9	E962.2	E982.9
kiln (carbon monoxide)	986	E868.8	–	E952.1	E962.2	E982.1
lead – *see* Lead						
specified source NEC – (*see* also specific substance)	987.8	E869.8	–	E952.8	E962.2	E982.8
Varidase	964.4	E858.2	E934.4	E950.4	E962.0	E980.4
Varnish	989.89	E861.6	–	E950.9	E962.1	E980.9
cleaner	982.8	E862.9	–	E950.9	E962.1	E980.9
Vaseline	976.3	E858.7	E946.3	E950.4	E962.0	E980.4
Vasodilan	972.5	E858.3	E942.5	E950.4	E962.0	E980.4
Vasodilators NEC	972.5	E858.3	E942.5	E950.4	E962.0	E980.4
coronary	972.4	E858.3	E942.4	E950.4	E962.0	E980.4
Vasopressin	962.5	E858.0	E932.5	E950.4	E962.0	E980.4
Vasopressor drugs	962.5	E858.0	E932.5	E950.4	E962.0	E980.4
Venom, venomous (bite) (sting)	989.5	E905.9	–	E950.9	E962.1	E980.9
arthropod NEC	989.5	E905.5	–	E950.9	E962.1	E980.9
bee	989.5	E905.3	–	E950.9	E962.1	E980.9
centipede	989.5	E905.4	–	E950.9	E962.1	E980.9
hornet	989.5	E905.3	–	E950.9	E962.1	E980.9
lizard	989.5	E905.0	–	E950.9	E962.1	E980.9
marine animals or plants	989.5	E905.6	–	E950.9	E962.1	E980.9
millipede (tropical)	989.5	E905.4	–	E950.9	E962.1	E980.9
plant NEC	989.5	E905.7	–	E950.9	E962.1	E980.9
marine	989.5	E905.6	–	E950.9	E962.1	E980.9
scorpion	989.5	E905.2	–	E950.9	E962.1	E980.9
snake	989.5	E905.0	–	E950.9	E962.1	E980.9
specified NEC	989.5	E905.8	–	E950.9	E962.1	E980.9
spider	989.5	E905.1	–	E950.9	E962.1	E980.9
wasp	989.5	E905.3	–	E950.9	E962.1	E980.9
Ventolin – *see* Salbutamol sulfate						
Veramon	967.0	E851	E937.0	E950.1	E962.0	E980.1
Veratrum						
album	988.2	E865.4	–	E950.9	E962.1	E980.9
alkaloids	972.6	E858.3	E942.6	E950.4	E962.0	E980.4
viride	988.2	E865.4	–	E950.9	E962.1	E980.9
Verdigris (*see also* Copper)	985.8	E866.4	–	E950.9	E962.1	E980.9
Veronal	967.0	E851	E937.0	E950.1	E962.0	E980.1
Veroxil	961.6	E857	E931.6	E950.4	E962.0	E980.4
Versidyne	965.7	E850.7	E935.7	E950.0	E962.0	E980.0
Viagra	972.5	E858.3	E942.5	E950.4	E962.0	E980.4
Vienna						
green	985.1	E866.3	–	E950.8	E962.1	E980.8
insecticide	985.1	E863.4	–	E950.6	E962.1	E980.7
red	989.89	E866.8	–	E950.9	E962.1	E980.9
pharmaceutical dye	977.4	E858.8	E947.4	E950.4	E962.0	E980.4
Vinbarbital, vinbarbitone	967.0	E851	E937.0	E950.1	E962.0	E980.1
Vinblastine	963.1	E858.1	E933.1	E950.4	E962.0	E980.4
Vincristine	963.1	E858.1	E933.1	E950.4	E962.0	E980.4
Vinesthene, vinethene	968.2	E855.1	E938.2	E950.4	E962.0	E980.4
Vinyl						
bital	967.0	E851	E937.0	E950.1	E962.0	E980.1
ether	968.2	E855.1	E938.2	E950.4	E962.0	E980.4
Vioform	961.3	E857	E931.3	E950.4	E962.0	E980.4
topical	976.0	E858.7	E946.0	E950.4	E962.0	E980.4
Viomycin	960.6	E856	E930.6	E950.4	E962.0	E980.4
Viosterol	963.5	E858.1	E933.5	E950.4	E962.0	E980.4
Viper (venom)	989.5	E905.0	–	E950.9	E962.1	E980.9
Viprynium (embonate)	961.6	E857	E931.6	E950.4	E962.0	E980.4
Virugon	961.7	E857	E931.7	E950.4	E962.0	E980.4
Visine	976.5	E858.7	E946.5	E950.4	E962.0	E980.4
Vitamins NEC	963.5	E858.1	E933.5	E950.4	E962.0	E980.4
B_{12}	964.1	E858.2	E934.1	E950.4	E962.0	E980.4
hematopoietic	964.1	E858.2	E934.1	E950.4	E962.0	E980.4
K	964.3	E858.2	E934.3	E950.4	E962.0	E980.4
Vleminckx's solution	976.4	E858.7	E946.4	E950.4	E962.0	E980.4
Voltaren – *see* Diclofenac sodium						
Warfarin (potassium) (sodium)	964.2	E858.2	E934.2	E950.4	E962.0	E980.4
rodenticide	989.4	E863.7	–	E950.6	E962.1	E980.7
Wasp (sting)	989.5	E905.3	–	E950.9	E962.1	E980.9
Water						
balance agents NEC	974.5	E858.5	E944.5	E950.4	E962.0	E980.4
gas	987.1	E868.1	–	E951.8	E962.2	E981.8
incomplete combustion of – *see* Carbon, monoxide, fuel, utility						
hemlock	988.2	E865.4	–	E950.9	E962.1	E980.9
moccasin (venom)	989.5	E905.0	–	E950.9	E962.1	E980.9
Wax (paraffin) (petroleum)	981	E862.3	–	E950.9	E962.1	E980.9
automobile	989.89	E861.2	–	E950.9	E962.1	E980.9
floor	981	E862.0	–	E950.9	E962.1	E980.9
Weed killers NEC	989.4	E863.5	–	E950.6	E962.1	E980.7
Welldorm	967.1	E852.0	E937.1	E950.2	E962.0	E980.2
White						
arsenic – *see* Arsenic						
hellebore	988.2	E865.4	–	E950.9	E962.1	E980.9
lotion (keratolytic)	976.4	E858.7	E946.4	E950.4	E962.0	E980.4
spirit	981	E862.0	–	E950.9	E962.1	E980.9
Whitewashes	989.89	E861.6	–	E950.9	E962.1	E980.9
Whole blood	964.7	E858.2	E934.7	E950.4	E962.0	E980.4
Wild						
black cherry	988.2	E865.4	–	E950.9	E962.1	E980.9
poisonous plants NEC	988.2	E865.4	–	E950.9	E962.1	E980.9
Window cleaning fluid	989.89	E861.3	–	E950.9	E962.1	E980.9
Wintergreen (oil)	976.3	E858.7	E946.3	E950.4	E962.0	E980.4
Witch hazel	976.2	E858.7	E946.2	E950.4	E962.0	E980.4
Wood						
alcohol	980.1	E860.2	–	E950.9	E962.1	E980.9
spirit	980.1	E860.2	–	E950.9	E962.1	E980.9
Woorali	975.2	E858.6	E945.2	E950.4	E962.0	E980.4
Wormseed, American	961.6	E857	E931.6	E950.4	E962.0	E980.4
Xanthine diuretics	974.1	E858.5	E944.1	E950.4	E962.0	E980.4
Xanthocillin	960.0	E856	E930.0	E950.4	E962.0	E980.4
Xanthotoxin	976.3	E858.7	E946.3	E950.4	E962.0	E980.4
Xigris	964.2	E858.2	E934.2	E950.4	E962.0	E980.4
Xylene (liquid) (vapor)	982.0	E862.4	–	E950.9	E962.1	E980.9
Xylocaine (infiltration) (topical)	968.5	E855.2	E938.5	E950.4	E962.0	E980.4
nerve block (peripheral) (plexus)	968.6	E855.2	E938.6	E950.4	E962.0	E980.4
spinal	968.7	E855.2	E938.7	E950.4	E962.0	E980.4
Xylol (liquid) (vapor)	982.0	E862.4	–	E950.9	E962.1	E980.9
Xylometazoline	971.2	E855.5	E941.2	E950.4	E962.0	E980.4
Yellow						
fever vaccine	979.3	E858.8	E949.3	E950.4	E962.0	E980.4
jasmine	988.2	E865.4	–	E950.9	E962.1	E980.9
Yew	988.2	E865.4	–	E950.9	E962.1	E980.9
Zactane	965.7	E850.7	E935.7	E950.0	E962.0	E980.0
Zaroxolyn	974.3	E858.5	E944.3	E950.4	E962.0	E980.4
Zephiran (topical)	976.0	E858.7	E946.0	E950.4	E962.0	E980.4
ophthalmic preparation	976.5	E858.7	E946.5	E950.4	E962.0	E980.4
Zerone	980.1	E860.2	–	E950.9	E962.1	E980.9
Zinc (compounds) (fumes) (salts) (vapor) NEC	985.8	E866.4	–	E950.9	E962.1	E980.9
anti-infectives	976.0	E858.7	E946.0	E950.4	E962.0	E980.4
antivaricose	972.7	E858.3	E942.7	E950.4	E962.0	E980.4
bacitracin	976.0	E858.7	E946.0	E950.4	E962.0	E980.4
chloride	976.2	E858.7	E946.2	E950.4	E962.0	E980.4
gelatin	976.3	E858.7	E946.3	E950.4	E962.0	E980.4
oxide	976.3	E858.7	E946.3	E950.4	E962.0	E980.4
peroxide	976.0	E858.7	E946.0	E950.4	E962.0	E980.4
pesticides	985.8	E863.4	–	E950.6	E962.1	E980.7

Drug, chemical	Poisoning	External Cause (E Code) Accident	Therapeutic Use	Suicide Attempt	Assault	Undetermined
Zinc – *continued*						
phosphide (rodenticide)	985.8	E863.7	–	E950.6	E962.1	E980.7
stearate	976.3	E858.7	E946.3	E950.4	E962.0	E980.4
sulfate (antivaricose)	972.7	E858.3	E942.7	E950.4	E962.0	E980.4
ENT agent	976.6	E858.7	E946.6	E950.4	E962.0	E980.4
ophthalmic solution	976.5	E858.7	E946.5	E950.4	E962.0	E980.4
topical NEC	976.0	E858.7	E946.0	E950.4	E962.0	E980.4
undecylenate	976.0	E858.7	E946.0	E950.4	E962.0	E980.4
Zovant	964.2	E858.2	E934.2	E950.4	E962.0	E980.4
Zoxazolamine	968.0	E855.1	E938.0	E950.4	E962.0	E980.4
Zygadenus (venenosus)	988.2	E865.4	–	E950.9	E962.1	E980.9

INDEX TO EXTERNAL CAUSES OF INJURY (E CODE)

The section beginning on the next page contains the index to the codes which classify environmental events, circumstances, and other conditions as the cause of injury and other adverse effects. Where a code from the section Supplementary Classification of External Causes of Injury and Poisoning (E800-E998) is applicable, it is intended that the E code shall be used in addition to a code from the main body of the classification, Chapters 1 to 17.

The alphabetic index to the E codes is organized by main terms which describe the accident, circumstance, event, or specific agent which caused the injury or other adverse effect.

Note *Transport accidents (E800-E848) include accidents involving:*

aircraft and space craft (E840-E845)
watercraft (E830-E838)
motor vehicle (E810-E825)
railway (E800-E807)
other road vehicles (E826-E829)

For definitions and examples related to transport accidents - see Supplementary Classification of External Causes of Injury and Poisoning (E800-E999).

The fourth-digit subdivisions for use with categories E800-E848 to identify the injured person are found at the beginning of the E code section in the Tabular List (Volume 1-311).

For identifying the place in which an accident or poisoning occurred (circumstances classifiable to categories E850-E869 and E880-E928) - see the listing in this section under "Accident, occurring."

See the Table of Drugs and Chemicals (Section 2 of this volume) for identifying the specific agent involved in drug overdose or a wrong substance given or taken in error, and for intoxication or poisoning by a drug or other chemical substance.

The specific adverse effect, reaction, or localized toxic effect to a correct drug or substance properly administered in therapeutic or prophylactic dosage should be classified according to the nature of the adverse effect (e.g., allergy, dermatitis, tachycardia) listed in Section I of this volume.

A

Barotitis, barodontalgia, berosinusitis, barotrauma (otitic) (sinus) - *see* Effects of, air pressure
Battered
  baby or child (syndrome) - *see* Abuse, child; category E967
  person other than baby or child - *see* Assault
Bayonet wound (*see also* Cut, by bayonet) E920.3
  in
    legal intervention E974
    terrorism E979.8
    war operations E995.2 ▲
Bean in nose E912
Bed set on fire NEC E898.0
Beheading (by guillotine)
  homicide E966
  legal execution E978
Bending, injury in E927.8
Bends E902.0
Bite
  animal NEC E906.5
    other specified (except arthropod) E906.3
    venomous NEC E905.9
  arthropod (nonvenomous) NEC E906.4
    venomous - *see* Sting
  black widow spider E905.1
  cat E906.3
  centipede E905.4
  cobra E905.0
  copperhead snake E905.0
  coral snake E905.0
  dog E906.0
  fer de lance E905.0
  gila monster E905.0
  human being
    accidental E928.3
    assault E968.7
  insect (nonvenomous) E906.4
    venomous - *see* Sting
  krait E905.0
  late effect of - *see* Late effect
  lizard E906.2
    venomous E905.0
  mamba E905.0
  marine animal
    nonvenomous E906.3
      snake E906.2
    venomous E905.6
      snake E905.0
  millipede E906.4
    venomous E905.4
  moray eel E906.3
  rat E906.1
  rattlesnake E905.0
  rodent, except rat E906.3
  serpent - *see* Bite, snake
  shark E906.3
  snake (venomous) E905.0
    nonvenomous E906.2
    sea E905.0
  spider E905.1
    nonvenomous E906.4
  tarantula (venomous) E905.1
  venomous NEC E905.9
    by specific animal - *see* category E905
  viper E905.0
  water moccasin E905.0
Blast (air)
  in
    terrorism E979.2
      from nuclear explosion E979.5
      underwater E979.0
    war operations E993.9 ▲
      from nuclear explosion (*see also* War operations, injury due to, nuclear weapons) E996.0 ▲
      underwater E992.9 ▲
Blizzard E908.3
Blow E928.9
  by law-enforcing agent, police (on duty) E975
    with blunt object (baton) (nightstick) (stave) (truncheon) E973
Blowing up (*see also* Explosion) E923.9
Brawl (hand) (fists) (foot) E960.0
Breakage (accidental)
  cable of cable car not on rails E847
  ladder (causing fall) E881.0
  part (any) of
    animal-drawn vehicle E827 4th
    ladder (causing fall) E881.0
    motor vehicle
      in motion (on public highway) E818 4th
        not on public highway E825 4th
    nonmotor road vehicle, except animal-drawn vehicle or pedal cycle E829 4th
    off-road type motor vehicle (not on public highway) NEC E821 4th
      on public highway E818 4th
    pedal cycle E826 4th
    scaffolding (causing fall) E881.1
    snow vehicle, motor-driven (not on public highway) E820 4th
      on public highway E818 4th
    vehicle NEC - *see* Accident, vehicle
Broken
  glass
    fall on E888.0
    injury by E920.8
  power line (causing electric shock) E925.1
Bumping against, into (accidentally)
  object (moving) E917.9
    caused by crowd E917.1
      with subsequent fall E917.6
    furniture E917.3
      with subsequent fall E917.7
    in
      running water E917.2
      sports E917.0
        with subsequent fall E917.5
    stationary E917.4
      with subsequent fall E917.8
  person(s) E917.9
    with fall E886.9
      in sports E886.0
    as, or caused by, a crowd E917.1
      with subsequent fall E917.6
    in sports E917.0
      with fall E886.0
Burning, burns (accidental) (by) (from) (on) E899
  acid (any kind) E924.1
    swallowed - *see* Table of Drugs and Chemicals
  airgun E928.7 ●
  bedclothes (*see also* Fire, specified NEC) E898.0
  blowlamp (*see also* Fire, specified NEC) E898.1
  blowtorch (*see also* Fire, specified NEC) E898.1
  boat, ship, watercraft - *see* categories E830, E831, E837
  bonfire (controlled) E897
    uncontrolled E892
  candle (*see also* Fire, specified NEC) E898.1
  caustic liquid, substance E924.1
    swallowed - *see* Table of Drugs and Chemicals
  chemical E924.1
    from swallowing caustic, corrosive substance - *see* Table of Drugs and Chemicals
    in
      terrorism E979.7
      war operations E997.2
  cigar(s) or cigarette(s) (*see also* Fire, specified NEC) E898.1
Burning, burns – *continued*
  clothes, clothing, nightdress - *see* Ignition, clothes
    with conflagration - *see* Conflagration
  conflagration - *see* Conflagration
  corrosive liquid, substance E924.1
    swallowed - *see* Table of Drugs and Chemicals
  electric current (*see also* Electric shock) E925.9
  fire, flames (*see also* Fire) E899
  firearm E928.7 ●
  flare, Verey pistol E922.8
  heat
    from appliance (electrical) E924.8
    in local application, or packing during medical or surgical procedure E873.5
  homicide (attempt) (*see also* Assault, burning) E968.0
  hot
    liquid E924.0
      caustic or corrosive E924.1
    object (not producing fire or flames) E924.8
    substance E924.9
      caustic or corrosive E924.1
      liquid (metal) NEC E924.0
      specified type NEC E924.8
    tap water E924.2
  ignition - *see also* Ignition
    clothes, clothing, nightdress - *see also* Ignition, clothes
      with conflagration - *see* Conflagration
    highly inflammable material (benzine) (fat) (gasoline) (kerosine) (paraffin) (petrol) E894
  in
    terrorism E979.3
      from nuclear explosion E979.5
      petrol bomb E979.3
    war operations (from fire-producing device or conventional weapon) E990.9
      from nuclear explosion (*see also* War operations, injury due to, nuclear weapons) E996.2 ▲
      incendiary bomb E990.0 ●
      petrol bomb E990.0
  inflicted by other person
    stated as
      homicidal, intentional (*see also* Assault, burning) E968.0
      undetermined whether accidental or intentional (*see also* Burn, stated as undetermined whether accidental or intentional) E988.1
  internal, from swallowed caustic, corrosive liquid, substance - *see* Table of Drugs and Chemicals
  lamp (*see also* Fire, specified NEC) E898.1
  late effect of NEC E929.4
  lighter (cigar) (cigarette) (*see also* Fire, specified NEC) E898.1
  lightning E907
  liquid (boiling) (hot) (molten) E924.0
    caustic, corrosive (external) E924.1
      swallowed - *see* Table of Drugs and Chemicals
  local application of externally applied substance in medical or surgical care E873.5
  machinery - *see* Accident, machine
  matches (*see also* Fire, specified NEC) E898.1
  medicament, externally applied E873.5
  metal, molten E924.0
  object (hot) E924.8
    producing fire or flames - *see* Fire
  oven (electric) (gas) E924.8
Burning, burns – *continued*
  pipe (smoking) (*see also* Fire, specified NEC) E898.1
  radiation - *see* Radiation
  railway engine, locomotive, train (*see also* Explosion, railway engine) E803 4th
  self-inflicted (unspecified whether accidental or intentional) E988.1
    caustic or corrosive substance NEC E988.7
    stated as intentional, purposeful E958.1
      caustic or corrosive substance NEC E958.7
  stated as undetermined whether accidental or intentional E988.1
    caustic or corrosive substance NEC or E988.7
  steam E924.0
    pipe E924.8
  substance (hot) E924.9
    boiling or molten E924.0
    caustic, corrosive (external) E924.1
      swallowed - *see* Table of Drugs and Chemicals
  suicidal (attempt) NEC E958.1
    caustic substance E958.7
    late effect of E959
  tanning bed E926.2
  therapeutic misadventure
    overdose of radiation E873.2
  torch, welding (*see also* Fire, specified NEC) E898.1
  trash fire (*see also* Burning, bonfire) E897
  vapor E924.0
  vitriol E924.1
  x-rays E926.3
    in medical, surgical procedure - *see* Misadventure, failure, in dosage, radiation operations
Butted by animal E906.8

Cachexia, lead or saturnine E866.0
  from pesticide NEC (*see also* Table of Drugs and Chemicals) E863.4
Caisson disease E902.2
Capital punishment (any means) E978
Car sickness E903
Casualty (not due to war) NEC E928.9
  terrorism E979.8
  war (*see also* War operations) E995.9 ▲
Cat
  bite E906.3
  scratch E906.8
Cataclysmic (any injury)
  earth surface movement or eruption E909.9
    specified type NEC E909.8
  storm or flood resulting from storm E908.9
    specified type NEC E909.8
Catching fire - *see* Ignition
Caught
  between
    objects (moving) (stationary and moving) E918
      and machinery - *see* Accident, machine
  by cable car, not on rails E847
  in
    machinery (moving parts of) - *see* Accident, machine
    object E918

Note: *In the case of collisions between different types of vehicles, persons and objects, priority in classification is in the following order:*

Aircraft
Watercraft
Motor vehicle
Railway vehicle
Pedal Cycle
Animal-drawn vehicle
Animal being ridden
Streetcar or other nonmotor road vehicle
Other vehicle
Pedestrian or person using pedestrian conveyance
Object (except where falling from or set in motion by vehicle etc. listed above)

In the listing below, the combinations are listed only under the vehicle, etc., having priority. For definitions, see Supplementary Classification of External Causes of Injury and Poisoning (E800-E999).

Cave-in – Collision

Cut, cutting – Explosion

- **Explosion** – *continued*
  - grenade – *continued*
    - in – *continued*
      - war operations E993.8 ▲
        - injury by fragments from E991.4 ▲
  - homicide (attempt) - *see* Assault, explosive
  - hot water heater, tank (in machinery) E921.0
  - in mine (of explosive gases) NEC E923.2
  - late effect of NEC E929.8
  - machinery - *see also* Accident, machine
    - pressure vessel - *see* Explosion, pressure vessel
  - methane E923.2
  - missile E923.8
    - in
      - terrorism E979.2
      - war operations E993.1 ▲
        - injury by fragments from E991.4 ▲
  - motor vehicle (part of)
    - in motion (on public highway) E818 [4th]
      - not on public highway E825 [4th]
  - munitions (dump) (factory) E923.8
    - in
      - terrorism E979.2
      - war operations E993.9 ▲
  - of mine E923.8
    - in
      - terrorism
        - at sea or in harbor E979.0
        - land E979.2
        - marine E979.0
      - war operations
        - after cessation of hostilities E998.0 ▲
        - at sea or in harbor E992.2 ▲
        - land E993.8 ▲
          - after cessation of hostilities E998.0 ▲
          - injury by fragments from E991.4 ▲
        - marine E992.2 ▲
  - own weapons
    - in
      - terrorism (*see also* Suicide) E979.2
      - war operations E993.7 ▲
        - injury by fragments from E991.9
          - antipersonnel bomb E991.3
  - pressure
    - cooker E921.8
    - gas tank (in machinery) E921.1
    - vessel (in machinery) E921.9
      - on transport vehicle - *see* categories E800-E848
      - specified type NEC E921.8
  - propane E923.2
  - railway engine, locomotive, train (boiler) (with subsequent collision, derailment, fall) E803 [4th]
    - with
      - collision (antecedent) (*see also* Collision, railway) E800 [4th]
      - derailment (antecedent) E802 [4th]
      - fire (without antecedent collision or derailment) E803 [4th]
  - secondary fire resulting from - *see* Fire
  - self-inflicted (unspecified whether accidental or intentional) E985.5
    - stated as intentional, purposeful E955.5
  - shell (artillery) E923.8
    - in
      - terrorism E979.2
      - war operations E993.2 ▲
        - injury by fragments from E991.4 ▲
  - stated as undetermined whether caused accidentally or purposely inflicted E985.5
  - steam or water lines (in machinery) E921.0

- **Explosion** – *continued*
  - suicide (attempted) E955.5
  - torpedo E923.8
    - in
      - terrorism E979.0
      - war operations E992.0 ▲
  - transport accident - *see* categories E800-E848
  - terrorism - *see* Terrorism, explosion
  - war operations - *see* War operations, explosion
  - watercraft (boiler) E837 [4th]
    - causing drowning, submersion (after jumping from watercraft) E830 [4th]
- **Exposure** (weather) (conditions) (rain) (wind) E904.3
  - with homicidal intent E968.4
  - environmental
    - to
      - algae bloom E928.6
      - blue-green algae bloom E928.6
      - brown tide E928.6
      - cyanobacteria bloom E928.6
      - Florida red tide E928.6
      - harmful algae
        - and toxins E928.6
        - bloom E928.6
      - pfiesteria piscicida E928.6
      - red tide E928.6
  - excessive E904.3
    - cold (*see also* Cold, exposure to) E901.9
      - self-inflicted - *see* Cold, exposure to, self-inflicted
    - heat (*see also* Heat) E900.9
  - helpless person, infant, newborn due to abandonment or neglect E904.0
  - noise E928.1
  - prolonged in deep-freeze unit or refrigerator E901.1
  - radiation - *see* Radiation
  - resulting from transport accident - *see* categories E800-E848
  - smoke from, due to
    - fire - *see* Fire
    - tobacco, second-hand E869.4
  - vibration E928.2
- **External cause status** E000.9 ●
  - civilian ●
    - done for ●
      - financial or other compensation E000.0 ●
      - pay or income E000.0 ●
  - for income E000.0 ●
  - hobby or leisure E000.8 ●
  - off duty military E000.8 ●
  - military E000.1 ●
    - off duty E000.8 ●
  - recreation E000.8 ●
  - specified NEC E000.8 ●
  - sport not for income E000.8 ●
  - student E000.8 ●
  - volunteer E000.8 ●

F

- **Fall, falling** (accidental) E888.9
  - building E916
    - burning E891.8
      - private E890.8
  - down
    - escalator E880.0
    - ladder E881.0
      - in boat, ship, watercraft E833
    - staircase E880.9
    - stairs, steps - *see* Fall, from, stairs
  - earth (with asphyxia or suffocation (by pressure)) (*see also* Earth, falling) E913.3

- **Fall, falling** – *continued*
  - from, off
    - aircraft (at landing, take-off) (in-transit) (while alighting, boarding) E843 [4th]
      - resulting from accident to aircraft - *see* categories E840-E842
    - animal (in sport or transport) E828 [4th]
    - animal-drawn vehicle E827 [4th]
    - balcony E882
    - bed E884.4
    - bicycle E826 [4th]
    - boat, ship, watercraft (into water) E832 [4th]
      - after accident to, collision, fire on E830 [4th]
        - and subsequently struck by (part of) boat E831 [4th]
      - and subsequently struck by (part of) while alighting, boat E838 [4th]
      - burning, crushed, sinking E830 [4th]
        - and subsequently struck by (part of) boat E831 [4th]
    - bridge E882
    - building E882
      - burning (uncontrolled fire) E891.8
        - in terrorism E979.3
      - private E890.8
    - bunk in boat, ship, watercraft E834 [4th]
      - due to accident to watercraft E831 [4th]
    - cable car (not on rails) E847
      - on rails E829 [4th]
    - car - *see* Fall from motor vehicle E884.9
    - chair E884.2
    - cliff E884.1
    - commode E884.6
    - curb (sidewalk) E880.1
    - elevation aboard ship E834 [4th]
      - due to accident to ship E831 [4th]
    - embankment E884.9
    - escalator E880.0
    - fire escape E882
    - flagpole E882
    - furniture NEC E884.5
    - gangplank (into water) (*see also* Fall, from, boat) E832 [4th]
      - to deck, dock E834 [4th]
    - hammock on ship E834 [4th]
      - due to accident to watercraft E831 [4th]
    - haystack E884.9
    - heelies E885.1
    - high place NEC E884.9
      - stated as undetermined whether accidental or intentional - *see* Jumping, from, high place
    - horse (in sport or transport) E828 [4th]
    - in-line skates E885.1
    - ladder E881.0
      - in boat, ship, watercraft E833 [4th]
        - due to accident to watercraft E831 [4th]
    - machinery - *see also* Accident, machine
      - not in operation E884.9
    - motor vehicle (in motion) (on public highway) E818 [4th]
      - not on public highway E825 [4th]
        - stationary, except while alighting, boarding, entering, leaving E884.9
        - while alighting, boarding, entering, leaving E824 [4th]
      - stationary, except while alighting, boarding, entering, leaving E884.9
      - while alighting, boarding, entering, leaving, except off-road type motor vehicle E817 [4th]
        - off-toad type - *see* Fall, from, off-road type motor vehicle

- **Fall, falling** – *continued*
  - from, off – *continued*
    - nonmotor road vehicle (while alighting, boarding) NEC E829 [4th]
      - stationary, except while alighting, boarding, entering, leaving E884.9
    - off road type motor vehicle (not on public highway) NEC E821 [4th]
      - on public highway E818 [4th]
        - while alighting, boarding, entering, leaving E817 [4th]
      - snow vehicle - *see* Fall from snow vehicle, motor-driven
    - one
      - deck to another on ship E834 [4th]
        - due to accident to ship E831 [4th]
      - level to another NEC E884.9
        - boat, ship, or watercraft E834 [4th]
          - due to accident to watercraft E831 [4th]
    - pedal cycle E826 [4th]
    - playground equipment E884.0
    - railway rolling stock, train, vehicle (while alighting, boarding) E804 [4th]
      - with
        - collision (*see also* Collision, railway) E800 [4th]
        - derailment (*see also* Derailment, railway) E802 [4th]
        - explosion (*see also* Explosion, railway engine) E803 [4th]
    - rigging (aboard ship) E834 [4th]
      - due to accident to watercraft E831 [4th]
    - roller skates E885.1
    - scaffolding E881.1
    - scooter (nonmotorized) E885.0
    - sidewalk (curb) E880.1
      - moving E885.9
    - skateboard E885.2
    - skis E885.3
    - snowboard E885.4
    - snow vehicle, motor-driven (not on public highway) E820 [4th]
      - on public highway E818 [4th]
        - while alighting. boarding, entering, leaving E817 [4th]
    - stairs, steps E880.9
      - boat, ship, watercraft E833 [4th]
        - due to accident to watercraft E831 [4th]
      - motor bus, motor vehicle - *see* Fall, from, motor vehicle, while alighting, boarding
      - street car E829 [4th]
    - stationary vehicle NEC E884.9
    - stepladder E881.0
    - street car (while boarding, alighting) E829 [4th]
      - stationary, except while boarding or alighting E884.9
    - structure NEC E882
      - burning (uncontrolled fire) E891.8
        - in terrorism E979.3
    - table E884.9
    - toilet E884.6
    - tower E882
    - tree E884.9
    - turret E882
    - vehicle NEC - *see also* Accident, vehicle NEC
      - stationary E884.9
    - viaduct E882
    - wall E882
    - wheelchair E884.3
    - wheelies E885.1
    - window E882

Fall, falling – *continued*
- in, on
  - aircraft (at landing, take-off) (in-transit) E843 4th
    - resulting from accident to aircraft - *see* categories E840-E842
  - boat, ship, watercraft E835 4th
    - due to accident to watercraft E831 4th
    - one level to another NEC E834 4th
    - on ladder, stairs E833 4th
  - cutting or piercing instrument machine E888.0
  - deck (of boat, ship, watercraft) E835 4th
    - due to accident to watercraft E831 4th
  - escalator E880.0
  - gangplank E835 4th
  - glass, broken E888.0
  - knife E888.0
  - ladder E881.0
    - in boat, ship, watercraft E833 4th
      - due to accident to watercraft E831 4th
  - object
    - edged, pointed or sharp E888.0
    - other E888.1
  - pitchfork E888.0
  - railway rolling stock, train, vehicle (while alighting, boarding) E804 4th
    - with
      - collision (*see also* Collision, railway) E800 4th
      - derailment (*see also* Derailment, railway) E802 4th
      - explosion (*see also* Explosion, railway engine) E803 4th
  - scaffolding E881.1
  - scissors E888.0
  - staircase, stairs, steps (*see also* Fall, from, stairs) E880.9
  - street car E829 4th
  - water transport (*see also* Fall, in, boat) E835 4th
- into
  - cavity E883.9
  - dock E883.9
    - from boat, ship, watercraft (*see also* Fall, from, boat) E832 4th
  - hold (of ship) E834 4th
    - due to accident to watercraft E831 4th
  - hole E883.9
  - manhole E883.2
  - moving part of machinery - *see* Accident, machine
  - opening in surface NEC E883.9
  - pit E883.9
  - quarry E883.9
  - shaft E883.9
  - storm drain E883.2
  - tank E883.9
  - water (with drowning or submersion) E910.9
  - well E883.1
- late effect of NEC E929.3
- object (*see also* Hit by, object, falling) E916
- other E888.8
- over
  - animal E885.9
  - cliff E884.1
  - embankment E884.9
  - small object E885.9
- overboard (*see also* Fall, from, boat) E832 4th
- resulting in striking against object E888.1
  - sharp E888.0
- rock E916
- same level NEC E888.9
  - aircraft (any kind) E843 4th
    - resulting from accident to aircraft - *see* categories E840-E842

Fall, falling – *continued*
- same level – *continued*
  - boat, ship, watercraft E835 4th
    - due to accident to, collision, watercraft E831 4th
  - from
    - collision, pushing, shoving, by or with other person(s) E886.9
      - as, or caused by, a crowd E917.6
      - in sports E886.0
    - in-line skates E885.1
    - roller skates E885.1
    - scooter (nonmotorized) E885.0
    - skateboard E885.2
    - skis E885.3
    - slipping, stumbling, tripping E885.9
    - snowboard E885.4
- snowslide E916
  - as avalanche E909.2
- stone E916
- through
  - hatch (on ship) E834 4th
    - due to accident to watercraft E831 4th
  - roof E882
  - window E882
- timber E916
- while alighting from, boarding, entering, leaving
  - aircraft (any kind) E843 4th
  - motor bus, motor vehicle - *see* Fall, from, motor vehicle, while alighting, boarding
  - nonmotor road vehicle NEC E829 4th
  - railway train E804 4th
  - street car E829 4th

Fallen on by
- animal (horse) (not being ridden) E906.8
  - being ridden (in sport or transport) E828 4th

Fell or jumped from high place, so stated - *see* Jumping, from, high place

Felo-de-se (*see also* Suicide) E958.9

Fever
- heat - *see* Heat
- thermic - *see* Heat

Fight (hand) (fist) (foot) (*see also* Assault, fight) E960.0

Fire (accidental) (caused by great heat from appliance (electrical), hot object or hot substance) (secondary, resulting from explosion) E899
- conflagration - *see* Conflagration E892
- controlled, normal (in brazier, fireplace, furnace, or stove) (charcoal) (coal) (coke) (electric) (gas) (wood)
  - bonfire E897
  - brazier, not in building or structure E897
  - in building or structure, except private dwelling (barn) (church) (convalescent or residential home) (factory) (farm outbuilding) (hospital) (hotel) (institution (educational) (dormitory) (residential)) (private garage)(school) (shop) (store) (theatre) E896
  - in private dwelling (apartment) (boarding house) (camping place)(caravan) (farmhouse) (home (private)) (house) (lodging house) (rooming house) (tenement) E895
  - not in building or structure E897
  - trash E897
- forest (uncontrolled) E892
- grass (uncontrolled) E892
- hay (uncontrolled) E892
- homicide (attempt) E968.0
  - late effect of E969
- in, of, on, starting in E892
  - aircraft (in transit) (powered) E841 4th
    - at landing. take-off E840 4th

Fire – *continued*
- in, of, on, starting in – *continued*
  - aircraft – *continued*
    - stationary E892
    - unpowered (balloon) (glider) E842 4th
  - balloon E842 4th
  - boat, ship, watercraft - *see* categories E830, E831, E837
  - building or structure, except private dwelling (barn) (church) (convalescent or residential home) (factory) (farm outbuilding) (hospital) (hotel) (institution (educational) (dormitory) (residential)) (school) (shop) (store) (theatre) (*see also* Conflagration, building or structure, except private dwelling) E891.9
  - forest (uncontrolled) E892
  - glider E842 4th
  - grass (uncontrolled) E892
  - hay (uncontrolled) E892
  - lumber (uncontrolled) E892
  - machinery - *see* Accident, machine
  - mine (uncontrolled) E892
  - motor vehicle (in motion) (on public highway) E818 4th
    - not on public highway E825 4th
    - stationary E892
  - prairie (uncontrolled) E892
  - private dwelling (apartment) (boarding house) (camping place) (caravan) (farmhouse) (home (private)) (house) (lodging house) (private garage) (rooming house) (tenement) (*see also* Conflagration, private dwelling) E890.9
  - railway rolling stock, train, vehicle (*see also* Explosion, railway engine) E803 4th
    - stationary E892
  - room NEC E898.1
  - street car (in motion) E829 4th
    - stationary E892
  - terrorism (by fire-producing device) E979.3
    - fittings or furniture (burning building) (uncontrolled fire) E979.3
    - from nuclear explosion E979.5
  - transport vehicle, stationary NEC E892
  - tunnel (uncontrolled) E892
  - war operations (by fire-producing device or conventional weapon) E990.9
    - from nuclear explosion (*see also* War operations, injury due to, nuclear weapons) E996.2 ▲
    - incendiary bomb E990.0 ●
    - petrol bomb E990.0
- late effect of NEC E929.4
- lumber (uncontrolled) E892
- mine (uncontrolled) E892
- prairie (uncontrolled) E892
- self-inflicted (unspecified whether accidental or intentional) E988.1
  - stated as intentional, purposeful E958.1
- specified NEC E898.1
  - with
    - conflagration - *see* Conflagration
    - ignition (of)
      - clothing - *see* Ignition, clothes
      - highly inflammable material (benzine) (fat) (gasoline) (kerosene) (paraffin) (petrol) E894
- started by other person
  - stated as
    - with intent to injure or kill E968.0

Fire – *continued*
- started by other person – *continued*
  - stated as – *continued*
    - undetermined whether or not with intent to injure or kill E988.1
- suicide (attempted) E958.1
  - late effect of E959
- tunnel (uncontrolled) E892

Fireball effects from nuclear explosion
- in
  - terrorism E979.5
  - war operations (*see also* War operations, injury due to, nuclear weapons) E996.2 ▲

Fireworks (explosion) E923.0

Flash burns from explosion (*see also* Explosion) E923.9

Flood (any injury) (resulting from storm) E908.2
- caused by collapse of dam or manmade structure E909.3

Forced landing (aircraft) E840 4th

Foreign body, object or material (entrance into (accidental))
- air passage (causing injury) E915
  - with asphyxia, obstruction, suffocation E912
    - food or vomitus E911
  - nose (with asphyxia, obstruction, suffocation) E912
    - causing injury without asphyxia, obstruction, suffocation E915
- alimentary canal (causing injury) (with obstruction) E915
  - with asphyxia, obstruction respiratory passage, suffocation E912
    - food E911
  - mouth E915
    - with asphyxia, obstruction, suffocation E912
      - food E911
  - pharynx E915
    - with asphyxia, obstruction, suffocation E912
      - food E911
- aspiration (with asphyxia, obstruction respiratory passage, suffocation) E912
  - causing injury without asphyxia, obstruction respiratory passage, suffocation E915
  - food (regurgitated) (vomited) E911
    - causing injury without asphyxia, obstruction respiratory passage, suffocation E915
  - mucus (not of newborn) E912
  - phlegm E912
- bladder (causing injury or obstruction) E915
- bronchus, bronchi - *see* Foreign body, air passages
- conjunctival sac E914
- digestive system - *see* Foreign body, alimentary canal
- ear (causing injury or obstruction) E915
- esophagus (causing injury or obstruction) (*see also* Foreign body, alimentary canal) E915
- eye (any part) E914
- eyelid E914
- hairball (stomach) (with obstruction) E915
- ingestion - *see* Foreign body, alimentary canal
- inhalation - *see* Foreign body, aspiration
- intestine (causing injury or obstruction) E915
- iris E914
- lacrimal apparatus E914
- larynx - *see* Foreign body, air passage
- late effect of NEC E929.8
- lung - *see* Foreign body, air passage
- mouth - *see* Foreign body, alimentary canal, mouth

Fall, falling – Foreign body, object or material

Foreign body, object or material – *continued*
- nasal passage - *see* Foreign body, air passage, nose
- nose - *see* Foreign body, air passage, nose
- ocular muscle E914
- operation wound (left in) - *see* Misadventure, foreign object
- orbit E914
- pharynx - *see* Foreign body, alimentary canal, pharynx
- rectum (causing injury or obstruction) E915
- stomach (hairball) (causing injury or obstruction) E915
- tear ducts or glands E914
- trachea - *see* Foreign body, air passage
- urethra (causing injury or obstruction) E915
- vagina (causing injury or obstruction) E915

Found dead, injured
- from exposure (to) - *see* Exposure
- on
  - public highway E819 4th
  - railway right of way E807 4th

Fracture (circumstances unknown or unspecified) E887
- due to specified external means - *see* manner of accident
- late effect of NEC E929.3
- occurring in water transport NEC E835 4th

Freezing - *see* Cold, exposure to

Frostbite E901.0
- due to manmade conditions E901.1

Frozen - *see* Cold, exposure to

G

Garrotting, homicidal (attempted) E963

Gored E906.8

Gunshot wound (*see also* Shooting) E922.9

H

Hailstones, injury by E904.3

Hairball (stomach) (with obstruction) E915

Hanged himself (*see also* Hanging, self-inflicted) E983.0

Hang gliding E842

Hanging (accidental) E913.8
- caused by other person
  - in accidental circumstances E913.8
  - stated as
    - intentional, homicidal E963
    - undetermined whether accidental or intentional E983.0
- homicide (attempt) E963
- in bed or cradle E913.0
- legal execution E978
- self-inflicted (unspecified whether accidental or intentional) E983.0
  - in accidental circumstances E913.8
  - stated as intentional, purposeful E953.0
- stated as undetermined whether accidental or intentional E983.0
- suicidal (attempt) E953.0

Heat (apoplexy) (collapse) (cramps) (effects of) (excessive) (exhaustion) (fever) (prostration) (stroke) E900.9
- due to
  - manmade conditions (as listed in E900.1, except boat, ship, watercraft) E900.1
  - weather (conditions) E900.0
- from
  - electric heating apparatus causing burning E924.8

Heat – *continued*
- from – *continued*
  - nuclear explosion
    - in
      - terrorism E979.5
      - war operations <u>(*see also* War operations, injury due to, nuclear weapons)</u> E996<u>.2</u> ▲
- generated in, boiler, engine, evaporator, fire room of boat, ship, watercraft E838 4th
- inappropriate in local application or packing in medical or surgical procedure E873.5
- late effect of NEC E989

Hemorrhage
- delayed following medical or surgical treatment without mention of misadventure - *see* Reaction, abnormal
- during medical or surgical treatment as misadventure - *see* Misadventure, cut

High
- altitude, effects E902.9
- level of radioactivity, effects - *see* Radiation
- pressure effects - *see also* Effects of, air pressure
  - from rapid descent in water (causing caisson or divers' disease, palsy, or paralysis) E902.2
- temperature, effects - *see* Heat

Hit, hitting (accidental) **by**
- aircraft (propeller) (without accident to aircraft) E844 4th
  - unpowered E842 4th
- avalanche E909.2
- being thrown against object in or part of
  - motor vehicle (in motion) (on public highway) E818 4th
    - not on public highway E825 4th
  - nonmotor road vehicle NEC E829 4th
  - street car E829 4th
- boat. ship, watercraft
  - after fall from watercraft E838 4th
    - damaged, involved in accident E831 4th
  - while swimming, water skiing E838 4th
- bullet (*see also* shooting) E922.9
  - from air gun E922.4
  - in
    - terrorism E979.4
    - war operations E991.2
      - rubber E991.0
- flare, Verey pistol (*see also* Shooting) E922.8
- hailstones E904.3
- landslide E909.2
- law-enforcing agent (on duty) E975
  - with blunt object (baton) (night stick) (stave) (truncheon) E973
- machine - *see* Accident, machine
- missile
  - firearm (*see also* shooting) E922.9
  - in
    - terrorism - *see* Terrorism, missile
    - war operations - *see* War operations, missile
- motor vehicle (on public highway) (traffic accident) E814 4th
  - not on public highway, nontraffic accident E822 4th
- nonmotor road vehicle NEC E829 4th
- object
  - falling E916
    - from, in, on
      - aircraft E844 4th
        - due to accident to aircraft - *see* categories E840-E842
        - unpowered E842 4th

Hit, hitting (accidental) **by** – *continued*
- object – *continued*
  - falling – *continued*
    - from, in, on – *continued*
      - boat, ship, watercraft E838 4th
        - due to accident to watercraft E831 4th
      - building E916
        - burning E891.8
          - in terrorism E979.3
          - private E890.8
      - cataclysmic
        - earth surface movement or eruption E909.9
        - storm E908.9
      - cave-in E916
        - with asphyxiation or suffocation (*see also* Suffocation, due to, cave-in) E913.3
      - earthquake E909.0
      - motor vehicle (in motion) (on public highway) E818 4th
        - not on public highway E825 4th
        - stationary E916
      - nonmotor road vehicle NEC E829 4th
      - pedal cycle E826 4th
      - railway rolling stock, train, vehicle E806 4th
      - street car E829 4th
      - structure, burning NEC E891.8
      - vehicle, stationary E916
  - moving NEC - *see* Striking against, object
  - projected NEC - *see* Striking against, object
  - set in motion by
    - compressed air or gas, spring, striking, throwing - *see* Striking against, object
    - explosion - *see* Explosion
  - thrown into, on, or towards
    - motor vehicle (in motion) (on public highway) E818 4th
      - not on public highway E825 4th
    - nonmotor road vehicle NEC E829 4th
    - pedal cycle E826 4th
    - street car E829 4th
- off-road type motor vehicle (not on public highway) E821 4th
  - on public highway E814 4th
- other person(s) E917.9
  - with blunt or thrown object E917.9
    - in sports E917.0
      - with subsequent fall E917.5
    - intentionally, homicidal E968.2
  - as, or caused by, a crowd E917.1
    - with subsequent fall E917.6
  - in sports E917.0
- pedal cycle E826 4th
- police (on duty) E975
  - with blunt object (baton) (nightstick) (stave) (truncheon) E973
- railway, rolling stock, train, vehicle (part of) E805 4th
- shot - *see* Shooting
- snow vehicle, motor-driven (not on public highway) E820 4th
  - on public highway E814 4th
- street car E829 4th
- vehicle NEC - *see* Accident, vehicle NEC

Homicide, homicidal (attempt) (justifiable) (*see also* Assault) E968.9

Hot
- liquid, object, substance, accident caused by - *see also* Accident, caused by, hot, by type of substance
  - late effect of E929.8
- place, effects - *see* Heat
- weather, effects E900.0

Humidity, causing problem E904.3

Hunger E904.1
- resulting from
  - abandonment or neglect E904.0
  - transport accident - *see* categories E800-E848

Hurricane (any injury) E908.0

Hypobarism, hypobaropethy - *see* Effects of, air pressure

Hypothermia - *see* Cold, exposure to

I

Ictus
- caloris - *see* Heat
- solaris E900.0

Ignition (accidental)
- anesthetic gas in operating theatre E923.2
- bedclothes
  - with
    - conflagration - *see* Conflagration
    - ignition (of)
      - clothing - *see* Ignition, clothes
      - highly inflammable material
        - obstruction (benzine) (fat) (gasoline) (kerosene) (paraffin) (petrol) E894
- benzine E894
- clothes, clothing (from controlled fire) (in building) E893.9
  - with conflagration - *see* Conflagration
  - from
    - bonfire E893.2
    - highly inflammable material E894
    - sources or material as listed in E893.8
    - trash fire E893.2
    - uncontrolled fire - *see* Conflagration
  - in
    - private dwelling E893.0
    - specified building or structure, except of private dwelling E893.1
  - not in building or structure E893.2
- explosive material - *see* Explosion
- fat E894
- gasoline E894
- kerosene E894
- material
  - explosive - *see* Explosion
  - highly inflammable E894
    - with conflagration - *see* Conflagration
    - with explosion E923.2
- nightdress - *see* Ignition, clothes
- paraffin E894
- petrol E894

Immersion - *see* Submersion

Implantation of quills of porcupine E906.8

Inanition (from) E904.9
- hunger - *see* Lack of, food
- resulting from homicidal intent E968.4
- thirst - *see* Lack of, water

Inattention after, at birth E904.0
- homicidal, infanticidal intent E968.4

Infanticide (*see also* Assault)

Ingestion
- foreign body (causing injury) (with obstruction) - *see* Foreign body, alimentary canal
- poisonous substance NEC - *see* Table of Drugs and Chemicals

Inhalation
- excessively cold substance, manmade E901.1
- foreign body - *see* Foreign body, aspiration
- liquid air, hydrogen, nitrogen E901.1
- mucus, not of newborn (with asphyxia, obstruction respiratory passage, suffocation) E912
- phlegm (with asphyxia, obstruction respiratory passage, suffocation) E912

Foreign body, object or material – Inhalation

- **Inhalation** – *continued*
  - poisonous gas - *see* Table of Drugs and Chemicals
  - smoke from, due to
    - fire - *see* Fire
    - tobacco, second-hand E869.4
  - vomitus (with asphyxia, obstruction respiratory passage, suffocation) E911
- **Injury, injured** (accidental(ly)) NEC E928.9
  - by, caused by, from
    - air rifle (B-B gun) E922.4
    - animal (not being ridden) NEC E906.9
      - being ridden (in sport or transport) E828 [4th]
    - assault (*see also* Assault) E968.9
    - avalanche E909.2
    - bayonet (*see also* Bayonet wound) E920.3
    - being thrown against some part of, or object in
      - motor vehicle (in motion) (on public highway) E818 [4th]
        - not on public highway E825 [4th]
      - nonmotor road vehicle NEC E829 [4th]
      - off-road motor vehicle NEC E821 [4th]
      - railway train E806 [4th]
      - snow vehicle, motor-driven E820 [4th]
      - street car E829 [4th]
    - bending E927.8
    - bite, human E928.3
    - broken glass E920.8
    - bullet - *see* Shooting
    - cave-in (*see also* Suffocation, due to, cave-in) E913.3
      - earth surface movement or eruption E909.9
      - storm E908.9
      - without asphyxiation or suffocation E916
    - cloudburst E908.8
    - component of firearm or air gun E928.7 ●
    - cutting or piercing instrument (*see also* Cut) E920.9
    - cyclone E908.1
    - earth surface movement or eruption E909.9
    - earthquake E909.0
    - electric current (*see also* Electric shock) E925.9
    - explosion (*see also* Explosion) E923.9
      - of gun part E928.7 ●
    - fire - *see* Fire
    - flare, Verey pistol E922.8
    - flood E908.2
    - foreign body - *see* Foreign body
    - gun recoil E928.7 ●
    - hailstones E904.3
    - hurricane E908.0
    - landslide E909.2
    - law-enforcing agent, police, in course of legal intervention - *see* Legal intervention
    - lightning E907
    - live rail or live wire - *see* Electric shock
    - machinery - *see also* Accident, machine
      - aircraft, without accident to aircraft E844 [4th]
      - boat, ship, watercraft (deck) (engine room) (galley) (laundry) (loading) E836 [4th]
    - mechanism of firearm or air gun E928.7 ●
    - missile
      - explosive E923.8
      - firearm - *see* Shooting
      - in
        - terrorism - *see* Terrorism, missile

- **Injury, injured** – *continued*
  - by, caused by, from – *continued*
    - missile – *continued*
      - in – *continued*
        - war operations - *see* War operations, missile
    - moving part of motor vehicle (in motion) (on public highway) E818 [4th]
      - not on public highway, nontraffic accident E825 [4th]
      - while alighting, boarding, entering, leaving - *see* Fall, from, motor vehicle, while alighting, boarding
    - nail E920.8
    - needle (sewing) E920.4
      - hypodermic E920.5
    - noise E928.1
    - object
      - fallen on
        - motor vehicle (in motion) (on public highway) E818 [4th]
          - not on public highway E825 [4th]
      - falling-*see* Hit by, object, falling
    - paintball gun E922.5
    - radiation-*see* Radiation
    - railway rolling stock, train, vehicle (part of) E805 [4th]
      - door or window E806 [4th]
    - recoil of firearm E938.7 ●
    - rotating propeller, aircraft E844 [4th]
    - rough landing of off-road type motor vehicle (after leaving ground or rough terrain) E821 [4th]
      - snow vehicle E820 [4th]
    - saber (*see also* Wound, saber) E920.3
    - shot - *see* Shooting
    - sound waves E928.1
    - splinter or sliver, wood E920.8
    - straining E927.8
    - street car (door) E829 [4th]
    - suicide (attempt) E958.9
    - sword E920.3
    - terrorism - *see* Terrorism
    - third rail-*see* Electric shock
    - thunderbolt E907
    - tidal wave E909.4
      - caused by storm E908.0
    - tornado E908.1
    - torrential rain E908.2
    - twisting E927.8
    - vehicle NEC-*see* Accident, vehicle NEC
    - vibration E928.2
    - volcanic eruption E909.1
    - weapon burst, in war operations E993.9 ▲
    - weightlessness (in spacecraft, real or simulated) E928.0
    - wood splinter or sliver E920.8
  - due to
    - civil insurrection - *see* War operations
      - occurring after cessation of hostilities E998.9 ▲
    - terrorism - *see* Terrorism
    - war operations - *see* War operations
      - occurring after cessation of hostilities E998.9 ▲
    - weapon of mass destruction [WMD] E997.3 ●
  - homicidal (*see also* Assault) E968.9
  - in, on
    - civil insurrection - *see* War operations
    - fight E960.0
    - parachute descent (voluntary) (without accident to aircraft) E844 [4th]
      - with accident to aircraft-*see* categories E840-E842
    - public highway E819 [4th]
    - railway right of way E807 [4th]
    - terrorism - *see* Terrorism
    - war operations-*see* War operations

- **Injury, injured** – *continued*
  - inflicted (by)
    - in course of arrest (attempted), suppression of disturbance, maintenance of order, by law enforcing agents-*see* Legal intervention
    - law-enforcing agent (on duty)-*see* Legal intervention
    - other person
      - stated as
        - accidental E928.9
        - homicidal, intentional-*see* Assault
        - undetermined whether accidental or intentional-*see* Injury, stated as undetermined
    - police (on duty)-*see* Legal intervention
  - late effect of E929.9
  - purposely (inflicted) by other person(s) - *see* Assault
  - self-inflicted (unspecified whether accidental or intentional) E988.9
    - stated as
      - accidental E928.9
      - intentionally, purposely E958.9
  - specified cause NEC E928.8
  - stated as
    - hanging E983.0
    - knife E986
    - late effect of E989
    - puncture (any part of body) E986
    - shooting-*see* Shooting, stated as undetermined whether accidental or intentional
    - specified means NEC E988.8
    - stab (any part of body) E986
    - strangulation-*see* Suffocation, stated as undetermined whether accidental or intentional
    - submersion E984
    - suffocation-*see* Suffocation, stated as undetermined whether accidental or intentional
    - undetermined whether accidentally or purposely inflicted (by) E988.9
      - cut (any part of body) E986
      - cutting or piercing instrument (classifiable to E920) E986
      - drowning E984
      - explosive(s) (missile) E985.5
      - falling from high place E987.9
        - manmade structure, except residential E987.1
      - natural site E987.2
      - residential premises E987.0
  - to child due to criminal abortion E968.8
- **Insufficient nourishment** - *see also* Lack of, food
  - homicidal intent E968.4
- **Insulation, effects** - *see* Heat
- **Interruption of respiration by**
  - food lodged in esophagus E911
  - foreign body, except food, in esophagus E912
- **Intervention, legal** - *see* Legal intervention
- **Intoxication, drug or poison** - *see* Table of Drugs and Chemicals
- **Irradiation** - *see* Radiation

J

- **Jammed** (accidentally)
  - between objects (moving) (stationary and moving) E918
  - in object E918
- **Jumped or fell from high place, so stated** - *see* Jumping, from, high place, stated as in undetermined circumstances

- **Jumping**
  - before train, vehicle or other moving object (unspecified whether accidental or intentional) E988.0
    - stated as
      - intentional, purposeful E958.0
      - suicidal (attempt) E958.0
  - from
    - aircraft
      - by parachute (voluntarily) (without accident to aircraft) E844 [4th]
      - due to accident to aircraft-*see* categories E840-E842
    - boat, ship, watercraft (into water)
      - after accident to, fire on, watercraft E830 [4th]
        - and subsequently struck by (part of) boat E831 [4th]
      - burning, crushed, sinking E830 [4th]
        - and subsequently struck by (part of) boat E831 [4th]
      - voluntarily, without accident (to boat) with injury other than drowning or submersion E883.0
    - building - *see also* Jumping, from, high place
      - burning (uncontrolled fire) E891.8
        - in terrorism E979.3
        - private E890.8
    - cable car (not on rails) E847
      - on rails E829 [4th]
    - high place
      - in accidental circumstances or in sport-*see* categories E880-E884 [4th]
      - stated as
        - with intent to injure self E957.9
          - man-made structures NEC E957.1
          - natural sites E957.2
          - residential premises E957.0
        - in undetermined circumstances E987.9
          - man-made structures NEC E987.1
          - natural sites E987.2
          - residential premises E987.0
        - suicidal (attempt) E957.9
          - man-made structures NEC E957.1
          - natural sites E957.1
          - residential premises E957.0
    - motor vehicle (in motion) (on public highway) - *see* Fall, from, motor vehicle
    - nonmotor road vehicle NEC E829 [4th]
    - street car E829 [4th]
    - structure - *see also* Jumping, from, high place
      - burning NEC (uncontrolled fire) E891.8
        - in terrorism E979.3
  - into water
    - with injury other than drowning or submersion E883.0
      - drowning or submersion-*see* Submersion
    - from, off, watercraft - *see* Jumping, from, boat
- **Justifiable homicide** - *see* Assault

K

- **Kicked by**
  - animal E906.8
  - person(s) (accidentally) E917.9
    - with intent to injure or kill E960.0
    - as, or caused by a crowd E917.1
      - with subsequent fall E917.6
    - in fight E960.0
    - in sports E917.0
      - with subsequent fall E917.5

Inhalation – Kicked by

Kicking against – Misadventure(s) to patient(s) during surgical or medical care

Privation – *continued*
- helpless person, infant, newborn due to abandonment or neglect E904.0
- late effect of NEC E929.5
- resulting from transport accident - *see* categories E800-E848
- water (*see also* Lack of, water) E904.2

Projected objects, striking against or struck by - *see* Striking against, object

Prolonged stay in
- high attitude (causing conditions as listed in E902.0) E902.0
- weightless environment E928.0

Prostration
- heat - *see* Heat

Pulling, injury in E927.8

Puncture, puncturing (*see also* Cut) E920.9
- by
  - plant thorns or spines E920.8
    - toxic reaction E905.7
      - marine or sea plants E905.6
  - sea-urchin spine E905.6

Pushing (injury in) (overexertion) E927.8
- by other person(s) (accidental) E917.9
  - as, or caused by, a crowd, human stampede E917.1
    - with subsequent fall E917.6
  - before moving vehicle or object
    - stated as
      - intentional, homicidal E968.5
      - undetermined whether accidental or intentional E988.8
  - from
    - high place
      - in accidental circumstances - *see* categories E880-E884
      - stated as
        - intentional, homicidal E968.1
        - undetermined whether accidental or intentional E987.9
        - man-made structure, except residential E987.1
        - natural site E987.2
        - residential E987.0
    - motor vehicle (*see also* Fall, from, motor vehicle) E818 [4th]
      - stated as
        - intentional, homicidal E968.5
        - undetermined whether accidental or intentional E988.8
  - in sports E917.0
    - with fall E886.0
  - with fall E886.9
    - in sports E886.0

R

Radiation (exposure to) E926.9
- abnormal reaction to medical test or therapy E879.2
- arc lamps E926.2
- atomic power plant (malfunction) NEC E926.9
  - in water transport E838 [4th]
- electromagnetic, ionizing E926.3
- gamma rays E926.3
- in
  - terrorism (from or following nuclear explosion) (direct) (secondary) E979.5
    - laser E979.8
  - war operations <u>(*see also* War operations, injury due to, nuclear weapons)</u> ~~(from or following nuclear explosion) (direct) (secondary)~~ E996.<u>3</u> ▲
    - laser(s) E997.0
  - water transport E838 [4th]

Radiation (exposure to) – *continued*
- inadvertent exposure of patient (receiving test or therapy) E873.3
- infrared (heaters and lamps) E926.1
  - excessive heat E900.1
- ionized, ionizing (particles, artificially accelerated) E926.8
  - electromagnetic E926.3
- isotopes, radioactive - *see* Radiation, radioactive isotopes
- laser(s) E926.4
  - in
    - terrorism E979.8
    - war operations E997.0
  - misadventure in medical care - *see* Misadventure, failure, in dosage, radiation
- late effect of NEC E929.8
  - excessive heat from - *see* Heat
- light sources (visible) (ultraviolet) E926.2
- misadventure in medical or surgical procedure - *see* Misadventure, failure, in dosage, radiation
- overdose (in medical or surgical pacemaker) procedure) E873.2
- radar E926.0
- radioactive isotopes E926.5
  - atomic power plant malfunction E926.5
    - in water transport E838 [4th]
  - misadventure in medical or surgical treatment - *see* Misadventure, failure, in dosage, radiation
- radiobiologicals - *see* Radiation, radioactive isotopes
- radiofrequency E926.0
- radiopharmaceuticals - *see* Radiation, radioactive isotopes
- radium NEC E926.9
- sun E926.2
  - excessive heat from E900.0
- tanning bed E926.2
- welding arc or torch E926.2
  - excessive heat from E900.1
- x-rays (hard) (soft) E926.3
  - misadventure in medical or surgical treatment - *see* Misadventure, failure, in dosage, radiation

Rape E960.1

Reaction, abnormal to or following (medical or surgical procedure) E879.9
- amputation (of limbs) E878.5
- anastomosis (arteriovenous) (blood vessel) (gastrojejunal) (skin) (tendon) (natural, artificial material, tissue) E878.2
  - external stoma, creation of E878.3
- aspiration (of fluid) E879.4
  - tissue E879.8
- biopsy E879.8
- blood
  - sampling E879.7
  - transfusion
    - procedure E879.8
- bypass - *see* Reaction, abnormal, anastomosis
- catheterization
  - cardiac E879.0
  - urinary E879.6
- colostomy E878.3
- cystostomy E878.3
- dialysis (kidney) E879.1
- drugs or biologicals - *see* Table of Drugs and Chemicals
- duodenostomy E878.3
- electroshock therapy E879.3
- formation of external stoma E878.3
- gastrostomy E878.3
- graft - *see* Reaction, abnormal, anastomosis
- hypothermia E879.8

Reaction, abnormal to or following – *continued*
- implant, implantation (of)
  - artificial
    - internal device (cardiac pacemaker) (electrodes in brain) (heart valve prosthesis) (orthopedic) E878.1
    - material or tissue (for anastomosis or bypass) E878.2
      - with creation of external stoma E878.3
  - natural tissues (for anastomosis or bypass) E878.2
    - as transplantation - *see* Reaction, abnormal, transplant
    - with creation of external stoma E878.3
- infusion
  - procedure E879.8
- injection
  - procedure E879.8
- insertion of gastric or duodenal sound E879.5
- insulin-shock therapy E879.3
- lumbar puncture E879.4
- perfusion E879.1
- procedures other than surgical operation (*see also* Reaction, abnormal, by specific type of procedure) E879.9
  - specified procedure NEC E879.8
- radiological procedure or therapy E879.2
- removal of organ (partial) (total) NEC E878.6
  - with
    - anastomosis, bypass or graft E878.2
    - formation of external stoma E878.3
    - implant of artificial internal device E878.1
    - transplant(ation)
      - partial organ E878.4
      - whole organ E878.0
- sampling
  - blood E879.7
  - fluid NEC E879.4
  - tissue E879.8
- shock therapy E879.3
- surgical operation (*see also* Reaction, abnormal, by specified type of operation) E878.9
  - restorative NEC E878.4
    - with
      - anastomosis, bypass or graft E878.2
      - formation of external stoma E878.3
      - implant(ation) - *see* Reaction, abnormal, implant
      - transplantation) - *see* Reaction, abnormal, transplant
  - specified operation NEC E878.8
- thoracentesis E879.4
- transfusion
  - procedure E879.8
- transplant, transplantation (heart) (kidney) (liver) E878.0
  - partial organ E878.4
- ureterostomy E878.3
- vaccination E879.8

Reduction in
- atmospheric pressure - *see also* Effects of, air pressure
  - while surfacing from
    - deep water diving causing caisson or divers' disease, palsy or paralysis E902.2
    - underground E902.8

Residual (effect) - *see* Late effect

Rock falling on or hitting (accidentally)
- motor vehicle (in motion) (on public highway) E818 [4th]
  - not on public highway E825 [4th]
- nonmotor road vehicle NEC E829 [4th]
- pedal cycle E826 [4th]

Rock falling on or hitting – *continued*
- person E916
- railway rolling stock, train, vehicle E806 [4th]

Running off, away
- animal (being ridden) (in sport or transport) E828 [4th]
  - not being ridden E906.8
- animal-drawn vehicle E827 [4th]
- rails, railway (*see also* Derailment) E802 [4th]
- roadway
  - motor vehicle (without antecedent collision) E816 [4th]
    - with
      - antecedent collision - *see* Collision motor vehicle
      - subsequent collision
        - involving any object, person or vehicle not on public of highway E816 [4th]
        - on public highway E811 [4th]
    - nontraffic accident E825 [4th]
      - with antecedent collision - *see* categories Collision, motor vehicle, not on public highway
  - nonmotor road vehicle NEC E829 [4th]
  - pedal cycle E826 [4th]

Run over (accidentally) (by)
- animal (not being ridden) E906.8
  - being ridden (in sport or transport) E828 [4th]
- animal-drawn vehicle E827 [4th]
- machinery - *see* Accident, machine
- motor vehicle (on public highway) - *see* Hit by, motor vehicle
- nonmotor road vehicle NEC E829 [4th]
- railway train E805 [4th]
- street car E829 [4th]
- vehicle NEC E848

S

Saturnism E866.0
- from insecticide NEC E863.4

Scald, scalding (accidental) (by) (from) (in) E924.0
- acid - *see* Scald, caustic
- boiling tap water E924.2
- caustic or corrosive liquid, substance E924.1
  - swallowed - *see* Table of Drugs and Chemicals
- homicide (attempt) - *see* Assault, burning
- inflicted by other person
  - stated as
    - intentional or homicidal E968.3
    - undetermined whether accidental or intentional E988.2
- late effect of NEC E929.8
- liquid (boiling) (hot) E924.0
- local application of externally applied substance in medical or surgical care E873.5
- molten metal E924.0
- self-inflicted (unspecified whether accidental or intentional) E988.2
  - stated as intentional, purposeful E958.2
- stated as undetermined whether accidental or intentional E988.2
- steam E924.0
- tap water (boiling) E924.2
- transport accident - *see* categories E800-E848
- vapor E924.0

Scratch, cat E906.8

Sea
- sickness E903

Self-mutilation - *see* Suicide

Sequelae – Submersion

- **Submersion** (accidental) – *continued*
  - due to – *continued*
    - fall
      - from
        - boat, ship, watercraft (not involved in accident) E832 4th
          - burning, crushed E830 4th
          - involved in accident, collision E830 4th
        - gangplank (into water) E832 4th
      - overboard NEC E832 4th
    - flood E908.2
    - hurricane E908.0
    - jumping into water E910.8
      - from boat, ship, watercraft
        - burning, crushed, sinking E830 4th
        - involved in accident, collision E830 4th
        - not involved in accident, for swim E910.2
      - in recreational activity (without diving equipment) E910.2
        - with or using diving equipment E910.1
      - to rescue another person E910.3
  - homicide (attempt) E964
  - in
    - bathtub E910.4
    - specified activity, not sport, transport or recreational E910.3
    - sport or recreational activity (without diving equipment) E910.2
      - with or using diving equipment E910.1
        - water skiing E910.0
    - swimming pool NEC E910.8
    - terrorism E979.8
    - war operations E995.4 ▲
      - intentional E995.3 ●
    - water transport E832 4th
      - due to accident to boat, ship, watercraft E830 4th
  - landslide E909.2
    - overturning boat, ship, watercraft E909.2
    - sinking boat, ship, watercraft E909.2
    - submersion boat, ship, watercraft E909.2
    - tidal wave E909.4
      - caused by storm E908.0
    - torrential rain E908.2
  - late effect of NEC E929.8
  - quenching tank E910.8
  - self-inflicted (unspecified whether accidental or intentional) E984
    - in accidental circumstances - *see* category E910
  - stated as intentional, purposeful E954
      - stated as undetermined whether accidental or intentional E984
  - suicidal (attempted) E954
  - while
    - attempting rescue of another person E910.3
    - engaged in
      - marine salvage E910.3
      - underwater construction or repairs E910.3
    - fishing, not from boat E910.2
    - hunting, not from boat E910.2
    - ice skating E910.2
    - pearl diving E910.3
    - placing fishing nets E910.3
    - playing in water E910.2
    - scuba diving E910.1
      - nonrecreational E910.3
    - skin diving E910.1
    - snorkel diving E910.2
    - spear fishing underwater E910.1
    - surfboarding E910.2
    - swimming (swimming pool) E910.2
    - wading (in water) E910.2

- **Submersion** (accidental) – *continued*
  - while – *continued*
    - water skiing E910.0
- **Sucked**
  - into
    - jet (aircraft) E844 4th
- **Suffocation** (accidental) (by external means) (by pressure) (mechanical) E913.9
  - caused by other person
    - in accidental circumstances - *see* category E913
    - stated as
      - intentional, homicidal E963
      - undetermined whether accidental or intentional E983.9
        - by, in
          - hanging E983.0
          - plastic bag E983.1
          - specified means NEC E983.8
  - due to, by
    - avalanche E909.2
    - bedclothes E913.0
    - bib E913.0
    - blanket E913.0
    - cave-in E913.3
      - caused by cataclysmic earth surface movement or eruption E909.9
    - conflagration - *see* Conflagration E983.8
    - explosion - *see* Explosion
    - falling earth, other substance E913.3 (attempted) (by) E958.9
    - fire - *see* Fire
    - food, any type (ingestion) (inhalation) (regurgitated) (vomited) E911
    - foreign body, except food (ingestion) (inhalation) E912
    - ignition - *see* Ignition
    - landslide E909.2
    - machine(ry) - *see* Accident, machine
    - material, object except food entering by nose or mouth, ingested, inhaled E912
    - mucus (aspiration) (inhalation), not of newborn E912
    - phlegm (aspiration) (inhalation) E912
    - pillow E913.0
    - plastic bag - *see* Suffocation, in, plastic bag
    - sheet (plastic) E913.0
    - specified means NEC E913.8
    - vomitus (aspiration) (inhalation) E911
  - homicidal (attempt) E963
    - in war operations E995.3 ●
  - in
    - airtight enclosed place E913.2
    - baby carriage E913.0
    - bed E913.0
    - closed place E913.2
    - cot, cradle E913.0
    - perambulator E913.0
    - plastic bag (in accidental circumstances) E913.1
      - homicidal, purposely inflicted by other person E963
      - self-inflicted (unspecified whether accidental or intentional) E983.1
        - in accidental circumstances E913.1
        - intentional, suicidal E953.1
      - stated as undetermined whether accidentally or purposely inflicted E983.1
      - suicidal, purposely self-inflicted E953.1
    - refrigerator E913.2
    - war operations E995.3 ●
  - self-inflicted - *see also* Suffocation, stated as undetermined whether accidental or intentional E953.9
    - in accidental circumstances - *see* category E913

- **Suffocation** – *continued*
  - self-inflicted – *continued*
    - stated as intentional, purposeful - *see* Suicide, suffocation
  - stated as undetermined whether accidental or intentional E983.9
    - by, in
      - hanging E983.0
      - plastic bag E983.1
      - specified means NEC E983.8
  - suicidal - *see* Suicide, suffocation
- **Suicide, suicidal** (attempted) (by) E958.9
  - burning, bums E958.1
  - caustic substance E958.7
    - poisoning E950.7
    - swallowed E950.7
  - cold, extreme E958.3
  - cut (any part of body) E956
  - cutting or piercing instrument (classifiable to E920) E956
  - drowning E954
  - electrocution E958.4
  - explosive(s) (classifiable to E923) E955.5
  - fire E958.1
  - firearm (classifiable to E922) - *see* Shooting, suicidal
  - hanging E953.0
  - jumping
    - before moving object, train, vehicle E958.0
    - from high place - *see* Jumping, from, high place, stated as, suicidal
  - knife E956
  - late effect of E959
  - motor vehicle, crashing of E958.5
  - poisoning - *see* Table of Drugs and Chemicals
  - puncture (any part of body) E956
  - scald E958.2
  - shooting - *see* Shooting, suicidal
  - specified means NEC E958.8
  - stab (any part of body) E956
  - strangulation - *see* Suicide, suffocation
  - submersion E954
  - suffocation E953.9
    - by, in
      - hanging E953.0
      - plastic bag E953.1
      - specified means NEC E953.8
  - wound NEC E958.9
- **Sunburn** E926.2
- **Sunstroke** E900.0
- **Supersonic waves** (causing injury) E928.1
- **Surgical procedure, complication of**
  - delayed or as an abnormal reaction vehicle without mention of misadventure *see* Reaction, abnormal
  - due to or as a result of misadventure - *see* Misadventure
- **Swallowed, swallowing**
  - foreign body - *see* Foreign body, alimentary canal
  - poison - *see* Table of Drugs and Chemicals
  - substance
    - caustic - *see* Table of Drugs and Chemicals drugs
    - corrosive - *see* Table of Drugs and Chemicals
    - poisonous - *see* Table of Drugs and Chemicals
- **Swimmers cramp** (*see also* category E910) E910.2
  - not in recreation or sport E910.3
- **Syndrome, battered**
  - baby or child - *see* Abuse, child
  - wife - *see* Assault

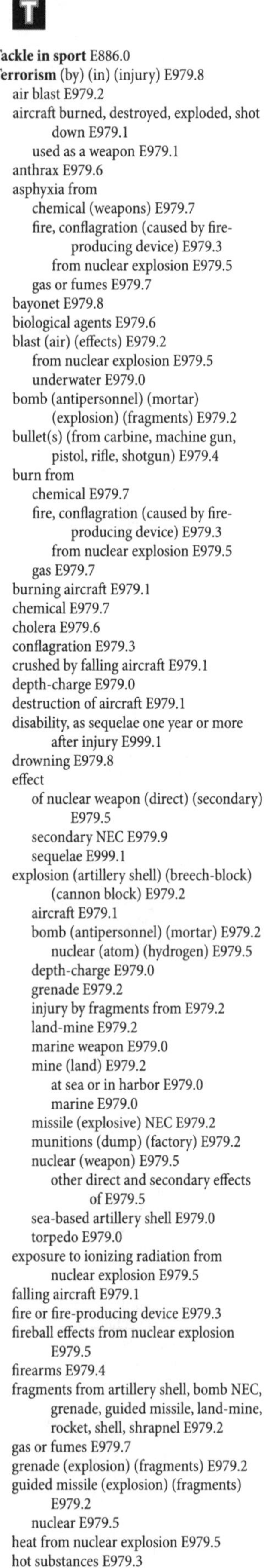

T

- **Tackle in sport** E886.0
- **Terrorism** (by) (in) (injury) E979.8
  - air blast E979.2
  - aircraft burned, destroyed, exploded, shot down E979.1
    - used as a weapon E979.1
  - anthrax E979.6
  - asphyxia from
    - chemical (weapons) E979.7
    - fire, conflagration (caused by fire-producing device) E979.3
      - from nuclear explosion E979.5
    - gas or fumes E979.7
  - bayonet E979.8
  - biological agents E979.6
  - blast (air) (effects) E979.2
    - from nuclear explosion E979.5
    - underwater E979.0
  - bomb (antipersonnel) (mortar) (explosion) (fragments) E979.2
  - bullet(s) (from carbine, machine gun, pistol, rifle, shotgun) E979.4
  - burn from
    - chemical E979.7
    - fire, conflagration (caused by fire-producing device) E979.3
      - from nuclear explosion E979.5
    - gas E979.7
  - burning aircraft E979.1
  - chemical E979.7
  - cholera E979.6
  - conflagration E979.3
  - crushed by falling aircraft E979.1
  - depth-charge E979.0
  - destruction of aircraft E979.1
  - disability, as sequelae one year or more after injury E999.1
  - drowning E979.8
  - effect
    - of nuclear weapon (direct) (secondary) E979.5
    - secondary NEC E979.9
    - sequelae E999.1
  - explosion (artillery shell) (breech-block) (cannon block) E979.2
    - aircraft E979.1
    - bomb (antipersonnel) (mortar) E979.2
      - nuclear (atom) (hydrogen) E979.5
    - depth-charge E979.0
    - grenade E979.2
    - injury by fragments from E979.2
    - land-mine E979.2
    - marine weapon E979.0
    - mine (land) E979.2
      - at sea or in harbor E979.0
      - marine E979.0
    - missile (explosive) NEC E979.2
    - munitions (dump) (factory) E979.2
    - nuclear (weapon) E979.5
      - other direct and secondary effects of E979.5
    - sea-based artillery shell E979.0
    - torpedo E979.0
  - exposure to ionizing radiation from nuclear explosion E979.5
  - falling aircraft E979.1
  - fire or fire-producing device E979.3
  - fireball effects from nuclear explosion E979.5
  - firearms E979.4
  - fragments from artillery shell, bomb NEC, grenade, guided missile, land-mine, rocket, shell, shrapnel E979.2
  - gas or fumes E979.7
  - grenade (explosion) (fragments) E979.2
  - guided missile (explosion) (fragments) E979.2
    - nuclear E979.5
  - heat from nuclear explosion E979.5
  - hot substances E979.3
  - hydrogen cyanide E979.7

Submersion – Terrorism

- **War operations** – *continued*
  - injury due to – *continued*
    - blast E993.9 ●
      - wave E993.9 ●
      - wind E993.9 ●
    - bomb E993.8 ●
    - but occurring after cessation of hostilities ●
      - explosion of bombs E998.1 ●
      - explosion of mines E998.0 ●
      - specified NEC E998.8 ●
    - conventional warfare E995.9 ●
      - specified form NEC E995.8 ●
    - depth charge E992.1 ●
    - destruction of aircraft E994.9 ●
      - due to ●
        - air to air missile E994.0 ●
        - collision with other aircraft E994.2 ●
        - enemy fire or explosives E994.0 ●
        - on board explosion (explosives) E994.1 ●
        - on board fire E994.3 ●
        - rocket propelled grenade [RPG] E994.0 ●
        - small arms fire E994.0 ●
        - surface to air missile E994.0 ●
      - specified NEC E994.8 ●
    - dirty bomb (see also War operations, injury due to, nuclear weapons) E996.9 ●
    - drowning E995.4 ●
    - explosion (direct pressure) (indirect pressure) (due to) E993.9 ●
      - depth charge E992.1 ●
      - improvised explosive device [IED] ●
        - person borne E993.3 ●
        - roadside E993.5 ●
        - specified NEC E993.5 ●
        - transport vehicle (air) (land) (water) borne E993.4 ●
        - vehicle (air) (land) (water) borne E993.4 ●
      - marine mines (in harbor) (at sea) E992.2 ●
      - marine weapons E992.9 ●
        - specified NEC E992.8 ●
      - sea based artillery shell E992.3 ●
      - specified NEC E993.8 ●
      - torpedo E992.0 ●
      - unintentional (of own) ●
        - autocannons E993.7 ●
        - automatic grenade launchers E993.7 ●
        - launch device discharge E993.7 ●
        - munitions detonation (ammunition) (artillery) (mortars) E993.6 ●
        - missile launchers E993.7 ●
        - small arms E993.7 ●

- **War operations** – *continued*
  - injury due to – *continued*
    - fragments (from) E991.9 ●
      - artillery E991.8 ●
      - artillery shells E991.4 ●
      - autocannons E991.8 ●
      - automatic grenade launchers [AGL] E991.8 ●
      - bombs E991.4 ●
        - antipersonnel E991.3 ●
      - detonation of unexploded ordnance [UXO] E991.4 ●
      - grenade E991.4 ●
      - guided missile E991.4 ●
      - improvised explosive device [IED] ●
        - person borne E991.5 ●
        - roadside E991.7 ●
        - specified NEC E991.7 ●
        - transport vehicle (air) (land) (water) borne E991.6 ●
        - vehicle (air) (land) (water) borne E991.6 ●
      - land mine E991.4 ●
      - missile launchers E991.8 ●
      - mortars E991.8 ●
      - munitions (artillery shells) (bombs) (grenades) (rockets) (shells) E991.4 ●
      - rockets E991.4 ●
      - shells E991.4 ●
      - small arms E991.8 ●
      - specified NEC E991.9 ●
      - weapons (artillery) (autocannons) (mortars) (small arms) E991.8 ●
    - grenade E993.8 ●
    - guided missile E993.1 ●
    - hand to hand combat, unarmed E995.0 ●
    - improvised explosive device [IED] ●
      - person borne E993.3 ●
      - roadside E993.5 ●
      - specified NEC E993.5 ●
      - transport vehicle (air) (land) (water) borne E993.4 ●
      - vehicle (air) (land) (water) borne E993.4 ●
    - inability to surface or obtain air E995.4 ●
    - land mine E993.8 ●
    - marine mines (in harbor) (at sea) E992.2 ●
    - marine weapons E992.9 ●
      - specified NEC E992.8 ●
    - mortar E993.2 ●
    - nuclear weapons E996.9 ●
      - beta burns E996.3 ●
      - blast debris E996.1 ●
      - blast pressure E996.0 ●
      - burns due to thermal radiation E996.2 ●
      - direct blast effect E996.0 ●
      - fallout exposure E996.3 ●
      - fireball effect E996.2 ●
      - flash burns E996.2 ●

- **War operations** – *continued*
  - injury due to – *continued*
    - nuclear weapons – *continued*
      - heat effect E996.2 ●
      - indirect blast effect E996.1 ●
      - nuclear radiation effects E996.3 ●
      - radiation exposure (acute) E996.3 ●
      - radiation sickness E996.3 ●
      - secondary effects E996.3 ●
      - specified effects NEC E996.8 ●
      - thermal radiation effect E996.2 ●
    - piercing object E995.2 ●
    - restriction of airway, intentional E995.3 ●
    - sea based artillery shell E992.3 ●
    - shrapnel E991.9 ●
    - stave E995.1 ●
    - strangulation E995.3 ●
    - strike by blunt object (baton) (nightstick) (stave) E995.1 ●
    - submersion (accidental) (unintentional) E995.4 ●
      - intentional E995.3 ●
    - suffocation E995.3 ●
      - accidental E995.4 ●
    - torpedo E992.0 ●
    - underwater blast E992.9 ●
    - weapon of mass destruction [WMD] E997.3 ●
  - knife E995.2 ●
  - lacrimator (gas) (chemical) E997.2
  - land mine (explosion) E993.8 ▲
    - after cessation of hostilities E998.0 ▲
    - fragments, injury by E991.4 ▲
  - laser(s) E997.0
  - late effect of E999.0
  - lewisite E997.2
  - lung irritant (chemical) (fumes) (gas) E997.2
  - marine mine E992.2 ▲
  - mine
    - after cessation of hostilities E998.0 ▲
    - at sea E992.2 ▲
    - in harbor E992.2 ▲
    - land (explosion) E993.8 ▲
      - fragments, injury by E991.4 ▲
    - marine E992.2 ▲
  - missile (guided) (explosion) E993.1 ▲
    - fragments, injury by E991.4 ▲
    - marine E992.8 ▲
    - nuclear (*see also* War operations, injury due to, nuclear weapons) E996.9 ▲
  - mortar bomb (explosion) E993.2 ▲
    - fragments, injury by E991.4 ▲
  - mustard gas E997.2
  - nerve gas E997.2
  - phosgene E997.2
  - piercing object E995.2 ●
  - poisoning (chemical) (fumes) (gas) E997.2
  - radiation, ionizing from nuclear explosion (*see also* War operations, injury due to, nuclear weapons) E996.3 ▲
  - rocket (explosion) E993.8 ▲
    - fragments, injury by E991.4 ▲

- **War operations** – *continued*
  - saber, sabre E995.2 ▲
  - screening smoke E997.8
  - shell (aircraft) (artillery) (cannon) (land based) (explosion) E993.2 ▲
    - fragments, injury by E991.4 ▲
    - sea-based E992.3 ▲
  - shooting E991.2
    - after cessation of hostilities E998.8 ▲
    - bullet(s) E991.2
      - rubber E991.0
    - pellet(s) (rifle) E991.1
    - shrapnel E991.9
  - stave E995.2 ●
  - strike by blunt object (baton) (nightstick) (stave) E995.1 ●
  - submersion E995.4 ▲
    - intentional E995.3 ●
  - sword E995.2 ●
  - torpedo E992.0 ▲
  - unconventional warfare, except by nuclear weapon E997.9
    - biological (warfare) E997.1
    - gas, fumes, chemicals E997.2
    - laser(s) E997.0
    - specified type NEC E997.8
  - underwater blast E992.9 ▲
  - vesicant (chemical) (fumes) (gas) E997.2
  - weapon burst E993.9 ▲
- **Washed**
  - away by flood - *see* Flood
  - away by tidal wave - *see* Tidal wave
  - off road by storm (transport vehicle) E908.9
  - overboard E832 4th
- **Weapon of mass destruction** [WMD] E997.3 ●
- **Weather exposure** - *see also* Exposure
  - cold E901.0
  - hot E900.0
- **Weightlessness** (causing injury) (effects of) (in spacecraft, real or simulated) E928.0
- **Wound** (accidental) NEC (*see also* Injury) E928.9
  - battle (*see also* War operations) E995.9 ▲
  - bayonet E920.3
    - in
      - legal intervention E974
      - war operations E995.2 ▲
  - gunshot - *see* Shooting
  - incised - *see* Cut
  - saber, sabre E920.3
    - in war operations E995.2 ▲
- **Wrong** ●
  - body part, performance of correct operation (procedure) on E876.7 ●
  - device implanted into correct surgical site E876.5 ●
  - patient, performance of operation (procedure) on E876.6 ●
  - procedure (operation) performed on correct patient E876.5 ●
  - side, performance of correct operation (procedure) on E876.7 ●
  - site, performance of correct operation (procedure) on E876.7 ●

1. INFECTIOUS AND PARASITIC DISEASES (001-139)

Note: *Categories for "late effects" of infectious and parasitic diseases are to be found at 137-139.*

Includes diseases generally recognized as communicable or transmissible as well as a few diseases of unknown but possibly infectious origin

Excludes *acute respiratory infections (460-466)*
carrier or suspected carrier of infectious organism (V02.0-V02.9)
certain localized infections
influenza (487.0-487.8, 488.0-488.1)

INTESTINAL INFECTIOUS DISEASES (001-009)

Excludes *helminthiases (120.0-129)*

4th **001 Cholera**
- **001.0 Due to Vibrio cholerae**
- **001.1 Due to Vibrio cholerae el tor**
- **001.9 Cholera, unspecified**

4th **002 Typhoid and paratyphoid fevers**
- **002.0 Typhoid fever**
  Typhoid (fever) (infection) [any site]
- **002.1 Paratyphoid fever A**
- **002.2 Paratyphoid fever B**
- **002.3 Paratyphoid fever C**
- **002.9 Paratyphoid fever, unspecified**

4th **003 Other salmonella infections**

Includes infection or food poisoning by Salmonella [any serotype]

- **003.0 Salmonella gastroenteritis**
  Salmonellosis
- **003.1 Salmonella septicemia**
- 5th **003.2 Localized salmonella infections**
  - **003.20 Localized salmonella infection, unspecified**
  - **003.21 Salmonella meningitis**
  - **003.22 Salmonella pneumonia**
  - **003.23 Salmonella arthritis**
  - **003.24 Salmonella osteomyelitis**
  - **003.29 Other**
- **003.8 Other specified salmonella infections**
- **003.9 Salmonella infection, unspecified**

4th **004 Shigellosis**

Includes bacillary dysentery

- **004.0 Shigella dysenteriae**
  Infection by group A Shigella (Schmitz) (Shiga)
- **004.1 Shigella flexneri**
  Infection by group B Shigella
- **004.2 Shigella boydii**
  Infection by group C Shigella
- **004.3 Shigella sonnei**
  Infection by group D Shigella
- **004.8 Other specified shigella infections**
- **004.9 Shigellosis, unspecified**

4th **005 Other food poisoning (bacterial)**

Excludes *salmonella infections (003.0-003.9)*
toxic effect of:
food contaminants (989.7)
noxious foodstuffs (988.0-988.9)

- **005.0 Staphylococcal food poisoning**
  Staphylococcal toxemia specified as due to food
- **005.1 Botulism food poisoning**
  Botulism NOS
  Food poisoning due to Clostridium botulinum
  Excludes *infant botulism (040.41)*
  wound botulism (040.42)
- **005.2 Food poisoning due to Clostridium perfringens [C. welchii]**
  Enteritis necroticans
- **005.3 Food poisoning due to other Clostridia**
- **005.4 Food poisoning due to Vibrio parahaemolyticus**
- 5th **005.8 Other bacterial food poisoning**
  Excludes *salmonella food poisoning (003.0-003.9)*
  - **005.81 Food poisoning due to Vibrio vulnificus**
  - **005.89 Other bacterial food poisoning**
    Food poisoning due to Bacillus cereus
- **005.9 Food poisoning, unspecified**

4th **006 Amebiasis**

Includes infection due to Entamoeba histolytica

Excludes *amebiasis due to organisms other than Entamoeba histolytica (007.8)*

- **006.0 Acute amebic dysentery without mention of abscess**
  Acute amebiasis
- **006.1 Chronic intestinal amebiasis without mention of abscess**
  Chronic:
  amebiasis
  amebic dysentery
- **006.2 Amebic nondysenteric colitis**
- **006.3 Amebic liver abscess**
  Hepatic amebiasis
- **006.4 Amebic lung abscess**
  Amebic abscess of lung (and liver)
- **006.5 Amebic brain abscess**
  Amebic abscess of brain (and liver) (and lung)
- **006.6 Amebic skin ulceration**
  Cutaneous amebiasis
- **006.8 Amebic infection of other sites**
  Amebic:
  appendicitis
  balanitis
  Ameboma
  Excludes *specific infections by free-living amebae (136.21-136.29)*
- **006.9 Amebiasis, unspecified**
  Amebiasis NOS

4th **007 Other protozoal intestinal diseases**

Includes protozoal:
colitis
diarrhea
dysentery

- **007.0 Balantidiasis**
  Infection by Balantidium coli
- **007.1 Giardiasis**
  Infection by Giardia lamblia
  Lambliasis
- **007.2 Coccidiosis**
  Infection by Isospora belli and Isospora hominis
  Isosporiasis
- **007.3 Intestinal trichomoniasis**
- **007.4 Cryptosporidiosis**
- **007.5 Cyclosporiasis**
- **007.8 Other specified protozoal intestinal diseases**
  Amebiasis due to organisms other than Entamoeba histolytica

007.9 Unspecified protozoal intestinal disease
Flagellate diarrhea
Protozoal dysentery NOS

4th 008 Intestinal infections due to other organisms
Includes any condition classifiable to 009.0-009.3 with mention of the responsible organisms
Excludes *food poisoning by these organisms (005.0-005.9)*

5th 008.0 Escherichia coli [E. coli]
008.00 E. coli, unspecified
E. coli enteritis NOS
008.01 Enteropathogenic E. coli
008.02 Enterotoxigenic E. coli
008.03 Enteroinvasive E. coli
008.04 Enterohemorrhagic E. coli
008.09 Other intestinal E. coli infections

008.1 Arizona group of paracolon bacilli

008.2 Aerobacter aerogenes
Enterobacter aerogenes

008.3 Proteus (mirabilis) (morganii)

5th 008.4 Other specified bacteria
008.41 Staphylococcus
Staphylococcal enterocolitis
008.42 Pseudomonas
008.43 Campylobacter
008.44 Yersinia enterocolitica
008.45 Clostridium difficile
Pseudomembranous colitis
Layman's: *C. difficile is a bacteria that occurs naturally in the colon, but can run amok in patients taking antibiotics. Reviewing documentation for onset soon after antibiotic use by the patient can help determine if 008.45 is a more appropriate code to use than the other infectious and autoimmune colitis codes.*
008.46 Other anaerobes
Anaerobic enteritis NOS
Bacteroides (fragilis)
Gram-negative anaerobes
008.47 Other gram-negative bacteria
Gram-negative enteritis NOS
Excludes *gram-negative anaerobes (008.46)*
008.49 Other

008.5 Bacterial enteritis, unspecified

5th 008.6 Enteritis due to specified virus
008.61 Rotavirus
008.62 Adenovirus
008.63 Norwalk virus
Norovirus
Norwalk-like agent
008.64 Other small round viruses [SRVs]
Small round virus NOS
▲008.65 Calicivirus
008.66 Astrovirus
008.67 Enterovirus NEC
Coxsackie virus
Echovirus
Excludes *poliovirus (045.0-045.9)*
008.69 Other viral enteritis
Torovirus

008.8 Other organism, not elsewhere classified
Viral:
enteritis NOS
gastroenteritis
Excludes *influenza with involvement of gastrointestinal tract (487.8)*

4th 009 Ill-defined intestinal infections
Excludes *diarrhea following gastrointestinal surgery (564.4)*
diarrheal disease or intestinal infection due to specified organism (001.0-008.8)
intestinal malabsorption (579.0-579.9)
ischemic enteritis (557.0-557.9)
other noninfectious gastroenteritis and colitis (558.1-558.9)
regional enteritis (555.0-555.9)
ulcerative colitis (556)

009.0 Infectious colitis, enteritis, and gastroenteritis
Colitis (septic)
Dysentery:
NOS
catarrhal
hemorrhagic
Enteritis (septic)
Gastroenteritis (septic)

009.1 Colitis, enteritis, and gastroenteritis of presumed infectious origin
Excludes *colitis NOS (558.9)*
enteritis NOS (558.9)
gastroenteritis NOS (558.9)

009.2 Infectious diarrhea
Diarrhea:
dysenteric
epidemic
Infectious diarrheal disease NOS

009.3 Diarrhea of presumed infectious origin
Excludes *diarrhea NOS (787.91)*

TUBERCULOSIS (010-018)

Includes infection by Mycobacterium tuberculosis (human) (bovine)
Excludes *congenital tuberculosis (771.2)*
late effects of tuberculosis (137.0-137.4)

The following fifth-digit subclassification is for use with categories 010-018:
0 unspecified
1 bacteriological or histological examination not done
2 bacteriological or histological examination unknown (at present)
3 tubercle bacilli found (in sputum) by microscopy
4 tubercle bacilli not found (in sputum) by microscopy, but found by bacterial culture
5 tubercle bacilli not found by bacteriological examination, but tuberculosis confirmed histologically
6 tubercle bacilli not found by bacteriological or histological examination, but tuberculosis confirmed by other methods [inoculation of animals]

4th 010 Primary tuberculous infection
Requires fifth digit. See beginning of section 010-018 for codes and definitions.

5th 010.0 Primary tuberculous infection
[0-6]
Excludes *nonspecific reaction to tuberculin skin test without active tuberculosis (795.5)*
positive PPD (795.5)
positive tuberculin skin test without active tuberculosis (795.5)

5th 010.1 **Tuberculous pleurisy in primary progressive tuberculosis**
[0-6]

5th 010.8 **Other primary progressive tuberculosis**
[0-6]

Excludes *tuberculous erythema nodosum (017.1)*

5th 010.9 **Primary tuberculous infection, unspecified**
[0-6]

4th 011 **Pulmonary tuberculosis**
Requires fifth digit. See beginning of section 010-018 for codes and definitions.
Use additional code to identify any associated silicosis (502)

5th 011.0 **Tuberculosis of lung, infiltrative**
[0-6]

5th 011.1 **Tuberculosis of lung, nodular**
[0-6]

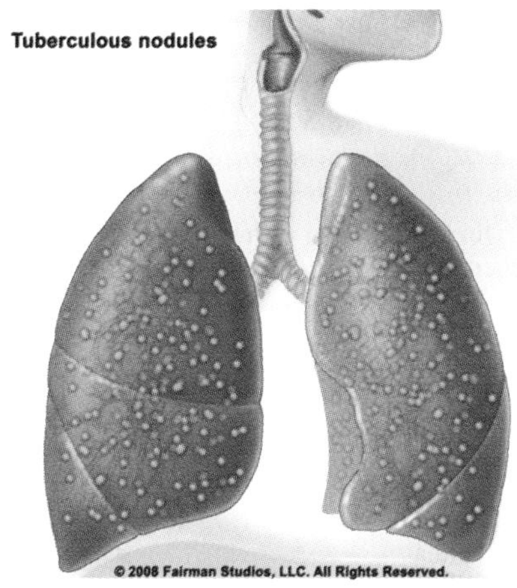

5th 011.2 **Tuberculosis of lung with cavitation**
[0-6]

5th 011.3 **Tuberculosis of bronchus**
[0-6]

Excludes *isolated bronchial tuberculosis (012.2)*

5th 011.4 **Tuberculous fibrosis of lung**
[0-6]

5th 011.5 **Tuberculous bronchiectasis**
[0-6]

5th 011.6 **Tuberculous pneumonia [any form]**
[0-6]

5th 011.7 **Tuberculous pneumothorax**
[0-6]

5th 011.8 **Other specified pulmonary tuberculosis**
[0-6]

5th 011.9 **Pulmonary tuberculosis, unspecified**
[0-6] Respiratory tuberculosis NOS
Tuberculosis of lung NOS

4th 012 **Other respiratory tuberculosis**
Requires fifth digit. See beginning of section 010-018 for codes and definitions.

Excludes *respiratory tuberculosis, unspecified (011.9)*

5th 012.0 **Tuberculous pleurisy**
[0-6] Tuberculosis of pleura
Tuberculous empyema
Tuberculous hydrothorax

Excludes *pleurisy with effusion without mention of cause (511.9)*
tuberculous pleurisy in primary progressive tuberculosis (010.1)

5th 012.1 **Tuberculosis of intrathoracic lymph nodes**
[0-6] Tuberculosis of lymph nodes:
hilar
mediastinal
tracheobronchial
Tuberculous tracheobronchial adenopathy

Excludes *that specified as primary (010.0-010.9)*

5th 012.2 **Isolated tracheal or bronchial tuberculosis**
[0-6]

5th 012.3 **Tuberculous laryngitis**
[0-6] Tuberculosis of glottis

5th 012.8 **Other specified respiratory tuberculosis**
[0-6] Tuberculosis of:
mediastinum
nasopharynx
nose (septum)
sinus [any nasal]

4th 013 **Tuberculosis of meninges and central nervous system**
Requires fifth digit. See beginning of section 010-018 for codes and definitions.

5th 013.0 **Tuberculous meningitis**
[0-6] Tuberculosis of meninges (cerebral) (spinal)
Tuberculous:
leptomeningitis
meningoencephalitis

Excludes *tuberculoma of meninges (013.1)*

5th 013.1 **Tuberculoma of meninges**
[0-6]

5th 013.2 **Tuberculoma of brain**
[0-6] Tuberculosis of brain (current disease)

5th 013.3 **Tuberculous abscess of brain**
[0-6]

5th 013.4 **Tuberculoma of spinal cord**
[0-6]

5th 013.5 **Tuberculous abscess of spinal cord**
[0-6]

5th 013.6 **Tuberculous encephalitis or myelitis**
[0-6]

5th 013.8 **Other specified tuberculosis of central nervous system**
[0-6]

5th 013.9 **Unspecified tuberculosis of central nervous system**
[0-6] Tuberculosis of central nervous system NOS

4th 014 **Tuberculosis of intestines, peritoneum, and mesenteric glands**
Requires fifth digit. See beginning of section 010-018 for codes and definitions.

5th 014.0 **Tuberculous peritonitis**
[0-6] Tuberculous ascites

5th 014.8 **Other**
[0-6] Tuberculosis (of):
anus
intestine (large) (small)
mesenteric glands
rectum
rectoperitoneal (lymph nodes)
Tuberculous enteritis

4th 015 Tuberculosis of bones and joints

Requires fifth digit. See beginning of section 010-018 for codes and definitions.

Use additional code to identify manifestation, as:
- tuberculous:
  - arthropathy (711.4)
  - necrosis of bone (730.8)
  - osteitis (730.8)
  - osteomyelitis (730.8)
  - synovitis (727.01)
  - tenosynovitis (727.01)

5th 015.0 Vertebral column
[0-6] Pott's disease

Use additional code to identify manifestation, as:
- curvature of spine [Pott's] (737.4)
- kyphosis (737.4)
- spondylitis (720.81)

5th 015.1 Hip
[0-6]

5th 015.2 Knee
[0-6]

5th 015.5 Limb bones
[0-6] Tuberculous dactylitis

5th 015.6 Mastoid
[0-6] Tuberculous mastoiditis

5th 015.7 Other specified bone
[0-6]

5th 015.8 Other specified joint
[0-6]

5th 015.9 Tuberculosis of unspecified bones and joints
[0-6]

4th 016 Tuberculosis of genitourinary system

Requires fifth digit. See beginning of section 010-018 for codes and definitions.

5th 016.0 Kidney
[0-6] Renal tuberculosis

Use additional code to identify manifestation, as:
- tuberculous:
  - nephropathy (583.81)
  - pyelitis (590.81)
  - pyelonephritis (590.81)

5th 016.1 Bladder
[0-6]

5th 016.2 Ureter
[0-6]

5th 016.3 Other urinary organs
[0-6]

5th 016.4 Epididymis ♂
[0-6]

5th 016.5 Other male genital organs ♂
[0-6]

Use additional code to identify manifestation, as:
- tuberculosis of:
  - prostate (601.4)
  - seminal vesicle (608.81)
  - testis (608.81)

5th 016.6 Tuberculous oophoritis and salpingitis ♀
[0-6]

5th 016.7 Other female genital organs ♀
[0-6] Tuberculous:
- cervicitis
- endometritis

5th 016.9 Genitourinary tuberculosis, unspecified
[0-6]

4th 017 Tuberculosis of other organs

Requires fifth digit. See beginning of section 010-018 for codes and definitions.

5th 017.0 Skin and subcutaneous cellular tissue
[0-6] Lupus:
- exedens
- vulgaris

Scrofuloderma

Tuberculosis:
- colliquativa
- cutis
- lichenoides
- papulonecrotica
- verrucosa cutis

Excludes *lupus erythematosus (695.4)*
disseminated (710.0)
lupus NOS (710.0)
nonspecific reaction to tuberculin skin test without active tuberculosis (795.5)
positive PPD (795.5)
positive tuberculin skin test without active tuberculosis (795.5)

5th 017.1 Erythema nodosum with hypersensitivity reaction in tuberculosis
[0-6] Bazin's disease

Erythema:
- induratum
- nodosum, tuberculous

Tuberculosis indurativa

Excludes *erythema nodosum NOS (695.2)*

5th 017.2 Peripheral lymph nodes
[0-6] Scrofula

Scrofulous abscess

Tuberculous adenitis

Excludes *tuberculosis of lymph nodes:*
bronchial and mediastinal (012.1)
mesenteric and retroperitoneal (014.8)
tuberculous tracheobronchial adenopathy (012.1)

5th 017.3 Eye
[0-6]

Use additional code to identify manifestation, as:
- tuberculous:
  - episcleritis (379.09)
  - interstitial keratitis (370.59)
  - iridocyclitis, chronic (364.11)
  - keratoconjunctivitis (phlyctenular) (370.31)

5th 017.4 Ear
[0-6] Tuberculosis of ear

Tuberculous otitis media

Excludes *tuberculous mastoiditis (015.6)*

5th 017.5 Thyroid gland
[0-6]

5th 017.6 Adrenal glands
[0-6] Addison's disease, tuberculous

5th 017.7 Spleen
[0-6]

5th 017.8 Esophagus
[0-6]

5th 017.9 Other specified organs
[0-6]

Use additional code to identify manifestation, as:
- tuberculosis of:
  - endocardium [any valve] (424.91)
  - myocardium (422.0)
  - pericardium (420.0)

4th **018 Miliary tuberculosis**
Includes tuberculosis:
disseminated
generalized
miliary, whether of a single specified site, multiple sites, or unspecified site
polyserositis

5th **018.0 Acute miliary tuberculosis**
[0-6]

5th **018.8 Other specified miliary tuberculosis**
[0-6]

5th **018.9 Miliary tuberculosis, unspecified**
[0-6]

ZOONOTIC BACTERIAL DISEASES (020-027)

4th **020 Plague**
Includes infection by Yersinia [Pasteurella] pestis

020.0 Bubonic

020.1 Cellulocutaneous

020.2 Septicemic

020.3 Primary pneumonic

020.4 Secondary pneumonic

020.5 Pneumonic, unspecified

020.8 Other specified types of plague
Abortive plague
Ambulatory plague
Pestis minor

020.9 Plague, unspecified

4th **021 Tularemia**
Includes deerfly fever
infection by Francisella [Pasteurella] tularensis
rabbit fever

021.0 Ulceroglandular tularemia

021.1 Enteric tularemia
Tularemia:
cryptogenic
intestinal
typhoidal

021.2 Pulmonary tularemia
Bronchopneumonic tularemia

021.3 Oculoglandular tularemia

021.8 Other specified tularemia
Tularemia:
generalized or disseminated
glandular

021.9 Unspecified tularemia

4th **022 Anthrax**

022.0 Cutaneous anthrax
Malignant pustule

022.1 Pulmonary anthrax
Respiratory anthrax
Wool-sorters' disease

022.2 Gastrointestinal anthrax

022.3 Anthrax septicemia

022.8 Other specified manifestations of anthrax

022.9 Anthrax, unspecified

4th **023 Brucellosis**
Includes fever:
Malta
Mediterranean
undulant

023.0 Brucella melitensis

023.1 Brucella abortus

023.2 Brucella suis

023.3 Brucella canis

023.8 Other brucellosis
Infection by more than one organism

023.9 Brucellosis, unspecified

024 Glanders
Farcy
Infection by:
Actinobacillus mallei
Malleomyces mallei
Pseudomonas mallei
Malleus

025 Melioidosis
Infection by:
Malleomyces pseudomallei
Pseudomonas pseudomallei
Whitmore's bacillus
Pseudoglanders

4th **026 Rat-bite fever**

026.0 Spirillary fever
Rat-bite fever due to Spirillum minor [S. minus]
Sodoku

026.1 Streptobacillary fever
Epidemic arthritic erythema
Haverhill fever
Rat-bite fever due to Streptobacillus moniliformis

026.9 Unspecified rat-bite fever

4th **027 Other zoonotic bacterial diseases**

027.0 Listeriosis
Infection by Listeria monocytogenes
Septicemia by Listeria monocytogenes
Use additional code to identify manifestations, as meningitis (320.7)
Excludes *congenital listeriosis (771.2)*

027.1 Erysipelothrix infection
Erysipeloid (of Rosenbach)
Infection by Erysipelothrix insidiosa [E. rhusiopathiae]
Septicemia by Erysipelothrix insidiosa [E. rhusiopathiae]

027.2 Pasteurellosis
Pasteurella pseudotuberculosis infection by Pasteurella multocida [P. septica]
Mesenteric adenitis by Pasteurella multocida [P. septica]
Septic infection (cat bite) (dog bite) by Pasteurella multocida [P. septica]
Excludes *infection by:*
Francisella [Pasteurella] tularensis (021.0-021.9)
Yersinia [Pasteurella] pestis (020.0-020.9)

027.8 Other specified zoonotic bacterial diseases

027.9 Unspecified zoonotic bacterial disease

OTHER BACTERIAL DISEASES (030-041)

Excludes *bacterial venereal diseases (098.0-099.9)*
bartonellosis (088.0)

4th **030 Leprosy**
Includes Hansen's disease
infection by Mycobacterium leprae

030.0 Lepromatous [type L]
Lepromatous leprosy (macular) (diffuse) (infiltrated) (nodular) (neuritic)

030.1 Tuberculoid [type T]
Tuberculoid leprosy (macular) (maculoanesthetic) (major) (minor) (neuritic)

030.2 Indeterminate [group I]
Indeterminate [uncharacteristic] leprosy (macular) (neuritic)

030.3 Borderline [group B]
Borderline or dimorphous leprosy (infiltrated) (neuritic)

030.8 **Other specified leprosy**

030.9 **Leprosy, unspecified**

4th 031 **Diseases due to other mycobacteria**

031.0 **Pulmonary**
Battey disease
Infection by Mycobacterium:
avium
intracellulare [Battey bacillus]
kansasii

031.1 **Cutaneous**
Buruli ulcer
Infection by Mycobacterium:
marinum [M. balnei]
ulcerans

031.2 **Disseminated**
Disseminated mycobacterium avium-intracellulare complex (DMAC)
Mycobacterium avium-intracellulare complex (MAC) bacteremia

031.8 **Other specified mycobacterial diseases**

031.9 **Unspecified diseases due to mycobacteria**
Atypical mycobacterium infection NOS

4th 032 **Diphtheria**
Includes infection by Corynebacterium diphtheriae

032.0 **Faucial diphtheria**
Membranous angina, diphtheritic

032.1 **Nasopharyngeal diphtheria**

032.2 **Anterior nasal diphtheria**

032.3 **Laryngeal diphtheria**
Laryngotracheitis, diphtheritic

5th 032.8 **Other specified diphtheria**

032.81 **Conjunctival diphtheria**
Pseudomembranous diphtheritic conjunctivitis

032.82 **Diphtheritic myocarditis**

032.83 **Diphtheritic peritonitis**

032.84 **Diphtheritic cystitis**

032.85 **Cutaneous diphtheria**

032.89 **Other**

032.9 **Diphtheria, unspecified**

4th 033 **Whooping cough**
Includes pertussis
Use additional code to identify any associated pneumonia (484.3)

033.0 **Bordetella pertussis [B. pertussis]**

033.1 **Bordetella parapertussis [B. parapertussis]**

033.8 **Whooping cough due to other specified organism**
Bordetella bronchiseptica [B. bronchiseptica]

033.9 **Whooping cough, unspecified organism**

4th 034 **Streptococcal sore throat and scarlet fever**

034.0 **Streptococcal sore throat** 6 6
Septic:
angina
sore throat
Streptococcal:
angina
laryngitis
pharyngitis
tonsillitis

034.1 **Scarlet fever**
Scarlatina
Excludes *parascarlatina (057.8)*

035 **Erysipelas**
Excludes *postpartum or puerperal erysipelas (670.8)*

4th 036 **Meningococcal infection**

036.0 **Meningococcal meningitis**
Cerebrospinal fever (meningococcal)
Meningitis:
cerebrospinal
epidemic

036.1 **Meningococcal encephalitis**

036.2 **Meningococcemia**
Meningococcal septicemia

036.3 **Waterhouse-Friderichsen syndrome, meningococcal**
Meningococcal hemorrhagic adrenalitis
Meningococcic adrenal syndrome
Waterhouse-Friderichsen syndrome NOS

5th 036.4 **Meningococcal carditis**

036.40 **Meningococcal carditis, unspecified**

036.41 **Meningococcal pericarditis**

036.42 **Meningococcal endocarditis**

036.43 **Meningococcal myocarditis**

5th 036.8 **Other specified meningococcal infections**

036.81 **Meningococcal optic neuritis**

036.82 **Meningococcal arthropathy**

036.89 **Other**

036.9 **Meningococcal infection, unspecified**
Meningococcal infection NOS

037 **Tetanus**
Excludes *tetanus:*
complicating:
abortion (634-638 with .0, 639.0)
ectopic or molar pregnancy (639.0)
neonatorum (771.3)
puerperal (670.8)

4th 038 **Septicemia**

ICD-9-CM Official Guidelines (Chapter 1b):

1) SIRS, Septicemia, and Sepsis

(a) The terms septicemia and sepsis are often used interchangeably by providers, however they are not considered synonymous terms. The following descriptions are provided for reference but do not preclude querying the provider for clarification about terms used in the documentation:

(i) Septicemia generally refers to a systemic disease associated with the presence of pathological microorganisms or toxins in the blood, which can include bacteria, viruses, fungi or other organisms.

(ii) Systemic inflammatory response syndrome (SIRS) generally refers to the systemic response to infection, trauma/burns, or other insult (such as cancer) with symptoms including fever, tachycardia, tachypnea, and leukocytosis.

(iii) Sepsis generally refers to SIRS due to infection.

(iv) Severe sepsis generally refers to sepsis with associated acute organ dysfunction.

(b) The Coding of SIRS, sepsis and severe sepsis

The coding of SIRS, sepsis and severe sepsis requires a minimum of 2 codes: a code for the underlying cause (such as infection or trauma) and a code from subcategory 995.9 Systemic inflammatory response syndrome (SIRS).

(i) The code for the underlying cause (such as infection or trauma) must be sequenced before the code from subcategory 995.9 Systemic inflammatory response syndrome (SIRS).

(ii) Sepsis and severe sepsis require a code for the systemic infection (038.xx, 112.5, etc.) and either code 995.91, Sepsis, or 995.92, Severe sepsis. If the causal organism is not documented, assign code 038.9, Unspecified septicemia.

(iii) Severe sepsis requires additional code(s) for the associated acute organ dysfunction(s).

(iv) If a patient has sepsis with multiple organ dysfunctions, follow the instructions for coding severe sepsis.

(v) Either the term sepsis or SIRS must be documented to assign a code from subcategory 995.9.

(vi) See Section I.C.17.g), Injury and poisoning, for information regarding systemic inflammatory response syndrome (SIRS) due to trauma/burns and other non-infectious processes.

(c) Due to the complex nature of sepsis and severe sepsis, some cases may require querying the provider prior to assignment of the codes.

2) Sequencing sepsis and severe sepsis

(a) Sepsis and severe sepsis as principal diagnosis

If sepsis or severe sepsis is present on admission, and meets the definition of principal diagnosis, the systemic infection code (e.g., 038.xx, 112.5, etc) should be assigned as the principal diagnosis, followed by code 995.91, Sepsis, or 995.92, Severe sepsis, as required by the sequencing rules in the Tabular List. Codes from subcategory 995.9 can never be assigned as a principal diagnosis. A code should also be assigned for any localized infection, if present.

If the sepsis or severe sepsis is due to a postprocedural infection, see Section I.C.10 for guidelines related to sepsis due to postprocedural infection.

(b) Sepsis and severe sepsis as secondary diagnoses

When sepsis or severe sepsis develops during the encounter (it was not present on admission), the systemic infection code and code 995.91 or 995.92 should be assigned as secondary diagnoses.

(c) Documentation unclear as to whether sepsis or severe sepsis is present on admission

Sepsis or severe sepsis may be present on admission but the diagnosis may not be confirmed until sometime after admission. If the documentation is not clear whether the sepsis or severe sepsis was present on admission, the provider should be queried.

3) Sepsis/SIRS with Localized Infection

If the reason for admission is both sepsis, severe sepsis, or SIRS and a localized infection, such as pneumonia or cellulitis, a code for the systemic infection (038.xx, 112.5, etc) should be assigned first, then code 995.91 or 995.92, followed by the code for the localized infection. If the patient is admitted with a localized infection, such as pneumonia, and sepsis/SIRS doesn't develop until after admission, see guideline I.C.1.b.2.b).

If the localized infection is postprocedural, see Section I.C.10 for guidelines related to sepsis due to postprocedural infection.

Note: The term urosepsis is a nonspecific term. If that is the only term documented then only code 599.0 should be assigned based on the default for the term in the ICD-9-CM index, in addition to the code for the causal organism if known.

4) Bacterial Sepsis and Septicemia

In most cases, it will be a code from category 038, Septicemia, that will be used in conjunction with a code from subcategory 995.9 such as the following:

(a) Streptococcal sepsis

If the documentation in the record states streptococcal sepsis, codes 038.0, Streptococcal septicemia, and code 995.91 should be used, in that sequence.

(b) Streptococcal septicemia

If the documentation states streptococcal septicemia, only code 038.0 should be assigned, however, the provider should be queried whether the patient has sepsis, an infection with SIRS.

ICD-9-CM Official Guidelines (Chapter 15):

*j. **Newborn sepsis***

Code 771.81, Septicemia [sepsis] of newborn, should be assigned with a secondary code from category 041, Bacterial infections in conditions classified elsewhere and of unspecified site, to identify the organism. It is not necessary to use a code from subcategory 995.9, Systemic inflammatory response syndrome (SIRS), on a newborn record. A code from category 038, Septicemia, should not be used on a newborn record. Code 771.81 describes the sepsis.

Use additional code for systemic inflammatory response syndrome (SIRS) (995.91-995.92)

Excludes *bacteremia (790.7)*
septicemia (sepsis) of newborn (771.81)

038.0 Streptococcal septicemia

5th **038.1 Staphylococcal septicemia**

038.10 Staphylococcal septicemia, unspecified

038.11 Methycillin susceptible Staphylococcus aureus septicemia

MSSA septicemia
Staphylococcus aureus septicemia NOS

038.12 Methicillin resistant Staphylococcus aureus septicemia

038.19 Other staphylococcal septicemia

038.2 Pneumococcal septicemia [Streptococcus pneumoniae septicemia]

038.3 Septicemia due to anaerobes

Septicemia due to bacteroides

Excludes *gas gangrene (040.0)*
that due to anaerobic streptococci (038.0)

5th **038.4 Septicemia due to other gram-negative organisms**

038.40 Gram-negative organism, unspecified

Gram-negative septicemia NOS

038.41 Hemophilus influenzae [H. influenzae]

038.42 Escherichia coli [E. coli]

038.43 Pseudomonas

038.44 Serratia

038.49 Other

038.8 Other specified septicemias

Excludes *septicemia (due to):*
anthrax (022.3)
gonococcal (098.89)
herpetic (054.5)
meningococcal (036.2)
septicemic plague (020.2)

038.9 Unspecified septicemia

A41.9 Sepsis, unspecified

Septicemia NOS

Excludes *bacteremia NOS (790.7)*

4th **039 Actinomycotic infections**

Includes actinomycotic mycetoma
infection by Actinomycetales, such as species of Actinomyces, Actinomadura, Nocardia, Streptomyces
maduromycosis (actinomycotic)
schizomycetoma (actinomycotic)

039.0 Cutaneous

Erythrasma
Trichomycosis axillaris

039.1 Pulmonary

Thoracic actinomycosis

039.2 Abdominal

039.3 Cervicofacial

039.4 Madura foot

Excludes *madura foot due to mycotic infection (117.4)*

039.8 Of other specified sites

039.9 Of unspecified site

Actinomycosis NOS
Maduromycosis NOS
Nocardiosis NOS

4th **040 Other bacterial diseases**

Excludes *bacteremia NOS (790.7)*
bacterial infection NOS (041.9)

040.0 Gas gangrene
Gas bacillus infection or gangrene
Infection by Clostridium:
histolyticum
oedematiens
perfringens [welchii]
septicum
sordellii
Malignant edema
Myonecrosis, clostridial
Myositis, clostridial

040.1 Rhinoscleroma

040.2 Whipple's disease
Intestinal lipodystrophy

040.3 Necrobacillosis

5th **040.4 Other specified botulism**
Non-foodborne intoxication due to toxins of Clostridium botulinum [C. botulinum]

Excludes *botulism NOS (005.1)*
food poisoning due to toxins of Clostridium botulinum (005.1)

040.41 Infant botulism P

040.42 Wound botulism
Non-foodborne botulism NOS
Use additional code to identify complicated open wound

5th **040.8 Other specified bacterial diseases**

040.81 Tropical pyomyositis

040.82 Toxic shock syndrome
Use additional code to identify the organism

040.89 Other

4th **041 Bacterial infection in conditions classified elsewhere and of unspecified site**

Note: *This category is provided to be used as an additional code to identify the bacterial agent in diseases classified elsewhere. This category will also be used to classify bacterial infections of unspecified nature or site.*

Excludes *septicemia (038.0-038.9)*

ICD-9-CM Official Guidelines (Chapter 15):

j. Newborn sepsis

Code 771.81, Septicemia [sepsis] of newborn, should be assigned with a secondary code from category 041, Bacterial infections in conditions classified elsewhere and of unspecified site, to identify the organism. It is not necessary to use a code from subcategory 995.9, Systemic inflammatory response syndrome (SIRS), on a newborn record. A code from category 038, Septicemia, should not be used on a newborn record. Code 771.81 describes the sepsis.

5th **041.0 Streptococcus**

041.00 Streptococcus, unspecified

041.01 Group A

041.02 Group B

041.03 Group C

041.04 Group D [Enterococcus]

041.05 Group G

041.09 Other Streptococcus

5th **041.1 Staphylococcus**

041.10 Staphylococcus, unspecified

041.11 Methicillin susceptible Staphylococcus aureus
MSSA
Staphylococcus aureus NOS

ICD-9-CM Official Guidelines (Chapter 1)

c. Methicillin Resistant Staphylococcus aureus (MRSA) Conditions

1) Selection and sequencing of MRSA codes

(a) Combination codes for MRSA infection

When a patient is diagnosed with an infection that is due to methicillin resistant Staphylococcus aureus (MRSA), and that infection has a combination code that includes the causal organism (e.g., septicemia, pneumonia) assign the appropriate code for the condition (e.g., code 038.12, Methicillin resistant Staphylococcus aureus septicemia or code 482.42, Methicillin resistant pneumonia due to Staphylococcus aureus). Do not assign code 041.12, Methicillin resistant Staphylococcus aureus, as an additional code because the code includes the type of infection and the MRSA organism. Do not assign a code from subcategory V09.0, Infection with microorganisms resistant to penicillins, as an additional diagnosis.

See Section C.1.b.1 for instructions on coding and sequencing of septicemia.

(b) Other codes for MRSA infection

When there is documentation of a current infection (e.g., wound infection, stitch abscess, urinary tract infection) due to MRSA, and that infection does not have a combination code that includes the causal organism, select the appropriate code to identify the condition along with code 041.12, Methicillin resistant Staphylococcus aureus, for the MRSA infection. Do not assign a code from subcategory V09.0, Infection with microorganisms resistant to penicillins.

041.12 Methicillin resistant Staphylococcus aureus
Methicillin-resistant staphylococcus aureus (MRSA)

041.19 Other Staphylococcus

041.2 Pneumococcus

▲**041.3 Klebsiella pneumoniae** ~~Friedländer's bacillus~~
~~Infection by Klebsiella pneumoniae~~

041.4 Escherichia coli [E.coli]

041.5 Hemophilus influenzae [H. influenzae]

041.6 Proteus (mirabilis) (morganii)

041.7 Pseudomonas

5th **041.8 Other specified bacterial infections**

041.81 Mycoplasma
Eaton's agent
Pleuropneumonia-like organisms [PPLO]

041.82 Bacteroides fragilis

041.83 Clostridium perfringens

041.84 Other anaerobes
Gram-negative anaerobes

Excludes *Helicobacter pylori (041.86)*

041.85 Other gram-negative organisms
Aerobacter aerogenes
Gram-negative bacteria NOS
Mima polymorpha
Serratia

Excludes *gram-negative anaerobes (041.84)*

▲**041.86 Helicobacter pylori [H. pylori]**

041.89 Other specified bacteria

041.9 Bacterial infection, unspecified

HUMAN IMMUNODEFICIENCY VIRUS (HIV) INFECTION (042)

ICD-9-CM Official Guidelines (Chapter 1a):

1) *Code only confirmed cases*

Code only confirmed cases of HIV infection/illness. This is an exception to the hospital inpatient guideline Section II, H.

In this context, "confirmation" does not require documentation of positive serology or culture for HIV; the provider's diagnostic statement that the patient is HIV positive, or has an HIV-related illness is sufficient.

2) *Selection and sequencing of HIV codes*

(a) ***Patient admitted for HIV-related condition***

If a patient is admitted for an HIV-related condition, the principal diagnosis should be 042, followed by additional diagnosis codes for all reported HIV-related conditions.

(b) ***Patient with HIV disease admitted for unrelated condition***

If a patient with HIV disease is admitted for an unrelated condition (such as a traumatic injury), the code for the unrelated condition (e.g., the nature of injury code) should be the principal diagnosis. Other diagnoses would be 042 followed by additional diagnosis codes for all reported HIV-related conditions.

(c) ***Whether the patient is newly diagnosed***

Whether the patient is newly diagnosed or has had previous admissions/encounters for HIV conditions is irrelevant to the sequencing decision.

(d) ***Asymptomatic human immunodeficiency virus***

V08 Asymptomatic human immunodeficiency virus [HIV] infection, is to be applied when the patient without any documentation of symptoms is listed as being "HIV positive," "known HIV," "HIV test positive," or similar terminology. Do not use this code if the term "AIDS" is used or if the patient is treated for any HIV-related illness or is described as having any condition(s) resulting from his/her HIV positive status; use 042 in these cases.

(e) ***Patients with inconclusive HIV serology***

Patients with inconclusive HIV serology, but no definitive diagnosis or manifestations of the illness, may be assigned code 795.71, Inconclusive serologic test for Human Immunodeficiency Virus [HIV].

(f) ***Previously diagnosed HIV-related illness***

Patients with any known prior diagnosis of an HIV-related illness should be coded to 042. Once a patient has developed an HIV-related illness, the patient should always be assigned code 042 on every subsequent admission/encounter. Patients previously diagnosed with any HIV illness (042) should never be assigned to 795.71 or V08.

(g) ***HIV Infection in Pregnancy, Childbirth and the Puerperium***

During pregnancy, childbirth or the puerperium, a patient admitted (or presenting for a health care encounter) because of an HIV-related illness should receive a principal diagnosis code of 647.6X, Other specified infectious and parasitic diseases in the mother classifiable elsewhere, but complicating the pregnancy, childbirth or the puerperium, followed by 042 and the code(s) for the HIV-related illness(es). Codes from Chapter 15 always take sequencing priority.

Patients with asymptomatic HIV infection status admitted (or presenting for a health care encounter) during pregnancy, childbirth, or the puerperium should receive codes of 647.6X and V08.

(h) ***Encounters for testing for HIV***

If a patient is being seen to determine his/her HIV status, use code V73.89, Screening for other specified viral disease. Use code V69.8, Other problems related to lifestyle, as a secondary code if an asymptomatic patient is in a known high risk group for HIV. Should a patient with signs or symptoms or illness, or a confirmed HIV related diagnosis be tested for HIV, code the signs and symptoms or the diagnosis. An additional counseling code V65.44 may be used if counseling is provided during the encounter for the test.

When a patient returns to be informed of his/her HIV test results use code V65.44, HIV counseling, if the results of the test are negative.

If the results are positive but the patient is asymptomatic use code V08, Asymptomatic HIV infection. If the results are positive and the patient is symptomatic use code 042, HIV infection, with codes for the HIV related symptoms or diagnosis. The HIV counseling code may also be used if counseling is provided for patients with positive test results.

042 Human immunodeficiency virus [HIV] disease 159, 160, 161, 162

B20 Human immunodeficiency virus [HIV] disease

Acquired immune deficiency syndrome
Acquired immunodeficiency syndrome
AIDS
AIDS-like syndrome
AIDS-related complex
ARC
HIV infection, symptomatic

Use additional code(s) to identify all manifestations of HIV
Use additional code to identify HIV-2 infection (079.53)

Excludes *asymptomatic HIV infection status (V08)*
exposure to HIV virus (V01.79)
nonspecific serologic evidence of HIV (795.71)

POLIOMYELITIS AND OTHER NON-ARTHROPOD-BORNE VIRAL DISEASES AND PRION DISEASES OF CENTRAL NERVOUS SYSTEM (045-049)

4th **045 Acute poliomyelitis**

Excludes *late effects of acute poliomyelitis (138)*

The following fifth-digit subclassification is for use with category 045:

0 poliovirus, unspecified type
1 poliovirus type I
2 poliovirus type II
3 poliovirus type III

5th **045.0 Acute paralytic poliomyelitis specified as bulbar**
[0-3]
Infantile paralysis (acute) specified as bulbar
Polioencephalitis (acute) (bulbar)
Polioencephalomyelitis (acute) (anterior) (bulbar)
Poliomyelitis (acute) (anterior) specified as bulbar

5th **045.1 Acute poliomyelitis with other paralysis**
[0-3]
Paralysis:
acute atrophic, spinal
infantile, paralytic
Poliomyelitis (acute) with paralysis except bulbar:
anterior
epidemic

5th **045.2 Acute nonparalytic poliomyelitis**
[0-3]
Poliomyelitis (acute) specified as nonparalytic:
anterior
epidemic

5th **045.9 Acute poliomyelitis, unspecified**
[0-3]
Infantile paralysis unspecified whether paralytic or nonparalytic
Poliomyelitis (acute) unspecified whether paralytic or nonparalytic:
anterior
epidemic

4th **046 Slow virus infections and prion diseases of central nervous system**

046.0 Kuru

5th **046.1 Jakob-Creutzfeldt disease**
Use additional code to identify dementia:
with behavioral disturbance (294.11)
without behavioral disturbance (294.10)

046.11 Variant Creutzfeldt-Jakob disease
vCJD

046.19 Other and unspecified Creutzfeldt-Jakob disease
CJD
Familial Creutzfeldt-Jakob disease
Iatrogenic Creutzfeldt-Jakob disease
Jakob-Creutzfeldt disease, unspecified
Sporadic Creutzfeldt-Jakob disease
Subacute spongiform encephalopathy
Excludes *variant Creutzfeldt-Jakob disease (vCJD) (046.11)*

046.2 Subacute sclerosing panencephalitis
Dawson's inclusion body encephalitis
Van Bogaert's sclerosing leukoencephalitis

046.3 Progressive multifocal leukoencephalopathy
Multifocal leukoencephalopathy NOS

5th **046.7 Other specified prion diseases of central nervous system**
Excludes *Creutzfeldt-Jakob disease (046.11-046.19)*
Jakob-Creutzfeldt disease (046.11-046.19)
kuru (046.0)
variant Creutzfeldt-Jakob disease (vCJD) (046.11)

046.71 Gerstmann-Sträussler-Scheinker syndrome
GSS syndrome

046.72 Fatal familial insomnia
FFI

046.79 Other and unspecified prion disease of central nervous system

046.8 Other specified slow virus infection of central nervous system

046.9 Unspecified slow virus infection of central nervous system

4th **047 Meningitis due to enterovirus**
Includes meningitis:
abacterial
aseptic
viral
Excludes *meningitis due to:*
adenovirus (049.1)
arthropod-borne virus (060.0-066.9)
leptospira (100.81)
virus of:
herpes simplex (054.72)
herpes zoster (053.0)
lymphocytic choriomeningitis (049.0)
mumps (072.1)
poliomyelitis (045.0-045.9)
any other infection specifically classified elsewhere

047.0 Coxsackie virus

047.1 ECHO virus
Meningo-eruptive syndrome

047.8 Other specified viral meningitis

047.9 Unspecified viral meningitis
Viral meningitis NOS

048 Other enterovirus diseases of central nervous system
Boston exanthem

4th **049 Other non-arthropod-borne viral diseases of central nervous system**
Excludes *late effects of viral encephalitis (139.0)*

049.0 Lymphocytic choriomeningitis
Lymphocytic:
meningitis (serous) (benign)
meningoencephalitis (serous) (benign)

049.1 Meningitis due to adenovirus

049.8 Other specified non-arthropod-borne viral diseases of central nervous system
Encephalitis:
acute:
inclusion body
necrotizing
epidemic
lethargica
Rio Bravo
von Economo's disease
Excludes *human herpesvirus 6 encephalitis (058.21)*
other human herpesvirus encephalitis (058.29)

049.9 Unspecified non-arthropod-borne viral diseases of central nervous system
Viral encephalitis NOS

VIRAL DISEASES GENERALLY ACCOMPANIED BY EXANTHEM (050-059)

Excludes *arthropod-borne viral diseases (060.0-066.9)*
Boston exanthem (048)

4th **050 Smallpox**

050.0 Variola major
Hemorrhagic (pustular) smallpox
Malignant smallpox
Purpura variolosa

050.1 Alastrim
Variola minor

050.2 Modified smallpox
Varioloid

050.9 Smallpox, unspecified

4th **051 Cowpox and paravaccinia**

5th **051.0 Cowpox and vaccinia not from vaccination**

051.01 Cowpox

051.02 Vaccinia not from vaccination
Excludes *vaccinia (generalized) (from vaccination) (999.0)*

051.1 Pseudocowpox
Milkers' node

051.2 Contagious pustular dermatitis
Ecthyma contagiosum
Orf

051.9 Paravaccinia, unspecified

4th **052 Chickenpox**

052.0 Postvaricella encephalitis
Postchickenpox encephalitis

052.1 Varicella (hemorrhagic) pneumonitis

052.2 Postvaricella myelitis
Postchickenpox myelitis

052.7 With other specified complications

052.8 With unspecified complication

052.9 Varicella without mention of complication
Chickenpox NOS
Varicella NOS

4th **053 Herpes zoster**
Includes shingles
zona

053.0 With meningitis

5th **053.1 With other nervous system complications**

053.10 With unspecified nervous system complication

053.11 Geniculate herpes zoster
Herpetic geniculate ganglionitis

053.12 Postherpetic trigeminal neuralgia

053.13 Postherpetic polyneuropathy

053.14 Herpes zoster myelitis

053.19 Other

5th 053.2 With ophthalmic complications

053.20 Herpes zoster dermatitis of eyelid
Herpes zoster ophthalmicus

053.21 Herpes zoster keratoconjunctivitis

053.22 Herpes zoster iridocyclitis

053.29 Other

5th 053.7 With other specified complications

053.71 Otitis externa due to herpes zoster

053.79 Other

053.8 With unspecified complication

053.9 Herpes zoster without mention of complication

B02.9 Zoster without complications

Herpes zoster NOS

4th 054 Herpes simplex

Excludes *congenital herpes simplex (771.2)*

054.0 Eczema herpeticum
Kaposi's varicelliform eruption

5th 054.1 Genital herpes

054.10 Genital herpes, unspecified
Herpes progenitalis

054.11 Herpetic vulvovaginitis ♀

054.12 Herpetic ulceration of vulva ♀

054.13 Herpetic infection of penis ♂

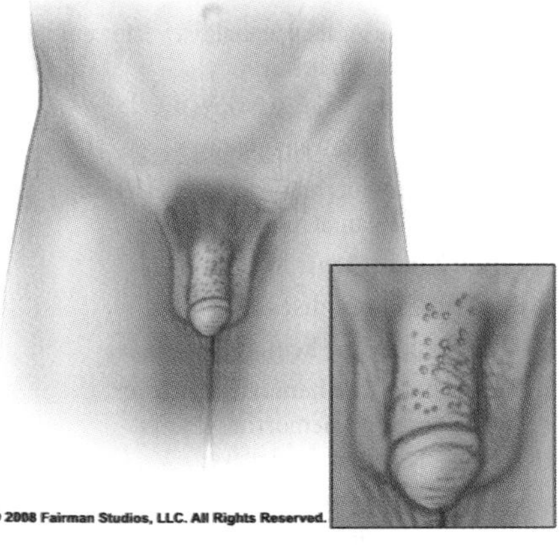
© 2008 Fairman Studios, LLC. All Rights Reserved.

054.19 Other

054.2 Herpetic gingivostomatitis

054.3 Herpetic meningoencephalitis
Herpes encephalitis
Simian B disease

Excludes *human herpesvirus 6 encephalitis (058.21)*
other human herpesvirus encephalitis (058.29)

5th 054.4 With ophthalmic complications

054.40 With unspecified ophthalmic complication

054.41 Herpes simplex dermatitis of eyelid

054.42 Dendritic keratitis

[illegible]54.43 Herpes simplex disciform keratitis

[illegible].44 Herpes simplex iridocyclitis

[illegible]9 Other

He[illegible]c septicemia

[illegible] H[illegible]hitlow

[illegible]erp[illegible]lon

[illegible]ith o[illegible]cified complications

[illegible]isc[illegible]erpes simplex

Her[illegible]lex meningitis

054.73 Herpes simplex otitis externa

054.74 Herpes simplex myelitis

054.79 Other

054.8 With unspecified complication

054.9 Herpes simplex without mention of complication

4th 055 Measles

Includes morbilli
rubeola

055.0 Postmeasles encephalitis

055.1 Postmeasles pneumonia

055.2 Postmeasles otitis media

5th 055.7 With other specified complications

055.71 Measles keratoconjunctivitis
Measles keratitis

055.79 Other

055.8 With unspecified complication

055.9 Measles without mention of complication

4th 056 Rubella

Includes German measles

Excludes *congenital rubella (771.0)*

5th 056.0 With neurological complications

056.00 With unspecified neurological complication

056.01 Encephalomyelitis due to rubella
Encephalitis due to rubella
Meningoencephalitis due to rubella

056.09 Other

5th 056.7 With other specified complications

056.71 Arthritis due to rubella

056.79 Other

056.8 With unspecified complications

056.9 Rubella without mention of complication

4th 057 Other viral exanthemata

057.0 Erythema infectiosum [fifth disease]

057.8 Other specified viral exanthemata
Dukes (-Filatow) disease
Fourth disease
Parascarlatina
Pseudoscarlatina

Excludes *exanthema subitum [sixth disease] (058.10-058.12)*
roseola infantum (058.10-058.12)

057.9 Viral exanthem, unspecified

4th 058 Other human herpesvirus

Excludes *congenital herpes (771.2)*
cytomegalovirus (078.5)
Epstein-Barr virus (075)
herpes NOS (054.0-054.9)
herpes simplex (054.0-054.9)
herpes zoster (053.0-053.9)
human herpesvirus NOS (054.0-054.9)
human herpesvirus 1 (054.0-054.9)
human herpesvirus 2 (054.0-054.9)
human herpesvirus 3 (052.0-053.9)
human herpesvirus 4 (075)
human herpesvirus 5 (078.5)
varicella (052.0-052.9)
varicella-zoster virus (052.0-053.9)

5th 058.1 Roseola infantum
Exanthema subitum [sixth disease]

058.10 Roseola infantum, unspecified P
Exanthema subitum [sixth disease], unspecified

058.11 Roseola infantum due to human herpesvirus 6 P
Exanthema subitum [sixth disease] due to human herpesvirus 6

053.14 – 058.11

058.12 **Roseola infantum due to human herpesvirus 7** P
Exanthema subitum [sixth disease] due to human herpesvirus 7

5th 058.2 **Other human herpesvirus encephalitis**
Excludes *herpes encephalitis NOS (054.3)*
herpes simplex encephalitis (054.3)
human herpesvirus encephalitis NOS (054.3)
simian B herpes virus encephalitis (054.3)

058.21 **Human herpesvirus 6 encephalitis**

058.29 **Other human herpesvirus encephalitis**
Human herpesvirus 7 encephalitis

5th 058.8 **Other human herpesvirus infections**

058.81 **Human herpesvirus 6 infection**

058.82 **Human herpesvirus 7 infection**

058.89 **Other human herpesvirus infection**
Human herpesvirus 8 infection
Kaposi's sarcoma-associated herpesvirus infection

4th 059 **Other poxvirus infections**
Excludes *contagious pustular dermatitis (051.2)*
cowpox (051.01)
ecthyma contagiosum (051.2)
milker's nodule (051.1)
orf (051.2)
paravaccinia NOS (051.9)
pseudocowpox (051.1)
smallpox (050.0-050.9)
vaccinia (generalized) (from vaccination) (999.0)
vaccinia not from vaccination (051.02)

5th 059.0 **Other orthopoxvirus infections**

059.00 **Orthopoxvirus infection, unspecified**

059.01 **Monkeypox**

059.09 **Other orthopoxvirus infection**

5th 059.1 **Other parapoxvirus infections**

059.10 **Parapoxvirus infection, unspecified**

059.11 **Bovine stomatitis**

059.12 **Sealpox**

059.19 **Other parapoxvirus infections**

5th 059.2 **Yatapoxvirus infections**

059.20 **Yatapoxvirus infection, unspecified**

059.21 **Tanapox**

059.22 **Yaba monkey tumor virus**

059.8 **Other poxvirus infections**

059.9 **Poxvirus infections, unspecified**

ARTHROPOD-BORNE VIRAL DISEASES (060-066)

Use additional code to identify any associated meningitis (321.2)
Excludes *late effects of viral encephalitis (139.0)*

4th 060 **Yellow fever**

060.0 **Sylvatic**
Yellow fever:
jungle
sylvan

060.1 **Urban**

060.9 **Yellow fever, unspecified**

061 **Dengue**
Breakbone fever
Excludes *hemorrhagic fever caused by dengue virus (065.4)*

4th 062 **Mosquito-borne viral encephalitis**

062.0 **Japanese encephalitis**
Japanese B encephalitis

062.1 **Western equine encephalitis**

062.2 **Eastern equine encephalitis**
Excludes *Venezuelan equine encephalitis (066.2)*

062.3 **St. Louis encephalitis**

062.4 **Australian encephalitis**
Australian arboencephalitis
Australian X disease
Murray Valley encephalitis

062.5 **California virus encephalitis**
Encephalitis:
California
La Crosse
Tahyna fever

062.8 **Other specified mosquito-borne viral encephalitis**
Encephalitis by Ilheus virus
Excludes *West Nile virus (066.40-066.49)*

062.9 **Mosquito-borne viral encephalitis, unspecified**

4th 063 **Tick-borne viral encephalitis**
Includes iphasic meningoencephalitis

063.0 **Russian spring-summer [taiga] encephalitis**

063.1 **Louping ill**

063.2 **Central European encephalitis**

063.8 **Other specified tick-borne viral encephalitis**
Langat encephalitis
Powassan encephalitis

063.9 **Tick-borne viral encephalitis, unspecified**

064 **Viral encephalitis transmitted by other and unspecified arthropods**
Arthropod-borne viral encephalitis, vector unknown
Negishi virus encephalitis
Excludes *viral encephalitis NOS (049.9)*

4th 065 **Arthropod-borne hemorrhagic fever**

065.0 **Crimean hemorrhagic fever [CHF Congo virus]**
Central Asian hemorrhagic fever

065.1 **Omsk hemorrhagic fever**

065.2 **Kyasanur Forest disease**

065.3 **Other tick-borne hemorrhagic fever**

065.4 **Mosquito-borne hemorrhagic fever**
Chikungunya hemorrhagic fever
Dengue hemorrhagic fever
Excludes *Chikungunya fever (066.3)*
dengue (061)
yellow fever (060.0-060.9)

065.8 **Other specified arthropod-borne hemorrhagic fever**
Mite-borne hemorrhagic fever

065.9 **Arthropod-borne hemorrhagic fever, unspecified**
Arbovirus hemorrhagic fever NOS

4th 066 **Other arthropod-borne viral diseases**

066.0 **Phlebotomus fever**
Changuinola fever
Sandfly fever

066.1 **Tick-borne fever**
Nairobi sheep disease
Tick fever:
American mountain
Colorado
Kemerovo
Quaranfil

066.2 **Venezuelan equine fever**
Venezuelan equine encephalitis

066.3 Other mosquito-borne fever
Fever (viral):
Bunyamwera
Bwamba
Chikungunya
Guama
Mayaro
Mucambo
O'Nyong-Nyong
Oropouche
Pixuna
Rift valley
Ross river
Wesselsbron
Zika
Excludes *dengue (061)*
yellow fever (060.0-060.9)

5th **066.4 West Nile fever**
066.40 West Nile fever, unspecified
West Nile fever NOS
West Nile fever without complications
West Nile virus NOS
066.41 West Nile fever with encephalitis
West Nile encephalitis
West Nile encephalomyelitis
066.42 West Nile fever with other neurologic manifestations
Use additional codes to specify the neurologic manifestation
066.49 West Nile fever with other complications
Use additional codes to specify the other conditions

066.8 Other specified arthropod-borne viral diseases
Chandipura fever
Piry fever

066.9 Arthropod-borne viral disease, unspecified
Arbovirus infection NOS

OTHER DISEASES DUE TO VIRUSES AND CHLAMYDIAE (070-079)

4th **070 Viral hepatitis**
Includes viral hepatitis (acute) (chronic)
Excludes *cytomegalic inclusion virus hepatitis (078.5)*

The following fifth-digit subclassification is for use with categories 070.2 and 070.3:
0 acute or unspecified, without mention of hepatitis delta
1 acute or unspecified, with hepatitis delta
2 chronic, without mention of hepatitis delta
3 chronic, with hepatitis delta

070.0 Viral hepatitis A with hepatic coma
070.1 Viral hepatitis A without mention of hepatic coma
Infectious hepatitis
5th **070.2 Viral hepatitis B with hepatic coma**
[0-3]
5th **070.3 Viral hepatitis B without mention of hepatic coma**
[0-3] Serum hepatitis
5th **070.4 Other specified viral hepatitis with hepatic coma**
070.41 Acute hepatitis C with hepatic coma
070.42 Hepatitis delta without mention of active hepatitis B disease with hepatic coma
Hepatitis delta with hepatitis B carrier state
070.43 Hepatitis E with hepatic coma
070.44 Chronic hepatitis C with hepatic coma
070.49 Other specified viral hepatitis with hepatic coma
5th **070.5 Other specified viral hepatitis without mention of hepatic coma**
070.51 Acute hepatitis C without mention of hepatic coma 83, 89, 183, 184
070.52 Hepatitis delta without mention of active hepatitis B disease or hepatic coma
070.53 Hepatitis E without mention of hepatic coma
070.54 Chronic hepatitis C without mention of hepatic coma 83, 89, 183, 184
B18.2 Chronic viral hepatitis C
070.59 Other specified viral hepatitis without mention of hepatic coma
070.6 Unspecified viral hepatitis with hepatic coma
Excludes *unspecified viral hepatitis C with hepatic coma (070.71)*
5th **070.7 Unspecified viral hepatitis C**
070.70 Unspecified viral hepatitis C without hepatic coma 83, 89, 183, 184
Unspecified viral hepatitis C NOS
070.71 Unspecified viral hepatitis C with hepatic coma
070.9 Unspecified viral hepatitis without mention of hepatic coma
Viral hepatitis NOS
Excludes *unspecified viral hepatitis C without hepatic coma (070.70)*

071 Rabies
Hydrophobia
Lyssa

4th **072 Mumps**
072.0 Mumps orchitis ♂
072.1 Mumps meningitis
072.2 Mumps encephalitis
Mumps meningoencephalitis
072.3 Mumps pancreatitis
5th **072.7 Mumps with other specified complications**
072.71 Mumps hepatitis
072.72 Mumps polyneuropathy
072.79 Other
072.8 Mumps with unspecified complication
072.9 Mumps without mention of complication
Epidemic parotitis
Infectious parotitis

4th **073 Ornithosis**
Includes parrot fever
psittacosis
073.0 With pneumonia
Lobular pneumonitis due to ornithosis
073.7 With other specified complications
073.8 With unspecified complication
073.9 Ornithosis, unspecified

4th **074 Specific diseases due to Coxsackie virus**
Excludes *Coxsackie virus:*
infection NOS (079.2)
meningitis (047.0)
074.0 Herpangina
Vesicular pharyngitis
074.1 Epidemic pleurodynia
Bornholm disease
Devil's grip
Epidemic:
myalgia
myositis

5th 074.2 **Coxsackie carditis**

074.20 **Coxsackie carditis, unspecified**

074.21 **Coxsackie pericarditis**

074.22 **Coxsackie endocarditis**

074.23 **Coxsackie myocarditis**
Aseptic myocarditis of newborn

074.3 **Hand, foot, and mouth disease**
Vesicular stomatitis and exanthema

074.8 **Other specified diseases due to Coxsackie virus**
Acute lymphonodular pharyngitis

075 **Infectious mononucleosis**
Glandular fever
Monocytic angina
Pfeiffer's disease

4th 076 **Trachoma**
Excludes *late effect of trachoma (139.1)*

076.0 **Initial stage**
Trachoma dubium

076.1 **Active stage**
Granular conjunctivitis (trachomatous)
Trachomatous:
follicular conjunctivitis
pannus

076.9 **Trachoma, unspecified**
Trachoma NOS

4th 077 **Other diseases of conjunctiva due to viruses and Chlamydiae**
Excludes *ophthalmic complications of viral diseases classified elsewhere*

077.0 **Inclusion conjunctivitis**
Paratrachoma
Swimming pool conjunctivitis
Excludes *inclusion blennorrhea (neonatal) (771.6)*

077.1 **Epidemic keratoconjunctivitis**
Shipyard eye

077.2 **Pharyngoconjunctival fever**
Viral pharyngoconjunctivitis

077.3 **Other adenoviral conjunctivitis**
Acute adenoviral follicular conjunctivitis

077.4 **Epidemic hemorrhagic conjunctivitis**
Apollo:
conjunctivitis
disease
Conjunctivitis due to enterovirus type 70
Hemorrhagic conjunctivitis (acute) (epidemic)

077.8 **Other viral conjunctivitis**
Newcastle conjunctivitis

5th 077.9 **Unspecified diseases of conjunctiva due to viruses and Chlamydiae**

077.98 **Due to Chlamydiae**

077.99 **Due to viruses**
Viral conjunctivitis NOS

4th 078 **Other diseases due to viruses and Chlamydiae**
Excludes *viral infection NOS (079.0-079.9)*
viremia NOS (790.8)

078.0 **Molluscum contagiosum**

5th 078.1 **Viral warts**
Viral warts due to human papillomavirus

078.10 **Viral warts, unspecified**
B07 Viral warts
Verruca:
NOS
vulgaris
Warts (infectious)

078.11 **Condyloma acuminatum**
Condyloma NOS
Genital warts NOS

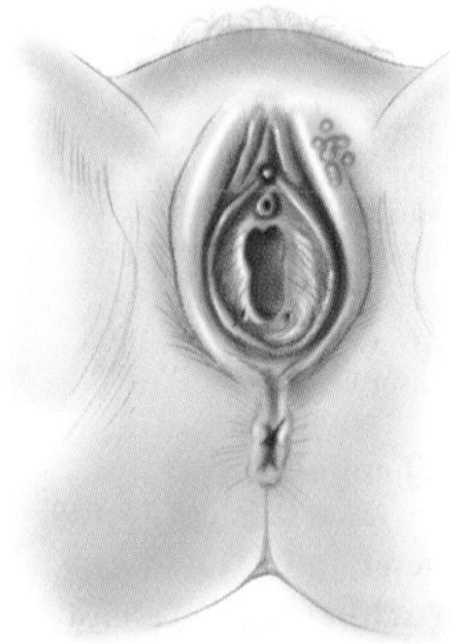

© 2008 Fairman Studios, LLC. All Rights Reserved.

078.12 **Plantar wart**

078.19 **Other specified viral warts**
Common wart
Flat wart
Verruca plana

078.2 **Sweating fever**
Miliary fever
Sweating disease

078.3 **Cat-scratch disease**
Benign lymphoreticulosis (of inoculation)
Cat-scratch fever

078.4 **Foot and mouth disease**
Aphthous fever
Epizootic:
aphthae
stomatitis

078.5 **Cytomegaloviral disease**
Cytomegalic inclusion disease
Salivary gland virus disease
Use additional code to identify manifestation, as:
cytomegalic inclusion virus:
hepatitis (573.1)
pneumonia (484.1)
Excludes *congenital cytomegalovirus infection (771.1)*

078.6 **Hemorrhagic nephrosonephritis**
Hemorrhagic fever:
epidemic
Korean
Russian with renal syndrome

078.7 **Arenaviral hemorrhagic fever**
Hemorrhagic fever:
Argentine
Bolivian
Junin virus
Machupo virus

5th 078.8 **Other specified diseases due to viruses and Chlamydiae**
Excludes *epidemic diarrhea (009.2)*
lymphogranuloma venereum (099.1)

078.81 **Epidemic vertigo**

078.82 **Epidemic vomiting syndrome**
Winter vomiting disease

078.88 **Other specified diseases due to Chlamydiae**

078.89 **Other specified diseases due to viruses**
Epidemic cervical myalgia
Marburg disease
~~Tanapox~~

4th **079 Viral and chlamydial infection in conditions classified elsewhere and of unspecified site**

Note: *This category is provided to be used as an additional code to identify the viral agent in diseases classifiable elsewhere. This category will also be used to classify virus infection of unspecified nature or site.*

079.0 Adenovirus

079.1 ECHO virus

079.2 Coxsackie virus

079.3 Rhinovirus

079.4 Human papillomavirus

5th **079.5 Retrovirus**

Excludes *human immunodeficiency virus, type 1 [HIV-1] (042)*
human T-cell lymphotrophic virus, type III [HTLV-III] (042)
lymphadenopathy-associated virus [LAV] (042)

079.50 Retrovirus, unspecified

079.51 Human T-cell lymphotrophic virus, type I [HTLV-I]

079.52 Human T-cell lymphotrophic virus, type II [HTLV-II]

079.53 Human immunodeficiency virus, type 2 [HIV-2] 159, 160, 161, 162

079.59 Other specified retrovirus

079.6 Respiratory syncytial virus (RSV)

5th **079.8 Other specified viral and chlamydial infections**

079.81 Hantavirus

079.82 SARS-associated coronavirus

079.83 Parvovirus B19
Human parvovirus
Parvovirus NOS

Excludes *erythema infectiosum [fifth disease] (057.0)*

079.88 Other specified chlamydial infection

079.89 Other specified viral infection

5th **079.9 Unspecified viral and chlamydial infections**

Excludes *viremia NOS (790.8)*

079.98 Unspecified chlamydial infection
Chlamydial infection NOS

079.99 Unspecified viral infection

B97.8 Other viral agents as the cause of diseases classified elsewhere

Viral infection NOS

RICKETTSIOSES AND OTHER ARTHROPOD-BORNE DISEASES (080-088)

Excludes *arthropod-borne viral diseases (060.0-066.9)*

080 Louse-borne [epidemic] typhus
Typhus (fever):
classical
epidemic
exanthematic NOS
louse-borne

4th **081 Other typhus**

081.0 Murine [endemic] typhus
Typhus (fever):
endemic
flea-borne

081.1 Brill's disease
Brill-Zinsser disease
Recrudescent typhus (fever)

081.2 Scrub typhus
Japanese river fever
Kedani fever
Mite-borne typhus
Tsutsugamushi

081.9 Typhus, unspecified
Typhus (fever) NOS

4th **082 Tick-borne rickettsioses**

082.0 Spotted fevers
Rocky mountain spotted fever
Sao Paulo fever

082.1 Boutonneuse fever
African tick typhus
India tick typhus
Kenya tick typhus
Marseilles fever
Mediterranean tick fever

082.2 North Asian tick fever
Siberian tick typhus

082.3 Queensland tick typhus

5th **082.4 Ehrlichiosis**

082.40 Ehrlichiosis, unspecified

082.41 Ehrlichiosis chaffeensis [E. chaffeensis]

082.49 Other ehrlichiosis

082.8 Other specified tick-borne rickettsioses
Lone star fever

082.9 Tick-borne rickettsiosis, unspecified
Tick-borne typhus NOS

4th **083 Other rickettsioses**

083.0 Q fever

083.1 Trench fever
Quintan fever
Wolhynian fever

083.2 Rickettsialpox
Vesicular rickettsiosis

083.8 Other specified rickettsioses

083.9 Rickettsiosis, unspecified

4th **084 Malaria**

Note: *Subcategories 084.0-084.6 exclude the listed conditions with mention of pernicious complications (084.8-084.9).*

Excludes *congenital malaria (771.2)*

084.0 Falciparum malaria [malignant tertian]
Malaria (fever):
by Plasmodium falciparum
subtertian

084.1 Vivax malaria [benign tertian]
Malaria (fever) by Plasmodium vivax

084.2 Quartan malaria
Malaria (fever) by Plasmodium malariae
Malariae malaria

084.3 Ovale malaria
Malaria (fever) by Plasmodium ovale

084.4 Other malaria
Monkey malaria

084.5 Mixed malaria
Malaria (fever) by more than one parasite

084.6 Malaria, unspecified
Malaria (fever) NOS

084.7 Induced malaria
Therapeutically induced malaria

Excludes *accidental infection from syringe, blood transfusion, etc. (084.0-084.6, above, according to parasite species)*
transmission from mother to child during delivery (771.2)

084.8 Blackwater fever
Hemoglobinuric:
fever (bilious)
malaria
Malarial hemoglobinuria

079 – 084.8

084.9 Other pernicious complications of malaria
Algid malaria
Cerebral malaria
Use additional code to identify complication, as:
malarial:
hepatitis (573.2)
nephrosis (581.81)

4th **085 Leishmaniasis**

085.0 Visceral [kala-azar]
Dumdum fever
Infection by Leishmania:
donovani
infantum
Leishmaniasis:
dermal, post-kala-azar
Mediterranean
visceral (Indian)

085.1 Cutaneous, urban
Aleppo boil
Baghdad boil
Delhi boil
Infection by Leishmania tropica (minor)
Leishmaniasis, cutaneous:
dry form
late
recurrent
ulcerating
Oriental sore

085.2 Cutaneous, Asian desert
Infection by Leishmania tropica major
Leishmaniasis, cutaneous:
acute necrotizing
rural
wet form
zoonotic form

085.3 Cutaneous, Ethiopian
Infection by Leishmania ethiopica
Leishmaniasis, cutaneous:
diffuse
lepromatous

085.4 Cutaneous, American
Chiclero ulcer
Infection by Leishmania mexicana
Leishmaniasis tegumentaria diffusa

085.5 Mucocutaneous (American)
Espundia
Infection by Leishmania braziliensis
Uta

085.9 Leishmaniasis, unspecified

4th **086 Trypanosomiasis**
Use additional code to identify manifestations, as:
trypanosomiasis:
encephalitis (323.2)
meningitis (321.3)

086.0 Chagas' disease with heart involvement
American trypanosomiasis with heart involvement
Infection by Trypanosoma cruzi with heart involvement
Any condition classifiable to 086.2 with heart involvement

086.1 Chagas' disease with other organ involvement
American trypanosomiasis with involvement of organ other than heart
Infection by Trypanosoma cruzi with involvement of organ other than heart
Any condition classifiable to 086.2 with involvement of organ other than heart

086.2 Chagas' disease without mention of organ involvement
American trypanosomiasis
Infection by Trypanosoma cruzi

086.3 Gambian trypanosomiasis
Gambian sleeping sickness
Infection by Trypanosoma gambiense

086.4 Rhodesian trypanosomiasis
Infection by Trypanosoma rhodesiense
Rhodesian sleeping sickness

086.5 African trypanosomiasis, unspecified
Sleeping sickness NOS

086.9 Trypanosomiasis, unspecified

4th **087 Relapsing fever**
Includes recurrent fever

087.0 Louse-borne

087.1 Tick-borne

087.9 Relapsing fever, unspecified

4th **088 Other arthropod-borne diseases**

088.0 Bartonellosis
Carrión's disease
Oroya fever
Verruga peruana

5th **088.8 Other specified arthropod-borne diseases**

088.81 Lyme disease
Erythema chronicum migrans
Layman's: *Untreated Lyme disease can present similarly to rheumatoid arthritis and is identified through serological testing.*

088.82 Babesiosis
Babesiasis

088.89 Other

088.9 Arthropod-borne disease, unspecified

SYPHILIS AND OTHER VENEREAL DISEASES (090-099)

Excludes *nonvenereal endemic syphilis (104.0)*
urogenital trichomoniasis (131.0)

4th **090 Congenital syphilis**

090.0 Early congenital syphilis, symptomatic
Congenital syphilitic:
choroiditis
coryza (chronic)
hepatomegaly
mucous patches
periostitis
splenomegaly
Syphilitic (congenital):
epiphysitis
osteochondritis
pemphigus
Any congenital syphilitic condition specified as early or manifest less than two years after birth

090.1 Early congenital syphilis, latent
Congenital syphilis without clinical manifestations, with positive serological reaction and negative spinal fluid test, less than two years after birth

090.2 Early congenital syphilis, unspecified
Congenital syphilis NOS, less than two years after birth

090.3 Syphilitic interstitial keratitis
Syphilitic keratitis:
parenchymatous
punctata profunda
Excludes *interstitial keratitis NOS (370.50)*

5th **090.4 Juvenile neurosyphilis**
Use additional code to identify any associated mental disorder

090.40 Juvenile neurosyphilis, unspecified
Congenital neurosyphilis
Dementia paralytica juvenilis
Juvenile:
general paresis
tabes
taboparesis

090.41 Congenital syphilitic encephalitis

090.42 Congenital syphilitic meningitis

090.49 Other

090.5 Other late congenital syphilis, symptomatic
Gumma due to congenital syphilis
Hutchinson's teeth
Syphilitic saddle nose
Any congenital syphilitic condition specified as late or manifest two years or more after birth

090.6 Late congenital syphilis, latent
Congenital syphilis without clinical manifestations, with positive serological reaction and negative spinal fluid test, two years or more after birth

090.7 Late congenital syphilis, unspecified
Congenital syphilis NOS, two years or more after birth

090.9 Congenital syphilis, unspecified

4th **091 Early syphilis, symptomatic**
Excludes *early cardiovascular syphilis (093.0-093.9)*
early neurosyphilis (094.0-094.9)

091.0 Genital syphilis (primary)
Genital chancre

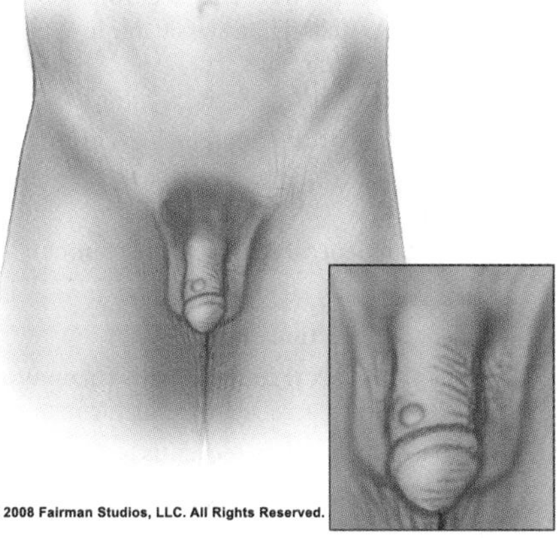
© 2008 Fairman Studios, LLC. All Rights Reserved.

091.1 Primary anal syphilis

091.2 Other primary syphilis
Primary syphilis of:
breast
fingers
lip
tonsils

091.3 Secondary syphilis of skin or mucous membranes
Condyloma latum
Secondary syphilis of:
anus
mouth
pharynx
skin
tonsils
vulva

091.4 Adenopathy due to secondary syphilis
Syphilitic adenopathy (secondary)
Syphilitic lymphadenitis (secondary)

5th **091.5 Uveitis due to secondary syphilis**

091.50 Syphilitic uveitis, unspecified

091.51 Syphilitic chorioretinitis (secondary)

091.52 Syphilitic iridocyclitis (secondary)

5th **091.6 Secondary syphilis of viscera and bone**

091.61 Secondary syphilitic periostitis

091.62 Secondary syphilitic hepatitis
Secondary syphilis of liver

091.69 Other viscera

091.7 Secondary syphilis, relapse
Secondary syphilis, relapse (treated) (untreated)

5th **091.8 Other forms of secondary syphilis**

091.81 Acute syphilitic meningitis (secondary)

091.82 Syphilitic alopecia

091.89 Other

091.9 Unspecified secondary syphilis

4th **092 Early syphilis, latent**
Includes syphilis (acquired) without clinical manifestations, with positive serological reaction and negative spinal fluid test, less than two years after infection

092.0 Early syphilis, latent, serological relapse after treatment

092.9 Early syphilis, latent, unspecified

4th **093 Cardiovascular syphilis**

093.0 Aneurysm of aorta, specified as syphilitic
Dilatation of aorta, specified as syphilitic

093.1 Syphilitic aortitis

5th **093.2 Syphilitic endocarditis**

093.20 Valve, unspecified
Syphilitic ostial coronary disease

093.21 Mitral valve

093.22 Aortic valve
Syphilitic aortic incompetence or stenosis

093.23 Tricuspid valve

093.24 Pulmonary valve

5th **093.8 Other specified cardiovascular syphilis**

093.81 Syphilitic pericarditis

093.82 Syphilitic myocarditis

093.89 Other

093.9 Cardiovascular syphilis, unspecified

4th **094 Neurosyphilis**
Use additional code to identify any associated mental disorder

094.0 Tabes dorsalis
Locomotor ataxia (progressive)
Posterior spinal sclerosis (syphilitic)
Tabetic neurosyphilis
Use additional code to identify manifestation, as:
neurogenic arthropathy [Charcot's joint disease] (713.5)

094.1 General paresis
Dementia paralytica
General paralysis (of the insane) (progressive)
Paretic neurosyphilis
Taboparesis

094.2 Syphilitic meningitis
Meningovascular syphilis
Excludes *acute syphilitic meningitis (secondary) (091.81)*

094.3 Asymptomatic neurosyphilis

5th **094.8 Other specified neurosyphilis**

094.81 Syphilitic encephalitis

094.82 Syphilitic Parkinsonism

094.83 Syphilitic disseminated retinochoroiditis

094.84 Syphilitic optic atrophy

094.85 Syphilitic retrobulbar neuritis

094.86 Syphilitic acoustic neuritis

094.87 Syphilitic ruptured cerebral aneurysm

094.89 Other

094.9 Neurosyphilis, unspecified
Gumma (syphilitic) of central nervous system NOS
Syphilis (early) (late) of central nervous system NOS
Syphiloma of central nervous system NOS

4th **095 Other forms of late syphilis, with symptoms**
Includes gumma (syphilitic)
tertiary, or unspecified stage

095.0 Syphilitic episcleritis

095.1 Syphilis of lung

095.2 Syphilitic peritonitis

095.3 Syphilis of liver

095.4 Syphilis of kidney

095.5 Syphilis of bone

095.6 Syphilis of muscle
Syphilitic myositis

095.7 Syphilis of synovium, tendon, and bursa
Syphilitic:
bursitis
synovitis

095.8 Other specified forms of late symptomatic syphilis
Excludes *cardiovascular syphilis (093.0-093.9)*
neurosyphilis (094.0-094.9)

095.9 Late symptomatic syphilis, unspecified

096 Late syphilis, latent
Syphilis (acquired) without clinical manifestations, with positive serological reaction and negative spinal fluid test, two years or more after infection

4th **097 Other and unspecified syphilis**

097.0 Late syphilis, unspecified

097.1 Latent syphilis, unspecified
Positive serological reaction for syphilis

097.9 Syphilis, unspecified
Syphilis (acquired) NOS
Excludes *syphilis NOS causing death under two years of age (090.9)*

4th **098 Gonococcal infections**

098.0 Acute, of lower genitourinary tract
Gonococcal:
Bartholinitis (acute)
urethritis (acute)
vulvovaginitis (acute)
Gonorrhea (acute):
NOS
genitourinary (tract) NOS

5th **098.1 Acute, of upper genitourinary tract**

098.10 Gonococcal infection (acute) of upper genitourinary tract, site unspecified

098.11 Gonococcal cystitis (acute)
Gonorrhea (acute) of bladder

098.12 Gonococcal prostatitis (acute) ♂

098.13 Gonococcal epididymo-orchitis (acute) ♂
Gonococcal orchitis (acute)

098.14 Gonococcal seminal vesiculitis (acute) ♂
Gonorrhea (acute) of seminal vesicle

098.15 Gonococcal cervicitis (acute) ♀
Gonorrhea (acute) of cervix

098.16 Gonococcal endometritis (acute) ♀
Gonorrhea (acute) of uterus

098.17 Gonococcal salpingitis, specified as acute ♀

098.19 Other

098.2 Chronic, of lower genitourinary tract
Gonococcal specified as chronic or with duration of two months or more:
Bartholinitis
urethritis
vulvovaginitis
Gonorrhea specified as chronic or with duration of two months or more:
NOS
genitourinary (tract)
Any condition classifiable to 098.0 specified as chronic or with duration two months or more

5th **098.3 Chronic, of upper genitourinary tract**
Any condition classifiable to 098.1 stated as chronic or with a duration two months or more

098.30 Chronic gonococcal infection of upper genitourinary tract, site unspecified

098.31 Gonococcal cystitis, chronic
Any condition classifiable to 098.11, specified as chronic
Gonorrhea of bladder, chronic

098.32 Gonococcal prostatitis, chronic ♂
Any condition classifiable to 098.12, specified as chronic

098.33 Gonococcal epididymo-orchitis, chronic ♂
Any condition classifiable to 098.13, specified as chronic
Chronic gonococcal orchitis

098.34 Gonococcal seminal vesiculitis, chronic ♂
Any condition classifiable to 098.14, specified as chronic
Gonorrhea of seminal vesicle, chronic

098.35 Gonococcal cervicitis, chronic ♀
Any condition classifiable to 098.15, specified as chronic
Gonorrhea of cervix, chronic

098.36 Gonococcal endometritis, chronic ♀
Any condition classifiable to 098.16, specified as chronic

098.37 Gonococcal salpingitis (chronic) ♀

098.39 Other

5th **098.4 Gonococcal infection of eye**

098.40 Gonococcal conjunctivitis (neonatorum)
Gonococcal ophthalmia (neonatorum)

098.41 Gonococcal iridocyclitis

098.42 Gonococcal endophthalmia

098.43 Gonococcal keratitis

098.49 Other

5th **098.5 Gonococcal infection of joint**

098.50 Gonococcal arthritis
Gonococcal infection of joint NOS

098.51 Gonococcal synovitis and tenosynovitis

098.52 Gonococcal bursitis

098.53 Gonococcal spondylitis

098.59 Other
Gonococcal rheumatism

098.6 Gonococcal infection of pharynx

098.7 Gonococcal infection of anus and rectum
Gonococcal proctitis

5th **098.8 Gonococcal infection of other specified sites**

098.81 Gonococcal keratosis (blennorrhagica)

098.82 Gonococcal meningitis

098.83 Gonococcal pericarditis

098.84 Gonococcal endocarditis

098.85 **Other gonococcal heart disease**

098.86 **Gonococcal peritonitis**

098.89 **Other**
Gonococcemia

4th 099 **Other venereal diseases**

099.0 **Chancroid**
Bubo (inguinal):
chancroidal
due to Hemophilus ducreyi
Chancre:
Ducrey's
simple
soft
Ulcus molle (cutis) (skin)

099.1 **Lymphogranuloma venereum**
Climatic or tropical bubo
(Durand-) Nicolas-Favre disease
Esthiomene
Lymphogranuloma inguinale

099.2 **Granuloma inguinale**
Donovanosis
Granuloma pudendi (ulcerating)
Granuloma venereum
Pudendal ulcer

099.3 **Reiter's disease**
Reiter's syndrome
Use additional code for associated:
arthropathy (711.1)
conjunctivitis (372.33)

5th 099.4 **Other nongonococcal urethritis [NGU]**

099.40 **Unspecified**
Nonspecific urethritis

099.41 **Chlamydia trachomatis**

099.49 **Other specified organism**

5th 099.5 **Other venereal diseases due to Chlamydia trachomatis**
Excludes *Chlamydia trachomatis infection of conjunctiva (076.0-076.9, 077.0, 077.9)*
Lymphogranuloma venereum (099.1)

099.50 **Unspecified site**

099.51 **Pharynx**

099.52 **Anus and rectum**

099.53 **Lower genitourinary sites**
Use additional code to specify site of infection, such as:
bladder (595.4)
cervix (616.0)
vagina and vulva (616.11)
Excludes *urethra (099.41)*

099.54 **Other genitourinary sites**
Use additional code to specify site of infection, such as:
pelvic inflammatory disease NOS (614.9)
testis and epididymis (604.91)

099.55 **Unspecified genitourinary site**

099.56 **Peritoneum**
Perihepatitis

099.59 **Other specified site**

099.8 **Other specified venereal diseases**

099.9 **Venereal disease, unspecified**

OTHER SPIROCHETAL DISEASES (100-104)

4th 100 **Leptospirosis**

100.0 **Leptospirosis icterohemorrhagica**
Leptospiral or spirochetal jaundice (hemorrhagic)
Weil's disease

5th 100.8 **Other specified leptospiral infections**

100.81 **Leptospiral meningitis (aseptic)**

100.89 **Other**
Fever:
Fort Bragg
pretibial
swamp
Infection by Leptospira:
Australis
bataviae
pyrogenes

100.9 **Leptospirosis, unspecified**

101 **Vincent's angina**
Acute necrotizing ulcerative:
gingivitis
stomatitis
Fusospirochetal pharyngitis
Spirochetal stomatitis
Trench mouth
Vincent's:
gingivitis
infection [any site]

4th 102 **Yaws**
Includes frambesia
pian

102.0 **Initial lesions**
Chancre of yaws
Frambesia, initial or primary
Initial frambesial ulcer
Mother yaw

102.1 **Multiple papillomata and wet crab yaws**
Butter yaws
Frambesioma
Pianoma
Plantar or palmar papilloma of yaws

102.2 **Other early skin lesions**
Cutaneous yaws, less than five years after infection
Early yaws (cutaneous) (macular) (papular) (maculopapular) (micropapular)
Frambeside of early yaws

102.3 **Hyperkeratosis**
Ghoul hand
Hyperkeratosis, palmar or plantar (early) (late) due to yaws
Worm-eaten soles

102.4 **Gummata and ulcers**
Gummatous frambeside
Nodular late yaws (ulcerated)

102.5 **Gangosa**
Rhinopharyngitis mutilans

102.6 **Bone and joint lesions**
Goundou of yaws (late)
Gumma, bone of yaws (late)
Gummatous osteitis or periostitis of yaws (late)
Hydrarthrosis of yaws (early) (late)
Osteitis of yaws (early) (late)
Periostitis (hypertrophic) of yaws (early) (late)

102.7 **Other manifestations**
Juxta-articular nodules of yaws
Mucosal yaws

102.8 **Latent yaws**
Yaws without clinical manifestations, with positive serology

102.9 **Yaws, unspecified**

4th 103 **Pinta**

103.0 **Primary lesions**
Chancre (primary) of pinta [carate]
Papule (primary) of pinta [carate]
Pintid of pinta [carate]

103.1 Intermediate lesions
Erythematous plaques of pinta [carate]
Hyperchromic lesions of pinta [carate]
Hyperkeratosis of pinta [carate]

103.2 Late lesions
Cardiovascular lesions of pinta [carate]
Skin lesions of pinta [carate]:
achromic
cicatricial
dyschromic
Vitiligo of pinta [carate]

103.3 Mixed lesions
Achromic and hyperchromic skin lesions of pinta [carate]

103.9 Pinta, unspecified

4th **104 Other spirochetal infection**

104.0 Nonvenereal endemic syphilis
Bejel
Njovera

104.8 Other specified spirochetal infections
Excludes *relapsing fever (087.0-087.9)*
syphilis (090.0-097.9)

104.9 Spirochetal infection, unspecified

MYCOSES (110-118)

Use additional code to identify manifestation, as:
arthropathy (711.6)
meningitis (321.0-321.1)
otitis externa (380.15)

Excludes *infection by Actinomycetales, such as species of Actinomyces, Actinomadura, Nocardia, Streptomyces (039.0-039.9)*

4th **110 Dermatophytosis**
Includes infection by species of Epidermophyton, Microsporum, and Trichophyton
tinea, any type except those in 111

110.0 Of scalp and beard
Kerion
Sycosis, mycotic
Trichophytic tinea [black dot tinea], scalp

110.1 Of nail
B35.1 Tinea unguium
Dermatophytic onychia
Onychomycosis
Tinea unguium

110.2 Of hand
Tinea manuum

110.3 Of groin and perianal area
Dhobie itch
Eczema marginatum
Tinea cruris

110.4 Of foot
Athlete's foot
Tinea pedis

Athlete's Foot

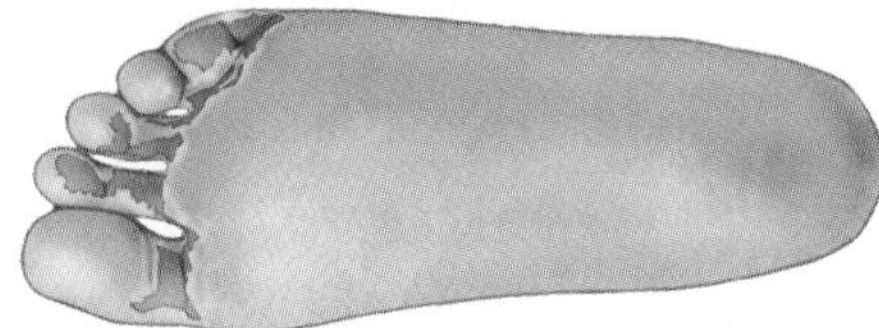

© 2008 Fairman Studios, LLC. All Rights Reserved.

110.5 Of the body
Herpes circinatus
Tinea imbricata [Tokelau]

110.6 Deep seated dermatophytosis
Granuloma trichophyticum
Majocchi's granuloma

110.8 Of other specified sites

110.9 Of unspecified site
Favus NOS
Microsporic tinea NOS
Ringworm NOS

4th **111 Dermatomycosis, other and unspecified**

111.0 Pityriasis versicolor
Infection by Malassezia [Pityrosporum] furfur
Tinea flava
Tinea versicolor

111.1 Tinea nigra
Infection by Cladosporium species
Keratomycosis nigricans
Microsporosis nigra
Pityriasis nigra
Tinea palmaris nigra

111.2 Tinea blanca
Infection by Trichosporon (beigelii) cutaneum
White piedra

111.3 Black piedra
Infection by Piedraia hortai

111.8 Other specified dermatomycoses

111.9 Dermatomycosis, unspecified

4th **112 Candidiasis**
Includes infection by Candida species
moniliasis
Excludes *neonatal monilial infection (771.7)*

112.0 Of mouth
Thrush (oral)

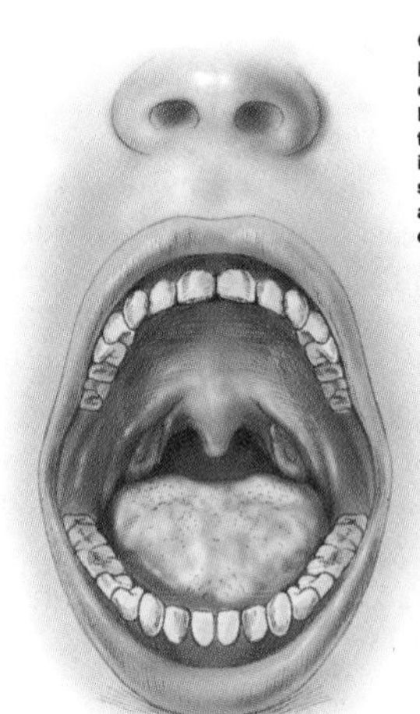

Oral thrush presents as creamy white lesions on the tongue, inner cheeks, soft palate and other oral structures

© 2008 Fairman Studios, LLC. All Rights Reserved.

112.1 Of vulva and vagina ♀
Candidal vulvovaginitis
Monilial vulvovaginitis

112.2 Of other urogenital sites
Candidal balanitis

112.3 Of skin and nails
Candidal intertrigo
Candidal onychia
Candidal perionyxis [paronychia]

112.4 Of lung
Candidal pneumonia

112.5 Disseminated
Systemic candidiasis

5th **112.8 Of other specified sites**

112.81 Candidal endocarditis

112.82 Candidal otitis externa
Otomycosis in moniliasis

112.83 Candidal meningitis

112.84 **Candidal esophagitis**

112.85 **Candidal enteritis**

112.89 **Other**

112.9 **Of unspecified site**

4th **114 Coccidioidomycosis**

Includes infection by Coccidioides (immitis)
Posada-Wernicke disease

114.0 **Primary coccidioidomycosis (pulmonary)**
Acute pulmonary coccidioidomycosis
Coccidioidomycotic pneumonitis
Desert rheumatism
Pulmonary coccidioidomycosis
San Joaquin Valley fever

114.1 **Primary extrapulmonary coccidioidomycosis**
Chancriform syndrome
Primary cutaneous coccidioidomycosis

114.2 **Coccidioidal meningitis**

114.3 **Other forms of progressive coccidioidomycosis**
Coccidioidal granuloma
Disseminated coccidioidomycosis

114.4 **Chronic pulmonary coccidioidomycosis**

114.5 **Pulmonary coccidioidomycosis, unspecified**

114.9 **Coccidioidomycosis, unspecified**

4th **115 Histoplasmosis**

The following fifth-digit subclassification is for use with category 115:

0 **without mention of manifestation**
1 **meningitis**
2 **retinitis**
3 **pericarditis**
4 **endocarditis**
5 **pneumonia**
9 **other**

5th **115.0 Infection by Histoplasma capsulatum**
[0-5,9] American histoplasmosis
Darling's disease
Reticuloendothelial cytomycosis
Small form histoplasmosis

5th **115.1 Infection by Histoplasma duboisii**
[0-5,9] African histoplasmosis
Large form histoplasmosis

5th **115.9 Histoplasmosis, unspecified**
[0-5,9] Histoplasmosis NOS

4th **116 Blastomycotic infection**

116.0 **Blastomycosis**
Blastomycotic dermatitis
Chicago disease
Cutaneous blastomycosis
Disseminated blastomycosis
Gilchrist's disease
Infection by Blastomyces [Ajellomyces] dermatitidis
North American blastomycosis
Primary pulmonary blastomycosis

116.1 **Paracoccidioidomycosis**
Brazilian blastomycosis
Infection by Paracoccidioides [Blastomyces] brasiliensis
Lutz-Splendore-Almeida disease
Mucocutaneous-lymphangitic paracoccidioidomycosis
Pulmonary paracoccidioidomycosis
South American blastomycosis
Visceral paracoccidioidomycosis

116.2 **Lobomycosis**
Infections by Loboa [Blastomyces] loboi
Keloidal blastomycosis
Lobo's disease

4th **117 Other mycoses**

117.0 **Rhinosporidiosis**
Infection by Rhinosporidium seeberi

117.1 **Sporotrichosis**
Cutaneous sporotrichosis
Disseminated sporotrichosis
Infection by Sporothrix [Sporotrichum] schenckii
Lymphocutaneous sporotrichosis
Pulmonary sporotrichosis
Sporotrichosis of the bones

117.2 **Chromoblastomycosis**
Chromomycosis
Infection by Cladosporidium carrionii, Fonsecaea compactum, Fonsecaea pedrosoi, Phialophora verrucosa

117.3 **Aspergillosis**
Infection by Aspergillus species, mainly A. fumigatus, A. flavus group, A. terreus group

117.4 **Mycotic mycetomas**
Infection by various genera and species of Ascomycetes and Deuteromycetes, such as Acremonium [Cephalosporium] falciforme, Neotestudina rosatii, Madurella grisea, Madurella mycetomii, Pyrenochaeta romeroi, Zopfia [Leptosphaeria] senegalensis
Madura foot, mycotic
Maduromycosis, mycotic
Excludes *actinomycotic mycetomas (039.0-039.9)*

117.5 **Cryptococcosis**
Busse-Buschke's disease
European cryptococcosis
Infection by Cryptococcus neoformans
Pulmonary cryptococcosis
Systemic cryptococcosis
Torula

117.6 **Allescheriosis [Petriellidosis]**
Infections by Allescheria [Petriellidium] boydii [Monosporium apiospermum]
Excludes *mycotic mycetoma (117.4)*

117.7 **Zygomycosis [Phycomycosis or Mucormycosis]**
Infection by species of Absidia, Basidiobolus, Conidiobolus, Cunninghamella, Entomophthora, Mucor, Rhizopus, Saksenaea

117.8 **Infection by dematiacious fungi [Phaehyphomycosis]**
Infection by dematiacious fungi, such as Cladosporium trichoides [bantianum], Dreschlera hawaiiensis, Phialophora gougerotii, Phialophora jeanselmi

117.9 **Other and unspecified mycoses**

118 Opportunistic mycoses
Infection of skin, subcutaneous tissues, and/or organs by a wide variety of fungi generally considered to be pathogenic to compromised hosts only (e.g., infection by species of Alternaria, Dreschlera, Fusarium)
Use additional code to identify manifestation, such as:
keratitis (370.8)

HELMINTHIASES (120-129)

4th **120 Schistosomiasis [bilharziasis]**

120.0 **Schistosoma haematobium**
Vesical schistosomiasis NOS

120.1 **Schistosoma mansoni**
Intestinal schistosomiasis NOS

120.2 **Schistosoma japonicum**
Asiatic schistosomiasis NOS
Katayama disease or fever

120.3 Cutaneous
Cercarial dermatitis
Infection by cercariae of Schistosoma
Schistosome dermatitis
Swimmers' itch

120.8 Other specified schistosomiasis
Infection by Schistosoma:
bovis
intercalatum
mattheii
spindale
Schistosomiasis chestermani

120.9 Schistosomiasis, unspecified
Blood flukes NOS
Hemic distomiasis

4th 121 Other trematode infections

121.0 Opisthorchiasis
Infection by:
cat liver fluke
Opisthorchis (felineus) (tenuicollis) (viverrini)

121.1 Clonorchiasis
Biliary cirrhosis due to clonorchiasis
Chinese liver fluke disease
Hepatic distomiasis due to Clonorchis sinensis
Oriental liver fluke disease

121.2 Paragonimiasis
Infection by Paragonimus
Lung fluke disease (oriental)
Pulmonary distomiasis

121.3 Fascioliasis
Infection by Fasciola:
gigantica
hepatica
Liver flukes NOS
Sheep liver fluke infection

121.4 Fasciolopsiasis
Infection by Fasciolopsis (buski)
Intestinal distomiasis

121.5 Metagonimiasis
Infection by Metagonimus yokogawai

121.6 Heterophyiasis
Infection by:
Heterophyes heterophyes
Stellantchasmus falcatus

121.8 Other specified trematode infections
Infection by:
Dicrocoelium dendriticum
Echinostoma ilocanum
Gastrodiscoides hominis

121.9 Trematode infection, unspecified
Distomiasis NOS
Fluke disease NOS

4th 122 Echinococcosis

Includes echinococciasis
hydatid disease
hydatidosis

122.0 Echinococcus granulosus infection of liver

122.1 Echinococcus granulosus infection of lung

122.2 Echinococcus granulosus infection of thyroid

122.3 Echinococcus granulosus infection, other

122.4 Echinococcus granulosus infection, unspecified

122.5 Echinococcus multilocularis infection of liver

122.6 Echinococcus multilocularis infection, other

122.7 Echinococcus multilocularis infection, unspecified

122.8 Echinococcosis, unspecified, of liver

122.9 Echinococcosis, other and unspecified

4th 123 Other cestode infection

123.0 Taenia solium infection, intestinal form
Pork tapeworm (adult) (infection)

123.1 Cysticercosis
Cysticerciasis
Infection by Cysticercus cellulosae [larval form of Taenia solium]

123.2 Taenia saginata infection
Beef tapeworm (infection)
Infection by Taeniarhynchus saginatus

123.3 Taeniasis, unspecified

123.4 Diphyllobothriasis, intestinal
Diphyllobothrium (adult) (latum) (pacificum) infection
Fish tapeworm (infection)

123.5 Sparganosis [larval diphyllobothriasis]
Infection by:
Diphyllobothrium larvae
Sparganum (mansoni) (proliferum)
Spirometra larvae

123.6 Hymenolepiasis
Dwarf tapeworm (infection)
Hymenolepis (diminuta) (nana) infection
Rat tapeworm (infection)

123.8 Other specified cestode infection
Diplogonoporus (grandis) infection
Dipylidium (caninum) infection
Dog tapeworm (infection)

123.9 Cestode infection, unspecified
Tapeworm (infection) NOS

124 Trichinosis
Trichinella spiralis infection
Trichinellosis
Trichiniasis

4th 125 Filarial infection and dracontiasis

125.0 Bancroftian filariasis
Chyluria due to Wuchereria bancrofti
Elephantiasis due to Wuchereria bancrofti
Infection due to Wuchereria bancrofti
Lymphadenitis due to Wuchereria bancrofti
Lymphangitis due to Wuchereria bancrofti
Wuchereriasis

125.1 Malayan filariasis
Brugia filariasis due to Brugia [Wuchereria] malayi
Chyluria due to Brugia [Wuchereria] malayi
Elephantiasis due to Brugia [Wuchereria] malayi
Infection due to Brugia [Wuchereria] malayi
Lymphadenitis due to Brugia [Wuchereria] malayi
Lymphangitis due to Brugia [Wuchereria] malayi

125.2 Loiasis
Eyeworm disease of Africa
Loa loa infection

125.3 Onchocerciasis
Onchocerca volvulus infection
Onchocercosis

125.4 Dipetalonemiasis
Infection by:
Acanthocheilonema perstans
Dipetalonema perstans

125.5 Mansonella ozzardi infection
Filariasis ozzardi

125.6 Other specified filariasis
Dirofilaria infection
Infection by:
Acanthocheilonema streptocerca
Dipetalonema streptocerca

125.7 **Dracontiasis**
Guinea-worm infection
Infection by Dracunculus medinensis

125.9 **Unspecified filariasis**

4th 126 **Ancylostomiasis and necatoriasis**
Includes cutaneous larva migrans due to Ancylostoma
hookworm (disease) (infection)
uncinariasis

126.0 **Ancylostoma duodenale**

126.1 **Necator americanus**

126.2 **Ancylostoma braziliense**

126.3 **Ancylostoma ceylanicum**

126.8 **Other specified Ancylostoma**

126.9 **Ancylostomiasis and necatoriasis, unspecified**
Creeping eruption NOS
Cutaneous larva migrans NOS

4th 127 **Other intestinal helminthiases**

127.0 **Ascariasis**
Ascaridiasis
Infection by Ascaris lumbricoides
Roundworm infection

127.1 **Anisakiasis**
Infection by Anisakis larva

127.2 **Strongyloidiasis**
Infection by Strongyloides stercoralis
Excludes *trichostrongyliasis (127.6)*

127.3 **Trichuriasis**
Infection by Trichuris trichiuria
Trichocephaliasis
Whipworm (disease) (infection)

127.4 **Enterobiasis**
Infection by Enterobius vermicularis
Oxyuriasis
Oxyuris vermicularis infection
Pinworm (disease) (infection)
Threadworm infection

127.5 **Capillariasis**
Infection by Capillaria philippinensis
Excludes *infection by Capillaria hepatica (128.8)*

127.6 **Trichostrongyliasis**
Infection by Trichostrongylus species

127.7 **Other specified intestinal helminthiasis**
Infection by:
Oesophagostomum apiostomum and related species
Ternidens diminutus
other specified intestinal helminth
Physalopteriasis

127.8 **Mixed intestinal helminthiasis**
Infection by intestinal helminths classified to more than one of the categories 120.0-127.7
Mixed helminthiasis NOS

127.9 **Intestinal helminthiasis, unspecified**

4th 128 **Other and unspecified helminthiases**

128.0 **Toxocariasis**
Larva migrans visceralis
Toxocara (canis) (cati) infection
Visceral larva migrans syndrome

128.1 **Gnathostomiasis**
Infection by Gnathostoma spinigerum and related species

128.8 **Other specified helminthiasis**
Infection by:
Angiostrongylus cantonensis
Capillaria hepatica
other specified helminth

128.9 **Helminth infection, unspecified**
Helminthiasis NOS
Worms NOS

129 **Intestinal parasitism, unspecified**

OTHER INFECTIOUS AND PARASITIC DISEASES (130-136)

4th 130 **Toxoplasmosis**
Includes infection by toxoplasma gondii
toxoplasmosis (acquired)
Excludes *congenital toxoplasmosis (771.2)*

130.0 **Meningoencephalitis due to toxoplasmosis**
Encephalitis due to acquired toxoplasmosis

130.1 **Conjunctivitis due to toxoplasmosis**

130.2 **Chorioretinitis due to toxoplasmosis**
Focal retinochoroiditis due to acquired toxoplasmosis

130.3 **Myocarditis due to toxoplasmosis**

130.4 **Pneumonitis due to toxoplasmosis**

130.5 **Hepatitis due to toxoplasmosis**

130.7 **Toxoplasmosis of other specified sites**

130.8 **Multisystemic disseminated toxoplasmosis**
Toxoplasmosis of multiple sites

130.9 **Toxoplasmosis, unspecified**

4th 131 **Trichomoniasis**
Includes infection due to Trichomonas (vaginalis)

5th 131.0 **Urogenital trichomoniasis**

131.00 **Urogenital trichomoniasis, unspecified**
Fluor (vaginalis) trichomonal or due to Trichomonas (vaginalis)
Leukorrhea (vaginalis) trichomonal or due to Trichomonas (vaginalis)

131.01 **Trichomonal vulvovaginitis** ♀
Vaginitis, trichomonal or due to Trichomonas (vaginalis)

131.02 **Trichomonal urethritis**

131.03 **Trichomonal prostatitis** ♂

131.09 **Other**

131.8 **Other specified sites**
Excludes *intestinal (007.3)*

131.9 **Trichomoniasis, unspecified**

4th 132 **Pediculosis and phthirus infestation**

132.0 **Pediculus capitis [head louse]**

Head Louse

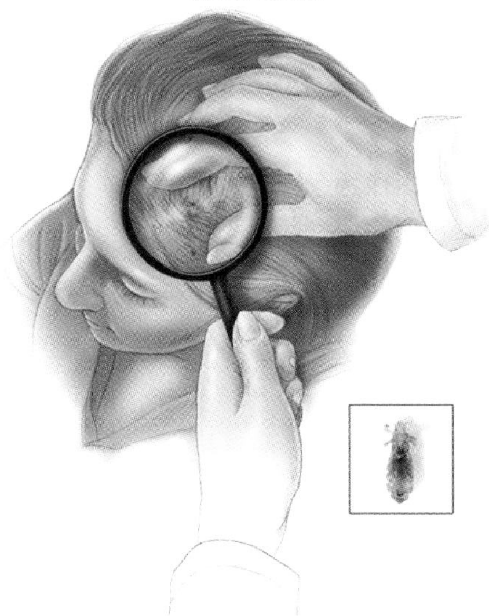

© 2008 Fairman Studios, LLC. All Rights Reserved.

132.1 **Pediculus corporis [body louse]**

132.2 Phthirus pubis [pubic louse]
Pediculus pubis

132.3 Mixed infestation
Infestation classifiable to more than one of the categories 132.0-132.2

132.9 Pediculosis, unspecified

4th **133 Acariasis**

133.0 Scabies
Infestation by Sarcoptes scabiei
Norwegian scabies
Sarcoptic itch

133.8 Other acariasis
Chiggers
Infestation by:
Demodex folliculorum
Trombicula

133.9 Acariasis, unspecified
Infestation by mites NOS

4th **134 Other infestation**

134.0 Myiasis
Infestation by:
Dermatobia (hominis)
fly larvae
Gasterophilus (intestinalis)
maggots
Oestrus ovis

134.1 Other arthropod infestation
Infestation by:
chigoe
sand flea
Jigger disease
Scarabiasis
Tunga penetrans
Tungiasis

134.2 Hirudiniasis
Hirudiniasis (external) (internal)
Leeches (aquatic) (land)

134.8 Other specified infestations

134.9 Infestation, unspecified
Infestation (skin) NOS
Skin parasites NOS

135 Sarcoidosis
Besnier-Boeck-Schaumann disease
Lupoid (miliary) of Boeck
Lupus pernio (Besnier)
Lymphogranulomatosis, benign (Schaumann's)
Sarcoid (any site):
NOS
Boeck
Darier-Roussy
Uveoparotid fever

4th **136 Other and unspecified infectious and parasitic diseases**

136.0 Ainhum
Dactylolysis spontanea

136.1 Behçet's syndrome

5th **136.2 Specific infections by free-living amebae**

136.21 Specific infection due to acanthamoeba
Use additional code to identify manifestation, such as:
keratitis (370.8)

136.29 Other specific infections by free-living amebae
Meningoencephalitis due to Naegleria

136.3 Pneumocystosis
Pneumonia due to Pneumocystis carinii
Pneumonia due to Pneumocystis jiroveci

136.4 Psorospermiasis

136.5 Sarcosporidiosis
Infection by Sarcocystis lindemanni

136.8 Other specified infectious and parasitic diseases
Candiru infestation

136.9 Unspecified infectious and parasitic diseases
Infectious disease NOS
Parasitic disease NOS

LATE EFFECTS OF INFECTIOUS AND PARASITIC DISEASES (137-139)

4th **137 Late effects of tuberculosis**

Note: *This category is to be used to indicate conditions classifiable to 010-018 as the cause of late effects, which are themselves classified elsewhere. The "late effects" include those specified as such, as sequelae, or as due to old or inactive tuberculosis, without evidence of active disease.*

137.0 Late effects of respiratory or unspecified tuberculosis

137.1 Late effects of central nervous system tuberculosis

137.2 Late effects of genitourinary tuberculosis

137.3 Late effects of tuberculosis of bones and joints

137.4 Late effects of tuberculosis of other specified organs

138 Late effects of acute poliomyelitis

Note: *This category is to be used to indicate conditions classifiable to 045 as the cause of late effects, which are themselves classified elsewhere. The "late effects" include conditions specified as such, or as sequelae, or as due to old or inactive poliomyelitis, without evidence of active disease.*

4th **139 Late effects of other infectious and parasitic diseases**

Note: *This category is to be used to indicate conditions classifiable to categories 001-009, 020-041, 046-136 as the cause of late effects, which are themselves classified elsewhere. The "late effects" include conditions specified as such; they also include sequela of diseases classifiable to the above categories if there is evidence that the disease itself is no longer present.*

139.0 Late effects of viral encephalitis
Late effects of conditions classifiable to 049.8-049.9, 062-064

139.1 Late effects of trachoma
Late effects of conditions classifiable to 076

139.8 Late effects of other and unspecified infectious and parasitic diseases

2. NEOPLASMS (140-239)

1. Content

This chapter contains the following broad groups:

140-195	Malignant neoplasms, stated or presumed to be primary, of specified sites, except of lymphatic and hematopoietic tissue
196-198	Malignant neoplasms, stated or presumed to be secondary, of specified sites
199	Malignant neoplasms, without specification of site
200-208	Malignant neoplasms, stated or presumed to be primary, of lymphatic and hematopoietic tissue
209	Neuroendocrine tumors
210-229	Benign neoplasms
230-234	Carcinoma in situ
235-238	Neoplasms of uncertain behavior [see **Note**, at beginning of section 235-238]
239	Neoplasms of unspecified nature

2. Functional activity

All neoplasms are classified in this chapter, whether or not functionally active. An additional code from Chapter 3 may be used to identify such functional activity associated with any neoplasm, e.g.:

catecholamine-producing malignant pheochromocytoma of adrenal:
code 194.0, additional code 255.6

basophil adenoma of pituitary with Cushing's syndrome:
code 227.3, additional code 255.0

3. Morphology [Histology]

For those wishing to identify the histological type of neoplasms, a comprehensive coded nomenclature, which comprises the morphology rubrics of the ICD-Oncology, is given after the E-code chapter.

4. Malignant neoplasms overlapping site boundaries

Categories 140-195 are for the classification of primary malignant neoplasms according to their point of origin. A malignant neoplasm that overlaps two or more subcategories within a three-digit rubric and whose point of origin cannot be determined should be classified to the subcategory .8 "Other." For example, "carcinoma involving tip and ventral surface of tongue" should be assigned to 141.8. On the other hand, "carcinoma of tip of tongue, extending to involve the ventral surface" should be coded to 141.2, as the point of origin, the tip, is known. Three subcategories (149.8, 159.8, 165.8) have been provided for malignant neoplasms that overlap the boundaries of three-digit rubrics within certain systems. Overlapping malignant neoplasms that cannot be classified as indicated above should be assigned to the appropriate subdivision of category 195 (Malignant neoplasm of other and ill-defined sites).

ICD-9-CM Official Guidelines (Chapter 2):

General guidelines

Chapter 2 of the ICD-9-CM contains the codes for most benign and all malignant neoplasms. Certain benign neoplasms, such as prostatic adenomas, may be found in the specific body system chapters. To properly code a neoplasm it is necessary to determine from the record if the neoplasm is benign, in-situ, malignant, or of uncertain histologic behavior. If malignant, any secondary (metastatic) sites should also be determined.

The neoplasm table in the Alphabetic Index should be referenced first. However, if the histological term is documented, that term should be referenced first, rather than going immediately to the Neoplasm Table, in order to determine which column in the Neoplasm Table is appropriate. For example, if the documentation indicates "adenoma," refer to the term in the Alphabetic Index to review the entries under this term and the instructional note to "see also neoplasm, by site, benign." The table provides the proper code based on the type of neoplasm and the site. It is important to select the proper column in the table that corresponds to the type of neoplasm. The tabular should then be referenced to verify that the correct code has been selected from the table and that a more specific site code does not exist.

See Section I. C. 18.d.4. for information regarding V codes for genetic susceptibility to cancer.

a. Treatment directed at the malignancy

If the treatment is directed at the malignancy, designate the malignancy as the principal diagnosis.

The only exception to this guideline is if a patient admission/encounter is solely for the administration of chemotherapy, immunotherapy or radiation therapy, assign the appropriate V58.x code as the first-listed or principal diagnosis, and the diagnosis or problem for which the service is being performed as a secondary diagnosis.

b. Treatment of secondary site

When a patient is admitted because of a primary neoplasm with metastasis and treatment is directed toward the secondary site only, the secondary neoplasm is designated as the principal diagnosis even though the primary malignancy is still present.

c. Coding and sequencing of complications

Coding and sequencing of complications associated with the malignancies or with the therapy thereof are subject to the following guidelines:

1) Anemia associated with malignancy

When admission/encounter is for management of an anemia associated with the malignancy, and the treatment is only for anemia, the appropriate anemia code (such as code 285.22, Anemia in neoplastic disease) is designated as the principal diagnosis and is followed by the appropriate code(s) for the malignancy.

Code 285.22 may also be used as a secondary code if the patient suffers from anemia and is being treated for the malignancy.

2) Anemia associated with chemotherapy, immunotherapy and radiation therapy

When the admission/encounter is for management of an anemia associated with chemotherapy, immunotherapy or radiotherapy and the only treatment is for the anemia, the anemia is sequenced first followed by code E933.1. The appropriate neoplasm code should be assigned as an additional code.

3) Management of dehydration due to the malignancy

When the admission/encounter is for management of dehydration due to the malignancy or the therapy, or a combination of both, and only the dehydration is being treated (intravenous rehydration), the dehydration is sequenced first, followed by the code(s) for the malignancy.

4) Treatment of a complication resulting from a surgical procedure

When the admission/encounter is for treatment of a complication resulting from a surgical procedure, designate the complication as the principal or first-listed diagnosis if treatment is directed at resolving the complication.

d. Primary malignancy previously excised

When a primary malignancy has been previously excised or eradicated from its site and there is no further treatment directed to that site and there is no evidence of any existing primary malignancy, a code from category V10, Personal history of malignant neoplasm, should be used to indicate the former site of the malignancy. Any mention of extension, invasion, or metastasis to another site is coded as a secondary malignant neoplasm to that site. The secondary site may be the principal or first-listed with the V10 code used as a secondary code.

e. Admissions/Encounters involving chemotherapy, immunotherapy and radiation therapy

1) Episode of care involves surgical removal of neoplasm

When an episode of care involves the surgical removal of a neoplasm, primary or secondary site, followed by adjunct chemotherapy or radiation treatment during the same episode of care, the neoplasm code should be assigned as principal or first-listed diagnosis, using codes in the 140-198 series or where appropriate in the 200-203 series.

Neoplasms

2) ***Patient admission/encounter solely for administration of chemotherapy, immunotherapy and radiation therapy***

If a patient admission/encounter is solely for the administration of chemotherapy, immunotherapy or radiation therapy assign code V58.0, Encounter for radiation therapy, or V58.11, Encounter for antineoplastic chemotherapy, or V58.12, Encounter for antineoplastic immunotherapy as the first-listed or principal diagnosis. If a patient receives more than one of these therapies during the same admission more than one of these codes may be assigned, in any sequence.

3) ***Patient admitted for radiotherapy/chemotherapy and immunotherapy and develops complications***

When a patient is admitted for the purpose of radiotherapy, immunotherapy or chemotherapy and develops complications such as uncontrolled nausea and vomiting or dehydration, the principal or first-listed diagnosis is V58.0, Encounter for radiotherapy, or V58.11, Encounter for antineoplastic chemotherapy, or V58.12, Encounter for antineoplastic immunotherapy followed by any codes for the complications.

f. ***Admission/encounter to determine extent of malignancy***

When the reason for admission/encounter is to determine the extent of the malignancy, or for a procedure such as paracentesis or thoracentesis, the primary malignancy or appropriate metastatic site is designated as the principal or first-listed diagnosis, even though chemotherapy or radiotherapy is administered.

g. ***Symptoms, signs, and ill-defined conditions listed in Chapter 16 associated with neoplasms***

Symptoms, signs, and ill-defined conditions listed in Chapter 16 characteristic of, or associated with, an existing primary or secondary site malignancy cannot be used to replace the malignancy as principal or first-listed diagnosis, regardless of the number of admissions or encounters for treatment and care of the neoplasm.

See section I.C.18.d.14, Encounter for prophylactic organ removal.

h. ***Admission/encounter for pain control/management***

See Section I.C.6.a.5 for information on coding admission/encounter for pain control/management.

MALIGNANT NEOPLASM OF LIP, ORAL CAVITY, AND PHARYNX (140-149)

Excludes *carcinoma in situ (230.0)*

4th **140 Malignant neoplasm of lip**

Excludes *skin of lip (173.0)*

140.0 Upper lip, vermilion border I 43, I 44
- Upper lip:
  - NOS
  - external
  - lipstick area

140.1 Lower lip, vermilion border I 43, I 44
- Lower lip:
  - NOS
  - external
  - lipstick area

140.3 Upper lip, inner aspect
- Upper lip:
  - buccal aspect
  - frenulum
  - mucosa
  - oral aspect

140.4 Lower lip, inner aspect I 43, I 44
- Lower lip:
  - buccal aspect
  - frenulum
  - mucosa
  - oral aspect

140.5 Lip, unspecified, inner aspect I 43, I 44
- Lip, not specified whether upper or lower:
  - buccal aspect
  - frenulum
  - mucosa
  - oral aspect

140.6 Commissure of lip I 43, I 44
- Labial commissure

140.8 Other sites of lip I 43, I 44
- Malignant neoplasm of contiguous or overlapping sites of lip whose point of origin cannot be determined

140.9 Lip, unspecified, vermilion border I 43, I 44
- Lip, not specified as upper or lower:
  - NOS
  - external
  - lipstick area

4th **141 Malignant neoplasm of tongue**

141.0 Base of tongue I 43, I 44
- Dorsal surface of base of tongue
- Fixed part of tongue NOS

141.1 Dorsal surface of tongue I 43, I 44
- Anterior two-thirds of tongue, dorsal surface
- Dorsal tongue NOS
- Midline of tongue

Excludes *dorsal surface of base of tongue (141.0)*

141.2 Tip and lateral border of tongue I 43, I 44

141.3 Ventral surface of tongue I 43, I 44
- Anterior two-thirds of tongue, ventral surface
- Frenulum linguae

141.4 Anterior two-thirds of tongue, part unspecified I 43, I 44
- Mobile part of tongue NOS

141.5 Junctional zone I 43, I 44
- Border of tongue at junction of fixed and mobile parts at insertion of anterior tonsillar pillar

141.6 Lingual tonsil I 43, I 44

141.8 Other sites of tongue I 43, I 44
- Malignant neoplasm of contiguous or overlapping sites of tongue whose point of origin cannot be determined

141.9 Tongue, unspecified I 43, I 44
- Tongue NOS

4th **142 Malignant neoplasm of major salivary glands**

Includes salivary ducts

Excludes *malignant neoplasm of minor salivary glands:*
- *NOS (145.9)*
- *buccal mucosa (145.0)*
- *soft palate (145.3)*
- *tongue (141.0-141.9)*
- *tonsil, palatine (146.0)*

142.0 Parotid gland I 43, I 44

142.1 Submandibular gland I 43, I 44
- Submaxillary gland

142.2 Sublingual gland I 43, I 44

142.8 Other major salivary glands I 43, I 44
- Malignant neoplasm of contiguous or overlapping sites of salivary glands and ducts whose point of origin cannot be determined

142.9 Salivary gland, unspecified I 43, I 44
- Salivary gland (major) NOS

4th **143 Malignant neoplasm of gum**

Includes alveolar (ridge) mucosa
- gingiva (alveolar) (marginal)
- interdental papillae

Excludes *malignant odontogenic neoplasms (170.0-170.1)*

143.0 Upper gum I 43, I 44

143.1 Lower gum 143, 144

143.8 Other sites of gum 143, 144
Malignant neoplasm of contiguous or overlapping sites of gum whose point of origin cannot be determined

143.9 Gum, unspecified 143, 144

4th **144 Malignant neoplasm of floor of mouth**

144.0 Anterior portion 143, 144
Anterior to the premolar-canine junction

144.1 Lateral portion 143, 144

144.8 Other sites of floor of mouth 143, 144
Malignant neoplasm of contiguous or overlapping sites of floor of mouth whose point of origin cannot be determined

144.9 Floor of mouth, part unspecified 143, 144

4th **145 Malignant neoplasm of other and unspecified parts of mouth**
Excludes *mucosa of lips (140.0-140.9)*

145.0 Cheek mucosa 143, 144
Buccal mucosa
Cheek, inner aspect

145.1 Vestibule of mouth 143, 144
Buccal sulcus (upper) (lower)
Labial sulcus (upper) (lower)

145.2 Hard palate 143, 144

145.3 Soft palate 143, 144
Excludes *nasopharyngeal [posterior] [superior] surface of soft palate (147.3)*

145.4 Uvula 143, 144

145.5 Palate, unspecified 143, 144
Junction of hard and soft palate
Roof of mouth

145.6 Retromolar area 143, 144

145.8 Other specified parts of mouth 143, 144
Malignant neoplasm of contiguous or overlapping sites of mouth whose point of origin cannot be determined

145.9 Mouth, unspecified 143, 144
Buccal cavity NOS
Minor salivary gland, unspecified site
Oral cavity NOS

4th **146 Malignant neoplasm of oropharynx**

146.0 Tonsil 143, 144
Tonsil:
NOS
faucial
palatine
Excludes *lingual tonsil (141.6)*
pharyngeal tonsil (147.1)

146.1 Tonsillar fossa 143, 144

146.2 Tonsillar pillars (anterior) (posterior) 143, 144
Faucial pillar
Glossopalatine fold
Palatoglossal arch
Palatopharyngeal arch

146.3 Vallecula 143, 144
Anterior and medial surface of the pharyngoepiglottic fold

146.4 Anterior aspect of epiglottis 143, 144
Epiglottis, free border [margin]
Glossoepiglottic fold(s)
Excludes *epiglottis:*
NOS (161.1)
suprahyoid portion (161.1)

146.5 Junctional region 143, 144
Junction of the free margin of the epiglottis, the aryepiglottic fold, and the pharyngoepiglottic fold

146.6 Lateral wall of oropharynx 143, 144

146.7 Posterior wall of oropharynx 143, 144

146.8 Other specified sites of oropharynx 143, 144
Branchial cleft
Malignant neoplasm of contiguous or overlapping sites of oropharynx whose point of origin cannot be determined

146.9 Oropharynx, unspecified 143, 144

4th **147 Malignant neoplasm of nasopharynx**

147.0 Superior wall 143, 144
Roof of nasopharynx

147.1 Posterior wall 143, 144
Adenoid
Pharyngeal tonsil

147.2 Lateral wall 143, 144
Fossa of Rosenmüller
Opening of auditory tube
Pharyngeal recess

147.3 Anterior wall 143, 144
Floor of nasopharynx
Nasopharyngeal [posterior] [superior] surface of soft palate
Posterior margin of nasal septum and choanae

147.8 Other specified sites of nasopharynx 143, 144
Malignant neoplasm of contiguous or overlapping sites of nasopharynx whose point of origin cannot be determined

147.9 Nasopharynx, unspecified 143, 144
Nasopharyngeal wall NOS

4th **148 Malignant neoplasm of hypopharynx**

148.0 Postcricoid region 143, 144

148.1 Pyriform sinus 143, 144
Pyriform fossa

148.2 Aryepiglottic fold, hypopharyngeal aspect 143, 144
Aryepiglottic fold or interarytenoid fold:
NOS
marginal zone
Excludes *aryepiglottic fold or interarytenoid fold, laryngeal aspect (161.1)*

148.3 Posterior hypopharyngeal wall 143, 144

148.8 Other specified sites of hypopharynx 143, 144
Malignant neoplasm of contiguous or overlapping sites of hypopharynx whose point of origin cannot be determined

148.9 Hypopharynx, unspecified 143, 144
Hypopharyngeal wall NOS
Hypopharynx NOS

4th **149 Malignant neoplasm of other and ill-defined sites within the lip, oral cavity, and pharynx**

149.0 Pharynx, unspecified 143, 144

149.1 Waldeyer's ring 143, 144

149.8 Other 143, 144
Malignant neoplasms of lip, oral cavity, and pharynx whose point of origin cannot be assigned to any one of the categories 140-148
Excludes *"book leaf" neoplasm [ventral surface of tongue and floor of mouth] (145.8)*

149.9 Ill-defined 143, 144

MALIGNANT NEOPLASM OF DIGESTIVE ORGANS AND PERITONEUM (150-159)

Excludes *carcinoma in situ (230.1-230.9)*

4th **150 Malignant neoplasm of esophagus**

150.0 Cervical esophagus 143, 144

150.1 Thoracic esophagus 143, 144

150.2 Abdominal esophagus 143, 144
Excludes *adenocarcinoma (151.0)*
cardio-esophageal junction (151.0)

143.1 – 150.2

150.3 Upper third of esophagus 143, 144
Proximal third of esophagus

150.4 Middle third of esophagus 143, 144

150.5 Lower third of esophagus 143, 144
Distal third of esophagus
Excludes *adenocarcinoma (151.0)*
cardio-esophageal junction (151.0)

150.8 Other specified part 143, 144
Malignant neoplasm of contiguous or overlapping sites of esophagus whose point of origin cannot be determined

150.9 Esophagus, unspecified 143, 144
C15.9 Malignant neoplasm of esophagus, unspecified

4th **151 Malignant neoplasm of stomach**
Excludes *benign carcinoid tumor of stomach (209.63)*
malignant carcinoid tumor of stomach (209.23)

151.0 Cardia 143, 144
Cardiac orifice
Cardio-esophageal junction
Excludes *squamous cell carcinoma (150.2, 150.5)*

151.1 Pylorus 143, 144
Prepylorus
Pyloric canal

151.2 Pyloric antrum 143, 144
Antrum of stomach NOS

151.3 Fundus of stomach 143, 144

151.4 Body of stomach 143, 144

151.5 Lesser curvature, unspecified 143, 144
Lesser curvature, not classifiable to 151.1-151.4

151.6 Greater curvature, unspecified 143, 144
Greater curvature, not classifiable to 151.0-151.4

151.8 Other specified sites of stomach 143, 144
Anterior wall, not classifiable to 151.0-151.4
Posterior wall, not classifiable to 151.0-151.4
Malignant neoplasm of contiguous or overlapping sites of stomach whose point of origin cannot be determined

151.9 Stomach, unspecified 143, 144
C16.9 Malignant neoplasm of stomach, unspecified
Carcinoma ventriculi
Gastric cancer

4th **152 Malignant neoplasm of small intestine, including duodenum**
Excludes *benign carcinoid tumor of small intestine and duodenum (209.40-209.43)*
malignant carcinoid tumor of small intestine and duodenum (209.00-209.03)

152.0 Duodenum 143, 144

152.1 Jejunum 143, 144

152.2 Ileum 143, 144
Excludes *ileocecal valve (153.4)*

152.3 Meckel's diverticulum 143, 144

152.8 Other specified sites of small intestine 143, 144
Duodenojejunal junction
Malignant neoplasm of contiguous or overlapping sites of small intestine whose point of origin cannot be determined

152.9 Small intestine, unspecified 143, 144

4th **153 Malignant neoplasm of colon**
Excludes *benign carcinoid tumor of colon (209.50-209.56)*
malignant carcinoid tumor of colon (209.10-209.16)

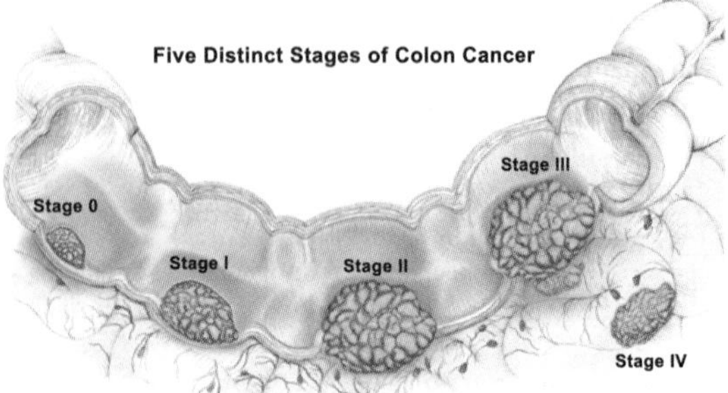

153.0 Hepatic flexure 72, 100, 143, 144

153.1 Transverse colon 72, 100, 143, 144

153.2 Descending colon 72, 100, 143, 144
Left colon

153.3 Sigmoid colon 72, 100, 143, 144
C18.7 Malignant neoplasm of sigmoid colon
Sigmoid (flexure)
Excludes *rectosigmoid junction (154.0)*

153.4 Cecum 72, 100, 143, 144
Ileocecal valve

153.5 Appendix 72, 100, 143, 144

153.6 Ascending colon 72, 100, 143, 144
Right colon

153.7 Splenic flexure 72, 100, 143, 144

153.8 Other specified sites of large intestine 72, 100, 143, 144
C18.8 Malignant neoplasm of overlapping sites of colon
Malignant neoplasm of contiguous or overlapping sites of colon whose point of origin cannot be determined
Excludes *ileocecal valve (153.4)*
rectosigmoid junction (154.0)

153.9 Colon, unspecified 72, 100, 143, 144
C18.9 Malignant neoplasm of colon, unspecified
Large intestine NOS

4th **154 Malignant neoplasm of rectum, rectosigmoid junction, and anus**
Excludes *benign carcinoid tumor of rectum (209.57)*
malignant carcinoid tumor of rectum (209.17)

154.0 Rectosigmoid junction 100, 143, 144
C19 Malignant neoplasm of rectosigmoid junction
Colon with rectum
Rectosigmoid (colon)

154.1 Rectum 100, 143, 144
C20 Malignant neoplasm of rectum
Rectal ampulla

154.2 Anal canal 143, 144
Anal sphincter
Excludes *skin of anus (172.5, 173.5)*

154.3 Anus, unspecified 143, 144
Excludes *anus:*
margin (172.5, 173.5)
skin (172.5, 173.5)
perianal skin (172.5, 173.5)

154.8 Other 100, 143, 144
Anorectum
Cloacogenic zone
Malignant neoplasm of contiguous or overlapping sites of rectum, rectosigmoid junction, and anus whose point of origin cannot be determined

4th 155 Malignant neoplasm of liver and intrahepatic bile ducts

155.0 Liver, primary I 43, I 44
Carcinoma:
hepatocellular
liver cell
liver, specified as primary
Hepatoblastoma

155.1 Intrahepatic bile ducts I 43, I 44
Canaliculi biliferi
Interlobular:
bile ducts
biliary canals
Intrahepatic:
biliary passages
canaliculi
gall duct
Excludes *hepatic duct (156.1)*

155.2 Liver, not specified as primary or secondary I 43, I 44

4th 156 Malignant neoplasm of gallbladder and extrahepatic bile ducts

156.0 Gallbladder I 43, I 44

156.1 Extrahepatic bile ducts I 43, I 44
Biliary duct or passage NOS
Common bile duct
Cystic duct
Hepatic duct
Sphincter of Oddi

156.2 Ampulla of Vater I 43, I 44

156.8 Other specified sites of gallbladder and extrahepatic bile ducts I 43, I 44
Malignant neoplasm of contiguous or overlapping sites of gallbladder and extrahepatic bile ducts whose point of origin cannot be determined

156.9 Biliary tract, part unspecified I 43, I 44
Malignant neoplasm involving both intrahepatic and extrahepatic bile ducts

4th 157 Malignant neoplasm of pancreas

157.0 Head of pancreas I 43, I 44, I 56

157.1 Body of pancreas I 43, I 44, I 56

157.2 Tail of pancreas I 43, I 44, I 56

157.3 Pancreatic duct I 43, I 44, I 56
Duct of:
Santorini
Wirsung

157.4 Islets of Langerhans I 43, I 44, I 56
Islets of Langerhans, any part of pancreas
Use additional code to identify any functional activity

157.8 Other specified sites of pancreas I 43, I 44, I 56
Ectopic pancreatic tissue
Malignant neoplasm of contiguous or overlapping sites of pancreas whose point of origin cannot be determined

157.9 Pancreas, part unspecified I 43, I 44, I 56
C25.9 Malignant neoplasm of pancreas, unspecified

4th 158 Malignant neoplasm of retroperitoneum and peritoneum

158.0 Retroperitoneum I 43, I 44
Periadrenal tissue
Perinephric tissue
Perirenal tissue
Retrocecal tissue

158.8 Specified parts of peritoneum I 43, I 44
Cul-de-sac (of Douglas)
Mesentery
Mesocolon
Omentum
Peritoneum:
parietal
pelvic
Rectouterine pouch
Malignant neoplasm of contiguous or overlapping sites of retroperitoneum and peritoneum whose point of origin cannot be determined

158.9 Peritoneum, unspecified I 43, I 44

4th 159 Malignant neoplasm of other and ill-defined sites within the digestive organs and peritoneum

159.0 Intestinal tract, part unspecified I 43, I 44
Intestine NOS

159.1 Spleen, not elsewhere classified I 43, I 44
Angiosarcoma of spleen
Fibrosarcoma of spleen
Excludes *Hodgkin's disease (201.0-201.9)*
lymphosarcoma (200.1)
reticulosarcoma (200.0)

159.8 Other sites of digestive system and intra-abdominal organs I 43, I 44
Malignant neoplasm of digestive organs and peritoneum whose point of origin cannot be assigned to any one of the categories 150-158
Excludes *anus and rectum (154.8)*
cardio-esophageal junction (151.0)
colon and rectum (154.0)

159.9 Ill-defined I 43, I 44
Alimentary canal or tract NOS
Gastrointestinal tract NOS
Excludes *abdominal NOS (195.2)*
intra-abdominal NOS (195.2)

MALIGNANT NEOPLASM OF RESPIRATORY AND INTRATHORACIC ORGANS (160-165)

Excludes *carcinoma in situ (231.0-231.9)*

4th 160 Malignant neoplasm of nasal cavities, middle ear, and accessory sinuses

160.0 Nasal cavities I 43, I 44
Cartilage of nose
Conchae, nasal
Internal nose
Septum of nose
Vestibule of nose
Excludes *nasal bone (170.0)*
nose NOS (195.0)
olfactory bulb (192.0)
posterior margin of septum and choanae (147.3)
skin of nose (172.3, 173.3)
turbinates (170.0)

160.1 Auditory tube, middle ear, and mastoid air cells I 43, I 44
Antrum tympanicum
Eustachian tube
Tympanic cavity
Excludes *auditory canal (external) (172.2, 173.2)*
bone of ear (meatus) (170.0)
cartilage of ear (171.0)
ear (external) (skin) (172.2, 173.2)

160.2 Maxillary sinus I 43, I 44
Antrum (Highmore) (maxillary)

160.3 Ethmoidal sinus I 43, I 44

160.4 Frontal sinus I 43, I 44

160.5 **Sphenoidal sinus** I 43, I 44

160.8 **Other** I 43, I 44
Malignant neoplasm of contiguous or overlapping sites of nasal cavities, middle ear, and accessory sinuses whose point of origin cannot be determined

160.9 **Accessory sinus, unspecified** I 43, I 44

4th 161 **Malignant neoplasm of larynx**

161.0 **Glottis** I 43, I 44
Intrinsic larynx
Laryngeal commissure (anterior) (posterior)
True vocal cord
Vocal cord NOS

161.1 **Supraglottis** I 43, I 44
Aryepiglottic fold or interarytenoid fold, laryngeal aspect
Epiglottis (suprahyoid portion) NOS
Extrinsic larynx
False vocal cords
Posterior (laryngeal) surface of epiglottis
Ventricular bands
Excludes *anterior aspect of epiglottis (146.4)*
aryepiglottic fold or interarytenoid fold:
NOS (148.2)
hypopharyngeal aspect (148.2)
marginal zone (148.2)

161.2 **Subglottis** I 43, I 44

161.3 **Laryngeal cartilages** I 43, I 44
Cartilage:
arytenoid
cricoid
cuneiform
thyroid

161.8 **Other specified sites of larynx** I 43, I 44
Malignant neoplasm of contiguous or overlapping sites of larynx whose point of origin cannot be determined

161.9 **Larynx, unspecified** I 43, I 44

4th 162 **Malignant neoplasm of trachea, bronchus, and lung**
Excludes *benign carcinoid tumor of bronchus (209.61)*
malignant carcinoid tumor of bronchus (209.21)

162.0 **Trachea** I 43, I 44, I 56
Cartilage of trachea
Mucosa of trachea

162.2 **Main bronchus** I 43, I 44, I 56, I 57
Carina
Hilus of lung

162.3 **Upper lobe, bronchus or lung** I 43, I 44, I 56, I 57
C34.10 Malignant neoplasm of upper lobe, bronchus or lung, unspecified side

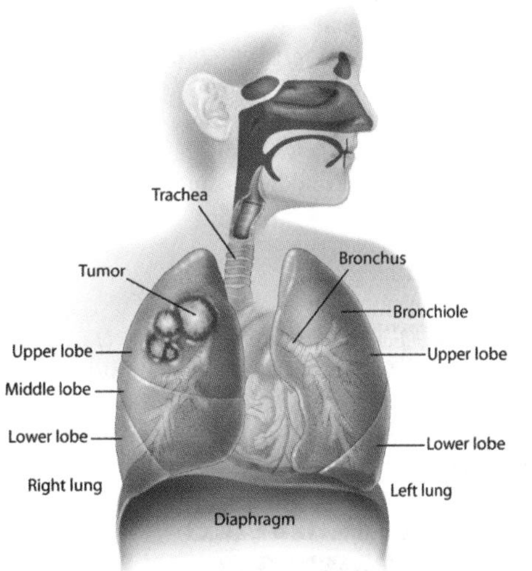

162.4 **Middle lobe, bronchus or lung** I 43, I 44, I 56, I 57

162.5 **Lower lobe, bronchus or lung** I 43, I 44, I 56, I 57
C34.30 Malignant neoplasm of lower lobe, bronchus or lung, unspecified side

162.8 **Other parts of bronchus or lung** I 43, I 44, I 56
C34.80 Malignant neoplasm of overlapping sites of bronchus and lung, unspecified side
Malignant neoplasm of contiguous or overlapping sites of bronchus or lung whose point of origin cannot be determined

162.9 **Bronchus and lung, unspecified** I 43, I 44, I 56
C34.90 Malignant neoplasm of bronchus or lung, unspecified, unspecified side

4th 163 **Malignant neoplasm of pleura**

163.0 **Parietal pleura** I 43, I 44

163.1 **Visceral pleura** I 43, I 44

163.8 **Other specified sites of pleura** I 43, I 44
Malignant neoplasm of contiguous or overlapping sites of pleura whose point of origin cannot be determined

163.9 **Pleura, unspecified** I 43, I 44

4th 164 **Malignant neoplasm of thymus, heart, and mediastinum**

164.0 **Thymus** I 43, I 44
Excludes *benign carcinoid tumor of the thymus (209.62)*
malignant carcinoid tumor of the thymus (209.22)

164.1 **Heart** I 43, I 44
Endocardium
Epicardium
Myocardium
Pericardium
Excludes *great vessels (171.4)*

164.2 **Anterior mediastinum** I 43, I 44

164.3 **Posterior mediastinum** I 43, I 44

164.8 **Other** I 43, I 44
Malignant neoplasm of contiguous or overlapping sites of thymus, heart, and mediastinum whose point of origin cannot be determined

164.9 **Mediastinum, part unspecified** I 43, I 44

4th 165 **Malignant neoplasm of other and ill-defined sites within the respiratory system and intrathoracic organs**

165.0 **Upper respiratory tract, part unspecified** I 43, I 44

165.8 **Other** I 43, I 44
Malignant neoplasm of respiratory and intrathoracic organs whose point of origin cannot be assigned to any one of the categories 160-164

165.9 **Ill-defined sites within the respiratory system** I 43, I 44
Respiratory tract NOS
Excludes *intrathoracic NOS (195.1)*
thoracic NOS (195.1)

160.5 – 165.9

MALIGNANT NEOPLASM OF BONE, CONNECTIVE TISSUE, SKIN, AND BREAST (170-176)

Excludes *carcinoma in situ:*
breast (233.0)
skin (232.0-232.9)

4th 170 Malignant neoplasm of bone and articular cartilage

Includes cartilage (articular) (joint)
periosteum

Excludes *bone marrow NOS (202.9)*
cartilage:
ear (171.0)
eyelid (171.0)
larynx (161.3)
nose (160.0)
synovia (171.0-171.9)

170.0 Bones of skull and face, except mandible I 43, I 44
Bone:
ethmoid
frontal
malar
nasal
occipital
orbital
parietal
sphenoid
temporal
zygomatic
Maxilla (superior)
Turbinate
Upper jaw bone
Vomer

Excludes *carcinoma, any type except intraosseous or odontogenic:*
jaw bone (lower) (170.1)
maxilla, maxillary (sinus) (160.2)
upper jaw bone (143.0)

170.1 Mandible I 43, I 44
Inferior maxilla
Jaw bone NOS
Lower jaw bone

Excludes *carcinoma, any type except intraosseous or odontogenic:*
jaw bone NOS (143.9)
lower (143.1)
upper jaw bone (170.0)

170.2 Vertebral column, excluding sacrum and coccyx I 43, I 44
Spinal column
Spine
Vertebra

Excludes *sacrum and coccyx (170.6)*

170.3 Ribs, sternum, and clavicle I 43, I 44
Costal cartilage
Costovertebral joint
Xiphoid process

170.4 Scapula and long bones of upper limb I 43, I 44
Acromion
Bones NOS of upper limb
Humerus
Radius
Ulna

170.5 Short bones of upper limb I 43, I 44
Carpal
Cuneiform, wrist
Metacarpal
Navicular, of hand
Phalanges of hand
Pisiform
Scaphoid (of hand)
Semilunar or lunate
Trapezium
Trapezoid
Unciform

170.6 Pelvic bones, sacrum, and coccyx I 43, I 44
Coccygeal vertebra
Ilium
Ischium
Pubic bone
Sacral vertebra

170.7 Long bones of lower limb I 43, I 44
Bones NOS of lower limb
Femur
Fibula
Tibia

170.8 Short bones of lower limb I 43, I 44
Astragalus [talus]
Calcaneus
Cuboid
Cuneiform, ankle
Metatarsal
Navicular (of ankle)
Patella
Phalanges of foot
Tarsal

170.9 Bone and articular cartilage, site unspecified I 43, I 44

4th 171 Malignant neoplasm of connective and other soft tissue

Includes blood vessel
bursa
fascia
fat,
ligament, except uterine
muscle
peripheral, sympathetic, and parasympathetic nerves and ganglia
synovia
tendon (sheath)

Excludes *cartilage (of):*
articular (170.0-170.9)
larynx (161.3)
nose (160.0)
connective tissue:
breast (174.0-175.9)
internal organs – code to malignant neoplasm of the site [e.g., leiomyosarcoma of stomach, 151.9]
heart (164.1)
uterine ligament (183.4)

171.0 Head, face, and neck I 43, I 44
Cartilage of:
ear
eyelid

171.2 Upper limb, including shoulder I 43, I 44
Arm
Finger
Forearm
Hand

171.3 Lower limb, including hip I43, I44
Foot
Leg
Popliteal space
Thigh
Toe

171.4 Thorax I43, I44
Axilla
Diaphragm
Great vessels
Excludes *heart (164.1)*
mediastinum (164.2-164.9)
thymus (164.0)

171.5 Abdomen I43, I44
Abdominal wall
Hypochondrium
Excludes *peritoneum (158.8)*
retroperitoneum (158.0)

171.6 Pelvis I43, I44
Buttock
Groin
Inguinal region
Perineum
Excludes *pelvic peritoneum (158.8)*
retroperitoneum (158.0)
uterine ligament, any (183.3-183.5)

171.7 Trunk, unspecified I43, I44
Back NOS
Flank NOS

171.8 Other specified sites of connective and other soft tissue I43, I44
Malignant neoplasm of contiguous or overlapping sites of connective tissue whose point of origin cannot be determined

171.9 Connective and other soft tissue, site unspecified I43, I44

4th **172 Malignant melanoma of skin**
Includes melanocarcinoma
melanoma in situ of skin
melanoma (skin) NOS
Excludes *skin of genital organs (184.0-184.9, 187.1-187.9)*
sites other than skincode to malignant neoplasm of the site

172.0 Lip I36, I37, I38, I43, I44
Excludes *vermilion border of lip (140.0-140.1, 140.9)*

172.1 Eyelid, including canthus I36, I37, I38, I43, I44

172.2 Ear and external auditory canal I36, I37, I38, I43, I44
Auricle (ear)
Auricular canal, external
External [acoustic] meatus
Pinna

172.3 Other and unspecified parts of face I36, I37, I38, I43, I44
Cheek (external)
Chin
Eyebrow
Forehead
Nose, external
Temple

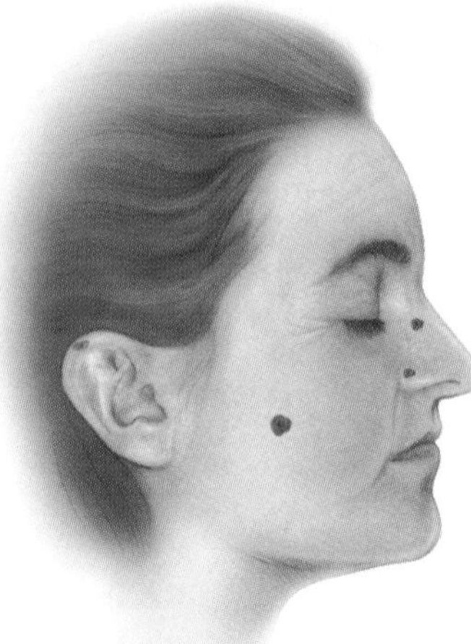

© 2008 Fairman Studios, LLC. All Rights Reserved.

172.4 Scalp and neck I36, I37, I38, I43, I44

172.5 Trunk, except scrotum I36, I37, I38, I43, I44
Axilla
Breast
Buttock
Groin
Perianal skin
Perineum
Umbilicus
Excludes *anal canal (154.2)*
anus NOS (154.3)
scrotum (187.7)

172.6 Upper limb, including shoulder I36, I37, I38, I43, I44
Arm
Finger
Forearm
Hand

172.7 Lower limb, including hip I36, I37, I38, I43, I44
Ankle
Foot
Heel
Knee
Leg
Popliteal area
Thigh
Toe

172.8 Other specified sites of skin I36, I37, I38, I43, I44
Malignant melanoma of contiguous or overlapping sites of skin whose point of origin cannot be determined

172.9 Melanoma of skin, site unspecified I36, I37, I38, I43, I44

4th 173 Other malignant neoplasm of skin

Includes malignant neoplasm of:
sebaceous glands
sudoriferous, sudoriparous glands
sweat glands

Excludes *Kaposi's sarcoma (176.0-176.9)*
malignant melanoma of skin (172.0-172.9)
skin of genital organs (184.0-184.9, 187.1-187.9)

173.0 Skin of lip 143, 144

Excludes *vermilion border of lip (140.0-140.1, 140.9)*

173.1 Eyelid, including canthus 143, 144

Excludes *cartilage of eyelid (171.0)*

173.2 Skin of ear and external auditory canal 143, 144

C44.20 Malignant neoplasm of skin of ear and external auricular canal, unspecified side

Auricle (ear)
Auricular canal, external
External meatus
Pinna

Excludes *cartilage of ear (171.0)*

173.3 Skin of other and unspecified parts of face 143, 144

C44.30 Malignant neoplasm of skin of unspecified part of face
C44.31 Malignant neoplasm of skin of nose
C44.39 Malignant neoplasm of skin of other parts of face

Cheek, external
Chin
Eyebrow
Forehead
Nose, external
Temple

173.4 Scalp and skin of neck 143, 144

C44.4 Malignant neoplasm of skin of scalp and neck

173.5 Skin of trunk, except scrotum 143, 144

C44.59 Malignant neoplasm of other part of trunk

Axillary fold
Perianal skin
Skin of:
abdominal wall
anus
back
breast
buttock
chest wall
groin
perineum
Umbilicus

Excludes *anal canal (154.2)*
anus NOS (154.3)
skin of scrotum (187.7)

173.6 Skin of upper limb, including shoulder 143, 144

C44.60 Malignant neoplasm of skin of upper limb, including shoulder, unspecified side

Arm
Finger
Forearm
Hand

173.7 Skin of lower limb, including hip 143, 144

Ankle
Foot
Heel
Knee
Leg
Popliteal area
Thigh
Toe

173.8 Other specified sites of skin 143, 144

Malignant neoplasm of contiguous or overlapping sites of skin whose point of origin cannot be determined

173.9 Skin, site unspecified 143, 144

C44.9 Malignant neoplasm of skin, unspecified

4th 174 Malignant neoplasm of female breast

Includes breast (female)
connective tissue
soft parts
Paget's disease of:
breast
nipple

Use additional code to identify estrogen receptor status (V86.0, V86.1)

Excludes *skin of breast (172.5, 173.5)*

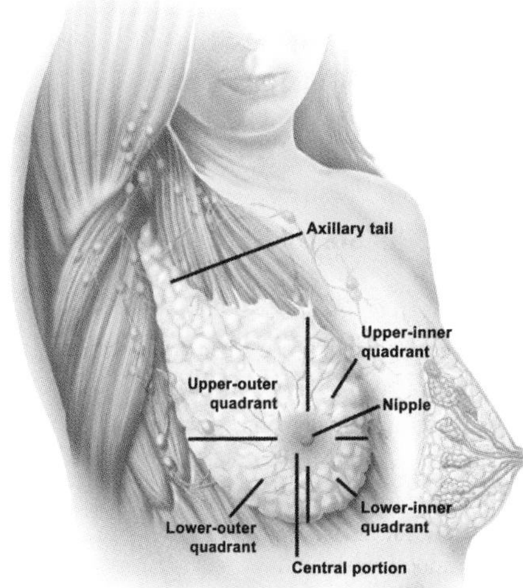

174.0 Nipple and areola ♀ 71, 99, 143, 144

174.1 Central portion ♀ 71, 99, 143, 144

174.2 Upper-inner quadrant ♀ 71, 99, 143, 144

174.3 Lower-inner quadrant ♀ 71, 99, 143, 144

174.4 Upper-outer quadrant ♀ 71, 99, 143, 144

C50.419 Malignant neoplasm of upper-outer quadrant of unspecified female breast

174.5 Lower-outer quadrant ♀ 71, 99, 143, 144

174.6 Axillary tail ♀ 71, 99, 143, 144

174.8 Other specified sites of female breast ♀ 71, 99, 143, 144

C50.819 Malignant neoplasm of overlapping sites of unspecified female breast

Ectopic sites
Inner breast
Lower breast
Midline of breast
Outer breast
Upper breast
Malignant neoplasm of contiguous or overlapping sites of breast whose point of origin cannot be determined

174.9 Breast (female), unspecified ♀ 71, 99, 143, 144

C50.919 Malignant neoplasm of unspecified site of unspecified female breast

4th 175 Malignant neoplasm of male breast

Use additional code to identify estrogen receptor status (V86.0, V86.1)

Excludes *skin of breast (172.5, 173.5)*

175.0 Nipple and areola ♂ 99, 143, 144

175.9 **Other and unspecified sites of male breast** ♂ 99, 143, 144
Ectopic breast tissue, male

4th 176 **Kaposi's sarcoma**
176.0 **Skin** 143, 144
176.1 **Soft tissue** 143, 144
Blood vessel
Connective tissue
Fascia
Ligament
Lymphatic(s) NEC
Muscle
Excludes *lymph glands and nodes (176.5)*
176.2 **Palate** 143, 144
176.3 **Gastrointestinal sites** 143, 144
176.4 **Lung** 143, 144
176.5 **Lymph nodes** 143, 144
176.8 **Other specified sites** 143, 144
Oral cavity NEC
176.9 **Unspecified** 143, 144
Viscera NOS

MALIGNANT NEOPLASM OF GENITOURINARY ORGANS (179-189)

Excludes *carcinoma in situ (233.1-233.9)*

179 **Malignant neoplasm of uterus, part unspecified** ♀ 143, 144

4th 180 **Malignant neoplasm of cervix uteri**
Includes invasive malignancy [carcinoma]
Excludes *carcinoma in situ (233.1)*
180.0 **Endocervix** ♀ 143, 144
Cervical canal NOS
Endocervical canal
Endocervical gland
180.1 **Exocervix** ♀ 143, 144
180.8 **Other specified sites of cervix** ♀ 143, 144
Cervical stump
Squamocolumnar junction of cervix
Malignant neoplasm of contiguous or overlapping sites of cervix uteri whose point of origin cannot be determined
180.9 **Cervix uteri, unspecified** ♀ 143, 144

181 **Malignant neoplasm of placenta** ♀ 143, 144
Choriocarcinoma NOS
Chorioepithelioma NOS
Excludes *chorioadenoma (destruens) (236.1)*
hydatidiform mole (630)
malignant (236.1)
invasive mole (236.1)
male choriocarcinoma NOS (186.0-186.9)

4th 182 **Malignant neoplasm of body of uterus**
Excludes *carcinoma in situ (233.2)*
182.0 **Corpus uteri, except isthmus** ♀ 143, 144
C54.1 Malignant neoplasm of endometrium
C54.2 Malignant neoplasm of myometrium
C54.3 Malignant neoplasm of fundus uteri
C54.9 Malignant neoplasm of corpus uteri, unspecified
Cornu
Endometrium
Fundus
Myometrium
182.1 **Isthmus** ♀ 143, 144
Lower uterine segment
182.8 **Other specified sites of body of uterus** ♀ 143, 144
Malignant neoplasm of contiguous or overlapping sites of body of uterus whose point of origin cannot be determined
Excludes *uterus NOS (179)*

4th 183 **Malignant neoplasm of ovary and other uterine adnexa**
Excludes *Douglas' cul-de-sac (158.8)*
183.0 **Ovary** ♀ 143, 144
C56.9 Malignant neoplasm of ovary, unspecified side
Use additional code to identify any functional activity
183.2 **Fallopian tube** ♀ 143, 144
Oviduct
Uterine tube
183.3 **Broad ligament** ♀ 143, 144
Mesovarium
Parovarian region
183.4 **Parametrium** ♀ 143, 144
Uterine ligament NOS
Uterosacral ligament
183.5 **Round ligament** ♀ 143, 144
183.8 **Other specified sites of uterine adnexa** ♀ 143, 144
Tubo-ovarian
Utero-ovarian
Malignant neoplasm of contiguous or overlapping sites of ovary and other uterine adnexa whose point of origin cannot be determined
183.9 **Uterine adnexa, unspecified** ♀ 143, 144

4th 184 **Malignant neoplasm of other and unspecified female genital organs**
Excludes *carcinoma in situ (233.30-233.39)*
184.0 **Vagina** ♀ 143, 144
Gartner's duct
Vaginal vault
184.1 **Labia majora** ♀ 143, 144
Greater vestibular [Bartholin's] gland
184.2 **Labia minora** ♀ 143, 144
184.3 **Clitoris** ♀ 143, 144
184.4 **Vulva, unspecified** ♀ 143, 144
External female genitalia NOS
Pudendum
184.8 **Other specified sites of female genital organs** ♀ 143, 144
Malignant neoplasm of contiguous or overlapping sites of female genital organs whose point of origin cannot be determined
184.9 **Female genital organ, site unspecified** ♀ 143, 144
Female genitourinary tract NOS

185 **Malignant neoplasm of prostate** ♂ 102, 104, 105, 143, 144
C61 Malignant neoplasm of prostate
Excludes *seminal vesicles (187.8)*

4th 186 **Malignant neoplasm of testis**
Use additional code to identify any functional activity
186.0 **Undescended testis** ♂ 143, 144
Ectopic testis
Retained testis
186.9 **Other and unspecified testis** ♂ 143, 144
Testis:
NOS
descended
scrotal

4th 187 **Malignant neoplasm of penis and other male genital organs**
187.1 **Prepuce** ♂ 143, 144
Foreskin
187.2 **Glans penis** ♂ 143, 144

187.3 **Body of penis** ♂ I 43, I 44
Corpus cavernosum

187.4 **Penis, part unspecified** ♂ I 43, I 44
Skin of penis NOS

187.5 **Epididymis** ♂ I 43, I 44

187.6 **Spermatic cord** ♂ I 43, I 44
Vas deferens

187.7 **Scrotum** ♂ I 43, I 44
Skin of scrotum

187.8 **Other specified sites of male genital organs** ♂ I 43, I 44
Seminal vesicle
Tunica vaginalis
Malignant neoplasm of contiguous or overlapping sites of penis and other male genital organs whose point of origin cannot be determined

187.9 **Male genital organ, site unspecified** ♂ I 43, I 44
Male genital organ or tract NOS

4th 188 **Malignant neoplasm of bladder**
Excludes *carcinoma in situ (233.7)*

188.0 **Trigone of urinary bladder** I 43, I 44

188.1 **Dome of urinary bladder** I 43, I 44

188.2 **Lateral wall of urinary bladder** I 43, I 44

188.3 **Anterior wall of urinary bladder** I 43, I 44

188.4 **Posterior wall of urinary bladder** I 43, I 44

188.5 **Bladder neck** I 43, I 44
Internal urethral orifice

188.6 **Ureteric orifice** I 43, I 44

188.7 **Urachus** I 43, I 44

188.8 **Other specified sites of bladder** I 43, I 44
Malignant neoplasm of contiguous or overlapping sites of bladder whose point of origin cannot be determined

188.9 **Bladder, part unspecified** I 43, I 44
C67.9 Malignant neoplasm of bladder, unspecified
Bladder wall NOS

4th 189 **Malignant neoplasm of kidney and other and unspecified urinary organs**
Excludes *benign carcinoid tumor of kidney (209.64)*
malignant carcinoid tumor of kidney (209.24)

189.0 **Kidney, except pelvis** I 43, I 44
C64.9 Malignant neoplasm of kidney, except renal pelvis, unspecified side
Kidney NOS
Kidney parenchyma

189.1 **Renal pelvis** I 43, I 44
Renal calyces
Ureteropelvic junction

189.2 **Ureter** I 43, I 44
Excludes *ureteric orifice of bladder (188.6)*

189.3 **Urethra** I 43, I 44
Excludes *urethral orifice of bladder (188.5)*

189.4 **Paraurethral glands** I 43, I 44

189.8 **Other specified sites of urinary organs** I 43, I 44
Malignant neoplasm of contiguous or overlapping sites of kidney and other urinary organs whose point of origin cannot be determined

189.9 **Urinary organ, site unspecified** I 43, I 44
Urinary system NOS

MALIGNANT NEOPLASM OF OTHER AND UNSPECIFIED SITES (190-199)

Excludes *carcinoma in situ (234.0-234.9)*

4th 190 **Malignant neoplasm of eye**
Excludes *carcinoma in situ (234.0)*
dark area on retina and choroid (239.81)
eyelid (skin) (172.1, 173.1)
cartilage (171.0)
optic nerve (192.0)
orbital bone (170.0)
retinal freckle (239.81)

190.0 **Eyeball, except conjunctiva, cornea, retina, and choroid** I 43, I 44
Ciliary body
Crystalline lens
Iris
Sclera
Uveal tract

190.1 **Orbit** I 43, I 44
Connective tissue of orbit
Extraocular muscle
Retrobulbar
Excludes *bone of orbit (170.0)*

190.2 **Lacrimal gland** I 43, I 44

190.3 **Conjunctiva** I 43, I 44

190.4 **Cornea** I 43, I 44

190.5 **Retina** I 43, I 44

190.6 **Choroid** I 43, I 44

190.7 **Lacrimal duct** I 43, I 44
Lacrimal sac
Nasolacrimal duct

190.8 **Other specified sites of eye** I 43, I 44
Malignant neoplasm of contiguous or overlapping sites of eye whose point of origin cannot be determined

190.9 **Eye, part unspecified** I 43, I 44

4th 191 **Malignant neoplasm of brain**
Excludes *cranial nerves (192.0)*
retrobulbar area (190.1)

191.0 **Cerebrum, except lobes and ventricles** I 43, I 44
Basal ganglia
Cerebral cortex
Corpus striatum
Globus pallidus
Hypothalamus
Thalamus

191.1 **Frontal lobe** I 43, I 44

191.2 **Temporal lobe** I 43, I 44
Hippocampus
Uncus

191.3 **Parietal lobe** I 43, I 44

191.4 **Occipital lobe** I 43, I 44

191.5 **Ventricles** I 43, I 44
Choroid plexus
Floor of ventricle

191.6 **Cerebellum NOS** I 43, I 44
Cerebellopontine angle

191.7 **Brain stem** I 43, I 44
Cerebral peduncle
Medulla oblongata
Midbrain
Pons

191.8 **Other parts of brain** I 43, I 44
Corpus callosum
Tapetum
Malignant neoplasm of contiguous or overlapping sites of brain whose point of origin cannot be determined

187.3 – 191.8

191.9 Brain, unspecified I 43, I 44
Cranial fossa NOS

4th **192 Malignant neoplasm of other and unspecified parts of nervous system**
Excludes *peripheral, sympathetic, and parasympathetic nerves and ganglia (171.0-171.9)*

192.0 Cranial nerves I 43, I 44
Olfactory bulb

192.1 Cerebral meninges I 43, I 44
Dura (mater)
Falx (cerebelli) (cerebri)
Meninges NOS
Tentorium

192.2 Spinal cord I 43, I 44
Cauda equina

192.3 Spinal meninges I 43, I 44

192.8 Other specified sites of nervous system I 43, I 44
Malignant neoplasm of contiguous or overlapping sites of other parts of nervous system whose point of origin cannot be determined

192.9 Nervous system, part unspecified I 43, I 44
Nervous system (central) NOS
Excludes *meninges NOS (192.1)*

193 Malignant neoplasm of thyroid gland I 43, I 44
Thyroglossal duct
Use additional code to identify any functional activity

4th **194 Malignant neoplasm of other endocrine glands and related structures**
Excludes *islets of Langerhans (157.4)*
neuroendocrine tumors (209.00-209.69)
ovary (183.0)
testis (186.0-186.9)
thymus (164.0)

194.0 Adrenal gland I 43, I 44
Adrenal cortex
Adrenal medulla
Suprarenal gland

194.1 Parathyroid gland I 43, I 44

194.3 Pituitary gland and craniopharyngeal duct I 43, I 44
Craniobuccal pouch
Hypophysis
Rathke's pouch
Sella turcica

194.4 Pineal gland I 43, I 44

194.5 Carotid body I 43, I 44

194.6 Aortic body and other paraganglia I 43, I 44
Coccygeal body
Glomus jugulare
Para-aortic body

194.8 Other I 43, I 44
Pluriglandular involvement NOS
Note: *If the sites of multiple involvements are known, they should be coded separately.*

194.9 Endocrine gland, site unspecified I 43, I 44

4th **195 Malignant neoplasm of other and ill-defined sites**
Includes malignant neoplasms of contiguous sites, not elsewhere classified, whose point of origin cannot be determined
Excludes *malignant neoplasm:*
lymphatic and hematopoietic tissue (200.0-208.9)
secondary sites (196.0-198.8)
unspecified site (199.0-199.1)

195.0 Head, face, and neck I 43, I 44
Cheek NOS
Jaw NOS
Nose NOS
Supraclavicular region NOS

195.1 Thorax I 43, I 44
Axilla
Chest (wall) NOS
Intrathoracic NOS

195.2 Abdomen I 43, I 44
Intra-abdominal NOS

195.3 Pelvis I 43, I 44
Groin
Inguinal region NOS
Presacral region
Sacrococcygeal region
Sites overlapping systems within pelvis, as:
rectovaginal (septum)
rectovesical (septum)

195.4 Upper limb I 43, I 44

195.5 Lower limb I 43, I 44

195.8 Other specified sites I 43, I 44
Back NOS
Flank NOS
Trunk NOS

4th **196 Secondary and unspecified malignant neoplasm of lymph nodes**
Excludes *any malignant neoplasm of lymph nodes, specified as primary (200.0-202.9)*
Hodgkin's disease (201.0-201.9)
lymphosarcoma (200.1)
reticulosarcoma (200.0)
other forms of lymphoma (202.0-202.9)
secondary neuroendocrine tumor of (distant) lymph nodes (209.71)

196.0 Lymph nodes of head, face, and neck I 43, I 44
Cervical
Cervicofacial
Scalene
Supraclavicular

196.1 Intrathoracic lymph nodes I 43, I 44
Bronchopulmonary
Intercostal
Mediastinal
Tracheobronchial

196.2 Intra-abdominal lymph nodes I 43, I 44
Intestinal
Mesenteric
Retroperitoneal

196.3 Lymph nodes of axilla and upper limb I 43, I 44
Brachial
Epitrochlear
Infraclavicular
Pectoral

196.5 Lymph nodes of inguinal region and lower limb I 43, I 44
Femoral
Groin
Popliteal
Tibial

196.6 **Intrapelvic lymph nodes** I 43, I 44
Hypogastric
Iliac
Obturator
Parametrial

196.8 **Lymph nodes of multiple sites** I 43, I 44

196.9 **Site unspecified** I 43, I 44
Lymph nodes NOS

4th 197 **Secondary malignant neoplasm of respiratory and digestive systems**
Excludes *lymph node metastasis (196.0-196.9)*
secondary neuroendocrine tumor of liver (209.72)
secondary neuroendocrine tumor of respiratory organs (209.79)

197.0 **Lung** I 43, I 44
Bronchus

197.1 **Mediastinum** I 43, I 44

197.2 **Pleura** I 43, I 44

197.3 **Other respiratory organs** I 43, I 44
Trachea

197.4 **Small intestine, including duodenum** I 43, I 44

197.5 **Large intestine and rectum** I 43, I 44

197.6 **Retroperitoneum and peritoneum** I 43, I 44

197.7 **Liver, specified as secondary** I 43, I 44

197.8 **Other digestive organs and spleen** I 43, I 44

4th 198 **Secondary malignant neoplasm of other specified sites**
Excludes *lymph node metastasis (196.0-196.9)*
secondary neuroendocrine tumor of other specified sites (209.79)

198.0 **Kidney** I 43, I 44

198.1 **Other urinary organs** I 43, I 44

198.2 **Skin** I 43, I 44
Skin of breast

198.3 **Brain and spinal cord** I 43, I 44

198.4 **Other parts of nervous system** I 43, I 44
Meninges (cerebral) (spinal)

198.5 **Bone and bone marrow** I 43, I 44
C79.51 Secondary malignant neoplasm of bone
C79.52 Secondary malignant neoplasm of bone marrow

198.6 **Ovary** ♀ I 43, I 44

198.7 **Adrenal gland** I 43, I 44
Suprarenal gland

5th 198.8 **Other specified sites**

198.81 **Breast** I 43, I 44
Excludes *skin of breast (198.2)*

198.82 **Genital organs** I 43, I 44

198.89 **Other** I 43, I 44
Excludes *retroperitoneal lymph nodes (196.2)*

4th 199 **Malignant neoplasm without specification of site**
Excludes *malignant carcinoid tumor of unknown primary site (209.20)*
malignant (poorly differentiated) neuroendocrine carcinoma, any site (209.30)
malignant (poorly differentiated) neuroendocrine tumor, any site (209.30)
neuroendocrine carcinoma (high grade), any site (209.30)

199.0 **Disseminated** I 43, I 44
Carcinomatosis unspecified site (primary) (secondary)
Generalized:
cancer unspecified site (primary) (secondary)
malignancy unspecified site (primary) (secondary)
Multiple cancer unspecified site (primary) (secondary)

199.1 **Other** I 43, I 44
C80.1 Malignant neoplasm, unspecified
Cancer unspecified site (primary) (secondary)
Carcinoma unspecified site (primary) (secondary)
Malignancy unspecified site (primary) (secondary)

ICD-9-CM Official Guidelines (Chapter 2)

i. ***Malignant neoplasm associated with transplanted organ***
A malignant neoplasm of a transplanted organ should be coded as a transplant complication. Assign first the appropriate code from subcategory 996.8, Complications of transplanted organ, followed by code 199.2, Malignant neoplasm associated with transplanted organ. Use an additional code for the specific malignancy.

199.2 **Malignant neoplasm associated with transplanted organ** I 43, I 44
Code first complication of transplanted organ (996.80-996.89)
Use additional code for specific malignancy ~~site~~

MALIGNANT NEOPLASM OF LYMPHATIC AND HEMATOPOIETIC TISSUE (200-208)

Excludes *autoimmune lymphoproliferative syndrome (279.41)*
secondary neoplasm of:
bone marrow (198.5)
spleen (197.8)
secondary and unspecified neoplasm of lymph nodes (196.0-196.9)

The following fifth-digit subclassification is for use with categories 200-202:

0 unspecified site, extranodal and solid organ sites
1 lymph nodes of head, face, and neck
2 intrathoracic lymph nodes
3 intra-abdominal lymph nodes
4 lymph nodes of axilla and upper limb
5 lymph nodes of inguinal region and lower limb
6 intrapelvic lymph nodes
7 spleen
8 lymph nodes of multiple sites

4th 200 **Lymphosarcoma and reticulosarcoma and other specified malignant tumors of lymphatic tissue**
Requires fifth digit. See note before section 200 for codes and definitions.

5th 200.0 **Reticulosarcoma** I 43, I 44
[0-8] Lymphoma (malignant):
histiocytic (diffuse):
nodular
pleomorphic cell type
reticulum cell type
Reticulum cell sarcoma:
NOS
pleomorphic cell type

5th 200.1 **Lymphosarcoma** I 43, I 44
[0-8] Lymphoblastoma (diffuse)
Lymphoma (malignant):
lymphoblastic (diffuse)
lymphocytic (cell type) (diffuse)
lymphosarcoma type
Lymphosarcoma:
NOS
diffuse NOS
lymphoblastic (diffuse)
lymphocytic (diffuse)
prolymphocytic
Excludes *lymphosarcoma:*
follicular or nodular (202.0)
mixed cell type (200.8)
lymphosarcoma cell leukemia (207.8)

5th **200.2 Burkitt's tumor or lymphoma** I43, I44
[0-8] Malignant lymphoma, Burkitt's type

5th **200.3 Marginal zone lymphoma** I43, I44
[0-8] Extranodal marginal zone B-cell lymphoma
Mucosa associated lymphoid tissue [MALT]
Nodal marginal zone B-cell lymphoma
Splenic marginal zone B-cell lymphoma

5th **200.4 Mantle cell lymphoma** I43, I44
[0-8]

5th **200.5 Primary central nervous system lymphoma** I43, I44
[0-8]

5th **200.6 Anaplastic large cell lymphoma** I43, I44
[0-8]

5th **200.7 Large cell lymphoma** I43, I44
[0-8]

5th **200.8 Other named variants** I43, I44
[0-8] Lymphoma (malignant):
lymphoplasmacytoid type
mixed lymphocytic-histiocytic (diffuse)
Lymphosarcoma, mixed cell type (diffuse)
Reticulolymphosarcoma (diffuse)

4th **201 Hodgkin's disease**

Requires fifth digit. See Note before section 200 for codes and definitions.

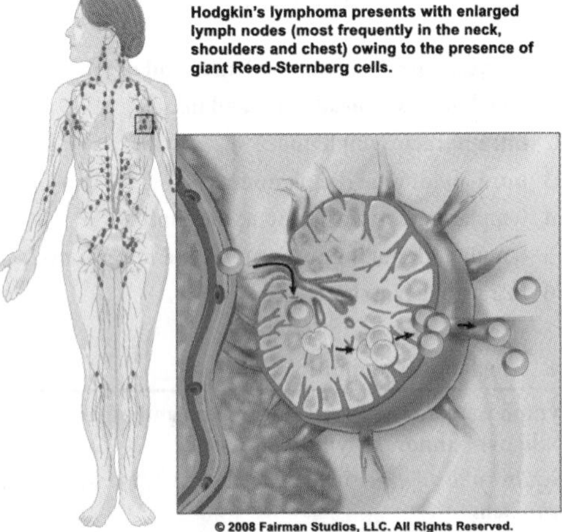

5th **201.0 Hodgkin's paragranuloma** I43, I44
[0-8]

5th **201.1 Hodgkin's granuloma** I43, I44
[0-8]

5th **201.2 Hodgkin's sarcoma** I43, I44
[0-8]

5th **201.4 Lymphocytic-histiocytic predominance** I43, I44
[0-8]

5th **201.5 Nodular sclerosis** I43, I44
[0-8] Hodgkin's disease, nodular sclerosis:
NOS
cellular phase

5th **201.6 Mixed cellularity** I43, I44
[0-8]

5th **201.7 Lymphocytic depletion** I43, I44
[0-8] Hodgkin's disease, lymphocytic depletion:
NOS
diffuse fibrosis
reticular type

5th **201.9 Hodgkin's disease, unspecified** I43, I44
[0-8] Hodgkin's:
disease NOS
lymphoma NOS
Malignant:
lymphogranuloma
lymphogranulomatosis

4th **202 Other malignant neoplasms of lymphoid and histiocytic tissue**

Requires fifth digit. See note before section 200 for codes and definitions.

5th **202.0 Nodular lymphoma** I43, I44
[0-8] Brill-Symmers disease
Lymphoma:
follicular (giant) (large cell)
lymphocytic, nodular
Lymphosarcoma:
follicular (giant)
nodular

5th **202.1 Mycosis fungoides** I43, I44
[0-8]

Excludes *peripheral T-cell lymphoma (202.7)*

5th **202.2 Sézary's disease** I43, I44
[0-8]

5th **202.3 Malignant histiocytosis** I43, I44
[0-8] Histiocytic medullary reticulosis
Malignant:
reticuloendotheliosis
reticulosis

5th **202.4 Leukemic reticuloendotheliosis** I43, I44
[0-8] Hairy-cell leukemia

5th **202.5 Letterer-Siwe disease** I43, I44
[0-8] Acute:
differentiated progressive histiocytosis
histiocytosis X (progressive)
infantile reticuloendotheliosis
reticulosis of infancy

Excludes *Hand-Schüller-Christian disease (277.89)*
histiocytosis (acute) (chronic) (277.89)
histiocytosis X (chronic) (277.89)

5th **202.6 Malignant mast cell tumors** I43, I44
[0-8] Malignant:
mastocytoma
mastocytosis
Mast cell sarcoma
Systemic tissue mast cell disease

Excludes *mast cell leukemia (207.8)*

5th **202.7 Peripheral T-cell lymphoma** I43, I44
[0-8]

5th **202.8 Other lymphomas** I43, I44
[0-8] Lymphoma (malignant):
NOS
diffuse

Excludes *benign lymphoma (229.0)*

5th **202.9 Other and unspecified malignant neoplasms of lymphoid and histiocytic tissue** I43, I44
[0-8] Follicular dendritic cell sarcoma
Interdigitating dendritic cell sarcoma
Langerhans cell sarcoma
Malignant neoplasm of bone marrow NOS

4th 203 **Multiple myeloma and immunoproliferative neoplasms**

The following fifth-digit subclassification is for use with category 203:

0 **without mention of having achieved remission**
failed remission

1 **in remission**

2 **in relapse**

5th 203.0 **Multiple myeloma** 69, I 43, I 44
[0-2]
69 is only valid for 5th digits "0" and "2"
Kahler's disease
Myelomatosis
Excludes *solitary myeloma (238.6)*

5th 203.1 **Plasma cell leukemia** I 43, I 44
[0-2] Plasmacytic leukemia

5th 203.8 **Other immunoproliferative neoplasms** I 43, I 44
[0-2]

4th 204 **Lymphoid leukemia**

Includes leukemia:
lymphatic
lymphoblastic
lymphocytic
lymphogenous

The following fifth-digit subclassification is for use with category 204:

0 **without mention of having achieved remission**
failed remission

1 **in remission**

2 **in relapse**

5th 204.0 **Acute** 67, I 43, I 44
[0-2]
67 is only valid for 5th digits "0" and "2"
Excludes *acute exacerbation of chronic lymphoid leukemia (204.1)*

5th 204.1 **Chronic** 70, I 43, I 44
[0-2]
70 is only valid for 5th digits "0" and "2"

5th 204.2 **Subacute** I 43, I 44
[0-2]

5th 204.8 **Other lymphoid leukemia** I 43, I 44
[0-2] Aleukemic leukemia:
lymphatic
lymphocytic
lymphoid

5th 204.9 **Unspecified lymphoid leukemia** I 43, I 44
[0-2]

4th 205 **Myeloid leukemia**

Includes leukemia:
granulocytic
myeloblastic
myelocytic
myelogenous
myelomonocytic
myelosclerotic
myelosis

The following fifth-digit subclassification is for use with category 205:

0 **without mention of having achieved remission**
failed remission

1 **in remission**

2 **in relapse**

5th 205.0 **Acute** 67, I 43, I 44
[0-2]
67 is only valid for 5th digits "0" and "2"
Acute promyelocytic leukemia
Excludes *acute exacerbation of chronic myeloid leukemia (205.1)*

5th 205.1 **Chronic** I 43, I 44
[0-2] Eosinophilic leukemia
Neutrophilic leukemia

5th 205.2 **Subacute** I 43, I 44
[0-2]

5th 205.3 **Myeloid sarcoma** I 43, I 44
[0-2] Chloroma
Granulocytic sarcoma

5th 205.8 **Other myeloid leukemia** I 43, I 44
[0-2] Aleukemic leukemia:
granulocytic
myelogenous
myeloid
Aleukemic myelosis

5th 205.9 **Unspecified myeloid leukemia** I 43, I 44
[0-2]

4th 206 **Monocytic leukemia**

Includes leukemia:
histiocytic
monoblastic
monocytoid

The following fifth-digit subclassification is for use with category 206:

0 **without mention of having achieved remission**
failed remission

1 **in remission**

2 **in relapse**

5th 206.0 **Acute** 67, I 43, I 44
[0-2]
67 is only valid for 5th digits "0" and "2"
Excludes *acute exacerbation of chronic monocytic leukemia (206.1)*

5th 206.1 **Chronic** I 43, I 44
[0-2]

5th 206.2 **Subacute** I 43, I 44
[0-2]

5th 206.8 **Other monocytic leukemia** I 43, I 44
[0-2] Aleukemic:
monocytic leukemia
monocytoid leukemia

5th 206.9 **Unspecified monocytic leukemia** I 43, I 44
[0-2]

4th 207 **Other specified leukemia**

Excludes *leukemic reticuloendotheliosis (202.4)*
plasma cell leukemia (203.1)

The following fifth-digit subclassification is for use with category 207:

0 **without mention of having achieved remission**
failed remission

1 **in remission**

2 **in relapse**

5th 207.0 **Acute erythremia and erythroleukemia** 67, I 43, I 44
[0-2]
67 is only valid for 5th digits "0" and "2"
Acute erythremic myelosis
Di Guglielmo's disease
Erythremic myelosis

5th 207.1 **Chronic erythremia** I 43, I 44
[0-2] Heilmeyer-Schöner disease

5th 207.2 **Megakaryocytic leukemia** 67, I 43, I 44
[0-2]
67 is only valid for 5th digits "0" and "2"
Megakaryocytic myelosis
Thrombocytic leukemia

5th 207.8 **Other specified leukemia** I 43, I 44
[0-2] Lymphosarcoma cell leukemia

203 – 207.8

4th 208 **Leukemia of unspecified cell type**

The following fifth-digit subclassification is for use with category 208:

0 **without mention of having achieved remission**
failed remission

1 **in remission**

2 **in relapse**

5th 208.0 **Acute** 67, 143, 144
[0-2]
67 is only valid for 5th digits "0" and "2"
Acute leukemia NOS
Blast cell leukemia
Stem cell leukemia
Excludes *acute exacerbation of chronic unspecified leukemia (208.1)*

5th 208.1 **Chronic** 143, 144
[0-2] Chronic leukemia NOS

5th 208.2 **Subacute** 143, 144
[0-2] Subacute leukemia NOS

5th 208.8 **Other leukemia of unspecified cell type** 143, 144
[0-2]

5th 208.9 **Unspecified leukemia** 143, 144
[0-2] Leukemia NOS

NEUROENDOCRINE TUMORS (209)

4th 209 **Neuroendocrine tumors**

Use additional code to identify associated endocrine syndrome, such as:
carcinoid syndrome (259.2)

Code first any associated multiple endocrine neoplasia syndrome (258.01-258.03)

Excludes benign pancreatic islet cell tumors (211.7)
malignant pancreatic islet cell tumors (157.4)

5th 209.0 **Malignant carcinoid tumors of the small intestine**

209.00 **Malignant carcinoid tumor of the small intestine, unspecified portion** 143, 144

209.01 **Malignant carcinoid tumor of the duodenum** 143, 144

209.02 **Malignant carcinoid tumor of the jejunum** 143, 144

209.03 **Malignant carcinoid tumor of the ileum** 143, 144

5th 209.1 **Malignant carcinoid tumors of the appendix, large intestine, and rectum**

209.10 **Malignant carcinoid tumor of the large intestine, unspecified portion** 143, 144
Malignant carcinoid tumor of the colon NOS

209.11 **Malignant carcinoid tumor of the appendix** 143, 144

209.12 **Malignant carcinoid tumor of the cecum** 143, 144

209.13 **Malignant carcinoid tumor of the ascending colon** 143, 144

209.14 **Malignant carcinoid tumor of the transverse colon** 143, 144

209.15 **Malignant carcinoid tumor of the descending colon** 143, 144

209.16 **Malignant carcinoid tumor of the sigmoid colon** 143, 144

209.17 **Malignant carcinoid tumor of the rectum** 143, 144

5th 209.2 **Malignant carcinoid tumors of other and unspecified sites**

209.20 **Malignant carcinoid tumor of unknown primary site** 143, 144

209.21 **Malignant carcinoid tumor of the bronchus and lung** 143, 144

209.22 **Malignant carcinoid tumor of the thymus** 143, 144

209.23 **Malignant carcinoid tumor of the stomach** 143, 144

209.24 **Malignant carcinoid tumor of the kidney** 143, 144

209.25 **Malignant carcinoid tumor of the foregut NOS** 143, 144

209.26 **Malignant carcinoid tumor of the midgut NOS** 143, 144

209.27 **Malignant carcinoid tumor of the hindgut NOS** 143, 144

209.29 **Malignant carcinoid tumors of other sites** 143, 144

5th 209.3 **Malignant poorly differentiated neuroendocrine tumors**

209.30 **Malignant poorly differentiated neuroendocrine carcinoma, any site** 143, 144
High grade neuroendocrine carcinoma, any site
Malignant poorly differentiated neuroendocrine tumor NOS

Excludes Merkel cell carcinoma (209.31-209.36)

Rationale: *Merkel cell carcinoma is an aggressive neuroendocrine skin cancer with a rising incidence. In the United States there are about 1,500 new cases per year, approximating cutaneous T-cell lymphoma. This lethal cancer of the skin has a 33% disease specific mortality which is much higher than that of melanoma (~15%) making it the most common cause of non-melanoma skin cancer death in the United States. The incidence of Merkel cell carcinoma has more than tripled in the past 20 years. Both melanoma and cutaneous T-cell lymphoma (CTCL/mycosis fungoides) have their own ICD-9-CM codes.*

Previously the index directed the coder to code Merkel cell carcinoma to malignant neoplasm, by site which for the skin is category 173, "Other malignant neoplasm of the skin." This category is also used for far more common skin tumors such as basal and squamous cell carcinoma. This made it difficult for Merkel cell carcinoma patients to be tracked and receive appropriate medical care needed for this more aggressive cancer.

● 209.31 **Merkel cell carcinoma of the face**
Merkel cell carcinoma of the ear
Merkel cell carcinoma of the eyelid, including canthus
Merkel cell carcinoma of the lip

● 209.32 **Merkel cell carcinoma of the scalp and neck**

● 209.33 **Merkel cell carcinoma of the upper limb**

● 209.34 **Merkel cell carcinoma of the lower limb**

● 209.35 **Merkel cell carcinoma of the trunk**

● 209.36 **Merkel cell carcinoma of other sites**
Merkel cell carcinoma of the buttock
Merkel cell carcinoma of the genitals
Merkel cell carcinoma NOS

5th 209.4 **Benign carcinoid tumors of the small intestine**

209.40 **Benign carcinoid tumor of the small intestine, unspecified portion**

209.41 **Benign carcinoid tumor of the duodenum**

209.42 **Benign carcinoid tumor of the jejunum**

209.43 **Benign carcinoid tumor of the ileum**

5th 209.5 **Benign carcinoid tumors of the appendix, large intestine, and rectum**

209.50 **Benign carcinoid tumor of the large intestine, unspecified portion**
Benign carcinoid tumor of the colon NOS

209.51 **Benign carcinoid tumor of the appendix**

209.52 **Benign carcinoid tumor of the cecum**

209.53 **Benign carcinoid tumor of the ascending colon**

209.54 **Benign carcinoid tumor of the transverse colon**

209.55 **Benign carcinoid tumor of the descending colon**

209.56 **Benign carcinoid tumor of the sigmoid colon**

209.57 **Benign carcinoid tumor of the rectum**

5th 209.6 **Benign carcinoid tumors of other and unspecified sites**

209.60 **Benign carcinoid tumor of unknown primary site**
Carcinoid tumor NOS
Neuroendocrine tumor NOS

209.61 **Benign carcinoid tumor of the bronchus and lung**

209.62 **Benign carcinoid tumor of the thymus**

209.63 **Benign carcinoid tumor of the stomach**

209.64 **Benign carcinoid tumor of the kidney**

209.65 **Benign carcinoid tumor of the foregut NOS**

209.66 **Benign carcinoid tumor of the midgut NOS**

209.67 **Benign carcinoid tumor of the hindgut NOS**

209.69 **Benign carcinoid tumors of other sites**

● 5th 209.7 **Secondary neuroendocrine tumors**
Secondary carcinoid tumors

Rationale: *On October 1, 2008 category 209, "Neuroendocrine tumors," became effective. This category includes codes for primary neuroendocrine tumors. The facility that requested the category asked that additional codes be created for secondary neuroendocrine tumors and personal history of neuroendocrine tumors to fully classify these types of neoplasms.*

This additional subcategory under 209 was created for the secondary sites, and a new code V10.91, "Personal history of malignant neuroendocrine tumor," was also created. The use of these codes follows the same guidelines as for all malignant neoplasms.

● 209.70 **Secondary neuroendocrine tumor, unspecified site**

● 209.71 **Secondary neuroendocrine tumor of distant lymph nodes**
Mesentery metastasis of neuroendocrine tumor

● 209.72 **Secondary neuroendocrine tumor of liver**

● 209.73 **Secondary neuroendocrine tumor of bone**

● 209.74 **Secondary neuroendocrine tumor of peritoneum**

● 209.75 **Secondary Merkel cell carcinoma**
Merkel cell carcinoma nodal presentation
Merkel cell carcinoma visceral metastatic presentation
Secondary Merkel cell carcinoma, any site

● 209.79 **Secondary neuroendocrine tumor of other sites**

BENIGN NEOPLASMS (210-229)

4th 210 **Benign neoplasm of lip, oral cavity, and pharynx**

Excludes *cyst (of):*
jaw (526.0-526.2, 526.89)
oral soft tissue (528.4)
radicular (522.8)

210.0 **Lip**
Frenulum labii
Lip (inner aspect) (mucosa) (vermilion border)

Excludes *labial commissure (210.4)*
skin of lip (216.0)

210.1 **Tongue**
Lingual tonsil

210.2 **Major salivary glands**
Gland:
parotid
sublingual
submandibular

Excludes *benign neoplasms of minor salivary glands:*
NOS (210.4)
buccal mucosa (210.4)
lips (210.0)
palate (hard) (soft) (210.4)
tongue (210.1)
tonsil, palatine (210.5)

210.3 **Floor of mouth**

210.4 **Other and unspecified parts of mouth**
Gingiva
Gum (upper) (lower)
Labial commissure
Oral cavity NOS
Oral mucosa
Palate (hard) (soft)
Uvula

Excludes *benign odontogenic neoplasms of bone (213.0-213.1)*
developmental odontogenic cysts (526.0)
mucosa of lips (210.0)
nasopharyngeal [posterior] [superior] surface of soft palate (210.7)

210.5 **Tonsil**
Tonsil (faucial) (palatine)

Excludes *lingual tonsil (210.1)*
pharyngeal tonsil (210.7)
tonsillar:
fossa (210.6)
pillars (210.6)

210.6 **Other parts of oropharynx**
Branchial cleft or vestiges
Epiglottis, anterior aspect
Fauces NOS
Mesopharynx NOS
Tonsillar:
fossa
pillars
Vallecula

Excludes *epiglottis:*
NOS (212.1)
suprahyoid portion (212.1)

210.7 **Nasopharynx**
Adenoid tissue
Lymphadenoid tissue
Pharyngeal tonsil
Posterior nasal septum

210.8 **Hypopharynx**
Arytenoid fold
Laryngopharynx
Postcricoid region
Pyriform fossa

210.9 **Pharynx, unspecified**
Throat NOS

209.52 – 210.9

4th 211 Benign neoplasm of other parts of digestive system

Excludes *benign stromal tumors of digestive system (215.5)*

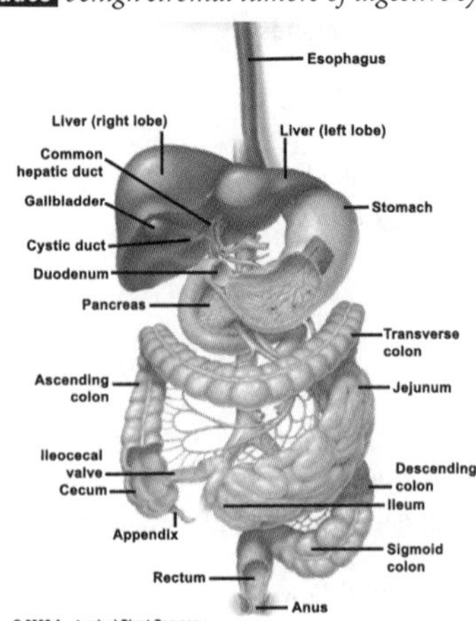

211.0 Esophagus

211.1 Stomach
Body of stomach
Cardiac orifice
Cardia of stomach
Fundus of stomach
Pylorus
Excludes *benign carcinoid tumors of the stomach (209.63)*

211.2 Duodenum, jejunum, and ileum
Small intestine NOS
Excludes *ampulla of Vater (211.5)*
benign carcinoid tumors of the small intestine (209.40-209.43)
ileocecal valve (211.3)

211.3 Colon
D12.0 Benign neoplasm of cecum
D12.1 Benign neoplasm of appendix
D12.6 Benign neoplasm of colon, unspecified
Appendix
Cecum
Ileocecal valve
Large intestine NOS
Excludes *benign carcinoid tumors of the large intestine (209.50-209.56)*
rectosigmoid junction (211.4)

211.4 Rectum and anal canal
Anal canal or sphincter
Anus NOS
Rectosigmoid junction
Excludes *anus:*
margin (216.5)
skin (216.5)
perianal skin (216.5)
benign carcinoid tumors of the rectum (209.57)

211.5 Liver and biliary passages
Ampulla of Vater
Common bile duct
Cystic duct
Gallbladder
Hepatic duct
Sphincter of Oddi

211.6 Pancreas, except islets of Langerhans

211.7 Islets of Langerhans
Islet cell tumor
Use additional code to identify any functional activity

211.8 Retroperitoneum and peritoneum
Mesentery
Mesocolon
Omentum
Retroperitoneal tissue

211.9 Other and unspecified site
Alimentary tract NOS
Digestive system NOS
Gastrointestinal tract NOS
Intestinal tract NOS
Intestine NOS
Spleen, not elsewhere classified

4th 212 Benign neoplasm of respiratory and intrathoracic organs

212.0 Nasal cavities, middle ear, and accessory sinuses
Cartilage of nose
Eustachian tube
Nares
Septum of nose
Sinus:
ethmoidal
frontal
maxillary
sphenoidal
Excludes *auditory canal (external) (216.2)*
bone of:
ear (213.0)
nose [turbinates] (213.0)
cartilage of ear (215.0)
ear (external) (skin) (216.2)
nose NOS (229.8)
skin (216.3)
olfactory bulb (225.1)
polyp of:
accessory sinus (471.8)
ear (385.30-385.35)
nasal cavity (471.0)
posterior margin of septum and choanae (210.7)

212.1 Larynx
Cartilage:
arytenoid
cricoid
cuneiform
thyroid
Epiglottis (suprahyoid portion) NOS
Glottis
Vocal cords (false) (true)
Excludes *epiglottis, anterior aspect (210.6)*
polyp of vocal cord or larynx (478.4)

212.2 Trachea

212.3 Bronchus and lung
Carina
Hilus of lung
Excludes *benign carcinoid tumors of bronchus and lung (209.61)*

212.4 Pleura

212.5 Mediastinum

212.6 Thymus
Excludes *benign carcinoid tumors of thymus (209.62)*

212.7 Heart
Excludes *great vessels (215.4)*

212.8 Other specified sites

212.9 Site unspecified
Respiratory organ NOS
Upper respiratory tract NOS
Excludes *intrathoracic NOS (229.8)*
thoracic NOS (229.8)

4th 213 Benign neoplasm of bone and articular cartilage

Includes cartilage (articular) (joint)
periosteum

Excludes *cartilage of:*
ear (215.0)
eyelid (215.0)
larynx (212.1)
nose (212.0)
exostosis NOS (726.91)
synovia (215.0-215.9)

213.0 Bones of skull and face

Excludes *lower jaw bone (213.1)*

213.1 Lower jaw bone

213.2 Vertebral column, excluding sacrum and coccyx

213.3 Ribs, sternum, and clavicle

213.4 Scapula and long bones of upper limb

213.5 Short bones of upper limb

213.6 Pelvic bones, sacrum, and coccyx

213.7 Long bones of lower limb

213.8 Short bones of lower limb

213.9 Bone and articular cartilage, site unspecified

4th 214 Lipoma

Includes angiolipoma
fibrolipoma
hibernoma
lipoma (fetal) (infiltrating) (intramuscular)
myelolipoma
myxolipoma

214.0 Skin and subcutaneous tissue of face

214.1 Other skin and subcutaneous tissue

214.2 Intrathoracic organs

214.3 Intra-abdominal organs

214.4 Spermatic cord ♂

214.8 Other specified sites

214.9 Lipoma, unspecified site

4th 215 Other benign neoplasm of connective and other soft tissue

Includes blood vessel
bursa
fascia
ligament
muscle
peripheral, sympathetic, and parasympathetic nerves and ganglia
synovia tendon (sheath)

Excludes *cartilage:*
articular (213.0-213.9)
larynx (212.1)
nose (212.0)
connective tissue of:
breast (217)
internal organ, except lipoma and hemangioma – code to benign neoplasm of the site
lipoma (214.0-214.9)

215.0 Head, face, and neck

215.2 Upper limb, including shoulder

215.3 Lower limb, including hip

215.4 Thorax

Excludes *heart (212.7)*
mediastinum (212.5)
thymus (212.6)

215.5 Abdomen

Abdominal wall
Benign stromal tumors of abdomen
Hypochondrium

215.6 Pelvis

Buttock
Groin
Inguinal region
Perineum

Excludes *uterine:*
leiomyoma (218.0-218.9)
ligament, any (221.0)

215.7 Trunk, unspecified

Back NOS
Flank NOS

215.8 Other specified sites

215.9 Site unspecified

4th 216 Benign neoplasm of skin

Includes blue nevus
dermatofibroma
hydrocystoma
pigmented nevus
syringoadenoma
syringoma

Excludes *skin of genital organs (221.0-222.9)*

216.0 Skin of lip

Excludes *vermilion border of lip (210.0)*

216.1 Eyelid, including canthus

Excludes *cartilage of eyelid (215.0)*

216.2 Ear and external auditory canal

Auricle (ear)
Auricular canal, external
External meatus
Pinna

Excludes *cartilage of ear (215.0)*

216.3 Skin of other and unspecified parts of face

D23.30 Other benign neoplasm of skin of unspecified part of face

D23.39 Other benign neoplasm of skin of other parts of face

Cheek, external
Eyebrow
Nose, external
Temple

216.4 Scalp and skin of neck

216.5 Skin of trunk, except scrotum

D23.5 Other benign neoplasm of skin of trunk

Axillary fold
Perianal skin
Skin of:
abdominal wall
anus
back
breast
buttock
chest wall
groin
perineum
Umbilicus

Excludes *anal canal (211.4)*
anus NOS (211.4)
skin of scrotum (222.4)

216.6 Skin of upper limb, including shoulder

216.7 Skin of lower limb, including hip

216.8 Other specified sites of skin

216.9 Skin, site unspecified

213 – 216.9

217 Benign neoplasm of breast
Breast (male) (female):
connective tissue
glandular tissue
soft parts
Excludes *adenofibrosis (610.2)*
benign cyst of breast (610.0)
fibrocystic disease (610.1)
skin of breast (216.5)

4th **218 Uterine leiomyoma**
Includes fibroid (bleeding) (uterine)
uterine:
fibromyoma
myoma

218.0 Submucous leiomyoma of uterus ♀
218.1 Intramural leiomyoma of uterus ♀
Interstitial leiomyoma of uterus
218.2 Subserous leiomyoma of uterus ♀
Subperitoneal leiomyoma of uterus
218.9 Leiomyoma of uterus, unspecified ♀

4th **219 Other benign neoplasm of uterus**
219.0 Cervix uteri ♀
219.1 Corpus uteri ♀
Endometrium
Fundus
Myometrium
219.8 Other specified parts of uterus ♀
219.9 Uterus, part unspecified ♀

220 Benign neoplasm of ovary ♀
Use additional code to identify any functional activity (256.0-256.1)
Excludes *cyst:*
corpus albicans (620.2)
corpus luteum (620.1)
endometrial (617.1)
follicular (atretic) (620.0)
graafian follicle (620.0)
ovarian NOS (620.2)
retention (620.2)

4th **221 Benign neoplasm of other female genital organs**
Includes adenomatous polyp
benign teratoma
Excludes *cyst:*
epoophoron (752.11)
fimbrial (752.11)
Gartner's duct (752.11)
parovarian (752.11)

221.0 Fallopian tube and uterine ligaments ♀
Oviduct
Parametrium
Uterine ligament (broad) (round) (uterosacral)
Uterine tube
221.1 Vagina ♀
221.2 Vulva ♀
Clitoris
External female genitalia NOS
Greater vestibular [Bartholin's] gland
Labia (majora) (minora)
Pudendum
Excludes *Bartholin's (duct) (gland) cyst (616.2)*
221.8 Other specified sites of female genital organs ♀
221.9 Female genital organ, site unspecified ♀
Female genitourinary tract NOS

4th **222 Benign neoplasm of male genital organs**
222.0 Testis ♂
Use additional code to identify any functional activity
222.1 Penis ♂
Corpus cavernosum
Glans penis
Prepuce
222.2 Prostate ♂
Excludes *adenomatous hyperplasia of prostate (600.20-600.21)*
prostatic:
adenoma (600.20-600.21)
enlargement (600.00-600.01)
hypertrophy (600.00-600.01)
222.3 Epididymis ♂
222.4 Scrotum ♂
Skin of scrotum
222.8 Other specified sites of male genital organs ♂
Seminal vesicle
Spermatic cord
222.9 Male genital organ, site unspecified ♂
Male genitourinary tract NOS

4th **223 Benign neoplasm of kidney and other urinary organs**
223.0 Kidney, except pelvis
Kidney NOS
Excludes *benign carcinoid tumors of kidney (209.64)*
renal:
calyces (223.1)
pelvis (223.1)
223.1 Renal pelvis
223.2 Ureter
Excludes *ureteric orifice of bladder (223.3)*
223.3 Bladder
5th **223.8 Other specified sites of urinary organs**
223.81 Urethra
Excludes *urethral orifice of bladder (223.3)*
223.89 Other
Paraurethral glands
223.9 Urinary organ, site unspecified
Urinary system NOS

4th **224 Benign neoplasm of eye**
Excludes *cartilage of eyelid (215.0)*
eyelid (skin) (216.1)
optic nerve (225.1)
orbital bone (213.0)
224.0 Eyeball, except conjunctiva, cornea, retina, and choroid
Ciliary body
Iris
Sclera
Uveal tract
224.1 Orbit
Excludes *bone of orbit (213.0)*
224.2 Lacrimal gland
224.3 Conjunctiva
224.4 Cornea
224.5 Retina
Excludes *hemangioma of retina (228.03)*
224.6 Choroid
224.7 Lacrimal duct
Lacrimal sac
Nasolacrimal duct
224.8 Other specified parts of eye
224.9 Eye, part unspecified

4th 225 **Benign neoplasm of brain and other parts of nervous system**
Excludes *hemangioma (228.02)*
neurofibromatosis (237.7)
peripheral, sympathetic, and parasympathetic nerves and ganglia (215.0-215.9)
retrobulbar (224.1)

225.0 **Brain**

225.1 **Cranial nerves**

225.2 **Cerebral meninges**
Meninges NOS
Meningioma (cerebral)

225.3 **Spinal cord**
Cauda equina

225.4 **Spinal meninges**
Spinal meningioma

225.8 **Other specified sites of nervous system**

225.9 **Nervous system, part unspecified**
Nervous system (central) NOS
Excludes *meninges NOS (225.2)*

226 **Benign neoplasm of thyroid glands**
Use additional code to identify any functional activity

4th 227 **Benign neoplasm of other endocrine glands and related structures**
Use additional code to identify any functional activity
Excludes *ovary (220)*
pancreas (211.6)
testis (222.0)

227.0 **Adrenal gland**
Suprarenal gland

227.1 **Parathyroid gland**

227.3 **Pituitary gland and craniopharyngeal duct (pouch)**
Craniobuccal pouch
Hypophysis
Rathke's pouch
Sella turcica

227.4 **Pineal gland**
Pineal body

227.5 **Carotid body**

227.6 **Aortic body and other paraganglia**
Coccygeal body
Glomus jugulare
Para-aortic body

227.8 **Other**

227.9 **Endocrine gland, site unspecified**

4th 228 **Hemangioma and lymphangioma, any site**
Includes angioma (benign) (cavernous) (congenital) NOS
cavernous nevus
glomus tumor
hemangioma (benign) (congenital)
Excludes *benign neoplasm of spleen, except hemangioma and lymphangioma (211.9)*
glomus jugulare (227.6)
nevus:
NOS (216.0-216.9)
blue or pigmented (216.0-216.9)
vascular (757.32)

5th 228.0 **Hemangioma, any site**
Layman's: *Hemangiomas are benign tumors of the cells that line the blood vessels. Despite a similar appearance, they are distinct from vascular nevus (port wine stains) in that they generally resolve without intervention prior to the patient reaching puberty. Hemangiomas predominantly occur on the face and neck, rarely develop in adults and are significantly more likely to present in females than males.*

228.00 **Of unspecified site**

228.01 **Of skin and subcutaneous tissue**

228.02 **Of intracranial structures**

228.03 **Of retina**

228.04 **Of intra-abdominal structures**
Peritoneum
Retroperitoneal tissue

228.09 **Of other sites**
Systemic angiomatosis

228.1 **Lymphangioma, any site**
Congenital lymphangioma
Lymphatic nevus

4th 229 **Benign neoplasm of other and unspecified sites**

229.0 **Lymph nodes**
Excludes *lymphangioma (228.1)*

229.8 **Other specified sites**
Intrathoracic NOS
Thoracic NOS

229.9 **Site unspecified**

CARCINOMA IN SITU (230-234)

Includes Bowen's disease
erythroplasia
Queyrat's erythroplasia
Excludes *leukoplakia – see Alphabetic Index*

4th 230 **Carcinoma in situ of digestive organs**

230.0 **Lip, oral cavity, and pharynx**
Gingiva
Hypopharynx
Mouth [any part]
Nasopharynx
Oropharynx
Salivary gland or duct
Tongue
Excludes *aryepiglottic fold or interarytenoid fold, laryngeal aspect (231.0)*
epiglottis:
NOS (231.0)
suprahyoid portion (231.0)
skin of lip (232.0)

230.1 **Esophagus**

230.2 **Stomach**
Body of stomach
Cardiac orifice
Cardia of stomach
Fundus of stomach
Pylorus

230.3 **Colon**
Appendix
Cecum
Ileocecal valve
Large intestine NOS
Excludes *rectosigmoid junction (230.4)*

230.4 **Rectum**
Rectosigmoid junction

230.5 **Anal canal**
Anal sphincter

230.6 **Anus, unspecified**
Excludes *anus:*
margin (232.5)
skin (232.5)
perianal skin (232.5)

230.7 **Other and unspecified parts of intestine**
Duodenum
Ileum
Jejunum
Small intestine NOS
Excludes *ampulla of Vater (230.8)*

230.8 Liver and biliary system
Ampulla of Vater
Common bile duct
Cystic duct
Gallbladder
Hepatic duct
Sphincter of Oddi

230.9 Other and unspecified digestive organs
Digestive organ NOS
Gastrointestinal tract NOS
Pancreas
Spleen

4th 231 Carcinoma in situ of respiratory system

231.0 Larynx
Cartilage:
arytenoid
cricoid
cuneiform
thyroid
Epiglottis:
NOS
posterior surface
suprahyoid portion
Vocal cords (false) (true)

Excludes *aryepiglottic fold or interarytenoid fold:*
NOS (230.0)
hypopharyngeal aspect (230.0)
marginal zone (230.0)

231.1 Trachea

231.2 Bronchus and lung
Carina
Hilus of lung

231.8 Other specified parts of respiratory system
Accessory sinuses
Middle ear
Nasal cavities
Pleura

Excludes *ear (external) (skin) (232.2)*
nose NOS (234.8)
skin (232.3)

231.9 Respiratory system, part unspecified
Respiratory organ NOS

4th 232 Carcinoma in situ of skin

Includes pigment cells

Excludes *melanoma in situ of skin (172.0-172.9)*

232.0 Skin of lip

Excludes *vermilion border of lip (230.0)*

232.1 Eyelid, including canthus

232.2 Ear and external auditory canal

232.3 Skin of other and unspecified parts of face

232.4 Scalp and skin of neck

232.5 Skin of trunk, except scrotum
Anus, margin
Axillary fold
Perianal skin
Skin of:
abdominal wall
anus
back
breast
buttock
chest wall
groin
perineum
Umbilicus

Excludes *anal canal (230.5)*
anus NOS (230.6)
skin of genital organs (233.30-233.39, 233.5-233.6)

232.6 Skin of upper limb, including shoulder

232.7 Skin of lower limb, including hip

232.8 Other specified sites of skin

232.9 Skin, site unspecified

4th 233 Carcinoma in situ of breast and genitourinary system

233.0 Breast

Excludes *Paget's disease (174.0-174.9)*
skin of breast (232.5)

Ductal Carcinoma in Situ (DCIS) | Invasive Ductal Carcinoma (IDC)

© 2006 Anatomical Chart Company

233.1 Cervix uteri ♀
Adenocarcinoma in situ of cervix
Cervical intraepithelial glandular neoplasia, grade III
Cervical intraepithelial neoplasia III [CIN III]
Severe dysplasia of cervix

Excludes *cervical intraepithelial neoplasia II [CIN II] (622.12)*
cytologic evidence of mailgnancy without histologic confirmation(795.06)
high grade squamous intraepithelial lesion (HGSIL) (795.04)
moderate dysplasia of cervix (622.12)

233.2 Other and unspecified parts of uterus ♀

5th 233.3 Other and unspecified female genital organs

233.30 Unspecified female genital organ ♀

233.31 Vagina ♀
Severe dysplasia of vagina
Vaginal intraepithelial neoplasia III [VAIN III]

233.32 Vulva ♀
Severe dysplasia of vulva
Vulvar intraepithelial neoplasia III [VAIN III]

233.39 Other female genital organ ♀

233.4 Prostate ♂

233.5 Penis ♂

233.6 Other and unspecified male genital organs ♂

233.7 Bladder

233.9 Other and unspecified urinary organs

4th 234 Carcinoma in situ of other and unspecified sites

234.0 Eye

Excludes *cartilage of eyelid (234.8)*
eyelid (skin) (232.1)
optic nerve (234.8)
orbital bone (234.8)

234.8 Other specified sites
Endocrine gland [any]

234.9 Site unspecified
Carcinoma in situ NOS

NEOPLASMS OF UNCERTAIN BEHAVIOR (235-238)

Note: *Categories 235-238 classify by site certain histo-morphologically well-defined neoplasms, the subsequent behavior of which cannot be predicted from the present appearance.*

4th **235 Neoplasm of uncertain behavior of digestive and respiratory systems**

Excludes *stromal tumors of uncertain behavior of digestive system (238.1)*

235.0 Major salivary glands I43, I44

Gland:
- parotid
- sublingual
- submandibular

Excludes *minor salivary glands (235.1)*

235.1 Lip, oral cavity, and pharynx I43, I44

Gingiva
Hypopharynx
Minor salivary glands
Mouth
Nasopharynx
Oropharynx
Tongue

Excludes *aryepiglottic fold or interarytenoid fold, laryngeal aspect (235.6)*
epiglottis:
NOS (235.6)
suprahyoid portion (235.6)
skin of lip (238.2)

235.2 Stomach, intestines, and rectum I43, I44

235.3 Liver and biliary passages I43, I44

Ampulla of Vater
Bile ducts [any]
Gallbladder
Liver

235.4 Retroperitoneum and peritoneum I43, I44

235.5 Other and unspecified digestive organs I43, I44

Anal:
- canal
- sphincter

Anus NOS
Esophagus
Pancreas
Spleen

Excludes *anus:*
margin (238.2)
skin (238.2)
perianal skin (238.2)

235.6 Larynx I43, I44

Excludes *aryepiglottic fold or interarytenoid fold:*
NOS (235.1)
hypopharyngeal aspect (235.1)
marginal zone (235.1)

235.7 Trachea, bronchus, and lung I43, I44

235.8 Pleura, thymus, and mediastinum I43, I44

235.9 Other and unspecified respiratory organs I43, I44

Accessory sinuses
Middle ear
Nasal cavities
Respiratory organ NOS

Excludes *ear (external) (skin) (238.2)*
nose (238.8)
skin (238.2)

4th **236 Neoplasm of uncertain behavior of genitourinary organs**

236.0 Uterus ♀ I43, I44

236.1 Placenta ♀ I43, I44

Chorioadenoma (destruens)
Invasive mole
Malignant hydatid(iform) mole

236.2 Ovary ♀ I43, I44

Use additional code to identify any functional activity

236.3 Other and unspecified female genital organs ♀ I43, I44

236.4 Testis ♂ I43, I44

Use additional code to identify any functional activity

236.5 Prostate ♂ I43, I44

236.6 Other and unspecified male genital organs ♂ I43, I44

236.7 Bladder I43, I44

5th **236.9 Other and unspecified urinary organs**

236.90 Urinary organ, unspecified I43, I44

236.91 Kidney and ureter I43, I44

236.99 Other I43, I44

4th **237 Neoplasm of uncertain behavior of endocrine glands and nervous system**

237.0 Pituitary gland and craniopharyngeal duct I43, I44

Use additional code to identify any functional activity

237.1 Pineal gland I43, I44

237.2 Adrenal gland I43, I44

Suprarenal gland
Use additional code to identify any functional activity

237.3 Paraganglia I43, I44

Aortic body
Carotid body
Coccygeal body
Glomus jugulare

237.4 Other and unspecified endocrine glands I43, I44

Parathyroid gland
Thyroid gland

237.5 Brain and spinal cord I43, I44

237.6 Meninges I43, I44

Meninges:
- NOS
- cerebral
- spinal

5th **237.7 Neurofibromatosis**

von Recklinghausen's disease

237.70 Neurofibromatosis, unspecified I43, I44

237.71 Neurofibromatosis, type 1 [von Recklinghausen's disease] I43, I44

237.72 Neurofibromatosis, type 2 [acoustic neurofibromatosis] I43, I44

237.9 Other and unspecified parts of nervous system I43, I44

Cranial nerves

Excludes *peripheral, sympathetic, and parasympathetic nerves and ganglia (238.1)*

4th **238 Neoplasm of uncertain behavior of other and unspecified sites and tissues**

238.0 Bone and articular cartilage I43, I44

Excludes *cartilage:*
ear (238.1)
eyelid (238.1)
larynx (235.6)
nose (235.9)
synovia (238.1)

238.1 Connective and other soft tissue I 4 3, I 4 4
Peripheral, sympathetic, and parasympathetic nerves and ganglia
Stromal tumors of digestive system
Excludes *cartilage (of):*
articular (238.0)
larynx (235.6)
nose (235.9)
connective tissue of breast (238.3)

238.2 Skin I 4 3, I 4 4
D48.5 Neoplasm of uncertain behavior of skin
Excludes *anus NOS (235.5)*
skin of genital organs (236.3, 236.6)
vermilion border of lip (235.1)

238.3 Breast I 4 3, I 4 4
Excludes *skin of breast (238.2)*

238.4 Polycythemia vera I 4 3, I 4 4
D45 Polycythemia vera

238.5 Histiocytic and mast cells I 4 3, I 4 4
Mast cell tumor NOS
Mastocytoma NOS

238.6 Plasma cells I 4 3, I 4 4
Plasmacytoma NOS
Solitary myeloma

5th **238.7 Other lymphatic and hematopoietic tissues**
Excludes *acute myelogenous leukemia (205.0)*
chronic myelomonocytic leukemia (205.1)
myelosclerosis NOS (289.89)
myelosis:
NOS (205.9)
megakaryocytic (207.2)

238.71 Essential thrombocythemia I 4 3, I 4 4
Essential hemorrhagic thrombocythemia
Essential thrombocytosis
Idiopathic (hemorrhagic) thrombocythemia
Primary thrombocytosis

238.72 Low grade myelodysplastic syndrome lesions 6 7, 6 8, I 4 3, I 4 4
Refractory anemia (RA)
Refractory anemia with excess blasts-1 (RAEB-1)
Refractory anemia with ringed sideroblasts (RARS)
Refractory cytopenia with multilineage dysplasia (RCMD)
Refractory cytopenia with multilineage dysplasia and ringed sideroblasts (RCMD-RS)

238.73 High grade myelodysplastic syndrome lesions 6 7, 6 8, I 4 3, I 4 4
~~Refractory anemia with excess blasts-1 (RAEB-1)~~
Refractory anemia with excess blasts-2 (RAEB-2)

238.74 Myelodysplastic syndrome with 5q deletion 6 7, 6 8, I 4 3, I 4 4
5q minus syndrome NOS
Excludes *constitutional 5q deletion (758.39)*
high grade myelodysplastic syndrome with 5q deletion (238.73)

238.75 Myelodysplastic syndrome, unspecified 6 7, 6 8, I 4 3, I 4 4

238.76 Myelofibrosis with myeloid metaplasia I 4 3, I 4 4
Agnogenic myeloid metaplasia
Idiopathic myelofibrosis (chronic)
Myelosclerosis with myeloid metaplasia
Primary myelofibrosis
Excludes *myelofibrosis NOS (289.83)*
myelophthisic anemia (284.2)
myelophthisis (284.2)
secondary myelofibrosis (289.83)

238.77 Post-transplant lymphoproliferative disorder (PTLD) I 4 3, I 4 4
Code first complications of transplant (996.80-996.89)

238.79 Other lymphatic and hematopoietic tissues I 4 3, I 4 4
C94.40 Acute panmyelosis, not in remission
C94.41 Acute panmyelosis, in remission
C94.50 Acute myelofibrosis, not in remission
C94.51 Acute myelofibrosis, in remission
D47.7 Other specified neoplasms of uncertain behavior of lymphoid, hematopoietic and related tissue
Lymphoproliferative disease (chronic) NOS
Megakaryocytic myelosclerosis
Myeloproliferative disease (chronic) NOS
Panmyelosis (acute)

238.8 Other specified sites I 4 3, I 4 4
Eye
Heart
Excludes *eyelid (skin) (238.2)*
cartilage (238.1)

238.9 Site unspecified I 4 3, I 4 4

NEOPLASMS OF UNSPECIFIED NATURE (239)

4th **239 Neoplasms of unspecified nature**
Note: *Category 239 classifies by site neoplasms of unspecified morphology and behavior. The term "mass," unless otherwise stated, is not to be regarded as a neoplastic growth.*
Includes "growth" NOS
neoplasm NOS
new growth NOS
tumor NOS

239.0 Digestive system I 4 3, I 4 4
Excludes *anus:*
margin (239.2)
skin (239.2)
perianal skin (239.2)

239.1 Respiratory system I 4 3, I 4 4

239.2 Bone, soft tissue, and skin I 4 3, I 4 4
D49.2 Neoplasm of unspecified behavior of bone, soft tissue, and skin
Excludes *anal canal (239.0)*
anus NOS (239.0)
bone marrow (202.9)
cartilage:
larynx (239.1)
nose (239.1)
connective tissue of breast (239.3)
skin of genital organs (239.5)
vermilion border of lip (239.0)

239.3 Breast I 43, I 44

Excludes *skin of breast (239.2)*

239.4 Bladder I 43, I 44

239.5 Other genitourinary organs I 43, I 44

239.6 Brain I 43, I 44

Excludes *cerebral meninges (239.7)*
cranial nerves (239.7)

239.7 Endocrine glands and other parts of nervous system I 43, I 44

Excludes *peripheral, sympathetic, and parasympathetic nerves and ganglia (239.2)*

5th **239.8 Other specified sites**

Excludes *eyelid (skin) (239.2)*
cartilage (239.2)
great vessels (239.2)
optic nerve (239.7)

● **239.81 Retina and choroid** I 43, I 44

Dark area on retina
Retinal freckle

Rationale: *Not uncommonly, an eye examination will reveal a black or dark area or spot within the retina. Ophthalmologists must continue to evaluate these areas as they are suspicious of a retinal melanoma. Previously there was no unique code that allowed for the identification of these suspicious areas on the retina.*

Assignment of codes from Chapter 2, "Neoplasms," generally requires histologic confirmation. Although these dark areas are correctly referred to as neoplasms or "suspected melanoma," a biopsy of the retina is difficult and poses a risk to the eye, and done only after such an area or spot grows, so there is generally no tissue sample to confirm the diagnosis.

To allow for the identification of this condition within the structure of the classification, a new code in Chapter 2 under category 239, "Neoplasms of unspecified nature," was created. Histologic confirmation is not required for codes in this category. Inclusion terms also were added to validate for opthalmologists and coders that this is the correct code for this condition since users may not realize to look for the code in the Neoplasm table or in the index.

● **239.89 Other specified sites** I 43, I 44

239.9 Site unspecified I 43, I 44

3. ENDOCRINE, NUTRITIONAL AND METABOLIC DISEASES, AND IMMUNITY DISORDERS (240-279)

Excludes *endocrine and metabolic disturbances specific to the fetus and newborn (775.0-775.9)*

Note: *All neoplasms, whether functionally active or not, are classified in Chapter 2. Codes in Chapter 3 (i.e., 242.8, 246.0, 251-253, 255-259) may be used to identify such functional activity associated with any neoplasm, or by ectopic endocrine tissue.*

DISORDERS OF THYROID GLAND (240-246)

4th **240 Simple and unspecified goiter**

240.0 Goiter, specified as simple

Any condition classifiable to 240.9, specified as simple

240.9 Goiter, unspecified

Enlargement of thyroid
Goiter or struma:
NOS
diffuse colloid
endemic
hyperplastic
nontoxic (diffuse)
parenchymatous
sporadic

Excludes *congenital (dyshormonogenic) goiter (246.1)*

4th **241 Nontoxic nodular goiter**

Excludes *adenoma of thyroid (226)*
cystadenoma of thyroid (226)

241.0 Nontoxic uninodular goiter

E04.1 Nontoxic single thyroid nodule

Thyroid nodule
Uninodular goiter (nontoxic)

241.1 Nontoxic multinodular goiter

Multinodular goiter (nontoxic)

241.9 Unspecified nontoxic nodular goiter

Adenomatous goiter
Nodular goiter (nontoxic) NOS
Struma nodosa (simplex)

4th **242 Thyrotoxicosis with or without goiter**

Excludes *neonatal thyrotoxicosis (775.3)*

The following fifth-digit subclassification is for use with category 242:

0 **without mention of thyrotoxic crisis or storm**
1 **with mention of thyrotoxic crisis or storm**

5th **242.0 Toxic diffuse goiter**

[0-1] Basedow's disease
Exophthalmic or toxic goiter NOS
Graves' disease
Primary thyroid hyperplasia

5th **242.1 Toxic uninodular goiter**

[0-1] Thyroid nodule, toxic or with hyperthyroidism
Uninodular goiter, toxic or with hyperthyroidism

5th **242.2 Toxic multinodular goiter**

[0-1] Secondary thyroid hyperplasia

5th **242.3 Toxic nodular goiter, unspecified**

[0-1] Adenomatous goiter, toxic or with hyperthyroidism
Nodular goiter, toxic or with hyperthyroidism
Struma nodosa, toxic or with hyperthyroidism
Any condition classifiable to 241.9 specified as toxic or with hyperthyroidism

5th **242.4 Thyrotoxicosis from ectopic thyroid nodule**

[0-1]

5th **242.8 Thyrotoxicosis of other specified origin**

[0-1] Overproduction of thyroid-stimulating hormone [TSH]
Thyrotoxicosis:
factitia from ingestion of excessive thyroid material
Use additional E code to identify cause, if drug-induced

5th **242.9 Thyrotoxicosis without mention of goiter or other cause**
[0-1] Hyperthyroidism NOS
Thyrotoxicosis NOS

243 Congenital hypothyroidism
Congenital thyroid insufficiency
Cretinism (athyrotic) (endemic)
Use additional code to identify associated mental retardation
Excludes *congenital (dyshormonogenic) goiter (246.1)*

4th **244 Acquired hypothyroidism**
Includes athyroidism (acquired)
hypothyroidism (acquired)
myxedema (adult) (juvenile)
thyroid (gland) insufficiency (acquired)

244.0 Postsurgical hypothyroidism

244.1 Other postablative hypothyroidism
Hypothyroidism following therapy, such as irradiation

244.2 Iodine hypothyroidism
Hypothyroidism resulting from administration or ingestion of iodide
Use additional E to identify drug

244.3 Other iatrogenic hypothyroidism
Hypothyroidism resulting from:
P-aminosalicylic acid [PAS]
Phenylbutazone
Resorcinol
Iatrogenic hypothyroidism NOS
Use additional E to identify drug

244.8 Other specified acquired hypothyroidism
E01.8 Other iodine-deficiency related thyroid disorders and allied conditions
Secondary hypothyroidism NEC

244.9 Unspecified hypothyroidism
E03.9 Hypothyroidism, unspecified
Hypothyroidism, primary or NOS
Myxedema, primary or NOS

4th **245 Thyroiditis**

245.0 Acute thyroiditis
Abscess of thyroid
Thyroiditis:
nonsuppurative, acute
pyogenic
suppurative
Use additional code to identify organism

245.1 Subacute thyroiditis
Thyroiditis:
de Quervain's
giant cell
granulomatous
viral

245.2 Chronic lymphocytic thyroiditis
Hashimoto's disease
Struma lymphomatosa
Thyroiditis:
autoimmune
lymphocytic (chronic)

245.3 Chronic fibrous thyroiditis
Struma fibrosa
Thyroiditis:
invasive (fibrous)
ligneous
Riedel's

245.4 Iatrogenic thyroiditis
Use additional E to identify cause

245.8 Other and unspecified chronic thyroiditis
Chronic thyroiditis:
NOS
nonspecific

245.9 Thyroiditis, unspecified
Thyroiditis NOS

4th **246 Other disorders of thyroid**

246.0 Disorders of thyrocalcitonin secretion
Hypersecretion of calcitonin or thyrocalcitonin

246.1 Dyshormonogenic goiter
Congenital (dyshormonogenic) goiter
Goiter due to enzyme defect in synthesis of thyroid hormone
Goitrous cretinism (sporadic)

246.2 Cyst of thyroid
Excludes *cystadenoma of thyroid (226)*

246.3 Hemorrhage and infarction of thyroid

246.8 Other specified disorders of thyroid
Abnormality of thyroid-binding globulin
Atrophy of thyroid
Hyper-TBG-nemia
Hypo-TBG-nemia

246.9 Unspecified disorder of thyroid

DISEASES OF OTHER ENDOCRINE GLANDS (249-259)

ICD-9-CM Official Guidelines (Chapter 3)

7) ***Secondary Diabetes Mellitus***

Codes under category 249, Secondary diabetes mellitus, identify complications/manifestations associated with secondary diabetes mellitus. Secondary diabetes is always caused by another condition or event (e.g., cystic fibrosis, malignant neoplasm of pancreas, pancreatectomy, adverse effect of drug, or poisoning).

(a) ***Fifth-digits for category 249:***

A fifth-digit is required for all category 249 codes to identify whether the diabetes is controlled or uncontrolled.

(b) ***Secondary diabetes mellitus and the use of insulin***

For patients who routinely use insulin, code V58.67, Long-term (current) use of insulin, should also be assigned. Code V58.67 should not be assigned if insulin is given temporarily to bring a patient's blood sugar under control during an encounter.

(c) ***Assigning and sequencing secondary diabetes codes and associated conditions***

When assigning codes for secondary diabetes and its associated conditions (e.g. renal manifestations), the code(s) from category 249 must be sequenced before the codes for the associated conditions. The secondary diabetes codes and the diabetic manifestation codes that correspond to them are paired codes that follow the etiology/manifestation convention of the classification. Assign as many codes from category 249 as needed to identify all of the associated conditions that the patient has. The corresponding codes for the associated conditions are listed under each of the secondary diabetes codes. For example, secondary diabetes with diabetic nephrosis is assigned to code 249.40, followed by 581.81.

(d) ***Assigning and sequencing secondary diabetes codes and its causes***

The sequencing of the secondary diabetes codes in relationship to codes for the cause of the diabetes is based on the reason for the encounter, applicable ICD-9-CM sequencing conventions, and chapter-specific guidelines.

If a patient is seen for treatment of the secondary diabetes or one of its associated conditions, a code from category 249 is sequenced as the principal or first-listed diagnosis, with the cause of the secondary diabetes (e.g. cystic fibrosis) sequenced as an additional diagnosis.

If, however, the patient is seen for the treatment of the condition causing the secondary diabetes (e.g., malignant neoplasm of pancreas), the code for the cause of the secondary diabetes should be sequenced as the principal or first-listed diagnosis followed by a code from category 249.

(i) Secondary diabetes mellitus due to pancreatectomy

For postpancreatectomy diabetes mellitus (lack of insulin due to the surgical removal of all or part of the pancreas), assign code 251.3, Postsurgical hypoinsulinemia. A code from subcategory 249 should not be assigned for secondary diabetes mellitus due to pancreatectomy. Code also any diabetic manifestations (e.g. diabetic nephrosis 581.81).

(ii) Secondary diabetes due to drugs

Secondary diabetes may be caused by an adverse effect of correctly administered medications, poisoning or late effect of poisoning.

See section I.C.17.e for coding of adverse effects and poisoning, and section I.C.19 for E code reporting.

4th **249 Secondary diabetes mellitus**

Includes diabetes mellitus (due to) (in) (secondary) (with):
drug-induced or chemical induced
infection

Excludes *gestational diabetes (648.8)*
hyperglycemia NOS (790.29)
neonatal diabetes mellitus (775.1)
nonclinical diabetes (790.29)
Type I diabetes – see category 250
Type II diabetes – see category 250

The following fifth-digit subclassification is for use with category 249:

0 **not stated as uncontrolled, or unspecified**
1 **uncontrolled**

Use additional code to identify any associated insulin use (V58.67)

5th **249.0 Secondary diabetes mellitus without mention of complication**
[0-1] Secondary diabetes mellitus without mention of complication or manifestation classifiable to 249.1-249.9
Secondary diabetes mellitus NOS

5th **249.1 Secondary diabetes mellitus with ketoacidosis**
[0-1] Secondary diabetes mellitus with diabetic acidosis without mention of coma
Secondary diabetes mellitus with diabetic ketosis without mention of coma

5th **249.2 Secondary diabetes mellitus with hyperosmolarity**
[0-1] Secondary diabetes mellitus with hyperosmolar (nonketotic) coma

5th **249.3 Secondary diabetes mellitus with other coma**
[0-1] Secondary diabetes mellitus with diabetic coma (with ketoacidosis)
Secondary diabetes mellitus with diabetic hypoglycemic coma
Secondary diabetes mellitus with insulin coma NOS
Excludes *secondary diabetes mellitus with hyperosmolar coma (249.2)*

5th **249.4 Secondary diabetes mellitus with renal manifestations**
[0-1]
Use additional code to identify manifestation, as:
chronic kidney disease (585.1-585.9)
diabetic nephropathy NOS (583.81)
diabetic nephrosis (581.81)
intercapillary glomerulosclerosis (581.81)
Kimmelstiel-Wilson syndrome (581.81)

5th **249.5 Secondary diabetes mellitus with ophthalmic manifestations**
[0-1]
Use additional code to identify manifestation, as:
diabetic blindness (369.00-369.9)
diabetic cataract (366.41)
diabetic glaucoma (365.44)
diabetic macular edema (362.07)
diabetic retinal edema (362.07)
diabetic retinopathy (362.01-362.07)

5th **249.6 Secondary diabetes mellitus with neurological manifestations**
[0-1]
Use additional code to identify manifestation, as:
diabetic amyotrophy (353.5)
diabetic gastroparalysis (536.3)
diabetic gastroparesis (536.3)
diabetic mononeuropathy (354.0-355.9)
diabetic neurogenic arthropathy (713.5)
diabetic peripheral autonomic neuropathy (337.1)
diabetic polyneuropathy (357.2)

5th **249.7 Secondary diabetes mellitus with peripheral circulatory disorders**
[0-1]
Use additional code to identify manifestation, as:
diabetic gangrene (785.4)
diabetic peripheral angiopathy (443.81)

5th **249.8 Secondary diabetes mellitus with other specified manifestations**
[0-1] Secondary diabetic hypoglycemia in diabetes mellitus
Secondary hypoglycemic shock in diabetes mellitus
Use additional code to identify manifestation, as:
any associated ulceration (707.10-707.9)
diabetic bone changes (731.8)

5th **249.9 Secondary diabetes mellitus with unspecified complication**
[0-1]

ICD-9-CM Official Guidelines (Chapter 3):

a. Diabetes mellitus

Codes under category 250, Diabetes mellitus, identify complications/manifestations associated with diabetes mellitus. A fifth-digit is required for all category 250 codes to identify the type of diabetes mellitus and whether the diabetes is controlled or uncontrolled.

*1) **Fifth-digits for category 250:***

The following are the fifth-digits for the codes under category 250:

0 type II or unspecified type, not stated as uncontrolled
1 type I, [juvenile type], not stated as uncontrolled
2 type II or unspecified type, uncontrolled
3 type I, [juvenile type], uncontrolled

The age of a patient is not the sole determining factor, though most type I diabetics develop the condition before reaching puberty. For this reason type I diabetes mellitus is also referred to as juvenile diabetes.

*2) **Type of diabetes mellitus not documented***

If the type of diabetes mellitus is not documented in the medical record the default is type II.

*3) **Diabetes mellitus and the use of insulin***

All type I diabetics must use insulin to replace what their bodies do not produce. However, the use of insulin does not mean that a patient is a type I diabetic. Some patients with type II diabetes mellitus are unable to control their blood sugar through diet and oral medication alone and do require insulin. If the documentation in a medical record does not indicate the type of diabetes but does indicate that the patient uses insulin, the appropriate fifth-digit for type II must be used. For type II patients who routinely use insulin, code V58.67, Long-term (current) use of insulin, should also be assigned to indicate that the patient uses insulin. Code V58.67 should not be assigned

249 – 249.9

if insulin is given temporarily to bring a type II patient's blood sugar under control during an encounter.

4) Assigning and sequencing diabetes codes and associated conditions

When assigning codes for diabetes and its associated conditions, the code(s) from category 250 must be sequenced before the codes for the associated conditions. The diabetes codes and the secondary codes that correspond to them are paired codes that follow the etiology/manifestation convention of the classification (See Section I.A.6., Etiology/manifestation convention). Assign as many codes from category 250 as needed to identify all of the associated conditions that the patient has. The corresponding secondary codes are listed under each of the diabetes codes.

(a) Diabetic retinopathy/diabetic macular edema

Diabetic macular edema, code 362.07, is only present with diabetic retinopathy. Another code from subcategory 362.0, Diabetic retinopathy, must be used with code 362.07. Codes under subcategory 362.0 are diabetes manifestation codes, so they must be used following the appropriate diabetes code.

4th **250 Diabetes mellitus**

Excludes *gestational diabetes (648.8)*
hyperglycemia NOS (790.29)
neonatal diabetes mellitus (775.1)
nonclinical diabetes (790.29)
secondary diabetes (249.0-249.9)

The following fifth-digit subclassification is for use with category 250:

0 type II or unspecified type, not stated as uncontrolled
Fifth-digit 0 is for use for type II patients, even if the patient requires insulin
Use additional code, if applicable, for associated long-term (current) insulin use V58.67

1 type I [juvenile type], not stated as uncontrolled

2 type II or unspecified type, uncontrolled
Fifth-digit 2 is for use for type II patients, even if the patient requires insulin
Use additional code, if applicable, for associated long-term (current) insulin use V58.67

3 type I [juvenile type], uncontrolled

Layman's: *Despite the use of the term "juvenile" when referring to type I diabetes, age is not the sole determining factor of whether a patient has type I or type II diabetes. Rather, the bodies of type I diabetics are unable to produce insulin on their own, whereas the bodies of type II diabetics cannot process insulin properly. Around 90-95% of Americans with diabetes have type II diabetes.*

5th **250.0 Diabetes mellitus without mention of complication** 1, 2, 3, 117, 118, 119, 126, 127, 163

E11.9 Type 2 diabetes mellitus without complications
E10.9 Type 1 diabetes mellitus without complications

[0-3] Diabetes mellitus without mention of complication or manifestation classifiable to 250.1-250.9
Diabetes (mellitus) NOS

5th **250.1 Diabetes with ketoacidosis** 1, 2, 3, 117, 118, 119, 126, 127, 163

[0-3] Diabetic:
acidosis without mention of coma
ketosis without mention of coma

5th **250.2 Diabetes with hyperosmolarity** 1, 2, 3, 117, 118, 119, 126, 127, 163

[0-3] Hyperosmolar (nonketotic) coma

5th **250.3 Diabetes with other coma** 1, 2, 3, 117, 118, 119, 126, 127, 163

[0-3] Diabetic coma (with ketoacidosis)
Diabetic hypoglycemic coma
Insulin coma NOS

Excludes *diabetes with hyperosmolar coma (250.2)*

5th **250.4 Diabetes with renal manifestations** 1, 2, 3, 117, 118, 119, 126, 127, 163

[0-3]
Use additional code to identify manifestation, as:
chronic kidney disease (585.1-585.9)
diabetic:
nephropathy NOS (583.81)
nephrosis (581.81)
intercapillary glomerulosclerosis (581.81)
Kimmelstiel-Wilson syndrome (581.81)

5th **250.5 Diabetes with ophthalmic manifestations** 1, 2, 3, 117, 118, 119, 126, 127, 163

[0-3]
Use additional code to identify manifestation, as:
diabetic:
blindness (369.00-369.9)
cataract (366.41)
glaucoma (365.44)
macular edema (362.07)
retinal edema (362.07)
retinopathy (362.01-362.07)

5th **250.6 Diabetes with neurological manifestations** 1, 2, 3, 117, 118, 119, 126, 127, 163

[0-3]
Use additional code to identify manifestation, as:
diabetic:
amyotrophy (353.5)
gastroparalysis (536.3)
gastroparesis (536.3)
mononeuropathy (354.0-355.9)
neurogenic arthropathy (713.5)
peripheral autonomic neuropathy (337.1)
polyneuropathy (357.2)

5th **250.7 Diabetes with peripheral circulatory disorders** 1, 2, 3, 117, 118, 119, 126, 127, 163

[0-3]
Use additional code to identify manifestation, as:
diabetic:
gangrene (785.4)
peripheral angiopathy (443.81)

5th **250.8 Diabetes with other specified manifestations** 1, 2, 3, 117, 118, 119, 126, 127, 163

[0-3] Diabetic hypoglycemia NOS
Hypoglycemic shock NOS
Use additional code to identify manifestation, as:
any associated ulceration (707.10-707.9)
diabetic bone changes (731.8)

5th **250.9 Diabetes with unspecified complication** 1, 2, 3, 117, 118, 119, 126, 127, 163

[0-3]

4th **251 Other disorders of pancreatic internal secretion**

251.0 Hypoglycemic coma
Iatrogenic hyperinsulinism
Non-diabetic insulin coma
Use additional E code to identify cause, if drug-induced

Excludes *hypoglycemic coma in diabetes mellitus (249.3, 250.3)*

251.1 Other specified hypoglycemia
Hyperinsulinism:
NOS
ectopic
functional
Hyperplasia of pancreatic islet beta cells NOS
Use additional E code to identify cause, if drug-induced

Excludes *hypoglycemia in diabetes mellitus (249.8, 250.8)*
hypoglycemia in infant of diabetic mother (775.0)
hypoglycemic coma (251.0)
neonatal hypoglycemia (775.6)

251.2 Hypoglycemia, unspecified
E16.2 Hypoglycemia, unspecified
Hypoglycemia:
NOS
reactive
spontaneous
Excludes *hypoglycemia:*
with coma (251.0)
in diabetes mellitus (249.8, 250.8)
leucine-induced (270.3)

251.3 Postsurgical hypoinsulinemia
Hypoinsulinemia following complete or partial pancreatectomy
Postpancreatectomy hyperglycemia
Use additional code to identify (any associated):
acquired absence of pancreas (V45.79)
insulin use (V58.67)
secondary diabetes mellitus (249.00-249.91)
Excludes *transient hyperglycemia post procedure (790.29)*
transient hypoglycemia post procedure (251.2)

251.4 Abnormality of secretion of glucagon
Hyperplasia of pancreatic islet alpha cells with glucagon excess

251.5 Abnormality of secretion of gastrin
Hyperplasia of pancreatic alpha cells with gastrin excess
Zollinger-Ellison syndrome

251.8 Other specified disorders of pancreatic internal secretion

251.9 Unspecified disorder of pancreatic internal secretion
Islet cell hyperplasia NOS

4th **252 Disorders of parathyroid gland**
Excludes *hungry bone syndrome (275.5)*

5th **252.0 Hyperparathyroidism**
Excludes *ectopic hyperparathyroidism (259.3)*

252.00 Hyperparathyroidism, unspecified
E21.3 Hyperparathyroidism, unspecified

252.01 Primary hyperparathyroidism
Hyperplasia of parathyroid

252.02 Secondary hyperparathyroidism, non-renal
Excludes *secondary hyperparathyroidism (of renal origin) (588.81)*

252.08 Other hyperparathyroidism
Tertiary hyperparathyroidism

252.1 Hypoparathyroidism
Parathyroiditis (autoimmune)
Tetany:
parathyroid
parathyroprival
Excludes *pseudohypoparathyroidism (275.49)*
pseudopseudohypoparathyroidism (275.49)
tetany NOS (781.7)
transitory neonatal hypoparathyroidism (775.4)

252.8 Other specified disorders of parathyroid gland
Cyst of parathyroid gland
Hemorrhage of parathyroid gland

252.9 Unspecified disorder of parathyroid gland

4th **253 Disorders of the pituitary gland and its hypothalamic control**
Includes the listed conditions whether the disorder is in the pituitary or the hypothalamus
Excludes *Cushing's syndrome (255.0)*

253.0 Acromegaly and gigantism
Overproduction of growth hormone

253.1 Other and unspecified anterior pituitary hyperfunction
Forbes-Albright syndrome
Excludes *overproduction of:*
ACTH (255.3)
thyroid-stimulating hormone [TSH] (242.8)

253.2 Panhypopituitarism
Cachexia, pituitary
Necrosis of pituitary (postpartum)
Pituitary insufficiency NOS
Sheehan's syndrome
Simmonds' disease
Excludes *iatrogenic hypopituitarism (253.7)*

253.3 Pituitary dwarfism
Isolated deficiency of (human) growth hormone [HGH]
Lorain-Levi dwarfism

253.4 Other anterior pituitary disorders
Isolated or partial deficiency of an anterior pituitary hormone, other than growth hormone
Prolactin deficiency

253.5 Diabetes insipidus
Vasopressin deficiency
Excludes *nephrogenic diabetes insipidus (588.1)*

253.6 Other disorders of neurohypophysis
Syndrome of inappropriate secretion of antidiuretic hormone [ADH]
Excludes *ectopic antidiuretic hormone secretion (259.3)*

253.7 Iatrogenic pituitary disorders
Hypopituitarism:
hormone-induced
hypophysectomy-induced
postablative
radiotherapy-induced
Use additional E code to identify cause

253.8 Other disorders of the pituitary and other syndromes of diencephalohypophyseal origin
Abscess of pituitary
Adiposogenital dystrophy
Cyst of Rathke's pouch
Fröhlich's syndrome
Excludes *craniopharyngioma (237.0)*

253.9 Unspecified
Dyspituitarism

4th **254 Diseases of thymus gland**
Excludes *aplasia or dysplasia with immunodeficiency (279.2)*
hypoplasia with immunodeficiency (279.2)
myasthenia gravis (358.00-358.01)

254.0 Persistent hyperplasia of thymus
Hypertrophy of thymus

254.1 Abscess of thymus

254.8 Other specified diseases of thymus gland
Atrophy of thymus
Cyst of thymus
Excludes *thymoma (212.6)*

254.9 Unspecified disease of thymus gland

4th **255 Disorders of adrenal glands**
Includes the listed conditions whether the basic disorder is in the adrenals or is pituitary-induced

255.0 Cushing's syndrome
Adrenal hyperplasia due to excess ACTH
Cushing's syndrome:
NOS
iatrogenic
idiopathic
pituitary-dependent
Ectopic ACTH syndrome
Iatrogenic syndrome of excess cortisol
Overproduction of cortisol
Use additional E code to identify cause, if drug-induced
Excludes *congenital adrenal hyperplasia (255.2)*

251.2 – 255.0

5th 255.1 **Hyperaldosteronism**

255.10 **Hyperaldosteronism, unspecified**
Aldosteronism NOS
Primary aldosteronism, unspecified
Excludes *Conn's syndrome (255.12)*

255.11 **Glucocorticoid-remediable aldosteronism**
Familial aldosteronism type I
Excludes *Conn's syndrome (255.12)*

255.12 **Conn's syndrome**

255.13 **Bartter's syndrome**

255.14 **Other secondary aldosteronism**

255.2 **Adrenogenital disorders**
Achard-Thiers syndrome
Adrenogenital syndromes, virilizing or feminizing, whether acquired or associated with congenital adrenal hyperplasia consequent on inborn enzyme defects in hormone synthesis
Congenital adrenal hyperplasia
Female adrenal pseudohermaphroditism
Male:
macrogenitosomia praecox
sexual precocity with adrenal hyperplasia
Virilization (female) (suprarenal)
Excludes *adrenal hyperplasia due to excess ACTH (255.0)*
isosexual virilization (256.4)

255.3 **Other corticoadrenal overactivity**
Acquired benign adrenal androgenic overactivity
Overproduction of ACTH

5th 255.4 **Corticoadrenal insufficiency**
Excludes *tuberculous Addison's disease (017.6)*

255.41 **Glucocorticoid deficiency**
Addisonian crisis
Addison's disease NOS
Adrenal atrophy (autoimmune)
Adrenal calcification
Adrenal crisis
Adrenal hemorrhage
Adrenal infarction
Adrenal insufficiency NOS
Combined glucocorticoid and mineralocorticoid deficiency
Corticoadrenal insufficiency NOS

255.42 **Mineralocorticoid deficiency**
Hypoaldosteronism
Excludes *combined glucocorticoid and mineralocorticoid deficiency (255.41)*

255.5 **Other adrenal hypofunction**
Adrenal medullary insufficiency
Excludes *Waterhouse-Friderichsen syndrome (meningococcal) (036.3)*

255.6 **Medulloadrenal hyperfunction**
Catecholamine secretion by pheochromocytoma

255.8 **Other specified disorders of adrenal glands**
Abnormality of cortisol-binding globulin

255.9 **Unspecified disorder of adrenal glands**

4th 256 **Ovarian dysfunction**

256.0 **Hyperestrogenism** ♀

256.1 **Other ovarian hyperfunction** ♀
Hypersecretion of ovarian androgens

256.2 **Postablative ovarian failure** ♀
Ovarian failure:
iatrogenic
postirradiation
postsurgical
Use additional code for states associated with artificial menopause (627.4)
Excludes *acquired absence of ovary (V45.77)*
asymptomatic age-related (natural) postmenopausal status (V49.81)

5th 256.3 **Other ovarian failure**
Use additional code for states associated with natural menopause (627.2)
Excludes *asymptomatic age-related (natural) postmenopausal status (V49.81)*

256.31 **Premature menopause** A ♀

256.39 **Other ovarian failure** ♀
Delayed menarche
Ovarian hypofunction
Primary ovarian failure NOS

256.4 **Polycystic ovaries** ♀
Isosexual virilization
Stein-Leventhal syndrome

256.8 **Other ovarian dysfunction** ♀

256.9 **Unspecified ovarian dysfunction** ♀

4th 257 **Testicular dysfunction**

257.0 **Testicular hyperfunction** ♂
Hypersecretion of testicular hormones

257.1 **Postablative testicular hypofunction** ♂
Testicular hypofunction:
iatrogenic
postirradiation
postsurgical

257.2 **Other testicular hypofunction**
E29.1 Testicular hypofunction
Defective biosynthesis of testicular androgen
Eunuchoidism:
NOS
hypogonadotropic
Failure:
Leydig's cell, adult
seminiferous tubule, adult
Testicular hypogonadism
Excludes *azoospermia (606.0)*

257.8 **Other testicular dysfunction**
Excludes *androgen insensitivity syndromes (259.50-259.52)*

257.9 **Unspecified testicular dysfunction** ♂

4th 258 **Polyglandular dysfunction and related disorders**

5th 258.0 **Polyglandular activity in multiple endocrine adenomatosis**
Multiple endocrine neoplasia [MEN] syndromes
Use additional codes to identify any malignancies and other conditions associated with the syndromes

258.01 **Multiple endocrine neoplasia [MEN] type I**
Wermer's syndrome

258.02 **Multiple endocrine neoplasia [MEN] type IIA**
Sipple's syndrome

258.03 **Multiple endocrine neoplasia [MEN] type IIB**

258.1 **Other combinations of endocrine dysfunction**
Lloyd's syndrome
Schmidt's syndrome

258.8 **Other specified polyglandular dysfunction**

258.9 **Polyglandular dysfunction, unspecified**

4th 259 **Other endocrine disorders**

259.0 **Delay in sexual development and puberty, not elsewhere classified**
Delayed puberty

259.1 **Precocious sexual development and puberty, not elsewhere classified** P
Sexual precocity:
NOS
constitutional
cryptogenic
idiopathic

259.2 **Carcinoid syndrome**
Hormone secretion by carcinoid tumors

259.3 **Ectopic hormone secretion, not elsewhere classified**
Ectopic:
antidiuretic hormone secretion [ADH]
hyperparathyroidism
Excludes *ectopic ACTH syndrome (255.0)*

259.4 **Dwarfism, not elsewhere classified**
Dwarfism:
NOS
constitutional
Excludes *dwarfism:*
achondroplastic (756.4)
intrauterine (759.7)
nutritional (263.2)
pituitary (253.3)
renal (588.0)
progeria (259.8)

5th 259.5 **Androgen insensitivity syndrome**

259.50 **Androgen insensitivity, unspecified**

259.51 **Androgen insensitivity syndrome**
Complete androgen insensitivity
de Quervain's syndrome
Goldberg-Maxwell Syndrome

259.52 **Partial androgen insensitivity**
Partial androgen insensitivity syndrome
Reifenstein syndrome

259.8 **Other specified endocrine disorders**
Pineal gland dysfunction
Progeria
Werner's syndrome

259.9 **Unspecified endocrine disorder**
Disturbance:
endocrine NOS
hormone NOS
Infantilism NOS

NUTRITIONAL DEFICIENCIES (260-269)

Excludes *deficiency anemias (280.0-281.9)*

260 **Kwashiorkor**
Nutritional edema with dyspigmentation of skin and hair

261 **Nutritional marasmus**
Nutritional atrophy
Severe calorie deficiency
Severe malnutrition NOS

262 **Other severe protein-calorie malnutrition**
Nutritional edema without mention of dyspigmentation of skin and hair

4th 263 **Other and unspecified protein-calorie malnutrition**

263.0 **Malnutrition of moderate degree**

263.1 **Malnutrition of mild degree**

263.2 **Arrested development following protein-calorie malnutrition**
Nutritional dwarfism
Physical retardation due to malnutrition

263.8 **Other protein-calorie malnutrition**

263.9 **Unspecified protein-calorie malnutrition**
E46 Unspecified protein-calorie malnutrition
Dystrophy due to malnutrition
Malnutrition (calorie) NOS
Excludes *nutritional deficiency NOS (269.9)*

4th 264 **Vitamin A deficiency**

264.0 **With conjunctival xerosis**

264.1 **With conjunctival xerosis and Bitot's spot**
Bitot's spot in the young child

264.2 **With corneal xerosis**

264.3 **With corneal ulceration and xerosis**

264.4 **With keratomalacia**

264.5 **With night blindness**

264.6 **With xerophthalmic scars of cornea**

264.7 **Other ocular manifestations of vitamin A deficiency**
Xerophthalmia due to vitamin A deficiency

264.8 **Other manifestations of vitamin A deficiency**
Follicular keratosis due to vitamin A deficiency
Xeroderma due to vitamin A deficiency

264.9 **Unspecified vitamin A deficiency**
Hypovitaminosis A NOS

4th 265 **Thiamine and niacin deficiency states**

265.0 **Beriberi**

265.1 **Other and unspecified manifestations of thiamine deficiency**
Other vitamin B_1 deficiency states

265.2 **Pellagra**
Deficiency:
niacin (-tryptophan)
nicotinamide
nicotinic acid
vitamin PP
Pellagra (alcoholic)

4th 266 **Deficiency of B-complex components**

266.0 **Ariboflavinosis**
Riboflavin [vitamin B_2] deficiency

266.1 **Vitamin B_6 deficiency**
Deficiency:
pyridoxal
pyridoxamine
pyridoxine
Vitamin B_6 deficiency syndrome
Excludes *vitamin B_6-responsive sideroblastic anemia (285.0)*

266.2 **Other B-complex deficiencies**
E53.8 Deficiency of other specified B group vitamins
Deficiency:
cyanocobalamin
folic acid
vitamin B_{12}
Excludes *combined system disease with anemia (281.0-281.1)*
deficiency anemias (281.0-281.9)
subacute degeneration of spinal cord with anemia (281.0-281.1)

266.9 **Unspecified vitamin B deficiency**

267 **Ascorbic acid deficiency**
Deficiency of vitamin C
Scurvy
Excludes *scorbutic anemia (281.8)*

259 – 267

4th 268 Vitamin D deficiency

Excludes *vitamin D-resistant:*
osteomalacia (275.3)
rickets (275.3)

268.0 Rickets, active

Excludes *celiac rickets (579.0)*
renal rickets (588.0)

268.1 Rickets, late effect

Any condition specified as due to rickets and stated to be a late effect or sequela of rickets

Code first the nature of late effect

268.2 Osteomalacia, unspecified

268.9 Unspecified vitamin D deficiency

Avitaminosis D

4th 269 Other nutritional deficiencies

269.0 Deficiency of vitamin K

Excludes *deficiency of coagulation factor due to vitamin K deficiency (286.7)*
vitamin K deficiency of newborn (776.0)

269.1 Deficiency of other vitamins

Deficiency:
vitamin E
vitamin P

269.2 Unspecified vitamin deficiency

Multiple vitamin deficiency NOS

269.3 Mineral deficiency, not elsewhere classified

Deficiency:
calcium, dietary
iodine

Excludes *deficiency:*
calcium NOS (275.40)
potassium (276.8)
sodium (276.1)

269.8 Other nutritional deficiency

Excludes *adult failure to thrive (783.7)*
failure to thrive in childhood (783.41)
feeding problems (783.3)
newborn (779.31-779.34)

269.9 Unspecified nutritional deficiency

OTHER METABOLIC AND IMMUNITY DISORDERS (270-279)

Use additional code to identify any associated mental retardation

4th 270 Disorders of amino-acid transport and metabolism

Excludes *abnormal findings without manifest disease (790.0-796.9)*
disorders of purine and pyrimidine metabolism (277.1-277.2)
gout (274.00-274.9)

270.0 Disturbances of amino-acid transport

Cystinosis
Cystinuria
Fanconi (-de Toni) (-Debré) syndrome
Glycinuria (renal)
Hartnup disease

270.1 Phenylketonuria [PKU]

Hyperphenylalaninemia

270.2 Other disturbances of aromatic amino-acid metabolism

Albinism
Alkaptonuria
Alkaptonuric ochronosis
Disturbances of metabolism of tyrosine and tryptophan
Homogentisic acid defects
Hydroxykynureninuria
Hypertyrosinemia
Indicanuria
Kynureninase defects
Oasthouse urine disease
Ochronosis
Tyrosinosis
Tyrosinuria
Waardenburg syndrome

Excludes *vitamin B_6-deficiency syndrome (266.1)*

270.3 Disturbances of branched-chain amino-acid metabolism

Disturbances of metabolism of leucine, isoleucine, and valine
Hypervalinemia
Intermittent branched-chain ketonuria
Leucine-induced hypoglycemia
Leucinosis
Maple syrup urine disease

270.4 Disturbances of sulphur-bearing amino-acid metabolism

Cystathioninemia
Cystathioninuria
Disturbances of metabolism of methionine, homocystine, and cystathionine
Homocystinuria
Hypermethioninemia
Methioninemia

270.5 Disturbances of histidine metabolism

Carnosinemia
Histidinemia
Hyperhistidinemia
Imidazole aminoaciduria

270.6 Disorders of urea cycle metabolism

Argininosuccinic aciduria
Citrullinemia
Disorders of metabolism of ornithine, citrulline, argininosuccinic acid, arginine, and ammonia
Hyperammonemia
Hyperornithinemia

270.7 Other disturbances of straight-chain amino-acid metabolism

Glucoglycinuria
Glycinemia (with methylmalonic acidemia)
Hyperglycinemia
Hyperlysinemia
Other disturbances of metabolism of glycine, threonine, serine, glutamine, and lysine
Pipecolic acidemia
Saccharopinuria

270.8 Other specified disorders of amino-acid metabolism

Alaninemia
Ethanolaminuria
Glycoprolinuria
Hydroxyprolinemia
Hyperprolinemia
Iminoacidopathy
Prolinemia
Prolinuria
Sarcosinemia

270.9 Unspecified disorder of amino-acid metabolism

4th 271 Disorders of carbohydrate transport and metabolism

Excludes *abnormality of secretion of glucagon (251.4)*
diabetes mellitus (249.0-249.9, 250.0-250.9)
hypoglycemia NOS (251.2)
mucopolysaccharidosis (277.5)

271.0 Glycogenosis
Amylopectinosis
Glucose-6-phosphatase deficiency
Glycogen storage disease
McArdle's disease
Pompe's disease
von Gierke's disease

271.1 Galactosemia
Galactose-1-phosphate uridyl transferase deficiency
Galactosuria

271.2 Hereditary fructose intolerance
Essential benign fructosuria
Fructosemia

271.3 Intestinal disaccharidase deficiencies and disaccharide malabsorption
Intolerance or malabsorption (congenital) (of):
glucose-galactose
lactose
sucrose-isomaltose

271.4 Renal glycosuria
Renal diabetes

271.8 Other specified disorders of carbohydrate transport and metabolism
Essential benign pentosuria
Fucosidosis
Glycolic aciduria
Hyperoxaluria (primary)
Mannosidosis
Oxalosis
Xylosuria
Xylulosuria

271.9 Unspecified disorder of carbohydrate transport and metabolism

4th 272 Disorders of lipoid metabolism

Excludes *localized cerebral lipidoses (330.1)*

272.0 Pure hypercholesterolemia
E78.0 Pure hypercholesterolemia
Familial hypercholesterolemia
Fredrickson Type IIa hyperlipoproteinemia
Hyperbetalipoproteinemia
Hyperlipidemia, Group A
Low-density-lipoid-type [LDL] hyperlipoproteinemia
Layman's: *Raised total cholesterol, exhibiting significantly high LDL, but HDL and triglycerides at normal levels.*

272.1 Pure hyperglyceridemia
E78.1 Pure hyperglyceridemia
Endogenous hyperglyceridemia
Fredrickson Type IV hyperlipoproteinemia
Hyperlipidemia, Group B
Hyperprebetalipoproteinemia
Hypertriglyceridemia, essential
Very-low-density-lipoid-type [VLDL] hyperlipoproteinemia

272.2 Mixed hyperlipidemia
E78.2 Mixed hyperlipidemia
Broad- or floating-betalipoproteinemia
Combined hyperlipidemia
Elevated cholesterol with elevated triglycerides NEC
Fredrickson Type IIb or III hyperlipoproteinemia
Hypercholesterolemia with endogenous hyperglyceridemia
Hyperbetalipoproteinemia with prebetalipoproteinemia
Tubo-eruptive xanthoma
Xanthoma tuberosum

272.3 Hyperchylomicronemia
Bürger-Grütz syndrome
Fredrickson type I or V hyperlipoproteinemia
Hyperlipidemia, Group D
Mixed hyperglyceridemia

272.4 Other and unspecified hyperlipidemia
E78.4 Other hyperlipidemia
Alpha-lipoproteinemia
~~Combined hyperlipidemia~~
Hyperlipidemia NOS
Hyperlipoproteinemia NOS
Layman's: *When it is presumed that a patient is experiencing abnormally high levels of fats and/or cholesterol, but the actual levels are still undetermined, code 272.4 is more appropriate than the more specific codes in the 272.x range.*

272.5 Lipoprotein deficiencies
Abetalipoproteinemia
Bassen-Kornzweig syndrome
High-density lipoid deficiency
Hypoalphalipoproteinemia
Hypobetalipoproteinemia (familial)

272.6 Lipodystrophy
Barraquer-Simons disease
Progressive lipodystrophy
Use additional E code to identify cause, if iatrogenic
Excludes *intestinal lipodystrophy (040.2)*

272.7 Lipidoses
Chemically induced lipidosis
Disease:
Anderson's
Fabry's
Gaucher's
I cell [mucolipidosis I]
lipoid storage NOS
Niemann-Pick
pseudo-Hurler's or mucolipidosis III
triglyceride storage, Type I or II
Wolman's or triglyceride storage, Type III
Mucolipidosis II
Primary familial xanthomatosis
Excludes *cerebral lipidoses (330.1)*
Tay-Sachs disease (330.1)

272.8 Other disorders of lipoid metabolism
Hoffa's disease or liposynovitis prepatellaris
Launois-Bensaude's lipomatosis
Lipoid dermatoarthritis

272.9 Unspecified disorder of lipoid metabolism
E78.9 Disorder of lipoprotein metabolism, unspecified

4th 273 Disorders of plasma protein metabolism

Excludes *agammaglobulinemia and hypogammaglobulinemia (279.0-279.2)*
coagulation defects (286.0-286.9)
hereditary hemolytic anemias (282.0-282.9)

273.0 Polyclonal hypergammaglobulinemia
Hypergammaglobulinemic purpura:
benign primary
Waldenström's

271 – 273.0

273.1 **Monoclonal paraproteinemia**
D47.2 Monoclonal gammopathy
Benign monoclonal hypergammaglobulinemia [BMH]
Monoclonal gammopathy:
NOS
associated with lymphoplasmacytic dyscrasias
benign
Paraproteinemia:
benign (familial)
secondary to malignant or inflammatory disease

273.2 **Other paraproteinemias**
Cryoglobulinemic:
purpura
vasculitis
Mixed cryoglobulinemia

273.3 **Macroglobulinemia**
Macroglobulinemia (idiopathic) (primary)
Waldenström's macroglobulinemia

273.4 **Alpha-1-antitrypsin deficiency**
AAT deficiency

273.8 **Other disorders of plasma protein metabolism**
Abnormality of transport protein
Bisalbuminemia

273.9 **Unspecified disorder of plasma protein metabolism**

4th 274 **Gout**
Excludes *lead gout (984.0-984.9)*

5th 274.0 **Gouty arthropathy**

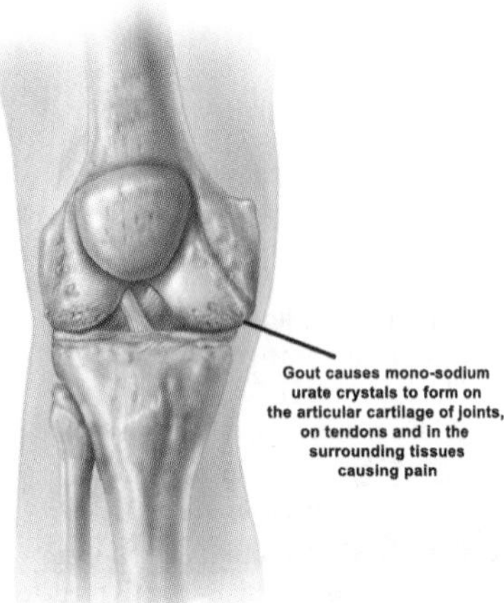

© 2008 Fairman Studios, LLC. All Rights Reserved.

● 274.00 **Gouty arthropathy, unspecified**

● 274.01 **Acute gouty arthropathy**
Acute gout
Gout attack
Gout flare
Podagra

● 274.02 **Chronic gouty arthropathy without mention of tophus (tophi)**
Chronic gout

● 274.03 **Chronic gouty arthropathy with tophus (tophi)**
Chronic tophaceous gout
Gout with tophi NOS

5th 274.1 **Gouty nephropathy**

274.10 **Gouty nephropathy, unspecified**

274.11 **Uric acid nephrolithiasis**

274.19 **Other**

5th 274.8 **Gout with other specified manifestations**

274.81 **Gouty tophi of ear**

274.82 **Gouty tophi of other sites**
Gouty tophi of heart
Excludes *gout with tophi NOS (274.03)*
gouty arthropathy with tophi (274.03)

274.89 **Other**
Use additional code to identify manifestations, as:
gouty:
iritis (364.11)
neuritis (357.4)

274.9 **Gout, unspecified**
M10.9 Gout, unspecified

4th 275 **Disorders of mineral metabolism**
Excludes *abnormal findings without manifest disease (790.0-796.9)*

275.0 **Disorders of iron metabolism**
Bronzed diabetes
Hemochromatosis
Pigmentary cirrhosis (of liver)
Excludes *anemia:*
iron deficiency (280.0-280.9)
sideroblastic (285.0)

275.1 **Disorders of copper metabolism**
Hepatolenticular degeneration
Wilson's disease

275.2 **Disorders of magnesium metabolism**
Hypermagnesemia
Hypomagnesemia

275.3 **Disorders of phosphorus metabolism**
Familial hypophosphatemia
Hypophosphatasia
Vitamin D-resistant:
osteomalacia
rickets

5th 275.4 **Disorders of calcium metabolism**
Excludes *hungry bone syndrome (275.5)*
parathyroid disorders (252.00-252.9)
vitamin D deficiency (268.0-268.9)

275.40 **Unspecified disorder of calcium metabolism**

275.41 **Hypocalcemia**

275.42 **Hypercalcemia**
E83.52 Hypercalcemia

275.49 **Other disorders of calcium metabolism**
Nephrocalcinosis
Pseudohypoparathyroidism
Pseudopseudohypoparathyroidism

275.5 **Hungry bone syndrome**

275.8 **Other specified disorders of mineral metabolism**

275.9 **Unspecified disorder of mineral metabolism**

4th 276 **Disorders of fluid, electrolyte, and acid-base balance**
Excludes *diabetes insipidus (253.5)*
familial periodic paralysis (359.3)

276.0 **Hyperosmolality and/or hypernatremia**
Sodium [Na] excess
Sodium [Na] overload

276.1 **Hyposmolality and/or hyponatremia**
E87.1 Hypo-osmolality and hyponatremia
Sodium [Na] deficiency

276.2 **Acidosis**
Acidosis:
NOS
lactic
metabolic
respiratory
Excludes *diabetic acidosis (249.1, 250.1)*

276.3 Alkalosis
Alkalosis:
NOS
metabolic
respiratory

276.4 Mixed acid-base balance disorder
Hypercapnia with mixed acid-base disorder

5th **276.5 Volume depletion**
Excludes *hypovolemic shock:*
postoperative (998.0)
traumatic (958.4)

Layman's: *A patient can be dehydrated (deficient in intracellular water volume) without being hypovolemic (deficient in extracellular blood volume) as the body will pull fluid from the cells in an attempt to maintain homeostasis. This, in turn, can cause hypovolemia as the fluid balance is upset. Hypovolemia can also be caused by more direct means of blood volume depletion such as hemorrhage, taking blood pressure medication and vomiting.*

276.50 Volume depletion, unspecified
E86.9 Volume depletion, unspecified

276.51 Dehydration

276.52 Hypovolemia
Depletion of volume of plasma

276.6 Fluid overload
Fluid retention
Excludes *ascites (789.51-789.59)*
localized edema (782.3)

276.7 Hyperpotassemia
E87.5 Hyperkalemia
Hyperkalemia
Potassium [K]:
excess
intoxication
overload

276.8 Hypopotassemia
E87.6 Hypokalemia
Hypokalemia
Potassium [K] deficiency

276.9 Electrolyte and fluid disorders not elsewhere classified
E87.8 Other disorders of electrolyte and fluid balance, not elsewhere classified
Electrolyte imbalance
Hyperchloremia
Hypochloremia
Excludes *electrolyte imbalance:*
associated with hyperemesis gravidarum (643.1)
complicating labor and delivery (669.0)
following abortion and ectopic or molar pregnancy (634-638 with .4, 639.4)

4th **277 Other and unspecified disorders of metabolism**

5th **277.0 Cystic fibrosis**
Fibrocystic disease of the pancreas
Mucoviscidosis

277.00 Without mention of meconium ileus
Cystic fibrosis NOS

277.01 With meconium ileus N
Meconium:
ileus (of newborn)
obstruction of intestine in mucoviscidosis

277.02 With pulmonary manifestations
Cystic fibrosis with pulmonary exacerbation
Use additional code to identify any infectious organism present, such as:
pseudomonas (041.7)

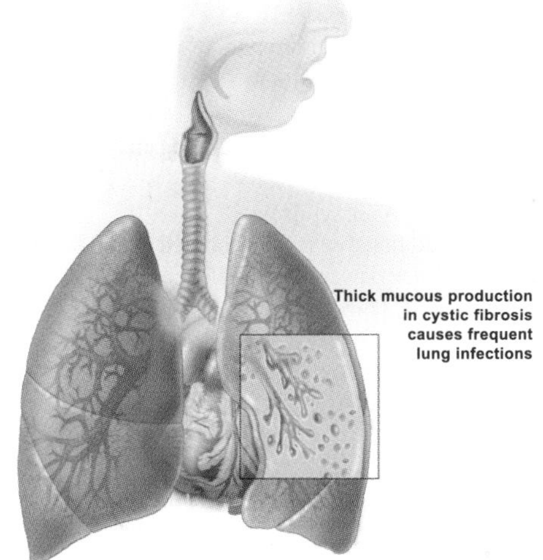

© 2008 Fairman Studios, LLC. All Rights Reserved.

277.03 With gastrointestinal manifestations
Excludes *with meconium ileus (277.01)*

277.09 With other manifestations

277.1 Disorders of porphyrin metabolism
Hematoporphyria
Hematoporphyrinuria
Hereditary coproporphyria
Porphyria
Porphyrinuria
Protocoproporphyria
Protoporphyria
Pyrroloporphyria

277.2 Other disorders of purine and pyrimidine metabolism
Hypoxanthine-guanine-phosphoribosyltransferase deficiency [HG-PRT deficiency]
Lesch-Nyhan syndrome
Xanthinuria
Excludes *gout (274.00-274.9)*
orotic aciduric anemia (281.4)

5th **277.3 Amyloidosis**

277.30 Amyloidosis, unspecified
Amyloidosis NOS

277.31 Familial Mediterranean fever
Benign paroxysmal peritonitis
Hereditary amyloid nephropathy
Periodic familial polyserositis
Recurrent polyserositis

277.39 Other amyloidosis
Hereditary cardiac amyloidosis
Inherited systemic amyloidosis
Neuropathic (Portuguese) (Swiss) amyloidosis
Secondary amyloidosis

277.4 Disorders of bilirubin excretion
Hyperbilirubinemia:
congenital
constitutional
Syndrome:
Crigler-Najjar
Dubin-Johnson
Gilbert's
Rotor's
Excludes *hyperbilirubinemias specific to the perinatal period (774.0-774.7)*

277.5 Mucopolysaccharidosis
Gargoylism
Hunter's syndrome
Hurler's syndrome
Lipochondrodystrophy
Maroteaux-Lamy syndrome
Morquio-Brailsford disease
Osteochondrodystrophy
Sanfilippo's syndrome
Scheie's syndrome

277.6 Other deficiencies of circulating enzymes
Hereditary angioedema

277.7 Dysmetabolic syndrome X
Use additional code for associated manifestation, such as:
cardiovascular disease (414.00-414.07)
obesity (278.00-278.01)

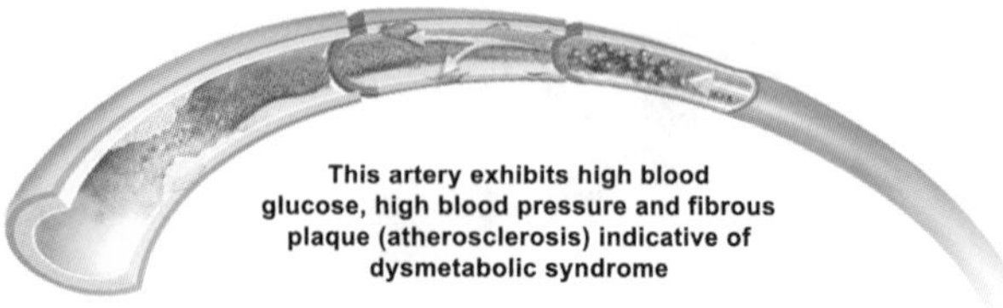
This artery exhibits high blood glucose, high blood pressure and fibrous plaque (atherosclerosis) indicative of dysmetabolic syndrome

© 2006 Anatomical Chart Company

5th **277.8 Other specified disorders of metabolism**

277.81 Primary carnitine deficiency

277.82 Carnitine deficiency due to inborn errors of metabolism

277.83 Iatrogenic carnitine deficiency
Carnitine deficiency due to:
hemodialysis
valproic acid therapy

277.84 Other secondary carnitine deficiency

277.85 Disorders of fatty acid oxidation
Carnitine palmitoyltransferase deficiencies (CPT1, CPT2)
Glutaric aciduria type II (type IIA, IIB, IIC)
Long chain 3-hydroxyacyl CoA dehydrogenase deficiency (LCHAD)
Long chain/very long chain acyl CoA dehydrogenase deficiency (LCAD, VLCAD)
Medium chain acyl CoA dehydrogenase deficiency (MCAD)
Short chain acyl CoA dehydrogenase deficiency (SCAD)
Excludes *primary carnitine deficiency (277.81)*

277.86 Peroxisomal disorders
Adrenomyeloneuropathy
Neonatal adrenoleukodystrophy
Rhizomelic chrondrodysplasia punctata
X-linked adrenoleukodystrophy
Zellweger syndrome
Excludes *infantile Refsum disease (356.3)*

277.87 Disorders of mitochondrial metabolism
Kearns-Sayre syndrome
Mitochondrial Encephalopathy, Lactic Acidosis and Stroke-like episodes (MELAS syndrome)
Mitochondrial Neurogastrointestinal Encephalopathy syndrome (MNGIE)
Myoclonus with Epilepsy and Ragged Red Fibers (MERRF syndrome)
Neuropathy, Ataxia and Retinitis Pigmentosa (NARP Syndrome)
Use additional code for associated conditions
Excludes *disorders of pyruvate metabolism (271.8)*
Leber's optic atrophy (377.16)
Leigh's subacute necrotizing encephalopathy (330.8)
Reye's syndrome (331.81)

● **277.88 Tumor lysis syndrome**
Spontaneous tumor lysis syndrome
Tumor lysis syndrome following antineoplastic drug therapy
Use additional E code to identify cause, if drug-induced

Rationale: *Tumor lysis syndrome is a very serious and sometimes life-threatening complication of cancer therapy. Prior to 2010, it was not specifically indexed in ICD-9-CM. Advice given in the American Hospital Association's Coding Clinic for ICD-9-CM. (Nov/Dec 1985, page 1) advised coders to use code 584.8, "Acute renal failure with other specified pathological lesion in kidney," along with external cause code E933.1, "Adverse effects of antineoplastic and immunosuppressive drugs," if the tumor lysis syndrome is post-chemotherapy.*

Recent literature shows that tumor lysis syndrome is a group of metabolic complications that can occur after treatment of cancer, usually lymphomas and leukemias, and sometimes even without treatment. These complications are caused by the breakdown products of dying cancer cells and include hyperkalemia, hyperphosphatemia, hyperuricemia, hypocalcemia and acute renal failure. Furthermore, pretreatment spontaneous tumor lysis syndrome is associated with acute renal failure due to uric acid nephropathy prior to the institution of chemotherapy. The important distinction between this syndrome and the post-chemotherapy syndrome is that spontaneous tumor lysis syndrome is not associated with hyperphosphatemia.

277.89 Other specified disorders of metabolism
Hand-Schüller-Christian disease
Histiocytosis (acute) (chronic)
Histiocytosis X (chronic)
Excludes *histiocytosis:*
acute differentiated progressive (202.5)
X, acute (progressive) (202.5)

277.9 Unspecified disorder of metabolism
Enzymopathy NOS

4th **278 Overweight, obesity and other hyperalimentation**

Excludes *hyperalimentation NOS (783.6)*
poisoning by vitamins NOS (963.5)
polyphagia (783.6)

5th **278.0 Overweight and obesity**

Use additional code to identify Body Mass Index (BMI), if known (V85.0-V85.54)

Excludes *adiposogenital dystrophy (253.8)*
obesity of endocrine origin NOS (259.9)

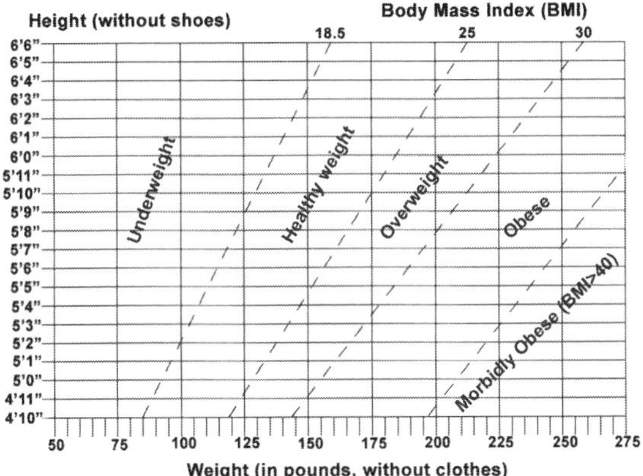

278.00 Obesity, unspecified
Obesity NOS

278.01 Morbid obesity
Severe obesity

278.02 Overweight

278.1 Localized adiposity
Fat pad

278.2 Hypervitaminosis A

278.3 Hypercarotinemia

278.4 Hypervitaminosis D

278.8 Other hyperalimentation

4th **279 Disorders involving the immune mechanism**

5th **279.0 Deficiency of humoral immunity**

279.00 Hypogammaglobulinemia, unspecified
Agammaglobulinemia NOS

279.01 Selective IgA immunodeficiency

279.02 Selective IgM immunodeficiency

279.03 Other selective immunoglobulin deficiencies
Selective deficiency of IgG

279.04 Congenital hypogammaglobulinemia
Agammaglobulinemia:
Bruton's type
X-linked

279.05 Immunodeficiency with increased IgM
Immunodeficiency with hyper-IgM:
autosomal recessive
X-linked

279.06 Common variable immunodeficiency
Dysgammaglobulinemia (acquired) (congenital) (primary)
Hypogammaglobulinemia:
acquired primary
congenital non-sex-linked
sporadic

Layman's: *CVID has come to be viewed as an overused (or even "trashcan") diagnosis. While it is valid if adequate testing of immuneglobulin levels are performed, it should not be assumed that any immune deficiency is CVID, rather it can be used as a diagnosis of exclusion when other possibilities are ruled out.*

279.09 Other
Transient hypogammaglobulinemia of infancy

5th **279.1 Deficiency of cell-mediated immunity**

279.10 Immunodeficiency with predominant T-cell defect, unspecified

279.11 DiGeorge's syndrome
Pharyngeal pouch syndrome
Thymic hypoplasia

279.12 Wiskott-Aldrich syndrome

279.13 Nezelof's syndrome
Cellular immunodeficiency with abnormal immunoglobulin deficiency

279.19 Other
Excludes *ataxia-telangiectasia (334.8)*

279.2 Combined immunity deficiency
Agammaglobulinemia:
autosomal recessive
Swiss-type
X-linked recessive
Severe combined immunodeficiency [SCID]
Thymic:
alymphoplasia
aplasia or dysplasia with immunodeficiency
Excludes *thymic hypoplasia (279.11)*

279.3 Unspecified immunity deficiency

5th **279.4 Autoimmune disease, not elsewhere classified**
~~Autoimmune disease NOS~~
Excludes *transplant failure or rejection (996.80-996.89)*

● **279.41 Autoimmune lymphoproliferative syndrome**
ALPS

Rationale: *Autoimmune lymphoproliferative syndrome (ALPS) is a rare disease that affects both children and adults. It has only recently been understood. It is caused by a genetic defect which results in lymphocytes not dying off as they should, resulting in an overabundance of lymphocytes in many tissues. Clinical features of the syndrome present in early childhood or even at birth and include chronic multifocal lymphadenopathy, splenomegaly, autoimmune hemolytic anemia and often other immune cytopenias. Though the majority of patients improve with steroid therapy, and generally, autoimmune complications lessen in severity as a patient gets older, they have a greater risk of developing lymphoma.*

● **279.49 Autoimmune disease, not elsewhere classified**
Autoimmune disease NOS

5th **279.5 Graft-versus-host disease**
Code first underlying cause, such as:
complication of blood transfusion (999.89)
complication of transplanted organ ~~(bone marrow)~~ (996.80-996.89)
Use additional code to identify associated manifestations, such as:
desquamative dermatitis (695.89)
diarrhea (787.91)
elevated bilirubin (782.4)
hair loss (704.09)

279.50 Graft-versus-host disease, unspecified

279.51 Acute graft-versus-host disease

279.52 Chronic graft-versus-host disease

279.53 Acute on chronic graft-versus-host disease

279.8 Other specified disorders involving the immune mechanism
Single complement [C1-C9] deficiency or dysfunction

279.9 Unspecified disorder of immune mechanism

278 – 279.9

4. DISEASES OF THE BLOOD AND BLOOD-FORMING ORGANS (280-289)

4th 280 Iron deficiency anemias

Includes anemia:
- asiderotic
- hypochromic-microcytic
- sideropenic

Excludes *familial microcytic anemia (282.49)*

280.0 Secondary to blood loss (chronic)

D50.0 Iron deficiency anemia secondary to blood loss (chronic)

Normocytic anemia due to blood loss

Excludes *acute posthemorrhagic anemia (285.1)*

280.1 Secondary to inadequate dietary iron intake

280.8 Other specified iron deficiency anemias

Paterson-Kelly syndrome
Plummer-Vinson syndrome
Sideropenic dysphagia

280.9 Iron deficiency anemia, unspecified

D50.9 Iron deficiency anemia, unspecified

Anemia:
- achlorhydric
- chlorotic
- idiopathic hypochromic
- iron [Fe] deficiency NOS

4th 281 Other deficiency anemias

281.0 Pernicious anemia

D51.0 Vitamin B_{12} deficiency anemia due to intrinsic factor deficiency

Anemia:
- Addison's
- Biermer's
- congenital pernicious

Congenital intrinsic factor [Castle's] deficiency

Excludes *combined system disease without mention of anemia (266.2)*
subacute degeneration of spinal cord without mention of anemia (266.2)

Layman's: *Pernicious anemia is differentiated from other forms of B_{12} deficiency and megaloblastic anemias in that it is specifically due to the absence of intrinsic factor which assists in the absorption of B_{12} that is necessary for blood cell synthesis.*

281.1 Other vitamin B_{12} deficiency anemia

D51.1 Vitamin B_{12} deficiency anemia due to selective vitamin B_{12} malabsorption with proteinuria
D51.3 Other dietary vitamin B_{12} deficiency anemia
D51.8 Other vitamin B_{12} deficiency anemias

Anemia:
- vegan's
- vitamin B_{12} deficiency (dietary)
- due to selective vitamin B_{12} malabsorption with proteinuria

Syndrome:
- Imerslund's
- Imerslund-Gräsbeck

Excludes *combined system disease without mention of anemia (266.2)*
subacute degeneration of spinal cord without mention of anemia (266.2)

281.2 Folate-deficiency anemia

Congenital folate malabsorption
Folate or folic acid deficiency anemia:
- NOS
- dietary
- drug-induced

Goat's milk anemia
Nutritional megaloblastic anemia (of infancy)
Use additional E code to identify drug

281.3 Other specified megaloblastic anemias, not elsewhere classified

Combined B_{12} and folate-deficiency anemia
Refractory megaloblastic anemia

281.4 Protein-deficiency anemia

Amino-acid-deficiency anemia

281.8 Anemia associated with other specified nutritional deficiency

Scorbutic anemia

281.9 Unspecified deficiency anemia

D53.9 Nutritional anemia, unspecified

Anemia:
- dimorphic
- macrocytic
- megaloblastic NOS
- nutritional NOS
- simple chronic

4th 282 Hereditary hemolytic anemias

282.0 Hereditary spherocytosis

Acholuric (familial) jaundice
Congenital hemolytic anemia (spherocytic)
Congenital spherocytosis
Minkowski-Chauffard syndrome
Spherocytosis (familial)

Excludes *hemolytic anemia of newborn (773.0-773.5)*

282.1 Hereditary elliptocytosis

Elliptocytosis (congenital)
Ovalocytosis (congenital) (hereditary)

282.2 Anemias due to disorders of glutathione metabolism

Anemia:
- 6-phosphogluconic dehydrogenase deficiency
- enzyme deficiency, drug-induced
- erythrocytic glutathione deficiency
- glucose-6-phosphate dehydrogenase [G-6-PD] deficiency
- glutathione-reductase deficiency
- hemolytic nonspherocytic (hereditary), type I

Disorder of pentose phosphate pathway
Favism

282.3 Other hemolytic anemias due to enzyme deficiency

Anemia:
- hemolytic nonspherocytic (hereditary), type II
- hexokinase deficiency
- pyruvate kinase [PK] deficiency
- triosephosphate isomerase deficiency

5th 282.4 Thalassemias

Excludes *sickle-cell:*
disease (282.60-282.69)
trait (282.5)

282.41 Sickle-cell thalassemia without crisis

Sickle-cell thalassemia NOS
Thalassemia Hb-S disease without crisis

282.42 Sickle-cell thalassemia with crisis

Sickle-cell thalassemia with vaso-occlusive pain
Thalassemia Hb-S disease with crisis
Use additional code for type of crisis, such as:
- acute chest syndrome (517.3)
- splenic sequestration (289.52)

282.49 **Other thalassemia**
Cooley's anemia
Hb-Bart's disease
Hereditary leptocytosis
Mediterranean anemia (with other hemoglobinopathy)
Microdrepanocytosis
Thalassemia (alpha) (beta) (intermedia) (major) (minima) (minor) (mixed) (trait) (with other hemoglobinopathy)
Thalassemia NOS

282.5 Sickle-cell trait
Hb-AS genotype
Hemoglobin S [Hb-S] trait
Heterozygous:
Hb-S
hemoglobin S
Excludes *that with other hemoglobinopathy (282.60-282.69)*
that with thalassemia (282.49)

5th **282.6 Sickle-cell disease**
Sickle-cell anemia
Excludes *sickle-cell thalassemia (282.41-282.42)*
sickle-cell trait (282.5)

282.60 Sickle-cell disease, unspecified
Sickle-cell anemia NOS

282.61 Hb-SS disease without crisis

282.62 Hb-SS disease with crisis
Hb-SS disease with vaso-occlusive pain
Sickle-cell crisis NOS
Use additional code for type of crisis, such as:
acute chest syndrome (517.3)
splenic sequestration (289.52)

282.63 Sickle-cell/Hb-C disease without crisis
Hb-S/Hb-C disease without crisis

282.64 Sickle-cell/HB-C disease with crisis
Hb-S/Hb-C disease with crisis
Sickle-cell/Hb-C disease with vaso-occlusive pain
Use additional code for types of crisis, such as:
acute chest syndrome (517.3)
splenic sequestration (289.52)

282.68 Other sickle-cell disease without crisis
Hb-S/Hb-D disease without crisis
Hb-S/Hb-E disease without crisis
Sickle-cell/Hb-D disease without crisis
Sickle-cell/Hb-E disease without crisis

282.69 Other sickle-cell disease with crisis
Hb-S/Hb-D disease with crisis
Hb-S/Hb-E disease with crisis
Sickle-cell/Hb-D disease with crisis
Sickle-cell/Hb-E disease with crisis
Other sickle-cell disease with vaso-occlusive pain
Use additional code for type of crisis, such as:
acute chest syndrome (517.3)
splenic sequestration (289.52)

282.7 Other hemoglobinopathies
Abnormal hemoglobin NOS
Congenital Heinz-body anemia
Disease:
hemoglobin C [Hb-C]
hemoglobin D [Hb-D]
hemoglobin E [Hb-E]
hemoglobin Zurich [Hb-Zurich]
Hemoglobinopathy NOS
Hereditary persistence of fetal hemoglobin [HPFH]
Unstable hemoglobin hemolytic disease
Excludes *familial polycythemia (289.6)*
hemoglobin M [Hb-M] disease (289.7)
high-oxygen-affinity hemoglobin (289.0)

282.8 Other specified hereditary hemolytic anemias
Stomatocytosis

282.9 Hereditary hemolytic anemia, unspecified
Hereditary hemolytic anemia NOS

4th **283 Acquired hemolytic anemias**

283.0 Autoimmune hemolytic anemias
Autoimmune hemolytic disease (cold type) (warm type)
Chronic cold hemagglutinin disease
Cold agglutinin disease or hemoglobinuria
Hemolytic anemia:
cold type (secondary) (symptomatic)
drug-induced
warm type (secondary) (symptomatic)
Use additional E code to identify cause, if drug-induced
Excludes *Evans' syndrome (287.32)*
hemolytic disease of newborn (773.0-773.5)

5th **283.1 Non-autoimmune hemolytic anemias**

283.10 Non-autoimmune hemolytic anemia, unspecified

283.11 Hemolytic-uremic syndrome

283.19 Other non-autoimmune hemolytic anemias
Hemolytic anemia:
mechanical
microangiopathic
toxic
Use additional E code to identify cause

283.2 Hemoglobinuria due to hemolysis from external causes
Acute intravascular hemolysis
Hemoglobinuria:
from exertion
march
paroxysmal (cold) (nocturnal)
due to other hemolysis
Marchiafava-Micheli syndrome
Use additional E code to identify cause

283.9 Acquired hemolytic anemia, unspecified
Acquired hemolytic anemia NOS
Chronic idiopathic hemolytic anemia

4th **284 Aplastic anemia and other bone marrow failure syndromes**

5th **284.0 Constitutional aplastic anemia**

284.01 Constitutional red blood cell aplasia
Aplasia, (pure) red cell:
congenital
of infants
primary
Blackfan-Diamond syndrome
Familial hypoplastic anemia

284.09 Other constitutional aplastic anemia
Fanconi's anemia
Pancytopenia with malformations

284.1 Pancytopenia
Excludes *pancytopenia (due to) (with):*
aplastic anemia NOS (284.9)
bone marrow infiltration (284.2)
constitutional red blood cell aplasia (284.01)
drug induced (284.89)
hairy cell leukemia (202.4)
human immunodeficiency virus disease (042)
leukoerythroblastic anemia (284.2)
malformations (284.09)
myelodysplastic syndromes (238.72-238.75)
myeloproliferative disease (238.79)
other constitutional aplastic anemia (284.09)

284.2 Myelophthisis
Leukoerythroblastic anemia
Myelophthisic anemia
Code first the underlying disorder, such as:
malignant neoplasm of breast (174.0-174.9, 175.0-175.9)
tuberculosis (015.0-015.9)
Excludes *idiopathic myelofibrosis (238.76)*
myelofibrosis NOS (289.83)
myelofibrosis with myeloid metaplasia (238.76)
primary myelofibrosis (238.76)
secondary myelofibrosis (289.83)

5th **284.8 Other specified aplastic anemias**

284.81 Red cell aplasia (acquired) (adult) (with thymoma)
Red cell aplasia NOS

284.89 Other specified aplastic anemias
D61.89 Other specified aplastic anemias and other bone marrow failure syndromes
Aplastic anemia (due to):
chronic systemic disease
drugs
infection
radiation
toxic (paralytic)
Use additional E code to identify cause

284.9 Aplastic anemia, unspecified
Anemia:
aplastic (idiopathic) NOS
aregenerative
hypoplastic NOS
nonregenerative
Medullary hypoplasia
Excludes *refractory anemia (238.72)*

4th **285 Other and unspecified anemias**

285.0 Sideroblastic anemia
Anemia:
hypochromic with iron loading
sideroachrestic
sideroblastic:
acquired
congenital
hereditary
primary
secondary (drug-induced) (due to disease)
sex-linked hypochromic
vitamin B_6-responsive
Pyridoxine-responsive (hypochromic) anemia
Use additional E code to identify cause, if drug-induced
Excludes *refractory sideroblastic anemia (238.72)*

285.1 Acute posthemorrhagic anemia
Anemia due to acute blood loss
Excludes *anemia due to chronic blood loss (280.0)*
blood loss anemia NOS (280.0)

ICD-9-CM Official Guidelines (Chapter 4):

*a. **Anemia of chronic disease***

Subcategory 285.2, Anemia in chronic illness, has codes for anemia in chronic kidney disease, code 285.21; anemia in neoplastic disease, code 285.22; and anemia in other chronic illness, code 285.29. These codes can be used as the principal/first listed code if the reason for the encounter is to treat the anemia. They may also be used as secondary codes if treatment of the anemia is a component of an encounter, but not the primary reason for the encounter. When using a code from subcategory 285 it is also necessary to use the code for the chronic condition causing the anemia.

*1) **Anemia in chronic kidney disease***

When assigning code 285.21, Anemia in chronic kidney disease, it is also necessary to assign a code from category 585, Chronic kidney disease, to indicate the stage of chronic kidney disease.

See I.C.10.a. Chronic kidney disease (CKD).

*2) **Anemia in neoplastic disease***

When assigning code 285.22, Anemia in neoplastic disease, it is also necessary to assign the neoplasm code that is responsible for the anemia. Code 285.22 is for use for anemia that is due to the malignancy, not for anemia due to antineoplastic chemotherapy drugs, which is an adverse effect.

See I.C.2.c.1 Anemia associated with malignancy. See I.C.2.c.2 Anemia associated with chemotherapy, immunotherapy and radiation therapy. See I.C.17.e.1. Adverse effects.

5th **285.2 Anemia of chronic disease**
Anemia in (due to) (with) chronic illness

285.21 Anemia in chronic kidney disease
D63.1 Anemia in chronic kidney disease
Anemia in end stage renal disease
Erythropoietin-resistant anemia (EPO resistant anemia)

285.22 Anemia in neoplastic disease
D63.0 Anemia in neoplastic disease
Excludes *anemia due to antineoplastic chemotherapy (285.3)*

285.29 Anemia of other chronic disease
D63.8 Anemia in other chronic diseases classified elsewhere
Anemia in other chronic illness

● **285.3 Antineoplastic chemotherapy induced anemia**
Anemia due to antineoplastic chemotherapy
Excludes *anemia due to drug NEC – code to type of anemia*
anemia in neoplastic disease (285.22)
aplastic anemia due to antineoplastic chemotherapy (284.89)

Rationale: *Antineoplastic chemotherapy induced anemia is anemia acquired secondary to the administration of antineoplastic chemotherapy. Cancer and its treatment can interfere with the supply of red blood cells by inhibiting the production of bone marrow. This type of anemia is only rarely a hemolytic process and is not truly an aplastic process, aplasia implying that the bone marrow is "wiped out". Antineoplastic chemotherapy induced changes are usually short-term and they do not commonly reduce the marrow cellularity to a point of aplasia. This type of anemia can be diagnosed with a blood test which measures the volume of red blood cells in whole blood.*

It is estimated that chemotherapy-induced anemia is one of the most common side effects caused by treatment with antineoplastic chemotherapy, affecting between 20%-60% of cancer patients. Patients afflicted with antineoplastic chemotherapy induced anemia often have a lower quality of life resulting in fatigue and an inability to perform everyday activities including work, social and leisure activities.

Prior to 2010, there were no ICD-9-CM codes to differentiate antineoplastic chemotherapy induced anemia from other anemias. This void lead to a lack of specificity in coding that causes limitations in the specificity of the reporting of both chemotherapy induced anemia and other anemia.

285.8 Other specified anemias
D64.8 Other specified anemias
Anemia:
dyserythropoietic (congenital)
dyshematopoietic (congenital)
von Jaksch's
Infantile pseudoleukemia

285.9 Anemia, unspecified

D64.9 Anemia, unspecified

Anemia:
- NOS
- essential
- normocytic, not due to blood loss
- profound
- progressive
- secondary

Oligocythemia

Excludes *anemia (due to):*
blood loss:
acute (285.1)
chronic or unspecified (280.0)
iron deficiency (280.0-280.9)

4th 286 Coagulation defects

286.0 Congenital factor VIII disorder

Antihemophilic globulin [AHG] deficiency
Factor VIII (functional) deficiency
Hemophilia:
- NOS
- A
- classical
- familial
- hereditary

Subhemophilia

Excludes *factor VIII deficiency with vascular defect (286.4)*

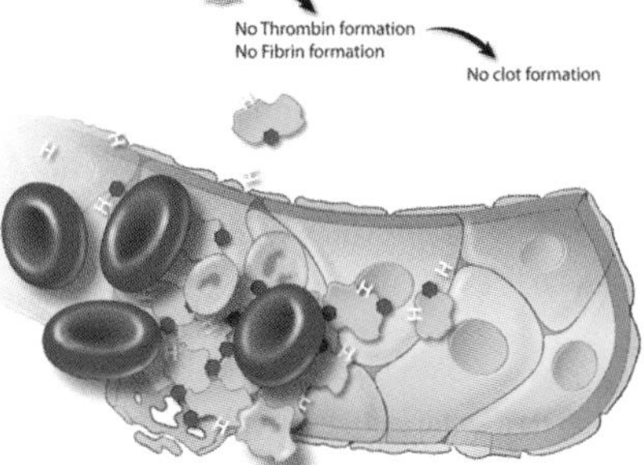

The lack of clotting factor VIII causes an inability for injuries to clot on their own resulting in increased blood loss, easy and extensive bruising, internal bleeding and swelling

© 2008 Fairman Studios, LLC. All Rights Reserved.

286.1 Congenital factor IX disorder

Christmas disease
Deficiency:
- factor IX (functional)
- plasma thromboplastin component [PTC]

Hemophilia B

286.2 Congenital factor XI deficiency

Hemophilia C
Plasma thromboplastin antecedent [PTA] deficiency
Rosenthal's disease

286.3 Congenital deficiency of other clotting factors

Congenital afibrinogenemia
Deficiency:
- AC globulin factor:
  - I [fibrinogen]
  - II [prothrombin]
  - V [labile]
  - VII [stable]
  - X [Stuart-Prower]
  - XII [Hageman]
  - XIII [fibrin stabilizing]
- Laki-Lorand factor
- proaccelerin

Disease:
- Owren's
- Stuart-Prower

Dysfibrinogenemia (congenital)
Dysprothrombinemia (constitutional)
Hypoproconvertinemia
Hypoprothrombinemia (hereditary)
Parahemophilia

286.4 von Willebrand's disease

Angiohemophilia (A) (B)
Constitutional thrombopathy
Factor VIII deficiency with vascular defect
Pseudohemophilia type B
Vascular hemophilia
von Willebrand's (-Jürgens') disease

Excludes *factor VIII deficiency:*
NOS (286.0)
with functional defect (286.0)
hereditary capillary fragility (287.8)

286.5 Hemorrhagic disorder due to intrinsic circulating anticoagulants

D68.31 Hemorrhagic disorder due to intrinsic circulating anticoagulants

Antithrombinemia
Antithromboplastinemia
Antithromboplastino-genemia
Hyperheparinemia
Increase in:
- anti-VIIIa
- anti-IXa
- anti-Xa
- anti-XIa
- antithrombin

Secondary hemophilia
Systemic lupus erythematosus [SLE] inhibitor

286.6 Defibrination syndrome

Afibrinogenemia, acquired
Consumption coagulopathy
Diffuse or disseminated intravascular coagulation [DIC syndrome]
Fibrinolytic hemorrhage, acquired
Hemorrhagic fibrinogenolysis
Pathologic fibrinolysis
Purpura:
- fibrinolytic
- fulminans

Excludes *disseminated intravascular coagulation in newborn (776.2)*
that complicating:
abortion (634-638 with .1, 639.1)
pregnancy or the puerperium (641.3, 666.3)

285.9 – 286.6

286.7 Acquired coagulation factor deficiency
Deficiency of coagulation factor due to:
liver disease
vitamin K deficiency
Hypoprothrombinemia, acquired
Use additional E-code to identify cause, if drug-induced
Excludes *vitamin K deficiency of newborn (776.0)*

286.9 Other and unspecified coagulation defects
D68.8 Other specified coagulation defects
D68.9 Coagulation defect, unspecified
Defective coagulation NOS
Deficiency, coagulation factor NOS
Delay, coagulation
Disorder:
coagulation
hemostasis
Excludes *abnormal coagulation profile (790.92)*
hemorrhagic disease of newborn (776.0)
that complicating:
abortion (634-638 with .1, 639.1)
pregnancy or the puerperium (641.3, 666.3)

4th **287 Purpura and other hemorrhagic conditions**
Excludes *hemorrhagic thrombocythemia (238.79)*
purpura fulminans (286.6)

287.0 Allergic purpura
Peliosis rheumatica
Purpura:
anaphylactoid
autoimmune
Henoch's
nonthrombocytopenic:
hemorrhagic
idiopathic
rheumatica
Schönlein-Henoch
vascular
Vasculitis, allergic
Excludes *hemorrhagic purpura (287.39)*
purpura annularis telangiectodes (709.1)

287.1 Qualitative platelet defects
Thrombasthenia (hemorrhagic) (hereditary)
Thrombocytasthenia
Thrombocytopathy (dystrophic)
Thrombopathy (Bernard-Soulier)
Excludes *von Willebrand's disease (286.4)*

287.2 Other nonthrombocytopenic purpuras
Purpura:
NOS
senile
simplex

5th **287.3 Primary thrombocytopenia**
Excludes *thrombotic thrombocytopenic purpura (446.6)*
transient thrombocytopenia of newborn (776.1)

287.30 Primary thrombocytopenia, unspecified
D69.6 Thrombocytopenia, unspecified
Megakaryocytic hypoplasia

287.31 Immune thrombocytopenic purpura
Idiopathic thrombocytopenic purpura
Tidal platelet dysgenesis

287.32 Evans' syndrome

287.33 Congenital and hereditary thrombocytopenia purpura
Congenital and hereditary thrombocytopenia
Thrombocytopenia with absent radii (TAR) syndrome
Excludes *Wiskott-Aldrich syndrome (279.12)*

287.39 Other primary thrombocytopenia

287.4 Secondary thrombocytopenia
Posttransfusion purpura
Thrombocytopenia (due to):
dilutional
drugs
extracorporeal circulation of blood
massive blood transfusion
platelet alloimmunization
Use additional E code to identify cause
Excludes *heparin-induced thrombocytopenia (HIT) (289.84)*
transient thrombocytopenia of newborn (776.1)

287.5 Thrombocytopenia, unspecified
D69.6 Thrombocytopenia, unspecified

287.8 Other specified hemorrhagic conditions
Capillary fragility (hereditary)
Vascular pseudohemophilia

287.9 Unspecified hemorrhagic conditions
Hemorrhagic diathesis (familial)

4th **288 Diseases of white blood cells**
Excludes *leukemia (204.0-208.9)*

5th **288.0 Neutropenia**
Decreased Absolute Neutrophil Count (ANC)
Use additional code for any associated:
fever (780.61)
mucositis (478.11, 528.00-528.09, 538, 616.81)
Excludes *neutropenic splenomegaly (289.53)*
transitory neonatal neutropenia (776.7)

288.00 Neutropenia, unspecified
D70.9 Neutropenia, unspecified

288.01 Congenital neutropenia
Congenital agranulocytosis
Infantile genetic agranulocytosis
Kostmann's syndrome

288.02 Cyclic neutropenia
Cyclic hematopoiesis
Periodic neutropenia

288.03 Drug induced neutropenia
Use additional E code to identify drug

288.04 Neutropenia due to infection

288.09 Other neutropenia
Agranulocytosis
Neutropenia:
immune
toxic

288.1 Functional disorders of polymorphonuclear neutrophils
Chronic (childhood) granulomatous disease
Congenital dysphagocytosis
Job's syndrome
Lipochrome histiocytosis (familial)
Progressive septic granulomatosis

288.2 Genetic anomalies of leukocytes
Anomaly (granulation) (granulocyte) or syndrome:
Alder's (-Reilly)
Chédiak-Steinbrinck (-Higashi)
Jordan's
May-Hegglin
Pelger-Huet
Hereditary:
hypersegmentation
hyposegmentation
leukomelanopathy

288.3 Eosinophilia
Eosinophilia
allergic
hereditary
idiopathic
secondary
Eosinophilic leukocytosis
Excludes *Löffler's syndrome (518.3)*
pulmonary eosinophilia (518.3)

288.4 Hemophagocytic syndromes
Familial hemophagocytic lymphohistiocytosis
Familial hemophagocytic reticulosis
Hemophagocytic syndrome, infection-associated
Histiocytic syndromes
Macrophage activation syndrome

5th **288.5 Decreased white blood cell count**
Excludes *neutropenia (288.01-288.09)*

288.50 Leukocytopenia, unspecified
Decreased leukocytes, unspecified
Decreased white blood cell count, unspecified
Leukopenia NOS

288.51 Lymphocytopenia
Decreased lymphocytes

288.59 Other decreased white blood cell count
Basophilic leukopenia
Eosinophilic leukopenia
Monocytopenia
Plasmacytopenia

5th **288.6 Elevated white blood cell count**
Excludes *eosinophilia (288.3)*

288.60 Leukocytosis, unspecified
Elevated leukocytes, unspecified
Elevated white blood cell count, unspecified

288.61 Lymphocytosis (symptomatic)
Elevated lymphocytes

288.62 Leukemoid reaction
Basophilic leukemoid reaction
Lymphocytic leukemoid reaction
Monocytic leukemoid reaction
Myelocytic leukemoid reaction
Neutrophilic leukemoid reaction

288.63 Monocytosis (symptomatic)
Excludes *infectious mononucleosis (075)*

288.64 Plasmacytosis

288.65 Basophilia

288.66 Bandemia
Bandemia without diagnosis of specific infection
Excludes *confirmed infection – code to infection*
leukemia (204.00-208.9)

288.69 Other elevated white blood cell count

288.8 Other specified disease of white blood cells
D72.89 Other specified disorders of white blood cells
Excludes *decreased white blood cell counts (288.50-288.59)*
elevated white blood cell counts (288.60-288.69)
immunity disorders (279.0-279.9)

288.9 Unspecified disease of white blood cells

4th **289 Other diseases of blood and blood-forming organs**

289.0 Polycythemia, secondary
High-oxygen-affinity hemoglobin
Polycythemia:
acquired
benign
due to:
fall in plasma volume
high altitude
emotional
erythropoietin
hypoxemic
nephrogenous
relative
spurious
stress
Excludes *polycythemia:*
neonatal (776.4)
primary (238.4)
vera (238.4)

289.1 Chronic lymphadenitis
Chronic:
adenitis any lymph node, except mesenteric
lymphadenitis any lymph node, except mesenteric
Excludes *acute lymphadenitis (683)*
mesenteric (289.2)
enlarged glands NOS (785.6)

289.2 Nonspecific mesenteric lymphadenitis
Mesenteric lymphadenitis (acute) (chronic)

289.3 Lymphadenitis, unspecified, except mesenteric

289.4 Hypersplenism
"Big spleen" syndrome
Dyssplenism
Hypersplenia
Excludes *primary splenic neutropenia (289.53)*

5th **289.5 Other diseases of spleen**

289.50 Disease of spleen, unspecified

289.51 Chronic congestive splenomegaly

289.52 Splenic sequestration
Code first sickle-cell disease in crisis (282.42, 282.62, 282.64, 282.69)

289.53 Neutropenic splenomegaly

289.59 Other
Lien migrans
Perisplenitis
Splenic:
abscess
atrophy
cyst
fibrosis
infarction
rupture, nontraumatic
Splenitis
Wandering spleen
Excludes *bilharzial splenic fibrosis (120.0-120.9)*
hepatolienal fibrosis (571.5)
splenomegaly NOS (789.2)

288.3 – 289.59

289.6 Familial polycythemia
Familial:
benign polycythemia
erythrocytosis

289.7 Methemoglobinemia
Congenital NADH [DPNH]-methemoglobin-reductase deficiency
Hemoglobin M [Hb-M] disease
Methemoglobinemia:
NOS
acquired (with sulfhemoglobinemia)
hereditary
toxic
Stokvis' disease
Sulfhemoglobinemia
Use additional E code to identify cause

5th **289.8 Other specified diseases of blood and blood-forming organs**

289.81 Primary hypercoagulable state
Activated protein C resistance
Antithrombin III deficiency
Factor V Leiden mutation
Lupus anticoagulant
Protein C deficiency
Protein S deficiency
Prothrombin gene mutation

289.82 Secondary hypercoagulable state
Excludes *heparin-induced thrombocytopenia (HIT) (289.84)*

289.83 *Myelofibrosis*
Myelofibrosis NOS
Secondary myelofibrosis
Code first the underlying disorder, such as:
malignant neoplasm of breast (174.0-174.9, 175.0-175.9)
Use additional code for associated therapy-related myelodysplastic syndrome, if applicable (238.72, 238.73)
Use additional external cause code if due to anti-neoplastic chemotherapy (E933.1)
Excludes *idiopathic myelofibrosis (238.76)*
leukoerythroblastic anemia (284.2)
myelofibrosis with myeloid metaplasia (238.76)
myelophthisic anemia (284.2)
myelophthisis (284.2)
primary myelofibrosis (238.76)

289.84 Heparin-induced thrombocytopenia (HIT)

289.89 Other specified diseases of blood and blood-forming organs
Hypergammaglobulinemia
Pseudocholinesterase deficiency

289.9 Unspecified diseases of blood and blood-forming organs
D75.9 Disease of blood and blood-forming organs, unspecified
Blood dyscrasia NOS
Erythroid hyperplasia

5. MENTAL DISORDERS (290-319)

PSYCHOSES (290-299)

Excludes *mental retardation (317-319)*

ORGANIC PSYCHOTIC CONDITIONS (290-294)

Includes psychotic organic brain syndrome
Excludes *nonpsychotic syndromes of organic etiology (310.0-310.9)*
psychoses classifiable to 295-298 and without impairment of orientation, comprehension, calculation, learning capacity, and judgement, but associated with physical disease, injury, or condition affecting the brain [e.g., following childbirth] (295.0-298.8)

4th **290 Dementias**
Code first the associated neurological condition
Excludes *dementia due to alcohol (291.0-291.2)*
dementia due to drugs (292.82)
dementia not classified as senile, presenile, or arteriosclerotic (294.10-294.11)
psychoses classifiable to 295-298 occurring in the senium without dementia or delirium (295.0-298.8)
senility with mental changes of nonpsychotic severity (310.1)
transient organic psychotic conditions (293.0-293.9)

Layman's: *Senile (≥ 65 years of age) and presenile (<65 years) dementia are differentiated solely by the age of the patient.*

290.0 Senile dementia, uncomplicated A
F03 Unspecified dementia
Senile dementia:
NOS
simple type
Excludes *mild memory disturbances, not amounting to dementia, associated with senile brain disease (310.8)*
senile dementia with:
delirium or confusion (290.3)
delusional [paranoid] features (290.20)
depressive features (290.21)

5th **290.1 Presenile dementia**
Brain syndrome with presenile brain disease
Excludes *arteriosclerotic dementia (290.40-290.43)*
dementia associated with other cerebral conditions (294.10-294.11)

290.10 Presenile dementia, uncomplicated A
Presenile dementia:
NOS
simple type

290.11 Presenile dementia with delirium A
Presenile dementia with acute confusional state

290.12 Presenile dementia with delusional features A
Presenile dementia, paranoid type

290.13 Presenile dementia with depressive features A
Presenile dementia, depressed type

5th **290.2 Senile dementia with delusional or depressive features**
Excludes *senile dementia:*
NOS (290.0)
with delirium and/or confusion (290.3)

290.20 Senile dementia with delusional features A
F03 Unspecified dementia
F05 Delirium due to known physiological condition
Senile dementia, paranoid type
Senile psychosis NOS

290.21 Senile dementia with depressive features A
F03 Unspecified dementia

290.3 Senile dementia with delirium A
Senile dementia with acute confusional state
Excludes *senile:*
dementia NOS (290.0)
psychosis NOS (290.20)

5th **290.4 Vascular dementia**
Multi-infarct dementia or psychosis
Use additional code to identify cerebral atherosclerosis (437.0)
Excludes *suspected cases with no clear evidence of arteriosclerosis (290.9)*

290.40 Vascular dementia,uncomplicated A
Arteriosclerotic dementia:
NOS
simple type

290.41 Vascular dementia, with delirium A
Arteriosclerotic dementia with acute confusional state

290.42 Vascular dementia, with delusions A
Arteriosclerotic dementia, paranoid type

290.43 Vascular dementia, with depressed mood A
Arteriosclerotic dementia, depressed type

290.8 Other specified senile psychotic conditions
Presbyophrenic psychosis

290.9 Unspecified senile psychotic condition A

4th **291 Alcohol-induced mental disorders**
Excludes *alcoholism without psychosis (303.0-303.9)*

291.0 Alcohol withdrawal delirium
Alcoholic delirium
Delirium tremens
Excludes *alcohol withdrawal (291.81)*

291.1 Alcohol-induced persisting amnestic disorder
Alcoholic polyneuritic psychosis
Korsakoff's psychosis, alcoholic
Wernicke-Korsakoff syndrome (alcoholic)

291.2 Alcohol-induced persisting dementia
Alcoholic dementia NOS
Alcoholism associated with dementia NOS
Chronic alcoholic brain syndrome

291.3 Alcohol-induced psychotic disorder with hallucinations
Alcoholic:
hallucinosis (acute)
psychosis with hallucinosis
Excludes *alcohol withdrawal with delirium (291.0)*
schizophrenia (295.0-295.9) and paranoid states (297.0-297.9) taking the form of chronic hallucinosis with clear consciousness in an alcoholic

291.4 Idiosyncratic alcohol intoxication
Pathologic:
alcohol intoxication
drunkenness
Excludes *acute alcohol intoxication (305.0)*
in alcoholism (303.0)
simple drunkenness (305.0)

291.5 Alcohol-induced psychotic disorder with delusions
Alcoholic:
paranoia
psychosis, paranoid type
Excludes *nonalcoholic paranoid states (297.0-297.9)*
schizophrenia, paranoid type (295.3)

5th **291.8 Other specified alcohol-induced mental disorders**

291.81 Alcohol withdrawal
Alcohol:
abstinence syndrome or symptoms
withdrawal syndrome or symptoms
Excludes *alcohol withdrawal:*
delirium (291.0)
hallucinosis (291.3)
delirium tremens (291.0)

291.82 Alcohol induced sleep disorders
Alcohol induced circadian rhythm sleep disorders
Alcohol induced hypersomnia
Alcohol induced insomnia
Alcohol induced parasomnia

291.89 Other
Alcohol-induced anxiety disorder
Alcohol-induced mood disorder
Alcohol-induced sexual dysfunction

291.9 Unspecified alcohol-induced mental disorders
Alcoholic:
mania NOS
psychosis NOS
Alcoholism (chronic) with psychosis
Alcohol-related disorder NOS

4th **292 Drug-induced mental disorders**
Includes organic brain syndrome associated with consumption of drugs
Use additional code for any associated drug dependence (304.0-304.9)
Use additional E code to identify drug

292.0 Drug withdrawal
Drug:
abstinence syndrome or symptoms
withdrawal syndrome or symptoms

5th **292.1 Drug-induced psychotic disorders**

292.11 Drug-induced psychotic disorder with delusions
Paranoid state induced by drugs

292.12 Drug-induced psychotic disorder with hallucintions
Excludes *states following LSD or other hallucinogens, lasting only a few days or less ["bad trips"] (305.3)*

292.2 Pathological drug intoxication
Drug reaction resulting in brief psychotic states
NOS
idiosyncratic
pathologic
Excludes *expected brief psychotic reactions to hallucinogens ["bad trips"] (305.3)*
physiological side-effects of drugs (e.g., dystonias)

5th **292.8 Other specified drug-induced mental disorders**

292.81 Drug-induced delirium

292.82 Drug-induced persisting dementia

292.83 Drug-induced persisting amnestic disorder

292.84 Drug-induced mood disorder
Depressive state induced by drugs

292.85 Drug induced sleep disorders
Drug induced circadian rhythm sleep disorder
Drug induced hypersomnia
Drug induced insomnia
Drug induced parasomnia

292.89 Other
Drug-induced anxiety disorder
Drug-induced organic personality syndrome
Drug-induced sexual dysfunction
Drug intoxication

292.9 Unspecified drug-induced mental disorder
Drug-related disorder NOS
Organic psychosis NOS due to or associated with drugs

4th 293 Transient mental disorders due to conditions classified elsewhere
Includes transient organic mental disorders not associated with alcohol or drugs
Code first the associated physical or neurological condition
Excludes confusional state or delirium superimposed on senile dementia (290.3)
dementia due to:
alcohol (291.0-291.9)
arteriosclerosis (290.40-290.43)
drugs (292.82)
senility (290.0)

293.0 Delirium due to conditions classified elsewhere
Acute:
confusional state
infective psychosis
organic reaction
posttraumatic organic psychosis
psycho-organic syndrome
Acute psychosis associated with endocrine, metabolic, or cerebrovascular disorder
Epileptic:
confusional state
twilight state

293.1 Subacute delirium
Subacute:
confusional state
infective psychosis
organic reaction
posttraumatic organic psychosis
psycho-organic syndrome
psychosis associated with endocrine or metabolic disorder

5th 293.8 Other specified transient mental disorders due to conditions classified elsewhere

293.81 Psychotic disorder with delusions in conditions classified elsewhere
Transient organic psychotic condition, paranoid type

293.82 Psychotic disorder with hallucinations in conditions classified elsewhere
Transient organic psychotic condition, hallucinatory type

293.83 Mood disorder in conditions classified elsewhere
Transient organic psychotic condition, depressive type

293.84 Anxiety disorder in conditions classified elsewhere

293.89 Other
Catatonic disorder in conditions classified elsewhere

293.9 Unspecified transient mental disorder in conditions classified elsewhere
Organic psychosis:
infective NOS
posttraumatic NOS
transient NOS
Psycho-organic syndrome

4th 294 Persistent mental disorders due to conditions classified elsewhere
Includes organic psychotic brain syndromes (chronic), not elsewhere classified

294.0 Amnestic disorder in conditions classified elsewhere
Korsakoff's psychosis or syndrome (nonalcoholic)
Code first underlying condition
Excludes alcoholic:
amnestic syndrome (291.1)
Korsakoff's psychosis (291.1)

5th 294.1 Dementia in conditions classified elsewhere
Dementia of the Alzheimer's type
Code first any underlying physical condition as:
dementia in:
Alzheimer's disease (331.0)
cerebral lipidoses (330.1)
dementia with Lewy bodies (331.82)
dementia with Parkinsonism (331.82)
epilepsy (345.0-345.9)
frontal dementia (331.19)
frontotemporal dementia (331.19)
general paresis [syphilis] (094.1)
hepatolenticular degeneration (275.1)
Huntington's chorea (333.4)
Jakob-Creutzfeldt disease (046.11-046.19)
multiple sclerosis (340)
Pick's disease of the brain (331.11)
polyarteritis nodosa (446.0)
syphilis (094.1)
Excludes dementia:
arteriosclerotic (290.40-290.43)
presenile (290.10-290.13)
senile (290.0)
epileptic psychosis NOS (294.8)

294.10 *Dementia in conditions classified elsewhere without behavioral disturbance*
Dementia in conditions classified elsewhere NOS

294.11 *Dementia in conditions classified elsewhere with behavioral disturbance*
Aggressive behavior
Combative behavior
Violent behavior
Wandering off

294.8 Other persistent mental disorders due to conditions classified elsewhere
F06.0 Psychotic disorder with hallucinations due to known physiological condition
F06.8 Other specified mental disorders due to known physiological condition
Amnestic disorder NOS
Dementia NOS
Epileptic psychosis NOS
Mixed paranoid and affective organic psychotic states
Use additional code for associated epilepsy (345.0-345.9)
Excludes mild memory disturbances, not amounting to dementia (310.8)

294.9 Unspecified persistent mental disorders due to conditions classified elsewhere
Cognitive disorder NOS
Organic psychosis (chronic)

OTHER PSYCHOSES (295-299)

Use additional code to identify any associated physical disease, injury, or condition affecting the brain with psychoses classifiable to 295-298

4th 295 Schizophrenic disorders

Includes schizophrenia of the types described in 295.0-295.9 occurring in children

Excludes *childhood type schizophrenia (299.9)*
infantile autism (299.0)

The following fifth-digit subclassification is for use with category 295:

- 0 unspecified
- 1 subchronic
- 2 chronic
- 3 subchronic with acute exacerbation
- 4 chronic with acute exacerbation
- 5 in remission

5th 295.0 Simple type
[0-5] Schizophrenia simplex
Excludes *latent schizophrenia (295.5)*

5th 295.1 Disorganized type
[0-5] Hebephrenia
Hebephrenic type schizophrenia

5th 295.2 Catatonic type
[0-5] Catatonic (schizophrenia):
agitation
excitation
excited type
stupor
withdrawn type
Schizophrenic:
catalepsy
catatonia
flexibilitas cerea

5th 295.3 Paranoid type
F20.0 Paranoid schizophrenia
[0-5] Paraphrenic schizophrenia
Excludes *involutional paranoid state (297.2)*
paranoia (297.1)
paraphrenia (297.2)

5th 295.4 Schizophreniform disorder
[0-5] Oneirophrenia
Schizophreniform:
attack
psychosis, confusional type
Excludes *acute forms of schizophrenia of:*
catatonic type (295.2)
hebephrenic type (295.1)
paranoid type (295.3)
simple type (295.0)
undifferentiated type (295.8)

5th 295.5 Latent schizophrenia
[0-5] Latent schizophrenic reaction
Schizophrenia:
borderline
incipient
prepsychotic
prodromal
pseudoneurotic
pseudopsychopathic
Excludes *schizoid personality (301.20-301.22)*

5th 295.6 Residual type
[0-5] Chronic undifferentiated schizophrenia
Restzustand (schizophrenic)
Schizophrenic residual state

5th 295.7 Schizoaffective disorder
F25.9 Schizoaffective disorder, unspecified
[0-5] Cyclic schizophrenia
Mixed schizophrenic and affective psychosis
Schizo-affective psychosis
Schizophreniform psychosis, affective type

Layman's: *In simplest terms, patients diagnosed with schizoaffective disorder exhibit both the psychotic symptoms of schizophrenia and the episodic nature of mood disorders. As such, schizophrenia without mood disorder and mood disorder in the absence of schizophrenia should be ruled out prior to assigning a code in the 295.7x range.*

5th 295.8 Other specified types of schizophrenia
[0-5] Acute (undifferentiated) schizophrenia
Atypical schizophrenia
Cenesthopathic schizophrenia
Excludes *infantile autism (299.0)*

5th 295.9 Unspecified schizophrenia
F20.9 Schizophrenia, unspecified
[0-5] Schizophrenia:
NOS
mixed NOS
undifferentiated NOS
undifferentiated type
Schizophrenic reaction NOS
Schizophreniform psychosis NOS

4th 296 Episodic mood disorders

Includes episodic affective disorders

Excludes *neurotic depression (300.4)*
reactive depressive psychosis (298.0)
reactive excitation (298.1)

The following fifth-digit subclassification is for use with categories 296.0-296.6:

- 0 unspecified
- 1 mild
- 2 moderate
- 3 severe, without mention of psychotic behavior
- 4 severe, specified as with psychotic behavior
- 5 in partial or unspecified remission
- 6 in full remission

5th 296.0 Bipolar I disorder, single manic episode
[0-6] Hypomania (mild) NOS single episode or unspecified
Hypomanic psychosis single episode or unspecified
Mania (monopolar) NOS single episode or unspecified
Manic-depressive psychosis or reaction, single episode or unspecified:
hypomanic, single episode or unspecified
manic, single episode or unspecified
Excludes *circular type, if there was a previous attack of depression (296.4)*

5th 296.1 Manic disorder, recurrent episode
[0-6] Any condition classifiable to 296.0, stated to be recurrent
Excludes *circular type, if there was a previous attack of depression (296.4)*

5th **296.2 Major depressive disorder, single episode** 9, 106, 107
[0-6]

9, 106, 107 are only valid for 5th digits "0," "1," "2," "3," "4," and "5"

Depressive psychosis, single episode or unspecified
Endogenous depression, single episode or unspecified
Involutional melancholia, single episode or unspecified
Manic-depressive psychosis or reaction, depressed type, single episode or unspecified
Monopolar depression, single episode or unspecified
Psychotic depression, single episode or unspecified

Excludes *circular type, if previous attack was of manic type (296.5)*
depression NOS (311)
reactive depression (neurotic) (300.4)
psychotic (298.0)

5th **296.3 Major depressive disorder, recurrent episode** 9, 106, 107
[0-6]

9, 106, 107 are only valid for 5th digits "0," "1," "2," "3," "4," and "5"

Any condition classifiable to 296.2, stated to be recurrent

Excludes *circular type, if previous attack was of manic type (296.5)*
depression NOS (311)
reactive depression (neurotic) (300.4)
psychotic (298.0)

5th **296.4 Bipolar I disorder, most recent episode (or current) manic**
[0-6] Bipolar disorder, now manic
Manic-depressive psychosis, circular type but currently manic

Excludes *brief compensatory or rebound mood swings (296.99)*

5th **296.5 Bipolar I disorder, most recent episode (or current) depressed**
[0-6] Bipolar disorder, now depressed
Manic-depressive psychosis, circular type but currently depressed

Excludes *brief compensatory or rebound mood swings (296.99)*

5th **296.6 Bipolar I disorder, most recent episode (or current) mixed**
[0-6] Manic-depressive psychosis, circular type, mixed

296.7 Bipolar I disorder, most recent episode (or current) unspecified

F31.60 Bipolar disorder, current episode mixed, unspecified

Atypical bipolar affective disorder NOS
Manic-depressive psychosis, circular type, current condition not specified as either manic or depressive

5th **296.8 Other and unspecified bipolar disorders**

296.80 Bipolar disorder, unspecified
Bipolar disorder NOS
Manic-depressive:
reaction NOS
syndrome NOS

296.81 Atypical manic disorder

296.82 Atypical depressive disorder

296.89 Other
Bipolar II disorder
Manic-depressive psychosis, mixed type

5th **296.9 Other and unspecified episodic mood disorder**

Excludes *psychogenic affective psychoses (298.0-298.8)*

296.90 Unspecified episodic mood disorder
Affective psychosis NOS
Melancholia NOS
Mood disorder NOS

296.99 Other specified episodic mood disorder
Mood swings:
brief compensatory
rebound

4th **297 Delusional disorders**

Includes paranoid disorders

Excludes *acute paranoid reaction (298.3)*
alcoholic jealousy or paranoid state (291.5)
paranoid schizophrenia (295.3)

297.0 Paranoid state, simple

297.1 Delusional disorder
Chronic paranoid psychosis
Sander's disease
Systematized delusions

Excludes *paranoid personality disorder (301.0)*

297.2 Paraphrenia
Involutional paranoid state
Late paraphrenia
Paraphrenia (involutional)

297.3 Shared psychotic disorder
Folie à deux
Induced psychosis or paranoid disorder

297.8 Other specified paranoid states
Paranoia querulans
Sensitiver Beziehungswahn

Excludes *acute paranoid reaction or state (298.3)*
senile paranoid state (290.20)

297.9 Unspecified paranoid state
Paranoid:
disorder NOS
psychosis NOS
reaction NOS
state NOS

4th **298 Other nonorganic psychoses**

Includes psychotic conditions due to or provoked by:
emotional stress
environmental factors as major part of etiology

298.0 Depressive type psychosis 9
Psychogenic depressive psychosis
Psychotic reactive depression
Reactive depressive psychosis

Excludes *manic-depressive psychosis, depressed type (296.2-296.3)*
neurotic depression (300.4)
reactive depression NOS (300.4)

298.1 Excitative type psychosis
Acute hysterical psychosis
Psychogenic excitation
Reactive excitation

Excludes *manic-depressive psychosis, manic type (296.0-296.1)*

298.2 Reactive confusion
Psychogenic confusion
Psychogenic twilight state

Excludes *acute confusional state (293.0)*

298.3 Acute paranoid reaction
Acute psychogenic paranoid psychosis
Bouffée délirante

Excludes *paranoid states (297.0-297.9)*

298.4 Psychogenic paranoid psychosis
Protracted reactive paranoid psychosis

298.8 Other and unspecified reactive psychosis
Brief psychotic disorder
Brief reactive psychosis NOS
Hysterical psychosis
Psychogenic psychosis NOS
Psychogenic stupor
Excludes *acute hysterical psychosis (298.1)*

298.9 Unspecified psychosis
F29 Unspecified psychosis not due to a substance or known physiological condition
Atypical psychosis
Psychosis NOS
Psychotic disorder NOS

4th **299 Pervasive developmental disorders**
Excludes *adult type psychoses occurring in childhood, as:*
affective disorders (296.0-296.9)
manic-depressive disorders (296.0-296.9)
schizophrenia (295.0-295.9)

The following fifth-digit subclassification is for use with category 299:
0 current or active state
1 residual state

5th **299.0 Autistic disorder**
[0-1] Childhood autism
Infantile psychosis
Kanner's syndrome
Excludes *disintegrative psychosis (299.1)*
Heller's syndrome (299.1)
schizophrenic syndrome of childhood (299.9)

5th **299.1 Childhood disintegrative disorder**
[0-1] Heller's syndrome
Use additional code to identify any associated neurological disorder
Excludes *infantile autism (299.0)*
schizophrenic syndrome of childhood (299.9)

5th **299.8 Other specified pervasive developmental disorders**
[0-1] Asperger's disorder
Atypical childhood psychosis
Borderline psychosis of childhood
Excludes *simple stereotypes without psychotic disturbance (307.3)*

5th **299.9 Unspecified pervasive developmental disorder**
[0-1] Child psychosis NOS
Pervasive developmental disorder NOS
Schizophrenia, childhood type NOS
Schizophrenic syndrome of childhood NOS
Excludes *schizophrenia of adult type occurring in childhood (295.0-295.9)*

NEUROTIC DISORDERS, PERSONALITY DISORDERS, AND OTHER NONPSYCHOTIC MENTAL DISORDERS (300-316)

4th **300 Anxiety, dissociative and somatoform disorders**

5th **300.0 Anxiety states**
Excludes *anxiety in:*
acute stress reaction (308.0)
transient adjustment reaction (309.24)
neurasthenia (300.5)
psychophysiological disorders (306.0-306.9)
separation anxiety (309.21)

300.00 Anxiety state, unspecified
F41.9 Anxiety disorder, unspecified
Anxiety:
neurosis
reaction
state (neurotic)
Atypical anxiety disorder

300.01 Panic disorder without agoraphobia
Panic:
attack
state
Excludes *panic disorder without agoraphobia (300.21)*

300.02 Generalized anxiety disorder
F41.1 Generalized anxiety disorder

300.09 Other

5th **300.1 Dissociative, conversion and factitious disorders**
Excludes *adjustment reaction (309.0-309.9)*
anorexia nervosa (307.1)
gross stress reaction (308.0-308.9)
hysterical personality (301.50-301.59)
psychophysiologic disorders (306.0-306.9)

300.10 Hysteria, unspecified

300.11 Conversion disorder
Astasia-abasia, hysterical
Conversion hysteria or reaction
Hysterical:
blindness
deafness
paralysis

300.12 Dissociative amnesia
Hysterical amnesia

300.13 Dissociative fugue
Hysterical fugue

300.14 Dissociative identity disorder

300.15 Dissociative disorder or reaction, unspecified

300.16 Factitious disorder with predominantly psychological signs and symptoms
Compensation neurosis
Ganser's syndrome, hysterical

300.19 Other and unspecified factitious illness
Factitious disorder (with combined psychological and physical signs and symptoms)(with predominantly physical signs and symptoms) NOS
Excludes *multiple operations or hospital addiction syndrome (301.51)*

5th **300.2 Phobic disorders**
Excludes *anxiety state not associated with a specific situation or object (300.00-300.09)*
obsessional phobias (300.3)

300.20 Phobia, unspecified
Anxiety-hysteria NOS
Phobia NOS

300.21 Agoraphobia with panic disorder
Fear of:
open spaces with panic attacks
streets with panic attacks
travel with panic attacks
Panic disorder with agoraphobia
Excludes *agoraphobia without panic disorder (300.22)*
panic disorder without agoraphobia (300.01)

300.22 Agoraphobia without mention of panic attacks
Any condition classifiable to 300.21 without mention of panic attacks

300.23 Social phobia
Fear of:
eating in public
public speaking
washing in public

300.29 **Other isolated or specific phobias**
Acrophobia
Animal phobias
Claustrophobia
Fear of crowds

300.3 **Obsessive-compulsive disorders**
Anancastic neurosis
Compulsive neurosis
Obsessional phobia [any]
Excludes *obsessive-compulsive symptoms occurring in:*
endogenous depression (296.2-296.3)
organic states (e.g., encephalitis)
schizophrenia (295.0-295.9)

300.4 **Dysthymic disorder** 9
F34.1 Dysthymic disorder
Anxiety depression
Depression with anxiety
Depressive reaction
Neurotic depressive state
Reactive depression
Excludes *adjustment reaction with depressive symptoms (309.0-309.1)*
depression NOS (311)
manic-depressive psychosis, depressed type (296.2-296.3)
reactive depressive psychosis (298.0)

Layman's: *Dysthymic disorder differs from other major depressive disorders in that it is considered less severe. Although it is common to think of dysthymia as "reactive" or spurred by an event, it is actually considered a chronic disorder.*

300.5 **Neurasthenia**
Fatigue neurosis
Nervous debility
Psychogenic:
asthenia
general fatigue
Use additional code to identify any associated physical disorder
Excludes *anxiety state (300.00-300.09)*
neurotic depression (300.4)
psychophysiological disorders (306.0-306.9)
specific nonpsychotic mental disorders following organic brain damage (310.0-310.9)

300.6 **Depersonalization disorder**
Derealization (neurotic)
Neurotic state with depersonalization episode
Excludes *depersonalization associated with:*
anxiety (300.00-300.09)
depression (300.4)
manic-depressive disorder or psychosis (296.0-296.9)
schizophrenia (295.0-295.9)

300.7 **Hypochondriasis**
Body dysmorphic disorder
Excludes *hypochondriasis in:*
hysteria (300.10-300.19)
manic-depressive psychosis, depressed type (296.2-296.3)
neurasthenia (300.5)
obsessional disorder (300.3)
schizophrenia (295.0-295.9)

5th 300.8 **Somatoform disorders**

300.81 **Somatization disorder**
Briquet's disorder
Severe somatoform disorder

300.82 **Undifferentiated somatoform disorder**
Atypical somatoform disorder
Somatoform disorder NOS

300.89 **Other somatoform disorders**
Occupational neurosis, including writers' cramp
Psychasthenia
Psychasthenic neurosis

300.9 **Unspecified nonpsychotic mental disorder**
Psychoneurosis NOS

4th 301 **Personality disorders**
Includes character neurosis
Use additional code to identify any associated neurosis or psychosis, or physical condition
Excludes *nonpsychotic personality disorder associated with organic brain syndromes (310.0-310.9)*

301.0 **Paranoid personality disorder**
Fanatic personality
Paranoid personality (disorder)
Paranoid traits
Excludes *acute paranoid reaction (298.3)*
alcoholic paranoia (291.5)
paranoid schizophrenia (295.3)
paranoid states (297.0-297.9)

5th 301.1 **Affective personality disorder**
Excludes *affective psychotic disorders (296.0-296.9)*
neurasthenia (300.5)
neurotic depression (300.4)

301.10 **Affective personality disorder, unspecified**

301.11 **Chronic hypomanic personality disorder**
Chronic hypomanic disorder
Hypomanic personality

301.12 **Chronic depressive personality disorder**
Chronic depressive disorder
Depressive character or personality

301.13 **Cyclothymic disorder**
Cycloid personality
Cyclothymia
Cyclothymic personality

5th 301.2 **Schizoid personality disorder**
Excludes *schizophrenia (295.0-295.9)*

301.20 **Schizoid personality disorder, unspecified**

301.21 **Introverted personality**

301.22 **Schizotypal personality disorder**

301.3 **Explosive personality disorder**
Aggressive:
personality
reaction
Aggressiveness
Emotional instability (excessive)
Pathological emotionality
Quarrelsomeness
Excludes *dyssocial personality (301.7)*
hysterical neurosis (300.10-300.19)

301.4 **Obsessive-compulsive personality disorder**
Anancastic personality
Obsessional personality
Excludes *obsessive-compulsive disorder (300.3)*
phobic state (300.20-300.29)

5th 301.5 **Histrionic personality disorder**
Excludes *hysterical neurosis (300.10-300.19)*

301.50 **Histrionic personality disorder, unspecified**
Hysterical personality NOS

301.51 **Chronic factitious illness with physical symptoms**
Hospital addiction syndrome
Multiple operations syndrome
Munchausen syndrome

301.59 **Other histrionic personality disorder**
Personality:
emotionally unstable
labile
psychoinfantile

301.6 **Dependent personality disorder**
Asthenic personality
Inadequate personality
Passive personality
Excludes *neurasthenia (300.5)*
passive-aggressive personality (301.84)

301.7 **Antisocial personality disorder**
Amoral personality
Asocial personality
Dyssocial personality
Personality disorder with predominantly sociopathic or asocial manifestation
Excludes *disturbance of conduct without specifiable personality disorder (312.0-312.9)*
explosive personality (301.3)

5th 301.8 **Other personality disorders**
301.81 **Narcissistic personality disorder**
301.82 **Avoidant personality disorder**
301.83 **Borderline personality disorder**
301.84 **Passive-aggressive personality**
301.89 **Other**
Personality:
eccentric
"haltlose" type
immature
masochistic
psychoneurotic
Excludes *psychoinfantile personality (301.59)*

301.9 **Unspecified personality disorder**
Pathological personality NOS
Personality disorder NOS
Psychopathic:
constitutional state
personality (disorder)

4th 302 **Sexual and gender identity disorders**
Excludes *sexual disorder manifest in:*
organic brain syndrome (290.0-294.9, 310.0-310.9)
psychosis (295.0-298.9)

302.0 **Ego-dystonic sexual orientation**
Ego-dystonic lesbianism
Sexual orientation conflict disorder
Excludes *homosexual pedophilia (302.2)*

302.1 **Zoophilia**
Bestiality

302.2 **Pedophilia**

302.3 **Transvestic fetishism**
Excludes *trans-sexualism (302.5)*

302.4 **Exhibitionism**

5th 302.5 **Trans-sexualism**
Sex reassignment surgery status
Excludes *transvestism (302.3)*
302.50 **With unspecified sexual history**
302.51 **With asexual history**
302.52 **With homosexual history**
302.53 **With heterosexual history**

302.6 **Gender identity disorder in children**
Feminism in boys
Gender indentity disorder NOS
Excludes *gender identity disorder in adult (302.85)*
trans-sexualism (302.50-302.53)
transvestism (302.3)

5th 302.7 **Psychosexual dysfunction**
Excludes *decreased sexual desire NOS (799.81)*
impotence of organic origin (607.84)
normal transient symptoms from ruptured hymen
transient or occasional failures of erection due to fatigue, anxiety, alcohol, or drugs
302.70 **Psychosexual dysfunction, unspecified**
Sexual dysfunction NOS
302.71 **Hypoactive sexual desire disorder**
Excludes *decreased sexual desire NOS (799.81)*
302.72 **With inhibited sexual excitement**
Female sexual arousal disorder
Frigidity
Male erectile disorder
Impotence
302.73 **Female orgasmic disorder** ♀
302.74 **Male orgasmic disorder** ♂
302.75 **Premature ejaculation** ♂
302.76 **Dyspareunia, psychogenic** ♀
302.79 **With other specified psychosexual dysfunctions**
Sexual aversion disorder

5th 302.8 **Other specified psychosexual disorders**
302.81 **Fetishism**
302.82 **Voyeurism**
302.83 **Sexual masochism**
302.84 **Sexual sadism**
302.85 **Gender identity disorder in adolescents or adults**
Use additional code to identify sex reassignment surgery status (302.5)
Excludes *gender identity disorder NOS (302.6)*
gender identity disorder in children (302.6)
302.89 **Other**
Frotteurism
Nymphomania
Satyriasis

302.9 **Unspecified psychosexual disorder**
Paraphilia NOS
Pathologic sexuality NOS
Sexual deviation NOS
Sexual disorder NOS

4th 303 Alcohol dependence syndrome

Use additional code to identify any associated condition, as:
alcoholic psychoses (291.0-291.9)
drug dependence (304.0-304.9)
physical complications of alcohol, such as:
cerebral degeneration (331.7)
cirrhosis of liver (571.2)
epilepsy (345.0-345.9)
gastritis (535.3)
hepatitis (571.1)
liver damage NOS (571.3)

Excludes *drunkenness NOS (305.0)*

The following fifth-digit subclassification is for use with category 303:

0 unspecified
1 continuous
2 episodic
3 in remission

5th 303.0 Acute alcoholic intoxication
[0-3] Acute drunkenness in alcoholism

5th 303.9 Other and unspecified alcohol dependence
[0-3] Chronic alcoholism
Dipsomania

4th 304 Drug dependence

Excludes *nondependent abuse of drugs (305.1-305.9)*

The following fifth-digit subclassification is for use with category 304:

0 unspecified
1 continuous
2 episodic
3 in remission

5th 304.0 Opioid type dependence
[0-3] Heroin
Meperidine
Methadone
Morphine
Opium
Opium alkaloids and their derivatives
Synthetics with morphine-like effects

5th 304.1 Sedative, hypnotic or anxiolytic dependence
[0-3] Barbiturates
Nonbarbiturate sedatives and tranquilizers with a similar effect:
chlordiazepoxide
diazepam
glutethimide
meprobamate
methaqualone

5th 304.2 Cocaine dependence
[0-3] Coca leaves and derivatives

5th 304.3 Cannabis dependence
[0-3] Hashish
Hemp
Marihuana

5th 304.4 Amphetamine and other psychostimulant dependence
[0-3] Methylphenidate
Phenmetrazine

5th 304.5 Hallucinogen dependence
[0-3] Dimethyltryptamine [DMT]
Lysergic acid diethylamide [LSD] and derivatives
Mescaline
Psilocybin

5th 304.6 Other specified drug dependence
[0-3] Absinthe addiction
Glue sniffing
Inhalant dependence
Phencyclidine dependence

Excludes *tobacco dependence (305.1)*

5th 304.7 Combinations of opioid type drug with any other
[0-3]

5th 304.8 Combinations of drug dependence excluding opioid type drug
[0-3]

5th 304.9 Unspecified drug dependence
[0-3] Drug addiction NOS
Drug dependence NOS

4th 305 Nondependent abuse of drugs

Note: *Includes cases where a person, for whom no other diagnosis is possible, has come under medical care because of the maladaptive effect of a drug on which he is not dependent and that he has taken on his own initiative to the detriment of his health or social functioning.*

Excludes *alcohol dependence syndrome (303.0-303.9)*
drug dependence (304.0-304.9)
drug withdrawal syndrome (292.0)
poisoning by drugs or medicinal substances (960.0-979.9)

The following fifth-digit subclassification is for use with codes 305.0, 305.2-305.9

0 unspecified
1 continuous
2 episodic
3 in remission

5th 305.0 Alcohol abuse
[0-3] Drunkenness NOS
Excessive drinking of alcohol NOS
"Hangover" (alcohol)
Inebriety NOS

Excludes *acute alcohol intoxication in alcoholism (303.0)*
alcoholic psychoses (291.0-291.9)

305.1 Tobacco use disorder
Tobacco dependence

Excludes *history of tobacco use (V15.82)*
smoking complicating pregnancy (649.0)
tobacco use disorder complicating pregnancy (649.0)

5th 305.2 Cannabis abuse
[0-3]

5th 305.3 Hallucinogen abuse
[0-3] Acute intoxication from hallucinogens ["bad trips"]
LSD reaction

5th 305.4 Sedative, hypnotic or anxiolytic abuse
[0-3]

5th 305.5 Opioid abuse
[0-3]

5th 305.6 Cocaine abuse
[0-3]

5th 305.7 Amphetamine or related acting sympathomimetic abuse
[0-3]

5th 305.8 Antidepressant type abuse
[0-3]

5th 305.9 Other, mixed, or unspecified drug abuse
[0-3] Caffeine intoxication
Inhalant abuse
"Laxative habit"
Misuse of drugs NOS
Nonprescribed use of drugs or patent medicinals
Phencyclidine abuse

4th 306 Physiological malfunction arising from mental factors

Includes psychogenic:
physical symptoms not involving tissue damage
physiological manifestations not involving tissue damage

Excludes *hysteria (300.11-300.19)*
physical symptoms secondary to a psychiatric disorder classified elsewhere
psychic factors associated with physical conditions involving tissue damage classified elsewhere (316)
specific nonpsychotic mental disorders following organic brain damage (310.0-310.9)

306.0 Musculoskeletal
Psychogenic paralysis
Psychogenic torticollis
Excludes *Gilles de la Tourette's syndrome (307.23)*
paralysis as hysterical or conversion reaction (300.11)
tics (307.20-307.22)

306.1 Respiratory
Psychogenic:
air hunger
cough
hiccough
hyperventilation
yawning
Excludes *psychogenic asthma (316 and 493.9)*

306.2 Cardiovascular
Cardiac neurosis
Cardiovascular neurosis
Neurocirculatory asthenia
Psychogenic cardiovascular disorder
Excludes *psychogenic paroxysmal tachycardia (316 and 427.2)*

306.3 Skin
Psychogenic pruritus
Excludes *psychogenic:*
alopecia (316 and 704.00)
dermatitis (316 and 692.9)
eczema (316 and 691.8 or 692.9)
urticaria (316 and 708.0-708.9)

306.4 Gastrointestinal
Aerophagy
Cyclical vomiting, psychogenic
Diarrhea, psychogenic
Nervous gastritis
Psychogenic dyspepsia
Excludes *cyclical vomiting NOS (536.2)*
associated with migraine (346.2)
globus hystericus (300.11)
mucous colitis (316 and 564.9)
psychogenic:
cardiospasm (316 and 530.0)
duodenal ulcer (316 and 532.0-532.9)
gastric ulcer (316 and 531.0-531.9)
peptic ulcer NOS (316 and 533.0-533.9)
vomiting NOS (307.54)

5th 306.5 Genitourinary
Excludes *enuresis, psychogenic (307.6)*
frigidity (302.72)
impotence (302.72)
psychogenic dyspareunia (302.76)

306.50 Psychogenic genitourinary malfunction, unspecified

306.51 Psychogenic vaginismus ♀
Functional vaginismus

306.52 Psychogenic dysmenorrhea ♀

306.53 Psychogenic dysuria

306.59 Other

306.6 Endocrine

306.7 Organs of special sense
Excludes *hysterical blindness or deafness (300.11)*
psychophysical visual disturbances (368.16)

306.8 Other specified psychophysiological malfunction
Bruxism
Teeth grinding

306.9 Unspecified psychophysiological malfunction
Psychophysiologic disorder NOS
Psychosomatic disorder NOS

4th 307 Special symptoms or syndromes, not elsewhere classified

Note: *This category is intended for use if the psychopathology is manifested by a single specific symptom or group of symptoms which is not part of an organic illness or other mental disorder classifiable elsewhere.*

Excludes *those due to mental disorders classified elsewhere*
those of organic origin

307.0 Stuttering
Excludes *dysphasia (784.59)*
lisping or lalling (307.9)
retarded development of speech (315.31-315.39)
stuttering (fluency disorder) due to late effect of cerebrovascular accident (438.14)

307.1 Anorexia nervosa
Excludes *eating disturbance NOS (307.50)*
feeding problem (783.3)
of nonorganic origin (307.59)
loss of appetite (783.0)
of nonorganic origin (307.59)

5th 307.2 Tics
Excludes *nail-biting or thumb-sucking (307.9)*
stereotypes occurring in isolation (307.3)
tics of organic origin (333.3)

307.20 Tic disorder, unspecified
Tic disorder NOS

307.21 Transient tic disorder

307.22 Chronic motor or vocal tic disorder

307.23 Tourette's disorder
Motor-verbal tic disorder

307.3 Stereotypic movement disorder
Body-rocking
Head banging
Spasmus nutans
Stereotypes NOS
Excludes *tics (307.20-307.23)*
of organic origin (333.3)

5th 307.4 Specific disorders of sleep of nonorganic origin
Excludes *narcolepsy (347.00-347.11)*
organic hypersomnia (327.10-327.19)
organic insomnia (327.00-327.09)
those of unspecified cause (780.50-780.59)

307.40 Nonorganic sleep disorder, unspecified

307.41 Transient disorder of initiating or maintaining sleep
Adjustment insomnia
Hyposomnia associated with acute or intermittent emotional reactions or conflicts
Insomnia associated with acute or intermittent emotional reactions or conflicts
Sleeplessness associated with acute or intermittent emotional reactions or conflicts

307.42 Persistent disorder of initiating or maintaining sleep
Hyposomnia, insomnia, or sleeplessness associated with:
anxiety
conditioned arousal
depression (major) (minor)
psychosis
Idiopathic insomnia
Paradoxical insomnia
Primary insomnia
Psychophysiological insomnia

307.43 Transient disorder of initiating or maintaining wakefulness
Hypersomnia associated with acute or intermittent emotional reactions or conflicts

307.44 Persistent disorder of initiating or maintaining wakefulness
Hypersomnia associated with depression (major) (minor)
Insufficient sleep syndrome
Primary hypersomnia
Excludes *sleep deprivation (V69.4)*

307.45 Circadian rhythm sleep disorder of nonorganic origin

307.46 Sleep arousal disorder
Night terror disorder
Night terrors
Sleep terror disorder
Sleepwalking
Somnambulism

307.47 Other dysfunctions of sleep stages or arousal from sleep
Nightmare disorder
Nightmares:
NOS
REM-sleep type
Sleep drunkenness

307.48 Repetitive intrusions of sleep
Repetitive intrusion of sleep with:
atypical polysomnographic features
environmental disturbances
repeated REM-sleep interruptions

307.49 Other
"Short-sleeper"
Subjective insomnia complaint

5th **307.5 Other and unspecified disorders of eating**
Excludes *anorexia:*
nervosa (307.1)
of unspecified cause (783.0)
overeating, of unspecified cause (783.6)
vomiting:
NOS (787.03)
cyclical (536.2)
associated with migraine (346.2)
psychogenic (306.4)

307.50 Eating disorder, unspecified
Eating disorder NOS

307.51 Bulimia nervosa
Overeating of nonorganic origin

307.52 Pica
Perverted appetite of nonorganic origin

307.53 Rumination disorder
Regurgitation, of nonorganic origin, of food with reswallowing
Excludes *obsessional rumination (300.3)*

307.54 Psychogenic vomiting

307.59 Other
Feeding disorder of infancy or early childhood of nonorganic origin
Infantile feeding disturbances of nonorganic origin
Loss of appetite of nonorganic origin

307.6 Enuresis 49, 50
Enuresis (primary) (secondary) of nonorganic origin
Excludes *enuresis of unspecified cause (788.3)*

307.7 Encopresis
Encopresis (continuous) (discontinuous) of nonorganic origin
Excludes *encopresis of unspecified cause (787.6)*

5th **307.8 Pain disorders related to psycholgical factors**

307.80 Psychogenic pain, site unspecified

307.81 Tension headache
Excludes *headache:*
NOS (784.0)
migraine (346.0-346.9)
syndromes (339.00-339.89)
tension type (339.10-339.12)

307.89 Other
Code first to type or site of pain
Excludes *pain disorder exclusively attributed to psychological factors (307.80)*
psychogenic pain (307.80)

307.9 Other and unspecified special symptoms or syndromes, not elsewhere classified
Communication disorder NOS
Hair plucking
Lalling
Lisping
Masturbation
Nail-biting
Thumb-sucking

4th **308 Acute reaction to stress**
Includes catastrophic stress
combat fatigue
gross stress reaction (acute)
transient disorders in response to exceptional physical or mental stress which usually subside within hours or days
Excludes *adjustment reaction or disorder (309.0-309.9)*
chronic stress reaction (309.1-309.9)

308.0 Predominant disturbance of emotions
Anxiety as acute reaction to exceptional [gross] stress
Emotional crisis as acute reaction to exceptional [gross] stress
Panic state as acute reaction to exceptional [gross] stress

308.1 Predominant disturbance of consciousness
Fugues as acute reaction to exceptional [gross] stress

308.2 Predominant psychomotor disturbance
Agitation states as acute reaction to exceptional [gross] stress
Stupor as acute reaction to exceptional [gross] stress

308.3 Other acute reactions to stress
Acute situational disturbance
Acute stress disorder
Excludes *prolonged posttraumatic emotional disturbance (309.81)*

308.4 Mixed disorders as reaction to stress

308.9 Unspecified acute reaction to stress

4th 309 Adjustment reaction

Includes adjustment disorders
reaction (adjustment) to chronic stress

Excludes *acute reaction to major stress (308.0-308.9)*
neurotic disorders (300.0-300.9)

309.0 Adjustment disorder with depressed mood 9

F43.21 Adjustment disorder with depressed mood

Grief reaction

Excludes *affective psychoses (296.0-296.9)*
neurotic depression (300.4)
prolonged depressive reaction (309.1)
psychogenic depressive psychosis (298.0)

309.1 Prolonged depressive reaction 9

Excludes *affective psychoses (296.0-296.9)*
brief depressive reaction (309.0)
neurotic depression (300.4)
psychogenic depressive psychosis (298.0)

5th 309.2 With predominant disturbance of other emotions

309.21 Separation anxiety disorder

309.22 Emancipation disorder of adolescence and early adult life

309.23 Specific academic or work inhibition

309.24 Adjustment disorder with anxiety

309.28 Adjustment disorder with mixed anxiety and depressed mood

F43.23 Adjustment disorder with mixed anxiety and depressed mood

Adjustment reaction with anxiety and depression

309.29 Other

Culture shock

309.3 Adjustment disorder with disturbance of conduct

Conduct disturbance as adjustment reaction
Destructiveness as adjustment reaction

Excludes *destructiveness in child (312.9)*
disturbance of conduct NOS (312.9)
dyssocial behavior without manifest psychiatric disorder (V71.01-V71.02)
personality disorder with predominantly sociopathic or asocial manifestations (301.7)

309.4 Adjustment disorder with mixed disturbance of emotions and conduct

5th 309.8 Other specified adjustment reactions

309.81 Posttraumatic stress disorder

Chronic posttraumatic stress disorder
Concentration camp syndrome
Posttraumatic stress disorder NOS
Post-traumatic stress disorder (PTSD)

Excludes *acute stress disorder (308.3)*
posttraumatic brain syndrome:
nonpsychotic (310.2)
psychotic (293.0-293.9)

309.82 Adjustment reaction with physical symptoms

309.83 Adjustment reaction with withdrawal

Elective mutism as adjustment reaction
Hospitalism (in children) NOS

309.89 Other

309.9 Unspecified adjustment reaction

Adaptation reaction NOS
Adjustment reaction NOS

4th 310 Specific nonpsychotic mental disorders due to brain damage

Excludes *neuroses, personality disorders, or other nonpsychotic conditions occurring in a form similar to that seen with functional disorders but in association with a physical condition (300.0-300.9, 301.0-301.9)*

310.0 Frontal lobe syndrome

Lobotomy syndrome
Postleucotomy syndrome [state]

Excludes *postcontusion syndrome (310.2)*

310.1 Personality change due to conditions classified elsewhere

Cognitive or personality change of other type, of nonpsychotic severity
Organic psychosyndrome of nonpsychotic severity
Presbyophrenia NOS
Senility with mental changes of nonpsychotic severity

Excludes ~~*memory loss of unknown cause (780.93)*~~
mild cognitive impairment (331.83)
postconcussion syndrome (310.2)
signs and symptoms involving emotional state (799.21-799.29)

310.2 Postconcussion syndrome

Postcontusion syndrome or encephalopathy
Posttraumatic brain syndrome, nonpsychotic
Status postcommotio cerebri

Use additional code to identify associated post-traumatic headache, if applicable (339.20-339.22)

Excludes *any organic psychotic conditions following head injury (293.0-294.0)*
frontal lobe syndrome (310.0)
postencephalitic syndrome (310.8)

310.8 Other specified nonpsychotic mental disorders following organic brain damage

Mild memory disturbance
Postencephalitic syndrome
Other focal (partial) organic psychosyndromes

Excludes *memory loss of unknown cause (780.93)*

310.9 Unspecified nonpsychotic mental disorder following organic brain damage

311 Depressive disorder, not elsewhere classified 9

F33.9 Major depressive disorder, recurrent, unspecified

Depressive disorder NOS
Depressive state NOS
Depression NOS

Excludes *acute reaction to major stress with depressive symptoms (308.0)*
affective personality disorder (301.10-301.13)
affective psychoses (296.0-296.9)
brief depressive reaction (309.0)
depressive states associated with stressful events (309.0-309.1)
disturbance of emotions specific to childhood and adolescence, with misery and unhappiness (313.1)
mixed adjustment reaction with depressive symptoms (309.4)
neurotic depression (300.4)
prolonged depressive adjustment reaction (309.1)
psychogenic depressive psychosis (298.0)

309 – 311

4th **312 Disturbance of conduct, not elsewhere classified**

Excludes *adjustment reaction with disturbance of conduct (309.3)*
drug dependence (304.0-304.9)
dyssocial behavior without manifest psychiatric disorder (V71.01-V71.02)
personality disorder with predominantly sociopathic or asocial manifestations (301.7)
sexual deviations (302.0-302.9)

The following fifth-digit subclassification is for use with categories 312.0-312.2:

0 unspecified
1 mild
2 moderate
3 severe

5th **312.0 Undersocialized conduct disorder, aggressive type**
[0-3] Aggressive outburst
Anger reaction
Unsocialized aggressive disorder

5th **312.1 Undersocialized conduct disorder, unaggressive type**
[0-3] Childhood truancy, unsocialized
Solitary stealing
Tantrums

5th **312.2 Socialized conduct disorder**
[0-3] Childhood truancy, socialized
Group delinquency
Excludes *gang activity without manifest psychiatric disorder (V71.01)*

5th **312.3 Disorders of impulse control, not elsewhere classified**

312.30 Impulse control disorder, unspecified

312.31 Pathological gambling

312.32 Kleptomania

312.33 Pyromania

312.34 Intermittent explosive disorder

312.35 Isolated explosive disorder

312.39 Other
Trichotillomania

312.4 Mixed disturbance of conduct and emotions
Neurotic delinquency
Excludes *compulsive conduct disorder (312.3)*

5th **312.8 Other specified disturbances of conduct, not elsewhere classified**

312.81 Conduct disorder, childhood onset type

312.82 Conduct disorder, adolescent onset type

312.89 Other conduct disorder
Conduct disorder of unspecified onset

312.9 Unspecified disturbance of conduct
Delinquency (juvenile)
Disruptive behavior disorder NOS

4th **313 Disturbance of emotions specific to childhood and adolescence**

Excludes *adjustment reaction (309.0-309.9)*
emotional disorder of neurotic type (300.0-300.9)
masturbation, nail-biting, thumb-sucking, and other isolated symptoms (307.0-307.9)

313.0 Overanxious disorder
Anxiety and fearfulness of childhood and adolescence
Overanxious disorder of childhood and adolescence
Excludes *abnormal separation anxiety (309.21)*
anxiety states (300.00-300.09)
hospitalism in children (309.83)
phobic state (300.20-300.29)

313.1 Misery and unhappiness disorder
Excludes *depressive neurosis (300.4)*

5th **313.2 Sensitivity, shyness, and social withdrawal disorder**
Excludes *infantile autism (299.0)*
schizoid personality (301.20-301.22)
schizophrenia (295.0-295.9)

313.21 Shyness disorder of childhood
Sensitivity reaction of childhood or adolescence

313.22 Introverted disorder of childhood
Social withdrawal of childhood or adolescence
Withdrawal reaction of childhood or adolescence

313.23 Selective mutism
Excludes *elective mutism as adjustment reaction (309.83)*

313.3 Relationship problems
Sibling jealousy
Excludes *relationship problems associated with aggression, destruction, or other forms of conduct disturbance (312.0-312.9)*

5th **313.8 Other or mixed emotional disturbances of childhood or adolescence**

313.81 Oppositional defiant disorder

313.82 Identity disorder
Identity problem

313.83 Academic underachievement disorder

313.89 Other P
Reactive attachment disorder of infancy or early childhood

313.9 Unspecified emotional disturbance of childhood or adolescence P
Mental disorder of infancy, childhood or adolescence NOS

4th **314 Hyperkinetic syndrome of childhood**

Excludes *hyperkinesis as symptom of underlying disorder – code the underlying disorder*

5th **314.0 Attention deficit disorder**
Adult
Child

314.00 Without mention of hyperactivity
Predominantly inattentive type

314.01 With hyperactivity
Combined type
Overactivity NOS
Predominantly hyperactive/impulsive type
Simple disturbance of attention with overactivity

314.1 Hyperkinesis with developmental delay
Developmental disorder of hyperkinesis
Use additional code to identify any associated neurological disorder

314.2 Hyperkinetic conduct disorder
Hyperkinetic conduct disorder without developmental delay
Excludes *hyperkinesis with significant delays in specific skills (314.1)*

314.8 Other specified manifestations of hyperkinetic syndrome

314.9 Unspecified hyperkinetic syndrome
Hyperkinetic reaction of childhood or adolescence NOS
Hyperkinetic syndrome NOS

4th **315 Specific delays in development**

Excludes *that due to a neurological disorder (320.0-389.9)*

5th **315.0 Specific reading disorder**

315.00 Reading disorder, unspecified

315.01 Alexia

315.02 Developmental dyslexia

315.09 Other
Specific spelling difficulty

312 – 315.09

315.1 Mathematics disorder
Dyscalculia

315.2 Other specific learning difficulties
Disorder of written expression
Excludes *specific arithmetical disorder (315.1)*
specific reading disorder (315.00-315.09)

5th **315.3 Developmental speech or language disorder**

315.31 Expressive language disorder
Developmental aphasia
Word deafness
Excludes *acquired aphasia (784.3)*
elective mutism (309.83, 313.0, 313.23)

315.32 Mixed receptive-expressive language disorder
Central auditory processing disorder
Excludes *acquired auditory processing disorder (388.45)*

315.34 Speech and language developmental delay due to hearing loss

315.39 Other
Developmental articulation disorder
Dyslalia
Phonological disorder
Excludes *lisping and lalling (307.9)*
stammering and stuttering (307.0)

315.4 Developmental coordination disorder
Clumsiness syndrome
Dyspraxia syndrome
Specific motor development disorder

315.5 Mixed development disorder

315.8 Other specified delays in development

315.9 Unspecified delay in development
Developmental disorder NOS
Learning disorder NOS

316 Psychic factors associated with diseases classified elsewhere
Psychologic factors in physical conditions classified elsewhere
Use additional code to identify the associated physical condition, as:
psychogenic:
asthma (493.9)
dermatitis (692.9)
duodenal ulcer (532.0-532.9)
eczema (691.8, 692.9)
gastric ulcer (531.0-531.9)
mucous colitis (564.9)
paroxysmal tachycardia (427.2)
ulcerative colitis (556)
urticaria (708.0-708.9)
psychosocial dwarfism (259.4)
Excludes *physical symptoms and physiological malfunctions, not involving tissue damage, of mental origin (306.0-306.9)*

MENTAL RETARDATION (317-319)

Use additional code(s) to identify any associated psychiatric or physical condition(s)

317 Mild mental retardation
High-grade defect
IQ 50-70
Mild mental subnormality

4th **318 Other specified mental retardation**

318.0 Moderate mental retardation
IQ 35-49
Moderate mental subnormality

318.1 Severe mental retardation
IQ 20-34
Severe mental subnormality

318.2 Profound mental retardation
IQ under 20
Profound mental subnormality

319 Unspecified mental retardation
Mental deficiency NOS
Mental subnormality NOS

6. DISEASES OF THE NERVOUS SYSTEM AND SENSE ORGANS (320-389)

INFLAMMATORY DISEASES OF THE CENTRAL NERVOUS SYSTEM (320-326)

4th 320 **Bacterial meningitis**

Includes arachnoiditis bacterial
leptomeningitis bacterial
meningitis bacterial
meningoencephalitis bacterial
meningomyelitis bacterial
pachymeningitis bacterial

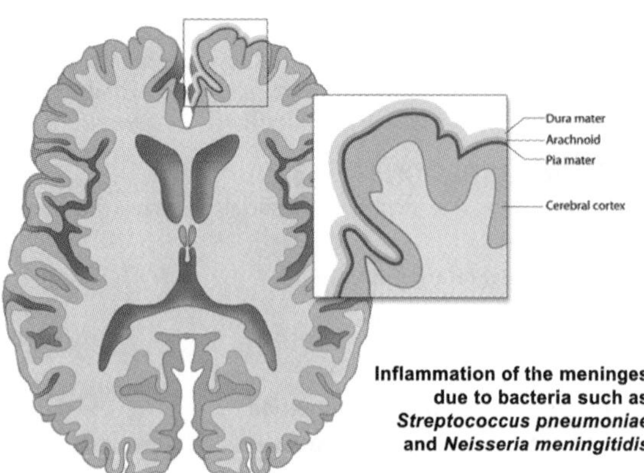

Inflammation of the meninges due to bacteria such as ***Streptococcus pneumoniae*** and ***Neisseria meningitidis***

© 2008 Fairman Studios, LLC. All Rights Reserved.

320.0 **Hemophilus meningitis**
Meningitis due to Hemophilus influenzae [H. influenzae]

320.1 **Pneumococcal meningitis**

320.2 **Streptococcal meningitis**

320.3 **Staphylococcal meningitis**

320.7 ***Meningitis in other bacterial diseases classified elsewhere***
Code first underlying disease as:
actinomycosis (039.8)
listeriosis (027.0)
typhoid fever (002.0)
whooping cough (033.0-033.9)
Excludes *meningitis (in):*
epidemic (036.0)
gonococcal (098.82)
meningococcal (036.0)
salmonellosis (003.21)
syphilis:
NOS (094.2)
congenital (090.42)
meningovascular (094.2)
secondary (091.81)
tuberculosis (013.0)

5th 320.8 **Meningitis due to other specified bacteria**

320.81 **Anaerobic meningitis**
Bacteroides (fragilis)
Gram-negative anaerobes

320.82 **Meningitis due to gram-negative bacteria, not elsewhere classified**
Aerobacter aerogenes
Escherichia coli [E. coli]
Friedländer bacillus
Klebsiella pneumoniae
Proteus morganii
Pseudomonas
Excludes *gram-negative anaerobes (320.81)*

320.89 **Meningitis due to other specified bacteria**
Bacillus pyocyaneus

320.9 **Meningitis due to unspecified bacterium**
Meningitis:
bacterial NOS
purulent NOS
pyogenic NOS
suppurative NOS

4th 321 **Meningitis due to other organisms**

Includes arachnoiditis due to organisms other than bacteria
leptomeningitis due to organisms other than bacteria
meningitis due to organisms other than bacteria
pachymeningitis due to organisms other than bacteria

321.0 ***Cryptococcal meningitis***
Code first underlying disease (117.5)

321.1 ***Meningitis in other fungal diseases***
Code first underlying disease (110.0-118)
Excludes *meningitis in:*
candidiasis (112.83)
coccidioidomycosis (114.2)
histoplasmosis (115.01, 115.11, 115.91)

321.2 ***Meningitis due to viruses not elsewhere classified***
Code first underlying disease, as:
meningitis due to arbovirus (060.0-066.9)
Excludes *meningitis (due to):*
abacterial (047.0-047.9)
adenovirus (049.1)
aseptic NOS (047.9)
Coxsackie (virus) (047.0)
ECHO virus (047.1)
enterovirus (047.0-047.9)
herpes simplex virus (054.72)
herpes zoster virus (053.0)
lymphocytic choriomeningitis virus (049.0)
mumps (072.1)
viral NOS (047.9)
meningo-eruptive syndrome (047.1)

321.3 ***Meningitis due to trypanosomiasis***
Code first underlying disease (086.0-086.9)

321.4 ***Meningitis in sarcoidosis***
Code first underlying disease (135)

321.8 ***Meningitis due to other nonbacterial organisms classified elsewhere***
Code first underlying disease
Excludes *leptospiral meningitis (100.81)*

4th 322 **Meningitis of unspecified cause**

Includes arachnoiditis with no organism specified as cause
leptomeningitis with no organism specified as cause
meningitis with no organism specified as cause
pachymeningitis with no organism specified as cause

322.0 **Nonpyogenic meningitis**
Meningitis with clear cerebrospinal fluid

322.1 **Eosinophilic meningitis**

322.2 **Chronic meningitis**

322.9 **Meningitis, unspecified**

4th 323 **Encephalitis, myelitis, and encephalomyelitis**

Includes acute disseminated encephalomyelitis
meningoencephalitis, except bacterial
meningomyelitis, except bacterial
myelitis:
ascending
transverse

Excludes *acute transverse myelitis NOS (341.20)*
acute transverse myelitis in conditions classified elsewhere (341.21)
bacterial:
meningoencephalitis (320.0-320.9)
meningomyelitis (320.0-320.9)
idiopathic transverse myelitis (341.22)

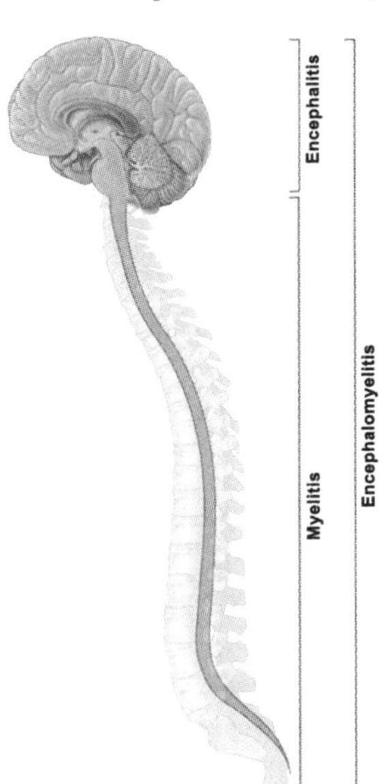

© 2008 Fairman Studios, LLC. All Rights Reserved.

5th 323.0 **Encephalitis myelitis, and encephalomyelitis in viral diseases classified elsewhere**
Code first underlying disease, as:
cat-scratch disease (078.3)
infectious mononucleosis (075)
ornithosis (073.7)

323.01 ***Encephalitis and encephalomyelitis in viral diseases classified elsewhere***
Excludes *encephalitis (in):*
arthropod-borne viral (062.0-064)
herpes simplex (054.3)
mumps (072.2)
poliomyelitis (045.0-045.9)
rubella (056.01)
slow virus infections of central nervous system (046.0-046.9)
other viral diseases of central nervous system (049.8-049.9)
viral NOS (049.9)
West Nile (066.41)

323.02 ***Myelitis in viral diseases classified elsewhere***
Excludes *myelitis (in):*
herpes simplex (054.74)
herpes zoster (053.14)
poliomyelitis (045.0-045.9)
rubella (056.01)
other viral diseases of central nervous system (049.8-049.9)

323.1 ***Encephalitis, myelitis, and encephalomyelitis in rickettsial diseases classified elsewhere***
Code first underlying disease (080-083.9)

323.2 ***Encephalitis, myelitis, and encephalomyelitis in protozoal diseases classified elsewhere***
Code first underlying disease, as:
malaria (084.0-084.9)
trypanosomiasis (086.0-086.9)

5th 323.4 **Other encephalitis, myelitis, and encephalomyelitis due to infection classified elsewhere**
Code first underlying disease

323.41 ***Other encephalitis and encephalomyelitis due to infection classified elsewhere***
Excludes *encephalitis (in):*
meningococcal (036.1)
syphilis:
NOS (094.81)
congenital (090.41)
toxoplasmosis (130.0)
tuberculosis (013.6)
meningoencephalitis due to free-living ameba [Naegleria] (136.29)

323.42 ***Other myelitis due to infection classified elsewhere***
Excludes *myelitis (in):*
syphilis (094.89)
tuberculosis (013.6)

5th 323.5 **Encephalitis, myelitis, and encephalomyelitis following immunization procedures**
Use additional E code to identify vaccine

323.51 **Encephalitis and encephalomyelitis following immunization procedures**
Encephalitis postimmunization or postvaccinal
Encephalomyelitis postimmunization or postvaccinal

323.52 **Myelitis following immunization procedures**
Myelitis postimmunization or postvaccinal

5th 323.6 **Postinfectious encephalitis**
Code first underlying disease

323.61 ***Infectious acute disseminated encephalomyelitis (ADEM)***
Acute necrotizing hemorrhagic encephalopathy
Excludes *noninfectious acute disseminated encephalomyelitis (ADEM) (323.81)*

323.62 ***Other postinfectious encephalitis and encephalomyelitis***
Excludes *encephalitis:*
postchickenpox (052.0)
postmeasles (055.0)

323.63 ***Postinfectious myelitis***

5th 323.7 **Toxic encephalitis, myelitis, and encephalomyelitis**
Code first underlying cause, as:
carbon tetrachloride (982.1)
hydroxyquinoline derivatives (961.3)
lead (984.0-984.9)
mercury (985.0)
thallium (985.8)

323.71 ***Toxic encephalitis and encephalomyelitis***

323.72 ***Toxic myelitis***

5th 323.8 **Other causes of encephalitis, myelitis, and encephalomyelitis**

323.81 **Other causes of encephalitis and encephalomyelitis**
Noninfectious acute disseminated encephalomyelitis (ADEM)

323.82 **Other causes of myelitis**
Transverse myelitis NOS

323.9 **Unspecified cause of encephalitis, myelitis, and encephalomyelitis**

4th **324 Intracranial and intraspinal abscess**

324.0 Intracranial abscess

Abscess (embolic):
- cerebellar
- cerebral

Abscess (embolic) of brain [any part]:
- epidural
- extradural
- otogenic
- subdural

Excludes *tuberculous (013.3)*

324.1 Intraspinal abscess

Abscess (embolic) of spinal cord [any part]:
- epidural
- extradural
- subdural

Excludes *tuberculous (013.5)*

324.9 Of unspecified site

Extradural or subdural abscess NOS

325 Phlebitis and thrombophlebitis of intracranial venous sinuses

Embolism of cavernous, lateral, or other intracranial or unspecified intracranial venous sinus

Endophlebitis of cavernous, lateral, or other intracranial or unspecified intracranial venous sinus

Phlebitis, septic or suppurative of cavernous, lateral, or other intracranial or unspecified intracranial venous sinus

Thrombophlebitis of cavernous, lateral, or other intracranial or unspecified intracranial venous sinus

Thrombosis of cavernous, lateral, or other intracranial or unspecified intracranial venous sinus

Excludes *that specified as:*
- *complicating pregnancy, childbirth, or the puerperium (671.5)*
- *of nonpyogenic origin (437.6)*

326 Late effects of intracranial abscess or pyogenic infection

Note: *This category is to be used to indicate conditions whose primary classification is to 320-325 [excluding 320.7, 321.0-321.8, 323.01-323.42, 323.6-323.7] as the cause of late effects, themselves classifiable elsewhere. The "late effects" include conditions specified as such, or as sequelae, which may occur at any time after the resolution of the causal condition.*

Use additional code to identify condition, as:
- hydrocephalus (331.4)
- paralysis (342.0-342.9, 344.0-344.9)

ORGANIC SLEEP DISORDERS (327)

4th **327 Organic sleep disorders**

5th **327.0 Organic disorders of initiating and maintaining sleep [Organic insomnia]**

Excludes *insomnia NOS (780.52)*
insomnia not due to a substance or known physiological condition (307.41-307.42)
insomnia with sleep apnea NOS (780.51)

327.00 Organic insomnia, unspecified

327.01 *Insomnia due to medical condition classified elsewhere*

Code first underlying condition

Excludes *insomnia due to mental disorder (327.02)*

327.02 *Insomnia due to mental disorder*

Code first mental disorder

Excludes *alcohol induced insomnia (291.82)*
drug induced insomnia (292.85)

327.09 Other organic insomnia

5th **327.1 Organic disorder of excessive somnolence [Organic hypersomnia]**

Excludes *hypersomnia NOS (780.54)*
hypersomnia not due to a substance or known physiological condition (307.43-307.44)
hypersomnia with sleep apnea NOS (780.53)

327.10 Organic hypersomnia, unspecified

327.11 Idiopathic hypersomnia with long sleep time

327.12 Idiopathic hypersomnia without long sleep time

327.13 Recurrent hypersomnia

Kleine-Levin syndrome
Menstrual related hypersomnia

327.14 *Hypersomnia due to medical condition classified elsewhere*

Code first underlying condition

Excludes *hypersomnia due to mental disorder (327.15)*

327.15 *Hypersomnia due to mental disorder*

Code first mental disorder

Excludes *alcohol induced hypersomnia (291.82)*
drug induced hypersomnia (292.85)

327.19 Other organic hypersomnia

5th **327.2 Organic sleep apnea**

Excludes *Cheyne-Stokes breathing (786.04)*
hypersomnia with sleep apnea NOS (780.53)
insomnia with sleep apnea NOS (780.51)
sleep apnea in newborn (770.81-770.81)
sleep apnea NOS (780.57)

327.20 Organic sleep apnea, unspecified

327.21 Primary central sleep apnea

327.22 High altitude periodic breathing

327.23 Obstructive sleep apnea (adult) (pediatric)

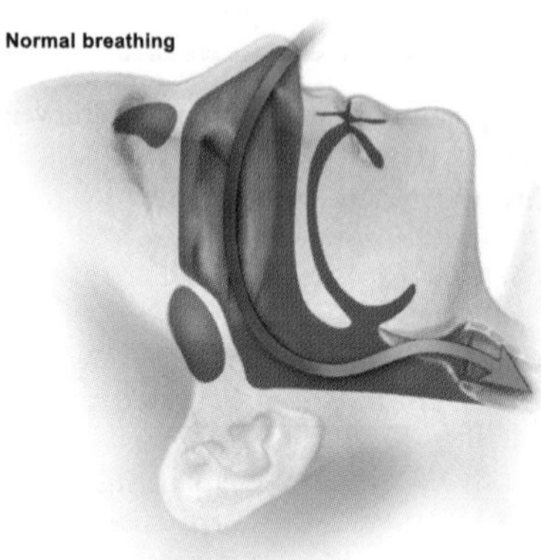

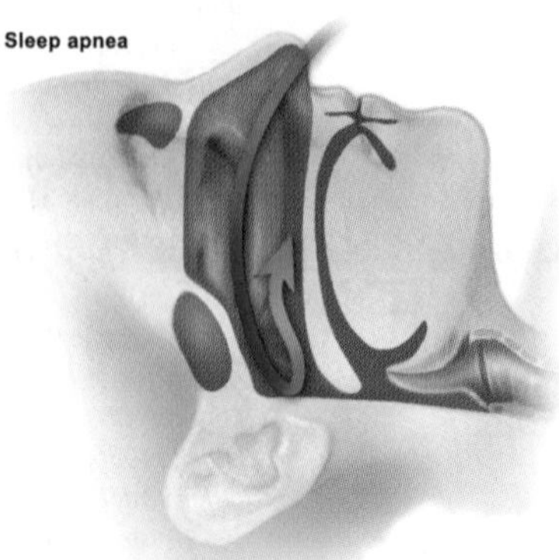

© 2008 Fairman Studios, LLC. All Rights Reserved.

327.24 **Idiopathic sleep related nonobstructive alveolar hypoventilation**
Sleep related hypoxia

327.25 **Congenital central alveolar hypoventilation syndrome**

327.26 ***Sleep related hypoventilation/hypoxemia in conditions classifiable elsewhere***
Code first underlying condition

327.27 ***Central sleep apnea in conditions classified elsewhere***
Code first underlying condition

327.29 **Other organic sleep apnea**

5th 327.3 **Circadian rhythm sleep disorder**
Organic disorder of sleep wake cycle
Organic disorder of sleep wake schedule
Excludes *alcohol induced circadian rhythm sleep disorder (291.82)*
circadian rhythm sleep disorder of nonorganic origin (307.45)
disruption of 24 hour sleep wake cycle NOS (780.55)
drug induced circadian rhythm sleep disorder (292.85)

327.30 **Circadian rhythm sleep disorder, unspecified**

327.31 **Circadian rhythm sleep disorder, delayed sleep phase type**

327.32 **Circadian rhythm sleep disorder, advanced sleep phase type**

327.33 **Circadian rhythm sleep disorder, irregular sleep-wake type**

327.34 **Circadian rhythm sleep disorder, free-running type**

327.35 **Circadian rhythm sleep disorder, jet lag type**

327.36 **Circadian rhythm sleep disorder, shift work type**

327.37 ***Circadian rhythm sleep disorder in conditions classified elsewhere***
Code first underlying condition

327.39 **Other circadian rhythm sleep disorder**

5th 327.4 **Organic parasomnia**
Excludes *alcohol induced parasomnia (291.82)*
drug induced parasomnia (292.85)
parasomnia not due to a known physiological conditions (307.47)

327.40 **Organic parasomnia, unspecified**

327.41 **Confusional arousals**

327.42 **REM sleep behavior disorder**

327.43 **Recurrent isolated sleep paralysis**

327.44 ***Parasomnia in conditions classified elsewhere***
Code first underlying condition

327.49 **Other organic parasomnia**

5th 327.5 **Organic sleep related movement disorders**
Excludes *restless legs syndrome (333.94)*
sleep related movement disorder NOS (780.58)

327.51 **Periodic limb movement disorder**
Periodic limb movement sleep disorder

327.52 **Sleep related leg cramps**

327.53 **Sleep related bruxism**

327.59 **Other organic sleep related movement disorders**

327.8 **Other organic sleep disorders**

HEREDITARY AND DEGENERATIVE DISEASES OF THE CENTRAL NERVOUS SYSTEM (330-337)

Excludes *hepatolenticular degeneration (275.1)*
multiple sclerosis (340)
other demyelinating diseases of central nervous system (341.0-341.9)

4th 330 **Cerebral degenerations usually manifest in childhood**
Use additional code to identify associated mental retardation

330.0 **Leukodystrophy**
Krabbe's disease
Leukodystrophy:
NOS
globoid cell
metachromatic
sudanophilic
Pelizaeus-Merzbacher disease
Sulfatide lipidosis

330.1 **Cerebral lipidoses**
Amaurotic (familial) idiocy
Disease:
Batten
Jansky-Bielschowsky
Kufs'
Spielmeyer-Vogt
Tay-Sachs
Gangliosidosis

330.2 ***Cerebral degeneration in generalized lipidoses***
Code first underlying disease, as:
Fabry's disease (272.7)
Gaucher's disease (272.7)
Niemann-Pick disease (272.7)
sphingolipidosis (272.7)

330.3 ***Cerebral degeneration of childhood in other diseases classified elsewhere***
Code first underlying disease, as:
Hunter's disease (277.5)
mucopolysaccharidosis (277.5)

330.8 **Other specified cerebral degenerations in childhood**
Alpers' disease or gray-matter degeneration
Infantile necrotizing encephalomyelopathy
Leigh's disease
Subacute necrotizing encephalopathy or encephalomyelopathy

330.9 **Unspecified cerebral degeneration in childhood**

4th 331 **Other cerebral degenerations**
Use additional code, where applicable, to identify dementia:
with behavioral disturbance (294.11)
without behavioral disturbance (294.10)

331.0 **Alzheimer's disease**
G30.9 Alzheimer's disease, unspecified

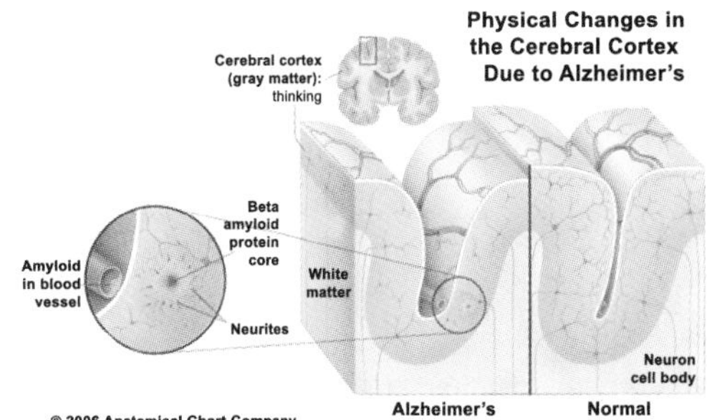

5th 331.1 **Frontotemporal dementia**

331.11 **Pick's disease**

331.19 **Other frontotemporal dementia**
Frontal dementia

331.2 Senile degeneration of brain
Excludes *senility NOS (797)*

331.3 Communicating hydrocephalus
Secondary normal pressure hydrocephalus
Excludes *congenital hydrocephalus (742.3)*
idiopathic normal pressure hydrocephalus (331.5)
normal pressure hydrocephalus (331.5)
spina bifida with hydrocephalus (741.0)

331.4 Obstructive hydrocephalus
Acquired hydrocephalus NOS
Excludes *congenital hydrocephalus (742.3)*
idiopathic normal pressure hydrocephalus (331.5)
normal pressure hydrocephalus (331.5)
spina bifida with hydrocephalus (741.0)

331.5 Idiopathic normal pressure hydrocephalus (INPH)
Normal pressure hydrocephalus NOS
Excludes *congenital hydrocephalus (742.3)*
secondary normal pressure hydrocephalus (331.3)
spina bifida with hydrocephalus (741.0)

331.7 *Cerebral degeneration in diseases classified elsewhere*
Code first underlying disease, as:
alcoholism (303.0-303.9)
beriberi (265.0)
cerebrovascular disease (430-438)
congenital hydrocephalus (741.0, 742.3)
neoplastic disease (140.0-239.9)
myxedema (244.0-244.9)
vitamin B_{12} deficiency (266.2)
Excludes *cerebral degeneration in:*
Jakob-Creutzfeldt disease (046.11-046.19)
progressive multifocal leukoencephalopathy (046.3)
subacute spongiform encephalopathy (046.1)

5th **331.8 Other cerebral degeneration**

331.81 Reye's syndrome P

331.82 Dementia with Lewy bodies
Dementia with Parkinsonism
Lewy body dementia
Lewy body disease

331.83 Mild cognitive impairment, so stated
Excludes *altered mental status (780.97)*
cerebral degeneration (331.0-331.9)
change in mental status (780.97)
cognitive deficits following (late effects of) cerebral hemorrhage or infarction (438.0)
cognitive impairment due to intracranial or head injury (850-854, 959.01)
cognitive impairment due to late effect of intracranial injury (907.0)
cognitive impairment due to skull fracture (800-801, 803-804)
dementia (290.0-290.43, 294.8)
mild memory disturbance (310.8)
neurologic neglect syndrome (781.8)
personality change, nonpsychotic (310.1)

331.89 Other
Cerebral ataxia

331.9 Cerebral degeneration, unspecified
G31.9 Degenerative disease of nervous system, unspecified

4th **332 Parkinson's disease**
Excludes *dementia with Parkinsonism (331.82)*

332.0 Paralysis agitans
G20 Parkinson's disease
Parkinsonism or Parkinson's disease:
NOS
idiopathic
primary

332.1 Secondary Parkinsonism
Neuroleptic-induced Parkinsonism
Parkinsonism due to drugs
Use additional E code to identify drug, if drug-induced
Excludes *Parkinsonism (in):*
Huntington's disease (333.4)
progressive supranuclear palsy (333.0)
Shy-Drager syndrome (333.0)
syphilitic (094.82)

4th **333 Other extrapyramidal disease and abnormal movement disorders**
Includes other forms of extrapyramidal, basal ganglia, or striatopallidal disease
Excludes *abnormal movements of head NOS (781.0)*
sleep related movement disorders (327.51-327.59)

333.0 Other degenerative diseases of the basal ganglia
Atrophy or degeneration:
olivopontocerebellar [Déjérine-Thomas syndrome]
pigmentary pallidal [Hallervorden-Spatz disease]
striatonigral
Parkinsonian syndrome associated with:
idiopathic orthostatic hypotension
symptomatic orthostatic hypotension
Progressive supranuclear ophthalmoplegia
Shy-Drager syndrome

333.1 Essential and other specified forms of tremor
Benign essential tremor
Familial tremor
Medication-induced postural tremor
Use additional E code to identify drug, if drug-induced
Excludes *tremor NOS (781.0)*

Layman's: *Tremors are distinct from convulsions/seizures in that their origin is a primary neuromuscular dysfunction, rather than a symptom of another neurologic condition (e.g., Parkinson's disease, epilepsy, dystonia, etc.).*

333.2 Myoclonus
Familial essential myoclonus
Palatal myoclonus
~~Progressive myoclonic epilepsy~~
~~Unverricht-Lundborg disease~~
Use additional E code to identify drug, if drug-induced
Excludes *progressive myoclonic epilepsy (345.1)*
Unverricht-Lundborg disease (345.1)

333.3 Tics of organic origin
Use additional E code to identify drug, if drug-induced
Excludes *Gilles de la Tourette's syndrome (307.23)*
habit spasm (307.22)
tic NOS (307.20)

333.4 Huntington's chorea

333.5 Other choreas
Hemiballism(us)
Paroxysmal choreo-athetosis
Use additional E code to identify drug, if drug-induced
Excludes *Sydenham's or rheumatic chorea (392.0-392.9)*

333.6 Genetic torsion dystonia
Dystonia:
deformans progressiva
musculorum deformans
(Schwalbe-) Ziehen-Oppenheim disease

331.2 – 333.6

5th 333.7 **Acquired torsion dystonia**

333.71 **Athetoid cerebral palsy**
Double athetosis (syndrome)
Vogt's disease
Excludes *infantile cerebral palsy (343.0-343.9)*

333.72 **Acute dystonia due to drugs**
Acute dystonic reaction due to drugs
Neuroleptic induced acute dystonia
Use additional E code to identify drug
Excludes *blepharospasm due to drugs (333.85)*
orofacial dyskinesia due to drugs (333.85)
secondary Parkinsonism (332.1)
subacute dyskinesia due to drugs (333.85)
tardive dyskinesia (333.85)

333.79 **Other acquired torsion dystonia**

5th 333.8 **Fragments of torsion dystonia**
Use additional E code to identify drug, if drug-induced

333.81 **Blepharospasm**
Excludes *blepharospasm due to drugs (333.85)*

333.82 **Orofacial dyskinesia**
Excludes *orofacial dyskinesia due to drugs (333.85)*

333.83 **Spasmodic torticollis**
Excludes *torticollis:*
NOS (723.5)
hysterical (300.11)
psychogenic (306.0)

333.84 **Organic writers' cramp**
Excludes *psychogenic (300.89)*

333.85 **Subacute dyskinesia due to drugs**
Blepharospasm due to drugs
Orofacial dyskinesia due to drugs
Tardive dyskinesia
Use additional E code to identify drug
Excludes *acute dystonia due to drugs (333.72)*
acute dystonic reaction due to drugs (333.72)
secondary Parkinsonism (332.1)

333.89 **Other**

5th 333.9 **Other and unspecified extrapyramidal diseases and abnormal movement disorders**

333.90 **Unspecified extrapyramidal disease and abnormal movement disorder**
Medication-induced movement disorders NOS
Use additional E code to identify drug, if drug induced

333.91 **Stiff-man syndrome**

333.92 **Neuroleptic malignant syndrome**
Use additional E to identify drug
Excludes *neuroleptic induced Parkinsonism (332.1)*

333.93 **Benign shuddering attacks**

333.94 **Restless legs syndrome (RLS)**

333.99 **Other**
Neuroleptic-induced acute akathisia
Use additional E code to identify drug, if drug-induced

4th 334 **Spinocerebellar disease**
Excludes *olivopontocerebellar degeneration (333.0)*
peroneal muscular atrophy (356.1)

334.0 **Friedreich's ataxia**

334.1 **Hereditary spastic paraplegia**

334.2 **Primary cerebellar degeneration**
Cerebellar ataxia:
Marie's
Sanger-Brown
Dyssynergia cerebellaris myoclonica
Primary cerebellar degeneration:
NOS
hereditary
sporadic

334.3 **Other cerebellar ataxia**
Cerebellar ataxia NOS
Use additional E code to identify drug, if drug-induced

334.4 ***Cerebellar ataxia in diseases classified elsewhere***
Code first underlying disease, as:
alcoholism (303.0-303.9)
myxedema (244.0-244.9)
neoplastic disease (140.0-239.9)

334.8 **Other spinocerebellar diseases**
Ataxia-telangiectasia [Louis-Bar syndrome]
Corticostriatal-spinal degeneration

334.9 **Spinocerebellar disease, unspecified**

4th 335 **Anterior horn cell disease**

335.0 **Werdnig-Hoffmann disease**
Infantile spinal muscular atrophy
Progressive muscular atrophy of infancy

5th 335.1 **Spinal muscular atrophy**

335.10 **Spinal muscular atrophy, unspecified**

335.11 **Kugelberg-Welander disease**
Spinal muscular atrophy:
familial
juvenile

335.19 **Other**
Adult spinal muscular atrophy

5th 335.2 **Motor neuron disease**

335.20 **Amyotrophic lateral sclerosis** A
Motor neuron disease (bulbar) (mixed type)

335.21 **Progressive muscular atrophy**
Duchenne-Aran muscular atrophy
Progressive muscular atrophy (pure)

335.22 **Progressive bulbar palsy**

335.23 **Pseudobulbar palsy**

335.24 **Primary lateral sclerosis**

335.29 **Other**

335.8 **Other anterior horn cell diseases**

335.9 **Anterior horn cell disease, unspecified**

4th 336 **Other diseases of spinal cord**

336.0 **Syringomyelia and syringobulbia**

336.1 **Vascular myelopathies**
Acute infarction of spinal cord (embolic) (nonembolic)
Arterial thrombosis of spinal cord
Edema of spinal cord
Hematomyelia
Subacute necrotic myelopathy

336.2 ***Subacute combined degeneration of spinal cord in diseases classified elsewhere***
Code first underlying disease, as:
pernicious anemia (281.0)
other vitamin B_{12} deficiency anemia (281.1)
vitamin B_{12} deficiency (266.2)

336.3 ***Myelopathy in other diseases classified elsewhere***
Code first underlying disease, as:
myelopathy in neoplastic disease (140.0-239.9)
Excludes *myelopathy in:*
intervertebral disc disorder (722.70-722.73)
spondylosis (721.1, 721.41-721.42, 721.91)

333.7 – 336.3

336.8 Other myelopathy
Myelopathy:
drug-induced
radiation-induced
Use additional E code to identify cause

336.9 Unspecified disease of spinal cord
Cord compression NOS
Myelopathy NOS
Excludes *myelitis (323.02, 323.1, 323.2, 323.42, 323.52, 323.63, 323.72, 323.82, 323.9)*
spinal (canal) stenosis (723.0, 724.00-724.09)

4th **337 Disorders of the autonomic nervous system**
Includes disorders of peripheral autonomic, sympathetic, parasympathetic, or vegetative system
Excludes *familial dysautonomia [Riley-Day syndrome] (742.8)*

5th **337.0 Idiopathic peripheral autonomic neuropathy**

337.00 Idiopathic peripheral autonomic neuropathy, unspecified

337.01 Carotid sinus syndrome
Carotid sinus syncope

337.09 Other idiopathic peripheral autonomic neuropathy
Cervical sympathetic dystrophy or paralysis

337.1 *Peripheral autonomic neuropathy in disorders classified elsewhere*
Code first underlying disease, as:
amyloidosis (277.30-277.39)
diabetes (249.6, 250.6)

5th **337.2 Reflex sympathetic dystrophy**

337.20 Reflex sympathetic dystrophy, unspecified
Complex regional pain syndrome type I, unspecified

337.21 Reflex sympathetic dystrophy of the upper limb
Complex regional pain syndrome type I of the upper limb

337.22 Reflex sympathetic dystrophy of the lower limb
Complex regional pain syndrome type I of the lower limb

337.29 Reflex sympathetic dystrophy of other specified site
Complex regional pain syndrome type I of other specified site

337.3 Autonomic dysreflexia
Use additional code to identify the cause, such as:
fecal impaction (560.39)
pressure ulcer (707.00-707.09)
urinary tract infection (599.0)

337.9 Unspecified disorder of autonomic nervous system

PAIN (338)

ICD-9-CM Official Guidelines (Chapter 6a):

1) General coding information

Codes in category 338 may be used in conjunction with codes from other categories and chapters to provide more detail about acute or chronic pain and neoplasm-related pain, unless otherwise indicated below.

If the pain is not specified as acute or chronic, do not assign codes from category 338, except for post-thoracotomy pain, postoperative pain, neoplasm related pain, or central pain syndrome.

A code from subcategories 338.1 and 338.2 should not be assigned if the underlying (definitive) diagnosis is known, unless the reason for the encounter is pain control/ management and not management of the underlying condition.

(a) Category 338 Codes as Principal or First-Listed Diagnosis

Category 338 codes are acceptable as principal diagnosis or the first-listed code:

- *When pain control or pain management is the reason for the admission/encounter (e.g., a patient with displaced intervertebral disc, nerve impingement and severe back pain presents for injection of steroid into the spinal canal). The underlying cause of the pain should be reported as an additional diagnosis, if known.*
- *When an admission or encounter is for a procedure aimed at treating the underlying condition (e.g., spinal fusion, kyphoplasty), a code for the underlying condition (e.g., vertebral fracture, spinal stenosis) should be assigned as the principal diagnosis. No code from category 338 should be assigned.*
- *When a patient is admitted for the insertion of a neurostimulator for pain control, assign the appropriate pain code as the principal or first listed diagnosis. When an admission or encounter is for a procedure aimed at treating the underlying condition and a neurostimulator is inserted for pain control during the same admission/encounter, a code for the underlying condition should be assigned as the principal diagnosis and the appropriate pain code should be assigned as a secondary diagnosis.*

(b) Use of Category 338 Codes in Conjunction with Site Specific Pain Codes

(i) Assigning Category 338 Codes and Site-Specific Pain Codes

Codes from category 338 may be used in conjunction with codes that identify the site of pain (including codes from chapter 16) if the category 338 code provides additional information. For example, if the code describes the site of the pain, but does not fully describe whether the pain is acute or chronic, then both codes should be assigned.

(ii) Sequencing of Category 338 Codes with Site-Specific Pain Codes

The sequencing of category 338 codes with site-specific pain codes (including chapter 16 codes), is dependent on the circumstances of the encounter/admission as follows:

- *If the encounter is for pain control or pain management, assign the code from category 338 followed by the code identifying the specific site of pain (e.g., encounter for pain management for acute neck pain from trauma is assigned code 338.11, Acute pain due to trauma, followed by code 723.1, Cervicalgia, to identify the site of pain).*
- *If the encounter is for any other reason except pain control or pain management, and a related definitive diagnosis has not been established (confirmed) by the provider, assign the code for the specific site of pain first, followed by the appropriate code from category 338.*

2) Pain due to devices, implants and grafts

Pain associated with devices, implants or grafts left in a surgical site (for example painful hip prosthesis) is assigned to the appropriate code(s) found in Chapter 17, Injury and Poisoning. Use additional code(s) from category 338 to identify acute or chronic pain due to presence of the device, implant or graft (338.18-338.19 or 338.28-338.29).

3) ***Postoperative Pain***

Post-thoracotomy pain and other postoperative pain are classified to subcategories 338.1 and 338.2, depending on whether the pain is acute or chronic. The default for post-thoracotomy and other postoperative pain not specified as acute or chronic is the code for the acute form.

Routine or expected postoperative pain immediately after surgery should not be coded.

(a) ***Postoperative pain not associated with specific postoperative complication***

Postoperative pain not associated with a specific postoperative complication is assigned to the appropriate postoperative pain code in category 338.

(b) ***Postoperative pain associated with specific postoperative complication***

Postoperative pain associated with a specific postoperative complication (such as painful wire sutures) is assigned to the appropriate code(s) found in Chapter 17, Injury and Poisoning. If appropriate, use additional code(s) from category 338 to identify acute or chronic pain (338.18 or 338.28). If pain control/management is the reason for the encounter, a code from category 338 should be assigned as the principal or first-listed diagnosis in accordance with Section I.C.6.a.1.a above.

(c) ***Postoperative pain as principal or first-listed diagnosis***

Postoperative pain may be reported as the principal or first-listed diagnosis when the stated reason for the admission/encounter is documented as postoperative pain control/management.

(d) ***Postoperative pain as secondary diagnosis***

Postoperative pain may be reported as a secondary diagnosis code when a patient presents for outpatient surgery and develops an unusual or inordinate amount of postoperative pain.

The provider's documentation should be used to guide the coding of postoperative pain, as well as Section III. Reporting Additional Diagnoses and Section IV. Diagnostic Coding and Reporting in the Outpatient Setting.

See Section II.I.2 for information on sequencing of diagnoses for patients admitted to hospital inpatient care following post-operative observation.

See Section II.J for information on sequencing of diagnoses for patients admitted to hospital inpatient care from outpatient surgery.

See Section IV.A.2 for information on sequencing of diagnoses for patients admitted for observation.

4) ***Chronic pain***

Chronic pain is classified to subcategory 338.2. There is no time frame defining when pain becomes chronic pain. The provider's documentation should be used to guide use of these codes.

5) ***Neoplasm Related Pain***

Code 338.3 is assigned to pain documented as being related, associated or due to cancer, primary or secondary malignancy, or tumor. This code is assigned regardless of whether the pain is acute or chronic.

This code may be assigned as the principal or first-listed code when the stated reason for the admission/encounter is documented as pain control/pain management. The underlying neoplasm should be reported as an additional diagnosis.

When the reason for the admission/encounter is management of the neoplasm and the pain associated with the neoplasm is also documented, code 338.3 may be assigned as an additional diagnosis.

See Section I.C.2 for instructions on the sequencing of neoplasms for all other stated reasons for the admission/encounter (except for pain control/pain management).

6) ***Chronic pain syndrome***

This condition is different than the term "chronic pain," and therefore this code should only be used when the provider has specifically documented this condition.

4th **338 Pain, not elsewhere classified**

Use additional code to identify:
pain associated with psychological factors (307.89)

Excludes *generalized pain (780.96)*
headache syndromes (339.00-339.89)
localized pain, unspecified type - code to pain by site
migraines (346.0-346.9)
pain disorder exclusively attributed to psychological factors (307.80)
vulvar vestibulitis (625.71)
vulvodynia (625.70-625.79)

338.0 Central pain syndrome
Déjérine-Roussy syndrome
Myelopathic pain syndrome
Thalamic pain syndrome (hyperesthetic)

5th **338.1 Acute pain category**

338.11 Acute pain due to trauma

338.12 Acute post-thoracotomy pain
Post-thoracotomy pain NOS

338.18 Other acute postoperative pain
Postoperative pain NOS

338.19 Other acute pain
Excludes *neoplasm related acute pain (338.3)*

5th **338.2 Chronic pain**

Excludes *causalgia (355.9)*
lower limb (355.71)
upper limb (354.4)
chronic pain syndrome (338.4)
myofascial pain syndrome (729.1)
neoplasm related chronic pain (338.3)
reflex sympathetic dystrophy (337.20-337.29)

338.21 Chronic pain due to trauma

338.22 Chronic post-thoracotomy pain

338.28 Other chronic postoperative pain

338.29 Other chronic pain

338.3 Neoplasm related pain (acute) (chronic)
Cancer associated pain
Pain due to malignancy (primary) (secondary)
Tumor associated pain

338.4 Chronic pain syndrome
Chronic pain associated with significant psychosocial dysfunction

OTHER HEADACHE SYNDROMES (339)

4th **339 Other headache syndromes**

Excludes *headache:*
NOS (784.0)
due to lumbar puncture (349.0)
migraine (346.0-346.9)

5th **339.0 Cluster headaches and other trigeminal autonomic cephalgias**
TACS

339.00 Cluster headache syndrome, unspecified
Ciliary neuralgia
Cluster headache NOS
Histamine cephalgia
Lower half migraine
Migrainous neuralgia

339.01 Episodic cluster headache

339.02 Chronic cluster headache

339.03 Episodic paroxysmal hemicrania
Paroxysmal hemicrania NOS

338 – 339.03

339.04 Chronic paroxysmal hemicrania

339.05 Short lasting unilateral neuralgiform headache with conjunctival injection and tearing
SUNCT

339.09 Other trigeminal autonomic cephalgias

5th 339.1 Tension type headache

Excludes *tension headache NOS (307.81)*
tension headache related to psychological factors (307.81)

339.10 Tension type headache, unspecified

339.11 Episodic tension type headache

339.12 Chronic tension type headache

5th 339.2 Post-traumatic headache

339.20 Post-traumatic headache, unspecified

339.21 Acute post-traumatic headache

339.22 Chronic post-traumatic headache

339.3 Drug induced headache, not elsewhere classified
Medication overuse headache
Rebound headache

5th 339.4 Complicated headache syndromes

339.41 Hemicrania continua

339.42 New daily persistent headache
NDPH

339.43 Primary thunderclap headache

339.44 Other complicated headache syndrome

5th 339.8 Other specified headache syndromes

339.81 Hypnic headache

339.82 Headache associated with sexual activity
Orgasmic headache
Preorgasmic headache

339.83 Primary cough headache

339.84 Primary exertional headache

339.85 Primary stabbing headache

339.89 Other specified headache syndromes

OTHER DISORDERS OF THE CENTRAL NERVOUS SYSTEM (340-349)

340 Multiple sclerosis

G35 Multiple sclerosis

Disseminated or multiple sclerosis:
NOS
brain stem
cord
generalized

4th 341 Other demyelinating diseases of central nervous system

341.0 Neuromyelitis optica

341.1 Schilder's disease
Baló's concentric sclerosis
Encephalitis periaxialis:
concentrica [Baló's]
diffusa [Schilder's]

5th 341.2 Acute (transverse) myelitis

Excludes *acute (transverse) myelitis (in) (due to):*
following immunization procedures (323.52)
infection classified elsewhere (323.42)
postinfectious (323.63)
protozoal diseases classified elsewhere (323.2)
rickettsial diseases classified elsewhere (323.1)
toxic (323.72)
viral diseases classified elsewhere (323.02)
transverse myelitis NOS (323.82)

341.20 Acute (transverse) myelitis NOS

341.21 *Acute (transverse) myelitis in conditions classified elsewhere*
Code first underlying condition

341.22 Idiopathic transverse myelitis

341.8 Other demyelinating diseases of central nervous system
Central demyelination of corpus callosum
Central pontine myelinosis
Marchiafava (-Bignami) disease

341.9 Demyelinating disease of central nervous system, unspecified

4th 342 Hemiplegia and hemiparesis

Note: *This category is to be used when hemiplegia (complete) (incomplete) is reported without further specification, or is stated to be old or long-standing but of unspecified cause. The category is also for use in multiple coding to identify these types of hemiplegia resulting from any cause.*

Excludes *congenital (343.1)*
hemiplegia due to late effect of cerebrovascular accident (438.20-438.22)
infantile NOS (343.4)

The following fifth-digits are for use with codes 342.0-342.9
0 affecting unspecified side
1 affecting dominant side
2 affecting nondominant side

5th 342.0 Flaccid hemiplegia
[0-2]

5th 342.1 Spastic hemiplegia
[0-2]

5th 342.8 Other specified hemiplegia
[0-2]

5th 342.9 Hemiplegia, unspecified
[0-2]

4th 343 Infantile cerebral palsy

Includes cerebral:
palsy NOS
spastic infantile paralysis
congenital spastic paralysis (cerebral)
Little's disease
paralysis (spastic) due to birth injury:
intracranial
spinal

Excludes *athetoid cerebral palsy (333.71)*
hereditary cerebral paralysis, such as:
hereditary spastic paraplegia (334.1)
Vogt's disease (333.71)
spastic paralysis specified as noncongenital or noninfantile (344.0-344.9)

343.0 Diplegic
Congenital diplegia
Congenital paraplegia

343.1 Hemiplegic
Congenital hemiplegia
Excludes *infantile hemiplegia NOS (343.4)*

343.2 Quadriplegic
Tetraplegic

343.3 Monoplegic

343.4 Infantile hemiplegia
Infantile hemiplegia (postnatal) NOS

343.8 Other specified infantile cerebral palsy

343.9 Infantile cerebral palsy, unspecified
Cerebral palsy NOS

4th 344 Other paralytic syndromes

Note: *This category is to be used when the listed conditions are reported without further specification or are stated to be old or long-standing but of unspecified cause. The category is also for use in multiple coding to identify these conditions resulting from any cause.*

Includes paralysis (complete) (incomplete), except as classifiable to 342 and 343

Excludes *congenital or infantile cerebral palsy (343.0-343.9)*
hemiplegia (342.0-342.9)
congenital or infantile (343.1, 343.4)

5th 344.0 Quadriplegia and quadriparesis

344.00 Quadriplegia, unspecified

344.01 C_1-C_4, complete

344.02 C_1-C_4, incomplete

344.03 C_5-C_7, complete

344.04 C_5-C_7, incomplete

344.09 Other

344.1 Paraplegia
Paralysis of both lower limbs
Paraplegia (lower)

344.2 Diplegia of upper limbs
Diplegia (upper)
Paralysis of both upper limbs

5th 344.3 Monoplegia of lower limb
Paralysis of lower limb
Excludes *monoplegia of lower limb due to late effect of cerebrovascular accident (438.40-438.42)*

344.30 Affecting unspecified side

344.31 Affecting dominant side

344.32 Affecting nondominant side

5th 344.4 Monoplegia of upper limb
Paralysis of upper limb
Excludes *monoplegia of upper limb due to late effect of cerebrovascular accident (438.30-438.32)*

344.40 Affecting unspecified side

344.41 Affecting dominant side

344.42 Affecting nondominant side

344.5 Unspecified monoplegia

5th 344.6 Cauda equina syndrome

344.60 Without mention of neurogenic bladder

344.61 With neurogenic bladder
Acontractile bladder
Autonomic hyperreflexia of bladder
Cord bladder
Detrusor hyperreflexia

5th 344.8 Other specified paralytic syndromes

344.81 Locked-in state

344.89 Other specified paralytic syndrome

344.9 Paralysis, unspecified

4th 345 Epilepsy and recurrent seizures

Excludes *progressive myoclonic epilepsy (333.2)*

The following fifth-digit subclassification is for use with categories 345.0, .1, .4-.9:

0 without mention of intractable epilepsy

1 with intractable epilepsy
pharmacoresistant (pharmacologically resistant)
poorly controlled
refractory (medically)
treatment resistant
Excludes *hippocampal sclerosis (348.81)*
mesial temporal sclerosis (348.81)
temporal sclerosis (348.81)

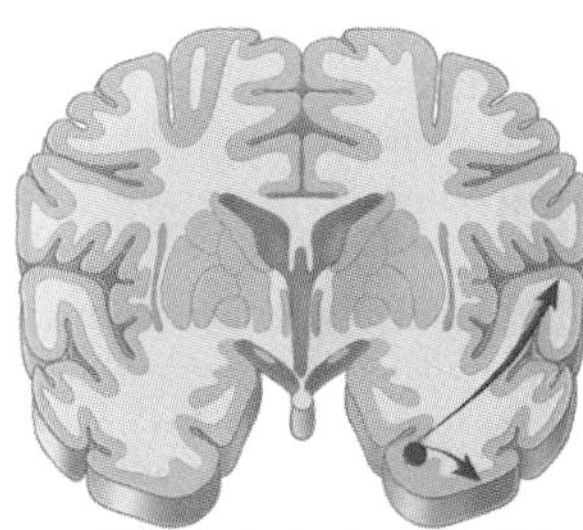

Partial seizure - localized to temporal lobe

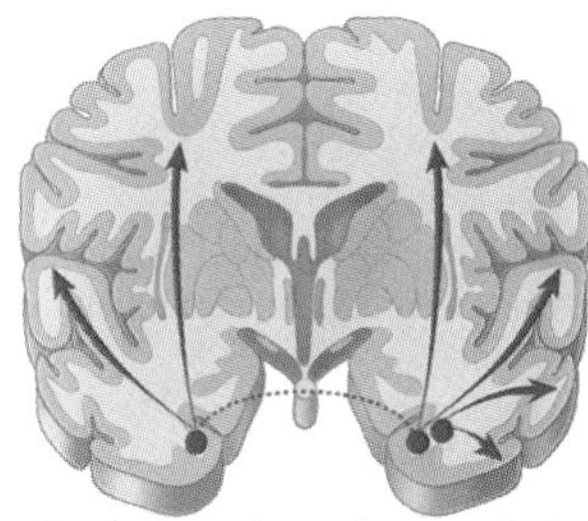

Partial seizure with secondary generalization

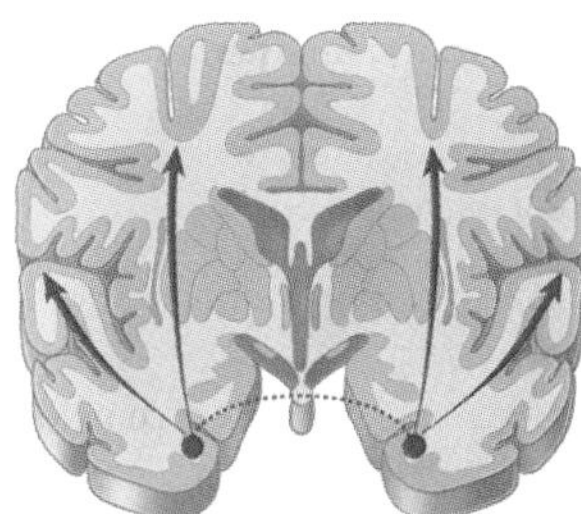

Primarily generalized seizure

© 2008 Fairman Studios, LLC. All Rights Reserved.

5th 345.0 Generalized nonconvulsive epilepsy
[0-1]
Absences:
atonic
typical
Minor epilepsy
Petit mal
Pykno-epilepsy
Seizures:
akinetic
atonic

344 – 345.0

5th **345.1 Generalized convulsive epilepsy**
[0-1] Epileptic seizures:
clonic
myoclonic
tonic
tonic-clonic
Grand mal
Major epilepsy
Progressive myoclonic epilepsy
Unverricht-Lundborg disease
Excludes *convulsions:*
NOS (780.39)
infantile (780.39)
newborn (779.0)
infantile spasms (345.6)

345.2 Petit mal status
Epileptic absence status

345.3 Grand mal status
Status epilepticus NOS
Excludes *epilepsia partialis continua (345.7)*
status:
psychomotor (345.7)
temporal lobe (345.7)

5th **345.4 Localization-related (focal) (partial) epilepsy and epileptic syndromes with complex partial seizures**
[0-1] Epilepsy:
limbic system
partial:
secondarily generalized
with impairment of consciousness
with memory and ideational disturbances
psychomotor
psychosensory
temporal lobe
Epileptic automatism

5th **345.5 Localization-related (focal) (partial) epilepsy and epileptic syndromes with simple partial seizures**
[0-1] Epilepsy:
Bravais-Jacksonian NOS
focal (motor) NOS
Jacksonian NOS
motor partial
partial NOS:
without impairment of consciousness
sensory-induced
somatomotor
somatosensory
visceral
visual

5th **345.6 Infantile spasms**
[0-1] Hypsarrhythmia
Lightning spasms
Salaam attacks
Excludes *salaam tic (781.0)*

5th **345.7 Epilepsia partialis continua**
[0-1] Kojevnikov's epilepsy

5th **345.8 Other forms of epilepsy and recurrent seizures**
[0-1] Epilepsy:
cursive [running]
gelastic

5th **345.9 Epilepsy, unspecified**
[0-1] Epileptic convulsions, fits, or seizures NOS
Recurrent seizures NOS
Seizure disorder NOS
Excludes *convulsion (convulsive) disorder (780.39)*
convulsive seizure or fit NOS (780.39)
recurrent convulsions (780.39)

4th **346 Migraine**
Excludes *headache:*
NOS (784.0)
syndromes (339.00-339.89)

The following fifth-digit subclassification is for use with category 346:
0 **without mention of intractable migraine without mention of status migrainosus**
1 **with intractable migraine, so stated without mention of status migrainosus**
2 **without mention of intractable migraine with status migrainosus**
3 **with intractable migraine, so stated, with status migrainosus**

Layman's: *Signs and symptoms that are seen in migraines that are rarely or never present in tension headaches and other headache syndromes include: prolonged unilateral focus, sensitivity to light and/or sound, nausea or vomiting and aura. Dull head pain with a lack of these symptoms typically indicates tension headache (307.81) or a less severe headache syndrome (339.xx).*

5th **346.0 Migraine with aura**
[0-3] Basilar migraine
Classic migraine
Migraine preceded or accompanied by transient focal neurological phenomena
Migraine triggered seizures
Migraine with acute-onset aura
Migraine with aura without headache (migraine equivalents)
Migraine with prolonged aura
Migraine with typical aura
Retinal migraine
Excludes *persistent migraine aura (346.5, 346.6)*

5th **346.1 Migraine without aura**
[0-3] Common migraine

5th **346.2 Variants of migraine, not elsewhere classified**
[0-3] Abdominal migraine
Cyclical vomiting associated with migraine
Ophthalmoplegic migraine
Periodic headache syndromes in child or adolescent
Excludes *cyclical vomiting NOS (536.2)*
psychogenic cyclical vomiting (306.4)

5th **346.3 Hemiplegic migraine**
[0-3] Familial migraine
Sporadic migraine

5th **346.4 Menstrual migraine** ♀
[0-3] Menstrual headache
Menstrually related migraine
Premenstrual headache
Premenstrual migraine
Pure menstrual migraine

5th **346.5 Persistent migraine aura without cerebral infarction**
[0-3] Persistent migraine aura NOS

5th **346.6 Persistent migraine aura with cerebral infarction**
[0-3]

5th **346.7 Chronic migraine without aura**
[0-3] Transformed migraine without aura

5th **346.8 Other forms of migraine**
[0-3]

5th **346.9 Migraine, unspecified**
[0-3]

4th **347 Cataplexy and narcolepsy**

5th **347.0 Narcolepsy**
347.00 Without cataplexy
Narcolepsy NOS
347.01 With cataplexy

5th 347.1 **Narcolepsy in conditions classified elsewhere**
Code first underlying condition
347.10 ***Without cataplexy***
347.11 ***With cataplexy***

4th 348 **Other conditions of brain**

348.0 **Cerebral cysts**
Arachnoid cyst
Porencephalic cyst
Porencephaly, acquired
Pseudoporencephaly

348.1 **Anoxic brain damage**
Use additional E code to identify cause
Excludes *that occurring in:*
abortion (634-638 with .7, 639.8)
ectopic or molar pregnancy (639.8)
labor or delivery (668.2, 669.4)
that of newborn (767.0, 768.0-768.9, 772.1-772.2)

348.2 **Benign intracranial hypertension**
Pseudotumor cerebri
Excludes *hypertensive encephalopathy (437.2)*

5th 348.3 **Encephalopathy, not elsewhere classified**
348.30 **Encephalopathy, unspecified**
G93.40 Encephalopathy, unspecified
348.31 **Metabolic encephalopathy**
Septic encephalopathy
Excludes *toxic metabolic encephalopathy (349.82)*
348.39 **Other encephalopathy**
Excludes *encephalopathy:*
alcoholic (291.2)
hepatic (572.2)
hypertensive (437.2)
toxic (349.82)

348.4 **Compression of brain**
Compression brain (stem)
Herniation brain (stem)
Posterior fossa compression syndrome

348.5 **Cerebral edema**

5th 348.8 **Other conditions of brain**
~~Cerebral:~~
~~calcification~~
~~fungus~~

● 348.81 **Temporal sclerosis**
Hippocampal sclerosis
Mesial temporal sclerosis

Rationale: *Localization related epilepsy can be an acquired condition, and by far the largest numbers of focal seizures arise from the temporal lobes. These, in turn, are often found to be due to structural changes in the brain, including, but not limited to: tumors; vascular malformations; developmental cortical malformations; and scarring. There are structures in this region that are particularly prone to both traumatic injury and hypoxic injury, resulting in sclerosis. The most common of these is mesial temporal sclerosis (or hippocampal sclerosis). Both of these are frequent discharge diagnoses from epilepsy units, particularly because both are potentially amenable to surgical removal to reduce the frequency of or eliminate seizures.*

Previously, the default for sclerosis of the brain was to code 341.9, "Demyelinating disease of central nervous system, unspecified." However, neither of these conditions is a demylenating disease.

● 348.89 **Other conditions of brain**
Cerebral:
calcification
fungus

348.9 **Unspecified condition of brain**

4th 349 **Other and unspecified disorders of the nervous system**

349.0 **Reaction to spinal or lumbar puncture**
Headache following lumbar puncture

349.1 **Nervous system complications from surgically implanted device**
Excludes *immediate postoperative complications (997.00-997.09)*
mechanical complications of nervous system device (996.2)

349.2 **Disorders of meninges, not elsewhere classified**
Adhesions, meningeal (cerebral) (spinal)
Cyst, spinal meninges
Meningocele, acquired
Pseudomeningocele, acquired

5th 349.3 **Dural tear**
349.31 **Accidental puncture or laceration of dura during a procedure**
Incidental (inadvertent) durotomy
349.39 **Other dural tear**

5th 349.8 **Other specified disorders of nervous system**
349.81 **Cerebrospinal fluid rhinorrhea**
Excludes *cerebrospinal fluid otorrhea (388.61)*
349.82 **Toxic encephalopathy**
Toxic metabolic encephalopathy
Use additional E code to identify cause
349.89 **Other**

349.9 **Unspecified disorders of nervous system**
Disorder of nervous system (central) NOS

DISORDERS OF THE PERIPHERAL NERVOUS SYSTEM (350-359)

Excludes *diseases of:*
acoustic [8th] nerve (388.5)
neuralgia NOS or "rheumatic" (729.2)
neuritis NOS or "rheumatic" (729.2)
oculomotor [3rd, 4th, 6th] nerves (378.0-378.9)
optic [2nd] nerve (377.0-377.9)
peripheral autonomic nerves (337.0-337.9)
peripheral neuritis in pregnancy (646.4)
radiculitis NOS or "rheumatic" (729.2)

4th 350 **Trigeminal nerve disorders**
Includes disorders of 5th cranial nerve

350.1 **Trigeminal neuralgia**
Tic douloureux
Trifacial neuralgia
Trigeminal neuralgia NOS
Excludes *postherpetic (053.12)*

350.2 **Atypical face pain**
350.8 **Other specified trigeminal nerve disorders**
350.9 **Trigeminal nerve disorder, unspecified**

4th 351 **Facial nerve disorders**
Includes disorders of 7th cranial nerve
Excludes *that in newborn (767.5)*

351.0 **Bell's palsy**
Facial palsy

351.1 **Geniculate ganglionitis**
Geniculate ganglionitis NOS
Excludes *herpetic (053.11)*

347.1 – 351.1

351.8 **Other facial nerve disorders**
Facial myokymia
Melkersson's syndrome

351.9 **Facial nerve disorder, unspecified**

4th 352 **Disorders of other cranial nerves**

352.0 **Disorders of olfactory [1st] nerve**

352.1 **Glossopharyngeal neuralgia**

352.2 **Other disorders of glossopharyngeal [9th] nerve**

352.3 **Disorders of pneumogastric [10th] nerve**
Disorders of vagal nerve
Excludes *paralysis of vocal cords or larynx (478.30-478.34)*

352.4 **Disorders of accessory [11th] nerve**

352.5 **Disorders of hypoglossal [12th] nerve**

352.6 **Multiple cranial nerve palsies**
Collet-Sicard syndrome
Polyneuritis cranialis

352.9 **Unspecified disorder of cranial nerves**

4th 353 **Nerve root and plexus disorders**
Excludes *conditions due to:*
intervertebral disc disorders (722.0-722.9)
spondylosis (720.0-721.9)
vertebrogenic disorders (723.0-724.9)

353.0 **Brachial plexus lesions**
Cervical rib syndrome
Costoclavicular syndrome
Scalenus anticus syndrome
Thoracic outlet syndrome
Excludes *brachial neuritis or radiculitis NOS (723.4)*
that in newborn (767.6)

353.1 **Lumbosacral plexus lesions**

353.2 **Cervical root lesions, not elsewhere classified**

353.3 **Thoracic root lesions, not elsewhere classified**

353.4 **Lumbosacral root lesions, not elsewhere classified**

353.5 **Neuralgic amyotrophy**
Parsonage-Aldren-Turner syndrome
Code first any associated underlying disease, such as:
diabetes mellitus (249.6, 250.6)

353.6 **Phantom limb (syndrome)**

353.8 **Other nerve root and plexus disorders**

353.9 **Unspecified nerve root and plexus disorder**

4th 354 **Mononeuritis of upper limb and mononeuritis multiplex**

354.0 **Carpal tunnel syndrome**
G56.00 Carpal tunnel syndrome, unspecified side
Median nerve entrapment
Partial thenar atrophy

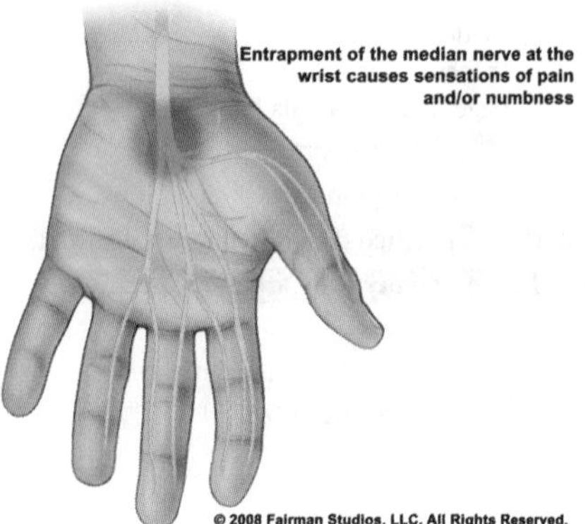

354.1 **Other lesion of median nerve**
Median nerve neuritis

354.2 **Lesion of ulnar nerve**
Cubital tunnel syndrome
Tardy ulnar nerve palsy

354.3 **Lesion of radial nerve**
Acute radial nerve palsy

354.4 **Causalgia of upper limb**
Complex regional pain syndrome type II of the upper limb
Excludes *causalgia:*
NOS (355.9)
lower limb (355.71)
complex regional pain syndrome type II of the lower limb (355.71)

354.5 **Mononeuritis multiplex**
Combinations of single conditions classifiable to 354 or 355

354.8 **Other mononeuritis of upper limb**

354.9 **Mononeuritis of upper limb, unspecified**

4th 355 **Mononeuritis of lower limb**

355.0 **Lesion of sciatic nerve**
Excludes *sciatica NOS (724.3)*

355.1 **Meralgia paresthetica**
Lateral cutaneous femoral nerve of thigh compression or syndrome

355.2 **Other lesion of femoral nerve**

355.3 **Lesion of lateral popliteal nerve**
Lesion of common peroneal nerve

355.4 **Lesion of medial popliteal nerve**

355.5 **Tarsal tunnel syndrome**

355.6 **Lesion of plantar nerve**
G57.60 Lesion of plantar nerve, unspecified side
Morton's metatarsalgia, neuralgia, or neuroma

5th 355.7 **Other mononeuritis of lower limb**

355.71 **Causalgia of lower limb**
Excludes *causalgia:*
NOS (355.9)
upper limb (354.4)
complex regional pain syndrome type II of upper limb (354.4)

355.79 **Other mononeuritis of lower limb**

355.8 **Mononeuritis of lower limb, unspecified**

355.9 **Mononeuritis of unspecified site**
Causalgia NOS
Complex regional pain syndrome NOS
Excludes *causalgia:*
lower limb (355.71)
upper limb (354.4)
complex regional pain syndrome:
lower limb (355.71)
upper limb (354.4)

4th 356 **Hereditary and idiopathic peripheral neuropathy**

356.0 **Hereditary peripheral neuropathy**
Déjérine-Sottas disease

356.1 **Peroneal muscular atrophy**
Charcôt-Marie-Tooth disease
Neuropathic muscular atrophy

356.2 **Hereditary sensory neuropathy**

356.3 **Refsum's disease**
Heredopathia atactica polyneuritiformis

356.4 **Idiopathic progressive polyneuropathy**

356.8 **Other specified idiopathic peripheral neuropathy**
Supranuclear paralysis

356.9 **Unspecified**
G60.9 Hereditary and idiopathic neuropathy, unspecified

4th 357 **Inflammatory and toxic neuropathy**

357.0 **Acute infective polyneuritis**
Guillain-Barré syndrome
Postinfectious polyneuritis

357.1 ***Polyneuropathy in collagen vascular disease***
Code first underlying disease, as:
disseminated lupus erythematosus (710.0)
polyarteritis nodosa (446.0)
rheumatoid arthritis (714.0)

357.2 ***Polyneuropathy in diabetes*** I, 117, 119, 163
Code first underlying disease (249.6, 250.6)

357.3 ***Polyneuropathy in malignant disease***
Code first underlying disease (140.0-208.9)

357.4 ***Polyneuropathy in other diseases classified elsewhere***
Code first underlying disease, as:
amyloidosis (277.30-277.39)
beriberi (265.0)
chronic uremia (585.9)
deficiency of B vitamins (266.0-266.9)
diphtheria (032.0-032.9)
hypoglycemia (251.2)
pellagra (265.2)
porphyria (277.1)
sarcoidosis (135)
uremia NOS (586)
Excludes *polyneuropathy in:*
herpes zoster (053.13)
mumps (072.72)

357.5 **Alcoholic polyneuropathy**

357.6 **Polyneuropathy due to drugs**
Use additional E code to identify drug

357.7 **Polyneuropathy due to other toxic agents**
Use additional E code to identify toxic agent

5th 357.8 **Other**

357.81 **Chronic inflammatory demyelinating polyneuritis**

357.82 **Critical illness polyneuropathy**
Acute motor neuropathy

357.89 **Other inflammatory and toxic neuropathy**

357.9 **Unspecified**

4th 358 **Myoneural disorders**

5th 358.0 **Myasthenia gravis**

358.00 **Myasthenia gravis without (acute) exacerbation**

358.01 **Myasthenia gravis with (acute) exacerbation**
Myasthenia gravis in crisis

358.1 ***Myasthenic syndromes in diseases classified elsewhere***
Eaton-Lambert syndrome from stated cause classified elsewhere
Code first underlying disease, as:
botulism (005.1, 040.41-041.42)
hypothyroidism (244.0-244.9)
malignant neoplasm (140.0-208.9)
pernicious anemia (281.0)
thyrotoxicosis (242.0-242.9)

358.2 **Toxic myoneural disorders**
Use additional E code to identify toxic agent

358.8 **Other specified myoneural disorders**

358.9 **Myoneural disorders, unspecified**

4th 359 **Muscular dystrophies and other myopathies**
Excludes *idiopathic polymyositis (710.4)*

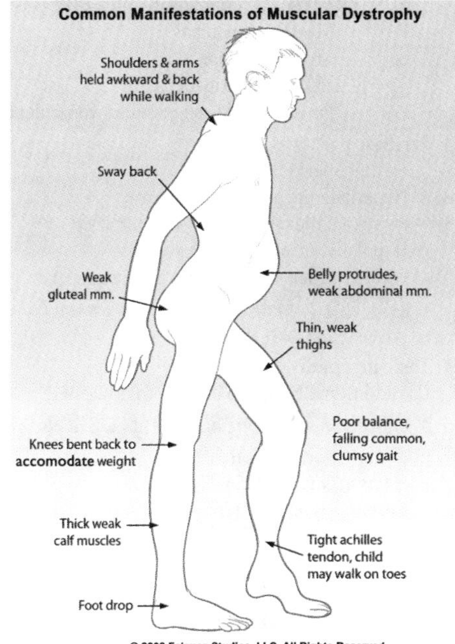

359.0 **Congenital hereditary muscular dystrophy**
Benign congenital myopathy
Central core disease
Centronuclear myopathy
Myotubular myopathy
Nemaline body disease
Excludes *arthrogryposis multiplex congenita (754.89)*

359.1 **Hereditary progressive muscular dystrophy**
Muscular dystrophy:
NOS
distal
Duchenne
Erb's
fascioscapulohumeral
Gower's
Landouzy-Déjérine
limb-girdle
ocular
oculopharyngeal

5th 359.2 **Myotonic disorders**
Excludes *periodic paralysis (359.3)*

359.21 **Myotonic muscular dystrophy**
Dystrophia myotonica
Myotonia atrophica
Myotonic dystrophy
Proximal myotonic myopathy (PROMM)
Steinert's disease

359.22 **Myotonia congenita**
Acetazolamide responsive myotonia congenita
Dominant form (Thomsen's disease)
Myotonia levior
Recessive form (Becker's disease)

359.23 **Myotonic chondrodystrophy**
Congenital myotonic chondrodystrophy
Schwartz-Jampel disease

357 – 359.23

359.24 **Drug-induced myotonia**
Use additional E code to identify drug

359.29 **Other specified myotonic disorder**
Myotonia fluctuans
~~Myotonia levior~~
Myotonia permanens
Paramyotonia congenita (of von Eulenburg)

359.3 **Periodic paralysis**
Familial periodic paralysis
Hyperkalemic periodic paralysis
Hypokalemic familial periodic paralysis
Hypokalemic periodic paralysis
Potassium sensitive periodic paralysis
Excludes *paramyotonia congenita (of von Eulenburg) (359.29)*

359.4 **Toxic myopathy**
Use additional E code to identify toxic agent

359.5 ***Myopathy in endocrine diseases classified elsewhere***
Code first underlying disease, as:
Addison's disease (255.41)
Cushing's syndrome (255.0)
hypopituitarism (253.2)
myxedema (244.0-244.9)
thyrotoxicosis (242.0-242.9)

359.6 ***Symptomatic inflammatory myopathy in diseases classified elsewhere***
Code first underlying disease, as:
amyloidosis (277.30-277.39)
disseminated lupus erythematosus (710.0)
malignant neoplasm (140.0-208.9)
polyarteritis nodosa (446.0)
rheumatoid arthritis (714.0)
sarcoidosis (135)
scleroderma (710.1)
Sjögren's disease (710.2)

● 5th 359.7 **Inflammatory and immune myopathies, NEC**

● 359.71 **Inclusion body myositis**
IBM

Rationale: *The American Academy of Neurology (AAN) requested a new code for inclusion body myositis (IBM). IBM is an inflammatory myopathy that is not due to some other identifiable disease.*

● 359.79 **Other inflammatory and immune myopathies, NEC**
Inflammatory myopathy NOS

5th 359.8 **Other myopathies**

359.81 **Critical illness myopathy**
Acute necrotizing myopathy
Acute quadriplegic myopathy
Intensive care (ICU) myopathy
Myopathy of critical illness

359.89 **Other myopathies**

359.9 **Myopathy, unspecified**

DISORDERS OF THE EYE AND ADNEXA (360-379)

Use additional external cause code, if applicable, to identify the cause of the eye condition

4th 360 **Disorders of the globe**
Includes disorders affecting multiple structures of eye

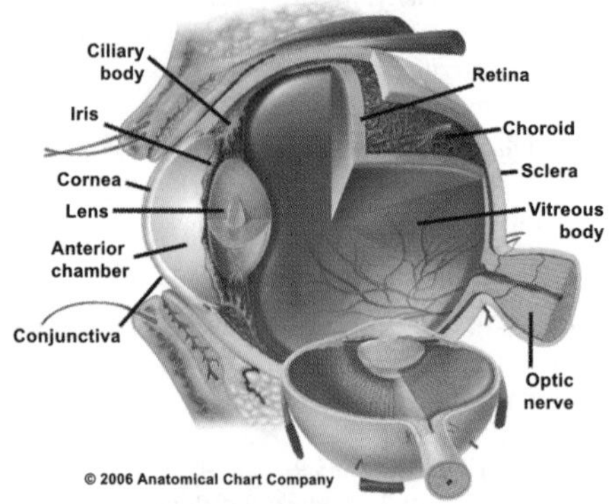

5th 360.0 **Purulent endophthalmitis**
Excludes *bleb associated endophthalmitis (379.63)*

360.00 **Purulent endophthalmitis, unspecified**
360.01 **Acute endophthalmitis**
360.02 **Panophthalmitis**
360.03 **Chronic endophthalmitis**
360.04 **Vitreous abscess**

5th 360.1 **Other endophthalmitis**
Excludes *bleb associated endophthalmitis (379.63)*

360.11 **Sympathetic uveitis**
360.12 **Panuveitis**
360.13 **Parasitic endophthalmitis NOS**
360.14 **Ophthalmia nodosa**
360.19 **Other**
Phacoanaphylactic endophthalmitis

5th 360.2 **Degenerative disorders of globe**

360.20 **Degenerative disorder of globe, unspecified**
360.21 **Progressive high (degenerative) myopia**
Malignant myopia
360.23 **Siderosis**
360.24 **Other metallosis**
Chalcosis
360.29 **Other**
Excludes *xerophthalmia (264.7)*

5th 360.3 **Hypotony of eye**

360.30 **Hypotony, unspecified**
360.31 **Primary hypotony**
360.32 **Ocular fistula causing hypotony**
360.33 **Hypotony associated with other ocular disorders**
360.34 **Flat anterior chamber**

5th 360.4 **Degenerated conditions of globe**

360.40 **Degenerated globe or eye, unspecified**
360.41 **Blind hypotensive eye**
Atrophy of globe
Phthisis bulbi
360.42 **Blind hypertensive eye**
Absolute glaucoma
360.43 **Hemophthalmos, except current injury**
Excludes *traumatic (871.0-871.9, 921.0-921.9)*
360.44 **Leucocoria**

5th **360.5 Retained (old) intraocular foreign body, magnetic**

Excludes *current penetrating injury with magnetic foreign body (871.5)*
retained (old) foreign body of orbit (376.6)

360.50 Foreign body, magnetic, intraocular, unspecified
360.51 Foreign body, magnetic, in anterior chamber
360.52 Foreign body, magnetic, in iris or ciliary body
360.53 Foreign body, magnetic, in lens
360.54 Foreign body, magnetic, in vitreous
360.55 Foreign body, magnetic, in posterior wall
360.59 Foreign body, magnetic, in other or multiple sites

5th **360.6 Retained (old) intraocular foreign body, nonmagnetic**

Retained (old) foreign body:
NOS
nonmagnetic

Excludes *current penetrating injury with (nonmagnetic) foreign body (871.6)*
retained (old) foreign body in orbit (376.6)

360.60 Foreign body, intraocular, unspecified
360.61 Foreign body in anterior chamber
360.62 Foreign body in iris or ciliary body
360.63 Foreign body in lens
360.64 Foreign body in vitreous
360.65 Foreign body in posterior wall
360.69 Foreign body in other or multiple sites

5th **360.8 Other disorders of globe**

360.81 Luxation of globe
360.89 Other

360.9 Unspecified disorder of globe

4th **361 Retinal detachments and defects**

5th **361.0 Retinal detachment with retinal defect**

Rhegmatogenous retinal detachment

Excludes *detachment of retinal pigment epithelium (362.42-362.43)*
retinal detachment (serous) (without defect) (361.2)

361.00 Retinal detachment with retinal defect, unspecified
361.01 Recent detachment, partial, with single defect
361.02 Recent detachment, partial, with multiple defects
361.03 Recent detachment, partial, with giant tear

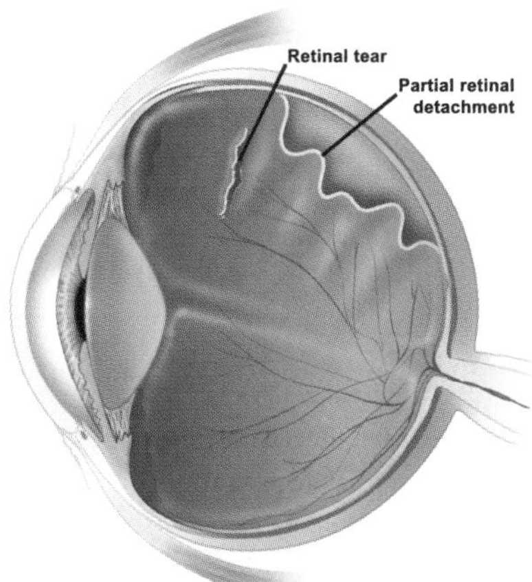

© 2008 Fairman Studios, LLC. All Rights Reserved.

361.04 Recent detachment, partial, with retinal dialysis
Dialysis (juvenile) of retina (with detachment)

361.05 Recent detachment, total or subtotal
361.06 Old detachment, partial
Delimited old retinal detachment

361.07 Old detachment, total or subtotal

5th **361.1 Retinoschisis and retinal cysts**

Excludes *juvenile retinoschisis (362.73)*
microcystoid degeneration of retina (362.62)
parasitic cyst of retina (360.13)

361.10 Retinoschisis, unspecified
361.11 Flat retinoschisis
361.12 Bullous retinoschisis
361.13 Primary retinal cysts
361.14 Secondary retinal cysts
361.19 Other
Pseudocyst of retina

361.2 Serous retinal detachment

Retinal detachment without retinal defect

Excludes *central serous retinopathy (362.41)*
retinal pigment epithelium detachment (362.42-362.43)

5th **361.3 Retinal defects without detachment**

Excludes *chorioretinal scars after surgery for detachment (363.30-363.35)*
peripheral retinal degeneration without defect (362.60-362.66)

361.30 Retinal defect, unspecified
Retinal break(s) NOS

361.31 Round hole of retina without detachment
361.32 Horseshoe tear of retina without detachment
Operculum of retina without mention of detachment

361.33 Multiple defects of retina without detachment

5th **361.8 Other forms of retinal detachment**

361.81 Traction detachment of retina
Traction detachment with vitreoretinal organization

361.89 Other

361.9 Unspecified retinal detachment

4th **362 Other retinal disorders**

Excludes *chorioretinal scars (363.30-363.35)*
chorioretinitis (363.0-363.2)

5th **362.0 Diabetic retinopathy**

Code first diabetes (249.5, 250.5)

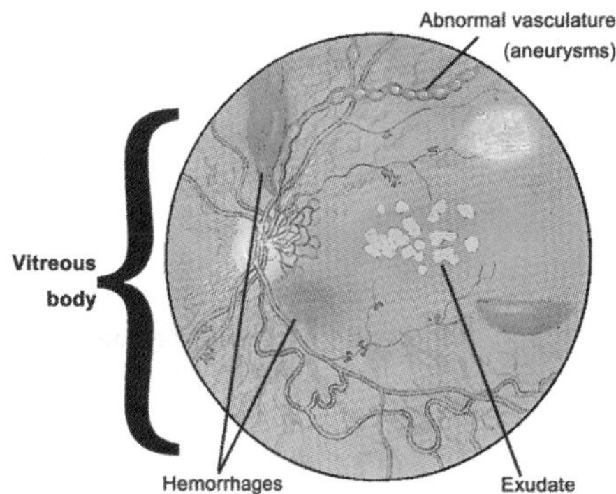

© 2006 Anatomical Chart Company

362.01 *Background diabetic retinopathy* 1, 2, 3, 18, 19, 117, 119, 163

E11.319 Type 2 diabetes mellitus with unspecified diabetic retinopathy without macular edema

Diabetic retinal microaneurysms
Diabetic retinopathy NOS

360.5 – 362.01

362.02 *Proliferative diabetic retinopathy* 1, 2, 3, 18, 19, 117, 119, 163

E11.359 Type 2 diabetes mellitus with proliferative diabetic retinopathy without macular edema

362.03 *Nonproliferative diabetic retinopathy NOS* 1, 2, 3, 18, 19, 117, 119, 163

362.04 *Mild nonproliferative diabetic retinopathy* 1, 2, 3, 18, 19, 117, 119, 163

362.05 *Moderate nonproliferative diabetic retinopathy* 1, 2, 3, 18, 19, 117, 119, 163

362.06 *Severe nonproliferatve diabetic retinopathy* 1, 2, 3, 18, 19, 117, 119, 163

362.07 *Diabetic macular edema* 1, 2, 3, 117, 119, 163

Note: *Code 362.07 must be used with a code for diabetic retinopathy (362.01-362.06)*

Diabetic retinal edema

5th 362.1 **Other background retinopathy and retinal vascular changes**

362.10 **Background retinopathy, unspecified**

362.11 **Hypertensive retinopathy**

ICD-9-CM Official Guidelines (Chapter 7a):

6) Hypertensive Retinopathy

Two codes are necessary to identify the condition. First assign the code from subcategory 362.11, Hypertensive retinopathy, then the appropriate code from categories 401-405 to indicate the type of hypertension.

362.12 **Exudative retinopathy**
Coats' syndrome

362.13 **Changes in vascular appearance**
Vascular sheathing of retina
Use additional code for any associated atherosclerosis (440.8)

362.14 **Retinal microaneurysms NOS**

362.15 **Retinal telangiectasia**

362.16 **Retinal neovascularization NOS**
Neovascularization:
choroidal
subretinal

362.17 **Other intraretinal microvascular abnormalities**
Retinal varices

362.18 **Retinal vasculitis**
Eales' disease
Retinal:
arteritis
endarteritis
perivasculitis
phlebitis

5th 362.2 **Other proliferative retinopathy**

362.20 **Retinopathy of prematurity, unspecified**
Retinopathy of prematurity NOS

362.21 **Retrolental fibroplasia**
Cicatricial retinopathy of prematurity

362.22 **Retinopathy of prematurity, stage 0**

362.23 **Retinopathy of prematurity, stage 1**

362.24 **Retinopathy of prematurity, stage 2**

362.25 **Retinopathy of prematurity, stage 3**

362.26 **Retinopathy of prematurity, stage 4**

362.27 **Retinopathy of prematurity, stage 5**

362.29 **Other nondiabetic proliferative retinopathy**

5th 362.3 **Retinal vascular occlusion**

362.30 **Retinal vascular occlusion, unspecified**

362.31 **Central retinal artery occlusion**

362.32 **Arterial branch occlusion**

362.33 **Partial arterial occlusion**
Hollenhorst plaque
Retinal microembolism

362.34 **Transient arterial occlusion**
Amaurosis fugax

362.35 **Central retinal vein occlusion**

362.36 **Venous tributary (branch) occlusion**

362.37 **Venous engorgement**
Occlusion:
incipient of retinal vein
of retinal vein
partial of retinal vein

5th 362.4 **Separation of retinal layers**

Excludes *retinal detachment (serous) (361.2)*
rhegmatogenous (361.00-361.07)

362.40 **Retinal layer separation, unspecified**

362.41 **Central serous retinopathy**

362.42 **Serous detachment of retinal pigment epithelium**
Exudative detachment of retinal pigment epithelium

362.43 **Hemorrhagic detachment of retinal pigment epithelium**

5th 362.5 **Degeneration of macula and posterior pole**

Excludes *degeneration of optic disc (377.21-377.24)*
hereditary retinal degeneration [dystrophy] (362.70-362.77)

362.50 **Macular degeneration (senile), unspecified** 14, 140

H35.30 Unspecified macular degeneration (age-related)

362.51 **Nonexudative senile macular degeneration** 14, 140

H35.31 Nonexudative age-related macular degeneration

Senile macular degeneration:
atrophic
dry

362.52 **Exudative senile macular degeneration** 14, 140

H35.32 Exudative age-related macular degeneration

Kuhnt-Junius degeneration
Senile macular degeneration:
disciform
wet

362.53 **Cystoid macular degeneration**
Cystoid macular edema

362.54 **Macular cyst, hole, or pseudohole**

362.55 **Toxic maculopathy**
Use additional E to identify drug, if drug induced

362.56 **Macular puckering**

H35.379 Puckering of macula, unspecified eye

Preretinal fibrosis

362.57 **Drusen (degenerative)**

5th 362.6 **Peripheral retinal degenerations**

Excludes *hereditary retinal degeneration [dystrophy] (362.70-362.77)*
retinal degeneration with retinal defect (361.00-361.07)

362.60 **Peripheral retinal degeneration, unspecified**

362.61 **Paving stone degeneration**

362.62 **Microcystoid degeneration**
Blessig's cysts
Iwanoff's cysts

362.63 Lattice degeneration
Palisade degeneration of retina

362.64 Senile reticular degeneration

362.65 Secondary pigmentary degeneration
Pseudoretinitis pigmentosa

362.66 Secondary vitreoretinal degeneration

5th **362.7 Hereditary retinal dystrophies**

362.70 Hereditary retinal dystrophy, unspecified

362.71 *Retinal dystrophy in systemic or cerebroretinal lipidoses*
Code first underlying disease, as:
cerebroretinal lipidoses (330.1)
systemic lipidoses (272.7)

362.72 *Retinal dystrophy in other systemic disorders and syndromes*
Code first underlying disease, as:
Bassen-Kornzweig syndrome (272.5)
Refsum's disease (356.3)

362.73 Vitreoretinal dystrophies
Juvenile retinoschisis

362.74 Pigmentary retinal dystrophy
Retinal dystrophy, albipunctate
Retinitis pigmentosa

362.75 Other dystrophies primarily involving the sensory retina
Progressive cone(-rod) dystrophy
Stargardt's disease

362.76 Dystrophies primarily involving the retinal pigment epithelium
Fundus flavimaculatus
Vitelliform dystrophy

362.77 Dystrophies primarily involving Bruch's membrane
Dystrophy:
hyaline
pseudoinflammatory foveal
Hereditary drusen

5th **362.8 Other retinal disorders**
Excludes *chorioretinal inflammations (363.0-363.2)*
chorioretinal scars (363.30-363.35)

362.81 Retinal hemorrhage
Hemorrhage:
preretinal
retinal (deep) (superficial)
subretinal

362.82 Retinal exudates and deposits

362.83 Retinal edema
H35.81 Retinal edema
Retinal:
cotton wool spots
edema (localized) (macular) (peripheral)

362.84 Retinal ischemia

362.85 Retinal nerve fiber bundle defects

362.89 Other retinal disorders

362.9 Unspecified retinal disorder

4th **363 Chorioretinal inflammations, scars, and other disorders of choroid**

5th **363.0 Focal chorioretinitis and focal retinochoroiditis**
Excludes *focal chorioretinitis or retinochoroiditis in:*
histoplasmosis (115.02, 115.12, 115.92)
toxoplasmosis (130.2)
congenital infection (771.2)

363.00 Focal chorioretinitis, unspecified
Focal:
choroiditis or chorioretinitis NOS
retinitis or retinochoroiditis NOS

363.01 Focal choroiditis and chorioretinitis, juxtapapillary

363.03 Focal choroiditis and chorioretinitis of other posterior pole

363.04 Focal choroiditis and chorioretinitis, peripheral

363.05 Focal retinitis and retinochoroiditis, juxtapapillary
Neuroretinitis

363.06 Focal retinitis and retinochoroiditis, macular or paramacular

363.07 Focal retinitis and retinochoroiditis of other posterior pole

363.08 Focal retinitis and retinochoroiditis, peripheral

5th **363.1 Disseminated chorioretinitis and disseminated retinochoroiditis**
Excludes *disseminated choroiditis or chorioretinitis in secondary syphilis (091.51)*
neurosyphilitic disseminated retinitis or retinochoroiditis (094.83)
retinal (peri)vasculitis (362.18)

363.10 Disseminated chorioretinitis, unspecified
Disseminated:
choroiditis or chorioretinitis NOS
retinitis or retinochoroiditis NOS

363.11 Disseminated choroiditis and chorioretinitis, posterior pole

363.12 Disseminated choroiditis and chorioretinitis, peripheral

363.13 Disseminated choroiditis and chorioretinitis, generalized
Code first any underlying disease, as:
tuberculosis (017.3)

363.14 Disseminated retinitis and retinochoroiditis, metastatic

363.15 Disseminated retinitis and retinochoroiditis, pigment epitheliopathy
Acute posterior multifocal placoid pigment epitheliopathy

5th **363.2 Other and unspecified forms of chorioretinitis and retinochoroiditis**
Excludes *panophthalmitis (360.02)*
sympathetic uveitis (360.11)
uveitis NOS (364.3)

363.20 Chorioretinitis, unspecified
Choroiditis NOS
Retinitis NOS
Uveitis, posterior NOS

363.21 Pars planitis
Posterior cyclitis

363.22 Harada's disease

5th **363.3 Chorioretinal scars**
Scar (postinflammatory) (postsurgical) (posttraumatic):
choroid
retina

363.30 Chorioretinal scar, unspecified

363.31 **Solar retinopathy**

363.32 **Other macular scars**

363.33 **Other scars of posterior pole**

363.34 **Peripheral scars**

363.35 **Disseminated scars**

5th 363.4 **Choroidal degenerations**

363.40 **Choroidal degeneration, unspecified**
Choroidal sclerosis NOS

363.41 **Senile atrophy of choroid**

363.42 **Diffuse secondary atrophy of choroid**

363.43 **Angioid streaks of choroid**

5th 363.5 **Hereditary choroidal dystrophies**
Hereditary choroidal atrophy:
partial [choriocapillaris]
total [all vessels]

363.50 **Hereditary choroidal dystrophy or atrophy, unspecified**

363.51 **Circumpapillary dystrophy of choroid, partial**

363.52 **Circumpapillary dystrophy of choroid, total**
Helicoid dystrophy of choroid

363.53 **Central dystrophy of choroid, partial**
Dystrophy, choroidal:
central areolar
circinate

363.54 **Central choroidal atrophy, total**
Dystrophy, choroidal:
central gyrate
serpiginous

363.55 **Choroideremia**

363.56 **Other diffuse or generalized dystrophy, partial**
Diffuse choroidal sclerosis

363.57 **Other diffuse or generalized dystrophy, total**
Generalized gyrate atrophy, choroid

5th 363.6 **Choroidal hemorrhage and rupture**

363.61 **Choroidal hemorrhage, unspecified**

363.62 **Expulsive choroidal hemorrhage**

363.63 **Choroidal rupture**

5th 363.7 **Choroidal detachment**

363.70 **Choroidal detachment, unspecified**

363.71 **Serous choroidal detachment**

363.72 **Hemorrhagic choroidal detachment**

363.8 **Other disorders of choroid**

363.9 **Unspecified disorder of choroid**

4th 364 **Disorders of iris and ciliary body**

5th 364.0 **Acute and subacute iridocyclitis**
Anterior uveitis, acute, subacute
Cyclitis, acute, subacute
Iridocyclitis, acute, subacute
Iritis, acute, subacute
Excludes *gonococcal (098.41)*
herpes simplex (054.44)
herpes zoster (053.22)

364.00 **Acute and subacute iridocyclitis, unspecified**

364.01 **Primary iridocyclitis**

364.02 **Recurrent iridocyclitis**

364.03 **Secondary iridocyclitis, infectious**

364.04 **Secondary iridocyclitis, noninfectious**
Aqueous:
cells
fibrin
flare

364.05 **Hypopyon**

5th 364.1 **Chronic iridocyclitis**
Excludes *posterior cyclitis (363.21)*

364.10 **Chronic iridocyclitis, unspecified**

364.11 ***Chronic iridocyclitis in diseases classified elsewhere***
Code first underlying disease, as:
sarcoidosis (135)
tuberculosis (017.3)
Excludes *syphilitic iridocyclitis (091.52)*

5th 364.2 **Certain types of iridocyclitis**
Excludes *posterior cyclitis (363.21)*
sympathetic uveitis (360.11)

364.21 **Fuchs' heterochromic cyclitis**

364.22 **Glaucomatocyclitic crises**

364.23 **Lens-induced iridocyclitis**

364.24 **Vogt-Koyanagi syndrome**

364.3 **Unspecified iridocyclitis**
Uveitis NOS

5th 364.4 **Vascular disorders of iris and ciliary body**

364.41 **Hyphema**
Hemorrhage of iris or ciliary body

364.42 **Rubeosis iridis**
Neovascularization of iris or ciliary body

5th 364.5 **Degenerations of iris and ciliary body**

364.51 **Essential or progressive iris atrophy**

364.52 **Iridoschisis**

364.53 **Pigmentary iris degeneration**
Acquired heterochromia of iris
Pigment dispersion syndrome of iris
Translucency of iris

364.54 **Degeneration of pupillary margin**
Atrophy of sphincter of iris
Ectropion of pigment epithelium of iris

364.55 **Miotic cysts of pupillary margin**

364.56 **Degenerative changes of chamber angle**

364.57 **Degenerative changes of ciliary body**

364.59 **Other iris atrophy**
Iris atrophy (generalized) (sector shaped)

5th 364.6 **Cysts of iris, ciliary body, and anterior chamber**
Excludes *miotic pupillary cyst (364.55)*
parasitic cyst (360.13)

364.60 **Idiopathic cysts**

364.61 **Implantation cysts**
Epithelial down-growth, anterior chamber
Implantation cysts (surgical) (traumatic)

364.62 **Exudative cysts of iris or anterior chamber**

364.63 **Primary cyst of pars plana**

364.64 **Exudative cyst of pars plana**

5th 364.7 **Adhesions and disruptions of iris and ciliary body**
Excludes *flat anterior chamber (360.34)*

364.70 **Adhesions of iris, unspecified**
Synechiae (iris) NOS

364.71 **Posterior synechiae**

364.72 **Anterior synechiae**

364.73 **Goniosynechiae**
Peripheral anterior synechiae

364.74 **Pupillary membranes**
Iris bombé
Pupillary:
occlusion
seclusion

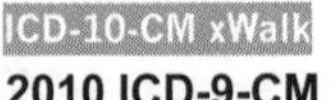

364.75 **Pupillary abnormalities**
Deformed pupil
Ectopic pupil
Rupture of sphincter, pupil

364.76 **Iridodialysis**

364.77 **Recession of chamber angle**

5th 364.8 **Other disorders of iris and ciliary body**

364.81 **Floppy iris syndrome**
Intraoperative floppy iris syndrome (IFIS)
Use additional E code to identify cause, such as:
sympatholytics [antiadrenergics] causing adverse effect in therapeutic use (E941.3)

364.82 **Plateau iris syndrome**

364.89 **Other disorders of iris and ciliary body**
Prolapse of iris NOS
Excludes *prolapse of iris in recent wound (871.1)*

364.9 **Unspecified disorder of iris and ciliary body**

4th 365 **Glaucoma**

Excludes *blind hypertensive eye [absolute glaucoma] (360.42)*
congenital glaucoma (743.20-743.22)

5th 365.0 **Borderline glaucoma [glaucoma suspect]**

365.00 **Preglaucoma, unspecified**
H40.0 Glaucoma suspect

365.01 **Open angle with borderline findings** I 2
H40.0 Glaucoma suspect
Open angle with:
borderline intraocular pressure
cupping of optic discs

365.02 **Anatomical narrow angle**

365.03 **Steroid responders**

365.04 **Ocular hypertension**
H40.0 Glaucoma suspect

5th 365.1 **Open-angle glaucoma**

365.10 **Open-angle glaucoma, unspecified** I 2, I 4 1
H40.10 Unspecified open-angle glaucoma
Wide-angle glaucoma NOS

365.11 **Primary open angle glaucoma** I 2, I 4 1
H40.11 Primary open-angle glaucoma
Chronic simple glaucoma

365.12 **Low tension glaucoma** I 2, I 4 1

365.13 **Pigmentary glaucoma**

365.14 **Glaucoma of childhood**
Infantile or juvenile glaucoma

365.15 **Residual stage of open angle glaucoma** I 2, I 4 1

5th 365.2 **Primary angle-closure glaucoma**

365.20 **Primary angle-closure glaucoma, unspecified**

365.21 **Intermittent angle-closure glaucoma**
Angle-closure glaucoma:
interval
subacute

365.22 **Acute angle-closure glaucoma**

365.23 **Chronic angle-closure glaucoma**

365.24 **Residual stage of angle-closure glaucoma**

5th 365.3 **Corticosteroid-induced glaucoma**

365.31 **Glaucomatous stage**

365.32 **Residual stage**

5th 365.4 **Glaucoma associated with congenital anomalies, dystrophies, and systemic syndromes**

365.41 **Glaucoma associated with chamber angle anomalies**

365.42 **Glaucoma associated with anomalies of iris**

365.43 **Glaucoma associated with other anterior segment anomalies**

365.44 ***Glaucoma associated with systemic syndromes***
Code first associated disease, as:
neurofibromatosis (237.7)
Sturge-Weber (-Dimitri) syndrome (759.6)

5th 365.5 **Glaucoma associated with disorders of the lens**

365.51 **Phacolytic glaucoma**

365.52 **Pseudoexfoliation glaucoma**

365.59 **Glaucoma associated with other lens disorders**

5th 365.6 **Glaucoma associated with other ocular disorders**

365.60 **Glaucoma associated with unspecified ocular disorder**

365.61 **Glaucoma associated with pupillary block**

365.62 **Glaucoma associated with ocular inflammations**

365.63 **Glaucoma associated with vascular disorders**

365.64 **Glaucoma associated with tumors or cysts**

365.65 **Glaucoma associated with ocular trauma**

5th 365.8 **Other specified forms of glaucoma**

365.81 **Hypersecretion glaucoma**

365.82 **Glaucoma with increased episcleral venous pressure**

365.83 **Aqueous misdirection**
Malignant glaucoma

365.89 **Other specified glaucoma**

365.9 **Unspecified glaucoma**

364.75 – 365.9

4th 366 Cataract

Excludes congenital cataract (743.30-743.34)

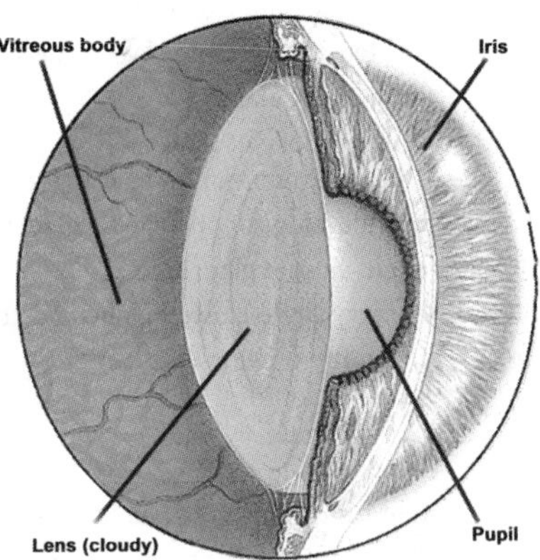

Layman's: *Acquired cataracts are categorized primarily by their location in the lens, though mixed morphology is common:*

Nuclear: *located in the interior of the lens; the most common type*

Cortical: *originate at the outer rim of the lens and radiate inward; common in diabetics*

Subcapsular: *located on the surface of the lens in the front (anterior) or rear (posterior)*

5th 366.0 Infantile, juvenile, and presenile cataract

366.00 Nonsenile cataract, unspecified

366.01 Anterior subcapsular polar cataract

366.02 Posterior subcapsular polar cataract

366.03 Cortical, lamellar, or zonular cataract

366.04 Nuclear cataract

366.09 Other and combined forms of nonsenile cataract

5th 366.1 Senile cataract

366.10 Senile cataract, unspecified A

H25.9 Unspecified age-related cataract

366.11 Pseudoexfoliation of lens capsule A

366.12 Incipient cataract A

H25.099 Other age-related incipient cataract, unspecified eye

Cataract:
- coronary
- immature NOS
- punctate

Water clefts

366.13 Anterior subcapsular polar senile cataract A

366.14 Posterior subcapsular polar senile cataract A

H25.049 Posterior subcapsular polar age-related cataract, unspecified eye

366.15 Cortical senile cataract A

H25.019 Cortical age-related cataract, unspecified eye

366.16 Nuclear sclerosis A

H25.13 Age-related nuclear cataract, bilateral

Cataracta brunescens
Nuclear cataract

366.17 Total or mature cataract A

H25.89 Other age-related cataract

366.18 Hypermature cataract A

Morgagni cataract

366.19 Other and combined forms of senile cataract A

H25.819 Combined forms of age-related cataract, unspecified eye

H25.89 Other age-related cataract

5th 366.2 Traumatic cataract

366.20 Traumatic cataract, unspecified

366.21 Localized traumatic opacities

Vossius' ring

366.22 Total traumatic cataract

366.23 Partially resolved traumatic cataract

5th 366.3 Cataract secondary to ocular disorders

366.30 Cataracta complicata, unspecified

366.31 Glaucomatous flecks (subcapsular)

Code first underlying glaucoma (365.0-365.9)

366.32 Cataract in inflammatory disorders

Code first underlying condition, as:
chronic choroiditis (363.0-363.2)

366.33 Cataract with neovascularization

Code first underlying condition, as:
chronic iridocyclitis (364.10)

366.34 Cataract in degenerative disorders

Sunflower cataract

Code first underlying condition, as:
chalcosis (360.24)
degenerative myopia (360.21)
pigmentary retinal dystrophy (362.74)

5th 366.4 Cataract associated with other disorders

366.41 *Diabetic cataract* 1, 2, 3, 117, 118, 163

Code first diabetes (249.5, 250.5)

366.42 *Tetanic cataract*

Code first underlying disease as:
calcinosis (275.40)
hypoparathyroidism (252.1)

366.43 *Myotonic cataract*

Code first underlying disorder (359.21, 359.23)

366.44 *Cataract associated with other syndromes*

Code first underlying condition, as:
craniofacial dysostosis (756.0)
galactosemia (271.1)

366.45 Toxic cataract

Drug-induced cataract

Use additional E to identify drug or other toxic substance

366.46 Cataract associated with radiation and other physical influences

Use additional E to identify cause

5th 366.5 After-cataract

366.50 After-cataract, unspecified

Secondary cataract NOS

366.51 Soemmering's ring

366.52 Other after-cataract, not obscuring vision

366.53 After-cataract, obscuring vision

H26.499 Other secondary cataract, unspecified eye

366.8 Other cataract

Calcification of lens

366.9 Unspecified cataract

H26.9 Unspecified cataract

4th 367 Disorders of refraction and accommodation

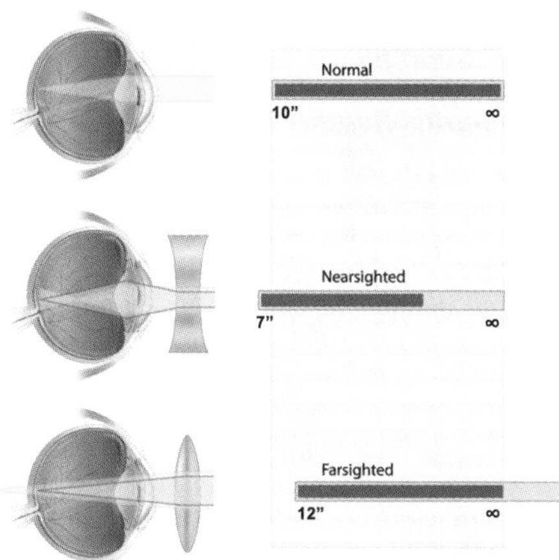

In myopia (nearsightedness), the point of focus (intersection of the yellow lines) falls short of the retina. A concave lens can correct the focus (red lines). Hypermetropia (farsightedness) can be corrected with a convex lens.

© 2008 Fairman Studios, LLC. All Rights Reserved.

367.0 Hypermetropia
Far-sightedness
Hyperopia

367.1 Myopia
Near-sightedness

5th **367.2 Astigmatism**

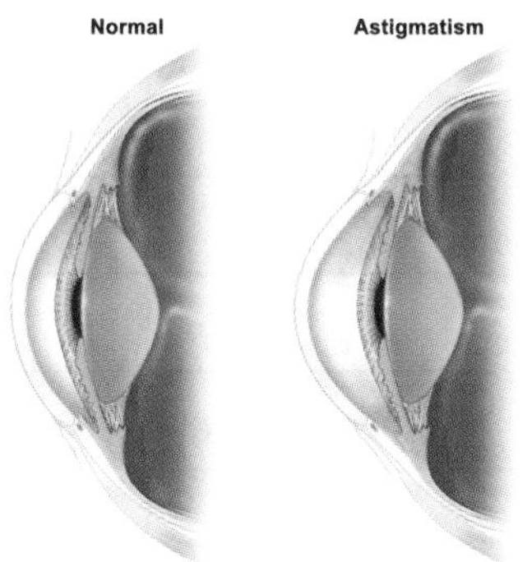

© 2008 Fairman Studios, LLC. All Rights Reserved.

367.20 Astigmatism, unspecified

367.21 Regular astigmatism

367.22 Irregular astigmatism

5th **367.3 Anisometropia and aniseikonia**

367.31 Anisometropia

367.32 Aniseikonia

367.4 Presbyopia
H52.4 Presbyopia

5th **367.5 Disorders of accommodation**

367.51 Paresis of accommodation
Cycloplegia

367.52 Total or complete internal ophthalmoplegia

367.53 Spasm of accommodation

5th **367.8 Other disorders of refraction and accommodation**

367.81 Transient refractive change

367.89 Other
Drug-induced disorders of refraction and accommodation
Toxic disorders of refraction and accommodation

367.9 Unspecified disorder of refraction and accommodation

4th 368 Visual disturbances

Excludes *electrophysiological disturbances (794.11-794.14)*

5th **368.0 Amblyopia ex anopsia**

368.00 Amblyopia, unspecified

368.01 Strabismic amblyopia
Suppression amblyopia

368.02 Deprivation amblyopia

368.03 Refractive amblyopia

5th **368.1 Subjective visual disturbances**

368.10 Subjective visual disturbance, unspecified

368.11 Sudden visual loss

368.12 Transient visual loss I 0
Concentric fading
Scintillating scotoma

368.13 Visual discomfort
Asthenopia
Eye strain
Photophobia

368.14 Visual distortions of shape and size
Macropsia
Metamorphopsia
Micropsia

368.15 Other visual distortions and entoptic phenomena
Photopsia
Refractive:
diplopia
polyopia
Visual halos

368.16 Psychophysical visual disturbances
Prosopagnosia
Visual:
agnosia
disorientation syndrome
hallucinations
object agnosia

368.2 Diplopia I 0
Double vision

5th **368.3 Other disorders of binocular vision**

368.30 Binocular vision disorder, unspecified

368.31 Suppression of binocular vision

368.32 Simultaneous visual perception without fusion

368.33 Fusion with defective stereopsis

368.34 Abnormal retinal correspondence

5th **368.4 Visual field defects**

368.40 Visual field defect, unspecified

368.41 Scotoma involving central area
Scotoma:
central
centrocecal
paracentral

368.42 Scotoma of blind spot area
Enlarged:
angioscotoma
blind spot
Paracecal scotoma

368.43 Sector or arcuate defects
Scotoma:
arcuate
Bjerrum
Seidel

368.44 Other localized visual field defect
Scotoma:
NOS
ring
Visual field defect:
nasal step
peripheral

368.45 Generalized contraction or constriction

368.46 Homonymous bilateral field defects
Hemianopsia (altitudinal) (homonymous)
Quadrant anopia

368.47 Heteronymous bilateral field defects
Hemianopsia:
binasal
bitemporal

5th **368.5 Color vision deficiencies**
Color blindness

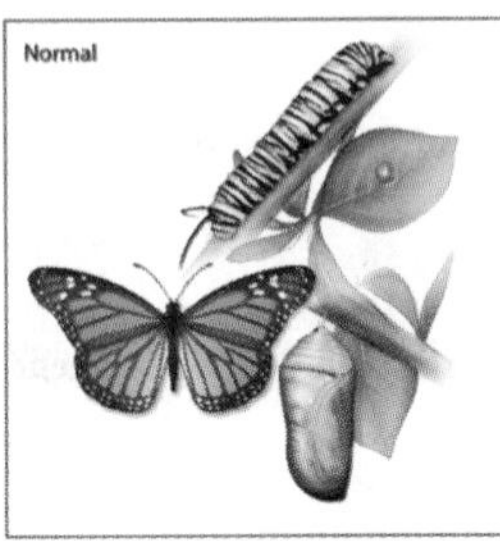

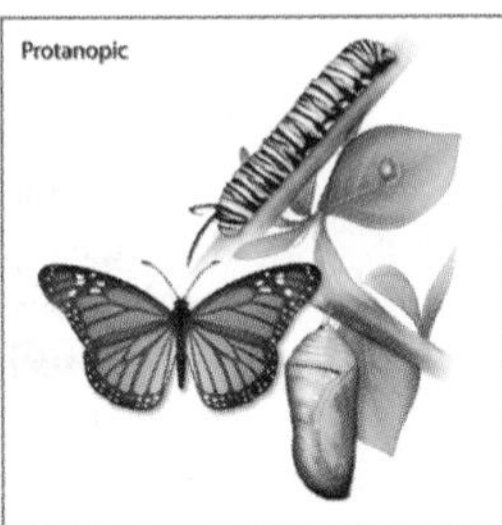

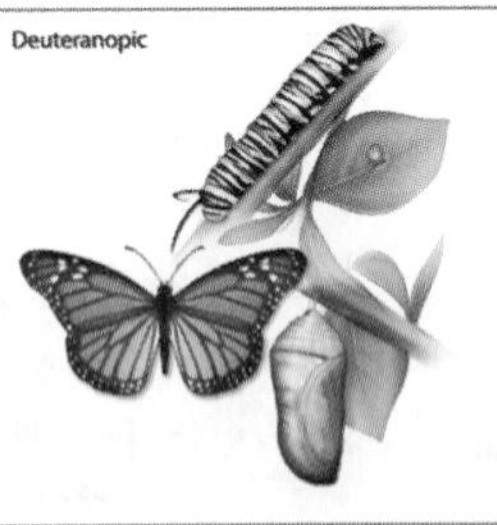

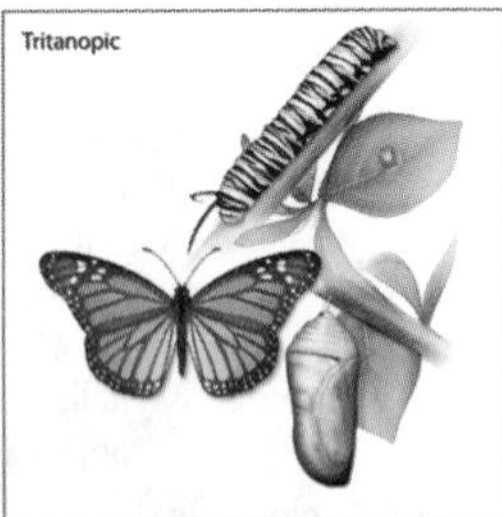

Protanopia is caused by the absence of red retinal photoreceptors. Deuteranopia is caused by the absence of green retinal photoreceptors. Tritanopia is caused by the absence of blue retinal photoreceptors. Monochromatism is caused by the absence of 2 or 3 cone pigments resulting in total color blindness.

© 2008 Fairman Studios, LLC. All Rights Reserved.

368.51 Protan defect
Protanomaly
Protanopia

368.52 Deutan defect
Deuteranomaly
Deuteranopia

368.53 Tritan defect
Tritanomaly
Tritanopia

368.54 Achromatopsia
Monochromatism (cone) (rod)

368.55 Acquired color vision deficiencies

368.59 Other color vision deficiencies

5th **368.6 Night blindness**

368.60 Night blindness, unspecified

368.61 Congenital night blindness
Hereditary night blindness
Oguchi's disease

368.62 Acquired night blindness
Excludes *that due to vitamin A deficiency (264.5)*

368.63 Abnormal dark adaptation curve
Abnormal threshold of cones or rods
Delayed adaptation of cones or rods

368.69 Other night blindness

368.8 Other specified visual disturbances
H53.8 Other visual disturbances
Blurred vision NOS

368.9 Unspecified visual disturbance

4th **369 Blindness and low vision**

Note: *Visual impairment refers to a functional limitation of the eye (e.g., limited visual acuity or visual field). It should be distinguished from visual disability, indicating a limitation of the abilities of the individual (e.g., limited reading skills, vocational skills), and from visual handicap, indicating a limitation of personal and socioeconomic independence (e.g., limited mobility, limited employability).*

The levels of impairment defined in the table below are based on the recommendations of the WHO Study Group on Prevention of Blindness, and of the International Council of Ophthalmology.

Note that definitions of blindness vary in different settings.

For international reporting, WHO defines blindness as profound impairment. This definition can be applied to blindness of one eye (369.1, 369.6) and to blindness of the individual (369.0).

For determination of benefits in the U.S.A., the definition of legal blindness as severe impairment is often used. This definition applies to blindness of the individual only.

Excludes *correctable impaired vision due to refractive errors (367.0-367.9)*

ICD-9-CM Defined Levels of Visual Impairment (defined by the *worse* of patient's visual acuity and visual field limitation)*	**Other Classifications**	
	World Health Organization (WHO)	"Legal blindness" in the USA
"Normal vision" Visual acuity > 20/30 (0.7)	Normal vision	Not legally blind
"Near normal vision" Visual acuity > 20/70 (0.286) but ≤ 20/30 (0.7)	Near-normal vision	
"Moderate impairment" Visual acuity > 20/200 (0.1) but ≤ 20/70 (0.286)	Low vision	
"Severe impairment" Visual acuity > 20/500 (0.04) but ≤ 20/200 (0.1) *or* Visual field > 10 degrees but ≤ 20 degrees		Legally blind (both eyes)
"Profound impairment" Visual acuity > 20/1000 (0.02) but ≤ 20/500 (0.04) *or* Visual field > 5 degrees but ≤ 10 degrees	Blindness (one or both eyes)	
"Near-total impairment" Visual acuity ≤ 20/1000 with light perception *or* Visual field ≤5 degrees		
"Total impairment" No light perception (NLP)		

* Visual acuity should be measured as the best achievable acuity with vision correction.
* Visual field measurements refer to largest field diameter for Goldman isopter III4e, 1/100 white test object or equivalent.

5th **369.0 Profound impairment, both eyes**

369.00 Impairment level not further specified
Blindness:
NOS according to WHO definition
both eyes

369.01 Better eye: total impairment; lesser eye: total impairment

369.02 Better eye: near-total impairment; lesser eye: not further specified

369.03 Better eye: near-total impairment; lesser eye: total impairment

369.04 Better eye: near-total impairment; lesser eye: near-total impairment

369.05 Better eye: profound impairment; lesser eye: not further specified

369.06 Better eye: profound impairment; lesser eye: total impairment

369.07 Better eye: profound impairment; lesser eye: near-total impairment

369.08 Better eye: profound impairment; lesser eye: profound impairment

5th 369.1 Moderate or severe impairment, better eye, profound impairment lesser eye

369.10 Impairment level not further specified
Blindness, one eye, low vision other eye

369.11 Better eye: severe impairment; lesser eye: blind, not further specified

369.12 Better eye: severe impairment; lesser eye: total impairment

369.13 Better eye: severe impairment; lesser eye: near-total impairment

369.14 Better eye: severe impairment; lesser eye: profound impairment

369.15 Better eye: moderate impairment; lesser eye: blind, not further specified

369.16 Better eye: moderate impairment; lesser eye: total impairment

369.17 Better eye: moderate impairment; lesser eye: near-total impairment

369.18 Better eye: moderate impairment; lesser eye: profound impairment

5th 369.2 Moderate or severe impairment, both eyes

369.20 Impairment level not further specified
Low vision, both eyes NOS

369.21 Better eye: severe impairment; lesser eye: not further specified

369.22 Better eye: severe impairment; lesser eye: severe impairment

369.23 Better eye: moderate impairment; lesser eye: not further specified

369.24 Better eye: moderate impairment; lesser eye: severe impairment

369.25 Better eye: moderate impairment; lesser eye: moderate impairment

369.3 Unqualified visual loss, both eyes

Excludes *blindness NOS:*
legal [U.S.A. definition] (369.4)
WHO definition (369.00)

369.4 Legal blindness, as defined in U.S.A.
Blindness NOS according to U.S.A. definition

Excludes *legal blindness with specification of impairment level (369.01-369.08, 369.11-369.14, 369.21-369.22)*

5th 369.6 Profound impairment, one eye

369.60 Impairment level not further specified
Blindness, one eye

369.61 One eye: total impairment; other eye: not specified

369.62 One eye: total impairment; other eye: near-normal vision

369.63 One eye: total impairment; other eye: normal vision

369.64 One eye: near-total impairment; other eye: not specified

369.65 One eye: near-total impairment; other eye: near-normal vision

369.66 One eye: near-total impairment; other eye: normal vision

369.67 One eye: profound impairment; other eye: not specified

369.68 One eye: profound impairment; other eye: near-normal vision

369.69 One eye: profound impairment; other eye: normal vision

5th 369.7 Moderate or severe impairment, one eye

369.70 Impairment level not further specified
Low vision, one eye

369.71 One eye: severe impairment; other eye: not specified

369.72 One eye: severe impairment; other eye: near-normal vision

369.73 One eye: severe impairment; other eye: normal vision

369.74 One eye: moderate impairment; other eye: not specified

369.75 One eye: moderate impairment; other eye: near-normal vision

369.76 One eye: moderate impairment; other eye: normal vision

369.8 Unqualified visual loss, one eye

369.9 Unspecified visual loss

4th 370 Keratitis

5th 370.0 Corneal ulcer

Excludes *that due to vitamin A deficiency (264.3)*

370.00 Corneal ulcer, unspecified

370.01 Marginal corneal ulcer

370.02 Ring corneal ulcer

370.03 Central corneal ulcer

370.04 Hypopyon ulcer
Serpiginous ulcer

370.05 Mycotic corneal ulcer

370.06 Perforated corneal ulcer

370.07 Mooren's ulcer

5th 370.2 Superficial keratitis without conjunctivitis

Excludes *dendritic [herpes simplex] keratitis (054.42)*

370.20 Superficial keratitis, unspecified

370.21 Punctate keratitis
Thygeson's superficial punctate keratitis

370.22 Macular keratitis
Keratitis:
areolar
nummular
stellate
striate

370.23 Filamentary keratitis

370.24 Photokeratitis
Snow blindness
Welders' keratitis

5th 370.3 Certain types of keratoconjunctivitis

370.31 Phlyctenular keratoconjunctivitis
Phlyctenulosis
Use additional code for any associated tuberculosis (017.3)

370.32 Limbar and corneal involvement in vernal conjunctivitis
Use additional code for vernal conjunctivitis (372.13)

370.33 Keratoconjunctivitis sicca, not specified as Sjögren's
Excludes *Sjögren's syndrome (710.2)*
370.34 Exposure keratoconjunctivitis
370.35 Neurotrophic keratoconjunctivitis
5th 370.4 Other and unspecified keratoconjunctivitis
370.40 Keratoconjunctivitis, unspecified
Superficial keratitis with conjunctivitis NOS
370.44 *Keratitis or keratoconjunctivitis in exanthema*
Code first underlying condition (050.0-052.9)
Excludes *herpes simplex (054.43)*
herpes zoster (053.21)
measles (055.71)
370.49 Other
Excludes *epidemic keratoconjunctivitis (077.1)*
5th 370.5 Interstitial and deep keratitis
370.50 Interstitial keratitis, unspecified
370.52 Diffuse interstitial keratitis
Cogan's syndrome
370.54 Sclerosing keratitis
370.55 Corneal abscess
370.59 Other
Excludes *disciform herpes simplex keratitis (054.43)*
syphilitic keratitis (090.3)
5th 370.6 Corneal neovascularization
370.60 Corneal neovascularization, unspecified
370.61 Localized vascularization of cornea
370.62 Pannus (corneal)
370.63 Deep vascularization of cornea
370.64 Ghost vessels (corneal)
370.8 Other forms of keratitis
Code first underlying condition, such as:
Acanthamoeba (136.21)
Fusarium (118)
370.9 Unspecified keratitis
4th 371 Corneal opacity and other disorders of cornea
5th 371.0 Corneal scars and opacities
Excludes *that due to vitamin A deficiency (264.6)*
371.00 Corneal opacity, unspecified
Corneal scar NOS
371.01 Minor opacity of cornea
Corneal nebula
371.02 Peripheral opacity of cornea
Corneal macula not interfering with central vision
371.03 Central opacity of cornea
Corneal:
leucoma interfering with central vision
macula interfering with central vision
371.04 Adherent leucoma
371.05 *Phthisical cornea*
Code first underlying tuberculosis (017.3)
5th 371.1 Corneal pigmentations and deposits
371.10 Corneal deposit, unspecified
371.11 Anterior pigmentations
Stähli's lines
371.12 Stromal pigmentations
Hematocornea
371.13 Posterior pigmentations
Krukenberg spindle
371.14 Kayser-Fleischer ring
371.15 Other deposits associated with metabolic disorders
371.16 Argentous deposits
5th 371.2 Corneal edema
371.20 Corneal edema, unspecified
371.21 Idiopathic corneal edema
371.22 Secondary corneal edema
371.23 Bullous keratopathy
371.24 Corneal edema due to wearing of contact lenses
5th 371.3 Changes of corneal membranes
371.30 Corneal membrane change, unspecified
371.31 Folds and rupture of Bowman's membrane
371.32 Folds in Descemet's membrane
371.33 Rupture in Descemet's membrane
5th 371.4 Corneal degenerations
371.40 Corneal degeneration, unspecified
371.41 Senile corneal changes
Arcus senilis
Hassall-Henle bodies
371.42 Recurrent erosion of cornea
Excludes *Mooren's ulcer (370.07)*
371.43 Band-shaped keratopathy
371.44 Other calcerous degenerations of cornea
371.45 Keratomalacia NOS
Excludes *that due to vitamin A deficiency (264.4)*
371.46 Nodular degeneration of cornea
Salzmann's nodular dystrophy
371.48 Peripheral degenerations of cornea
Marginal degeneration of cornea [Terrien's]
371.49 Other
Discrete colliquative keratopathy
5th 371.5 Hereditary corneal dystrophies
371.50 Corneal dystrophy, unspecified
371.51 Juvenile epithelial corneal dystrophy
371.52 Other anterior corneal dystrophies
Corneal dystrophy:
microscopic cystic
ring-like
371.53 Granular corneal dystrophy
371.54 Lattice corneal dystrophy
371.55 Macular corneal dystrophy
371.56 Other stromal corneal dystrophies
Crystalline corneal dystrophy
371.57 Endothelial corneal dystrophy
Combined corneal dystrophy
Cornea guttata
Fuchs' endothelial dystrophy
371.58 Other posterior corneal dystrophies
Polymorphous corneal dystrophy
5th 371.6 Keratoconus
371.60 Keratoconus, unspecified
371.61 Keratoconus, stable condition
371.62 Keratoconus, acute hydrops
5th 371.7 Other corneal deformities
371.70 Corneal deformity, unspecified
371.71 Corneal ectasia
371.72 Descemetocele
371.73 Corneal staphyloma
5th 371.8 Other corneal disorders
371.81 Corneal anesthesia and hypoesthesia

371.82 Corneal disorder due to contact lens
Excludes *corneal edema due to contact lens (371.24)*

371.89 Other

371.9 Unspecified corneal disorder

4th 372 Disorders of conjunctiva
Excludes *keratoconjunctivitis (370.3-370.4)*

5th 372.0 Acute conjunctivitis

372.00 Acute conjunctivitis, unspecified

372.01 Serous conjunctivitis, except viral
Excludes *viral conjunctivitis NOS (077.9)*

372.02 Acute follicular conjunctivitis
Conjunctival folliculosis NOS
Excludes *conjunctivitis:*
adenoviral (acute follicular) (077.3)
epidemic hemorrhagic (077.4)
inclusion (077.0)
Newcastle (077.8)
epidemic keratoconjunctivitis (077.1)
pharyngoconjunctival fever (077.2)

372.03 Other mucopurulent conjunctivitis
Catarrhal conjunctivitis
Excludes *blennorrhea neonatorum (gonococcal) (098.40)*
neonatal conjunctivitis (771.6)
ophthalmia neonatorum NOS (771.6)

372.04 Pseudomembranous conjunctivitis
Membranous conjunctivitis
Excludes *diphtheritic conjunctivitis (032.81)*

372.05 Acute atopic conjunctivitis

● 372.06 Acute chemical conjunctivitis
Acute toxic conjunctivitis
Use additional E code to identify the chemical or toxic agent
Excludes *burn of eye and adnexa (940.0-940.9)*
chemical corrosion injury of eye (940.2-940.3)

Rationale: *Chemical conjunctivitis (pink eye) may place a patient's vision at significant risk, but not be as serious as an alkaline (940.2) or acid (940.3) eye burn. It can result when any irritating substance enters the eyes. Common irritants include household cleaners, sprays, smoke, smog, industrial pollutants, and chlorine in swimming pools.*

The American Academy of Pediatrics proposed the addition of a new code for acute chemical conjunctivitis, due to concerns that the 2009 ICD-9-CM code set did not allow for adequate monitoring of this condition as the ICD-9-CM index pointed chemical conjunctivitis to 372.01, "Serous conjunctivitis (except viral)."

5th 372.1 Chronic conjunctivitis

372.10 Chronic conjunctivitis, unspecified

372.11 Simple chronic conjunctivitis

372.12 Chronic follicular conjunctivitis

372.13 Vernal conjunctivitis

372.14 Other chronic allergic conjunctivitis

372.15 *Parasitic conjunctivitis*
Code first underlying disease as:
filariasis (125.0-125.9)
mucocutaneous leishmaniasis (085.5)

5th 372.2 Blepharoconjunctivitis

372.20 Blepharoconjunctivitis, unspecified

372.21 Angular blepharoconjunctivitis

372.22 Contact blepharoconjunctivitis

5th 372.3 Other and unspecified conjunctivitis

372.30 Conjunctivitis, unspecified

372.31 *Rosacea conjunctivitis*
Code first underlying rosacea dermatitis (695.3)

372.33 *Conjunctivitis in mucocutaneous disease*
Code first underlying disease as:
erythema multiforme (695.10-695.19)
Reiter's disease (099.3)
Excludes *ocular pemphigoid (694.61)*

372.34 Pingueculitis
Excludes *pinguecula (372.51)*

372.39 Other

5th 372.4 Pterygium
Excludes *pseudopterygium (372.52)*

372.40 Pterygium, unspecified

372.41 Peripheral pterygium, stationary

372.42 Peripheral pterygium, progressive

372.43 Central pterygium

372.44 Double pterygium

372.45 Recurrent pterygium

5th 372.5 Conjunctival degenerations and deposits

372.50 Conjunctival degeneration, unspecified

372.51 Pinguecula
Excludes *pingueculitis (372.34)*

372.52 Pseudopterygium

372.53 Conjunctival xerosis
Excludes *conjunctival xerosis due to vitamin A deficiency (264.0, 264.1, 264.7)*

372.54 Conjunctival concretions

372.55 Conjunctival pigmentations
Conjunctival argyrosis

372.56 Conjunctival deposits

5th 372.6 Conjunctival scars

372.61 Granuloma of conjunctiva

372.62 Localized adhesions and strands of conjunctiva

372.63 Symblepharon
Extensive adhesions of conjunctiva

372.64 Scarring of conjunctiva
Contraction of eye socket (after enucleation)

5th 372.7 Conjunctival vascular disorders and cysts

372.71 Hyperemia of conjunctiva

372.72 Conjunctival hemorrhage
Hyposphagma
Subconjunctival hemorrhage

372.73 Conjunctival edema
Chemosis of conjunctiva
Subconjunctival edema

372.74 Vascular abnormalities of conjunctiva
Aneurysm(ata) of conjunctiva

372.75 Conjunctival cysts

5th 372.8 Other disorders of conjunctiva

372.81 Conjunctivochalasis

372.89 Other disorders of conjunctiva

372.9 Unspecified disorder of conjunctiva

4th 373 Inflammation of eyelids

5th 373.0 Blepharitis
Excludes *blepharoconjunctivitis (372.20-372.22)*

373.00 Blepharitis, unspecified

373.01 Ulcerative blepharitis

373.02 Squamous blepharitis

5th 373.1 **Hordeolum and other deep inflammation of eyelid**

373.11 **Hordeolum externum**
Hordeolum NOS
Stye

373.12 **Hordeolum internum**
Infection of meibomian gland

373.13 **Abscess of eyelid**
Furuncle of eyelid

373.2 **Chalazion**
Meibomian (gland) cyst
Excludes *infected meibomian gland (373.12)*

373.3 **Noninfectious dermatoses of eyelid**

373.31 **Eczematous dermatitis of eyelid**

373.32 **Contact and allergic dermatitis of eyelid**

373.33 **Xeroderma of eyelid**

373.34 **Discoid lupus erythematosus of eyelid**

373.4 ***Infective dermatitis of eyelid of types resulting in deformity***
Code first underlying disease, as:
leprosy (030.0-030.9)
lupus vulgaris (tuberculous) (017.0)
yaws (102.0-102.9)

373.5 ***Other infective dermatitis of eyelid***
Code first underlying disease, as:
actinomycosis (039.3)
impetigo (684)
mycotic dermatitis (110.0-111.9)
vaccinia (051.0)
postvaccination (999.0)
Excludes *herpes:*
simplex (054.41)
zoster (053.20)

373.6 ***Parasitic infestation of eyelid***
Code first underlying disease, as:
leishmaniasis (085.0-085.9)
loiasis (125.2)
onchocerciasis (125.3)
pediculosis (132.0)

373.8 **Other inflammations of eyelids**

373.9 **Unspecified inflammation of eyelid**

4th 374 **Other disorders of eyelids**

5th 374.0 **Entropion and trichiasis of eyelid**

374.00 **Entropion, unspecified**

374.01 **Senile entropion** A

374.02 **Mechanical entropion**

374.03 **Spastic entropion**

374.04 **Cicatricial entropion**

374.05 **Trichiasis without entropion**

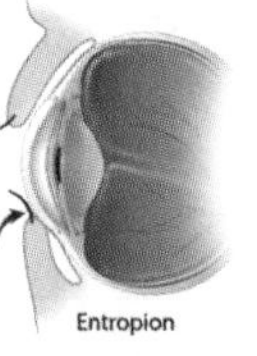

5th 374.1 **Ectropion**

374.10 **Ectropion, unspecified**

374.11 **Senile ectropion** A

374.12 **Mechanical ectropion**

374.13 **Spastic ectropion**

374.14 **Cicatricial ectropion**

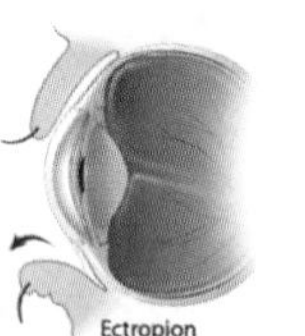

© 2008 Fairman Studios, LLC. All Rights Reserved.

5th 374.2 **Lagophthalmos**

374.20 **Lagophthalmos, unspecified**

374.21 **Paralytic lagophthalmos**

374.22 **Mechanical lagophthalmos**

374.23 **Cicatricial lagophthalmos**

5th 374.3 **Ptosis of eyelid**

374.30 **Ptosis of eyelid, unspecified**

374.31 **Paralytic ptosis**

374.32 **Myogenic ptosis**

374.33 **Mechanical ptosis**

374.34 **Blepharochalasis**
Pseudoptosis

5th 374.4 **Other disorders affecting eyelid function**
Excludes *blepharoclonus (333.81)*
blepharospasm (333.81)
facial nerve palsy (351.0)
third nerve palsy or paralysis (378.51-378.52)
tic (psychogenic) (307.20-307.23)
organic (333.3)

374.41 **Lid retraction or lag**

374.43 **Abnormal innervation syndrome**
Jaw-blinking
Paradoxical facial movements

374.44 **Sensory disorders**

374.45 **Other sensorimotor disorders**
Deficient blink reflex

374.46 **Blepharophimosis**
Ankyloblepharon

5th 374.5 **Degenerative disorders of eyelid and periocular area**

374.50 **Degenerative disorder of eyelid, unspecified**

374.51 ***Xanthelasma***
Xanthoma (planum) (tuberosum) of eyelid
Code first underlying condition (272.0-272.9)

374.52 **Hyperpigmentation of eyelid**
Chloasma
Dyspigmentation

374.53 **Hypopigmentation of eyelid**
Vitiligo of eyelid

374.54 **Hypertrichosis of eyelid**

374.55 **Hypotrichosis of eyelid**
Madarosis of eyelid

374.56 **Other degenerative disorders of skin affecting eyelid**

5th 374.8 **Other disorders of eyelid**

374.81 **Hemorrhage of eyelid**
Excludes *black eye (921.0)*

374.82 **Edema of eyelid**
Hyperemia of eyelid

374.83 **Elephantiasis of eyelid**

374.84 **Cysts of eyelids**
Sebaceous cyst of eyelid

374.85 **Vascular anomalies of eyelid**

374.86 **Retained foreign body of eyelid**

374.87 **Dermatochalasis**

374.89 **Other disorders of eyelid**

374.9 **Unspecified disorder of eyelid**

4th 375 **Disorders of lacrimal system**

5th 375.0 **Dacryoadenitis**

375.00 **Dacryoadenitis, unspecified**

375.01 **Acute dacryoadenitis**

375.02 **Chronic dacryoadenitis**

375.03 **Chronic enlargement of lacrimal gland**

5th 375.1 **Other disorders of lacrimal gland**

375.11 **Dacryops**

375.12 **Other lacrimal cysts and cystic degeneration**

375.13 **Primary lacrimal atrophy**

375.14 **Secondary lacrimal atrophy**

375.15 **Tear film insufficiency, unspecified**
H04.129 Dry eye syndrome of unspecified lacrimal gland
Dry eye syndrome

375.16 Dislocation of lacrimal gland

5th 375.2 Epiphora

375.20 Epiphora, unspecified as to cause

375.21 Epiphora due to excess lacrimation

375.22 Epiphora due to insufficient drainage

5th 375.3 Acute and unspecified inflammation of lacrimal passages

Excludes *neonatal dacryocystitis (771.6)*

375.30 Dacryocystitis, unspecified

375.31 Acute canaliculitis, lacrimal

375.32 Acute dacryocystitis

Acute peridacryocystitis

375.33 Phlegmonous dacryocystitis

5th 375.4 Chronic inflammation of lacrimal passages

375.41 Chronic canaliculitis

375.42 Chronic dacryocystitis

375.43 Lacrimal mucocele

5th 375.5 Stenosis and insufficiency of lacrimal passages

375.51 Eversion of lacrimal punctum

375.52 Stenosis of lacrimal punctum

375.53 Stenosis of lacrimal canaliculi

375.54 Stenosis of lacrimal sac

375.55 Obstruction of nasolacrimal duct, neonatal

Excludes *congenital anomaly of nasolacrimal duct (743.65)*

375.56 Stenosis of nasolacrimal duct, acquired

375.57 Dacryolith

5th 375.6 Other changes of lacrimal passages

375.61 Lacrimal fistula

375.69 Other

5th 375.8 Other disorders of lacrimal system

375.81 Granuloma of lacrimal passages

375.89 Other

375.9 Unspecified disorder of lacrimal system

4th 376 Disorders of the orbit

5th 376.0 Acute inflammation of orbit

376.00 Acute inflammation of orbit, unspecified

376.01 Orbital cellulitis

Abscess of orbit

376.02 Orbital periostitis

376.03 Orbital osteomyelitis

376.04 Tenonitis

5th 376.1 Chronic inflammatory disorders of orbit

376.10 Chronic inflammation of orbit, unspecified

376.11 Orbital granuloma

Pseudotumor (inflammatory) of orbit

376.12 Orbital myositis

376.13 *Parasitic infestation of orbit*

Code first underlying disease, as:
hydatid infestation of orbit (122.3, 122.6, 122.9)
myiasis of orbit (134.0)

5th 376.2 Endocrine exophthalmos

Code first underlying thyroid disorder (242.0-242.9)

376.21 *Thyrotoxic exophthalmos*

376.22 *Exophthalmic ophthalmoplegia*

5th 376.3 Other exophthalmic conditions

376.30 Exophthalmos, unspecified

376.31 Constant exophthalmos

376.32 Orbital hemorrhage

376.33 Orbital edema or congestion

376.34 Intermittent exophthalmos

376.35 Pulsating exophthalmos

376.36 Lateral displacement of globe

5th 376.4 Deformity of orbit

376.40 Deformity of orbit, unspecified

376.41 Hypertelorism of orbit

376.42 Exostosis of orbit

376.43 Local deformities due to bone disease

376.44 Orbital deformities associated with craniofacial deformities

376.45 Atrophy of orbit

376.46 Enlargement of orbit

376.47 Deformity due to trauma or surgery

5th 376.5 Enophthalmos

376.50 Enophthalmos, unspecified as to cause

376.51 Enophthalmos due to atrophy of orbital tissue

376.52 Enophthalmos due to trauma or surgery

376.6 Retained (old) foreign body following penetrating wound of orbit

Retrobulbar foreign body

5th 376.8 Other orbital disorders

376.81 Orbital cysts

Encephalocele of orbit

376.82 Myopathy of extraocular muscles

376.89 Other

376.9 Unspecified disorder of orbit

4th 377 Disorders of optic nerve and visual pathways

5th 377.0 Papilledema

377.00 Papilledema, unspecified

377.01 Papilledema associated with increased intracranial pressure

377.02 Papilledema associated with decreased ocular pressure

377.03 Papilledema associated with retinal disorder

377.04 Foster-Kennedy syndrome

5th 377.1 Optic atrophy

377.10 Optic atrophy, unspecified

377.11 Primary optic atrophy

Excludes *neurosyphilitic optic atrophy (094.84)*

377.12 Postinflammatory optic atrophy

377.13 Optic atrophy associated with retinal dystrophies

377.14 Glaucomatous atrophy [cupping] of optic disc

377.15 Partial optic atrophy

Temporal pallor of optic disc

377.16 Hereditary optic atrophy

Optic atrophy:
dominant hereditary
Leber's

5th 377.2 Other disorders of optic disc

377.21 Drusen of optic disc

377.22 Crater-like holes of optic disc

377.23 Coloboma of optic disc

377.24 Pseudopapilledema

5th 377.3 Optic neuritis

Excludes *meningococcal optic neuritis (036.81)*

377.30 Optic neuritis, unspecified

377.31 Optic papillitis

377.32 Retrobulbar neuritis (acute)

Excludes *syphilitic retrobulbar neuritis (094.85)*

377.33 Nutritional optic neuropathy

377.34 Toxic optic neuropathy

Toxic amblyopia

375.16 – 377.34

377.39 Other
Excludes *ischemic optic neuropathy (377.41)*

5th 377.4 Other disorders of optic nerve
377.41 Ischemic optic neuropathy
377.42 Hemorrhage in optic nerve sheaths
377.43 Optic nerve hypoplasia
377.49 Other
Compression of optic nerve

5th 377.5 Disorders of optic chiasm
377.51 Associated with pituitary neoplasms and disorders
377.52 Associated with other neoplasms
377.53 Associated with vascular disorders
377.54 Associated with inflammatory disorders

5th 377.6 Disorders of other visual pathways
377.61 Associated with neoplasms
377.62 Associated with vascular disorders
377.63 Associated with inflammatory disorders

5th 377.7 Disorders of visual cortex
Excludes *visual:*
agnosia (368.16)
hallucinations (368.16)
halos (368.15)
377.71 Associated with neoplasms
377.72 Associated with vascular disorders
377.73 Associated with inflammatory disorders
377.75 Cortical blindness

377.9 Unspecified disorder of optic nerve and visual pathways

4th 378 Strabismus and other disorders of binocular eye movements
Excludes *nystagmus and other irregular eye movements (379.50-379.59)*

5th 378.0 Esotropia
Convergent concomitant strabismus
Excludes *intermittent esotropia (378.20-378.22)*
378.00 Esotropia, unspecified
378.01 Monocular esotropia
378.02 Monocular esotropia with A pattern
378.03 Monocular esotropia with V pattern
378.04 Monocular esotropia with other noncomitancies
Monocular esotropia with X or Y pattern
378.05 Alternating esotropia
378.06 Alternating esotropia with A pattern
378.07 Alternating esotropia with V pattern
378.08 Alternating esotropia with other noncomitancies
Alternating esotropia with X or Y pattern

5th 378.1 Exotropia
Divergent concomitant strabismus
Excludes *intermittent exotropia (378.20, 378.23-378.24)*
378.10 Exotropia, unspecified
378.11 Monocular exotropia
378.12 Monocular exotropia with A pattern
378.13 Monocular exotropia with V pattern
378.14 Monocular exotropia with other noncomitancies
Monocular exotropia with X or Y pattern
378.15 Alternating exotropia
378.16 Alternating exotropia with A pattern
378.17 Alternating exotropia with V pattern
378.18 Alternating exotropia with other noncomitancies
Alternating exotropia with X or Y pattern

5th 378.2 Intermittent heterotropia
Excludes *vertical heterotropia (intermittent) (378.31)*
378.20 Intermittent heterotropia, unspecified
Intermittent:
esotropia NOS
exotropia NOS
378.21 Intermittent esotropia, monocular
378.22 Intermittent esotropia, alternating
378.23 Intermittent exotropia, monocular
378.24 Intermittent exotropia, alternating

5th 378.3 Other and unspecified heterotropia
378.30 Heterotropia, unspecified
378.31 Hypertropia
Vertical heterotropia (constant) (intermittent)
378.32 Hypotropia
378.33 Cyclotropia
378.34 Monofixation syndrome
Microtropia
378.35 Accommodative component in esotropia

5th 378.4 Heterophoria
378.40 Heterophoria, unspecified
378.41 Esophoria
378.42 Exophoria
378.43 Vertical heterophoria
378.44 Cyclophoria
378.45 Alternating hyperphoria

5th 378.5 Paralytic strabismus
378.50 Paralytic strabismus, unspecified
378.51 Third or oculomotor nerve palsy, partial
378.52 Third or oculomotor nerve palsy, total
378.53 Fourth or trochlear nerve palsy
378.54 Sixth or abducens nerve palsy
378.55 External ophthalmoplegia
378.56 Total ophthalmoplegia

5th 378.6 Mechanical strabismus
378.60 Mechanical strabismus, unspecified
378.61 Brown's (tendon) sheath syndrome
378.62 Mechanical strabismus from other musculofascial disorders
378.63 Limited duction associated with other conditions

5th 378.7 Other specified strabismus
378.71 Duane's syndrome
378.72 Progressive external ophthalmoplegia
378.73 Strabismus in other neuromuscular disorders

5th 378.8 Other disorders of binocular eye movements
Excludes *nystagmus (379.50-379.56)*
378.81 Palsy of conjugate gaze
378.82 Spasm of conjugate gaze
378.83 Convergence insufficiency or palsy
378.84 Convergence excess or spasm
378.85 Anomalies of divergence
378.86 Internuclear ophthalmoplegia
378.87 Other dissociated deviation of eye movements
Skew deviation

378.9 Unspecified disorder of eye movements
Ophthalmoplegia NOS
Strabismus NOS

4th 379 Other disorders of eye

5th 379.0 Scleritis and episcleritis

Excludes *syphilitic episcleritis (095.0)*

379.00 **Scleritis, unspecified**
Episcleritis NOS

379.01 Episcleritis periodica fugax

379.02 Nodular episcleritis

379.03 Anterior scleritis

379.04 Scleromalacia perforans

379.05 Scleritis with corneal involvement
Scleroperikeratitis

379.06 Brawny scleritis

379.07 Posterior scleritis
Sclerotenonitis

379.09 **Other**
Scleral abscess

5th 379.1 Other disorders of sclera

Excludes *blue sclera (743.47)*

379.11 Scleral ectasia
Scleral staphyloma NOS

379.12 Staphyloma posticum

379.13 Equatorial staphyloma

379.14 Anterior staphyloma, localized

379.15 Ring staphyloma

379.16 **Other degenerative disorders of sclera**

379.19 **Other**

5th 379.2 Disorders of vitreous body

379.21 Vitreous degeneration

H43.819 Vitreous degeneration, unspecified eye

Vitreous:
cavitation
detachment
liquefaction

379.22 Crystalline deposits in vitreous
Asteroid hyalitis
Synchysis scintillans

379.23 Vitreous hemorrhage

379.24 **Other vitreous opacities**

H43.399 Other vitreous opacities, unspecified eye

Vitreous floaters

379.25 Vitreous membranes and strands

379.26 Vitreous prolapse

379.29 **Other disorders of vitreous**

Excludes *vitreous abscess (360.04)*

5th 379.3 Aphakia and other disorders of lens

Excludes *after-cataract (366.50-366.53)*

379.31 Aphakia

Excludes *cataract extraction status (V45.61)*

379.32 Subluxation of lens

379.33 Anterior dislocation of lens

379.34 Posterior dislocation of lens

379.39 **Other disorders of lens**

5th 379.4 Anomalies of pupillary function

379.40 **Abnormal pupillary function, unspecified**

379.41 Anisocoria

Normal Anisocoria

© 2008 Fairman Studios, LLC. All Rights Reserved.

379.42 Miosis (persistent), not due to miotics

379.43 Mydriasis (persistent), not due to mydriatics

379.45 Argyll Robertson pupil, atypical
Argyll Robertson phenomenon or pupil, nonsyphilitic

Excludes *Argyll Robertson pupil (syphilitic) (094.89)*

379.46 Tonic pupillary reaction
Adie's pupil or syndrome

379.49 **Other**
Hippus
Pupillary paralysis

5th 379.5 Nystagmus and other irregular eye movements

379.50 **Nystagmus, unspecified**

379.51 Congenital nystagmus

379.52 Latent nystagmus

379.53 Visual deprivation nystagmus

379.54 Nystagmus associated with disorders of the vestibular system

379.55 Dissociated nystagmus

379.56 **Other forms of nystagmus**

379.57 Deficiencies of saccadic eye movements
Abnormal optokinetic response

379.58 Deficiencies of smooth pursuit movements

379.59 **Other irregularities of eye movements**
Opsoclonus

5th 379.6 Inflammation (infection) of postprocedural bleb
Postprocedural blebitis

379.60 **Inflammation (infection) of postprocedural bleb, unspecified**

379.61 Inflammation (infection) of postprocedural bleb, stage 1

379.62 Inflammation (infection) of postprocedural bleb, stage 2

379.63 Inflammation (infection) of postprocedural bleb, stage 3
Bleb associated endophthalmitis

379.8 **Other specified disorders of eye and adnexa**

5th 379.9 Unspecified disorder of eye and adnexa

379.90 **Disorder of eye, unspecified**

379.91 Pain in or around eye

379.92 Swelling or mass of eye

379.93 Redness or discharge of eye

379.99 **Other ill-defined disorders of eye**

Excludes *blurred vision NOS (368.8)*

DISEASES OF THE EAR AND MASTOID PROCESS (380-389)

Use additional external cause code, if applicable, to identify the cause of the ear condition

4th 380 Disorders of external ear

5th 380.0 Perichondritis and chondritis of pinna
Chondritis of auricle
Perichondritis of auricle

380.00 **Perichondritis of pinna, unspecified**

380.01 **Acute perichondritis of pinna**

380.02 **Chronic perichondritis of pinna**

380.03 **Chondritis of pinna**

5th 380.1 **Infective otitis externa**

380.10 **Infective otitis externa, unspecified** 91, 92, 93

Otitis externa (acute):
- NOS
- circumscribed
- diffuse
- hemorrhagica
- infective NOS

380.11 **Acute infection of pinna** 91, 92, 93

Excludes *furuncular otitis externa (680.0)*

380.12 **Acute swimmers' ear** 91, 92, 93

Beach ear
Tank ear

380.13 ***Other acute infections of external ear*** 91, 92, 93

Code first underlying disease, as:
- *erysipelas (035)*
- *impetigo (684)*
- *seborrheic dermatitis (690.10-690.18)*

Excludes *herpes simplex (054.73)*
herpes zoster (053.71)

380.14 **Malignant otitis externa**

380.15 ***Chronic mycotic otitis externa***

Code first underlying disease, as:
- *aspergillosis (117.3)*
- *otomycosis NOS (111.9)*

Excludes *candidal otitis externa (112.82)*

380.16 **Other chronic infective otitis externa**

Chronic infective otitis externa NOS

5th 380.2 **Other otitis externa**

380.21 **Cholesteatoma of external ear**

Keratosis obturans of external ear (canal)

Excludes *cholesteatoma NOS (385.30-385.35)*
postmastoidectomy (383.32)

380.22 **Other acute otitis externa** 91, 92, 93

Acute otitis externa:
- actinic
- chemical
- contact
- eczematoid
- reactive

380.23 **Other chronic otitis externa**

Chronic otitis externa NOS

5th 380.3 **Noninfectious disorders of pinna**

380.30 **Disorder of pinna, unspecified**

380.31 **Hematoma of auricle or pinna**

380.32 **Acquired deformities of auricle or pinna**

Excludes *cauliflower ear (738.7)*

380.39 **Other**

Excludes *gouty tophi of ear (274.81)*

380.4 **Impacted cerumen**

H61.23 Impacted cerumen, bilateral

Wax in ear

Layman's: *Earwax is only considered impacted if it is tightly packed and causes blockage of the ear canal, generally requiring instruments to remove. Because most payers reimburse at a higher rate for the removal of impacted cerumen (CPT® code 69210) than they do for a low level office visit, it is critical that the severity of impaction be documented when submitting claims for 69210.*

5th 380.5 **Acquired stenosis of external ear canal**

Collapse of external ear canal

380.50 **Acquired stenosis of external ear canal, unspecified as to cause**

380.51 **Secondary to trauma**

380.52 **Secondary to surgery**

380.53 **Secondary to inflammation**

5th 380.8 **Other disorders of external ear**

380.81 **Exostosis of external ear canal**

380.89 **Other**

380.9 **Unspecified disorder of external ear**

4th 381 **Nonsuppurative otitis media and Eustachian tube disorders**

5th 381.0 **Acute nonsuppurative otitis media**

Acute tubotympanic catarrh
Otitis media, acute or subacute:
- catarrhal
- exudative
- transudative
- with effusion

Excludes *otitic barotrauma (993.0)*

381.00 **Acute nonsuppurative otitis media, unspecified**

381.01 **Acute serous otitis media**

Acute or subacute secretory otitis media

381.02 **Acute mucoid otitis media**

Acute or subacute seromucinous otitis media
Blue drum syndrome

381.03 **Acute sanguinous otitis media**

381.04 **Acute allergic serous otitis media**

381.05 **Acute allergic mucoid otitis media**

381.06 **Acute allergic sanguinous otitis media**

5th 381.1 **Chronic serous otitis media**

Chronic tubotympanic catarrh

381.10 **Chronic serous otitis media, simple or unspecified** 94, 95

381.19 **Other** 94, 95

Serosanguinous chronic otitis media

5th 381.2 **Chronic mucoid otitis media**

Glue ear

Excludes *adhesive middle ear disease (385.10-385.19)*

381.20 **Chronic mucoid otitis media, simple or unspecified** 94, 95

381.29 **Other** 94, 95

Mucosanguinous chronic otitis media

381.3 **Other and unspecified chronic nonsuppurative otitis media** 94, 95

Otitis media, chronic:
- with effusion
- allergic
- exudative
- secretory
- seromucinous
- transudative

381.4 **Nonsuppurative otitis media, not specified as acute or chronic** 94, 95

Otitis media:
- with effusion
- allergic
- catarrhal
- exudative
- mucoid
- secretory
- seromucinous
- serous
- transudative

5th 381.5 Eustachian salpingitis
381.50 Eustachian salpingitis, unspecified
381.51 Acute Eustachian salpingitis
381.52 Chronic Eustachian salpingitis

5th 381.6 Obstruction of Eustachian tube
Stenosis of Eustachian tube
Stricture of Eustachian tube
381.60 Obstruction of Eustachian tube, unspecified
381.61 Osseous obstruction of Eustachian tube
Obstruction of Eustachian tube from cholesteatoma, polyp, or other osseous lesion
381.62 Intrinsic cartilagenous obstruction of Eustachian tube
381.63 Extrinsic cartilagenous obstruction of Eustachian tube
Compression of Eustachian tube

381.7 Patulous Eustachian tube

5th 381.8 Other disorders of Eustachian tube
381.81 Dysfunction of Eustachian tube
381.89 Other

381.9 Unspecified Eustachian tube disorder

4th 382 Suppurative and unspecified otitis media

5th 382.0 Acute suppurative otitis media
Otitis media, acute:
necrotizing NOS
purulent
382.00 Acute suppurative otitis media without spontaneous rupture of ear drum
382.01 Acute suppurative otitis media with spontaneous rupture of ear drum
382.02 *Acute suppurative otitis media in diseases classified elsewhere*
Code first underlying disease, as:
influenza (487.8)
scarlet fever (034.1)
Excludes *postmeasles otitis (055.2)*

382.1 Chronic tubotympanic suppurative otitis media
Benign chronic suppurative otitis media (with anterior perforation of ear drum)
Chronic tubotympanic disease (with anterior perforation of ear drum)

382.2 Chronic atticoantral suppurative otitis media
Chronic atticoantral disease (with posterior or superior marginal perforation of ear drum)
Persistent mucosal disease (with posterior or superior marginal perforation of ear drum)

382.3 Unspecified chronic suppurative otitis media
Chronic purulent otitis media
Excludes *tuberculous otitis media (017.4)*

382.4 Unspecified suppurative otitis media
Purulent otitis media NOS

382.9 Unspecified otitis media
Otitis media:
NOS
acute NOS
chronic NOS

4th 383 Mastoiditis and related conditions

5th 383.0 Acute mastoiditis
Abscess of mastoid
Empyema of mastoid
383.00 Acute mastoiditis without complications
383.01 Subperiosteal abscess of mastoid
383.02 Acute mastoiditis with other complications
Gradenigo's syndrome

383.1 Chronic mastoiditis
Caries of mastoid
Fistula of mastoid
Excludes *tuberculous mastoiditis (015.6)*

5th 383.2 Petrositis
Coalescing osteitis of petrous bone
Inflammation of petrous bone
Osteomyelitis of petrous bone
383.20 Petrositis, unspecified
383.21 Acute petrositis
383.22 Chronic petrositis

5th 383.3 Complications following mastoidectomy
383.30 Postmastoidectomy complication, unspecified
383.31 Mucosal cyst of postmastoidectomy cavity
383.32 Recurrent cholesteatoma of postmastoidectomy cavity
383.33 Granulations of postmastoidectomy cavity
Chronic inflammation of postmastoidectomy cavity

5th 383.8 Other disorders of mastoid
383.81 Postauricular fistula
383.89 Other

383.9 Unspecified mastoiditis

4th 384 Other disorders of tympanic membrane

5th 384.0 Acute myringitis without mention of otitis media
384.00 Acute myringitis, unspecified
Acute tympanitis NOS
384.01 Bullous myringitis
Myringitis bullosa hemorrhagica
384.09 Other

384.1 Chronic myringitis without mention of otitis media
Chronic tympanitis

5th 384.2 Perforation of tympanic membrane
Perforation of ear drum:
NOS
persistent posttraumatic
postinflammatory
Excludes *otitis media with perforation of tympanic membrane (382.00-382.9)*
traumatic perforation [current injury] (872.61)

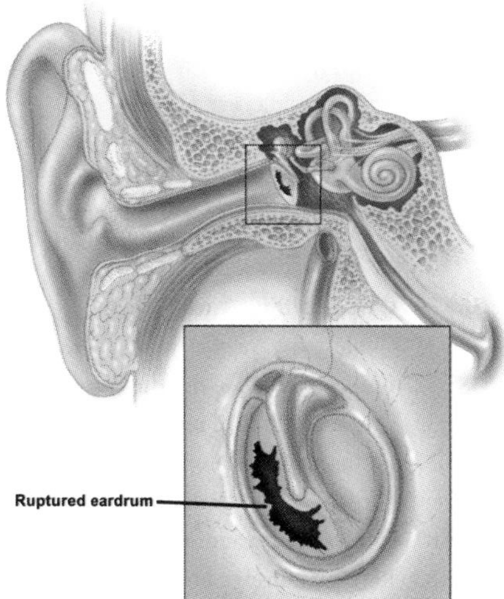

© 2008 Fairman Studios, LLC. All Rights Reserved.

384.20 Perforation of tympanic membrane, unspecified
384.21 Central perforation of tympanic membrane
384.22 Attic perforation of tympanic membrane
Pars flaccida

384.23 Other marginal perforation of tympanic membrane

384.24 Multiple perforations of tympanic membrane

384.25 Total perforation of tympanic membrane

5th 384.8 Other specified disorders of tympanic membrane

384.81 Atrophic flaccid tympanic membrane
Healed perforation of ear drum

384.82 Atrophic nonflaccid tympanic membrane

384.9 Unspecified disorder of tympanic membrane

4th 385 Other disorders of middle ear and mastoid
Excludes *mastoiditis (383.0-383.9)*

5th 385.0 Tympanosclerosis

385.00 Tympanosclerosis, unspecified as to involvement

385.01 Tympanosclerosis involving tympanic membrane only

385.02 Tympanosclerosis involving tympanic membrane and ear ossicles

385.03 Tympanosclerosis involving tympanic membrane, ear ossicles, and middle ear

385.09 Tympanosclerosis involving other combination of structures

5th 385.1 Adhesive middle ear disease
Adhesive otitis
Otitis media:
chronic adhesive
fibrotic
Excludes *glue ear (381.20-381.29)*

385.10 Adhesive middle ear disease, unspecified as to involvement

385.11 Adhesions of drum head to incus

385.12 Adhesions of drum head to stapes

385.13 Adhesions of drum head to promontorium

385.19 Other adhesions and combinations

5th 385.2 Other acquired abnormality of ear ossicles

385.21 Impaired mobility of malleus
Ankylosis of malleus

385.22 Impaired mobility of other ear ossicles
Ankylosis of ear ossicles, except malleus

385.23 Discontinuity or dislocation of ear ossicles

385.24 Partial loss or necrosis of ear ossicles

5th 385.3 Cholesteatoma of middle ear and mastoid
Cholesterosis of (middle) ear
Epidermosis of (middle) ear
Keratosis of (middle) ear
Polyp of (middle) ear
Excludes *cholesteatoma:*
external ear canal (380.21)
recurrent of postmastoidectomy cavity (383.32)

385.30 Cholesteatoma, unspecified

385.31 Cholesteatoma of attic

385.32 Cholesteatoma of middle ear

385.33 Cholesteatoma of middle ear and mastoid

385.35 Diffuse cholesteatosis

5th 385.8 Other disorders of middle ear and mastoid

385.82 Cholesterin granuloma

385.83 Retained foreign body of middle ear

385.89 Other

385.9 Unspecified disorder of middle ear and mastoid

4th 386 Vertiginous syndromes and other disorders of vestibular system
Excludes *vertigo NOS (780.4)*

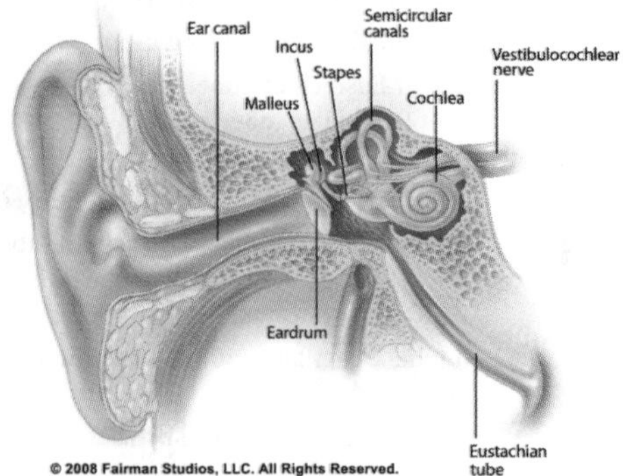

© 2008 Fairman Studios, LLC. All Rights Reserved.

5th 386.0 Ménière's disease
Endolymphatic hydrops
Lermoyez's syndrome
Ménière's syndrome or vertigo

386.00 Ménière's disease, unspecified
Ménière's disease (active)

386.01 Active Ménière's disease, cochleovestibular

386.02 Active Ménière's disease, cochlear

386.03 Active Ménière's disease, vestibular

386.04 Inactive Ménière's disease
Ménière's disease in remission

5th 386.1 Other and unspecified peripheral vertigo
Excludes *epidemic vertigo (078.81)*

386.10 Peripheral vertigo, unspecified

386.11 Benign paroxysmal positional vertigo
Benign paroxysmal positional nystagmus

386.12 Vestibular neuronitis
Acute (and recurrent) peripheral vestibulopathy

386.19 Other
Aural vertigo
Otogenic vertigo

386.2 Vertigo of central origin I-10
Central positional nystagmus
Malignant positional vertigo

5th 386.3 Labyrinthitis

386.30 Labyrinthitis, unspecified

386.31 Serous labyrinthitis
Diffuse labyrinthitis

386.32 Circumscribed labyrinthitis
Focal labyrinthitis

386.33 Suppurative labyrinthitis
Purulent labyrinthitis

386.34 Toxic labyrinthitis

386.35 Viral labyrinthitis

5th 386.4 Labyrinthine fistula

386.40 Labyrinthine fistula, unspecified

386.41 Round window fistula

386.42 Oval window fistula

386.43 Semicircular canal fistula

386.48 Labyrinthine fistula of combined sites

5th 386.5 Labyrinthine dysfunction

386.50 Labyrinthine dysfunction, unspecified

386.51 Hyperactive labyrinth, unilateral

386.52 Hyperactive labyrinth, bilateral

386.53 Hypoactive labyrinth, unilateral

386.54 Hypoactive labyrinth, bilateral

386.55 Loss of labyrinthine reactivity, unilateral

386.56 Loss of labyrinthine reactivity, bilateral

386.58 Other forms and combinations

386.8 Other disorders of labyrinth

386.9 Unspecified vertiginous syndromes and labyrinthine disorders

4th 387 Otosclerosis

Includes otospongiosis

387.0 Otosclerosis involving oval window, nonobliterative

387.1 Otosclerosis involving oval window, obliterative

387.2 Cochlear otosclerosis
Otosclerosis involving:
otic capsule
round window

387.8 Other otosclerosis

387.9 Otosclerosis, unspecified

4th 388 Other disorders of ear

5th 388.0 Degenerative and vascular disorders of ear

388.00 Degenerative and vascular disorders, unspecified

388.01 Presbyacusis

388.02 Transient ischemic deafness

5th 388.1 Noise effects on inner ear

388.10 Noise effects on inner ear, unspecified

388.11 Acoustic trauma (explosive) to ear
Otitic blast injury

388.12 Noise-induced hearing loss

388.2 Sudden hearing loss, unspecified

5th 388.3 Tinnitus

Layman's: *Objective tinnitus is generally caused by a structural defect and can be detected by the examiner, whereas subjective tinnitus is mainly idiopathic and can only be heard by the patient. Cases of subjective tinnitus are significantly more common than objective, however objective is considered more treatable.*

388.30 Tinnitus, unspecified

388.31 Subjective tinnitus

388.32 Objective tinnitus

5th 388.4 Other abnormal auditory perception

388.40 Abnormal auditory perception, unspecified

388.41 Diplacusis

388.42 Hyperacusis

388.43 Impairment of auditory discrimination

388.44 Recruitment

388.45 Acquired auditory processing disorder
Auditory processing disorder NOS

Excludes *cerebrospinal fluid rhinorrhea (349.81)*

388.5 Disorders of acoustic nerve
Acoustic neuritis
Degeneration of acoustic or eighth nerve
Disorder of acoustic or eighth nerve

Excludes *acoustic neuroma (225.1)*
syphilitic acoustic neuritis (094.86)

5th 388.6 Otorrhea

388.60 Otorrhea, unspecified
Discharging ear NOS

388.61 Cerebrospinal fluid otorrhea

Excludes *cerebrospinal fluid rhinorrhea (349.81)*

388.69 Other
Otorrhagia

5th 388.7 Otalgia

388.70 Otalgia, unspecified
Earache NOS

388.71 Otogenic pain

388.72 Referred pain

388.8 Other disorders of ear

388.9 Unspecified disorder of ear

4th 389 Hearing loss

Layman's: *The critical factors when making the determination on the appropriate hearing loss diagnosis are: 1) the nature of the impairment as structural (conductive [non-cochlear]) or functional (sensory [cochlear], neural [auditory nerve] or central [brain]); 2) laterality of the hearing loss (i.e., one ear or both); and 3) in the case of conductive hearing loss, the site of the structural defect or damage.*

5th 389.0 Conductive hearing loss
Conductive deafness

Excludes *mixed conductive and sensorineural hearing loss (389.20-389.22)*

389.00 Conductive hearing loss, unspecified

389.01 Conductive hearing loss, external ear

389.02 Conductive hearing loss, tympanic membrane

389.03 Conductive hearing loss, middle ear

389.04 Conductive hearing loss, inner ear

389.05 Conductive hearing loss, unilateral

389.06 Conductive hearing loss, bilateral

389.08 Conductive hearing loss of combined types

5th 389.1 Sensorineural hearing loss
Perceptive hearing loss or deafness

Excludes *abnormal auditory perception (388.40-388.44)*
mixed conductive and sensorineural hearing loss (389.20-389.22)
psychogenic deafness (306.7)

389.10 Sensorineural hearing loss, unspecified

H90.5 Unspecified sensorineural hearing loss

389.11 Sensory hearing loss, bilateral

389.12 Neural hearing loss, bilateral

389.13 Neural hearing loss, unilateral

389.14 Central hearing loss

389.15 Sensorineural hearing loss, unilateral

389.16 Sensorineural hearing loss, asymmetrical

389.17 Sensory hearing loss, unilateral

389.18 Sensorineural hearing loss, bilateral

5th 389.2 Mixed conductive and sensorineural hearing loss
Deafness or hearing loss of type classifiable to 389.00-389.08 with type classifiable to 389.10-389.18

389.20 Mixed hearing loss, unspecified

389.21 Mixed hearing loss, unilateral

389.22 Mixed hearing loss, bilateral

389.7 Deaf nonspeaking, not elsewhere classifiable

389.8 Other specified forms of hearing loss

389.9 Unspecified hearing loss
Deafness NOS

386.56 – 389.9

7. DISEASES OF THE CIRCULATORY SYSTEM (390-459)

ACUTE RHEUMATIC FEVER (390-392)

390 Rheumatic fever without mention of heart involvement

Arthritis, rheumatic, acute or subacute
Rheumatic fever (active) (acute)
Rheumatism, articular, acute or subacute

Excludes *that with heart involvement (391.0-391.9)*

4th **391 Rheumatic fever with heart involvement**

Excludes *chronic heart diseases of rheumatic origin (393-398.99) unless rheumatic fever is also present or there is evidence of recrudescence or activity of the rheumatic process*

Heart Anatomy

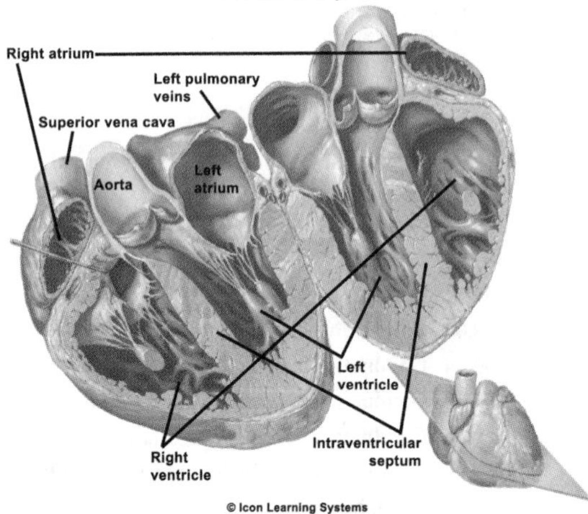

© Icon Learning Systems

391.0 Acute rheumatic pericarditis

Rheumatic:
- fever (active) (acute) with pericarditis
- pericarditis (acute)

Any condition classifiable to 390 with pericarditis

Excludes *that not specified as rheumatic (420.0-420.9)*

391.1 Acute rheumatic endocarditis

Rheumatic:
- endocarditis, acute
- fever (active) (acute) with endocarditis or valvulitis
- valvulitis acute

Any condition classifiable to 390 with endocarditis or valvulitis

391.2 Acute rheumatic myocarditis

Rheumatic fever (active) (acute) with myocarditis
Any condition classifiable to 390 with myocarditis

391.8 Other acute rheumatic heart disease

Rheumatic:
- fever (active) (acute) with other or multiple types of heart involvement
- pancarditis, acute

Any condition classifiable to 390 with other or multiple types of heart involvement

391.9 Acute rheumatic heart disease, unspecified

Rheumatic:
- carditis, acute
- fever (active) (acute) with unspecified type of heart involvement
- heart disease, active or acute

Any condition classifiable to 390 with unspecified type of heart involvement

4th **392 Rheumatic chorea**

Includes Sydenham's chorea

Excludes *chorea:*
- *NOS (333.5)*
- *Huntington's (333.4)*

392.0 With heart involvement

Rheumatic chorea with heart involvement of any type classifiable to 391

392.9 Without mention of heart involvement

CHRONIC RHEUMATIC HEART DISEASE (393-398)

393 Chronic rheumatic pericarditis

Adherent pericardium, rheumatic
Chronic rheumatic:
- mediastinopericarditis
- myopericarditis

Excludes *pericarditis NOS or not specified as rheumatic (423.0-423.9)*

4th **394 Diseases of mitral valve**

Excludes *that with aortic valve involvement (396.0-396.9)*

394.0 Mitral stenosis

Mitral (valve):
- obstruction (rheumatic)
- stenosis NOS

394.1 Rheumatic mitral insufficiency

Rheumatic mitral:
- incompetence
- regurgitation

Excludes *that not specified as rheumatic (424.0)*

394.2 Mitral stenosis with insufficiency

Mitral stenosis with incompetence or regurgitation

394.9 Other and unspecified mitral valve diseases

Mitral (valve):
- disease (chronic)
- failure

4th **395 Diseases of aortic valve**

Excludes *that not specified as rheumatic (424.1)*
that with mitral valve involvement (396.0-396.9)

395.0 Rheumatic aortic stenosis

Rheumatic aortic (valve) obstruction

395.1 Rheumatic aortic insufficiency

Rheumatic aortic:
- incompetence
- regurgitation

395.2 Rheumatic aortic stenosis with insufficiency

Rheumatic aortic stenosis with incompetence or regurgitation

395.9 Other and unspecified rheumatic aortic diseases

Rheumatic aortic (valve) disease

4th 396 **Diseases of mitral and aortic valves**

Includes involvement of both mitral and aortic valves, whether specified as rheumatic or not

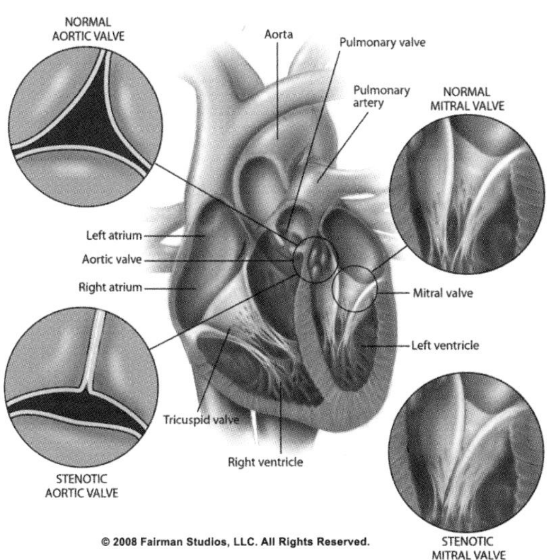

© 2008 Fairman Studios, LLC. All Rights Reserved.

396.0 Mitral valve stenosis and aortic valve stenosis
Atypical aortic (valve) stenosis
Mitral and aortic (valve) obstruction (rheumatic)

396.1 Mitral valve stenosis and aortic valve insufficiency

396.2 Mitral valve insufficiency and aortic valve stenosis

396.3 Mitral valve insufficiency and aortic valve insufficiency
Mitral and aortic (valve):
- incompetence
- regurgitation

396.8 Multiple involvement of mitral and aortic valves
Stenosis and insufficiency of mitral or aortic valve with stenosis or insufficiency, or both, of the other valve

396.9 Mitral and aortic valve diseases, unspecified

4th 397 **Diseases of other endocardial structures**

397.0 Diseases of tricuspid valve
Tricuspid (valve) (rheumatic):
- disease
- insufficiency
- obstruction
- regurgitation
- stenosis

397.1 Rheumatic diseases of pulmonary valve
Excludes *that not specified as rheumatic (424.3)*

397.9 Rheumatic diseases of endocardium, valve unspecified
Rheumatic:
- endocarditis (chronic)
- valvulitis (chronic)

Excludes *that not specified as rheumatic (424.90-424.99)*

4th 398 **Other rheumatic heart disease**

398.0 Rheumatic myocarditis
Rheumatic degeneration of myocardium
Excludes *myocarditis not specified as rheumatic (429.0)*

5th **398.9 Other and unspecified rheumatic heart diseases**

398.90 Rheumatic heart disease, unspecified
Rheumatic:
- carditis
- heart disease NOS

Excludes *carditis not specified as rheumatic (429.89)*
heart disease NOS not specified as rheumatic (429.9)

398.91 Rheumatic heart failure (congestive)
Rheumatic left ventricular failure

398.99 Other

HYPERTENSIVE DISEASE (401-405)

Excludes *that complicating pregnancy, childbirth, or the puerperium (642.0-642.9)*
that involving coronary vessels (410.00-414.9)

ICD-9-CM Official Guidelines (Chapter 7):

a. Hypertension

Hypertension Table

The Hypertension Table, found under the main term, "Hypertension", in the Alphabetic Index, contains a complete listing of all conditions due to or associated with hypertension and classifies them according to malignant, benign, and unspecified....

6) Hypertensive Retinopathy

Two codes are necessary to identify the condition. First assign the code from subcategory 362.11, Hypertensive retinopathy, then the appropriate code from categories 401-405 to indicate the type of hypertension....

8) Hypertension, Transient

Assign code 796.2, Elevated blood pressure reading without diagnosis of hypertension, unless patient has an established diagnosis of hypertension. Assign code 642.3x for transient hypertension of pregnancy.

9) Hypertension, Controlled

Assign appropriate code from categories 401-405. This diagnostic statement usually refers to an existing state of hypertension under control by therapy.

10) Hypertension, Uncontrolled

Uncontrolled hypertension may refer to untreated hypertension or hypertension not responding to current therapeutic regimen. In either case, assign the appropriate code from categories 401-405 to designate the stage and type of hypertension. Code to the type of hypertension.

4th 401 **Essential hypertension**

Includes high blood pressure
hyperpiesia
hyperpiesis
hypertension (arterial) (essential) (primary) (systemic)
hypertensive vascular:
- degeneration
- disease

Excludes *elevated blood pressure without diagnosis of hypertension (796.2)*
pulmonary hypertension (416.0-416.9)
that involving vessels of:
- *brain (430-438)*
- *eye (362.11)*

ICD-9-CM Official Guidelines (Chapter 7a):

1) Hypertension, Essential, or NOS

Assign hypertension (arterial) (essential) (primary) (systemic) (NOS) to category code 401 with the appropriate fourth digit to indicate malignant (.0), benign (.1), or unspecified (.9). Do not use either .0 malignant or .1 benign unless medical record documentation supports such a designation....

11) Elevated Blood Pressure

For a statement of elevated blood pressure without further specificity, assign code 796.2, Elevated blood pressure reading without diagnosis of hypertension, rather than a code from category 401.

401.0 Malignant

I10 Essential (primary) hypertension

Layman's: *Malignant hypertension is generally defined as repeated adult systolic BP readings of > 220 mmHg and diastolic readings of > 120 mmHg. It is rare, affecting around 1% of all hypertension sufferers.*

401.1 **Benign**

I10 Essential (primary) hypertension

Layman's: *Benign hypertension is generally defined as repeated adult systolic BP readings of > 140 mmHg and a diastolic readings of > 90 mmHg.*

401.9 **Unspecified**

I10 Essential (primary) hypertension

4th **402 Hypertensive heart disease**

Includes hypertensive:
- cardiomegaly
- cardiopathy
- cardiovascular disease
- heart (disease) (failure)

any condition classifiable to 429.0-429.3, 429.8, 429.9 due to hypertension

Use additional code to specify type of heart failure (428.0-428.43), if known

ICD-9-CM Official Guidelines (Chapter 7):

a. Hypertension

2) Hypertension with Heart Disease

Heart conditions (425.8, 429.0-429.3, 429.8, 429.9) are assigned to a code from category 402 when a causal relationship is stated (due to hypertension) or implied (hypertensive). Use an additional code from category 428 to identify the type of heart failure in those patients with heart failure. More than one code from category 428 may be assigned if the patient has systolic or diastolic failure and congestive heart failure.

The same heart conditions (425.8, 429.0-429.3, 429.8, 429.9) with hypertension, but without a stated causal relationship, are coded separately. Sequence according to the circumstances of the admission/encounter.

5th **402.0 Malignant**

402.00 Without heart failure

402.01 With heart failure 5, 8

5th **402.1 Benign**

402.10 Without heart failure

I11.9 Hypertensive heart disease without heart failure

402.11 With heart failure 5, 8

5th **402.9 Unspecified**

402.90 Without heart failure

I11.9 Hypertensive heart disease without heart failure

402.91 With heart failure 5, 8

4th **403 Hypertensive chronic kidney disease**

Includes arteriolar nephritis
arteriosclerosis of:
- kidney
- renal arterioles

arteriosclerotic nephritis (chronic) (interstitial)
hypertensive:
- nephropathy
- renal failure
- uremia (chronic)

nephrosclerosis
renal sclerosis with hypertension
any condition classifiable to 585 with any condition classifiable to 401

Excludes *acute kidney ~~renal~~ failure (584.5-584.9)*
renal disease stated as not due to hypertension
renovascular hypertension (405.0-405.9 with fifth digit 1)

The following fifth-digit subclassification is for use with category 403:

0 **with chronic kidney disease stage I through stage IV, or unspecified**
Use additional code to identify the stage of chronic kidney disease (585.1-585.4, 585.9)

1 **with chronic kidney disease stage V or end stage renal disease**
Use additional code to identify the stage of chronic kidney disease (585.5, 585.6)

ICD-9-CM Official Guidelines (Chapter 7):

a. Hypertension

3) Hypertensive Chronic Kidney Disease

Assign codes from category 403, Hypertensive chronic kidney disease, when conditions classified to categories 585-587 are present. Unlike hypertension with heart disease, ICD-9-CM presumes a cause-and-effect relationship and classifies chronic kidney disease (CKD) with hypertension as hypertensive chronic kidney disease.

Fifth digits for category 403 should be assigned as follows:
- *0 with CKD stage I through stage IV, or unspecified.*
- *1 with CKD stage V or end stage renal disease. The appropriate code from category 585, Chronic kidney disease, should be used as a secondary code with a code from category 403 to identify the stage of chronic kidney disease.*

See Section I.C.10.a for information on the coding of chronic kidney disease.

5th **403.0 Malignant**
[0-1]

5th **403.1 Benign**
[0-1]

5th **403.9 Unspecified**
[0-1]

4th **404 Hypertensive heart and chronic kidney disease**

Includes disease:
cardiorenal
cardiovascular renal
any condition classifiable to 402 with any condition classifiable to 403

Use additional code to specify type of heart failure (428.0-428.43), if known

The following fifth-digit subclassification is for use with category 404:

0 **without heart failure or chronic kidney disease and with chronic kidney disease stage I through stage IV, or unspecified**
Use additional code to identify the stage of chronic kidney disease (585.1-585.4, 585.9)

1 **with heart failure and with chronic kidney disease stage I through stage IV, or unspecified** 5, 8
Use additional code to identify the stage of chronic kidney disease (585.1-585.4, 585.9)

2 **without heart failure and with chronic kidney disease stage V or end stage renal disease**
Use additional code to identify the stage of chronic kidney disease (585.5, 585.6)

3 **with heart failure and chronic kidney disease stage V or end stage renal disease** 5, 8
Use additional code to identify the stage of chronic kidney disease (585.5-585.6) Use additional code to specify type of heart failure (428.0, 428.20-428.23, 428.30-428.33, 428.40-428.43)

ICD-9-CM Official Guidelines (Chapter 7):

a. Hypertension

4) Hypertensive Heart and Chronic Kidney Disease

Assign codes from combination category 404, Hypertensive heart and chronic kidney disease, when both hypertensive kidney disease and hypertensive heart disease are stated in the diagnosis. Assume a relationship between the hypertension and the chronic kidney disease, whether or not the condition is so designated. Assign an additional code from category 428, to identify the type of heart failure. More than one code from category 428 may be assigned if the patient has systolic or diastolic failure and congestive heart failure.

Fifth digits for category 404 should be assigned as follows:

- *0 without heart failure and with chronic kidney disease (CKD) stage I through stage IV, or unspecified*
- *1 with heart failure and with CKD stage I through stage IV, or unspecified*
- *2 without heart failure and with CKD stage V or end stage renal disease*
- *3 with heart failure and with CKD stage V or end stage renal disease*

The appropriate code from category 585, Chronic kidney disease, should be used as a secondary code with a code from category 404 to identify the stage of kidney disease.

See Section I.C.10.a for information on the coding of chronic kidney disease.

5th **404.0 Malignant**
[0-3]

5th **404.1 Benign**
[0-3]

5th **404.9 Unspecified**
[0-3]

4th **405 Secondary hypertension**

ICD-9-CM Official Guidelines (Chapter 7):

a. Hypertension

7) Hypertension, Secondary

Two codes are required: one to identify the underlying etiology and one from category 405 to identify the hypertension. Sequencing of codes is determined by the reason for admission/encounter.

5th **405.0 Malignant**
405.01 Renovascular
405.09 Other

5th **405.1 Benign**
405.11 Renovascular
405.19 Other

5th **405.9 Unspecified**
405.91 Renovascular
405.99 Other

ISCHEMIC HEART DISEASE (410-414)

Includes that with mention of hypertension

Use additional code to identify presence of hypertension (401.0-405.9)

4th **410 Acute myocardial infarction**

ST elevation (STEMI) and non-ST elevation (NSTEMI) myocardial infarction

Includes cardiac infarction
coronary (artery):
embolism
occlusion
rupture
thrombosis
infarction of heart, myocardium, or ventricle
rupture of heart, myocardium, or ventricle
ST elevation (STEMI) and non-ST elevation (NSTEMI) myocardial infarction
any condition classifiable to 414.1-414.9 specified as acute or with a stated duration of 8 weeks or less

The following fifth-digit subclassification is for use with category 410:

0 **episode of care unspecified**
Use when the source document does not contain sufficient information for the assignment of fifth-digit 1 or 2.

1 **initial episode of care** 2 8
Use fifth-digit 1 to designate the first episode of care (regardless of facility site) for a newly diagnosed myocardial infarction. The fifth-digit 1 is assigned regardless of the number of times a patient may be transferred during the initial episode of care.

2 **subsequent episode of care**
Use fifth-digit 2 to designate an episode of care following the initial episode when the patient is admitted for further observation, evaluation or treatment for a myocardial infarction that has received initial treatment, but is still less than 8 weeks old.

5th **410.0 Of anterolateral wall** 6, 7, 118, 152
[0-2]

ICD-9-CM Official Guidelines (Chapter 7):

e. Acute myocardial infarction (AMI)

1) ST elevation myocardial infarction (STEMI) and non ST elevation myocardial infarction (NSTEMI)

The ICD-9-CM codes for acute myocardial infarction (AMI) identify the site, such as anterolateral wall or true posterior wall. Subcategories 410.0-410.6 and 410.8 are used for ST elevation myocardial infarction (STEMI). Subcategory 410.7, Subendocardial infarction, is used for non ST elevation myocardial infarction (NSTEMI) and nontransmural MIs.

2) *Acute myocardial infarction, unspecified*

Subcategory 410.9 is the default for the unspecified term acute myocardial infarction. If only STEMI or transmural MI without the site is documented, query the provider as to the site, or assign a code from subcategory 410.9.

3) *AMI documented as nontransmural or subendocardial but site provided*

If an AMI is documented as nontransmural or subendocardial, but the site is provided, it is still coded as a subendocardial AMI. If NSTEMI evolves to STEMI, assign the STEMI code. If STEMI converts to NSTEMI due to thrombolytic therapy, it is still coded as STEMI.

5th **410.1 Of other anterior wall** 6, 7, 118, 152

[0-2] Infarction:
- anterior (wall) NOS (with contiguous portion of intraventricular septum)
- anteroapical (with contiguous portion of intraventricular septum)
- anterseptal (with contiguous portion of intraventricular septum)
- ST elevation myocardial infarction (STEMI) of anterolateral wall

5th **410.2 Of inferolateral wall** 6, 7, 118, 152

[0-2] ST elevation myocardial infarction (STEMI) of inferolateral wall

5th **410.3 Of inferoposterior wall** 6, 7, 118, 152

[0-2] ST elevation myocardial infarction (STEMI) of inferoposterior wall

5th **410.4 Of other inferior wall** 6, 7, 118, 152

[0-2] Infarction:
- diaphragmatic wall NOS (with contiguous portion of intraventricular septum)
- inferior (wall) NOS (with contiguous portion of intraventricular septum)
- ST elevation myocardial infarction (STEMI) of other inferior wall

5th **410.5 Of other lateral wall** 6, 7, 118, 152

[0-2] Infarction:
- apical-lateral
- basal-lateral
- high lateral
- posterolateral

ST elevation myocardial infarction (STEMI) of other lateral wall

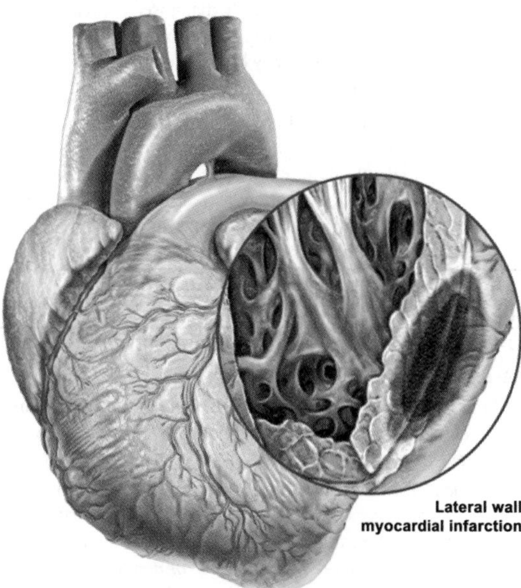

Lateral wall myocardial infarction

© 2006 Anatomical Chart Company

5th **410.6 True posterior wall infarction** 6, 7, 118, 152

[0-2] Infarction:
- posterobasal
- strictly posterior

ST elevation myocardial infarction (STEMI) of true posterior wall

5th **410.7 Subendocardial infarction** 6, 7, 118, 152

I21.4 Non-ST elevation (NSTEMI) myocardial infarction

[0-2] Non-ST elevation myocardial infarction (NSTEMI)
Nontransmural infarction

5th **410.8 Of other specified sites** 6, 7, 118, 152

[0-2] Infarction of:
- atrium
- papillary muscle
- septum alone

ST elevation myocardial infarction (STEMI) of other specified sites

5th **410.9 Unspecified site** 6, 7, 118, 152

I21.3 ST elevation (STEMI) myocardial infarction of unspecified site

[0-2] Acute myocardial infarction NOS
Coronary occlusion NOS
Myocardial infarcation NOS

4th **411 Other acute and subacute forms of ischemic heart disease**

411.0 Postmyocardial infarction syndrome 6, 7, 118, 152

Dressler's syndrome

411.1 Intermediate coronary syndrome 6, 7, 118, 152

I20.0 Unstable angina

Impending infarction
Preinfarction angina
Preinfarction syndrome
Unstable angina

Excludes *angina (pectoris) (413.9)*
decubitus (413.0)

Layman's: *Unstable angina differs from stable angina and other angina pectoris (413.x) in that it: 1) is not tied to exercise or stress, 2) is severe and acute (as opposed to dull and regular in presentation), and 3) it gets worse (in severity, duration and/or frequency) over time due to movement of clots and commonly culminates in infarction.*

5th **411.8 Other**

481.81 Acute coronary occlusion without myocardial infarction 6, 7, 118, 152

Acute coronary (artery):
- embolism without or not resulting in myocardial infarction
- obstruction without or not resulting in myocardial infarction
- occlusion without or not resulting in myocardial infarction
- thrombosis without or not resulting in myocardial infarction

Excludes *obstruction without infarction due to atherosclerosis (414.00-414.07)*
occlusion without infarction due to atherosclerosis (414.00-414.07)

411.89 Other 6, 7, 118, 152

Coronary insufficiency (acute)
Subendocardial ischemia

412 Old myocardial infarction 6, 7, 118, 152

I25.2 Old myocardial infarction

Healed myocardial infarction
Past myocardial infarction diagnosed on ECG [EKG] or other special investigation, but currently presenting no symptoms

4th **413 Angina pectoris**

413.0 Angina decubitus 6, 7, 54, 118, 152

Nocturnal angina

413.1 **Prinzmetal angina** 6, 7, 54, 118, 152
Variant angina pectoris

413.9 **Other and unspecified angina pectoris** 6, 7, 54, 118, 152

I20.8 Other forms of angina pectoris
I20.9 Angina pectoris, unspecified

Angina:
NOS
cardiac
equivalent
of effort
Anginal syndrome
Status anginosus
Stenocardia
Syncope anginosa
Use additional code(s) for symptoms associated with angina equivalent

Excludes *preinfarction angina (411.1)*

4th 414 **Other forms of chronic ischemic heart disease**

Excludes *arteriosclerotic cardiovascular disease [ASCVD] (429.2)*
cardiovascular:
arteriosclerosis or sclerosis (429.2)
degeneration or disease (429.2)

5th 414.0 **Coronary atherosclerosis**
Arteriosclerotic heart disease [ASHD]
Atherosclerotic heart disease
Coronary (artery):
arteriosclerosis
arteritis or endarteritis
atheroma
sclerosis
stricture
Use additional code, if applicable, to identify chronic total occlusion of coronary artery (414.2)

Excludes *embolism of graft (996.72)*
occlusion NOS of graft (996.72)
thrombus of graft (996.72)

Layman's: *Atherosclerosis is commonly referred to as the hardening of the arteries due to fatty plaques like cholesterol. If there is no documented history of the patient having received a coronary artery bypass graft (CABG), a deeper check of the medical history should be performed before selecting code 414.00. Technically, 414.00 should only be used if it is known that the patient has had a CABG, but the documentation does not state whether the atherosclerosis was localized in the CABG or a native artery.*

414.00 **Of unspecified type of vessel, native or graft** 6, 7, 118, 152 A

I25.10 Atherosclerotic heart disease of native coronary artery without angina pectoris

414.01 **Of native coronary artery** 6, 7, 118, 152 A

I25.10 Atherosclerotic heart disease of native coronary artery without angina pectoris

414.02 **Of autologous biological bypass graft** 6, 7, 118, 152 A

I25.810 Atherosclerosis of coronary artery bypass graft(s) without angina pectoris

414.03 **Of nonautologous biological bypass graft** 6, 7, 118, 152 A

414.04 **Of artery bypass graft** 6, 7, 118, 152 A
Internal mammary artery

414.05 **Of unspecified type of bypass graft** 6, 7, 118, 152 A
Bypass graft NOS

414.06 **Of native coronary artery of transplanted heart** 6, 7, 118, 152

414.07 **Of bypass graft (artery) (vein) of transplanted heart** 6, 7, 118, 152 A

5th 414.1 **Aneurysm and dissection of heart**

414.10 **Aneurysm of heart (wall)**
Aneurysm (arteriovenous):
mural
ventricular

414.11 **Aneurysm of coronary vessels**
Aneurysm (arteriovenous) of coronary vessels

414.12 **Dissection of coronary artery**

414.19 **Other aneurysm of heart**
Arteriovenous fistula, acquired, of heart

414.2 **Chronic total occlusion of coronary artery**
Complete occlusion of coronary artery
Total occlusion of coronary artery
Code first coronary atherosclerosis (414.00-414.07)

Excludes *acute coronary occlusion with myocardial infarction (410.00-410.92)*
acute coronary occlusion without myocardial infarction (411.81)

414.3 **Coronary atherosclerosis due to lipid rich plaque** A
Code first coronary atherosclerosis (414.00-414.07)

414.8 **Other specified forms of chronic ischemic heart disease** 6, 7, 118, 152

I25.5 Ischemic cardiomyopathy
I25.89 Other forms of chronic ischemic heart disease

Chronic coronary insufficiency
Ischemia, myocardial (chronic)
Any condition classifiable to 410 specified as chronic, or presenting with symptoms after 8 weeks from date of infarction

Excludes *coronary insufficiency (acute) (411.89)*

414.9 **Chronic ischemic heart disease, unspecified** 6, 7, 118, 152

I25.9 Chronic ischemic heart disease, unspecified

Ischemic heart disease NOS

DISEASES OF PULMONARY CIRCULATION (415-417)

4th 415 **Acute pulmonary heart disease**

415.0 **Acute cor pulmonale**

Excludes *cor pulmonale NOS (416.9)*

5th 415.1 **Pulmonary embolism and infarction**
Pulmonary (artery) (vein):
apoplexy
embolism
infarction (hemorrhagic)
thrombosis

Excludes *chronic pulmonary embolism (416.2)*
personal history of pulmonary embolism (V12.51)
that complicating:
abortion (634-638 with .6, 639.6)
ectopic or molar pregnancy (639.6)
pregnancy, childbirth, or the puerperium (673.0-673.8)

415.11 **Iatrogenic pulmonary embolism and infarction**
Use additional code for associated septic pulmonary embolism, if applicable, 415.12

415.12 **Septic pulmonary embolism**
Septic embolism NOS
Code first underlying infection, such as:
septicemia (038.0-038.9)

Excludes *septic arterial embolism (449)*

415.19 Other

I26.99 Other pulmonary embolism without acute cor pulmonale

4th 416 **Chronic pulmonary heart disease**

416.0 **Primary pulmonary hypertension**

Idiopathic pulmonary arteriosclerosis

Pulmonary hypertension (essential) (idiopathic) (primary)

416.1 **Kyphoscoliotic heart disease**

● 416.2 **Chronic pulmonary embolism**

Use additional code, if applicable, for associated long-term (current) use of anticoagulants (V58.61)

Excludes *personal history of pulmonary embolism (V12.51)*

Rationale: *It has been deemed to be beneficial to be able to identify patients with chronic pulmonary embolism who are receiving anticoagulation treatment but are no longer in the initial episode of care. Patients with venous thromboembolic disease often require a subsequent hospital admission for treatment of a complication, such as extension of the initial embolus or anticoagulant-related bleeding. In addition, when these patients are readmitted for treatment of an underlying surgical problem, their pulmonary embolus is frequently coded as an "active" embolus, presumably because they are still receiving ongoing anticoagulant treatment.*

416.8 **Other chronic pulmonary heart diseases**

Pulmonary hypertension, secondary

416.9 **Chronic pulmonary heart disease, unspecified**

Chronic cardiopulmonary disease

Cor pulmonale (chronic) NOS

4th 417 **Other diseases of pulmonary circulation**

417.0 **Arteriovenous fistula of pulmonary vessels**

Excludes *congenital arteriovenous fistula (747.3)*

417.1 **Aneurysm of pulmonary artery**

Excludes *congenital aneurysm (747.3)*

417.8 **Other specified diseases of pulmonary circulation**

Pulmonary:
- arteritis
- endarteritis

Rupture of pulmonary vessel

Stricture of pulmonary vessel

417.9 **Unspecified disease of pulmonary circulation**

OTHER FORMS OF HEART DISEASE (420-429)

4th 420 **Acute pericarditis**

Includes acute:
- mediastinopericarditis
- myopericarditis
- pericardial effusion
- pleuropericarditis
- pneumopericarditis

Excludes *acute rheumatic pericarditis (391.0)*
postmyocardial infarction syndrome [Dressler's] (411.0)

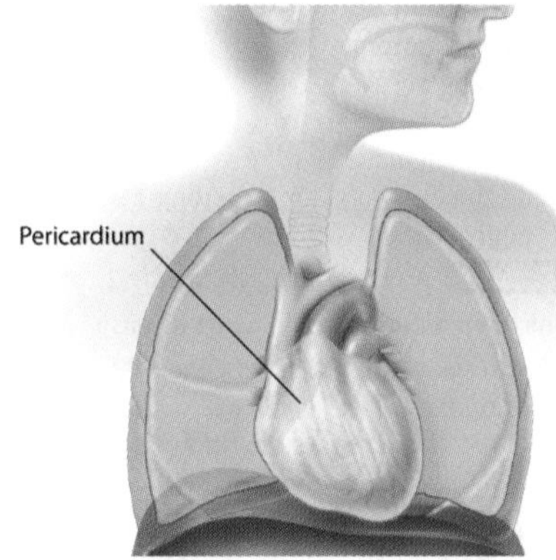

© 2008 Fairman Studios, LLC. All Rights Reserved.

420.0 ***Acute pericarditis in diseases classified elsewhere***

Code first underlying disease, as:
- *actinomycosis (039.8)*
- *amebiasis (006.8)*
- *chronic uremia (585.9)*
- *nocardiosis (039.8)*
- *tuberculosis (017.9)*
- *uremia NOS (586)*

Excludes *pericarditis (acute) (in):*
- *Coxsackie (virus) (074.21)*
- *gonococcal (098.83)*
- *histoplasmosis (115.0-115.9 with fifth-digit 3)*
- *meningococcal infection (036.41)*
- *syphilitic (093.81)*

5th 420.9 **Other and unspecified acute pericarditis**

420.90 **Acute pericarditis, unspecified**

Pericarditis (acute):
- NOS
- infective NOS
- sicca

420.91 **Acute idiopathic pericarditis**

Pericarditis, acute:
- benign
- nonspecific
- viral

420.99 **Other**

Pericarditis (acute):
- pneumococcal
- purulent
- staphylococcal
- streptococcal
- suppurative

Pneumopyopericardium

Pyopericardium

Excludes *pericarditis in diseases classified elsewhere (420.0)*

4th 421 Acute and subacute endocarditis

421.0 Acute and subacute bacterial endocarditis

Endocarditis (acute) (chronic) (subacute):
- bacterial
- infective NOS
- lenta
- malignant
- purulent
- septic
- ulcerative
- vegetative

Infective aneurysm
Subacute bacterial endocarditis [SBE]

Use additional code, if desired, to identify infectious organism [e.g., Streptococcus 041.0, Staphylococcus 041.1]

421.1 *Acute and subacute infective endocarditis in diseases classified elsewhere*

Code first underlying disease, as:
- *blastomycosis (116.0)*
- *Q fever (083.0)*
- *typhoid (fever) (002.0)*

Excludes *endocarditis (in):*
- *Coxsackie (virus) (074.22)*
- *gonococcal (098.84)*
- *histoplasmosis (115.0-115.9 with fifth-digit 4)*
- *meningococcal infection (036.42)*
- *monilial (112.81)*

421.9 Acute endocarditis, unspecified

Endocarditis, acute or subacute
Myoendocarditis, acute or subacute
Periendocarditis, acute or subacute

Excludes *acute rheumatic endocarditis (391.1)*

4th 422 Acute myocarditis

Excludes *acute rheumatic myocarditis (391.2)*

422.0 *Acute myocarditis in diseases classified elsewhere*

Code first underlying disease, as:
- *myocarditis (acute):*
  - *influenzal (487.8)*
  - *tuberculous (017.9)*

Excludes *myocarditis (acute) (due to):*
- *aseptic, of newborn (074.23)*
- *Coxsackie (virus) (074.23)*
- *diphtheritic (032.82)*
- *meningococcal infection (036.43)*
- *syphilitic (093.82)*
- *toxoplasmosis (130.3)*

5th 422.9 Other and unspecified acute myocarditis

422.90 Acute myocarditis, unspecified

Acute or subacute (interstitial) myocarditis

422.91 Idiopathic myocarditis

Myocarditis (acute or subacute):
- Fiedler's
- giant cell
- isolated (diffuse) (granulomatous)
- nonspecific granulomatous

422.92 Septic myocarditis

Myocarditis, acute or subacute:
- pneumococcal
- staphylococcal

Use additional code to identify infectious organism [e.g., Staphylococcus 041.1]

Excludes *myocarditis, acute or subacute:*
- *in bacterial diseases classified elsewhere (422.0)*
- *streptococcal (391.2)*

422.93 Toxic myocarditis

422.99 Other

4th 423 Other diseases of pericardium

Excludes *that specified as rheumatic (393)*

423.0 Hemopericardium

423.1 Adhesive pericarditis

Adherent pericardium
Fibrosis of pericardium
Milk spots
Pericarditis:
- adhesive
- obliterative

Soldiers' patches

423.2 Constrictive pericarditis

Concato's disease
Pick's disease of heart (and liver)

423.3 Cardiac tamponade

Code first the underlying cause

423.8 Other specified diseases of pericardium

Calcification of pericardium
Fistula of pericardium

423.9 Unspecified disease of pericardium

4th 424 Other diseases of endocardium

Excludes *bacterial endocarditis (421.0-421.9)*
rheumatic endocarditis (391.1, 394.0-397.9)
syphilitic endocarditis (093.20-093.24)

424.0 Mitral valve disorders

I34.0 Nonrheumatic mitral (valve) insufficiency
I34.8 Other nonrheumatic mitral valve disorders

Mitral (valve):
- incompetence NOS of specified cause, except rheumatic
- insufficiency NOS of specified cause, except rheumatic
- regurgitation NOS of specified cause, except rheumatic

Excludes *mitral (valve):*
- *disease (394.9)*
- *failure (394.9)*
- *stenosis (394.0)*

the listed conditions:
- *specified as rheumatic (394.1)*
- *unspecified as to cause but with mention of:*
  - *diseases of aortic valve (396.0-396.9)*
  - *mitral stenosis or obstruction (394.2)*

424.1 Aortic valve disorders

I35.0 Nonrheumatic aortic (valve) stenosis
I35.8 Other nonrheumatic aortic valve disorders

Aortic (valve):
- incompetence NOS of specified cause, except rheumatic
- insufficiency NOS of specified cause, except rheumatic
- regurgitation NOS of specified cause, except rheumatic
- stenosis NOS of specified cause, except rheumatic

Excludes *hypertrophic subaortic stenosis (425.1)*
that specified as rheumatic (395.0-395.9)
that of unspecified cause but with mention of diseases of mitral valve (396.0-396.9)

424.2 Tricuspid valve disorders, specified as nonrheumatic

I36.0 Nonrheumatic tricuspid (valve) stenosis
I36.8 Other nonrheumatic tricuspid valve disorders

Tricuspid (valve):
- incompetence of specified cause, except rheumatic
- insufficiency of specified cause, except rheumatic
- regurgitation of specified cause, except rheumatic
- stenosis of specified cause, except rheumatic

Excludes *rheumatic or of unspecified cause (397.0)*

424.3 Pulmonary valve disorders
Pulmonic:
incompetence NOS
insufficiency NOS
regurgitation NOS
stenosis NOS
Excludes *that specified as rheumatic (397.1)*

5th **424.9 Endocarditis, valve unspecified**

424.90 Endocarditis, valve unspecified, unspecified cause
Endocarditis (chronic):
NOS
nonbacterial thrombotic
Valvular:
incompetence of unspecified valve, unspecified cause
insufficiency of unspecified valve, unspecified cause
regurgitation of unspecified valve, unspecified cause
stenosis of unspecified valve, unspecified cause
Valvulitis (chronic) of unspecified valve, unspecified cause

424.91 *Endocarditis in diseases classified elsewhere*
Code first underlying disease, as:
atypical verrucous endocarditis [Libman-Sacks] (710.0)
disseminated lupus erythematosus (710.0)
tuberculosis (017.9)
Excludes *syphilitic (093.20-093.24)*

424.99 Other
Any condition classifiable to 424.90 with specified cause, except rheumatic
Excludes *endocardial fibroelastosis (425.3)*
that specified as rheumatic (397.9)

4th **425 Cardiomyopathy**
Includes myocardiopathy

425.0 Endomyocardial fibrosis

425.1 Hypertrophic obstructive cardiomyopathy
Hypertrophic subaortic stenosis (idiopathic)

425.2 Obscure cardiomyopathy of Africa
Becker's disease
Idiopathic mural endomyocardial disease

425.3 Endocardial fibroelastosis
Elastomyofibrosis

425.4 Other primary cardiomyopathies
I42.2 Other hypertrophic cardiomyopathy
I42.5 Other restrictive cardiomyopathy
I42.8 Other cardiomyopathies
Cardiomyopathy:
NOS
congestive
constrictive
familial
hypertrophic
idiopathic
nonobstructive
obstructive
restrictive
Cardiovascular collagenosis

425.5 Alcoholic cardiomyopathy

425.7 *Nutritional and metabolic cardiomyopathy*
Code first underlying disease, as:
amyloidosis (277.30-277.39)
beriberi (265.0)
cardiac glycogenosis (271.0)
mucopolysaccharidosis (277.5)
thyrotoxicosis (242.0-242.9)
Excludes *gouty tophi of heart (274.82)*

425.8 *Cardiomyopathy in other diseases classified elsewhere*
Code first underlying disease, as:
Friedreich's ataxia (334.0)
myotonia atrophica (359.21)
progressive muscular dystrophy (359.1)
sarcoidosis (135)
Excludes *cardiomyopathy in Chagas' disease (086.0)*

425.9 Secondary cardiomyopathy, unspecified

4th **426 Conduction disorders**

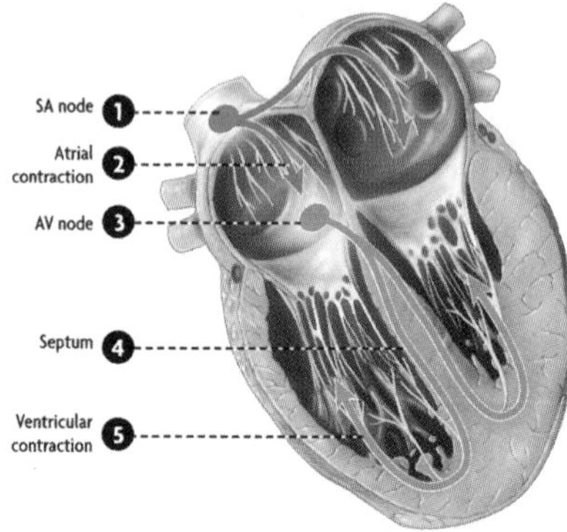

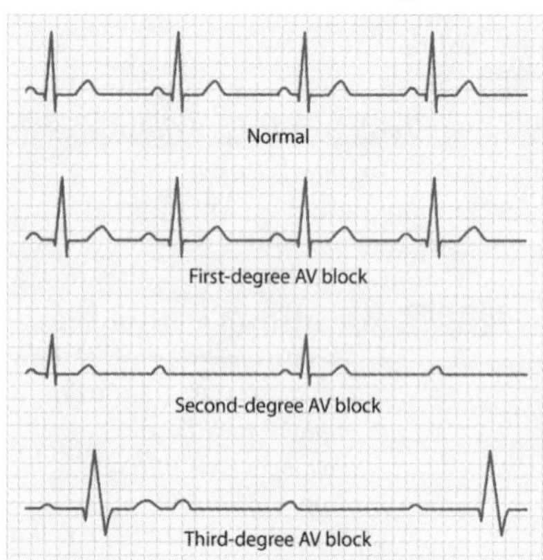

© 2008 Fairman Studios, LLC. All Rights Reserved.

426.0 Atrioventricular block, complete
I44.2 Atrioventricular block, complete
Third degree atrioventricular block

5th **426.1 Atrioventricular block, other and unspecified**

426.10 Atrioventricular block, unspecified
Atrioventricular [AV] block (incomplete) (partial)

426.11 First degree atrioventricular block
Incomplete atrioventricular block, first degree
Prolonged P-R interval NOS

426.12 Mobitz (type) II atrioventricular block
Incomplete atrioventricular block:
Mobitz (type) II
second degree, Mobitz (type) II

426.13 Other second degree atrioventricular block
Incomplete atrioventricular block:
Mobitz (type) I [Wenckebach's]
second degree:
NOS
Mobitz (type) I
with 2:1 atrioventricular response [block]
Wenckebach's phenomenon

426.2 Left bundle branch hemiblock
Block:
left anterior fascicular
left posterior fascicular

426.3 Other left bundle branch block
Left bundle branch block:
NOS
anterior fascicular with posterior fascicular
complete
main stem

426.4 Right bundle branch block

5th **426.5 Bundle branch block, other and unspecified**

426.50 Bundle branch block, unspecified

426.51 Right bundle branch block and left posterior fascicular block

426.52 Right bundle branch block and left anterior fascicular block

426.53 Other bilateral bundle branch block
Bifascicular block NOS
Bilateral bundle branch block NOS
Right bundle branch with left bundle branch block (incomplete) (main stem)

426.54 Trifascicular block

426.6 Other heart block
Intraventricular block:
NOS
diffuse
myofibrillar
Sinoatrial block
Sinoauricular block

426.7 Anomalous atrioventricular excitation
Atrioventricular conduction:
accelerated
accessory
pre-excitation
Ventricular pre-excitation
Wolff-Parkinson-White syndrome

5th **426.8 Other specified conduction disorders**

426.81 Lown-Ganong-Levine syndrome
Syndrome of short P-R interval, normal QRS complexes, and supraventricular tachycardias

426.82 Long QT syndrome

426.89 Other
Dissociation:
atrioventricular [AV]
interference
isorhythmic
Nonparoxysmal AV nodal tachycardia

426.9 Conduction disorder, unspecified
Heart block NOS
Stokes-Adams syndrome

4th **427 Cardiac dysrhythmias**
Excludes *that complicating:*
abortion (634-638 with .7, 639.8)
ectopic or molar pregnancy (639.8)
labor or delivery (668.1, 669.4)

427.0 Paroxysmal supraventricular tachycardia
I47.1 Supraventricular tachycardia
Paroxysmal tachycardia:
atrial [PAT]
atrioventricular [AV]
junctional
nodal

427.1 Paroxysmal ventricular tachycardia
I47.2 Ventricular tachycardia
Ventricular tachycardia (paroxysmal)

427.2 Paroxysmal tachycardia, unspecified
Bouveret-Hoffmann syndrome
Paroxysmal tachycardia:
NOS
essential

5th **427.3 Atrial fibrillation and flutter**
Layman's: *In the most general sense, the difference between fibrillation and flutter is the irregularity of the pattern. Although both imply irregular heart beats, fibrillation is commonly referred to as "irregularly irregular," whereas flutter is a more organized irregularity (i.e., the classic "saw-tooth" pattern is still shown on an ECG, although the heart rate is obviously irregular).*

427.31 Atrial fibrillation
I48.0 Atrial fibrillation

427.32 Atrial flutter
I48.0 Atrial fibrillation

5th **427.4 Ventricular fibrillation and flutter**

427.41 Ventricular fibrillation

427.42 Ventricular flutter

427.5 Cardiac arrest
I46.9 Cardiac arrest, cause unspecified
Cardiorespiratory arrest

5th **427.6 Premature beats**

427.60 Premature beats, unspecified
Ectopic beats
Extrasystoles
Extrasystolic arrhythmia
Premature contractions or systoles NOS

427.61 Supraventricular premature beats
Atrial premature beats, contractions, or systoles

427.69 Other
I49.49 Other premature depolarization
Ventricular premature beats, contractions, or systoles

5th **427.8 Other specified cardiac dysrhythmias**

427.81 Sinoatrial node dysfunction
I49.5 Sick sinus syndrome
Sinus bradycardia:
persistent
severe
Syndrome:
sick sinus
tachycardia-bradycardia
Excludes *sinus bradycardia NOS (427.89)*

427.89 **Other**
I49.8 Other specified cardiac arrhythmias
Rhythm disorder:
coronary sinus
ectopic
nodal
Wandering (atrial) pacemaker
Excludes *carotid sinus syncope (337.0)*
neonatal bradycardia (779.81)
neonatal tachycardia (779.82)
reflex bradycardia (337.0)
tachycardia NOS (785.0)

427.9 **Cardiac dysrhythmia, unspecified**
I49.9 Cardiac arrhythmia, unspecified
Arrhythmia (cardiac) NOS

4th **428 Heart failure**
Code, if applicable, heart failure due to hypertension first (402.0-402.9, with fifth-digit 1 or 404.0-404.9 with fifth-digit 1 or 3)
Excludes *rheumatic (398.91)*
that complicating:
abortion (634-638 with .7, 639.8)
ectopic or molar pregnancy (639.8)
labor or delivery (668.1, 669.4)

428.0 **Congestive heart failure, unspecified** 5, 8
I50.9 Heart failure, unspecified
Congestive heart disease
Right heart failure (secondary to left heart failure)
Excludes *fluid overload NOS (276.6)*

428.1 **Left heart failure** 5, 8
I50.1 Left ventricular failure
Acute edema of lung with heart disease NOS or heart failure
Acute pulmonary edema with heart disease NOS or heart failure
Cardiac asthma
Left ventricular failure

5th 428.2 **Systolic heart failure**
Excludes *combined systolic and diastolic heart failure (428.40-428.43)*
428.20 **Unspecified** 5, 8
428.21 **Acute** 5, 8
428.22 **Chronic** 5, 8
428.23 **Acute on chronic** 5, 8

5th 428.3 **Diastolic heart failure**
Excludes *combined systolic and diastolic heart failure (428.40-428.43)*
428.30 **Unspecified** 5, 8
428.31 **Acute** 5, 8
428.32 **Chronic** 5, 8
428.33 **Acute on chronic** 5, 8

5th 428.4 **Combined systolic and diastolic heart failure**
428.40 **Unspecified** 5, 8
428.41 **Acute** 5, 8
428.42 **Chronic** 5, 8
428.43 **Acute on chronic** 5, 8

428.9 **Heart failure, unspecified** 5, 8
Cardiac failure NOS
Heart failure NOS
Myocardial failure NOS
Weak heart

4th **429 Ill-defined descriptions and complications of heart disease**

429.0 **Myocarditis, unspecified**
Myocarditis (with mention of arteriosclerosis):
NOS (with mention of arteriosclerosis)
chronic (interstitial) (with mention of arteriosclerosis)
fibroid (with mention of arteriosclerosis)
senile (with mention of arteriosclerosis)
Use additional code to identify presence of arteriosclerosis
Excludes *acute or subacute (422.0-422.9)*
rheumatic (398.0)
acute (391.2)
that due to hypertension (402.0-402.9)

429.1 **Myocardial degeneration**
Degeneration of heart or myocardium (with mention of arteriosclerosis):
fatty (with mention of arteriosclerosis)
mural (with mention of arteriosclerosis)
muscular (with mention of arteriosclerosis)
Myocardial (with mention of arteriosclerosis):
degeneration (with mention of arteriosclerosis)
disease (with mention of arteriosclerosis)
Use additional code to identify presence of arteriosclerosis
Excludes *that due to hypertension (402.0-402.9)*

429.2 **Cardiovascular disease, unspecified**
I51.9 Heart disease, unspecified
Arteriosclerotic cardiovascular disease [ASCVD]
Cardiovascular arteriosclerosis
Cardiovascular:
degeneration (with mention of arteriosclerosis)
disease (with mention of arteriosclerosis)
sclerosis (with mention of arteriosclerosis)
Use additional code to identify presence of arteriosclerosis
Excludes *that due to hypertension (402.0-402.9)*

429.3 **Cardiomegaly**
I51.7 Cardiomegaly
Cardiac:
dilatation
hypertrophy
Ventricular dilatation
Excludes *that due to hypertension (402.0-402.9)*

429.4 **Functional disturbances following cardiac surgery**
Cardiac insufficiency following cardiac surgery or due to prosthesis
Heart failure following cardiac surgery or due to prosthesis
Postcardiotomy syndrome
Postvalvulotomy syndrome
Excludes *cardiac failure in the immediate postoperative period (997.1)*

429.5 **Rupture of chordae tendineae**

429.6 **Rupture of papillary muscle**

5th 429.7 **Certain sequelae of myocardial infarction, not elsewhere classified**
Use additional code to identify the associated myocardial infarction:
with onset of 8 weeks or less (410.00-410.92)
with onset of more than 8 weeks (414.8)
Excludes *congenital defects of heart (745, 746)*
coronary aneurysm (414.11)
disorders of papillary muscle (429.6, 429.81)
postmyocardial infarction syndrome (411.0)
rupture of chordae tendineae (429.5)

429.71 **Acquired cardiac septal defect** A
Excludes *acute septal infarction (410.00-410.92)*

429.79 **Other** A
Mural thrombus (atrial) (ventricular) acquired, following myocardial infarction

427.89 – 429.79

5th 429.8 **Other ill-defined heart diseases**

429.81 **Other disorders of papillary muscle**
Papillary muscle:
atrophy
degeneration
dysfunction
incompetence
incoordination
scarring

429.82 **Hyperkinetic heart disease**

429.83 **Takotsubo syndrome**
Broken heart syndrome
Reversible left ventricular dysfunction following sudden emotional stress
Stress induced cardiomyopathy
Transient left ventricular apical ballooning syndrome

429.89 **Other**
Carditis
Excludes *that due to hypertension (402.0-402.9)*

429.9 **Heart disease, unspecified**
Heart disease (organic) NOS
Morbus cordis NOS
Excludes *that due to hypertension (402.0-402.9)*

CEREBROVASCULAR DISEASE (430-438)

Includes with mention of hypertension (conditions classifiable to 401-405)

Use additional code to identify presence of hypertension

Excludes *any condition classifiable to 430-434, 436, 437 occurring during pregnancy, childbirth, or the puerperium, or specified as puerperal (674.0)*
iatrogenic cerebrovascular infarction or hemorrhage (997.02)

ICD-9-CM Official Guidelines (Chapter 7):

a. Hypertension

5) Hypertensive Cerebrovascular Disease

First assign codes from 430-438, Cerebrovascular disease, then the appropriate hypertension code from categories 401-405....

c. Postoperative cerebrovascular accident

A cerebrovascular hemorrhage or infarction that occurs as a result of medical intervention is coded to 997.02, Iatrogenic cerebrovascular infarction or hemorrhage. Medical record documentation should clearly specify the cause- and-effect relationship between the medical intervention and the cerebrovascular accident in order to assign this code. A secondary code from the code range 430-432 or from a code from subcategories 433 or 434 with a fifth digit of "1" should also be used to identify the type of hemorrhage or infarct.

This guideline conforms to the use additional code note instruction at category 997. Code 436, Acute, but ill-defined, cerebrovascular disease, should not be used as a secondary code with code 997.02.

430 **Subarachnoid hemorrhage**
Meningeal hemorrhage
Ruptured:
berry aneurysm
(congenital) cerebral aneurysm NOS
Excludes *syphilitic ruptured cerebral aneurysm (094.87)*

431 **Intracerebral hemorrhage** 10, 31, 35, 36

I61.9 Nontraumatic intracerebral hemorrhage, unspecified

Hemorrhage (of):
basilar
bulbar
cerebellar
cerebral
cerebromeningeal
cortical
internal capsule
intrapontine
pontine
subcortical
ventricular
Rupture of blood vessel in brain

4th 432 **Other and unspecified intracranial hemorrhage**

432.0 **Nontraumatic extradural hemorrhage**
Nontraumatic epidural hemorrhage

432.1 **Subdural hemorrhage**
Subdural hematoma, nontraumatic

432.9 **Unspecified intracranial hemorrhage**
Intracranial hemorrhage NOS

Etiologies of Stroke

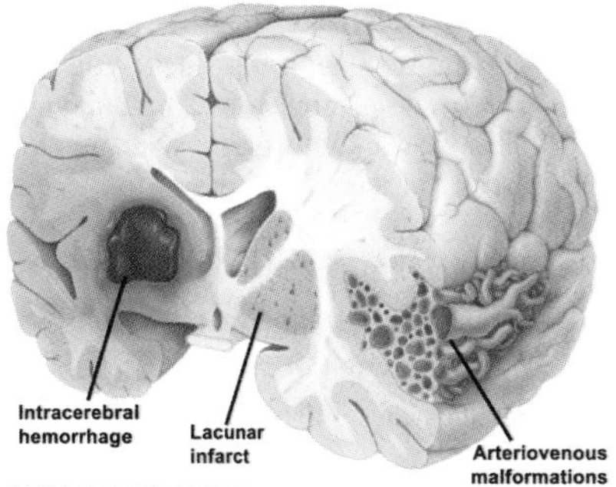

4th 433 **Occlusion and stenosis of precerebral arteries**

Includes embolism of basilar, carotid, and vertebral arteries
narrowing of basilar, carotid, and vertebral arteries
obstruction of basilar, carotid, and vertebral arteries
thrombosis of basilar, carotid, and vertebral arteries

Use additional code, if applicable, to identify status post administration of tPA (rtPA) in a different facility within the last 24 hours prior to admission to current facility (V45.88)

Excludes *insufficiency NOS of precerebral arteries (435.0-435.9)*

The following fifth-digit subclassification is for use with category 433:

0 **without mention of cerebral infarction**
1 **with cerebral infarction** 10, 11, 31, 32, 33, 34, 35, 36

5th 433.0 **Basilar artery**
[0-1]

5th 433.1 **Carotid artery**
[0-1]

5th 433.2 **Vertebral artery**
[0-1]

5th 433.3 **Multiple and bilateral**
[0-1]

5th 433.8 **Other specified precerebral artery**
[0-1]

5th 433.9 **Unspecified precerebral artery**
[0-1] Precerebral artery NOS

4th 434 Occlusion of cerebral arteries

Use additional code, if applicable, to identify status post administration of tPA (rtPA) in a different facility within the last 24 hours prior to admission to current facility (V45.88)

The following fifth-digit subclassification is for use with category 434:

- 0 without mention of cerebral infarction
- 1 with cerebral infarction 10, 11, 31, 32, 33, 34, 35, 36

5th 434.0 Cerebral thrombosis
[0-1] Thrombosis of cerebral arteries

5th 434.1 Cerebral embolism
[0-1]

5th 434.9 Cerebral artery occlusion, unspecified
[0-1]

ICD-9-CM Official Guidelines (Chapter 7):

b. Cerebral infarction/stroke/cerebrovascular accident (CVA)

The terms stroke and CVA are often used interchangeably to refer to a cerebral infarction. The terms stroke, CVA, and cerebral infarction NOS are all indexed to the default code 434.91, Cerebral artery occlusion, unspecified, with infarction. Code 436, Acute, but ill-defined, cerebrovascular disease, should not be used when the documentation states stroke or CVA.

4th 435 Transient cerebral ischemia

Includes cerebrovascular insufficiency (acute) with transient focal neurological signs and symptoms
insufficiency of basilar, carotid, and vertebral arteries
spasm of cerebral arteries

Excludes *acute cerebrovascular insufficiency NOS (437.1)*
that due to any condition classifiable to 433 (433.0-433.9)

435.0 Basilar artery syndrome 10, 11, 32, 33

435.1 Vertebral artery syndrome 10, 11, 32, 33

435.2 Subclavian steal syndrome 10, 11, 32, 33

435.3 Vertebrobasilar artery syndrome 10, 11, 32, 33

435.8 Other specified transient cerebral ischemias 10, 11, 32, 33

435.9 Unspecified transient cerebral ischemia 10, 11, 32, 33

G45.9 Transient cerebral ischemic attack, unspecified

Impending cerebrovascular accident
Intermittent cerebral ischemia
Transient ischemic attack [TIA]

436 Acute, but ill-defined cerebrovascular disease

I67.8 Other specified cerebrovascular diseases

Apoplexy, apoplectic:
- NOS
- attack
- cerebral
- seizure

Cerebral seizure

Excludes *any condition classifiable to categories 430-435*
cerebrovascular accident (434.91)
CVA (ischemic) (434.91)
embolic (434.11)
hemorrhagic (430, 431,432.0-432.9)
thrombotic (434.01)
postoperative cerebrovascular accident (997.02)
stroke (ischemic) (434.91)
embolic (434.11)
hemorrhagic (430, 431, 432.0-432.9)
thrombotic (434.01)

ICD-9-CM Official Guidelines (Chapter 7):

b. Cerebral infarction/stroke/cerebrovascular accident (CVA)

The terms stroke and CVA are often used interchangeably to refer to a cerebral infarction. The terms stroke, CVA, and cerebral infarction NOS are all indexed to the default code 434.91, Cerebral artery occlusion, unspecified, with infarction. Code 436, Acute, but ill-defined, cerebrovascular disease, should not be used when the documentation states stroke or CVA.

c. Postoperative cerebrovascular accident

A cerebrovascular hemorrhage or infarction that occurs as a result of medical intervention is coded to 997.02, Iatrogenic cerebrovascular infarction or hemorrhage. Medical record documentation should clearly specify the cause- and-effect relationship between the medical intervention and the cerebrovascular accident in order to assign this code. A secondary code from the code range 430-432 or from a code from subcategories 433 or 434 with a fifth digit of "1" should also be used to identify the type of hemorrhage or infarct.

This guideline conforms to the use additional code note instruction at category 997. Code 436, Acute, but ill-defined, cerebrovascular disease, should not be used as a secondary code with code 997.02.

4th 437 Other and ill-defined cerebrovascular disease

437.0 Cerebral atherosclerosis A
Atheroma of cerebral arteries
Cerebral arteriosclerosis

437.1 Other generalized ischemic cerebrovascular disease

I67.8 Other specified cerebrovascular diseases

Acute cerebrovascular insufficiency NOS
Cerebral ischemia (chronic)

437.2 Hypertensive encephalopathy

437.3 Cerebral aneurysm, nonruptured
Internal carotid artery, intracranial portion
Internal carotid artery NOS

Excludes *congenital cerebral aneurysm, nonruptured (747.81)*
internal carotid artery, extracranial portion (442.81)

437.4 Cerebral arteritis

437.5 Moyamoya disease

437.6 Nonpyogenic thrombosis of intracranial venous sinus

Excludes *pyogenic (325)*

437.7 Transient global amnesia 10

437.8 Other

437.9 Unspecified
Cerebrovascular disease or lesion NOS

4th 438 Late effects of cerebrovascular disease

Note: *This category is to be used to indicate conditions in 430-437 as the cause of late effects. The "late effects" include conditions specified as such, or as sequelae, which may occur at any time after the onset of the causal condition.*

Excludes *personal history of:*
cerebral infarction without residual deficits (V12.54)
PRIND (Prolonged reversible ischemic neurologic deficit) (V12.54)
RIND (Reversible ischemic neurological deficit) (V12.54)
transient ischemic attack (TIA) (V12.54)

ICD-9-CM Official Guidelines (Chapter 7):

d. Late Effects of Cerebrovascular Disease

1) Category 438, Late Effects of Cerebrovascular disease

Category 438 is used to indicate conditions classifiable to categories 430-437 as the causes of late effects (neurologic deficits), themselves classified elsewhere. These "late effects" include neurologic deficits that persist after initial onset of conditions classifiable to 430-437. The neurologic deficits caused by cerebrovascular disease may be present from the onset or may arise at any time after the onset of the condition classifiable to 430-437.

2) Codes from category 438 with codes from 430-437

Codes from category 438 may be assigned on a health care record with codes from 430-437, if the patient has a current cerebrovascular accident (CVA) and deficits from an old CVA.

3) Code V12.54

Assign code V12.54, Transient ischemic attack (TIA), and cerebral infarction without residual deficits (and not a code from category 438) as an additional code for history of cerebrovascular disease when no neurologic deficits are present.

438.0 Cognitive deficits

5th **438.1 Speech and language deficits**

438.10 Speech and language deficit, unspecified

438.11 Aphasia

438.12 Dysphasia

● **438.13 Dysarthria**

Rationale: *The American Speech-Language-Hearing Association (ASHA) recommended additions and revisions to the ICD-9-CM so that diagnostic information can be coded that clarifies and augments the nature and description of a variety of fluency disorders, including stuttering.*

Stuttering is defined as a disruption in speech production characterized by primary behavioral symptoms that include sound and syllable repetitions, blocks (articulatory fixations that prevent the speaker from moving forward in his or her speech), and inappropriate prolongations of speech sounds. The speaker's inability to initiate or continue speaking may cause secondary reactions characterized by visible signs of awareness, tension and struggle.

Presently, there are three major recognized forms of stuttering: stuttering with onset in early childhood, psychogenic stuttering and fluency disorder subsequent to brain lesion or disease, most typically as a result of cerebral vascular events (sometimes called neurogenic stuttering).

The prevalence of stuttering in the general population, both in the United States and in other surveyed regions, is approximately 1% of the general population. There is a higher incidence, approximately 4%, with onset in early childhood that spontaneously resolves. It is not currently possible to predict which children will experience remission or become persistent stutterers. Persistent stuttering is a potentially handicapping and disabling condition with significant educational, social and vocational consequences

In contrast, psychogenic stuttering and neurogenic stuttering are much less frequently observed speech fluency disorders. Psychogenic stuttering, a form of conversion reaction, has been documented in relatively few published reports with virtually all reported cases showing onset in adulthood. The number of documented cases of stuttering secondary to central nervous system damage or disease is growing. Stuttering is most commonly observed subsequent to cerebral vascular events, but may be seen in neurodegenerative diseases, among a variety of causes.

Previously, the only code in ICD-9-CM for stuttering was in Chapter 5, Mental Disorders. ASHA recognized the appropriateness of this code for individuals showing post-childhood onset of stuttering symptoms secondary to emotional stress or trauma, but proposed adding codes for stuttering to categories 438 and 784. It is hoped that epidemiological, research, and treatment efforts could improve considerably with the increased specificity available in the 2010 ICD-9-CM to distinguish among types of fluency disturbances.

● **438.14 Fluency disorder**

Stuttering

438.19 Other speech and language deficits

5th **438.2 Hemiplegia/hemiparesis**

438.20 Hemiplegia affecting unspecified side

438.21 Hemiplegia affecting dominant side

438.22 Hemiplegia affecting nondominant side

5th **438.3 Monoplegia of upper limb**

438.30 Monoplegia of upper limb affecting unspecified side

438.31 Monoplegia of upper limb affecting dominant side

438.32 Monoplegia of upper limb affecting nondominant side

5th **438.4 Monoplegia of lower limb**

438.40 Monoplegia of lower limb affecting unspecified side

438.41 Monoplegia of lower limb affecting dominant side

438.42 Monoplegia of lower limb affecting nondominant side

5th **438.5 Other paralytic syndrome**

Use additional code to identify type of paralytic syndrome, such as:

locked-in state (344.81)

quadriplegia (344.00-344.09)

Excludes *late effects of cerebrovascular accident with:*
hemiplegia/hemiparesis (438.20-438.22)
monoplegia of lower limb (438.40-438.42)
monoplegia of upper limb (438.40-438.42)

438.50 Other paralytic syndrome affecting unspecified side

438.51 Other paralytic syndrome affecting dominant side

438.52 Other paralytic syndrome affecting nondominant side

438.53 Other paralytic syndrome, bilateral

438.6 Alterations of sensations

Use additional code to identify the altered sensation

438.7 Disturbances of vision

Use additional code to identify the visual disturbance

5th **438.8 Other late effects of cerebrovascular disease**

438.81 Apraxia

438.82 Dysphagia

Use additional code to identify the type of dysphagia, if known (787.20-787.29)

438.83 Facial weakness

Facial droop

438.84 Ataxia

438.85 Vertigo

438.89 Other late effects of cerebrovascular disease

Use additional code to identify the late effect

438.9 Unspecified late effects of cerebrovascular disease

DISEASES OF ARTERIES, ARTERIOLES, AND CAPILLARIES (440-449)

Major Arteries

Brachiocephalic trunk
Common carotid arteries
Axillary artery
Left subclavian artery
Axillary artery
Brachial artery
Aortic arch
Thoracic aorta
Superior mesenteric artery
Abdominal aorta
Celiac trunk
Inferior mesenteric artery
Renal arteries
Common iliac arteries
Radial artery
Ulnar artery
External iliac arteries
Superficial palmar arch
Internal iliac arteries
Femoral arteries
Descending genicular arteries
Popliteal arteries
Anterior tibial arteries
Dorsalis pedis artery
Arcuate artery

© Icon Learning Systems

4th **440 Atherosclerosis**

Includes arteriolosclerosis
arteriosclerosis (obliterans) (senile)
arteriosclerotic vascular disease
atheroma
degeneration:
  arterial
  arteriovascular
  vascular
endarteritis deformans or obliterans
senile:
  arteritis
  endarteritis

Excludes *atheroembolism (445.01-445.89)*
atherosclerosis of bypass graft of the extremities (440.30-440.32)

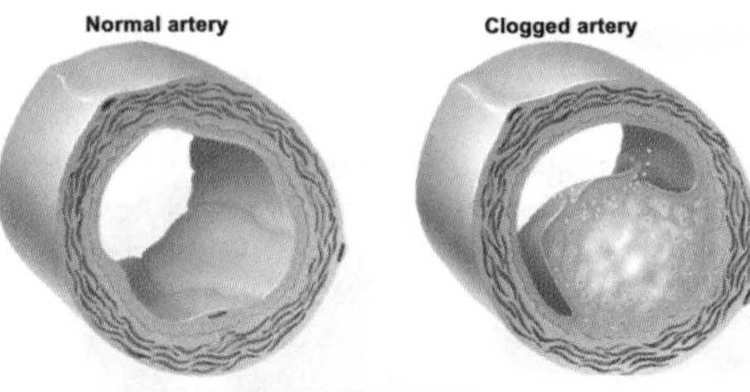

440.0 Of aorta A

440.1 Of renal artery A

Excludes *atherosclerosis of renal arterioles (403.00-403.91)*

5th **440.2 Of native arteries of the extremities**

Use additional code, if applicable, to identify chronic total occlusion of artery of the extremities (440.4)

Excludes *atherosclerosis of bypass graft of the extremities (440.30-440.32)*

440.20 Atherosclerosis of the extremities, unspecified A

I70.209 Unspecified atherosclerosis of native arteries of extremities, unspecified extremity

440.21 Atherosclerosis of the extremities with intermittent claudication A

I70.219 Atherosclerosis of native arteries of extremities with intermittent claudication, unspecified extremity

Layman's: *If the pain and/or cramping of the legs due to atherosclerosis resolves with rest, code to 440.21. If it persists, 440.22 is more appropriate.*

440.22 Atherosclerosis of the extremities with rest pain

Includes any condition classifiable to 440.21

440.23 Atherosclerosis of the extremities with ulceration A

Includes any condition classifiable to 440.21-440.22

Use additional code for any associated ulceration (707.10-707.9)

440.24 Atherosclerosis of the extremities with gangrene

Includes any condition classifiable to 440.21, 440.22, and 440.23 with ischemic gangrene 785.4

Use additional code for any associated ulceration (707.10-707.9)

Excludes *gas gangrene 040.0*

440.29 Other A

5th 440.3 **Of bypass graft of the extremities**

Excludes *atherosclerosis of native artery of the extremity (440.21-440.24)*
embolism [occlusion NOS] [thrombus] of graft (996.74)

440.30 **Of unspecified graft** A

440.31 **Of autologous vein bypass graft** A

440.32 **Of nonautologous vein bypass graft** A

440.4 **Chronic total occlusion of artery of the extremities**

Complete occlusion of artery of the extremities
Total occlusion of artery of the extremities

Code first atherosclerosis of arteries of the extremities (440.20-440.29, 440.30-440.32)

Excludes *acute occlusion of artery of extremity (444.21-444.22)*

440.8 **Of other specified arteries** A

Excludes *basilar (433.0)*
carotid (433.1)
cerebral (437.0)
coronary (414.00-414.07)
mesenteric (557.1)
precerebral (433.0-433.9)
pulmonary (416.0)
vertebral (433.2)

440.9 **Generalized and unspecified atherosclerosis** A

Arteriosclerotic vascular disease NOS

Excludes *arteriosclerotic cardiovascular disease [ASCVD] (429.2)*

4th 441 **Aortic aneurysm and dissection**

Excludes *syphilitic aortic aneurysm (093.0)*
traumatic aortic aneurysm (901.0, 902.0)

5th 441.0 **Dissection of aorta**

441.00 **Unspecified site**

441.01 **Thoracic**

441.02 **Abdominal**

441.03 **Thoracoabdominal**

441.1 **Thoracic aneurysm, ruptured**

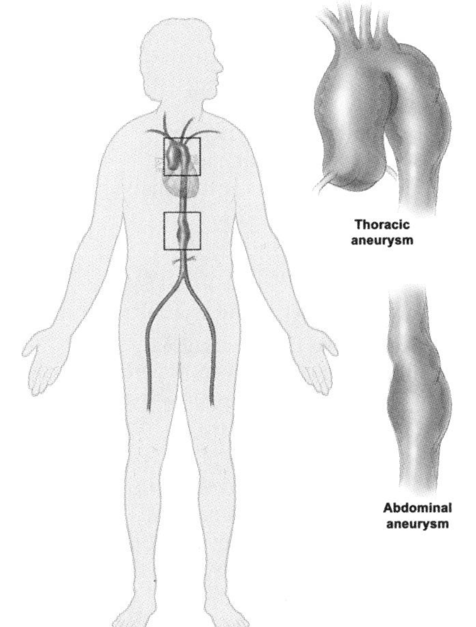

© 2008 Fairman Studios, LLC. All Rights Reserved.

441.2 **Thoracic aneurysm without mention of rupture**

441.3 **Abdominal aneurysm, ruptured**

441.4 **Abdominal aneurysm without mention of rupture**

I71.4 Abdominal aortic aneurysm, without rupture

441.5 **Aortic aneurysm of unspecified site, ruptured**

Rupture of aorta NOS

441.6 **Thoracoabdominal aneurysm, ruptured**

441.7 **Thoracoabdominal aneurysm, without mention of rupture**

441.9 **Aortic aneurysm of unspecified site without mention of rupture**

Aneurysm
Dilatation of aorta
Hyaline necrosis of aorta

4th 442 **Other aneurysm**

Includes aneurysm (ruptured) (cirsoid) (false) (varicose)
aneurysmal varix

Excludes *arteriovenous aneurysm or fistula:*
acquired (447.0)
congenital (747.60-747.69)
traumatic (900.0-904.9)

442.0 **Of artery of upper extremity**

442.1 **Of renal artery**

442.2 **Of iliac artery**

442.3 **Of artery of lower extremity**

Aneurysm:
femoral artery
popliteal artery

5th 442.8 **Of other specified artery**

442.81 **Artery of neck**

Aneurysm of carotid artery (common) (external) (internal, extracranial portion)

Excludes *internal carotid artery, intracranial portion (437.3)*

442.82 **Subclavian artery**

442.83 **Splenic artery**

442.84 **Other visceral artery**

Aneurysm:
celiac artery
gastroduodenal artery
gastroepiploic artery
hepatic artery
pancreaticoduodenal artery
superior mesenteric artery

442.89 **Other**

Aneurysm:
mediastinal artery
spinal artery

Excludes *cerebral (nonruptured) (437.3)*
congenital (747.81)
ruptured (430)
coronary (414.11)
heart (414.10)
pulmonary (417.1)

442.9 **Of unspecified site**

4th 443 **Other peripheral vascular disease**

443.0 **Raynaud's syndrome**

Raynaud's:
disease
phenomenon (secondary)

Use additional code to identify gangrene (785.4)

443.1 **Thromboangiitis obliterans [Buerger's disease]**

Presenile gangrene

5th 443.2 **Other arterial dissection**

Excludes *dissection of aorta (441.00-441.03)*
dissection of coronary arteries (414.12)

443.21 **Dissection of carotid artery**

443.22 **Dissection of iliac artery**

443.23 **Dissection of renal artery**

443.24 **Dissection of vertebral artery**

443.29 **Dissection of other artery**

440.3 – 443.29

5th 443.8 **Other specified peripheral vascular diseases**

443.81 ***Peripheral angiopathy in diseases classified elsewhere***

Code first underlying disease, as:
diabetes mellitus (249.7, 250.7)

443.82 **Erythromelalgia**

443.89 **Other**

Acrocyanosis
Acroparesthesia:
simple [Schultze's type]
vasomotor [Nothnagel's type]
Erythrocyanosis

Excludes *chilblains (991.5)*
frostbite (991.0-991.3)
immersion foot (991.4)

443.9 **Peripheral vascular disease, unspecified**

I73.9 Peripheral vascular disease, unspecified

Intermittent claudication NOS
Peripheral:
angiopathy NOS
vascular disease NOS
Spasm of artery

Excludes *atherosclerosis of the arteries of the extremities (440.20-440.22)*
spasm of cerebral artery (435.0-435.9)

4th 444 **Arterial embolism and thrombosis**

Includes infarction:
embolic
thrombotic
occlusion

Excludes *atheroembolism (445.01-445.89)*
septic arterial embolism (449)
that complicating:
abortion (634-638 with .6, 639.6)
ectopic or molar pregnancy (639.6)
pregnancy, childbirth, or the puerperium (673.0-673.8)

444.0 **Of abdominal aorta**

Aortic bifurcation syndrome
Aortoiliac obstruction
Leriche's syndrome
Saddle embolus

444.1 **Of thoracic aorta**

Embolism or thrombosis of aorta (thoracic)

5th 444.2 **Of arteries of the extremities**

444.21 **Upper extremity**

444.22 **Lower extremity**

I74.3 Embolism and thrombosis of arteries of the lower extremities

Arterial embolism or thrombosis:
femoral
peripheral NOS
popliteal

Excludes *iliofemoral (444.81)*

5th 444.8 **Of other specified artery**

444.81 **Iliac artery**

444.89 **Other**

Excludes *basilar (433.0)*
carotid (433.1)
cerebral (434.0-434.9)
coronary (410.00-410.92)
mesenteric (557.0)
ophthalmic (362.30-362.34)
precerebral (433.0-433.9)
pulmonary (415.19)
renal (593.81)
retinal (362.30-362.34)
vertebral (433.2)

444.9 **Of unspecified artery**

4th 445 **Atheroembolism**

Includes atherothrombotic microembolism
cholesterol embolism

5th 445.0 **Of extremities**

445.01 **Upper extremity**

445.02 **Lower extremity**

5th 445.8 **Of other sites**

445.81 **Kidney**

Use additional code for any associated acute kidney ~~renal~~ failure or chronic kidney disease (584, 585)

445.89 **Other site**

4th 446 **Polyarteritis nodosa and allied conditions**

446.0 **Polyarteritis nodosa**

Disseminated necrotizing periarteritis
Necrotizing angiitis
Panarteritis (nodosa)
Periarteritis (nodosa)

446.1 **Acute febrile mucocutaneous lymph node syndrome [MCLS]**

Kawasaki disease

5th 446.2 **Hypersensitivity angiitis**

Excludes *antiglomerular basement membrane disease without pulmonary hemorrhage (583.89)*

446.20 **Hypersensitivity angiitis, unspecified**

446.21 **Goodpasture's syndrome**

Antiglomerular basement membrane antibody-mediated nephritis with pulmonary hemorrhage
Use additional code to identify renal disease (583.81)

446.29 **Other specified hypersensitivity angiitis**

446.3 **Lethal midline granuloma**

Malignant granuloma of face

446.4 **Wegener's granulomatosis**

Necrotizing respiratory granulomatosis
Wegener's syndrome

446.5 **Giant cell arteritis**

Cranial arteritis
Horton's disease
Temporal arteritis

446.6 **Thrombotic microangiopathy**

Moschcowitz's syndrome
Thrombotic thrombocytopenic purpura

446.7 **Takayasu's disease**

Aortic arch arteritis
Pulseless disease

4th 447 **Other disorders of arteries and arterioles**

447.0 **Arteriovenous fistula, acquired**

Arteriovenous aneurysm, acquired

Excludes *cerebrovascular (437.3)*
coronary (414.19)
pulmonary (417.0)
surgically created arteriovenous shunt or fistula:
complication (996.1, 996.61-996.62)
status or presence (V45.11)
traumatic (900.0-904.9)

447.1 **Stricture of artery**

447.2 **Rupture of artery**

Erosion of artery
Fistula, except arteriovenous of artery
Ulcer of artery

Excludes *traumatic rupture of artery (900.0-904.9)*

447.3 **Hyperplasia of renal artery**

Fibromuscular hyperplasia of renal artery

447.4 **Celiac artery compression syndrome**
Celiac axis syndrome
Marable's syndrome

447.5 **Necrosis of artery**

447.6 **Arteritis, unspecified**
Aortitis NOS
Endarteritis NOS
Excludes *arteritis, endarteritis:*
aortic arch (446.7)
cerebral (437.4)
coronary (414.00-414.07)
deformans (440.0-440.9)
obliterans (440.0-440.9)
pulmonary (417.8)
senile (440.0-440.9)
polyarteritis NOS
syphilitic aortitis (093.1)

447.8 **Other specified disorders of arteries and arterioles**
Fibromuscular hyperplasia of arteries, except renal

447.9 **Unspecified disorders of arteries and arterioles**

4th 448 **Disease of capillaries**

448.0 **Hereditary hemorrhagic telangiectasia**
Rendu-Osler-Weber disease

448.1 **Nevus, non-neoplastic**
Nevus:
araneus
senile
spider
stellar
Excludes *neoplastic (216.0-216.9)*
port wine (757.32)
strawberry (757.32)

448.9 **Other and unspecified capillary diseases**
Capillary:
hemorrhage
hyperpermeability
thrombosis
Excludes *capillary fragility (hereditary) (287.8)*

449 **Septic arterial embolism**
Code first underlying infection, such as:
infective endocarditis (421.0)
lung abscess (513.0)
Use additional code to identify the site of the embolism (433.0-433.9, 444.0-444.9)
Excludes *septic pulmonary embolism (415.12)*

DISEASES OF VEINS AND LYMPHATICS, AND OTHER DISEASES OF CIRCULATORY SYSTEM (451-459)

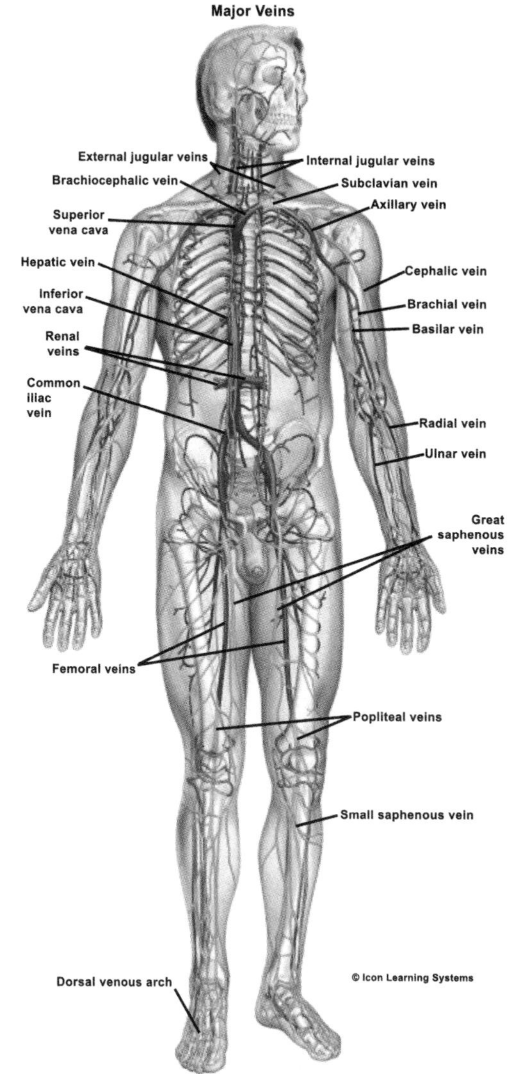

4th 451 **Phlebitis and thrombophlebitis**
Includes endophlebitis
inflammation, vein
periphlebitis
suppurative phlebitis
Use additional E code to identify drug if drug-induced
Excludes *that complicating:*
abortion (634-638 with .7, 639.8)
ectopic or molar pregnancy (639.8)
pregnancy, childbirth, or the puerperium (671.0-671.9)
that due to or following:
implant or catheter device (996.61-996.62)
infusion, perfusion, or transfusion (999.2)

451.0 **Of superficial vessels of lower extremities**
Saphenous vein (greater) (lesser)

5th 451.1 **Of deep vessels of lower extremities**

451.11 **Femoral vein (deep) (superficial)**

451.19 **Other**
I80.209 Phlebitis and thrombophlebitis of unspecified deep vessels of unspecified lower extremity
Femoropopliteal vein
Popliteal vein
Tibial vein

451.2 **Of lower extremities, unspecified**

5th 451.8 **Of other sites**

Excludes *intracranial venous sinus (325)*
nonpyogenic (437.6)
portal (vein) (572.1)

451.81 **Iliac vein**

451.82 **Of superficial veins of upper extremities**
Antecubital vein
Basilic vein
Cephalic vein

451.83 **Of deep veins of upper extremities**
Brachial vein
Radial vein
Ulnar vein

451.84 **Of upper extremities, unspecified**

451.89 **Other**
Axillary vein
Jugular vein
Subclavian vein
Thrombophlebitis of breast (Mondor's disease)

451.9 **Of unspecified site**

452 **Portal vein thrombosis**
Portal (vein) obstruction

Excludes *hepatic vein thrombosis (453.0)*
phlebitis of portal vein (572.1)

4th 453 **Other venous embolism and thrombosis**

Excludes *that complicating:*
abortion (634-638 with .7, 639.8)
ectopic or molar pregnancy (639.8)
pregnancy, childbirth, or the puerperium (671.0-671.9)
~~*that with inflammation, phlebitis, and thrombophlebitis (451.0-451.9)*~~

453.0 **Budd-Chiari syndrome**
Hepatic vein thrombosis

453.1 **Thrombophlebitis migrans**

▲453.2 **Of inferior vena cava**

453.3 **Of renal vein**

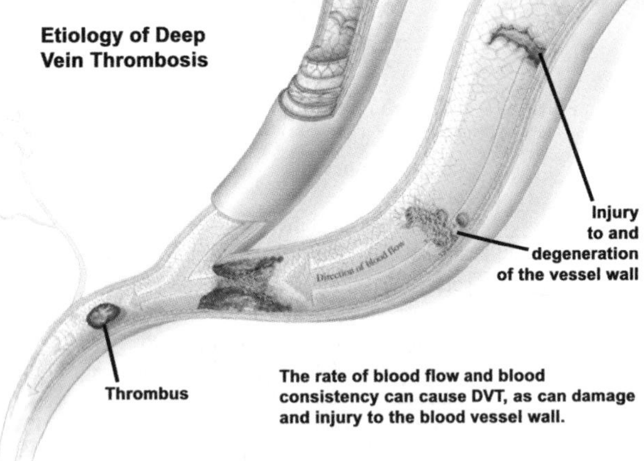

▲ 5th 453.4 **Acute venous embolism and thrombosis of deep vessels of lower extremity**

Rationale: It has been deemed to be beneficial to be able to identify patients with sub-acute or chronic deep vein thrombosis who are receiving anticoagulation treatment but are no longer in the initial episode of care. Patients with venous thromboembolic disease often require a subsequent hospital admission for treatment of a complication, such as extension of the initial thrombosis or anticoagulant related bleeding. In addition, when these patients are readmitted for treatment of an underlying surgical problem, their deep-vein thrombosis is frequently coded as an "active" thrombosis, presumably because they are still receiving ongoing anticoagulant treatment.

The revisions to 453.40-453.42 and the creation of new codes 453.40-453.89 are modeled after the modifications of acute myocardial infarction codes, which distinguish between "initial episode of care," "subsequent episode of care," and "episode of care unspecified." The use of the terms "acute", "sub-acute" and "chronic" are consistent with similar terms used in the 2002 modifications to the heart failure codes.

▲453.40 **Acute venous embolism and thrombosis of unspecified deep vessels of lower extremity**
Deep vein thrombosis NOS
DVT NOS

▲453.41 **Acute venous embolism and thrombosis of deep vessels of proximal lower extremity**
Femoral
Iliac
Popliteal
Thigh
Upper leg NOS

▲453.42 **Acute venous embolism and thrombosis of deep vessels of distal lower extremity**
Calf
Lower leg NOS
Peroneal
Tibial

● 5th 453.5 **Chronic venous embolism and thrombosis of deep vessels of lower extremity**
Use additional code, if applicable, for associated long-term (current) use of anticoagulants (V58.61)

Excludes *personal history of venous thrombosis and embolism (V12.51)*

●453.50 **Chronic venous embolism and thrombosis of unspecified deep vessels of lower extremity**

●453.51 **Chronic venous embolism and thrombosis of deep vessels of proximal lower extremity**

●453.52 **Chronic venous embolism and thrombosis of deep vessels of distal lower extremity**

●453.6 **Venous embolism and thrombosis of superficial vessels of lower extremity**
Saphenous vein (greater) (lesser)

Rationale: On October 1, 2004 codes for venous embolism and thrombosis of deep vessels of lower extremity, were implemented (codes 453.40-453.42). These changes did not address the problem of superficial thromboses of lower extremities and there is a need to define thromboses affecting those sites. Previously, many of these sites were indexed to one code, 453.8, "Other venous embolism and thrombosis of other specified veins."

● 5th 453.7 **Chronic venous embolism and thrombosis of other specified vessels**
Use additional code, if applicable, for associated long-term (current) use of anticoagulants (V58.61)
Excludes *personal history of venous thrombosis and embolism (V12.51)*

Rationale: *On October 1, 1993, codes were implemented to describe phlebitis and thrombophlebitis of veins of the upper extremities (codes 451.82-451.84). However, no corresponding codes were created to distinguish venous embolism and thrombosis affecting the upper extremities. Additionally, the term thrombophlebitis is outdated terminology. The presence of phlebitis (inflammation of the vein) in association with thrombosis has no clinical or prognostic significance. Patients with venous thrombosis are now categorized as having superficial or deep venous thrombosis affecting a specified vein defined by name or location. There was a need to create codes to define venous thrombosis affecting the vessels in the thorax, neck and upper extremities. With the increasing use of PICC lines, central catheters, tunnel dialysis catheters and wired cardiac devices, deep vein thrombosis of the major veins in the thorax and upper extremities has become very common. Previously, the terms "thrombosis, arm," "thrombosis, upper extremity," or "thrombosis, vein, upper extremity" were not represented in the diagnosis index or tabular. In addition, thromboses resulting from indwelling central venous catheters, which typically affect the axillary, subclavian, and/or brachiocephalic veins, were not specifically indexed.*

● 453.71 **Chronic venous embolism and thrombosis of superficial veins of upper extremity**
Antecubital vein
Basilic vein
Cephalic vein

● 453.72 **Chronic venous embolism and thrombosis of deep veins of upper extremity**
Brachial vein
Radial vein
Ulnar vein

● 453.73 **Chronic venous embolism and thrombosis of upper extremity, unspecified**

● 453.74 **Chronic venous embolism and thrombosis of axillary veins**

● 453.75 **Chronic venous embolism and thrombosis of subclavian veins**

● 453.76 **Chronic venous embolism and thrombosis of internal jugular veins**

● 453.77 **Chronic venous embolism and thrombosis of other thoracic veins**
Brachiocephalic (innominate)
Superior vena cava

● 453.79 **Chronic venous embolism and thrombosis of other specified veins**

▲ 5th 453.8 **Acute venous embolism and thrombosis of other specified veins**
Excludes *cerebral (434.0-434.9)*
coronary (410.00-410.92)
intracranial venous sinus (325)
nonpyogenic (437.6)
mesenteric (557.0)
portal (452)
precerebral (433.0-433.9)
pulmonary (415.19)

● 453.81 **Acute venous embolism and thrombosis of superficial veins of upper extremity**
Antecubital vein
Basilic vein
Cephalic vein

● 453.82 **Acute venous embolism and thrombosis of deep veins of upper extremity**
Brachial vein
Radial vein
Ulnar vein

● 453.83 **Acute venous embolism and thrombosis of upper extremity, unspecified**

● 453.84 **Acute venous embolism and thrombosis of axillary veins**

● 453.85 **Acute venous embolism and thrombosis of subclavian veins**

● 453.86 **Acute venous embolism and thrombosis of internal jugular veins**

● 453.87 **Acute venous embolism and thrombosis of other thoracic veins**
Brachiocephalic (innominate)
Superior vena cava

● 453.89 **Acute venous embolism and thrombosis of other specified veins**

453.9 **Of unspecified site**
I82.9 Embolism and thrombosis of unspecified vein
Embolism of vein
Thrombosis (vein)

4th 454 **Varicose veins of lower extremities**
Excludes *that complicating pregnancy, childbirth, or the puerperium (671.0)*

454.0 **With ulcer** A
Varicose ulcer (lower extremity, any part)
Varicose veins with ulcer of lower extremity [any part] or of unspecified site
Any condition classifiable to 454.9 with ulcer or specified as ulcerated

454.1 **With inflammation** A
Stasis dermatitis
Varicose veins with inflammation of lower extremity [any part] or of unspecified site
Any condition classifiable to 454.9 with inflammation or specified as inflamed

454.2 **With ulcer and inflammation** A
Varicose veins with ulcer and inflammation of lower extremity [any part] or of unspecified site
Any condition classifiable to 454.9 with ulcer and inflammation

454.8 **With other complications**
Edema
Pain
Swelling

454.9 **Asymptomatic varicose veins** A
Phlebectasia of lower extremity [any part] or of unspecified site
Varicose veins NOS
Varicose veins of lower extremity [any part] or of unspecified site
Varix of lower extremity [any part] or of unspecified site

4th 455 **Hemorrhoids**
Includes hemorrhoids (anus) (rectum)
piles
varicose veins, anus or rectum
Excludes *that complicating pregnancy, childbirth, or the puerperium (671.8)*

455.0 **Internal hemorrhoids without mention of complication**

455.1 **Internal thrombosed hemorrhoids**

455.2 **Internal hemorrhoids with other complication**
Internal hemorrhoids:
bleeding
prolapsed
strangulated
ulcerated

455.3 **External hemorrhoids without mention of complication**
I84.22 External hemorrhoids without complication

455.4 **External thrombosed hemorrhoids**

455.5 **External hemorrhoids with other complication**
External hemorrhoids:
bleeding
prolapsed
strangulated
ulcerated

455.6 **Unspecified hemorrhoids without mention of complication**
Hemorrhoids NOS

455.7 **Unspecified thrombosed hemorrhoids**
Thrombosed hemorrhoids, unspecified whether internal or external

455.8 **Unspecified hemorrhoids with other complication**
Hemorrhoids, unspecified whether internal or external:
bleeding
prolapsed
strangulated
ulcerated

455.9 **Residual hemorrhoidal skin tags**
Skin tags, anus or rectum

4th **456 Varicose veins of other sites**

456.0 **Esophageal varices with bleeding**

456.1 **Esophageal varices without mention of bleeding**

5th **456.2 Esophageal varices in diseases classified elsewhere**
Code first underlying disease, as:
cirrhosis of liver (571.0-571.9)
portal hypertension (572.3)

456.20 ***With bleeding***

456.21 ***Without mention of bleeding***

456.3 **Sublingual varices**

456.4 **Scrotal varices** ♂
Varicocele

456.5 **Pelvic varices**
Varices of broad ligament

456.6 **Vulval varices** ♀
Varices of perineum
Excludes *that complicating pregnancy, childbirth, or the puerperium (671.1)*

456.8 **Varices of other sites**
Varicose veins of nasal septum (with ulcer)
Excludes *placental varices (656.7)*
retinal varices (362.17)
varicose ulcer of unspecified site (454.0)
varicose veins of unspecified site (454.9)

4th **457 Noninfectious disorders of lymphatic channels**

457.0 **Postmastectomy lymphedema syndrome** A
Elephantiasis due to mastectomy
Obliteration of lymphatic vessel due to mastectomy

457.1 **Other lymphedema**
Elephantiasis (nonfilarial) NOS
Lymphangiectasis
Lymphedema:
acquired (chronic)
praecox
secondary
Obliteration, lymphatic vessel
Excludes *elephantiasis (nonfilarial):*
congenital (757.0)
eyelid (374.83)
vulva (624.8)

457.2 **Lymphangitis**
Lymphangitis:
NOS
chronic
subacute
Excludes *acute lymphangitis (682.0-682.9)*

457.8 **Other noninfectious disorders of lymphatic channels**
Chylocele (nonfilarial)
Chylous:
ascites
cyst
Lymph node or vessel:
fistula
infarction
rupture
Excludes *chylocele:*
filarial (125.0-125.9)
tunica vaginalis (nonfilarial) (608.84)

457.9 **Unspecified noninfectious disorder of lymphatic channels**

4th **458 Hypotension**
Includes hypopiesis
Excludes *cardiovascular collapse (785.50)*
maternal hypotension syndrome (669.2)
shock (785.50-785.59)
Shy-Drager syndrome (333.0)

458.0 **Orthostatic hypotension**
Hypotension:
orthostatic (chronic)
postural

458.1 **Chronic hypotension**
Permanent idiopathic hypotension

5th **458.2 Iatrogenic hypotension**

458.21 **Hypotension of hemodialysis**
Intra-dialytic hypotension

458.29 **Other iatrogenic hypotension**
Postoperative hypotension

458.8 **Other specified hypotension**

458.9 **Hypotension, unspecified**
I95.9 Hypotension, unspecified
Hypotension (arterial) NOS

4th **459 Other disorders of circulatory system**

459.0 **Hemorrhage, unspecified**
Rupture of blood vessel NOS
Spontaneous hemorrhage NEC
Excludes *hemorrhage:*
gastrointestinal NOS (578.9)
in newborn NOS (772.9)
nontraumatic hematoma of soft tissue (729.92)
secondary or recurrent following trauma (958.2)
traumatic rupture of blood vessel (900.0-904.9)

5th **459.1 Postphlebitic syndrome**

Chronic venous hypertension due to deep vein thrombosis

Excludes *chronic venous hypertension without deep vein thrombosis (459.30-459.39)*

459.10 Postphlebitic syndrome without complications

Asymptomatic postphlebitic syndrome
Postphlebitic syndrome NOS

459.11 Postphlebitic syndrome with ulcer

459.12 Postphlebitic syndrome with inflammation

459.13 Postphlebitic syndrome with ulcer and inflammation

459.19 Postphlebitic syndrome with other complication

459.2 Compression of vein

Stricture of vein
Vena cava syndrome (inferior) (superior)

5th **459.3 Chronic venous hypertension (idiopathic)**

Stasis edema

Excludes *chronic venous hypertension due to deep vein thrombosis (459.10-459.19)*
varicose veins (454.0-454.9)

459.30 Chronic venous hypertension without complications

Asymptomatic chronic venous hypertension
Chronic venous hypertension NOS

459.31 Chronic venous hypertension with ulcer I 8 6

459.32 Chronic venous hypertension with inflammation

459.33 Chronic venous hypertension with ulcer and inflammation I 8 6

459.39 Chronic venous hypertension with other complication

5th **459.8 Other specified disorders of circulatory system**

459.81 Venous (peripheral) insufficiency, unspecified I 8 6

I87.2 Venous insufficiency (chronic) (peripheral)

Chronic venous insufficiency NOS
Use additional code for any associated ulceration (707.10-707.9)

459.89 Other

Collateral circulation (venous), any site
Phlebosclerosis
Venofibrosis

459.9 Unspecified circulatory system disorder

8. DISEASES OF THE RESPIRATORY SYSTEM (460-519)

Use additional code to identify infectious organism

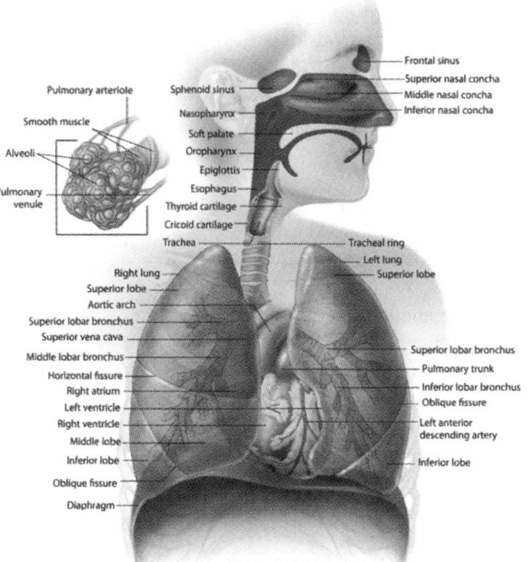

ACUTE RESPIRATORY INFECTIONS (460-466)

Excludes *pneumonia and influenza (480.0-488)*

460 Acute nasopharyngitis [common cold] 6 5

Coryza (acute)
Nasal catarrh, acute
Nasopharyngitis:
NOS
acute
infective NOS
Rhinitis:
acute
infective

Excludes *nasopharyngitis, chronic (472.2)*
pharyngitis:
acute or unspecified (462)
chronic (472.1)
rhinitis:
allergic (477.0-477.9)
chronic or unspecified (472.0)
sore throat:
acute or unspecified (462)
chronic (472.1)

4th **461 Acute sinusitis**

Includes abscess, acute, of sinus (accessory) (nasal)
empyema, acute, of sinus (accessory) (nasal)
infection, acute, of sinus (accessory) (nasal)
inflammation, acute, of sinus (accessory) (nasal)
suppuration, acute, of sinus (accessory) (nasal)

Excludes *chronic or unspecified sinusitis (473.0-473.9)*

The Facial Sinuses

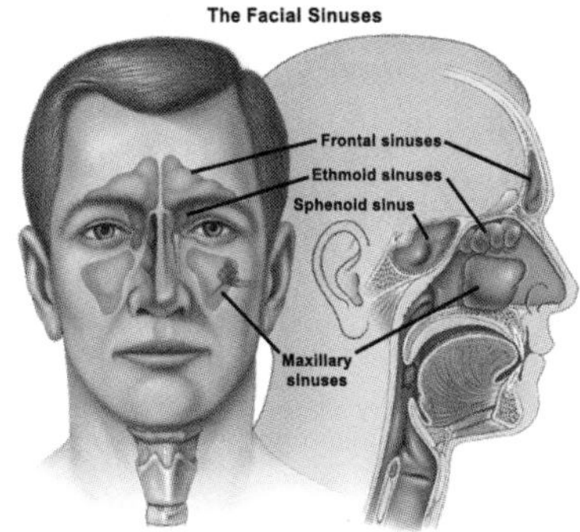

461.0 Maxillary

Acute antritis

459.1 – 461.0

461.1 Frontal

461.2 Ethmoidal

461.3 Sphenoidal

461.8 Other acute sinusitis
Acute pansinusitis

461.9 Acute sinusitis, unspecified
J01.90 Acute sinusitis, unspecified
Acute sinusitis NOS

462 Acute pharyngitis 6 6
J02.9 Acute pharyngitis, unspecified
Acute sore throat NOS
Pharyngitis (acute):
NOS
gangrenous
infective
phlegmonous
pneumococcal
staphylococcal
suppurative
ulcerative
Sore throat (viral) NOS
Viral pharyngitis
Excludes *abscess:*
peritonsillar [quinsy] (475)
pharyngeal NOS (478.29)
retropharyngeal (478.24)
chronic pharyngitis (472.1)
infectious mononucleosis (075)
that specified as (due to):
Coxsackie (virus) (074.0)
gonococcus (098.6)
herpes simplex (054.79)
influenza (487.1)
septic (034.0)
streptococcal (034.0)

463 Acute tonsillitis 6 6
Tonsillitis (acute):
NOS
follicular
gangrenous
infective
pneumococcal
septic
staphylococcal
suppurative
ulcerative
viral
Excludes *chronic tonsillitis (474.0)*
hypertrophy of tonsils (474.1)
peritonsillar abscess [quinsy] (475)
sore throat:
acute or NOS (462)
septic (034.0)
streptococcal tonsillitis (034.0)

4th **464 Acute laryngitis and tracheitis**
Excludes *that associated with influenza (487.1)*
that due to Streptococcus (034.0)

5th **464.0 Acute laryngitis**
Laryngitis (acute):
NOS
edematous
Hemophilus influenzae [H. influenzae]
pneumococcal
septic
suppurative
ulcerative
Excludes *chronic laryngitis (476.0-476.1)*
influenzal laryngitis (487.1)

464.00 Without mention of obstruction

464.01 With obstruction

5th **464.1 Acute tracheitis**
Tracheitis (acute):
NOS
catarrhal
viral
Excludes *chronic tracheitis (491.8)*

464.10 Without mention of obstruction

464.11 With obstruction

5th **464.2 Acute laryngotracheitis**
Laryngotracheitis (acute)
Tracheitis (acute) with laryngitis (acute)
Excludes *chronic laryngotracheitis (476.1)*

464.20 Without mention of obstruction

464.21 With obstruction

5th **464.3 Acute epiglottitis**
Viral epiglottitis
Excludes *epiglottitis, chronic (476.1)*

464.30 Without mention of obstruction

464.31 With obstruction

464.4 Croup
Croup syndrome

5th **464.5 Supraglottitis, unspecified**

464.50 Without mention of obstruction

464.51 With obstruction

4th **465 Acute upper respiratory infections of multiple or unspecified sites**
Excludes *upper respiratory infection due to:*
influenza (487.1)
Streptococcus (034.0)

465.0 Acute laryngopharyngitis 6 5

465.8 Other multiple sites 6 5
Multiple URI

465.9 Unspecified site 6 5
J06.9 Acute upper respiratory infection, unspecified
Acute URI NOS
Upper respiratory infection (acute)

4th / 5th Fourth/Fifth Digit Required | ● New Code ▲ Revised Code | Unspecified Code Other Specified Code Manifestation Code ICD-10-CM xWalk

4th 466 **Acute bronchitis and bronchiolitis**

Includes that with:
bronchospasm
obstruction

466.0 **Acute bronchitis** I 1 6

J20.9 Acute bronchitis, unspecified

Bronchitis, acute or subacute:
fibrinous
membranous
pneumococcal
purulent
septic
viral
with tracheitis
Croupous bronchitis
Tracheobronchitis, acute

Excludes *acute bronchitis with chronic obstructive pulmonary disease (491.22)*

ICD-9-CM Official Guidelines (Chapter 8):

b. Chronic Obstructive Pulmonary Disease [COPD] and Bronchitis

1) Acute bronchitis with COPD

Acute bronchitis, code 466.0, is due to an infectious organism. When acute bronchitis is documented with COPD, code 491.22, Obstructive chronic bronchitis with acute bronchitis, should be assigned. It is not necessary to also assign code 466.0. If a medical record documents acute bronchitis with COPD with acute exacerbation, only code 491.22 should be assigned. The acute bronchitis included in code 491.22 supersedes the acute exacerbation. If a medical record documents COPD with acute exacerbation without mention of acute bronchitis, only code 491.21 should be assigned.

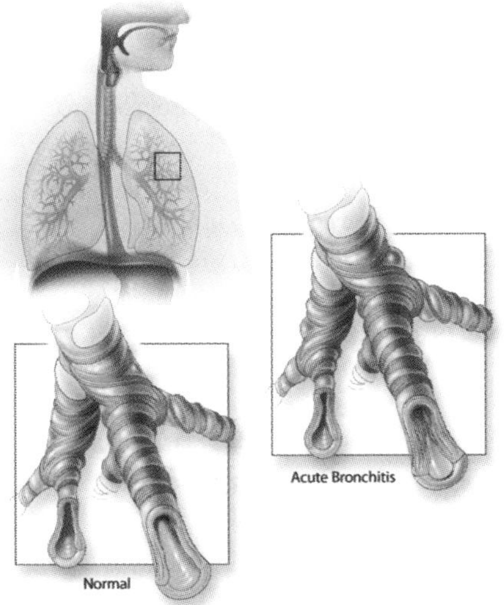

© 2008 Fairman Studios, LLC. All Rights Reserved.

5th 466.1 **Acute bronchiolitis**

Bronchiolitis (acute)
Capillary pneumonia

466.11 **Acute bronchiolitis due to respiratory syncytial virus (RSV)**

466.19 **Acute bronchiolitis due to other infectious organisms**

Use additional code to identify organism

OTHER DISEASES OF THE UPPER RESPIRATORY TRACT (470-478)

Upper Respiratory Tract

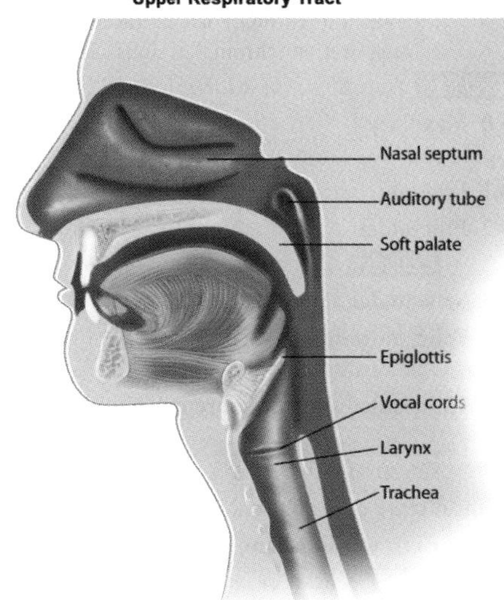

© 2008 Fairman Studios, LLC. All Rights Reserved.

470 **Deviated nasal septum**

Deflected septum (nasal) (acquired)

Excludes *congenital (754.0)*

4th 471 **Nasal polyps**

Excludes *adenomatous polyps (212.0)*

471.0 **Polyp of nasal cavity**

Polyp:
choanal
nasopharyngeal

471.1 **Polypoid sinus degeneration**

Woakes' syndrome or ethmoiditis

471.8 **Other polyp of sinus**

Polyp of sinus:
accessory
ethmoidal
maxillary
sphenoidal

471.9 **Unspecified nasal polyp**

Nasal polyp NOS

4th 472 **Chronic pharyngitis and nasopharyngitis**

472.0 **Chronic rhinitis**

Ozena
Rhinitis:
NOS
atrophic
granulomatous
hypertrophic
obstructive
purulent
ulcerative

Excludes *allergic rhinitis (477.0-477.9)*

472.1 **Chronic pharyngitis**

Chronic sore throat
Pharyngitis:
atrophic
granular (chronic)
hypertrophic

472.2 **Chronic nasopharyngitis**

Excludes *acute or unspecified nasopharyngitis (460)*

466 – 472.2

4th 473 Chronic sinusitis

Includes abscess (chronic) of sinus (accessory) (nasal)
empyema (chronic) of sinus (accessory) (nasal)
infection (chronic) of sinus (accessory) (nasal)
suppuration (chronic) of sinus (accessory) (nasal)

Excludes *acute sinusitis (461.0-461.9)*

473.0 Maxillary
Antritis (chronic)

473.1 Frontal

473.2 Ethmoidal
Excludes *Woakes' ethmoiditis (471.1)*

473.3 Sphenoidal

473.8 Other chronic sinusitis
Pansinusitis (chronic)

473.9 Unspecified sinusitis (chronic)
J32.9 Chronic sinusitis, unspecified
Sinusitis (chronic) NOS

4th 474 Chronic disease of tonsils and adenoids

5th 474.0 Chronic tonsillitis and adenoiditis
Excludes *acute or unspecified tonsillitis (463)*

474.00 Chronic tonsillitis

474.01 Chronic adenoiditis

474.02 Chronic tonsillitis and adenoiditis

5th 474.1 Hypertrophy of tonsils and adenoids
Enlargement of tonsils or adenoids
Hyperplasia of tonsils or adenoids
Hypertrophy of tonsils or adenoids
Excludes *that with:*
adenoiditis (474.01)
adenoiditis and tonsillitis (474.02)
tonsillitis (474.00)

474.10 Tonsils with adenoids

474.11 Tonsils alone

474.12 Adenoids alone

474.2 Adenoid vegetations

474.8 Other chronic disease of tonsils and adenoids
Amygdalolith
Calculus, tonsil
Cicatrix of tonsil (and adenoid)
Tonsillar tag
Ulcer, tonsil

474.9 Unspecified chronic disease of tonsils and adenoids
Disease (chronic) of tonsils (and adenoids)

475 Peritonsillar abscess
Abscess of tonsil
Peritonsillar cellulitis
Quinsy
Excludes *tonsillitis:*
acute or NOS (463)
chronic (474.0)

4th 476 Chronic laryngitis and laryngotracheitis

476.0 Chronic laryngitis
Laryngitis:
catarrhal
hypertrophic
sicca

476.1 Chronic laryngotracheitis
Laryngitis, chronic, with tracheitis (chronic)
Tracheitis, chronic, with laryngitis
Excludes *chronic tracheitis (491.8)*
laryngitis and tracheitis, acute or unspecified (464.00-464.51)

4th 477 Allergic rhinitis

Includes allergic rhinitis (nonseasonal) (seasonal)
hay fever
spasmodic rhinorrhea

Excludes *allergic rhinitis with asthma (bronchial) (493.0)*

477.0 Due to pollen
J30.1 Allergic rhinitis due to pollen
Pollinosis

477.1 Due to food

477.2 Due to animal (cat) (dog) hair and dander

477.8 Due to other allergen
J30.2 Other seasonal allergic rhinitis
J30.89 Other allergic rhinitis

477.9 Cause unspecified
J30.0 Vasomotor rhinitis
J30.9 Allergic rhinitis, unspecified

4th 478 Other diseases of upper respiratory tract

478.0 Hypertrophy of nasal turbinates

5th 478.1 Other diseases of nasal cavity and sinuses
Excludes *varicose ulcer of nasal septum (456.8)*

478.11 Nasal mucositis (ulcerative)
Use additional E code to identify adverse effects of therapy, such as:
antineoplastic and immunosuppressive drugs (E930.7, E933.1)
radiation therapy (E879.2)

478.19 Other diseases of nasal cavity and sinuses
Abscess of nose (septum)
Cyst or mucocele of sinus (nasal)
Necrosis of nose (septum)
Rhinolith
Ulcer of nose (septum)

5th 478.2 Other diseases of pharynx, not elsewhere classified

478.20 Unspecified disease of pharynx

478.21 Cellulitis of pharynx or nasopharynx

478.22 Parapharyngeal abscess

478.24 Retropharyngeal abscess

478.25 Edema of pharynx or nasopharynx

478.26 Cyst of pharynx or nasopharynx

478.29 Other
Abscess of pharynx or nasopharynx
Excludes *ulcerative pharyngitis (462)*

5th 478.3 Paralysis of vocal cords or larynx

478.30 Paralysis, unspecified
Laryngoplegia
Paralysis of glottis

478.31 Unilateral, partial

478.32 Unilateral, complete

478.33 Bilateral, partial

478.34 Bilateral, complete

478.4 Polyp of vocal cord or larynx
Excludes *adenomatous polyps (212.1)*

478.5 Other diseases of vocal cords
Abscess of vocal cords
Cellulitis of vocal cords
Chorditis (fibrinous) (nodosa) (tuberosa)
Granuloma of vocal cords
Leukoplakia of vocal cords
Singers' nodes

478.6 Edema of larynx
Edema (of):
glottis
subglottic
supraglottic

5th 478.7 **Other diseases of larynx, not elsewhere classified**

478.70 **Unspecified disease of larynx**

478.71 **Cellulitis and perichondritis of larynx**

478.74 **Stenosis of larynx**

478.75 **Laryngeal spasm**
Laryngismus (stridulus)

478.79 **Other**
Abscess of larynx
Necrosis of larynx
Obstruction of larynx
Pachyderma of larynx
Ulcer of larynx
Excludes *ulcerative laryngitis (464.00-464.01)*

478.8 **Upper respiratory tract hypersensitivity reaction, site unspecified**
Excludes *hypersensitivity reaction of lower respiratory tract, as:*
extrinsic allergic alveolitis (495.0-495.9)
pneumoconiosis (500-505)

478.9 **Other and unspecified diseases of upper respiratory tract**
Abscess of trachea
Cicatrix of trachea

PNEUMONIA AND INFLUENZA (480-488)

Excludes *pneumonia:*
allergic or eosinophilic (518.3)
aspiration:
NOS (507.0)
newborn (770.18)
solids and liquids (507.0-507.8)
congenital (770.0)
lipoid (507.1)
passive (514)
rheumatic (390)
ventilator-associated (997.31)

4th 480 **Viral pneumonia**

480.0 **Pneumonia due to adenovirus**

480.1 **Pneumonia due to respiratory syncytial virus**

480.2 **Pneumonia due to parainfluenza virus**

480.3 **Pneumonia due to SARS-associated coronavirus**

480.8 **Pneumonia due to other virus not elsewhere classified**
Excludes *congenital rubella pneumonitis (771.0)*
influenza with pneumonia, any form (487.0)
pneumonia complicating viral diseases classified elsewhere (484.1-484.8)

480.9 **Viral pneumonia, unspecified**

481 **Pneumococcal pneumonia [Streptococcus pneumoniae pneumonia]** 56, 57, 58, 59
Lobar pneumonia, organism unspecified

4th 482 **Other bacterial pneumonia**

482.0 **Pneumonia due to Klebsiella pneumoniae** 56, 57, 58, 59

482.1 **Pneumonia due to Pseudomonas** 56, 57, 58, 59

482.2 **Pneumonia due to Hemophilus influenzae [H. influenzae]** 56, 57, 58, 59

5th 482.3 **Pneumonia due to Streptococcus**
Excludes *Streptococcus pneumoniae pneumonia (481)*

482.30 **Streptococcus, unspecified** 56, 57, 58, 59

482.31 **Group A** 56, 57, 58, 59

482.32 **Group B** 56, 57, 58, 59

482.39 **Other Streptococcus** 56, 57, 58, 59

5th 482.4 **Pneumonia due to Staphylococcus**

482.40 **Pneumonia due to Staphylococcus, unspecified** 56, 57, 58, 59

482.41 **Methicillin susceptible pneumonia due to Staphylococcus aureus** 56, 57, 58, 59
MSSA pneumonia
Pneumonia due to Staphylococcus aureus NOS

482.42 **Methicillin resistant pneumonia due to Staphylococcus aureus** 56, 57, 58, 59

482.49 **Other Staphylococcus pneumonia** 56, 57, 58, 59

5th 482.8 **Pneumonia due to other specified bacteria**
Excludes *pneumonia complicating infectious disease classified elsewhere (484.1-484.8)*

482.81 **Anaerobes** 56, 57, 58, 59
Bacteroides (melaninogenicus)
Gram-negative anaerobes

482.82 **Escherichia coli [E. coli]** 56, 57, 58, 59

482.83 **Other gram-negative bacteria** 56, 57, 58, 59
Gram-negative pneumonia NOS
Proteus
Serratia marcescens
Excludes *gram-negative anaerobes (482.81)*
Legionnaires' disease (482.84)

482.84 **Legionnaires' disease** 56, 57, 58, 59

482.89 **Other specified bacteria** 56, 57, 58, 59

482.9 **Bacterial pneumonia, unspecified** 56, 57, 58, 59
J15.9 Unspecified bacterial pneumonia

4th 483 **Pneumonia due to other specified organism**

483.0 **Mycoplasma pneumoniae** 56, 57, 58, 59
Eaton's agent
Pleuropneumonia-like organisms [PPLO]

483.1 **Chlamydia** 56, 57, 58, 59

483.8 **Other specified organism** 56, 57, 58, 59

4th 484 **Pneumonia in infectious diseases classified elsewhere**
Excludes *influenza with pneumonia, any form (487.0)*

484.1 ***Pneumonia in cytomegalic inclusion disease***
Code first underlying disease, as: (078.5)

484.3 ***Pneumonia in whooping cough***
Code first underlying disease, as: (033.0-033.9)

484.5 ***Pneumonia in anthrax***
Code first underlying disease (022.1)

484.6 ***Pneumonia in aspergillosis***
Code first underlying disease (117.3)

484.7 ***Pneumonia in other systemic mycoses***
Code first underlying disease
Excludes *pneumonia in:*
candidiasis (112.4)
coccidioidomycosis (114.0)
histoplasmosis (115.0-115.9 with fifth-digit 5)

484.8 ***Pneumonia in other infectious diseases classified elsewhere***
Code first underlying disease, as:
Q fever (083.0)
typhoid fever (002.0)
Excludes *pneumonia in:*
actinomycosis (039.1)
measles (055.1)
nocardiosis (039.1)
ornithosis (073.0)
Pneumocystis carinii (136.3)
salmonellosis (003.22)
toxoplasmosis (130.4)
tuberculosis (011.6)
tularemia (021.2)
varicella (052.1)

485 Bronchopneumonia, organism unspecified 5 6, 5 7, 5 8, 5 9

Bronchopneumonia:
hemorrhagic
terminal
Pleurobronchopneumonia
Pneumonia:
lobular
segmental

Excludes *bronchiolitis (acute) (466.11- 466.19)*
chronic (491.8)
lipoid pneumonia (507.1)

486 Pneumonia, organism unspecified 5 6, 5 7, 5 8, 5 9

J18.9 Pneumonia, unspecified organism

Excludes *hypostatic or passive pneumonia (514)*
influenza with pneumonia, any form (487.0)
inhalation or aspiration pneumonia due to foreign materials (507.0-507.8)
pneumonitis due to fumes and vapors (506.0)

4th **487 Influenza**

Influenza caused by unspecified influenza virus

Excludes *Hemophilus influenzae [H. influenzae]:*
infection NOS (041.5)
laryngitis (464.00-464.01)
meningitis (320.0)
influenza due to 2009 H1N1 [swine] influenza virus (488.1)
influenza due to identified avian influenza virus (488.0)
influenza due to identified novel H1N1 influenza virus (488.1)

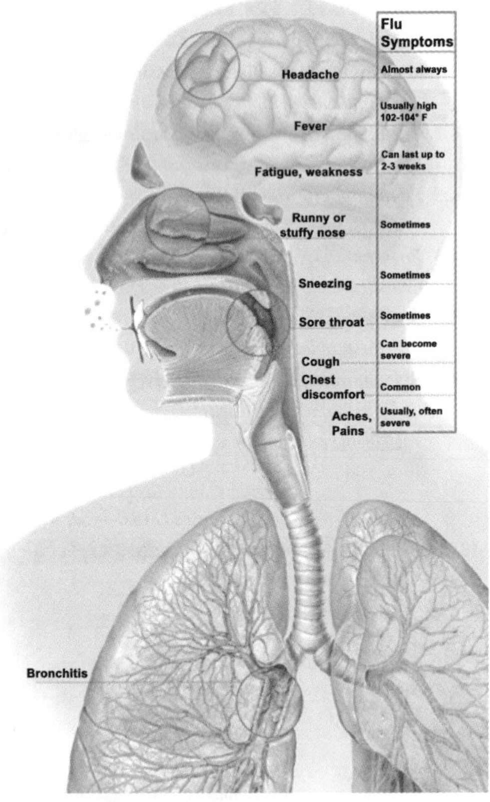

487.0 With pneumonia 5 6, 5 7, 5 8, 5 9

Influenza with pneumonia, any form
Influenzal:
bronchopneumonia
pneumonia
Use additional code to identify the type of pneumonia (480.0-480.9, 481, 482.0-482.9, 483.0-483.8, 485)

487.1 With other respiratory manifestations

Influenza NOS
Influenzal:
laryngitis
pharyngitis
respiratory infection (upper) (acute)

487.8 With other manifestations

Encephalopathy due to influenza
Influenza with involvement of gastrointestinal tract

Excludes *"intestinal flu" [viral gastroenteritis] (008.8)*

▲4th **488 Influenza due to certain identified ~~avian~~ influenza viruses**

~~**Note:** *Influenza caused by influenza viruses that normally infect only birds and, less commonly, other animals*~~

Excludes *influenza caused by ~~other~~ unspecified influenza viruses (487.0-487.8)*

Rationale: *An expansion has been made changing the three digit code 488 to a category, with two new codes added: 488.0, "Influenza due to identified avian influenza virus," and 488.1, "Influenza due to identified novel H1N1 influenza virus. These codes have been created to provide data capture for the novel H1N1 influenza virus (swine flu virus), which was first identified in April, after the March 2009 ICD-9-CM Coordination and Maintenance Committee meeting.*

● **488.0 Influenza due to identified avian influenza virus**

Avian influenza
Bird flu
Influenza A/H5N1

ICD-9-CM Official Guidelines (Chapter 8):

d. Influenza due to identified avian influenza virus (avian influenza)

Code only confirmed cases of avian influenza. This is an exception to the hospital inpatient guideline Section II, H. (Uncertain Diagnosis).

In this context, "confirmation" does not require documentation of positive laboratory testing specific for avian influenza. However, coding should be based on the provider's diagnostic statement that the patient has avian influenza.

If the provider records "suspected or possible or probable avian influenza," the appropriate influenza code from category 487 should be assigned. Code 488, Influenza due to identified avian influenza virus, should not be assigned.

● **488.1 Influenza due to identified novel H1N1 influenza virus**

2009 H1N1 [swine] influenza virus
Novel 2009 influenza H1N1
Novel H1N1 influenza
Novel influenza A/H1N1
Swine flu

CHRONIC OBSTRUCTIVE PULMONARY DISEASE AND ALLIED CONDITIONS (490-496)

490 Bronchitis, not specified as acute or chronic

J40 Bronchitis, not specified as acute or chronic

Bronchitis NOS:
catarrhal
with tracheitis NOS
Tracheobronchitis NOS

Excludes *bronchitis:*
allergic NOS (493.9)
asthmatic NOS (493.9)
due to fumes and vapors (506.0)

4th **491 Chronic bronchitis**

Excludes *chronic obstructive asthma (493.2)*

491.0 Simple chronic bronchitis 5 1, 5 2

Catarrhal bronchitis, chronic
Smokers' cough

491.1 Mucopurulent chronic bronchitis 5 1 , 5 2
Bronchitis (chronic) (recurrent):
fetid
mucopurulent
purulent

5th **491.2 Obstructive chronic bronchitis**
Bronchitis:
emphysematous
obstructive (chronic) (diffuse)
Bronchitis with:
chronic airway obstruction
emphysema
Excludes *asthmatic bronchitis (acute) (NOS) 493.9*
chronic obstructive asthma 493.2

491.20 Without exacerbation 5 1 , 5 2
J44.9 Chronic obstructive pulmonary disease, unspecified
Emphysema with chronic bronchitis

ICD-9-CM Official Guidelines (Chapter 8):

*a. **Chronic Obstructive Pulmonary Disease [COPD] and Asthma***

*1) **Conditions that comprise COPD and Asthma***

The conditions that comprise COPD are obstructive chronic bronchitis, subcategory 491.2, and emphysema, category 492. All asthma codes are under category 493, Asthma. Code 496, Chronic airway obstruction, not elsewhere classified, is a nonspecific code that should only be used when the documentation in a medical record does not specify the type of COPD being treated.

*2) **Acute exacerbation of chronic obstructive bronchitis and asthma***

The codes for chronic obstructive bronchitis and asthma distinguish between uncomplicated cases and those in acute exacerbation. An acute exacerbation is a worsening or a decompensation of a chronic condition. An acute exacerbation is not equivalent to an infection superimposed on a chronic condition, though an exacerbation may be triggered by an infection.

*3) **Overlapping nature of the conditions that comprise COPD and asthma***

Due to the overlapping nature of the conditions that make up COPD and asthma, there are many variations in the way these conditions are documented. Code selection must be based on the terms as documented. When selecting the correct code for the documented type of COPD and asthma, it is essential to first review the index, and then verify the code in the tabular list. There are many instructional notes under the different COPD subcategories and codes. It is important that all such notes be reviewed to assure correct code assignment.

*4) **Acute exacerbation of asthma and status asthmaticus***

An acute exacerbation of asthma is an increased severity of the asthma symptoms, such as wheezing and shortness of breath. Status asthmaticus refers to a patient's failure to respond to therapy administered during an asthmatic episode and is a life threatening complication that requires emergency care. If status asthmaticus is documented by the provider with any type of COPD or with acute bronchitis, the status asthmaticus should be sequenced first. It supersedes any type of COPD including that with acute exacerbation or acute bronchitis. It is inappropriate to assign an asthma code with 5th digit 2, with acute exacerbation, together with an asthma code with 5th digit 1, with status asthmatics. Only the 5th digit 1 should be assigned.

*b. **Chronic Obstructive Pulmonary Disease [COPD] and Bronchitis***

*1) **Acute bronchitis with COPD***

Acute bronchitis, code 466.0, is due to an infectious organism. When acute bronchitis is documented with COPD, code 491.22, Obstructive chronic bronchitis with acute bronchitis, should be assigned. It is not necessary to also assign code 466.0. If a medical record documents acute bronchitis with COPD with acute exacerbation, only code 491.22 should be assigned. The acute bronchitis included in code 491.22 supersedes the acute exacerbation. If a medical record documents COPD with acute exacerbation without mention of acute bronchitis, only code 491.21 should be assigned.

491.21 With (acute) exacerbation 5 1 , 5 2
J44.1 Chronic obstructive pulmonary disease with (acute) exacerbation
Acute exacerbation of chronic obstructive pulmonary disease [COPD]
Decompensated chronic obstructive pulmonary disease [COPD]
Decompensated chronic obstructive pulmonary disease [COPD] with exacerbation
Excludes *chronic obstructive asthma with acute exacerbation 493.22*

491.22 With acute bronchitis 5 1 , 5 2

491.8 Other chronic bronchitis 5 1 , 5 2
Chronic:
tracheitis
tracheobronchitis

491.9 Unspecified chronic bronchitis 5 1 , 5 2

4th **492 Emphysema**

492.0 Emphysematous bleb 5 1 , 5 2
Giant bullous emphysema
Ruptured emphysematous bleb
Tension pneumatocele
Vanishing lung

492.8 Other emphysema 5 1 , 5 2
J43.9 Emphysema, unspecified
Emphysema (lung or pulmonary):
NOS
centriacinar
centrilobular
obstructive
panacinar
panlobular
unilateral
vesicular
MacLeod's syndrome
Swyer-James syndrome
Unilateral hyperlucent lung
Excludes *emphysema:*
with chronic bronchitis (491.20-491.22)
compensatory (518.2)
due to fumes and vapors (506.4)
interstitial (518.1)
newborn (770.2)
mediastinal (518.1)
surgical (subcutaneous) (998.81)
traumatic (958.7)

491.1 – 492.8

4th **493 Asthma**

Excludes *wheezing NOS (786.07)*

The following fifth-digit subclassification is for use with category 493.0-493.2, 493.9:

0 unspecified
1 with status asthmaticus
2 with (acute) exacerbation

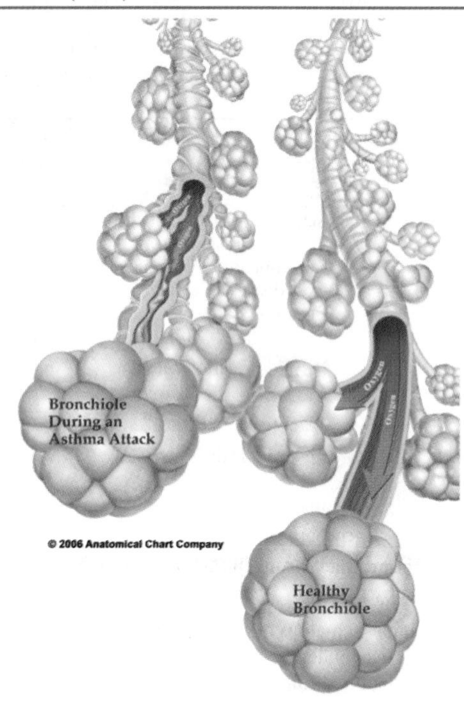

ICD-9-CM Official Guidelines (Chapter 8):

a. Chronic Obstructive Pulmonary Disease [COPD] and Asthma

1) Conditions that comprise COPD and Asthma

The conditions that comprise COPD are obstructive chronic bronchitis, subcategory 491.2, and emphysema, category 492. All asthma codes are under category 493, Asthma. Code 496, Chronic airway obstruction, not elsewhere classified, is a nonspecific code that should only be used when the documentation in a medical record does not specify the type of COPD being treated.

2) Acute exacerbation of chronic obstructive bronchitis and asthma

The codes for chronic obstructive bronchitis and asthma distinguish between uncomplicated cases and those in acute exacerbation. An acute exacerbation is a worsening or a decompensation of a chronic condition. An acute exacerbation is not equivalent to an infection superimposed on a chronic condition, though an exacerbation may be triggered by an infection.

3) Overlapping nature of the conditions that comprise COPD and asthma

Due to the overlapping nature of the conditions that make up COPD and asthma, there are many variations in the way these conditions are documented. Code selection must be based on the terms as documented. When selecting the correct code for the documented type of COPD and asthma, it is essential to first review the index, and then verify the code in the tabular list. There are many instructional notes under the different COPD subcategories and codes. It is important that all such notes be reviewed to assure correct code assignment.

4) Acute exacerbation of asthma and status asthmaticus

An acute exacerbation of asthma is an increased severity of the asthma symptoms, such as wheezing and shortness of breath. Status asthmaticus refers to a patient's failure to respond to therapy administered during an asthmatic episode and is a life threatening complication that requires emergency care. If status asthmaticus is documented by the provider with any type of COPD or with acute bronchitis, the status asthmaticus should be sequenced first. It supersedes any type of COPD including that with acute exacerbation or acute bronchitis. It is inappropriate to assign an asthma code with 5th digit 2, with acute exacerbation, together with an asthma code with 5th digit 1, with status asthmatics. Only the 5th digit 1 should be assigned.

Layman's: *The key difference between extrinsic (allergic) and intrinsic (non-allergic) are its triggers being external stimuli or internal processes, respectively. Typically, extrinsic asthma manifests in childhood and intrinsic develops in people over the age of 30, though most patients with extrinsic asthma are also presumed to have internal triggers.*

5th **493.0 Extrinsic asthma** 53, 64
[0-2] Asthma:
allergic with stated cause
atopic
childhood
hay
platinum
Hay fever with asthma

Excludes *asthma:*
allergic NOS (493.9)
detergent (507.8)
miners' (500)
wood (495.8)

5th **493.1 Intrinsic asthma** 53, 64
[0-2] Late-onset asthma

5th **493.2 Chronic obstructive asthma** 53, 64
[0-2] Asthma with chronic obstructive pulmonary disease [COPD]
Chronic asthmatic bronchitis

Excludes *acute bronchitis (466.0)*
chronic obstructive bronchitis (491.20-491.22)

5th **493.8 Other forms of asthma**

493.81 Exercise induced bronchospasm 53, 64

493.82 Cough variant asthma 53, 64

5th **493.9 Asthma, unspecified** 53, 64
[0-2] Asthma (bronchial) (allergic NOS)
Bronchitis:
allergic
asthmatic

4th **494 Bronchiectasis**

Bronchiectasis (fusiform) (postinfectious) (recurrent)
Bronchiolectasis

Excludes *congenital (748.61)*
tuberculous bronchiectasis (current disease) (011.5)

494.0 Bronchiectasis without acute exacerbation

494.1 Bronchiectasis with acute exacerbation

4th **495 Extrinsic allergic alveolitis**

Includes allergic alveolitis and pneumonitis due to inhaled organic dust particles of fungal, thermophilic actinomycete, or other origin

495.0 Farmers' lung

495.1 Bagassosis

495.2 Bird-fanciers' lung
Budgerigar-fanciers' disease or lung
Pigeon-fanciers' disease or lung

495.3 Suberosis
Cork-handlers' disease or lung

495.4 Malt workers' lung
Alveolitis due to Aspergillus clavatus

495.5 Mushroom workers' lung

495.6 Maple bark-strippers' lung
Alveolitis due to Cryptostroma corticale

495.7 **"Ventilation" pneumonitis**
Allergic alveolitis due to fungal, thermophilic actinomycete, and other organisms growing in ventilation [air conditioning] systems

495.8 **Other specified allergic alveolitis and pneumonitis**
Cheese-washers' lung
Coffee workers' lung
Fish-meal workers' lung
Furriers' lung
Grain-handlers' disease or lung
Pituitary snuff-takers' disease
Sequoiosis or red-cedar asthma
Wood asthma

495.9 **Unspecified allergic alveolitis and pneumonitis**
Alveolitis, allergic (extrinsic)
Hypersensitivity pneumonitis

496 **Chronic airway obstruction, not elsewhere classified** 51, 52
J44.9 Chronic obstructive pulmonary disease, unspecified
Note: *This code is not to be used with any code from categories 491-493*
Chronic:
nonspecific lung disease
obstructive lung disease
obstructive pulmonary disease [COPD] NOS
Excludes *chronic obstructive lung disease [COPD] specified (as) (with):*
allergic alveolitis (495.0-495.9)
asthma (493.2)
bronchiectasis (494.0-494.1)
bronchitis (491.20-491.22)
with emphysema (491.20-491.22)
decompensated (491.21)
emphysema (492.0-492.8)

PNEUMOCONIOSES AND OTHER LUNG DISEASES DUE TO EXTERNAL AGENTS (500-508)

500 **Coal workers' pneumoconiosis** A
Anthracosilicosis
Anthracosis
Black lung disease
Coal workers' lung
Miners' asthma

501 **Asbestosis** A

502 **Pneumoconiosis due to other silica or silicates**
Pneumoconiosis due to talc
Silicosis (simple) (complicated)
Silicotic fibrosis (massive) of lung

503 **Pneumoconiosis due to other inorganic dust**
Aluminosis (of lung)
Bauxite fibrosis (of lung)
Berylliosis
Graphite fibrosis (of lung)
Siderosis
Stannosis

504 **Pneumonopathy due to inhalation of other dust**
Byssinosis
Cannabinosis
Flax-dressers' disease
Excludes *allergic alveolitis (495.0-495.9)*
asbestosis (501)
bagassosis (495.1)
farmers' lung (495.0)

505 **Pneumoconiosis, unspecified**

4th 506 **Respiratory conditions due to chemical fumes and vapors**
Use additional E code to identify cause

506.0 **Bronchitis and pneumonitis due to fumes and vapors**
Chemical bronchitis (acute)

506.1 **Acute pulmonary edema due to fumes and vapors**
Chemical pulmonary edema (acute)
Excludes *acute pulmonary edema NOS (518.4)*
chronic or unspecified pulmonary edema (514)

506.2 **Upper respiratory inflammation due to fumes and vapors**

506.3 **Other acute and subacute respiratory conditions due to fumes and vapors**

506.4 **Chronic respiratory conditions due to fumes and vapors**
Emphysema (diffuse) (chronic) due to inhalation of chemical fumes and vapors
Obliterative bronchiolitis (chronic) (subacute) due to inhalation of chemical fumes and vapors
Pulmonary fibrosis (chronic) due to inhalation of chemical fumes and vapors

506.9 **Unspecified respiratory conditions due to fumes and vapors**
Silo-fillers' disease

4th 507 **Pneumonitis due to solids and liquids**
Excludes *fetal aspiration pneumonitis (770.18)*

507.0 **Due to inhalation of food or vomitus**
J69.0 Pneumonitis due to inhalation of food and vomit
Aspiration pneumonia (due to):
NOS
food (regurgitated)
gastric secretions
milk
saliva
vomitus

507.1 **Due to inhalation of oils and essences**
Lipoid pneumonia (exogenous)
Excludes *endogenous lipoid pneumonia (516.8)*

507.8 **Due to other solids and liquids**
Detergent asthma

4th 508 **Respiratory conditions due to other and unspecified external agents**
Use additional E code to identify cause

508.0 **Acute pulmonary manifestations due to radiation**
Radiation pneumonitis

508.1 **Chronic and other pulmonary manifestations due to radiation**
Fibrosis of lung following radiation

508.8 **Respiratory conditions due to other specified external agents**

508.9 **Respiratory conditions due to unspecified external agent**

OTHER DISEASES OF RESPIRATORY SYSTEM (510-519)

4th 510 **Empyema**
Use additional code to identify infectious organism (041.0-041.9)
Excludes *abscess of lung (513.0)*

510.0 **With fistula**
Fistula:
bronchocutaneous
bronchopleural
hepatopleural
mediastinal
pleural
thoracic
Any condition classifiable to 510.9 with fistula

510.9 Without mention of fistula
Abscess:
pleura
thorax
Empyema (chest) (lung) (pleura)
Fibrinopurulent pleurisy
Pleurisy:
purulent
septic
seropurulent
suppurative
Pyopneumothorax
Pyothorax

4th **511 Pleurisy**
Excludes *pleurisy with mention of tuberculosis, current disease (012.0)*

511.0 Without mention of effusion or current tuberculosis
Adhesion, lung or pleura
Calcification of pleura
Pleurisy (acute) (sterile):
diaphragmatic
fibrinous
interlobar
Pleurisy:
NOS
pneumococcal
staphylococcal
streptococcal
Thickening of pleura

511.1 With effusion, with mention of a bacterial cause other than tuberculosis
Pleurisy with effusion (exudative) (serous):
pneumococcal
staphylococcal
streptococcal
other specified nontuberculous bacterial cause

5th **511.8 Other specified forms of effusion, except tuberculous**
Excludes *traumatic (860.2-860.5, 862.29, 862.39)*

511.81 Malignant pleural effusion
Code first malignant neoplasm, if known

511.89 Other specified forms of effusion, except tuberculous
Encysted pleurisy
Hemopneumothorax
Hemothorax
Hydropneumothorax
Hydrothorax

511.9 Unspecified pleural effusion
J90 Pleural effusion, not elsewhere classified
J91.8 Pleural effusion in other conditions classified elsewhere
Pleural effusion NOS
Pleurisy:
exudative
serofibrinous
serous
with effusion NOS

4th **512 Pneumothorax**

512.0 Spontaneous tension pneumothorax

512.1 Iatrogenic pneumothorax
Postoperative pneumothorax

512.8 Other spontaneous pneumothorax
Pneumothorax:
NOS
acute
chronic
Excludes *pneumothorax:*
congenital (770.2)
traumatic (860.0-860.1, 860.4-860.5)
tuberculous, current disease (011.7)

4th **513 Abscess of lung and mediastinum**

513.0 Abscess of lung
Abscess (multiple) of lung
Gangrenous or necrotic pneumonia
Pulmonary gangrene or necrosis

513.1 Abscess of mediastinum

514 Pulmonary congestion and hypostasis
J18.2 Hypostatic pneumonia, unspecified organism
J81.1 Chronic pulmonary edema
Hypostatic:
bronchopneumonia
pneumonia
Passive pneumonia
Pulmonary congestion (chronic) (passive)
Pulmonary edema:
NOS
chronic
Excludes *acute pulmonary edema:*
NOS (518.4)
with mention of heart disease or failure (428.1)
hypostatic pneumonia due to or specified as a specific type of pneumonia – code to the type of pneumonia (480.0-480.9, 481, 482.0-482.49, 483.0-483.8, 485, 486, 487.0)

515 Postinflammatory pulmonary fibrosis
J84.1 Other interstitial pulmonary diseases with fibrosis
Cirrhosis of lung chronic or unspecified
Fibrosis of lung (atrophic) (confluent) (massive) (perialveolar) (peribronchial) chronic or unspecified
Induration of lung chronic or unspecified

4th **516 Other alveolar and parietoalveolar pneumonopathy**

516.0 Pulmonary alveolar proteinosis

516.1 *Idiopathic pulmonary hemosiderosis*
Essential brown induration of lung
Code first underlying disease (275.0)

516.2 Pulmonary alveolar microlithiasis

516.3 Idiopathic fibrosing alveolitis
Alveolar capillary block
Diffuse (idiopathic) (interstitial) pulmonary fibrosis
Hamman-Rich syndrome

516.8 Other specified alveolar and parietoalveolar pneumonopathies
Endogenous lipoid pneumonia
Interstitial pneumonia (desquamative) (lymphoid)
Excludes *lipoid pneumonia, exogenous or unspecified (507.1)*

516.9 Unspecified alveolar and parietoalveolar pneumonopathy

4th **517 Lung involvement in conditions classified elsewhere**
Excludes *rheumatoid lung (714.81)*

517.1 *Rheumatic pneumonia*
Code first underlying disease (390)

517.2 *Lung involvement in systemic sclerosis*
Code first underlying disease (710.1)

517.3 *Acute chest syndrome*
Code first sickle-cell disease in crisis (282.42, 282.62, 282.64, 282.69)

517.8 **Lung involvement in other diseases classified elsewhere**

Code first underlying disease, as:
amyloidosis (277.30-277.39)
polymyositis (710.4)
sarcoidosis (135)
Sjögren's disease (710.2)
systemic lupus erythematosus (710.0)

Excludes *syphilis (095.1)*

4th **518 Other diseases of lung**

518.0 Pulmonary collapse

J98.11 Atelectasis

J98.19 Other pulmonary collapse

Atelectasis
Collapse of lung
Middle lobe syndrome

Excludes *atelectasis:*
congenital (partial) (770.5)
primary (770.4)
tuberculous, current disease (011.8)

518.1 Interstitial emphysema

Mediastinal emphysema

Excludes *surgical (subcutaneous) emphysema (998.81)*
that in fetus or newborn (770.2)
traumatic emphysema (958.7)

518.2 Compensatory emphysema

518.3 Pulmonary eosinophilia

J82 Pulmonary eosinophilia, not elsewhere classified

Eosinophilic asthma
Löffler's syndrome
Pneumonia:
allergic
eosinophilic
Tropical eosinophilia

518.4 Acute edema of lung, unspecified

Acute pulmonary edema NOS
Pulmonary edema, postoperative

Excludes *pulmonary edema:*
acute, with mention of heart disease or failure (428.1)
chronic or unspecified (514)
due to external agents (506.0-508.9)

518.5 Pulmonary insufficiency following trauma and surgery

Adult respiratory distress syndrome
Pulmonary insufficiency following:
shock
surgery
trauma
Shock lung

Excludes *adult respiratory distress syndrome associated with other conditions (518.82)*
pneumonia:
aspiration (507.0)
hypostatic (514)
respiratory failure in other conditions (518.81, 518.83-518.84)

518.6 Allergic bronchopulmonary aspergillosis

518.7 Transfusion related acute lung injury (TRALI)

5th **518.8 Other diseases of lung**

518.81 Acute respiratory failure

J96.0 Acute respiratory failure

Respiratory failure NOS

Excludes *acute and chronic respiratory failure (518.84)*
acute respiratory distress (518.82)
chronic respiratory failure (518.83)
respiratory arrest (799.1)
respiratory failure, newborn (770.84)

ICD-9-CM Official Guidelines (Chapter 8):

c. Acute Respiratory Failure

*1) **Acute respiratory failure as principal diagnosis***

Code 518.81, Acute respiratory failure, may be assigned as a principal diagnosis when it is the condition established after study to be chiefly responsible for occasioning the admission to the hospital, and the selection is supported by the Alphabetic Index and Tabular List. However, chapter-specific coding guidelines (such as obstetrics, poisoning, HIV, newborn) that provide sequencing direction take precedence.

*2) **Acute respiratory failure as secondary diagnosis***

Respiratory failure may be listed as a secondary diagnosis if it occurs after admission, or if it is present on admission, but does not meet the definition of principal diagnosis.

*3) **Sequencing of acute respiratory failure and another acute condition***

When a patient is admitted with respiratory failure and another acute condition, (e.g., myocardial infarction, cerebrovascular accident, aspiration pneumonia), the principal diagnosis will not be the same in every situation. This applies whether the other acute condition is a respiratory or nonrespiratory condition. Selection of the principal diagnosis will be dependent on the circumstances of admission. If both the respiratory failure and the other acute condition are equally responsible for occasioning the admission to the hospital, and there are no chapter-specific sequencing rules, the guideline regarding two or more diagnoses that equally meet the definition for principal diagnosis (Section II, C.) may be applied in these situations.

If the documentation is not clear as to whether acute respiratory failure and another condition are equally responsible for occasioning the admission, query the provider for clarification.

ICD-9-CM Official Guidelines (Chapter 17c1):

c. When a patient is admitted for burn injuries and other related conditions such as smoke inhalation and/or respiratory failure, the circumstances of admission govern the selection of the principal or first-listed diagnosis.

518.82 Other pulmonary insufficiency, not elsewhere classified

J80 Acute respiratory distress syndrome

Acute respiratory distress
Acute respiratory insufficiency
Adult respiratory distress syndrome NEC

Excludes *adult respiratory distress syndrome associated with trauma or surgery (518.5)*
pulmonary insufficiency following trauma or surgery (518.5)
respiratory distress:
NOS (786.09)
newborn (770.89)
syndrome, newborn (769)
shock lung (518.5)

518.83 **Chronic respiratory failure**

518.84 **Acute and chronic respiratory failure**
Acute on chronic respiratory failure

518.89 **Other diseases of lung, not elsewhere classified**
J98.4 Other disorders of lung
Broncholithiasis
Calcification of lung
Lung disease NOS
Pulmolithiasis

4th 519 **Other diseases of respiratory system**

5th 519.0 **Tracheostomy complications**

519.00 **Tracheostomy complication, unspecified**

519.01 **Infection of tracheostomy**
Use additional code to identify type of infection, such as:
abscess or cellulitis of neck (682.1)
septicemia (038.0-038.9)
Use additional code to identify organism (041.00-041.9)

519.02 **Mechanical complication of tracheostomy**
Tracheal stenosis due to tracheostomy

519.09 **Other tracheostomy complications**
Hemorrhage due to tracheostomy
Tracheoesophageal fistula due to tracheostomy

519.1 **Other diseases of trachea and bronchus, not elsewhere classified**

519.11 **Acute bronchospasm**
Bronchospasm NOS
Excludes *acute bronchitis with bronchospasm (466.0)*
asthma (493.00-493.92)
exercise induced bronchospasm (493.81)

519.19 **Other diseases of trachea and bronchus**
Calcification of bronchus or trachea
Stenosis of bronchus or trachea
Ulcer of bronchus or trachea

519.2 **Mediastinitis**

519.3 **Other diseases of mediastinum, not elsewhere classified**
Fibrosis of mediastinum
Hernia of mediastinum
Retraction of mediastinum

519.4 **Disorders of diaphragm**
Diaphragmitis
Paralysis of diaphragm
Relaxation of diaphragm
Excludes *congenital defect of diaphragm (756.6)*
diaphragmatic hernia (551-553 with .3)
congenital (756.6)

519.8 **Other diseases of respiratory system, not elsewhere classified**

519.9 **Unspecified disease of respiratory system**
Respiratory disease (chronic) NOS

9. DISEASES OF THE DIGESTIVE SYSTEM (520-579)

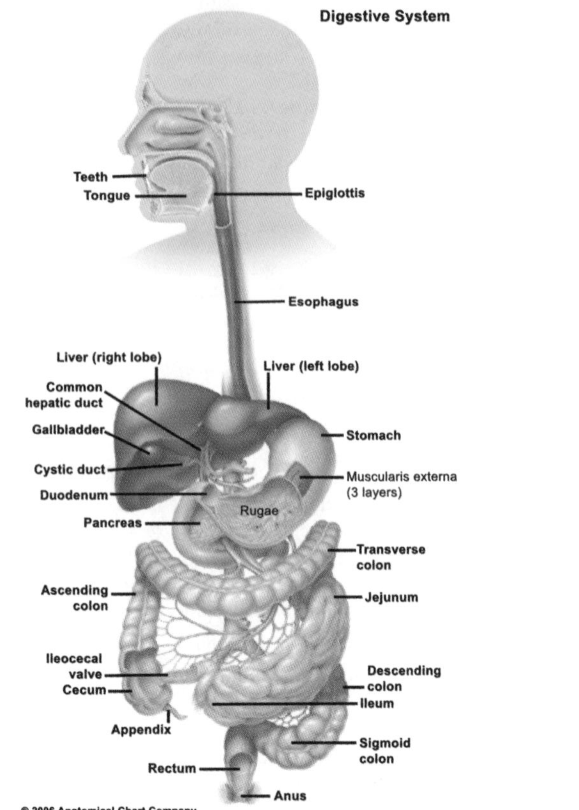

DISEASES OF ORAL CAVITY, SALIVARY GLANDS, AND JAWS (520-529)

4th 520 **Disorders of tooth development and eruption**

520.0 **Anodontia**
Absence of teeth (complete) (congenital) (partial)
Hypodontia
Oligodontia
Excludes *acquired absence of teeth (525.10-525.19)*

520.1 **Supernumerary teeth**
Distomolar
Fourth molar
Mesiodens
Paramolar
Supplemental teeth
Excludes *supernumerary roots (520.2)*

520.2 **Abnormalities of size and form**
Concrescence of teeth
Dens evaginatus
Dens in dente
Dens invaginatus
Enamel pearls
Fusion of teeth
Gemination of teeth
Macrodontia
Microdontia
Peg-shaped [conical] teeth
Supernumerary roots
Taurodontism
Tuberculum paramolare
Excludes *that due to congenital syphilis (090.5)*
tuberculum Carabelli, which is regarded as a normal variation

520.3 **Mottled teeth**
Dental fluorosis
Mottling of enamel
Nonfluoride enamel opacities

520.4 Disturbances of tooth formation
Aplasia and hypoplasia of cementum
Dilaceration of tooth
Enamel hypoplasia (neonatal) (postnatal) (prenatal)
Horner's teeth
Hypocalcification of teeth
Regional odontodysplasia
Turner's tooth
Excludes *Hutchinson's teeth and mulberry molars in congenital syphilis (090.5)*
mottled teeth (520.3)

520.5 Hereditary disturbances in tooth structure, not elsewhere classified
Amelogenesis imperfecta
Dentinal dysplasia
Dentinogenesis imperfecta
Odontogenesis imperfecta
Shell teeth

520.6 Disturbances in tooth eruption
Teeth:
- embedded
- impacted
- natal
- neonatal
- prenatal
- primary [deciduous]:
  - persistent
  - shedding, premature

Tooth eruption:
- late
- obstructed
- premature

Excludes *exfoliation of teeth (attributable to disease of surrounding tissues) (525.0-525.19)*

520.7 Teething syndrome

520.8 Other specified disorders of tooth development and eruption
Color changes during tooth formation
Pre-eruptive color changes
Excludes *posteruptive color changes (521.7)*

520.9 Unspecified disorder of tooth development and eruption

4th **521 Diseases of hard tissues of teeth**

5th **521.0 Dental caries**

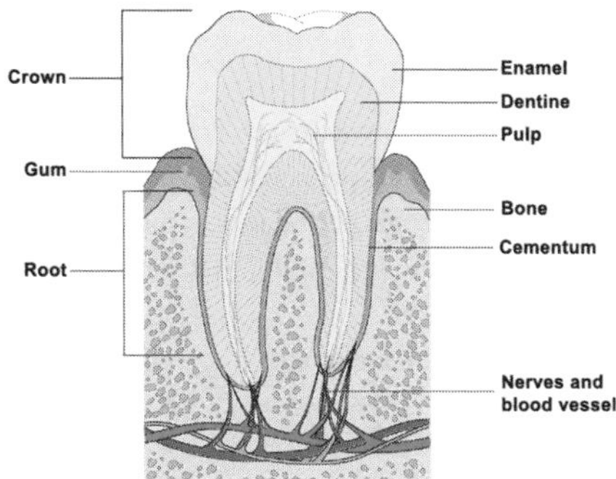

521.00 Dental caries, unspecified

521.01 Dental caries limited to enamel
Initial caries
White spot lesion

521.02 Dental caries extending into dentine

521.03 Dental caries extending into pulp

521.04 Arrested dental caries

521.05 Odontoclasia
Infantile melanodontia
Melanodontoclasia
Excludes *internal and external resorption of teeth (521.40-521.49)*

521.06 Dental caries pit and fissure
Primary dental caries, pit and fissure origin

521.07 Dental caries of smooth surface
Primary dental caries, smooth surface origin

521.08 Dental caries of root surface
Primary dental caries, root surface

521.09 Other dental caries

5th **521.1 Excessive attrition (approximal wear) (occlusal wear)**

521.10 Excessive attrition, unspecified

521.11 Excessive attrition, limited to enamel

521.12 Excessive attrition, extending into dentine

521.13 Excessive attrition, extending into pulp

521.14 Excessive attrition, localized

521.15 Excessive attrition, generalized

5th **521.2 Abrasion**
Abrasion of teeth:
- dentifrice
- habitual
- occupational
- ritual
- traditional

Wedge defect NOS of teeth

521.20 Abrasion, unspecified

521.21 Abrasion, limited to enamel

521.22 Abrasion, extending into dentine

521.23 Abrasion, extending into pulp

521.24 Abrasion, localized

521.25 Abrasion, generalized

5th **521.3 Erosion**
Erosion of teeth:
- NOS
- due to:
  - medicine
  - persistent vomiting
- idiopathic
- occupational

521.30 Erosion, unspecified

521.31 Erosion, limited to enamel

521.32 Erosion, extending into dentine

521.33 Erosion, extending into pulp

521.34 Erosion, localized

521.35 Erosion, generalized

5th **521.4 Pathological resorption**

521.40 Pathological resorption, unspecified

521.41 Pathological resorption, internal

521.42 Pathological resorption, external

521.49 Other pathological resorption
Internal granuloma of pulp

521.5 Hypercementosis
Cementation hyperplasia

521.6 Ankylosis of teeth

521.7 Intrinsic posteruptive color changes
Staining [discoloration] of teeth:
NOS
due to:
drugs
metals
pulpal bleeding
Excludes *accretions [deposits] on teeth (523.6)*
extrinsic color changes (523.6)
pre-eruptive color changes (520.8)

5th **521.8 Other specified diseases of hard tissues of teeth**

521.81 Cracked tooth
Excludes *asymptomatic craze lines in enamel – omit code*
broken tooth due to trauma (873.63, 873.73)
fractured tooth due to trauma (873.63, 873.73)

521.89 Other specified diseases of hard tissues of teeth
Irradiated enamel
Sensitive dentin

521.9 Unspecified disease of hard tissues of teeth

4th **522 Diseases of pulp and periapical tissues**

522.0 Pulpitis
Pulpal:
abscess
polyp
Pulpitis:
acute
chronic (hyperplastic) (ulcerative)
suppurative

522.1 Necrosis of the pulp
Pulp gangrene

522.2 Pulp degeneration
Denticles
Pulp calcifications
Pulp stones

522.3 Abnormal hard tissue formation in pulp
Secondary or irregular dentin

522.4 Acute apical periodontitis of pulpal origin

522.5 Periapical abscess without sinus
Abscess:
dental
dentoalveolar
Excludes *periapical abscess with sinus (522.7)*

522.6 Chronic apical periodontitis
Apical or periapical granuloma
Apical periodontitis NOS

522.7 Periapical abscess with sinus
Fistula:
alveolar process
dental

522.8 Radicular cyst
Cyst:
apical (periodontal)
periapical
radiculodental
residual radicular
Excludes *lateral developmental or lateral periodontal cyst (526.0)*

522.9 Other and unspecified diseases of pulp and periapical tissues

4th **523 Gingival and periodontal diseases**

5th **523.0 Acute gingivitis**
Excludes *acute necrotizing ulcerative gingivitis (101)*
herpetic gingivostomatitis (054.2)

523.00 Acute gingivitis, plaque induced
Acute gingivitis NOS

523.01 Acute gingivitis, non-plaque induced

5th **523.1 Chronic gingivitis**
Gingivitis (chronic):
desquamative
hyperplastic
simple marginal
ulcerative
Excludes *herpetic gingivostomatitis (054.2)*

523.10 Chronic gingivitis, plaque induced
Chronic gingivitis NOS
Gingivitis NOS

523.11 Chronic gingivitis, non-plaque induced

5th **523.2 Gingival recession**
Gingival recession (postinfective) (postoperative)

523.20 Gingival recession, unspecified

523.21 Gingival recession, minimal

523.22 Gingival recession, moderate

523.23 Gingival recession, severe

523.24 Gingival recession, localized

523.25 Gingival recession, generalized

5th **523.3 Aggressive and acute periodontitis**
Acute:
pericementitis
pericoronitis
Excludes *acute apical periodontitis (522.4)*
periapical abscess (522.5, 522.7)

523.30 Aggressive periodontitis, unspecified

523.31 Aggressive periodontitis, localized
Periodontal abscess

523.32 Aggressive periodontitis, generalized

523.33 Acute periodontitis

5th **523.4 Chronic periodontitis**
Chronic pericoronitis
Pericementitis (chronic)
Periodontitis:
NOS
complex
simplex
Excludes *chronic apical periodontitis (522.6)*

523.40 Chronic periodontitis, unspecified

523.41 Chronic periodontitis, localized

523.42 Chronic periodontitis, generalized

523.5 Periodontosis

523.6 Accretions on teeth
Dental calculus:
subgingival
supragingival
Deposits on teeth:
betel
materia alba
soft
tartar
tobacco
Extrinsic discoloration of teeth
Excludes *intrinsic discoloration of teeth (521.7)*

523.8 **Other specified periodontal diseases**
Giant cell:
epulis
peripheral granuloma
Gingival:
cysts
enlargement NOS
fibromatosis
Gingival polyp
Periodontal lesions due to traumatic occlusion
Peripheral giant cell granuloma
Excludes *leukoplakia of gingiva (528.6)*

523.9 **Unspecified gingival and periodontal disease**

4th 524 **Dentofacial anomalies, including malocclusion**

5th 524.0 **Major anomalies of jaw size**
Excludes *hemifacial atrophy or hypertrophy (754.0)*
unilateral condylar hyperplasia or hypoplasia of mandible

524.00 **Unspecified anomaly**
524.01 **Maxillary hyperplasia**
524.02 **Mandibular hyperplasia**
524.03 **Maxillary hypoplasia**
524.04 **Mandibular hypoplasia**
524.05 **Macrogenia**
524.06 **Microgenia**
524.07 **Excessive tuberosity of jaw**
Entire maxillary tuberosity
524.09 **Other specified anomaly**

5th 524.1 **Anomalies of relationship of jaw to cranial base**
524.10 **Unspecified anomaly**
Prognathism
Retrognathism
524.11 **Maxillary asymmetry**
524.12 **Other jaw asymmetry**
524.19 **Other specified anomaly**

5th 524.2 **Anomalies of dental arch relationship**
Anomaly of dental arch
Excludes *hemifacial atrophy or hypertrophy (754.0)*
soft tissue impingement (524.81-524.82)
unilateral condylar hyperplasia or hypoplasia of mandible (526.89)

524.20 **Unspecified anomaly of dental arch relationship**
524.21 **Malocclusion, Angle's class I**
Neutro-occlusion
524.22 **Malocclusion, Angle's class II**
Disto-occlusion Division I
Disto-occlusion Division II
524.23 **Malocclusion, Angle's class III**
Mesio-occlusion
524.24 **Open anterior occlusal relationship**
Anterior open bite
524.25 **Open posterior occlusal relationship**
Posterior open bite
524.26 **Excessive horizontal overlap**
Excessive horizontal overjet
524.27 **Reverse articulation**
Anterior articulation
Crossbite
Posterior articulation
524.28 **Anomalies of interarch distance**
Excessive interarch distance
Inadequate interarch distance
524.29 **Other anomalies of dental arch relationship**
Other anomalies of dental arch

5th 524.3 **Anomalies of tooth position of fully erupted teeth**
Excludes *impacted or embedded teeth with abnormal position of such teeth or adjacent teeth (520.6)*

524.30 **Unspecified anomaly of tooth position**
Diastema of teeth NOS
Displacement of teeth NOS
Transposition of teeth NOS
524.31 **Crowding of teeth**
524.32 **Excessive spacing of teeth**
524.33 **Horizontal displacement of teeth**
Tipped teeth
Tipping of teeth
524.34 **Vertical displacement of teeth**
Extruded tooth
Infraeruption of teeth
Intruded tooth
Supraeruption of teeth
524.35 **Rotation of tooth/teeth**
524.36 **Insufficient interocclusal distance of teeth (ridge)**
Lack of adequate intermaxillary vertical dimension
524.37 **Excessive interocclusal distance of teeth**
Excessive intermaxillary vertical dimension
Loss of occlusal vertical dimension
524.39 **Other anomalies of tooth position**

524.4 **Malocclusion, unspecified**

5th 524.5 **Dentofacial functional abnormalities**
524.50 **Dentofacial functional abnormality, unspecified**
524.51 **Abnormal jaw closure**
524.52 **Limited mandibular range of motion**
524.53 **Deviation in opening and closing of the mandible**
524.54 **Insufficient anterior guidance**
Insufficient anterior occlusal guidance
524.55 **Centric occlusion maximum intercuspation discrepancy**
Centric occlusion of teeth discrepancy
524.56 **Non-working side interference**
Balancing side interference
524.57 **Lack of posterior occlusal support**
524.59 **Other dentofacial functional abnormalities**
Abnormal swallowing
Mouth breathing
Sleep postures
Tongue, lip, or finger habits

5th 524.6 **Temporomandibular joint disorders**
Excludes *current temporomandibular joint:*
dislocation (830.0-830.1)
strain (848.1)

524.60 **Temporomandibular joint disorders, unspecified**
Temporomandibular joint-pain-dysfunction syndrome [TMJ]
524.61 **Adhesions and ankylosis (bony or fibrous)**
524.62 **Arthralgia of temporomandibular joint**
524.63 **Articular disc disorder (reducing or nonreducing)**
524.64 **Temporomandibular joint sounds on opening and/or closing the jaw**
524.69 **Other specified temporomandibular joint disorders**

5th 524.7 **Dental alveolar anomalies**
524.70 **Unspecified alveolar anomaly**
524.71 **Alveolar maxillary hyperplasia**
524.72 **Alveolar mandibular hyperplasia**
524.73 **Alveolar maxillary hypoplasia**

524.74 **Alveolar mandibular hypoplasia**

524.75 **Vertical displacement of alveolus and teeth**
Extrusion of alveolus and teeth

524.76 **Occlusal plane deviation**

524.79 **Other specified alveolar anomaly**

5th 524.8 **Other specified dentofacial anomalies**

524.81 **Anterior soft tissue impingement**

524.82 **Posterior soft tissue impingement**

524.89 **Other specified dentofacial anomalies**

524.9 **Unspecified dentofacial anomalies**

4th 525 **Other diseases and conditions of the teeth and supporting structures**

525.0 **Exfoliation of teeth due to systemic causes**

5th 525.1 **Loss of teeth due to trauma, extraction, or periodontal disease**
Code first class of edentulism (525.40-525.44, 525.50-525.54)

525.10 ***Acquired absence of teeth, unspecified***
Tooth extraction status, NOS

525.11 ***Loss of teeth due to trauma***

525.12 ***Loss of teeth due to periodontal disease***

525.13 ***Loss of teeth due to caries***

525.19 ***Other loss of teeth***

5th 525.2 **Atrophy of edentulous alveolar ridge**

525.20 **Unspecified atrophy of edentulous alveolar ridge**
Atrophy of the mandible NOS
Atrophy of the maxilla NOS

525.21 **Minimal atrophy of the mandible**

525.22 **Moderate atrophy of the mandible**

525.23 **Severe atrophy of the mandible**

525.24 **Minimal atrophy of the maxilla**

525.25 **Moderate atrophy of the maxilla**

525.26 **Severe atrophy of the maxilla**

525.3 **Retained dental root**

5th 525.4 **Complete edentulism**
Use additional code to identify cause of edentulism (525.10-525.19)

525.40 **Complete edentulism, unspecified**
Edentulism NOS

525.41 **Complete edentulism, class I**

525.42 **Complete edentulism, class II**

525.43 **Complete edentulism, class III**

525.44 **Complete edentulism, class IV**

5th 525.5 **Partial edentulism**
Use additional code to identify cause of edentulism (525.10-525.19)

525.50 **Partial edentulism, unspecified**

525.51 **Partial edentulism, class I**

525.52 **Partial edentulism, class II**

525.53 **Partial edentulism, class III**

525.54 **Partial edentulism, class IV**

5th 525.6 **Unsatisfactory restoration of tooth**
Defective bridge, crown, fillings
Defective dental restoration
Excludes *dental restoration status (V45.84)*
unsatisfactory endodontic treatment (526.61-526.69)

525.60 **Unspecified unsatisfactory restoration of tooth**
Unspecified defective dental restoration

525.61 **Open restoration margins**
Dental restoration failure of marginal integrity
Open margin on tooth restoration

525.62 **Unrepairable overhanging of dental restorative materials**
Overhanging of tooth restoration

525.63 **Fractured dental restorative material without loss of material**
Excludes *cracked tooth (521.81)*
fractured tooth (873.63, 873.73)

525.64 **Fractured dental restorative material with loss of material**
Excludes *cracked tooth (521.81)*
fractured tooth (873.63, 873.73)

525.65 **Contour of existing restoration of tooth biologically incompatible with oral health**
Dental restoration failure of periodontal anatomical integrity
Unacceptable contours of existing restoration
Unacceptable morphology of existing restoration

525.66 **Allergy to existing dental restorative material**
Use additional code to identify the specific type of allergy

525.67 **Poor aesthetics of existing restoration**
Dental restoration aesthetically inadequate or displeasing

525.69 **Other unsatisfactory restoration of existing tooth**

5th 525.7 **Endosseous dental implant failure**

525.71 **Osseointegration failure of dental implant**
Failure of dental implant due to infection
Failure of dental implant due to unintentional loading
Failure of dental implant osseointegration due to premature loading
Failure of dental implant to osseointegrate prior to intentional prosthetic loading
Hemorrhagic complications of dental implant placement
Iatrogenic osseointegration failure of dental implant
Osseointegration failure of dental implant due to complications of systemic disease
Osseointegration failure of dental implant due to poor bone quality
Pre-integration failure of dental implant NOS
Pre-osseointegration failure of dental implant

525.72 **Post-osseointegration biological failure of dental implant**
Failure of dental implant due to lack of attached gingiva
Failure of dental implant due to occlusal trauma (caused by poor prosthetic design)
Failure of dental implant due to parafunctional habits
Failure of dental implant due to periodontal infection (peri-implantitis)
Failure of dental implant due to poor oral hygiene
Failure of dental implant to osseointegrate following intentional prosthetic loading
Iatrogenic post-osseointegration failure of dental implant
Post-osseointegration failure of dental implant due to complications of systemic disease

525.73 **Post-osseointegration mechanical failure of dental implant**
Failure of dental prosthesis causing loss of dental implant
Fracture of dental implant
Mechanical failure of dental implant NOS
Excludes *cracked tooth (521.81)*
fractured dental restorative material with loss of material (525.64)
fractured dental restorative material without loss of material (525.63)
fractured tooth (873.63, 873.73)

525.79 **Other endosseous dental implant failure**
Dental implant failure NOS

525.8 **Other specified disorders of the teeth and supporting structures**
Enlargement of alveolar ridge NOS
Irregular alveolar process

525.9 **Unspecified disorder of the teeth and supporting structures**

4th 526 **Diseases of the jaws**

526.0 **Developmental odontogenic cysts**
Cyst:
dentigerous
eruption
follicular
lateral developmental
lateral periodontal
primordial
Keratocyst
Excludes *radicular cyst (522.8)*

526.1 **Fissural cysts of jaw**
Cyst:
globulomaxillary
incisor canal
median anterior maxillary
median palatal
nasopalatine
palatine of papilla
Excludes *cysts of oral soft tissues (528.4)*

526.2 **Other cysts of jaws**
Cyst of jaw:
NOS
aneurysmal
hemorrhagic
traumatic

526.3 **Central giant cell (reparative) granuloma**
Excludes *peripheral giant cell granuloma (523.8)*

526.4 **Inflammatory conditions**
Abscess of jaw (acute) (chronic) (suppurative)
Osteitis of jaw (acute) (chronic) (suppurative)
Osteomyelitis (neonatal) of jaw (acute) (chronic) (suppurative)
Periostitis of jaw (acute) (chronic) (suppurative)
Sequestrum of jaw bone
Excludes *alveolar osteitis (526.5)*
osteonecrosis of jaw (733.45)

526.5 **Alveolitis of jaw**
Alveolar osteitis
Dry socket

5th 526.6 **Periradicular pathology associated with previous endodontic treatment**

526.61 **Perforation of root canal space**

526.62 **Endodontic overfill**

526.63 **Endodontic underfill**

526.69 **Other periradicular pathology associated with previous endodontic treatment**

5th 526.8 **Other specified diseases of the jaws**

526.81 **Exostosis of jaw**
Torus mandibularis
Torus palatinus

526.89 **Other**
Cherubism
Fibrous dysplasia of jaw(s)
Latent bone cyst of jaw(s)
Osteoradionecrosis of jaw(s)
Unilateral condylar hyperplasia or hypoplasia of mandible

526.9 **Unspecified disease of the jaws**

4th 527 **Diseases of the salivary glands**

527.0 **Atrophy**

527.1 **Hypertrophy**

527.2 **Sialoadenitis**
Parotitis:
NOS
allergic
toxic
Sialoangitis
Sialodochitis
Excludes *epidemic or infectious parotitis (072.0-072.9)*
uveoparotid fever (135)

527.3 **Abscess**

527.4 **Fistula**
Excludes *congenital fistula of salivary gland (750.24)*

527.5 **Sialolithiasis**
Calculus of salivary gland or duct
Stone of salivary gland or duct
Sialodocholithiasis

527.6 **Mucocele**
Mucous:
extravasation cyst of salivary gland
retention cyst of salivary gland
Ranula

527.7 **Disturbance of salivary secretion**
Hyposecretion
Ptyalism
Sialorrhea
Xerostomia

527.8 **Other specified diseases of the salivary glands**
Benign lymphoepithelial lesion of salivary gland
Sialectasia
Sialosis
Stenosis of salivary duct
Stricture of salivary duct

527.9 **Unspecified disease of the salivary glands**

4th 528 **Diseases of the oral soft tissues, excluding lesions specific for gingiva and tongue**

5th 528.0 **Stomatitis and mucositis (ulcerative)**
Excludes *cellulitis and abscess of mouth (528.3)*
diphtheritic stomatitis (032.0)
epizootic stomatitis (078.4)
gingivitis (523.0-523.1)
oral thrush (112.0)
Stevens-Johnson syndrome (695.13)
stomatitis:
acute necrotizing ulcerative (101)
aphthous (528.2)
gangrenous (528.1)
herpetic (054.2)
Vincent's (101)

528.00 **Stomatitis and mucositis, unspecified**
Mucositis NOS
Ulcerative mucositis NOS
Ulcerative stomatitis NOS
Vesicular stomatitis NOS

528.01 **Mucositis (ulcerative) due to antineoplastic therapy**
Use additional E code to identify adverse effects of therapy, such as:
antineoplastic and immunosuppressive drugs (E930.7, E933.1)
radiation therapy (E879.2)

528.02 **Mucositis (ulcerative) due to other drugs**
Use additional E code to identify drug

528.09 **Other stomatitis and mucositis (ulcerative)**

528.1 **Cancrum oris**
Gangrenous stomatitis
Noma

528.2 **Oral aphthae**
Aphthous stomatitis
Canker sore
Periadenitis mucosa necrotica recurrens
Recurrent aphthous ulcer
Stomatitis herpetiformis
Excludes *herpetic stomatitis (054.2)*

528.3 **Cellulitis and abscess**
Cellulitis of mouth (floor)
Ludwig's angina
Oral fistula
Excludes *abscess of tongue (529.0)*
cellulitis or abscess of lip (528.5)
fistula (of):
dental (522.7)
lip (528.5)
gingivitis (523.00-523.11)

528.4 **Cysts**
Dermoid cyst of mouth
Epidermoid cyst of mouth
Epstein's pearl of mouth
Lymphoepithelial cyst of mouth
Nasoalveolar cyst of mouth
Nasolabial cyst of mouth
Excludes *cyst:*
gingiva (523.8)
tongue (529.8)

528.5 **Diseases of lips**
Abscess of lip(s)
Cellulitis of lip(s)
Cheilitis:
NOS
angular
Cheilodynia
Cheilosis
Fistula of lip(s)
Hypertrophy of lip(s)
Excludes *actinic cheilitis (692.79)*
congenital fistula of lip (750.25)
leukoplakia of lips (528.6)

528.6 **Leukoplakia of oral mucosa, including tongue**
Leukokeratosis of oral mucosa
Leukoplakia of:
gingiva
lips
tongue
Excludes *carcinoma in situ (230.0, 232.0)*
leukokeratosis nicotina palati (528.79)

5th 528.7 **Other disturbances of oral epithelium, including tongue**
Excludes *carcinoma in situ (230.0, 232.0)*
leukokeratosis NOS (702.8)

528.71 **Minimal keratinized residual ridge mucosa**
Minimal keratinization of alveolar ridge mucosa

528.72 **Excessive keratinized residual ridge mucosa**
Excessive keratinization of alveolar ridge mucosa

528.79 **Other disturbances of oral epithelium, including tongue**
Erythroplakia of mouth or tongue
Focal epithelial hyperplasia of mouth or tongue
Leukoedema of mouth or tongue
Leukokeratosis nicotina palate
Other oral epithelium disturbances

528.8 **Oral submucosal fibrosis, including of tongue**

528.9 **Other and unspecified diseases of the oral soft tissues**
Cheek and lip biting
Denture sore mouth
Denture stomatitis
Eosinophilic granuloma of oral mucosa
Irritative hyperplasia of oral mucosa
Melanoplakia
Papillary hyperplasia of palate
Pyogenic granuloma of oral mucosa
Ulcer (traumatic) of oral mucosa

4th 529 **Diseases and other conditions of the tongue**

529.0 **Glossitis**
Abscess of tongue
Ulceration (traumatic) of tongue
Excludes *glossitis:*
benign migratory (529.1)
Hunter's (529.4)
median rhomboid (529.2)
Moeller's (529.4)

529.1 **Geographic tongue**
Benign migratory glossitis
Glossitis areata exfoliativa

529.2 **Median rhomboid glossitis**

529.3 **Hypertrophy of tongue papillae**
Black hairy tongue
Coated tongue
Hypertrophy of foliate papillae
Lingua villosa nigra

529.4 **Atrophy of tongue papillae**
Bald tongue
Glazed tongue
Glossitis:
Hunter's
Moeller's
Glossodynia exfoliativa
Smooth atrophic tongue

529.5 **Plicated tongue**
Fissured tongue
Furrowed tongue
Scrotal tongue
Excludes *fissure of tongue, congenital (750.13)*

529.6 **Glossodynia**
Glossopyrosis
Painful tongue
Excludes *glossodynia exfoliativa (529.4)*

529.8 **Other specified conditions of the tongue**
Atrophy (of) tongue
Crenated (of) tongue
Enlargement (of) tongue
Glossocele
Glossoptosis
Hypertrophy (of) tongue
Excludes *erythroplasia of tongue (528.79)*
leukoplakia of tongue (528.6)
macroglossia (congenital) (750.15)
microglossia (congenital) (750.16)
oral submucosal fibrosis (528.8)

529.9 **Unspecified condition of the tongue**

DISEASES OF ESOPHAGUS, STOMACH, AND DUODENUM (530-538)

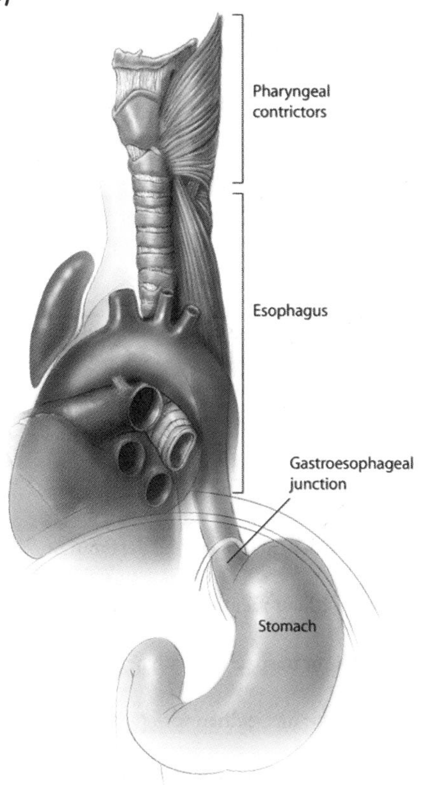

© 2008 Fairman Studios, LLC. All Rights Reserved.

4th 530 **Diseases of esophagus**

Excludes *esophageal varices (456.0-456.2)*

530.0 **Achalasia and cardiospasm**
Achalasia (of cardia)
Aperistalsis of esophagus
Megaesophagus
Excludes *congenital cardiospasm (750.7)*

5th 530.1 **Esophagitis**
Esophagitis:
chemical
peptic
postoperative
regurgitant
Use additional E code to identify cause, if induced by chemical
Excludes *tuberculous esophagitis (017.8)*

530.10 **Esophagitis, unspecified**
Esophagitis NOS

530.11 **Reflux esophagitis**
K21.0 Gastro-esophageal reflux disease with esophagitis
Layman's: *As the ICD-10-CM crosswalks for 530.11 and 530.81 indicate, the key differentiator between these two codes is the GERD causing irritation in the esophagus (530.11) or causing the acid reflux, but without resulting esophageal irritation (530.81).*

530.12 **Acute esophagitis**

530.13 **Eosinophilic esophagitis**

530.19 **Other esophagitis**
Abscess of esophagus

5th 530.2 **Ulcer of esophagus**
Ulcer of esophagus
fungal
peptic
Ulcer of esophagus due to ingestion of:
aspirin
chemicals
medicines
Use additional E code to identify cause, if induced by chemical or drug

530.20 **Ulcer of esophagus without bleeding**
Ulcer of esophagus NOS

530.21 **Ulcer of esophagus with bleeding**
Excludes *bleeding esophageal varices (456.0, 456.20)*

530.3 **Stricture and stenosis of esophagus**
Compression of esophagus
Obstruction of esophagus
Excludes *congenital stricture of esophagus (750.3)*

530.4 **Perforation of esophagus**
Rupture of esophagus
Excludes *traumatic perforation of esophagus (862.22, 862.32, 874.4-874.5)*

530.5 **Dyskinesia of esophagus**
Corkscrew esophagus
Curling esophagus
Esophagospasm
Spasm of esophagus
Excludes *cardiospasm (530.0)*

530.6 **Diverticulum of esophagus, acquired**
Diverticulum, acquired:
epiphrenic
pharyngoesophageal
pulsion
subdiaphragmatic
traction
Zenker's (hypopharyngeal)
Esophageal pouch, acquired
Esophagocele, acquired
Excludes *congenital diverticulum of esophagus (750.4)*

530.7 **Gastroesophageal laceration-hemorrhage syndrome**
Mallory-Weiss syndrome

5th 530.8 **Other specified disorders of esophagus**

530.81 **Esophageal reflux**
K21.9 Gastro-esophageal reflux disease without esophagitis
Gastroesophageal reflux
Excludes *reflux esophagitis (530.11)*

530.82 **Esophageal hemorrhage**
Excludes *hemorrhage due to esophageal varices (456.0-456.2)*

530.83 **Esophageal leukoplakia**

530.84 **Tracheoesophageal fistula**
Excludes *congenital tracheoesophageal fistula (750.3)*

530.85 **Barrett's esophagus**

530.86 **Infection of esophagostomy**
Use additional code to specify infection

530.87 **Mechanical complication of esophagostomy**
Malfunction of esophagostomy

530.89 **Other**
Excludes *Paterson-Kelly syndrome (280.8)*

530.9 **Unspecified disorder of esophagus**

4th 531 **Gastric ulcer**

Includes ulcer (peptic):
prepyloric
pylorus
stomach

Use additional E code to identify drug, if drug-induced

Excludes *peptic ulcer NOS (533.0-533.9)*

The following fifth-digit subclassification is for use with category 531:

0 **without mention of obstruction**
1 **with obstruction**

5th 531.0 **Acute with hemorrhage**
[0-1]

5th 531.1 **Acute with perforation**
[0-1]

5th 531.2 **Acute with hemorrhage and perforation**
[0-1]

5th 531.3 **Acute without mention of hemorrhage or perforation**
[0-1]

Gastric Ulcers

Acute ulcer
Erosion
Chronic ulcer

© 2006 Anatomical Chart Company

5th 531.4 **Chronic or unspecified with hemorrhage**
[0-1]

5th 531.5 **Chronic or unspecified with perforation**
[0-1]

5th 531.6 **Chronic or unspecified with hemorrhage and perforation**
[0-1]

5th 531.7 **Chronic without mention of hemorrhage or perforation**
[0-1]

5th 531.9 **Unspecified as acute or chronic, without mention of hemorrhage or perforation**
[0-1]

4th 532 **Duodenal ulcer**

Includes erosion (acute) of duodenum
ulcer (peptic):
duodenum
postpyloric

Use additional E code to identify drug, if drug-induced

Excludes *peptic ulcer NOS (533.0-533.9)*

The following fifth-digit subclassification is for use with category 532:

0 **without mention of obstruction**
1 **with obstruction**

5th 532.0 **Acute with hemorrhage**
[0-1]

5th 532.1 **Acute with perforation**
[0-1]

5th 532.2 **Acute with hemorrhage and perforation**
[0-1]

5th 532.3 **Acute without mention of hemorrhage or perforation**
[0-1]

5th 532.4 **Chronic or unspecified with hemorrhage**
[0-1]

5th 532.5 **Chronic or unspecified with perforation**
[0-1]

5th 532.6 **Chronic or unspecified with hemorrhage and perforation**
[0-1]

5th 532.7 **Chronic without mention of hemorrhage or perforation**
[0-1]

5th 532.9 **Unspecified as acute or chronic, without mention of hemorrhage or perforation**
[0-1]

4th 533 **Peptic ulcer, site unspecified**

Includes gastroduodenal ulcer NOS
peptic ulcer NOS
stress ulcer NOS

Use additional E code to identify drug, if drug-induced

Excludes *peptic ulcer:*
duodenal (532.0-532.9)
gastric (531.0-531.9)

The following fifth-digit subclassification is for use with category 533:

0 **without mention of obstruction**
1 **with obstruction**

5th 533.0 **Acute with hemorrhage**
[0-1]

5th 533.1 **Acute with perforation**
[0-1]

5th 533.2 **Acute with hemorrhage and perforation**
[0-1]

5th 533.3 **Acute without mention of hemorrhage and perforation**
[0-1]

5th 533.4 **Chronic or unspecified with hemorrhage**
[0-1]

5th 533.5 **Chronic or unspecified with perforation**
[0-1]

5th 533.6 **Chronic or unspecified with hemorrhage and perforation**
[0-1]

5th 533.7 **Chronic without mention of hemorrhage or perforation**
[0-1]

5th 533.9 **Unspecified as acute or chronic, without mention of hemorrhage or perforation**
[0-1]

4th 534 **Gastrojejunal ulcer**

Includes ulcer (peptic) or erosion:
anastomotic
gastrocolic
gastrointestinal
gastrojejunal
jejunal
marginal
stomal

Excludes *primary ulcer of small intestine (569.82)*

The following fifth-digit subclassification is for use with category 534:

0 **without mention of obstruction**
1 **with obstruction**

5th 534.0 **Acute with hemorrhage**
[0-1]

5th 534.1 **Acute with perforation**
[0-1]

5th 534.2 **Acute with hemorrhage and perforation**
[0-1]

5th 534.3 **Acute without mention of hemorrhage or perforation**
[0-1]

5th 534.4 **Chronic or unspecified with hemorrhage**
[0-1]

5th 534.5 **Chronic or unspecified with perforation**
[0-1]

5th 534.6 **Chronic or unspecified with hemorrhage and perforation**
[0-1]

5th 534.7 **Chronic without mention of hemorrhage or perforation**
[0-1]

5th 534.9 **Unspecified as acute or chronic, without mention of hemorrhage or perforation**
[0-1]

4th 535 **Gastritis and duodenitis**

The following fifth-digit subclassification is for use with category 535:
0 without mention of hemorrhage
1 with hemorrhage

5th 535.0 **Acute gastritis**
[0-1]

5th 535.1 **Atrophic gastritis**
[0-1] Gastritis:
atrophic-hyperplastic
chronic (atrophic)

5th 535.2 **Gastric mucosal hypertrophy**
[0-1] Hypertrophic gastritis

5th 535.3 **Alcoholic gastritis**
[0-1]

5th 535.4 **Other specified gastritis**
[0-1] Gastritis:
allergic
bile induced
irritant
superficial
toxic
Excludes *eosinophilic gastritis (535.7)*

5th 535.5 **Unspecified gastritis and gastroduodenitis**
[0-1]

5th 535.6 **Duodenitis**
[0-1]

5th 535.7 **Eosinophilic gastritis**
[0-1]

4th 536 **Disorders of function of stomach**
Excludes *functional disorders of stomach specified as psychogenic (306.4)*

536.0 **Achlorhydria**

536.1 **Acute dilatation of stomach**
Acute distention of stomach

536.2 **Persistent vomiting**
Cyclical vomiting
Habit vomiting
Persistent vomiting [not of pregnancy]
Uncontrollable vomiting
Excludes *bilious emesis (vomiting) (787.04)*
excessive vomiting in pregnancy (643.0-643.9)
vomiting NOS (787.03)
cyclical, associated with migraine (346.2)
vomiting of fecal matter (569.87)

536.3 **Gastroparesis**
Gastroparalysis
Code first underlying disease, such as:
diabetes mellitus (249.6, 250.6)

5th 536.4 **Gastrostomy complications**

536.40 **Gastrostomy complication, unspecified**

536.41 **Infection of gastrostomy**
Use additional code to identify type of infection, such as:
abscess or cellulitis of abdomen (682.2)
septicemia (038.0-038.9)
Use additional code to identify organism (041.00-041.9)

536.42 **Mechanical complication of gastrostomy**

536.49 **Other gastrostomy complications**

536.8 **Dyspepsia and other specified disorders of function of stomach**
Achylia gastrica
Hourglass contraction of stomach
Hyperacidity
Hyperchlorhydria
Hypochlorhydria
Indigestion
Tachygastria
Excludes *achlorhydria (536.0)*
heartburn (787.1)

536.9 **Unspecified functional disorder of stomach**
Functional gastrointestinal:
disorder
disturbance
irritation

4th 537 **Other disorders of stomach and duodenum**

537.0 **Acquired hypertrophic pyloric stenosis**
Constriction of pylorus, acquired or adult
Obstruction of pylorus, acquired or adult
Stricture of pylorus, acquired or adult
Excludes *congenital or infantile pyloric stenosis (750.5)*

537.1 **Gastric diverticulum**
Excludes *congenital diverticulum of stomach (750.7)*

537.2 **Chronic duodenal ileus**

537.3 **Other obstruction of duodenum**
Cicatrix of duodenum
Stenosis of duodenum
Stricture of duodenum
Volvulus of duodenum
Excludes *congenital obstruction of duodenum (751.1)*

537.4 **Fistula of stomach or duodenum**
Gastrocolic fistula
Gastrojejunocolic fistula

537.5 **Gastroptosis**

537.6 **Hourglass stricture or stenosis of stomach**
Cascade stomach
Excludes *congenital hourglass stomach (750.7)*
hourglass contraction of stomach (536.8)

5th 537.8 **Other specified disorders of stomach and duodenum**

537.81 **Pylorospasm**
Excludes *congenital pylorospasm (750.5)*

537.82 **Angiodysplasia of stomach and duodenum without mention of hemorrhage**

537.83 **Angiodysplasia of stomach and duodenum with hemorrhage**

537.84 **Dieulafoy lesion (hemorrhagic) of stomach and duodenum**

537.89 **Other**
Gastric or duodenal:
prolapse
rupture
Intestinal metaplasia of gastric mucosa
Passive congestion of stomach
Excludes *diverticula of duodenum (562.00-562.01)*
gastrointestinal hemorrhage (578.0-578.9)

537.9 **Unspecified disorder of stomach and duodenum**

538 **Gastrointestinal mucositis (ulcerative)**
Use additional E code to identify adverse effects of therapy, such as:
antineoplastic and immunosuppressive drugs (E930.7, E933.1)
radiation therapy (E879.2)
Excludes *mucositis (ulcerative) of mouth and oral soft tissue (528.00- 528.09)*

534.9 – 538

APPENDICITIS (540-543)

4th **540 Acute appendicitis**

540.0 With generalized peritonitis
Appendicitis (acute) with:
perforation, peritonitis (generalized), rupture:
fulminating
gangrenous
obstructive
Cecitis (acute) with:
perforation, peritonitis (generalized), rupture
Rupture of appendix
Excludes *acute appendicitis with peritoneal abscess (540.1)*

540.1 With peritoneal abscess
Abscess of appendix with generalized peritonitis

540.9 Without mention of peritonitis
Acute:
appendicitis without mention of perforation, peritonitis, or rupture:
fulminating
gangrenous
inflamed
obstructive
cecitis without mention of perforation, peritonitis, or rupture

541 Appendicitis, unqualified

542 Other appendicitis
Appendicitis:
chronic
recurrent
relapsing
subacute
Excludes *hyperplasia (lymphoid) of appendix (543.0)*

4th **543 Other diseases of appendix**

543.0 Hyperplasia of appendix (lymphoid)

543.9 Other and unspecified diseases of appendix
Appendicular or appendiceal:
colic
concretion
fistula
Diverticulum of appendix
Fecalith of appendix
Intussusception of appendix
Mucocele of appendix
Stercolith of appendix

HERNIA OF ABDOMINAL CAVITY (550-553)

Includes hernia:
acquired
congenital, except diaphragmatic or hiatal

Layman's: *Inguinal and femoral hernias both present as lumps in the groin with the difference being the occurance above (inguinal) or below (femoral) the inguinal ligament. Because of the differences in male and female anatomy, inguinal hernias are much more likely to occur in men, while femoral hernia are more common in females.*

4th **550 Inguinal hernia**
Includes bubonocele
inguinal hernia (direct) (double) (indirect) (oblique) (sliding)
scrotal hernia

The following fifth-digit subclassification is for use with category 550:
0 **unilateral or unspecified (not specified as recurrent)**
Unilateral NOS
1 **unilateral or unspecified, recurrent**
2 **bilateral (not specified as recurrent)**
Bilateral NOS
3 **bilateral, recurrent**

5th **550.0 Inguinal hernia, with gangrene**
[0-3] Inguinal hernia with gangrene (and obstruction)

5th **550.1 Inguinal hernia, with obstruction, without mention of gangrene**
[0-3] Inguinal hernia with mention of incarceration, irreducibility, or strangulation

5th **550.9 Inguinal hernia, without mention of obstruction or gangrene**
[0-3] Inguinal hernia NOS

4th **551 Other hernia of abdominal cavity, with gangrene**
Includes that with gangrene (and obstruction)

5th **551.0 Femoral hernia with gangrene**
551.00 Unilateral or unspecified (not specified as recurrent)
Femoral hernia NOS with gangrene
551.01 Unilateral or unspecified, recurrent
551.02 Bilateral (not specified as recurrent)
551.03 Bilateral, recurrent

551.1 Umbilical hernia with gangrene
Parumbilical hernia specified as gangrenous

5th **551.2 Ventral hernia with gangrene**
551.20 Ventral, unspecified, with gangrene
551.21 Incisional, with gangrene
Hernia:
postoperative specified as gangrenous
recurrent, ventral specified as gangrenous
551.29 Other
Epigastric hernia specified gangrenous

551.3 Diaphragmatic hernia with gangrene
Hernia:
hiatal (esophageal) (sliding) specified as gangrenous
paraesophageal specified as gangrenous
Thoracic stomach specified as gangrenous
Excludes *congenital diaphragmatic hernia (756.6)*

551.8 Hernia of other specified sites, with gangrene
Any condition classifiable to 553.8 if specified as gangrenous

551.9 Hernia of unspecified site, with gangrene
Any condition classifiable to 553.9 if specified as gangrenous

4th **552 Other hernia of abdominal cavity, with obstruction, but without mention of gangrene**
Excludes *that with mention of gangrene (551.0-551.9)*

5th **552.0 Femoral hernia with obstruction**
Femoral hernia specified as incarcerated, irreducible, strangulated, or causing obstruction
552.00 Unilateral or unspecified (not specified as recurrent)
552.01 Unilateral or unspecified, recurrent
552.02 Bilateral (not specified as recurrent)
552.03 Bilateral, recurrent

552.1 Umbilical hernia with obstruction
Parumbilical hernia specified as incarcerated, irreducible, strangulated, or causing obstruction

5th **552.2 Ventral hernia with obstruction**
Ventral hernia specified as incarcerated, irreducible, strangulated, or causing obstruction
552.20 Ventral, unspecified, with obstruction
552.21 Incisional, with obstruction
Hernia:
postoperative specified as incarcerated, irreducible, strangulated, or causing obstruction
recurrent, ventral specified as incarcerated, irreducible, strangulated, or causing obstruction
552.29 Other
Epigastric hernia specified as incarcerated, irreducible, strangulated, or causing obstruction

552.3 **Diaphragmatic hernia with obstruction**
Hernia:
hiatal (esophageal) (sliding) specified as incarcerated, irreducible, strangulated, or causing obstruction
paraesophageal specified as incarcerated, irreducible, strangulated, or causing obstruction
Thoracic stomach specified as incarcerated, irreducible, strangulated, or causing obstruction
Excludes *congenital diaphragmatic hernia (756.6)*

552.8 **Hernia of other specified sites, with obstruction**
Any condition classifiable to 553.8 if specified as incarcerated, irreducible, strangulated, or causing obstruction
Excludes *hernia due to adhesion with obstruction (560.81)*

552.9 **Hernia of unspecified site, with obstruction**
Any condition classifiable to 553.9 if specified as incarcerated, irreducible, strangulated, or causing obstruction

4th 553 **Other hernia of abdominal cavity without mention of obstruction or gangrene**
Excludes *the listed conditions with mention of:*
gangrene (and obstruction) (551.0-551.9)
obstruction (552.0-552.9)

5th 553.0 **Femoral hernia**
553.00 **Unilateral or unspecified (not specified as recurrent)**
Femoral hernia NOS
553.01 **Unilateral or unspecified, recurrent**
553.02 **Bilateral (not specified as recurrent)**
553.03 **Bilateral, recurrent**

553.1 **Umbilical hernia**
Parumbilical hernia

5th 553.2 **Ventral hernia**
553.20 **Ventral, unspecified**
553.21 **Incisional**
Hernia:
postoperative
recurrent, ventral
553.29 **Other**
Hernia:
epigastric
spigelian

553.3 **Diaphragmatic hernia**
K44.9 Diaphragmatic hernia without obstruction or gangrene
Hernia:
hiatal (esophageal) (sliding)
paraesophageal
Thoracic stomach
Excludes *congenital:*
diaphragmatic hernia (756.6)
hiatal hernia (750.6)
esophagocele (530.6)

553.8 **Hernia of other specified sites**
Hernia:
ischiatic
ischiorectal
lumbar
obturator
pudendal
retroperitoneal
sciatic
Other abdominal hernia of specified site
Excludes *vaginal enterocele (618.6)*

553.9 **Hernia of unspecified site**
Enterocele
Epiplocele
Hernia:
NOS
interstitial
intestinal
intra-abdominal
Rupture (nontraumatic)
Sarcoepiplocele

NONINFECTIOUS ENTERITIS AND COLITIS (555-558)

4th 555 **Regional enteritis**
Includes Crohn's disease
Granulomatous enteritis
Excludes *ulcerative colitis (556)*

555.0 **Small intestine**
Ileitis:
regional
segmental
terminal
Regional enteritis or Crohn's disease of:
duodenum
ileum
jejunum

555.1 **Large intestine**
Colitis:
granulomatous
regional
transmural
Regional enteritis or Crohn's disease of:
colon
large bowel
rectum

555.2 **Small intestine with large intestine**
Regional ileocolitis

555.9 **Unspecified site**
Crohn's disease NOS
Regional enteritis NOS

4th 556 **Ulcerative colitis**

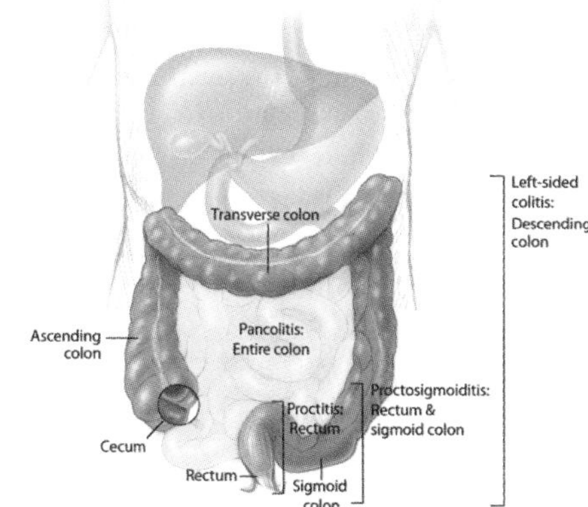

© 2008 Fairman Studios, LLC. All Rights Reserved.

556.0 **Ulcerative (chronic) enterocolitis**
556.1 **Ulcerative (chronic) ileocolitis**
556.2 **Ulcerative (chronic) proctitis**
556.3 **Ulcerative (chronic) proctosigmoiditis**
556.4 **Pseudopolyposis of colon**
556.5 **Left-sided ulcerative (chronic) colitis**
556.6 **Universal ulcerative (chronic) colitis**
Pancolitis
556.8 **Other ulcerative colitis**
556.9 **Ulcerative colitis, unspecified**
Ulcerative enteritis NOS

552.3 – 556.9

4th 557 **Vascular insufficiency of intestine**

Excludes *necrotizing enterocolitis of the newborn (777.50-777.53)*

557.0 **Acute vascular insufficiency of intestine**

Acute:
- hemorrhagic enterocolitis
- ischemic colitis, enteritis, or enterocolitis
- massive necrosis of intestine

Bowel infarction
Embolism of mesenteric artery
Fulminant enterocolitis
Hemorrhagic necrosis of intestine
Infarction of appendices epiploicae
Intestinal gangrene
Intestinal infarction (acute) (agnogenic) (hemorrhagic) (nonocclusive)
Mesenteric infarction (embolic) (thrombotic)
Necrosis of intestine
Terminal hemorrhagic enteropathy
Thrombosis of mesenteric artery

557.1 **Chronic vascular insufficiency of intestine**

Angina, abdominal
Chronic ischemic colitis, enteritis, or enterocolitis
Ischemic stricture of intestine
Mesenteric:
- angina
- artery syndrome (superior)
- vascular insufficiency

557.9 **Unspecified vascular insufficiency of intestine**

Alimentary pain due to vascular insufficiency
Ischemic colitis, enteritis, or enterocolitis NOS

4th 558 **Other and unspecified noninfectious gastroenteritis and colitis**

Excludes *infectious:*
- *colitis, enteritis, or gastroenteritis (009.0-009.1)*
- *diarrhea (009.2-009.3)*

558.1 **Gastroenteritis and colitis due to radiation**

Radiation enterocolitis

558.2 **Toxic gastroenteritis and colitis**

Use additional E code to identify cause

558.3 **Allergic gastroenteritis and colitis**

Use additional code to identify type of food allergy (V15.01-V15.05)

5th 558.4 **Eosinophilic gastroenteritis and colitis**

558.41 **Eosinophilic gastroenteritis**

Eosinophilic enteritis

558.42 **Eosinophilic colitis**

558.9 **Other and unspecified noninfectious gastroenteritis and colitis**

K52.8 Other specified noninfective gastroenteritis and colitis
K52.9 Noninfective gastroenteritis and colitis, unspecified

Colitis, NOS, dietetic, or noninfectious
Enteritis, NOS, dietetic, or noninfectious
Gastroenteritis, NOS, dietetic, or noninfectious
Ileitis, NOS, dietetic or noninfectious
Jejunitis, NOS, dietetic, or noninfectious
Sigmoiditis, NOS, dietetic, or noninfectious

OTHER DISEASES OF INTESTINES & PERITONEUM (560-569)

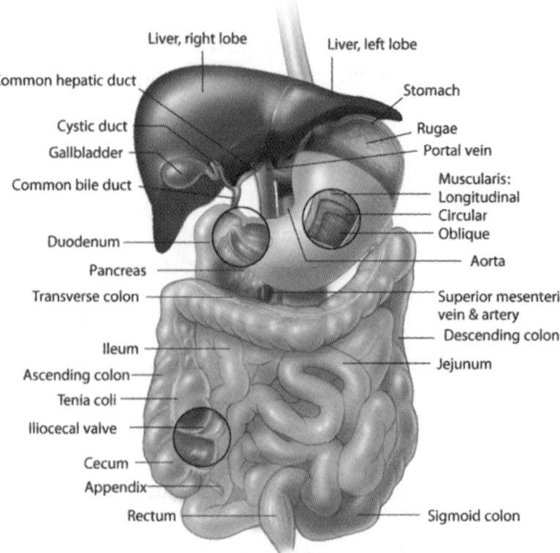

© 2008 Fairman Studios, LLC. All Rights Reserved.

4th 560 **Intestinal obstruction without mention of hernia**

Excludes *duodenum (537.2-537.3)*
- *inguinal hernia with obstruction (550.1)*
- *intestinal obstruction complicating hernia (552.0-552.9)*
- *mesenteric:*
  - *embolism (557.0)*
  - *infarction (557.0)*
  - *thrombosis (557.0)*
- *neonatal intestinal obstruction (277.01, 777.1-777.2, 777.4)*

560.0 **Intussusception**

Intussusception (colon) (intestine) (rectum)
Invagination of intestine or colon

Excludes *intussusception of appendix (543.9)*

560.1 **Paralytic ileus**

K56.0 Paralytic ileus

Adynamic ileus
Ileus (of intestine) (of bowel) (of colon)
Paralysis of intestine or colon

Excludes *gallstone ileus (560.31)*

560.2 **Volvulus**

Knotting of intestine, bowel, or colon
Strangulation of intestine, bowel, or colon
Torsion of intestine, bowel, or colon
Twist of intestine, bowel, or colon

5th 560.3 **Impaction of intestine**

560.30 **Impaction of intestine, unspecified**

Impaction of colon

560.31 **Gallstone ileus**

Obstruction of intestine by gallstone

560.39 **Other**

Concretion of intestine
Enterolith
Fecal impaction

5th 560.8 **Other specified intestinal obstruction**

560.81 **Intestinal or peritoneal adhesions with obstruction (postoperative) (postinfection)**

Excludes *adhesions without obstruction (568.0)*

560.89 **Other**

Acute psuedo-obstruction of intestine
Mural thickening causing obstruction

Excludes *ischemic stricture of intestine (557.1)*

560.9 **Unspecified intestinal obstruction**
K56.60 Unspecified intestinal obstruction
Enterostenosis
Obstruction of intestine or colon
Occlusion of intestine or colon
Stenosis of intestine or colon
Stricture of intestine or colon
Excludes *congenital stricture or stenosis of intestine (751.1-751.2)*

4th **562 Diverticula of intestine**
Use additional code to identify any associated:
peritonitis (567.0-567.9)
Excludes *congenital diverticulum of colon (751.5)*
diverticulum of appendix (543.9)
Meckel's diverticulum (751.0)

Layman's: *Diverticulosis is the condition of having small pouches in the intestines that are often asymptomatic. If these diverticula become inflamed, the condition is referred to as diverticulitis.*

5th **562.0 Small intestine**
562.00 Diverticulosis of small intestine (without mention of hemorrhage)
Diverticulosis:
duodenum without mention of diverticulitis
ileum without mention of diverticulitis
jejunum without mention of diverticulitis
562.01 Diverticulitis of small intestine (without mention of hemorrhage)
Diverticulitis (with diverticulosis):
duodenum
ileum
jejunum
small intestine
562.02 Diverticulosis of small intestine with hemorrhage
562.03 Diverticulitis of small intestine with hemorrhage

5th **562.1 Colon**
562.10 Diverticulosis of colon (without mention of hemorrhage)
K57.30 Diverticulosis of large intestine without perforation or abscess without bleeding
Diverticulosis without mention of diverticulitis:
NOS
intestine (large)
Diverticular disease (colon) without mention of diverticulitis
562.11 Diverticulitis of colon without mention of hemorrhage
K57.80 Diverticulitis of intestine, part unspecified, with perforation and abscess without bleeding
Diverticulitis (with diverticulosis):
NOS
colon
intestine (large)
562.12 Diverticulosis of colon with hemorrhage
562.13 Diverticulitis of colon with hemorrhage

4th **564 Functional digestive disorders, not elsewhere classified**
Excludes *functional disorders of stomach (536.0-536.9)*
those specified as psychogenic (306.4)

5th **564.0 Constipation**
Excludes *psychogenic constipation (306.4)*
564.00 Constipation, unspecified
K59.00 Constipation, unspecified
564.01 Slow transit constipation
564.02 Outlet dysfunction constipation
564.09 Other constipation

564.1 Irritable bowel syndrome
K58.9 Irritable bowel syndrome without diarrhea
Irritable colon
Spastic colon

564.2 Postgastric surgery syndromes
Dumping syndrome
Jejunal syndrome
Postgastrectomy syndrome
Postvagotomy syndrome
Excludes *malnutrition following gastrointestinal surgery (579.3)*
postgastrojejunostomy ulcer (534.0-534.9)

564.3 Vomiting following gastrointestinal surgery
Vomiting (bilious) following gastrointestinal surgery

564.4 Other postoperative functional disorders
Diarrhea following gastrointestinal surgery
Excludes *colostomy and enterostomy complications (569.60-569.69)*

564.5 Functional diarrhea
Excludes *diarrhea:*
NOS (787.91)
psychogenic (306.4)

564.6 Anal spasm
Proctalgia fugax

564.7 Megacolon, other than Hirschsprung's
Dilatation of colon
Excludes *megacolon:*
congenital [Hirschsprung's] (751.3)
toxic (556)

5th **564.8 Other specified functional disorders of intestine**
Excludes *malabsorption (579.0-579.9)*
564.81 Neurogenic bowel
564.89 Other functional disorders of intestine
Atony of colon

564.9 Unspecified functional disorder of intestine

4th **565 Anal fissure and fistula**
565.0 Anal fissure
Excludes *anal sphincter tear (healed) (non-traumatic) (old) (569.43)*
traumatic (863.89, 863.99)

565.1 Anal fistula
Fistula:
anorectal
rectal
rectum to skin
Excludes *fistula of rectum to internal organs – see Alphabetic Index*
ischiorectal fistula (566)
rectovaginal fistula (619.1)

566 Abscess of anal and rectal regions
Abscess:
ischiorectal
perianal
perirectal
Cellulitis:
anal
perirectal
rectal
Ischiorectal fistula

560.9 – 566

4th 567 **Peritonitis and retroperitoneal infections**

Excludes *peritonitis:*
benign paroxysmal (277.31)
pelvic, female (614.5, 614.7)
periodic familial (277.31)
puerperal (670.8)
with or following:
abortion (634-638 with .0, 639.0)
appendicitis (540.0-540.1)
ectopic or molar pregnancy (639.0)

567.0 ***Peritonitis in infectious diseases classified elsewhere***
Code first underlying disease
Excludes *peritonitis:*
gonococcal (098.86)
syphilitic (095.2)
tuberculous (014.0)

567.1 **Pneumococcal peritonitis**

5th 567.2 **Other suppurative peritonitis**
Excludes *bacterial peritonitis NOS (567.29)*

567.21 **Peritonitis (acute) generalized**
Pelvic peritonitis, male

567.22 **Peritoneal abscess**
Abscess (of):
abdominopelvic
mesenteric
omentum
peritoneum
retrocecal
subdiaphragmatic
subhepatic
subphrenic

567.23 **Spontaneous bacterial peritonitis**

567.29 **Other suppurative peritonitis**
Subphrenic peritonitis

5th 567.3 **Retroperitoneal infections**

567.31 **Psoas muscle abscess**

567.38 **Other retroperitoneal abscess**

567.39 **Other retroperitoneal infections**

5th 567.8 **Other specified peritonitis**

567.81 **Choleperitonitis**
Peritonitis due to bile

567.82 **Sclerosing mesenteritis**
Fat necrosis of peritoneum
(Idiopathic) sclerosing mesenteric fibrosis
Mesenteric lipodystrophy
Mesenteric panniculitis
Retractile mesenteritis

567.89 **Other specified peritonitis**
Other specified peritonitis
Mesenteric saponification
Peritonitis due to urine

567.9 **Unspecified peritonitis**
Peritonitis:
NOS
of unspecified cause

4th 568 **Other disorders of peritoneum**

568.0 **Peritoneal adhesions (postoperative) (postinfection)**
Adhesions (of):
abdominal (wall)
diaphragm
intestine
male pelvis
mesenteric
omentum
stomach
Adhesive bands
Excludes *adhesions:*
pelvic, female (614.6)
with obstruction:
duodenum (537.3)
intestine (560.81)

5th 568.8 **Other specified disorders of peritoneum**

568.81 **Hemoperitoneum (nontraumatic)**

568.82 **Peritoneal effusion (chronic)**
Excludes *ascites NOS (789.51-789.59)*

568.89 **Other**
Peritoneal:
cyst
granuloma

568.9 **Unspecified disorder of peritoneum**

4th 569 **Other disorders of intestine**

569.0 **Anal and rectal polyp**
Anal and rectal polyp NOS
Excludes *adenomatous anal and rectal polyp (211.4)*

569.1 **Rectal prolapse**
Procidentia:
anus (sphincter)
rectum (sphincter)
Proctoptosis
Prolapse:
anal canal
rectal mucosa
Excludes *prolapsed hemorrhoids (455.2, 455.5)*

569.2 **Stenosis of rectum and anus**
Stricture of anus (sphincter)

569.3 **Hemorrhage of rectum and anus**
K62.5 Hemorrhage of anus and rectum
Excludes *gastrointestinal bleeding NOS (578.9)*
melena (578.1)

5th 569.4 **Other specified disorders of rectum and anus**

569.41 **Ulcer of anus and rectum**
Solitary ulcer of anus (sphincter) or rectum (sphincter)
Stercoral ulcer of anus (sphincter) or rectum (sphincter)

569.42 **Anal or rectal pain**

569.43 **Anal sphincter tear (healed) (old)**
Tear of anus, nontraumatic
Use additional code for any associated fecal incontinence (787.6)
Excludes *anal fissure (565.0)*
anal sphincter tear (healed) (old) complicating delivery (654.8)

569.44 Dysplasia of anus
Anal intraepithelial neoplasia I and II (AIN I and II) (histologically confirmed)
Dysplasia of anus NOS
Mild and moderate dysplasia of anus (histologically confirmed)
Excludes *abnormal results from anal cytologic examination without histologic confirmation (796.70-796.79)*
anal intraepithelial neoplasia III (230.5, 230.6)
carcinoma in situ of anus (230.5, 230.6)
HGSIL of anus (796.74)
severe dysplasia of anus (230.5, 230.6)

569.49 Other
Granuloma of rectum (sphincter)
Hypertrophy of anal papillae
Proctitis NOS
Rupture of rectum (sphincter)
Excludes *fistula of rectum to:*
internal organs – see Alphabetic Index
skin (565.1)
hemorrhoids (455.0-455.9)
incontinence of sphincter ani (787.6)

569.5 Abscess of intestine
Excludes *appendiceal abscess (540.1)*

5th **569.6 Colostomy and enterostomy complications**

569.60 Colostomy and enterostomy complication, unspecified

569.61 Infection of colostomy and enterostomy
Use additional code to identify organism (041.00-041.9)
Use additional code to specify type of infection, such as:
abscess or cellulits of abdomen (682.2)
septicemia (038.0-038.9)

569.62 Mechanical complication of colostomy and enterostomy
Malfunction of colostomy and enterostomy

569.69 Other complication
Fistula
Hernia
Prolapse

● 5th **569.7 Complications of intestinal pouch**

● **569.71 Pouchitis**
Inflammation of internal ileoanal pouch

Rationale: *Pouchitis is a nonspecific inflammation of an internal ileoanal pouch, which has been created following removal of part of the colon. The surgical procedure is a restorative proctocolectomy with ileal pouch anal anastomosis, and it may be done for treatment of ulcerative colitis or familial adenomatous polyposis. Creation of the pouch means that the patient does not need a permanent ileostomy, but can have preserved continence.*

One of the most common complications of the pouch is pouchitis. Presenting symptoms of pouchitis include diarrhea, which may be bloody, along with urgency and incontinence. This may be accompanied by abdominal pain, fever, loss of appetite, and general malaise. Pouchitis may usually be treated successfully with antibiotics; however, relapse is common. The cause of pouchitis is not understood.

● **569.79 Other complications of intestinal pouch**

5th **569.8 Other specified disorders of intestine**

569.81 Fistula of intestine, excluding rectum and anus
Fistula:
abdominal wall
enterocolic
enteroenteric
ileorectal
Excludes *fistula of intestine to internal organs – see Alphabetic Index*
persistent postoperative fistula (998.6)

569.82 Ulceration of intestine
Primary ulcer of intestine
Ulceration of colon
Excludes *that with perforation (569.83)*

Layman's: *Although most ulcerative digestive disorder codes are divided by "with hemorrhage" or "without mention of hemorrhage," it is notable that 569.82 (Ulceration of intestine) is not subdivided. As such, code 578.9 should be used in conjunction with 569.82 in cases of a hemorrhagic intestinal ulcer.*

569.83 Perforation of intestine

569.84 Angiodysplasia of intestine (without mention of hemorrhage)

569.85 Angiodysplasia of intestine with hemorrhage

569.86 Dieulafoy lesion (hemorrhagic) of intestine

● **569.87 Vomiting of fecal matter**

Rationale: *Vomiting can be a very non-specific complaint with many different conditions. However, in the same way that persistent vomiting (536.2) can indicate a more significant problem, vomiting of fecal matter can also be indicative of a serious condition that may require an extensive evaluation. Previously, vomiting fecal matter was indexed to a non-specific code, "Other disorders of intestine, other" (569.89).*

569.89 Other
Enteroptosis
Granuloma of intestine
Pericolitis
Perisigmoiditis
Prolapse of intestine
Visceroptosis
Excludes *gangrene of intestine, mesentery, or omentum (557.0)*
hemorrhage of intestine NOS (578.9)
obstruction of intestine (560.0-560.9)

569.9 Unspecified disorder of intestine

OTHER DISEASES OF DIGESTIVE SYSTEM (570-579)

570 Acute and subacute necrosis of liver
Acute hepatic failure
Acute or subacute hepatitis, not specified as infective
Necrosis of liver (acute) (diffuse) (massive) (subacute)
Parenchymatous degeneration of liver
Yellow atrophy (liver) (acute) (subacute)
Excludes *icterus gravis of newborn (773.0-773.2)*
serum hepatitis (070.2-070.3)
that with:
abortion (634-638 with .7, 639.8)
ectopic or molar pregnancy (639.8)
pregnancy, childbirth, or the puerperium (646.7)
viral hepatitis (070.0-070.9)

4th **571 Chronic liver disease and cirrhosis**

571.0 Alcoholic fatty liver A

571.1 Acute alcoholic hepatitis A
Acute alcoholic liver disease

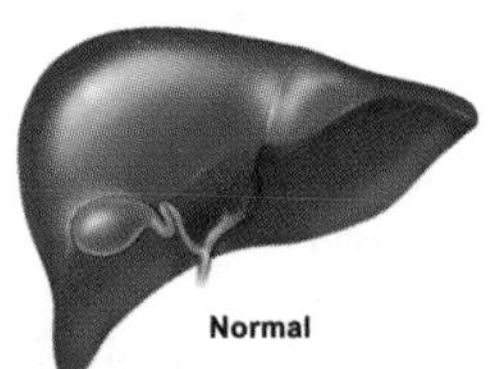

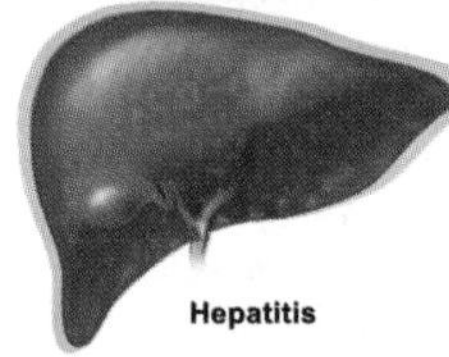

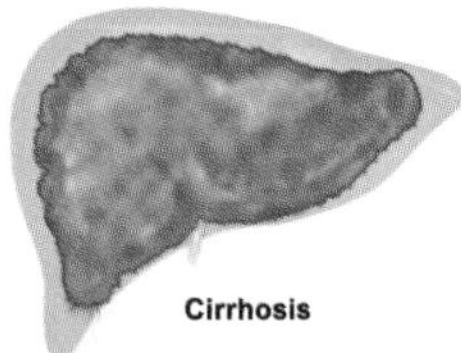

© 2008 Fairman Studios, LLC. All Rights Reserved.

571.2 Alcoholic cirrhosis of liver A
Florid cirrhosis
Laennec's cirrhosis (alcoholic)

571.3 Alcoholic liver damage, unspecified A

5th **571.4 Chronic hepatitis**
Excludes *viral hepatitis (acute) (chronic) (070.0-070.9)*

571.40 Chronic hepatitis, unspecified

571.41 Chronic persistent hepatitis

571.42 Autoimmune hepatitis

571.49 Other
Chronic hepatitis:
active
aggressive
Recurrent hepatitis

571.5 Cirrhosis of liver without mention of alcohol
K74.0 Hepatic fibrosis
Cirrhosis of liver:
NOS
cryptogenic
macronodular
micronodular
posthepatitic
postnecrotic
Healed yellow atrophy (liver)
Portal cirrhosis
Code first, if applicable, viral hepatitis (acute) (chronic) (070.0-070.9)

571.6 Biliary cirrhosis
Chronic nonsuppurative destructive cholangitis
Cirrhosis:
cholangitic
cholestatic

571.8 Other chronic nonalcoholic liver disease
Chronic yellow atrophy (liver)
Fatty liver, without mention of alcohol

571.9 Unspecified chronic liver disease without mention of alcohol

4th **572 Liver abscess and sequelae of chronic liver disease**

572.0 Abscess of liver
Excludes *amebic liver abscess (006.3)*

572.1 Portal pyemia
Phlebitis of portal vein
Portal thrombophlebitis
Pylephlebitis
Pylethrombophlebitis

▲**572.2 Hepatic encephalopathy ~~coma~~**
Hepatic coma
~~Hepatic encephalopathy~~
Hepatocerebral intoxication
Portal-systemic encephalopathy
Excludes *hepatic coma associated with viral hepatitis – see category 070*

572.3 Portal hypertension

572.4 Hepatorenal syndrome
Excludes *that following delivery (674.8)*

572.8 Other sequelae of chronic liver disease

4th **573 Other disorders of liver**
Excludes *amyloid or lardaceous degeneration of liver (277.39)*
congenital cystic disease of liver (751.62)
glycogen infiltration of liver (271.0)
hepatomegaly NOS (789.1)
portal vein obstruction (452)

573.0 Chronic passive congestion of liver

573.1 *Hepatitis in viral diseases classified elsewhere*
Code first underlying disease, as:
Coxsackie virus disease (074.8)
cytomegalic inclusion virus disease (078.5)
infectious mononucleosis (075)
Excludes *hepatitis (in):*
mumps (072.71)
viral (070.0-070.9)
yellow fever (060.0-060.9)

573.2 *Hepatitis in other infectious diseases classified elsewhere*
Code first underlying disease, as:
malaria (084.9)
Excludes *hepatitis in:*
late syphilis (095.3)
secondary syphilis (091.62)
toxoplasmosis (130.5)

573.3 Hepatitis, unspecified
K71.9 Toxic liver disease, unspecified
Toxic (noninfectious) hepatitis
Use additional E code to identify cause

573.4 Hepatic infarction

573.8 Other specified disorders of liver
Hepatoptosis

573.9 Unspecified disorder of liver
K76.9 Liver disease, unspecified

4th 574 Cholelithiasis

The following fifth-digit subclassification is for use with category 574:

0 **without mention of obstruction**
1 **with obstruction**

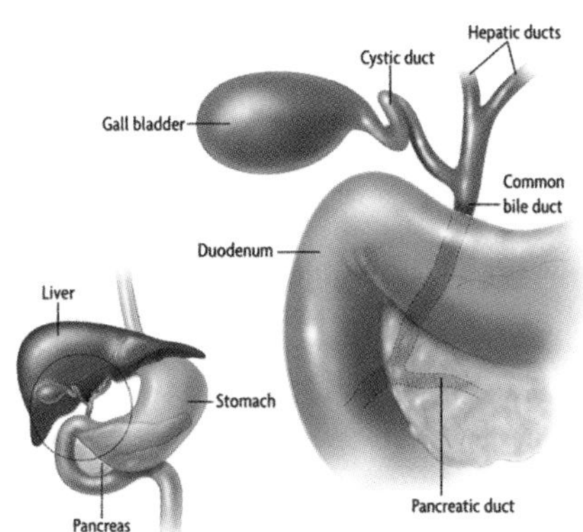

© 2008 Fairman Studios, LLC. All Rights Reserved.

Layman's: *Cholelithiasis is the clinical term for gallstones. Codes in the 574.xx series are differentiated by the location of the stone and the acuteness of inflammation of the gallbladder (cholecystitis).*

5th **574.0 Calculus of gallbladder with acute cholecystitis**
[0-1] Biliary calculus with acute cholecystitis
Calculus of cystic duct with acute cholecystitis
Cholelithiasis with acute cholecystitis
Any condition classifiable to 574.2 with acute cholecystitis

5th **574.1 Calculus of gallbladder with other cholecystitis**
[0-1] Biliary calculus with cholecystitis
Calculus of cystic duct with cholecystitis
Cholecystitis with cholelithiasis NOS
Cholelithiasis with cholecystitis
Any condition classifiable to 574.2 with cholecystitis (chronic)

5th **574.2 Calculus of gallbladder without mention of cholecystitis**
[0-1] Biliary:
calculus NOS
colic NOS
Calculus of cystic duct
Cholelithiasis NOS
Colic (recurrent) of gallbladder
Gallstone (impacted)

5th **574.3 Calculus of bile duct with acute cholecystitis**
[0-1] Calculus of bile duct [any] with acute cholecystitis
Choledocholithiasis with acute cholecystitis
Any condition classifiable to 574.5 with acute cholecystitis

5th **574.4 Calculus of bile duct with other cholecystitis**
[0-1] Calculus of bile duct [any] with cholecystitis (chronic)
Choledocholithiasis with cholecystitis (chronic)
Any condition classifiable to 574.5 with cholecystitis (chronic)

5th **574.5 Calculus of bile duct without mention of cholecystitis**
[0-1] Calculus of:
bile duct [any]
common duct
hepatic duct
Choledocholithiasis
Hepatic:
colic (recurrent)
lithiasis

5th **574.6 Calculus of gallbladder and bile duct with acute cholecystitis**
[0-1] Any condition classifiable to 574.0 and 574.3

5th **574.7 Calculus of gallbladder and bile duct with other cholecystitis**
[0-1] Any condition classifiable to 574.1 and 574.4

5th **574.8 Calculus of gallbladder and bile duct with acute and chronic cholecystitis**
[0-1] Any condition classifiable to 574.6 and 574.7

5th **574.9 Calculus of gallbladder and bile duct without cholecystitis**
[0-1] Any condition classifiable to 574.2 and 574.5

4th 575 Other disorders of gallbladder

575.0 Acute cholecystitis
Abscess of gallbladder without mention of calculus
Angiocholecystitis without mention of calculus
Cholecystitis without mention of calculus:
emphysematous (acute)
gangrenous
suppurative
Empyema of gallbladder without mention of calculus
Gangrene of gallbladder without mention of calculus

Excludes *that with:*
acute and chronic cholecystitis (575.12)
choledocholithiasis (574.3)
choledocholithiasis and cholelithiasis (574.6)
cholelithiasis (574.0)

5th **575.1 Other cholecystitis**
Cholecystitis without mention of calculus:
NOS
chronic

Excludes *that with:*
choledocholithiasis (574.4)
choledocholithiasis and cholelithiasis (574.8)
cholelithiasis (574.1)

575.10 Cholecystitis, unspecified
Cholecystitis NOS

575.11 Chronic cholecystitis

575.12 Acute and chronic cholecystitis

575.2 Obstruction of gallbladder
Occlusion of cystic duct or gallbladder without mention of calculus
Stenosis of cystic duct or gallbladder without mention of calculus
Stricture of cystic duct or gallbladder without mention of calculus

575.3 Hydrops of gallbladder
Mucocele of gallbladder

575.4 Perforation of gallbladder
Rupture of cystic duct or gallbladder

575.5 Fistula of gallbladder
Fistula:
cholecystoduodenal
cholecystoenteric

575.6 Cholesterolosis of gallbladder
Strawberry gallbladder

575.8 Other specified disorders of gallbladder
Adhesions (of) cystic duct gallbladder
Atrophy (of) cystic duct gallbladder
Biliary dyskinesia
Cyst (of) cystic duct gallbladder
Hypertrophy (of) cystic duct gallbladder
Nonfunctioning (of) cystic duct gallbladder
Ulcer (of) cystic duct gallbladder

Excludes *Hartmann's pouch of intestine (V44.3)*
nonvisualization of gallbladder (793.3)

575.9 Unspecified disorder of gallbladder

4th 576 Other disorders of biliary tract

Excludes *that involving the:*
cystic duct (575.0-575.9)
gallbladder (575.0-575.9)

576.0 Postcholecystectomy syndrome

574 – 576.0

576.1 Cholangitis
Cholangitis:
NOS
acute
ascending
chronic
primary
recurrent
sclerosing
secondary
stenosing
suppurative

576.2 Obstruction of bile duct
Occlusion of bile duct, except cystic duct, without mention of calculus
Stenosis of bile duct, except cystic duct, without mention of calculus
Stricture of bile duct, except cystic duct, without mention of calculus
Excludes *congenital (751.61)*
that with calculus (574.3-574.5 with fifth-digit 1)

576.3 Perforation of bile duct
Rupture of bile duct, except cystic duct

576.4 Fistula of bile duct
Choledochoduodenal fistula

576.5 Spasm of sphincter of Oddi

576.8 Other specified disorders of biliary tract
Adhesions of bile duct [any]
Atrophy of bile duct [any]
Cyst of bile duct [any]
Hypertrophy of bile duct [any]
Stasis of bile duct [any]
Ulcer of bile duct [any]
Excludes *congenital choledochal cyst (751.69)*

576.9 Unspecified disorder of biliary tract

4th **577 Diseases of pancreas**

577.0 Acute pancreatitis
K85.9 Acute pancreatitis, unspecified
Abscess of pancreas
Necrosis of pancreas:
acute
infective
Pancreatitis:
NOS
acute (recurrent)
apoplectic
hemorrhagic
subacute
suppurative
Excludes *mumps pancreatitis (072.3)*

577.1 Chronic pancreatitis
Chronic pancreatitis:
NOS
infectious
interstitial
Pancreatitis:
painless
recurrent
relapsing

577.2 Cyst and pseudocyst of pancreas

577.8 Other specified diseases of pancreas
Atrophy of pancreas
Calculus of pancreas
Cirrhosis of pancreas
Fibrosis of pancreas
Pancreatic:
infantilism
necrosis:
NOS
aseptic
fat
Pancreatolithiasis
Excludes *fibrocystic disease of pancreas (277.00-277.09)*
islet cell tumor of pancreas (211.7)
pancreatic steatorrhea (579.4)

577.9 Unspecified disease of pancreas

4th **578 Gastrointestinal hemorrhage**
Excludes *that with mention of:*
angiodysplasia of stomach and duodenum (537.83)
angiodysplasia of intestine (569.85)
diverticulitis, intestine:
large (562.13)
small (562.03)
diverticulosis, intestine:
large (562.12)
small (562.02)
gastritis and duodenitis (535.0-535.6)
ulcer, duodenal, gastric, gastrojejunal, or peptic (531.00-534.91)

578.0 Hematemesis
Vomiting of blood

578.1 Blood in stool
K92.1 Melena
Melena
Excludes *melena of the newborn (772.4, 777.3)*
occult blood (792.1)

578.9 Hemorrhage of gastrointestinal tract, unspecified
K92.2 Gastrointestinal hemorrhage, unspecified
Gastric hemorrhage
Intestinal hemorrhage

4th **579 Intestinal malabsorption**

579.0 Celiac disease
Celiac:
crisis
infantilism
rickets
Gee (-Herter) disease
Gluten enteropathy
Idiopathic steatorrhea
Nontropical sprue

579.1 Tropical sprue
Sprue:
NOS
tropical
Tropical steatorrhea

579.2 Blind loop syndrome
Postoperative blind loop syndrome

579.3 Other and unspecified postsurgical nonabsorption
Hypoglycemia following gastrointestinal surgery
Malnutrition following gastrointestinal surgery

579.4 Pancreatic steatorrhea

579.8 Other specified intestinal malabsorption
Enteropathy:
exudative
protein-losing
Steatorrhea (chronic)

579.9 Unspecified intestinal malabsorption
Malabsorption syndrome NOS

10. DISEASES OF THE GENITOURINARY SYSTEM (580-629)

NEPHRITIS, NEPHROTIC SYNDROME, AND NEPHROSIS (580-589)

Excludes *hypertensive chronic kidney disease (403.00-403.91, 404.00-404.93)*

4th **580 Acute glomerulonephritis**
Includes acute nephritis

580.0 With lesion of proliferative glomerulonephritis
Acute (diffuse) proliferative glomerulonephritis
Acute poststreptococcal glomerulonephritis

580.4 With lesion of rapidly progressive glomerulonephritis
Acute nephritis with lesion of necrotizing glomerulitis

5th **580.8 With other specified pathological lesion in kidney**

580.81 *Acute glomerulonephritis in diseases classified elsewhere*
Code first underlying disease, as:
infectious hepatitis (070.0-070.9)
mumps (072.79)
subacute bacterial endocarditis (421.0)
typhoid fever (002.0)

580.89 Other
Glomerulonephritis, acute, with lesion of:
exudative nephritis
interstitial (diffuse) (focal) nephritis

580.9 Acute glomerulonephritis with unspecified pathological lesion in kidney
Glomerulonephritis:
NOS specified as acute
hemorrhagic specified as acute
Nephritis specified as acute
Nephropathy specified as acute

4th **581 Nephrotic syndrome**

581.0 With lesion of proliferative glomerulonephritis

581.1 With lesion of membranous glomerulonephritis
Epimembranous nephritis
Idiopathic membranous glomerular disease
Nephrotic syndrome with lesion of:
focal glomerulosclerosis
sclerosing membranous glomerulonephritis
segmental hyalinosis

581.2 With lesion of membranoproliferative glomerulonephritis
Nephrotic syndrome with lesion (of):
endothelial glomerulonephritis
hypocomplementemic glomerulonephritis
persistent glomerulonephritis
lobular glomerulonephritis
mesangiocapillary glomerulonephritis
mixed membranous and proliferative glomerulonephritis

581.3 With lesion of minimal change glomerulonephritis
Foot process disease
Lipoid nephrosis
Minimal change:
glomerular disease
glomerulitis
nephrotic syndrome

5th **581.8 With other specified pathological lesion in kidney**

581.81 *Nephrotic syndrome in diseases classified elsewhere*
Code first underlying disease, as:
amyloidosis (277.30-277.39)
diabetes mellitus (249.4, 250.4)
malaria (084.9)
polyarteritis (446.0)
systemic lupus erythematosus (710.0)
Excludes *nephrosis in epidemic hemorrhagic fever (078.6)*

581.89 Other
Glomerulonephritis with edema and lesion of:
exudative nephritis
interstitial (diffuse) (focal) nephritis

581.9 Nephrotic syndrome with unspecified pathological lesion in kidney
Glomerulonephritis with edema NOS
Nephritis:
nephrotic NOS
with edema NOS
Nephrosis NOS
Renal disease with edema NOS

4th **582 Chronic glomerulonephritis**
Includes chronic nephritis

582.0 With lesion of proliferative glomerulonephritis
Chronic (diffuse) proliferative glomerulonephritis

582.1 With lesion of membranous glomerulonephritis
Chronic glomerulonephritis:
membranous
sclerosing
Focal glomerulosclerosis
Segmental hyalinosis

582.2 With lesion of membranoproliferative glomerulonephritis
Chronic glomerulonephritis:
endothelial
hypocomplementemic persistent
lobular
membranoproliferative
mesangiocapillary
mixed membranous and proliferative

582.4 With lesion of rapidly progressive glomerulonephritis
Chronic nephritis with lesion of necrotizing glomerulitis

5th **582.8 With other specified pathological lesion in kidney**

582.81 *Chronic glomerulonephritis in diseases classified elsewhere*
Code first underlying disease, as:
amyloidosis (277.30-277.39)
systemic lupus erythematosus (710.0)

582.89 Other
Chronic glomerulonephritis with lesion of:
exudative nephritis
interstitial (diffuse) (focal) nephritis

582.9 Chronic glomerulonephritis with unspecified pathological lesion in kidney
Glomerulonephritis specified as chronic:
NOS
hemorrhagic
Nephritis specified as chronic
Nephropathy specified as chronic

4th **583 Nephritis and nephropathy, not specified as acute or chronic**
Includes "renal disease" so stated, not specified as acute or chronic but with stated pathology or cause

583.0 With lesion of proliferative glomerulonephritis
Proliferative:
glomerulonephritis (diffuse) NOS
nephritis NOS
nephropathy NOS

583.1 With lesion of membranous glomerulonephritis
Membranous:
glomerulonephritis NOS
nephritis NOS
Membranous nephropathy NOS

583.2 With lesion of membranoproliferative glomerulonephritis
Membranoproliferative:
glomerulonephritis NOS
nephritis NOS
nephropathy NOS
Nephritis NOS, with lesion of:
hypocomplementemic persistent glomerulonephritis
lobular glomerulonephritis
mesangiocapillary glomerulonephritis
mixed membranous and proliferative glomerulonephritis

583.4 With lesion of rapidly progressive glomerulonephritis
Necrotizing or rapidly progressive:
glomerulitis NOS
glomerulonephritis NOS
nephritis NOS
nephropathy NOS
Nephritis, unspecified, with lesion of necrotizing glomerulitis

583.6 With lesion of renal cortical necrosis
Nephritis NOS with (renal) cortical necrosis
Nephropathy NOS with (renal) cortical necrosisc
Renal cortical necrosis NOS

583.7 With lesion of renal medullary necrosis
Nephritis NOS with (renal) medullary [papillary] necrosis
Nephropathy NOS with (renal) medullary [papillary] necrosis

5th **583.8 With other specified pathological lesion in kidney**

583.81 ***Nephritis and nephropathy, not specified as acute or chronic, in diseases classified elsewhere***
Code first underlying disease, as:
amyloidosis (277.30-277.39)
diabetes mellitus (249.4, 250.4)
gonococcal infection (098.19)
Goodpasture's syndrome (446.21)
systemic lupus erythematosus (710.0)
tuberculosis (016.0)
Excludes *gouty nephropathy (274.10)*
syphilitic nephritis (095.4)

583.89 Other
Glomerulitis with lesion of:
exudative nephritis
interstitial nephritis
Glomerulonephritis with lesion of:
exudative nephritis
interstitial nephritis
Nephritis with lesion of:
exudative nephritis
interstitial nephritis
Nephropathy with lesion of:
exudative nephritis
interstitial nephritis
Renal disease with lesion of:
exudative nephritis
interstitial nephritis

583.9 With unspecified pathological lesion in kidney
Glomerulitis NOS
Glomerulonephritis NOS
Nephritis NOS
Nephropathy NOS
Excludes *nephropathy complicating pregnancy, labor, or the puerperium (642.0-642.9, 646.2)*
renal disease NOS with no stated cause (593.9)

▲4th **584 Acute kidney ~~renal~~ failure**
Includes acute renal failure
Excludes *following labor and delivery (669.3)*
posttraumatic (958.5)
that complicating:
abortion (634-638 with .3, 639.3)
ectopic or molar pregnancy (639.3)

▲584.5 Acute kidney failure with lesion of tubular necrosis
Lower nephron nephrosis
Renal failure with (acute) tubular necrosis
Tubular necrosis:
NOS
acute

▲584.6 Acute kidney failure with lesion of renal cortical necrosis

▲584.7 Acute kidney failure with lesion of renal medullary [papillary] necrosis
Necrotizing renal papillitis

▲584.8 Acute kidney failure with other specified pathological lesion in kidney

▲584.9 Acute kidney failure, with unspecified type of lesion
N17.9 Acute renal failure, unspecified
Excludes *traumatic kidney injury (866.00-866.13)*

4th **585 Chronic kidney disease (CKD)**
Includes chronic uremia
Code first hypertensive chronic kidney disease, if applicable (403.00-403.91, 404.00-404.93)
Use additional code to identify:
kidney transplant status, if applicable (V42.0)
manifestation as:
uremic:
neuropathy (357.4)
pericarditis (420.0)

ICD-9-CM Official Guidelines (Chapter 10):

a. Chronic kidney disease

*1) **Stages of chronic kidney disease (CKD)***

The ICD-9-CM classifies CKD based on severity. The severity of CKD is designated by stages I-V. Stage II, code 585.2, equates to mild CKD; stage III, code 585.3, equates to moderate CKD; and stage IV, code 585.4, equates to severe CKD. Code 585.6, End stage renal disease (ESRD), is assigned when the provider has documented end-stage-renal disease (ESRD).

If both a stage of CKD and ESRD are documented, assign code 585.6 only.

*2) **Chronic kidney disease and kidney transplant status***

Patients who have undergone kidney transplant may still have some form of CKD, because the kidney transplant may not fully restore kidney function. Therefore, the presence of CKD alone does not constitute a transplant complication. Assign the appropriate 585 code for the patient's stage of CKD and code V42.0. If a transplant complication such as failure or rejection is documented, see section I.C.17.f.1.b for information on coding complications of a kidney transplant. If the documentation is unclear as to whether the patient has a complication of the transplant, query the provider.

*3) **Chronic kidney disease with other conditions***

Patients with CKD may also suffer from other serious conditions, most commonly diabetes mellitus and hypertension. The sequencing of the CKD code in relationship to codes for other

contributing conditions is based on the conventions in the tabular list.
See I.C.3.a.4 for sequencing instructions for diabetes.
See I.C.4.a.1 for anemia in CKD.
See I.C.7.a.3 for hypertensive chronic kidney disease.
See I.C.17.f.1.b, Kidney transplant complications, for instructions on coding of documented rejection or failure.

Layman's: *The stages of CKD are differentiated by the glomerular filtration rate (GFR) of the patient, as follows:*

Stage I: GFR >90 ml/min/1.73 m^2
Stage II: GFR 60-89 ml/min/1.73 m^2
Stage III: GFR 30-59 ml/min/1.73 m^2
Stage IV: GFR 15-29 ml/min/1.73 m^2
Stage V: GFR <15 ml/min/1.73 m^2
ESRD: GFR <15 ml/min/1.73 m^2 and patient is on dialysis or undergoing kidney transplantation

585.1 **Chronic kidney disease, Stage I**
N18.1 Chronic kidney disease, stage I

585.2 **Chronic kidney disease, Stage II (mild)**
N18.2 Chronic kidney disease, stage II (mild)

585.3 **Chronic kidney disease, Stage III (moderate)**
N18.3 Chronic kidney disease, stage III (moderate)

585.4 **Chronic kidney disease, Stage IV (severe)** 121, 122, 123, 135, 153, 172
N18.4 Chronic kidney disease, stage IV (severe)

585.5 **Chronic kidney disease, Stage V** 121, 122, 123, 135, 153, 172
N18.5 Chronic kidney disease, stage V
Excludes *chronic kidney disease, stage V requiring chronic dialysis (585.6)*

585.6 **End stage renal disease** 79, 81, 82, 172, 174, 175
N18.6 End stage renal disease
Chronic kidney disease requiring chronic dialysis

585.9 **Chronic kidney disease, unspecified**
Chronic renal disease
Chronic renal failure, NOS
Chronic renal insufficiency

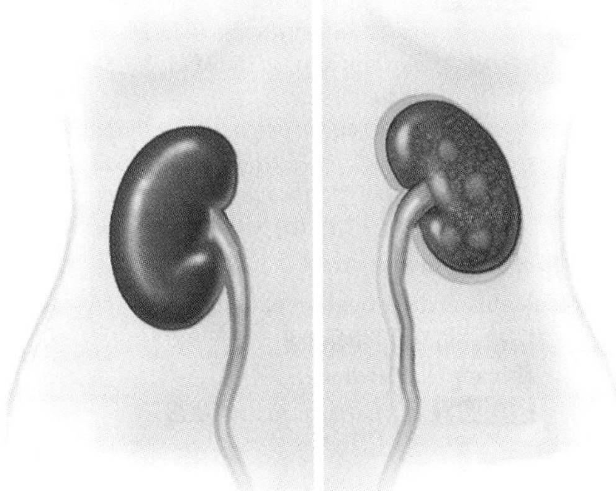

Normal

Chronic Kidney Disease

© 2008 Fairman Studios, LLC. All Rights Reserved.

586 **Renal failure, unspecified**
N19 Unspecified renal failure
Uremia NOS
Excludes *following labor and delivery (669.3)*
posttraumatic renal failure (958.5)
that complicating:
abortion (634-638 with .3, 639.3)
ectopic or molar pregnancy (639.3)
uremia:
extrarenal (788.9)
prerenal (788.9)

587 **Renal sclerosis, unspecified**
Includes atrophy of kidney
~~Atrophy of kidney~~
Contracted kidney
Renal:
cirrhosis
fibrosis

4th 588 **Disorders resulting from impaired renal function**
Excludes *secondary hypertension (405.0-405.9)*

588.0 **Renal osteodystrophy**
Azotemic osteodystrophy
Phosphate-losing tubular disorders
Renal:
dwarfism
infantilism
rickets

588.1 **Nephrogenic diabetes insipidus**
Excludes *diabetes insipidus NOS (253.5)*

5th 588.8 **Other specified disorders resulting from impaired renal function**

588.81 **Secondary hyperparathyroidism (of renal origin)**
N25.81 Secondary hyperparathyroidism of renal origin
Secondary hyperparathyroidism NOS

588.89 **Other specified disorders resulting from impaired renal function**
N25.89 Other disorders resulting from impaired renal tubular function
Hypokalemic nephropathy

588.9 **Unspecified disorder resulting from impaired renal function**

4th 589 **Small kidney of unknown cause**
589.0 **Unilateral small kidney**
589.1 **Bilateral small kidneys**
589.9 **Small kidney, unspecified**

OTHER DISEASES OF URINARY SYSTEM (590-599)

4th 590 **Infections of kidney**
Use additional code to identify organism, such as Escherichia coli [E. coli] (041.4)

5th 590.0 **Chronic pyelonephritis**
Chronic pyelitis
Chronic pyonephrosis
Code, if applicable, any causal condition first
590.00 **Without lesion of renal medullary necrosis**
590.01 **With lesion of renal medullary necrosis**

5th 590.1 **Acute pyelonephritis**
Acute pyelitis
Acute pyonephrosis
590.10 **Without lesion of renal medullary necrosis**
590.11 **With lesion of renal medullary necrosis**

585.1 – 590.11

590.2 Renal and perinephric abscess
Abscess:
kidney
nephritic
perirenal
Carbuncle of kidney

590.3 Pyeloureteritis cystica
Infection of renal pelvis and ureter
Ureteritis cystica

5th **590.8 Other pyelonephritis or pyonephrosis, not specified as acute or chronic**

590.80 Pyelonephritis, unspecified
Pyelitis NOS
Pyelonephritis NOS

590.81 Pyelitis or pyelonephritis in diseases classified elsewhere
Code first underlying disease, as:
tuberculosis (016.0)

590.9 Infection of kidney, unspecified
Excludes *urinary tract infection NOS (599.0)*

591 Hydronephrosis
N13.30 Unspecified hydronephrosis
Hydrocalycosis
Hydronephrosis
Hydroureteronephrosis
Excludes *congenital hydronephrosis (753.29)*
hydroureter (593.5)

Layman's: *Hydronephrosis is the enlargement of the kidney due to a blockage of the urinary tract. It often presents with loin and flank pain and sometimes can be felt upon palpation. Left untreated, it can lead to progressive kidney atrophy or infection.*

4th **592 Calculus of kidney and ureter**
Excludes *nephrocalcinosis (275.49)*

592.0 Calculus of kidney
N20.0 Calculus of kidney
Nephrolithiasis NOS
Renal calculus or stone
Staghorn calculus
Stone in kidney
Excludes *uric acid nephrolithiasis (274.11)*

Calculi
© Icon Learning Systems

592.1 Calculus of ureter
N20.1 Calculus of ureter
Ureteric stone
Ureterolithiasis

592.9 Urinary calculus, unspecified

4th **593 Other disorders of kidney and ureter**

593.0 Nephroptosis
Floating kidney
Mobile kidney

593.1 Hypertrophy of kidney

593.2 Cyst of kidney, acquired
N28.1 Cyst of kidney, acquired
Cyst (multiple) (solitary) of kidney, not congenital
Peripelvic (lymphatic) cyst
Excludes *calyceal or pyelogenic cyst of kidney (591)*
congenital cyst of kidney (753.1)
polycystic (disease of) kidney (753.1)

593.3 Stricture or kinking of ureter
Angulation of ureter (postoperative)
Constriction of ureter (postoperative)
Stricture of pelviureteric junction

593.4 Other ureteric obstruction
Idiopathic retroperitoneal fibrosis
Occlusion NOS of ureter
Excludes *that due to calculus (592.1)*

593.5 Hydroureter
Excludes *congenital hydroureter (753.22)*
hydroureteronephrosis (591)

593.6 Postural proteinuria
Benign postural proteinuria
Orthostatic proteinuria
Excludes *proteinuria NOS (791.0)*

5th **593.7 Vesicoureteral reflux**

593.70 Unspecified or without reflux nephropathy

593.71 With reflux nephropathy, unilateral

593.72 With reflux nephropathy, bilateral

593.73 With reflux nephropathy NOS

5th **593.8 Other specified disorders of kidney and ureter**

593.81 Vascular disorders of kidney
Renal (artery):
embolism
hemorrhage
thrombosis
Renal infarction

593.82 Ureteral fistula
Intestinoureteral fistula
Excludes *fistula between ureter and female genital tract (619.0)*

593.89 Other
Adhesions, kidney or ureter
Periureteritis
Polyp of ureter
Pyelectasia
Ureterocele
Excludes *tuberculosis of ureter (016.2)*
ureteritis cystica (590.3)

593.9 Unspecified disorder of kidney and ureter
N28.9 Disorder of kidney and ureter, unspecified
Acute renal disease
Acute renal insufficiency
Renal disease NOS
Salt-losing nephritis or syndrome
Excludes *chronic renal insufficiency (585.9)*
cystic kidney disease (753.1)
nephropathy, so stated (583.0-583.9)
renal disease:
arising in pregnancy or the puerperium (642.1-642.2, 642.4-642.7, 646.2)
not specified as acute or chronic, but with stated pathology or cause (583.0-583.9)

4th **594 Calculus of lower urinary tract**

594.0 Calculus in diverticulum of bladder

594.1 Other calculus in bladder
Urinary bladder stone
Excludes *staghorn calculus (592.0)*

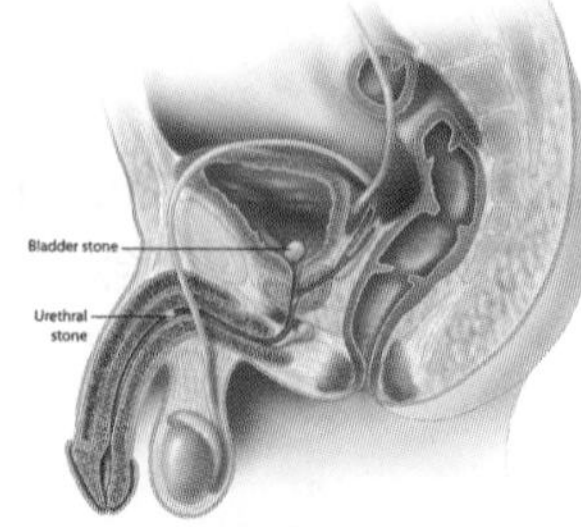

594.2 Calculus in urethra

594.8 Other lower urinary tract calculus

594.9 Calculus of lower urinary tract, unspecified

Excludes *calculus of urinary tract NOS (592.9)*

4th 595 Cystitis

Use additional code to identify organism, such as Escherichia coli [E. coli] (041.4)

Excludes *prostatocystitis (601.3)*

595.0 Acute cystitis

N30.00 Acute cystitis without hematuria

N30.01 Acute cystitis with hematuria

Excludes *trigonitis (595.3)*

595.1 Chronic interstitial cystitis

Hunner's ulcer
Panmural fibrosis of bladder
Submucous cystitis

595.2 Other chronic cystitis

Chronic cystitis NOS
Subacute cystitis

Excludes *trigonitis (595.3)*

595.3 Trigonitis

Follicular cystitis
Trigonitis (acute) (chronic)
Urethrotrigonitis

595.4 *Cystitis in diseases classified elsewhere*

Code first underlying disease, as:
actinomycosis (039.8)
amebiasis (006.8)
bilharziasis (120.0-120.9)
Echinococcus infestation (122.3, 122.6)

Excludes *cystitis:*
diphtheritic (032.84)
gonococcal (098.11, 098.31)
monilial (112.2)
trichomonal (131.09)
tuberculous (016.1)

5th 595.8 Other specified types of cystitis

595.81 Cystitis cystica

595.82 Irradiation cystitis

Use additional E-Code to identify cause

595.89 Other

Abscess of bladder
Cystitis:
bullous
emphysematous
glandularis

595.9 Cystitis, unspecified

4th 596 Other disorders of bladder

Use additional code to identify urinary incontinence (625.6, 788.30-788.39)

596.0 Bladder neck obstruction

N32.0 Bladder-neck obstruction

Contracture (acquired) of bladder neck or vesicourethral orifice
Obstruction (acquired) of bladder neck or vesicourethral orifice
Stenosis (acquired) of bladder neck or vesicourethral orifice

Excludes *congenital (753.6)*

596.1 Intestinovesical fistula

Fistula:
enterovesical
vesicocolic
vesicoenteric
vesicorectal

596.2 Vesical fistula, not elsewhere classified

Fistula:
bladder NOS
urethrovesical
vesicocutaneous
vesicoperineal

Excludes *fistula between bladder and female genital tract (619.0)*

596.3 Diverticulum of bladder

Diverticulitis of bladder
Diverticulum (acquired) (false) of bladder

Excludes *that with calculus in diverticulum of bladder (594.0)*

596.4 Atony of bladder

High compliance bladder
Hypotonicity of bladder
Inertia of bladder

Excludes *neurogenic bladder (596.54)*

5th 596.5 Other functional disorders of bladder

Excludes *cauda equina syndrome with neurogenic bladder (344.61)*

596.51 Hypertonicity of bladder

Hyperactivity
Overactive bladder

596.52 Low bladder compliance

596.53 Paralysis of bladder

596.54 Neurogenic bladder NOS

Layman's: *Neurogenic bladder is a dysfunction of the bladder that is directly attributable to a disease of the CNS or peripheral nerves that control urination. Typically, it causes difficulty or complete inability to pass urine without catheterization or other methods of facilitation.*

596.55 Detrusor sphincter dyssynergia

596.59 Other functional disorder of bladder

Detrusor instability

596.6 Rupture of bladder, nontraumatic

596.7 Hemorrhage into bladder wall

Hyperemia of bladder

Excludes *acute hemorrhagic cystitis (595.0)*

596.8 Other specified disorders of bladder

Bladder:
calcified
contracted
hemorrhage
hypertrophy

Excludes *cystocele, female (618.01- 618.02, 618.09, 618.2-618.4)*
hernia or prolapse of bladder, female (618.01-618.02, 618.09, 618.2-618.4)

596.9 Unspecified disorder of bladder

4th 597 Urethritis, not sexually transmitted, and urethral syndrome

Excludes *nonspecific urethritis, so stated (099.4)*

597.0 Urethral abscess

Abscess:
periurethral
urethral (gland)
Abscess of:
bulbourethral gland
Cowper's gland
Littré's gland
Periurethral cellulitis

Excludes *urethral caruncle (599.3)*

5th 597.8 Other urethritis

597.80 Urethritis, unspecified

597.81 Urethral syndrome NOS

597.89 **Other**
Adenitis, Skene's glands
Cowperitis
Meatitis, urethral
Ulcer, urethra (meatus)
Verumontanitis
Excludes *trichomonal (131.02)*

4th 598 **Urethral stricture**
Includes pinhole meatus
stricture of urinary meatus
Use additional code to identify urinary incontinence (625.6, 788.30-788.39)
Excludes *congenital stricture of urethra and urinary meatus (753.6)*

5th 598.0 **Urethral stricture due to infection**
598.00 **Due to unspecified infection**
598.01 ***Due to infective diseases classified elsewhere***
Code first underlying disease, as:
gonococcal infection (098.2)
schistosomiasis (120.0-120.9)
syphilis (095.8)

598.1 **Traumatic urethral stricture**
Stricture of urethra:
late effect of injury
postobstetric
Excludes *postoperative following surgery on genitourinary tract (598.2)*

598.2 **Postoperative urethral stricture**
Postcatheterization stricture of urethra

598.8 **Other specified causes of urethral stricture**

598.9 **Urethral stricture, unspecified**

4th 599 **Other disorders of urethra and urinary tract**

599.0 **Urinary tract infection, site not specified**
N39.0 Urinary tract infection, site not specified
Excludes *candidiasis of urinary tract (112.2)*
urinary tract infection of newborn (771.82)
Use additional code to identify organism, such as Escherichia coli [E. coli] (041.4)
Layman's: *It is important that documentation be reviewed to see if the site of the UTI (e.g., kidney, bladder, urethra, etc.) is mentioned. If so, the site-specific code (e.g., 590.1x, 595.0, 597.80, etc.) is more appropriate than 599.0.*

599.1 **Urethral fistula**
Fistula:
urethroperineal
urethrorectal
Urinary fistula NOS
Excludes *fistula:*
urethroscrotal (608.89)
urethrovaginal (619.0)
urethrovesicovaginal (619.0)

599.2 **Urethral diverticulum**

599.3 **Urethral caruncle**
Polyp of urethra

599.4 **Urethral false passage**

599.5 **Prolapsed urethral mucosa**
Prolapse of urethra
Urethrocele
Excludes *urethrocele, female (618.03, 618.09, 618.2-618.4)*

5th 599.6 **Urinary obstruction**
Use additional code to identify urinary incontinence (625.6, 788.30-788.39)
Excludes *obstructive nephropathy NOS (593.89)*

599.60 **Urinary obstruction, unspecified**
Obstructive uropathy NOS
Urinary (tract) obstruction NOS

599.69 **Urinary obstruction, not elsewhere classified**
Code, if applicable, any causal condition first, such as:
hyperplasia of prostate (600.0-600.9 with fifth-digit 1)

5th 599.7 **Hematuria**
Hematuria (benign) (essential)
Excludes *hemoglobinuria (791.2)*

599.70 **Hematuria, unspecified**
R31.9 Hematuria, unspecified

599.71 **Gross hematuria**

599.72 **Microscopic hematuria**

5th 599.8 **Other specified disorders of urethra and urinary tract**
Use additional code to identify urinary incontinence (625.6, 788.30-788.39)
Excludes *symptoms and other conditions classifiable to 788.0-788.2, 788.4-788.9, 791.0-791.9*

599.81 **Urethral hypermobility**

599.82 **Intrinsic (urethral) sphincter deficiency [ISD]**

599.83 **Urethral instability**

599.84 **Other specified disorders of urethra**
Rupture of urethra (nontraumatic)
Urethral:
cyst
granuloma

599.89 **Other specified disorders of urinary tract**

599.9 **Unspecified disorder of urethra and urinary tract**

DISEASES OF MALE GENITAL ORGANS (600-608)

4th 600 **Hyperplasia of prostate**
Includes enlarged prostate

Normal Prostate

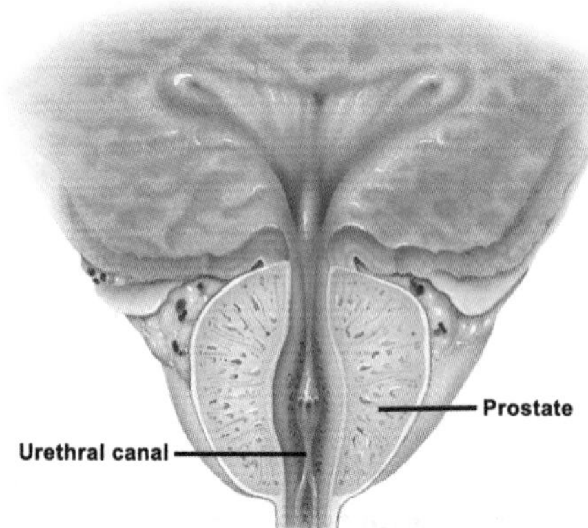

Hyperplasia of the prostate causes impingement of the urethral canal and urinary symptoms.
© 2006 Anatomical Chart Company

5th 600.0 **Hypertrophy (benign) of prostate**
Benign prostatic hypertrophy
Enlargement of prostate
Smooth enlarged prostate
Soft enlarged prostate

600.00 **Hypertrophy (benign) of prostate without urinary obstruction and other lower urinary tract symptoms (LUTS)** A ♂
N40.0 Enlarged prostate without lower urinary tract symptoms (LUTS)
Hypertrophy (benign) of prostate NOS

600.01 Hypertrophy (benign) of prostate with urinary obstruction and other lower urinary tract symptoms (LUTS) A ♂

N40.1 Enlarged prostate with lower urinary tract symptoms (LUTS)

Hypertrophy (benign) of prostate with urinary retention

Use additional code to identify symptoms:
- incomplete bladder emptying (788.21)
- nocturia (788.43)
- straining on urination (788.65)
- urinary frequency (788.41)
- urinary hesitancy (788.64)
- urinary incontinence (788.30-788.39)
- urinary obstruction (599.69)
- urinary retention (788.20)
- urinary urgency (788.63)
- weak urinary stream (788.62)

5th **600.1 Nodular prostate**

Hard, firm prostate
Multinodular prostate

Excludes *malignant neoplasm of prostate (185)*

600.10 Nodular prostate without urinary obstruction A ♂

Nodular prostate NOS

600.11 Nodular prostate with urinary obstruction A ♂

Nodular prostate with urinary retention

5th **600.2 Benign localized hyperplasia of prostate**

Adenofibromatous hypertrophy of prostate
Adenoma of prostate
Fibroadenoma of prostate
Fibroma of prostate
Myoma of prostate
Polyp of prostate

Excludes *benign neoplasms of prostate (222.2)*
hypertrophy of prostate (600.00-600.01)
malignant neoplasm of prostate (185)

600.20 Benign localized hyperplasia of prostate without urinary obstruction and other lower urinary tract symptoms (LUTS) A ♂

Benign localized hyperplasia of prostate NOS

600.21 Benign localized hyperplasia of prostate with urinary obstruction and other lower urinary tract symptoms (LUTS) A ♂

Benign localized hyperplasia of prostate with urinary retention

Use additional code to identify symptoms:
- incomplete bladder emptying (788.21)
- nocturia (788.43)
- straining on urination (788.65)
- urinary frequency (788.41)
- urinary hesitancy (788.64)
- urinary incontinence (788.30-788.39)
- urinary obstruction (599.69)
- urinary retention (788.20)
- urinary urgency (788.63)
- weak urinary stream (788.62)

600.3 Cyst of prostate A ♂

5th **600.9 Hyperplasia of prostate, unspecified**

Median bar
Prostatic obstruction NOS

600.90 Hyperplasia of prostate, unspecified, without urinary obstruction and other lower urinary tract symptoms (LUTS) A ♂

Hyperplasia of prostate NOS

600.91 Hyperplasia of prostate, unspecified, with urinary obstruction and other lower urinary tract symptoms (LUTS) A ♂

Hyperplasia of prostate, unspecified, with urinary retention

Use additional code to identify symptoms:
- incomplete bladder emptying (788.21)
- nocturia (788.43)
- straining on urination (788.65)
- urinary frequency (788.41)
- urinary hesitancy (788.64)
- urinary incontinence (788.30-788.39)
- urinary obstruction (599.69)
- urinary retention (788.20)
- urinary urgency (788.63)
- weak urinary stream (788.62)

4th **601 Inflammatory diseases of prostate**

Use additional code to identify organism, such as Staphylococcus (041.1), or Streptococcus (041.0)

601.0 Acute prostatitis A ♂

601.1 Chronic prostatitis A ♂

601.2 Abscess of prostate A ♂

601.3 Prostatocystitis A ♂

601.4 *Prostatitis in diseases classified elsewhere* A ♂

Code first underlying disease, as:
- *actinomycosis (039.8)*
- *blastomycosis (116.0)*
- *syphilis (095.8)*
- *tuberculosis (016.5)*

Excludes *prostatitis:*
- *gonococcal (098.12, 098.32)*
- *monilial (112.2)*
- *trichomonal (131.03)*

601.8 Other specified inflammatory diseases of prostate A ♂

Prostatitis:
- cavitary
- diverticular
- granulomatous

601.9 Prostatitis, unspecified A ♂

N41.9 Inflammatory disease of prostate, unspecified

Prostatitis NOS

4th **602 Other disorders of prostate**

602.0 Calculus of prostate A ♂

Prostatic stone

602.1 Congestion or hemorrhage of prostate A ♂

602.2 Atrophy of prostate A ♂

602.3 Dysplasia of prostate ♂

Prostatic intraepithelial neoplasia I (PIN I)
Prostatic intraepithelial neoplasia II (PIN II)

Excludes *prostatic intraepithelial neoplasia III (PIN III) (233.4)*

602.8 Other specified disorders of prostate A ♂

Fistula of prostate
Infarction of prostate
Periprostatic adhesions
Stricture of prostate

602.9 Unspecified disorder of prostate A ♂

N42.9 Disorder of prostate, unspecified

4th **603 Hydrocele**

Includes hydrocele of spermatic cord, testis, or tunica vaginalis

Excludes *congenital (778.6)*

603.0 Encysted hydrocele ♂

603.1 Infected hydrocele ♂

Use additional code to identify organism

603.8 Other specified types of hydrocele ♂

603.9 Hydrocele, unspecified ♂

4th **604 Orchitis and epididymitis**
Use additional code to identify organism such as Escherichia coli [E. coli] (041.4), Staphylococcus (041.1), or Streptococcus (041.0)

604.0 Orchitis, epididymitis, and epididymo-orchitis, with abscess ♂
Abscess of epididymis or testis

5th **604.9 Other orchitis, epididymitis, and epididymo-orchitis, without mention of abscess**

604.90 Orchitis and epididymitis, unspecified ♂

604.91 *Orchitis and epididymitis in diseases classified elsewhere* ♂
Code first underlying disease, as:
diphtheria (032.89)
filariasis (125.0-125.9)
syphilis (095.8)
Excludes *orchitis:*
gonococcal (098.13, 098.33)
mumps (072.0)
tuberculous (016.5)
tuberculous epididymitis (016.4)

604.99 Other ♂

605 Redundant prepuce and phimosis ♂
Adherent prepuce
Paraphimosis
Phimosis (congenital)
Tight foreskin

4th **606 Infertility, male**

606.0 Azoospermia A ♂
Absolute infertility
Infertility due to:
germinal (cell) aplasia
spermatogenic arrest (complete)

606.1 Oligospermia A ♂
Infertility due to:
germinal cell desquamation
hypospermatogenesis
incomplete spermatogenic arrest

606.8 Infertility due to extratesticular causes A ♂
Infertility due to:
drug therapy
infection
obstruction of efferent ducts
radiation
systemic disease

606.9 Male infertility, unspecified A ♂

4th **607 Disorders of penis**
Excludes *phimosis (605)*

607.0 Leukoplakia of penis ♂
Kraurosis of penis
Excludes *carcinoma in situ of penis (233.5)*
erythroplasia of Queyrat (233.5)

607.1 Balanoposthitis ♂
Balanitis
Use additional code to identify organism

607.2 Other inflammatory disorders of penis ♂
Abscess of corpus cavernosum or penis
Boil of corpus cavernosum or penis
Carbuncle of corpus cavernosum or penis
Cavernitis (penis)
Cellulitis of corpus cavernosum or penis
Use additional code to identify organism
Excludes *herpetic infection (054.13)*

607.3 Priapism ♂
Painful erection

5th **607.8 Other specified disorders of penis**

607.81 Balanitis xerotica obliterans ♂
Induratio penis plastica

607.82 Vascular disorders of penis ♂
Embolism of corpus cavernosum or penis
Hematoma (nontraumatic) of corpus cavernosum or penis
Hemorrhage of corpus cavernosum or penis
Thrombosis of corpus cavernosum or penis

607.83 Edema of penis ♂

607.84 Impotence of organic origin A ♂
N52.8 Other male erectile dysfunction
Excludes *nonorganic (302.72)*

607.85 Peyronie's disease ♂

607.89 Other ♂
Atrophy of corpus cavernosum or penis
Fibrosis of corpus cavernosum or penis
Hypertrophy of corpus cavernosum or penis
Ulcer (chronic) of corpus cavernosum or penis

607.9 Unspecified disorder of penis ♂

4th **608 Other disorders of male genital organs**

608.0 Seminal vesiculitis ♂
Abscess of seminal vesicle
Cellulitis of seminal vesicle
Vesiculitis (seminal)
Use additional code to identify organism
Excludes *gonococcal infection (098.14, 098.34)*

608.1 Spermatocele ♂

5th **608.2 Torsion of testis**

608.20 Torsion of testis, unspecified ♂

608.21 Extravaginal torsion of spermatic cord ♂

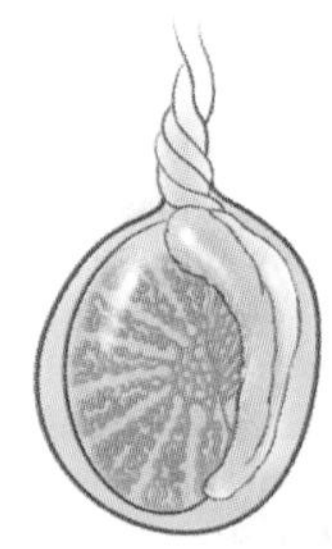
Extravaginal torsion

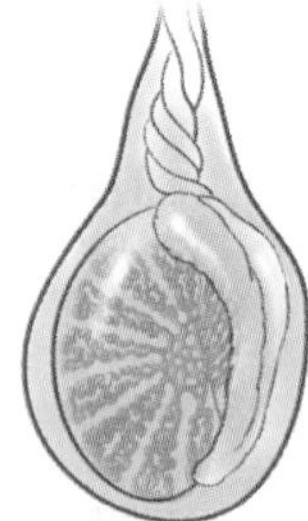
Intravaginal torsion

© 2008 Fairman Studios, LLC. All Rights Reserved.

608.22 Intravaginal torsion of spermatic cord ♂
Torsion of spermatic cord NOS

608.23 Torsion of appendix testis ♂

608.24 Torsion of appendix epididymis ♂

608.3 Atrophy of testis ♂

608.4 Other inflammatory disorders of male genital organs ♂
Abscess of scrotum, spermatic cord, testis [except abscess], tunica vaginalis, or vas deferens
Boil of scrotum, spermatic cord, testis [except abscess], tunica vaginalis, or vas deferens
Carbuncle of scrotum, spermatic cord, testis [except abscess], tunica vaginalis, or vas deferens
Cellulitis of scrotum, spermatic cord, testis [except abscess], tunica vaginalis, or vas deferens
Vasitis
Use additional code to identify organism
Excludes *abscess of testis (604.0)*

5th 608.8 Other specified disorders of male genital organs

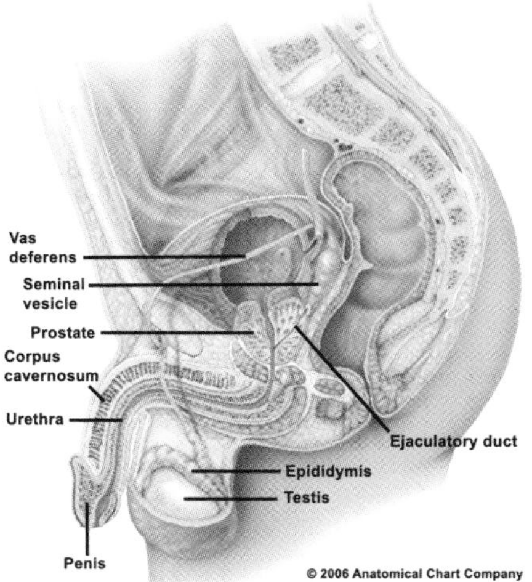

608.81 *Disorders of male genital organs in diseases classified elsewhere* ♂

Code first underlying disease, as:
filariasis (125.0-125.9)
tuberculosis (016.5)

608.82 **Hematospermia** ♂

608.83 **Vascular disorders** ♂

Hematocele NOS, male
Hematoma (nontraumatic) of seminal vesicle, spermatic cord, testis, scrotum, tunica vaginalis, or vas deferens
Hemorrhage of seminal vesicle, spermatic cord, testis, scrotum, tunica vaginalis, or vas deferens
Thrombosis of seminal vesicle, spermatic cord, testis, scrotum, tunica vaginalis, or vas deferens

608.84 **Chylocele of tunica vaginalis** ♂

608.85 **Stricture** ♂

Stricture of:
spermatic cord
tunica vaginalis
vas deferens

608.86 **Edema** ♂

608.87 **Retrograde ejaculation** ♂

608.89 **Other** ♂

Atrophy of seminal vesicle, spermatic cord, testis, scrotum tunica vaginalis, or vas deferens
Fibrosis of seminal vesicle, spermatic cord, testis, scrotum tunica vaginalis, or vas deferens
Hypertrophy of seminal vesicle, spermatic cord, testis, scrotum tunica vaginalis, or vas deferens
Ulcer of seminal vesicle, spermatic cord, testis, scrotum tunica vaginalis, or vas deferens

Excludes *atrophy of testis (608.3)*

608.9 **Unspecified disorder of male genital organs** ♂

DISORDERS OF BREAST (610-612)

4th 610 **Benign mammary dysplasias**

610.0 **Solitary cyst of breast**

Cyst (solitary) of breast

610.1 **Diffuse cystic mastopathy** A

N60.19 Diffuse cystic mastopathy of unspecified breast

Chronic cystic mastitis
Cystic breast
Fibrocystic disease of breast

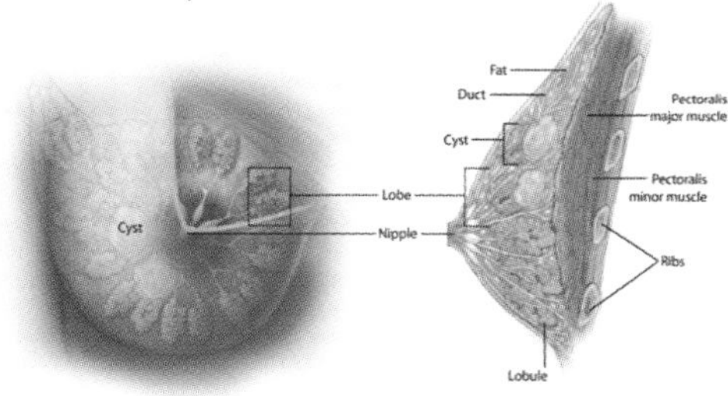

© 2008 Fairman Studios, LLC. All Rights Reserved.

610.2 **Fibroadenosis of breast**

Fibroadenosis of breast:
NOS
chronic
cystic
diffuse
periodic
segmental

610.3 **Fibrosclerosis of breast**

610.4 **Mammary duct ectasia**

Comedomastitis
Duct ectasia
Mastitis:
periductal
plasma cell

610.8 **Other specified benign mammary dysplasias**

Mazoplasia
Sebaceous cyst of breast

610.9 **Benign mammary dysplasia, unspecified**

4th 611 **Other disorders of breast**

Excludes *that associated with lactation or the puerperium (675.0-676.9)*

611.0 **Inflammatory disease of breast**

Abscess (acute) (chronic) (nonpuerperal) of:
areola
breast
Mammillary fistula
Mastitis (acute) (subacute) (nonpuerperal):
NOS
infective
retromammary
submammary

Excludes *carbuncle of breast (680.2)*
chronic cystic mastitis (610.1)
neonatal infective mastitis (771.5)
thrombophlebitis of breast [Mondor's disease] (451.89)

611.1 **Hypertrophy of breast**

Gynecomastia
Hypertrophy of breast:
NOS
massive pubertal

Excludes *breast engorgement in newborn (778.7)*
disproportion of reconstructed breast (612.1)

611.2 **Fissure of nipple**

611.3 **Fat necrosis of breast**

Fat necrosis (segmental) of breast

Code first breast necrosis due to breast graft (996.79)

611.4 **Atrophy of breast**

I - 186 PQRI Measure | ♂ Male ♀ Female | N Newborn Age (0) P Pediatric Age (0-17) M Maternity Age (12-55) A Adult Age (15-124)

611.5 **Galactocele**

611.6 **Galactorrhea not associated with childbirth**

5th 611.7 **Signs and symptoms in breast**

611.71 **Mastodynia**
Pain in breast

611.72 **Lump or mass in breast**
N63 Unspecified lump in breast
Layman's: *611.72 is a nonspecific diagnosis code that is most appropriate if the billing for a scan or other procedure is being submitted prior to receiving the results of a biopsy or other diagnostic test. If the test results are received prior to billing, it is appropriate to use the definitive diagnosis of the findings (e.g., one of the codes in the 610.x series) in lieu of 611.72, especially if there are further procedures that need to be performed based on the findings.*

611.79 **Other**
Induration of breast
Inversion of nipple
Nipple discharge
Retraction of nipple

5th 611.8 **Other specified disorders of breast**

611.81 **Ptosis of breast** A
Excludes *ptosis of native breast in relation to reconstructed breast (612.1)*

611.82 **Hypoplasia of breast** A
Micromastia
Excludes *congenital absence of breast (757.6)*
hypoplasia of native breast in relation to reconstructed breast (612.1)

611.83 **Capsular contracture of breast implant** A

611.89 **Other specified disorders of breast**
Hematoma (nontraumatic) of breast
Infarction of breast
Occlusion of breast duct
Subinvolution of breast (postlactational) (postpartum)

611.9 **Unspecified breast disorder**

4th 612 **Deformity and disproportion of reconstructed breast**

612.0 **Deformity of reconstructed breast** A
Contour irregularity in reconstructed breast
Excess tissue in reconstructed breast
Misshapen reconstructed breast

612.1 **Disproportion of reconstructed breast** A
Breast asymmetry between native breast and reconstructed breast
Disproportion between native breast and reconstructed breast

INFLAMMATORY DISEASE OF FEMALE PELVIC ORGANS (614-616)

Use additional code to identify organism, such as Staphylococcus (041.1), or Streptococcus (041.0)

Excludes *that associated with pregnancy, abortion, childbirth, or the puerperium (630-676.9)*

4th 614 **Inflammatory disease of ovary, fallopian tube, pelvic cellular tissue, and peritoneum**

Excludes *endometritis (615.0-615.9)*
major infection following delivery (670.0-670.8)
that complicating:
abortion (634-638 with .0, 639.0)
ectopic or molar pregnancy (639.0)
pregnancy or labor (646.6)

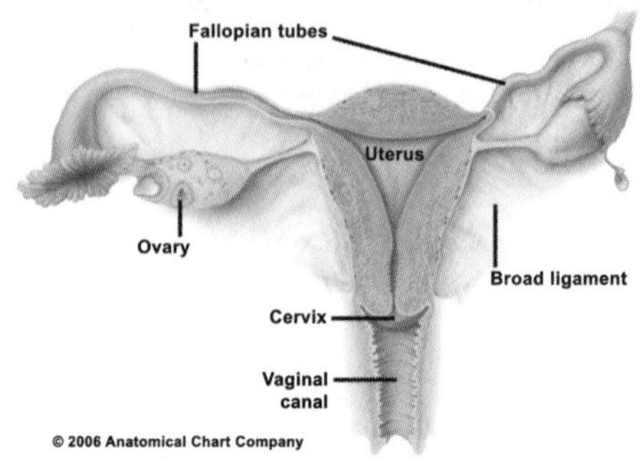

614.0 **Acute salpingitis and oophoritis** ♀
Any condition classifiable to 614.2, specified as acute or subacute

614.1 **Chronic salpingitis and oophoritis** ♀
Hydrosalpinx
Salpingitis:
follicularis
isthmica nodosa
Any condition classifiable to 614.2, specified as chronic

614.2 **Salpingitis and oophoritis not specified as acute, subacute, or chronic** ♀
Abscess (of):
fallopian tube
ovary
tubo-ovarian
Oophoritis
Perioophoritis
Perisalpingitis
Pyosalpinx
Salpingitis
Salpingo-oophoritis
Tubo-ovarian inflammatory disease
Excludes *gonococcal infection (chronic) (098.37)*
acute (098.17)
tuberculous (016.6)

614.3 **Acute parametritis and pelvic cellulitis** ♀
Acute inflammatory pelvic disease
Any condition classifiable to 614.4, specified as acute

614.4 **Chronic or unspecified parametritis and pelvic cellulitis** ♀
Abscess (of):
broad ligament chronic or NOS
parametrium chronic or NOS
pelvis, female chronic or NOS
pouch of Douglas chronic or NOS
Chronic inflammatory pelvic disease
Pelvic cellulitis, female
Excludes *tuberculous (016.7)*

614.5 **Acute or unspecified pelvic peritonitis, female** ♀

614.6 Pelvic peritoneal adhesions, female (postoperative) (postinfection) ♀
Adhesions:
peritubal
tubo-ovarian
Use additional code to identify any associated infertility (628.2)

614.7 Other chronic pelvic peritonitis, female ♀
Excludes *tuberculous (016.7)*

614.8 Other specified inflammatory disease of female pelvic organs and tissues ♀

614.9 Unspecified inflammatory disease of female pelvic organs and tissues ♀
Pelvic infection or inflammation, female NOS
Pelvic inflammatory disease [PID]

4th 615 Inflammatory diseases of uterus, except cervix
Excludes *following delivery (670.0-670.8)*
hyperplastic endometritis (621.30-621.35)
that complicating:
abortion (634-638 with .0, 639.0)
ectopic or molar pregnancy (639.0)
pregnancy or labor (646.6)

615.0 Acute ♀
Any condition classifiable to 615.9, specified as acute or subacute

615.1 Chronic ♀
Any condition classifiable to 615.9, specified as chronic

615.9 Unspecified inflammatory disease of uterus ♀
Endometritis
Endomyometritis
Metritis
Myometritis
Perimetritis
Pyometra
Uterine abscess

4th 616 Inflammatory disease of cervix, vagina, and vulva
Excludes *that complicating:*
abortion (634-638 with .0, 639.0)
ectopic or molar pregnancy (639.0)
pregnancy, childbirth, or the puerperium (646.6)

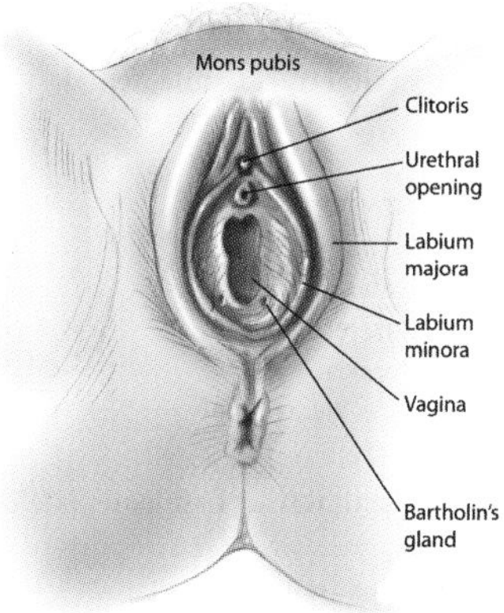

© 2008 Fairman Studios, LLC. All Rights Reserved.

616.0 Cervicitis and endocervicitis ♀
N76.0 Acute vaginitis
N76.1 Subacute and chronic vaginitis
N76.2 Acute vulvitis
N76.3 Subacute and chronic vulvitis
Cervicitis with or without mention of erosion or ectropion
Endocervicitis with or without mention of erosion or ectropion
Nabothian (gland) cyst or follicle
Excludes *erosion or ectropion without mention of cervicitis (622.0)*

5th 616.1 Vaginitis and vulvovaginitis
Excludes *vulvar vestibulitis (625.71)*

616.10 Vaginitis and vulvovaginitis, unspecified ♀
Vaginitis:
NOS
postirradiation
Vulvitis NOS
Vulvovaginitis NOS
Use additional code to identify organism, such as Escherichia coli [E. coli] (041.4), Staphylococcus (041.1), or Streptococcus (041.0)
Excludes *noninfective leukorrhea (623.5)*
postmenopausal or senile vaginitis (627.3)

616.11 Vaginitis and vulvovaginitis in diseases classified elsewhere ♀
Code first underlying disease, as:
pinworm vaginitis (127.4)
Excludes *herpetic vulvovaginitis (054.11)*
monilial vulvovaginitis (112.1)
trichomonal vaginitis or vulvovaginitis (131.01)

616.2 Cyst of Bartholin's gland ♀
Bartholin's duct cyst

616.3 Abscess of Bartholin's gland ♀
Vulvovaginal gland abscess

616.4 Other abscess of vulva ♀
Abscess of vulva
Carbuncle of vulva
Furuncle of vulva

5th 616.5 Ulceration of vulva

616.50 Ulceration of vulva, unspecified ♀
Ulcer NOS of vulva

616.51 Ulceration of vulva in diseases classified elsewhere ♀
Code first underlying disease, as:
Behçet's syndrome (136.1)
tuberculosis (016.7)
Excludes *vulvar ulcer (in):*
gonococcal (098.0)
herpes simplex (054.12)
syphilitic (091.0)

5th 616.8 Other specified inflammatory diseases of cervix, vagina, and vulva ♀
Excludes *noninflammatory disorders of:*
cervix (622.0-622.9)
vagina (623.0-623.9)
vulva (624.0-624.9)

616.81 Mucositis (ulcerative) of cervix, vagina, and vulva ♀
Use additional E code to identify adverse effects of therapy, such as:
antineoplastic and immunosuppressive drugs (E930.7, E933.1)
radiation therapy (E879.2)

616.89 Other inflammatory disease of cervix, vagina and vulva ♀
Caruncle, vagina or labium
Ulcer, vagina

616.9 Unspecified inflammatory disease of cervix, vagina, and vulva ♀

614.6 – 616.9

OTHER DISORDERS OF FEMALE GENITAL TRACT (617-629)

4th 617 Endometriosis

617.0 **Endometriosis of uterus** ♀
Adenomyosis
Endometriosis:
cervix
internal
myometrium
Excludes *stromal endometriosis (236.0)*

617.1 **Endometriosis of ovary** ♀
Chocolate cyst of ovary
Endometrial cystoma of ovary

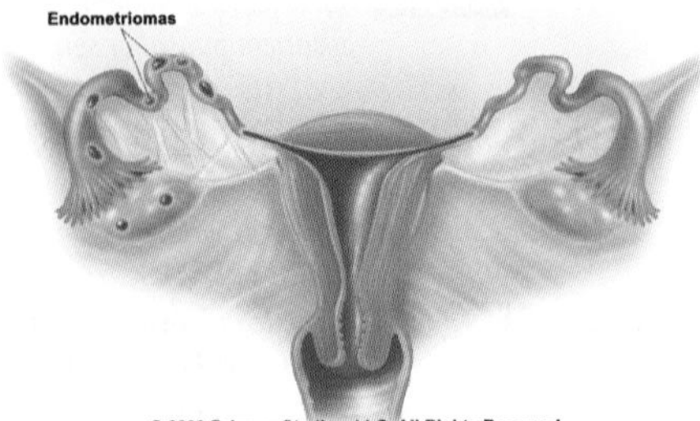

© 2008 Fairman Studios, LLC. All Rights Reserved.

617.2 **Endometriosis of fallopian tube** ♀

617.3 **Endometriosis of pelvic peritoneum** ♀
Endometriosis:
broad ligament
cul-de-sac (Douglas')
parametrium
round ligament

617.4 **Endometriosis of rectovaginal septum and vagina** ♀

617.5 **Endometriosis of intestine** ♀
Endometriosis:
appendix
colon
rectum

617.6 **Endometriosis in scar of skin** ♀

617.8 **Endometriosis of other specified sites** ♀
Endometriosis:
bladder
lung
umbilicus
vulva

617.9 **Endometriosis, site unspecified** ♀

4th 618 **Genital prolapse**
Use additional code to identify urinary incontinence (625.6, 788.31, 788.33-788.39)
Excludes *that complicating pregnancy, labor, or delivery (654.4)*

5th 618.0 **Prolapse of vaginal walls without mention of uterine prolapse**
Excludes *that with uterine prolapse (618.2-618.4)*
enterocele (618.6)
vaginal vault prolapse following hysterectomy (618.5)

Layman's: *Non-uterine vaginal prolapse is classified according to the organ(s) encroaching on the vaginal walls:*
Cystocele: *bladder*
Urethrocele: *urethra*
Rectocele: *rectum*
Perineocele: *perineal region*

618.00 **Unspecified prolapse of vaginal walls** ♀
N81.9 Female genital prolapse, unspecified
Vaginal prolapse NOS

618.01 **Cystocele, midline** ♀
Cystocele NOS

618.02 **Cystocele, lateral** ♀
Paravaginal

618.03 **Urethrocele** ♀

618.04 **Rectocele** ♀
Proctocele

618.05 **Perineocele** ♀

618.09 **Other prolapse of vaginal walls without mention of uterine prolapse** ♀
Cystourethrocele

618.1 **Uterine prolapse without mention of vaginal wall prolapse** ♀
Descensus uteri
Uterine prolapse:
NOS
complete
first degree
second degree
third degree
Excludes *that with mention of cystocele, urethrocele, or rectocele (618.2-618.4)*

618.2 **Uterovaginal prolapse, incomplete** ♀

618.3 **Uterovaginal prolapse, complete** ♀

618.4 **Uterovaginal prolapse, unspecified** ♀

618.5 **Prolapse of vaginal vault after hysterectomy** ♀

618.6 **Vaginal enterocele, congenital or acquired** ♀
Pelvic enterocele, congenital or acquired

618.7 **Old laceration of muscles of pelvic floor** ♀

5th 618.8 **Other specified genital prolapse**

618.81 **Incompetence or weakening of pubocervical tissue** ♀

618.82 **Incompetence or weakening of rectovaginal tissue** ♀

618.83 **Pelvic muscle wasting** ♀
Disuse atrophy of pelvic muscles and anal sphincter

618.84 **Cervical stump prolapse** ♀

618.89 **Other specified genital prolapse** ♀

618.9 **Unspecified genital prolapse** ♀

4th 619 **Fistula involving female genital tract**
Excludes *vesicorectal and intestinovesical fistula (596.1)*

619.0 **Urinary-genital tract fistula, female** ♀
Fistula:
cervicovesical
ureterovaginal
urethrovaginal
urethrovesicovaginal
uteroureteric
uterovesical
vesicocervicovaginal
vesicovaginal

619.1 **Digestive-genital tract fistula, female** ♀
Fistula:
intestinouterine
intestinovaginal
rectovaginal
rectovulval
sigmoidovaginal
uterorectal

619.2 **Genital tract-skin fistula, female** ♀
Fistula:
uterus to abdominal wall
vaginoperineal

619.8 Other specified fistulas involving female genital tract ♀
Fistula:
cervix
cul-de-sac (Douglas')
uterus
vagina

619.9 Unspecified fistula involving female genital tract ♀

4th **620 Noninflammatory disorders of ovary, fallopian tube, and broad ligament**
Excludes *hydrosalpinx (614.1)*

620.0 Follicular cyst of ovary ♀
Cyst of graafian follicle

620.1 Corpus luteum cyst or hematoma ♀
Corpus luteum hemorrhage or rupture
Lutein cyst

620.2 Other and unspecified ovarian cyst ♀
Cyst of ovary:
NOS
corpus albicans
retention NOS
serous
theca-lutein
Simple cystoma of ovary
Excludes *cystadenoma (benign) (serous) (220)*
developmental cysts (752.0)
neoplastic cysts (220)
polycystic ovaries (256.4)
Stein-Leventhal syndrome (256.4)

620.3 Acquired atrophy of ovary and fallopian tube ♀
Senile involution of ovary

620.4 Prolapse or hernia of ovary and fallopian tube ♀
Displacement of ovary and fallopian tube
Salpingocele

620.5 Torsion of ovary, ovarian pedicle, or fallopian tube ♀
Torsion:
accessory tube
hydatid of Morgagni

620.6 Broad ligament laceration syndrome ♀
Masters-Allen syndrome

620.7 Hematoma of broad ligament ♀
Hematocele, broad ligament

620.8 Other noninflammatory disorders of ovary, fallopian tube, and broad ligament ♀
Cyst of broad ligament or fallopian tube
Hematosalpinx of ovary or fallopian tube
Infarction of ovary or fallopian tube
Polyp of broad ligament or fallopian tube
Rupture of ovary or fallopian tube
Excludes *hematosalpinx in ectopic pregnancy (639.2)*
peritubal adhesions (614.6)
torsion of ovary, ovarian pedicle, or fallopian tube (620.5)

620.9 Unspecified noninflammatory disorder of ovary, fallopian tube, and broad ligament ♀

4th **621 Disorders of uterus, not elsewhere classified**

621.0 Polyp of corpus uteri ♀
Polyp:
endometrium
uterus NOS
Excludes *cervical polyp NOS (622.7)*

621.1 Chronic subinvolution of uterus ♀
Excludes *puerperal (674.8)*

621.2 Hypertrophy of uterus ♀
Bulky or enlarged uterus
Excludes *puerperal (674.8)*

5th **621.3 Endometrial hyperplasia**
~~Hyperplasia (adenomatous) (cystic) (glandular) of endometrium~~
~~Hyperplastic endometritis~~

621.30 Endometrial hyperplasia, unspecified ♀
Endometrial hyperplasia NOS
Hyperplasia (adenomatous) (cystic) (glandular) of endometrium
Hyperplastic endometritis

621.31 Simple endometrial hyperplasia without atypia ♀
Excludes *benign endometrial hyperplasia (621.34)*

621.32 Complex endometrial hyperplasia without atypia ♀
Excludes *benign endometrial hyperplasia (621.34)*

621.33 Endometrial hyperplasia with atypia ♀
Excludes *endometrial intraepithelial neoplasia [EIN] (621.35)*

● **621.34 Benign endometrial hyperplasia**

Rationale: *In the past, both generalized endometrial hormonal responses and localized premalignant lesions were lumped under the general term "endometrial hyperplasia" with various modifiers such as mild, moderate, severe and atypical that had no uniform meaning. The 1994 4-class WHO hyperplasia diagnostic system which is based on a classic 1985 study (but in which some subsets of patients had very small numbers), subdivided "hyperplasias" by architectural complexity (simple versus complex) and cytologic atypia (present or absent). Although this practice has been widespread, and has had a benefit of unifying terminology, it fails to optimally stratify patients according to those pathologic mechanisms and cancer risks necessary to appropriate therapeutic triaging. Diagnoses are poorly reproducible. Recent molecular studies have shown that bona fide premalignant lesions are mutation-bearing monoclonal neoplasms, and computerized image analysis has defined new histologic features for their accurate diagnosis. For these reasons, pathologists and gynecologists are increasingly using a practically oriented disease classification that distinguishes the benign hormonal effects of unopposed estrogens (benign hyperplasia) from emergent precancerous lesions (endometrial intraepithelial neoplasia [EIN]) through the use of non-overlapping terminology and discrete criteria. The subset of largely polyclonal proliferations that result from a physiologic response of the endometrium to an abnormal estrogenic stimulus precisely fits the general definition of hyperplasia and is a benign process. In contrast, the clonal subset has the characteristics of a non-invasive neoplasm, and should be diagnosed as EIN. Compelling genetic, biologic, and histologic evidence supports the use of two diagnostic entities in lieu of a 4-group hyperplasia strategy.*

Revised diagnostic criteria must be associated with the new diagnostic terms to avoid confusion with legacy methods. This is the main reason that simple rebundling of subsets of the old "hyperplasias" into two clinicopathologic entities is not appropriate. Differing diagnostic criteria cannot be directly extrapolated to a contemporary diagnosis of EIN or benign endometrial hyperplasia. Additionally, ICD conventions and the need for longitudinal data integrity prohibit the deletion of existing ICD-9-CM codes or the changing of meaning of existing codes. And though EIN, rather than the 1994 hyperplasia schema, is what is now taught to pathologists and gynecologists in training, the old terminology is still used by older practicing physicians. For these reasons, two new codes have been added to subcategory 621.3, "Endometrial hyperplasia," for benign endometrial hyperplasia, and endometrial intraepithelial neoplasia [EIN]. These new codes are excluded from the previously appropriate existing codes. It is hoped that over time

619.8 – 621.34

documentation would migrate over to the use of the new terminology.

● **621.35 Endometrial intraepithelial neoplasia [EIN]**
Excludes *malignant neoplasm of endometrium with endometrial intraepithelial neoplasia [EIN] (182.0)*

621.4 Hematometra
Hemometra
Excludes *that in congenital anomaly (752.2-752.3)*

621.5 Intrauterine synechiae ♀
Adhesions of uterus
Band(s) of uterus

621.6 Malposition of uterus ♀
Anteversion of uterus
Retroflexion of uterus
Retroversion of uterus
Excludes *malposition complicating pregnancy, labor, or delivery (654.3-654.4)*
prolapse of uterus (618.1-618.4)

621.7 Chronic inversion of uterus ♀
Excludes *current obstetrical trauma (665.2)*
prolapse of uterus (618.1-618.4)

621.8 Other specified disorders of uterus, not elsewhere classified ♀
Atrophy, acquired of uterus
Cyst of uterus
Fibrosis NOS of uterus
Old laceration (postpartum) of uterus
Ulcer of uterus
Excludes *bilharzial fibrosis (120.0-120.9)*
endometriosis (617.0)
fistulas (619.0-619.8)
inflammatory diseases (615.0-615.9)

621.9 Unspecified disorder of uterus ♀

4th **622 Noninflammatory disorders of cervix**
Excludes *abnormality of cervix complicating pregnancy, labor, or delivery (654.5-654.6)*
fistula (619.0-619.8)

622.0 Erosion and ectropion of cervix ♀
Eversion of cervix
Ulcer of cervix
Excludes *that in chronic cervicitis (616.0)*

5th **622.1 Dysplasia of cervix (uteri)**
Excludes *abnormal results from cervical cytologic examination without histologic confirmation (795.00-795.09)*
carcinoma in situ of cervix (233.1)
cervical intraepithelial neoplasia III [CIN III] (233.1)
HGSIL of cervix (795.04)

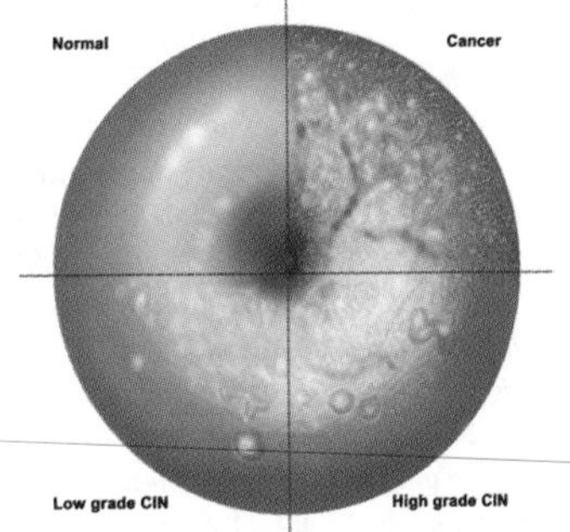

© 2008 Fairman Studios, LLC. All Rights Reserved.

622.10 Dysplasia of cervix, unspecified ♀
Anaplasia of cervix
Cervical atypism
Cervical dysplasia NOS

622.11 Mild dysplasia of cervix ♀
Cervical intraepithelial neoplasia I [CIN I]

622.12 Moderate dysplasia of cervix ♀
Cervical intraepithelial neoplasia II [CIN II]
Excludes *carcinoma in situ of cervix (233.1)*
cervical intraepithelial neoplasia III [CIN III] (233.1)
severe dysplasia (233.1)

622.2 Leukoplakia of cervix (uteri) ♀
Excludes *carcinoma in situ of cervix (233.1)*

622.3 Old laceration of cervix ♀
Adhesions of cervix
Band(s) of cervix
Cicatrix (postpartum) of cervix
Excludes *current obstetrical trauma (665.3)*

622.4 Stricture and stenosis of cervix ♀
Atresia (acquired) of cervix
Contracture of cervix
Occlusion of cervix
Pinpoint os uteri
Excludes *congenital (752.49)*
that complicating labor (654.6)

622.5 Incompetence of cervix ♀
Excludes *complicating pregnancy (654.5)*
that affecting fetus or newborn (761.0)

622.6 Hypertrophic elongation of cervix ♀

622.7 Mucous polyp of cervix ♀
Polyp NOS of cervix
Excludes *adenomatous polyp of cervix (219.0)*

622.8 Other specified noninflammatory disorders of cervix ♀
Atrophy (senile) of cervix
Cyst of cervix
Fibrosis of cervix
Hemorrhage of cervix
Excludes *endometriosis (617.0)*
fistula (619.0-619.8)
inflammatory diseases (616.0)

622.9 Unspecified noninflammatory disorder of cervix ♀

4th **623 Noninflammatory disorders of vagina**
Excludes *abnormality of vagina complicating pregnancy, labor, or delivery (654.7)*
congenital absence of vagina (752.49)
congenital diaphragm or bands (752.49)
fistulas involving vagina (619.0-619.8)

623.0 Dysplasia of vagina ♀
Mild and moderate dysplasia of vagina
Vaginal intraepithelial neoplasia I and II [VAIN I and II]
Excludes *abnormal results from vaginal cytological examination without histologic confirmation (795.10-795.19)*
carcinoma in situ of vagina (233.31)
HGSIL of vagina (795.14)
severe dysplasia of vagina (233.31)
vaginal intraepithelial neoplasia III [VAIN III] (233.31)

623.1 Leukoplakia of vagina ♀

623.2 Stricture or atresia of vagina ♀
Adhesions (postoperative) (postradiation) of vagina
Occlusion of vagina
Stenosis, vagina
Use additional E code to identify any external cause
Excludes *congenital atresia or stricture (752.49)*

623.3 **Tight hymenal ring** ♀
Rigid hymen acquired or congenital
Tight hymenal ring acquired or congenital
Tight introitus acquired or congenital
Excludes *imperforate hymen (752.42)*

623.4 **Old vaginal laceration** ♀
Excludes *old laceration involving muscles of pelvic floor (618.7)*

623.5 **Leukorrhea, not specified as infective** ♀
Leukorrhea NOS of vagina
Vaginal discharge NOS
Excludes *trichomonal (131.00)*

623.6 **Vaginal hematoma** ♀
Excludes *current obstetrical trauma (665.7)*

623.7 **Polyp of vagina** ♀

623.8 **Other specified noninflammatory disorders of vagina** ♀
Cyst of vagina
Hemorrhage of vagina

623.9 **Unspecified noninflammatory disorder of vagina**

4th 624 **Noninflammatory disorders of vulva and perineum**
Excludes *abnormality of vulva and perineum complicating pregnancy, labor, or delivery (654.8)*
condyloma acuminatum (078.11)
fistulas involving:
perineum – see Alphabetic Index
vulva (619.0-619.8)
vulval varices (456.6)
vulvar involvement in skin conditions (690-709.9)

5th 624.0 **Dystrophy of vulva**
Excludes *carcinoma in situ of vulva (233.32)*
severe dysplasia of vulva (233.32)
vulvar intraepithelial neoplasia III [VIN III] (233.32)

624.01 **Vulvar intraepithelial neoplasia I [VIN I]** ♀
Mild dysplasia of vulva

624.02 **Vulvar intraepithelial neoplasia II [VIN II]** ♀
Moderate dysplasia of vulva

624.09 **Other dystrophy of vulva** ♀
Kraurosis of vulva
Leukoplakia of vulva

624.1 **Atrophy of vulva** ♀

624.2 **Hypertrophy of clitoris** ♀
Excludes *that in endocrine disorders (255.2, 256.1)*

624.3 **Hypertrophy of labia** ♀
Hypertrophy of vulva NOS

624.4 **Old laceration or scarring of vulva** ♀

624.5 **Hematoma of vulva** ♀
Excludes *that complicating delivery (664.5)*

624.6 **Polyp of labia and vulva** ♀

624.8 **Other specified noninflammatory disorders of vulva and perineum** ♀
Cyst of vulva
Edema of vulva
Stricture of vulva

624.9 **Unspecified noninflammatory disorder of vulva and perineum** ♀

4th 625 **Pain and other symptoms associated with female genital organs**

625.0 **Dyspareunia** ♀
Excludes *psychogenic dyspareunia (302.76)*

625.1 **Vaginismus** ♀
Colpospasm
Vulvismus
Excludes *psychogenic vaginismus (306.51)*

625.2 **Mittelschmerz** ♀
Intermenstrual pain
Ovulation pain

625.3 **Dysmenorrhea** ♀
Painful menstruation
Excludes *psychogenic dysmenorrhea (306.52)*

625.4 **Premenstrual tension syndromes** ♀
Menstrual:
molimen
Premenstrual dysphoric disorder
Premenstrual syndrome
Premenstrual tension NOS
Excludes *menstrual migraine (346.4)*

625.5 **Pelvic congestion syndrome** ♀
Congestion-fibrosis syndrome
Taylor's syndrome

625.6 **Stress incontinence, female** 49, 50 ♀
N39.3 Stress incontinence (female) (male)
Excludes *mixed incontinence (788.33)*
stress incontinence, male (788.32)

© 2008 Fairman Studios, LLC. All Rights Reserved.

5th 625.7 **Vulvodynia**

625.70 **Vulvodynia, unspecified** ♀
Vulvodynia NOS

625.71 **Vulvar vestibulitis** ♀

625.79 **Other vulvodynia** ♀

625.8 **Other specified symptoms associated female genital organs** ♀

625.9 **Unspecified symptom associated with female genital organs** ♀
R39.8 Other symptoms and signs involving the genitourinary system

4th 626 **Disorders of menstruation and other abnormal bleeding from female genital tract**
Excludes *menopausal and premenopausal bleeding (627.0)*
pain and other symptoms associated with menstrual cycle (625.2-625.4)
postmenopausal bleeding (627.1)

626.0 **Absence of menstruation** ♀
Amenorrhea (primary) (secondary)

626.1 **Scanty or infrequent menstruation** ♀
Hypomenorrhea
Oligomenorrhea

626.2 **Excessive or frequent menstruation** ♀
Heavy periods
Menometrorrhagia
Menorrhagia
Polymenorrhea
Excludes *premenopausal (627.0)*
that in puberty (626.3)

623.3 – 626.2

626.3 **Puberty bleeding** ♀
Excessive bleeding associated with onset of menstrual periods
Pubertal menorrhagia

626.4 **Irregular menstrual cycle** ♀
Irregular:
bleeding NOS
menstruation
periods

626.5 **Ovulation bleeding** ♀
Regular intermenstrual bleeding

626.6 **Metrorrhagia** ♀
Bleeding unrelated to menstrual cycle
Irregular intermenstrual bleeding

626.7 **Postcoital bleeding** ♀

626.8 **Other** ♀
Dysfunctional or functional uterine hemorrhage NOS
Menstruation:
retained
suppression of

626.9 **Unspecified** ♀

4th 627 **Menopausal and postmenopausal disorders**
Excludes *asymptomatic age-related (natural) postmenopausal status (V49.81)*

627.0 **Premenopausal menorrhagia** ♀
Excessive bleeding associated with onset of menopause
Menorrhagia:
climacteric
menopausal
preclimacteric

627.1 **Postmenopausal bleeding** ♀
N95.0 Postmenopausal bleeding

627.2 **Symptomatic menopausal or female climacteric states** ♀
N95.11 Symptomatic menopausal state
Symptoms, such as flushing, sleeplessness, headache, lack of concentration, associated with the menopause
Layman's: *"Hot flashes," "night sweats" and mood swings attributed to menopause are some of the most common symptoms properly coded with 627.2.*

627.3 **Postmenopausal atrophic vaginitis** ♀
N95.2 Postmenopausal atrophic vaginitis
Senile (atrophic) vaginitis

627.4 **Symptomatic states associated with artificial menopause** ♀
Postartificial menopause syndromes
Any condition classifiable to 627.1, 627.2, or 627.3 which follows induced menopause

627.8 **Other specified menopausal and postmenopausal disorders** ♀
Excludes *premature menopause NOS (256.31)*

627.9 **Unspecified menopausal and postmenopausal disorder** ♀

4th 628 **Infertility, female**
Includes primary and secondary sterility

628.0 **Associated with anovulation** ♀
Anovulatory cycle
Use additional code for any associated Stein-Leventhal syndrome (256.4)

628.1 ***Of pituitary-hypothalamic origin*** ♀
Code first underlying disease, as:
adiposogenital dystrophy (253.8)
anterior pituitary disorder (253.0-253.4)

628.2 **Of tubal origin** ♀
Infertility associated with congenital anomaly of tube
Tubal:
block
occlusion
stenosis
Use additional code for any associated peritubal adhesions (614.6)

628.3 **Of uterine origin** ♀
Infertility associated with congenital anomaly of uterus
Nonimplantation
Use additional code for any associated tuberculous endometritis (016.7)

628.4 **Of cervical or vaginal origin** ♀
Infertility associated with:
anomaly or cervical mucus
congenital structural anomaly
dysmucorrhea

628.8 **Of other specified origin** ♀

628.9 **Of unspecified origin** ♀

4th 629 **Other disorders of female genital organs**

629.0 **Hematocele, female, not elsewhere classified** ♀
Excludes *hematocele or hematoma:*
broad ligament (620.7)
fallopian tube (620.8)
that associated with ectopic pregnancy (633.00-633.91)
uterus (621.4)
vagina (623.6)
vulva (624.5)

629.1 **Hydrocele, canal of Nuck** ♀
Cyst of canal of Nuck (acquired)
Excludes *congenital (752.41)*

5th 629.2 **Female genital mutilation status**
Female circumsion status
Female genital cutting

629.20 **Female genital mutilation status, unspecified** ♀
Female genital mutilation status NOS
Female genital cutting status, unspecified

629.21 **Female genital mutilation Type I status** ♀
Clitorectomy status
Female genital cutting Type I status

629.22 **Female genital mutilation Type II status** ♀
Clitorectomy with excision of labia minora status
Female genital cutting Type II status

629.23 **Female genital mutilation Type III status** ♀
Female genital cutting Type III status
Infibulation status

629.29 **Other female genital mutilation status** ♀
Female genital cutting Type IV status
Female genital mutilation Type IV status
Other female genital cutting status

5th 629.8 **Other specified disorders of female genital organs**

629.81 **Habitual aborter without current pregnancy** ♀
Excludes *habitual aborter with current pregnancy (646.3)*

629.89 **Other specified disorders of female genital organs** ♀

629.9 **Unspecified disorder of female genital organs** ♀

11. COMPLICATIONS OF PREGNANCY, CHILDBIRTH, AND THE PUERPERIUM (630-679)

ICD-9-CM Official Guidelines (Chapter 11):

a. General Rules for Obstetric Cases

1) Codes from chapter 11 and sequencing priority

Obstetric cases require codes from chapter 11, codes in the range 630-677, Complications of Pregnancy, Childbirth, and the Puerperium. Chapter 11 codes have sequencing priority over codes from other chapters. Additional codes from other chapters may be used in conjunction with chapter 11 codes to further specify conditions. Should the provider document that the pregnancy is incidental to the encounter, then code V22.2 should be used in place of any chapter 11 codes. It is the provider's responsibility to state that the condition being treated is not affecting the pregnancy.

2) Chapter 11 codes used only on the maternal record

Chapter 11 codes are to be used only on the maternal record, never on the record of the newborn....

b. Selection of OB Principal or First-listed Diagnosis

1) Routine outpatient prenatal visits

For routine outpatient prenatal visits when no complications are present codes V22.0, Supervision of normal first pregnancy, and V22.1, Supervision of other normal pregnancy, should be used as the first-listed diagnoses. These codes should not be used in conjunction with chapter 11 codes.

2) Prenatal outpatient visits for high-risk patients

For prenatal outpatient visits for patients with high-risk pregnancies, a code from category V23, Supervision of high-risk pregnancy, should be used as the first-listed diagnosis. Secondary chapter 11 codes may be used in conjunction with these codes if appropriate.

3) Episodes when no delivery occurs

In episodes when no delivery occurs, the principal diagnosis should correspond to the principal complication of the pregnancy, which necessitated the encounter. Should more than one complication exist, all of which are treated or monitored, any of the complications codes may be sequenced first.

4) When a delivery occurs

When a delivery occurs, the principal diagnosis should correspond to the main circumstances or complication of the delivery. In cases of cesarean delivery, the selection of the principal diagnosis should correspond to the reason the cesarean delivery was performed unless the reason for admission/ encounter was unrelated to the condition resulting in the cesarean delivery.

5) Outcome of delivery

An outcome of delivery code, V27.0-V27.9, should be included on every maternal record when a delivery has occurred. These codes are not to be used on subsequent records or on the newborn record.

ECTOPIC AND MOLAR PREGNANCY (630-633)

Use additional code from category 639 to identify any complications

630 Hydatidiform mole M ♀
- Trophoblastic disease NOS
- Vesicular mole

Excludes *chorioadenoma (destruens) (236.1)*
chorionepithelioma (181)
malignant hydatidiform mole (236.1)

631 Other abnormal product of conception M ♀
- Blighted ovum
- Mole:
  - NOS
  - carneous
  - fleshy
  - stone

632 Missed abortion M ♀
- Early fetal death before completion of 22 weeks' gestation with retention of dead fetus
- Retained products of conception, not following spontaneous or induced abortion or delivery

Excludes *failed induced abortion (638.0-638.9)*
fetal death (intrauterine) (late) (656.4)
missed delivery (656.4)
that with abnormal product of conception (630, 631)

4th **633 Ectopic pregnancy**

Includes ruptured ectopic pregnancy

5th **633.0 Abdominal pregnancy** M ♀
- Intraperitoneal pregnancy

633.00 Abdominal pregnancy without intrauterine pregnancy

633.01 Abdominal pregnancy with intrauterine pregnancy

5th **633.1 Tubal pregnancy**
- Fallopian pregnancy
- Rupture of (fallopian) tube due to pregnancy
- Tubal abortion

633.10 Tubal pregnancy without intrauterine pregnancy M ♀

633.11 Tubal pregnancy with intrauterine pregnancy M ♀

5th **633.2 Ovarian pregnancy**

633.20 Ovarian pregnancy without intrauterine pregnancy M ♀

633.21 Ovarian pregnancy with intrauterine pregnancy M ♀

5th **633.8 Other ectopic pregnancy**
- Pregnancy:
  - cervical
  - combined
  - cornual
  - intraligamentous
  - mesometric
  - mural

633.80 Other ectopic pregnancy without intrauterine pregnancy M ♀

633.81 Other ectopic pregnancy with intrauterine pregnancy M ♀

5th **633.9 Unspecified ectopic pregnancy**

633.90 Unspecified ectopic pregnancy without intrauterine pregnancy M ♀

633.91 Unspecified ectopic pregnancy with intrauterine pregnancy M ♀

630 – 633.91

OTHER PREGNANCY WITH ABORTIVE OUTCOME (634-639)

The following fourth digit subdivisions are for use with categories 634-638:

.0 Complicated by genital tract and pelvic infection
Endometritis
Salpingo-oophoritis
Sepsis NOS
Septicemia NOS
Any condition classifiable to 639.0, with condition classifiable to 634-638
Excludes *urinary tract infection (634-638 with .7)*

.1 Complicated by delayed or excessive hemorrhage
Afibrinogenemia
Defibrination syndrome
Intravascular hemolysis
Any condition classifiable to 639.1, with condition classifiable to 634-638

.2 Complicated by damage to pelvic organs and tissues
Laceration, perforation, or tear of:
bladder
uterus
Any condition classifiable to 639.2, with condition classifiable to 634-638

.3 Complicated by renal failure
Oliguria
Uremia
Any condition classifiable to 639.3, with condition classifiable to 634-638

.4 Complicated by metabolic disorder
Electrolyte imbalance with conditions classifiable to 634-638

.5 Complicated by shock
Circulatory collapse
Shock (postoperative) (septic)
Any condition classifiable to 639.5, with condition classifiable to 634-638

.6 Complicated by embolism
Embolism:
NOS
amniotic fluid
pulmonary
Any condition classifiable to 639.6, with condition classifiable to 634-638

.7 With other specified complications
Cardiac arrest or failure
Urinary tract infection
Any condition classifiable to 639.8, with condition classifiable to 634-638

.8 With unspecified complications

.9 Without mention of complication

ICD-9-CM Official Guidelines (Chapter 11):

k. Abortions

*1) **Fifth-digits required for abortion categories***
Fifth-digits are required for abortion categories 634-637. Fifth-digit 1, incomplete, indicates that all of the products of conception have not been expelled from the uterus. Fifth-digit 2, complete, indicates that all products of conception have been expelled from the uterus prior to the episode of care.

*2) **Code from categories 640-648 and 651-659***
A code from categories 640-648 and 651-659 may be used as additional codes with an abortion code to indicate the complication leading to the abortion....

*3) **Code 639 for complications***
Code 639 is to be used for all complications following abortion. Code 639 cannot be assigned with codes from categories 634-638....

*5) **Retained Products of Conception following an abortion***
Subsequent admissions for retained products of conception following a spontaneous or legally induced abortion are assigned the appropriate code from category 634, Spontaneous abortion, or 635 Legally induced abortion, with a fifth digit of "1" (incomplete). This advice is appropriate even when the patient was discharged previously with a discharge diagnosis of complete abortion.

4th 634 Spontaneous abortion
Includes miscarriage
spontaneous abortion

Requires fifth digit to identify stage:
0 unspecified
1 incomplete
2 complete

5th **634.0 Complicated by genital tract and pelvic infection** M ♀
[0-2]
5th **634.1 Complicated by delayed or excessive hemorrhage** M ♀
[0-2]
5th **634.2 Complicated by damage to pelvic organs or tissues** M ♀
[0-2]
5th **634.3 Complicated by renal failure** M ♀
[0-2]
5th **634.4 Complicated by metabolic disorder** M ♀
[0-2]
5th **634.5 Complicated by shock** M ♀
[0-2]
5th **634.6 Complicated by embolism** M ♀
[0-2]
5th **634.7 With other specified complications** M ♀
[0-2]
5th **634.8 With unspecified complication** M ♀
[0-2]
5th **634.9 Without mention of complication** M ♀
[0-2]

4th 635 Legally induced abortion
Includes abortion or termination of pregnancy:
elective
legal
therapeutic
Excludes *menstrual extraction or regulation (V25.3)*

Requires fifth digit to identify stage:
0 unspecified
1 incomplete
2 complete

5th **635.0 Complicated by genital tract and pelvic infection** M ♀
[0-2]
5th **635.1 Complicated by delayed or excessive hemorrhage** M ♀
[0-2]
5th **635.2 Complicated by damage to pelvic organs or tissues** M ♀
[0-2]
5th **635.3 Complicated by renal failure** M ♀
[0-2]
5th **635.4 Complicated by metabolic disorder** M ♀
[0-2]
5th **635.5 Complicated by shock** M ♀
[0-2]
5th **635.6 Complicated by embolism** M ♀
[0-2]
5th **635.7 With other specified complications** M ♀
[0-2]
5th **635.8 With unspecified complication** M ♀
[0-2]

5th 635.9 **Without mention of complication** M ♀
[0-2]

4th 636 **Illegally induced abortion**

Includes abortion:
criminal
illegal
self-induced

Requires fifth digit to identify stage:
0 unspecified
1 incomplete
2 complete

5th 636.0 **Complicated by genital tract and pelvic infection** M ♀
[0-2]

5th 636.1 **Complicated by delayed or excessive hemorrhage** M ♀
[0-2]

5th 636.2 **Complicated by damage to pelvic organs or tissues** M ♀
[0-2]

5th 636.3 **Complicated by renal failure** M ♀
[0-2]

5th 636.4 **Complicated by metabolic disorder** M ♀
[0-2]

5th 636.5 **Complicated by shock** M ♀
[0-2]

5th 636.6 **Complicated by embolism** M ♀
[0-2]

5th 636.7 **With other specified complications** M ♀
[0-2]

5th 636.8 **With unspecified complication** M ♀
[0-2]

5th 636.9 **Without mention of complication** M ♀
[0-2]

4th 637 **Unspecified abortion**

Includes abortion NOS
retained products of conception following abortion, not classifiable elsewhere

Requires fifth digit to identify stage:
0 unspecified
1 incomplete
2 complete

5th 637.0 **Complicated by genital tract and pelvic infection** M ♀
[0-2]

5th 637.1 **Complicated by delayed or excessive hemorrhage** M ♀
[0-2]

5th 637.2 **Complicated by damage to pelvic organs or tissues** M ♀
[0-2]

5th 637.3 **Complicated by renal failure** M ♀
[0-2]

5th 637.4 **Complicated by metabolic disorder** M ♀
[0-2]

5th 637.5 **Complicated by shock** M ♀
[0-2]

5th 637.6 **Complicated by embolism** M ♀
[0-2]

5th 637.7 **With other specified complications** M ♀
[0-2]

5th 637.8 **With unspecified complication** M ♀
[0-2]

5th 637.9 **Without mention of complication** M ♀
[0-2]

4th 638 **Failed attempted abortion**

Includes failure of attempted induction of (legal) abortion

Excludes *incomplete abortion (634.0-637.9)*

638.0 **Complicated by genital tract and pelvic infection** M ♀

638.1 **Complicated by delayed or excessive hemorrhage** M ♀

638.2 **Complicated by damage to pelvic organs or tissues** M ♀

638.3 **Complicated by renal failure** M ♀

638.4 **Complicated by metabolic disorder** M ♀

638.5 **Complicated by shock** M ♀

638.6 **Complicated by embolism** M ♀

638.7 **With other specified complications** M ♀

638.8 **With unspecified complication** M ♀

638.9 **Without mention of complication** M ♀

4th 639 **Complications following abortion and ectopic and molar pregnancies**

Note: *This category is provided for use when it is required to classify separately the complications classifiable to the fourth digit level in categories 634-638; for example:*

a) when the complication itself was responsible for an episode of medical care, the abortion, ectopic or molar pregnancy itself having been dealt with at a previous episode

b) when these conditions are immediate complications of ectopic or molar pregnancies classifiable to 630-633 where they cannot be identified at fourth digit level.

ICD-9-CM Official Guidelines (Chapter 11):

k. Abortions

3) Code 639 for complications

Code 639 is to be used for all complications following abortion. Code 639 cannot be assigned with codes from categories 634-638.

639.0 **Genital tract and pelvic infection** M ♀

Endometritis following conditions classifiable to 630-638
Parametritis following conditions classifiable to 630-638
Pelvic peritonitis following conditions classifiable to 630-638
Salpingitis following conditions classifiable to 630-638
Salpingo-oophoritis following conditions classifiable to 630-638
Sepsis NOS following conditions classifiable to 630-638
Septicemia NOS following conditions classifiable to 630-638

Excludes *urinary tract infection (639.8)*

639.1 **Delayed or excessive hemorrhage** M ♀

Afibrinogenemia following conditions classifiable to 630-638
Defibrination syndrome following conditions classifiable to 630-638
Intravascular hemolysis following conditions classifiable to 630-638

639.2 **Damage to pelvic organs and tissues** M ♀

Laceration, perforation, or tear of:
bladder following conditions classifiable to 630-638
bowel following conditions classifiable to 630-638
broad ligament following conditions classifiable to 630-638
cervix following conditions classifiable to 630-638
periurethral tissue following conditions classifiable to 630-638
uterus following conditions classifiable to 630-638
vagina following conditions classifiable to 630-638

▲639.3 **Kidney ~~renal~~ failure** M ♀
Oliguria following conditions classifiable to 630-638
Renal (kidney):
failure (acute) following conditions classifiable to 630-638
shutdown following conditions classifiable to 630-638
tubular necrosis following conditions classifiable to 630-638
Uremia following conditions classifiable to 630-638

639.4 **Metabolic disorders** M ♀
Electrolyte imbalance following conditions classifiable to 630-638

639.5 **Shock** M ♀
Circulatory collapse following conditions classifiable to 630-638
Shock (postoperative) (septic) following conditions classifiable to 630-638

639.6 **Embolism** M ♀
Embolism:
NOS following conditions classifiable to 630-638
air following conditions classifiable to 630-638
amniotic fluid following conditions classifiable to 630-638
blood-clot following conditions classifiable to 630-638
fat following conditions classifiable to 630-638
pulmonary following conditions classifiable to 630-638
pyemic following conditions classifiable to 630-638
septic following conditions classifiable to 630-638
soap following conditions classifiable to 630-638

639.8 **Other specified complications following abortion or ectopic and molar pregnancy** M ♀
Acute yellow atrophy or necrosis of liver following conditions classifiable to 630-638
Cardiac arrest or failure following conditions classifiable to 630-638
Cerebral anoxia following conditions classifiable to 630-638
Urinary tract infection following conditions classifiable to 630-638

639.9 **Unspecified complication following abortion or ectopic and molar pregnancy** M ♀
Complication(s) not further specified following conditions classifiable to 630-638

COMPLICATIONS MAINLY RELATED TO PREGNANCY (640-649)

Includes the listed conditions even if they arose or were present during labor, delivery, or the puerperium

The following fifth-digit subclassification is for use with categories 640-649 to denote the current episode of care:

0 **unspecified as to episode of care or not applicable**
1 **delivered, with or without mention of antepartum condition**
Antepartum condition with delivery
Delivery NOS (with mention of antepartum complication during current episode of care)
Intrapartum obstetric condition (with mention of antepartum complication during current episode of care)
Pregnancy, delivered (with mention of antepartum complication during current episode of care)
2 **delivered, with mention of postpartum complication**
Delivery with mention of puerperal complication during current episode of care
3 **antepartum condition or complication**
Antepartum obstetric condition, not delivered during the current episode of care
4 **postpartum condition or complication**
Postpartum or puerperal obstetric condition or complication following delivery that occurred:
during previous episode of care
outside hospital, with subsequent admission for observation or care

ICD-9-CM Official Guidelines (Chapter 11):

a. General Rules for Obstetric Cases

3) Chapter 11 fifth-digits

Categories 640-649, 651-676 have required fifth-digits, which indicate whether the encounter is antepartum, postpartum and whether a delivery has also occurred.

4) Fifth-digits, appropriate for each code

The fifth-digits, which are appropriate for each code number, are listed in brackets under each code. The fifth-digits on each code should all be consistent with each other. That is, should a delivery occur all of the fifth-digits should indicate the delivery.

k. Abortions

2) Code from categories 640-648 and 651-659

A code from categories 640-648 and 651-659 may be used as additional codes with an abortion code to indicate the complication leading to the abortion.

Fifth digit 3 is assigned with codes from these categories when used with an abortion code because the other fifth digits will not apply.

4th 640 **Hemorrhage in early pregnancy**
Requires fifth digit; valid digits are in [brackets] under each code. See beginning of section 640-649 for definitions.
Includes hemorrhage before completion of 22 weeks' gestation

5th 640.0 **Threatened abortion** M ♀
[0,1,3]

5th 640.8 **Other specified hemorrhage in early pregnancy** M ♀
[0,1,3]

5th 640.9 **Unspecified hemorrhage in early pregnancy** M ♀
[0,1,3]

4th 641 Antepartum hemorrhage, abruptio placentae, and placenta previa

Requires fifth digit; valid digits are in [brackets] under each code. See beginning of section 640-649 for definitions.

5th 641.0 Placenta previa without hemorrhage M ♀

[0,1,3] Low implantation of placenta without hemorrhage
Placenta previa noted:
during pregnancy without hemorrhage
before labor (and delivered by cesarean delivery) without hemorrhage

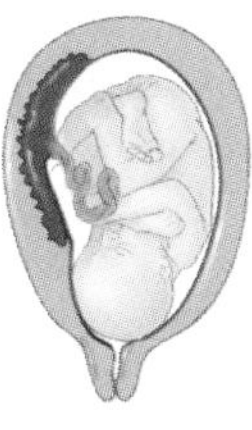

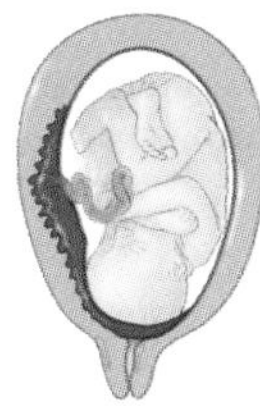

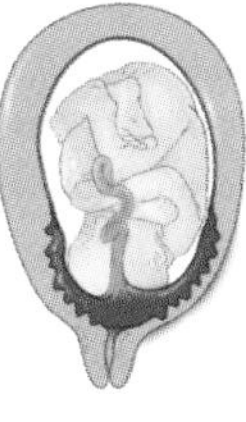

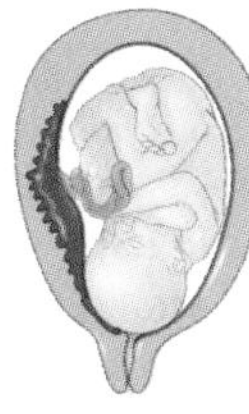

© 2008 Fairman Studios, LLC. All Rights Reserved.

5th 641.1 Hemorrhage from placenta previa M ♀

[0,1,3] Low implantation of placenta NOS or with hemorrhage (intrapartum)
Placenta previa:
incomplete NOS or with hemorrhage (intrapartum)
marginal NOS or with hemorrhage (intrapartum)
partial NOS or with hemorrhage (intrapartum)
total NOS or with hemorrhage (intrapartum)

Excludes *hemorrhage from vasa previa (663.5)*

5th 641.2 Premature separation of placenta M ♀

[0,1,3] Ablatio placentae
Abruptio placentae
Accidental antepartum hemorrhage
Couvelaire uterus
Detachment of placenta (premature)
Premature separation of normally implanted placenta

5th 641.3 Antepartum hemorrhage associated with coagulation defects M ♀

[0,1,3] Antepartum or intrapartum hemorrhage associated with:
afibrinogenemia
hyperfibrinolysis
hypofibrinogenemia

Excludes *coagulation defects not associated with antepartum hemorrhage (649.3)*

5th 641.8 Other antepartum hemorrhage M ♀

[0,1,3] Antepartum or intrapartum hemorrhage associated with:
trauma
uterine leiomyoma

5th 641.9 Unspecified antepartum hemorrhage M ♀

[0,1,3] Hemorrhage:
antepartum NOS
intrapartum NOS
of pregnancy NOS

4th 642 Hypertension complicating pregnancy, childbirth, and the puerperium

Requires fifth digit; valid digits are in [brackets] under each code. See beginning of section 640-649 for definitions.

5th 642.0 Benign essential hypertension complicating pregnancy, childbirth, and the puerperium M ♀

[0-4] Hypertension:
benign essential specified as complicating, or as a reason for obstetric care during pregnancy, childbirth, or the puerperium
chronic NOS specified as complicating, or as a reason for obstetric care during pregnancy, childbirth, or the puerperium
essential specified as complicating, or as a reason for obstetric care during pregnancy, childbirth, or the puerperium
pre-existing NOS specified as complicating, or as a reason for obstetric care during pregnancy, childbirth, or the puerperium

5th 642.1 Hypertension secondary to renal disease, complicating pregnancy, childbirth, and the puerperium M ♀

[0-4] Hypertension secondary to renal disease, specified as complicating, or as a reason for obstetric care during pregnancy, childbirth, or the puerperium

5th 642.2 Other pre-existing hypertension complicating pregnancy, childbirth, and the puerperium M ♀

[0-4] Hypertensive:
chronic kidney disease specified as complicating, or as a reason for obstetric care during pregnancy, childbirth, or the puerperium
heart and chronic kidney disease specified as complicating, or as a reason for obstetric care during pregnancy, childbirth, or the puerperium
heart disease specified as complicating, or as a reason for obstetric care during pregnancy, childbirth, or the puerperium
Malignant hypertension specified as complicating, or as a reason for obstetric care during pregnancy, childbirth, or the puerperium

5th 642.3 Transient hypertension of pregnancy M ♀

[0-4] Gestational hypertension
Transient hypertension, so described, in pregnancy, childbirth, or the puerperium

5th 642.4 Mild or unspecified pre-eclampsia M ♀

[0-4] Hypertension in pregnancy, childbirth, or the puerperium, not specified as pre-existing, with either albuminuria or edema, or both; mild or unspecified
Pre-eclampsia:
NOS
mild
Toxemia (pre-eclamptic):
NOS
mild

Excludes *albuminuria in pregnancy, without mention of hypertension (646.2)*
edema in pregnancy, without mention of hypertension (646.1)

5th 642.5 Severe pre-eclampsia M ♀

[0-4] Hypertension in pregnancy, childbirth, or the puerperium, not specified as pre-existing, with either albuminuria or edema, or both; specified as severe
Pre-eclampsia, severe
Toxemia (pre-eclamptic), severe

5th 642.6 Eclampsia M ♀

[0-4] Toxemia:
eclamptic
with convulsions

5th 642.7 **Pre-eclampsia or eclampsia superimposed on pre-existing hypertension** M ♀
[0-4] Conditions classifiable to 642.4-642.6, with conditions classifiable to 642.0-642.2

5th 642.9 **Unspecified hypertension complicating pregnancy, childbirth, or the puerperium** M ♀
[0-4] Hypertension NOS, without mention of albuminuria or edema, complicating pregnancy, childbirth, or the puerperium

4th 643 **Excessive vomiting in pregnancy**
Requires fifth digit; valid digits are in [brackets] under each code. See beginning of section 640-649 for definitions.
Includes hyperemesis arising during pregnancy
hyperemesis gravidarum
vomiting:
persistent arising during pregnancy
vicious arising during pregnancy

5th 643.0 **Mild hyperemesis gravidarum** M ♀
[0,1,3] Hyperemesis gravidarum, mild or unspecified, starting before the end of the 22nd week of gestation

5th 643.1 **Hyperemesis gravidarum with metabolic disturbance** M ♀
[0,1,3] Hyperemesis gravidarum, starting before the end of the 22nd week of gestation, with metabolic disturbance, such as:
carbohydrate depletion
dehydration
electrolyte imbalance

5th 643.2 **Late vomiting of pregnancy** M ♀
[0,1,3] Excessive vomiting starting after 22 completed weeks of gestation

5th 643.8 **Other vomiting complicating pregnancy** M ♀
[0,1,3] Vomiting due to organic disease or other cause, specified as complicating pregnancy, or as a reason for obstetric care during pregnancy
Use additional code to specify cause

5th 643.9 **Unspecified vomiting of pregnancy** M ♀
[0,1,3] Vomiting as a reason for care during pregnancy, length of gestation unspecified

4th 644 **Early or threatened labor**
Requires fifth digit; valid digits are in [brackets] under each code. See beginning of section 640-649 for definitions.

5th 644.0 **Threatened premature labor** M ♀
[0,3] Premature labor after 22 weeks, but before 37 completed weeks of gestation without delivery
Excludes *that occurring before 22 completed weeks of gestation (640.0)*

5th 644.1 **Other threatened labor** M ♀
[0,3] False labor:
NOS without delivery
after 37 completed weeks of gestation without delivery
Threatened labor NOS without delivery

5th 644.2 **Early onset of delivery** M ♀
[0-1] Onset (spontaneous) of delivery before 37 completed weeks of gestation
Premature labor with onset of delivery before 37 completed weeks of gestation

ICD-9-CM Official Guidelines (Chapter 11):
k. Abortions
4) Abortion with Liveborn Fetus
When an attempted termination of pregnancy results in a liveborn fetus assign code 644.21, Early onset of delivery, with an appropriate code from category V27, Outcome of Delivery. The procedure code for the attempted termination of pregnancy should also be assigned.

4th 645 **Late pregnancy**
Requires fifth digit; valid digits are in [brackets] under each code. See beginning of section 640-649 for definitions.

5th 645.1 **Post term pregnancy** M ♀
[0,1,3] Pregnancy over 40 completed weeks to 42 completed weeks gestation

5th 645.2 **Prolonged pregnancy** M ♀
[0,1,3] Pregnancy which has advanced beyond 42 completed weeks of gestation

4th 646 **Other complications of pregnancy, not elsewhere classified**
Use additional code(s) to further specify complication
Requires fifth digit; valid digits are in [brackets] under each code. See beginning of section 640-649 for definitions.

5th 646.0 **Papyraceous fetus** M ♀
[0,1,3]

5th 646.1 **Edema or excessive weight gain in pregnancy, without mention of hypertension** M ♀
[0-4] Gestational edema
Maternal obesity syndrome
Excludes *that with mention of hypertension (642.0-642.9)*

5th 646.2 **Unspecified renal disease in pregnancy, without mention of hypertension** M ♀
[0-4] Albuminuria in pregnancy or the puerperium, without mention of hypertension
Gestational proteinuria
Nephropathy NOS in pregnancy or the puerperium, without mention of hypertension
Renal disease NOS in pregnancy or the puerperium, without mention of hypertension
Uremia in pregnancy or the puerperium, without mention of hypertension
Excludes *that with mention of hypertension (642.0-642.9)*

5th 646.3 **Habitual aborter** M ♀
[0,1,3]
Excludes *with current abortion (634.0-634.9)*
without current pregnancy (629.81)

5th 646.4 **Peripheral neuritis in pregnancy** M ♀
[0-4]

5th 646.5 **Asymptomatic bacteriuria in pregnancy** M ♀
[0-4]

5th 646.6 **Infections of genitourinary tract in pregnancy** M ♀
[0-4] Conditions classifiable to 590, 595, 597, 599.0, 616 complicating pregnancy, childbirth, or the puerperium
Conditions classifiable to 614.0-614.5, 614.7-614.9, 615 complicating pregnancy or labor
Excludes *major puerperal infection (670.0-670.8)*

5th 646.7 **Liver disorders in pregnancy** M ♀
[0,1,3] Acute yellow atrophy of liver (obstetric) (true) of pregnancy
Icterus gravis of pregnancy
Necrosis of liver of pregnancy
Excludes *hepatorenal syndrome following delivery (674.8)*
viral hepatitis (647.6)

5th 646.8 **Other specified complications of pregnancy** M ♀
[0-4] Fatigue during pregnancy
Herpes gestationis
Insufficient weight gain of pregnancy

5th 646.9 **Unspecified complication of pregnancy** M ♀
[0,1,3]

4th 647 Infectious and parasitic conditions in the mother classifiable elsewhere, but complicating pregnancy, childbirth, or the puerperium

Requires fifth digit; valid digits are in [brackets] under each code. See beginning of section 640-649 for definitions.

Includes the listed conditions when complicating the pregnant state, aggravated by the pregnancy, or when a main reason for obstetric care

Use additional code(s) to further specify complication

Excludes *those conditions in the mother known or suspected to have affected the fetus (655.0-655.9)*

5th 647.0 Syphilis M ♀
[0-4] Conditions classifiable to 090-097

5th 647.1 Gonorrhea M ♀
[0-4] Conditions classifiable to 098

5th 647.2 Other venereal diseases M ♀
[0-4] Conditions classifiable to 099

5th 647.3 Tuberculosis M ♀
[0-4] Conditions classifiable to 010-018

5th 647.4 Malaria M ♀
[0-4] Conditions classifiable to 084

5th 647.5 Rubella M ♀
[0-4] Conditions classifiable to 056

5th 647.6 Other viral diseases M ♀
[0-4] Conditions classifiable to 042 and 050-055, 057-079, 795.05, 795.15, 796.75

ICD-9-CM Official Guidelines (Chapter 11):

d. HIV Infection in Pregnancy, Childbirth and the Puerperium

During pregnancy, childbirth or the puerperium, a patient admitted because of an HIV-related illness should receive a principal diagnosis of 647.6x, Other specified infectious and parasitic diseases in the mother classifiable elsewhere, but complicating the pregnancy, childbirth or the puerperium, followed by 042 and the code(s) for the HIV-related illness(es).

Patients with asymptomatic HIV infection status admitted during pregnancy, childbirth, or the puerperium should receive codes of 647.6x and V08.

5th 647.8 Other specified infectious and parasitic diseases M ♀
[0-4]

5th 647.9 Unspecified infection or infestation M ♀
[0-4]

4th 648 Other current conditions in the mother classifiable elsewhere, but complicating pregnancy, childbirth, or the puerperium

Requires fifth digit; valid digits are in [brackets] under each code. See beginning of section 640-649 for definitions.

Includes the listed conditions when complicating the pregnant state, aggravated by the pregnancy, or when a main reason for obstetric care

Use additional code(s) to identify the condition

Excludes *those conditions in the mother known or suspected to have affected the fetus (655.0-655.9)*

ICD-9-CM Official Guidelines (Chapter 11):

e. Current Conditions Complicating Pregnancy

Assign a code from subcategory 648.x for patients that have current conditions when the condition affects the management of the pregnancy, childbirth, or the puerperium. Use additional secondary codes from other chapters to identify the conditions, as appropriate.

5th 648.0 Diabetes mellitus 1, 2, 3, 117, 118, 119, 163 M ♀
[0-4] Conditions classifiable to 249, 250

Excludes *gestational diabetes (648.8)*

ICD-9-CM Official Guidelines (Chapter 11):

f. Diabetes mellitus in pregnancy

Diabetes mellitus is a significant complicating factor in pregnancy. Pregnant women who are diabetic should be assigned code 648.0x, Diabetes mellitus complicating pregnancy, and a secondary code from category 250, Diabetes mellitus, or category 249, Secondary diabetes to identify the type of diabetes.

Code V58.67, Long-term (current) use of insulin, should also be assigned if the diabetes mellitus is being treated with insulin.

5th 648.1 Thyroid dysfunction M ♀
[0-4] Conditions classifiable to 240-246

5th 648.2 Anemia M ♀
[0-4] Conditions classifiable to 280-285

5th 648.3 Drug dependence M ♀
[0-4] Conditions classifiable to 304

5th 648.4 Mental disorders M ♀
[0-4] Conditions classifiable to 290-303, 305.0, 305.2-305.9, 306-316, 317-319

5th 648.5 Congenital cardiovascular disorders M ♀
[0-4] Conditions classifiable to 745-747

5th 648.6 Other cardiovascular diseases M ♀
[0-4] Conditions classifiable to 390-398, 410-429

Excludes *cerebrovascular disorders in the puerperium (674.0)*
peripartum cardiomyopathy (674.5)
venous complications (671.0-671.9)

5th 648.7 Bone and joint disorders of back, pelvis, and lower limbs M ♀
[0-4] Conditions classifiable to 720-724, and those classifiable to 711-719 or 725-738, specified as affecting the lower limbs

5th 648.8 Abnormal glucose tolerance M ♀
[0-4] Conditions classifiable to 790.21-790.29
Gestational diabetes

Use additional code, if applicable, for associated long-term (current) insulin use (V58.67)

ICD-9-CM Official Guidelines (Chapter 11):

g. Gestational diabetes

Gestational diabetes can occur during the second and third trimester of pregnancy in women who were not diabetic prior to pregnancy. Gestational diabetes can cause complications in the pregnancy similar to those of pre-existing diabetes mellitus. It also puts the woman at greater risk of developing diabetes after the pregnancy. Gestational diabetes is coded to 648.8x, Abnormal glucose tolerance. Codes 648.0x and 648.8x should never be used together on the same record.

Code V58.67, Long-term (current) use of insulin, should also be assigned if the gestational diabetes is being treated with insulin.

5th 648.9 Other current conditions classifiable elsewhere M ♀
[0-4] Conditions classifiable to 440-459, 795.01-795.04, 795.06, 795.10-795.14, 795.16, 796.70-796.74, 796.76
Nutritional deficiencies [conditions classifiable to 260-269]

4th 649 Other conditions or status of the mother complicating pregnancy, childbirth, or the puerperium

Requires fifth digit; valid digits are in [brackets] under each code. See beginning of section 640-649 for definitions.

5th 649.0 Tobacco use disorder complicating pregnancy, childbirth, or the puerperium M ♀
[0-4] Smoking complicating pregnancy, childbirth, or the puerperium

5th 649.1 Obesity complicating pregnancy, childbirth, or the puerperium M ♀
[0-4]

Use additional code to identify the obesity (278.00, 278.01)

647 – 649.1

5th **649.2 Bariatric surgery status complicating pregnancy, childbirth, or the puerperium** M ♀
[0-4] Gastric banding status complicating pregnancy, childbirth, or the puerperium
Gastric bypass status for obesity complicating pregnancy, childbirth, or the puerperium
Obesity surgery status complicating pregnancy, childbirth, or the puerperium

5th **649.3 Coagulation defects complicating pregnancy, childbirth, or the puerperium** M ♀
[0-4] Conditions classifiable to 286, 287, 289
Use additional code to identify the specific coagulation defect (286.0-286.9, 287.0-287.9, 289.0-289.9)
Excludes *coagulation defects causing antepartum hemorrhage (641.3)*
postpartum coagulation defects (666.3)

5th **649.4 Epilepsy complicating pregnancy, childbirth, or the puerperium** M ♀
[0-4] Conditions classifiable to 345
Use additional code to identify the specific type of epilepsy (345.00-345.91)
Excludes *eclampsia (642.6)*

5th **649.5 Spotting complicating pregnancy** M ♀
[0,1,3]
Excludes *antepartum hemorrhage (641.0-641.9)*
hemorrhage in early pregnancy (640.0-640.9)

5th **649.6 Uterine size date discrepancy** M ♀
[0-4]
Excludes *suspected problem with fetal growth not found (V89.04)*

5th **649.7 Cervical shortening** M ♀
[0,1,3]
Excludes *suspected cervical shortening not found (V89.05)*

NORMAL DELIVERY, AND OTHER INDICATIONS FOR CARE IN PREGNANCY, LABOR, AND DELIVERY (650-659)

ICD-9-CM Official Guidelines (Chapter 11i):

1) ***Postpartum and peripartum periods***

The postpartum period begins immediately after delivery and continues for six weeks following delivery. The peripartum period is defined as the last month of pregnancy to five months postpartum.

2) ***Postpartum complication***

A postpartum complication is any complication occurring within the six-week period.

3) ***Pregnancy-related complications after 6 week period***

Chapter 11 codes may also be used to describe pregnancy-related complications after the six-week period should the provider document that a condition is pregnancy related.

4) ***Postpartum complications occurring during the same admission as delivery***

Postpartum complications that occur during the same admission as the delivery are identified with a fifth digit of "2." Subsequent admissions/encounters for postpartum complications should be identified with a fifth digit of "4."

5) ***Admission for routine postpartum care following delivery outside hospital***

When the mother delivers outside the hospital prior to admission and is admitted for routine postpartum care and no complications are noted, code V24.0, Postpartum care and examination immediately after delivery, should be assigned as the principal diagnosis.

6) ***Admission following delivery outside hospital with postpartum conditions***

A delivery diagnosis code should not be used for a woman who has delivered prior to admission to the hospital. Any postpartum conditions and/or postpartum procedures should be coded.

650 Normal delivery
Delivery requiring minimal or no assistance, with or without episiotomy, without fetal manipulation [e.g., rotation version] or instrumentation [forceps] of a spontaneous, cephalic, vaginal, full-term, single, live-born infant. This code is for use as a single diagnosis code and is not to be used with any other code in the range 630-676.
Use additional code to indicate outcome of delivery (V27.0)
Excludes *breech delivery (assisted) (spontaneous) NOS (652.2)*
delivery by vacuum extractor, forceps, cesarean section, or breech extraction, without specified complication (669.5-669.7)

ICD-9-CM Official Guidelines (Chapter 11):

h. ***Normal Delivery, Code 650***

1) ***Normal delivery***

Code 650 is for use in cases when a woman is admitted for a full-term normal delivery and delivers a single, healthy infant without any complications antepartum, during the delivery, or postpartum during the delivery episode. Code 650 is always a principal diagnosis. It is not to be used if any other code from chapter 11 is needed to describe a current complication of the antenatal, delivery, or perinatal period. Additional codes from other chapters may be used with code 650 if they are not related to or are in any way complicating the pregnancy.

2) ***Normal delivery with resolved antepartum complication***

Code 650 may be used if the patient had a complication at some point during her pregnancy, but the complication is not present at the time of the admission for delivery.

3) ***V27.0, Single liveborn, outcome of delivery***

V27.0, Single liveborn, is the only outcome of delivery code appropriate for use with 650.

The following fifth-digit subclassification is for use with categories 651-659 to denote the current episode of care:

0 unspecified as to episode of care or not applicable
1 delivered, with or without mention of antepartum condition
2 delivered, with mention of postpartum complication
3 antepartum condition or complication
4 postpartum condition or complication

4th **651 Multiple gestation**

5th **651.0 Twin pregnancy** M ♀
[0,1,3]
Excludes *fetal conjoined twins (678.1)*

5th **651.1 Triplet pregnancy** M ♀
[0,1,3]

5th **651.2 Quadruplet pregnancy** M ♀
[0,1,3]

5th **651.3 Twin pregnancy with fetal loss and retention of one fetus** M ♀
[0,1,3]

5th **651.4 Triplet pregnancy with fetal loss and retention of one or more fetus(es)** M ♀
[0,1,3]

5th **651.5 Quadruplet pregnancy with fetal loss and retention of one or more fetus(es)** M ♀
[0,1,3]

5th **651.6 Other multiple pregnancy with fetal loss and retention of one or more fetus(es)** M ♀
[0,1,3]

5th **651.7 Multiple gestation following (elective) fetal reduction** M ♀
[0,1,3] Fetal reduction of multiple fetuses reduced to single fetus

5th **651.8 Other specified multiple gestation** M ♀
[0,1,3]

5th **651.9 Unspecified multiple gestation** M ♀
[0,1,3]

4th 652 **Malposition and malpresentation of fetus**

Requires fifth digit; valid digits are in [brackets] under each code. See prior to category 651 for definitions.

Code first any associated obstructed labor (660.0)

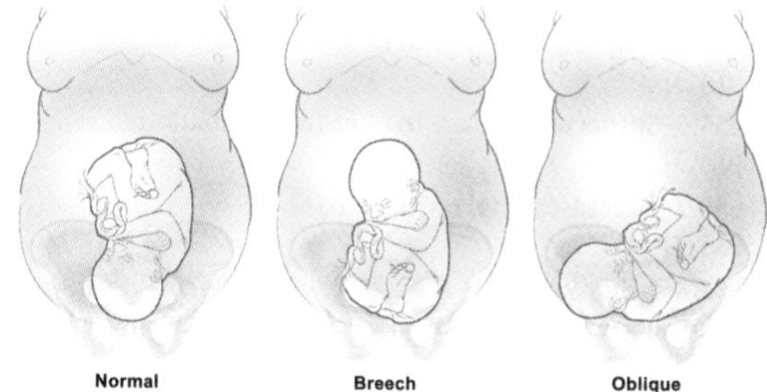

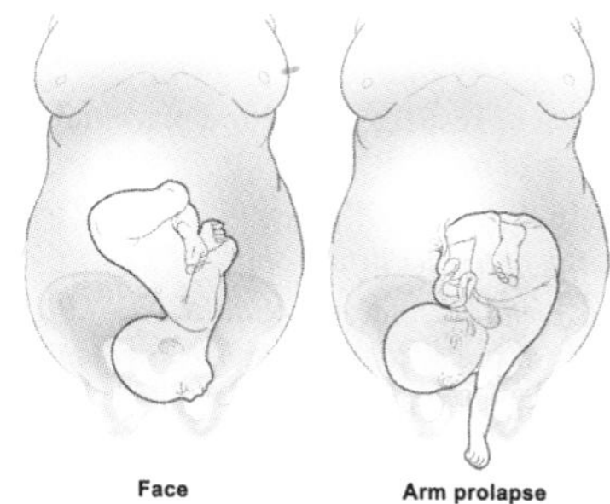

© 2008 Fairman Studios, LLC. All Rights Reserved.

5th 652.0 **Unstable lie** M ♀
[0,1,3]

5th 652.1 **Breech or other malpresentation successfully converted to cephalic presentation** M ♀
[0,1,3] Cephalic version NOS

5th 652.2 **Breech presentation without mention of version** M ♀
[0,1,3] Breech delivery (assisted) (spontaneous) NOS
Buttocks presentation
Complete breech
Frank breech
Excludes *footling presentation (652.8)*
incomplete breech (652.8)

5th 652.3 **Transverse or oblique presentation** M ♀
[0,1,3] Oblique lie
Transverse lie
Excludes *transverse arrest of fetal head (660.3)*

5th 652.4 **Face or brow presentation** M ♀
[0,1,3] Mentum presentation

5th 652.5 **High head at term** M ♀
[0,1,3] Failure of head to enter pelvic brim

5th 652.6 **Multiple gestation with malpresentation of one fetus or more** M ♀
[0,1,3]

5th 652.7 **Prolapsed arm** M ♀
[0,1,3]

5th 652.8 **Other specified malposition or malpresentation** M ♀
[0,1,3] Compound presentation

5th 652.9 **Unspecified malposition or malpresentation** M ♀
[0,1,3]

4th 653 **Disproportion**

Requires fifth digit; valid digits are in [brackets] under each code. See prior to category 651 for definitions.

Code first any associated obstructed labor (660.1)

5th 653.0 **Major abnormality of bony pelvis, not further specified** M ♀
[0,1,3] Pelvic deformity NOS

5th 653.1 **Generally contracted pelvis** M ♀
[0,1,3] Contracted pelvis NOS

5th 653.2 **Inlet contraction of pelvis** M ♀
[0,1,3] Inlet contraction (pelvis)

5th 653.3 **Outlet contraction of pelvis** M ♀
[0,1,3] Outlet contraction (pelvis)

5th 653.4 **Fetopelvic disproportion** M ♀
[0,1,3] Cephalopelvic disproportion NOS
Disproportion of mixed maternal and fetal origin, with normally formed fetus

5th 653.5 **Unusually large fetus causing disproportion** M ♀
[0,1,3] Disproportion of fetal origin with normally formed fetus
Fetal disproportion NOS
Excludes *that when the reason for medical care was concern for the fetus (656.6)*

5th 653.6 **Hydrocephalic fetus causing disproportion** M ♀
[0,1,3]
Excludes *that when the reason for medical care was concern for the fetus (655.0)*

5th 653.7 **Other fetal abnormality causing disproportion** M ♀
[0,1,3] Fetal:
ascites
hydrops
myelomeningocele
sacral teratoma
tumor
Excludes *conjoined twins causing disproportion (678.1)*

5th 653.8 **Disproportion of other origin** M ♀
[0,1,3]
Excludes *shoulder (girdle) dystocia (660.4)*

5th 653.9 **Unspecified disproportion** M ♀
[0,1,3]

4th 654 **Abnormality of organs and soft tissues of pelvis**

Requires fifth digit; valid digits are in [brackets] under each code. See prior to category 651 for definitions.

Includes the listed conditions during pregnancy, childbirth, or the puerperium

Code first any associated obstructed labor (660.2)

Excludes *trauma to perineum and vulva complicating current delivery (664.0-664.9)*

5th 654.0 **Congenital abnormalities of uterus** M ♀
[0-4] Double uterus
Uterus bicornis

5th 654.1 **Tumors of body of uterus** M ♀
[0-4] Uterine fibroids

5th 654.2 **Previous cesarean delivery** M ♀
[0,1,3] Uterine scar from previous cesarean delivery

5th 654.3 **Retroverted and incarcerated gravid uterus** M ♀
[0-4]

5th 654.4 **Other abnormalities in shape or position of gravid uterus and of neighboring structures** M ♀
[0-4] Cystocele
Pelvic floor repair
Pendulous abdomen
Prolapse of gravid uterus
Rectocele
Rigid pelvic floor

5th 654.5 **Cervical incompetence** M ♀
[0-4] Presence of Shirodkar suture with or without mention of cervical incompetence

5th 654.6 **Other congenital or acquired abnormality of cervix** M ♀
[0-4] Cicatricial cervix
Polyp of cervix
Previous surgery to cervix
Rigid cervix (uteri)
Stenosis or stricture of cervix
Tumor of cervix

5th 654.7 **Congenital or acquired abnormality of vagina** M ♀
[0-4] Previous surgery to vagina
Septate vagina
Stenosis of vagina (acquired) (congenital)
Sricture of vagina
Tumor of vagina

5th 654.8 **Congenital or acquired abnormality of vulva** M ♀
[0-4] Anal sphincter tear (healed) (old) complicating delivery
Fibrosis of perineum
Persistent hymen
Previous surgery to perineum or vulva
Rigid perineum
Tumor of vulva
Excludes *anal sphincter tear (healed) (old) not associated with delivery (569.43)*
varicose veins of vulva (671.1)

5th 654.9 **Other and unspecified** M ♀
[0-4] Uterine scar NEC

4th 655 **Known or suspected fetal abnormality affecting management of mother**
Requires fifth digit; valid digits are in [brackets] under each code. See prior to category 651 for definitions.
Includes the listed conditions in the fetus as a reason for observation or obstetrical care of the mother, or for termination of pregnancy

ICD-9-CM Official Guidelines (Chapter 11):
c. Fetal Conditions Affecting the Management of the Mother
1) Codes from category 655
Known or suspected fetal abnormality affecting management of the mother, and category 656, Other fetal and placental problems affecting the management of the mother, are assigned only when the fetal condition is actually responsible for modifying the management of the mother, i.e., by requiring diagnostic studies, additional observation, special care, or termination of pregnancy. The fact that the fetal condition exists does not justify assigning a code from this series to the mother's record.
2) In utero surgery
In cases when surgery is performed on the fetus, a diagnosis code from category 655, Known or suspected fetal abnormalities affecting management of the mother, should be assigned identifying the fetal condition. Procedure code 75.36, Correction of fetal defect, should be assigned on the hospital inpatient record.
No code from Chapter 15, the perinatal codes, should be used on the mother's record to identify fetal conditions. Surgery performed in utero on a fetus is still to be coded as an obstetric encounter.

5th 655.0 **Central nervous system malformation in fetus** M ♀
[0,1,3] Fetal or suspected fetal:
anencephaly
hydrocephalus
spina bifida (with myelomeningocele)

5th 655.1 **Chromosomal abnormality in fetus** M ♀
[0,1,3]

5th 655.2 **Hereditary disease in family possibly affecting fetus** M ♀
[0,1,3]

5th 655.3 **Suspected damage to fetus from viral disease in the mother** M ♀
[0,1,3] Suspected damage to fetus from maternal rubella

5th 655.4 **Suspected damage to fetus from other disease in the mother** M ♀
[0,1,3] Suspected damage to fetus from maternal:
alcohol addiction
listeriosis
toxoplasmosis

5th 655.5 **Suspected damage to fetus from drugs** M ♀
[0,1,3]

5th 655.6 **Suspected damage to fetus from radiation** M ♀
[0,1,3]

5th 655.7 **Decreased fetal movements** M ♀
[0,1,3]

5th 655.8 **Other known or suspected fetal abnormality, not elsewhere classified** M ♀
[0,1,3] Suspected damage to fetus from:
environmental toxins
intrauterine contraceptive device

5th 655.9 **Unspecified** M ♀
[0,1,3]

4th 656 **Other known or suspected fetal and placental problems affecting management of mother**
Requires fifth digit; valid digits are in [brackets] under each code. See prior to category 651 for definitions.
Excludes *fetal hematologic conditions (678.0)*
suspected placental problems not found (V89.02)

5th 656.0 **Fetal-maternal hemorrhage** M ♀
[0,1,3] Leakage (microscopic) of fetal blood into maternal circulation

5th 656.1 **Rhesus isoimmunization** M ♀
[0,1,3] Anti-D [Rh] antibodies
Rh incompatibility

5th 656.2 **Isoimmunization from other and unspecified blood-group incompatibility** M ♀
[0,1,3] ABO isoimmunization

5th 656.3 **Fetal distress** M ♀
[0,1,3] Fetal metabolic acidemia
Excludes *abnormal fetal acid-base balance (656.8)*
abnormality in fetal heart rate or rhythm (659.7)
fetal bradycardia (659.7)
fetal tachycardia (659.7)
meconium in liquor (656.8)

5th 656.4 **Intrauterine death** M ♀
[0,1,3] Fetal death:
NOS
after completion of 22 weeks' gestation
late
Missed delivery
Excludes *missed abortion (632)*

5th 656.5 **Poor fetal growth** M ♀
[0,1,3] "Light-for-dates"
"Placental insufficiency"
"Small-for-dates"

5th 656.6 **Excessive fetal growth** M ♀
[0,1,3] "Large-for-dates"

5th 656.7 **Other placental conditions** M ♀
[0,1,3] Abnormal placenta
Placental infarct
Excludes *placental polyp (674.4)*
placentitis (658.4)

5th 656.8 **Other specified fetal and placental problems** M ♀
[0,1,3] Abnormal acid-base balance
Intrauterine acidosis
Lithopedian
Meconium in liquor
Subchorionic hematoma

5th 656.9 **Unspecified fetal and placental problem** M ♀
[0,1,3]

654.6 – 656.9

4th 657 Polyhydramnios

Requires fifth digit; valid digits are in [brackets] under each code. See prior to category 651 for definitions.

Excludes *suspected polyhydramnios not found (V89.01)*

5th Use 0 as fourth digit for category 657 M ♀

[0,1,3] Hydramnios

4th 658 Other problems associated with amniotic cavity and membranes

Requires fifth digit; valid digits are in [brackets] under each code. See prior to category 651 for definitions.

Excludes *amniotic fluid embolism (673.1)*
suspected problems with amniotic cavity and membranes not found (V89.01)

5th 658.0 Oligohydramnios M ♀

[0,1,3] Oligohydramnios without mention of rupture of membranes

5th 658.1 Premature rupture of membranes M ♀

[0,1,3] Rupture of amniotic sac less than 24 hours prior to the onset of labor

5th 658.2 Delayed delivery after spontaneous or unspecified rupture of membranes M ♀

[0,1,3] Prolonged rupture of membranes NOS
Rupture of amniotic sac 24 hours or more prior to the onset of labor

5th 658.3 Delayed delivery after artificial rupture of membranes M ♀

[0,1,3]

5th 658.4 Infection of amniotic cavity M ♀

[0,1,3] Amnionitis
Chorioamnionitis
Membranitis
Placentitis

5th 658.8 Other M ♀

[0,1,3] Amnion nodosum
Amniotic cyst

5th 658.9 Unspecified M ♀

[0,1,3]

4th 659 Other indications for care or intervention related to labor and delivery, not elsewhere classified

Requires fifth digit; valid digits are in [brackets] under each code. See prior to category 651 for definitions.

5th 659.0 Failed mechanical induction M ♀

[0,1,3] Failure of induction of labor by surgical or other instrumental methods

5th 659.1 Failed medical or unspecified induction M ♀

[0,1,3] Failed induction NOS
Failure of induction of labor by medical methods, such as oxytocic drugs

5th 659.2 Maternal pyrexia during labor, unspecified M ♀

[0,1,3]

5th 659.3 Generalized infection during labor M ♀

[0,1,3] Septicemia during labor

5th 659.4 Grand multiparity M ♀

[0,1,3]

Excludes *supervision only, in pregnancy (V23.3)*
without current pregnancy (V61.5)

5th 659.5 Elderly primigravida M ♀

[0,1,3] First pregnancy in a woman who will be 35 years of age or older at expected date of delivery

Excludes *supervision only, in pregnancy (V23.81)*

5th 659.6 Elderly multigravida M ♀

[0,1,3] Second or more pregnancy in a woman who will be 35 years of age or older at expected date of delivery

Excludes *elderly primigravida (659.5)*
supervision only, in pregnancy (V23.82)

5th 659.7 Abnormality in fetal heart rate or rhythm M ♀

[0,1,3] Depressed fetal heart tones
Fetal:
bradycardia
tachycardia
Fetal heart rate decelerations
Non-reassuring fetal heart rate or rhythm

5th 659.8 Other specified indications for care or intervention related to labor and delivery M ♀

[0,1,3] Pregnancy in a female less than 16 years of age at expected date of delivery
Very young maternal age

5th 659.9 Unspecified indication for care or intervention related to labor and delivery M ♀

[0,1,3]

COMPLICATIONS OCCURRING MAINLY IN THE COURSE OF LABOR AND DELIVERY (660-669)

The following fifth-digit subclassification is for use with categories 660-669 to denote the current episode of care:

0 unspecified as to episode of care or not applicable
1 delivered, with or without mention of antepartum condition
2 delivered, with mention of postpartum complication
3 antepartum condition or complication
4 postpartum condition or complication

ICD-9-CM Official Guidelines (Chapter 11):

k. Abortions

2) Code from categories 640-648 and 651-659

.... Codes from the 660-669 series are not to be used for complications of abortion.

4th 660 Obstructed labor

Requires fifth digit; valid digits are in [brackets] under each code. See beginning of section 660-669 for definitions.

5th 660.0 Obstruction caused by malposition of fetus at onset of labor M ♀

[0,1,3] Any condition classifiable to 652, causing obstruction during labor
Use additional code from 652.0-652.9 to identify condition

5th 660.1 Obstruction by bony pelvis M ♀

[0,1,3] Any condition classifiable to 653, causing obstruction during labor
Use additional code from 653.0-653.9 to identify condition

5th 660.2 Obstruction by abnormal pelvic soft tissues M ♀

[0,1,3] Prolapse of anterior lip of cervix
Any condition classifiable to 654, causing obstruction during labor
Use additional code from 654.0-654.9 to identify condition

5th 660.3 Deep transverse arrest and persistent occipitoposterior position M ♀

[0,1,3]

5th 660.4 Shoulder (girdle) dystocia M ♀

[0,1,3] Impacted shoulders

5th 660.5 Locked twins M ♀

[0,1,3]

5th 660.6 Failed trial of labor, unspecified M ♀

[0,1,3] Failed trial of labor, without mention of condition or suspected condition

5th 660.7 Failed forceps or vacuum extractor, unspecified M ♀

[0,1,3] Application of ventouse or forceps, without mention of condition

5th 660.8 Other causes of obstructed labor M ♀

[0,1,3]
Use additional code to identify condition

5th **660.9 Unspecified obstructed labor** M ♀
[0,1,3] Dystocia:
NOS
fetal NOS
maternal NOS

4th **661 Abnormality of forces of labor**
Requires fifth digit; valid digits are in [brackets] under each code. See beginning of section 660-669 for definitions.

5th **661.0 Primary uterine inertia** M ♀
[0,1,3] Failure of cervical dilation
Hypotonic uterine dysfunction, primary
Prolonged latent phase of labor

5th **661.1 Secondary uterine inertia** M ♀
[0,1,3] Arrested active phase of labor
Hypotonic uterine dysfunction, secondary

5th **661.2 Other and unspecified uterine inertia** M ♀
[0,1,3] Atony of uterus without hemorrhage
Desultory labor
Irregular labor
Poor contractions
Slow slope active phase of labor
Excludes *atony of uterus with hemorrhage (666.1)*
postpartum atony of uterus without hemorrhage (669.8)

5th **661.3 Precipitate labor** M ♀
[0,1,3]

5th **661.4 Hypertonic, incoordinate, or prolonged uterine contractions** M ♀
[0,1,3] Cervical spasm
Contraction ring (dystocia)
Dyscoordinate labor
Hourglass contraction of uterus
Hypertonic uterine dysfunction
Incoordinate uterine action
Retraction ring (Bandl's) (pathological)
Tetanic contractions
Uterine dystocia NOS
Uterine spasm

5th **661.9 Unspecified abnormality of labor** M ♀
[0,1,3]

4th **662 Long labor**
Requires fifth digit; valid digits are in [brackets] under each code. See beginning of section 660-669 for definitions.

The Three Stages of Labor

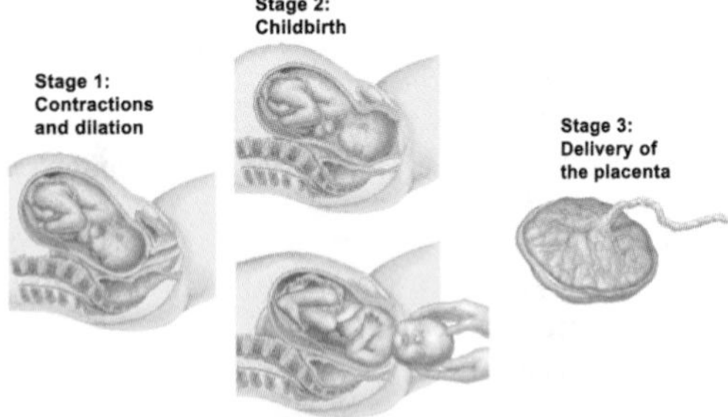

© 2006 Anatomical Chart Company

5th **662.0 Prolonged first stage** M ♀
[0,1,3]

5th **662.1 Prolonged labor, unspecified** M ♀
[0,1,3]

5th **662.2 Prolonged second stage** M ♀
[0,1,3]

5th **662.3 Delayed delivery of second twin, triplet, etc.** M ♀
[0,1,3]

4th **663 Umbilical cord complications**
Requires fifth digit; valid digits are in [brackets] under each code. See beginning of section 660-669 for definitions.

5th **663.0 Prolapse of cord** M ♀
[0,1,3] Presentation of cord

5th **663.1 Cord around neck, with compression** M ♀
[0,1,3] Cord tightly around neck

5th **663.2 Other and unspecified cord entanglement, with compression** M ♀
[0,1,3] Entanglement of cords of twins in mono-amniotic sac
Knot in cord (with compression)

5th **663.3 Other and unspecified cord entanglement, without mention of compression** M ♀
[0,1,3]

5th **663.4 Short cord** M ♀
[0,1,3]

5th **663.5 Vasa previa** M ♀
[0,1,3]

5th **663.6 Vascular lesions of cord** M ♀
[0,1,3] Bruising of cord
Hematoma of cord
Thrombosis of vessels of cord

5th **663.8 Other umbilical cord complications** M ♀
[0,1,3] Velamentous insertion of umbilical cord

5th **663.9 Unspecified umbilical cord complication** M ♀
[0,1,3]

4th **664 Trauma to perineum and vulva during delivery**
Requires fifth digit; valid digits are in [brackets] under each code. See beginning of section 660-669 for definitions.
Includes damage from instruments
that from extension of episiotomy

5th **664.0 First-degree perineal laceration** M ♀
[0,1,4] Perineal laceration, rupture, or tear involving:
fourchette
hymen
labia
skin
vagina
vulva

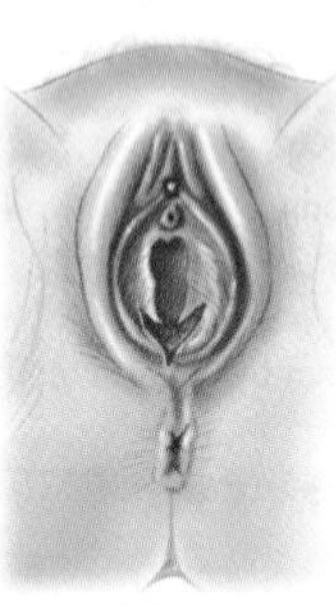

First degree Laceration
Vaginal Laceration
Perineal skin torn

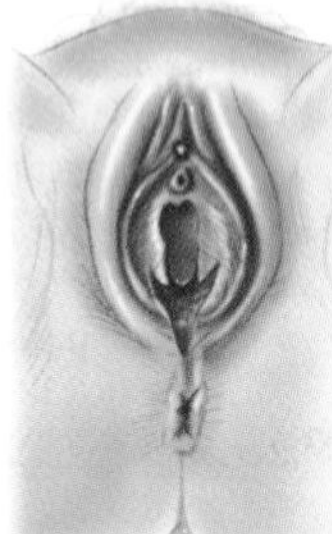

Second degree Laceration
Vaginal Laceration
Perineal skin torn
Perineal muscles torn

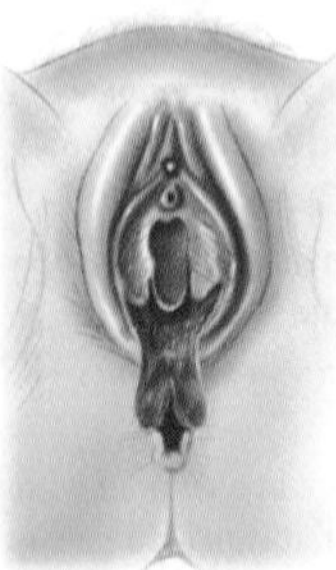

Third degree Laceration
Vaginal Laceration
Perineal skin torn
Perineal muscles torn
External anal sphincter torn

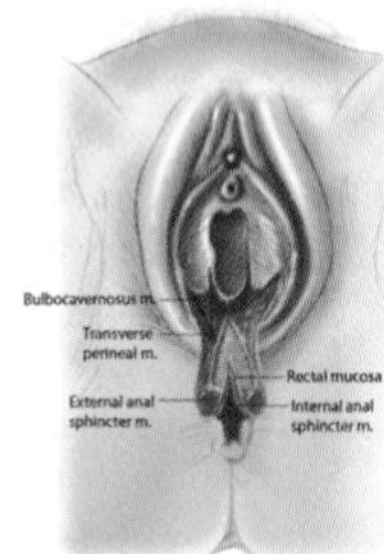

Fourth degree Laceration
Vaginal Laceration
Perineal skin torn
Perineal muscles torn
External anal sphincter torn
Complete anal sphincter tear and
Rectal mucosa may also be torn

© 2008 Fairman Studios, LLC. All Rights Reserved.

5th 664.1 **Second-degree perineal laceration** M ♀
[0,1,4] Perineal laceration, rupture, or tear (following episiotomy) involving:
pelvic floor
perineal muscles
vaginal muscles
Excludes *that involving anal sphincter (664.2)*

5th 664.2 **Third-degree perineal laceration** M ♀
[0,1,4] Perineal laceration, rupture, or tear (following episiotomy) involving:
anal sphincter
rectovaginal septum
sphincter NOS
Excludes *anal sphincter tear during delivery not associated with third-degree perineal laceration (664.6)*
that with anal or rectal mucosal laceration (664.3)

5th 664.3 **Fourth-degree perineal laceration** M ♀
[0,1,4] Perineal laceration, rupture, or tear as classifiable to 664.2 and involving also:
anal mucosa
rectal mucosa

5th 664.4 **Unspecified perineal laceration** M ♀
[0,1,4] Central laceration

5th 664.5 **Vulval and perineal hematoma** M ♀
[0,1,4]

5th 664.6 **Anal sphincter tear complicating delivery, not associated with third-degree perineal laceration** M ♀
[0,1,4]
Excludes *third-degree perineal laceration (664.2)*

5th 664.8 **Other specified trauma to perineum and vulva** M ♀
[0,1,4]

5th 664.9 **Unspecified trauma to perineum and vulva** M ♀
[0,1,4]

4th 665 **Other obstetrical trauma**
Requires fifth digit; valid digits are in [brackets] under each code. See beginning of section 660-669 for definitions.
Includes damage from instruments

5th 665.0 **Rupture of uterus before onset of labor** M ♀
[0,1,3]

5th 665.1 **Rupture of uterus during labor** M ♀
[0,1] Rupture of uterus NOS

5th 665.2 **Inversion of uterus** M ♀
[0,2,4]

5th 665.3 **Laceration of cervix** M ♀
[0,1,4]

5th 665.4 **High vaginal laceration** M ♀
[0,1,4] Laceration of vaginal wall or sulcus without mention of perineal laceration

5th 665.5 **Other injury to pelvic organs** M ♀
[0,1,4] Injury to:
bladder
urethra

5th 665.6 **Damage to pelvic joints and ligaments** M ♀
[0,1,4] Avulsion of inner symphyseal cartilage
Damage to coccyx
Separation of symphysis (pubis)

5th 665.7 **Pelvic hematoma** M ♀
[0-2,4] Hematoma of vagina

5th 665.8 **Other specified obstetrical trauma** M ♀
[0-4]

5th 665.9 **Unspecified obstetrical trauma** M ♀
[0-4]

4th 666 **Postpartum hemorrhage**
Requires fifth digit; valid digits are in [brackets] under each code. See beginning of section 660-669 for definitions.

5th 666.0 **Third-stage hemorrhage** M ♀
[0,2,4] Hemorrhage associated with retained, trapped, or adherent placenta
Retained placenta NOS

5th 666.1 **Other immediate postpartum hemorrhage** M ♀
[0,2,4] Atony of uterus with hemorrhage
Hemorrhage within the first 24 hours following delivery of placenta
Postpartum atony of uterus with hemorrhage
Postpartum hemorrhage (atonic) NOS
Excludes *atony of uterus without hemorrhage (661.2)*
postpartum atony of uterus without hemorrhage (669.8)

5th 666.2 **Delayed and secondary postpartum hemorrhage** M ♀
[0,2,4] Hemorrhage:
after the first 24 hours following delivery
associated with retained portions of placenta or membranes
Postpartum hemorrhage specified as delayed or secondary
Retained products of conception NOS, following delivery

5th 666.3 **Postpartum coagulation defects** M ♀
[0,2,4] Postpartum:
afibrinogenemia
fibrinolysis

4th 667 **Retained placenta without hemorrhage**
Requires fifth digit; valid digits are in [brackets] under each code. See beginning of section 660-669 for definitions.

5th 667.0 **Retained placenta without hemorrhage** M ♀
[0,2,4] Placenta accreta without hemorrhage
Retained placenta:
NOS without hemorrhage
total without hemorrhage

5th 667.1 **Retained portions of placenta or membranes, without hemorrhage** M ♀
[0,2,4] Retained products of conception following delivery, without hemorrhage

4th 668 **Complications of the administration of anesthetic or other sedation in labor and delivery**
Requires fifth digit; valid digits are in [brackets] under each code. See beginning of section 660-669 for definitions.
Includes complications arising from the administration of a general or local anesthetic, analgesic, or other sedation in labor and delivery
Use additional code(s) to further specify complication
Excludes *reaction to spinal or lumbar puncture (349.0)*
spinal headache (349.0)

5th 668.0 **Pulmonary complications** M ♀
[0-4] Inhalation [aspiration] of stomach contents or secretions following anesthesia or other sedation in labor or delivery
Mendelson's syndrome following anesthesia or other sedation in labor or delivery
Pressure collapse of lung following anesthesia or other sedation in labor or delivery

5th 668.1 **Cardiac complications** M ♀
[0-4] Cardiac arrest or failure following anesthesia or other sedation in labor and delivery

5th 668.2 **Central nervous system complications** M ♀
[0-4] Cerebral anoxia following anesthesia or other sedation in labor and delivery

5th 668.8 **Other complications of anesthesia or other sedation in labor and delivery** M ♀
[0-4]

5th **668.9 Unspecified complication of anesthesia and other sedation** M ♀
[0-4]

4th **669 Other complications of labor and delivery, not elsewhere classified**

Requires fifth digit; valid digits are in [brackets] under each code. See beginning of section 660-669 for definitions.

5th **669.0 Maternal distress** M ♀
[0-4] Metabolic disturbance in labor and delivery

5th **669.1 Shock during or following labor and delivery** M ♀
[0-4] Obstetric shock

5th **669.2 Maternal hypotension syndrome** M ♀
[0-4]

▲ 5th **669.3 Acute kidney ~~renal~~ failure following labor and delivery** M ♀
[0,2,4]

5th **669.4 Other complications of obstetrical surgery and procedures** M ♀
[0-4] Cardiac:
arrest following cesarean or other obstetrical surgery or procedure, including delivery NOS
failure following cesarean or other obstetrical surgery or procedure, including delivery NOS
Cerebral anoxia following cesarean or other obstetrical surgery or procedure, including delivery NOS

Excludes *complications of obstetrical surgical wounds (674.1-674.3)*

5th **669.5 Forceps or vacuum extractor delivery without mention of indication** M ♀
[0,1] Delivery by ventouse, without mention of indication

5th **669.6 Breech extraction, without mention of indication** M ♀
[0,1]

Excludes *breech delivery NOS (652.2)*

5th **669.7 Cesarean delivery, without mention of indication** M ♀
[0,1]

5th **669.8 Other complications of labor and delivery** M ♀
[0-4]

5th **669.9 Unspecified complication of labor and delivery** M ♀
[0-4]

COMPLICATIONS OF THE PUERPERIUM (670-677)

Note: *Categories 671 and 673-676 include the listed conditions even if they occur during pregnancy or childbirth.*

The following fifth-digit subclassification is for use with categories 670-676 to denote the current episode of care:

0 **unspecified as to episode of care or not applicable**
1 **delivered, with or without mention of antepartum condition**
2 **delivered, with mention of postpartum complication**
3 **antepartum condition or complication**
4 **postpartum condition or complication**

4th **670 Major puerperal infection**

Requires fifth digit; valid digits are in [brackets] under each code. See beginning of section 670-676 for definitions.

5th ~~**Use 0 as fourth digit for category 670**~~
~~[0,2,4] Puerperal:~~
~~endometritis~~
~~fever (septic)~~
~~pelvic:~~
~~cellulitis~~
~~sepsis~~
~~peritonitis~~
~~pyemia~~
~~salpingitis~~
~~septicemia~~

Excludes *infection following abortion (639.0)*
minor genital tract infection following delivery (646.6)
puerperal fever NOS (672)
puerperal pyrexia NOS (672)
puerperal pyrexia of unknown origin (672)
urinary tract infection following delivery (646.6)

Rationale: *The Agency for Healthcare Research and Quality (AHRQ) proposed that changes be made for venous complications in pregnancy and the puerperium to improve the specificity of ICD-9-CM codes used to define deep vein thrombosis and pulmonary embolism in pregnant and postpartum women. The most critical issue is the inclusion of both venous thrombosis and septic pelvic thrombophlebitis under one single subcategory/code, 671.4 (with either a 2 or a 4 selected as the 5th digit). Septic pelvic thrombophlebitis is an inflammatory condition that affects the adnexa in the pelvis. It is thought to be an infectious complication that follows delivery, especially after cesarean delivery. This condition does not commonly respond to heparin treatment. Thus, a new code for septic pelvic thrombophlebitis was needed to distinguish it from postpartum deep vein thrombosis.*

New codes under existing category 670 were added to specifically identify the three most serious manifestations of major puerperal infection: postpartum endometritis, postpartum sepsis, and postpartum septic pelvic thrombophlebitis. The existing fifth digits still apply.

▲ 5th **670.0 Major puerperal infection, unspecified** M ♀
[0,2,4]

● 5th **670.1 Puerperal endometritis** M ♀
[0,2,4]

● 5th **670.2 Puerperal sepsis** M ♀
[0,2,4] Puerperal pyemia

● 5th **670.3 Puerperal septic thrombophlebitis** M ♀
[0,2,4]

● 5th **670.8 Other major puerperal infection** M ♀
[0,2,4] Puerperal:
pelvic cellulitis
peritonitis
salpingitis

4th 671 Venous complications in pregnancy and the puerperium

Requires fifth digit; valid digits are in [brackets] under each code. See beginning of section 670-676 for definitions.

Excludes *personal history of venous complications prior to pregnancy, such as:*
thrombophlebitis (V12.52)
thrombosis and embolism (V12.51)

5th 671.0 Varicose veins of legs M ♀
[0-4] Varicose veins NOS

5th 671.1 Varicose veins of vulva and perineum M ♀
[0-4]

5th 671.2 Superficial thrombophlebitis M ♀
[0-4] Phlebitis NOS
Thrombophlebitis (superficial)
Thrombosis NOS

5th 671.3 Deep phlebothrombosis, antepartum M ♀
[0,1,3] Deep-vein thrombosis, antepartum
Use additional code to identify the deep vein thrombosis (453.40-453.42, 453.50-453.52, 453.72-453.79, 453.82-453.89)
Use additional code for long term (current) use of anticoagulants, if applicable (V58.61)

5th 671.4 Deep phlebothrombosis, postpartum M ♀
[0,2,4] Deep-vein thrombosis, postpartum
Pelvic thrombophlebitis, postpartum
Phlegmasia alba dolens (puerperal)
Use additional code to identify the deep vein thrombosis (453.40-453.42, 453.50-453.52, 453.72-453.79, 453.82-453.89)
Use additional code for long term (current) use of anticoagulants, if applicable (V58.61)

5th 671.5 Other phlebitis and thrombosis M ♀
[0-4] Cerebral venous thrombosis
Thrombosis of intracranial venous sinus

5th 671.8 Other venous complications M ♀
[0-4] Hemorrhoids

5th 671.9 Unspecified venous complication M ♀
[0-4] ~~Phlebitis NOS~~
~~Thrombosis NOS~~

4th 672 Pyrexia of unknown origin during the puerperium

Requires fifth digit; valid digits are in [brackets] under each code. See beginning of section 670-676 for definitions.

5th Use 0 as fourth digit for category 672 M ♀
[0,2,4] Postpartum fever NOS
Puerperal fever NOS
Puerperal pyrexia NOS

4th 673 Obstetrical pulmonary embolism

Requires fifth digit; valid digits are in [brackets] under each code. See beginning of section 670-676 for definitions.

Includes pulmonary emboli in pregnancy, childbirth, or the puerperium, or specified as puerperal

Excludes *embolism following abortion (639.6)*

5th 673.0 Obstetrical air embolism M ♀
[0-4]

5th 673.1 Amniotic fluid embolism M ♀
[0-4]

5th 673.2 Obstetrical blood-clot embolism M ♀
[0-4] Puerperal pulmonary embolism NOS

5th 673.3 Obstetrical pyemic and septic embolism M ♀
[0-4]

5th 673.8 Other pulmonary embolism M ♀
[0-4] Fat embolism

4th 674 Other and unspecified complications of the puerperium, not elsewhere classified

Requires fifth digit; valid digits are in [brackets] under each code. See beginning of section 670-676 for definitions.

5th 674.0 Cerebrovascular disorders in the puerperium M ♀
[0-4] Any condition classifiable to 430-434, 436-437 occurring during pregnancy, childbirth, or the puerperium, or specified as puerperal
Excludes *intracranial venous sinus thrombosis (671.5)*

5th 674.1 Disruption of cesarean wound M ♀
[0,2,4] Dehiscence or disruption of uterine wound
Excludes *uterine rupture before onset of labor (665.0)*
uterine rupture during labor (665.1)

5th 674.2 Disruption of perineal wound M ♀
[0,2,4] Breakdown of perineum
Disruption of wound of:
episiotomy
perineal laceration
Secondary perineal tear

5th 674.3 Other complications of obstetrical surgical wounds M ♀
[0,2,4] Hematoma of cesarean section or perineal wound
Hemorrhage of cesarean section or perineal wound
Infection of cesarean section or perineal wound
Excludes *damage from instruments in delivery (664.0-665.9)*

5th 674.4 Placental polyp M ♀
[0,2,4]

5th 674.5 Peripartum cardiomyopathy M ♀
[0-4] Postpartum cardiomyopathy

5th 674.8 Other M ♀
[0,2,4] Hepatorenal syndrome, following delivery
Postpartum:
subinvolution of uterus
uterine hypertrophy

5th 674.9 Unspecified M ♀
[0,2,4] Sudden death of unknown cause during the puerperium

4th 675 Infections of the breast and nipple associated with childbirth

Requires fifth digit; valid digits are in [brackets] under each code. See beginning of section 670-676 for definitions.

Includes the listed conditions during pregnancy, childbirth, or the puerperium

5th 675.0 Infections of nipple M ♀
[0-4] Abscess of nipple

5th 675.1 Abscess of breast M ♀
[0-4] Abscess:
mammary
subareolar
submammary
Mastitis:
purulent
retromammary
submammary

5th 675.2 Nonpurulent mastitis M ♀
[0-4] Lymphangitis of breast
Mastitis:
NOS
interstitial
parenchymatous

5th 675.8 Other specified infections of the breast and nipple M ♀
[0-4]

5th 675.9 Unspecified infection of the breast and nipple M ♀
[0-4]

671 – 675.9

4th **676 Other disorders of the breast associated with childbirth and disorders of lactation**

Requires fifth digit; valid digits are in [brackets] under each code. See beginning of section 670-676 for definitions.

Includes the listed conditions during pregnancy, the puerperium, or lactation

5th **676.0 Retracted nipple** M ♀
[0-4]

5th **676.1 Cracked nipple** M ♀
[0-4] Fissure of nipple

5th **676.2 Engorgement of breasts** M ♀
[0-4]

5th **676.3 Other and unspecified disorder of breast** M ♀
[0-4]

5th **676.4 Failure of lactation** M ♀
[0-4] Agalactia

5th **676.5 Suppressed lactation** M ♀
[0-4]

5th **676.6 Galactorrhea** M ♀
[0-4]

Excludes *galactorrhea not associated with childbirth (611.6)*

5th **676.8 Other disorders of lactation** M ♀
[0-4] Galactocele

5th **676.9 Unspecified disorder of lactation** M ♀
[0-4]

677 Late effect of complication of pregnancy, childbirth, and the puerperium M ♀

Note: *This category is to be used to indicate conditions in 632-648.9 and 651-676.9 as the cause of the late effect, themselves classifiable elsewhere. The "late effects" include conditions specified as such, or as sequelae, which may occur at any time after the puerperium.*

Code first any sequelae

ICD-9-CM Official Guidelines (Chapter 11):

j. Code 677, Late effect of complication of pregnancy

1) Code 677

Code 677, Late effect of complication of pregnancy, childbirth, and the puerperium is for use in those cases when an initial complication of a pregnancy develops a sequelae requiring care or treatment at a future date.

2) After the initial postpartum period

This code may be used at any time after the initial postpartum period.

3) Sequencing of Code 677

This code, like all late effect codes, is to be sequenced following the code describing the sequelae of the complication.

OTHER MATERNAL AND FETAL COMPLICATIONS (678-679)

The following fifth-digit subclassification is for use with categories 678-679 to denote the current episode of care:

- **0 unspecified as to episode of care or not applicable**
- **1 delivered, with or without mention of antepartum condition**
- **2 delivered, with mention of postpartum complication**
- **3 antepartum condition or complication**
- **4 postpartum condition or complication**

4th **678 Other fetal conditions**

Requires fifth digit; valid digits are in [brackets] under each code. See beginning of section 678-679 for definitions.

5th **678.0 Fetal hematologic conditions** M ♀
[0,1,3] Fetal anemia
Fetal thrombocytopenia
Fetal twin to twin transfusion

Excludes *fetal and neonatal hemorrhage (772.0-772.9)*
fetal hematologic disorders affecting newborn (776.0-776.9)
fetal-maternal hemorrhage (656.00-656.03)
isoimmunization incompatibility (656.10-656.13, 656.20-656.23)

5th **678.1 Fetal conjoined twins** M ♀
[0,1,3]

4th **679 Complications of in utero procedures**

Requires fifth digit; valid digits are in [brackets] under each code. See beginning of section 678-679 for definitions.

5th **679.0 Maternal complications from in utero procedure** M ♀
[0-4]

Excludes *maternal history of in utero procedure during previous pregnancy (V23.86)*

5th **679.1 Fetal complications from in utero procedure** M ♀
[0-4] Fetal complications from amniocentesis

Excludes *newborn affected by in utero procedure (760.61-760.64)*

12. DISEASES OF THE SKIN AND SUBCUTANEOUS TISSUE (680-709)

INFECTIONS OF SKIN AND SUBCUTANEOUS TISSUE (680-686)

Excludes *certain infections of skin classified under "Infectious and Parasitic Diseases," such as:*
erysipelas (035)
erysipeloid of Rosenbach (027.1)
herpes:
simplex (054.0-054.9)
zoster (053.0-053.9)
molluscum contagiosum (078.0)
viral warts (078.10-078.19)

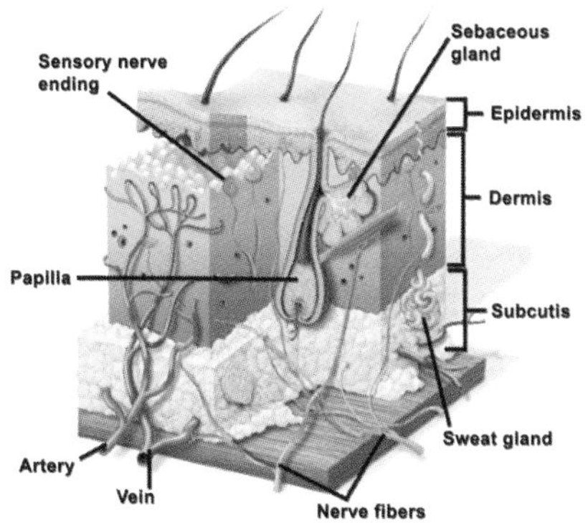

4th **680 Carbuncle and furuncle**
Includes boil
furunculosis

680.0 Face
Ear [any part]
Face [any part, except eye]
Nose (septum)
Temple (region)
Excludes *eyelid (373.13)*
lacrimal apparatus (375.31)
orbit (376.01)

680.1 Neck

680.2 Trunk
Abdominal wall
Back [any part, except buttocks]
Breast
Chest wall
Flank
Groin
Pectoral region
Perineum
Umbilicus
Excludes *buttocks (680.5)*
external genital organs:
female (616.4)
male (607.2, 608.4)

680.3 Upper arm and forearm
Arm [any part, except hand]
Axilla
Shoulder

680.4 Hand
Finger [any]
Thumb
Wrist

680.5 Buttock
Anus
Gluteal region

680.6 Leg, except foot
Ankle
Hip
Knee
Thigh

680.7 Foot
Heel
Toe

680.8 Other specified sites
Head [any part, except face]
Scalp
Excludes *external genital organs:*
female (616.4)
male (607.2, 608.4)

680.9 Unspecified site
Boil NOS
Carbuncle NOS
Furuncle NOS

4th **681 Cellulitis and abscess of finger and toe**
Includes that with lymphangitis
Use additional code to identify organism, such as Staphylococcus (041.1)

5th **681.0 Finger**

681.00 Cellulitis and abscess, unspecified

681.01 Felon
Pulp abscess
Whitlow
Excludes *herpetic whitlow (054.6)*

681.02 Onychia and paronychia of finger
Panaritium of finger
Perionychia of finger

5th **681.1 Toe**

681.10 Cellulitis and abscess, unspecified
L03.039 Cellulitis of unspecified toe
L03.049 Acute lymphangitis of unspecified toe

681.11 Onychia and paronychia of toe
L03.039 Cellulitis of unspecified toe
Panaritium of toe
Perionychia of toe

681.9 Cellulitis and abscess of unspecified digit
Infection of nail NOS

4th **682 Other cellulitis and abscess**
Includes abscess (acute) (with lymphangitis) except of finger or toe
cellulitis (diffuse) (with lymphangitis) except of finger or toe
lymphangitis, acute (with lymphangitis) except of finger or toe
Use additional code to identify organism, such as Staphylococcus (041.1)
Excludes *lymphangitis (chronic) (subacute) (457.2)*

682.0 Face
Cheek, external
Chin
Forehead
Nose, external
Submandibular
Temple (region)
Excludes *ear [any part] (380.10-380.16)*
eyelid (373.13)
lacrimal apparatus (375.31)
lip (528.5)
mouth (528.3)
nose (internal) (478.1)
orbit (376.01)

682.1 Neck

682.2 Trunk

L03.319 Cellulitis of trunk, unspecified

L03.329 Acute lymphangitis of trunk, unspecified

Abdominal wall
Back [any part, except buttock]
Chest wall
Flank
Groin
Pectoral region
Perineum
Umbilicus, except newborn

Excludes *anal and rectal regions (566)*
breast:
NOS (611.0)
puerperal (675.1)
external genital organs:
female (616.3-616.4)
male (604.0, 607.2, 608.4)
umbilicus, newborn (771.4)

682.3 Upper arm and forearm

Arm [any part, except hand]
Axilla
Shoulder

Excludes *hand (682.4)*

682.4 Hand, except fingers and thumb

Wrist

Excludes *finger and thumb (681.00-681.02)*

682.5 Buttock

Gluteal region

Excludes *anal and rectal regions (566)*

682.6 Leg, except foot

L03.119 Cellulitis of unspecified part of limb

L03.129 Acute lymphangitis of unspecified part of limb

Ankle
Hip
Knee
Thigh

682.7 Foot, except toes

L03.119 Cellulitis of unspecified part of limb

L03.129 Acute lymphangitis of unspecified part of limb

Heel

Excludes *toe (681.10-681.11)*

682.8 Other specified sites

Head [except face]
Scalp

Excludes *face (682.0)*

682.9 Unspecified site

L03.90 Cellulitis, unspecified

L03.91 Acute lymphangitis, unspecified

Abscess NOS
Cellulitis NOS
Lymphangitis, acute NOS

Excludes *lymphangitis NOS (457.2)*

683 Acute lymphadenitis

Abscess (acute) lymph gland or node, except mesenteric
Adenitis, acute lymph gland or node, except mesenteric
Lymphadenitis, acute lymph gland or node, except mesenteric
Use additional code to identify organism such as Staphylococcus (041.1)

Excludes *enlarged glands NOS (785.6)*
lymphadenitis:
chronic or subacute, except mesenteric (289.1)
mesenteric (acute) (chronic) (subacute) (289.2)
unspecified (289.3)

684 Impetigo

Impetiginization of other dermatoses
Impetigo (contagiosa) [any site] [any organism]:
bullous
circinate
neonatorum
simplex
Pemphigus neonatorum

Excludes *impetigo herpetiformis (694.3)*

4th **685 Pilonidal cyst**

Includes fistula, coccygeal or pilonidal
sinus, coccygeal or pilonidal

685.0 With abscess

685.1 Without mention of abscess

4th **686 Other local infections of skin and subcutaneous tissue**

Use additional code to identify any infectious organism (041.0-041.8)

5th **686.0 Pyoderma**

Dermatitis:
purulent
septic
suppurative

686.00 Pyoderma, unspecified

686.01 Pyoderma gangrenosum

686.09 Other pyoderma

686.1 Pyogenic granuloma

Granuloma:
septic
suppurative
telangiectaticum

Excludes *pyogenic granuloma of oral mucosa (528.9)*

686.8 Other specified local infections of skin and subcutaneous tissue

Bacterid (pustular)
Dermatitis vegetans
Ecthyma
Perlèche

Excludes *dermatitis infectiosa eczematoides (690.8)*
panniculitis (729.30-729.39)

686.9 Unspecified local infection of skin and subcutaneous tissue

L08.9 Local infection of the skin and subcutaneous tissue, unspecified

Fistula of skin NOS
Skin infection NOS

Excludes *fistula to skin from internal organs – see Alphabetic Index*

OTHER INFLAMMATORY CONDITIONS OF SKIN AND SUBCUTANEOUS TISSUE (690-698)

Excludes *panniculitis (729.30-729.39)*

4th **690 Erythematosquamous dermatosis**

Excludes *eczematous dermatitis of eyelid (373.31)*
parakeratosis variegata (696.2)
psoriasis (696.0-696.1)
seborrheic keratosis (702.11-702.19)

5th **690.1 Seborrheic dermatitis**

Layman's: *Seborrheic dermatitis in adults and adolescents is non-clinically referred to as dandruff.*

690.10 Seborheic dermatitis, unspecified

Seborrheic dermatitis NOS

690.11 Seborrhea capitis P

Cradle cap

690.12 Seborrheic infantile dermatitis P

690.18 Other seborrheic dermatitis

690.8 Other erythematosquamous dermatosis

682.2 – 690.8

4th 691 Atopic dermatitis and related conditions

691.0 Diaper or napkin rash
Ammonia dermatitis
Diaper or napkin:
dermatitis
erythema
rash
Psoriasiform napkin eruption

691.8 Other atopic dermatitis and related conditions
Atopic dermatitis
Besnier's prurigo
Eczema:
atopic
flexural
intrinsic (allergic)
Neurodermatitis:
atopic
diffuse (of Brocq)

4th 692 Contact dermatitis and other eczema

Includes dermatitis:
NOS
contact
occupational
venenata
eczema (acute) (chronic):
NOS
allergic
erythematous
occupational

Excludes *allergy NOS (995.3)*
contact dermatitis of eyelids (373.32)
dermatitis due to substances taken internally (693.0-693.9)
eczema of external ear (380.22)
perioral dermatitis (695.3)
urticarial reactions (708.0-708.9, 995.1)

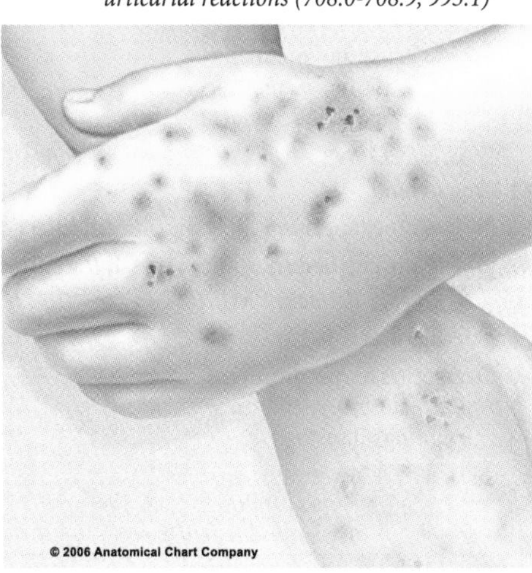

692.0 Due to detergents

692.1 Due to oils and greases

692.2 Due to solvents
Dermatitis due to solvents of:
chlorocompound group
cyclohexane group
ester group
glycol group
hydrocarbon group
ketone group

692.3 Due to drugs and medicines in contact with skin
Dermatitis (allergic) (contact) due to:
arnica
fungicides
iodine
keratolytics
mercurials
neomycin
pediculocides
phenols
scabicides
any drug applied to skin
Dermatitis medicamentosa due to drug applied to skin
Use additional E to identify drug

Excludes *allergy NOS due to drugs (995.27)*
dermatitis due to ingested drugs (693.0)
dermatitis medicamentosa NOS (693.0)

692.4 Due to other chemical products
Dermatitis due to:
acids
adhesive plaster
alkalis
caustics
dichromate
insecticide
nylon
plastic
rubber

692.5 Due to food in contact with skin
Dermatitis, contact, due to:
cereals
fish
flour
fruit
meat
milk

Excludes *dermatitis due to:*
dyes (692.89)
ingested foods (693.1)
preservatives (692.89)

692.6 Due to plants [except food]
Dermatitis due to:
lacquer tree [Rhus verniciflua]
poison:
ivy [Rhus toxicodendron]
oak [Rhus diversiloba]
sumac [Rhus venenata]
vine [Rhus radicans]
primrose [Primula]
ragweed [Senecio jacobae]
other plants in contact with the skin

Excludes *allergy NOS due to pollen (477.0)*
nettle rash (708.8)

5th 692.7 **Due to solar radiation**

Excludes *sunburn due to other ultraviolet radiation exposure (692.82)*

Degrees of Sunburn

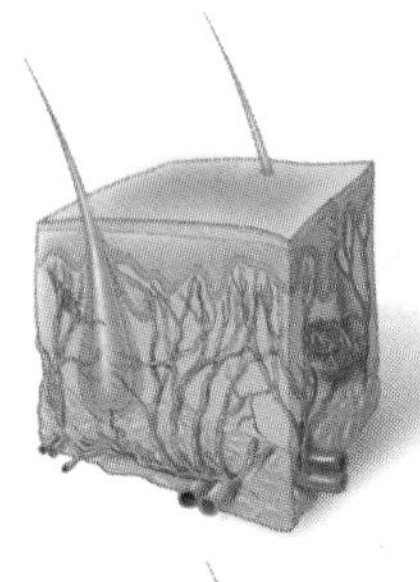

First degree sunburn is usually limited to redness and minor pain.

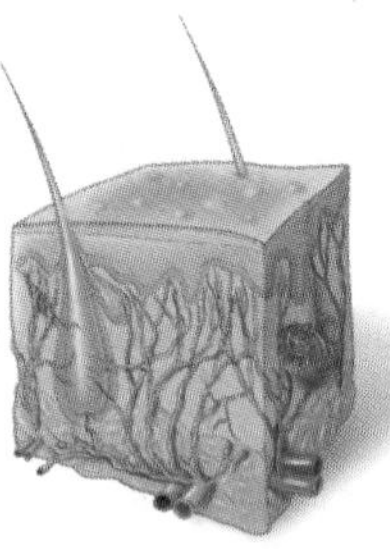

Second degree sunburn extends to the dermis and can involve nerves (thereby increasing pain). Additionally, blistering of the skin occurs.

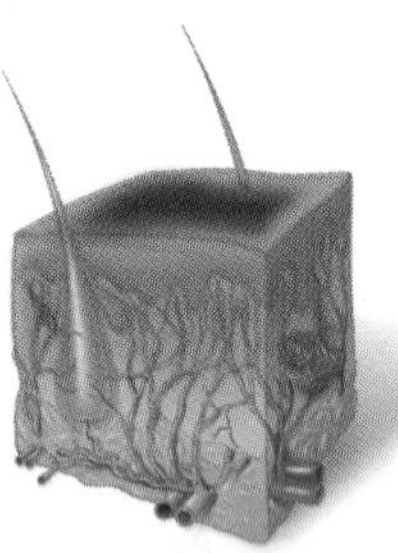

Third degree sunburn extends beyond the dermis and results in charred skin. Oftentimes, third degree sunburns is painless as nerve endings have been destroyed

© 2008 Fairman Studios, LLC. All Rights Reserved.

692.70 **Unspecified dermatitis due to sun**

692.71 **Sunburn**
- First degree sunburn
- Sunburn NOS

692.72 **Acute dermatitis due to solar radiation**
- Acute solar skin damage NOS
- Berloque dermatitis
- Photoallergic response
- Phototoxic response
- Polymorphous light eruption

Excludes *sunburn (692.71, 692.76-692.77)*

Use additional E code to identify drug, if drug induced

692.73 **Actinic reticuloid and actinic granuloma**

692.74 **Other chronic dermatitis due to solar radiation**
- Chronic solar skin damage NOS
- Solar elastosis

Excludes *actinic [solar] keratosis (702.0)*

692.75 **Disseminated superficial actinic porokeratosis (DSAP)**

692.76 **Sunburn of second degree**

692.77 **Sunburn of third degree**

692.79 **Other dermatitis due to solar radiation**
- Hydroa aestivale
- Photodermatitis (due to sun)
- Photosensitiveness (due to sun)
- Solar skin damage NOS

5th 692.8 **Due to other specified agents**

692.81 **Dermatitis due to cosmetics**

692.82 **Dermatitis due to other radiation**
- Infrared rays
- Light, except from sun
- Radiation NOS
- Tanning bed
- Ultraviolet rays, except from sun
- X-rays

Excludes *that due to solar radiation (692.70-692.79)*

692.83 **Dermatitis due to metals**
- Jewelry

692.84 **Due to animal (cat) (dog) dander**
- Due to animal (cat) (dog) hair

692.89 **Other**

Dermatitis due to:
- cold weather
- dyes
- hot weather
- preservatives

Excludes *allergy (NOS) (rhinitis) due to animal hair or dander(477.2)*
allergy to dust (477.8)
sunburn (692.71, 692.76-692.77)

692.9 **Unspecified cause**

L25.9 Unspecified contact dermatitis, unspecified cause

Dermatitis:
- NOS
- contact NOS
- venenata NOS

Eczema NOS

4th 693 **Dermatitis due to substances taken internally**

Excludes *adverse effect NOS of drugs and medicines (995.20)*
allergy NOS (995.3)
contact dermatitis (692.0-692.9)
urticarial reactions (708.0-708.9, 995.1)

693.0 **Due to drugs and medicines**

Dermatitis medicamentosa NOS

Use additional E code to identify drug

Excludes *that due to drugs in contact with skin (692.3)*

693.1 **Due to food**

693.8 **Due to other specified substances taken internally**

693.9 **Due to unspecified substance taken internally**

Excludes *dermatitis NOS (692.9)*

4th 694 **Bullous dermatoses**

694.0 **Dermatitis herpetiformis**
- Dermatosis herpetiformis
- Duhring's disease
- Hydroa herpetiformis

Excludes *herpes gestationis (646.8)*
dermatitis herpetiformis:
juvenile (694.2)
senile (694.5)

694.1 **Subcorneal pustular dermatosis**
- Sneddon-Wilkinson disease or syndrome

694.2 **Juvenile dermatitis herpetiformis**
- Juvenile pemphigoid

694.3 **Impetigo herpetiformis**

694.4 **Pemphigus**

Pemphigus:
- NOS
- erythematosus
- foliaceus
- malignant
- vegetans
- vulgaris

Excludes *pemphigus neonatorum (684)*

694.5 Pemphigoid
Benign pemphigus NOS
Bullous pemphigoid
Herpes circinatus bullosus
Senile dermatitis herpetiformis

5th **694.6 Benign mucous membrane pemphigoid**
Cicatricial pemphigoid
Mucosynechial atrophic bullous dermatitis

694.60 Without mention of ocular involvement

694.61 With ocular involvement
Ocular pemphigus

694.8 Other specified bullous dermatoses
Excludes *herpes gestationis (646.8)*

694.9 Unspecified bullous dermatoses

4th **695 Erythematous conditions**

695.0 Toxic erythema
Erythema venenatum

5th **695.1 Erythema multiforme**
Use additional code to identify associated manifestations, such as:
arthropathy associated with dermatological disorders (713.3)
conjunctival edema (372.73)
conjunctivitis (372.04, 372.33)
corneal scars and opacities (371.00-371.05)
corneal ulcer (370.00-370.07)
edema of eyelid (374.82)
inflammation of eyelid (373.8)
keratoconjunctivitis sicca (370.33)
mechanical lagophthalmos (374.22)
mucositis (478.11, 528.00, 538, 616.81)
stomatitis (528.00)
symblepharon (372.63)
Use additional E-code to identify drug, if drug-induced
Use additional code to identify percentage of skin exfoliation (695.50-695.59)
Excludes *(staphylococcal) scalded skin syndrome (695.81)*

695.10 Erythema multiforme, unspecified
Erythema iris
Herpes iris

695.11 Erythema multiforme minor

695.12 Erythema multiforme major

695.13 Stevens-Johnson syndrome

695.14 Stevens-Johnson syndrome-toxic epidermal necrolysis overlap syndrome
SJS-TEN overlap syndrome

695.15 Toxic epidermal necrolysis
Lyell's syndrome

695.19 Other erythema multiforme

695.2 Erythema nodosum
Excludes *tuberculous erythema nodosum (017.1)*

695.3 Rosacea
Acne:
erythematosa
rosacea
Perioral dermatitis
Rhinophyma

Layman's: *Rosacea is sometimes confused with common acne (vulgaris) because of its similar appearance. However, rosacea is most common in middle aged women, rather than teenagers, and is believed to have a neurovascular cause, rather than hormonal. Many acne medications actually have an adverse effect on rosacea.*

695.4 Lupus erythematosus
Lupus:
erythematodes (discoid)
erythematosus (discoid), not disseminated
Excludes *lupus (vulgaris) NOS (017.0)*
systemic [disseminated] lupus erythematosus (710.0)

5th **695.5 Exfoliation due to erythematous conditions according to extent of body surface involved**
Code first erythematous condition causing exfoliation, such as:
Ritter's disease (695.81)
(Staphylococcal) scalded skin syndrome (695.81)
Stevens-Johnson syndrome (695.13)
Stevens-Johnson syndrome-toxic epidermal necrolysis overlap syndrome (695.14)
toxic epidermal necrolysis (695.15)

695.50 ***Exfoliation due to erythematous condition involving less than 10 percent of body surface***
Exfoliation due to erythematous condition NOS

695.51 ***Exfoliation due to erythematous condition involving 10-19 percent of body surface***

695.52 ***Exfoliation due to erythematous condition involving 20-29 percent of body surface***

695.53 ***Exfoliation due to erythematous condition involving 30-39 percent of body surface***

695.54 ***Exfoliation due to erythematous condition involving 40-49 percent of body surface***

695.55 ***Exfoliation due to erythematous condition involving 50-59 percent of body surface***

695.56 ***Exfoliation due to erythematous condition involving 60-69 percent of body surface***

695.57 ***Exfoliation due to erythematous condition involving 70-79 percent of body surface***

695.58 ***Exfoliation due to erythematous condition involving 80-89 percent of body surface***

695.59 ***Exfoliation due to erythematous condition involving 90 percent or more of body surface***

5th **695.8 Other specified erythematous conditions**

695.81 Ritter's disease
Dermatitis exfoliativa neonatorum
(Staphylococcal) Scalded skin syndrome
Use additional code to identify percentage of skin exfoliation (695.50-695.59)

695.89 Other
Erythema intertrigo
Intertrigo
Pityriasis rubra (Hebra)
Excludes *mycotic intertrigo (111.0-111.9)*

695.9 Unspecified erythematous condition
Erythema NOS
Erythroderma (secondary)

4th **696 Psoriasis and similar disorders**

696.0 Psoriatic arthropathy

696.1 Other psoriasis
L40.0 Psoriasis vulgaris
L40.2 Acrodermatitis continua
L40.3 Pustulosis palmaris et plantaris
L40.4 Guttate psoriasis
L40.8 Other psoriasis
Acrodermatitis continua
Dermatitis repens
Psoriasis:
NOS
any type, except arthropathic
Excludes *psoriatic arthropathy (696.0)*

696.2 Parapsoriasis
Parakeratosis variegata
Parapsoriasis lichenoides chronica
Pityriasis lichenoides et varioliformis

696.3 Pityriasis rosea
Pityriasis circinata (et maculata)

696.4 Pityriasis rubra pilaris
Devergie's disease
Lichen ruber acuminatus
Excludes *pityriasis rubra (Hebra) (695.89)*

696.5 Other and unspecified pityriasis
Pityriasis:
NOS
alba
streptogenes
Excludes *pityriasis:*
simplex (690.18)
versicolor (111.0)

696.8 Other

4th **697 Lichen**
Excludes *lichen:*
obtusus corneus (698.3)
pilaris (congenital) (757.39)
ruber acuminatus (696.4)
sclerosus et atrophicus (701.0)
scrofulosus (017.0)
simplex chronicus (698.3)
spinulosus (congenital) (757.39)
urticatus (698.2)

697.0 Lichen planus
Lichen:
planopilaris
ruber planus

697.1 Lichen nitidus
Pinkus' disease

697.8 Other lichen, not elsewhere classified
Lichen:
ruber moniliforme
striata

697.9 Lichen, unspecified

4th **698 Pruritus and related conditions**
Excludes *pruritus specified as psychogenic (306.3)*

698.0 Pruritus ani
Perianal itch

698.1 Pruritus of genital organs

698.2 Prurigo
Lichen urticatus
Prurigo:
NOS
Hebra's
mitis
simplex
Urticaria papulosa (Hebra)
Excludes *prurigo nodularis (698.3)*

698.3 Lichenification and lichen simplex chronicus
Hyde's disease
Neurodermatitis (circumscripta) (local)
Prurigo nodularis
Excludes *neurodermatitis, diffuse (of Brocq) (691.8)*

698.4 Dermatitis factitia [artefacta]
Dermatitis ficta
Neurotic excoriation
Use additional code to identify any associated mental disorder

698.8 Other specified pruritic conditions
Pruritus:
hiemalis
senilis
Winter itch

698.9 Unspecified pruritic disorder
Itch NOS
Pruritus NOS

OTHER DISEASES OF SKIN AND SUBCUTANEOUS TISSUE (700-709)

Excludes *conditions confined to eyelids (373.0-374.9)*
congenital conditions of skin, hair, and nails (757.0-757.9)

700 Corns and callosities
L84 Corns and callosities
Callus
Clavus

4th **701 Other hypertrophic and atrophic conditions of skin**
Excludes *dermatomyositis (710.3)*
hereditary edema of legs (757.0)
scleroderma (generalized) (710.1)

701.0 Circumscribed scleroderma
Addison's keloid
Dermatosclerosis, localized
Lichen sclerosus et atrophicus
Morphea
Scleroderma, circumscribed or localized

701.1 Keratoderma, acquired
L85.0 Acquired ichthyosis
L85.1 Acquired keratosis [keratoderma] palmaris et plantaris
L87.0 Keratosis follicularis et parafollicularis in cutem penetrans
Acquired:
ichthyosis
keratoderma palmaris et plantaris
Elastosis perforans serpiginosa
Hyperkeratosis:
NOS
follicularis in cutem penetrans
palmoplantaris climacterica
Keratoderma:
climactericum
tylodes, progressive
Keratosis (blennorrhagica)
Excludes *Darier's disease [keratosis follicularis] (congenital) (757.39)*
keratosis:
arsenical (692.4)
gonococcal (098.81)

701.2 Acquired acanthosis nigricans
Keratosis nigricans

701.3 Striae atrophicae
Atrophic spots of skin
Atrophoderma maculatum
Atrophy blanche (of Milian)
Degenerative colloid atrophy
Senile degenerative atrophy
Striae distensae

701.4 Keloid scar
Cheloid
Hypertrophic scar
Keloid

701.5 Other abnormal granulation tissue
Excessive granulation

701.8 **Other specified hypertrophic and atrophic conditions of skin**
Acrodermatitis atrophicans chronica
Atrophia cutis senilis
Atrophoderma neuriticum
Confluent and reticulate papillomatosis
Cutis laxa senilis
Elastosis senilis
Folliculitis ulerythematosa reticulata
Gougerot-Carteaud syndrome or disease

701.9 **Unspecified hypertrophic and atrophic conditions of skin**
Atrophoderma

4th 702 **Other dermatoses**
Excludes *carcinoma in situ (232.0-232.9)*

Layman's: *Keratoses are distinguished from warts in that they are not caused by a virus. Actinic keratoses are specifically caused by exposure to sunlight, while use of the seborrheic keratosis (702.1x) codes should be limited to keratoses that are specifically documented to be unrelated to sun exposure.*

702.0 **Actinic keratosis**
L57.0 Actinic keratosis

5th 702.1 **Seborrheic keratosis**
Layman's: *Seborrheic keratoses are sometimes referred to as "barnacles" and commonly appear to be stuck on to the skin due to the involvement of only the epidermis.*

702.11 **Inflamed seborrheic keratosis**
L82.0 Inflamed seborrheic keratosis

702.19 **Other seborrheic keratosis**
L82.1 Other seborrheic keratosis
Seborrheic keratosis NOS

702.8 **Other specified dermatoses**

4th 703 **Diseases of nail**
Excludes *congenital anomalies (757.5)*
onychia and paronychia (681.02, 681.11)

703.0 **Ingrowing nail**
L60.0 Ingrowing nail
Ingrowing nail with infection
Unguis incarnatus
Excludes *infection, nail NOS (681.9)*

703.8 **Other specified diseases of nail**
L60.1 Onycholysis
L60.2 Onychogryphosis
L60.3 Nail dystrophy
L60.8 Other nail disorders
Dystrophia unguium
Hypertrophy of nail
Koilonychia
Leukonychia (punctata) (striata)
Onychauxis
Onychogryposis
Onycholysis

703.9 **Unspecified disease of nail**

4th 704 **Diseases of hair and hair follicles**
Excludes *congenital anomalies (757.4)*

5th 704.0 **Alopecia**
Excludes *madarosis (374.55)*
syphilitic alopecia (091.82)

704.00 **Alopecia, unspecified**
Baldness
Loss of hair

704.01 **Alopecia areata**
Ophiasis

704.02 **Telogen effluvium**

704.09 **Other**
Folliculitis decalvans
Hypotrichosis:
NOS
postinfectional NOS
Pseudopelade

704.1 **Hirsutism**
Hypertrichosis:
NOS
lanuginosa, acquired
Polytrichia
Excludes *hypertrichosis of eyelid (374.54)*

704.2 **Abnormalities of the hair**
Atrophic hair
Clastothrix
Fragilitas crinium
Trichiasis:
NOS
cicatrical
Trichorrhexis (nodosa)
Excludes *trichiasis of eyelid (374.05)*

704.3 **Variations in hair color**
Canities (premature)
Grayness, hair (premature)
Heterochromia of hair
Poliosis:
NOS
circumscripta, acquired

704.8 **Other specified diseases of hair and hair follicles**
Folliculitis:
NOS
abscedens et suffodiens
pustular
Perifolliculitis:
NOS
capitis abscedens et suffodiens
scalp
Sycosis:
NOS
barbae [not parasitic]
lupoid
vulgaris

704.9 **Unspecified disease of hair and hair follicles**

4th 705 **Disorders of sweat glands**

705.0 **Anhidrosis**
Hypohidrosis
Oligohidrosis

705.1 **Prickly heat**
Heat rash
Miliaria rubra (tropicalis)
Sudamina

5th 705.2 **Focal hyperhidrosis**
Excludes *generalized (secondary) hyperdrosis (780.8)*

705.21 **Primary focal hyperhidrosis**
Focal hyperhidrosis NOS
Hyperhidrosis NOS
Hyperhidrosis of:
axilla
face
palms
soles

705.22 **Secondary focal hyperhidrosis**
Frey's syndrome

5th 705.8 **Other specified disorders of sweat glands**

705.81 **Dyshidrosis**
Cheiropompholyx
Pompholyx

705.82 **Fox-Fordyce disease**

705.83 **Hidradenitis**
Hidradenitis suppurativa

705.89 **Other**
Bromhidrosis
Chromhidrosis
Granulosis rubra nasi
Urhidrosis
Excludes *generalized hidrocystoma (216.0-216.9)*
hyperhidrosis (780.8)

705.9 **Unspecified disorder of sweat glands**
Disorder of sweat glands NOS

4th 706 **Diseases of sebaceous glands**

706.0 **Acne varioliformis**
Acne:
frontalis
necrotica

706.1 **Other acne**
Acne:
NOS
conglobata
cystic
pustular
vulgaris
Blackhead
Comedo
Excludes *acne rosacea (695.3)*

706.2 **Sebaceous cyst**
L72.1 Trichodermal cyst
Atheroma, skin
Keratin cyst
Wen

706.3 **Seborrhea**
Excludes *seborrhea:*
capitis (690.11)
sicca (690.18)
seborrheic:
dermatitis (690.10)
keratosis (702.11-702.19)

706.8 **Other specified diseases of sebaceous glands**
Asteatosis (cutis)
Xerosis cutis

706.9 **Unspecified disease of sebaceous glands**

4th 707 **Chronic ulcer of skin**
Includes non-healing ulcer
non-infected sinus of skin
Excludes *varicose ulcer (454.0, 454.2)*

ICD-9-CM Official Guidelines (Chapter 12)

a. Pressure ulcer stage codes

1) Pressure ulcer stages

Two codes are needed to completely describe a pressure ulcer: A code from subcategory 707.0, Pressure ulcer, to identify the site of the pressure ulcer and a code from subcategory 707.2, Pressure ulcer stages.

The codes in subcategory 707.2, Pressure ulcer stages, are to be used as an additional diagnosis with a code(s) from subcategory 707.0, Pressure Ulcer. Codes from 707.2, Pressure ulcer stages, may not be assigned as a principal or first-listed diagnosis. The pressure ulcer stage codes should only be used with pressure ulcers and not with other types of ulcers (e.g., stasis ulcer).

The ICD-9-CM classifies pressure ulcer stages based on severity, which is designated by stages I-IV and unstageable.

3) Documented pressure ulcer stage

Assignment of the pressure ulcer stage code should be guided by clinical documentation of the stage or documentation of the terms found in the index. For clinical terms describing the stage that are not found in the index, and there is no documentation of the stage, the provider should be queried.

4) Bilateral pressure ulcers with same stage

When a patient has bilateral pressure ulcers (e.g., both buttocks) and both pressure ulcers are documented as being the same stage, only the code for the site and one code for the stage should be reported.

5) Bilateral pressure ulcers with different stages

When a patient has bilateral pressure ulcers at the same site (e.g., both buttocks) and each pressure ulcer is documented as being at a different stage, assign one code for the site and the appropriate codes for the pressure ulcer stage.

6) Multiple pressure ulcers of different sites and stages

When a patient has multiple pressure ulcers at different sites (e.g., buttock, heel, shoulder) and each pressure ulcer is documented as being at different stages (e.g., stage 3 and stage 4), assign the appropriate codes for each different site and a code for each different pressure ulcer stage.

7) Patients admitted with pressure ulcers documented as healed

No code is assigned if the documentation states that the pressure ulcer is completely healed.

8) Patients admitted with pressure ulcers documented as healing

Pressure ulcers described as healing should be assigned the appropriate pressure ulcer stage code based on the documentation in the medical record. If the documentation does not provide information about the stage of the healing pressure ulcer, assign code 707.20, Pressure ulcer stage, unspecified.

If the documentation is unclear as to whether the patient has a current (new) pressure ulcer or if the patient is being treated for a healing pressure ulcer, query the provider.

9) Patient admitted with pressure ulcer evolving into another stage during the admission

If a patient is admitted with a pressure ulcer at one stage and it progresses to a higher stage, assign the code for highest stage reported for that site.

5th 707.0 **Pressure ulcer**
Bed sore
Decubitus ulcer
Plaster ulcer
Use additional code to identify pressure ulcer stage (707.20-707.25)

707.00 **Unspecified site**
L89.90 Pressure ulcer of unspecified site, unspecified stage

707.01 **Elbow**
L89.009 Pressure ulcer of unspecified elbow, unspecified stage

707.02 **Upper back**
L89.109 Pressure ulcer of unspecified part of back, unspecified stage
Shoulder blades

707.03 **Lower back**
L89.159 Pressure ulcer of sacral region, unspecified stage
Coccyx
Sacrum

707.04 **Hip**
L89.209 Pressure ulcer of unspecified hip, unspecified stage

707.05 **Buttock**
L89.309 Pressure ulcer of unspecified buttock, unspecified stage

707.06 **Ankle**
L89.509 Pressure ulcer of unspecified ankle, unspecified stage

707.07 **Heel**
L89.609 Pressure ulcer of unspecified heel, unspecified stage

707.09 **Other site**
L89.819 Pressure ulcer of head, unspecified stage
L89.899 Pressure ulcer of other site, unspecified stage
Head

5th 707.1 **Ulcer of lower limbs, except pressure ulcer**
Ulcer, chronic, of lower limb:
neurogenic of lower limb
trophic of lower limb
Code, if applicable, any causal condition first:
atherosclerosis of the extremities with ulceration (440.23)
chronic venous hypertension with ulcer (459.31)
chronic venous hypertension with ulcer and inflammation (459.33)
diabetes mellitus (249.80-249.81, 250.80-250.83)
postphlebitic syndrome with ulcer (459.11)
postphlebitic syndrome with ulcer and inflammation (459.13)

707.10 **Ulcer of lower limb, unspecified**
L97.909 Non-pressure chronic ulcer of unspecified part of unspecified lower leg with unspecified severity

707.11 **Ulcer of thigh**

707.12 **Ulcer of calf** I 86

707.13 **Ulcer of ankle** I 86

707.14 **Ulcer of heel and midfoot** I 86
L97.409 Non-pressure chronic ulcer of unspecified heel and midfoot with unspecified severity
Plantar surface of midfoot

707.15 **Ulcer of other part of foot** I 86
L97.509 Non-pressure chronic ulcer of other part of unspecified foot with unspecified severity
Toes

707.19 **Ulcer of other part of lower limb** I 86

5th 707.2 **Pressure ulcer stages**
Code first site of pressure ulcer (707.00-707.09)

707.20 **Pressure ulcer, unspecified stage**
Healing pressure ulcer NOS
Healing pressure ulcer, unspecified stage

707.21 **Pressure ulcer stage I**
Healing pressure ulcer, stage I
Pressure pre-ulcer skin changes limited to persistent focal erythema

707.22 **Pressure ulcer stage II**
Healing pressure ulcer, stage II
Pressure ulcer with abrasion, blister, partial thickness skin loss involving epidermis and/or dermis

707.23 **Pressure ulcer stage III**
Healing pressure ulcer, stage III
Pressure ulcer with full thickness skin loss involving damage or necrosis of subcutaneous tissue

707.24 **Pressure ulcer stage IV**
Healing pressure ulcer, stage IV
Pressure ulcer with necrosis of soft tissues through to underlying muscle, tendon, or bone

ICD-9-CM Official Guidelines (Chapter 12)

a. Pressure ulcer stage codes

2) Unstageable pressure ulcers

Assignment of code 707.25, Pressure ulcer, unstageable, should be based on the clinical documentation. Code 707.25 is used for pressure ulcers whose stage cannot be clinically determined (e.g., the ulcer is covered by eschar or has been treated with a skin or muscle graft) and pressure ulcers that are documented as deep tissue injury but not documented as due to trauma. This code should not be confused with code 707.20, Pressure ulcer, stage unspecified. Code 707.20 should be assigned when there is no documentation regarding the stage of the pressure ulcer.

707.25 **Pressure ulcer, unstageable**

707.8 **Chronic ulcer of other specified sites**
Ulcer, chronic, of other specified sites:
neurogenic
trophic

707.9 **Chronic ulcer of unspecified site**
Chronic ulcer NOS
Trophic ulcer NOS
Tropical ulcer NOS
Ulcer of skin NOS

4th 708 **Urticaria**
Excludes *edema:*
angioneurotic (995.1)
Quincke's (995.1)
hereditary angioedema (277.6)
urticaria:
giant (995.1)
papulosa (Hebra) (698.2)
pigmentosa (juvenile) (congenital) (757.33)

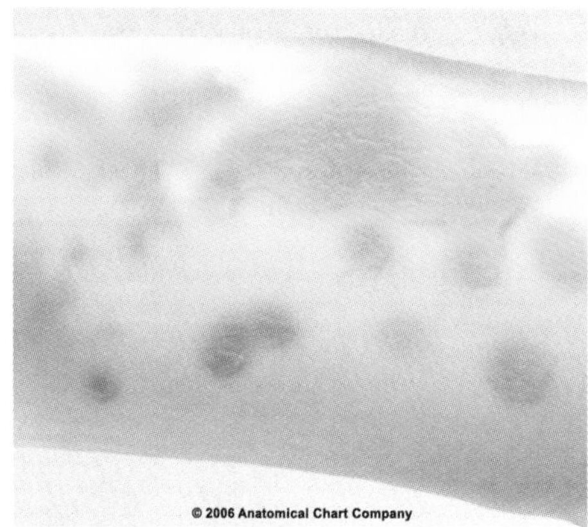
© 2006 Anatomical Chart Company

708.0 **Allergic urticaria**

708.1 **Idiopathic urticaria**

708.2 **Urticaria due to cold and heat**
Thermal urticaria

708.3 **Dermatographic urticaria**
Dermatographia
Factitial urticaria

708.4 **Vibratory urticaria**

708.5 **Cholinergic urticaria**

708.8 **Other specified urticaria**
Nettle rash
Urticaria:
chronic
recurrent periodic

708.9 **Urticaria, unspecified**
Hives NOS

707.06 – 708.9

4th 709 **Other disorders of skin and subcutaneous tissue**

5th 709.0 **Dyschromia**

Excludes *albinism (270.2)*
pigmented nevus (216.0-216.9)
that of eyelid (374.52-374.53)

709.00 **Dyschromia, unspecified**

709.01 **Vitiligo**

709.09 **Other**

709.1 **Vascular disorders of skin**

Angioma serpiginosum
Purpura (primary) annularis telangiectodes

709.2 **Scar conditions and fibrosis of skin**

Adherent scar (skin)
Cicatrix
Disfigurement (due to scar)
Fibrosis, skin NOS
Scar NOS

Excludes *keloid scar (701.4)*

709.3 **Degenerative skin disorders**

Calcinosis:
circumscripta
cutis
Colloid milium
Degeneration, skin
Deposits, skin
Senile dermatosis NOS
Subcutaneous calcification

709.4 **Foreign body granuloma of skin and subcutaneous tissue**

Excludes *residual foreign body without granuloma of skin and subcutaneous tissue (729.6)*
that of muscle (728.82)

709.8 **Other specified disorders of skin**

Epithelial hyperplasia
Menstrual dermatosis
Vesicular eruption

709.9 **Unspecified disorder of skin and subcutaneous tissue**

L98.9 Disorder of the skin and subcutaneous tissue, unspecified

Dermatosis NOS

13. DISEASES OF THE MUSCULOSKELETAL SYSTEM AND CONNECTIVE TISSUE (710-739)

Use additional external cause code, if applicable, to identify the cause of the musculoskeletal condition

The following fifth-digit subclassification is for use with categories 711-712, 715-716, 718-719, and 730:

0 **site unspecified**

1 **shoulder region**
Acromioclavicular joint(s)
Clavicle
Glenohumeral joint(s)
Scapula
Sternoclavicular joint(s)

2 **upper arm**
Elbow joint
Humerus

3 **forearm**
Radius
Ulna
Wrist joint

4 **hand**
Carpus
Metacarpus
Phalanges [fingers]

5 **pelvic region and thigh**
Buttock
Femur
Hip (joint)

6 **lower leg**
Fibula
Knee joint
Patella
Tibia

7 **ankle and foot**
Ankle joint
Digits [toes]
Metatarsus
Phalanges, foot
Tarsus
Other joints in foot

8 **other specified sites**
Head
Neck
Ribs
Skull
Trunk
Vertebral column

9 **multiple sites**

ARTHROPATHIES AND RELATED DISORDERS (710-719)

Excludes *disorders of spine (720.0-724.9)*

4th 710 **Diffuse diseases of connective tissue**

Includes all collagen diseases whose effects are not mainly confined to a single system

Excludes *those affecting mainly the cardiovascular system, i.e., polyarteritis nodosa and allied conditions (446.0-446.7)*

710.0 **Systemic lupus erythematosus**

M32.10 Systemic lupus erythematosus, organ or system involvement unspecified

Disseminated lupus erythematosus
Libman-Sacks disease

Use additional code to identify manifestation, as:
endocarditis (424.91)
nephritis (583.81)
chronic (582.81)
nephrotic syndrome (581.81)

Excludes *lupus erythematosus (discoid) NOS (695.4)*

710.1 Systemic sclerosis
Acrosclerosis
CRST syndrome
Progressive systemic sclerosis
Scleroderma
Use additional code to identify manifestation, as:
lung involvement (517.2)
myopathy (359.6)
Excludes *circumscribed scleroderma (701.0)*

710.2 Sicca syndrome
Keratoconjunctivitis sicca
Sjögren's disease

710.3 Dermatomyositis
Poikilodermatomyositis
Polymyositis with skin involvement

710.4 Polymyositis

710.5 Eosinophilia myalgia syndrome
Toxic oil syndrome
Use additional E to identify drug, if drug induced

710.8 Other specified diffuse diseases of connective tissue
Multifocal fibrosclerosis (idiopathic) NEC
Systemic fibrosclerosing syndrome

710.9 Unspecified diffuse connective tissue disease
Collagen disease NOS

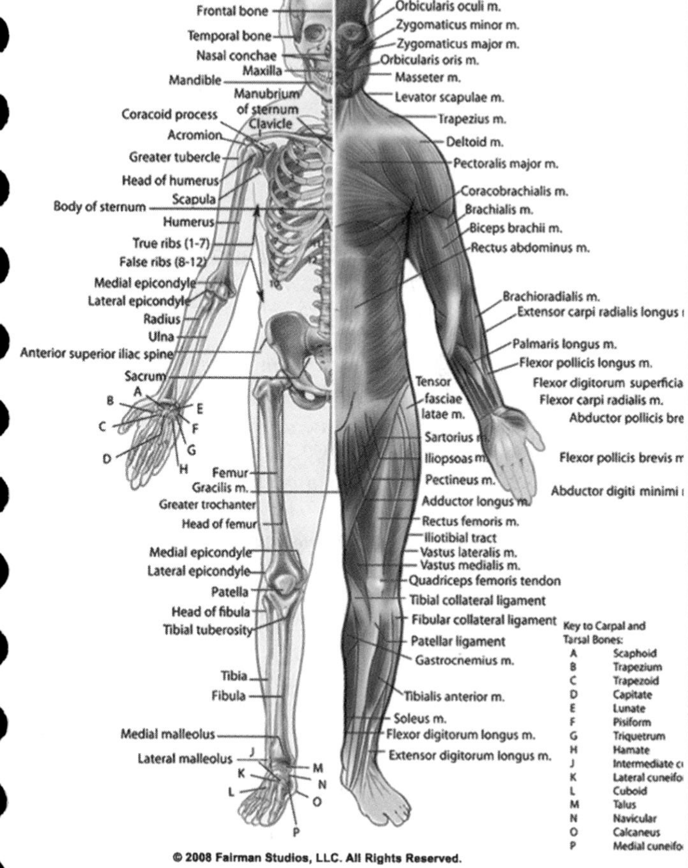

© 2008 Fairman Studios, LLC. All Rights Reserved.

4th 711 Arthropathy associated with infections
Includes arthritis associated with conditions classifiable below
arthropathy associated with conditions classifiable below
polyarthritis associated with conditions classifiable below
polyarthropathy associated with conditions classifiable below
Excludes *rheumatic fever (390)*

The following fifth-digit subclassification is for use with category 711; valid digits are in [brackets] under each code. See list at beginning of chapter for definitions:

0 **site unspecified**
1 **shoulder region**
2 **upper arm**
3 **forearm**
4 **hand**
5 **pelvic region and thigh**
6 **lower leg**
7 **ankle and foot**
8 **other specified sites**
9 **multiple sites**

5th 711.0 Pyogenic arthritis
[0-9]
Arthritis or polyarthritis (due to):
coliform [Escherichia coli]
Hemophilus influenzae [H. influenzae]
pneumococcal
Pseudomonas
staphylococcal
streptococcal
Pyarthrosis
Use additional code to identify infectious organism (041.0-041.8)

5th 711.1 *Arthropathy associated with Reiter's disease and nonspecific urethritis*
[0-9]
Code first underlying disease, as:
nonspecific urethritis (099.4)
Reiter's disease (099.3)

5th 711.2 *Arthropathy in Behçet's syndrome*
[0-9]
Code first underlying disease (136.1)

5th 711.3 *Postdysenteric arthropathy*
[0-9]
Code first underlying disease, as:
dysentery (009.0)
enteritis, infectious (008.0-009.3)
paratyphoid fever (002.1-002.9)
typhoid fever (002.0)
Excludes *salmonella arthritis (003.23)*

5th 711.4 *Arthropathy associated with other bacterial diseases*
[0-9]
Code first underlying disease, as:
diseases classifiable to 010-040, 090-099, except as in 711.1, 711.3, and 713.5
leprosy (030.0-030.9)
tuberculosis (015.0-015.9)
Excludes *gonococcal arthritis (098.50)*
meningococcal arthritis (036.82)

5th 711.5 *Arthropathy associated with other viral diseases*
[0-9]
Code first underlying disease, as:
diseases classifiable to 045-049. 050-079, 480, 487
O'nyong nyong (066.3)
Excludes *that due to rubella (056.71)*

5th 711.6 **Arthropathy associated with mycoses**
[0-9]

Code first underlying disease (110.0-118)

5th 711.7 **Arthropathy associated with helminthiasis**
[0-9]

Code first underlying disease, as:
filariasis (125.0-125.9)

5th 711.8 **Arthropathy associated with other infectious and parasitic diseases**
[0-9]

Code first underlying disease, as:
diseases classifiable to 080-088, 100-104, 130-136

Excludes *arthropathy associated with sarcoidosis (713.7)*

5th 711.9 **Unspecified infective arthritis**
[0-9] Infective arthritis or polyarthritis (acute) (chronic) (subacute) NOS

4th 712 **Crystal arthropathies**

Includes crystal-induced arthritis and synovitis

Excludes *gouty arthropathy (274.00-274.03)*

The following fifth-digit subclassification is for use with category 712; valid digits are in [brackets] under each code. See list at beginning of chapter for definitions:

0 site unspecified
1 shoulder region
2 upper arm
3 forearm
4 hand
5 pelvic region and thigh
6 lower leg
7 ankle and foot
8 other specified sites
9 multiple sites

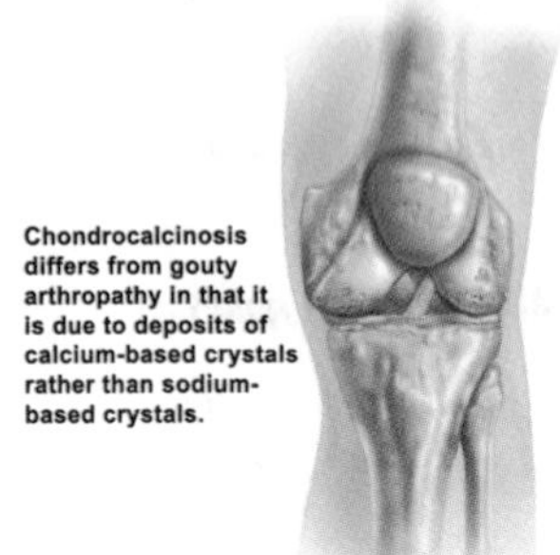

Chondrocalcinosis differs from gouty arthropathy in that it is due to deposits of calcium-based crystals rather than sodium-based crystals.

© 2008 Fairman Studios, LLC. All Rights Reserved.

5th 712.1 **Chondrocalcinosis due to dicalcium phosphate crystals**
[0-9] Chondrocalcinosis due to dicalcium phosphate crystals (with other crystals)

Code first underlying disease (275.49)

5th 712.2 **Chondrocalcinosis due to pyrophosphate crystals**
[0-9]

Code first underlying disease (275.49)

5th 712.3 **Chondrocalcinosis, unspecified**
[0-9]

Code first underlying disease (275.49)

5th 712.8 **Other specified crystal arthropathies**
[0-9]

5th 712.9 **Unspecified crystal arthropathy**
[0-9]

4th 713 **Arthropathy associated with other disorders classified elsewhere**

Includes arthritis associated with conditions classifiable below
arthropathy associated with conditions classifiable below
polyarthritis associated with conditions classifiable below
polyarthropathy associated with conditions classifiable below

713.0 **Arthropathy associated with other endocrine and metabolic disorders**

Code first underlying disease, as:
acromegaly (253.0)
hemochromatosis (275.0)
hyperparathyroidism (252.00-252.08)
hypogammaglobulinemia (279.00-279.09)
hypothyroidism (243-244.9)
lipoid metabolism disorder (272.0-272.9)
ochronosis (270.2)

Excludes *arthropathy associated with:*
amyloidosis (713.7)
crystal deposition disorders, except gout (712.1-712.9)
diabetic neuropathy (713.5)
gouty ~~arthropathy~~ (274.00-274.03)

713.1 **Arthropathy associated with gastrointestinal conditions other than infections**

Code first underlying disease, as:
regional enteritis (555.0-555.9)
ulcerative colitis (556)

713.2 **Arthropathy associated with hematological disorders**

Code first underlying disease, as:
hemoglobinopathy (282.4-282.7)
hemophilia (286.0-286.2)
leukemia (204.0-208.9)
malignant reticulosis (202.3)
multiple myelomatosis (203.0)

Excludes *arthropathy associated with Henoch-Schönlein purpura (713.6)*

713.3 **Arthropathy associated with dermatological disorders**

Code first underlying disease, as:
erythema multiforme (695.10-695.19)
erythema nodosum (695.2)

Excludes *psoriatic arthropathy (696.0)*

713.4 **Arthropathy associated with respiratory disorders**

Code first underlying disease, as:
diseases classifiable to 490-519

Excludes *arthropathy associated with respiratory infections (711.0, 711.4-711.8)*

713.5 **Arthropathy associated with neurological disorders**

Charcôt's arthropathy associated with diseases classifiable elsewhere
Neuropathic arthritis associated with diseases classifiable elsewhere

Code first underlying disease, as:
neuropathic joint disease [Charcôt's joints]:
NOS (094.0)
diabetic (249.6, 250.6)
syringomyelic (336.0)
tabetic [syphilitic] (094.0)

713.6 **Arthropathy associated with hypersensitivity reaction**

Code first underlying disease, as:
Henoch (-Schönlein) purpura (287.0)
serum sickness (999.5)

Excludes *allergic arthritis NOS (716.2)*

713.7 Other general diseases with articular involvement
Code first underlying disease, as:
amyloidosis (277.30-277.39)
familial Mediterranean fever (277.31)
sarcoidosis (135)

713.8 Arthropathy associated with other conditions classifiable elsewhere
Code first underlying disease, as:
conditions classifiable elsewhere except as in 711.1-711.8, 712, and 713.0-713.7

4th **714 Rheumatoid arthritis and other inflammatory polyarthropathies**
Excludes *rheumatic fever (390)*
rheumatoid arthritis of spine NOS (720.0)

Layman's: *According to the American College of Rheumatology, at least 4 of the following criteria must be met (i.e., documented) for a definitive diagnosis of rheumatoid arthritis: 1) joint stiffness of ≥1 hour on most mornings of a 6 week period, 2) arthritis and swelling of ≥3 of the 14 joint groups for at least 6 weeks, 3) arthritis of the hand joints for at least 6 weeks, 4) symmetric arthritis for at least 6 weeks, 5) subcutaneous nodules in specific joints, 6) rheumatoid factor levels of above 95%, and 7) radiological changes that suggest joint erosion.*

Osteoarthrosis (715.xx) differs from RA in that it: is not commonly symmetrical; is due to wear and tear, rather than an autoimmune process; tends to manifest in the larger joints (e.g., hips, knees) rather than smaller ones (e.g., hands feet); and is much more common (by a magnitude of 10:1).

714.0 Rheumatoid arthritis 108, 176, 177, 178, 179, 180
M06.9 Rheumatoid arthritis, unspecified
Arthritis or polyarthritis:
atrophic
rheumatic (chronic)
Use additional code to identify manifestation, as:
myopathy (359.6)
polyneuropathy (357.1)
Excludes *juvenile rheumatoid arthritis NOS (714.30)*

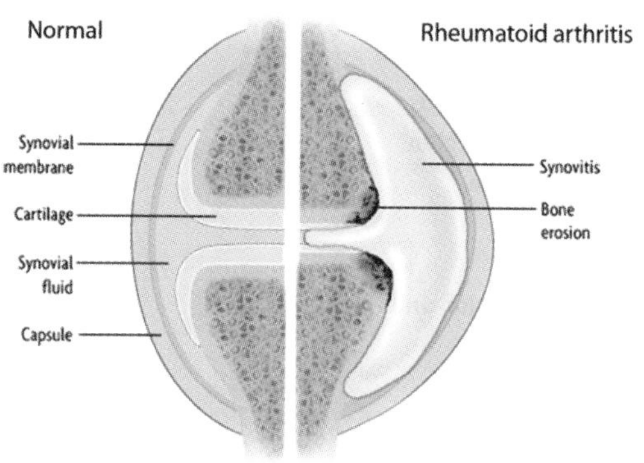

© 2008 Fairman Studios, LLC. All Rights Reserved.

714.1 Felty's syndrome 108, 176, 177, 178, 179, 180
Rheumatoid arthritis with splenoadenomegaly and leukopenia

714.2 Other rheumatoid arthritis with visceral or systemic involvement 108, 176, 177, 178, 179, 180
Rheumatoid carditis

5th **714.3 Juvenile chronic polyarthritis**

714.30 Polyarticular juvenile rheumatoid arthritis, chronic or unspecified
Juvenile rheumatoid arthritis NOS
Still's disease

714.31 Polyarticular juvenile rheumatoid arthritis, acute

714.32 Pauciarticular juvenile rheumatoid arthritis

714.33 Monoarticular juvenile rheumatoid arthritis

714.4 Chronic postrheumatic arthropathy
Chronic rheumatoid nodular fibrositis
Jaccoud's syndrome

5th **714.8 Other specified inflammatory polyarthropathies**

714.81 Rheumatoid lung 108, 176, 177, 178, 179, 180
Caplan's syndrome
Diffuse interstitial rheumatoid disease of lung
Fibrosing alveolitis, rheumatoid

714.89 Other

714.9 Unspecified inflammatory polyarthropathy
M06.4 Inflammatory polyarthropathy
Inflammatory polyarthropathy or polyarthritis NOS
Excludes *polyarthropathy NOS (716.5)*

4th **715 Osteoarthrosis and allied disorders**
Note: *Localized, in the subcategories below, includes bilateral involvement of the same site.*
Includes arthritis or polyarthritis:
degenerative
hypertrophic
degenerative joint disease
osteoarthritis
Excludes *Marie-Strümpell spondylitis (720.0)*
osteoarthrosis [osteoarthritis] of spine (721.0-721.9)

The following fifth-digit subclassification is for use with category 715; valid digits are in [brackets] under each code. See list at beginning of chapter for definitions:

0 site unspecified
1 shoulder region
2 upper arm
3 forearm
4 hand
5 pelvic region and thigh
6 lower leg
7 ankle and foot
8 other specified sites
9 multiple sites

Common sites for osteoarthrosis

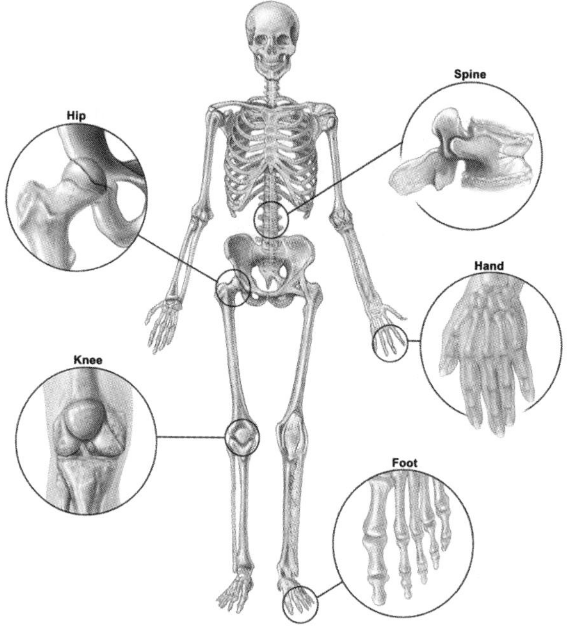

© 2008 Fairman Studios, LLC. All Rights Reserved.

5th **715.0 Osteoarthrosis, generalized** 109, 142
[0,4,9] Degenerative joint disease, involving multiple joints
Primary generalized hypertrophic osteoarthrosis

5th 715.1 **Osteoarthrosis, localized, primary** I09, I42
[0-8] Localized osteoarthropathy, idiopathic

5th 715.2 **Osteoarthrosis, localized, secondary** I09, I42
[0-8] Coxae malum senilis

5th 715.3 **Osteoarthrosis, localized, not specified whether primary or secondary** I09, I42
[0-8] Otto's pelvis

5th 715.8 **Osteoarthrosis involving, or with mention of more than one site, but not specified as generalized** I09, I42
[0,9]

5th 715.9 **Osteoarthrosis, unspecified whether generalized or localized** I09, I42
[0-8]

4th 716 **Other and unspecified arthropathies**

Excludes *cricoarytenoid arthropathy (478.79)*

The following fifth-digit subclassification is for use with category 716; valid digits are in [brackets] under each code. See list at beginning of chapter for definitions:

- 0 site unspecified
- 1 shoulder region
- 2 upper arm
- 3 forearm
- 4 hand
- 5 pelvic region and thigh
- 6 lower leg
- 7 ankle and foot
- 8 other specified sites
- 9 multiple sites

5th 716.0 **Kaschin-Beck disease**
[0-9] Endemic polyarthritis

5th 716.1 **Traumatic arthropathy**
[0-9]

5th 716.2 **Allergic arthritis**
[0-9]

Excludes *arthritis associated with Henoch-Schönlein purpura or serum sickness (713.6)*

5th 716.3 **Climacteric arthritis** ♀
[0-9] Menopausal arthritis

5th 716.4 **Transient arthropathy**
[0-9]

Excludes *palindromic rheumatism (719.3)*

5th 716.5 **Unspecified polyarthropathy or polyarthritis**
[0-9]

5th 716.6 **Unspecified monoarthritis**
[0-8] Coxitis

5th 716.8 **Other specified arthropathy**
[0-9]

5th 716.9 **Arthropathy, unspecified**
[0-9] Arthritis, (acute) (chronic) (subacute)
Arthropathy, (acute) (chronic) (subacute)
Articular rheumatism, (chronic)
Inflammation of joint, NOS

4th 717 **Internal derangement of knee**

Includes degeneration of articular cartilage or meniscus of knee
rupture, old of articular cartilage or meniscus of knee
tear, old of articular cartilage or meniscus of knee

Excludes *acute derangement of knee (836.0-836.6)*
ankylosis (718.5)
contracture (718.4)
current injury (836.0-836.6)
deformity (736.4-736.6)
recurrent dislocation (718.3)

717.0 **Old bucket handle tear of medial meniscus**
Old bucket handle tear of unspecified cartilage

717.1 **Derangement of anterior horn of medial meniscus**

717.2 **Derangement of posterior horn of medial meniscus**

717.3 **Other and unspecified derangement of medial meniscus**
Degeneration of internal semilunar cartilage

5th 717.4 **Derangement of lateral meniscus**

717.40 **Derangement of lateral meniscus, unspecified**

717.41 **Bucket handle tear of lateral meniscus**

717.42 **Derangement of anterior horn of lateral meniscus**

717.43 **Derangement of posterior horn of lateral meniscus**

717.49 **Other**

717.5 **Derangement of meniscus, not elsewhere classified**
Congenital discoid meniscus
Cyst of semilunar cartilage
Derangement of semilunar cartilage NOS

717.6 **Loose body in knee**
Joint mice, knee
Rice bodies, knee (joint)

717.7 **Chondromalacia of patella**
Chondromalacia patellae
Degeneration [softening] of articular cartilage of patella

5th 717.8 **Other internal derangement of knee**

717.81 **Old disruption of lateral collateral ligament**

717.82 **Old disruption of medial collateral ligament**

717.83 **Old disruption of anterior cruciate ligament**

717.84 **Old disruption of posterior cruciate ligament**

717.85 **Old disruption of other ligaments of knee**
Capsular ligament of knee

717.89 **Other**
Old disruption of ligaments of knee NOS

717.9 **Unspecified internal derangement of knee**
Derangement NOS of knee

4th 718 **Other derangement of joint**

Excludes *current injury (830.0-848.9)*
jaw (524.60-524.69)

The following fifth-digit subclassification is for use with category 718; valid digits are in [brackets] under each code. See list at beginning of chapter for definitions:

- 0 site unspecified
- 1 shoulder region
- 2 upper arm
- 3 forearm
- 4 hand
- 5 pelvic region and thigh
- 6 lower leg
- 7 ankle and foot
- 8 other specified sites
- 9 multiple sites

5th 718.0 **Articular cartilage disorder**
[0-5,7-9] Meniscus:
disorder
rupture, old
tear, old
Old rupture of ligament(s) of joint NOS

Excludes *articular cartilage disorder:*
in ochronosis (270.2)
knee (717.0-717.9)
chondrocalcinosis (275.49)
metastatic calcification (275.40)

5th 718.1 **Loose body in joint**
[0-5,7-9] Joint mice

Excludes *knee (717.6)*

5th 718.2 **Pathological dislocation**
[0-9] Dislocation or displacement of joint, not recurrent and not current

5th 718.3 **Recurrent dislocation of joint**
[0-9]

5th 718.4 **Contracture of joint**
[0-9]

5th 718.5 **Ankylosis of joint**
[0-9] Ankylosis of joint (fibrous) (osseous)
Excludes *spine (724.9)*
stiffness of joint without mention of ankylosis (719.5)

5th 718.6 **Unspecified intrapelvic protrusion of acetabulum**
[0,5] Protrusio acetabuli, unspecified

5th 718.7 **Developmental dislocation of joint**
[0-9]
Excludes *congenital dislocation of joint (754.0-755.8)*
traumatic dislocation of joint (830-839)

5th 718.8 **Other joint derangement, not elsewhere classified**
[0-9] Flail joint (paralytic)
Instability of joint
Excludes *deformities classifiable to 736 (736.0-736.9)*

5th 718.9 **Unspecified derangement of joint**
[0-5,7-9]
Excludes *knee (717.9)*

4th 719 **Other and unspecified disorders of joint**
Excludes *jaw (524.60-524.69)*

The following fifth-digit subclassification is for use with codes 719.0-719.6, 719.8-719.9; valid digits are in [brackets] under each code. See list at beginning of chapter for definitions:

0 site unspecified
1 shoulder region
2 upper arm
3 forearm
4 hand
5 pelvic region and thigh
6 lower leg
7 ankle and foot
8 other specified sites
9 multiple sites

5th 719.0 **Effusion of joint**
[0-9] Hydrarthrosis
Swelling of joint, with or without pain
Excludes *intermittent hydrarthrosis (719.3)*

5th 719.1 **Hemarthrosis**
[0-9]
Excludes *current injury (840.0-848.9)*

5th 719.2 **Villonodular synovitis**
[0-9]

5th 719.3 **Palindromic rheumatism**
[0-9] Hench-Rosenberg syndrome
Intermittent hydrarthrosis

5th 719.4 **Pain in joint**
[0-9] Arthralgia

5th 719.5 **Stiffness of joint, not elsewhere classified**
[0-9]

5th 719.6 **Other symptoms referable to joint**
[0-9] Joint crepitus
Snapping hip

719.7 **Difficulty in walking**
R26.2 Difficulty in walking, not elsewhere classified
Excludes *abnormality of gait (781.2)*

5th 719.8 **Other specified disorders of joint**
[0-9] Calcification of joint
Fistula of joint
Excludes *temporomandibular joint-pain-dysfunction syndrome [Costen's syndrome] (524.60)*

5th 719.9 **Unspecified disorder of joint**
[0-9]

DORSOPATHIES (720-724)

Excludes *curvature of spine (737.0-737.9)*
osteochondrosis of spine (juvenile) (732.0) adult (732.8)

4th 720 **Ankylosing spondylitis and other inflammatory spondylopathies**

720.0 **Ankylosing spondylitis**
Rheumatioid arthritis of spine NOS
Spondylitis:
Marie-Strümpell
rheumatoid

720.1 **Spinal enthesopathy**
Disorder of peripheral ligamentous or muscular attachments of spine
Romanus lesion

720.2 **Sacroiliitis, not elsewhere classified**
M46.1 Sacroiliitis, not elsewhere classified
Inflammation of sacroiliac joint NOS

5th 720.8 **Other inflammatory spondylopathies**

720.81 ***Inflammatory spondylopathies in diseases classified elsewhere***
Code first underlying disease, as:
tuberculosis (015.0)

720.89 **Other**

720.9 **Unspecified inflammatory spondylopathy**
Spondylitis NOS

4th 721 **Spondylosis and allied disorders**

721.0 **Cervical spondylosis without myelopathy**
M47.812 Spondylosis without myelopathy or radiculopathy, cervical region
Cervical or cervicodorsal:
arthritis
osteoarthritis
spondylarthritis

721.1 **Cervical spondylosis with myelopathy**
Anterior spinal artery compression syndrome
Spondylogenic compression of cervical spinal cord
Vertebral artery compression syndrome

721.2 **Thoracic spondylosis without myelopathy**
Thoracic:
arthritis
osteoarthritis
spondylarthritis

721.3 **Lumbosacral spondylosis without myelopathy** I 48, I 49, I 50, I 51
M47.817 Spondylosis without myelopathy or radiculopathy, lumbosacral region
Lumbar or lumbosacral:
arthritis
osteoarthritis
spondylarthritis

5th 721.4 **Thoracic or lumbar spondylosis with myelopathy**

721.41 **Thoracic region** I 48, I 49, I 50, I 51
Spondylogenic compression of thoracic spinal cord

721.42 **Lumbar region** I 48, I 49, I 50, I 51
Spondylogenic compression of lumbar spinal cord

721.5 **Kissing spine**
Baastrup's syndrome

721.6 **Ankylosing vertebral hyperostosis**

718.2 – 721.6

721.7 **Traumatic spondylopathy**
Kümmell's disease or spondylitis

721.8 **Other allied disorders of spine**

5th 721.9 **Spondylosis of unspecified site**

721.90 **Without mention of myelopathy** I 48, I 49, I 50, I 51

M47.819 Spondylosis without myelopathy or radiculopathy, site unspecified

Spinal:
arthritis (deformans) (degenerative) (hypertrophic)
osteoarthritis NOS
Spondylarthrosis NOS

721.91 **With myelopathy**
Spondylogenic compression of spinal cord NOS

4th 722 **Intervertebral disc disorders**

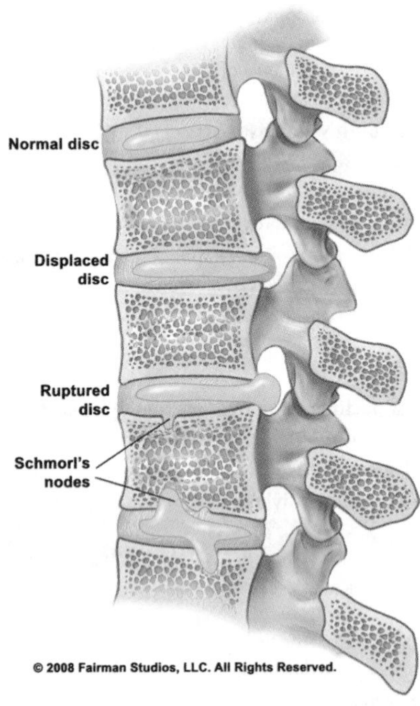

722.0 **Displacement of cervical intervertebral disc without myelopathy** I 48, I 49, I 50, I 51

M50.20 Other cervical disc displacement, unspecified cervical region

Neuritis (brachial) or radiculitis due to displacement or rupture of cervical intervertebral disc
Any condition classifiable to 722.2 of the cervical or cervicothoracic intervertebral disc

5th 722.1 **Displacement of thoracic or lumbar intervertebral disc without myelopathy**

722.10 **Lumbar intervertebral disc without myelopathy** I 48, I 49, I 50, I 51

M51.26 Other intervertebral disc displacement, lumbar region

Lumbago or sciatica due to displacement of intervertebral disc
Neuritis or radiculitis due to displacement or rupture of lumbar intervertebral disc
Any condition classifiable to 722.2 of the lumbar or lumbosacral intervertebral disc

722.11 **Thoracic intervertebral disc without myelopathy** I 48, I 49, I 50, I 51
Any condition classifiable to 722.2 of thoracic intervertebral disc

722.2 **Displacement of intervertebral disc, site unspecified, without myelopathy** I 48, I 49, I 50, I 51
Discogenic syndrome NOS
Herniation of nucleus pulposus NOS
Intervertebral disc NOS:
extrusion
prolapse
protrusion
rupture
Neuritis or radiculitis due to displacement or rupture of intervertebral disc

5th 722.3 **Schmorl's nodes**

722.30 **Unspecified region**

722.31 **Thoracic region** I 48, I 49, I 50, I 51

722.32 **Lumbar region** I 48, I 49, I 50, I 51

722.39 **Other** I 48, I 49, I 50, I 51

722.4 **Degeneration of cervical intervertebral disc** I 48, I 49, I 50, I 51

M50.30 Other cervical disc degeneration, unspecified cervical region

Degeneration of cervicothoracic intervertebral disc

5th 722.5 **Degeneration of thoracic or lumbar intervertebral disc**

722.51 **Thoracic or thoracolumbar intervertebral disc** I 48, I 49, I 50, I 51

722.52 **Lumbar or lumbosacral intervertebral disc** I 48, I 49, I 50, I 51

M51.36 Other intervertebral disc degeneration, lumbar region

M51.37 Other intervertebral disc degeneration, lumbosacral region

722.6 **Degeneration of intervertebral disc, site unspecified** I 48, I 49, I 50, I 51
Degenerative disc disease NOS
Narrowing of intervertebral disc or space NOS

5th 722.7 **Intervertebral disc disorder with myelopathy**

722.70 **Unspecified region** I 48, I 49, I 50, I 51

722.71 **Cervical region** I 48, I 49, I 50, I 51

722.72 **Thoracic region** I 48, I 49, I 50, I 51

722.73 **Lumbar region** I 48, I 49, I 50, I 51

5th 722.8 **Postlaminectomy syndrome**

722.80 **Unspecified region** I 48, I 49, I 50, I 51

722.81 **Cervical region** I 48, I 49, I 50, I 51

722.82 **Thoracic region** I 48, I 49, I 50, I 51

722.83 **Lumbar region** I 48, I 49, I 50, I 51

M96.1 Postlaminectomy syndrome, not elsewhere classified

5th 722.9 **Other and unspecified disc disorder**
Calcification of intervertebral cartilage or disc
Discitis

722.90 **Unspecified region** I 48, I 49, I 50, I 51

722.91 **Cervical region** I 48, I 49, I 50, I 51

722.92 **Thoracic region** I 48, I 49, I 50, I 51

722.93 **Lumbar region** I 48, I 49, I 50, I 51

4th 723 **Other disorders of cervical region**

Excludes *conditions due to:*
intervertebral disc disorders (722.0-722.9)
spondylosis (721.0-721.9)

723.0 **Spinal stenosis of cervical region** I 48, I 49, I 50, I 51

M48.02 Spinal stenosis, cervical region

723.1 **Cervicalgia**

M54.2 Cervicalgia

Pain in neck

721.7 – 723.1

723.2 **Cervicocranial syndrome**
Barré-Liéou syndrome
Posterior cervical sympathetic syndrome

723.3 **Cervicobrachial syndrome (diffuse)**

723.4 **Brachia neuritis or radiculitis NOS**
M54.12 Radiculopathy, cervical region
Cervical radiculitis
Radicular syndrome of upper limbs

723.5 **Torticollis, unspecified**
Contracture of neck
Excludes *congenital (754.1)*
due to birth injury (767.8)
hysterical (300.11)
ocular torticollis (781.93)
psychogenic (306.0)
spasmodic (333.83)
traumatic, current (847.0)

723.6 **Panniculitis specified as affecting neck**

723.7 **Ossification of posterior longitudinal ligament in cervical region**

723.8 **Other syndromes affecting cervical region**
Cervical syndrome NEC
Klippel's disease
Occipital neuralgia

723.9 **Unspecified musculoskeletal disorders and symptoms referable to neck**
Cervical (region) disorder NOS

4th 724 **Other and unspecified disorders of back**
Excludes *collapsed vertebra (code to cause, e.g., osteoporosis, 733.00-733.09)*
conditions due to:
intervertebral disc disorders (722.0-722.9)
spondylosis (721.0-721.9)

5th 724.0 **Spinal stenosis, other than cervical**

724.00 **Spinal stenosis, unspecified region** I 48, I 49, I 50, I 51
M48.00 Spinal stenosis, site unspecified

724.01 **Thoracic region** I 48, I 49, I 50, I 51

724.02 **Lumbar region** I 48, I 49, I 50, I 51
M48.06 Spinal stenosis, lumbar region

724.09 **Other** I 48, I 49, I 50, I 51

724.1 **Pain in thoracic spine**
M54.6 Pain in thoracic spine

724.2 **Lumbago** I 48, I 49, I 50, I 51
M54.5 Low back pain
Low back pain
Low back syndrome
Lumbalgia
Layman's: *Lumbago can be either acute or chronic, and is typically due to skeletal degeneration or trauma, though it also can be caused by inflammatory, mechanical, mental and neoplastic conditions. Its origin in the lumbar area differentiates code 724.2 from codes 723.1 and 724.1.*

724.3 **Sciatica** I 48, I 49, I 50, I 51
M54.30 Sciatica, unspecified side
Neuralgia or neuritis of sciatic nerve
Excludes *specified lesion of sciatic nerve (355.0)*

724.4 **Thoracic or lumbosacral neuritis or radiculitis, unspecified** I 48, I 49, I 50, I 51
M54.14 Radiculopathy, thoracic region
M54.15 Radiculopathy, thoracolumbar region
M54.16 Radiculopathy, lumbar region
M54.17 Radiculopathy, lumbosacral region
Radicular syndrome of lower limbs

724.5 **Backache, unspecified** I 48, I 49, I 50, I 51
M54.9 Dorsalgia, unspecified
Vertebrogenic (pain) syndrome NOS

724.6 **Disorders of sacrum** I 48, I 49, I 50, I 51
Ankylosis, lumbosacral or sacroiliac (joint)
Instability, lumbosacral or sacroiliac (joint)

5th 724.7 **Disorders of coccyx**

724.70 **Unspecified disorder of coccyx** I 48, I 49, I 50, I 51

724.71 **Hypermobility of coccyx** I 48, I 49, I 50, I 51

724.79 **Other** I 48, I 49, I 50, I 51
Coccygodynia

724.8 **Other symptoms referable to back**
Ossification of posterior longitudinal ligament NOS
Panniculitis specified as sacral or affecting back

724.9 **Other unspecified back disorders**
Ankylosis of spine NOS
Compression of spinal nerve root NEC
Spinal disorder NOS
Excludes *sacroiliitis (720.2)*

RHEUMATISM, EXCLUDING THE BACK (725-729)

Includes disorders of muscles and tendons and their attachments, and of other soft tissues

725 **Polymyalgia rheumatica**
M35.3 Polymyalgia rheumatica

4th 726 **Peripheral enthesopathies and allied syndromes**
Note: *Enthesopathies are disorders of peripheral ligamentous or muscular attachments.*
Excludes *spinal enthesopathy (720.1)*

726.0 **Adhesive capsulitis of shoulder**
M75.00 Adhesive capsulitis of unspecified shoulder

5th 726.1 **Rotator cuff syndrome of shoulder and allied disorders**

Rotator Cuff Tendons (anterior)

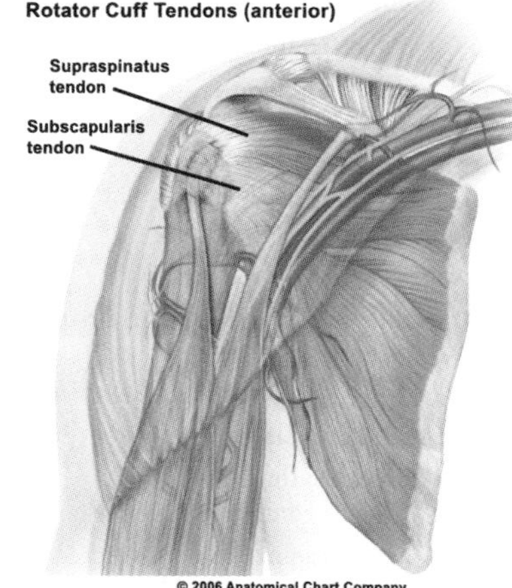

726.10 **Disorders of bursae and tendons in shoulder region, unspecified**
M75.10 Rotator cuff syndrome, unspecified shoulder
Rotator cuff syndrome NOS
Supraspinatus syndrome NOS

726.11 **Calcifying tendinitis of shoulder**

726.12 **Bicipital tenosynovitis**

726.19 **Other specified disorders**
Excludes *complete rupture of rotator cuff, nontraumatic (727.61)*

726.2 Other affections of shoulder region, not elsewhere classified
M75.80 Other shoulder lesions, unspecified shoulder
Periarthritis of shoulder
Scapulohumeral fibrositis

5th 726.3 Enthesopathy of elbow region
726.30 Enthesopathy of elbow, unspecified
726.31 Medial epicondylitis
726.32 Lateral epicondylitis
Epicondylitis NOS
Golfers' elbow
Tennis elbow
726.33 Olecranon bursitis
Bursitis of elbow
726.39 Other

726.4 Enthesopathy of wrist and carpus
Bursitis of hand or wrist
Periarthritis of wrist

726.5 Enthesopathy of hip region
M70.60 Trochanteric bursitis, unspecified hip
M70.70 Other bursitis of hip, unspecified hip
M76.10 Psoas tendinitis, unspecified side
M76.20 Iliac crest spur, unspecified hip
Bursitis of hip
Gluteal tendinitis
Iliac crest spur
Psoas tendinitis
Trochanteric tendinitis

5th 726.6 Enthesopathy of knee
726.60 Enthesopathy of knee, unspecified
Bursitis of knee NOS
726.61 Pes anserinus tendinitis or bursitis
726.62 Tibial collateral ligament bursitis
Pellegrini-Stieda syndrome
726.63 Fibular collateral ligament bursitis
726.64 Patellar tendinitis
726.65 Prepatellar bursitis
726.69 Other
Bursitis:
infrapatellar
subpatellar

5th 726.7 Enthesopathy of ankle and tarsus
726.70 Enthesopathy of ankle and tarsus, unspecified
Metatarsalgia NOS
Excludes *Morton's metatarsalgia (355.6)*
726.71 Achilles bursitis or tendinitis
726.72 Tibialis tendinitis
Tibialis (anterior) (posterior) tendinitis
726.73 Calcaneal spur
M77.30 Calcaneal spur, unspecified foot
726.79 Other
Peroneal tendinitis

726.8 Other peripheral enthesopathies

5th 726.9 Unspecified enthesopathy
726.90 Enthesopathy of unspecified site
M77.9 Enthesopathy, unspecified
Capsulitis NOS
Periarthritis NOS
Tendinitis NOS
726.91 Exostosis of unspecified site
Bone spur NOS

4th 727 Other disorders of synovium, tendon, and bursa

5th 727.0 Synovitis and tenosynovitis
727.00 Synovitis and tenosynovitis, unspecified
Synovitis NOS
Tenosynovitis NOS
727.01 *Synovitis and tenosynovitis in diseases classified elsewhere*
Code first underlying disease, as:
tuberculosis (015.0-015.9)
Excludes *crystal-induced (275.49)*
gonococcal (098.51)
gouty (274.00-274.03)
syphilitic (095.7)
727.02 Giant cell tumor of tendon sheath
727.03 Trigger finger (acquired)
M65.30 Trigger finger, unspecified finger
727.04 Radial styloid tenosynovitis
de Quervain's disease
727.05 Other tenosynovitis or hand and wrist
727.06 Tenosynovitis of foot and ankle
727.09 Other

727.1 Bunion

727.2 Specific bursitides often of occupational origin
Beat:
elbow
hand
knee
Chronic crepitant synovitis of wrist
Miners':
elbow
knee

727.3 Other bursitis
Bursitis NOS
Excludes *bursitis:*
gonococcal (098.52)
subacromial (726.19)
subcoracoid (726.19)
subdeltoid (726.19)
syphilitic (095.7)
"frozen shoulder" (726.0)

5th 727.4 Ganglion and cyst of synovium, tendon, and bursa
727.40 Synovial cyst, unspecified
Excludes *that of popliteal space (727.51)*
727.41 Ganglion of joint
727.42 Ganglion of tendon sheath
727.43 Ganglion, unspecified
727.49 Other
Cyst of bursa

5th 727.5 Rupture of synovium
727.50 Rupture of synovium, unspecified
727.51 Synovial cyst of popliteal space
Baker's cyst (knee)
727.59 Other

5th 727.6 Rupture of tendon, nontraumatic
727.60 Nontraumatic rupture of unspecified tendon
727.61 Complete rupture of rotator cuff
M75.10 Rotator cuff syndrome, unspecified shoulder
727.62 Tendons of biceps (long head)

727.63 **Extensor tendons of hand and wrist**

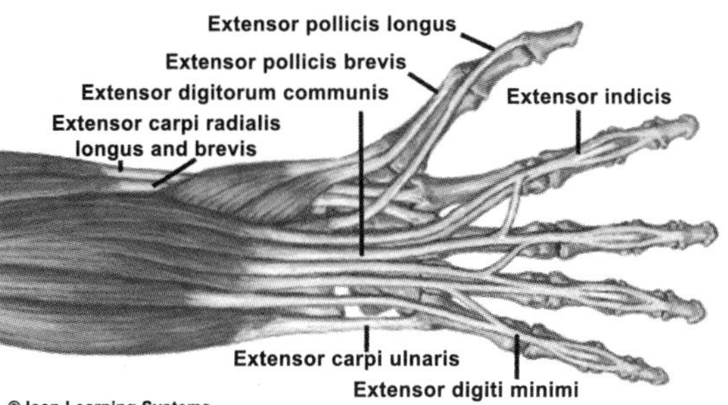

727.64 **Flexor tendons of hand and wrist**

727.65 **Quadriceps tendon**

727.66 **Patellar tendon**

727.67 **Achilles tendon**

727.68 **Other tendons of foot and ankle**

727.69 **Other**

5th 727.8 **Other disorders of synovium, tendon, and bursa**

727.81 **Contracture of tendon (sheath)**
Short Achilles tendon (acquired)

727.82 **Calcium deposits in tendon and bursa**
Calcification of tendon NOS
Calcific tendinitis NOS
Excludes *peripheral ligamentous or muscular attachments (726.0-726.9)*

727.83 **Plica syndrome**
Plica knee

727.89 **Other**
Abscess of bursa or tendon
Excludes *xanthomatosis localized to tendons (272.7)*

727.9 **Unspecified disorder of synovium, tendon, and bursa**

4th 728 **Disorders of muscle, ligament, and fascia**
Excludes *enthesopathies (726.0-726.9)*
muscular dystrophies (359.0-359.1)
myoneural disorders (358.00-358.9)
myopathies (359.2-359.9)
nontraumatic hematoma of muscle (729.92)
old disruption of ligaments of knee (717.81-717.89)

728.0 **Infective myositis**
Myositis:
purulent
suppurative
Excludes *myositis:*
epidemic (074.1)
interstitial (728.81)
myoneural disorder (358.00-358.9)
syphilitic (095.6)
tropical (040.81)

5th 728.1 **Muscular calcification and ossification**

728.10 **Calcification and ossification, unspecified**
Massive calcification (paraplegic)

728.11 **Progressive myositis ossificans**

728.12 **Traumatic myositis ossifications**
Myisitis ossificans (circumscripta)

728.13 **Postoperative heterotopic calcification**

728.19 **Other**
Polymyositis ossificans

728.2 **Muscular wasting and disuse atrophy, not elsewhere classified**
M62.50 Muscle wasting and atrophy, not elsewhere classified, unspecified site
Amyotrophia NOS
Myofibrosis
Excludes *neuralgic amyotrophy (353.5)*
pelvic muscle wasting and disuse atrophy (618.83)
progressive muscular atrophy (335.0-335.9)

728.3 **Other specific muscle disorders**
Arthrogryposis
Immobility syndrome (paraplegic)
Excludes *arthrogryposis multiplex congenita (754.89)*
stiff-man syndrome (333.91)

728.4 **Laxity of ligament**

728.5 **Hypermobility syndrome**

728.6 **Contracture of palmar fascia** A
Dupuytren's contracture

5th 728.7 **Other fibromatoses**

728.71 **Plantar fascial fibromatosis**
M72.2 Plantar fascial fibromatosis
Contracture of plantar fascia
Plantar fasciitis (traumatic)

728.79 **Other**
Garrod's or knuckle pads
Nodular fasciitis
Pseudosarcomatous fibromatosis (proliferative) (subcutaneous)

5th 728.8 **Other disorders of muscle, ligament, and fascia**

728.81 **Interstitial myositis**

728.82 **Foreign body granuloma of muscle**
Talc granuloma of muscle

728.83 **Rupture of muscle, nontraumatic**

728.84 **Diastasis of muscle**
Diastatsis recti (abdomen)
Excludes *diastatsis recti complicating pregnancy, labor, and delivery (665.8)*

728.85 **Spasm of muscle**
M62.40 Contracture of muscle, unspecified site

728.86 **Necrotizing fasciitis**
Use additional code to identify:
gangrene (785.4), if applicable
infectious organism (041.00-041.89)

728.87 **Muscle weakness (generalized)**
Excludes *generalized weakness (780.79)*

728.88 **Rhabdomyolysis**

728.89 **Other**
Eosinophilic fasciitis
Use additional E code to identify drug, if drug induced

728.9 **Unspecified disorder of muscle, ligament, and fascia**

4th 729 **Other disorders of soft tissues**
Excludes *acroparesthesia (443.89)*
carpal tunnel syndrome (354.0)
disorders of the back (720.0-724.9)
entrapment syndromes (354.0-355.9)
palindromic rheumatism (719.3)
periarthritis (726.0-726.9)
psychogenic rheumatism (306.0)

729.0 **Rheumatism, unspecified and fibrositis**
Layman's: *Fibrositis is commonly incorrectly referred to as fibromyalgia and is a family of disorders marked by chronic pain, stiffness and tenderness of the joints, tendons and muscles, with inflammation. It affects around 2% of the population of the US, of which, around 80% are female.*

727.63 – 729.0

729.1 **Myalgia and myositis, unspecified**
M60.9 Myositis, unspecified
M79.1 Myalgia
M79.7 Fibromyalgia
Fibromyositis NOS
Layman's: *Myalgia differs from fibrositis in that it affects the muscles only. Fibromyalgia affects the same sites as fibrositis, however is not accompanied by inflammation. Myositis is an inflammation of the skeletal (voluntary) muscles.*

729.2 **Neuralgia, neuritis, and radiculitis, unspecified**
M54.10 Radiculopathy, site unspecified
M79.2 Neuralgia and neuritis, unspecified
Excludes *brachia radiculitis (723.4)*
cervical radiculitis (723.4)
lumbosacral radiculitis (724.4)
mononeuritis (354.0-355.9)
radiculitis due to intervertebral disc involvement (722.0-722.2,722.7)
sciatica (724.3)

5th 729.3 **Panniculitis, unspecified**
729.30 **Panniculitis, unspecified site**
Weber-Christian disease
729.31 **Hypertrophy of fat pad, knee**
Hypertrophy of infrapatellar fat pad
729.39 **Other site**
Excludes *panniculitis specified as (affecting):*
back (724.8)
neck (723.6)
sacral (724.8)

729.4 **Fasciitis, unspecified**
Excludes *necrotizing fasciitis (728.86)*
nodular fasciitis (728.79)

729.5 **Pain in limb**
M79.609 Pain in unspecified limb

729.6 **Residual foreign body in soft tissue**
Excludes *foreign body granuloma:*
muscle (728.82)
skin and subcutaneous tissue (709.4)

5th 729.7 **Nontraumatic compartment syndrome**
Code first, if applicable, postprocedural complication (998.89)
Excludes *compartment syndrome NOS (958.90)*
traumatic compartment syndrome (958.90-958.99)
729.71 **Nontraumatic compartment syndrome of upper extremity**
Nontraumatic compartment syndrome of shoulder, arm, forearm, wrist, hand and fingers
729.72 **Nontraumatic compartment syndrome of lower extremity**
Nontraumatic compartment syndrome of hip, buttock, thigh, leg, foot and toes

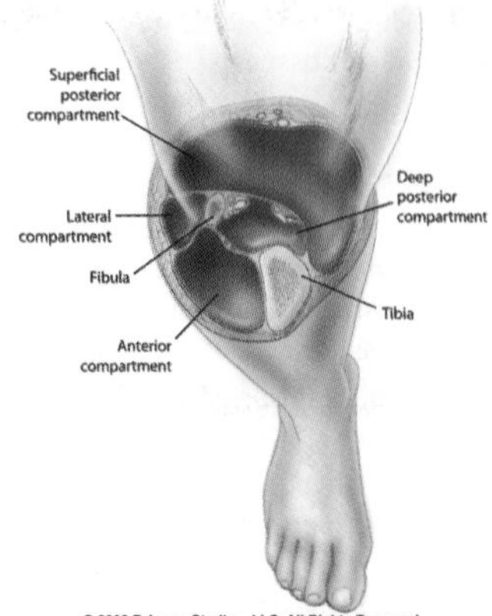

© 2008 Fairman Studios, LLC. All Rights Reserved.

729.73 **Nontraumatic compartment syndrome of abdomen**
729.79 **Nontraumatic compartment syndrome of other sites**

5th 729.8 **Other musculoskeletal symptoms referable to limbs**
729.81 **Swelling of limb**
M79.8 Other specified soft tissue disorders
729.82 **Cramp**
729.89 **Other**
Excludes *abnormality of gait (781.2)*
tetany (781.7)
transient paralysis of limb (781.4)

5th 729.9 **Other and unspecified disorders of soft tissue**
729.90 **Disorders of soft tissue, unspecified**
729.91 **Post-traumatic seroma**
Excludes *seroma complicating a procedure (998.13)*
729.92 **Nontraumatic hematoma of soft tissue**
Nontraumatic hematoma of muscle
729.99 **Other disorders of soft tissue**
Polyalgia

OSTEOPATHIES, CHONDROPATHIES, AND ACQUIRED MUSCULOSKELETAL DEFORMITIES (730-739)

4th 730 **Osteomyelitis, periostitis, and other infections involving bone**
Excludes *jaw (526.4-526.5)*
petrous bone (383.2)
Use additional code to identify organism, such as Staphylococcus (041.1)

The following fifth-digit subclassification is for use with category 730; valid digits are in [brackets] under each code. See list at beginning of chapter for definitions:

0 site unspecified
1 shoulder region
2 upper arm
3 forearm
4 hand
5 pelvic region and thigh
6 lower leg
7 ankle and foot
8 other specified sites
9 multiple sites

5th 730.0 **Acute osteomyelitis**
[0-9] Abscess of any bone except accessory sinus, jaw, or mastoid
Acute or subacute osteomyelitis, with or without mention of periostitis
Use additional code to identify major osseous defect, if applicable (731.3)

5th 730.1 **Chronic osteomyelitis**
[0-9] Brodie's abscess
Chronic or old osteomyelitis, with or without mention of periostitis
Sequestrum
Sclerosing osteomyelitis of Garré
Use additional code to identify major osseous defect, if applicable (731.3)
Excludes *aseptic necrosis of bone (733.40-733.49)*

5th 730.2 **Unspecified osteomyelitis**
[0-9] Osteitis or osteomyelitis NOS, with or without mention of periostitis
Use additional code to identify major osseous defect, if applicable (731.3)

5th **730.3 Periostitis without mention of ostemyelitis**
[0-9] Abscess of periosteum, without mention of osteomyelitis
Periostosis, without mention of osteomyelitis
Excludes *that in secondary syphilis (091.61)*

5th **730.7 *Osteopathy resulting from poliomyelitis***
[0-9]
Code first underlying disease (045.0-045.9)

5th **730.8 *Other infections involving bone in disease classified elsewhere***
[0-9]
Code first underlying disease, as:
tuberculosis (015.0-015.9)
typhoid fever (002.0)
Excludes *syphilitis of bone NOS (095.5)*

5th **730.9 Unspecified infection of bone**
[0-9]

4th **731 Osteitis deformans and osteopathies associated with other disorders classified elsewhere**

731.0 Osteitis deformans without mention of bone tumor
Paget's disease of bone

731.1 *Osteitis deformans in diseases classified elsewhere*
Code first underlying disease, as:
malignant neoplasm of bone (170.0-170.9)

731.2 Hypertrophic pulmonary osteoarthropathy
Bamberger-Marie disease

731.3 Major osseous defects
Code first underlying disease, if known, such as:
aseptic necrosis (733.40-733.49)
malignant neoplasm of bone (170.0-170.9)
osteomyelitis (730.00- 730.29)
osteoporosis (733.00-733.09)
peri-prosthetic osteolysis (996.45)

731.8 *Other bone involvement in diseases classified elsewhere*
Code first underlying disease, as:
diabetes mellitus (249.8, 250.8)
Use additional code to specify bone condition, such as:
acute osteomyelitis (730.00-730.09)

4th **732 Osteochondropathies**

732.0 Juvenile osteochondrosis of spine
Juvenile osteochondrosis (of):
marginal or vertebral ephiphysis (of Scheurermann)
spine NOS
Vertebral epiphysitis
Excludes *adolescent postural kyphosis (737.0)*

732.1 Juvenile osteochondrosis of hip and pelvis
Coxa plana
Ischiopubic synchondrosis (of van Neck)
Osteochondrosis (juvenile) of:
acetabulum
head of femur (of Legg-Calvé-Perthes)
iliac crest (of Buchanan)
symphysis pubis (of Pierson)
Pseudocoxalgia

732.2 Nontraumatic slipped upper femoral epiphysis
Slipped upper femoral epiphysis NOS

732.3 Juvenile osteochondrosis of upper extremity
Osteochondrosis (juvenile) of:
capitulum of humerus (of Panner)
carpal lunate (of Kienbock)
hand NOS
head of humerus (of Haas)
heads of metacarpas (of Mauclaire)
lower ulna (of Burns)
radial head (of Brailsford)
upper extremity NOS

732.4 Juvenile osteochondrosis of lower extremity, excluding foot
Osteochondrosis (juvenile) of:
lower extremity NOS
primary patellar center (of Köhler)
proximal tibia (of Blount)
secondary patellar center (of Sinding-Larsen)
tibial tubercle (of Osgood-Schlatter)
Tibia vara

732.5 Juvenile osteochondrosis of foot
Calcaneal apophysitis
Epiphysitis, os calcis
Osteochondrosis (juvenile) of:
astragalus (of Diaz)
calcaneum (of Sever)
foot NOS
metatarsal:
second (of Freilberg)
fifth (of Iselin)
os tibiale externum (of Haglund)
tarsal navicular (of Köhler)

732.6 Other juvenile osteochondrosis
Apophysitis specified as juvenile, of other site, or site NOS
Epiphysitis specified as juvenile, of other site, or site NOS
Osteochondritis specified as juvenile, of other site, or site NOS
Osteochondrosis specified as juvenile, of other site, or site NOS

732.7 Osteochondritis dissecans

732.8 Other specified forms of osteochondropathy
Adult osteochondrosis of spine

732.9 Unspecified osteochondropathy
Apophysitis
NOS
not specified as adult or juvenile, of unspecified site
Epiphysitis
NOS
not specified as adult or juvenile, of unspecified site
Osteochondritis
NOS
not specified as adult or juvenile, of unspecified site
Osteochondrosis
NOS
not specified as adult or juvenile, of unspecified site

4th **733 Other disorders of bone and cartilage**
Excludes *bone spur (726.91)*
cartilage of, or loose body in, joint (717.0-717.9, 718.0-718.9)
giant cell granuloma of jaw (526.3)
osteitis fibrosa cystica generalisata (252.01)
osteomalacia (268.2)
polyostotic fibrous dysplasia of bone (756.54)
prognathism, retrognathism (524.1)
xanthomatosis localized to bone (272.7)

5th **733.0 Osteoporosis**
Use additional code to identify major osseous defect, if applicable (731.3)
Use additional code to identify personal history of pathologic (healed) fracture (V13.51)

733.00 Osteoporosis, unspecified 41
M81.8 Other osteoporosis without current pathological fracture
Wedging of vertebra NOS

733.01 Senile osteoporosis 41
M81.0 Age-related osteoporosis without current pathological fracture
Postmenopausal osteoporosis

733.02 Idiopathic osteoporosis 41

733.03 Disuse osteoporosis 4 1

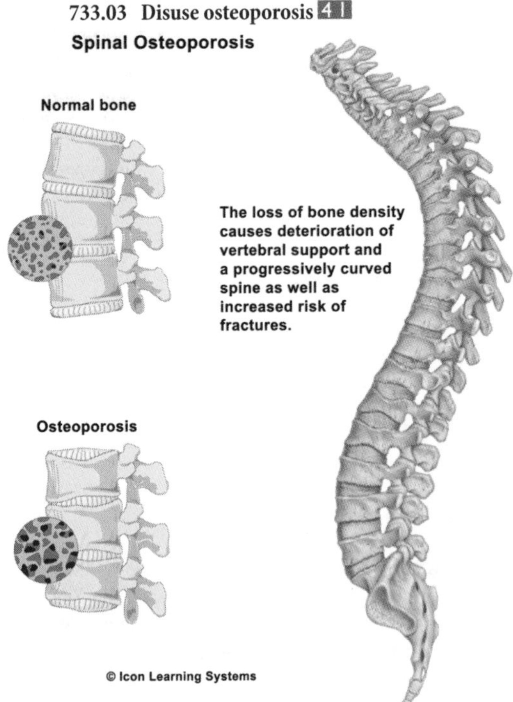

733.09 Other 4 1
Drug-induced osteoporosis
Use additional E code to identify drug

5th 733.1 **Pathologic fracture**
Chronic fracture
Spontaneous fracture
Excludes *stress fracture (733.93-733.95)*
traumatic fractures (800-829)

ICD-9-CM Official Guidelines (Chapter 13):

a. Coding of Pathologic Fractures

1) Acute Fractures vs. Aftercare

Pathologic fractures are reported using subcategory 733.1, when the fracture is newly diagnosed. Subcategory 733.1 may be used while the patient is receiving active treatment for the fracture. Examples of active treatment are: surgical treatment, emergency department encounter, evaluation and treatment by a new physician.

Fractures are coded using the aftercare codes (subcategories V54.0, V54.2, V54.8 or V54.9) for encounters after the patient has completed active treatment of the fracture and is receiving routine care for the fracture during the healing or recovery phase. Examples of fracture aftercare are: cast change or removal, removal of external or internal fixation device, medication adjustment, and follow up visits following fracture treatment.

Care for complications of surgical treatment for fracture repairs during the healing or recovery phase should be coded with the appropriate complication codes.

Care of complications of fractures, such as malunion and nonunion, should be reported with the appropriate codes.

See Section I. C. 17.b for information on the coding of traumatic fractures.

733.10 **Pathologic fracture, unspecified site**

733.11 **Pathologic fracture of humerus**

733.12 **Pathologic fracture of distal radius and ulna** 2 4, 4 0
Wrist NOS

733.13 **Pathologic fracture of vertebrae** 2 4, 4 0
M48.50xA Collapsed vertebra, not elsewhere classified, site specified , initial encounter for fracture
M48.50xG Collapsed vertebra, not elsewhere classified, site unspecified , subsequent encounter for fracture with delayed healing
M80.08xA Age-related osteoporosis with current pathological fracture, vertebra(e), initial encounter for fracture
M80.08xG Age-related osteoporosis with current pathological fracture, vertebra(e), subsequent encounter for fracture with delayed healing
M84.48xA Pathological fracture, other site, initial encounter for fracture
M84.48xG Pathological fracture, other site, subsequent encounter for fracture with delayed healing
M84.68xA Pathological fracture in other disease, other site, initial encounter for fracture
M84.68xG Pathological fracture in other disease, other site, subsequent encounter for fracture with delayed healing
Collapse of vertebra NOS

733.14 **Pathologic fracture of neck of femur** 2 4, 4 0
Femur NOS
Hip NOS

733.15 **Pathologic fracture of other specified part of femur**

733.16 **Pathologic fracture of tibia and fibula**
Ankle NOS

733.19 **Pathologic fracture of other specified site**

5th 733.2 **Cyst of bone**

733.20 **Cyst of bone (localized), unspecified**

733.21 **Solitary bone cyst**
Unicameral bone cyst

733.22 **Aneurysmal bone cyst**

733.29 **Other**
Fibrous dysplasia (monostotic)
Excludes *cyst of jaw (526.0-526.2, 526.89)*
osteitis fibrosa cystica (252.01)
polyostotic fibrous dysplasia of bone (756.54)

733.3 **Hyperostosis of skull**
Hyperostosis interna frontalis
Leontiasis ossium

5th 733.4 **Aseptic necrosis of bone**
Use additional code to identify major osseous defect, if applicable (731.3)
Excludes *osteochondropathies (732.0-732.9)*

733.40 **Aseptic necrosis of bone, site unspecified**

733.41 **Head of humerus**

733.42 **Head and neck of femur**
Femur NOS
Excludes *Legg-Calvé-Perthes disease (732.1)*

733.43 **Medial femoral condyle**

733.44 **Talus**

733.45 **Jaw**
Use additional E code to identify drug, if drug-induced
Excludes *osteoradionecrosis of jaw (526.89)*

733.49 **Other**

733.03 – 733.49

733.5 Osteitis condensans
Piriform sclerosis of ilium

733.6 Tietze's disease
Costochondral junction syndrome
Costochondritis

733.7 Algoneurodystrophy
Disuse atrophy of bone
Sudeck's atrophy

5th **733.8 Malunion and nonunion of fracture**

733.81 Malunion of fracture

733.82 Nonunion of fracture
Pseudoarthrosis (bone)

5th **733.9 Other and unspecified disorders of bone and cartilage**

733.90 Disorder of bone and cartilage, unspecified
M89.9 Disorder of bone, unspecified
M94.9 Disorder of cartilage, unspecified
Layman's: *Bone pain, low bone density, bone and cartilage degeneration and many other disorders that have not been directly linked to a injury (e.g., fracture, tear, etc.) or disorder (e.g., osteoporosis, etc.) are coded as 733.90.*

733.91 Arrest of bone development or growth
Epiphyseal arrest

733.92 Chondromalacia
Chondromalacia:
NOS
localized, except patella
systemic
tibial plateau
Excludes *chondromalacia of patella (717.7)*

733.93 Stress fracture of tibia or fibula
Stress reaction of tibia or fibula
Use additional external cause code(s) to identify the cause of the stress fracture

733.94 Stress fracture of the metatarsals
Stress reaction of metatarsals
Use additional external cause code(s) to identify the cause of the stress fracture

733.95 Stress fracture of other bone
Stress reaction of other bone
Use additional external cause code(s) to identify the cause of the stress fracture
Excludes *stress fracture of:*
femoral neck (733.96)
fibula (733.93)
metatarsals (733.94)
pelvis (733.98)
shaft of femur (733.97)
tibia (733.93)

733.96 Stress fracture of femoral neck
Stress reaction of femoral neck
Use additional external cause code(s) to identify the cause of the stress fracture

733.97 Stress fracture of shaft of femur
Stress reaction of shaft of femur
Use additional external cause code(s) to identify the cause of the stress fracture

733.98 Stress fracture of pelvis
Stress reaction of pelvis
Use additional external cause code(s) to identify the cause of the stress fracture

733.99 Other
Diaphysitis
Hypertrophy of bone
Relapsing polychondritis

734 Flat foot
Pes planus (acquired)
Talipes planus (acquired)
Excludes *congenital (754.61)*
rigid flat foot (754.61)
spastic (everted) flat foot (754.61)

4th **735 Acquired deformities of toe**
Excludes *congenital (754.60-754.69, 755.65-755.66)*

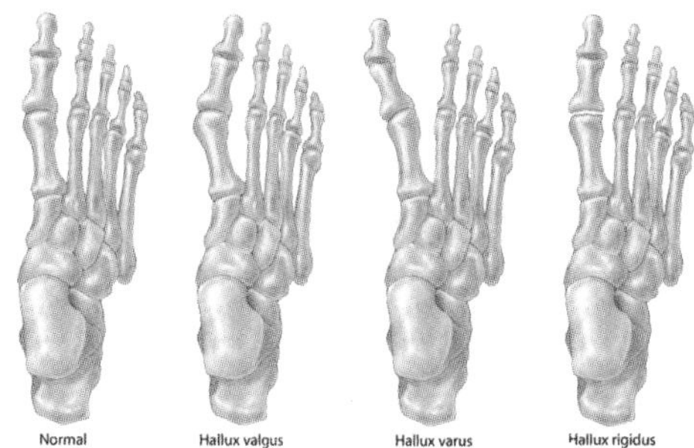

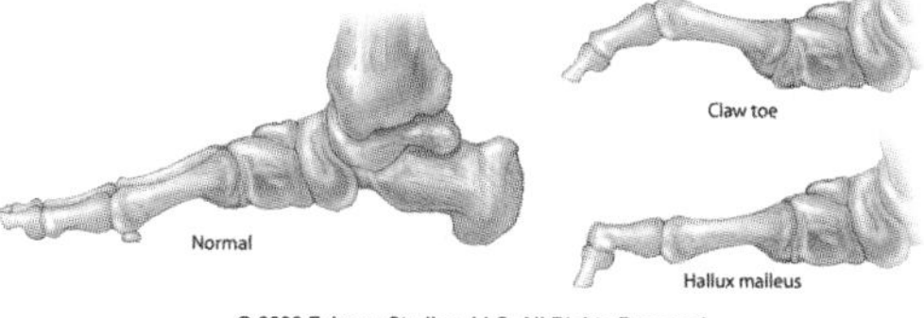

© 2008 Fairman Studios, LLC. All Rights Reserved.

735.0 Hallux valgus (acquired)
M20.10 Hallux valgus (acquired), unspecified foot

735.1 Hallux varus (acquired)

735.2 Hallux rigidus

735.3 Hallux malleus

735.4 Other hammer toe (acquired)
M20.40 Other hammer toe(s) (acquired), unspecified foot

735.5 Claw toe (acquired)

735.8 Other acquired deformities of toe

735.9 Unspecified acquired deformity of toe

4th **736 Other acquired deformities of limbs**
Excludes *congenital (754.3-755.9)*

5th **736.0 Acquired deformities of forearm, excluding fingers**

736.00 Unspecified deformity
Deformity of elbow, forearm, hand, or wrist (acquired) NOS

736.01 Cubitus valgus (acquired)

736.02 Cubitus varus (acquired)

736.03 Valgus deformity of wrist (acquired)

736.04 Varus deformity of wrist (acquired)

736.05 Wrist drop (acquired)

736.06 Claw hand (acquired)

736.07 Club hand (acquired)

736.09 Other

736.1 Mallet finger

5th **736.2 Other acquired deformities of finger**

736.20 Unspecified deformity
Deformity of finger (acquired) NOS

736.21 Boutonniere deformity

736.22 Swan-neck deformity

736.29 Other
Excludes *trigger finger (727.03)*

5th **736.3 Acquired deformities of hip**

736.30 Unspecified deformity
Deformity of hip (acquired) NOS

736.31 Coxa valga (acquired)

736.32 Coxa vara (acquired)

736.39 Other

5th 736.4 Genu valgum or varum (acquired)

736.41 Genu valgum (acquired)

736.42 Genu varum (acquired)

736.5 Genu recurvatum (acquired)

736.6 Other acquired deformities of knee
Deformity of knee (acquired) NOS

5th 736.7 Other acquired deformities of ankle and foot
Excludes *deformities of toe (acquired) (735.0-735.9)*
pes planu (acquired) (734)

736.70 Unspecified deformity of ankle and foot, acquired

736.71 Acquired equinovarus deformity
Clubfoot, acquired
Excludes *clubfoot not specified as acquired (754.5-754.7)*

736.72 Equinus deformity of foot, acquired

736.73 Cavus deformity of foot
Excludes *that with claw foot (736.74)*

736.74 Claw foot, acquired

736.75 Cavovarus deformity of foot, acquired

736.76 Other calcaneus deformity

736.79 Other
Acquired:
pes not elsewhere classified
talipes not elsewhere classified

5th 736.8 Acquired deformities of other parts of limbs

736.81 Unequal leg length (acquired)

736.89 Other
Deformity (acquired):
arm or leg, not elsewhere classified
shoulder

736.9 Acquired deformity of limb, site unspecified

4th 737 Curvature of spine
Excludes *congenital (754.2)*

Normal Lordosis Kyphosis Scoliosis

© 2008 Fairman Studios, LLC. All Rights Reserved.

737.0 Adolescent postural kyphosis
Excludes *osteochondrosis of spine (juvenile) (732.0)*
adult (732.8)

5th 737.1 Kyphosis (acquired)

737.10 Kyphosis (acquired) (postural)

737.11 Kyphosis due to radiation

737.12 Kyphosis, postlaminectomy

737.19 Other
Excludes *that associated with conditions classifiable elsewhere (737.41)*

5th 737.2 Lordosis (acquired)

737.20 Lordosis (acquired) (postural)

737.21 Lordosis, postlaminectomy

737.22 Other postsurgical lordosis

737.29 Other
Excludes *that associated with conditions classifiable elsewhere (737.42)*

5th 737.3 Kyphoscoliosis and scoliosis

737.30 Scoliosis [and kyphoscoliosis], idiopathic

737.31 Resolving infantile idiopathic scoliosis

737.32 Progressive infantile idiopathic scoliosis

737.33 Scoliosis due to radiation

737.34 Thoracogenic scoliosis

737.39 Other
Excludes *that associated with conditions classifiable elsewhere (737.43)*
that in kyphoscoliotic heart disease (416.1)

5th 737.4 Curvature of spine associated with other conditions
Code first associated condition, as:
Charcôt-Marie-Tooth disease (356.1)
mucopolysaccharidosis (277.5)
neurofibromatosis (237.7)
osteitis deformans (731.0)
osteitis fibrosa cystica (252.01)
osteoporosis (733.00-733.09)
poliomyelitis (138)
tuberculosis [Pott's curvature] (015.0)

737.40 *Curvature of spine, unspecified*

737.41 *Kyphosis*

737.42 *Lordosis*

737.43 *Scoliosis*

737.8 Other curvatures of spine

737.9 Unspecified curvature of spine
Curvature of spine (acquired) (idiopathic) NOS
Hunchback, acquired
Excludes *deformity of spine NOS (738.5)*

4th 738 Other acquired deformity
Excludes *congenital (754.0-756.9, 758.0-759.9)*
dentofacial anomalies (524.0-524.9)

738.0 Acquired deformity of nose
Deformity of nose (acquired)
Overdevelopment of nasal bones
Excludes *deflected of deviated nasal septum (470)*

5th 738.1 Other acquired deformity of head

738.10 Unspecified deformity

738.11 Zygomatic hyperplasia

738.12 Zygomatic hypoplasia

738.19 Other specified deformity

738.2 Acquired deformity of neck

738.3 Acquired deformity of chest and rib
Deformity:
chest (acquired)
rib (acquired)
Pectus:
carinatum, acquired
excavatum, acquired

738.4 Acquired spondylolisthesis I 48, I 49, I 50, I 51
Degenerative spondylolisthesis
Spondylolysis, acquired
Excludes *congenital (756.12)*

738.5 Other acquired deformity of back or spine I 48, I 49, I 50, I 51
Deformity of spine NOS
Excludes *curvature of spine (737.0-737.9)*

738.6 **Acquired deformity of pelvis**
Pelvic obliquity
Excludes *intrapelvic protrusion of acetabulum (718.6)*
that in relation to labor and delivery (653.0-653.4, 653.8-653.9)

738.7 **Cauliflower ear**

738.8 **Acquired deformity of other specified site**
Deformity of clavicle

738.9 **Acquired deformity of unspecified site**

4th 739 **Nonallopathic lesions, not elsewhere classified**
Includes segmental dysfunction
somatic dysfunction

739.0 **Head region**
Occipitocervical region

739.1 **Cervical region**
M99.01 Segmental and somatic dysfunction of cervical region
Cervicothoracic region

739.2 **Thoracic region**
M99.02 Segmental and somatic dysfunction of thoracic region
Thoracolumbar region

739.3 **Lumbar region** I 48, I 49, I 50, I 51
M99.03 Segmental and somatic dysfunction of lumbar region
Lumbosacral region

739.4 **Sacral region** I 48, I 49, I 50, I 51
M99.04 Segmental and somatic dysfunction of sacral region
Sacrococcygeal region
Sacroiliac region

739.5 **Pelvic region**
M99.05 Segmental and somatic dysfunction of pelvic region
Hip region
Pubic region

739.6 **Lower extremities**

739.7 **Upper extremities**
Acromioclavicular region
Sternoclavicular region

739.8 **Rib cage**
Costochondral region
Costovertebral region
Sternochondral region

739.9 **Abdomen and other**

14. CONGENITAL ANOMALIES (740-759)

ICD-9-CM Official Guidelines (Chapter 14):

a. ***Codes in categories 740-759, Congenital Anomalies***

Assign an appropriate code(s) from categories 740-759, Congenital Anomalies, when an anomaly is documented. A congenital anomaly may be the principal/first listed diagnosis on a record or a secondary diagnosis.

When a congenital anomaly does not have a unique code assignment, assign additional code(s) for any manifestations that may be present.

When the code assignment specifically identifies the congenital anomaly, manifestations that are an inherent component of the anomaly should not be coded separately. Additional codes should be assigned for manifestations that are not an inherent component.

Codes from Chapter 14 may be used throughout the life of the patient. If a congenital anomaly has been corrected, a personal history code should be used to identify the history of the anomaly. Although present at birth, a congenital anomaly may not be identified until later in life. Whenever the condition is diagnosed by the physician, it is appropriate to assign a code from codes 740-759.

For the birth admission, the appropriate code from category V30, Liveborn infants, according to type of birth should be sequenced as the principal diagnosis, followed by any congenital anomaly codes, 740-759.

4th 740 **Anencephalus and similar anomalies**

740.0 **Anencephalus**
Acrania
Amyelencephalus
Hemianencephaly
Hemicephaly

740.1 **Craniorachischisis**

740.2 **Iniencephaly**

4th 741 **Spina bifida**
Excludes *spina bifida occulta (756.17)*

The following fifth-digit subclassification is for use with category 741:
0 unspecified region
1 cervical region
2 dorsal (thoracic) region
3 lumbar region

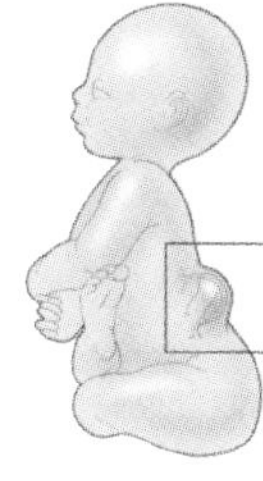
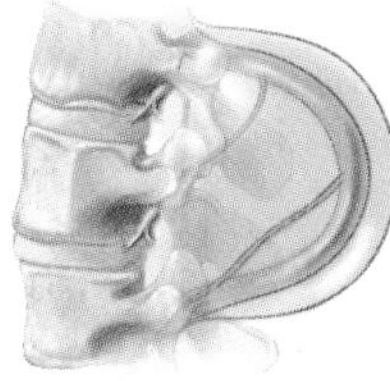

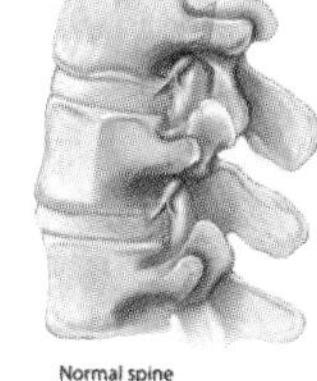

© 2008 Fairman Studios, LLC. All Rights Reserved.

5th 741.0 **With hydrocephalus**
[0-3] Arnold-Chiari syndrome, type II
Chiari malformation, type II
Any condition classifiable to 741.9 with any condition classifiable to 742.3

5th 741.9 **Without mention of hydrocephalus**
[0-3] Hydromeningocele (spinal)
Hydromyelocele
Meningocele (spinal)
Meningomyelocele
Myelocele
Myelocystocele
Rachischisis
Spina bifida (aperta)
Syringomyelocele

4th 742 **Other congenital anomalies of nervous system**

Excludes *congenital central alveolar hypoventilation syndrome (327.25)*

742.0 **Encephalocele**
- Encephalocystocele
- Encephalomyelocele
- Hydroencephalocele
- Hydromeningocele, cranial
- Meningocele, cerebral
- Meningoencephalocele

742.1 **Microcephalus**
- Hydromicrocephaly
- Micrencephaly

742.2 **Reduction deformities of brain**
- Absence of part of brain
- Agenesis of part of brain
- Agyria
- Aplasia of part of brain
- Arhinencephaly
- Holoprosencephaly
- Hypoplasia of part of brain
- Microgyria

742.3 **Congenital hydrocephalus**
- Aqueduct of Sylvius:
  - anomaly
  - obstruction, congenital
  - stenosis
- Atresia of foramina of Magendie and Luschka
- Hydrocephalus in newborn

Excludes *hydrocephalus:*
- *acquired (331.3-331.4)*
- *due to congenital toxoplasmosis (771.2)*
- *with any condition classifiable to 741.9 (741.0)*

742.4 **Other specified anomalies of brain**
- Congenital cerebral cyst
- Macroencephaly
- Macrogyria
- Megalencephaly
- Multiple anomalies of brain NOS
- Porencephaly
- Ulegyria

5th 742.5 **Other specified anomalies of spinal cord**

742.51 **Diastematomyelia**

742.53 **Hydromyelia**
- Hydrorhachis

742.59 **Other**
- Amyelia
- Atelomyelia
- Congenital anomaly of spinal meninges
- Defective development of cauda equina
- Hypoplasia of spinal cord
- Myelatelia
- Myelodysplasia

742.8 **Other specified anomalies of nervous system**
- Agenesis of nerve
- Displacement of brachial plexus
- Familial dysautonomia
- Jaw-winking syndrome
- Marcus-Gunn syndrome
- Riley-Day syndrome

Excludes *neurofibromatosis (237.7)*

742.9 **Unspecified anomaly of brain, spinal cord, and nervous system**
- Anomaly of brain, nervous system, and spinal cord
- Congenital
  - disease of brain, nervous system, and spinal cord
  - lesion of brain, nervous system, and spinal cord
- Deformity of brain, nervous system, and spinal cord

4th 743 **Congenital anomalies of eye**

5th 743.0 **Anophthalmos**

743.00 **Clinical anophthalmos, unspecified**
- Agenesis
- Anophthalmos NOS
- Congenital absence of eye

743.03 **Cystic eyeball, congenital**

743.06 **Cryptophthalmos**

5th 743.1 **Microphthalmos**
- Dysplasia of eye
- Hypoplasia of eye
- Rudimentary eye

743.10 **Microphthalmos, unspecified**

743.11 **Simple microphthalmos**

743.12 **Microphthalmos associated with other anomalies of eye and adnexa**

5th 743.2 **Buphthalmos**
- Glaucoma:
  - congenital
  - newborn
- Hydrophthalmos

Excludes *glaucoma of childhood (365.14)*
traumatic glaucoma due to birth injury (767.8)

743.20 **Buphthalmos, unspecified**

743.21 **Simple buphthalmos**

743.22 **Buphthalmos associated with other ocular anomalies**
- Keratoglobus, congenital, associated with buphthalmos
- Megalocornea associated with buphthalmos

5th 743.3 **Congenital cataract and lens anomalies**

Excludes *infantile cataract (366.00-366.09)*

743.30 **Congenital cataract, unspecified**

743.31 **Capsular and subcapsular cataract**

743.32 **Cortical and zonular cataract**

743.33 **Nuclear cataract**

743.34 **Total and subtotal cataract, congenital**

743.35 **Congenital aphakia**
- Congenital absence of lens

743.36 **Anomalies of lens shape**
- Microphakia
- Spherophakia

743.37 **Congenital ectopic lens**

743.39 **Other**

5th 743.4 **Coloboma and other anomalies of anterior segment**

743.41 **Anomalies of corneal size and shape**
- Microcornea

Excludes *that associated with buphthalmos (743.22)*

743.42 **Corneal opacities, interfering with vision, congenital**

743.43 **Other corneal opacities, congenital**

743.44 **Specified anomalies of anterior chamber, chamber angle, and related structures**
- Anomaly:
  - Axenfeld's
  - Peters'
  - Rieger's

743.45 **Aniridia**

743.46 **Other specified anomalies of iris and ciliary body**
- Anisocoria, congenital
- Atresia of pupil
- Coloboma of iris
- Corectopia

743.47 **Specified anomalies of sclera**

743.48 **Multiple and combined anomalies of anterior segment**

743.49 **Other**

5th 743.5 **Congenital anomalies of posterior segment**

743.51 **Vitreous anomalies**
Congenital vitreous opacity

743.52 **Fundus coloboma**

743.53 **Chorioretinal degeneration, congenital**

743.54 **Congenital folds and cysts of posterior segment**

743.55 **Congenital macular changes**

743.56 **Other retinal changes, congenital**

743.57 **Specified anomalies of optic disc**
Coloboma of optic disc (congenital)

743.58 **Vascular anomalies**
Congenital retinal aneurysm

743.59 **Other**

5th 743.6 **Congenital anomalies of eyelids, lacrimal system, and orbit**

743.61 **Congenital ptosis**

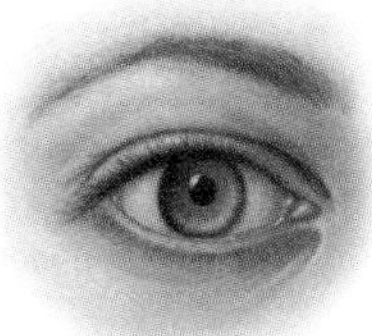
Normal

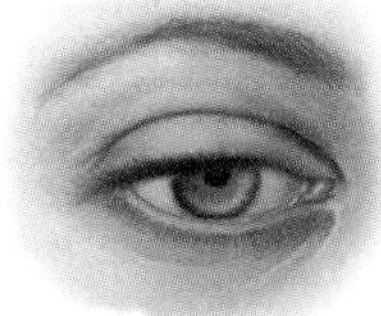
Ptosis

© 2008 Fairman Studios, LLC. All Rights Reserved.

743.62 **Congenital deformities of eyelids**
Ablepharon
Absence of eyelid
Accessory eyelid
Congenital:
ectropion
entropion

743.63 **Other specified congenital anomalies of eyelid**
Absence, agenesis, of cilia

743.64 **Specified congenital anomalies of lacrimal gland**

743.65 **Specified congenital anomalies of lacrimal passages**
Absence, agenesis of:
lacrimal apparatus
punctum lacrimale
Accessory lacrimal canal

743.66 **Specified congenital anomalies of orbit**

743.69 **Other**
Accessory eye muscles

743.8 **Other specified anomalies of eye**
Excludes *congenital nystagmus (379.51)*
ocular albinism (270.2)
optic nerve hypoplasia (377.43)
retinitis pigmentosa (362.74)

743.9 **Unspecified anomaly of eye**
Congenital:
anomaly NOS of eye [any part]
deformity NOS of eye [any part]

4th 744 **Congenital anomalies of ear, face, and neck**
Excludes *anomaly of:*
cervical spine (754.2, 756.10-756.19)
larynx (748.2-748.3)
nose (748.0-748.1)
parathyroid gland (759.2)
thyroid gland (759.2)
cleft lip (749.10-749.25)

5th 744.0 **Anomalies of ear causing impairment of hearing**
Excludes *congenital deafness without mention of cause (380.0-389.9)*

744.00 **Unspecified anomaly of ear with impairment of hearing**

744.01 **Absence of external ear**
Absence of:
auditory canal (external)
auricle (ear) (with stenosis or atresia of auditory canal)

744.02 **Other anomalies of external ear with impairment of hearing**
Atresia or stricture of auditory canal (external)

744.03 **Anomaly of middle ear, except ossicles**
Atresia or stricture of osseous meatus (ear)

744.04 **Anomalies of ear ossicles**
Fusion of ear ossicles

744.05 **Anomalies of inner ear**
Congenital anomaly of:
membranous labyrinth
organ of Corti

744.09 **Other**
Absence of ear, congenital

744.1 **Accessory auricle**
Accessory tragus
Polyotia
Preauricular appendage
Supernumerary:
ear
lobule

5th 744.2 **Other specified anomalies of ear**
Excludes *that with impairment of hearing (744.00-744.09)*

744.21 **Absence of ear lobe, congenital**

744.22 **Macrotia**

744.23 **Microtia**

744.24 **Specified anomalies of Eustachian tube**
Absence of Eustachian tube

744.29 **Other**
Bat ear
Darwin's tubercle
Pointed ear
Prominence of auricle
Ridge ear
Excludes *preauricular sinus (744.46)*

744.3 **Unspecified anomaly of ear**
Congenital:
anomaly NOS of ear, NEC
deformity NOS of ear, NEC

5th 744.4 **Branchial cleft cyst or fistula; preauricular sinus**

744.41 **Branchial cleft sinus or fistula**
Branchial:
sinus (external) (internal)
vestige

744.42 **Branchial cleft cyst**

744.43 **Cervical auricle**

744.46 **Preauricular sinus or fistula**

744.47 **Preauricular cyst**

743.47 – 744.47

744.49 **Other**
Fistula (of):
auricle, congenital
cervicoaural

744.5 **Webbing of neck**
Pterygium colli

5th 744.8 **Other specified anomalies of face and neck**

744.81 **Macrocheilia**
Hypertrophy of lip, congenital

744.82 **Microcheilia**

744.83 **Macrostomia**

744.84 **Microstomia**

744.89 **Other**
Excludes *congenital fistula of lip (750.25)*
musculoskeletal anomalies (754.0-754.1, 756.0)

744.9 **Unspecified anomalies of face and neck**
Congenital:
anomaly NOS of face [any part] or neck [any part]
deformity NOS of face [any part] or neck [any part]

4th 745 **Bulbus cordis anomalies and anomalies of cardiac septal closure**

745.0 **Common truncus**
Absent septum between aorta and pulmonary artery
Aortic septal defect
Common aortopulmonary trunk
Communication (abnormal) between aorta and pulmonary artery
Persistent truncus arteriosus

5th 745.1 **Transposition of great vessels**

745.10 **Complete transposition of great vessels**
Transposition of great vessels:
NOS
classical

745.11 **Double outlet right ventricle**
Dextratransposition of aorta
Incomplete transposition of great vessels
Origin of both great vessels from right ventricle
Taussig-Bing syndrome or defect

745.12 **Corrected transposition of great vessels**

745.19 **Other**

745.2 **Tetralogy of Fallot**
Fallot's pentalogy
Ventricular septal defect with pulmonary stenosis or atresia, dextraposition of aorta, and hypertrophy of right ventricle
Excludes *Fallot's triad (746.09)*

Layman's: *Tetralogy of Fallot occurs when all four of the following congenital cardiovascular defects are present: 1) VSD (745.4); 2) right ventricular hypertrophy (746.89); 3) pulmonary stenosis (746.02); and 4) overriding aorta (747.21). If all four of these conditions are present, 745.2 is a more appropriate code than the individual condition codes.*

745.3 **Common ventricle**
Cor triloculare biatriatum
Single ventricle

745.4 **Ventricular septal defect**
Eisenmenger's defect or complex
Gerbode defect
Interventricular septal defect
Left ventricular-right atrial communication
Roger's disease
Excludes *common atrioventricular canal type (745.69)*
single ventricle (745.3)

Layman's: *VSD occurs when the wall between the ventricles of the heart does not close completely during gestation. It is one of the most common congenital anomalies.*

745.5 **Ostium secundum type atrial septal defect**
Defect:
atrium secundum
fossa ovalis
Lutembacher's syndrome
Patent or persistent:
foramen ovale
ostium secundum

5th 745.6 **Endocardial cushion defects**

745.60 **Endocardial cushion defect, unspecified type**

745.61 **Ostium primum defect**
Persistent ostium primum

745.69 **Other**
Absence of atrial septum
Atrioventricular canal type ventricular septal defect
Common atrioventricular canal
Common atrium

745.7 **Cor biloculare**
Absence of atrial and ventricular septa

745.8 **Other**

745.9 **Unspecified defect of septal closure**
Septal defect NOS

4th 746 **Other congenital anomalies of heart**
Excludes *endocardial fibroelastosis (425.3)*

5th 746.0 **Anomalies of pulmonary valve**
Excludes *infundibular or subvalvular pulmonic stenosis (746.83)*
tetralogy of Fallot (745.2)

746.00 **Pulmonary valve anomaly, unspecified**

746.01 **Atresia, congenital**
Congenital absence of pulmonary valve

746.02 **Stenosis, congenital**

746.09 **Other**
Congenital insufficiency of pulmonary valve
Fallot's triad or trilogy

746.1 **Tricuspid atresia and stenosis, congenital**
Absence of tricuspid valve

746.2 **Ebstein's anomaly**

746.3 **Congenital stenosis of aortic valve**
Congenital aortic stenosis
Excludes *congenital:*
subaortic stenosis (746.81)
supravalvular aortic stenosis (747.22)

746.4 **Congenital insufficiency of aortic valve**
Bicuspid aortic valve
Congenital aortic insufficiency

746.5 **Congenital mitral stenosis**
Fused commissure of mitral valve
Parachute deformity of mitral valve
Supernumerary cusps of mitral valve

746.6 **Congenital mitral insufficiency**

746.7 **Hypoplastic left heart syndrome**
Atresia, or marked hypoplasia, of aortic orifice or valve, with hypoplasia of ascending aorta and defective development of left ventricle (with mitral valve atresia)

5th 746.8 **Other specified anomalies of heart**

746.81 **Subaortic stenosis**

746.82 **Cor triatriatum**

746.83 **Infundibular pulmonic stenosis**
Subvalvular pulmonic stenosis

746.84 **Obstructive anomalies of heart, NEC**
Shone's syndrome
Uhl's disease
Use additional code for associated anomalies, such as:
coarctation of aorta (747.10)
congenital mitral stenosis (746.5)
subaortic stenosis (746.81)

746.85 **Coronary artery anomaly**
Anomalous origin or communication of coronary artery
Arteriovenous malformation of coronary artery
Coronary artery:
absence
arising from aorta or pulmonary trunk
single

746.86 **Congenital heart block**
Complete or incomplete atrioventricular [AV] block

746.87 **Malposition of heart and cardiac apex**
Abdominal heart
Dextrocardia
Ectopia cordis
Levocardia (isolated)
Mesocardia
Excludes *dextrocardia with complete transposition of viscera (759.3)*

746.89 **Other**
Atresia of cardiac vein
Congenital:
cardiomegaly
diverticulum, left ventricle
pericardial defect
Hypoplasia of cardiac vein

746.9 **Unspecified anomaly of heart**
Congenital:
anomaly of heart NOS
heart disease NOS

4th 747 **Other congenital anomalies of circulatory system**

747.0 **Patent ductus arteriosus**
Patent ductus Botalli
Persistent ductus arteriosus

5th 747.1 **Coarctation of aorta**

747.10 **Coarctation of aorta (preductal) (postductal)**
Hypoplasia of aortic arch

747.11 **Interruption of aortic arch**

5th 747.2 **Other anomalies of aorta**

747.20 **Anomaly of aorta, unspecified**

747.21 **Anomalies of aortic arch**
Anomalous origin, right subclavian artery
Dextraposition of aorta
Double aortic arch
Kommerell's diverticulum
Overriding aorta
Persistent:
convolutions, aortic arch
right aortic arch
Vascular ring
Excludes *hypoplasia of aortic arch (747.10)*

747.22 **Atresia and stenosis of aorta**
Absence of aorta
Aplasia of aorta
Hypoplasia of aorta
Stricture of aorta
Supra (valvular)-aortic stenosis
Excludes *congenital aortic (valvular) stenosis or stricture, so stated (746.3)*
hypoplasia of aorta in hypoplastic left heart syndrome (746.7)

747.29 **Other**
Aneurysm of sinus of Valsalva
Congenital:
aneurysm of aorta
dilation of aorta

747.3 **Anomalies of pulmonary artery**
Agenesis of pulmonary artery
Anomaly of pulmonary artery
Atresia of pulmonary artery
Coarctation of pulmonary artery
Hypoplasia of pulmonary artery
Pulmonary arteriovenous aneurysm
Stenosis of pulmonary artery

5th 747.4 **Anomalies of great veins**

747.40 **Anomaly of great veins, unspecified**
Anomaly NOS of:
pulmonary veins
vena cava

747.41 **Total anomalous pulmonary venous connection**
Total anomalous pulmonary venous return [TAPVR]:
subdiaphragmatic
supradiaphragmatic

747.42 **Partial anomalous pulmonary venous connection**
Partial anomalous pulmonary venous return

747.49 **Other anomalies of great veins**
Absence of vena cava (inferior) (superior)
Congenital stenosis of vena cava (inferior) (superior)
Persistent:
left posterior cardinal vein
left superior vena cava
Scimitar syndrome
Transposition of pulmonary veins NOS

747.5 **Absence or hypoplasia of umbilical artery**
Single umbilical artery

5th 747.6 **Other anomalies of peripheral vascular system**
Absence of artery or vein, NEC
Anomaly of artery or vein, NEC
Arteriovenous aneurysm (peripheral)
Arteriovenous malformation of the peripheral vascular system
Atresia of artery or vein, NEC
Congenital:
aneurysm (peripheral)
phlebectasia
stricture, artery
varix
Multiple renal arteries
Excludes *anomalies of:*
cerebral vessels (747.81)
pulmonary artery (747.3)
congenital retinal aneurysm (743.58)
hemangioma (228.00-228.09)
lymphangioma (228.1)

747.60 **Anomaly of the peripheral vascular system, unspecified site**

747.61 **Gastrointestinal vessel anomaly**

747.62 **Renal vessel anomaly**

747.63 **Upper limb vessel anomaly**

747.64 **Lower limb vessel anomaly**

747.69 **Anomalies of other specified sites of peripheral vascular system**

746.84 – 747.69

5th 747.8 **Other specified anomalies of circulatory system**

747.81 Anomalies of cerebrovascular system
Arteriovenous malformation of brain
Cerebral arteriovenous aneurysm, congenital
Congenital anomalies of cerebral vessels
Excludes *ruptured cerebral (arteriovenous) aneurysm (430)*

747.82 Spinal vessel anomaly
Arteriovenous malformation of spinal vessel

747.83 Persistent fetal circulation N
Persistent pulmonary hypertension
Primary pulmonary hypertension of newborn

747.89 Other
Aneurysm, congenital, specified site not elsewhere classified
Excludes *congenital aneurysm:*
coronary (746.85)
peripheral (747.6)
pulmonary (747.3)
retinal (743.58)

747.9 Unspecified anomaly of circulatory system

4th 748 **Congenital anomalies of respiratory system**
Excludes *congenital central alveolar hypoventilation syndrome (327.25)*
congenital defect of diaphragm (756.6)

748.0 Choanal atresia
Atresia of nares (anterior) (posterior)
Congenital stenosis of nares (anterior) (posterior)

748.1 Other anomalies of nose
Absent nose
Accessory nose
Cleft nose
Congenital:
deformity of nose
notching of tip of nose
performation of wall of nasal sinus
Deformity of wall of nasal sinus
Excludes *congenital deviation of nasal septum (754.0)*

748.2 Web of larynx
Web of larynx:
NOS
glottic
subglottic

748.3 Other anomalies of larynx, trachea, and bronchus
Absence or agenesis of:
bronchus
larynx
trachea
Anomaly (of):
cricoid cartilage
epiglottis
thyroid cartilage
tracheal cartilage
Atresia (of):
epiglottis
glottis
larynx
trachea
Cleft thyroid, cartilage, congenital
Congenital:
dilation, trachea
stenosis:
larynx
trachea
tracheocele
Diverticulum:
bronchus
trachea
Fissure of epiglottis
Laryngocele
Posterior cleft of cricoid cartilage (congenital)
Rudimentary tracheal bronchus
Stridor, laryngeal, congenital

748.4 Congenital cystic lung
Disease, lung:
cystic, congenital
polycystic, congenital
Honeycomb lung, congenital
Excludes *acquired or unspecified cystic lung (518.89)*

748.5 Agenesis, hypoplasia, and dysplasia of lung
Absence of lung (fissures) (lobe)
Aplasia of lung
Hypoplasia of lung (lobe)
Sequestration of lung

5th 748.6 **Other anomalies of lung**

748.60 Anomaly of lung, unspecified

748.61 Congenital bronchiectasis

748.69 Other
Accessory lung (lobe)
Azygos lobe (fissure), lung

748.8 Other specified anomalies of respiratory system
Abnormal communication between pericardial and pleural sacs
Anomaly, pleural folds
Atresia of nasopharynx
Congenital cyst of mediastinum

748.9 Unspecified anomaly of respiratory system
Anomaly of respiratory system NOS

4th 749 Cleft palate and cleft lip

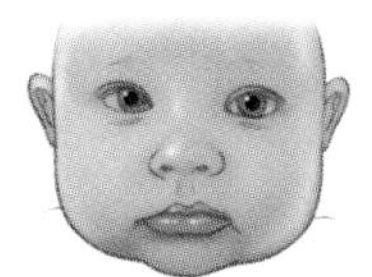
Normal lip

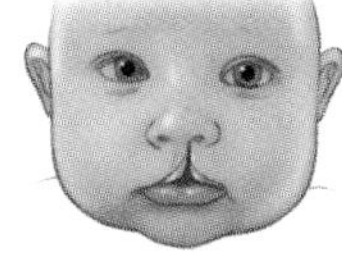
Cleft lip

Bilateral cleft lip

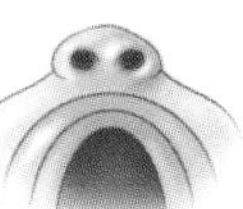
Normal palate and lip

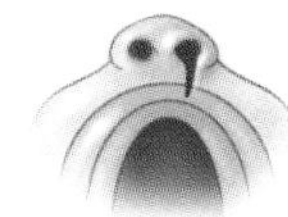
Cleft lip

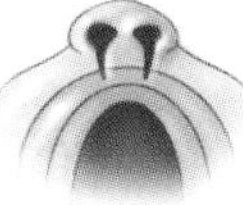
Bilateral cleft lip

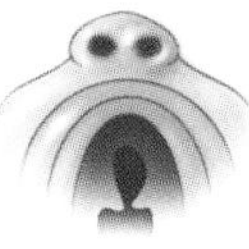
Cleft palate

Cleft lip with partial palate involvement

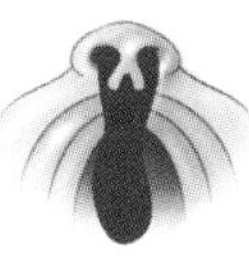
Bilateral cleft lip with full palate involvement

© 2008 Fairman Studios, LLC. All Rights Reserved.

5th 749.0 Cleft palate

749.00 Cleft palate, unspecified

749.01 Unilateral, complete

749.02 Unilateral, incomplete

Cleft uvula

749.03 Bilateral, complete

749.04 Bilateral, incomplete

5th 749.1 Cleft lip

Cheiloschisis
Congenital fissure of lip
Harelip
Labium leporinum

749.10 Cleft lip, unspecified

749.11 Unilateral, complete

749.12 Unilateral, incomplete

749.13 Bilateral, complete

749.14 Bilateral, incomplete

5th 749.2 Cleft palate with cleft lip

Cheilopalatoschisis

749.20 Cleft palate with cleft lip, unspecified

749.21 Unilateral, complete

749.22 Unilateral, incomplete

749.23 Bilateral, complete

749.24 Bilateral, incomplete

749.25 Other combinations

4th 750 Other congenital anomalies of upper alimentary tract

Excludes *dentofacial anomalies (524.0-524.9)*

750.0 Tongue tie

Ankyloglossia

5th 750.1 Other anomalies of tongue

750.10 Anomaly of tongue, unspecified

750.11 Aglossia

750.12 Congenital adhesions of tongue

750.13 Fissure of tongue

Bifid tongue
Double tongue

750.15 Macroglossia

Congenital hypertrophy of tongue

750.16 Microglossia

Hypoplasia of tongue

750.19 Other

5th 750.2 Other specified anomalies of mouth and pharynx

750.21 Absence of salivary gland

750.22 Accessory salivary gland

750.23 Atresia, salivary gland

Imperforate salivary duct

750.24 Congenital fistula of salivary gland

750.25 Congenital fistula of lip

Congenital (mucus) lip pits

750.26 Other specified anomalies of mouth

Absence of uvula

750.27 Diverticulum of pharynx

Pharyngeal pouch

750.29 Other specified anomalies of pharynx

Imperforate pharynx

750.3 Tracheoesophageal fistula, esophageal atresia and stenosis

Absent esophagus
Atresia of esophagus
Congenital:
- esophageal ring
- stenosis of esophagus
- stricture of esophagus

Congenital fistula:
- esophagobronchial
- esophagotracheal

Imperforate esophagus
Webbed esophagus

750.4 Other specified anomalies of esophagus

Dilatation, congenital, of esophagus
Displacement, congenital, of esophagus
Diverticulum of esophagus
Duplication of esophagus
Giant esophagus
Esophageal pouch

Excludes *congenital hiatus hernia (750.6)*

750.5 Congenital hypertrophic pyloric stenosis

Congenital or infantile:
- constriction of pylorus
- hypertrophy of pylorus
- spasm of pylorus
- stenosis of pylorus
- stricture of pylorus

750.6 Congenital hiatus hernia

Displacement of cardia through esophageal hiatus

Excludes *congenital diaphragmatic hernia (756.6)*

750.7 Other specified anomalies of stomach

Congenital:
- cardiospasm
- hourglass stomach

Displacement of stomach
Diverticulum of stomach, congenital
Duplication of stomach
Megalogastria
Microgastria
Transposition of stomach

750.8 Other specified anomalies of upper alimentary tract

750.9 Unspecified anomaly of upper alimentary tract

Congenital:
- anomaly NOS of upper alimentary tract [any part, except tongue]
- deformity NOS of upper alimentary tract [any part, except tongue]

4th 751 **Other congenital anomalies of digestive system**

751.0 Meckel's diverticulum

Meckel's diverticulum (displaced) (hypertrophic)
Persistent:
omphalomesenteric duct
vitelline duct

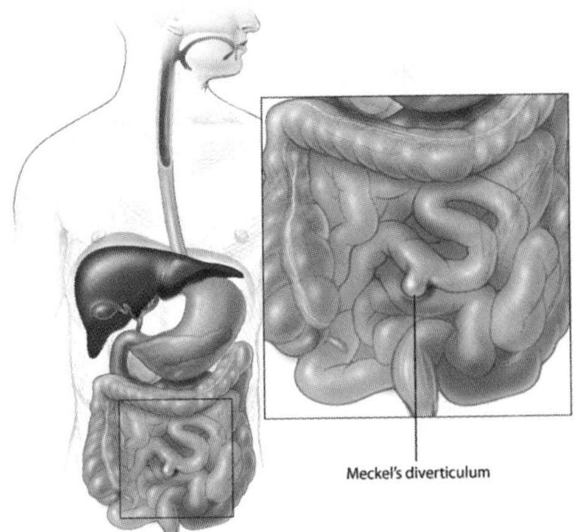

© 2008 Fairman Studios, LLC. All Rights Reserved.

751.1 Atresia and stenosis of small intestine P

Atresia of:
duodenum
ileum
intestine NOS
Congenital:
absence of small intestine or intestine NOS
obstruction of small intestine or intestine NOS
stenosis of small intestine or intestine NOS
stricture of small intestine or intestine NOS
Imperforate jejunum

751.2 Atresia and stenosis of large intestine, rectum, anal canal P

Absence:
anus (congenital)
appendix, congenital
large instestine, congenital
rectum
Atresia of:
anus
colon
rectum
Congenital or infantile:
obstruction of large intestine
occlusion of anus
stricture of anus
Imperforate:
anus
rectum
Stricture of rectum, congenital

751.3 Hirschsprung's disease and other congenital functional disorders of colon

Aganglionosis
Congenital dilation of colon
Congenital megacolon
Macrocolon

751.4 Anomalies of intestinal fixation

Congenital adhesions:
omental, anomalous
peritoneal
Jackson's membrane
Malrotation of colon
Rotation of cecum or colon:
failure of
incomplete
insufficient
Universal mesentery

751.5 Other anomalies of intestine

Congenital diverticulum, colon
Dolichocolon
Duplication of:
anus
appendix
cecum
intestine
Ectopic anus
Megaloappendix
Megaloduodenum
Microcolon
Persistent cloaca
Transposition of:
appendix
colon
intestine

5th **751.6 Anomalies of gallbladder, bile ducts, and liver**

751.60 Unspecified anomaly of gallbladder, bile ducts, and liver

751.61 Biliary atresia P

Congenital:
absence of bile duct (common) or passage
hypoplasia of bile duct (common) or passage
obstruction of bile duct (common) or passage
stricture of bile duct (common) or passage

751.62 Congenital cystic disease of liver

Congenital polycystic disease of liver
Fibrocystic disease of liver

751.69 Other anomalies of gallbladder, bile ducts, and liver

Absence of:
gallbladder, congenital
liver (lobe)
Accessory:
hepatic ducts
liver
Congenital:
choledochal cyst
hepatomegaly
Duplication of:
biliary duct
cystic duct
gallbladder
liver
Floating:
gallbladder
liver
Intrahepatic gallbladder

751.7 Anomalies of pancreas
Absence of pancreas
Accessory pancreas
Agenesis of pancreas
Annular pancreas
Ectopic pancreatic tissue
Hypoplasia of pancreas
Pancreatic heterotopia
Excludes *diabetes mellitus (249.0-249.9, 250.0-250.9)*
fibrocystic disease of pancreas (277.00-277.09)
neonatal diabetes mellitus (775.1)

751.8 Other specified anomalies of digestive system
Absence (complete) (partial) of alimentary tract NOS
Duplication of digestive organs NOS
Malposition, congenital of digestive organs NOS
Excludes *congenital diaphragmatic hernia (756.6)*
congenital hiatus hernia (750.6)

751.9 Unspecified anomaly of digestive system
Congenital:
anomaly NOS of digestive system NOS
deformity NOS of digestive system NOS

4th **752 Congenital anomalies of genital organs**
Excludes *syndromes associated with anomalies in the number and form of chromosomes (758.0-758.9)*

752.0 Anomalies of ovaries ♀
Absence, congenital, of ovary
Accessory ovary
Ectopic ovary
Streak of ovary

5th **752.1 Anomalies of fallopian tubes and broad ligaments**

752.10 Unspecified anomaly of fallopian tubes and broad ligaments ♀

752.11 Embryonic cyst of fallopian tubes and broad ligaments ♀
Cyst:
epoophoron
fimbrial
parovarian

752.19 Other ♀
Absence of fallopian tube or broad ligament
Accessory fallopian tube or broad ligament
Atresia of fallopian tube or broad ligament

752.2 Doubling of uterus ♀
Didelphic uterus
Doubling of uterus [any degree] (associated with doubling of cervix and vagina)

752.3 Other anomalies of uterus ♀
Absence, congenital, of uterus
Agenesis of uterus
Aplasia of uterus
Bicornuate uterus
Uterus unicornis
Uterus with only one functioning horn

5th **752.4 Anomalies of cervix, vagina, and external female genitalia**

752.40 Unspecified anomaly of cervix, vagina, and external female genitalia ♀

752.41 Embryonic cyst of cervix, vagina, and external female genitalia ♀
Cyst of:
canal of Nuck, congenital
Gartner's duct
vagina, embryonal
vulva, congenital

752.42 Imperforate hymen ♀

752.49 Other anomalies of cervix, vagina, and external female genitalia ♀
Absence of cervix, clitoris, vagina, or vulva
Agenesis of cervix, clitoris, vagina, or vulva
Congenital stenosis or stricture of:
cervical canal
vagina
Excludes *double vagina associated with total duplication (752.2)*

5th **752.5 Undescended and retractile testicle**

752.51 Undescended testis ♂
Cryptorchism
Ectopic testis

752.52 Retractile testis ♂

5th **752.6 Hypospadias and epispadias and other penile anomalies**

752.61 Hypospadias ♂

752.62 Epispadias ♂
Anaspadias

752.63 Congenital chordee ♂

752.64 Micropenis ♂

752.65 Hidden penis ♂

752.69 Other penile anomalies ♂

752.7 Indeterminate sex and pseudohermaphroditism
Gynandrism
Hermaphroditism
Ovotestis
Pseudohermaphroditism (male) (female)
Pure gonadal dysgenesis
Excludes *androgen insensitivity (259.50-259.52)*
pseudohermaphroditism:
female, with adrenocortical disorder (255.2)
male, with gonadal disorder (257.8)
with specified chromosomal anomaly (758.0-758.9)
testicular feminization syndrome (259.50-259.52)

5th **752.8 Other specified anomalies of genital organs**
Excludes *congenital hydrocele (778.6)*
penile anomalies (752.61-752.69)
phimosis or paraphimosis (605)

752.81 Scrotal transposition ♂

752.89 Other specified anomalies of genital organs
Absence of:
prostate
spermatic cord
vas deferens
Anorchism
Aplasia (congenital) of:
prostate
round ligament
testicle
Atresia of:
ejaculatory duct
vas deferens
Fusion of testes
Hypoplasia of testis
Monorchism
Polyorchism

752.9 Unspecified anomaly of genital organs
Congenital:
anomaly NOS of genital organ, NEC
deformity NOS of genital organ, NEC

4th 753 **Congenital anomalies of urinary system**

753.0 **Renal agenesis and dysgenesis**
Atrophy of kidney:
congenital
infantile
Congenital absence of kidney(s)
Hypoplasia of kidney(s)

5th 753.1 **Cystic kidney disease**
Excludes *acquired cyst of kidney (593.2)*

753.10 **Cystic kidney disease, unspecified**

753.11 **Congenital single renal cyst**

753.12 **Polycystic kidney, unspecified type**

753.13 **Polycystic kidney, autosomal dominant**

753.14 **Polycystic kidney, autosomal recessive**

753.15 **Renal dysplasia**

753.16 **Medullary cystic kidney**
Nephronopthisis

753.17 **Medullary sponge kidney**

753.19 **Other specified cystic kidney disease**
Multicystic kidney

5th 753.2 **Obstructive defects of renal pelvis and ureter**

753.20 **Unspecified obstructive defect of renal pelvis and ureter**

753.21 **Congenital obstruction of ureteropelvic junction**

753.22 **Congenital obstruction of ureterovesical junction**
Adynamic ureter
Congenital hydroureter

753.23 **Congenital ureterocele**

753.29 **Other**

753.3 **Other specified anomalies of kidney**
Accessory kidney
Congenital:
calculus of kidney
displaced kidney
Discoid kidney
Double kidney with double pelvis
Ectopic kidney
Fusion of kidneys
Giant kidney
Horseshoe kidney
Hyperplasia of kidney
Lobulation of kidney
Malrotation of kidney
Trifid kidney (pelvis)

753.4 **Other specified anomalies of ureter**
Absent ureter
Accessory ureter
Deviaton of ureter
Displaced ureteric orifice
Double ureter
Ectopic ureter
Implantation, anomalous, of ureter

753.5 **Exstrophy of urinary bladder**
Ectopia vesicae
Extroversion of bladder

753.6 **Atresia and stenosis of urethra and bladder neck**
Congenital obstruction:
bladder neck
urethra
Congenital stricture of:
urethra (valvular)
urinary meatus
vesicourethral orifice
Imperforate urinary meatus
Impervious urethra
Urethral valve formation

753.7 **Anomalies of urachus**
Cyst (of) urachus
Fistula (of) urachus
Patent (of) urachus
Persistent umbilical sinus

753.8 **Other specified anomalies of bladder and urethra**
Absence, congenital of:
bladder
urethra
Accessory:
bladder
urethra
Congenital:
diverticulum of bladder
hernia of bladder
Congenital urethrorectal fistula
Congenital prolapse of:
bladder (mucosa)
urethra
Double:
urethra
urinary meatus

753.9 **Unspecified anomaly of urinary system**
Congenital:
anomaly NOS of urinary system [any part, except urachus]
deformity NOS of urinary system [any part, except urachus]

4th 754 **Certain congenital musculoskeletal deformities**
Includes nonteratogenic deformities which are considered to be due to intrauterine malposition and pressure

754.0 **Of skull, face, and jaw**
Asymmetry of face
Compression facies
Depressions in skull
Deviation of nasal septum, congenital
Dolichocephaly
Plagiocephaly
Potter's facies
Squashed or bent nose, congenital
Excludes *dentofacial anomalies (524.0-524.9)*
syphilitic saddle nose (090.5)

754.1 **Of sternocleidomastoid muscle**
Congenital sternomastoid torticollis
Congenital wryneck
Contracture of sternocleidomastoid (muscle)
Sternomastoid tumor

754.2 **Of spine**
Congenital postural:
lordosis
scoliosis

5th 754.3 **Congenital dislocation of hip**

754.30 **Congenital dislocation of hip, unilateral**
Congenital dislocation of hip NOS

754.31 **Congenital dislocation of hip, bilateral**

754.32 **Congenital subluxation of hip, unilateral**
Congenital flexion deformity, hip or thigh
Predislocation status of hip at birth
Preluxation of hip, congenital

754.33 **Congenital subluxation of hip, bilateral**

754.35 **Congenital dislocation of one hip with subluxation of other hip**

5th 754.4 **Congenital genu recurvatum and bowing of long bones of leg**

754.40 **Genu recurvatum**

754.41 **Congenital dislocation of knee (with genu recurvatum)**

754.42 **Congenital bowing of femur**

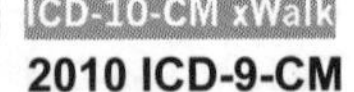

754.43 **Congenital bowing of tibia and fibula**

754.44 **Congenital bowing of unspecified long bones of leg**

5th 754.5 **Varus deformities of feet**

Excludes *acquired (736.71, 736.75, 736.79)*

754.50 **Talipes varus**
Congenital varus deformity of foot, unspecified
Pes varus

754.51 **Talipes equinovarus**
Equinovarus (congenital)

754.52 **Metatarsus primus varus**

754.53 **Metatarsus varus**

754.59 **Other**
Talipes calcaneovarus

5th 754.6 **Valgus deformities of feet**

Excludes *valgus deformity of foot (acquired) (736.79)*

754.60 **Talipes valgus**
Congenital valgus deformity of foot, unspecified

754.61 **Congenital pes planus**
Congenital rocker bottom flat foot
Flat foot, congenital

Excludes *pes planus (acquired) (734)*

754.62 **Talipes calcaneovalgus**

754.69 **Other**
Talipes:
equinovalgus
planovalgus

5th 754.7 **Other deformities of feet**

Excludes *acquired (736.70-736.79)*

754.70 **Talipes, unspecified**
Congenital deformity of foot NOS

754.71 **Talipes cavus**
Cavus foot (congenital)

754.79 **Other**
Asymmetric talipes
Talipes:
calcaneus
equinus

5th 754.8 **Other specified nonteratogenic anomalies**

754.81 **Pectus excavatum**
Congenital funnel chest

754.82 **Pectus carinatum**
Congenital pigeon chest [breast]

754.89 **Other**
Club hand (congenital)
Congenital:
deformity of chest wall
dislocation of elbow
Generalized flexion contractures of lower limb joints, congenital
Spade-like hand (congenital)

4th 755 **Other congenital anomalies of limbs**

Excludes *those deformities classifiable to 754.0-754.8*

5th 755.0 **Polydactyly**

755.00 **Polydactyly, unspecified digits**
Supernumerary digits

755.01 **Of fingers**
Accessory fingers

755.02 **Of toes**
Accessory toes

5th 755.1 **Syndactyly**
Symphalangy
Webbing of digits

755.10 **Of multiple and unspecified sites**

755.11 **Of fingers without fusion of bone**

755.12 **Of fingers with fusion of bone**

755.13 **Of toes without fusion of bone**

755.14 **Of toes with fusion of bone**

5th 755.2 **Reduction deformities of upper limb**

755.20 **Unspecified reduction deformity of upper limb**
Ectromelia NOS of upper limb
Hemimelia NOS of upper limb
Shortening of arm, congenital

755.21 **Transverse deficiency of upper limb**
Amelia of upper limb
Congenital absence of:
fingers, all (complete or partial)
forearm, including hand and fingers
upper limb, complete
Congenital amputation of upper limb
Transverse hemimelia of upper limb

755.22 **Longitudinal deficiency of upper limb, NEC**
Phocomelia NOS of upper limb
Rudimentary arm

755.23 **Longitudinal deficiency, combined, involving humerus, radius, and ulna (complete or incomplete)**
Congenital absence of arm and forearm (complete or incomplete) with or without metacarpal deficiency and/or phalangeal deficiency, incomplete
Phocomelia, complete, of upper limb

755.24 **Longitudinal deficiency, humeral, complete or partial (with or without distal deficiencies, incomplete)**
Congenital absence of humerus (with or without absence of some [but not all] distal elements)
Proximal phocomelia of upper limb

755.25 **Longitudinal deficiency, radioulnar, complete or partial (with or without distal deficiencies, incomplete)**
Congenital absence of radius and ulna (with or without absence of some [but not all] distal elements)
Distal phocomelia of upper limb

755.26 **Longitudinal deficiency, radial, complete or partial (with or without distal deficiencies, incomplete)**
Agenesis of radius
Congenital absence of radius (with or without absence of some [but not all] distal elements)

755.27 **Longitudinal deficiency, ulnar, complete or partial (with or without distal deficiencies, incomplete)**
Agenesis of ulna
Congenital absence of ulna (with or without absence of some [but not all] distal elements)

755.28 **Longitudinal deficiency, carpals or metacarpals, complete or partial (with or without incomplete phalangeal deficiency)**

755.29 **Longitudinal deficiency, phalanges, complete or partial**
Absence of finger, congenital
Aphalangia of upper limb, terminal, complete or partial

Excludes *terminal deficiency of all five digits (755.21)*
transverse deficiency of phalanges (755.21)

754.43 – 755.29

5th 755.3 **Reduction deformities of lower limb**

755.30 **Unspecified reduction deformity of lower limb**
Ectromelia NOS of lower limb
Hemimelia NOS of lower limb
Shortening of leg, congenital

755.31 **Transverse deficiency of lower limb**
Amelia of lower limb
Congenital absence of:
foot
leg, including foot and toes
lower limb, complete
toes, all, complete
Transverse hemimelia of lower limb

755.32 **Longitudinal deficiency of lower limb, NEC**
Phocomelia NOS of lower limb

755.33 **Longitudinal deficiency, combined, involving femur, tibia, and fibula (complete or incomplete)**
Congenital absence of thigh and (lower) leg (complete or incomplete) with or without metacarpal deficiency and/or phalangeal deficiency, incomplete
Phocomelia, complete, of lower limb

755.34 **Longitudinal deficiency, femoral, complete or partial (with or without distal deficiencies, incomplete)**
Congenital absence of femur (with or without absence of some [but not all] distal elements)
Proximal phocomelia of lower limb

755.35 **Longitudinal deficiency, tibiofibular, complete or partial (with or without distal deficiencies, incomplete)**
Congenital absence of tibia and fibula (with or without absence of some [but not all] distal elements)
Distal phocomelia of lower limb

755.36 **Longitudinal deficiency, tibia, complete or partial (with or without distal deficiencies, incomplete)**
Agenesis of tibia
Congenital absence of tibia (with or without absence of some [but not all] distal elements)

755.37 **Longitudinal deficiency, fibular, complete or partial (with or without distal deficiencies, incomplete)**
Agenesis of fibula
Congenital absence of fibula (with or without absence of some [but not all] distal elements)

755.38 **Longitudinal deficiency, tarsals or metatarsals, complete or partial (with or without incomplete phalangeal deficiency)**

755.39 **Longitudinal deficiency, phalanges, complete or partial**
Absence of toe, congenital
Aphalangia of lower limb, terminal, complete or partial
Excludes *terminal deficiency of all five digits (755.31)*
transverse deficiency of phalanges (755.31)

755.4 **Reduction deformities, unspecified limb**
Absence, congenital (complete or partial) of limb NOS
Amelia of unspecified limb
Ectromelia of unspecified limb
Hemimelia of unspecified limb
Phocomelia of unspecified limb

5th 755.5 **Other anomalies of upper limb, including shoulder girdle**

755.50 **Unspecified anomaly of upper limb**

755.51 **Congenital deformity of clavicle**

755.52 **Congenital elevation of scapula**
Sprengel's deformity

755.53 **Radioulnar synostosis**

755.54 **Madelung's deformity**

755.55 **Acrocephalosyndactyly**
Apert's syndrome

755.56 **Accessory carpal bones**

755.57 **Macrodactylia (fingers)**

755.58 **Cleft hand, congenital**
Lobster-claw hand

755.59 **Other**
Cleidocranial dysostosis
Cubitus:
valgus, congenital
varus, congenital
Excludes *club hand (congenital) (754.89)*
congenital dislocation of elbow (754.89)

5th 755.6 **Other anomalies of lower limb, including pelvic girdle**

755.60 **Unspecified anomaly of lower limb**

755.61 **Coxa valga, congenital**

755.62 **Coxa vara, congenital**

755.63 **Other congenital deformity of hip (joint)**
Congenital anteversion of femur (neck)
Excludes *congenital dislocation of hip (754.30-754.35)*

755.64 **Congenital deformity of knee (joint)**
Congenital:
absence of patella
genu valgum [knock-knee]
genu varum [bowleg]
Rudimentary patella

755.65 **Macrodactylia of toes**

755.66 **Other anomalies of toes**
Congenital:
hallux valgus
hallux varus
hammer toe

755.67 **Anomalies of foot, NEC**
Astragaloscaphoid synostosis
Calcaneonavicular bar
Coalition of calcaneus
Talonavicular synostosis
Tarsal coalitions

755.69 **Other**
Congenital:
angulation of tibia
deformity (of):
ankle (joint)
sacroiliac (joint)
fusion of sacroiliac joint

755.8 **Other specified anomalies of unspecified limb**

755.9 **Unspecified anomaly of unspecified limb**
Congenital:
anomaly NOS of unspecified limb
deformity NOS of unspecified limb
Excludes *reduction deformity of unspecified limb (755.4)*

755.3 – 755.9

4th 756 **Other congenital musculoskeletal anomalies**

Excludes *congenital myotonic chondrodystrophy (359.23)*
those deformities classifiable to 754.0-754.8

756.0 **Anomalies of skull and face bones**
Absence of skull bones
Acrocephaly
Congenital deformity of forehead
Craniosynostosis
Crouzon's disease
Hypertelorism
Imperfect fusion of skull
Oxycephaly
Platybasia
Premature closure of cranial sutures
Tower skull
Trigonocephaly
Excludes *acrocephalosyndactyly [Apert's syndrome] (755.55)*
dentofacial anomalies (524.0-524.9)
skull defects associated with brain anomalies, such as:
anencephalus (740.0)
encephalocele (742.0)
hydrocephalus (742.3)
microcephalus (742.1)

5th 756.1 **Anomalies of spine**

756.10 **Anomaly of spine, unspecified**

756.11 **Spondylolysis, lumbosacral region**
Prespondylolisthesis (lumbosacral)

756.12 **Spondylolisthesis** 148, 149, 150, 151

756.13 **Absence of vertebra, congenital**

756.14 **Hemivertebra**

756.15 **Fusion of spine [vertebra], congenital**

756.16 **Klippel-Feil syndrome**

756.17 **Spina bifida occulta**
Excludes *spina bifida (aperta) (741.0-741.9)*

756.19 **Other**
Platyspondylia
Supernumerary vertebra

756.2 **Cervical rib**
Supernumerary rib in the cervical region

756.3 **Other anomalies of ribs and sternum**
Congenital absence of:
rib
sternum
Congenital:
fissure of sternum
fusion of ribs
Sternum bifidum
Excludes *nonteratogenic deformity of chest wall (754.81-754.89)*

756.4 **Chondrodystrophy**
Achondroplasia
Chondrodystrophia (fetalis)
Dyschondroplasia
Enchondromatosis
Ollier's disease
Excludes *congenital myotonic chondrodystrophy (359.23)*
lipochondrodystrophy [Hurler's syndrome] (277.5)
Morquio's disease (277.5)

5th 756.5 **Osteodystrophies**

756.50 **Osteodystrophy, unspecified**

756.51 **Osteogenesis imperfecta**
Fragilitas ossium
Osteopsathyrosis

756.52 **Osteopetrosis**

756.53 **Osteopoikilosis**

756.54 **Polyostotic fibrous dysplasia of bone**

756.55 **Chondroectodermal dysplasia**
Ellis-van Creveld syndrome

756.56 **Multiple epiphyseal dysplasia**

756.59 **Other**
Albright (-McCune)-Sternberg syndrome

756.6 **Anomalies of diaphragm**
Absence of diaphragm
Congenital hernia:
diaphragmatic
foramen of Morgagni
Eventration of diaphragm
Excludes *congenital hiatus hernia (750.6)*

5th 756.7 **Anomalies of abdominal wall**

756.70 **Anomaly of abdominal wall, unspecified**

756.71 **Prune belly syndrome**
Eagle-Barrett syndrome
Prolapse of bladder mucosa

● 756.72 **Omphalocele**
Exomphalos

Rationale: *Omphalocele is a separately distinct ventral wall defect where the intestines are usually covered by a membranous sac with the intestine only being exposed if the sac ruptures. The incidence is 1-2 per 10,000 births. Unlike gastroschisis, omphalocele is frequently associated with other structural and chromosomal anomalies. More than half will have abnormalities of other organs or body parts and a third chromosomal abnormality, most commonly trisomy. This condition is more common in infants of mothers 35 and older.*

Previously, both of these conditions were indexed and included at code 756.79, "Other congenital anomalies of the abdominal wall. This made surveillance difficult to accurately separate these distinct defects. In order to improve better epidemiologic tracking of these two distinct entities the American Academy of Pediatrics (AAP) requested that new unique codes be established for each condition.

● 756.73 **Gastroschisis**

Rationale: *Gastroschisis, on the other hand, is a congenital ventral body wall defect, adjacent and usually to the right of the umbilical cord insertion that results from the failure of the developing abdomina'l wall to completely close. In turn this allows the extrusion of the fetal intestines from the defect. The exposed intestines are not covered by a membranous sac which results in a prolonged exposure to amniotic fluid. This results in a thick, swollen and inflamed intestine increasing the risk of heat and fluid loss and infection after birth. The incidence of this condition has been reported at 2-5 per 10,000 births with an increasing prevalence reported in many parts of the world (higher incidence in younger mothers). There are no associated syndromes with gastroschisis, but it may be associated with other gastrointestinal anomalies such as intestinal atresia, stenosis and malrotation.*

756.79 **Other congenital anomalies of abdominal wall**
~~Exomphalos~~
~~Gastroschisis~~
~~Omphalocele~~
Excludes *umbilical hernia (551-553 with .1)*

5th 756.8 **Other specified anomalies of muscle, tendon, fascia, and connective tissue**

756.81 **Absence of muscle and tendon**
Absence of muscle (pectoral)

756.82 **Accessory muscle**

756.83 **Ehlers-Danlos syndrome**

756.89 **Other**
Amyotrophia congenita
Congenital shortening of tendon

756.9 **Other and unspecified anomalies of musculoskeletal system**
Congenital:
anomaly NOS of musculoskeletal system, NEC
deformity NOS of musculoskeletal system, NEC

4th 757 **Congenital anomalies of the integument**
Includes anomalies of skin, subcutaneous tissue, hair, nails, and breast
Excludes *hemangioma (228.00-228.09)*
pigmented nevus (216.0-216.9)

757.0 **Hereditary edema of legs**
Congenital lymphedema
Hereditary trophedema
Milroy's disease

757.1 **Ichthyosis congenita**
Congenital ichthyosis
Harlequin fetus
Ichthyosiform erythroderma

757.2 **Dermatoglyphic anomalies**
Abnormal palmar creases

5th 757.3 **Other specified anomalies of skin**

757.31 **Congenital ectodermal dysplasia**

757.32 **Vascular hamartomas**
Birthmarks
Port-wine stain
Strawberry nevus

757.33 **Congenital pigmentary anomalies of skin**
Congenital poikiloderma
Urticaria pigmentosa
Xeroderma pigmentosum
Excludes *albinism (270.2)*

757.39 **Other**
Accessory skin tags, congenital
Congenital scar
Epidermolysis bullosa
Keratoderma (congenital)
Excludes *pilonidal cyst (685.0-685.1)*

757.4 **Specified anomalies of hair**
Congenital:
alopecia
atrichosis
beaded hair
hypertrichosis
monilethrix
Persistent lanugo

757.5 **Specified anomalies of nails**
Anonychia
Congenital:
clubnail
koilonychia
leukonychia
onychauxis
pachyonychia

▲757.6 **Specified congenital anomalies of breast**
Accessory breast or nipple
Congenital absent breast or nipple
Supernumerary breast or nipple
Excludes *absence of pectoral muscle (756.81)*
hypoplasia of breast (611.82)
micromastia (611.82)

757.8 **Other specified anomalies of the integument**

757.9 **Unspecified anomaly of the integument**
Congenital:
anomaly NOS of integument
deformity NOS of integument

4th 758 **Chromosomal anomalies**
Includes syndromes associated with anomalies in the number and form of chromosomes
Use additional codes for conditions associated with the chromosomal anomolies.

758.0 **Down's syndrome**
Mongolism
Translocation Down's syndrome
Trisomy:
21 or 22
G

758.1 **Patau's syndrome**
Trisomy:
13
D_1

758.2 **Edward's syndrome**
Trisomy:
18
E_3

5th 758.3 **Autosomal deletion syndromes**

758.31 **Cri-du-chat syndrome**
Deletion 5p

758.32 **Velo-cardio-facial syndrome**
Deletion 22q11.2

758.33 **Other microdeletions**
Miller-Dieker syndrome
Smith-Magenis syndrome

758.39 **Other autosomal deletions**

758.4 **Balanced autosomal translocation in normal individual**

758.5 **Other conditions due to autosomal anomalies**
Accessory autosomes NEC

758.6 **Gonadal dysgenesis**
Ovarian dysgenesis
Turner's syndrome
XO syndrome
Excludes *pure gonadal dysgenesis (752.7)*

758.7 **Klinefelter's syndrome** ♂
XXY syndrome

758.8 **Other conditions due to chromosome anomalies**

758.81 **Other conditions due to sex chromosome anomalies**

758.89 **Other**

758.9 **Conditions due to anomaly of unspecified chromosome**

4th 759 **Other and unspecified congenital anomalies**

759.0 **Anomalies of spleen**
Aberrant spleen
Absent spleen
Accessory spleen
Congenital splenomegaly
Ectopic spleen
Lobulation of spleen

759.1 **Anomalies of adrenal gland**
Aberrant adrenal gland
Absent adrenal gland
Accessory adrenal gland
Excludes *adrenogenital disorders (255.2)*
congenital disorders of steroid metabolism (255.2)

759.2 Anomalies of other endocrine glands
Absent parathyroid gland
Accessory thyroid gland
Persistent thyroglossal or thyrolingual duct
Thyroglossal (duct) cyst
Excludes *congenital:*
goiter (246.1)
hypothyroidism (243)

759.3 Situs inversus
Situs inversus or transversus:
abdominalis
thoracis
Transposition of viscera:
abdominal
thoracic
Excludes *dextrocardia without mention of complete transposition (746.87)*

759.4 Conjoined twins
Craniopagus
Dicephalus
Pygopagus
Thoracopagus
Xiphopagus

759.5 Tuberous sclerosis
Bourneville's disease
Epiloia

759.6 Other hamartoses, NEC
Syndrome:
Peutz-Jeghers
Sturge-Weber (-Dimitri)
von Hippel-Lindau
Excludes *neurofibromatosis (237.7)*

759.7 Multiple congenital anomalies, so described
Congenital:
anomaly, multiple NOS
deformity, multiple NOS

5th **759.8 Other specified anomalies**

759.81 Prader-Willi syndrome

759.82 Marfan syndrome

759.83 Fragile X syndrome

759.89 Other
Congenital malformation syndromes affecting multiple systems, NEC
Laurence-Moon-Biedl syndrome

759.9 Congenital anomaly, unspecified

15. CERTAIN CONDITIONS ORIGINATING IN THE PERINATAL PERIOD (760-779)

Includes conditions which have their origin in the perinatal period, before birth through the first 28 days after birth, even though death or morbidity occurs later

Use additional code(s) to further specify condition

ICD-9-CM Official Guidelines (Chapter 15):

For coding and reporting purposes the perinatal period is defined as before birth through the 28th day following birth. The following guidelines are provided for reporting purposes. Hospitals may record other diagnoses as needed for internal data use.

a. General Perinatal Rules

1) Chapter 15 Codes

They are never for use on the maternal record. Codes from Chapter 11, the obstetric chapter, are never permitted on the newborn record. Chapter 15 code may be used throughout the life of the patient if the condition is still present.

2) Sequencing of perinatal codes

Generally, codes from Chapter 15 should be sequenced as the principal/first-listed diagnosis on the newborn record, with the exception of the appropriate V30 code for the birth episode, followed by codes from any other chapter that provide additional detail. The "use additional code" note at the beginning of the chapter supports this guideline. If the index does not provide a specific code for a perinatal condition, assign code 779.89, Other specified conditions originating in the perinatal period, followed by the code from another chapter that specifies the condition. Codes for signs and symptoms may be assigned when a definitive diagnosis has not been established.

3) Birth process or community acquired conditions

If a newborn has a condition that may be either due to the birth process or community acquired and the documentation does not indicate which it is, the default is due to the birth process and the code from Chapter 15 should be used. If the condition is community-acquired, a code from Chapter 15 should not be assigned.

4) Code all clinically significant conditions

All clinically significant conditions noted on routine newborn examination should be coded. A condition is clinically significant if it requires:

- *clinical evaluation; or*
- *therapeutic treatment; or*
- *diagnostic procedures; or*
- *extended length of hospital stay; or*
- *increased nursing care and/or monitoring; or*
- *has implications for future health care needs*

Note: *The perinatal guidelines listed above are the same as the general coding guidelines for "additional diagnoses", except for the final point regarding implications for future health care needs. Codes should be assigned for conditions that have been specified by the provider as having implications for future health care needs. Codes from the perinatal chapter should not be assigned unless the provider has established a definitive diagnosis....*

g. Congenital Anomalies in Newborns

For the birth admission, the appropriate code from category V30, Liveborn infants according to type of birth, should be used, followed by any congenital anomaly codes, categories 740-759. Use additional secondary codes from other chapters to specify conditions associated with the anomaly, if applicable.

Also, see Section I.C.14 for information on the coding of congenital anomalies.

h. Coding Additional Perinatal Diagnoses

1) Assigning codes for conditions that require treatment

Assign codes for conditions that require treatment or further investigation, prolong the length of stay, or require resource utilization.

759.2 – 759.9

2) *Codes for conditions specified as having implications for future health care needs*

Assign codes for conditions that have been specified by the provider as having implications for future health care needs.

***Note:** This guideline should not be used for adult patients.*

3) *Codes for newborn conditions originating in the perinatal period*

Assign a code for newborn conditions originating in the perinatal period (categories 760-779), as well as complications arising during the current episode of care classified in other chapters, only if the diagnoses have been documented by the responsible provider at the time of transfer or discharge as having affected the fetus or newborn.

MATERNAL CAUSES OF PERINATAL MORBIDITY AND MORTALITY (760-763)

ICD-9-CM Official Guidelines (Chapter 15):

f. Maternal Causes of Perinatal Morbidity

Codes from categories 760-763, Maternal causes of perinatal morbidity and mortality, are assigned only when the maternal condition has actually affected the fetus or newborn. The fact that the mother has an associated medical condition or experiences some complication of pregnancy, labor or delivery does not justify the routine assignment of codes from these categories to the newborn record.

4th **760 Fetus or newborn affected by maternal conditions which may be unrelated to present pregnancy**

Includes the listed maternal conditions only when specified as a cause of mortality or morbidity of the fetus or newborn

Excludes *maternal endocrine and metabolic disorders affecting fetus or newborn (775.0-775.9)*

760.0 Maternal hypertensive disorders

Fetus or newborn affected by maternal conditions classifiable to 642

760.1 Maternal renal and urinary tract diseases

Fetus or newborn affected by maternal conditions classifiable to 580-599

760.2 Maternal infections

Fetus or newborn affected by maternal infectious disease classifiable to 001-136 and 487, but fetus or newborn not manifesting that disease

Excludes *congenital infectious diseases (771.0-771.8)*
maternal genital tract and other localized infections (760.8)

760.3 Other chronic maternal circulatory and respiratory diseases

Fetus or newborn affected by chronic maternal conditions classifiable to 390-459, 490-519, 745-748

760.4 Maternal nutritional disorders

Fetus or newborn affected by:
maternal disorders classifiable to 260-269
maternal malnutrition NOS

Excludes *fetal malnutrition (764.10-764.29)*

760.5 Maternal injury

Fetus or newborn affected by maternal conditions classifiable to 800-995

5th **760.6 Surgical operation on mother and fetus**

Excludes *cesarean section for present delivery (763.4)*
damage to placenta from amniocentesis, cesarean section, or surgical induction (762.1)

760.61 Newborn affected by amniocentesis N

Excludes *fetal complications from amniocentesis (679.1)*

760.62 Newborn affected by other in utero procedure N

Excludes *fetal complications of in utero procedure (679.1)*

760.63 Newborn affected by other surgical operations on mother during pregnancy N

Excludes *newborn affected by previous surgical procedure on mother not associated with pregnancy (760.64)*

760.64 Newborn affected by previous surgical procedure on mother not associated with pregnancy N

5th **760.7 Noxious influences affecting fetus or newborn via placenta or breast milk**

Fetus or newborn affected by noxious substance transmitted via placenta or breast milk

Excludes *anesthetic and analgesic drugs administered during labor and delivery (763.5)*
drug withdrawal syndrome in newborn (779.5)

760.70 Unspecified noxious substance

Fetus or newborn affected by:
drug NEC

760.71 Alcohol

Fetal alcohol syndrome

760.72 Narcotics

760.73 Hallucinogenic agents

760.74 Anti-infectives

Antibiotics
Antifungals

760.75 Cocaine

760.76 Diethylstilbestrol [DES]

760.77 Anticonvulsants N

Carbamazepine
Phenobarbital
Phenytoin
Valproic acid

760.78 Antimetabolic agents N

Methotrexate
Retinoic acid
Statins

760.79 Other

Fetus or newborn affected by:
immune sera transmitted via placenta or breast milk
medicinal agents NEC transmitted via placenta or breast milk
toxic substance NEC transmitted via placenta or breast milk

760.8 Other specified maternal conditions affecting fetus or newborn

Maternal genital tract and other localized infection affecting fetus or newborn, but fetus or newborn not manifesting that disease

Excludes *maternal urinary tract infection affecting fetus or newborn (760.1)*

760.9 Unspecified maternal condition affecting fetus or newborn

4th **761 Fetus or newborn affected by maternal complications of pregnancy**

Includes the listed maternal conditions only when specified as a cause of mortality or morbidity of the fetus or newborn

761.0 Incompetent cervix

761.1 Premature rupture of membranes

761.2 Oligohydramnios

Excludes *that due to premature rupture of membranes (761.1)*

761.3 Polyhydramnios

Hydramnios (acute) (chronic)

760 – 761.3

761.4 Ectopic pregnancy
Pregnancy:
abdominal
intraperitoneal
tubal

761.5 Multiple pregnancy
Triplet (pregnancy)
Twin (pregnancy)

761.6 Maternal death

761.7 Malpresentation before labor
Breech presentation before labor
External version before labor
Oblique lie before labor
Transverse lie before labor
Unstable lie before labor

761.8 Other specified maternal complications of pregnancy affecting fetus or newborn
Spontaneous abortion, fetus

761.9 Unspecified maternal complication of pregnancy affecting fetus or newborn

4th **762 Fetus or newborn affected by complications of placenta, cord, and membranes**

Includes the listed maternal conditions only when specified as a cause of mortality or morbidity in the fetus or newborn

762.0 Placenta previa N

762.1 Other forms of placental separation and hemorrhage N
Abruptio placentae
Antepartum hemorrhage
Damage to placenta from amniocentesis, cesarean section, or surgical induction
Maternal blood loss
Premature separation of placenta
Rupture of marginal sinus

762.2 Other and unspecified morphological and functional abnormalities of placenta N
Placental:
dysfunction
infarction
insufficiency

762.3 Placental transfusion syndromes N
Placental and cord abnormality resulting in twin-to-twin or other transplacental transfusion
Use additional code to indicate resultant condition in ~~fetus or~~ newborn:
fetal blood loss (772.0)
polycythemia neonatorum (776.4)

762.4 Prolapsed cord N
Cord presentation

762.5 Other compression of umbilical cord N
Cord around neck
Entanglement of cord
Knot in cord
Torsion of cord

762.6 Other and unspecified conditions of umbilical cord N
Short cord
Thrombosis of umbilical cord
Varices of umbilical cord
Vasa previa
Velamentous insertion of umbilical cord

Excludes *infection of umbilical cord (771.4)*
single umbilical artery (747.5)

762.7 Chorioamnionitis N
Amnionitis
Membranitis
Placentitis

762.8 Other specified abnormalities of chorion and amnion N

762.9 Unspecified abnormality of chorion and amnion N

4th **763 Fetus or newborn affected by other complications of labor and delivery**

Includes the listed conditions only when specified as a cause of mortality or morbidity in the fetus or newborn

Excludes *newborn affected by surgical procedures on mother (760.61-760.64)*

763.0 Breech delivery and extraction N

763.1 Other malpresentation, malposition, and disproportion during labor and delivery N
Fetus or newborn affected by:
abnormality of bony pelvis
contracted pelvis
persistent occipitoposterior position
shoulder presentation
transverse lie
conditions classifiable to 652, 653, and 660

763.2 Forceps delivery N
Fetus or newborn affected by forceps extraction

763.3 Delivery by vacuum extractor N

763.4 Cesarean delivery N

Excludes *placental separation or hemorrhage from cesarean section (762.1)*

763.5 Maternal anesthesia and analgesia N
Reactions and intoxications from maternal opiates and tranquilizers during labor and delivery

Excludes *drug withdrawal syndrome in newborn (779.5)*

763.6 Precipitate delivery N
Rapid second stage

763.7 Abnormal uterine contractions N
Fetus or newborn affected by:
contraction ring
hypertonic labor
hypotonic uterine dysfunction
uterine inertia or dysfunction
conditions classifiable to 661, except 661.3

5th **763.8 Other specified complications of labor and delivery affecting fetus or newborn**

763.81 Abnormality in fetal heart rate or rhythm before the onset of labor N

763.82 Abnormality in fetal heart rate or rhythm during labor N

763.83 Abnormality in fetal heart rate or rhythm, unspecified as to time of onset N

763.84 Meconium passage during delivery N

Excludes *meconium aspiration (770.11, 770.12)*
meconium staining (779.84)

763.89 Other specified complications of labor and delivery affecting fetus or newborn N
Fetus or newborn affected by:
abnormality of maternal soft tissues
destructive operation on live fetus to facilitate delivery
induction of labor (medical)
other conditions classifiable to 650-669
other procedures used in labor and delivery

763.9 Unspecified complication of labor and delivery affecting fetus or newborn N

761.4 – 763.9

OTHER CONDITIONS ORIGINATING IN THE PERINATAL PERIOD (764-779)

The following fifth-digit subclassification is for use with category 764 and codes 765.0 and 765.1 to denote birthweight:

0 unspecified [weight]
1 less than 500 grams
2 500-749 grams
3 750-999 grams
4 1,000-1,249 grams
5 1,250-1,499 grams
6 1,500-1,749 grams
7 1,750-1,999 grams
8 2,000-2,499 grams
9 2,500 grams and over

ICD-9-CM Official Guidelines (Chapter 15):

*i. **Prematurity and Fetal Growth Retardation***

Providers utilize different criteria in determining prematurity. A code for prematurity should not be assigned unless it is documented. The 5th digit assignment for codes from category 764 and subcategories 765.0 and 765.1 should be based on the recorded birth weight and estimated gestational age.

A code from subcategory 765.2, Weeks of gestation, should be assigned as an additional code with category 764 and codes from 765.0 and 765.1 to specify weeks of gestation as documented by the provider in the record.

4th **764 Slow fetal growth and fetal malnutrition**
Requires fifth digit. See beginning of section 764-779 for codes and definitions.

5th **764.0 "Light-for-dates" without mention of fetal malnutrition** N
[0-9] Infants underweight for gestational age
"Small-for-dates"

5th **764.1 "Light-for-dates" with signs of fetal malnutrition** N
[0-9] Infants "light-for-dates" classifiable to 764.0, who in addition show signs of fetal malnutrition, such as dry peeling skin and loss of subcutaneous tissue

5th **764.2 Fetal malnutrition without mention of "light-for-dates"** N
[0-9] Infants, not underweight for gestational age, showing signs of fetal malnutrition, such as dry peeling skin and loss of subcutaneous tissue
Intrauterine malnutrition

5th **764.9 Fetal growth retardation, unspecified** N
[0-9] Intrauterine growth retardation

4th **765 Disorders relating to short gestation and low birthweight**
Requires fifth digit. See beginning of section 764-779 for codes and definitions.
Includes the listed conditions, without further specification, as causes of mortality, morbidity, or additional care, in fetus or newborn

5th **765.0 Extreme immaturity** N
[0-9]
Note: *Usually implies a birthweight of less than 1,000 grams.*
Use additional code for weeks of gestation (765.20-765.29)

5th **765.1 Other preterm infants** N
[0-9]
Note: *Usually implies birthweight of 1,000-2,499 grams.*
Prematurity NOS
Prematurity or small size, not classifiable to 765.0 or as "light-for-dates" in 764
Use additional code for weeks of gestation (765.20-765.29)

5th **765.2 Weeks of gestation**
765.20 Unspecified weeks of gestation N
765.21 Less than 24 completed weeks of gestation N
765.22 24 weeks of gestation N
765.23 25-26 weeks of gestation N
765.24 27-28 weeks of gestation N
765.25 29-30 weeks of gestation N
765.26 31-32 weeks of gestation N
765.27 33-34 weeks of gestation N
765.28 35-36 weeks of gestation N
765.29 37 or more weeks of gestation N

4th **766 Disorders relating to long gestation and high birthweight**
Includes the listed conditions, without further specification, as causes of mortality, morbidity, or additional care, in fetus or newborn

766.0 Exceptionally large baby N
Note: *Usually implies a birthweight of 4,500 grams or more.*

766.1 Other "heavy-for-dates" infants N
Other fetus or infant "heavy-" or "large-for-dates" regardless of period of gestation

5th **766.2 Late infant, not "heavy-for-dates"**
766.21 Post-term infant N
Infant with gestation period over 40 completed weeks to 42 completed weeks
766.22 Prolonged gestation of infant N
Infant with gestation period over 42 completed weeks
Postmaturity NOS

4th **767 Birth trauma**

767.0 Subdural and cerebral hemorrhage N
Subdural and cerebral hemorrhage, whether described as due to birth trauma or to intrapartum anoxia or hypoxia
Subdural hematoma (localized)
Tentorial tear
Use additional code to identify cause
Excludes *intraventricular hemorrhage (772.10-772.14)*
subarachnoid hemorrhage (772.2)

5th **767.1 Injuries to scalp**
767.11 Epicranial subaponeurotic hemorrhage (massive) N
Subgaleal hemorrhage
767.19 Other injuries to scalp N
Caput succedaneum
Cephalhematoma
Chignon (from vacuum extraction)

767.2 Fracture of clavicle N

767.3 Other injuries to skeleton N
Fracture of:
long bones
skull
Excludes *congenital dislocation of hip (754.30-754.35)*
fracture of spine, congenital (767.4)

767.4 Injury to spine and spinal cord N
Dislocation of spine or spinal cord due to birth trauma
Fracture of spine or spinal cord due to birth trauma
Laceration of spine or spinal cord due to birth trauma
Rupture of spine or spinal cord due to birth trauma

767.5 Facial nerve injury N
Facial palsy

767.6 Injury to brachial plexus N
Palsy or paralysis:
brachial
Erb (-Duchenne)
Klumpke (-Déjérine)

767.7 Other cranial and peripheral nerve injuries N
Phrenic nerve paralysis

767.8 **Other specified birth trauma** N
Eye damage
Hematoma of:
liver (subcapsular)
testes
vulva
Rupture of:
liver
spleen
Scalpel wound
Traumatic glaucoma
Excludes *hemorrhage classifiable to 772.0-772.9*

767.9 **Birth trauma, unspecified** N
Birth injury NOS

4th **768 Intrauterine hypoxia and birth asphyxia**
Use only when associated with newborn morbidity classifiable elsewhere
Excludes *acidemia NOS of newborn (775.81)*
acidosis NOS of newborn (775.81)
cerebral ischemia NOS (779.2)
hypoxia NOS of newborn (770.88)
mixed metabolic and respiratory acidosis of newborn (775.81)
respiratory arrest of newborn (770.87)

768.0 **Fetal death from asphyxia or anoxia before onset of labor or at unspecified time** N

768.1 **Fetal death from asphyxia or anoxia during labor** N

768.2 **Fetal distress before onset of labor, in liveborn infant** N
Fetal metabolic acidemia before onset of labor, in liveborn infant

768.3 **Fetal distress first noted during labor and delivery, in liveborn infant** N
Fetal metabolic acidemia first noted during labor and delivery, in liveborn infant

768.4 **Fetal distress, unspecified as to time of onset, in liveborn infant** N
Fetal metabolic acidemia unspecified as to time of onset, in liveborn infant

768.5 **Severe birth asphyxia** N
Birth asphyxia with neurologic involvement
Excludes *hypoxic-ischemic encephalopathy (HIE) (768.70-768.73)*

768.6 **Mild or moderate birth asphyxia** N
Other specified birth asphyxia (without mention of neurologic involvement)
Excludes *hypoxic-ischemic encephalopathy (HIE) (768.70-768.73)*

5th 768.7 **Hypoxic-ischemic encephalopathy (HIE)**

Rationale: *Hypoxic-ischemic encephalopathy (HIE) has well defined clinical definitions (mild, moderate, severe) based on clinical presentation and imaging findings. Since code 768.7, "Hypoxic-ischemic encephalopathy (HIE)" was added in 2006, the lack of these specific diagnostic terms has made it difficult to track the specific clinical conditions. The American Academy of Pediatrics requested that this code be expanded to the 5th digit level to allow adding new codes for the specific clinical definitions.*

● 768.70 **Hypoxic-ischemic encephalopathy, unspecified** N

● 768.71 **Mild hypoxic-ischemic encephalopathy** N

● 768.72 **Moderate hypoxic-ischemic encephalopathy** N

● 768.73 **Severe hypoxic-ischemic encephalopathy** N

768.9 **Unspecified birth asphyxia in liveborn infant** N
Anoxia NOS, in liveborn infant
Asphyxia NOS, in liveborn infant

769 Respiratory distress syndrome N
Cardiorespiratory distress syndrome of newborn
Hyaline membrane disease (pulmonary)
Idiopathic respiratory distress syndrome [IRDS or RDS] of newborn
Pulmonary hypoperfusion syndrome
Excludes *transient tachypnea of newborn (770.6)*

4th **770 Other respiratory conditions of fetus and newborn**

770.0 **Congenital pneumonia** N
Infective pneumonia acquired prenatally
Excludes *pneumonia from infection acquired after birth (480.0-486)*

5th 770.1 **Fetal and newborn aspiration**
Excludes *aspiration of postnatal stomach contents (770.85, 770.86)*
meconium passage during delivery (763.84)
meconium staining (779.84)

770.10 **Fetal and newborn aspiration, unspecified** N

770.11 **Meconium aspiration without respiratory symptoms** N
Meconium aspiration NOS

770.12 **Meconium aspiration with respiratory symptoms** N
Meconium aspiration pneumonia
Meconium aspiration pneumonitis
Meconium aspiration syndrome NOS
Use additional code to identify any secondary pulmonary hypertension (416.8), if applicable

770.13 **Aspiration of clear amniotic fluid without respiratory symptoms** N
Aspiration of clear amniotic fluid NOS

770.14 **Aspiration of clear amniotic fluid with respiratory symptoms** N
Aspiration of clear amniotic fluid with pneumonia
Aspiration of clear amniotic fluid with pneumonitis
Use additional code to identify any secondary pulmonary hypertension (416.8), if applicable

770.15 **Aspiration of blood without respiratory symptoms** N
Aspiration of blood NOS

770.16 **Aspiration of blood with respiratory symptoms** N
Aspiration of blood with pneumonia
Aspiration of blood with pneumonitis
Use additional code to identify any secondary pulmonary hypertension (416.8), if applicable

770.17 **Other fetal and newborn aspiration without respiratory symptoms** N

770.18 **Other fetal and newborn aspiration with respiratory symptoms** N
Other aspiration pneumonia
Other aspiration pneumonitis
Use additional code to identify any secondary pulmonary hypertension (416.8), if applicable

770.2 **Interstitial emphysema and related conditions** N
Pneumomediastinum originating in the perinatal period
Pneumopericardium originating in the perinatal period
Pneumothorax originating in the perinatal period

770.3 **Pulmonary hemorrhage** N
Hemorrhage:
alveolar (lung) originating in the perinatal period
intra-alveolar (lung) originating in the perinatal period
massive pulmonary originating in the perinatal period

770.4 **Primary atelectasis** N
Pulmonary immaturity NOS

770.5 Other and unspecified atelectasis N
Atelectasis:
NOS originating in the perinatal period
partial originating in the perinatal period
secondary originating in the perinatal period
Pulmonary collapse originating in the perinatal period

770.6 Transitory tachypnea of newborn N
Ideopathic tachypnea of newborn
Wet lung syndrome
Excludes *respiratory distress syndrome (769)*

770.7 Chronic respiratory disease arising in the perinatal period
Bronchopulmonary dysplasia
Interstitial pulmonary fibrosis of prematurity
Wilson-Mikity syndrome

5th 770.8 Other respiratory problems after birth
Excludes *mixed metabolic and respiratory acidosis of newborn (775.81)*

770.81 Primary apnea of newborn N
Apneic spells of newborn NOS
Essential apnea of newborn
Sleep apnea of newborn

770.82 Other apnea of newborn N
Obstructive apnea of newborn

770.83 Cyanotic attacks of newborn N

770.84 Respiratory failure of newborn N
Excludes *respiratory distress syndrome (769)*

770.85 Aspiration of postnatal stomach contents without respiratory symptoms N
Aspiration of postnatal stomach contents NOS

770.86 Aspiration of postnatal stomach contents with respiratory symptoms N
Aspiration of postnatal stomach contents with pneumonia
Aspiration of postnatal stomach contents with pneumonitis
Use additional code to identify any secondary pulmonary hypertension (416.8), if applicable

770.87 Respiratory arrest of newborn N

770.88 Hypoxemia of newborn N
Hypoxia NOS of newborn

770.89 Other respiratory problems after birth N

770.9 Unspecified respiratory condition of fetus and newborn N

4th 771 Infections specific to the perinatal period
Includes infections acquired before or during birth via the umbilicus or during the first 28 days after birth
Excludes *congenital pneumonia (770.0)*
congenital syphilis (090.0-090.9)
infant botulism (040.41)
maternal infectious disease as a cause of mortality or morbidity in fetus or newborn, but fetus or newborn not manifesting the disease (760.2)
ophthalmia neonatorum due to gonococcus (098.40)
other infections not specifically classified to this category

771.0 Congenital rubella N
Congenital rubella pneumonitis

771.1 Congenital cytomegalovirus infection N
Congenital cytomegalic inclusion disease

771.2 Other congenital infections N
Congenital:
herpes simplex
listeriosis
malaria
toxoplasmosis
tuberculosis

771.3 Tetanus neonatorum N
Tetanus omphalitis
Excludes *hypocalcemic tetany (775.4)*

771.4 Omphalitis of the newborn N
Infection:
navel cord
umbilical stump
Excludes *tetanus omphalitis (771.3)*

771.5 Neonatal infective mastitis N
Excludes *noninfective neonatal mastitis (778.7)*

771.6 Neonatal conjunctivitis and dacryocystitis N
Ophthalmia neonatorum NOS
Excludes *ophthalmia neonatorum due to gonococcus (098.40)*

771.7 Neonatal Candida infection N
Neonatal moniliasis
Thrush in newborn

5th 771.8 Other infections specific to the perinatal period
Use additional code to identify organism (041.00-041.9)

771.81 Septicemia [sepsis] of newborn N
Use additional codes to identify severe sepsis (995.92) and any associated acute organ dysfunction, if applicable

ICD-9-CM Official Guidelines (Chapter 16)

j. Newborn sepsis

Code 771.81, Septicemia [sepsis] of newborn, should be assigned with a secondary code from category 041, Bacterial infections in conditions classified elsewhere and of unspecified site, to identify the organism. A code from category 038, Septicemia, should not be used on a newborn record. Do not assign code 995.91, Sepsis, as code 771.81 describes the sepsis. If applicable, use additional codes to identify severe sepsis (995.92) and any associated acute organ dysfunction.

771.82 Urinary tract infection of newborn N

771.83 Bacteremia of newborn N

771.89 Other infections specific to the perinatal period N
Intra-amniotic infection of fetus NOS
Infection of newborn NOS

4th 772 Fetal and neonatal hemorrhage
Excludes *fetal hematologic conditions complicating pregnancy (678.0)*
hematological disorders of fetus and newborn (776.0-776.9)

▲772.0 Fetal blood loss affecting newborn N
Fetal blood loss from:
cut end of co-twin's cord
placenta
ruptured cord
vasa previa
Fetal exsanguination
Fetal hemorrhage into:
co-twin
mother's circulation

5th 772.1 Intraventricular hemorrhage
Intraventricular hemorrhage from any perinatal cause

772.10 Unspecified grade N

772.11 Grade I N
Bleeding into germinal matrix

772.12 Grade II N
Bleeding into ventricle

772.13 Grade III N
Bleeding with enlargement of ventricle

772.14 Grade IV N
Bleeding into cerebral cortex

772.2 Subarachnoid hemorrhage N
Subarachnoid hemorrhage from any perinatal cause
Excludes *subdural and cerebral hemorrhage (767.0)*

772.3 Umbilical hemorrhage after birth N
Slipped umbilical ligature

772.4 Gastrointestinal hemorrhage N
Excludes *swallowed maternal blood (777.3)*

772.5 Adrenal hemorrhage N

772.6 Cutaneous hemorrhage N
Bruising in fetus or newborn
Ecchymoses in fetus or newborn
Petechiae in fetus or newborn
Superficial hematoma in fetus or newborn

772.8 Other specified hemorrhage of fetus or newborn N
Excludes *hemorrhagic disease of newborn (776.0)*
pulmonary hemorrhage (770.3)

772.9 Unspecified hemorrhage of newborn N

4th **773 Hemolytic disease of fetus or newborn, due to isoimmunization**

773.0 Hemolytic disease due to Rh isoimmunization N
Anemia due to Rh:
- antibodies
- isoimmunization
- maternal/fetal incompatibility

Erythroblastosis (fetalis) due to Rh:
- antibodies
- isoimmunization
- maternal/fetal incompatibility

Hemolytic disease (fetus) (newborn) due to Rh:
- antibodies
- isoimmunization
- maternal/fetal incompatibility

Jaundice due to Rh:
- antibodies
- isoimmunization
- maternal/fetal incompatibility

Rh hemolytic disease
Rh isoimmunization

773.1 Hemolytic disease due to ABO isoimmunization N
ABO hemolytic disease
ABO isoimmunization
Anemia due to ABO:
- antibodies
- isoimmunization
- maternal/fetal incompatibility

Erythroblastosis (fetalis) due to ABO:
- antibodies
- isoimmunization
- maternal/fetal incompatibility

Hemolytic disease (fetus) (newborn) due to ABO:
- antibodies
- isoimmunization
- maternal/fetal incompatibility

Jaundice due to ABO:
- antibodies
- isoimmunization
- maternal/fetal incompatibility

773.2 Hemolytic disease due to other and unspecified isoimmunization N
Erythroblastosis (fetalis) (neonatorum) NOS
Hemolytic disease (fetus) (newborn) NOS
Jaundice or anemia due to other and unspecified blood-group incompatibility

773.3 Hydrops fetalis due to isoimmunization N
Use additional code, if desired, to identify type of isoimmunization (773.0-773.2)

773.4 Kernicterus due to isoimmunization N
Use additional code, if desired, to identify type of isoimmunization (773.0-773.2)

773.5 Late anemia due to isoimmunization N

4th **774 Other perinatal jaundice**

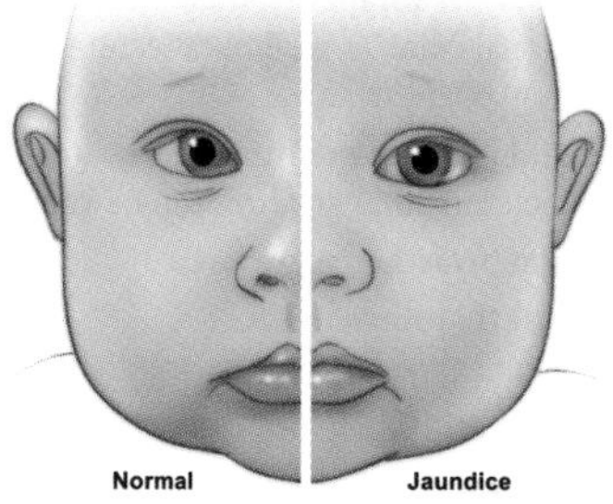

© 2008 Fairman Studios, LLC. All Rights Reserved.

774.0 ***Perinatal jaundice from hereditary hemolytic anemias*** N
Code first underlying disease (282.0-282.9)

774.1 Perinatal jaundice from other excessive hemolysis N
Fetal or neonatal jaundice from:
- bruising
- drugs or toxins transmitted from mother
- infection
- polycythemia
- swallowed maternal blood

Use additional code to identify cause
Excludes *jaundice due to isoimmunization (773.0-773.2)*

774.2 Neonatal jaundice associated with preterm delivery N
Hyperbilirubinemia of prematurity
Jaundice due to delayed conjugation associated with preterm delivery

5th **774.3 Neonatal jaundice due to delayed conjugation from other causes**

774.30 Neonatal jaundice due to delayed conjugation, cause unspecified N

774.31 ***Neonatal jaundice due to delayed conjugation in diseases classified elsewhere*** N
Code first underlying diseases, as:
- *congenital hypothyroidism (243)*
- *Crigler-Najjar syndrome (277.4)*
- *Gilbert's syndrome (277.4)*

774.39 Other N
Jaundice due to delayed conjugation from causes, such as:
- breast milk inhibitors
- delayed development of conjugating system

774.4 Perinatal jaundice due to hepatocellular damage N
Fetal or neonatal hepatitis
Giant cell hepatitis
Inspissated bile syndrome

774.5 ***Perinatal jaundice from other causes*** N
Code first underlying cause, as:
- *congenital obstruction of bile duct (751.61)*
- *galactosemia (271.1)*
- *mucoviscidosis (277.00-277.09)*

774.6 Unspecified fetal and neonatal jaundice N
Icterus neonatorum
Neonatal hyperbilirubinemia (transient)
Physiologic jaundice NOS in newborn
Excludes *that in preterm infants (774.2)*

774.7 Kernicterus not due to isoimmunization N
Bilirubin encephalopathy
Kernicterus of newborn NOS
Excludes *kernicterus due to isoimmunization (773.4)*

4th 775 **Endocrine and metabolic disturbances specific to the fetus and newborn**

Includes transitory endocrine and metabolic disturbances caused by the infant's response to maternal endocrine and metabolic factors, its removal from them, or its adjustment to extrauterine existence

775.0 **Syndrome of "infant of a diabetic mother"** N
Maternal diabetes mellitus affecting fetus or newborn (with hypoglycemia)

775.1 **Neonatal diabetes mellitus** N
Diabetes mellitus syndrome in newborn infant

775.2 **Neonatal myasthenia gravis** N

775.3 **Neonatal thyrotoxicosis** N
Neonatal hyperthyroidism (transient)

775.4 **Hypocalcemia and hypomagnesemia of newborn** N
Cow's milk hypocalcemia
Hypocalcemic tetany, neonatal
Neonatal hypoparathyroidism
Phosphate-loading hypocalcemia

775.5 **Other transitory neonatal electrolyte disturbances** N
Dehydration, neonatal

775.6 **Neonatal hypoglycemia** N
Excludes *infant of mother with diabetes mellitus (775.0)*

775.7 **Late metabolic acidosis of newborn** N

5th 775.8 **Other neonatal endocrine and metabolic disturbances**

775.81 **Other acidosis of newborn** N
Acidemia NOS of newborn
Acidosis of newborn NOS
Mixed metabolic and respiratory acidosis of newborn

775.89 **Other neonatal endocrine and metabolic disturbances** N
Amino-acid metabolic disorders described as transitory

775.9 **Unspecified endocrine and metabolic disturbances specific to the fetus and newborn** N

4th 776 **Hematological disorders of newborn**

Includes disorders specific to the newborn though possibly originating in utero

Excludes *fetal hematologic conditions (678.0)*

776.0 **Hemorrhagic disease of newborn** N
Hemorrhagic diathesis of newborn
Vitamin K deficiency of newborn
Excludes *fetal or neonatal hemorrhage (772.0-772.9)*

776.1 **Transient neonatal thrombocytopenia** N
Neonatal thrombocytopenia due to:
exchange transfusion
idiopathic maternal thrombocytopenia
isoimmunization

776.2 **Disseminated intravascular coagulation in newborn** N

776.3 **Other transient neonatal disorders of coagulation** N
Transient coagulation defect, newborn

776.4 **Polycythemia neonatorum** N
Plethora of newborn
Polycythemia due to:
donor twin transfusion
maternal-fetal transfusion

776.5 **Congenital anemia** N
Anemia following fetal blood loss
Excludes *anemia due to isoimmunization (773.0-.2, 773.5)*
hereditary hemolytic anemias (282.0-282.9)

776.6 **Anemia of prematurity** N

776.7 **Transient neonatal neutropenia** N
Isoimmune neutropenia
Maternal transfer neutropenia
Excludes *congenital neutropenia (nontransient) (288.01)*

776.8 **Other specified transient hematological disorders** N

▲776.9 **Unspecified hematological disorder specific to ~~fetus or~~ newborn** N

4th 777 **Perinatal disorders of digestive system**

Includes disorders specific to the fetus and newborn

Excludes *intestinal obstruction classifiable to 560.0-560.9*

777.1 **Meconium obstruction** N
Congenital fecaliths
Delayed passage of meconium
Meconium ileus NOS
Meconium plug syndrome
Excludes *meconium ileus in cystic fibrosis (277.01)*

777.2 **Intestinal obstruction due to inspissated milk** N

777.3 **Hematemesis and melena due to swallowed maternal blood** N
Swallowed blood syndrome in newborn
Excludes *that not due to swallowed maternal blood (772.4)*

777.4 **Transitory ileus of newborn** N
Excludes *Hirschsprung's disease (751.3)*

5th 777.5 **Necrotizing enterocolitis in newborn**
~~Pseudomembranous enterocolitis in newborn~~

777.50 **Necrotizing enterocolitis in newborn, unspecified** N
Necrotizing enterocolitis in newborn, NOS

777.51 **Stage I necrotizing enterocolitis in newborn** N
Necrotizing enterocolitis without pneumatosis, without perforation

777.52 **Stage II necrotizing enterocolitis in newborn** N
Necrotizing enterocolitis with pneumatosis, without perforation

777.53 **Stage III necrotizing enterocolitis in newborn** N
Necrotizing enterocolitis with perforation
Necrotizing enterocolitis with pneumatosis and perforation

777.6 **Perinatal intestinal perforation** N
Meconium peritonitis

777.8 **Other specified perinatal disorders of digestive system** N

777.9 **Unspecified perinatal disorder of digestive system** N

4th 778 **Conditions involving the integument and temperature regulation of fetus and newborn**

778.0 **Hydrops fetalis not due to isoimmunization** N
Idiopathic hydrops
Excludes *hydrops fetalis due to isoimmunization (773.3)*

778.1 **Sclerema neonatorum** N

778.2 **Cold injury syndrome of newborn** N

778.3 **Other hypothermia of newborn** N

778.4 **Other disturbances of temperature regulation of newborn** N
Dehydration fever in newborn
Environmentally induced pyrexia
Hyperthermia in newborn
Transitory fever of newborn

778.5 **Other and unspecified edema of newborn** N
Edema neonatorum

778.6 **Congenital hydrocele** N
Congenital hydrocele of tunica vaginalis

778.7 **Breast engorgement in newborn** N
Noninfective mastitis of newborn
Excludes *infective mastitis of newborn (771.5)*

778.8 **Other specified conditions involving the integument of fetus and newborn** N
Urticaria neonatorum
Excludes *impetigo neonatorum (684)*
pemphigus neonatorum (684)

778.9 **Unspecified condition involving the integument and temperature regulation of fetus and newborn** N

4th 779 **Other and ill-defined conditions originating in the perinatal period**

779.0 **Convulsions in newborn** N
Fits in newborn
Seizures in newborn

779.1 **Other and unspecified cerebral irritability in newborn** N

779.2 **Cerebral depression, coma, and other abnormal cerebral signs** N
Cerebral ischemia NOS of newborn
CNS dysfunction in newborn NOS
Excludes *cerebral ischemia due to birth trauma (767.0)*
intrauterine cerebral ischemia (768.2-768.9)
intraventricular hemorrhage (772.10-772.14)

▲ 5th 779.3 **Disorder of stomach function and feeding problems in newborn**
~~Regurgitation of food in newborn~~
~~Slow feeding in newborn~~
~~Vomiting in newborn~~

Rationale: *With the 2009 neonatal ICD-9-CM codes there was no ability to differentiate vomiting, bilious emesis or similar problems from other feeding issues in the newborn. The American Academy of Pediatrics requested ICD-9-CM modifications to enable better tracking of these conditions.*

● 779.31 **Feeding problems in newborn** N
Slow feeding in newborn
Excludes *feeding problem in child over 28 days old (783.3)*

● 779.32 **Bilious vomiting in newborn** N
Excludes *bilious vomiting in child over 28 days old (787.04)*

● 779.33 **Other vomiting in newborn** N
Regurgitation of food in newborn
Excludes *vomiting in child over 28 days old (536.2, 787.01-787.03, 787.04)*

● 779.34 **Failure to thrive in newborn** N
Excludes *failure to thrive in child over 28 days old (783.41)*

779.4 **Drug reactions and intoxications specific to newborn** N
Gray syndrome from chloramphenicol administration in newborn
Excludes *fetal alcohol syndrome (760.71)*
reactions and intoxications from maternal opiates and tranquilizers (763.5)

779.5 **Drug withdrawal syndrome in newborn** N
Drug withdrawal syndrome in infant of dependent mother
Excludes *fetal alcohol syndrome (760.71)*

779.6 **Termination of pregnancy (fetus)** N
Fetal death due to:
induced abortion
termination of pregnancy
Excludes *spontaneous abortion (fetus) (761.8)*

779.7 **Periventricular leukomalacia** N

5th 779.8 **Other specified conditions originating in the perinatal period**

779.81 **Neonatal bradycardia** N
Excludes *abnormality in fetal heart rate or rhythm complicating labor and delivery (763.81-763.83)*
bradycardia due to birth asphyxia (768.5-768.9)

779.82 **Neonatal tachycardia** N
Excludes *abnormality in fetal heart rate or rhythm complicating labor and delivery (763.81-763.83)*

779.83 **Delayed separation of umbilical cord** N

779.84 **Meconium staining** N
Excludes *meconium aspiration (770.11, 770.12)*
meconium passage during delivery (763.84)

779.85 **Cardiac arrest of newborn** N

779.89 **Other specified conditions originating in the perinatal period** N
Use additional code to specify condition

779.9 **Unspecified condition originating in the perinatal period** N
Congenital debility NOS
Stillbirth NEC

16. SYMPTOMS, SIGNS, AND ILL-DEFINED CONDITIONS (780-799)

This section includes symptoms, signs, abnormal results of laboratory or other investigative procedures, and ill-defined conditions regarding which no diagnosis classifiable elsewhere is recorded.

Signs and symptoms that point rather definitely to a given diagnosis are assigned to some category in the preceding part of the classification. In general, categories 780-796 include the more ill-defined conditions and symptoms that point with perhaps equal suspicion to two or more diseases or to two or more systems of the body, and without the necessary study of the case to make a final diagnosis. Practically all categories in this group could be designated as "not otherwise specified," or as "unknown etiology," or as "transient." The Alphabetic Index should be consulted to determine which symptoms and signs are to be allocated here and which to more specific sections of the classification; the residual subcategories numbered .9 are provided for other relevant symptoms which cannot be allocated elsewhere in the classification.

The conditions and signs or symptoms included in categories 780-796 consist of: (a) cases for which no more specific diagnosis can be made even after all facts bearing on the case have been investigated; (b) signs or symptoms existing at the time of initial encounter that proved to be transient and whose causes could not be determined; (c) provisional diagnoses in a patient who failed to return for further investigation or care; (d) cases referred elsewhere for investigation or treatment before the diagnosis was made; (e) cases in which a more precise diagnosis was not available for any other reason; (f) certain symptoms which represent important problems in medical care and which it might be desired to classify in addition to a known cause.

SYMPTOMS (780-789)

4th **780 General symptoms**

5th **780.0 Alteration of consciousness**

Excludes *alteration of consciousness due to:*
intracranial injuries (850.0-854.19)
skull fractures (800.00-801.99, 803.00-804.99)
coma:
diabetic (249.2-249.3, 250.2-250.3)
hepatic (572.2)
originating in the perinatal period (779.2)

780.01 Coma

780.02 Transient alteration of awareness 10

R40.4 Transient alteration of awareness

780.03 Persistent vegetative state

780.09 Other

R40.0 Somnolence

R40.1 Stupor

Drowsiness
Semicoma
Somnolence
Stupor
Unconsciousness

780.1 Hallucinations

Hallucinations:
NOS
auditory
gustatory
olfactory
tactile

Excludes *those associated with mental disorders, as functional psychoses (295.0-298.9)*
organic brain syndromes (290.0-294.9, 310.0-310.9)
visual hallucinations (368.16)

780.2 Syncope and collapse 55

R55 Syncope and collapse

Blackout
Fainting
(Near) (Pre) syncope
Vasovagal attack

Excludes *carotid sinus syncope (337.0)*
heat syncope (992.1)
neurocirculatory asthenia (306.2)
orthostatic hypotension (458.0)
shock NOS (785.50)

5th **780.3 Convulsions**

Excludes *convulsions:*
epileptic (345.10-345.91)
in newborn (779.0)

780.31 Febrile convulsions (simple), unspecified

Febrile seizures NOS

780.32 Complex febrile convulsions

Febrile seizure:
atypical
complex
complicated

Excludes *status epilepticus (345.3)*

780.39 Other convulsions

R56.9 Unspecified convulsions

Convulsive disorder NOS
Fits NOS
Recurrent convulsions NOS
Seizure NOS

Layman's: *Although 780.39 is often used to code for "unspecified" convusions, its designation as a "seizure NOS" technically necessitates the ruling out of seizures due to rapid onset fever (febrile) and epilepsy. Often, seizures coded appropriately to 780.39 are secondary to meningitis, encephalitis or some other inflammatory disease of the central nervous system.*

780.4 Dizziness and giddiness

R42 Dizziness and giddiness

Light-headedness
Vertigo NOS

Excludes *Ménière's disease and other specified vertiginous syndromes (386.0-386.9)*

5th **780.5 Sleep disturbances**

Excludes *circadian rhythm sleep disorders (327.30-327.39)*
organic hypersomnia (327.10-327.19)
organic insomnia (327.00-327.09)
organic sleep apnea (327.20-327.29)
organic sleep related movement disorders (327.51-327.59)
parasomnias (327.40-327.49)
that of nonorganic origin (307.40-307.49)

780.50 Sleep disturbance, unspecified

780.51 Insomnia with sleep apnea, unspecified

780.52 Insomnia, unspecified

780.53 Hypersomnia with sleep apnea, unspecified

G47.30 Sleep apnea, unspecified

780.54 Hypersomnia, unspecified

780.55 Disruptions of 24 hour sleep wake cycle, unspecified

780.56 Dysfunctions associated with sleep stages or arousal from sleep

780.57 Unspecified sleep apnea

780.58 Sleep related movement disorder, unspecified

Excludes *restless leg syndrome (333.94)*

780.59 Other

5th **780.6 Fever and other physiologic disturbances of temperature regulation**

Excludes *effects of reduced environmental temperature (991.0-991.9)*
effects of heat and light (992.0-992.9)
fever, chills or hypothermia associated with confirmed infection – code to infection

780.60 Fever, unspecified

R50.9 Fever, unspecified

Chills with fever
Fever NOS
Fever of unknown origin (FUO)
Hyperpyrexia NOS
Pyrexia NOS
Pyrexia of unknown origin

Excludes *chills without fever (780.64)*
neonatal fever (778.4)
pyrexia of unknown origin (during):
in newborn (778.4)
labor (659.2)
the puerperium (672)

780.61 *Fever presenting with conditions classified elsewhere*

Code first underlying condition when associated fever is present, such as with:
leukemia (conditions classifiable to 204-208)
neutropenia (288.00-288.09)
sickle-cell disease (282.60-282.69)

780.62 Postprocedural fever

Excludes *postvaccination fever (780.63)*

780.63 Postvaccination fever

Postimmunization fever

780.64 Chills (without fever)

Chills NOS

Excludes *chills with fever (780.60)*

780.65 Hypothermia not associated with low environmental temperature

Excludes *hypothermia:*
associated with low environmental temperature (991.6)
due to anesthesia (995.89)
of newborn (778.2, 778.3)

5th **780.7 Malaise and fatigue**

Excludes *debility, unspecified (799.3)*
fatigue (during):
combat (308.0-308.9)
heat (992.6)
pregnancy (646.8)
neurasthenia (300.5)
senile asthenia (797)

780.71 Chronic fatigue syndrome

R53.82 Chronic fatigue, unspecified

780.72 Functional quadriplegia

Complete immobility due to severe physical disability or frailty

Excludes *hysterical paralysis (300.11)*
immobility syndrome (728.3)
neurologic quadriplegia (344.00-344.09)
quadriplegia NOS (344.00)

780.79 Other malaise and fatigue

G 93.3 Postviral fatigue syndrome
R53.1 Weakness
R53.83 Other fatigue

Asthenia NOS
Lethargy
Postviral (asthenic) syndrome
Tiredness

780.8 Generalized hyperhidrosis

Diaphoresis
Excessive sweating
Secondary hyperhidrosis

Excludes *focal (localized) (primary) (secondary) hyperhidrosis (705.21-705.22)*
Frey's syndrome (705.22)

Sites commonly affected by hyperhidrosis

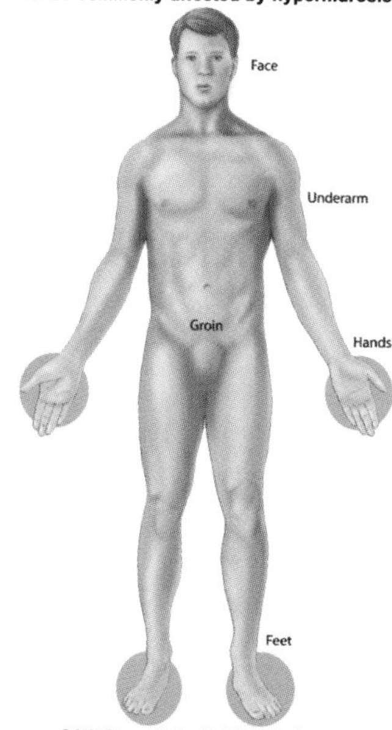

© 2008 Fairman Studios, LLC. All Rights Reserved.

5th **780.9 Other general symptoms**

Excludes *hypothermia:*
NOS (accidental) (991.6)
due to anesthesia (995.89)
of newborn (778.2-778.3)
memory disturbance as part of a pattern of mental disorder

780.91 Fussy infant (baby) P

780.92 Excessive crying of infant (baby) N

Excludes *excessive crying of child, adolescent or adult (780.95)*

780.93 Memory loss

Amnesia (retrograde)
Memory loss NOS

Excludes *memory loss due to:*
intracranial injuries (850.0-854.19)
skull fractures (800.00-801.99, 803.00-804.99)
mild memory disturbance due to organic brain damage (310.8)
transient global amnesia (437.7)

780.94 Early satiety

780.95 Excessive crying of child, adolescent, or adult

Excludes *excessive crying of infant (baby) (780.92)*

780.96 Generalized pain

Pain NOS

780.97 Altered mental status

Change in mental status

Excludes *altered level of consciousness (780.01-780.09)*
altered mental status due to known condition – code to condition
delirium NOS (780.09)

780.99 Other general symptoms

R68.89 Other general symptoms and signs

4th 781 Symptoms involving nervous and musculoskeletal systems

Excludes *depression NOS (311)*
disorders specifically relating to:
back (724.0-724.9)
hearing (388.0-389.9)
joint (718.0-719.9)
limb (729.0-729.9)
neck (723.0-723.9)
vision (368.0-369.9)
pain in limb (729.5)

781.0 Abnormal involuntary movements

Abnormal head movements
Fasciculation
Spasms NOS
Tremor NOS

Excludes *abnormal reflex (796.1)*
chorea NOS (333.5)
infantile spasms (345.60-345.61)
spastic paralysis (342.1, 343.0-344.9)
specified movement disorders classifiable to 333 (333.0-333.9)
that of nonorganic origin (307.2-307.3)

781.1 Disturbances of sensation of smell and taste

Anosmia
Parageusia
Parosmia

781.2 Abnormality of gait

R26.0 Ataxic gait
R26.1 Paralytic gait
R26.9 Unspecified abnormalities of gait and mobility

Gait:
ataxic
paralytic
spastic
staggering

Excludes *ataxia:*
NOS (781.3)
locomotor (progressive) (094.0)
difficulty in walking (719.7)

Layman's: *If the documentation does not definitively specify a gait abnormality in the absence of a disease or disorder, code 719.7 is more appropriate for use than 781.2.*

781.3 Lack of coordination I 0

R27.0 Ataxia, unspecified
R27.8 Other lack of coordination
R27.9 Unspecified lack of coordination

Ataxia NOS
Muscular incoordination

Excludes *ataxic gait (781.2)*
cerebellar ataxia (334.0-334.9)
difficulty in walking (719.7)
vertigo NOS (780.4)

781.4 Transient paralysis of limb I 0

Monoplegia, transient NOS

Excludes *paralysis (342.0-344.9)*

781.5 Clubbing of fingers

781.6 Meningismus

Dupré's syndrome
Meningism

781.7 Tetany

Carpopedal spasm

Excludes *tetanus neonatorum (771.3)*
tetany:
hysterical (300.11)
newborn (hypocalcemic) (775.4)
parathyroid (252.1)
psychogenic (306.0)

781.8 Neurologic neglect syndrome

Asomatognosia
Hemi-akinesia
Hemi-inattention
Hemispatial neglect
Left-sided neglect
Sensory extinction
Sensory neglect
Visuospatial neglect

5th 781.9 Other symptoms involving nervous and musculoskeletal systems

781.91 Loss of height

Excludes *osteoporosis (733.00-733.09)*

781.92 Abnormal posture

781.93 Ocular torticollis

781.94 Facial weakness I 0

Facial droop

Excludes *facial weakness due to late effect of cerebrovascular accident (438.83)*

781.99 Other symptoms involving nervous and musculoskeletal systems

4th 782 Symptoms involving skin and other integumentary tissue

Excludes *symptoms relating to breast (611.71-611.79)*

782.0 Disturbance of skin sensation I 0

R20.0 Anesthesia of skin
R20.1 Hypoesthesia of skin
R20.2 Paresthesia of skin
R20.3 Hyperesthesia
R20.8 Other disturbances of skin sensation
R20.9 Unspecified disturbances of skin sensation

Anesthesia of skin
Burning or prickling sensation
Hyperesthesia
Hypoesthesia
Numbness
Paresthesia
Tingling

782.1 Rash and other nonspecific skin eruption

R21 Rash and other nonspecific skin eruption

Exanthem

Excludes *vesicular eruption (709.8)*

782.2 Localized superficial swelling, mass, or lump

Subcutaneous nodules

Excludes *localized adiposity (278.1)*

782.3 Edema

R60.0 Localized edema

R60.1 Generalized edema

R60.9 Edema, unspecified

Anasarca
Dropsy
Localized edema NOS

Excludes *ascites (789.51-789.59)*
edema of:
newborn NOS (778.5)
pregnancy (642.0-642.9, 646.1)
fluid retention (276.6)
hydrops fetalis (773.3, 778.0)
hydrothorax (511.81-511.89)
nutritional edema (260, 262)

Normal Edema

© 2008 Fairman Studios, LLC. All Rights Reserved.

782.4 Jaundice, unspecified, not of newborn

Cholemia NOS
Icterus NOS

Excludes *jaundice in newborn (774.0-774.7)*
due to isoimmunization (773.0-773.2, 773.4)

782.5 Cyanosis

Excludes *newborn (770.83)*

5th **782.6 Pallor and flushing**

782.61 Pallor

782.62 Flushing

Excessive blushing

782.7 Spontaneous ecchymoses

Petechiae

Excludes *ecchymosis in fetus or newborn (772.6)*
purpura (287.0-287.9)

782.8 Changes in skin texture

Induration of skin
Thickening of skin

782.9 Other symptoms involving skin and integumentary tissues

4th **783 Symptoms concerning nutrition, metabolism, and development**

783.0 Anorexia

Loss of appetite

Excludes *anorexia nervosa (307.1)*
loss of appetite of nonorganic origin (307.59)

783.1 Abnormal weight gain

Excludes *excessive weight gain in pregnancy (646.1)*
obesity (278.00)
morbid (278.01)

5th **783.2 Abnormal loss of weight and underweight**

Use additional code to identify Body Mass Index (BMI), if known (V85.0-V85.54)

783.21 Loss of weight

R63.4 Abnormal weight loss

783.22 Underweight

Layman's: *Underweight is typically defined in America as an adult BMI of <18.5 and can be both an indicator of and precursor to other conditions.*

783.3 Feeding difficulties and mismanagement

Feeding problem (elderly) (infant)

Excludes *feeding disturbance or problems:*
in newborn (779.31-779.34)
of nonorganic origin (307.50-307.59)

5th **783.4 Lack of expected normal physiological development in childhood**

Excludes *delay in sexual development and puberty (259.0)*
gonadal dysgenesis (758.6)
pituitary dwarfism (253.3)
slow fetal growth and fetal malnutrition (764.00-764.99)
specific delays in mental development (315.0-315.9)

783.40 Lack of normal physiological development, unspecified

Inadequate development
Lack of development

783.41 Failure to thrive P

Failure to gain weight

Excludes *failure to thrive in newborn (779.34)*

783.42 Delayed milestones P

Late talker
Late walker

783.43 Short stature

Growth failure
Growth retardation
Lack of growth
Physical retardation

783.5 Polydipsia

Excessive thirst

783.6 Polyphagia

Excessive eating
Hyperalimentation NOS

Excludes *disorders of eating of nonorganic origin (307.50-307.59)*

783.7 Adult failure to thrive A

783.9 Other symptoms concerning nutrition, metabolism, and development

Hypometabolism

Excludes *abnormal basal metabolic rate (794.7)*
dehydration (276.51)
other disorders of fluid, electrolyte, and acid-base balance (276.0-276.9)

4th **784 Symptoms involving head and neck**

Excludes *encephalopathy NOS (348.30)*
specific symptoms involving neck classifiable to 723 (723.0-723.9)

784.0 Headache

G44.11 Vascular headache, not elsewhere classified, intractable

R51 Headache

Facial pain
Pain in head NOS

Excludes *atypical face pain (350.2)*
migraine (346.0-346.9)
tension headache (307.81)

784.1 Throat pain

Excludes *dysphagia (787.20 – 787.29)*
neck pain (723.1)
sore throat (462)
chronic (472.1)

784.2 Swelling, mass, or lump in head and neck
R22.0 Localized swelling, mass and lump, head
R22.1 Localized swelling, mass and lump, neck
Space-occupying lesion, intracranial NOS

784.3 Aphasia I10
Excludes *aphasia due to late effects of cerebrovascular disease (438.11)*
developmental aphasia (315.31)

▲ 5th **784.4 Voice ~~disturbance~~ and resonance disorders**

Rationale: The American Speech Language Hearing Association (ASHA) recommended changes to in ICD-9-CM so that diagnostic information may be coded that clarifies and delineates the disorders of phonation and resonance.

Prior to these changes, dysphonia, hoarseness, hypernasality, hyponasality, and change in voice all were included in code 784.49, "Other voice disturbance" (under subcategory 784.4, "Voice disturbance"). Voice disturbance is a disorder of phonation; whereas, hypernasality and hyponasality are disorders of resonance. Dysphonia and hyper/hyponasality are distinct manifestations and should not be grouped together as voice disturbances.

Dysphonia is a disorder of phonation; that is, voice production. Like aphonia, which is a complete loss of voice, dysphonia is a symptom of a laryngeal disorder affecting the structure and/or function of the larynx. Dysphonia is distinct and separate from impairments of resonance and nasal air flow.

Disorders of resonance and nasal air flow may be due to impairment(s) affecting the structure and/or function of the oral cavity, nasal airway, and/or the velopharyngeal port. Hypernasality is excessive nasality while hyponasality is diminished nasality.

▲ **784.40 Voice ~~disturbance~~ and resonance disorder, unspecified**

784.41 Aphonia
Loss of voice

● **784.42 Dysphonia**
Hoarseness

● **784.43 Hypernasality**

● **784.44 Hyponasality**

▲ **784.49 Other voice and resonance disorder**
Change in voice
~~Dysphonia~~
~~Hoarseness~~
~~Hypernasality~~
~~Hyponasality~~

5th **784.5 Other speech disturbance**
~~Dysarthria~~
~~Dysphasia~~
~~Slurred speech~~
Excludes *speech disorder due to late effect of cerebrovascular accident (438.10-438.19)*
stammering and stuttering (307.0)
that of nonorganic origin (307.0, 307.9)

● **784.51 Dysarthria**
Excludes *dysarthria due to late effect of cerebrovascular accident (438.13)*

Rationale: The American Speech-Language-Hearing Association (ASHA) recommended additions and revisions to the ICD-9-CM so that diagnostic information can be coded that clarifies and augments the nature and description of a variety of fluency disorders, including stuttering.

Stuttering is defined as a disruption in speech production characterized by primary behavioral symptoms that include sound and syllable repetitions, blocks (articulatory fixations that prevent the speaker from moving forward in his or her speech), and inappropriate prolongations of speech sounds. The speaker's inability to initiate or continue speaking may cause secondary reactions characterized by visible signs of awareness, tension and struggle.

Presently, there are three major recognized forms of stuttering: stuttering with onset in early childhood, psychogenic stuttering and fluency disorder subsequent to brain lesion or disease, most typically as a result of cerebral vascular events (sometimes called neurogenic stuttering).

The prevalence of stuttering in the general population, both in the United States and in other surveyed regions, is approximately 1% of the general population. There is a higher incidence, approximately 4%, with onset in early childhood that spontaneously resolves. It is not currently possible to predict which children will experience remission or become persistent stutterers. Persistent stuttering is a potentially handicapping and disabling condition with significant educational, social and vocational consequences

In contrast, psychogenic stuttering and neurogenic stuttering are much less frequently observed speech fluency disorders. Psychogenic stuttering, a form of conversion reaction, has been documented in relatively few published reports with virtually all reported cases showing onset in adulthood. The number of documented cases of stuttering secondary to central nervous system damage or disease is growing. Stuttering is most commonly observed subsequent to cerebral vascular events, but may be seen in neurodegenerative diseases, among a variety of causes.

Previously, the only code in ICD-9-CM for stuttering was in Chapter 5, Mental Disorders. ASHA recognized the appropriateness of this code for individuals showing post-childhood onset of stuttering symptoms secondary to emotional stress or trauma, but proposed adding codes for stuttering to categories 438 and 784. It is hoped that epidemiological, research, and treatment efforts could improve considerably with the increased specificity available in the 2010 ICD-9-CM to distinguish among types of fluency disturbances.

● **784.59 Other speech disturbance**
Dysphasia
Slurred speech
Speech disturbance NOS

5th **784.6 Other symbolic dysfunction**
Excludes *developmental learning delays (315.0-315.9)*

784.60 Symbolic dysfunction, unspecified

784.61 Alexia and dyslexia
Alexia (with agraphia)

784.69 Other
Acalculia
Agnosia
Agraphia NOS
Apraxia

784.7 Epistaxis
R04.0 Epistaxis
Hemorrhage from nose
Nosebleed

784.8 Hemorrhage from throat
Excludes *hemoptysis (786.3)*

5th **784.9 Other symptoms involving head and neck**

784.91 Postnasal drip

784.99 Other symptoms involving head and neck
Choking sensation
Feeling of foreign body in throat
Halitosis
Mouth breathing
Sneezing
Excludes *foreign body in throat (933.0)*

4th 785 Symptoms involving cardiovascular system

Excludes *heart failure NOS (428.9)*

785.0 Tachycardia, unspecified

R00.0 Tachycardia, unspecified

Rapid heart beat

Excludes *neonatal tachycardia (779.82)*
paroxysmal tachycardia (427.0-427.2)

785.1 Palpitations

R00.2 Palpitations

Awareness of heart beat

Excludes *specified dysrhythmias (427.0-427.9)*

785.2 Undiagnosed cardiac murmurs

R01.1 Cardiac murmur, unspecified

Heart murmur NOS

785.3 Other abnormal heart sounds

Cardiac dullness, increased or decreased
Friction fremitus, cardiac
Precordial friction

785.4 Gangrene

I96 Gangrene, not elsewhere classified

Gangrene:
NOS
spreading cutaneous
Gangrenous cellulitis
Phagedena

Code first any associated underlying condition

Excludes *gangrene of certain sites – see Alphabetic Index*
gangrene with atherosclerosis of the extremities (440.24)
gas gangrene (040.0)

5th 785.5 Shock without mention of trauma

785.50 Shock, unspecified

Failure of peripheral circulation

785.51 Cardiogenic shock

785.52 *Septic shock*

Shock:
endotoxic
gram-negative

Code first:
systemic inflammatory response syndrome due to infectious process with organ dysfunction (995.92)

785.59 Other

Shock:
hypovolemic

Excludes *shock (due to):*
anesthetic (995.4)
anaphylactic (995.0)
due to serum (999.4)
electric (994.8)
following abortion (639.5)
lightning (994.0)
obstetrical (669.1)
postoperative (998.0)
traumatic (958.4)

785.6 Enlargement of lymph nodes

R59.1 Generalized enlarged lymph nodes

Lymphadenopathy
"Swollen glands"

Excludes *lymphadenitis (chronic) (289.1-289.3)*
acute (683)

785.9 Other symptoms involving cardiovascular system

R09.89 Other specified symptoms and signs involving the circulatory and respiratory systems

Bruit (arterial)
Weak pulse

4th 786 Symptoms involving respiratory system and other chest symptoms

5th 786.0 Dyspnea and respiratory abnormalities

786.00 Respiratory abnormality, unspecified

R06.9 Unspecified abnormalities of breathing

786.01 Hyperventilation

Excludes *hyperventilation, psychogenic (306.1)*

786.02 Orthopnea

786.03 Apnea

Excludes *apnea of newborn (770.81, 770.82)*
sleep apnea (780.51, 780.53, 780.57)

786.04 Cheyne-Stokes respiration

786.05 Shortness of breath

R06.02 Shortness of breath

786.06 Tachypnea

Excludes *transitory tachypnea of newborn (770.6)*

Layman's: *Tachypnea is similar to hyperventilation (786.01) in that it is characterized by rapid breathing. However, tachypnea is characterized by rapid shallow breathing whereas hyperventilation manifests in rapid deep breathing. Tachypnea can also be necessitated for maintaining proper CO_2 levels in the body (e.g., after excercise), whereas hyperventilation is almost always exacerbating rather than palliative.*

786.07 Wheezing

Excludes *asthma (493.00-493.92)*

786.09 Other

R06.00 Dyspnea NOS
R06.09 Other forms of dyspnea
R06.89 Other abnormalities of breathing

Respiratory:
distress
insufficiency

Excludes *respiratory distress:*
following trauma and surgery (518.5)
newborn (770.89)
syndrome (newborn) (769)
adult (518.5)
respiratory failure (518.81, 518.83-518.84)
newborn (770.84)

786.1 Stridor

Excludes *congenital laryngeal stridor (748.3)*

786.2 Cough

R05 Cough

Excludes *cough:*
psychogenic (306.1)
smokers' (491.0)
with hemorrhage (786.3)

786.3 Hemoptysis

Cough with hemorrhage
Pulmonary hemorrhage NOS

Excludes *pulmonary hemorrhage of newborn (770.3)*

786.4 Abnormal sputum

Abnormal:
amount of sputum
color of sputum
odor of sputum
Excessive sputum

5th 786.5 Chest pain

786.50 Chest pain, unspecified 54

R07.9 Chest pain, unspecified

786.51 **Precordial pain** 5 4

R07.2 Precordial pain

Layman's: *Precordial pain differs from unstable angina (411.1) in that it 1) is often brought on by exertion rather than occurring at rest, 2) is sharp, stabbing and immediate, rather than "crushing" and increasing in severity, and 3) is often accompanied by a feeling of mental distress and anxiety.*

786.52 **Painful respiration** 5 4

R07.1 Chest pain on breathing

Pain:
anterior chest wall
pleuritic
Pleurodynia

Excludes *epidemic pleurodynia (074.1)*

786.59 **Other** 5 4

R07.89 Other chest pain

Discomfort in chest
Pressure in chest
Tightness in chest

Excludes *pain in breast (611.71)*

786.6 **Swelling, mass, or lump in chest**

R22.2 Localized swelling, mass and lump, trunk

Excludes *lump in breast (611.72)*

786.7 **Abnormal chest sounds**

Abnormal percussion, chest
Friction sounds, chest
Rales
Tympany, chest

Excludes *wheezing (786.07)*

786.8 **Hiccough**

Excludes *psychogenic hiccough (306.1)*

786.9 **Other symptoms involving respiratory system and chest**

Breath-holding spell

4th 787 **Symptoms involving digestive system**

Excludes *constipation (564.0-564.9)*
pylorospasm (537.81)
congenital (750.5)

5th 787.0 **Nausea and vomiting**

Emesis

Excludes *hematemesis NOS (578.0)*
vomiting:
bilious, following gastrointestinal surgery (564.3)
cyclical (536.2)
associated with migraine (346.2)
psychogenic (306.4)
excessive, in pregnancy (643.0-643.9)
fecal matter (569.87)
habit (536.2)
of newborn (779.32, 779.33)
persistent (536.2)
psychogenic NOS (307.54)

787.01 **Nausea with vomiting**

R11.0 Nausea with vomiting

787.02 **Nausea alone**

R11.1 Nausea alone

787.03 **Vomiting alone**

R11.3 Other vomiting without nausea

● 787.04 **Bilious emesis**

Bilious vomiting

Excludes *bilious emesis (vomiting) in newborn (779.32)*

Rationale: *Vomiting can be a very non-specific complaint with many different conditions. However, in the same way that persistent vomiting (536.2) can indicate a more significant problem, bilious emesis can also be indicative of a serious condition that may require an extensive evaluation.*

787.1 **Heartburn**

Pyrosis
Waterbrash

Excludes *dyspepsia or indigestion (536.8)*

5th 787.2 **Dysphagia**

Code first, if applicable, dysphagia due to late effect of cerebrovascular accident (438.82)

787.20 **Dysphagia, unspecified**

R13.10 Dysphagia, unspecified

Difficulty in swallowing NOS

787.21 **Dysphagia, oral phase**

787.22 **Dysphagia, oropharyngeal phase**

787.23 **Dysphagia, pharyngeal phase**

787.24 **Dysphagia, pharyngoesophageal phase**

787.29 **Other dysphagia**

Cervical dysphagia
Neurogenic dysphagia

787.3 **Flatulence, eructation, and gas pain**

R14.0 Abdominal distension (gaseous)
R14.1 Gas pain
R14.2 Eructation
R14.3 Flatulence

Abdominal distention (gaseous)
Bloating
Tympanites (abdominal) (intestinal)

Excludes *aerophagy (306.4)*

787.4 **Visible peristalsis**

Hyperperistalsis

787.5 **Abnormal bowel sounds**

Absent bowel sounds
Hyperactive bowel sounds

787.6 **Incontinence of feces**

Encopresis NOS
Incontinence of sphincter ani

Excludes *that of nonorganic origin (307.7)*

787.7 **Abnormal feces**

Bulky stools

Excludes *abnormal stool content (792.1)*
melena:
NOS (578.1)
newborn (772.4, 777.3)

5th 787.9 **Other symptoms involving digestive system**

Excludes *gastrointestinal hemorrhage (578.0-578.9)*
intestinal obstruction (560.0-560.9)
specific functional digestive disorders:
esophagus (530.0-530.9)
stomach and duodenum (536.0-536.9)
those not elsewhere classified (564.0-564.9)

787.91 **Diarrhea**

R19.7 Diarrhea, unspecified

Diarrhea NOS

787.99 **Other**

Change in bowel habits
Tenesmus (rectal)

4th **788 Symptoms involving urinary system**

Excludes *hematuria (599.70-599.72)*
nonspecific findings on examination of the urine (791.0-791.9)
small kidney of unknown cause (589.0-589.9)
uremia NOS (586)
urinary obstruction (599.60, 599.69)

788.0 Renal colic
Colic (recurrent) of:
kidney
ureter

788.1 Dysuria
R30.0 Dysuria
Painful urination
Strangury

5th **788.2 Retention of urine**
Code, if applicable, any causal condition first, such as:
hyperplasia of prostate (600.0-600.9 with fifth-digit 1)

788.20 Retention of urine, unspecified
R33.9 Retention of urine, unspecified

788.21 Incomplete bladder emptying
R39.14 Feeling of incomplete bladder emptying

788.29 Other specified retention of urine

5th **788.3 Urinary incontinence**
Code, if applicable, any causal condition first, such as:
congenital ureterocele (753.23)
genital prolapse (618.00-618.9)
hyperplasia of prostate (600.0-600.9 with fifth-digit 1)

Excludes *functional urinary incontinence (788.91)*
that of nonorganic origin (307.6)
urinary incontinence associated with cognitive impairment (788.91)

788.30 Urinary incontinence, unspecified 49, 50
R32 Unspecified urinary incontinence
Enuresis NOS

788.31 Urge incontinence 49, 50
N39.41 Urge incontinence

788.32 Stress incontinence, male ♂
Excludes *stress incontinence, female (625.6)*

788.33 Mixed incontinence (female) (male) 49, 50
Urge and stress

788.34 Incontinence without sensory awareness 49, 50

788.35 Post-void dribbling 49, 50

788.36 Nocturnal enuresis 49, 50

788.37 Continuous leakage 49, 50

788.38 Overflow incontinence 49, 50

788.39 Other urinary incontinence 49, 50

5th **788.4 Frequency of urination and polyuria**
Code, if applicable, any causal condition first, such as:
hyperplasia of prostate (600.0-600.9 with fifth-digit 1)

788.41 Urinary frequency
R35.0 Frequency of micturition
Frequency of micturition

788.42 Polyuria

788.43 Nocturia
R35.1 Nocturia

788.5 Oliguria and anuria
Deficient secretion of urine
Suppression of urinary secretion

Excludes *that complicating:*
abortion (634-638 with .3, 639.3)
ectopic or molar pregnancy (639.3)
pregnancy, childbirth, or the puerperium (642.0-642.9, 646.2)

5th **788.6 Other abnormality of urination**
Code, if applicable, any causal condition first, such as:
hyperplasia of prostate (600.0-600.9 with fifth-digit 1)

788.61 Splitting of urinary stream
Intermittent urinary stream

788.62 Slowing of urinary stream
Weak stream

788.63 Urgency of urination
Excludes *urge incontinence (788.31, 788.33)*

788.64 Urinary hesitancy

788.65 Straining on urination

788.69 Other

788.7 Urethral discharge
Penile discharge
Urethrorrhea

788.8 Extravasation of urine

5th **788.9 Other symptoms involving urinary system**

788.91 Functional urinary incontinence
Urinary incontinence due to cognitive impairment, or severe physical disability or immobility

Excludes *urinary incontinence due to physiologic condition (788.30-788.39)*

788.99 Other symptoms involving urinary system
Extrarenal uremia
Vesical:
pain
tenesmus

4th **789 Other symptoms involving abdomen and pelvis**

Excludes *symptoms referable to genital organs:*
female (625.0-625.9)
male (607.0-608.9)
psychogenic (302.70-302.79)

The following fifth-digit subclassification is to be used for codes 789.0, 789.3, 789.4, 789.6

0 **unspecified site**
1 **right upper quadrant**
2 **left upper quadrant**
3 **right lower quadrant**
4 **left lower quadrant**
5 **periumbilic**
6 **epigastric**
7 **generalized**
9 **other specified site**
Multiple sites

5th **789.0 Abdominal pain**
[0-7,9] ~~Colic:~~
~~NOS~~
~~infantile~~
Cramps, abdominal
~~**Excludes** *renal colic (788.0)*~~

789.1 Hepatomegaly
Enlargement of liver

789.2 Splenomegaly
Enlargement of spleen

5th **789.3 Abdominal or pelvic swelling, mass, or lump**
[0-7,9] Diffuse or generalized swelling or mass:
abdominal NOS
umbilical
Excludes *abdominal distention (gaseous) (787.3)*
ascites (789.51-789.59)

5th **789.4 Abdominal rigidity**
[0-7,9]

5th **789.5 Ascites**
Fluid in peritoneal cavity

789.51 *Malignant ascites*
Code first malignancy, such as:
malignant neoplasm of ovary (183.0)
secondary malignant neoplasm of retroperitoneum and peritoneum (197.6)

789.59 Other ascites

5th **789.6 Abdominal tenderness**
[0-7,9] Rebound tenderness

● **789.7 Colic**
Colic NOS
Infantile colic
Excludes *colic in adult and child over 12 months old (789.0)*
renal colic (788.0)

Rationale: *Colic generally affects newborns and infants between 3 and 12 weeks of age. While very concerning to most parents, it is a benign condition. The etiology is unclear. Previously, infantile colic was coded to 789.0x, "Abdominal pain," with a fifth-digit for site.*

The American Academy of Pediatrics (AAP) stated that this does not appear appropriate, especially since the underlying cause may not be related to abdominal pain. The AAP recommended removing the term colic as an inclusion term at code 789.0 and providing it with its own code to allow for better tracking of this condition.

789.9 Other symptoms involving abdomen and pelvis
Umbilical:
bleeding
discharge

NONSPECIFIC ABNORMAL FINDINGS (790-796)

4th **790 Nonspecific findings on examination of blood**
Excludes *abnormality of:*
platelets (287.0-287.9)
thrombocytes (287.0-287.9)
white blood cells (288.00-288.9)

5th **790.0 Abnormality of red blood cells**
Excludes *anemia:*
congenital (776.5)
newborn, due to isoimmunization (773.0-773.2, 773.5)
of premature infant (776.6)
other specified types (280.0-285.9)
hemoglobin disorders (282.5-282.7)
polycythemia:
familial (289.6)
neonatorum (776.4)
secondary (289.0)
vera (238.4)

790.01 Precipitous drop in hematocrit
Drop in hematocrit
Drop in hemoglobin

790.09 Other abnormality of red blood cells
Abnormal red cell morphology NOS
Abnormal red cell volume NOS
Anisocytosis
Poikilocytosis

790.1 Elevated sedimentation rate

5th **790.2 Abnormal glucose**
Excludes *diabetes mellitus (249.00-249.91, 250.00-250.93)*
dysmetabolic syndrome X (277.7)
gestational diabetes (648.8)
glycosuria (791.5)
hypoglycemia (251.2)
that complicating pregnancy, childbirth, or the puerperium (648.8)

790.21 Impaired fasting glucose
Elevated fasting glucose

790.22 Impaired glucose tolerance test (oral)
Elevated glucose tolerance test

790.29 Other abnormal glucose
Abnormal glucose NOS
Abnormal non-fasting glucose
Hyperglycemia NOS
Pre-diabetes NOS

790.3 Excessive blood level of alcohol
Elevated blood-alcohol

790.4 Nonspecific elevation of levels of transaminase or lactic acid dehydrogenase [LDH]
R74.0 Nonspecific elevation of levels of transaminase and lactic acid dehydrogenase [LDH]

790.5 Other nonspecific abnormal serum enzyme levels
Abnormal serum level of:
acid phosphatase
alkaline phosphatase
amylase
lipase
Excludes *deficiency of circulating enzymes (277.6)*

790.6 Other abnormal blood chemistry
R78.89 Finding of other specified substances, not normally found in blood
R79.0 Abnormal level of blood mineral
Abnormal blood levels of:
cobalt
copper
iron
lead
lithium
magnesium
mineral
zinc
Excludes *abnormality of electrolyte or acid-base balance (276.0-276.9)*
hypoglycemia NOS (251.2)
lead poisoning (984.0-984.9)
specific finding indicating abnormality of:
amino-acid transport and metabolism (270.0-270.9)
carbohydrate transport and metabolism (271.0-271.9)
lipid metabolism (272.0-272.9)
uremia NOS (586)

790.7 Bacteremia
R78.81 Bacteremia
Excludes *bacteremia of newborn (771.83)*
septicemia (038)
Use additional code to identify organism (041)

Layman's: *Bacteremia is a transient septic condition that is sometimes incorrectly used to refer to patients with septicemia or sepsis. Patients suffering solely from bacteremia typically recover with no medical intervention and are rarely admitted to an inpatient facility.*

790.8 Viremia, unspecified

5th 790.9 **Other nonspecific findings on examination of blood**

790.91 **Abnormal arterial blood gases**

790.92 **Abnormal coagulation profile**

R79.1 Abnormal coagulation profile

Abnormal or prolonged:
- bleeding time
- coagulation time
- partial thromboplastin time [PTT]
- prothrombin time [PT]

Excludes *coagulation (hemorrhagic) disorders (286.0-286.9)*

790.93 **Elevated prostate specific antigen [PSA]** A ♂

R97.2 Elevated prostate specific antigen [PSA]

790.94 **Euthyroid sick syndrome**

790.95 **Elevated C-reactive protein (CRP)**

790.99 **Other**

4th 791 **Nonspecific findings on examination of urine**

Excludes *hematuria NOS (599.70-599.72)*
specific findings indicating abnormality of:
amino-acid transport and metabolism (270.0-270.9)
carbohydrate transport and metabolism (271.0-271.9)

791.0 **Proteinuria**
- Albuminuria
- Bence-Jones proteinuria

Excludes *postural proteinuria (593.6)*
that arising during pregnancy or the puerperium (642.0-642.9, 646.2)

791.1 **Chyluria**

Excludes *filarial (125.0-125.9)*

791.2 **Hemoglobinuria**

791.3 **Myoglobinuria**

791.4 **Biliuria**

791.5 **Glycosuria**

Excludes *renal glycosuria (271.4)*

791.6 **Acetonuria**
- Ketonuria

791.7 **Other cells and casts in urine**

791.9 **Other nonspecific findings on examination of urine**
- Crystalluria
- Elevated urine levels of:
  - 17-ketosteroids
  - catecholamines
  - indolacetic acid
  - vanillylmandelic acid [VMA]
- Melanuria

4th 792 **Nonspecific abnormal findings in other body substances**

Excludes *that in chromosomal analysis (795.2)*

792.0 **Cerebrospinal fluid**

792.1 **Stool contents**
- Abnormal stool color
- Fat in stool
- Mucus in stool
- Occult blood
- Pus in stool

Excludes *blood in stool [melena] (578.1)*
newborn (772.4, 777.3)

792.2 **Semen** ♂
- Abnormal spermatozoa

Excludes *azoospermia (606.0)*
oligospermia (606.1)

792.3 **Amniotic fluid** M ♀

792.4 **Saliva**

Excludes *that in chromosomal analysis (795.2)*

792.5 **Cloudy (hemodialysis) (peritoneal) dialysis effluent**

792.9 **Other nonspecific abnormal findings in body substances**
- Peritoneal fluid
- Pleural fluid
- Synovial fluid
- Vaginal fluids

▲4th 793 **Nonspecific (abnormal) findings on radiological and other examination of body structure**

Includes nonspecific abnormal findings of:
- thermography
- ultrasound examination [echogram]
- x-ray examination

Excludes *abnormal results of function studies and radioisotope scans (794.0-794.9)*

Rationale: *Category 793, Nonspecific abnormal findings on radiological and other examination of body structure, was considered the best category for new code 793.82, but there were concerns that because dense breasts are not abnormal category 793 would not be correct. To remedy this potential conflict, it was decided that the title of category 793 be modified to have the term abnormal be nonessential allowing the inclusion of inconclusive, but not necessarily abnormal, test findings to be included in this category.*

▲793.0 **Skull and head**

Excludes *nonspecific abnormal echoencephalogram (794.01)*

▲793.1 **Lung field**

R91 Abnormal findings on diagnostic imaging of lung

- Coin lesion of lung
- Shadow, lung

▲793.2 **Other intrathoracic organ**
- Abnormal:
  - echocardiogram
  - heart shadow
  - ultrasound cardiogram
- Mediastinal shift

▲793.3 **Biliary tract**
- Nonvisualization of gallbladder

▲793.4 **Gastrointestinal tract**

▲793.5 **Genitourinary organs**
- Filling defect:
  - bladder
  - kidney
  - ureter

▲793.6 **Abdominal area, including retroperitoneum**

▲793.7 **Musculoskeletal system**

5th 793.8 **Breast**

793.80 **Abnormal mammogram, unspecified**

R92.8 Other abnormal findings on diagnostic imaging of breast

793.81 **Mammographic microcalcification**

Excludes *mammographic calcification (793.89)*
mammographic calculus (793.89)

● 793.82 **Inconclusive mammogram**
- Dense breasts NOS
- Inconclusive mammogram NEC
- Inconclusive mammography due to dense breasts
- Inconclusive mammography NEC

Rationale: *A routine mammogram may be deemed inconclusive due to what is termed dense breasts. This is not considered an abnormal condition, but one which requires further testing to confirm that no malignant condition exists that cannot be noted on mammogram. This new code was requested to explain this situation and to justify further testing.*

790.9 – 793.82

▲793.89 **Other (abnormal) findings on radiological examination of breast**
Mammographic calcification
Mammographic calculus

5th 793.9 **Other**
Excludes *abnormal finding by radioisotope localization of placenta (794.9)*

793.91 **Image test inconclusive due to excess body fat**
Use additional code to identify Body Mass Index (BMI), if known (V85.0-V85.54)

▲793.99 **Other nonspecific abnormal findings on radiological and other examinations of body structure**
Abnormal:
placental finding by x-ray or ultrasound method
radiological findings in skin and subcutaneous tissue

4th 794 **Nonspecific abnormal results of function studies**
Includes radioisotope:
scans
uptake studies
scintiphotography

5th 794.0 **Brain and central nervous system**

794.00 **Abnormal function study, unspecified**

794.01 **Abnormal echoencephalogram**

794.02 **Abnormal electroencephalogram [EEG]**

794.09 **Other**
Abnormal brain scan

5th 794.1 **Peripheral nervous system and special senses**

794.10 **Abnormal response to nerve stimulation, unspecified**

794.11 **Abnormal retinal function studies**
Abnormal electroretinogram [ERG]

794.12 **Abnormal electro-oculogram [EOG]**

794.13 **Abnormal visually evoked potential**

794.14 **Abnormal oculomotor studies**

794.15 **Abnormal auditory function studies**

794.16 **Abnormal vestibular function studies**

794.17 **Abnormal electromyogram [EMG]**
Excludes *that of eye (794.14)*

794.19 **Other**

794.2 **Pulmonary**
Abnormal lung scan
Reduced:
ventilatory capacity
vital capacity

5th 794.3 **Cardiovascular**

794.30 **Abnormal function study, unspecified**
R94.30 Abnormal result of cardiovascular function study, unspecified

794.31 **Abnormal electrocardiogram [ECG] [EKG]**
R94.31 Abnormal electrocardiogram [ECG] [EKG]
Excludes *long QT syndrome (426.82)*

794.39 **Other**
Abnormal:
ballistocardiogram
phonocardiogram
vectorcardiogram

794.4 **Kidney**
Abnormal renal function test

794.5 **Thyroid**
Abnormal thyroid:
scan
uptake

794.6 **Other endocrine function study**

794.7 **Basal metabolism**
Abnormal basal metabolic rate [BMR]

794.8 **Liver**
R94.5 Abnormal results of liver function studies
Abnormal liver scan

794.9 **Other**
Bladder
Pancreas
Placenta
Spleen

4th 795 **Other and nonspecific abnormal cytological, histological, immunological and DNA test findings**
Excludes *abnormal cytologic smear of anus and anal HPV (796.70-796.79)*
nonspecific abnormalities of red blood cells (790.01-790.09)

5th 795.0 **Abnormal Papanicolaou smear of cervix and cervical HPV**
Abnormal cervical cytology
Abnormal thin preparation smear of cervix
Excludes *abnormal cytologic smear of vagina and vaginal HPV (795.10-795.19)*
carcinoma in situ of cervix (233.1)
cervical intraepithelial neoplasia I (CIN I) (622.11)
cervical intraepithelial neoplasia II (CIN II) (622.12)
cervical intraepithelial neoplasia III (CIN III) (233.1)
dysplasia (histologically confirmed) of cervix (uteri) NOS (622.10)
mild cervical dysplasia (histologically confirmed) (622.11)
moderate cervical dysplasia (histologically confirmed) (622.12)
severe cervical dysplasia (histologically confirmed) (233.1)

795.00 **Abnormal glandular Papanicolaou smear of cervix** ♀
Atypical cervical glandular cells NOS
Atypical endocervical cells NOS
Atypical endometrial cells NOS

795.01 **Papanicolaou smear of cervix with atypical squamous cells of undetermined significance (ASC-US)** ♀

795.02 **Papanicolaou smear of cervix with atypical squamous cells cannot exclude high grade squamous intraepithelial lesion (ASC-H)** ♀

795.03 **Papanicolaou smear of cervix with low grade squamous intraepithelial lesion (LGSIL)** ♀

795.04 **Papanicolaou smear of cervix with high grade squamous intraepithelial lesion (HGSIL)** ♀

795.05 **Cervical high risk human papillomavirus (HPV) DNA test positive** ♀

795.06 **Papanicolaou smear of cervix with cytologic evidence of malignancy** ♀

795.07 **Satisfactory cervical smear but lacking transformation zone** ♀

795.08 **Unsatisfactory cervical cytology smear** ♀
Inadequate cervical cytology sample

795.09 **Other abnormal Papanicolaou smear of cervix and cervical HPV** ♀
Cervical low risk human papillomavirus (HPV) DNA test positive
Use additional code for associated human papillomavirus (079.4)
Excludes *encounter for Papanicolaou cervical smear to confirm findings of recent normal smear following initial abnormal smear (V72.32)*

5th 795.1 **Abnormal Papanicolaou smear of vagina and vaginal HPV**
Abnormal thin preparation smear of vagina NOS
Abnormal vaginal cytology NOS
Use additional code to identify acquired absence of uterus and cervix, if applicable (V88.01-V88.03)
Excludes *abnormal cytologic smear of cervix and cervical HPV (795.00-795.09)*
carcinoma in situ of vagina (233.31)
carcinoma in situ of vulva (233.32)
dysplasia (histologically confirmed) of vagina NOS (623.0, 233.31)
dysplasia (histologically confirmed) of vulva NOS (624.01, 624.02, 233.32)
mild vaginal dysplasia (histologically confirmed) (623.0)
mild vulvar dysplasia (histologically confirmed) (624.01)
moderate vaginal dysplasia (histologically confirmed) (623.0)
moderate vulvar dysplasia (histologically confirmed) (624.02)
severe vaginal dysplasia (histologically confirmed) (233.31)
severe vulvar dysplasia (histologically confirmed) (233.32)
vaginal intraepithelial neoplasia I (VAIN I) (623.0)
vaginal intraepithelial neoplasia II (VAIN II) (623.0)
vaginal intraepithelial neoplasia III (VAIN III) (233.31)
vulvar intraepithelial neoplasia I (VIN I) (624.01)
vulvar intraepithelial neoplasia II (VIN II) (624.02)
vulvar intraepithelial neoplasia III (VIN III) (233.32)

795.10 **Abnormal glandular Papanicolaou smear of vagina** ♀
Atypical vaginal glandular cells NOS

795.11 **Papanicolaou smear of vagina with atypical squamous cells of undetermined significance (ASC-US)** ♀

795.12 **Papanicolaou smear of vagina with atypical squamous cells cannot exclude high grade squamous intraepithelial lesion (ASC-H)** ♀

795.13 **Papanicolaou smear of vagina with low grade squamous intraepithelial lesion (LGSIL)** ♀

795.14 **Papanicolaou smear of vagina with high grade squamous intraepithelial lesion (HGSIL)** ♀

795.15 **Vaginal high risk human papillomavirus (HPV) DNA test positive** ♀
Excludes *condyloma acuminatum (078.11)*
genital warts (078.11)

795.16 **Papanicolaou smear of vagina with cytologic evidence of malignancy** ♀

795.18 **Unsatisfactory vaginal cytology smear** ♀
Inadequate vaginal cytology sample

795.19 **Other abnormal Papanicolaou smear of vagina and vaginal HPV** ♀
Vaginal low risk human papillomavirus (HPV) DNA test positive
Use additional code for associated human papillomavirus (079.4)

795.2 **Nonspecific abnormal findings on chromosomal analysis**
Abnormal karyotype

5th 795.3 **Nonspecific positive culture findings**
Positive culture findings in:
- nose
- sputum
- throat
- wound

Excludes *that of:*
blood (790.7-790.8)
urine (791.9)

795.31 **Nonspecific positive findings for anthrax**
Positive findings by nasal swab

795.39 **Other nonspecific positive culture findings**
Excludes *colonization status (V02.0-V02.9)*

795.4 **Other nonspecific abnormal histological findings**

795.5 **Nonspecific reaction to tuberculin skin test without active tuberculosis**
Abnormal result of Mantoux test
PPD positive
Tuberculin (skin test):
- positive
- reactor

795.6 **False positive serological test for syphilis**
False positive Wassermann reaction

5th 795.7 **Other nonspecific immunological findings**
Excludes *abnormal tumor markers (795.81-795.89)*
elevated prostate specific antigen [PSA] (790.93)
elevated tumor associated antigens (795.81-795.89)
isoimmunization, in pregnancy (656.1-656.2)
affecting fetus or newborn (773.0-773.2)

795.71 **Nonspecific serologic evidence of human immunodeficiency virus [HIV]**
Inconclusive human immunodeficiency virus [HIV] test (adult) (infant)
Note: *This code is ONLY to be used when a test finding is reported as nonspecific. Asymptomatic positive findings are coded to V08. If any HIV infection symptom or condition is present, see code 042. Negative findings are not coded.*
Excludes *acquired immunodeficiency syndrome [AIDS] (042)*
asymptomatic human immunodeficiency virus, [HIV] infection status (V08)
HIV infection, symptomatic (042)
human immunodeficiency virus [HIV] disease (042)
positive (status) NOS (V08)

795.79 **Other and unspecified nonspecific immunological findings**
Raised antibody titer
Raised level of immunoglobulins

5th 795.8 **Abnormal tumor markers**
Elevated tumor associated antigens [TAA]
Elevated tumor specific antigens [TSA]
Excludes *elevated prostate specific antigen [PSA] (790.93)*

795.81 **Elevated carcinoembryonic antigen [CEA]**

795.82 **Elevated cancer antigen 125 [CA 125]**

795.89 **Other abnormal tumor markers**

795.09 – 795.89

4th **796 Other nonspecific abnormal findings**

796.0 Nonspecific abnormal toxicological findings
Abnormal levels of heavy metals or drugs in blood, urine, or other tissue
Excludes *excessive blood level of alcohol (790.3)*

796.1 Abnormal reflex

796.2 Elevated blood pressure reading without diagnosis of hypertension
R03.0 Elevated blood-pressure reading, without diagnosis of hypertension
Note: *This category is to be used to record an episode of elevated blood pressure in a patient in whom no formal diagnosis of hypertension has been made, or as an incidental finding.*
Layman's: *796.2 is the appropriate code to submit for "white coat hypertension."*

796.3 Nonspecific low blood pressure reading

796.4 Other abnormal clinical findings
R68.89 Other general symptoms and signs

796.5 Abnormal finding on antenatal screening M ♀

796.6 Abnormal findings on neonatal screening N
Excludes *nonspecific serologic evidence of human immunodeficiency virus [HIV] (795.71)*

5th **796.7 Abnormal cytologic smear of anus and anal HPV**
Excludes *abnormal cytologic smear of cervix and cervical HPV (795.00-795.09)*
abnormal cytologic smear of vagina and vaginal HPV (795.10-795.19)
anal intraepithelial neoplasia I (AIN I) (569.44)
anal intraepithelial neoplasia II (AIN II) (569.44)
anal intraepithelial neoplasia III (AIN III) (230.5, 230.6)
carcinoma in situ of anus (230.5, 230.6)
dysplasia (histologically confirmed) of anus NOS (569.44)
mild anal dysplasia (histologically confirmed) (569.44)
moderate anal dysplasia (histologically confirmed) (569.44)
severe anal dysplasia (histologically confirmed) (230.5, 230.6 ~~569.44~~)

796.70 Abnormal glandular Papanicolaou smear of anus ♀
Atypical anal glandular cells NOS

796.71 Papanicolaou smear of anus with atypical squamous cells of undetermined significance (ASC-US) ♀

796.72 Papanicolaou smear of anus with atypical squamous cells cannot exclude high grade squamous intraepithelial lesion (ASC-H) ♀

796.73 Papanicolaou smear of anus with low grade squamous intraepithelial lesion (LGSIL) ♀

796.74 Papanicolaou smear of anus with high grade squamous intraepithelial lesion (HGSIL) ♀

796.75 Anal high risk human papillomavirus (HPV) DNA test positive ♀

796.76 Papanicolaou smear of anus with cytologic evidence of malignancy ♀

796.77 Satisfactory anal smear but lacking transformation zone ♀

796.78 Unsatisfactory anal cytology smear ♀
Inadequate anal cytology sample

796.79 Other abnormal Papanicolaou smear of anus and anal HPV ♀
Anal low risk human papillomavirus (HPV) DNA test positive
Use additional code for associated human papillomavirus (079.4)

796.9 Other

ILL-DEFINED AND UNKNOWN CAUSES OF MORBIDITY AND MORTALITY (797-799)

797 Senility without mention of psychosis
Frailty
Old age
Senescence
Senile asthenia
Senile:
debility
exhaustion
Excludes *senile psychoses (290.0-290.9)*

4th **798 Sudden death, cause unknown**

798.0 Sudden infant death syndrome P
Cot death
Crib death
Sudden death of nonspecific cause in infancy

798.1 Instantaneous death

798.2 Death occurring in less than 24 hours from onset of symptoms, not otherwise explained
Death known not to be violent or instantaneous, for which no cause could be discovered
Died without sign of disease

798.9 Unattended death
Death in circumstances where the body of the deceased was found and no cause could be discovered
Found dead

4th **799 Other ill-defined and unknown causes of morbidity and mortality**

5th **799.0 Asphyxia and hypoxemia**
Excludes *asphyxia and hypoxemia (due to):*
carbon monoxide (986)
hypercapnia (786.09)
inhalation of food or foreign body (932-934.9)
newborn (768.0-768.9)
traumatic (994.7)
Layman's: *Asphyxia is the cutting off of oxygen to the lungs by external sources, whereas hypoxemia (also called hypoxia or anoxia) is the same condition due to internal causes.*

799.01 Asphyxia
R09.01 Asphyxia

799.02 Hypoxemia

799.1 Respiratory arrest
Cardiorespiratory failure
Excludes *cardiac arrest (427.5)*
failure of peripheral circulation (785.50)
respiratory distress:
NOS (786.09)
acute (518.82)
following trauma or surgery (518.5)
newborn (770.89)
syndrome (newborn) (769)
adult (following trauma or surgery) (518.5)
other (518.82)
respiratory failure (518.81, 518.83-518.84)
newborn (770.84)
respiratory insufficiency (786.09)
acute (518.82)

▲ 5th 799.2 ~~Nervousness~~ Signs and symptoms involving emotional state

~~"Nerves"~~

Excludes *anxiety (293.84, 300.00-300.09)*
depression (311)

Rationale: *Codes in the 799.2x series are to be used to describe other symptoms associated with conditions classified elsewhere. This change adds new specificity to emotional/behavioral symptoms due to conditions classified elsewhere. These codes are not specific to traumatic brain injury and may be used to associate emotional/behavioral symptoms due to other conditions. These codes should be utilized when specific syndromes, disorders, or conditions were excluded, or while awaiting evaluations of their diagnostic significance by qualified professionals. When such symptoms are noted to be part of a a specific disorder or syndrome (such as a mental disorder or syndrome) the appropriate code for the disorder or syndrome would be assigned rather than the symptom code.*

● **799.21 Nervousness**
Nervous

● **799.22 Irritability**
Irritable

● **799.23 Impulsiveness**
Impulsive
Excludes *impulsive neurosis (300.3)*

● **799.24 Emotional lability**

● **799.25 Demoralization and apathy**
Apathetic

● **799.29 Other signs and symptoms involving emotional state**

799.3 Debility, unspecified

R53.81 Other malaise

Excludes *asthenia (780.79)*
nervous debility (300.5)
neurasthenia (300.5)
senile asthenia (797)

Layman's: *Debility is defined as weakness or feebleness, but is mainly associated with a declining state of overall health. As such, it is a common diagnosis for hospice patients, usually with other comorbidities.*

799.4 Cachexia
Wasting disease
Code first underlying condition, if known

5th **799.8 Other ill-defined conditions**

799.81 Decreased libido A
Decreased sexual desire
Excludes *psychosexual dysfunction with inhibited sexual desire (302.71)*

● **799.82 Apparent life threatening event in infant** N
ALTE
Apparent life threatening event in newborn and infant
Use additional code(s) for associated signs and symptoms
Excludes *signs and symptoms associated with a confirmed diagnosis - code to confirmed diagnosis*

Rationale: *An Apparent Life Threatening Event (ALTE) in an infant has been defined by a National Institutes of Health (NIH) Consensus Development Conference as, "An episode that is frightening to the observer and that is characterized by some combination of apnea (central or occasionally obstructive), color change (usually cyanotic or pallid but occasionally erythematous or plethoric), marked change in muscle tone (usually marked limpness), choking, or gagging. In some cases, the observer fears that the infant has died." Some previously used terms include "aborted crib death" and "near-miss SIDS," but according to the NIH Consensus Development Conference, such terminology "should be abandoned because it implies a possibly misleadingly close association between this type of spell and SIDS."*

The term ALTE describes a clinical syndrome. A variety of identifiable diseases or conditions can cause such episodes (e.g., gastroesophageal reflux, respiratory disease or seizures), but in approximately one-half of the cases, despite extensive workup, no cause can be identified. These episodes can occur during sleep, wakefulness, or feeding and are in infants who were generally born at greater than 37 weeks gestational age.

In one study of ALTE (by Davies and Gupta), cyanosis and apnea were the predominant presenting symptoms (71% and 70% respectively) while significant numbers of patient also presented with difficulty breathing, pallor, stiffness, floppiness, choking, red face, limb jerking and vomiting. Over half of the episodes (58%) occurred while the child was awake.

Infants on home cardiorespiratory monitoring for ALTEs have been shown to have an increased risk of repeated significant events. The American Academy of Pediatrics (AAP) has found that infants who have experienced an ALTE are one of the few groups in which use of a home monitor is appropriate.

Because of current reporting methods, the true incidence of ALTE is unknown. Reported incidence ranges from 0.05 to 6 percent in reports published in the medical literature. Current coding guidelines and Coding Clinic advice has directed that the particular signs and symptoms be used when coding for an ALTE. Because of the wide variety of presentations of this condition, prior coding recommendations did not allow this significant condition to be well tracked.

The AAP expressed strong concern that without an adequate method of tracking this condition, there would never be a truly good idea of its incidence, and that the only way that this condition can be properly monitored is through a unique code.

799.89 Other ill-defined conditions

799.9 Other unknown and unspecified cause
Undiagnosed disease, not specified as to site or system involved
Unknown cause of morbidity or mortality

17. INJURY AND POISONING (800-999)

Use E code(s) to identify the cause and intent of the injury or poisoning (E800-E999)

Note:

1. *The principle of multiple coding of injuries should be followed wherever possible. Combination categories for multiple injuries are provided for use when there is insufficient detail as to the nature of the individual conditions, or for primary tabulation purposes when it is more convenient to record a single code; otherwise, the component injuries should be coded separately.*

   Where multiple sites of injury are specified in the titles, the word "with" indicates involvement of both sites, and the word "and" indicates involvement of either or both sites. The word "finger" Includes thumb.
2. *Categories for "late effect" of injuries are to be found at 905-909.*

ICD-9-CM Official Guidelines (Chapter 17):

a. Coding of Injuries

When coding injuries, assign separate codes for each injury unless a combination code is provided, in which case the combination code is assigned. Multiple injury codes are provided in ICD-9-CM, but should not be assigned unless information for a more specific code is not available. These codes are not to be used for normal, healing surgical wounds or to identify complications of surgical wounds.

The code for the most serious injury, as determined by the provider and the focus of treatment, is sequenced first.

1) Superficial injuries

Superficial injuries such as abrasions or contusions are not coded when associated with more severe injuries of the same site.

2) Primary injury with damage to nerves/blood vessels

When a primary injury results in minor damage to peripheral nerves or blood vessels, the primary injury is sequenced first with additional code(s) from categories 950-957, Injury to nerves and spinal cord, and/or 900-904, Injury to blood vessels. When the primary injury is to the blood vessels or nerves, that injury should be sequenced first.

FRACTURES (800-829)

Excludes *malunion (733.81)*
nonunion (733.82)
pathologic or spontaneous fracture (733.10-733.19)
stress fracture (733.93-733.95)

The terms "condyle," "coronoid process," "ramus," and "symphysis" indicate the portion of the bone fractured, not the name of the bone involved.

The descriptions "closed" and "open" used in the fourth-digit subdivisions include the following terms:

closed *(with or without delayed healing):*
comminuted
depressed
elevated
fissured
fracture NOS
greenstick
impacted
linear
simple
slipped epiphysis
spiral

open *(with or without delayed healing):*
compound
infected
missile
puncture
with foreign body

Note: *A fracture not indicated as closed or open should be classified as closed.*

ICD-9-CM Official Guidelines (Chapter 17):

b. Coding of Traumatic Fractures

The principles of multiple coding of injuries should be followed in coding fractures. Fractures of specified sites are coded individually by site in accordance with both the provisions within categories 800-829 and the level of detail furnished by medical record content. Combination categories for multiple fractures are provided for use when there is insufficient detail in the medical record (such as trauma cases transferred to another hospital), when the reporting form limits the number of codes that can be used in reporting pertinent clinical data, or when there is insufficient specificity at the fourth-digit or fifth-digit level. More specific guidelines are as follows:

1) Acute Fractures vs. Aftercare

Traumatic fractures are coded using the acute fracture codes (800-829) while the patient is receiving active treatment for the fracture. Examples of active treatment are: surgical treatment, emergency department encounter, and evaluation and treatment by a new physician.

Fractures are coded using the aftercare codes (subcategories V54.0, V54.1, V54.8, or V54.9) for encounters after the patient has completed active treatment of the fracture and is receiving routine care for the fracture during the healing or recovery phase. Examples of fracture aftercare are: cast change or removal, removal of external or internal fixation device, medication adjustment, and follow up visits following fracture treatment.

Care for complications of surgical treatment for fracture repairs during the healing or recovery phase should be coded with the appropriate complication codes.

Care of complications of fractures, such as malunion and nonunion, should be reported with the appropriate codes.

Pathologic fractures are not coded in the 800-829 range, but instead are assigned to subcategory 733.1. See Section I.C.13.a for additional information.

2) Multiple fractures of same limb

Multiple fractures of same limb classifiable to the same three-digit or four-digit category are coded to that category.

3) Multiple unilateral or bilateral fractures of same bone

Multiple unilateral or bilateral fractures of same bone(s) but classified to different fourth-digit subdivisions (bone part) within the same three-digit category are coded individually by site.

4) Multiple fracture categories 819 and 828

Multiple fracture categories 819 and 828 classify bilateral fractures of both upper limbs (819) and both lower limbs (828), but without any detail at the fourth-digit level other than open and closed type of fractures.

5) Multiple fractures sequencing

Multiple fractures are sequenced in accordance with the severity of the fracture. The provider should be asked to list the fracture diagnoses in the order of severity.

Injury and Poisoning

FRACTURE OF SKULL (800-804)

Includes traumatic brain injury due to fracture of skull

The following fifth-digit subclassification is for use with the appropriate codes in categories 800, 801, 803, and 804:

0 unspecified state of consciousness
1 with no loss of consciousness
2 with brief [less than one hour] loss of consciousness
3 with moderate [1-24 hours] loss of consciousness
4 with prolonged [more than 24 hours] loss of consciousness and return to pre-existing conscious level
5 with prolonged [more than 24 hours] loss of consciousness, without return to pre-existing conscious level
Use fifth-digit 5 to designate when a patient is unconscious and dies before regaining consciousness, regardless of the duration of the loss of consciousness
6 with loss of consciousness of unspecified duration
9 with concussion, unspecified

4th 800 **Fracture of vault of skull**
Requires fifth digit. See beginning of section 800-804 for codes and definitions.
Includes frontal bone
parietal bone

5th 800.0 **Closed without mention of intracranial injury**
[0-6,9]
5th 800.1 **Closed with cerebral laceration and contusion**
[0-6,9]
5th 800.2 **Closed with subarachnoid, subdural, and extradural hemorrhage**
[0-6,9]
5th 800.3 **Closed with other and unspecified intracranial hemorrhage**
[0-6,9]
5th 800.4 **Closed with intracranialinjury of other and unspecified nature**
[0-6,9]
5th 800.5 **Open without mention of intracranial injury**
[0-6,9]
5th 800.6 **Open with cerebral laceration and contusion**
[0-6,9]
5th 800.7 **Open with subarachnoid, subdural, and extradural hemorrhage**
[0-6,9]
5th 800.8 **Open with other and unspecified intracranial hemorrhage**
[0-6,9]
5th 800.9 **Open with intracranial injury of other and unspecified nature**
[0-6,9]

4th 801 **Fracture of base of skull**
Requires fifth digit. See beginning of section 800-804 for codes and definitions.
Includes fossa:
anterior
middle
posterior
occiput bone
orbital roof
sinus:
ethmoid
frontal
sphenoid bone
temporal bone

5th 801.0 **Closed without mention of intracranial injury**
[0-6,9]
5th 801.1 **Closed with cerebral laceration and contusion**
[0-6,9]
5th 801.2 **Closed with subarachnoid, subdural, and extradural hemorrhage**
[0-6,9]
5th 801.3 **Closed with other and unspecified intracranial hemorrhage**
[0-6,9]
5th 801.4 **Closed with intracranial injury of other and unspecified nature**
[0-6,9]
5th 801.5 **Open without mention of intracranial injury**
[0-6,9]
5th 801.6 **Open with cerebral laceration and contusion**
[0-6,9]
5th 801.7 **Open with subarachnoid, subdural, and extradural hemorrhage**
[0-6,9]
5th 801.8 **Open with other and unspecified intracranial hemorrhage**
[0-6,9]
5th 801.9 **Open with intracranial injury of other and unspecified nature**
[0-6,9]

4th 802 **Fracture of face bones**
802.0 **Nasal bones, closed**
802.1 **Nasal bones, open**
5th 802.2 **Mandible, closed**
Inferior maxilla
Lower jaw (bone)
802.20 **Unspecified site**
802.21 **Condylar process**
802.22 **Subcondylar**
802.23 **Coronoid process**
802.24 **Ramus, unspecified**
802.25 **Angle of jaw**
802.26 **Symphysis of body**
802.27 **Alveolar border of body**
802.28 **Body, other and unspecified**
802.29 **Multiple sites**
5th 802.3 **Mandible, open**
802.30 **Unspecified site**
802.31 **Condylar process**
802.32 **Subcondylar**
802.33 **Coronoid process**
802.34 **Ramus, unspecified**
802.35 **Angle of jaw**
802.36 **Symphysis of body**
802.37 **Alveolar border of body**
802.38 **Body, other and unspecified**
802.39 **Multiple sites**
802.4 **Malar and maxillary bones, closed**
Superior maxilla
Upper jaw (bone)
Zygoma
Zygomatic arch
802.5 **Malar and maxillary bones, open**
802.6 **Orbital floor (blow-out), closed**
802.7 **Orbital floor (blow-out), open**

800 – 802.7

802.8 Other facial bones, closed
Alveolus
Orbit:
NOS
part other than roof or floor
Palate
Excludes *orbital:*
floor (802.6)
roof (801.0-801.9)

802.9 Other facial bones, open

4th 803 **Other and unqualified skull fractures**
Requires fifth digit. See beginning of section 800-804 for codes and definitions.
Includes skull NOS
skull multiple NOS

5th 803.0 **Closed without mention of intracranial injury** [0-6,9]

5th 803.1 **Closed with cerebral laceration and contusion** [0-6,9]

5th 803.2 **Closed with subarachnoid, subdural, and extradural hemorrhage** [0-6,9]

5th 803.3 **Closed with other and unspecified intracranial hemorrhage** [0-6,9]

5th 803.4 **Closed with intracranial injury of other and unspecified nature** [0-6,9]

5th 803.5 **Open without mention of intracranial injury** [0-6,9]

5th 803.6 **Open with cerebral laceration and contusion** [0-6,9]

5th 803.7 **Open with subarachnoid, subdural, and extradural hemorrhage** [0-6,9]

5th 803.8 **Open with other and unspecified intracranial hemorrhage** [0-6,9]

5th 803.9 **Open with intracranial injury of other and unspecified nature** [0-6,9]

4th 804 **Multiple fractures involving skull or face with other bones**
Requires fifth digit. See beginning of section 800-804 for codes and definitions.

5th 804.0 **Closed without mention of intracranial injury** [0-6,9]

5th 804.1 **Closed with cerebral laceration and contusion** [0-6,9]

5th 804.2 **Closed with subarachnoid, subdural, and extradural hemorrhage** [0-6,9]

5th 804.3 **Closed with other and unspecified intracranial hemorrhage** [0-6,9]

5th 804.4 **Closed with intracranial injury of other and unspecified nature** [0-6,9]

5th 804.5 **Open without mention of intracranial injury** [0-6,9]

5th 804.6 **Open with cerebral laceration and contusion** [0-6,9]

5th 804.7 **Open with subarachnoid, subdural, and extradural hemorrhage** [0-6,9]

5th 804.8 **Open with other and unspecified intracranial hemorrhage** [0-6,9]

5th 804.9 **Open with intracranial injury of other and unspecified nature** [0-6,9]

FRACTURE OF NECK AND TRUNK (805-809)

4th 805 **Fracture of vertebral column without mention of spinal cord injury**
Includes neural arch
spine
spinous process
transverse process
vertebra

The following fifth-digit subclassification is for use with codes 805.0-805.1:
- 0 cervical vertebra, unspecified level
- 1 first cervical vertebra
- 2 second cervical vertebra
- 3 third cervical vertebra
- 4 fourth cervical vertebra
- 5 fifth cervical vertebra
- 6 sixth cervical vertebra
- 7 seventh cervical vertebra
- 8 multiple cervical vertebrae

5th 805.0 **Cervical, closed** 24, 40
[0-8] Atlas
Axis

5th 805.1 **Cervical, open** [0-8]

805.2 **Dorsal [thoracic], closed** 24, 40

805.3 **Dorsal [thoracic], open**

805.4 **Lumbar, closed** 24, 40

805.5 **Lumbar, open**

805.6 **Sacrum and coccyx, closed** 24, 40

805.7 **Sacrum and coccyx, open**

805.8 **Unspecified, closed** 24, 40

805.9 **Unspecified, open**

4th **806 Fracture of vertebral column with spinal cord injury**

Includes any condition classifiable to 805 with:
complete or incomplete transverse lesion (of cord)
hematomyelia
injury to:
cauda equina
nerve
paralysis
paraplegia
quadriplegia
spinal concussion

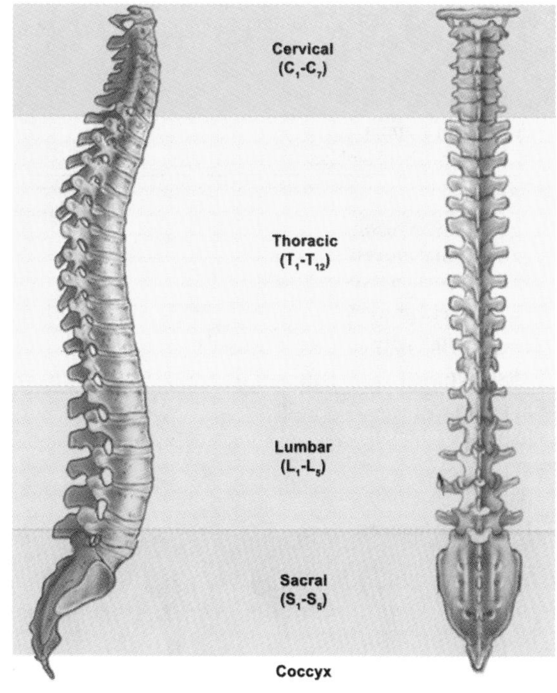

© 2008 Fairman Studios, LLC. All Rights Reserved.

5th **806.0 Cervical, closed**

806.00 C_1-C_4 level with unspecified spinal cord injury
Cervical region NOS with spinal cord injury NOS

806.01 C_1-C_4 level with complete lesion of cord

806.02 C_1-C_4 level with anterior cord syndrome

806.03 C_1-C_4 level with central cord syndrome

806.04 C_1-C_4 level with other specified spinal cord injury
C_1-C_4 level with:
incomplete spinal cord lesion NOS
posterior cord syndrome

806.05 C_5-C_7 level with unspecified spinal cord injury

806.06 C_5-C_7 level with complete lesion of cord

806.07 C_5-C_7 level with anterior cord syndrome

806.08 C_5-C_7 level with central cord syndrome

806.09 C_5-C_7 level with other specified spinal cord injury
C_5-C_7 level with:
incomplete spinal cord lesion NOS
posterior cord syndrome

5th **806.1 Cervical, open**

806.10 C_1-C_4 level with unspecified spinal cord injury

806.11 C_1-C_4 level with complete lesion of cord

806.12 C_1-C_4 level with anterior cord syndrome

806.13 C_1-C_4 level with central cord syndrome

806.14 C_1-C_4 level with other specified spinal cord injury
C_1-C_4 level with:
incomplete spinal cord lesion NOS
posterior cord syndrome

806.15 C_5-C_7 level with unspecified spinal cord injury

806.16 C_5-C_7 level with complete lesion of cord

806.17 C_5-C_7 level with anterior cord syndrome

806.18 C_5-C_7 level with central cord syndrome

806.19 C_5-C_7 level with other specified spinal cord injury
C_5-C_7 level with:
incomplete spinal cord lesion NOS
posterior cord syndrome

5th **806.2 Dorsal [thoracic], closed**

806.20 T_1-T_6 level with unspecified spinal cord injury
Thoracic region NOS with spinal cord injury NOS

806.21 T_1-T_6 level with complete lesion of cord

806.22 T_1-T_6 level with anterior cord syndrome

806.23 T_1-T_6 level with central cord syndrome

806.24 T_1-T_6 level with other specified spinal cord injury
T_1-T_6 level with:
incomplete spinal cord lesion NOS
posterior cord syndrome

806.25 T_7-T_{12} level with unspecified spinal cord injury

806.26 T_7-T_{12} level with complete lesion of cord

806.27 T_7-T_{12} level with anterior cord syndrome

806.28 T_7-T_{12} level with central cord syndrome

806.29 T_7-T_{12} level with other specified spinal cord injury
T_7-T_{12} level with:
incomplete spinal cord lesion NOS
posterior cord syndrome

5th **806.3 Dorsal [thoracic], open**

806.30 T_1-T_6 level with unspecified spinal cord injury

806.31 T_1-T_6 level with complete lesion of cord

806.32 T_1-T_6 level with anterior cord syndrome

806.33 T_1-T_6 level with central cord syndrome

806.34 T_1-T_6 level with other specified spinal cord injury
T_1-T_6 level with:
incomplete spinal cord lesion NOS
posterior cord syndrome

806.35 T_7-T_{12} level with unspecified spinal cord injury

806.36 T_7-T_{12} level with complete lesion of cord

806.37 T_7-T_{12} level with anterior cord syndrome

806.38 T_7-T_{12} level with central cord syndrome

806.39 T_7-T_{12} level with other specified spinal cord injury
T_7-T_{12} level with:
incomplete spinal cord lesion NOS
posterior cord syndrome

806.4 Lumbar, closed

806.5 Lumbar, open

5th **806.6 Sacrum and coccyx, closed**

806.60 With unspecified spinal cord injury

806.61 With complete cauda equina lesion

806.62 With other cauda equina injury

806.69 With other spinal cord injury

5th **806.7 Sacrum and coccyx, open**

806.70 With unspecified spinal cord injury

806.71 With complete cauda equina lesion

806.72 With other cauda equina injury

806.79 With other spinal cord injury

806.8 Unspecified, closed

806.9 Unspecified, open

4th 807 Fracture of rib(s), sternum, larynx, and trachea

The following fifth-digit subclassification is for use with codes 807.0-807.1:

- 0 **rib(s), unspecified**
- 1 **one rib**
- 2 **two ribs**
- 3 **three ribs**
- 4 **four ribs**
- 5 **five ribs**
- 6 **six ribs**
- 7 **seven ribs**
- 8 **eight or more ribs**
- 9 **multiple ribs, unspecified**

5th 807.0 Rib(s), closed
[0-9]

5th 807.1 Rib(s), open
[0-9]

807.2 Sternum, closed

807.3 Sternum, open

807.4 Flail chest

807.5 Larynx and trachea, closed
Hyoid bone
Thyroid cartilage
Trachea

807.6 Larynx and trachea, open

4th 808 Fracture of pelvis

808.0 Acetabulum, closed

808.1 Acetabulum, open

808.2 Pubis, closed

808.3 Pubis, open

5th 808.4 Other specified part, closed

808.41 Ilium

808.42 Ischium

808.43 Multiple pelvic fractures with disruption of pelvic circle

808.49 Other
Innominate bone
Pelvic rim

5th 808.5 Other specified part, open

808.51 Ilium

808.52 Ischium

808.53 Multiple pelvic fractures with disruption of pelvic circle

808.59 Other

808.8 Unspecified, closed

808.9 Unspecified, open

4th 809 Ill-defined fractures of bones of trunk

Includes bones of trunk with other bones except those of skull and face
multiple bones of trunk

Excludes *multiple fractures of:*
pelvic bones alone (808.0-808.9)
ribs alone (807.0-807.1, 807.4)
ribs or sternum with limb bones (819.0-819.1, 828.0-828.1)
skull or face with other bones (804.0-804.9)

809.0 Fracture of bones of trunk, closed

809.1 Fracture of bones of trunk, open

FRACTURE OF UPPER LIMB (810-819)

4th 810 Fracture of clavicle

Includes collar bone
interligamentous part of clavicle

The following fifth-digit subclassification is for use with category 810:

- 0 **unspecified part**
  Clavicle NOS
- 1 **sternal end of clavicle**
- 2 **shaft of clavicle**
- 3 **acromial end of clavicle**

5th 810.0 Closed
[0-3]

5th 810.1 Open
[0-3]

4th 811 Fracture of scapula

Includes shoulder blade

The following fifth-digit subclassification is for use with category 811:

- 0 **unspecified part**
- 1 **acromial process**
  Acromion (process)
- 2 **coracoid process**
- 3 **glenoid cavity and neck of scapula**
- 9 **other**

5th 811.0 Closed
[0-3,9]

5th 811.1 Open
[0-3,9]

4th 812 Fracture of humerus

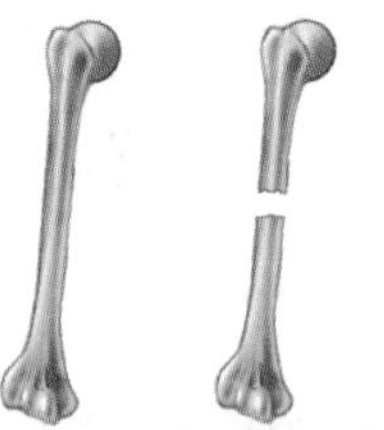
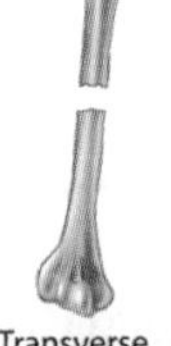
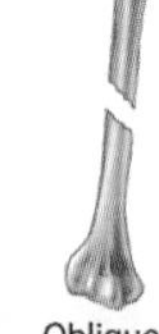
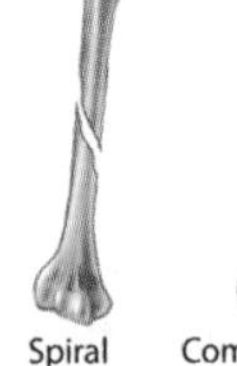

Normal Transverse Oblique Spiral Comminuted

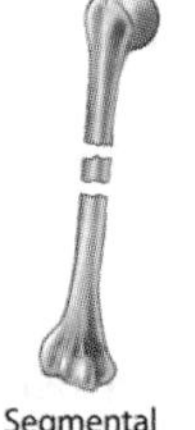
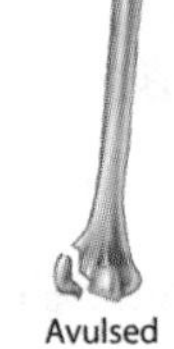
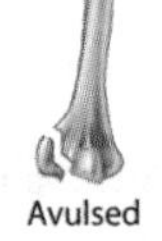
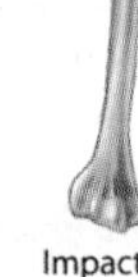
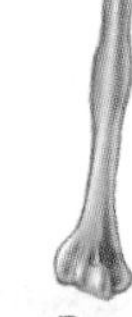
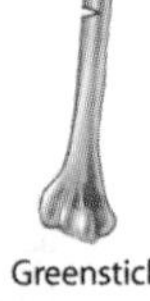

Segmental Avulsed Impacted Torus Greenstick

© 2008 Fairman Studios, LLC. All Rights Reserved.

5th 812.0 Upper end, closed

812.00 Upper end, unspecified part

S42.209A Unspecified fracture of upper end of unspecified humerus, initial encounter for closed fracture

S42.209G Unspecified fracture of upper end of unspecified humerus, subsequent encounter for fracture with delayed healing

Proximal end
Shoulder

812.01 Surgical neck
Neck of humerus NOS

812.02 Anatomical neck

812.03 Greater tuberosity

812.09 Other
Head
Upper epiphysis

5th 812.1 Upper end, open
812.10 Upper end, unspecified part
812.11 Surgical neck
812.12 Anatomical neck
812.13 Greater tuberosity
812.19 Other

5th 812.2 Shaft or unspecified part, closed
812.20 Unspecified part of humerus
Humerus NOS
Upper arm NOS
812.21 Shaft of humerus

5th 812.3 Shaft or unspecified part, open
812.30 Unspecified part of humerus
812.31 Shaft of humerus

5th 812.4 Lower end, closed
Distal end of humerus
Elbow
812.40 Lower end, unspecified part
812.41 Supracondylar fracture of humerus
812.42 Lateral condyle
External condyle
812.43 Medial condyle
Internal epicondyle
812.44 Condyle(s), unspecified
Articular process NOS
Lower epiphysis
812.49 Other
Multiple fractures of lower end
Trochlea

5th 812.5 Lower end, open
812.50 Lower end, unspecified part
812.51 Supracondylar fracture of humerus
812.52 Lateral condyle
812.53 Medial condyle
812.54 Condyle(s), unspecified
812.59 Other

4th 813 Fracture of radius and ulna

5th 813.0 Upper end, closed
Proximal end
813.00 Upper end of forearm, unspecified
813.01 Olecranon process of ulna
813.02 Coronoid process of ulna
813.03 Monteggia's fracture
813.04 Other and unspecified fractures of proximal end of ulna (alone)
Multiple fractures of ulna, upper end
813.05 Head of radius
813.06 Neck of radius
813.07 Other and unspecified fractures of proximal end of radius (alone)
Multiple fractures of radius, upper end
813.08 Radius with ulna, upper end [any part]

5th 813.1 Upper end, open
813.10 Upper end of forearm, unspecified
813.11 Olecranon process of ulna
813.12 Coronoid process of ulna
813.13 Monteggia's fracture
813.14 Other and unspecified fractures of proximal end of ulna (alone)
813.15 Head of radius
813.16 Neck of radius
813.17 Other and unspecified fractures of proximal end of radius (alone)
813.18 Radius with ulna, upper end [any part]

5th 813.2 Shaft, closed
813.20 Shaft, unspecified
813.21 Radius (alone)
813.22 Ulna (alone)
813.23 Radius with ulna

5th 813.3 Shaft, open
813.30 Shaft, unspecified
813.31 Radius (alone)
813.32 Ulna (alone)
813.33 Radius with ulna

5th 813.4 Lower end, closed
Distal end
813.40 Lower end of forearm, unspecified 24, 40
813.41 Colles' fracture 24, 40
S52.539A Colles' fracture of unspecified radius, initial encounter for closed fracture
Smith's fracture
813.42 Other fractures of distal end of radius (alone) 24, 40
S52.509A Unspecified fracture of the lower end of unspecified radius, initial encounter for closed fracture
Dupuytren's fracture, radius
Radius, lower end
813.43 Distal end of ulna (alone)
Ulna:
head
lower end
lower epiphysis
styloid process
813.44 Radius with ulna, lower end 24, 40
▲813.45 Torus fracture of radius (alone) 24, 40
Excludes *torus fracture of radius and ulna (813.47)*

Rationale: In 2002, a new code was added for "Torus fracture of radius," 813.45. Torus or buckle fractures generally occur from axial loading on a long bone of an extremity, such as falling on an outstretched arm. They are most common in children. While torus fractures are most common in the radius, they can also involve either the ulna alone, or both the radius and ulna. The American Academy of Pediatrics (AAP) requested that additional codes be created for torus fractures of these other sites.
The term buckle fracture had not been indexed, so it was indexed, referring to torus fracture. Also, as torus fractures can occur in the humerus, torus fractures of the humerus are now indexed to code 812.49, "Other fracture of lower end of the humerus, closed."

●813.46 Torus fracture of ulna (alone)
Excludes *torus fracture of radius and ulna (813.47)*
●813.47 Torus fracture of radius and ulna

5th 813.5 Lower end, open
813.50 Lower end of forearm, unspecified 24, 40
813.51 Colles' fracture 24, 40
813.52 Other fractures of distal end of radius (alone) 24, 40
813.53 Distal end of ulna (alone)
813.54 Radius with ulna, lower end 24, 40

812.09 – 813.54

5th 813.8 Unspecified part, closed
813.80 Forearm, unspecified
813.81 Radius (alone)
813.82 Ulna (alone)
813.83 Radius with ulna

5th 813.9 Unspecified part, open
813.90 Forearm, unspecified
813.91 Radius (alone)
813.92 Ulna (alone)
813.93 Radius with ulna

4th 814 Fracture of carpal bone(s)

The following fifth-digit subclassification is for use with category 814:
0 carpal bone, unspecified
Wrist NOS
1 navicular [scaphoid] of wrist
2 lunate [semilunar] bone of wrist
3 triquetral [cuneiform] bone of wrist
4 pisiform
5 trapezium bone [larger multangular]
6 trapezoid bone [smaller multangular]
7 capitate bone [os magnum]
8 hamate [unciform] bone
9 other

The Carpal Bones

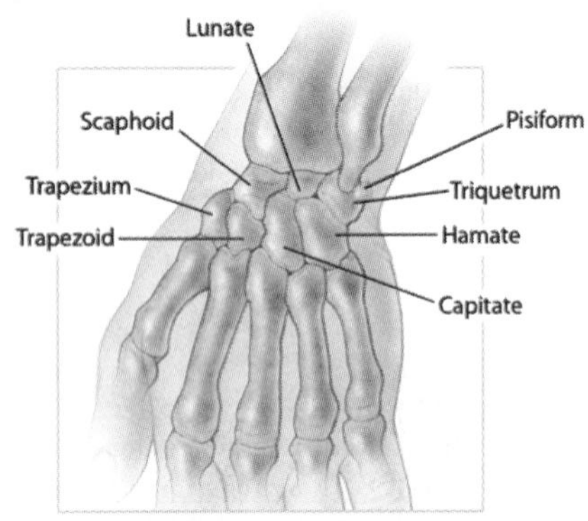

© 2008 Fairman Studios, LLC. All Rights Reserved.

5th 814.0 Closed
[0-9]

5th 814.1 Open
[0-9]

4th 815 Fracture of metacarpal bone(s)
Includes hand [except finger]
metacarpus

The following fifth-digit subclassification is for use with category 815:
0 metacarpal bone(s), site unspecified
1 base of thumb [first] metacarpal
Bennett's fracture
2 base of other metacarpal bone(s)
3 shaft of metacarpal bone(s)
4 neck of metacarpal bone(s)
9 multiple sites of metacarpus

5th 815.0 Closed
[0-4,9]

5th 815.1 Open
[0-4,9]

4th 816 Fracture of one or more phalanges of hand
Includes finger(s)
thumb

The following fifth-digit subclassification is for use with category 816:
0 phalanx or phalanges, unspecified
1 middle or proximal phalanx or phalanges
2 distal phalanx or phalanges
3 multiple sites

5th 816.0 Closed
[0-3]

5th 816.1 Open
[0-3]

4th 817 Multiple fractures of hand bones
Includes metacarpal bone(s) with phalanx or phalanges of same hand
817.0 Closed
817.1 Open

4th 818 Ill-defined fractures of upper limb
Includes arm NOS
multiple bones of same upper limb
Excludes *multiple fractures of:*
metacarpal bone(s) with phalanx or phalanges (817.0-817.1)
phalanges of hand alone (816.0-816.1)
radius with ulna (813.0-813.9)
818.0 Closed
818.1 Open

4th 819 Multiple fractures involving both upper limbs, and upper limb with rib(s) and sternum
Includes arm(s) with rib(s) or sternum
both arms [any bones]

ICD-9-CM Official Guidelines (Chapter 17):

b. Coding of Traumatic Fractures

4) Multiple fracture categories 819 and 828

Multiple fracture categories 819 and 828 classify bilateral fractures of both upper limbs (819) and both lower limbs (828), but without any detail at the fourth-digit level other than open and closed type of fractures.

819.0 Closed
819.1 Open

FRACTURE OF LOWER LIMB (820-829)

4th 820 Fracture of neck of femur

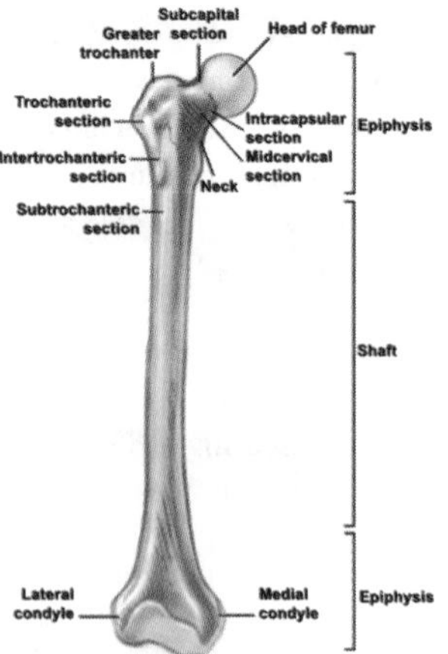

© 2008 Fairman Studios, LLC. All Rights Reserved.

5th 820.0 Transcervical fracture, closed
820.00 Intracapsular section, unspecified 24, 40
820.01 Epiphysis (separation) (upper) 24, 40
Transepiphyseal

820.02 **Midcervical section** 24, 40
Transcervical NOS

820.03 **Base of neck** 24, 40
Cervicotrochanteric section

820.09 **Other** 24, 40
Head of femur
Subcapital

5th 820.1 **Transcervical fracture, open**

820.10 **Intracapsular section, unspecified**

820.11 **Epiphysis (separation) (upper)**

820.12 **Midcervical section**

820.13 **Base of neck**

820.19 **Other**

5th 820.2 **Pertrochanteric fracture, closed**

820.20 **Trochanteric section, unspecified** 24, 40
Trochanter:
NOS
greater
lesser

820.21 **Intertrochanteric section** 24, 40
S72.143A Displaced intertrochanteric fracture of unspecified femur, initial encounter for closed fracture
S72.146A Nondisplaced intertrochanteric fracture of unspecified femur, initial encounter for closed fracture

820.22 **Subtrochanteric section** 24, 40

5th 820.3 **Pertrochanteric fracture, open**

820.30 **Trochanteric section, unspecified**

820.31 **Intertrochanteric section**

820.32 **Subtrochanteric section**

820.8 **Unspecified part of neck of femur, closed** 24, 40
S72.009A Fracture of unspecified part of neck of unspecified femur, initial encounter for closed fracture
Hip NOS
Neck of femur NOS

820.9 **Unspecified part of neck of femur, open**

4th 821 **Fracture of other and unspecified parts of femur**

5th 821.0 **Shaft or unspecified part, closed**

821.00 **Unspecified part of femur**
Thigh
Upper leg
Excludes *hip NOS (820.8)*

821.01 **Shaft**

5th 821.1 **Shaft or unspecified part, open**

821.10 **Unspecified part of femur**

821.11 **Shaft**

5th 821.2 **Lower end, closed**
Distal end

821.20 **Lower end, unspecified part**

821.21 **Condyle, femoral**

821.22 **Epiphysis, lower (separation)**

821.23 **Supracondylar fracture of femur**

821.29 **Other**
Multiple fractures of lower end

5th 821.3 **Lower end, open**

821.30 **Lower end, unspecified part**

821.31 **Condyle, femoral**

821.32 **Epiphysis, lower (separation)**

821.33 **Supracondylar fracture of femur**

821.39 **Other**

4th 822 **Fracture of patella**

822.0 **Closed**

822.1 **Open**

4th 823 **Fracture of tibia and fibula**
Excludes *Dupuytren's fracture (824.4-824.5)*
ankle (824.4-824.5)
radius (813.42, 813.52)
Pott's fracture (824.4-824.5)
that involving ankle (824.0-824.9)

The following fifth-digit subclassification is for use with category 823:
0 tibia alone
1 fibula alone
2 fibula with tibia

5th 823.0 **Upper end, closed**
[0-2] Head
Proximal end
Tibia:
condyles
tuberosity

5th 823.1 **Upper end, open**
[0-2]

5th 823.2 **Shaft, closed**
[0-2]

5th 823.3 **Shaft, open**
[0-2]

5th 823.4 **Torus fracture**
[0-2]

5th 823.8 **Unspecified part, closed**
[0-2] Lower leg NOS

5th 823.9 **Unspecified part, open**
[0-2]

4th 824 **Fracture of ankle**

824.0 **Medial malleolus, closed**
Tibia involving:
ankle
malleolus

824.1 **Medial malleolus, open**

824.2 **Lateral malleolus, closed**
Fibula involving:
ankle
malleolus

824.3 **Lateral malleolus, open**

824.4 **Bimalleolar, closed**
Dupuytren's fracture, fibula
Pott's fracture

824.5 **Bimalleolar, open**

824.6 **Trimalleolar, closed**
Lateral and medial malleolus with anterior or posterior lip of tibia

824.7 **Trimalleolar, open**

824.8 **Unspecified, closed**
Ankle NOS

824.9 **Unspecified, open**

4th 825 **Fracture of one or more tarsal and metatarsal bones**

The Tarsal Bones and Metatarsals

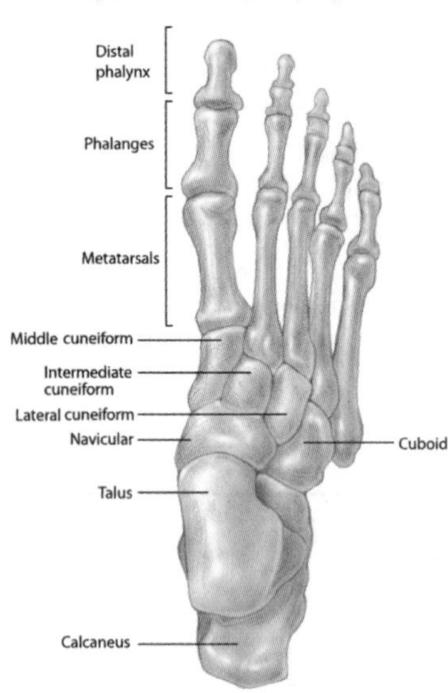

© 2008 Fairman Studios, LLC. All Rights Reserved.

825.0 Fracture of calcaneus, closed
Heel bone
Os calcis

825.1 Fracture of calcaneus, open

5th **825.2 Fracture of other tarsal and metatarsal bones, closed**

825.20 Unspecified bone(s) of foot [except toes]
Instep

825.21 Astragalus
Talus

825.22 Navicular [scaphoid], foot

825.23 Cuboid

825.24 Cuneiform, foot

825.25 Metatarsal bone(s)

825.29 Other
Tarsal with metatarsal bone(s) only
Excludes *calcaneus (825.0)*

5th **825.3 Fracture of other tarsal and metatarsal bones, open**

825.30 Unspecified bone(s) of foot [except toes]

825.31 Astragalus

825.32 Navicular [scaphoid], foot

825.33 Cuboid

825.34 Cuneiform, foot

825.35 Metatarsal bone(s)

825.39 Other

4th 826 **Fracture of one or more phalanges of foot**
Includes toe(s)

826.0 Closed

826.1 Open

4th 827 **Other, multiple, and ill-defined fractures of lower limb**
Includes leg NOS
multiple bones of same lower limb
Excludes *multiple fractures of:*
ankle bones alone (824.4-824.9)
phalanges of foot alone (826.0-826.1)
tarsal with metatarsal bones (825.29, 825.39)
tibia with fibula (823.0-823.9 with fifth-digit 2)

827.0 Closed

827.1 Open

4th 828 **Multiple fractures involving both lower limbs, lower with upper limb, and lower limb(s) with rib(s) and sternum**
Includes arm(s) with leg(s) [any bones]
both legs [any bones]
leg(s) with rib(s) or sternum

ICD-9-CM Official Guidelines (Chapter 17):
b. Coding of Traumatic Fractures
4) Multiple fracture categories 819 and 828
Multiple fracture categories 819 and 828 classify bilateral fractures of both upper limbs (819) and both lower limbs (828), but without any detail at the fourth-digit level other than open and closed type of fractures.

828.0 Closed

828.1 Open

4th 829 **Fracture of unspecified bones**

829.0 Unspecified bone, closed

829.1 Unspecified bone, open

DISLOCATION (830-839)

Includes displacement
subluxation

Excludes *congenital dislocation (754.0-755.8)*
pathological dislocation (718.2)
recurrent dislocation (718.3)

The descriptions "closed" and "open," used in the fourth-digit subdivisions, include the following terms:

closed:
complete
dislocation NOS
partial
simple
uncomplicated

open:
compound
infected
with foreign body

Note: *A dislocation not indicated as closed or open should be classified as closed.*

4th 830 **Dislocation of jaw**
Includes jaw (cartilage) (meniscus)
mandible
maxilla (inferior)
temporomandibular (joint)

830.0 Closed dislocation

830.1 Open dislocation

4th 831 **Dislocation of shoulder**
Excludes *sternoclavicular joint (839.61, 839.71)*
sternum (839.61, 839.71)

The following fifth-digit subclassification is for use with category 831:
0 **shoulder, unspecified**
Humerus NOS
1 **anterior dislocation of humerus**
2 **posterior dislocation of humerus**
3 **inferior dislocation of humerus**
4 **acromioclavicular (joint)**
Clavicle
9 **other**
Scapula

5th **831.0 Closed dislocation**
[0-4,9]

5th **831.1 Open dislocation**
[0-4,9]

4th 832 **Dislocation of elbow**

The following fifth-digit subclassification is for use with subcategories 832.0 and 832.1 ~~category 832~~:

0 **elbow unspecified**
1 **anterior dislocation of elbow**
2 **posterior dislocation of elbow**
3 **medial dislocation of elbow**
4 **lateral dislocation of elbow**
9 **other**

5th 832.0 **Closed dislocation**
[0-4,9]

5th 832.1 **Open dislocation**
[0-4,9]

● 832.2 **Nursemaid's elbow**
Subluxation of radial head

Rationale: *The American Academy of Pediatrics (AAP) requested a unique code for nursemaid's elbow. This condition is a subluxation of the radial head commonly seen in children under the age of five. Previously, the index of ICD-9-CM directed you to code this to dislocation of the elbow. It was decided that a new code be created in category 832, "Dislocation of elbow," to indicate subluxation.*

4th 833 **Dislocation of wrist**

The following fifth-digit subclassification is for use with category 833:

0 **wrist, unspecified part**
Carpal (bone)
Radius, distal end
1 **radioulnar (joint), distal**
2 **radiocarpal (joint)**
3 **midcarpal (joint)**
4 **carpometacarpal (joint)**
5 **metacarpal (bone), proximal end**
9 **other**
Ulna, distal end

5th 833.0 **Closed dislocation**
[0-5,9]

5th 833.1 **Open dislocation**
[0-5,9]

4th 834 **Dislocation of finger**

Includes finger(s)
phalanx of hand
thumb

The following fifth-digit subclassification is for use with category 834:

0 **finger, unspecified part**
1 **metacarpophalangeal (joint)**
Metacarpal (bone), distal end
2 **interphalangeal (joint), hand**

5th 834.0 **Closed dislocation**
[0-2]

5th 834.1 **Open dislocation**
[0-2]

4th 835 **Dislocation of hip**

The following fifth-digit subclassification is for use with category 835:

0 **dislocation of hip, unspecified**
1 **posterior dislocation**
2 **obturator dislocation**
3 **other anterior dislocation**

5th 835.0 **Closed dislocation**
[0-3]

5th 835.1 **Open dislocation**
[0-3]

4th 836 **Dislocation of knee**

Excludes *dislocation of knee:*
old or pathological (718.2)
recurrent (718.3)
internal derangement of knee joint (717.0-717.5, 717.8-717.9)
old tear of cartilage or meniscus of knee (717.0-717.5, 717.8-717.9)

836.0 **Tear of medial cartilage or meniscus of knee, current**

S83.211D Bucket-handle tear of medial meniscus, current injury, rightknee , subsequent encounter for fracture with routine healing
S83.212D Bucket-handle tear of medial meniscus, current injury, left knee, subsequent encounter for fracture with routine healing
S83.219A Bucket-handle tear of medial meniscus, current injury, unspecified knee, initial encounter for fracture
S83.219D Bucket-handle tear of medial meniscus, current injury, unspecified knee, subsequent encounter for fracture with routine healing
S83.221D Peripheral tear of medial meniscus, current injury, right knee, subsequent encounter for fracture with routine healing
S83.222D Peripheral tear of medial meniscus, current injury, left knee, subsequent encounter for fracture with routine healing
S83.229D Peripheral tear of medial meniscus, current injury, unspecified knee, subsequent encounter for fracture with routine healing
S83.231D Complex tear of medial meniscus, current injury, right knee, subsequent encounter for fracture with routine healing
S83.232D Complex tear of medial meniscus, current injury, left knee, subsequent encounter for fracture with routine healing
S83.239D Complex tear of medial meniscus, current injury, unspecified knee, subsequent encounter for fracture with routine healing
S83.241D Other tear of medial meniscus, current injury, right knee, subsequent encounter for fracture with routine healing
S83.242D Other tear of medial meniscus, current injury, left knee, subsequent encounter for fracture with routine healing
S83.249A Other tear of medial meniscus, current injury, unspecified knee, initial encounter for fracture
S83.249D Other tear of medial meniscus, current injury, unspecified knee, subsequent encounter for fracture with routine healing

Bucket handle tear:
NOS current injury
medial meniscus current injury

836.1 **Tear of lateral cartilage or meniscus of knee, current**

836.2 **Other tear of cartilage or meniscus of knee, current**
Tear of:
cartilage (semilunar) current injury, not specified as medial or lateral
meniscus current injury, not specified as medial or lateral

836.3 **Dislocation of patella, closed**

836.4 **Dislocation of patella, open**

5th 836.5 **Other dislocation of knee, closed**

836.50 **Dislocation of knee, unspecified**

836.51 **Anterior dislocation of tibia, proximal end**
Posterior dislocation of femur, distal end

832 – 836.51

836.52 **Posterior dislocation of tibia, proximal end**
Anterior dislocation of femur, distal end

836.53 **Medial dislocation of tibia, proximal end**

836.54 **Lateral dislocation of tibia, proximal end**

836.59 **Other**

5th 836.6 **Other dislocation of knee, open**

836.60 **Dislocation of knee, unspecified**

836.61 **Anterior dislocation of tibia, proximal end**

836.62 **Posterior dislocation of tibia, proximal end**

836.63 **Medial dislocation of tibia, proximal end**

836.64 **Lateral dislocation of tibia, proximal end**

836.69 **Other**

4th 837 **Dislocation of ankle**

Includes astragalus
fibula, distal end
navicular, foot
scaphoid, foot
tibia, distal end

837.0 **Closed dislocation**

837.1 **Open dislocation**

4th 838 **Dislocation of foot**

The following fifth-digit subclassification is for use with category 838:

0 foot, unspecified
1 tarsal (bone), joint unspecified
2 midtarsal (joint)
3 tarsometatarsal (joint)
4 metatarsal (bone), joint unspecified
5 metatarsophalangeal (joint)
6 interphalangeal (joint), foot
9 other

5th 838.0 **Closed dislocation**
[0-6,9]

5th 838.1 **Open dislocation**
[0-6,9]

4th 839 **Other, multiple, and ill-defined dislocations**

5th 839.0 **Cervical vertebra, closed**
Cervical spine
Neck

839.00 **Cervical vertebra, unspecified**

839.01 **First cervical vertebra**

839.02 **Second cervical vertebra**

839.03 **Third cervical vertebra**

839.04 **Fourth cervical vertebra**

839.05 **Fifth cervical vertebra**

839.06 **Sixth cervical vertebra**

839.07 **Seventh cervical vertebra**

839.08 **Multiple cervical vertebrae**

5th 839.1 **Cervical vertebra, open**

839.10 **Cervical vertebra, unspecified**

839.11 **First cervical vertebra**

839.12 **Second cervical vertebra**

839.13 **Third cervical vertebra**

839.14 **Fourth cervical vertebra**

839.15 **Fifth cervical vertebra**

839.16 **Sixth cervical vertebra**

839.17 **Seventh cervical vertebra**

839.18 **Multiple cervical vertebrae**

5th 839.2 **Thoracic and lumbar vertebra, closed**

839.20 **Lumbar vertebra**

S33.0xxD Traumatic rupture of lumbar intervertebral disc, subsequent encounter

S33.100D Subluxation of unspecified lumbar vertebra, subsequent encounter

S33.101A Dislocation of unspecified lumbar vertebra, initial encounter

S33.101D Dislocation of unspecified lumbar vertebra, subsequent encounter

S33.110D Subluxation of L_1/L_2 lumbar vertebra, subsequent encounter

S33.111D Dislocation of L_1/L_2 lumbar vertebra, subsequent encounter

S33.120D Subluxation of L_2/L_3 lumbar vertebra, subsequent encounter

S33.121.D Dislocation of L_2/L_3 lumbar vertebra, subsequent encounter

S33.130D Subluxation of L_3/L_4 lumbar vertebra, subsequent encounter

S33.131D Dislocation of L_3/L_4 lumbar vertebra, subsequent encounter

S33.140D Subluxation of L_4/L_5 lumbar vertebra, subsequent encounter

S33.141D Dislocation of L_4/L_5 lumbar vertebra, subsequent encounter

839.21 **Thoracic vertebra**
Dorsal [thoracic] vertebra

5th 839.3 **Thoracic and lumbar vertebra, open**

839.30 **Lumbar vertebra**

839.31 **Thoracic vertebra**

5th 839.4 **Other vertebra, closed**

839.40 **Vertebra, unspecified site**
Spine NOS

839.41 **Coccyx**

839.42 **Sacrum**
Sacroiliac (joint)

839.49 **Other**

5th 839.5 **Other vertebra, open**

839.50 **Vertebra, unspecified site**

839.51 **Coccyx**

839.52 **Sacrum**

839.59 **Other**

5th 839.6 **Other location, closed**

839.61 **Sternum**
Sternoclavicular joint

839.69 **Other**
Pelvis

5th 839.7 **Other location, open**

839.71 **Sternum**

839.79 **Other**

839.8 **Multiple and ill-defined, closed**
Arm
Back
Hand
Multiple locations, except fingers or toes alone
Other ill-defined locations
Unspecified location

839.9 **Multiple and ill-defined, open**

SPRAINS AND STRAINS OF JOINTS AND ADJACENT MUSCLES (840-848)

Includes avulsion of joint capsule, ligament, muscle, tendon
hemarthrosis of joint capsule, ligament, muscle, tendon
laceration of joint capsule, ligament, muscle, tendon
rupture of joint capsule, ligament, muscle, tendon
sprain of joint capsule, ligament, muscle, tendon
strain of joint capsule, ligament, muscle, tendon
tear of joint capsule, ligament, muscle, tendon

Excludes *laceration of tendon in open wounds (880-884 and 890-894 with .2)*

4th 840 Sprains and strains of shoulder and upper arm
- 840.0 Acromioclavicular (joint) (ligament)
- 840.1 Coracoclavicular (ligament)
- 840.2 Coracohumeral (ligament)
- 840.3 Infraspinatus (muscle) (tendon)
- 840.4 Rotator cuff (capsule)
  - S43.421D Sprain of right rotator cuff capsule, subsequent encounter
  - S43.422D Sprain of left rotator cuff capsule, subsequent encounter
  - S43.429A Sprain of unspecified rotator cuff capsule, initial encounter
  - S43.429D Sprain of unspecified rotator cuff capsule, subsequent encounter

  Excludes *complete rupture of rotator cuff, nontraumatic (727.61)*
- 840.5 Subscapularis (muscle)
- 840.6 Supraspinatus (muscle) (tendon)
- 840.7 Superior glenoid labrum lesion
  SLAP lesion
- 840.8 Other specified sites of shoulder and upper arm
- 840.9 Unspecified site of shoulder and upper arm
  - S43.401D Unspecified sprain of right shoulder joint, subsequent encounter
  - S43.402D Unspecified sprain of left shoulder joint, subsequent encounter
  - S43.409A Unspecified sprain of unspecified shoulder joint, initial encounter
  - S43.409D Unspecified sprain of unspecified shoulder joint, subsequent encounter
  - S43.90xD Sprain of unspecified parts of shoulder girdle, unspecified side, subsequent encounter
  - S43.91xD Sprain of unspecified parts of right shoulder girdle, subsequent encounter
  - S43.92xD Sprain of unspecified parts of left shoulder girdle, subsequent encounter

  Arm NOS
  Shoulder NOS

4th 841 Sprains and strains of elbow and forearm
- 841.0 Radial collateral ligament
- 841.1 Ulnar collateral ligament
- 841.2 Radiohumeral (joint)
- 841.3 Ulnohumeral (joint)
- 841.8 Other specified sites of elbow and forearm
- 841.9 Unspecified site of elbow and forearm
  Elbow NOS

4th 842 Sprains and strains of wrist and hand
- 5th 842.0 Wrist
  - 842.00 Unspecified site
  - 842.01 Carpal (joint)
  - 842.02 Radiocarpal (joint) (ligament)
  - 842.09 Other
    Radioulnar joint, distal
- 5th 842.1 Hand
  - 842.10 Unspecified site
  - 842.11 Carpometacarpal (joint)
  - 842.12 Metacarpophalangeal (joint)
  - 842.13 Interphalangeal (joint)
  - 842.19 Other
    Midcarpal (joint)

4th 843 Sprains and strains of hip and thigh
- 843.0 Iliofemoral (ligament)
- 843.1 Ischiocapsular (ligament)
- 843.8 Other specified sites of hip and thigh

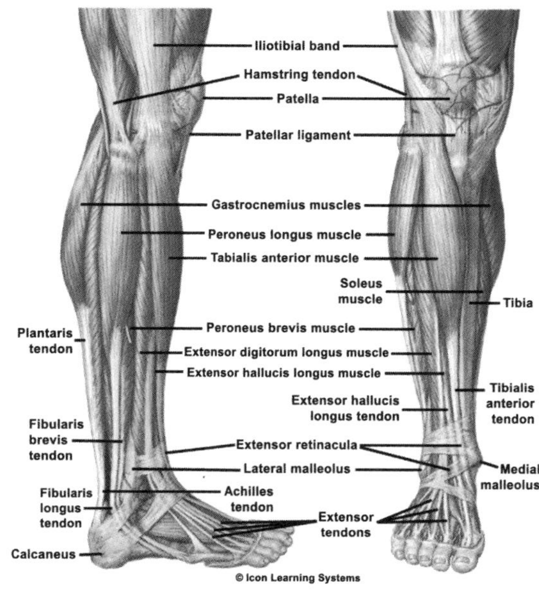

- 843.9 Unspecified site of hip and thigh
  Hip NOS
  Thigh NOS

4th 844 Sprains and strains of knee and leg
- 844.0 Lateral collateral ligament of knee
- 844.1 Medial collateral ligament of knee
- 844.2 Cruciate ligament of knee
- 844.3 Tibiofibular (joint) (ligament), superior
- 844.8 Other specified sites of knee and leg
- 844.9 Unspecified site of knee and leg
  - S83.90xA Sprain of unspecified site of knee, unspecified side, initial encounter
  - S83.90xD Sprain of unspecified site of knee, unspecified side, subsequent encounter
  - S83.91xD Sprain of unspecified site of right knee, subsequent encounter
  - S86.92xD Sprain of unspecified site of left knee, subsequent encounter
  - S86.911D Strain of unspecified muscle(s) and tendon(s) at lower leg level, right leg, subsequent encounter
  - S86.912D Strain of unspecified muscle(s) and tendon(s) at lower leg level, left leg, subsequent encounter
  - S86.919A Strain of unspecified muscle(s) and tendon(s) at lower leg level, unspecified leg, initial encounter
  - S86.919D Strain of unspecified muscle(s) and tendon(s) at lower leg level, unspecified leg, subsequent encounter

  Knee NOS
  Leg NOS

4th 845 **Sprains and strains of ankle and foot**

5th 845.0 **Ankle**

845.00 **Unspecified site**

S93.401D Sprain of unspecified ligament of right ankle, subsequent encounter

S93.402D Sprain of unspecified ligament of left ankle, subsequent encounter

S93.409A Sprain of unspecified ligament of unspecified ankle, initial encounter

S93.409D Sprain of unspecified ligament of unspecified ankle, subsequent encounter

845.01 **Deltoid (ligament), ankle**
Internal collateral (ligament), ankle

845.02 **Calcaneofibular (ligament)**

845.03 **Tibiofibular (ligament), distal**

845.09 **Other**
Achilles tendon

5th 845.1 **Foot**

845.10 **Unspecified site**

845.11 **Tarsometatarsal (joint) (ligament)**

845.12 **Metatarsophalangeal (joint)**

845.13 **Interphalangeal (joint), toe**

845.19 **Other**

4th 846 **Sprains and strains of sacroiliac region**

846.0 **Lumbosacral (joint) (ligament)** I 48, I 49, I 50, I 51

S33.8xxA Sprain of other parts of lumbar spine and pelvis, initial encounter

S33.8xxD Sprain of other parts of lumbar spine and pelvis, subsequent encounter

846.1 **Sacroiliac ligament** I 48, I 49, I 50, I 51

846.2 **Sacrospinatus (ligament)** I 48, I 49, I 50, I 51

846.3 **Sacrotuberous (ligament)** I 48, I 49, I 50, I 51

846.8 **Other specified sites of sacroiliac region** I 48, I 49, I 50, I 51

846.9 **Unspecified site of sacroiliac region** I 48, I 49, I 50, I 51

4th 847 **Sprains and strains of other and unspecified parts of back**

Excludes *lumbosacral (846.0)*

847.0 **Neck**

S13.4xxA Sprain of ligaments of cervical spine, initial encounter

S13.4xxD Sprain of ligaments of cervical spine, subsequent encounter

S13.8xxA Sprain of joints and ligaments of other parts of neck, initial encounter

S13.8xxD Sprain of joints and ligaments of other parts of neck, subsequent encounter

S16.1xxD Strain of muscle, fascia and tendon at neck level, subsequent encounter

Anterior longitudinal (ligament), cervical
Atlanto-axial (joints)
Atlanto-occipital (joints)
Whiplash injury

Excludes *neck injury NOS (959.09)*
thyroid region (848.2)

847.1 **Thoracic**

847.2 **Lumbar** I 48, I 49, I 50, I 51

S33.5xxA Sprain of ligaments of lumbar spine, initial encounter

S33.5xxD Sprain of ligaments of lumbar spine, subsequent encounter

847.3 **Sacrum**
Sacrococcygeal (ligament)

847.4 **Coccyx**

847.9 **Unspecified site of back**
Back NOS

4th 848 **Other and ill-defined sprains and strains**

848.0 **Septal cartilage of nose**

848.1 **Jaw**
Temporomandibular (joint) (ligament)

848.2 **Thyroid region**
Cricoarytenoid (joint) (ligament)
Cricothyroid (joint) (ligament)
Thyroid cartilage

848.3 **Ribs**
Chondrocostal (joint) without mention of injury to sternum
Costal cartilage without mention of injury to sternum

5th 848.4 **Sternum**

848.40 **Unspecified site**

848.41 **Sternoclavicular (joint) (ligament)**

848.42 **Chondrosternal (joint)**

848.49 **Other**
Xiphoid cartilage

848.5 **Pelvis**
Symphysis pubis

Excludes *that in childbirth (665.6)*

848.8 **Other specified sites of sprains and strains**

848.9 **Unspecified site of sprain and strain**

INTRACRANIAL INJURY, EXCLUDING THOSE WITH SKULL FRACTURE (850-854)

Includes traumatic brain injury without skull fracture

Excludes *intracranial injury with skull fracture (800-801 and 803-804, except .0 and .5)*
open wound of head without intracranial injury (870.0-873.9)
skull fracture alone (800-801 and 803-804 with .0, .5)

Note: *The description "with open intracranial wound," used in the fourth-digit subdivisions, includes those specified as open or with mention of infection or foreign body.*

4th 850 **Concussion**

Includes commotio cerebri

Excludes *concussion with:*
cerebral laceration or contusion (851.0-851.9)
cerebral hemorrhage (852-853)
head injury NOS (959.01)

850.0 **With no loss of consciousness**
Concussion with mental confusion or disorientation, without loss of consciousness

5th 850.1 **With brief loss of consciousness**
Loss of consciousness for less than one hour

850.11 **With loss of consciousness of 30 minutes or less**

850.12 **With loss of consciousness from 31 to 59 minutes**

850.2 **With moderate loss of consciousness**
Loss of consciousness for 1-24 hours

850.3 **With prolonged loss of consciousness and return to pre-existing conscious level**
Loss of consciousness for more than 24 hours with complete recovery

850.4 **With prolonged loss of consciousness, without return to pre-existing conscious level**

850.5 **With loss of consciousness of unspecified duration**

850.9 **Concussion, unspecified**

845 – 850.9

The following fifth-digit subclassification is for use with categories 851-854:

0 unspecified state of consciousness
1 with no loss of consciousness
2 with brief [less than one hour] loss of consciousness
3 with moderate [1-24 hours] loss of consciousness
4 with prolonged [more than 24 hours] loss of consciousness and return to pre-existing conscious level
5 with prolonged [more than 24 hours] loss of consciousness without return to pre-existing conscious level
Use fifth-digit 5 to designate when a patient is unconscious and dies before regaining consciousness, regardless of the duration of the loss of consciousness
6 with loss of consciousness of unspecified duration
9 with concussion, unspecified

4th **851 Cerebral laceration and contusion**

5th **851.0 Cortex (cerebral) contusion without mention of open intracranial wound**
[0-6,9]

5th **851.1 Cortex (cerebral) contusion with open intracranial wound**
[0-6,9]

5th **851.2 Cortex (cerebral) laceration without mention of open intracranial wound**
[0-6,9]

5th **851.3 Cortex (cerebral) laceration with open intracranial wound**
[0-6,9]

5th **851.4 Cerebellar or brain stem contusion without mention of open intracranial wound**
[0-6,9]

5th **851.5 Cerebellar or brain stem contusion with open intracranial wound**
[0-6,9]

5th **851.6 Cerebellar or brain stem laceration without mention of open intracranial wound**
[0-6,9]

5th **851.7 Cerebellar or brain stem laceration with open intracranial wound**
[0-6,9]

5th **851.8 Other and unspecified cerebral laceration and contusion, without mention of open intracranial wound**
[0-6,9] Brain (membrane) NOS

5th **851.9 Other and unspecified cerebral laceration and contusion, with open intracranial wound**
[0-6,9]

4th **852 Subarachnoid, subdural, and extradural hemorrhage, following injury**
Requires fifth digit. See prior to category 851 for codes and definitions.
Excludes *cerebral contusion or laceration (with hemorrhage) (851.0-851.9)*

5th **852.0 Subarachnoid hemorrhage following injury without mention of open intracranial wound**
[0-6,9] Middle meningeal hemorrhage following injury

5th **852.1 Subarachnoid hemorrhage following injury with open intracranial wound**
[0-6,9]

5th **852.2 Subdural hemorrhage following injury without mention of open intracranial wound**
[0-6,9]

5th **852.3 Subdural hemorrhage following injury with open intracranial wound**
[0-6,9]

5th **852.4 Extradural hemorrhage following injury without mention of open intracranial wound**
[0-6,9] Epidural hematoma following injury

5th **852.5 Extradural hemorrhage following injury with open intracranial wound**
[0-6,9]

4th **853 Other and unspecified intracranial hemorrhage following injury**
Requires fifth digit. See prior to category 851 for codes and definitions.

5th **853.0 Without mention of open intracranial wound**
[0-6,9] Cerebral compression due to injury
Intracranial hematoma following injury
Traumatic cerebral hemorrhage

5th **853.1 With open intracranial wound**
[0-6,9]

4th **854 Intracranial injury of other and unspecified nature**
Requires fifth digit. See prior to category 851 for codes and definitions.
Includes injury:
brain NOS
cavernous sinus
intracranial
traumatic brain NOS
Excludes *any condition classifiable to 850-853*
head injury NOS (959.01)

5th **854.0 Without mention of open intracranial wound**
[0-6,9]

5th **854.1 With open intracranial wound**
[0-6,9]

INTERNAL INJURY OF THORAX, ABDOMEN, AND PELVIS (860-869)

Includes blast injuries of internal organs
blunt trauma of internal organs
bruise of internal organs
concussion injuries (except cerebral) of internal organs
crushing of internal organs
hematoma of internal organs
laceration of internal organs
puncture of internal organs
tear of internal organs
traumatic rupture of internal organs

Excludes *concussion NOS (850.0-850.9)*
flail chest (807.4)
foreign body entering through orifice (930.0-939.9)
injury to blood vessels (901.0-902.9)

Note: *The description "with open wound," used in the fourth-digit subdivisions, includes those with mention of infection or foreign body.*

4th **860 Traumatic pneumothorax and hemothorax**

860.0 Pneumothorax without mention of open wound into thorax

860.1 Pneumothorax with open wound into thorax

860.2 Hemothorax without mention of open wound into thorax

860.3 Hemothorax with open wound into thorax

860.4 Pneumohemothorax without mention of open wound into thorax

860.5 Pneumohemothorax with open wound into thorax

4th **861 Injury to heart and lung**
Excludes *injury to blood vessels of thorax (901.0-901.9)*

5th **861.0 Heart, without mention of open wound into thorax**

861.00 Unspecified injury

861.01 Contusion
Cardiac contusion
Myocardial contusion

861.02 Laceration without penetration of heart chambers

861.03 Laceration with penetration of heart chambers

5th **861.1 Heart, with open wound into thorax**

861.10 Unspecified injury

861.11 Contusion

861.12 Laceration without penetration of heart chambers
861.13 Laceration with penetration of heart chambers

5th 861.2 Lung, without mention of open wound into thorax
861.20 Unspecified injury
861.21 Contusion
861.22 Laceration

5th 861.3 Lung, with open wound into thorax
861.30 Unspecified injury
861.31 Contusion
861.32 Laceration

4th 862 Injury to other and unspecified intrathoracic organs

Excludes *injury to blood vessels of thorax (901.0-901.9)*

862.0 Diaphragm, without mention of open wound into cavity
862.1 Diaphragm, with open wound into cavity

5th 862.2 Other specified intrathoracic organs, without mention of open wound into cavity
862.21 Bronchus
862.22 Esophagus
862.29 Other
Pleura
Thymus gland

5th 862.3 Other specified intrathoracic organs, with open wound into cavity
862.31 Bronchus
862.32 Esophagus
862.39 Other

862.8 Multiple and unspecified intrathoracic organs, without mention of open wound into cavity
Crushed chest
Multiple intrathoracic organs

862.9 Multiple and unspecified intrathoracic organs, with open wound into cavity

4th 863 Injury to gastrointestinal tract

Excludes *anal sphincter laceration during delivery (664.2)*
bile duct (868.0-868.1 with fifth-digit 2)
gallbladder (868.0-868.1 with fifth-digit 2)

863.0 Stomach, without mention of open wound into cavity
863.1 Stomach, with open wound into cavity

5th 863.2 Small intestine, without mention of open wound into cavity
863.20 Small intestine, unspecified site
863.21 Duodenum
863.29 Other

5th 863.3 Small intestine, with open wound into cavity
863.30 Small intestine, unspecified site
863.31 Duodenum
863.39 Other

5th 863.4 Colon or rectum, without mention of open wound into cavity
863.40 Colon, unspecified site
863.41 Ascending [right] colon
863.42 Transverse colon
863.43 Descending [left] colon
863.44 Sigmoid colon
863.45 Rectum
863.46 Multiple sites in colon and rectum
863.49 Other

5th 863.5 Colon or rectum, with open wound into cavity
863.50 Colon, unspecified site
863.51 Ascending [right] colon
863.52 Transverse colon
863.53 Descending [left] colon
863.54 Sigmoid colon
863.55 Rectum
863.56 Multiple sites in colon and rectum
863.59 Other

5th 863.8 Other and unspecified gastrointestinal sites, without mention of open wound into cavity
863.80 Gastrointestinal tract, unspecified site
863.81 Pancreas, head
863.82 Pancreas, body
863.83 Pancreas, tail
863.84 Pancreas, multiple and unspecified sites
863.85 Appendix
863.89 Other
Intestine NOS

5th 863.9 Other and unspecified gastrointestinal sites, with open wound into cavity
863.90 Gastrointestinal tract, unspecified site
863.91 Pancreas, head
863.92 Pancreas, body
863.93 Pancreas, tail
863.94 Pancreas, multiple and unspecified sites
863.95 Appendix
863.99 Other

4th 864 Injury to liver

The following fifth-digit subclassification is for use with category 864:
0 unspecified injury
1 hematoma and contusion
2 laceration, minor
Laceration involving capsule only, or without significant involvement of hepatic parenchyma [i.e., less than 1 cm deep]
3 laceration, moderate
Laceration involving parenchyma but without major disruption of parenchyma [i.e., less than 10 cm long and less than 3 cm deep]
4 laceration, major
Laceration with significant disruption of hepatic parenchyma [i.e., 10 cm long and 3 cm deep]
Multiple moderate lacerations, with or without hematoma
Stellate lacerations of liver
5 laceration, unspecified
9 other

5th 864.0 Without mention of open wound into cavity
[0-5,9]

5th 864.1 With open wound into cavity
[0-5,9]

4th 865 Injury to spleen

The following fifth-digit subclassification is for use with category 865:
0 unspecified injury
1 hematoma without rupture of capsule
2 capsular tears, without major disruption of parenchyma
3 laceration extending into parenchyma
4 massive parenchymal disruption
9 other

5th 865.0 Without mention of open wound into cavity
[0-4,9]

5th 865.1 With open wound into cavity
[0-4,9]

4th 866 **Injury to kidney**

Excludes *acute kidney injury (nontraumatic) (584.9)*

The following fifth-digit subclassification is for use with category 866:

- 0 unspecified injury
- 1 hematoma without rupture of capsule
- 2 laceration
- 3 complete disruption of kidney parenchyma

5th **866.0 Without mention of open wound into cavity**
[0-3]

5th **866.1 With open wound into cavity**
[0-3]

4th 867 **Injury to pelvic organs**

Excludes *injury during delivery (664.0-665.9)*

867.0 Bladder and urethra, without mention of open wound into cavity

867.1 Bladder and urethra, with open wound into cavity

867.2 Ureter, without mention of open wound into cavity

867.3 Ureter, with open wound into cavity

867.4 Uterus, without mention of open wound into cavity ♀

867.5 Uterus, with open wound into cavity ♀

867.6 Other specified pelvic organs, without mention of open wound into cavity

Fallopian tube
Ovary
Prostate
Seminal vesicle
Vas deferens

867.7 Other specified pelvic organs, with open wound into cavity

867.8 Unspecified pelvic organ, without mention of open wound into cavity

867.9 Unspecified pelvic organ, with open wound into cavity

4th 868 **Injury to other intra-abdominal organs**

The following fifth-digit subclassification is for use with category 868:

- 0 unspecified intra-abdominal organ
- 1 adrenal gland
- 2 bile duct and gallbladder
- 3 peritoneum
- 4 retroperitoneum
- 9 other and multiple intra-abdominal organs

5th **868.0 Without mention of open wound into cavity**
[0-4,9]

5th **868.1 With open wound into cavity**
[0-4,9]

4th 869 **Internal injury to unspecified or ill-defined organs**

Includes internal injury NOS
multiple internal injury NOS

869.0 Without mention of open wound into cavity

869.1 With open wound into cavity

OPEN WOUNDS (870-897)

Includes animal bite
avulsion
cut
laceration
puncture wound
traumatic amputation

Excludes *burn (940.0-949.5)*
crushing (925-929.9)
puncture of internal organs (860.0-869.1)
superficial injury (910.0-919.9)
that incidental to:
dislocation (830.0-839.9)
fracture (800.0-829.1)
internal injury (860.0-869.1)
intracranial injury (851.0-854.1)

Note: *The description "complicated" used in the fourth-digit subdivisions includes those with mention of delayed healing, delayed treatment, foreign body, or infection.*

~~Use additional code to identify infection~~

OPEN WOUND OF HEAD, NECK, AND TRUNK (870-879)

4th 870 **Open wound of ocular adnexa**

870.0 Laceration of skin of eyelid and periocular area

870.1 Laceration of eyelid, full-thickness, not involving lacrimal passages

870.2 Laceration of eyelid involving lacrimal passages

870.3 Penetrating wound of orbit, without mention of foreign body

870.4 Penetrating wound of orbit with foreign body

Excludes *retained (old) foreign body in orbit (376.6)*

870.8 Other specified open wounds of ocular adnexa

870.9 Unspecified open wound of ocular adnexa

4th 871 **Open wound of eyeball**

Excludes *2nd cranial nerve [optic] injury (950.0-950.9)*
3rd cranial nerve [oculomotor] injury (951.0)

871.0 Ocular laceration without prolapse of intraocular tissue

871.1 Ocular laceration with prolapse or exposure of intraocular tissue

871.2 Rupture of eye with partial loss of intraocular tissue

871.3 Avulsion of eye

Traumatic enucleation

871.4 Unspecified laceration of eye

871.5 Penetration of eyeball with magnetic foreign body

Excludes *retained (old) magnetic foreign body in globe (360.50-360.59)*

871.6 Penetration of eyeball with (nonmagnetic) foreign body

Excludes *retained (old) (nonmagnetic) foreign body in globe (360.60-360.69)*

871.7 Unspecified ocular penetration

871.9 Unspecified open wound of eyeball

4th 872 **Open wound of ear**

5th **872.0 External ear, without mention of complication**

872.00 External ear, unspecified site

872.01 Auricle, ear

Pinna

872.02 Auditory canal

5th **872.1 External ear, complicated**

872.10 External ear, unspecified site

872.11 Auricle, ear

872.12 Auditory canal

866 – 872.12

5th 872.6 Other specified parts of ear, without mention of complication
872.61 Ear drum
Drumhead
Tympanic membrane
872.62 Ossicles
872.63 Eustachian tube
872.64 Cochlea
872.69 Other and multiple sites
5th 872.7 Other specified parts of ear, complicated
872.71 Ear drum
872.72 Ossicles
872.73 Eustachian tube
872.74 Cochlea
872.79 Other and multiple sites
872.8 Ear, part unspecified, without mention of complication
Ear NOS
872.9 Ear, part unspecified, complicated
4th 873 Other open wound of head
873.0 Scalp, without mention of complication
873.1 Scalp, complicated
5th 873.2 Nose, without mention of complication
873.20 Nose, unspecified site
873.21 Nasal septum
873.22 Nasal cavity
873.23 Nasal sinus
873.29 Multiple sites
5th 873.3 Nose, complicated
873.30 Nose, unspecified site
873.31 Nasal septum
873.32 Nasal cavity
873.33 Nasal sinus
873.39 Multiple sites
5th 873.4 Face, without mention of complication
873.40 Face, unspecified site
873.41 Cheek
873.42 Forehead
Eyebrow
873.43 Lip
873.44 Jaw
873.49 Other and multiple sites
5th 873.5 Face, complicated
873.50 Face, unspecified site
873.51 Cheek
873.52 Forehead
873.53 Lip
873.54 Jaw
873.59 Other and multiple sites
5th 873.6 Internal structures of mouth, without mention of complication
873.60 Mouth, unspecified site
873.61 Buccal mucosa
873.62 Gum (alveolar process)
873.63 Tooth (broken) (fractured) (due to trauma)
Excludes *cracked tooth (521.81)*
873.64 Tongue and floor of mouth
873.65 Palate
873.69 Other and multiple sites
5th 873.7 Internal structures of mouth, complicated
873.70 Mouth, unspecified site
873.71 Buccal mucosa
873.72 Gum (alveolar process)
873.73 Tooth (broken) (fractured) (due to trauma)
Excludes *cracked tooth (521.81)*
873.74 Tongue and floor of mouth
873.75 Palate
873.79 Other and multiple sites
873.8 Other and unspecified open wound of head without mention of complication
Head NOS
873.9 Other and unspecified open wound of head, complicated
4th 874 Open wound of neck
5th 874.0 Larynx and trachea, without mention of complication
874.00 Larynx with trachea
874.01 Larynx
874.02 Trachea
5th 874.1 Larynx and trachea, complicated
874.10 Larynx with trachea
874.11 Larynx
874.12 Trachea
874.2 Thyroid gland, without mention of complication
874.3 Thyroid gland, complicated
874.4 Pharynx, without mention of complication
Cervical esophagus
874.5 Pharynx, complicated
874.8 Other and unspecified parts, without mention of complication
Nape of neck
Supraclavicular region
Throat NOS
874.9 Other and unspecified parts, complicated
4th 875 Open wound of chest (wall)
Excludes *open wound into thoracic cavity (860.0-862.9)*
traumatic pneumothorax and hemothorax (860.1, 860.3, 860.5)
875.0 Without mention of complication
875.1 Complicated
4th 876 Open wound of back
Includes loin
lumbar region
Excludes *open wound into thoracic cavity (860.0-862.9)*
traumatic pneumothorax and hemothorax (860.1, 860.3, 860.5)
876.0 Without mention of complication
876.1 Complicated
4th 877 Open wound of buttock
Includes sacroiliac region
877.0 Without mention of complication
877.1 Complicated
4th 878 Open wound of genital organs (external), including traumatic amputation
Excludes *injury during delivery (664.0-665.9)*
internal genital organs (867.0-867.9)
878.0 Penis, without mention of complication ♂
878.1 Penis, complicated ♂
878.2 Scrotum and testes, without mention of complication ♂
878.3 Scrotum and testes, complicated ♂
878.4 Vulva, without mention of complication ♀
Labium (majus) (minus)
878.5 Vulva, complicated ♀
878.6 Vagina, without mention of complication ♀

878.7 Vagina, complicated ♀

878.8 Other and unspecified parts, without mention of complication

878.9 Other and unspecified parts, complicated

4th 879 Open wound of other and unspecified sites, except limbs

879.0 Breast, without mention of complication

879.1 Breast, complicated

879.2 Abdominal wall, anterior, without mention of complication
- Abdominal wall NOS
- Epigastric region
- Hypogastric region
- Pubic region
- Umbilical region

879.3 Abdominal wall, anterior, complicated

879.4 Abdominal wall, lateral, without mention of complication
- Flank
- Groin
- Hypochondrium
- Iliac (region)
- Inguinal region

879.5 Abdominal wall, lateral, complicated

879.6 Other and unspecified parts of trunk, without mention of complication
- Pelvic region
- Perineum
- Trunk NOS

879.7 Other and unspecified parts of trunk, complicated

879.8 Open wound(s) (multiple) of unspecified site(s) without mention of complication
- Multiple open wounds NOS
- Open wound NOS

879.9 Open wound(s) (multiple) of unspecified site(s), complicated

OPEN WOUND OF UPPER LIMB (880-887)

4th 880 Open wound of shoulder and upper arm

The following fifth-digit subclassification is for use with category 880:
- 0 shoulder region
- 1 scapular region
- 2 axillary region
- 3 upper arm
- 9 multiple sites

5th 880.0 Without mention of complication

5th 880.1 Complicated

5th 880.2 With tendon involvement

4th 881 Open wound of elbow, forearm, and wrist

The following fifth-digit subclassification is for use with category 881:
- 0 forearm
- 1 elbow
- 2 wrist

5th 881.0 Without mention of complication

5th 881.1 Complicated

5th 881.2 With tendon involvement

4th 882 Open wound of hand except finger(s) alone

882.0 Without mention of complication

882.1 Complicated

882.2 With tendon involvement

4th 883 Open wound of finger(s)

Includes fingernail
thumb (nail)

883.0 Without mention of complication

883.1 Complicated

883.2 With tendon involvement

4th 884 Multiple and unspecified open wound of upper limb

Includes arm NOS
multiple sites of one upper limb
upper limb NOS

884.0 Without mention of complication

884.1 Complicated

884.2 With tendon involvement

4th 885 Traumatic amputation of thumb (complete) (partial)

Includes thumb(s) (with finger(s) of either hand)

885.0 Without mention of complication

885.1 Complicated

4th 886 Traumatic amputation of other finger(s) (complete) (partial)

Includes finger(s) of one or both hands, without mention of thumb(s)

886.0 Without mention of complication

886.1 Complicated

4th 887 Traumatic amputation of arm and hand (complete) (partial)

887.0 Unilateral, below elbow, without mention of complication

887.1 Unilateral, below elbow, complicated

887.2 Unilateral, at or above elbow, without mention of complication

887.3 Unilateral, at or above elbow, complicated

887.4 Unilateral, level not specified, without mention of complication

887.5 Unilateral, level not specified, complicated

887.6 Bilateral [any level], without mention of complication
- One hand and other arm

887.7 Bilateral [any level], complicated

OPEN WOUND OF LOWER LIMB (890-897)

4th 890 Open wound of hip and thigh

890.0 Without mention of complication

890.1 Complicated

890.2 With tendon involvement

4th 891 Open wound of knee, leg [except thigh], and ankle

Includes leg NOS
multiple sites of leg, except thigh

Excludes *that of thigh (890.0-890.2)*
with multiple sites of lower limb (894.0-894.2)

891.0 Without mention of complication

891.1 Complicated

891.2 With tendon involvement

4th 892 Open wound of foot except toe(s) alone

Includes heel

892.0 Without mention of complication

892.1 Complicated

892.2 With tendon involvement

4th 893 Open wound of toe(s)

Includes toenail

893.0 Without mention of complication

893.1 Complicated

893.2 With tendon involvement

4th 894 Multiple and unspecified open wound of lower limb

Includes lower limb NOS
multiple sites of one lower limb, with thigh

894.0 Without mention of complication

894.1 Complicated

894.2 With tendon involvement

878.7 – 894.2

4th 895 **Traumatic amputation of toe(s) (complete) (partial)**
Includes toe(s) of one or both feet
895.0 **Without mention of complication**
895.1 **Complicated**

4th 896 **Traumatic amputation of foot (complete) (partial)**
896.0 **Unilateral, without mention of complication**
896.1 **Unilateral, complicated**
896.2 **Bilateral, without mention of complication**
Excludes *one foot and other leg (897.6-897.7)*
896.3 **Bilateral, complicated**

4th 897 **Traumatic amputation of leg(s) (complete) (partial)**
897.0 **Unilateral, below knee, without mention of complication**
897.1 **Unilateral, below knee, complicated**
897.2 **Unilateral, at or above knee, without mention of complication**
897.3 **Unilateral, at or above knee, complicated**
897.4 **Unilateral, level not specified, without mention of complication**
897.5 **Unilateral, level not specified, complicated**
897.6 **Bilateral [any level], without mention of complication**
One foot and other leg
897.7 **Bilateral [any level], complicated**

INJURY TO BLOOD VESSELS (900-904)

Includes arterial hematoma of blood vessel, secondary to other injuries, e.g., fracture or open wound
avulsion of blood vessel, secondary to other injuries, e.g., fracture or open wound
cut of blood vessel, secondary to other injuries, e.g., fracture or open wound
laceration of blood vessel, secondary to other injuries, e.g., fracture or open wound
rupture of blood vessel, secondary to other injuries, e.g., fracture or open wound
traumatic aneurysm or fistula (arteriovenous) of blood vessel, secondary to other injuries, e.g., fracture or open wound

Excludes *accidental puncture or laceration during medical procedure (998.2)*
intracranial hemorrhage following injury (851.0-854.1)

ICD-9-CM Official Guidelines (Chapter 17):

a. Coding of Injuries

*2) **Primary injury with damage to nerves/blood vessels***
When a primary injury results in minor damage to peripheral nerves or blood vessels, the primary injury is sequenced first with additional code(s) from categories 950-957, Injury to nerves and spinal cord, and/or 900-904, Injury to blood vessels. When the primary injury is to the blood vessels or nerves, that injury should be sequenced first.

4th 900 **Injury to blood vessels of head and neck**
5th 900.0 **Carotid artery**
900.00 **Carotid artery, unspecified**
900.01 **Common carotid artery**
900.02 **External carotid artery**
900.03 **Internal carotid artery**
900.1 **Internal jugular vein**
5th 900.8 **Other specified blood vessels of head and neck**
900.81 **External jugular vein**
Jugular vein NOS
900.82 **Multiple blood vessels of head and neck**
900.89 **Other**
900.9 **Unspecified blood vessel of head and neck**

4th 901 **Injury to blood vessels of thorax**
Excludes *traumatic hemothorax (860.2-860.5)*
901.0 **Thoracic aorta**
901.1 **Innominate and subclavian arteries**
901.2 **Superior vena cava**
901.3 **Innominate and subclavian veins**
5th 901.4 **Pulmonary blood vessels**
901.40 **Pulmonary vessel(s), unspecified**
901.41 **Pulmonary artery**
901.42 **Pulmonary vein**
5th 901.8 **Other specified blood vessels of thorax**
901.81 **Intercostal artery or vein**
901.82 **Internal mammary artery or vein**
901.83 **Multiple blood vessels of thorax**
901.89 **Other**
Azygos vein
Hemiazygos vein
901.9 **Unspecified blood vessel of thorax**

4th 902 **Injury to blood vessels of abdomen and pelvis**
902.0 **Abdominal aorta**
5th 902.1 **Inferior vena cava**
902.10 **Inferior vena cava, unspecified**
902.11 **Hepatic veins**
902.19 **Other**
5th 902.2 **Celiac and mesenteric arteries**
902.20 **Celiac and mesenteric arteries, unspecified**
902.21 **Gastric artery**
902.22 **Hepatic artery**
902.23 **Splenic artery**
902.24 **Other specified branches of celiac axis**
902.25 **Superior mesenteric artery (trunk)**
902.26 **Primary branches of superior mesenteric artery**
Ileo-colic artery
902.27 **Inferior mesenteric artery**
902.29 **Other**
5th 902.3 **Portal and splenic veins**
902.31 **Superior mesenteric vein and primary subdivisions**
Ileo-colic vein
902.32 **Inferior mesenteric vein**
902.33 **Portal vein**
902.34 **Splenic vein**
902.39 **Other**
Cystic vein
Gastric vein
5th 902.4 **Renal blood vessels**
902.40 **Renal vessel(s), unspecified**
902.41 **Renal artery**
902.42 **Renal vein**
902.49 **Other**
Suprarenal arteries
5th 902.5 **Iliac blood vessels**
902.50 **Iliac vessel(s), unspecified**
902.51 **Hypogastric artery**
902.52 **Hypogastric vein**
902.53 **Iliac artery**
902.54 **Iliac vein**
902.55 **Uterine artery** ♀
902.56 **Uterine vein** ♀
902.59 **Other**

5th 902.8 Other specified blood vessels of abdomen and pelvis
902.81 Ovarian artery ♀
902.82 Ovarian vein ♀
902.87 Multiple blood vessels of abdomen and pelvis
902.89 Other
902.9 Unspecified blood vessel of abdomen and pelvis

4th 903 Injury to blood vessels of upper extremity
5th 903.0 Axillary blood vessels
903.00 Axillary vessel(s), unspecified
903.01 Axillary artery
903.02 Axillary vein
903.1 Brachial blood vessels
903.2 Radial blood vessels
903.3 Ulnar blood vessels
903.4 Palmar artery
903.5 Digital blood vessels
903.8 Other specified blood vessels of upper extremity
Multiple blood vessels of upper extremity
903.9 Unspecified blood vessel of upper extremity

4th 904 Injury to blood vessels of lower extremity and unspecified sites
904.0 Common femoral artery
Femoral artery above profunda origin
904.1 Superficial femoral artery
904.2 Femoral veins
904.3 Saphenous veins
Saphenous vein (greater) (lesser)
5th 904.4 Popliteal blood vessels
904.40 Popliteal vessel(s), unspecified
904.41 Popliteal artery
904.42 Popliteal vein
5th 904.5 Tibial blood vessels
904.50 Tibial vessel(s), unspecified
904.51 Anterior tibial artery
904.52 Anterior tibial vein
904.53 Posterior tibial artery
904.54 Posterior tibial vein
904.6 Deep plantar blood vessels
904.7 Other specified blood vessels of lower extremity
Multiple blood vessels of lower extremity
904.8 Unspecified blood vessel of lower extremity
904.9 Unspecified site
Injury to blood vessel NOS

LATE EFFECTS OF INJURIES, POISONINGS, TOXIC EFFECTS, AND OTHER EXTERNAL CAUSES (905-909)

Note: *These categories are to be used to indicate conditions classifiable to 800-999 as the cause of late effects, which are themselves classified elsewhere. The "late effects" include those specified as such, or as sequelae, which may occur at any time after the acute injury.*

4th 905 Late effects of musculoskeletal and connective tissue injuries
905.0 Late effect of fracture of skull and face bones
Late effect of injury classifiable to 800-804
905.1 Late effect of fracture of spine and trunk without mention of spinal cord lesion
Late effect of injury classifiable to 805, 807-809
905.2 Late effect of fracture of upper extremities
Late effect of injury classifiable to 810-819
905.3 Late effect of fracture of neck of femur
Late effect of injury classifiable to 820
905.4 Late effect of fracture of lower extremities
Late effect of injury classifiable to 821-827
905.5 Late effect of fracture of multiple and unspecified bones
Late effect of injury classifiable to 828-829
905.6 Late effect of dislocation
Late effect of injury classifiable to 830-839
905.7 Late effect of sprain and strain without mention of tendon injury
Late effect of injury classifiable to 840-848, except tendon injury
905.8 Late effect of tendon injury
Late effect of tendon injury due to:
open wound [injury classifiable to 880-884 with .2, 890-894 with .2]
sprain and strain [injury classifiable to 840-848]
905.9 Late effect of traumatic amputation
Late effect of injury classifiable to 885-887, 895-897
Excludes *late amputation stump complication (997.60-997.69)*

4th 906 Late effects of injuries to skin and subcutaneous tissues
906.0 Late effect of open wound of head, neck, and trunk
Late effect of injury classifiable to 870-879
906.1 Late effect of open wound of extremities without mention of tendon injury
Late effect of injury classifiable to 880-884, 890-894 except .2
906.2 Late effect of superficial injury
Late effect of injury classifiable to 910-919
906.3 Late effect of contusion
Late effect of injury classifiable to 920-924
906.4 Late effect of crushing
Late effect of injury classifiable to 925-929
906.5 Late effect of burn of eye, face, head, and neck
Late effect of injury classifiable to 940-941

ICD-9-CM Official Guidelines (Chapter 17):

c. Coding of Burns

7) Encounters for treatment of late effects of burns

Encounters for the treatment of the late effects of burns (i.e., scars or joint contractures) should be coded to the residual condition (sequelae) followed by the appropriate late effect code (906.5-906.9). A late effect E code may also be used, if desired.

8) Sequelae with a late effect code and current burn

When appropriate, both a sequelae with a late effect code, and a current burn code may be assigned on the same record (when both a current burn and sequelae of an old burn exist).

906.6 Late effect of burn of wrist and hand
Late effect of injury classifiable to 944
906.7 Late effect of burn of other extremities
Late effect of injury classifiable to 943 or 945
906.8 Late effect of burns of other specified sites
Late effect of injury classifiable to 942, 946-947
906.9 Late effect of burn of unspecified site
Late effect of injury classifiable to 948-949

4th 907 Late effects of injuries to the nervous system
907.0 Late effect of intracranial injury without mention of skull fracture
Late effect of injury classifiable to 850-854
907.1 Late effect of injury to cranial nerve
Late effect of injury classifiable to 950-951
907.2 Late effect of spinal cord injury
Late effect of injury classifiable to 806, 952
907.3 Late effect of injury to nerve root(s), spinal plexus(es), and other nerves of trunk
Late effect of injury classifiable to 953-954
907.4 Late effect of injury to peripheral nerve of shoulder girdle and upper limb
Late effect of injury classifiable to 955

907.5 **Late effect of injury to peripheral nerve of pelvic girdle and lower limb**
Late effect of injury classifiable to 956

907.9 **Late effect of injury to other and unspecified nerve**
Late effect of injury classifiable to 957

4th 908 **Late effects of other and unspecified injuries**

908.0 **Late effect of internal injury to chest**
Late effect of injury classifiable to 860-862

908.1 **Late effect of internal injury to intra-abdominal organs**
Late effect of injury classifiable to 863-866, 868

908.2 **Late effect of internal injury to other internal organs**
Late effect of injury classifiable to 867 or 869

908.3 **Late effect of injury to blood vessel of head, neck, and extremities**
Late effect of injury classifiable to 900, 903-904

908.4 **Late effect of injury to blood vessel of thorax, abdomen, and pelvis**
Late effect of injury classifiable to 901-902

908.5 **Late effect of foreign body in orifice**
Late effect of injury classifiable to 930-939

908.6 **Late effect of certain complications of trauma**
Late effect of complications classifiable to 958

908.9 **Late effect of unspecified injury**
Late effect of injury classifiable to 959

4th 909 **Late effects of other and unspecified external causes**

909.0 **Late effect of poisoning due to drug, medicinal or biological substance**
Late effect of conditions classifiable to 960-979
Excludes *late effect of adverse effect of drug, medicinal or biological substance (909.5)*

909.1 **Late effect of toxic effects of nonmedical substances**
Late effect of conditions classifiable to 980-989

909.2 **Late effect of radiation**
Late effect of conditions classifiable to 990

909.3 **Late effect of complications of surgical and medical care**
Late effect of conditions classifiable to 996-999

909.4 **Late effect of certain other external causes**
Late effect of conditions classifiable to 991-994

909.5 **Late effect of adverse effect of drug, medicinal or biological substance**
Excludes *late effect of poisoning due to drug, medicinal or biological substances (909.0)*

909.9 **Late effect of other and unspecified external causes**

SUPERFICIAL INJURY (910-919)

Excludes *burn (blisters) (940.0-949.5)*
contusion (920-924.9)
foreign body:
granuloma (728.82)
inadvertently left in operative wound (998.4)
residual, in soft tissue (729.6)
insect bite, venomous (989.5)
open wound with incidental foreign body (870.0-897.7)

ICD-9-CM Official Guidelines (Chapter 17):

a. *Coding of Injuries*

1) *Superficial injuries*

Superficial injuries such as abrasions or contusions are not coded when associated with more severe injuries of the same site.

4th 910 **Superficial injury of face, neck, and scalp except eye**

Includes cheek
ear
gum
lip
nose
throat

Excludes *eye and adnexa (918.0-918.9)*

910.0 **Abrasion or friction burn without mention of infection**

910.1 **Abrasion or friction burn, infected**

910.2 **Blister without mention of infection**

910.3 **Blister, infected**

910.4 **Insect bite, nonvenomous, without mention of infection**

910.5 **Insect bite, nonvenomous, infected**

910.6 **Superficial foreign body (splinter) without major open wound and without mention of infection**

910.7 **Superficial foreign body (splinter) without major open wound, infected**

910.8 **Other and unspecified superficial injury of face, neck, and scalp without mention of infection**

910.9 **Other and unspecified superficial injury of face, neck, and scalp, infected**

4th 911 **Superficial injury of trunk**

Includes abdominal wall
anus
back
breast
buttock
chest wall
flank
groin
interscapular region
labium (majus) (minus)
penis
perineum
scrotum
testis
vagina
vulva

Excludes *hip (916.0-916.9)*
scapular region (912.0-912.9)

911.0 **Abrasion or friction burn without mention of infection**

911.1 **Abrasion or friction burn, infected**

911.2 **Blister without mention of infection**

911.3 **Blister, infected**

911.4 **Insect bite, nonvenomous, without mention of infection**

911.5 **Insect bite, nonvenomous, infected**

911.6 **Superficial foreign body (splinter) without major open wound and without mention of infection**

911.7 **Superficial foreign body (splinter) without major open wound, infected**

911.8 Other and unspecified superficial injury of trunk without mention of infection

911.9 Other and unspecified superficial injury of trunk, infected

4th 912 Superficial injury of shoulder and upper arm

Includes axilla
scapular region

912.0 Abrasion or friction burn without mention of infection

912.1 Abrasion or friction burn, infected

912.2 Blister without mention of infection

912.3 Blister, infected

912.4 Insect bite, nonvenomous, without mention of infection

912.5 Insect bite, nonvenomous, infected

912.6 Superficial foreign body (splinter) without major open wound and without mention of infection

912.7 Superficial foreign body (splinter) without major open wound, infected

912.8 Other and unspecified superficial injury of shoulder and upper arm without mention of infection

912.9 Other and unspecified superficial injury of shoulder and upper arm, infected

4th 913 Superficial injury of elbow, forearm, and wrist

913.0 Abrasion or friction burn without mention of infection

913.1 Abrasion or friction burn, infected

913.2 Blister without mention of infection

913.3 Blister, infected

913.4 Insect bite, nonvenomous, without mention of infection

913.5 Insect bite, nonvenomous, infected

913.6 Superficial foreign body (splinter) without major open wound and without mention of infection

913.7 Superficial foreign body (splinter) without major open wound, infected

913.8 Other and unspecified superficial injury of elbow, forearm, and wrist without mention of infection

913.9 Other and unspecified superficial injury of elbow, forearm, and wrist, infected

4th 914 Superficial injury of hand(s) except finger(s) alone

914.0 Abrasion or friction burn without mention of infection

914.1 Abrasion or friction burn, infected

914.2 Blister without mention of infection

914.3 Blister, infected

914.4 Insect bite, nonvenomous, without mention of infection

914.5 Insect bite, nonvenomous, infected

914.6 Superficial foreign body (splinter) without major open wound and without mention of infection

914.7 Superficial foreign body (splinter) without major open wound, infected

914.8 Other and unspecified superficial injury of hand without mention of infection

914.9 Other and unspecified superficial injury of hand, infected

4th 915 Superficial injury of finger(s)

Includes fingernail
thumb (nail)

915.0 Abrasion or friction burn without mention of infection

915.1 Abrasion or friction burn, infected

915.2 Blister without mention of infection

915.3 Blister, infected

915.4 Insect bite, nonvenomous, without mention of infection

915.5 Insect bite, nonvenomous, infected

915.6 Superficial foreign body (splinter) without major open wound and without mention of infection

915.7 Superficial foreign body (splinter) without major open wound, infected

915.8 Other and unspecified superficial injury of fingers without mention of infection

915.9 Other and unspecified superficial injury of fingers, infected

4th 916 Superficial injury of hip, thigh, leg, and ankle

916.0 Abrasion or friction burn without mention of infection

916.1 Abrasion or friction burn, infected

916.2 Blister without mention of infection

916.3 Blister, infected

916.4 Insect bite, nonvenomous, without mention of infection

916.5 Insect bite, nonvenomous, infected

916.6 Superficial foreign body (splinter) without major open wound and without mention of infection

916.7 Superficial foreign body (splinter) without major open wound, infected

916.8 Other and unspecified superficial injury of hip, thigh, leg, and ankle without mention of infection

916.9 Other and unspecified superficial injury of hip, thigh, leg, and ankle, infected

4th 917 Superficial injury of foot and toe(s)

Includes heel
toenail

917.0 Abrasion or friction burn without mention of infection

917.1 Abrasion or friction burn, infected

917.2 Blister without mention of infection

917.3 Blister, infected

917.4 Insect bite, nonvenomous, without mention of infection

917.5 Insect bite, nonvenomous, infected

917.6 Superficial foreign body (splinter) without major open wound and without mention of infection

917.7 Superficial foreign body (splinter) without major open wound, infected

917.8 Other and unspecified superficial injury of foot and toes without mention of infection

917.9 Other and unspecified superficial injury of foot and toes, infected

4th 918 Superficial injury of eye and adnexa

Excludes *burn (940.0-940.9)*
foreign body on external eye (930.0-930.9)

918.0 Eyelids and periocular area
Abrasion
Insect bite
Superficial foreign body (splinter)

918.1 Cornea
Corneal abrasion
Superficial laceration
Excludes *corneal injury due to contact lens (371.82)*

918.2 Conjunctiva

918.9 Other and unspecified superficial injuries of eye
Eye (ball) NOS

4th 919 Superficial injury of other, multiple, and unspecified sites

Excludes *multiple sites classifiable to the same three-digit category (910.0-918.9)*

919.0 Abrasion or friction burn without mention of infection

919.1 Abrasion or friction burn, infected

919.2 Blister without mention of infection

919.3 Blister, infected

919.4 Insect bite, nonvenomous, without mention of infection

919.5 Insect bite, nonvenomous, infected

919.6 Superficial foreign body (splinter) without major open wound and without mention of infection

919.7 Superficial foreign body (splinter) without major open wound, infected

919.8 Other and unspecified superficial injury without mention of infection

919.9 Other and unspecified superficial injury, infected

CONTUSION WITH INTACT SKIN SURFACE (920-924)

Includes bruise without fracture or open wound
hematoma without fracture or open wound

Excludes *concussion (850.0-850.9)*
hemarthrosis (840.0-848.9)
internal organs (860.0-869.1)
that incidental to:
crushing injury (925-929.9)
dislocation (830.0-839.9)
fracture (800.0-829.1)
internal injury (860.0-869.1)
intracranial injury (850.0-854.1)
nerve injury (950.0-957.9)
open wound (870.0-897.7)

920 Contusion of face, scalp, and neck except eye(s)
Cheek
Ear (auricle)
Gum
Lip
Mandibular joint area
Nose
Throat

4th **921 Contusion of eye and adnexa**

921.0 Black eye, NOS

921.1 Contusion of eyelids and periocular area

921.2 Contusion of orbital tissues

921.3 Contusion of eyeball

921.9 Unspecified contusion of eye
Injury of eye NOS

4th **922 Contusion of trunk**

922.0 Breast

922.1 Chest wall

922.2 Abdominal wall
Flank
Groin

5th 922.3 Back

922.31 Back
Excludes *interscapular region (922.33)*

922.32 Buttock

922.33 Interscapular region
Excludes *scapular region (923.01)*

922.4 Genital organs
Labium (majus) (minus)
Penis
Perineum
Scrotum
Testis
Vagina
Vulva

922.8 Multiple sites of trunk

922.9 Unspecified part
Trunk NOS

4th **923 Contusion of upper limb**

5th 923.0 Shoulder and upper arm

923.00 Shoulder region

923.01 Scapular region

923.02 Axillary region

923.03 Upper arm

923.09 Multiple sites

5th 923.1 Elbow and forearm

923.10 Forearm

923.11 Elbow

5th 923.2 Wrist and hand(s), except finger(s) alone

923.20 Hand(s)

923.21 Wrist

923.3 Finger
Fingernail
Thumb (nail)

923.8 Multiple sites of upper limb

923.9 Unspecified part of upper limb
Arm NOS

4th **924 Contusion of lower limb and of other and unspecified sites**

5th 924.0 Hip and thigh

924.00 Thigh

924.01 Hip

5th 924.1 Knee and lower leg

924.10 Lower leg

924.11 Knee

5th 924.2 Ankle and foot, excluding toe(s)

924.20 Foot
Heel

924.21 Ankle

924.3 Toe
Toenail

924.4 Multiple sites of lower limb

924.5 Unspecified part of lower limb
Leg NOS

924.8 Multiple sites, not elsewhere classified

924.9 Unspecified site

CRUSHING INJURY (925-929)

Use additional code to identify any associated injuries, such as:
fractures (800-829)
internal injuries (860.0-869.1)
intracranial injury (850.0-854.1)

4th **925 Crushing injury of face, scalp, and neck**
Cheek
Ear
Larynx
Pharynx
Throat

925.1 Crushing injury of face and scalp
Cheek
Ear

925.2 Crushing injury of neck
Larynx
Pharynx
Throat

4th **926 Crushing injury of trunk**

926.0 External genitalia
Labium (majus) (minus)
Penis
Scrotum
Testis
Vulva

5th 926.1 Other specified sites

926.11 Back

926.12 Buttock

926.19 Other
Breast

926.8 Multiple sites of trunk

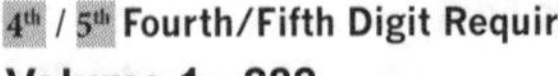

926.9 Unspecified site
Trunk NOS

4th 927 Crushing injury of upper limb

5th 927.0 Shoulder and upper arm
927.00 Shoulder region
927.01 Scapular region
927.02 Axillary region
927.03 Upper arm
927.09 Multiple sites

5th 927.1 Elbow and forearm
927.10 Forearm
927.11 Elbow

5th 927.2 Wrist and hand(s), except finger(s) alone
927.20 Hand(s)
927.21 Wrist

927.3 Finger(s)

927.8 Multiple sites of upper limb

927.9 Unspecified site
Arm NOS

4th 928 Crushing injury of lower limb

5th 928.0 Hip and thigh
928.00 Thigh
928.01 Hip

928.1 Knee and lower leg
928.10 Lower leg
928.11 Knee

928.2 Ankle and foot, excluding toe(s) alone
928.20 Foot
Heel
928.21 Ankle

928.3 Toe(s)

928.8 Multiple sites of lower limb

928.9 Unspecified site
Leg NOS

4th 929 Crushing injury of multiple and unspecified sites

929.0 Multiple sites, not elsewhere classified

929.9 Unspecified site

EFFECTS OF FOREIGN BODY ENTERING THROUGH ORIFICE (930-939)

Excludes *foreign body:*
granuloma (728.82)
inadvertently left in operative wound (998.4, 998.7)
in open wound (800-839, 851-897)
residual, in soft tissues (729.6)
superficial w/out major open wound (910-919 with .6 or .7)

4th 930 Foreign body on external eye

Excludes *foreign body in penetrating wound of:*
eyeball (871.5-871.6)
retained (old) (360.5-360.6)
ocular adnexa (870.4)
retained (old) (376.6)

930.0 Corneal foreign body

930.1 Foreign body in conjunctival sac

930.2 Foreign body in lacrimal punctum

930.8 Other and combined sites

930.9 Unspecified site
External eye NOS

931 Foreign body in ear
Auditory canal
Auricle

932 Foreign body in nose
Nasal sinus
Nostril

4th 933 Foreign body in pharynx and larynx

933.0 Pharynx
Nasopharynx
Throat NOS

933.1 Larynx
Asphyxia due to foreign body
Choking due to:
food (regurgitated)
phlegm

4th 934 Foreign body in trachea, bronchus, and lung

934.0 Trachea

934.1 Main bronchus

934.8 Other specified parts
Bronchioles
Lung

934.9 Respiratory tree, unspecified
Inhalation of liquid or vomitus, lower respiratory tract NOS

4th 935 Foreign body in mouth, esophagus, and stomach

935.0 Mouth

935.1 Esophagus

935.2 Stomach

936 Foreign body in intestine and colon

937 Foreign body in anus and rectum
Rectosigmoid (junction)

938 Foreign body in digestive system, unspecified
Alimentary tract NOS
Swallowed foreign body

4th 939 Foreign body in genitourinary tract

939.0 Bladder and urethra

939.1 Uterus, any part ♀

Excludes *intrauterine contraceptive device:*
complications from (996.32, 996.65)
presence of (V45.51)

939.2 Vulva and vagina ♀

939.3 Penis ♂

939.9 Unspecified site

BURNS (940-949)

Includes burns from:
electrical heating appliance
electricity
flame
hot object
lightning
radiation
chemical burns (external) (internal)
scalds

Excludes *friction burns (910-919 with .0, .1)*
sunburn (692.71, 692.76-692.77)

ICD-9-CM Official Guidelines (Chapter 17):

*c. **Coding of Burns***

Current burns (940-948) are classified by depth, extent and by agent (E code). Burns are classified by depth as first degree (erythema), second degree (blistering), and third degree (full-thickness involvement).

*1) **Sequencing of burn and related condition codes***

Sequence first the code that reflects the highest degree of burn when more than one burn is present.

a. When the reason for the admission or encounter is for treatment of external multiple burns, sequence first the code that reflects the burn of the highest degree.

b. When a patient has both internal and external burns, the circumstances of admission govern the selection of the principal diagnosis or first-listed diagnosis.

c. When a patient is admitted for burn injuries and other related conditions such as smoke inhalation and/or respiratory failure, the circumstances of admission govern the selection of the principal or first-listed diagnosis.

*2) **Burns of the same local site***

Classify burns of the same local site (three-digit category level, 940-947) but of different degrees to the subcategory identifying the highest degree recorded in the diagnosis.

*3) **Non-healing burns***

Non-healing burns are coded as acute burns.

Necrosis of burned skin should be coded as a non-healed burn.

*4) **Code 958.3, Posttraumatic wound infection***

Assign code 958.3, Posttraumatic wound infection, not elsewhere classified, as an additional code for any documented infected burn site.

*5) **Assign separate codes for each burn site***

When coding burns, assign separate codes for each burn site. Category 946 Burns of Multiple specified sites, should only be used if the location of the burns are not documented.

Category 949, Burn, unspecified, is extremely vague and should rarely be used.

*6) **Assign codes from category 948, Burns***

Burns classified according to extent of body surface involved, when the site of the burn is not specified or when there is a need for additional data. It is advisable to use category 948 as additional coding when needed to provide data for evaluating burn mortality, such as that needed by burn units. It is also advisable to use category 948 as an additional code for reporting purposes when there is mention of a third-degree burn involving 20 percent or more of the body surface.

In assigning a code from category 948:

- *Fourth-digit codes are used to identify the percentage of total body surface involved in a burn (all degree).*
- *Fifth-digits are assigned to identify the percentage of body surface involved in third-degree burn.*
- *Fifth-digit zero (0) is assigned when less than 10 percent or when no body surface is involved in a third-degree burn.*
- *Category 948 is based on the classic "rule of nines" in estimating body surface involved: head and neck are assigned nine percent, each arm nine percent, each leg 18 percent, the anterior trunk 18 percent, posterior trunk 18 percent, and genitalia one percent. Providers may change these percentage assignments where necessary to accommodate infants and children who have proportionately larger heads than adults and patients who have large buttocks, thighs, or abdomen that involve burns.*

*7) **Encounters for treatment of late effects of burns***

Encounters for the treatment of the late effects of burns (i.e., scars or joint contractures) should be coded to the residual condition (sequelae) followed by the appropriate late effect code (906.5-906.9). A late effect E code may also be used, if desired.

*8) **Sequelae with a late effect code and current burn***

When appropriate, both a sequelae with a late effect code, and a current burn code may be assigned on the same record (when both a current burn and sequelae of an old burn exist).

4th 940 Burn confined to eye and adnexa

940.0 Chemical burn of eyelids and periocular area

940.1 Other burns of eyelids and periocular area

940.2 Alkaline chemical burn of cornea and conjunctival sac

940.3 Acid chemical burn of cornea and conjunctival sac

940.4 Other burn of cornea and conjunctival sac

940.5 Burn with resulting rupture and destruction of eyeball

940.9 Unspecified burn of eye and adnexa

4th 941 Burn of face, head, and neck

Excludes *mouth (947.0)*

The following fifth-digit subclassification is for use with category 941:

0 face and head, unspecified site
1 ear [any part]
2 eye (with other parts of face, head, and neck)
3 lip(s)
4 chin
5 nose (septum)
6 scalp [any part]
Temple (region)
7 forehead and cheek
8 neck
9 multiple sites [except with eye] of face, head, and neck

5th 941.0 Unspecified degree
[0-9]

5th 941.1 Erythema [first degree]
[0-9]

5th 941.2 Blisters, epidermal loss [second degree]
[0-9]

5th 941.3 Full-thickness skin loss [third degree NOS]
[0-9]

5th 941.4 Deep necrosis of underlying tissues [deep third degree] without mention of loss of a body part
[0-9]

5th 941.5 Deep necrosis of underlying tissues [deep third degree] with loss of a body part
[0-9]

4th 942 Burn of trunk

Excludes *scapular region (943.0-943.5 with fifth-digit 6)*

The following fifth-digit subclassification is for use with category 942:

0 trunk, unspecified site
1 breast
2 chest wall, excluding breast and nipple
3 abdominal wall
Flank
Groin
4 back [any part]
Buttock
Interscapular region
5 genitalia
Labium (majus) (minus)
Penis
Perineum
Scrotum
Testis
Vulva
9 other and multiple sites of trunk

5th 942.0 Unspecified degree
[0-5,9]

5th 942.1 Erythema [first degree]
[0-5,9]

5th 942.2 Blisters, epidermal loss [second degree]
[0-5,9]

5th 942.3 Full-thickness skin loss [third degree NOS]
[0-5,9]

5th 942.4 Deep necrosis of underlying tissues [deep third degree] without mention of loss of a body part
[0-5,9]

5th 942.5 Deep necrosis of underlying tissues [deep third degree] with loss of a body part
[0-5,9]

4th 943 Burn of upper limb, except wrist and hand

The following fifth-digit subclassification is for use with category 943:

0 upper limb, unspecified site
1 forearm
2 elbow
3 upper arm
4 axilla
5 shoulder
6 scapular region
9 multiple sites of upper limb, except wrist and hand

5th 943.0 Unspecified degree
[0-6,9]

5th 943.1 Erythema [first degree]
[0-6,9]

5th 943.2 Blisters, epidermal loss [second degree]
[0-6,9]

5th 943.3 Full-thickness skin loss [third degree NOS]
[0-6,9]

5th 943.4 Deep necrosis of underlying tissues [deep third degree] without mention of loss of a body part
[0-6,9]

5th 943.5 Deep necrosis of underlying tissues [deep third degree] with loss of a body part
[0-6,9]

4th 944 Burn of wrist(s) and hand(s)

The following fifth-digit subclassification is for use with category 944:

0 hand, unspecified site
1 single digit [finger (nail)] other than thumb
2 thumb (nail)
3 two or more digits, not including thumb
4 two or more digits including thumb
5 palm
6 back of hand
7 wrist
8 multiple sites of wrist(s) and hand(s)

5th 944.0 Unspecified degree
[0-8]

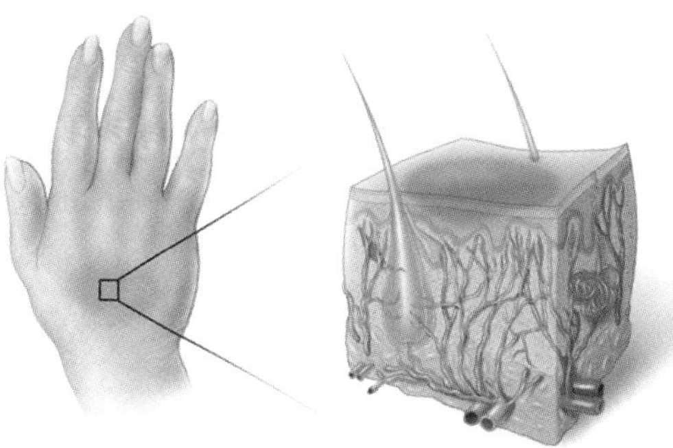

First degree burn

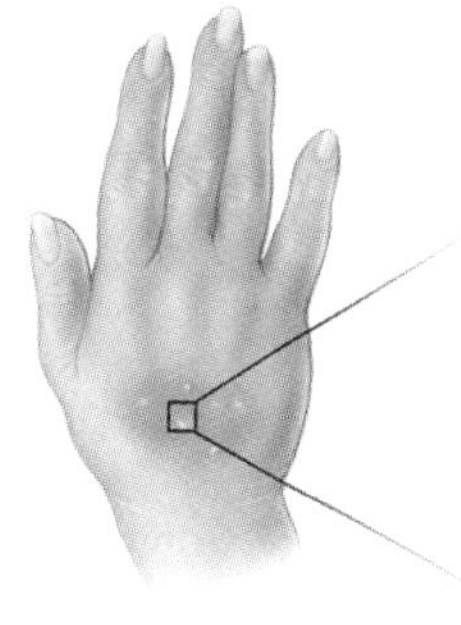

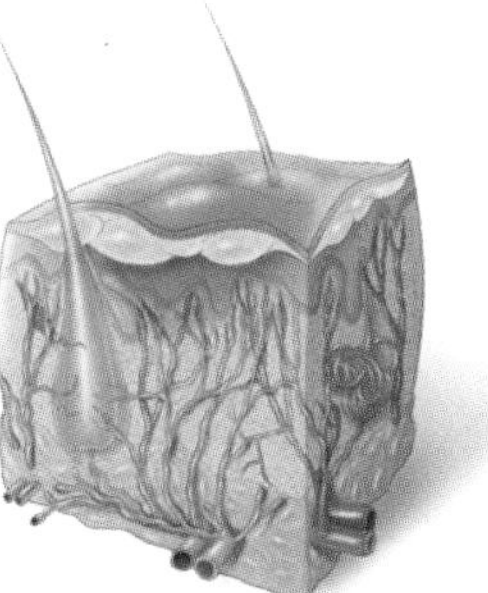

Second degree burn

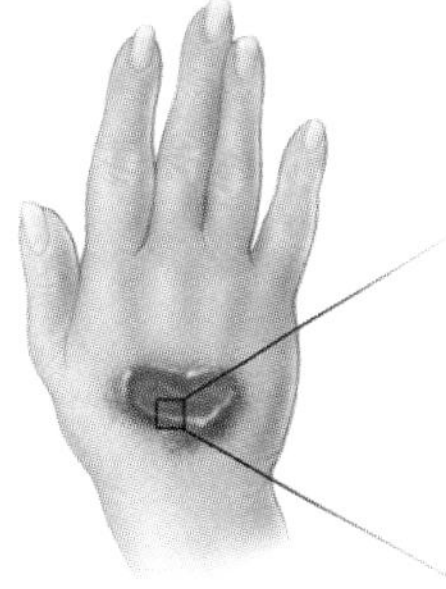

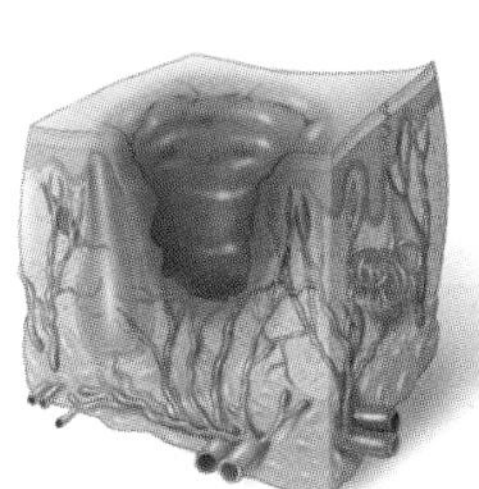

Third degree burn

© 2008 Fairman Studios, LLC. All Rights Reserved.

5th 944.1 Erythema [first degree]
[0-8]

5th 944.2 Blisters, epidermal loss [second degree]
[0-8]

5th 944.3 Full-thickness skin loss [third degree NOS]
[0-8]

5th 944.4 Deep necrosis of underlying tissues [deep third degree] without mention of loss of a body part
[0-8]

5th 944.5 Deep necrosis of underlying tissues [deep third degree] with loss of a body part
[0-8]

4th 945 Burn of lower limb(s)

The following fifth-digit subclassification is for use with category 945:

0 lower limb [leg], unspecified site
1 toe(s) (nail)
2 foot
3 ankle
4 lower leg
5 knee
6 thigh [any part]
9 multiple sites of lower limb(s)

5th 945.0 Unspecified degree
[0-6,9]

5th 945.1 Erythema [first degree]
[0-6,9]

5th 945.2 Blisters, epidermal loss [second degree]
[0-6,9]

5th 945.3 Full-thickness skin loss [third degree NOS]
[0-6,9]

5th 945.4 Deep necrosis of underlying tissues [deep third degree] without mention of loss of a body part
[0-6,9]

5th 945.5 Deep necrosis of underlying tissues [deep third degree] with loss of a body part
[0-6,9]

4th 946 Burns of multiple specified sites

Includes burns of sites classifiable to more than one three-digit category in 940-945

Excludes *multiple burns NOS (949.0-949.5)*

946.0 Unspecified degree

946.1 Erythema [first degree]

946.2 Blisters, epidermal loss [second degree]

946.3 Full-thickness skin loss [third degree NOS]

946.4 Deep necrosis of underlying tissues [deep third degree] without mention of loss of a body part

946.5 Deep necrosis of underlying tissues [deep third degree] with loss of a body part

4th 947 Burn of internal organs

Includes burns from chemical agents (ingested)

947.0 Mouth and pharynx
Gum
Tongue

947.1 Larynx, trachea, and lung

947.2 Esophagus

947.3 Gastrointestinal tract
Colon
Rectum
Small intestine
Stomach

947.4 Vagina and uterus ♀

947.8 Other specified sites

947.9 Unspecified site

4th 948 Burns classified according to extent of body surface involved

Note: *This category is to be used when the site of the burn is unspecified, or with categories 940-947 when the site is specified.*

Excludes *sunburn (692.71, 692.76-692.77)*

The following fifth-digit subclassification is for use with category 948 to indicate the percent of body surface with third degree burn; valid digits are in [brackets] under each code:

0 less than 10 percent or unspecified
1 10-19%
2 20-29%
3 30-39%
4 40-49%
5 50-59%
6 60-69%
7 70-79%
8 80-89%
9 90% or more of body surface

The "Rule of Nines"

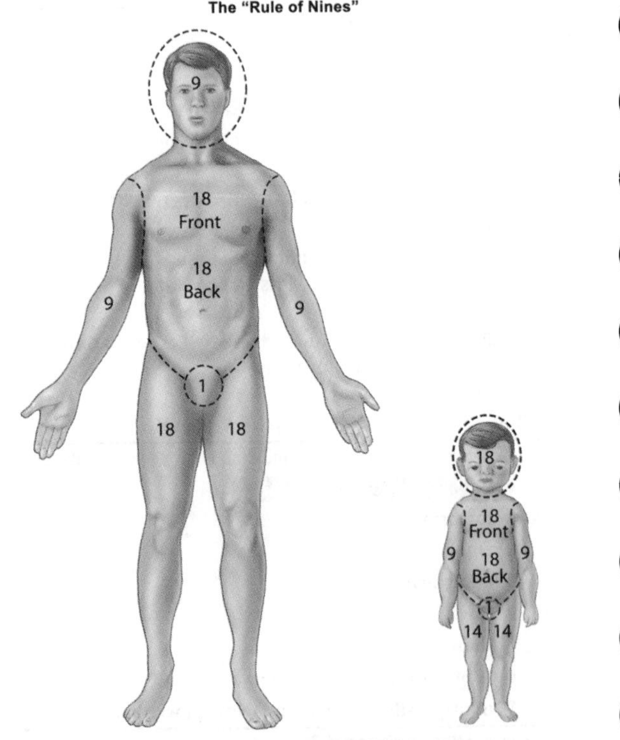

© 2008 Fairman Studios, LLC. All Rights Reserved.

ICD-9-CM Official Guidelines (Chapter 17):

c. Coding of Burns

6) Assign codes from category 948, Burns

Burns classified according to extent of body surface involved, when the site of the burn is not specified or when there is a need for additional data. It is advisable to use category 948 as additional coding when needed to provide data for evaluating burn mortality, such as that needed by burn units. It is also advisable to use category 948 as an additional code for reporting purposes when there is mention of a third-degree burn involving 20 percent or more of the body surface.

In assigning a code from category 948:

- *Fourth-digit codes are used to identify the percentage of total body surface involved in a burn (all degree).*
- *Fifth-digits are assigned to identify the percentage of body surface involved in third-degree burn.*
- *Fifth-digit zero (0) is assigned when less than 10 percent or*

when no body surface is involved in a third-degree burn.

- *Category 948 is based on the classic "rule of nines" in estimating body surface involved: head and neck are assigned nine percent, each arm nine percent, each leg 18 percent, the anterior trunk 18 percent, posterior trunk 18 percent, and genitalia one percent. Providers may change these percentage assignments where necessary to accommodate infants and children who have proportionately larger heads than adults and patients who have large buttocks, thighs, or abdomen that involve burns.*

5th **948.0 Burn [any degree] involving less than 10 percent of body surface**
[0]

5th **948.1 10-19 percent of body surface**
[0-1]

5th **948.2 20-29 percent of body surface**
[0-2]

5th **948.3 30-39 percent of body surface**
[0-3]

5th **948.4 40-49 percent of body surface**
[0-4]

5th **948.5 50-59 percent of body surface**
[0-5]

5th **948.6 60-69 percent of body surface**
[0-6]

5th **948.7 70-79 percent of body surface**
[0-7]

5th **948.8 80-89 percent of body surface**
[0-8]

5th **948.9 90 percent or more of body surface**
[0-9]

4th **949 Burn, unspecified**

Includes burn NOS
multiple burns NOS

Excludes *burn of unspecified site but with statement of the extent of body surface involved (948.0-948.9)*

949.0 Unspecified degree

949.1 Erythema [first degree]

949.2 Blisters, epidermal loss [second degree]

949.3 Full-thickness skin loss [third degree NOS]

949.4 Deep necrosis of underlying tissues [deep third degree] without mention of loss of a body part

949.5 Deep necrosis of underlying tissues [deep third degree] with loss of a body part

INJURY TO NERVES AND SPINAL CORD (950-957)

Includes division of nerve
lesion in continuity (with open wound)
traumatic neuroma (with open wound)
traumatic transient paralysis (with open wound)

Excludes *accidental puncture or laceration during medical procedure (998.2)*

ICD-9-CM Official Guidelines (Chapter 17):

a. *Coding of Injuries*

2) ***Primary injury with damage to nerves/blood vessels***

When a primary injury results in minor damage to peripheral nerves or blood vessels, the primary injury is sequenced first with additional code(s) from categories 950-957, Injury to nerves and spinal cord, and/or 900-904, Injury to blood vessels. When the primary injury is to the blood vessels or nerves, that injury should be sequenced first.

4th **950 Injury to optic nerve and pathways**

950.0 Optic nerve injury
Second cranial nerve

950.1 Injury to optic chiasm

950.2 Injury to optic pathways

950.3 Injury to visual cortex

950.9 Unspecified
Traumatic blindness NOS

4th **951 Injury to other cranial nerve(s)**

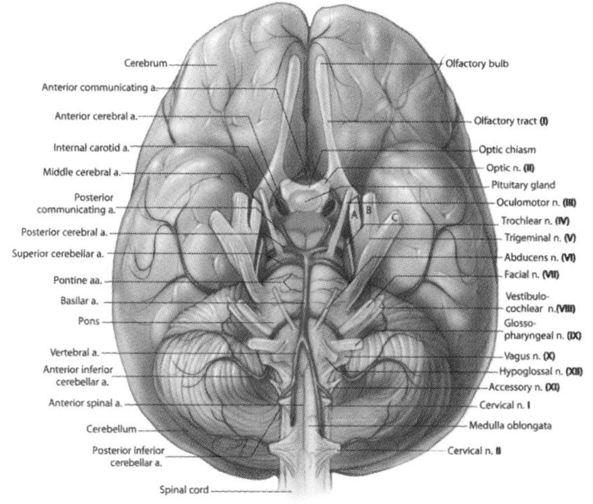

© 2008 Fairman Studios, LLC. All Rights Reserved.

951.0 Injury to oculomotor nerve
Third cranial nerve

951.1 Injury to trochlear nerve
Fourth cranial nerve

951.2 Injury to trigeminal nerve
Fifth cranial nerve

951.3 Injury to abducens nerve
Sixth cranial nerve

951.4 Injury to facial nerve
Seventh cranial nerve

951.5 Injury to acoustic nerve
Auditory nerve
Eighth cranial nerve
Traumatic deafness NOS

951.6 Injury to accessory nerve
Eleventh cranial nerve

951.7 Injury to hypoglossal nerve
Twelfth cranial nerve

951.8 Injury to other specified cranial nerves
Glossopharyngeal [9th cranial] nerve
Olfactory [1st cranial] nerve
Pneumogastric [10th cranial] nerve
Traumatic anosmia NOS
Vagus [10th cranial] nerve

951.9 Injury to unspecified cranial nerve

4th **952 Spinal cord injury without evidence of spinal bone injury**

5th **952.0 Cervical**

952.00 C_1-C_4 level with unspecified spinal cord injury
Spinal cord injury, cervical region NOS

952.01 C_1-C_4 level with complete lesion of spinal cord

952.02 C_1-C_4 level with anterior cord syndrome

952.03 C_1-C_4 level with central cord syndrome

952.04 C_1-C_4 level with other specified spinal cord injury
Incomplete spinal cord lesion at C_1-C_4 level:
NOS
with posterior cord syndrome

952.05 C_5-C_7 level with unspecified spinal cord injury

952.06 C_5-C_7 level with complete lesion of spinal cord

952.07 C_5-C_7 level with anterior cord syndrome

952.08 C_5-C_7 level with central cord syndrome

948.0 – 952.08

952.09 C_5-C_7 level with other specified spinal cord injury
Incomplete spinal cord lesion at C_5-C_7 level:
NOS
with posterior cord syndrome

5th 952.1 Dorsal [thoracic]

952.10 T_1-T_6 level with unspecified spinal cord injury
Spinal cord injury, thoracic region NOS

952.11 T_1-T_6 level with complete lesion of spinal cord

952.12 T_1-T_6 level with anterior cord syndrome

952.13 T_1-T_6 level with central cord syndrome

952.14 T_1-T_6 level with other specified spinal cord injury
Incomplete spinal cord lesion at T_1-T_6 level:
NOS
with posterior cord syndrome

952.15 T_7-T_{12} level with unspecified spinal cord injury

952.16 T_7-T_{12} level with complete lesion of spinal cord

952.17 T_7-T_{12} level with anterior cord syndrome

952.18 T_7-T_{12} level with central cord syndrome

952.19 T_7-T_{12} level with other specified spinal cord injury
Incomplete spinal cord lesion at T_7-T_{12} level:
NOS
with posterior cord syndrome

952.2 Lumbar

952.3 Sacral

952.4 Cauda equina

952.8 Multiple sites of spinal cord

952.9 Unspecified site of spinal cord

4th 953 Injury to nerve roots and spinal plexus

953.0 Cervical root

953.1 Dorsal root

953.2 Lumbar root

953.3 Sacral root

953.4 Brachial plexus

953.5 Lumbosacral plexus

953.8 Multiple sites

953.9 Unspecified site

4th 954 Injury to other nerve(s) of trunk, excluding shoulder and pelvic girdles

954.0 Cervical sympathetic

954.1 Other sympathetic
Celiac ganglion or plexus
Inferior mesenteric plexus
Splanchnic nerve(s)
Stellate ganglion

954.8 Other specified nerve(s) of trunk

954.9 Unspecified nerve of trunk

4th 955 Injury to peripheral nerve(s) of shoulder girdle and upper limb

955.0 Axillary nerve

955.1 Median nerve

955.2 Ulnar nerve

955.3 Radial nerve

955.4 Musculocutaneous nerve

955.5 Cutaneous sensory nerve, upper limb

955.6 Digital nerve

955.7 Other specified nerve(s) of shoulder girdle and upper limb

955.8 Multiple nerves of shoulder girdle and upper limb

955.9 Unspecified nerve of shoulder girdle and upper limb

4th 956 Injury to peripheral nerve(s) of pelvic girdle and lower limb

956.0 Sciatic nerve

956.1 Femoral nerve

956.2 Posterior tibial nerve

956.3 Peroneal nerve

956.4 Cutaneous sensory nerve, lower limb

956.5 Other specified nerve(s) of pelvic girdle and lower limb

956.8 Multiple nerves of pelvic girdle and lower limb

956.9 Unspecified nerve of pelvic girdle and lower limb

4th 957 Injury to other and unspecified nerves

957.0 Superficial nerves of head and neck

957.1 Other specified nerve(s)

957.8 Multiple nerves in several parts
Multiple nerve injury NOS

957.9 Unspecified site
Nerve injury NOS

CERTAIN TRAUMATIC COMPLICATIONS AND UNSPECIFIED INJURIES (958-959)

4th 958 Certain early complications of trauma

Excludes *adult respiratory distress syndrome (518.5)*
flail chest (807.4)
post-traumatic seroma (729.91)
shock lung (518.5)
that occurring during or following medical procedures (996.0-999.9)

958.0 Air embolism
Pneumathemia
Excludes *that complicating:*
abortion (634-638 with .6, 639.6)
ectopic or molar pregnancy (639.6)
pregnancy, childbirth, or the puerperium (673.0)

958.1 Fat embolism
Excludes *that complicating:*
abortion (634-638 with .6, 639.6)
pregnancy, childbirth, or the puerperium (673.8)

958.2 Secondary and recurrent hemorrhage

958.3 Posttraumatic wound infection, not elsewhere classified
Excludes *infected open wounds - code to complicated open wound of site*

ICD-9-CM Official Guidelines (Chapter 17):

c. Coding of Burns

4) Code 958.3, Posttraumatic wound infection

Assign code 958.3, Posttraumatic wound infection, not elsewhere classified, as an additional code for any documented infected burn site.

958.4 Traumatic shock
Shock (immediate) (delayed) following injury
Excludes *shock:*
anaphylactic (995.0)
due to serum (999.4)
anesthetic (995.4)
electric (994.8)
following abortion (639.5)
lightning (994.0)
nontraumatic NOS (785.50)
obstetric (669.1)
postoperative (998.0)

958.5 Traumatic anuria
Crush syndrome
Renal failure following crushing
Excludes *that due to a medical procedure (997.5)*

958.6 Volkmann's ischemic contracture
Posttraumatic muscle contracture

958.7 Traumatic subcutaneous emphysema
Excludes *subcutaneous emphysema resulting from a procedure (998.81)*

958.8 Other early complications of trauma

5th 958.9 **Traumatic compartment syndrome**

Excludes *nontraumatic compartment syndrome (729.71-729.79)*

958.90 **Compartment syndrome, unspecified**

958.91 **Traumatic compartment syndrome of upper extremity**

Traumatic compartment syndrome of shoulder, arm, forearm, wrist, hand, and fingers

958.92 **Traumatic compartment syndrome of lower extremity**

Traumatic compartment syndrome of hip, buttock, thigh, leg, foot, and toes

958.93 **Traumatic compartment syndrome of abdomen**

958.99 **Traumatic compartment syndrome of other sites**

4th 959 **Injury, other and unspecified**

Includes injury NOS

Excludes *injury NOS of:*
blood vessels (900.0-904.9)
eye (921.0-921.9)
internal organs (860.0-869.1)
intracranial sites (854.0-854.1)
nerves (950.0-951.9, 953.0-957.9)
spinal cord (952.0-952.9)

5th 959.0 **Head, face and neck**

959.01 **Head injury, unspecified**

S09.10xD Unspecified injury of muscle and tendon of head, subsequent encounter
S09.11xD Strain of muscle and tendon of head, subsequent encounter
S09.19xD Other injury of muscle and tendon of head, subsequent encounter
S09.8xxA Other specified injuries of head, initial encounter
S09.8xxD Other specified injuries of head, subsequent encounter
S09.90xA Unspecified injury of head, initial encounter
S09.90xD Unspecified injury of head, subsequent encounter

Excludes *concussion (850.0-850.9)*
with head injury NOS (850.0-850.9)
head injury NOS with loss of consciousness (850.1-850.5)
specified head injuries (850.0-854.1)

959.09 **Injury of face and neck**

5th 959.1 **Trunk**

Excludes *scapular region (959.2)*

959.11 **Other injury of chest wall**

959.12 **Other injury of abdomen**

959.13 **Fracture of corpus cavernosum penis** ♂

959.14 **Other injury of external genitals**

959.19 **Other injury of other sites of trunk**

Injury of trunk NOS

959.2 **Shoulder and upper arm**

Axilla
Scapular region

959.3 **Elbow, forearm, and wrist**

959.4 **Hand, except finger**

959.5 **Finger**

Fingernail
Thumb (nail)

959.6 **Hip and thigh**

Upper leg

959.7 **Knee, leg, ankle, and foot**

959.8 **Other specified sites, including multiple**

Excludes *multiple sites classifiable to the same four-digit category (959.0-959.7)*

959.9 **Unspecified site**

POISONING BY DRUGS, MEDICINAL AND BIOLOGICAL SUBSTANCES (960-979)

Includes overdose of these substances
wrong substance given or taken in error

Use additional code to specify the effects of the poisoning

Excludes *adverse effects ["hypersensitivity," "reaction," etc.] of correct substance properly administered. Such cases are to be classified according to the nature of the adverse effect, such as:*
adverse effect NOS (995.20)
allergic lymphadenitis (289.3)
aspirin gastritis (535.4)
blood disorders (280.0-289.9)
dermatitis:
contact (692.0-692.9)
due to ingestion (693.0-693.9)
nephropathy (583.9)
[The drug giving rise to the adverse effect may be identified by use of categories E930-E949.]
drug dependence (304.0-304.9)
drug reaction and poisoning affecting the newborn (760.0-779.9)
nondependent abuse of drugs (305.0-305.9)
pathological drug intoxication (292.2)

ICD-9-CM Official Guidelines (Chapter 17):

e. Adverse Effects, Poisoning and Toxic Effects

2) Poisoning

(a) Error was made in drug prescription

Errors made in drug prescription or in the administration of the drug by provider, nurse, patient, or other person, use the appropriate poisoning code from the 960-979 series.

(b) Overdose of a drug intentionally taken

If an overdose of a drug was intentionally taken or administered and resulted in drug toxicity, it would be coded as a poisoning (960-979 series).

(c) Nonprescribed drug taken with correctly prescribed and properly administered drug

If a nonprescribed drug or medicinal agent was taken in combination with a correctly prescribed and properly administered drug, any drug toxicity or other reaction resulting from the interaction of the two drugs would be classified as a poisoning.

(d) Sequencing of poisoning

When coding a poisoning or reaction to the improper use of a medication (e.g., wrong dose, wrong substance, wrong route of administration) the poisoning code is sequenced first, followed by a code for the manifestation. If there is also a diagnosis of drug abuse or dependence to the substance, the abuse or dependence is coded as an additional code.

See Section I.C.3.a.6.b. if poisoning is the result of insulin pump malfunctions and Section I.C.19 for general use of E-codes.

4th 960 **Poisoning by antibiotics**

Excludes *antibiotics:*
ear, nose, and throat (976.6)
eye (976.5)
local (976.0)

960.0 **Penicillins**

Ampicillin
Carbenicillin
Cloxacillin
Penicillin G

960.1 Antifungal antibiotics
Amphotericin B
Griseofulvin
Nystatin
Trichomycin
Excludes *preparations intended for topical use (976.0-976.9)*

960.2 Chloramphenicol group
Chloramphenicol
Thiamphenicol

960.3 Erythromycin and other macrolides
Oleandomycin
Spiramycin

960.4 Tetracycline group
Doxycycline
Minocycline
Oxytetracycline

960.5 Cephalosporin group
Cephalexin
Cephaloglycin
Cephaloridine
Cephalothin

960.6 Antimycobacterial antibiotics
Cycloserine
Kanamycin
Rifampin
Streptomycin

960.7 Antineoplastic antibiotics
Actinomycin such as:
Bleomycin
Cactinomycin
Dactinomycin
Daunorubicin
Mitomycin

960.8 Other specified antibiotics

960.9 Unspecified antibiotic

4th **961 Poisoning by other anti-infectives**
Excludes *anti-infectives:*
ear, nose, and throat (976.6)
eye (976.5)
local (976.0)

961.0 Sulfonamides
Sulfadiazine
Sulfafurazole
Sulfamethoxazole

961.1 Arsenical anti-infectives

961.2 Heavy metal anti-infectives
Compounds of:
antimony
bismuth
lead
mercury
Excludes *mercurial diuretics (974.0)*

961.3 Quinoline and hydroxyquinoline derivatives
Chiniofon
Diiodohydroxyquin
Excludes *antimalarial drugs (961.4)*

961.4 Antimalarials and drugs acting on other blood protozoa
Chloroquine
Cycloguanil
Primaquine
Proguanil [chloroguanide]
Pyrimethamine
Quinine

961.5 Other antiprotozoal drugs
Emetine

961.6 Anthelmintics
Hexylresorcinol
Piperazine
Thiabendazole

961.7 Antiviral drugs
Methisazone
Excludes *amantadine (966.4)*
cytarabine (963.1)
idoxuridine (976.5)

961.8 Other antimycobacterial drugs
Ethambutol
Ethionamide
Isoniazid
Para-aminosalicylic acid derivatives
Sulfones

961.9 Other and unspecified anti-infectives
Flucytosine
Nitrofuran derivatives

4th **962 Poisoning by hormones and synthetic substitutes**
Excludes *oxytocic hormones (975.0)*

962.0 Adrenal cortical steroids
Cortisone derivatives
Desoxycorticosterone derivatives
Fluorinated corticosteroids

962.1 Androgens and anabolic congeners
Methandriol
Nandrolone
Oxymetholone
Testosterone

962.2 Ovarian hormones and synthetic substitutes
Contraceptives, oral
Estrogens
Estrogens and progestogens, combined
Progestogens

962.3 Insulins and antidiabetic agents
Acetohexamide
Biguanide derivatives, oral
Chlorpropamide
Glucagon
Insulin
Phenformin
Sulfonylurea derivatives, oral
Tolbutamide

962.4 Anterior pituitary hormones
Corticotropin
Gonadotropin
Somatotropin [growth hormone]

962.5 Posterior pituitary hormones
Vasopressin
Excludes *oxytocic hormones (975.0)*

962.6 Parathyroid and parathyroid derivatives

962.7 Thyroid and thyroid derivatives
Dextrothyroxin
Levothyroxine sodium
Liothyronine
Thyroglobulin

962.8 Antithyroid agents
Iodides
Thiouracil
Thiourea

962.9 Other and unspecified hormones and synthetic substitutes

4th 963 **Poisoning by primarily systemic agents**

963.0 **Antiallergic and antiemetic drugs**
Antihistamines
Chlorpheniramine
Diphenhydramine
Diphenylpyraline
Thonzylamine
Tripelennamine
Excludes *phenothiazine-based tranquilizers (969.1)*

963.1 **Antineoplastic and immunosuppressive drugs**
Azathioprine
Busulfan
Chlorambucil
Cyclophosphamide
Cytarabine
Fluorouracil
Mercaptopurine
thio-TEPA
Excludes *antineoplastic antibiotics (960.7)*

963.2 **Acidifying agents**

963.3 **Alkalizing agents**

963.4 **Enzymes, not elsewhere classified**
Penicillinase

963.5 **Vitamins, not elsewhere classified**
Vitamin A
Vitamin D
Excludes *nicotinic acid (972.2)*
vitamin K (964.3)

963.8 **Other specified systemic agents**
Heavy metal antagonists

963.9 **Unspecified systemic agent**

4th 964 **Poisoning by agents primarily affecting blood constituents**

964.0 **Iron and its compounds**
Ferric salts
Ferrous sulfate and other ferrous salts

964.1 **Liver preparations and other antianemic agents**
Folic acid

964.2 **Anticoagulants**
Coumarin
Heparin
Phenindione
Warfarin sodium

964.3 **Vitamin K [phytonadione]**

964.4 **Fibrinolysis-affecting drugs**
Aminocaproic acid
Streptodornase
Streptokinase
Urokinase

964.5 **Anticoagulant antagonists and other coagulants**
Hexadimethrine
Protamine sulfate

964.6 **Gamma globulin**

964.7 **Natural blood and blood products**
Blood plasma
Human fibrinogen
Packed red cells
Whole blood
Excludes *transfusion reactions (999.4-999.8)*

964.8 **Other specified agents affecting blood constituents**
Macromolecular blood substitutes
Plasma expanders

964.9 **Unspecified agents affecting blood constituents**

4th 965 **Poisoning by analgesics, antipyretics, and antirheumatics**
Use additional code to identify:
drug dependence (304.0-304.9)
nondependent abuse (305.0-305.9)

5th 965.0 **Opiates and related narcotics**

965.00 **Opium (alkaloids), unspecified**

965.01 **Heroin**
Diacetylmorphine

965.02 **Methadone**

965.09 **Other**
Codeine [methylmorphine]
Meperidine [pethidine]
Morphine

965.1 **Salicylates**
Acetylsalicylic acid [aspirin]
Salicylic acid salts

965.4 **Aromatic analgesics, not elsewhere classified**
Acetanilid
Paracetamol [acetaminophen]
Phenacetin [acetophenetidin]

965.5 **Pyrazole derivatives**
Aminophenazone [aminopyrine]
Phenylbutazone

5th 965.6 **Antirheumatics [antiphlogistics]**
Excludes *salicylates (965.1)*
steroids (962.0-962.9)

965.61 **Propionic acid derivatives**
Fenoprofen
Flurbiprofen
Ibuprofen
Ketoprofen
Naproxen
Oxaprozin

965.69 **Other antirheumatics**
Gold salts
Indomethacin

965.7 **Other non-narcotic analgesics**
Pyrabital

965.8 **Other specified analgesics and antipyretics**
Pentazocine

965.9 **Unspecified analgesic and antipyretic**

4th 966 **Poisoning by anticonvulsants and anti-Parkinsonism drugs**

966.0 **Oxazolidine derivatives**
Paramethadione
Trimethadione

966.1 **Hydantoin derivatives**
Phenytoin

966.2 **Succinimides**
Ethosuximide
Phensuximide

966.3 **Other and unspecified anticonvulsants**
Primidone
Excludes *barbiturates (967.0)*
sulfonamides (961.0)

966.4 **Anti-Parkinsonism drugs**
Amantadine
Ethopropazine [profenamine]
Levodopa [L-dopa]

4th 967 **Poisoning by sedatives and hypnotics**
Use additional code to identify:
drug dependence (304.0-304.9)
nondependent abuse (305.0-305.9)

967.0 **Barbiturates**
Amobarbital [amylobarbitone]
Barbital [barbitone]
Butabarbital [butabarbitone]
Pentobarbital [pentobarbitone]
Phenobarbital [phenobarbitone]
Secobarbital [quinalbarbitone]
Excludes *thiobarbiturate anesthetics (968.3)*

967.1 **Chloral hydrate group**

967.2 **Paraldehyde**

967.3 **Bromine compounds**
Bromide
Carbromal (derivatives)

967.4 **Methaqualone compounds**

967.5 **Glutethimide group**

967.6 **Mixed sedatives, not elsewhere classified**

967.8 **Other sedatives and hypnotics**

967.9 **Unspecified sedative or hypnotic**
Sleeping:
drug NOS
pill NOS
tablet NOS

4th 968 **Poisoning by other central nervous system depressants and anesthetics**
Use additional code to identify:
drug dependence (304.0-304.9)
nondependent abuse (305.0-305.9)

968.0 **Central nervous system muscle-tone depressants**
Chlorphenesin (carbamate)
Mephenesin
Methocarbamol

968.1 **Halothane**

968.2 **Other gaseous anesthetics**
Ether
Halogenated hydrocarbon derivatives, except halothane
Nitrous oxide

968.3 **Intravenous anesthetics**
Ketamine
Methohexital [methohexitone]
Thiobarbiturates, such as thiopental sodium

968.4 **Other and unspecified general anesthetics**

968.5 **Surface [topical] and infiltration anesthetics**
Cocaine
Lidocaine [lignocaine]
Procaine
Tetracaine

968.6 **Peripheral nerve- and plexus-blocking anesthetics**

968.7 **Spinal anesthetics**

968.9 **Other and unspecified local anesthetics**

4th 969 **Poisoning by psychotropic agents**
Use additional code to identify:
drug dependence (304.0-304.9)
nondependent abuse (305.0-305.9)

5th 969.0 **Antidepressants**
~~Amitriptyline~~
~~Imipramine~~
~~Monoamine oxidase [MAO] inhibitors~~

Rationale: *Prior to 2010, poisoning by antidepressants had a single code, 969.0. All classes of antidepressants were grouped together at this code. This limited the utility of hospital discharge data to identify the substance responsible for the overdose. The Poison Workgroup of the State and Territorial Injury Prevention Directors Association requested that code 969.0 be expanded to provide a code for each of the 7 current classes of antidepressants.*

● 969.00 **Antidepressant, unspecified**

● 969.01 **Monoamine oxidase inhibitors**
MAOI

● 969.02 **Selective serotonin and norepinephrine reuptake inhibitors**
SSNRI antidepressants

● 969.03 **Selective serotonin reuptake inhibitors**
SSRI antidepressants

● 969.04 **Tetracyclic antidepressants**

● 969.05 **Tricyclic antidepressants**

● 969.09 **Other antidepressants**

969.1 **Phenothiazine-based tranquilizers**
Chlorpromazine
Fluphenazine
Prochlorperazine
Promazine

969.2 **Butyrophenone-based tranquilizers**
Haloperidol
Spiperone
Trifluperidol

969.3 **Other antipsychotics, neuroleptics, and major tranquilizers**

969.4 **Benzodiazepine-based tranquilizers**
Chlordiazepoxide
Diazepam
Flurazepam
Lorazepam
Medazepam
Nitrazepam

969.5 **Other tranquilizers**
Hydroxyzine
Meprobamate

969.6 **Psychodysleptics [hallucinogens]**
Cannabis (derivatives)
Lysergide [LSD]
Marihuana (derivatives)
Mescaline
Psilocin
Psilocybin

5th 969.7 **Psychostimulants**
~~Amphetamine~~
~~Caffeine~~
Excludes *central appetite depressants (977.0)*

Rationale: *Similar to code 969.0, caffeine and amphetamines were grouped together under code 969.7, "Poisoning by psychostimulants." Code 969.7 has been expanded to allow for the separation of caffeine from the other psychostimulants.*

● 969.70 **Psychostimulant, unspecified**

● 969.71 **Caffeine**

● 969.72 **Amphetamines**
Methamphetamines

● 969.73 Methylphenidate

● 969.79 Other psychostimulants

969.8 Other specified psychotropic agents

969.9 Unspecified psychotropic agent

4th 970 Poisoning by central nervous system stimulants

970.0 Analeptics
- Lobeline
- Nikethamide

970.1 Opiate antagonists
- Levallorphan
- Nalorphine
- Naloxone

970.8 Other specified central nervous system stimulants

970.9 Unspecified central nervous system stimulant

4th 971 Poisoning by drugs primarily affecting the autonomic nervous system

971.0 Parasympathomimetics [cholinergics]
- Acetylcholine
- Anticholinesterase:
  - organophosphorus
  - reversible
- Pilocarpine

971.1 Parasympatholytics [anticholinergics and antimuscarinics] and spasmolytics
- Atropine
- Homatropine
- Hyoscine [scopolamine]
- Quaternary ammonium derivatives

Excludes *papaverine (972.5)*

971.2 Sympathomimetics [adrenergics]
- Epinephrine [adrenalin]
- Levarterenol [noradrenalin]

971.3 Sympatholytics [antiadrenergics]
- Phenoxybenzamine
- Tolazoline hydrochloride

971.9 Unspecified drug primarily affecting autonomic nervous system

4th 972 Poisoning by agents primarily affecting the cardiovascular system

972.0 Cardiac rhythm regulators
- Practolol
- Procainamide
- Propranolol
- Quinidine

Excludes *lidocaine (968.5)*

972.1 Cardiotonic glycosides and drugs of similar action
- Digitalis glycosides
- Digoxin
- Strophanthins

972.2 Antilipemic and antiarteriosclerotic drugs
- Clofibrate
- Nicotinic acid derivatives

972.3 Ganglion-blocking agents
- Pentamethonium bromide

972.4 Coronary vasodilators
- Dipyridamole
- Nitrates [nitroglycerin]
- Nitrites

972.5 Other vasodilators
- Cyclandelate
- Diazoxide
- Papaverine

Excludes *nicotinic acid (972.2)*

972.6 Other antihypertensive agents
- Clonidine
- Guanethidine
- Rauwolfia alkaloids
- Reserpine

972.7 Antivaricose drugs, including sclerosing agents
- Sodium morrhuate
- Zinc salts

972.8 Capillary-active drugs
- Adrenochrome derivatives
- Metaraminol

972.9 Other and unspecified agents primarily affecting the cardiovascular system

4th 973 Poisoning by agents primarily affecting the gastrointestinal system

973.0 Antacids and antigastric secretion drugs
- Aluminum hydroxide
- Magnesium trisilicate

973.1 Irritant cathartics
- Bisacodyl
- Castor oil
- Phenolphthalein

973.2 Emollient cathartics
- Dioctyl sulfosuccinates

973.3 Other cathartics, including intestinal atonia drugs
- Magnesium sulfate

973.4 Digestants
- Pancreatin
- Papain
- Pepsin

973.5 Antidiarrheal drugs
- Kaolin
- Pectin

Excludes *anti-infectives (960.0-961.9)*

973.6 Emetics

973.8 Other specified agents primarily affecting the gastrointestinal system

973.9 Unspecified agent primarily affecting the gastrointestinal system

4th 974 Poisoning by water, mineral, and uric acid metabolism drugs

974.0 Mercurial diuretics
- Chlormerodrin
- Mercaptomerin
- Mersalyl

974.1 Purine derivative diuretics
- Theobromine
- Theophylline

Excludes *aminophylline [theophylline ethylenediamine] (975.7)*
caffeine (969.71)

974.2 Carbonic acid anhydrase inhibitors
- Acetazolamide

974.3 Saluretics
- Benzothiadiazides
- Chlorothiazide group

974.4 Other diuretics
- Ethacrynic acid
- Furosemide

974.5 Electrolytic, caloric, and water-balance agents

974.6 Other mineral salts, not elsewhere classified

974.7 Uric acid metabolism drugs
- Allopurinol
- Colchicine
- Probenecid

969.73 – 974.7

4th 975 **Poisoning by agents primarily acting on the smooth and skeletal muscles and respiratory system**

975.0 **Oxytocic agents**
Ergot alkaloids
Oxytocin
Prostaglandins

975.1 **Smooth muscle relaxants**
Adiphenine
Metaproterenol [orciprenaline]
Excludes *papaverine (972.5)*

975.2 **Skeletal muscle relaxants**

975.3 **Other and unspecified drugs acting on muscles**

975.4 **Antitussives**
Dextromethorphan
Pipazethate

975.5 **Expectorants**
Acetylcysteine
Guaifenesin
Terpin hydrate

975.6 **Anti-common cold drugs**

975.7 **Antiasthmatics**
Aminophylline [theophylline ethylenediamine]

975.8 **Other and unspecified respiratory drugs**

4th 976 **Poisoning by agents primarily affecting skin and mucous membrane, ophthalmological, otorhinolaryngological, and dental drugs**

976.0 **Local anti-infectives and anti-inflammatory drugs**

976.1 **Antipruritics**

976.2 **Local astringents and local detergents**

976.3 **Emollients, demulcents, and protectants**

976.4 **Keratolytics, keratoplastics, other hair treatment drugs and preparations**

976.5 **Eye anti-infectives and other eye drugs**
Idoxuridine

976.6 **Anti-infectives and other drugs and preparations for ear, nose, and throat**

976.7 **Dental drugs topically applied**
Excludes *anti-infectives (976.0)*
local anesthetics (968.5)

976.8 **Other agents primarily affecting skin and mucous membrane**
Spermicides [vaginal contraceptives]

976.9 **Unspecified agent primarily affecting skin and mucous membrane**

4th 977 **Poisoning by other and unspecified drugs and medicinal substances**

977.0 **Dietetics**
Central appetite depressants

977.1 **Lipotropic drugs**

977.2 **Antidotes and chelating agents, not elsewhere classified**

977.3 **Alcohol deterrents**

977.4 **Pharmaceutical excipients**
Pharmaceutical adjuncts

977.8 **Other specified drugs and medicinal substances**
Contrast media used for diagnostic x-ray procedures
Diagnostic agents and kits

977.9 **Unspecified drug or medicinal substance**

4th 978 **Poisoning by bacterial vaccines**

978.0 **BCG**

978.1 **Typhoid and paratyphoid**

978.2 **Cholera**

978.3 **Plague**

978.4 **Tetanus**

978.5 **Diphtheria**

978.6 **Pertussis vaccine, including combinations with a pertussis component**

978.8 **Other and unspecified bacterial vaccines**

978.9 **Mixed bacterial vaccines, except combinations with a pertussis component**

4th 979 **Poisoning by other vaccines and biological substances**
Excludes *gamma globulin (964.6)*

979.0 **Smallpox vaccine**

979.1 **Rabies vaccine**

979.2 **Typhus vaccine**

979.3 **Yellow fever vaccine**

979.4 **Measles vaccine**

979.5 **Poliomyelitis vaccine**

979.6 **Other and unspecified viral and rickettsial vaccines**
Mumps vaccine

979.7 **Mixed viral-rickettsial and bacterial vaccines, except combinations with a pertussis component**
Excludes *combinations with a pertussis component (978.6)*

979.9 **Other and unspecified vaccines and biological substances**

TOXIC EFFECTS OF SUBSTANCES CHIEFLY NONMEDICINAL AS TO SOURCE (980-989)

Excludes *burns from chemical agents (ingested) (947.0-947.9)*
localized toxic effects indexed elsewhere (001.0-799.9)
respiratory conditions due to external agents (506.0-508.9)

Use additional code to specify the nature of the toxic effect

ICD-9-CM Official Guidelines (Chapter 17):

e. Adverse Effects, Poisoning and Toxic Effects

3) Toxic Effects

(a) Toxic effect codes

When a harmful substance is ingested or comes in contact with a person, this is classified as a toxic effect. The toxic effect codes are in categories 980-989.

(b) Sequencing toxic effect codes

A toxic effect code should be sequenced first, followed by the code(s) that identify the result of the toxic effect.

(c) External cause codes for toxic effects

An external cause code from categories E860-E869 for accidental exposure, codes E950.6 or E950.7 for intentional self-harm, category E962 for assault, or categories E980-E982, for undetermined, should also be assigned to indicate intent.

4th 980 **Toxic effect of alcohol**

980.0 **Ethyl alcohol**
Denatured alcohol
Ethanol
Grain alcohol
Use additional code to identify any associated:
acute alcohol intoxication (305.0)
in alcoholism (303.0)
drunkenness (simple) (305.0)
pathological (291.4)

980.1 **Methyl alcohol**
Methanol
Wood alcohol

980.2 **Isopropyl alcohol**
Dimethyl carbinol
Isopropanol
Rubbing alcohol

980.3 **Fusel oil**
Alcohol:
amyl
butyl
propyl

980.8 **Other specified alcohols**

980.9 **Unspecified alcohol**

981 Toxic effect of petroleum products
Benzine
Gasoline
Kerosene
Paraffin wax
Petroleum:
ether
naphtha
spirit

4th **982 Toxic effect of solvents other than petroleum based**

982.0 **Benzene and homologues**

982.1 **Carbon tetrachloride**

982.2 **Carbon disulfide**
Carbon bisulfide

982.3 **Other chlorinated hydrocarbon solvents**
Tetrachloroethylene
Trichloroethylene
Excludes *chlorinated hydrocarbon preparations other than solvents (989.2)*

982.4 **Nitroglycol**

982.8 **Other nonpetroleum-based solvents**
Acetone

4th **983 Toxic effect of corrosive aromatics, acids, and caustic alkalis**

983.0 **Corrosive aromatics**
Carbolic acid or phenol
Cresol

983.1 **Acids**
Acid:
hydrochloric
nitric
sulfuric

983.2 **Caustic alkalis**
Lye
Potassium hydroxide
Sodium hydroxide

983.9 **Caustic, unspecified**

4th **984 Toxic effect of lead and its compounds (including fumes)**
Includes that from all sources except medicinal substances

984.0 **Inorganic lead compounds**
Lead dioxide
Lead salts

984.1 **Organic lead compounds**
Lead acetate
Tetraethyl lead

984.8 **Other lead compounds**

984.9 **Unspecified lead compound**

4th **985 Toxic effect of other metals**
Includes that from all sources except medicinal substances

985.0 **Mercury and its compounds**
Minamata disease

985.1 **Arsenic and its compounds**

985.2 **Manganese and its compounds**

985.3 **Beryllium and its compounds**

985.4 **Antimony and its compounds**

985.5 **Cadmium and its compounds**

985.6 **Chromium**

985.8 **Other specified metals**
Brass fumes
Copper salts
Iron compounds
Nickel compounds

985.9 **Unspecified metal**

986 Toxic effect of carbon monoxide

4th **987 Toxic effect of other gases, fumes, or vapors**

987.0 **Liquefied petroleum gases**
Butane
Propane

987.1 **Other hydrocarbon gas**

987.2 **Nitrogen oxides**
Nitrogen dioxide
Nitrous fumes

987.3 **Sulfur dioxide**

987.4 **Freon**
Dichloromonofluoromethane

987.5 **Lacrimogenic gas**
Bromobenzyl cyanide
Chloroacetophenone
Ethyliodoacetate

987.6 **Chlorine gas**

987.7 **Hydrocyanic acid gas**

987.8 **Other specified gases, fumes, or vapors**
Phosgene
Polyester fumes

987.9 **Unspecified gas, fume, or vapor**

4th **988 Toxic effect of noxious substances eaten as food**
Excludes *allergic reaction to food, such as:*
gastroenteritis (558.3)
rash (692.5, 693.1)
food poisoning (bacterial) (005.0-005.9)
toxic effects of food contaminants, such as:
aflatoxin and other mycotoxin (989.7)
mercury (985.0)

988.0 **Fish and shellfish**

988.1 **Mushrooms**

988.2 **Berries and other plants**

988.8 **Other specified noxious substances eaten as food**

988.9 **Unspecified noxious substance eaten as food**

4th **989 Toxic effect of other substances, chiefly nonmedicinal as to source**

989.0 **Hydrocyanic acid and cyanides**
Potassium cyanide
Sodium cyanide
Excludes *gas and fumes (987.7)*

989.1 **Strychnine and salts**

989.2 **Chlorinated hydrocarbons**
Aldrin
Chlordane
DDT
Dieldrin
Excludes *chlorinated hydrocarbon solvents (982.0-982.3)*

989.3 **Organophosphate and carbamate**
Carbaryl
Dichlorvos
Malathion
Parathion
Phorate
Phosdrin

989.4 **Other pesticides, not elsewhere classified**
Mixtures of insecticides

989.5 **Venom**
Bites of venomous snakes, lizards, and spiders
Tick paralysis

989.6 **Soaps and detergents**

989.7 **Aflatoxin and other mycotoxin [food contaminants]**

980.8 – 989.7

5th 989.8 **Other substances, chiefly nonmedicinal as to source**

989.81 **Asbestos**

Excludes *asbestosis (501)*
exposure to asbestos (V15.84)

989.82 **Latex**

989.83 **Silicone**

Excludes *silicone used in medical devices, implants and grafts (996.00-996.79)*

989.84 **Tobacco**

989.89 **Other**

989.9 **Unspecified substance, chiefly nonmedicinal as to source**

OTHER AND UNSPECIFIED EFFECTS OF EXTERNAL CAUSES (990-995)

990 **Effects of radiation, unspecified**

Complication of:
phototherapy
radiation therapy
Radiation sickness

Excludes *specified adverse effects of radiation. Such conditions are to be classified according to the nature of the adverse effect, as:*
burns (940.0-949.5)
dermatitis (692.7-692.8)
leukemia (204.0-208.9)
pneumonia (508.0)
sunburn (692.71, 692.76-692.77)
[The type of radiation giving rise to the adverse effect may be identified by use of the E codes.]

4th 991 **Effects of reduced temperature**

991.0 **Frostbite of face**

991.1 **Frostbite of hand**

991.2 **Frostbite of foot**

991.3 **Frostbite of other and unspecified sites**

991.4 **Immersion foot**

Trench foot

991.5 **Chilblains**

Erythema pernio
Perniosis

991.6 **Hypothermia**

Hypothermia (accidental)

Excludes *hypothermia following anesthesia (995.89)*
hypothermia not associated with low environmental temperature (780.65)

991.8 **Other specified effects of reduced temperature**

991.9 **Unspecified effect of reduced temperature**

Effects of freezing or excessive cold NOS

4th 992 **Effects of heat and light**

Excludes *burns (940.0-949.5)*
diseases of sweat glands due to heat (705.0-705.9)
malignant hyperpyrexia following anesthesia (995.86)
sunburn (692.71, 692.76-692.77)

992.0 **Heat stroke and sunstroke**

Heat apoplexy
Heat pyrexia
Ictus solaris
Siriasis
Thermoplegia

992.1 **Heat syncope**

Heat collapse

992.2 **Heat cramps**

992.3 **Heat exhaustion, anhydrotic**

Heat prostration due to water depletion

Excludes *that associated with salt depletion (992.4)*

992.4 **Heat exhaustion due to salt depletion**

Heat prostration due to salt (and water) depletion

992.5 **Heat exhaustion, unspecified**

Heat prostration NOS

992.6 **Heat fatigue, transient**

992.7 **Heat edema**

992.8 **Other specified heat effects**

992.9 **Unspecified**

4th 993 **Effects of air pressure**

993.0 **Barotrauma, otitic**

Aero-otitis media
Effects of high altitude on ears

993.1 **Barotrauma, sinus**

Aerosinusitis
Effects of high altitude on sinuses

993.2 **Other and unspecified effects of high altitude**

Alpine sickness
Andes disease
Anoxia due to high altitude
Hypobaropathy
Mountain sickness

993.3 **Caisson disease**

Bends
Compressed-air disease
Decompression sickness
Divers' palsy or paralysis

993.4 **Effects of air pressure caused by explosion**

993.8 **Other specified effects of air pressure**

993.9 **Unspecified effect of air pressure**

4th 994 **Effects of other external causes**

Excludes *certain adverse effects not elsewhere classified (995.0-995.8)*

994.0 **Effects of lightning**

Shock from lightning
Struck by lightning NOS

Excludes *burns (940.0-949.5)*

994.1 **Drowning and nonfatal submersion**

Bathing cramp
Immersion

994.2 **Effects of hunger**

Deprivation of food
Starvation

994.3 **Effects of thirst**

Deprivation of water

994.4 **Exhaustion due to exposure**

994.5 **Exhaustion due to excessive exertion**

Exhaustion due to overexertion

994.6 **Motion sickness**

Air sickness
Seasickness
Travel sickness

994.7 **Asphyxiation and strangulation**

Suffocation (by):
bedclothes
cave-in
constriction
mechanical
plastic bag
pressure
strangulation

Excludes *asphyxia from:*
carbon monoxide (986)
inhalation of food or foreign body (932-934.9)
other gases, fumes, and vapors (987.0-987.9)

989.8 – 994.7

994.8 Electrocution and nonfatal effects of electric current
Shock from electric current
Shock from electroshock gun (taser)
Excludes *electric burns (940.0-949.5)*

994.9 Other effects of external causes
Effects of:
abnormal gravitational [G] forces or states
weightlessness

4th 995 Certain adverse effects not elsewhere classified
Excludes *complications of surgical and medical care (996.0-999.9)*

995.0 Other anaphylactic shock
Allergic shock NOS or due to adverse effect of correct medicinal substance properly administered
Anaphylactic reaction NOS or due to adverse effect of correct medicinal substance properly administered
Anaphylaxis NOS or due to adverse effect of correct medicinal substance properly administered
Use additional E code to identify external cause, such as:
adverse effects of correct medicinal substance properly administered [E930-E949]
Excludes *anaphylactic reaction to serum (999.4)*
anaphylactic shock due to adverse food reaction (995.60-995.69)

995.1 Angioneurotic edema
Giant urticaria
Excludes *urticaria:*
due to serum (999.5)
other specified (698.2, 708.0-708.9, 757.33)

5th 995.2 Other and unspecified adverse effect of drug, medicinal and biological substance (due) to correct medicinal substance properly administered
Adverse effect to correct medicinal substance properly administered
Allergic reaction to correct medicinal substance properly administered
Drug:
hypersensitivity NOS
reaction NOS
Hypersensitivity to correct medicinal substance properly administered
Idiosyncrasy due to correct medicinal substance properly administered
Excludes *pathological drug intoxication (292.2)*

ICD-9-CM Official Guidelines (Chapter 17):

e. Adverse Effects, Poisoning and Toxic Effects

The properties of certain drugs, medicinal and biological substances or combinations of such substances, may cause toxic reactions. The occurrence of drug toxicity is classified in ICD-9-CM as follows:

1) Adverse Effect

When the drug was correctly prescribed and properly administered, code the reaction plus the appropriate code from the E930-E949 series. Codes from the E930-E949 series must be used to identify the causative substance for an adverse effect of drug, medicinal and biological substances, correctly prescribed and properly administered. The effect, such as tachycardia, delirium, gastrointestinal hemorrhaging, vomiting, hypokalemia, hepatitis, renal failure, or respiratory failure, is coded and followed by the appropriate code from the E930-E949 series.

Adverse effects of therapeutic substances correctly prescribed and properly administered (toxicity, synergistic reaction, side effect, and idiosyncratic reaction) may be due to (1) differences among patients, such as age, sex, disease, and genetic factors, and (2) drug-related factors, such as type of drug, route of administration, duration of therapy, dosage, and bioavailability.

995.20 Unspecified adverse effect of unspecified drug, medicinal and biological substance

995.21 Arthus phenomenon
Arthus reaction

995.22 Unspecified adverse effect of anesthesia

995.23 Unspecified adverse effect of insulin

● **995.24 Failed moderate sedation during procedure**
Failed conscious sedation during procedure

Rationale: *The American Society of Anesthesiologists (ASA) requested a unique ICD-9-CM diagnosis code to describe instances of failed sedation. Under some circumstances, moderate (conscious) sedation by non-anesthesia providers can be sufficient to provide safe and satisfactory pain relief and/or amnesia to patients undergoing noxious procedures that do not ordinarily require a full anesthetic. In some situations, however, this may produce inadequate sedation making the procedure more difficult to perform and less satisfactory to the patient or may also produce unsafe conditions for the patient. Reasons for this may include, but are not limited to, situations where, maximum prudent and safe medication doses are administered but the patient remains inadequately sedated for the procedure; patient exhibits idiosyncratic responses to the mediations administered; patient becomes more deeply sedated than intended; patient is unable to adequately maintain a patent airway but respirations are depressed such that adequate air exchange is compromised; hemodynamic changes occur posing potential risks to the patient; other situations arise that are beyond the experience or expertise of the provider administering sedation.*

Such situations may have arisen during a previous procedure performed under moderate (conscious) sedating, necessitating planned intervention during subsequent procedures. Alternatively this situation may occur during a procedure currently in progress, making urgent intervention necessary to ensure a safe outcome for the patient and satisfactory conditions for completion of the procedure. In such circumstances, it may be necessary to enlist the services of an anesthesiologist or other provider with the training to administer adequate moderate (conscious) sedation or to administer deep sedation and/or anesthesia.

995.27 Other drug allergy
Drug allergy NOS
Drug hypersensitivity NOS

995.29 Unspecified adverse effect of other drug, medicinal and biological substance

995.3 Allergy, unspecified
Allergic reaction NOS
Hypersensitivity NOS
Idiosyncrasy NOS
Excludes *allergic reaction NOS to correct medicinal substance properly administered (995.27)*
allergy to existing dental restorative materials (525.66)
specific types of allergic reaction, such as:
allergic diarrhea (558.3)
dermatitis (691.0-693.9)
hayfever (477.0-477.9)

995.4 Shock due to anesthesia
Shock due to anesthesia in which the correct substance was properly administered
Excludes *complications of anesthesia in labor or delivery (668.0-668.9)*
overdose or wrong substance given (968.0-969.9)
postoperative shock NOS (998.0)
specified adverse effects of anesthesia classified elsewhere, such as:
anoxic brain damage (348.1)
hepatitis (070.0-070.9), etc.
unspecified adverse effect of anesthesia (995.22)

994.8 – 995.4

5th **995.5 Child maltreatment syndrome**
Use additional code(s), if applicable, to identify any associated injuries
Use additional E code to identify:
nature of abuse (E960-E968)
perpetrator (E967.0-E967.9)

995.50 Child abuse, unspecified P

995.51 Child emotional/psychological abuse P

995.52 Child neglect (nutritional) P
Use additional code to identify intent of neglect (E904.0, E968.4)

995.53 Child sexual abuse P

995.54 Child physical abuse P
Battered baby or child syndrome
Excludes *shaken infant syndrome (995.55)*

995.55 Shaken infant syndrome P
Use additional code(s) to identify any associated injuries

995.59 Other child abuse and neglect P
Multiple forms of abuse
Use additional code to identify intent of neglect (E904.0, E968.4)

5th **995.6 Anaphylactic shock due to adverse food reaction**
Anaphylactic reaction due to food
Anaphylactic shock due to nonpoisonous foods

995.60 Due to unspecified food

995.61 Due to peanuts

995.62 Due to crustaceans

995.63 Due to fruits and vegetables

995.64 Due to tree nuts and seeds

995.65 Due to fish

995.66 Due to food additives

995.67 Due to milk products

995.68 Due to eggs

995.69 Due to other specified food

995.7 Other adverse food reactions, not elsewhere classified
Use additional code to identify the type of reaction, such as:
hives (708.0)
wheezing (786.07)
Excludes *anaphylactic shock due to adverse food reaction (995.6)*
asthma (493.0, 493.9)
dermatitis due to food (693.1)
in contact with the skin (692.5)
gastroenteritis and colitis due to food (558.3)
rhinitis due to food (477.1)

5th **995.8 Other specified adverse effects, not elsewhere classified**

995.80 Adult maltreatment, unspecified A
Abused person NOS
Use additional code to identify:
any associated injury
nature of abuse (E960-E968)
perpetrator (E967.0-E967.9)

995.81 Adult physical abuse A
Battered:
man
person syndrome NEC
spouse
woman
Use additional code to identify:
any associated injury
nature of abuse (E960-E968)
perpetrator (E967.0-E967.9)

995.82 Adult emotional/psychological abuse A
Use additional E code to identify perpetrator (E967.0-E967.9)

995.83 Adult sexual abuse A
Use additional code to identify:
any associated injury
perpetrator (E967.0-E967.9)

995.84 Adult neglect (nutritional) A
Use additional code to identify:
intent of neglect (E904.0-E968.4)
perpetrator (E967.0-E967.9)

995.85 Other adult abuse and neglect A
Multiple forms of abuse and neglect
Use additional code to identify:
any associated injury
intent of neglect (E904.0, E968.4)
nature of abuse (E960-E968)
perpetrator (E967.0-E967.9)

995.86 Malignant hyperthermia
Malignant hyperpyrexia due to anesthesia

995.89 Other
Hypothermia due to anesthesia

5th **995.9 Systemic inflammatory response syndrome (SIRS)**

ICD-9-CM Official Guidelines (Chapter 1):

b. Septicemia, Systemic Inflammatory Response Syndrome (SIRS), Sepsis, Severe Sepsis, and Septic Shock

12. Only one code from subcategory 995.9 should be assigned. Therefore, when a non-infectious condition leads to an infection resulting in sepsis or severe sepsis, assign either code 995.91 or 995.92. Do not additionally assign code 995.93, Systemic inflammatory response syndrome due to non-infectious process without acute organ dysfunction, or 995.94, Systemic inflammatory response syndrome with acute organ dysfunction.

ICD-9-CM Official Guidelines (Chapter 19):

a. General E Code Coding Guidelines

7) External cause code(s) with systemic inflammatory response syndrome (SIRS)

An external cause code is not appropriate with a code from subcategory 995.9, unless the patient also has an injury, poisoning, or adverse effect of drugs.

995.90 Systemic inflammatory response syndrome, unspecified
SIRS NOS

995.91 Sepsis
Systemic inflammatory response syndrome due to infectious process without acute organ dysfunction
Code first underlying infection
Excludes *sepsis with acute organ dysfunction (995.92)*
sepsis with multiple organ dysfunction (995.92)
severe sepsis (995.92)

995.92 Severe sepsis
Sepsis with acute organ dysfunction
Sepsis with multiple organ dysfunction (MOD)
Systemic inflammatory response syndrome due to infectious process with acute organ dysfunction
Code first underlying infection
Use additional code to specify acute organ dysfunction, such as:
acute kidney ~~renal~~ failure (584.5-584.9)
acute respiratory failure (518.81)
acute respiratory insufficiency (518.82)
acute vascular insufficiency of intestine (557.0)
critical illness myopathy (359.81)
critical illness polyneuropathy (357.82)
disseminated intravascular coagulopathy (DIC) syndrome (286.6)
encephalopathy (348.31)
hepatic failure (570)
necrosis of intestines (557.0)
septic shock (785.52)

ICD-9-CM Official Guidelines (Chapter 17):

g. SIRS due to Non-infectious Process

The systemic inflammatory response syndrome (SIRS) can develop as a result of certain non-infectious disease processes, such as trauma, malignant neoplasm, or pancreatitis. When SIRS is documented with a noninfectious condition, and no subsequent infection is documented, the code for the underlying condition, such as an injury, should be assigned, followed by code 995.93, Systemic inflammatory response syndrome due to noninfectious process without acute organ dysfunction, or 995.94, Systemic inflammatory response syndrome due to non-infectious process with acute organ dysfunction. If an acute organ dysfunction is documented, the appropriate code(s) for the associated acute organ dysfunction(s) should be assigned in addition to code 995.94. If acute organ dysfunction is documented, but it cannot be determined if the acute organ dysfunction is associated with SIRS or due to another condition (e.g., directly due to the trauma), the provider should be queried.

When the non-infectious condition has led to an infection that results in SIRS, see Section I.C.1.b.11 for the guideline for sepsis and severe sepsis associated with a non-infectious process.

995.93 Systemic inflammatory response syndrome due to non-infectious process without acute organ dysfunction
Code first underlying conditions, such as:
acute pancreatitis (577.0)
trauma
Excludes *systemic inflammatory response syndrome due to noninfectious process with acute organ dysfunction (995.94)*

995.94 Systemic inflammatory response syndrome due to non-infectious process with acute organ dysfunction
Code first underlying conditions, such as:
acute pancreatitis (577.0)
trauma
Use additional code to specify acute organ dysfunction, such as:
acute kidney ~~renal~~ failure (584.5-584.9)
acute respiratory failure (518.81)
acute respiratory insufficiency (518.82)
acute vascular insufficiency of intestine (557.0)
critical illness myopathy (359.81)
critical illness polyneuropathy (357.82)
disseminated intravascular coagulopathy (DIC) syndrome (286.6)
encephalopathy (348.31)
hepatic failure (570)
necrosis of intestines (557.0)
Excludes *severe sepsis (995.92)*

COMPLICATIONS OF SURGICAL AND MEDICAL CARE, NOT ELSEWHERE CLASSIFIED (996-999)

Excludes *adverse effects of medicinal agents (001.0-799.9, 995.0-995.8)*
burns from local applications and irradiation (940.0-949.5)
complications of:
conditions for which the procedure was performed
surgical procedures during abortion, labor, and delivery (630-676.9)
poisoning and toxic effects of drugs and chemicals (960.0-989.9)
postoperative conditions in which no complications are present, such as:
artificial opening status (V44.0-V44.9)
closure of external stoma (V55.0-V55.9)
fitting of prosthetic device (V52.0-V52.9)
specified complications classified elsewhere
anesthetic shock (995.4)
electrolyte imbalance (276.0-276.9)
postlaminectomy syndrome (722.80-722.83)
postmastectomy lymphedema syndrome (457.0)
postoperative psychosis (293.0-293.9)
any other condition classified elsewhere in the Alphabetic Index when described as due to a procedure

4th **996 Complications peculiar to certain specified procedures**
Includes complications, not elsewhere classified, in the use of artificial substitutes [e.g., Dacron, metal, Silastic, Teflon] or natural sources [e.g., bone] involving:
anastomosis (internal)
graft (bypass) (patch)
implant
internal device:
catheter
electronic
fixation
prosthetic
reimplant
transplant
Excludes *accidental puncture or laceration during procedure (998.2)*
capsular contracture of breast implant (611.83)
complications of internal anastomosis of:
gastrointestinal tract (997.4)
urinary tract (997.5)
endosseous dental implant failures (525.71-525.79)
intraoperative floppy iris syndrome (IFIS) (364.81)
mechanical complication of respirator (V46.14)
other specified complications classified elsewhere, such as:
hemolytic anemia (283.1)
functional cardiac disturbances (429.4)
serum hepatitis (070.2-070.3)

5th **996.0 Mechanical complication of cardiac device, implant, and graft**
Breakdown (mechanical)
Displacement
Leakage
Obstruction, mechanical
Perforation
Protrusion

996.00 Unspecified device, implant, and graft

996.01 Due to cardiac pacemaker (electrode)

996.02 Due to heart valve prosthesis

996.03 Due to coronary bypass graft
Excludes *atherosclerosis of graft (414.02, 414.03)*
embolism [occlusion NOS] [thrombus] of graft (996.72)

996.04 Due to automatic implantable cardiac defibrillator

996.09 Other

996.1 Mechanical complication of other vascular device, implant, and graft
Mechanical complications involving:
aortic (bifurcation) graft (replacement)
arteriovenous:
dialysis catheter
fistula surgically created
shunt surgically created
balloon (counterpulsation) device, intra-aortic
carotid artery bypass graft
femoral-popliteal bypass graft
umbrella device, vena cava
Excludes *atherosclerosis of biological graft (440.30-440.32)*
embolism [occlusion NOS] [thrombus] of (biological) (synthetic) graft (996.74)
peritoneal dialysis catheter (996.56)

996.2 Mechanical complication of nervous system device, implant, and graft
Mechanical complications involving:
dorsal column stimulator
electrodes implanted in brain [brain "pacemaker"]
peripheral nerve graft
ventricular (communicating) shunt

5th **996.3 Mechanical complication of genitourinary device, implant, and graft**
996.30 Unspecified device, implant, and graft
996.31 Due to urethral [indwelling] catheter
996.32 Due to intrauterine contraceptive device ♀
996.39 Other
Cystostomy catheter
Prosthetic reconstruction of vas deferens
Repair (graft) of ureter without mention of resection
Excludes *complications due to:*
external stoma of urinary tract (997.5)
internal anastomosis of urinary tract (997.5)

5th **996.4 Mechanical complication of internal orthopedic device, implant, and graft**
Mechanical complications involving:
external (fixation) device utilizing internal screw(s), pin(s) or other methods of fixation
grafts of bone, cartilage, muscle, or tendon
internal (fixation) device such as nail, plate, rod, etc.
Use additional code to identify prosthetic joint with mechanical complication (V43.60-V43.69)
Excludes *complications of external orthopedic device, such as:*
pressure ulcer due to cast (707.00-707.09)
996.40 Unspecified mechanical complication of internal orthopedic device, implant, and graft
996.41 Mechanical loosening of prosthetic joint
Aseptic loosening
996.42 Dislocation of prosthetic joint
Instability of prosthetic joint
Subluxation of prosthetic joint
▲**996.43 Broken prosthetic joint implant ~~failure~~**
Breakage (fracture) of prosthetic joint
996.44 Peri-prosthetic fracture around prosthetic joint
996.45 Peri-prosthetic osteolysis
Use additional code to identify major osseous defect, if applicable (731.3)
996.46 Articular bearing surface wear of prosthetic joint
996.47 Other mechanical complication of prosthetic joint implant
Mechanical complication of prosthetic joint NOS
Prosthetic joint implant failure NOS
996.49 Other mechanical complication of other internal orthopedic device, implant, and graft
Breakage of internal fixation device in bone
Dislocation of internal fixation device in bone
Excludes *mechanical complication of prosthetic joint implant (996.41-996.47)*

5th **996.5 Mechanical complication of other specified prosthetic device, implant, and graft**
Mechanical complications involving:
nonabsorbable surgical material NOS
prosthetic implant in:
bile duct
breast
chin
orbit of eye
other graft, implant, and internal device, not elsewhere classified
996.51 Due to corneal graft
996.52 Due to graft of other tissue, not elsewhere classified
Skin graft failure or rejection
Excludes *failure of artificial skin graft (996.55)*
failure of decellularized allodermis (996.55)
sloughing of temporary skin allografts or xenografts (pigskin) – omit code
996.53 Due to ocular lens prosthesis
Excludes *contact lenses – code to condition*
996.54 Due to breast prosthesis
Breast capsule (prosthesis)
Mammary implant
996.55 Due to artificial skin graft and decellularized allodermis
Dislodgement
Displacement
Failure
Non-adherence
Poor incorporation
Shearing
996.56 Due to peritoneal dialysis catheter
Excludes *mechancial complication of arteriovenous dialysis catheter (996.1)*
996.57 Due to insulin pump
996.59 Due to other implant and internal device, not elsewhere classified
Nonabsorbable surgical material NOS
Prosthetic implant in:
bile duct
chin
orbit of eye

5th **996.6 Infection and inflammatory reaction due to internal prosthetic device, implant, and graft**
Infection (causing obstruction) due to (presence of) any device, implant, and graft classifiable to 996.0-996.5
Inflammation due to (presence of) any device, implant, and graft classifiable to 996.0-996.5
Use additional code to identify specified infections
996.60 Due to unspecified device, implant and graft

996.61 Due to cardiac device, implant and graft
Cardiac pacemaker or defibrillator:
electrode(s), lead(s)
pulse generator
subcutaneous pocket
Coronary artery bypass graft
Heart valve prosthesis

996.62 Due to vascular device, implant and graft
Arterial graft
Arteriovenous fistula or shunt
Infusion pump
Vascular catheter (arterial) (dialysis) (peripheral venous)
Excludes *infection due to:*
central venous catheter (999.31)
Hickman catheter (999.31)
peripherally inserted central catheter (PICC) (999.31)
portacath (port-a-cath) (999.31)
triple lumen catheter (999.31)
umbilical venous catheter (999.31)

996.63 Due to nervous system device, implant and graft
Electrodes implanted in brain
Peripheral nerve graft
Spinal canal catheter
Ventricular (communicating) shunt (catheter)

996.64 Due to indwelling urinary catheter
Use additional code to identify specified infections, such as:
cystitis (595.0-595.9)
sepsis (038.0-038.9)

996.65 Due to other genitourinary device, implant and graft
Intrauterine contraceptive device

996.66 Due to internal joint prosthesis
Use additional code to identify infected prosthetic joint (V43.60-V43.69)

996.67 Due to other internal orthopedic device, implant and graft
Bone growth stimulator (electrode)
Internal fixation device (pin) (rod) (screw)

996.68 Due to peritoneal dialysis catheter
Exit-site infection or inflammation

996.69 Due to other internal prosthetic device, implant, and graft
Breast prosthesis
Ocular lens prosthesis
Prosthetic orbital implant

5th **996.7 Other complications of internal (biological) (synthetic) prosthetic device, implant, and graft**
Complication NOS due to (presence of) any device, implant, and graft classifiable to 996.0-996.5
Embolism due to (presence of) any device, implant, and graft classifiable to 996.0-996.5
Fibrosis due to (presence of) any device, implant, and graft classifiable to 996.0-996.5
Hemorrhage due to (presence of) any device, implant, and graft classifiable to 996.0-996.5
Occlusion NOS due to (presence of) any device, implant, and graft classifiable to 996.0-996.5
Pain due to (presence of) any device, implant, and graft classifiable to 996.0-996.5
Stenosis due to (presence of) any device, implant, and graft classifiable to 996.0-996.5
Thrombus due to (presence of) any device, implant, and graft classifiable to 996.0-996.5
Use additional code to identify complication, such as:
pain due to presence of device, implant or graft (338.18-338.19, 338.28-338.29)
venous embolism and thrombosis (453.2-453.9)
Excludes *disruption (dehiscence) of internal suture material (998.31)*
transplant rejection (996.8)

996.70 Due to unspecified device, implant, and graft

996.71 Due to heart valve prosthesis

996.72 Due to other cardiac device, implant, and graft
Cardiac pacemaker or defibrillator:
electrode(s), lead(s)
subcutaneous pocket
Coronary artery bypass (graft)
Excludes *occlusion due to atherosclerosis (414.00-414.07)*

996.73 Due to renal dialysis device, implant, and graft I 72

996.74 Due to vascular device, implant, and graft
Excludes *occlusion of biological graft due to atherosclerosis (440.30-440.32)*

996.75 Due to nervous system device, implant, and graft

996.76 Due to genitourinary device, implant, and graft

996.77 Due to internal joint prosthesis
Use additional code to identify prosthetic joint (V43.60 - V43.69)

996.78 Due to other internal orthopedic device, implant, and graft

996.79 Due to other internal prosthetic device, implant, and graft

5th 996.8 **Complications of transplanted organ**
Transplant failure or rejection
Use additional code to identify nature of complication, such as:
cytomegalovirus [CMV] infection (078.5)
graft-versus-host disease (279.50-279.53)
malignancy associated with organ transplant (199.2)
post-transplant lymphoproliferative disorder (PTLD) (238.77)

ICD-9-CM Official Guidelines (Chapter 17):

f. Complications of care

1) Transplant complications

(a) Transplant complications other than kidney

Codes under subcategory 996.8, Complications of transplanted organ, are for use for both complications and rejection of transplanted organs. A transplant complication code is only assigned if the complication affects the function of the transplanted organ. Two codes are required to fully describe a transplant complication, the appropriate code from subcategory 996.8 and a secondary code that identifies the complication.

Pre-existing conditions or conditions that develop after the transplant are not coded as complications unless they affect the function of the transplanted organs.

996.80 Transplanted organ, unspecified
996.81 Kidney

ICD-9-CM Official Guidelines (Chapter 17f)

2) Transplant complications

(b) Chronic kidney disease and kidney transplant complications

Patients who have undergone kidney transplant may still have some form of chronic kidney disease (CKD) because the kidney transplant may not fully restore kidney function. Code 996.81 should be assigned for documented complications of a kidney transplant, such as transplant failure or rejection or other transplant complication. Code 996.81 should not be assigned for post kidney transplant patients who have chronic kidney (CKD) unless a transplant complication such as transplant failure or rejection is documented. If the documentation is unclear as to whether the patient has a complication of the transplant, query the provider.

For patients with CKD following a kidney transplant, but who do not have a complication such as failure or rejection, see section I.C.10.a.2, Chronic kidney disease and kidney transplant status.

996.82 Liver
996.83 Heart
996.84 Lung
996.85 Bone marrow
996.86 Pancreas
996.87 Intestine
996.89 Other specified transplanted organ

5th 996.9 **Complications of reattached extremity or body part**
996.90 Unspecified extremity
996.91 Forearm
996.92 Hand
996.93 Finger(s)
996.94 Upper extremity, other and unspecified
996.95 Foot and toe(s)
996.96 Lower extremity, other and unspecified
996.99 Other specified body part

4th 997 **Complications affecting specified body systems, not elsewhere classified**
Use additional code to identify complication
Excludes *the listed conditions when specified as:*
causing shock (998.0)
complications of:
anesthesia:
adverse effect (001.0-799.9, 995.0-995.8)
in labor or delivery (668.0-668.9)
poisoning (968.0-969.9)
implanted device or graft (996.0-996.9)
obstetrical procedures (669.0-669.4)
reattached extremity (996.90-996.96)
transplanted organ (996.80-996.89)

5th 997.0 **Nervous system complications**
997.00 Nervous system complication, unspecified
997.01 Central nervous system complication
Anoxic brain damage
Cerebral hypoxia
Excludes *cerebrovascular hemorrhage or infarction (997.02)*
997.02 Iatrogenic cerebrovascular infarction or hemorrhage
Postoperative stroke
997.09 Other nervous system complications

997.1 Cardiac complications
Cardiac:
arrest during or resulting from a procedure
insufficiency during or resulting from a procedure
Cardiorespiratory failure during or resulting from a procedure
Heart failure during or resulting from a procedure
Excludes *the listed conditions as long-term effects of cardiac surgery or due to the presence of cardiac prosthetic device (429.4)*

997.2 Peripheral vascular complications
Phlebitis or thrombophlebitis during or resulting from a procedure
Excludes *the listed conditions due to:*
implant or catheter device (996.62)
infusion, perfusion, or transfusion (999.2)
complications affecting blood vessels (997.71-997.79)

5th 997.3 **Respiratory complications**
Excludes *iatrogenic [postoperative] pneumothorax (512.1)*
iatrogenic pulmonary embolism (415.11)
Mendelson's syndrome in labor and delivery (668.0)
specified complications classified elsewhere, such as:
adult respiratory distress syndrome (518.5)
pulmonary edema, postoperative (518.4)
respiratory insufficiency, acute, postoperative (518.5)
shock lung (518.5)
tracheostomy complications (519.00-519.09)
transfusion related acute lung injury (TRALI) (518.7)

ICD-9-CM Official Guidelines (Chapter 17f)

3) Ventilator associated pneumonia

(a) Documentation of Ventilator associated Pneumonia

As with all procedural or postprocedural complications, code assignment is based on the provider's documentation of the relationship between the condition and the procedure.

Code 997.31, Ventilator associated pneumonia, should be assigned only when the provider has documented ventilator associated pneumonia (VAP). An additional code to identify the organism (e.g., Pseudomonas aeruginosa, code 041.7) should also be assigned. Do not assign an additional code from categories 480-484 to identify the type of pneumonia.

Code 997.31 should not be assigned for cases where the patient has pneumonia and is on a mechanical ventilator but the provider has not specifically stated that the pneumonia is ventilator-associated pneumonia.

If the documentation is unclear as to whether the patient has a pneumonia that is a complication attributable to the mechanical ventilator, query the provider.

(b) Patient admitted with pneumonia and develops VAP

A patient may be admitted with one type of pneumonia (e.g., code 481, Pneumococcal pneumonia) and subsequently develop VAP. In this instance, the principal diagnosis would be the appropriate code from categories 480-484 for the pneumonia diagnosed at the time of admission. Code 997.31, Ventilator associated pneumonia, would be assigned as an additional diagnosis when the provider has also documented the presence of ventilator associated pneumonia.

997.31 Ventilator associated pneumonia
Ventilator associated pneumonitis
Use additional code to identify organism

997.39 Other respiratory complications
Mendelson's syndrome resulting from a procedure
Pneumonia (aspiration) resulting from a procedure

997.4 Digestive system complications
Complications of:
intestinal (internal) anastomosis and bypass, not elsewhere classified, except that involving urinary tract
Hepatic failure specified as due to a procedure
Hepatorenal syndrome specified as due to a procedure
Intestinal obstruction NOS specified as due to a procedure
Excludes *specified gastrointestinal complications classified elsewhere, such as:*
blind loop syndrome (579.2)
colostomy or enterostomy complications (569.60-569.69)
complications of intestinal pouch (569.71-569.79)
gastrojejunal ulcer (534.0-534.9)
gastrostomy complications (536.40-536.49)
infection of esophagostomy (530.86)
infection of external stoma (569.61)
mechanical complication of esophagostomy (530.87)
pelvic peritoneal adhesions, female (614.6)
peritoneal adhesions (568.0)
peritoneal adhesions with obstruction (560.81)
postcholecystectomy syndrome (576.0)
postgastric surgery syndromes (564.2)
pouchitis (569.71)
vomiting following gastrointestinal surgery (564.3)

997.5 Urinary complications
Complications of:
external stoma of urinary tract
internal anastomosis and bypass of urinary tract, including that involving intestinal tract
Oliguria or anuria specified as due to procedure
Renal (kidney):
failure (acute) specified as due to procedure
insufficiency (acute) specified as due to procedure
Tubular necrosis (acute) specified as due to procedure
Excludes *specified complications classified elsewhere, such as:*
postoperative stricture of:
ureter (593.3)
urethra (598.2)

5th **997.6 Amputation stump complication**
Excludes *admission for treatment for a current traumatic amputation – code to complicated traumatic amptutation*
phantom limb (syndrome) (353.6)

997.60 Unspecified complication

997.61 Neuroma of amputation stump

997.62 Infection (chronic)
Use additional code to identify the organism

997.69 Other

5th **997.7 Vascular complications of other vessels**
Excludes *peripheral vascular complications (997.2)*

997.71 Vascular complications of mesenteric artery

997.72 Vascular complications of renal artery

997.79 Vascular complications of other vessels

5th **997.9 Complications affecting other specified body systems, not elsewhere classified**
Excludes *specified complications classified elsewhere, such as:*
broad ligament laceration syndrome (620.6)
postartificial menopause syndrome (627.4)
postoperative stricture of vagina (623.2)

997.91 Hypertension
Excludes *essential hypertension (401.0-401.9)*

997.99 Other
Vitreous touch syndrome

4th **998 Other complications of procedures, NEC**

998.0 Postoperative shock
Collapse NOS during or resulting from a surgical procedure
Shock (endotoxic) (hypovolemic) (septic) during or resulting from a surgical procedure
Excludes *shock:*
anaphylactic due to serum (999.4)
anesthetic (995.4)
electric (994.8)
following abortion (639.5)
obstetric (669.1)
traumatic (958.4)

5th **998.1 Hemorrhage or hematoma or seroma complicating a procedure**
Excludes *hemorrhage, hematoma or seroma:*
complicating cesarean section or puerperal perineal wound (674.3)
due to implanted device or graft (996.70-996.79)

998.11 Hemorrhage complicating a procedure

998.12 Hematoma complicating a procedure

998.13 Seroma complicating a procedure

998.2 Accidental puncture or laceration during a procedure
Accidental perforation by catheter or other instrument during a procedure on:
blood vessel
nerve
organ
Excludes *dural tear (349.31)*
iatrogenic [postoperative] pneumothorax (512.1)
incidental durotomy (349.31)
puncture or laceration caused by implanted device intentionally left in operation wound (996.0-996.5)
specified complications classified elsewhere, such as:
broad ligament laceration syndrome (620.6)
trauma from instruments during delivery (664.0-665.9)

5th **998.3 Disruption of wound**
Dehiscence of operation wound
Disruption of any suture materials or other closure method
Disruption of postprocedural wound closure or post-traumatic wound repair
Rupture of operation wound
Excludes *disruption of:*
amputation stump (997.69)
cesarean wound (674.1)
perineal wound, puerperal (674.2)

998.30 Disruption of wound, unspecified
Disruption of wound NOS

998.31 Disruption of internal operation (surgical) wound
Deep disruption or dehiscence of operation wound NOS
Disruption or dehiscence of closure of:
fascia, superficial or muscular
internal organ
muscle or muscle flap
ribs or rib cage
skull or craniotomy
sternum or sternotomy
tendon or ligament
Excludes *complications of internal anastomosis of:*
gastrointestinal tract (997.4)
urinary tract (997.5)

998.32 Disruption of external operation (surgical) wound
Disruption of operation wound NOS
Disruption or dehiscence of closure of:
cornea
mucosa
skin
subcutaneous tissue
Full-thickness skin disruption or dehiscence
Superficial disruption or dehiscence of operation wound

998.33 Disruption of traumatic injury wound repair
Disruption or dehiscence of closure of traumatic laceration (external) (internal)

998.4 Foreign body accidentally left during a procedure
Adhesions due to foreign body accidentally left in operative wound or body cavity during a procedure
Obstruction due to foreign body accidentally left in operative wound or body cavity during a procedure
Perforation due to foreign body accidentally left in operative wound or body cavity during a procedure
Excludes *obstruction or perforation caused by implanted device intentionally left in body (996.0-996.5)*

5th **998.5 Postoperative infection**
Excludes *bleb associated endophthalmitis (379.63)*
infection due to:
implanted device (996.60-996.69)
infusion, perfusion, or transfusion (999.31-999.39)
postoperative obstetrical wound infection (674.3)

998.51 Infected postoperative seroma
Use additional code to identify organism

998.59 Other postoperative infection
Abscess:
intra-abdominal postoperative
stitch postoperative
subphrenic postoperative
wound postoperative
Septicemia postoperative
Use additional code to identify infection

998.6 Persistent postoperative fistula

998.7 Acute reaction to foreign substance accidentally left during a procedure
Peritonitis:
aseptic
chemical

5th **998.8 Other specified complications of procedures, not elsewhere classified**

998.81 Emphysema (subcutaneous) (surgical) resulting from a procedure

998.82 Cataract fragments in eye following cataract surgery

998.83 Non-healing surgical wound

998.89 Other specified complications

998.9 Unspecified complication of procedure, not elsewhere classified
Postoperative complication NOS
Excludes *complication NOS of obstetrical surgery or procedure (669.4)*

4th **999 Complications of medical care, not elsewhere classified**
Includes complications, not elsewhere classified, of:
dialysis (hemodialysis) (peritoneal) (renal)
extracorporeal circulation
hyperalimentation therapy
immunization
infusion
inhalation therapy
injection
inoculation
perfusion
transfusion
vaccination
ventilation therapy
Use additional code, where applicable, to identify specific complication
Excludes *specified complications classified elsewhere such as:*
complications of implanted device (996.0-996.9)
contact dermatitis due to drugs (692.3)
dementia dialysis (294.8)
transient (293.9)
dialysis disequilibrium syndrome (276.0-276.9)
poisoning and toxic effects of drugs and chemicals (960.0-989.9)
postvaccinal encephalitis (323.51)
water and electrolyte imbalance (276.0-276.9)

999.0 Generalized vaccinia
Excludes *vaccinia not from vaccine (051.02)*

999.1 Air embolism
Air embolism to any site following infusion, perfusion, or transfusion
Excludes *embolism specified as:*
complicating:
abortion (634-638 with .6, 639.6)
ectopic or molar pregnancy (639.6)
pregnancy, childbirth, or the puerperium (673.0)
due to implanted device (996.7)
traumatic (958.0)

999.2 Other vascular complications
Phlebitis following infusion, perfusion, or transfusion
Thromboembolism following infusion, perfusion, or transfusion
Thrombophlebitis following infusion, perfusion, or transfusion
Excludes *extravasation of vesicant drugs (999.81, 999.82)*
the listed conditions when specified as:
due to implanted device (996.61-996.62, 996.72-996.74)
postoperative NOS (997.2, 997.71-997.79)

5th **999.3 Other infection**
Infection following infusion, injection, transfusion, or vaccination
Sepsis following infusion, injection, transfusion, or vaccination
Septicemia following infusion, injection, transfusion, or vaccination
Use additional code to identify the specified infection, such as:
septicemia (038.0-038.9)
Excludes *the listed conditions when specified as:*
due to implanted device (996.60-996.69)
postoperative NOS (998.51-998.59)

999.31 Infection due to central venous catheter
Catheter-related bloodstream infection (CRBSI) NOS
Infection due to:
Hickman catheter
peripherally inserted central catheter (PICC)
portacath (port-a-cath)
triple lumen catheter
umbilical venous catheter
Excludes *infection due to:*
arterial catheter (996.62)
catheter NOS (996.69)
peripheral venous catheter (996.62)
urinary catheter (996.64)

999.39 Infection following other infusion, injection, transfusion, or vaccination

999.4 Anaphylactic shock due to serum
Anaphylactic reaction due to serum
Excludes *shock:*
allergic NOS (995.0)
anaphylactic:
NOS (995.0)
due to drugs and chemicals (995.0)

999.5 Other serum reaction
Intoxication by serum
Protein sickness
Serum rash
Serum sickness
Urticaria due to serum
Excludes *serum hepatitis (070.2-070.3)*

999.6 ABO incompatibility reaction
Incompatible blood transfusion
Reaction to blood group incompatibility in infusion or transfusion
Excludes *minor blood group antigens reactions (Duffy) (E) (K(ell)) (Kidd) (Lewis) (M) (N) (P) (S) (999.89)*

999.7 Rh incompatibility reaction
Reactions due to Rh factor in infusion or transfusion

5th **999.8 Other infusion and transfusion reaction**
Excludes *postoperative shock (998.0)*
transfusion related acute lung injury (TRALI) (518.7)

999.81 Extravasation of vesicant chemotherapy
Infiltration of vesicant chemotherapy

999.82 Extravasation of other vesicant agent
Infiltration of other vesicant agent

999.88 Other infusion reaction

999.89 Other transfusion reaction
Transfusion reaction NOS
Use additional code to identify graft-versus-host reaction (279.5)

999.9 Other and unspecified complications of medical care, not elsewhere classified
Complications, not elsewhere classified, of:
electroshock therapy
inhalation therapy
ultrasound therapy
ventilation therapy
Unspecified misadventure of medical care
Excludes *unspecified complication of:*
phototherapy (990)
radiation therapy (990)
ventilator associated pneumonia (997.31)

18. SUPPLEMENTARY CLASSIFICATION OF FACTORS INFLUENCING HEALTH STATUS AND CONTACT WITH HEALTH SERVICES (V01-V89)

This classification is provided to deal with occasions when circumstances other than a disease or injury classifiable to categories 001-999 (the main part of ICD) are recorded as "diagnoses" or "problems." This can arise mainly in three ways:

a) When a person who is not currently sick encounters the health services for some specific purpose, such as to act as a donor of an organ or tissue, to receive prophylactic vaccination, or to discuss a problem which is in itself not a disease or injury. This will be a fairly rare occurrence among hospital inpatients, but will be relatively more common among hospital outpatients and patients of family practitioners, health clinics, etc.

b) When a person with a known disease or injury, whether it is current or resolving, encounters the health care system for a specific treatment of that disease or injury (e.g., dialysis for renal disease; chemotherapy for malignancy; cast change).

c) When some circumstance or problem is present which influences the person's health status but is not in itself a current illness or injury. Such factors may be elicited during population surveys, when the person may or may not be currently sick, or be recorded as an additional factor to be borne in mind when the person is receiving care for some current illness or injury classifiable to categories 001-999.

In the latter circumstances the V code should be used only as a supplementary code and should not be the one selected for use in primary, single cause tabulations. Examples of these circumstances are a personal history of certain diseases, or a person with an artificial heart valve in situ.

ICD-9-CM Official Guidelines (Chapter 18):

Note: *The chapter specific guidelines provide additional information about the use of V codes for specified encounters.*

a. Introduction

ICD-9-CM provides codes to deal with encounters for circumstances other than a disease or injury. The Supplementary Classification of Factors Influencing Health Status and Contact with Health Services (V01.0 - V84.8) is provided to deal with occasions when circumstances other than a disease or injury (codes 001-999) are recorded as a diagnosis or problem.

There are four primary circumstances for the use of V codes:

1) *A person who is not currently sick encounters the health services for some specific reason, such as to act as an organ donor, to receive prophylactic care, such as inoculations or health screenings, or to receive counseling on health related issues.*
2) *A person with a resolving disease or injury, or a chronic, long-term condition requiring continuous care, encounters the health care system for specific aftercare of that disease or injury (e.g., dialysis for renal disease; chemotherapy for malignancy; cast change). A diagnosis/symptom code should be used whenever a current, acute, diagnosis is being treated or a sign or symptom is being studied.*
3) *Circumstances or problems influence a person's health status but are not in themselves a current illness or injury.*
4) *Newborns, to indicate birth status*

b. V codes use in any healthcare setting

V codes are for use in any healthcare setting. V codes may be used as either a first listed (principal diagnosis code in the inpatient setting) or secondary code, depending on the circumstances of the encounter. Certain V codes may only be used as first listed, others only as secondary codes.

See Section I.C.18.e, V Code Table.

c. V Codes indicate a reason for an encounter

They are not procedure codes. A corresponding procedure code must accompany a V code to describe the procedure performed.

d. Categories of V Codes...

3) Status

Status codes indicate that a patient is either a carrier of a disease or has the sequelae or residual of a past disease or condition. This includes such things as the presence of prosthetic or mechanical devices resulting from past treatment. A status code is informative, because the status may affect the course of treatment and its outcome. A status code is distinct from a history code. The history code indicates that the patient no longer has the condition.

A status code should not be used with a diagnosis code from one of the body system chapters, if the diagnosis code includes the information provided by the status code. For example, code V42.1, Heart transplant status, should not be used with code 996.83, Complications of transplanted heart. The status code does not provide additional information. The complication code indicates that the patient is a heart transplant patient.

The status V codes/categories are:

V02 Carrier or suspected carrier of infectious diseases

Carrier status indicates that a person harbors the specific organisms of a disease without manifest symptoms and is capable of transmitting the infection.

V08 Asymptomatic HIV infection status

This code indicates that a patient has tested positive for HIV but has manifested no signs or symptoms of the disease.

V09 Infection with drug-resistant microorganisms

This category indicates that a patient has an infection that is resistant to drug treatment. Sequence the infection code first.

V21 Constitutional states in development

V22.2 Pregnant state, incidental

This code is a secondary code only for use when the pregnancy is in no way complicating the reason for visit. Otherwise, a code from the obstetric chapter is required.

V26.5x Sterilization status

V42 Organ or tissue replaced by transplant

V43 Organ or tissue replaced by other means

V44 Artificial opening status

V45 Other postsurgical states

V46 Other dependence on machines

V49.6 Upper limb amputation status

V49.7 Lower limb amputation status

Note: *Categories V42-V46, and subcategories V49.6, V49.7 are for use only if there are no complications or malfunctions of the organ or tissue replaced, the amputation site or the equipment on which the patient is dependent.*

V49.81 Postmenopausal status

V49.82 Dental sealant status

V49.83 Awaiting organ transplant status

V58.6x Long-term (current) drug use

Codes from this subcategory indicate a patient's continuous use of a prescribed drug (including such things as aspirin therapy) for the long-term treatment of a condition or for prophylactic use. It is not for use for patients who have addictions to drugs.

Assign a code from subcategory V58.6, Long-term (current) drug use, if the patient is receiving a medication for an extended period as a prophylactic measure (such as for the prevention of deep vein thrombosis) or as treatment of a chronic condition (such as arthritis) or a disease requiring a lengthy course of treatment (such as cancer). Do not assign a code from subcategory V58.6 for medication being administered for a brief period of time to treat an acute illness or injury (such as a course of antibiotics to treat acute bronchitis).

V Codes

V83 Genetic carrier status

Genetic carrier status indicates that a person carries a gene, associated with a particular disease, which may be passed to offspring who may develop that disease. The person does not have the disease and is not at risk of developing the disease.

V84 Genetic susceptibility status

Genetic susceptibility indicates that a person has a gene that increases the risk of that person developing the disease.

Codes from category V84, Genetic susceptibility to disease, should not be used as principal or first-listed codes. If the patient has the condition to which he/she is susceptible, and that condition is the reason for the encounter, the code for the current condition should be sequenced first. If the patient is being seen for follow-up after completed treatment for this condition, and the condition no longer exists, a follow-up code should be sequenced first, followed by the appropriate personal history and genetic susceptibility codes. If the purpose of the encounter is genetic counseling associated with procreative management, a code from subcategory V26.3, Genetic counseling and testing, should be assigned as the first-listed code, followed by a code from category V84. Additional codes should be assigned for any applicable family or personal history.

See Section I.C. 18.d.14 for information on prophylactic organ removal due to a genetic susceptibility.

V86 Estrogen receptor status

10) Counseling

Counseling V codes are used when a patient or family member receives assistance in the aftermath of an illness or injury, or when support is required in coping with family or social problems. They are not necessary for use in conjunction with a diagnosis code when the counseling component of care is considered integral to standard treatment.

The counseling V categories/codes:

V25.0 General counseling and advice for contraceptive management
V26.3 Genetic counseling
V26.4 General counseling and advice for procreative management
V61 Other family circumstances
V65.1 Person consulted on behalf of another person
V65.3 Dietary surveillance and counseling
V65.4 Other counseling, not elsewhere classified

12) Newborn, infant and child

See Section I.C.15, the Newborn guidelines for further instruction on the use of these codes.

Newborn V code categories:

V20 Health supervision of infant or child
V29 Observation and evaluation of newborns for suspected condition not found
(See Section I.C.18.d.7, Observation)
V30-V39 Liveborn infant according to type of birth

14) Miscellaneous V codes

The miscellaneous V codes capture a number of other health care encounters that do not fall into one of the other categories. Certain of these codes identify the reason for the encounter, others are for use as additional codes that provide useful information on circumstances that may affect a patient's care and treatment.

Miscellaneous V code categories/codes:

V07 Need for isolation and other prophylactic measures
V50 Elective surgery for purposes other than remedying health states
V58.5 Orthodontics
V60 Housing, household, and economic circumstances
V62 Other psychosocial circumstances
V63 Unavailability of other medical facilities for care
V64 Persons encountering health services for specific procedures, not carried out
V66 Convalescence and Palliative Care
V68 Encounters for administrative purposes
V69 Problems related to lifestyle
V85 Body Mass Index

15) Nonspecific V codes

Certain V codes are so non-specific, or potentially redundant with other codes in the classification, that there can be little justification for their use in the inpatient setting. Their use in the outpatient setting should be limited to those instances when there is no further documentation to permit more precise coding. Otherwise, any sign or symptom or any other reason for visit that is captured in another code should be used.

Nonspecific V code categories/codes:

V11 Personal history of mental disorder A code from the mental disorders chapter, with an in remission fifth-digit, should be used.
V13.4 Personal history of arthritis
V13.6 Personal history of congenital malformations
V15.7 Personal history of contraception
V23.2 Pregnancy with history of abortion
V40 Mental and behavioral problems
V41 Problems with special senses and other special functions
V47 Other problems with internal organs
V48 Problems with head, neck, and trunk
V49 Problems with limbs and other problems

Exceptions:

V49.6 Upper limb amputation status
V49.7 Lower limb amputation status
V49.81 Postmenopausal status
V49.82 Dental sealant status
V49.83 Awaiting organ transplant status

V51 Aftercare involving the use of plastic surgery
V58.2 Blood transfusion, without reported diagnosis
V58.9 Unspecified aftercare

See Section IV.K. and Section IV.L. of the Outpatient guidelines.

PERSONS WITH POTENTIAL HEALTH HAZARDS RELATED TO COMMUNICABLE DISEASES (V01-V06)

Excludes *family history of infectious and parasitic diseases (V18.8)*
personal history of infectious and parasitic diseases (V12.0)

4th V01 Contact with or exposure to communicable diseases

ICD-9-CM Official Guidelines (Chapter 18):

d. Categories of V Codes

1) Contact/Exposure

Category V01 indicates contact with or exposure to communicable diseases. These codes are for patients who do not show any sign or symptom of a disease but have been exposed to it by close personal contact with an infected individual or are in an area where a disease is epidemic. These codes may be used as a first listed code to explain an encounter for testing, or, more commonly, as a secondary code to identify a potential risk.

V01.0 Cholera
Conditions classifiable to 001

V01.1 Tuberculosis
Conditions classifiable to 010-018

V01.2 Poliomyelitis
Conditions classifiable to 045

V01.3 Smallpox
Conditions classifiable to 050

V01.4 Rubella
Conditions classifiable to 056

V01.5 Rabies
Conditions classifiable to 071

V01.6 Venereal diseases
Conditions classifiable to 090-099

5th **V01.7 Other viral diseases**
Conditions classifiable to 042-078, and V08, except as above

V01.71 Varicella

V01.79 Other viral diseases

5th **V01.8 Other communicable diseases**
Conditions classifiable to 001-136, except as above

V01.81 Anthrax

V01.82 Exposure to SARS-associated coronavirus

V01.83 Escherichia coli (E. coli)

V01.84 Meningococcus

V01.89 Other communicable diseases

V01.9 Unspecified communicable disease

4th **V02 Carrier or suspected carrier of infectious diseases**
Includes colonization status

V02.0 Cholera

V02.1 Typhoid

V02.2 Amebiasis

V02.3 Other gastrointestinal pathogens

V02.4 Diphtheria

5th **V02.5 Other specified bacterial diseases**

V02.51 Group B streptococcus

V02.52 Other streptococcus

V02.53 Methicillin susceptible Staphylococcus aureus
MSSA colonization

ICD-9-CM Official Guidelines (Chapter 1c1)

(c) Methicillin susceptible Staphylococcus aureus (MSSA) and MRSA colonization

The condition or state of being colonized or carrying MSSA or MRSA is called colonization or carriage, while an individual person is described as being colonized or being a carrier. Colonization means that MSSA or MSRA is present on or in the body without necessarily causing illness. A positive MRSA colonization test might be documented by the provider as "MRSA screen positive" or "MRSA nasal swab positive".

Assign code V02.54, Carrier or suspected carrier, Methicillin resistant Staphylococcus aureus, for patients documented as having MRSA colonization. Assign code V02.53, Carrier or suspected carrier, Methicillin susceptible Staphylococcus aureus, for patient documented as having MSSA colonization. Colonization is not necessarily indicative of a disease process or as the cause of a specific condition the patient may have unless documented as such by the provider.

Code V02.59, Other specified bacterial diseases, should be assigned for other types of staphylococcal colonization (e.g., S. epidermidis, S. saprophyticus). Code V02.59 should not be assigned for colonization with any type of Staphylococcus aureus (MRSA, MSSA).

(d) MRSA colonization and infection

If a patient is documented as having both MRSA colonization and infection during a hospital admission, code V02.54, Carrier or suspected carrier, Methicillin resistant Staphylococcus aureus, and a code for the MRSA infection may both be assigned.

V02.54 Methicillin resistant Staphylococcus aureus
MRSA colonization

V02.59 Other specified bacterial diseases
Meningococcal
Staphylococcal

5th **V02.6 Viral hepatitis**

V02.60 Viral hepatitis carrier, unspecified

V02.61 Hepatitis B carrier

V02.62 Hepatitis C carrier

V02.69 Other viral hepatitis carrier

V02.7 Gonorrhea

V02.8 Other venereal diseases

V02.9 Other specified infectious organism

4th **V03 Need for prophylactic vaccination and inoculation against bacterial diseases**
Excludes *vaccination not carried out (V64.00-V64.09)*
vaccines against combinations of diseases (V06.0-V06.9)

ICD-9-CM Official Guidelines (Chapter 18):

d. Categories of V Codes

2) Inoculations and vaccinations

Categories V03-V06 are for encounters for inoculations and vaccinations. They indicate that a patient is being seen to receive a prophylactic inoculation against a disease. The injection itself must be represented by the appropriate procedure code. A code from V03-V06 may be used as a secondary code if the inoculation is given as a routine part of preventive health care, such as a well-baby visit.

V03.0 Cholera alone

V03.1 Typhoid-paratyphoid alone [TAB]

V03.2 Tuberculosis [BCG]

V03.3 Plague

V03.4 Tularemia

V03.5 Diphtheria alone

V03.6 Pertussis alone

V03.7 Tetanus toxoid alone

5th **V03.8 Other specified vaccinations against single bacterial diseases**

V03.81 Hemophilus influenza, type B [Hib]

V03.82 Streptococcus pneumoniae [pneumococcus]

Z23 Encounter for immunization

V03.89 Other specified vaccination

V03.9 Unspecified single bacterial disease

4th **V04 Need for prophylactic vaccination and inoculation against certain diseases**
Excludes *vaccines against combinations of diseases (V06.0-V06.9)*

V04.0 Poliomyelitis

V04.1 Smallpox

V04.2 Measles alone

V04.3 Rubella alone

V04.4 Yellow fever

V04.5 Rabies

V04.6 Mumps alone

V04.7 Common cold

5th **V04.8 Other viral diseases**

V04.81 Influenza

Z23 Encounter for immunization

V04.82 Respiratory syncytial virus (RSV)

V04.89 Other viral diseases

V01.3 – V04.89

4th **V05 Need for prophylactic vaccination and inoculation against single diseases**

Excludes *vaccines against combinations of diseases (V06.0-V06.9)*

V05.0 Arthropod-borne viral encephalitis

V05.1 Other arthropod-borne viral diseases

V05.2 Leishmaniasis

V05.3 Viral hepatitis

V05.4 Varicella

Chicken pox

V05.8 Other specified disease

V05.9 Unspecified single disease

4th **V06 Need for prophylactic vaccination and inoculation against combinations of diseases**

Note: *Use additional single vaccination codes from categories V03-V05 to identify any vaccinations not included in a combination code.*

V06.0 Cholera with typhoid-paratyphoid [cholera TAB]

V06.1 Diphtheria-tetanus-pertussis, combined [DTP] [DTaP]

V06.2 Diphtheria-tetanus-pertussis with typhoid-paratyphoid [DTP TAB]

V06.3 Diphtheria-tetanus-pertussis with poliomyelitis [DTP+polio]

V06.4 Measles-mumps-rubella [MMR]

V06.5 Tetanus-diphtheria [Td] [DT]

Z23 Encounter for immunization

V06.6 Streptococcus pneumoniae [pneumococcus] and influenza

V06.8 Other combinations

Excludes *multiple single vaccination codes (V03.0-V05.9)*

V06.9 Unspecified combined vaccine

PERSONS WITH NEED FOR ISOLATION, OTHER POTENTIAL HEALTH HAZARDS AND PROPHYLACTIC MEASURES (V07-V09)

4th **V07 Need for isolation and other prophylactic measures**

Excludes *prophylactic organ removal (V50.41-V50.49)*

V07.0 Isolation

Admission to protect the individual from his surroundings or for isolation of individual after contact with infectious diseases

V07.1 Desensitization to allergens

V07.2 Prophylactic immunotherapy

Administration of:
- antivenin
- immune sera [gamma globulin]
- RhoGAM
- tetanus antitoxin

5th **V07.3 Other prophylactic chemotherapy**

V07.31 Prophylactic fluoride administration

V07.39 Other prophylactic chemotherapy

Excludes *maintenance chemotherapy following disease (V58.11)*

V07.4 Hormone replacement therapy (postmenopausal) ♀ 2

5th **V07.5 Prophylactic use of agents affecting estrogen receptors and estrogen levels**

Code first, if applicable:
- *malignant neoplasm of breast (174.0-174.9, 175.0-175.9)*
- *malignant neoplasm of prostate (185)*

Use additional code, if applicable, to identify:
- estrogen receptor positive status (V86.0)
- family history of breast cancer (V16.3)
- genetic susceptibility to cancer (V84.01-V84.09)
- personal history of breast cancer (V10.3)
- personal history of prostate cancer (V10.46)
- postmenopausal status (V49.81)

Excludes *hormone replacement therapy (postmenopausal) (V07.4)*

V07.51 Prophylactic use of selective estrogen receptor modulators (SERMs) 2

Prophylactic use of:
- raloxifene (Evista)
- tamoxifen (Nolvadex)
- toremifene (Fareston)

V07.52 Prophylactic use of aromatase inhibitors 2

Prophylactic use of:
- anastrozole (Arimidex)
- exemestane (Aromasin)
- letrozole (Femara)

V07.59 Prophylactic use of other agents affecting estrogen receptors and estrogen levels 2

Prophylactic use of:
- estrogen receptor downregulators
- fulvestrant (Faslodex)
- gonadotropin-releasing hormone (GnRH) agonist
- goserelin acetate (Zoladex)
- leuprolide acetate (leuprorelin) (Lupron)
- megestrol acetate (Megace)

V07.8 Other specified prophylactic measure

V07.9 Unspecified prophylactic measure

V08 Asymptomatic human immunodeficiency virus [HIV] infection status 159, 160, 161, 162

HIV positive NOS

Note: *This code is ONLY to be used when NO HIV infection symptoms or conditions are present. If any HIV infection symptoms or conditions are present, see code 042.*

Excludes *AIDS (042)*
- *human immunodeficiency virus [HIV] disease (042)*
- *exposure to HIV (V01.79)*
- *nonspecific serologic evidence of HIV (795.71)*
- *symptomatic human immunodeficiency virus [HIV] infection (042)*

4th **V09 Infection with drug-resistant microorganisms**

Note: *This category is intended for use as an additional code for infectious conditions classified elsewhere to indicate the presence of drug-resistance of the infectious organism.*

V09.0 Infection with microorganisms resistant to penicillins 2

V09.1 Infection with microorganisms resistant to cephalosporins and other B-lactam antibiotics 2

V09.2 Infection with microorganisms resistant to macrolides 2

V09.3 Infection with microorganisms resistant to tetracyclines 2

V09.4 Infection with microorganisms resistant to aminoglycosides 2

5th **V09.5 Infection with microorganisms resistant to quinolones and fluoroquinolones**

V09.50 Without mention of resistance to multiple quinolones and fluoroquinoles 2

V09.51 With resistance to multiple quinolones and fluoroquinoles 2

V09.6 **Infection with microorganisms resistant to sulfonamides** 2

5th V09.7 **Infection with microorganisms resistant to other specified antimycobacterial agents**

Excludes *Amikacin (V09.4)*
Kanamycin (V09.4)
Streptomycin [SM] (V09.4)

V09.70 **Without mention of resistance to multiple antimycobacterial agents** 2

V09.71 **With resistance to multiple antimycobacterial agents** 2

5th V09.8 **Infection with microorganisms resistant to other specified drugs**

Vancomycin (glycopeptide) intermediate staphylococcus aureus (VISA/GISA)
Vancomycin (glycopeptide) resistant enterococcus (VRE)
Vancomycin (glycopeptide) resistant staphylococcus aureus (VRSA/GRSA)

V09.80 **Without mention of resistance to multiple drugs** 2

V09.81 **With resistance to multiple drugs** 2

5th V09.9 **Infection with drug-resistant microorganisms, unspecified**

Drug resistance NOS

V09.90 **Without mention of multiple drug resistance** 2

V09.91 **With multiple drug resistance** 2

Multiple drug resistance NOS

PERSONS WITH POTENTIAL HEALTH HAZARDS RELATED TO PERSONAL AND FAMILY HISTORY (V10-V19)

Excludes *obstetric patients where the possibility that the fetus might be affected is the reason for observation or management during pregnancy (655.0-655.9)*

ICD-9-CM Official Guidelines (Chapter 18):

d. Categories of V Codes

4) History (of)

There are two types of history V codes, personal and family. Personal history codes explain a patient's past medical condition that no longer exists and is not receiving any treatment, but that has the potential for recurrence, and therefore may require continued monitoring. The exceptions to this general rule are category V14, Personal history of allergy to medicinal agents, and subcategory V15.0, Allergy, other than to medicinal agents. A person who has had an allergic episode to a substance or food in the past should always be considered allergic to the substance.

Family history codes are for use when a patient has a family member(s) who has had a particular disease that causes the patient to be at higher risk of also contracting the disease.

Personal history codes may be used in conjunction with follow-up codes and family history codes may be used in conjunction with screening codes to explain the need for a test or procedure. History codes are also acceptable on any medical record regardless of the reason for visit. A history of an illness, even if no longer present, is important information that may alter the type of treatment ordered.

The history V code categories are:

V10 Personal history of malignant neoplasm
V12 Personal history of certain other diseases
V13 Personal history of other diseases
Except: *V13.4, Personal history of arthritis, and V13.6, Personal history of congenital malformations. These conditions are life-long so are not true history codes.*
V14 Personal history of allergy to medicinal agents
V15 Other personal history presenting hazards to health
Except: *V15.7, Personal history of contraception.*
V16 Family history of malignant neoplasm
V17 Family history of certain chronic disabling diseases
V18 Family history of certain other specific diseases
V19 Family history of other conditions

4th V10 **Personal history of malignant neoplasm**

~~*Code first any continuing functional activity, such as: carcinoid syndrome (259.2)*~~

5th V10.0 **Gastrointestinal tract**

History of conditions classifiable to 140-159

Excludes *personal history of malignant carcinoid tumor (V10.91)*
personal history of malignant neuroendocrine tumor (V10.91)

V10.00 **Gastrointestinal tract, unspecified**
V10.01 **Tongue**
V10.02 **Other and unspecified oral cavity and pharynx**
V10.03 **Esophagus**
V10.04 **Stomach**
V10.05 **Large intestine**
V10.06 **Rectum, rectosigmoid junction, and anus**
V10.07 **Liver**
V10.09 **Other**

5th V10.1 **Trachea, bronchus, and lung**

History of conditions classifiable to 162

Excludes *personal history of malignant carcinoid tumor (V10.91)*
personal history of malignant neuroendocrine tumor (V10.91)

V10.11 **Bronchus and lung**
V10.12 **Trachea**

5th V10.2 **Other respiratory and intrathoracic organs**

History of conditions classifiable to 160, 161, 163-165

V10.20 **Respiratory organ, unspecified**
V10.21 **Larynx**
V10.22 **Nasal cavities, middle ear, and accessory sinuses**
V10.29 **Other**

V10.3 **Breast**

Z85.3 **Personal history of primary malignant neoplasm of breast**

History of conditions classifiable to 174 and 175

5th V10.4 **Genital organs**

History of conditions classifiable to 179-187

V10.40 **Female genital organ, unspecified** ♀
V10.41 **Cervix uteri** ♀
V10.42 **Other parts of uterus** ♀
V10.43 **Ovary** ♀
V10.44 **Other female genital organs** ♀
V10.45 **Male genital organ, unspecified** ♂
V10.46 **Prostate** ♂
V10.47 **Testis** ♂
V10.48 **Epididymis** ♂
V10.49 **Other male genital organs** ♂

5th V10.5 **Urinary organs**

History of conditions classifiable to 188 and 189

V10.50 **Urinary organ, unspecified**
V10.51 **Bladder**
V10.52 **Kidney**

Excludes *renal pelvis (V10.53)*

V10.53 **Renal pelvis**
V10.59 **Other**

5th V10.6 Leukemia
Conditions classifiable to 204-208
Excludes *leukemia in remission (204-208)*
V10.60 Leukemia, unspecified
V10.61 Lymphoid leukemia
V10.62 Myeloid leukemia
V10.63 Monocytic leukemia
V10.69 Other
5th V10.7 Other lymphatic and hematopoietic neoplasms
Conditions classifiable to 200-203
Excludes *listed conditions in 200-203 in remission*
V10.71 Lymphosarcoma and reticulosarcoma
V10.72 Hodgkin's disease
V10.79 Other
5th V10.8 Personal history of malignant neoplasm of other sites
History of conditions classifiable to 170-173, 190-195
Excludes *personal history of malignant carcinoid tumor (V10.91)*
personal history of malignant neuroendocrine tumor (V10.91)
V10.81 Bone
V10.82 Malignant melanoma of skin 1 3 6, 1 3 7
V10.83 Other malignant neoplasm of skin
Z85.821 Personal history of other primary malignant neoplasm of skin
V10.84 Eye
V10.85 Brain
V10.86 Other parts of nervous system
Excludes *peripheral, sympathetic, and parasympathetic nerves (V10.89)*
V10.87 Thyroid
V10.88 Other endocrine glands and related structures
V10.89 Other
▲ 5th V10.9 Other and unspecified personal history of malignant neoplasm
● V10.90 Personal history of unspecified malignant neoplasm
Personal history of malignant neoplasm NOS
Excludes *personal history of malignant carcinoid tumor (V10.91)*
personal history of malignant neuroendocrine tumor (V10.91)
personal history of Merkel cell carcinoma (V10.91)
● V10.91 Personal history of malignant neuroendocrine tumor
Personal history of malignant carcinoid tumor NOS
Personal history of malignant neuroendocrine tumor NOS
Personal history of Merkel cell carcinoma NOS
Code first any continuing functional activity, such as: carcinoid syndrome (259.2)

4th V11 Personal history of mental disorder
V11.0 Schizophrenia
Excludes *that in remission (295.0-295.9 with fifth-digit 5)*
V11.1 Affective disorders
Personal history of manic-depressive psychosis
Excludes *that in remission (296.0-296.6 with fifth-digit 5, 6)*
V11.2 Neurosis
V11.3 Alcoholism
V11.8 Other mental disorders
V11.9 Unspecified mental disorder

4th V12 Personal history of certain other diseases
5th V12.0 Infectious and parasitic diseases
Excludes *personal history of infectious disease specific to a body system*
V12.00 Unspecified infectious and parasitic disease
V12.01 Tuberculosis
V12.02 Poliomyelitis
V12.03 Malaria
V12.04 Methicillin resistant Staphylococcus aureus
MRSA
V12.09 Other
V12.1 Nutritional deficiency
V12.2 Endocrine, metabolic, and immunity disorders
Excludes *history of allergy (V14.0-V14.9, V15.01-V15.09)*
V12.3 Diseases of blood and blood-forming organs
5th V12.4 Disorders of nervous system and sense organs
V12.40 Unspecified disorder of nervous system and sense organs
V12.41 Benign neoplasm of the brain
V12.42 Infections of the central nervous system
Encephalitis
Meningitis
V12.49 Other disorders of nervous system and sense organs
5th V12.5 Diseases of circulatory system
Excludes *old myocardial infarction (412)*
postmyocardial infarction syndrome (411.0)
V12.50 Unspecified circulatory disease
V12.51 Venous thrombosis and embolism
Pulmonary embolism
V12.52 Thrombophlebitis
V12.53 Sudden cardiac arrest
Sudden cardiac death successfully resuscitated
V12.54 Transient ischemic attack (TIA), and cerebral infarction without residual deficits
Prolonged reversible ischemic neurological deficit (PRIND)
Reversible ischemic neurologic deficit (RIND)
Stroke NOS without residual deficits
Excludes *history of traumatic brain injury (V15.52)*
late effects of cerebrovascular disease (438.0-438.9)
V12.59 Other
5th V12.6 Diseases of respiratory system
Excludes *tuberculosis (V12.01)*
V12.60 Unspecified disease of respiratory system
V12.61 Pneumonia (recurrent)
V12.69 Other disease of respiratory system
5th V12.7 Diseases of digestive system
V12.70 Unspecified digestive disease
V12.71 Peptic ulcer disease
V12.72 Colonic polyps 1 8 5
V12.79 Other

4th V13 Personal history of other diseases
5th V13.0 Disorders of urinary system
V13.00 Unspecified urinary disorder
V13.01 Urinary calculi
V13.02 Urinary (tract) infection
V13.03 Nephrotic syndrome
V13.09 Other

V13.1 Trophoblastic disease ♀
Excludes *supervision during a current pregnancy (V23.1)*

5th V13.2 Other genital system and obstetric disorders
Excludes *supervision during a current pregnancy of a woman with poor obstetric history (V23.0-V23.9)*
habitual aborter (646.3)
without current pregnancy (629.81)

V13.21 Personal history of pre-term labor ♀
Excludes *current pregnancy with history of pre-term labor (V23.41)*

V13.22 Personal history of cervical dysplasia ♀
Personal history of conditions classifiable to 622.10-622.12
Excludes *personal history of malignant neoplasm of cervix uteri (V10.41)*

V13.29 Other genital system and obstetric disorders ♀

V13.3 Diseases of skin and subcutaneous tissue

V13.4 Arthritis

5th V13.5 Other musculoskeletal disorders

V13.51 Pathologic fracture
Healed pathologic fracture
Excludes *personal history of traumatic fracture (V15.51)*

V13.52 Stress fracture
Healed stress fracture
Excludes *personal history of traumatic fracture (V15.51)*

V13.59 Other musculoskeletal disorders

5th V13.6 Congenital malformations

V13.61 Hypospadias ♂

V13.69 Other congenital malformations

V13.7 Perinatal problems
Excludes *low birth weight status (V21.30-V21.35)*

V13.8 Other specified diseases

V13.9 Unspecified disease

4th V14 Personal history of allergy to medicinal agents

V14.0 Penicillin 2

V14.1 Other antibiotic agent 2

V14.2 Sulfonamides 2

V14.3 Other anti-infective agent 2

V14.4 Anesthetic agent 2

V14.5 Narcotic agent 2

V14.6 Analgesic agent 2

V14.7 Serum or vaccine 2

V14.8 Other specified medicinal agents 2

V14.9 Unspecified medicinal agent 2

4th V15 Other personal history presenting hazards to health
Excludes *personal history of drug therapy (V87.41-V87.49)*

5th V15.0 Allergy, other than to medicinal agents
Excludes *allergy to food substance used as base for medicinal agent (V14.0-V14.9)*

V15.01 Allergy to peanuts 2

V15.02 Allergy to milk products 2
Excludes *lactose intolerance (271.3)*

V15.03 Allergy to eggs 2

V15.04 Allergy to seafood 2
Seafood (octopus) (squid) ink
Shellfish

V15.05 Allergy to other foods 2
Food additives
Nuts other than peanuts

▲ V15.06 Allergy to insects and arachnids 2
Bugs
Insect bites and stings
Spiders

V15.07 Allergy to latex 2
Latex sensitivity

V15.08 Allergy to radiographic dye 2
Contrast media used for diagnostic x-ray procedures

V15.09 Other allergy, other than to medicinal agents 2

V15.1 Surgery to heart and great vessels 2
Excludes *replacement by transplant or other means (V42.1-V42.2, V43.2-V43.4)*

5th V15.2 Surgery to other organs
Excludes *replacement by transplant or other means (V42.0-V43.8)*

V15.21 Personal history of undergoing in utero procedure during pregnancy M ♀ 2

V15.22 Personal history of undergoing in utero procedure while a fetus 2

V15.29 Surgery to other organs 2

V15.3 Irradiation 2
Previous exposure to therapeutic or other ionizing radiation

5th V15.4 Psychological trauma
Excludes *history of condition classifiable to 290-316 (V11.0-V11.9)*

V15.41 History of physical abuse 2
Rape

V15.42 History of emotional abuse 2
Neglect

V15.49 Other 2

5th V15.5 Injury

V15.51 Traumatic fracture 2
Healed traumatic fracture
Excludes *personal history of pathologic and stress fracture (V13.51, V13.52)*

● V15.52 History of traumatic brain injury 2
Excludes *personal history of cerebrovascular accident (cerebral infarction) without residual deficits (V12.54)*

V15.59 Other injury 2

V15.6 Poisoning 2

V15.7 Contraception 2
Excludes *current contraceptive management (V25.0-V25.4)*
presence of intrauterine contraceptive device as incidental finding (V45.5)

5th V15.8 Other specified personal history presenting hazards to health
Excludes *contact with and (suspected) exposure to:*
aromatic compounds and dyes (V87.11-V87.19)
arsenic and other metals (V87.01-V87.09)
molds (V87.31)

● V15.80 History of failed moderate sedation 2
History of failed conscious sedation

Rationale: *The American Society of Anesthesiologists (ASA) requested a unique ICD-9-CM diagnosis code to describe instances of failed sedation. Under some circumstances, moderate (conscious) sedation by non-anesthesia providers can be sufficient to provide safe and satisfactory pain relief and/or amnesia to patients undergoing noxious procedures that do not ordinarily require a full anesthetic. In some situations, however, this may produce inadequate* *sedation making the procedure more difficult to perform and less satisfactory to the patient or may also produce unsafe conditions for the patient. Reasons for this may include, but are not limited to, situations where, maximum prudent and safe medication doses are administered but the patient remains inadequately sedated for the procedure; patient exhibits idiosyncratic responses to the mediations administered; patient becomes more deeply sedated than intended; patient is unable to adequately maintain a patent airway but respirations are depressed such that adequate air exchange is compromised; hemodynamic changes occur posing potential risks to the patient; other situations arise that are beyond the experience or expertise of the provider administering sedation.*

Such situations may have arisen during a previous procedure performed under moderate (conscious) sedating, necessitating planned intervention during subsequent procedures. Alternatively this situation may occur during a procedure currently in progress, making urgent intervention necessary to ensure a safe outcome for the patient and satisfactory conditions for completion of the procedure. In such circumstances, it may be necessary to enlist the services of an anesthesiologist or other provider with the training to administer adequate moderate (conscious) sedation or to administer deep sedation and/or anesthesia.

V15.81 Noncompliance with medical treatment 2

Excludes *noncompliance with renal dialysis (V45.12)*

V15.82 History of tobacco use 2

Excludes *tobacco dependence (305.1)*

● **V15.83 Underimmunization status** 2

Delinquent immunization status
Lapsed immunization schedule status

Rationale: *Childhood immunization is a key element in the prevention of childhood illness. According to the 2006 National Immunization Survey, a significant number of children are "under immunized". T hey may have received none or only some of the recommended immunization schedule. Some common reasons identified for this include: persons immigrating to the United States; foreign adoptees who may not have been fully immunized according to U.S. scheduled recommendations; families moving without re-establishing with a new provider to continue the recommended vaccination schedule; as well as persons without health insurance coverage for immunizations.*

Studies show that there is a poor "catch-up" rate for delinquent immunizations in older children. While there were ICD-9-CM codes in the V64.0 sub-category to indicate why an immunization was not carried out when offered, there was no code to indicate the status of the person who is at risk due to being behind schedule on the recommended immunization schedule. These people place themselves and others at risk of contracting and spreading a given disease for which they are not immunized.

To help better track this at risk population the American Academy of Pediatrics (AAP) requested that a new unique status V code be established.

▲ **V15.84 Contact with and (suspected) exposure to asbestos** 2

▲ **V15.85 Contact with and (suspected) exposure to potentially hazardous body fluids** 2

▲ **V15.86 Contact with and (suspected) exposure to lead** 2

V15.87 History of extracorporeal membrane oxygenation [ECMO] 2

V15.88 History of fall

At risk for falling

V15.89 Other 2

Excludes *contact with and (suspected) exposure to other potentially hazardous chemicals (V87.2)*
contact with and (suspected) exposure to other potentially hazardous substances (V87.39)

Layman's: *For Medicare, V15.89 is used in lieu of V76.2 for patients who meet the specified criteria as at high risk for cervical or vaginal cancer. Other carriers may have different coding guidelines.*

V15.9 Unspecified personal history presenting hazards to health 2

4th **V16 Family history of malignant neoplasm**

V16.0 Gastrointestinal tract
Family history of condition classifiable to 140-159

V16.1 Trachea, bronchus, and lung
Family history of condition classifiable to 162

V16.2 Other respiratory and intrathoracic organs
Family history of condition classifiable to 160-161, 163-165

V16.3 Breast
Family history of condition classifiable to 174

5th **V16.4 Genital organs**
Family history of condition classifiable to 179-187

V16.40 Genital organ, unspecified

V16.41 Ovary

V16.42 Prostate

V16.43 Testis

V16.49 Other

5th **V16.5 Urinary organs**
Family history of condition classifiable to 188-189

V16.51 Kidney

V16.52 Bladder

V16.59 Other

V16.6 Leukemia
Family history of condition classifiable to 204-208

V16.7 Other lymphatic and hematopoietic neoplasms
Family history of condition classifiable to 200-203

V16.8 Other specified malignant neoplasm
Family history of other condition classifiable to 140-199

V16.9 Unspecified malignant neoplasm

4th **V17 Family history of certain chronic disabling diseases**

V17.0 Psychiatric condition

Excludes *family history of mental retardation (V18.4)*

V17.1 Stroke (cerebrovascular)

V17.2 Other neurological diseases
Epilepsy
Huntington's chorea

V17.3 Ischemic heart disease

5th **V17.4 Other cardiovascular diseases**

V17.41 Family history of sudden cardiac death (SCD)

Excludes *family history of ischemic heart disease (V17.3)*
family history of myocardial infarction (V17.3)

V17.49 Family history of other cardiovascular diseases
Family history of cardiovascular disease NOS

V17.5 Asthma

V17.6 Other chronic respiratory conditions

V17.7 Arthritis

5th **V17.8 Other musculoskeletal diseases**

V17.81 Osteoporosis

V17.89 Other musculoskeletal disease

4th V18 Family history of certain other specific conditions
- V18.0 Diabetes mellitus
- 5th V18.1 Other endocrine and metabolic diseases
  - V18.11 Multiple endocrine neoplasia [MEN] syndrome
  - V18.19 Other endocrine and metabolic diseases
- V18.2 Anemia
- V18.3 Other blood disorders
- V18.4 Mental retardation
- 5th V18.5 Digestive disorders
  - V18.51 Colonic polyps
    - **Excludes** *family history of malignant neoplasm of gastrointestinal tract (V16.0)*
  - V18.59 Other digestive disorders
- 5th V18.6 Kidney diseases
  - V18.61 Polycystic kidney
  - V18.69 Other kidney diseases
- V18.7 Other genitourinary diseases
- V18.8 Infectious and parasitic diseases
- V18.9 Genetic disease carrier

4th V19 Family history of other conditions
- V19.0 Blindness or visual loss
- V19.1 Other eye disorders
- V19.2 Deafness or hearing loss
- V19.3 Other ear disorders
- V19.4 Skin conditions
- V19.5 Congenital anomalies
- V19.6 Allergic disorders
- V19.7 Consanguinity
- V19.8 Other condition

PERSONS ENCOUNTERING HEALTH SERVICES IN CIRCUMSTANCES RELATED TO REPRODUCTION AND DEVELOPMENT (V20-V29)

4th V20 Health supervision of infant or child
- V20.0 Foundling P I
- V20.1 Other healthy infant or child receiving care P I
  - Medical or nursing care supervision of healthy infant in cases of:
    - maternal illness, physical or psychiatric
    - socioeconomic adverse condition at home
    - too many children at home preventing or interfering with normal care
- V20.2 Routine infant or child health check P I
  - Developmental testing of infant or child
  - Health check for child over 28 days old
  - Immunizations appropriate for age
  - ~~Initial and subsequent routine newborn check~~
  - Routine vision and hearing testing
  - Use additional code(s) to identify:
    - special screening examination(s) performed (V73.0-V82.9)
  - **Excludes** *health check for child under 29 days old (V20.31-V20.32)*
    - *newborn health supervision (V20.31-V20.32)*
    - *special screening for developmental handicaps (V79.3)*

ICD-9-CM Official Guidelines (Chapter 18):

d. Categories of V Codes

13) Routine and administrative examinations

The V codes allow for the description of encounters for routine examinations, such as, a general check-up, or, examinations for administrative purposes, such as, a pre-employment physical. The codes are not to be used if the examination is for diagnosis of a suspected condition or for treatment purposes. In such cases the diagnosis code is used. During a routine exam, should a diagnosis or condition be discovered, it should be coded as an additional code. Pre-existing and chronic conditions and history codes may also be included as additional codes as long as the examination is for administrative purposes and not focused on any particular condition.

Pre-operative examination V codes are for use only in those situations when a patient is being cleared for surgery and no treatment is given.

● 5th V20.3 Newborn health supervision
- Health check for child under 29 days old
- **Excludes** *health check for child over 28 days old (V20.2)*

Rationale: *The American Academy of Pediatrics (AAP) recommends that all otherwise healthy newborns that are discharged from the hospital less than 48 hours from delivery should be examined by their primary care provider within 2 days of that discharge.*

The purpose of the follow-up visit is to:

- *Weigh the infant; assess the infant's general health, hydration, and degree of jaundice; identify any new problems; review feeding pattern and technique, including observation of breastfeeding for adequacy of position, latch-on, and swallowing; and obtain historical evidence of adequate urination and defecation patterns for the infant.*
- *Assess quality of mother-infant interaction and details of infant behavior.*
- *Reinforce maternal or family education in infant care, particularly regarding infant feeding.*
- *Review the outstanding results of laboratory tests performed before discharge.*
- *Perform screening tests in accordance with state regulations and other tests that are clinically indicated, such as serum bilirubin.*
- *Verify the plan for health care maintenance, including a method for obtaining emergency services, preventive care and immunizations, periodic evaluations and physical examinations, and necessary screenings.*

AAP raised the concern that existing codes did not adequately describe the reason for the encounter, including codes for the well child exam (V20.2), observation for other specified condition (V29.8) and other specified aftercare (V58.89). Therefore, AAP asked that a new specific code be established for this type of visit. Based on recently published guidelines from AAP for post-hospital newborn care for both vaginal and caesarian deliveries, modifications to the previous proposal were made to delineate between infants in the first 7 days of life and those aged 8 to 28 days.

- ● V20.31 Health supervision for newborn under 8 days old N I
  - Health check for newborn under 8 days old
- ● V20.32 Health supervision for newborn 8 to 28 days old N I
  - Health check for newborn 8 to 28 days old
  - Newborn weight check

4th V21 Constitutional states in development
- V21.0 Period of rapid growth in childhood 2
- V21.1 Puberty 2
- V21.2 Other adolescence 2
- 5th V21.3 Low birth weight status
  - **Excludes** *history of perinatal problems (V13.7)*
  - V21.30 Low birth weight status, unspecified 2
  - V21.31 Low birth weight status, less than 500 grams 2
  - V21.32 Low birth weight status, 500-999 grams 2
  - V21.33 Low birth weight status, 1000-1499 grams 2
  - V21.34 Low birth weight status, 1500-1999 grams 2
  - V21.35 Low birth weight status, 2000-2500 grams 2

V21.8 Other specified constitutional states in development 2

V21.9 Unspecified constitutional state in development 2

4th V22 Normal pregnancy

Excludes *pregnancy examination or test, pregnancy unconfirmed (V72.40)*

ICD-9-CM Official Guidelines (Chapter 18):

d. Categories of V Codes

11) Obstetrics and related conditions

See Section I.C.11., the Obstetrics guidelines for further instruction on the use of these codes.

V codes for pregnancy are for use in those circumstances when none of the problems or complications included in the codes from the Obstetrics chapter exist (a routine prenatal visit or postpartum care). Codes V22.0, Supervision of normal first pregnancy, and V22.1, Supervision of other normal pregnancy, are always first listed and are not to be used with any other code from the OB chapter.

The outcome of delivery, category V27, should be included on all maternal delivery records. It is always a secondary code.

V codes for family planning (contraceptive) or procreative management and counseling should be included on an obstetric record either during the pregnancy or the postpartum stage, if applicable.

Obstetrics and related conditions V code categories:

V22 Normal pregnancy

V23 Supervision of high-risk pregnancy

***Except:** V23.2, Pregnancy with history of abortion. Code 646.3, Habitual aborter, from the OB chapter is required to indicate a history of abortion during a pregnancy.*

V24 Postpartum care and evaluation

V25 Encounter for contraceptive management

***Except:** V25.0x*

(See Section I.C.18.d.11, Counseling)

V26 Procreative management

***Except:** V26.5x, Sterilization status, V26.3 and V26.4*

(See Section I.C.18.d.11., Counseling)

V27 Outcome of delivery

V28 Antenatal screening

(See Section I.C.18.d.6., Screening)

V22.0 Supervision of normal first pregnancy ♀ I 6 1 1

V22.1 Supervision of other normal pregnancy ♀ I 6 1 1

V22.2 Pregnant state, incidental ♀ I 6 1 2

Pregnant state NOS

4th V23 Supervision of high-risk pregnancy

V23.0 Pregnancy with history of infertility M ♀ I 6 1

V23.1 Pregnancy with history of trophoblastic disease M ♀ I 6 1

Pregnancy with history of:

hydatidiform mole

vesicular mole

Excludes *that without current pregnancy (V13.1)*

V23.2 Pregnancy with history of abortion M ♀ I 6 1

Pregnancy with history of conditions classifiable to 634-638

Excludes *habitual aborter:*

care during pregnancy (646.3)

that without current pregnancy (629.81)

V23.3 Grand multiparity M ♀ I 6 1

Excludes *care in relation to labor and delivery (659.4)*

that without current pregnancy (V61.5)

5th V23.4 Pregnancy with other poor obstetric history

Pregnancy with history of other conditions classifiable to 630-676

V23.41 Pregnancy with history of pre-term labor M ♀ I 6 1

V23.49 Pregnancy with other poor obstetric history M ♀ I 6 1

V23.5 Pregnancy with other poor reproductive history M ♀ I 6 1

Pregnancy with history of stillbirth or neonatal death

V23.7 Insufficient prenatal care M ♀ I 6 1

History of little or no prenatal care

5th V23.8 Other high-risk pregnancy

V23.81 Elderly primigravida M ♀ I 6 1

First pregnancy in a woman who will be 35 years of age or older at expected date of delivery

Excludes *elderly primigravida complicating pregnancy (659.5)*

V23.82 Elderly multigravida M ♀ I 6 1

Second or more pregnancy in a woman who will be 35 years of age or older at expected date of delivery

Excludes *elderly multigravida complicating pregnancy (659.6)*

V23.83 Young primigravida M ♀ I 6 1

First pregnancy in a female less than 16 years old at expected date of delivery

Excludes *young primigravida complicating pregnancy (659.8)*

V23.84 Young multigravida M ♀ I 6 1

Second or more pregnancy in a female less than 16 years old at expected date of delivery

Excludes *young multigravida complicating pregnancy (659.8)*

V23.85 Pregnancy resulting from assisted reproductive technology M ♀

Pregnancy resulting from in vitro fertilization

V23.86 Pregnancy with history of in utero procedure during previous pregnancy M ♀

Excludes *management of pregnancy affected by in utero procedure during current pregnancy (679.0- 679.1)*

V23.89 Other high-risk pregnancy M ♀ I 6 1

V23.9 Unspecified high-risk pregnancy M ♀ I 6 1

4th V24 Postpartum care and examination

ICD-9-CM Official Guidelines (Chapter 18):

d. Categories of V Codes

8) Follow-up

The follow-up codes are used to explain continuing surveillance following completed treatment of a disease, condition, or injury. They imply that the condition has been fully treated and no longer exists. They should not be confused with aftercare codes that explain current treatment for a healing condition or its sequelae. Follow-up codes may be used in conjunction with history codes to provide the full picture of the healed condition and its treatment. The follow-up code is sequenced first, followed by the history code.

A follow-up code may be used to explain repeated visits. Should a condition be found to have recurred on the follow-up visit, then the diagnosis code should be used in place of the follow-up code.

V24.0 Immediately after delivery M ♀ 1

Care and observation in uncomplicated cases

V24.1 Lactating mother ♀ 1

Supervision of lactation

V24.2 Routine postpartum follow-up ♀ 1

4th V25 Encounter for contraceptive management

5th V25.0 General counseling and advice

V25.01 Prescription of oral contraceptives ♀

V25.02 **Initiation of other contraceptive measures**
Fitting of diaphragm
Prescription of foams, creams, or other agents

V25.03 **Encounter for emergency contraceptive counseling and prescription**
Encounter for postcoital contraceptive counseling and prescription

V25.04 **Counseling and instruction in natural family planning to avoid pregnancy**

V25.09 **Other**
Family planning advice

V25.1 **Insertion of intrauterine contraceptive device** ♀

V25.2 **Sterilization**
Admission for interruption of fallopian tubes or vas deferens

V25.3 **Menstrual extraction** ♀
Menstrual regulation

5th V25.4 **Surveillance of previously prescribed contraceptive methods**
Checking, reinsertion, or removal of contraceptive device
Repeat prescription for contraceptive method
Routine examination in connection with contraceptive maintenance

Excludes *presence of intrauterine contraceptive device as incidental finding (V45.5)*

V25.40 **Contraceptive surveillance, unspecified**

V25.41 **Contraceptive pill** ♀

V25.42 **Intrauterine contraceptive device** ♀
Checking, reinsertion, or removal of intrauterine device

V25.43 **Implantable subdermal contraceptive** ♀

V25.49 **Other contraceptive method**

V25.5 **Insertion of implantable subdermal contraceptive** ♀

V25.8 **Other specified contraceptive management**
Postvasectomy sperm count

Excludes *sperm count following sterilization reversal (V26.22)*
sperm count for fertility testing (V26.21)

V25.9 **Unspecified contraceptive management**

4th V26 **Procreative management**

V26.0 **Tuboplasty or vasoplasty after previous sterilization**

V26.1 **Artificial insemination** ♀

5th V26.2 **Investigation and testing**

Excludes *postvasectomy sperm count (V25.8)*

V26.21 **Fertility testing**
Fallopian insufflation
Sperm count for fertility testing

Excludes *genetic counseling and testing (V26.31-V26.39)*

V26.22 **Aftercare following sterilization reversal**
Fallopian insufflation following sterilization reversal
Sperm count following sterilization reversal

V26.29 **Other investigation and testing**

5th V26.3 **Genetic counseling and testing**

Excludes *fertility testing (V26.21)*
nonprocreative genetic screening (V82.71, V82.79)

V26.31 **Testing of female for genetic disease carrier status** ♀

V26.32 **Other genetic testing of female** ♀
Use additional code to identify habitual aborter (629.81, 646.3)

V26.33 **Genetic counseling**

V26.34 **Testing of male for genetic disease carrier status** ♂

V26.35 **Encounter for testing of male partner of habitual aborter** ♂

V26.39 **Other genetic testing of male** ♂

5th V26.4 **General counseling and advice**

V26.41 **Procreative counseling and advice using natural family planning**

● V26.42 **Encounter for fertility preservation counseling**
Encounter for fertility preservation counseling prior to cancer therapy
Encounter for fertility preservation counseling prior to surgical removal of gonads

Rationale: *More and more patients are living significant portions of their life following the diagnosis of cancer. Some types of cancer treatment can affect a person's ability to conceive a child or maintain a pregnancy. Infertility following cancer treatment may be temporary or permanent and may depend on the type and dose of drugs given, how drugs are given, dose of radiation therapy and the area being irradiated, type of cancer, patient's age and gender, and whether a patient had fertility problems before cancer treatment.*

The first goal is to cure the cancer, even if the treatment causes sterility. However since it may be possible to preserve fertility before and after cancer treatments patients are advised to talk with their doctor, or may be referred to a fertility specialist, to become informed about options available before starting treatment (chemotherapy, surgery or radiation). Discussion points may include: whether the patient should try to conceive before cancer treatment, should he/she try to bank sperm/eggs/ovarian tissue/embryos, should the surgery be modified so as to spare the uterus (possible in some types of cervical cancer), and the pros and cons of attempting to undergo fertility preservation or tissue/gamete banking.

The American Society for Reproductive Medicine (ASRM) in collaboration with the American College of OB-GYN (ACOG) requested codes for encounters for fertility preservation. The use of these codes need not be limited to those seeking this advice prior to cancer treatment. They may be applied to individuals seeking this advice prior to other treatments that could affect fertility.

V26.49 **Other procreative management counseling and advice**

5th V26.5 **Sterilization status**

V26.51 **Tubal ligation status** ♀ 2

Excludes *infertility not due to previous tubal ligation (628.0-628.9)*

V26.52 **Vasectomy status** ♂ 2

5th V26.8 **Other specified procreative management**

V26.81 **Encounter for assisted reproductive fertility procedure cycle** ♀ 1
Patient undergoing in vitro fertilization cycle
Use additional code to identify the type of infertility

Excludes *pre-cycle diagnosis and testing – code to reason for encounter*

● V26.82 **Encounter for fertility preservation procedure** 1
Encounter for fertility preservation procedure prior to cancer therapy
Encounter for fertility preservation procedure prior to surgical removal of gonads

V26.89 **Other specified procreative management**

V26.9 **Unspecified procreative management**

V25.02 – V26.9

4th V27 **Outcome of delivery**

Note: *This category is intended for the coding of the outcome of delivery on the mother's record.*

- V27.0 **Single liveborn** M ♀ 2
- V27.1 **Single stillborn** M ♀ 2
- V27.2 **Twins, both liveborn** M ♀ 2
- V27.3 **Twins, one liveborn and one stillborn** M ♀ 2
- V27.4 **Twins, both stillborn** M ♀ 2
- V27.5 **Other multiple birth, all liveborn** M ♀ 2
- V27.6 **Other multiple birth, some liveborn** M ♀ 2
- V27.7 **Other multiple birth, all stillborn** M ♀ 2
- V27.9 **Unspecified outcome of delivery** M ♀ 2

4th V28 **Encounter for antenatal screening of mother**

Excludes *abnormal findings on screening – code to findings*
routine prenatal care (V22.0-V23.9)
suspected fetal conditions affecting management of pregnancy (655.00-655.93, 656.00-656.93, 657.00-657.03, 658.00-658.93)
suspected fetal conditions not found (V89.01-V89.09)

ICD-9-CM Official Guidelines (Chapter 18):

d. Categories of V Codes

5) Screening

Screening is the testing for disease or disease precursors in seemingly well individuals so that early detection and treatment can be provided for those who test positive for the disease. Screenings that are recommended for many subgroups in a population include: routine mammograms for women over 40, a fecal occult blood test for everyone over 50, an amniocentesis to rule out a fetal anomaly for pregnant women over 35, because the incidence of breast cancer and colon cancer in these subgroups is higher than in the general population, as is the incidence of Down's syndrome in older mothers.

The testing of a person to rule out or confirm a suspected diagnosis because the patient has some sign or symptom is a diagnostic examination, not a screening. In these cases, the sign or symptom is used to explain the reason for the test.

A screening code may be a first listed code if the reason for the visit is specifically the screening exam. It may also be used as an additional code if the screening is done during an office visit for other health problems. A screening code is not necessary if the screening is inherent to a routine examination, such as a pap smear done during a routine pelvic examination.

Should a condition be discovered during the screening then the code for the condition may be assigned as an additional diagnosis.

The V code indicates that a screening exam is planned. A procedure code is required to confirm that the screening was performed.

- V28.0 **Screening for chromosomal anomalies by amniocentesis** M ♀
- V28.1 **Screening for raised alpha-fetoprotein levels in amniotic fluid** M ♀
- V28.2 **Other screening based on amniocentesis** M ♀
- V28.3 **Encounter for routine screening for malformation using ultrasonics** ♀
  Encounter for routine fetal ultrasound NOS
  Excludes *encounter for fetal anatomic survey (V28.81)*
  genetic counseling and testing (V26.31- V26.39)
- V28.4 **Screening for fetal growth retardation using ultrasonics** ♀
- V28.5 **Screening for isoimmunization** ♀
- V28.6 **Screening for Streptococcus B** M ♀

5th V28.8 **Other specified antenatal screening**

- V28.81 **Encounter for fetal anatomic survey** M ♀
- V28.82 **Encounter for screening for risk of pre-term labor** M ♀
- V28.89 **Other specified antenatal screening** M ♀
  Chorionic villus sampling
  Genomic screening
  Nuchal translucency testing
  Proteomic screening

V28.9 **Unspecified antenatal screening** ♀

4th V29 **Observation and evaluation of newborns for suspected condition not found**

Note: *This category is to be used for newborns, within the neonatal period (the first 28 days of life), who are suspected of having an abnormal condition resulting from exposure from the mother or the birth process, but without signs or symptoms, and which, after examination and observation, is found not to exist.*

Excludes *suspected fetal conditions not found (V89.01-V89.09)*

ICD-9-CM Official Guidelines (Chapter 18):

d. Categories of V Codes

6) Observation

There are two observation V code categories. They are for use in very limited circumstances when a person is being observed for a suspected condition that is ruled out. The observation codes are not for use if an injury or illness or any signs or symptoms related to the suspected condition are present. In such cases the diagnosis/symptom code is used with the corresponding E code to identify any external cause.

The observation codes are to be used as principal diagnosis only. The only exception to this is when the principal diagnosis is required to be a code from the V30, Live born infant, category. Then the V29 observation code is sequenced after the V30 code. Additional codes may be used in addition to the observation code but only if they are unrelated to the suspected condition being observed.

- V29.0 **Observation for suspected infectious condition** N 1
- V29.1 **Observation for suspected neurological condition** N 1
- V29.2 **Observation for suspected respiratory condition** N 1
- V29.3 **Observation for suspected genetic or metabolic condition** N 1
- V29.8 **Observation for other specified suspected condition** N 1
- V29.9 **Observation for unspecified suspected condition** N 1

LIVEBORN INFANTS ACCORDING TO TYPE OF BIRTH (V30-V39)

Note: *These categories are intended for the coding of liveborn infants who are consuming health care [e.g., crib or bassinet occupancy].*

The following fourth-digit subdivisions are for use with categories V30-V39:

5th .0 **Born in hospital** N
[0-1]
.1 **Born before admission to hospital** N
.2 **Born outside hospital and not hospitalized**

The following two fifth-digits are for use with the fourth-digit .0, Born in hospital:

0 delivered without mention of cesarean delivery
1 delivered by cesarean delivery

4th V30 **Single liveborn** 1
[.0-.2]

4th V31 **Twin, mate liveborn** 1
[.0-.2]

4th V32 **Twin, mate stillborn** 1
[.0-.2]

4th V33 **Twin, unspecified** 1
[.0-.2]

4th V34 **Other multiple, mates all liveborn** 1
[.0-.2]

4th V35 Other multiple, mates all stillborn
[.0-.2]

4th V36 Other multiple, mates live- and stillborn
[.0-.2]

4th V37 Other multiple, unspecified
[.0-.2]

4th V39 Unspecified
[.0-.2]

PERSONS WITH A CONDITION INFLUENCING THEIR HEALTH STATUS (V40-V49)

Note: *These categories are intended for use when these conditions are recorded as "diagnoses" or "problems."*

4th V40 Mental and behavioral problems
- V40.0 Problems with learning
- V40.1 Problems with communication [including speech]
- V40.2 Other mental problems
- V40.3 Other behavioral problems
- V40.9 Unspecified mental or behavioral problem

4th V41 Problems with special senses and other special functions
- V41.0 Problems with sight
- V41.1 Other eye problems
- V41.2 Problems with hearing
- V41.3 Other ear problems
- V41.4 Problems with voice production
- V41.5 Problems with smell and taste
- V41.6 Problems with swallowing and mastication
- V41.7 Problems with sexual function
  - Excludes *marital problems (V61.10)*
    psychosexual disorders (302.0-302.9)
- V41.8 Other problems with special functions
- V41.9 Unspecified problem with special functions

4th V42 Organ or tissue replaced by transplant
Includes homologous or heterologous (animal) (human) transplant organ status
- V42.0 Kidney 2
  - Z94.0 Kidney transplant status
- V42.1 Heart 2
- V42.2 Heart valve 2
- V42.3 Skin 2
- V42.4 Bone 2
- V42.5 Cornea 2
- V42.6 Lung 2
- V42.7 Liver 2
- 5th V42.8 Other specified organ or tissue
  - V42.81 Bone marrow 2
  - V42.82 Peripheral stem cells 2
  - V42.83 Pancreas 2
  - V42.84 Intestines 2
  - V42.89 Other 2
- V42.9 Unspecified organ or tissue 2

4th V43 Organ or tissue replaced by other means
Includes organ or tissue assisted by other means
replacement of organ by:
artificial device
mechanical device
prosthesis
Excludes *cardiac pacemaker in situ (V45.01)*
fitting and adjustment of prosthetic device (V52.0-V52.9)
renal dialysis status (V45.11)
- V43.0 Eye globe 2
- V43.1 Lens 2
  - Z96.1 Presence of intraocular lens
    Pseudophakos
- 5th V43.2 Heart
  - V43.21 Heart assist device 2
  - V43.22 Fully implantable artificial heart 2
- V43.3 Heart valve 2
  - Z95.2 Presence of prosthetic heart valve
- V43.4 Blood vessel 2
- V43.5 Bladder 2
- 5th V43.6 Joint
  - V43.60 Unspecified joint 2
  - V43.61 Shoulder 2
  - V43.62 Elbow 2
  - V43.63 Wrist 2
  - V43.64 Hip 2
    - Z96.649 Presence of unspecified artificial hip joint
  - V43.65 Knee 2
    - Z96.659 Presence of unspecified artificial knee joint
  - V43.66 Ankle 2
  - V43.69 Other 2
- V43.7 Limb 2
- 5th V43.8 Other organ or tissue
  - V43.81 Larynx 2
  - V43.82 Breast 2
  - V43.83 Artificial skin 2
  - V43.89 Other 2

4th V44 Artificial opening status
Excludes *artificial openings requiring attention or management (V55.0-V55.9)*
- V44.0 Tracheostomy 2
- V44.1 Gastrostomy 2
- V44.2 Ileostomy 2
- V44.3 Colostomy 2
- V44.4 Other artificial opening of gastrointestinal tract 2
- 5th V44.5 Cystostomy
  - V44.50 Cystostomy, unspecified 2
  - V44.51 Cutaneous-vesicostomy 2
  - V44.52 Appendico-vesicostomy 2
  - V44.59 Other cystostomy 2
- V44.6 Other artificial opening of urinary tract 2
  Nephrostomy
  Ureterostomy
  Urethrostomy
- V44.7 Artificial vagina 2
- V44.8 Other artificial opening status 2
- V44.9 Unspecified artificial opening status 2

4th V45 Other postprocedural states
Excludes *aftercare management (V51-V58.9)*
malfunction or other complicationcode to condition
- 5th V45.0 Cardiac device in situ
  - Excludes *artificial heart (V43.22)*
    heart assist device (V43.21)
  - V45.00 Unspecified cardiac device 2
  - V45.01 Cardiac pacemaker 2
    - Z95.0 Presence of cardiac pacemaker
  - V45.02 Automatic implantable cardiac defibrillator 2

V35 – V45.02

V45.09 Other specified cardiac device 2
Carotid sinus pacemaker in situ

5th V45.1 Renal dialysis status
Excludes *admission for dialysis treatment or session (V56.0)*

V45.11 Renal dialysis status 2
Hemodialysis status
Patient requiring intermittent renal dialysis
Peritoneal dialysis status
Presence of arterial-venous shunt (for dialysis)

V45.12 Noncompliance with renal dialysis 2

V45.2 Presence of cerebrospinal fluid drainage device 2
Cerebral ventricle (communicating) shunt, valve, or device in situ
Excludes *malfunction (996.2)*

V45.3 Intestinal bypass or anastomosis status 2
Excludes *bariatric surgery status (V45.86)*
gastric bypass status (V45.86)
obesity surgery status (V45.86)

V45.4 Arthrodesis status 2

5th V45.5 Presence of contraceptive device
Excludes *checking, reinsertion, or removal of device (V25.42)*
complication from device (996.32)
insertion of device (V25.1)

V45.51 Intrauterine contraceptive device ♀ 2

V45.52 Subdermal contraceptive implant 2

V45.59 Other 2

5th V45.6 States following surgery of eye and adnexa
Excludes *aphakia (379.31)*
artificial eye globe (V43.0)

V45.61 Cataract extraction status 2
Use additional code for associated artifical lens status (V43.1)

V45.69 Other states following surgery of eye and adnexa 2

5th V45.7 Acquired absence of organ

V45.71 Acquired absence of breast and nipple
Excludes *congenital absence of breast and nipple (757.6)*

V45.72 Acquired absence of intestine (large) (small)

V45.73 Acquired absence of kidney

V45.74 Other parts of urinary tract
Bladder

V45.75 Stomach

V45.76 Lung

V45.77 Genital organs
Excludes *acquired absence of cervix and uterus (V88.01-V88.03)*
female genital mutilation status (629.20-629.29)

V45.78 Eye

V45.79 Other acquired absence of organ

5th V45.8 Other postprocedural status

V45.81 Aortocoronary bypass status 6, 7, 118, 152 2

Z95.1 Presence of aortocoronary bypass graft

V45.82 Percutaneous transluminal coronary angioplasty status 6, 7, 118, 152 2

V45.83 Breast implant removal status 2

V45.84 Dental restoration status 2
Dental crowns status
Dental fillings status

V45.85 Insulin pump status 2

V45.86 Bariatric surgery status 2
Gastric banding status
Gastric bypass status for obesity
Obesity surgery status
Excludes *bariatric surgery status complicating pregnancy, childbirth or the puerperium (649.2)*
intestinal bypass or anastomosis status (V45.3)

V45.87 Transplanted organ removal status 2
Transplanted organ previously removed due to complication, failure, rejection or infection
Excludes *encounter for removal of transplanted organ – code to complication of transplanted organ (996.80-996.89)*

V45.88 Status post administration of tPA (rtPA) in a different facility within the last 24 hours prior to admission to current facility 2
Code first condition requiring tPA administration, such as:
acute cerebral infarction (433.0-433.9 with fifth-digit 1, 434.0-434.9 with fifth digit 1)
acute myocardial infarction (410.00-410.92)

V45.89 Other 2
Presence of neuropacemaker or other electronic device
Excludes *artificial heart valve in situ (V43.3)*
vascular prosthesis in situ (V43.4)

4th V46 Other dependence on machines and devices

V46.0 Aspirator 2

5th V46.1 Respirator [Ventilator]
Iron lung

V46.11 Dependence on respirator, status 2

V46.12 Encounter for respirator dependence during power failure 1

V46.13 Encounter for weaning from respirator [ventilator] 1

V46.14 Mechanical complication of respirator [ventilator] 2
Mechanical failure of respirator [ventilator]

V46.2 Supplemental oxygen 2
Long-term oxygen therapy

V46.3 Wheelchair dependence 2
Wheelchair confinement status
Code first cause of dependence, such as:
muscular dystrophy (359.1)
obesity (278.00, 278.01)

V46.8 Other enabling machines 2
Hyperbaric chamber
Possum [Patient-Operated-Selector-Mechanism]
Excludes *cardiac pacemaker (V45.0)*
kidney dialysis machine (V45.11)

V46.9 Unspecified machine dependence

4th V47 Other problems with internal organs

V47.0 Deficiencies of internal organs

V47.1 Mechanical and motor problems with internal organs

V47.2 Other cardiorespiratory problems
Cardiovascular exercise intolerance with pain (with):
at rest
less than ordinary activity
ordinary activity

V47.3 Other digestive problems

V47.4 Other urinary problems

V47.5 Other genital problems

V47.9 Unspecified
R68.89 Other general symptoms and signs

4th V48 Problems with head, neck, and trunk
V48.0 Deficiencies of head
Excludes *deficiencies of ears, eyelids, and nose (V48.8)*
V48.1 Deficiencies of neck and trunk
V48.2 Mechanical and motor problems with head
V48.3 Mechanical and motor problems with neck and trunk
V48.4 Sensory problem with head
V48.5 Sensory problem with neck and trunk
V48.6 Disfigurements of head
V48.7 Disfigurements of neck and trunk
V48.8 Other problems with head, neck, and trunk
V48.9 Unspecified problem with head, neck, or trunk

4th V49 Other conditions influencing health status
V49.0 Deficiencies of limbs
V49.1 Mechanical problems with limbs
V49.2 Motor problems with limbs
V49.3 Sensory problems with limbs
V49.4 Disfigurements of limbs
V49.5 Other problems of limbs
5th V49.6 Upper limb amputation status
V49.60 Unspecified level
V49.61 Thumb
V49.62 Other finger(s)
V49.63 Hand
V49.64 Wrist
Disarticulation of wrist
V49.65 Below elbow
V49.66 Above elbow
Disarticulation of elbow
V49.67 Shoulder
Disarticulation of shoulder
5th V49.7 Lower limb amputation status
V49.70 Unspecified level
V49.71 Great toe
V49.72 Other toe(s)
V49.73 Foot
V49.74 Ankle
Disarticulation of ankle
V49.75 Below knee
V49.76 Above knee
Disarticulation of knee
V49.77 Hip
Disarticulation of hip
5th V49.8 Other specified conditions influencing health status
V49.81 Asymptomatic postmenopausal status (age-related) (natural) A ♀
Excludes *menopausal and premenopausal disorders (627.0-627.9)*
postsurgical menopause (256.2)
premature menopause (256.31)
symptomatic menopause(627.0-627.9)
V49.82 Dental sealant status 2
V49.83 Awaiting organ trasplant status 2
V49.84 Bed confinement status
V49.85 Dual sensory impairment 2
Blindness with deafness
Combined visual hearing impairment
Code first:
hearing impairment (389.00-389.9)
visual impairment (369.00-369.9)
V49.89 Other specified conditions influencing health status
Z87.89 Personal history of other specified conditions
V49.9 Unspecified

PERSONS ENCOUNTERING HEALTH SERVICES FOR SPECIFIC PROCEDURES AND AFTERCARE (V50-V59)

Note: *Categories V51-V58 are intended for use to indicate a reason for care in patients who may have already been treated for some disease or injury not now present, or who are receiving care to consolidate the treatment, to deal with residual states, or to prevent recurrence.*

Excludes *follow-up examination for medical surveillance following treatment (V67.0-V67.9)*

4th V50 Elective surgery for purposes other than remedying health states
V50.0 Hair transplant
V50.1 Other plastic surgery for unacceptable cosmetic appearance
Breast augmentation or reduction
Face-lift
Excludes *encounter for breast reduction (611.1)*
plastic surgery following healed injury or operation (V51.0-V51.8)
V50.2 Routine or ritual circumcision ♂
Circumcision in the absence of significant medical indication
V50.3 Ear piercing
5th V50.4 Prophylactic organ removal
Excludes *organ donations (V59.0-V59.9)*
therapeutic organ removal – code to condition

ICD-9-CM Official Guidelines (Chapter 18):

d. Categories of V Codes

14) Miscellaneous V codes

Prophylactic Organ Removal

For encounters specifically for prophylactic removal of breasts, ovaries, or another organ due to a genetic susceptibility to cancer or a family history of cancer, the principal or first listed code should be a code from subcategory V50.4, Prophylactic organ removal, followed by the appropriate genetic susceptibility code and the appropriate family history code.

If the patient has a malignancy of one site and is having prophylactic removal at another site to prevent either a new primary malignancy or metastatic disease, a code for the malignancy should also be assigned in addition to a code from subcategory V50.4. A V50.4 code should not be assigned if the patient is having organ removal for treatment of a malignancy, such as the removal of the testes for the treatment of prostate cancer.

V50.41 Breast
V50.42 Ovary ♀
V50.49 Other
V50.8 Other
V50.9 Unspecified

V47.9 – V50.9

4th V51 **Aftercare involving the use of plastic surgery**
Plastic surgery following healed injury or operation
Excludes *cosmetic plastic surgery (V50.1)*
plastic surgery as treatment for current condition or injury – code to condition or injury
repair of scar tissue – code to scar

V51.0 **Encounter for breast reconstruction following mastectomy** A I
Excludes *deformity and disproportion of reconstructed breast (612.0-612.1)*

V51.8 **Other aftercare involving the use of plastic surgery**

4th V52 **Fitting and adjustment of prosthetic device and implant**
Includes removal of device
Excludes *malfunction or complication of prosthetic device (996.0-996.7)*
status only, without need for care (V43.0-V43.8)

ICD-9-CM Official Guidelines (Chapter 18):

d. Categories of V Codes

7) Aftercare

Aftercare visit codes cover situations when the initial treatment of a disease or injury has been performed and the patient requires continued care during the healing or recovery phase, or for the long-term consequences of the disease. The aftercare V code should not be used if treatment is directed at a current, acute disease or injury. The diagnosis code is to be used in these cases. Exceptions to this rule are codes V58.0, Radiotherapy, and codes from subcategory V58.1, Encounter for chemotherapy and immunotherapy for neoplastic conditions. These codes are to be first listed, followed by the diagnosis code when a patient's encounter is solely to receive radiation therapy or chemotherapy for the treatment of a neoplasm. Should a patient receive both chemotherapy and radiation therapy during the same encounter code V58.0 and V58.1 may be used together on a record with either one being sequenced first.

The aftercare codes are generally first listed to explain the specific reason for the encounter. An aftercare code may be used as an additional code when some type of aftercare is provided in addition to the reason for admission and no diagnosis code is applicable. An example of this would be the closure of a colostomy during an encounter for treatment of another condition.

Certain aftercare V code categories need a secondary diagnosis code to describe the resolving condition or sequelae, for others, the condition is inherent in the code title.

Additional V code aftercare category terms include, fitting and adjustment, and attention to artificial openings.

Status V codes may be used with aftercare V codes to indicate the nature of the aftercare. For example code V45.81, Aortocoronary bypass status, may be used with code V58.73, Aftercare following surgery of the circulatory system, NEC, to indicate the surgery for which the aftercare is being performed.

Also, a transplant status code may be used following code V58.44, Aftercare following organ transplant, to identify the organ transplanted. A status code should not be used when the aftercare code indicates the type of status, such as using V55.0, Attention to tracheostomy with V44.0, Tracheostomy status.

The aftercare V category/codes:

V52 Fitting and adjustment of prosthetic device and implant
V53 Fitting and adjustment of other device
V54 Other orthopedic aftercare
V55 Attention to artificial openings
V56 Encounter for dialysis and dialysis catheter care
V57 Care involving the use of rehabilitation procedures
V58.0 Radiotherapy
V58.11 Encounter for antineoplastic chemotherapy
V58.12 Encounter for antineoplastic immunotherapy
V58.3x Attention to dressings and sutures
V58.41 Encounter for planned post-operative wound closure
V58.42 Aftercare, surgery, neoplasm
V58.43 Aftercare, surgery, trauma
V58.44 Aftercare involving organ transplant
V58.49 Other specified aftercare following surgery
V58.7x Aftercare following surgery
V58.81 Fitting and adjustment of vascular catheter
V58.82 Fitting and adjustment of non-vascular catheter
V58.83 Monitoring therapeutic drug
V58.89 Other specified aftercare

V52.0 **Artificial arm (complete) (partial)**

V52.1 **Artificial leg (complete) (partial)**

V52.2 **Artificial eye**

V52.3 **Dental prosthetic device**

V52.4 **Breast prosthesis and implant** ♀
Elective implant exchange (different material) (different size)
Removal of tissue expander without synchronous insertion of permanent implant
Excludes *admission for initial breast implant insertion for breast augmentation (V50.1)*
complications of breast implant (996.54, 996.69, 996.79)
encounter for breast reconstruction following mastectomy (V51.0)

V52.8 **Other specified prosthetic device**

V52.9 **Unspecified prosthetic device**

4th V53 **Fitting and adjustment of other device**
Includes removal of device
replacement of device
Excludes *status only, without need for care (V45.0-V45.8)*

5th V53.0 **Devices related to nervous system and special senses**

V53.01 **Fitting and adjustment of cerebral ventricle (communicating) shunt**

V53.02 **Neuropacemaker (brain) (peripheral nerve) (spinal cord)**

V53.09 **Fitting and adjustment of other devices related to nervous system and special senses**
Auditory substitution device
Visual substitution device

V53.1 **Spectacles and contact lenses**

V53.2 **Hearing aid**

5th V53.3 **Cardiac device**
Reprogramming

V53.31 **Cardiac pacemaker**
Excludes *mechanical complication of cardiac pacemaker (996.01)*

V53.32 **Automatic implantable cardiac defibrillator**

V53.39 **Other cardiac device**

V53.4 **Orthodontic devices**

▲ 5th V53.5 **Other gastrointestinal appliance and device**
Excludes *colostomy (V55.3)*
ileostomy (V55.2)
other artifical opening of digestive tract (V55.4)

● V53.50 **Fitting and adjustment of intestinal appliance and device**

● V53.51 **Fitting and adjustment of gastric lap band**

Rationale: *Gastric banding ("lap band") is a type of bariatric surgery used to treat obesity. The restrictive device, which is an inflatable silicone prosthesis, is placed around the top portion of the stomach. This reduces the size of the stomach, thus restricting food intake and causing weight loss. The band may be periodically adjusted to achieve the optimal restriction of food intake necessary for weight loss while still allowing adequate nutrition. During pregnancy,* *a gastric lap band patient may need to adjust the band to allow additional intake to assure optimal nutrition for mother and baby. Although a port is inserted to allow patients to "self-adjust" the band, often a physician office visit is required to achieve optimal adjustments described above.*

Previously there was no unique code for these encounters and it was advised, through the American Hospital Association's Coding Clinic for ICD-9-CM Editorial Advisory Board to use existing code V53.5, "Fitting and adjustment of other intestinal appliance or device." For 2010 it was decided to expand this code to allow for creation of a unique code for these encounters.

● **V53.59 Fitting and adjustment of other gastrointestinal appliance and device**

V53.6 Urinary devices
Urinary catheter
Excludes *cystostomy (V55.5)*
nephrostomy (V55.6)
ureterostomy (V55.6)
urethrostomy (V55.6)

V53.7 Orthopedic devices
Orthopedic:
brace
cast
corset
shoes
Excludes *other orthopedic aftercare (V54)*

V53.8 Wheelchair

5th **V53.9 Other and unspecified device**

V53.90 Unspecified device

V53.91 Fitting and adjustment of insulin pump
Insulin pump titration

V53.99 Other device

4th **V54 Other orthopedic aftercare**
Excludes *fitting and adjustment of orthopedic devices (V53.7)*
malfunction of internal orthopedic device (996.40-996.49)
other complication of nonmechanical nature (996.60-996.79)

5th **V54.0 Aftercare involving internal fixation device**
Excludes *malfunction of internal orthopedic device (996.40-996.49)*
other complication of nonmechanical nature (996.60-996.79)
removal of external fixation device (V54.89)

V54.01 Encounter for removal of internal fixation device

V54.02 Encounter for lengthening/adjustment of growth rod

V54.09 Other aftercare involving internal fixation device

5th **V54.1 Aftercare for healing traumatic fracture**
Excludes *aftercare for amputation stump (V54.89)*
aftercare following joint replacement (V54.81)

V54.10 Aftercare for healing traumatic fracture of arm, unspecified

V54.11 Aftercare for healing traumatic fracture of upper arm

V54.12 Aftercare for healing traumatic fracture of lower arm

V54.13 Aftercare for healing traumatic fracture of hip

V54.14 Aftercare for healing traumatic fracture of leg, unspecified

V54.15 Aftercare for healing traumatic fracture of upper leg
Excludes *aftercare for healing traumatic fracture of hip (V54.13)*

V54.16 Aftercare for healing traumatic fracture of lower leg

V54.17 Aftercare for healing traumatic fracture of vertebrae

V54.19 Aftercare for healing traumatic fracture of other bone

5th **V54.2 Aftercare for healing pathologic fracture**
Excludes *aftercare following joint replacement (V54.81)*

V54.20 Aftercare for healing pathologic fracture of arm, unspecified

V54.21 Aftercare for healing pathologic fracture of upper arm

V54.22 Aftercare for healing pathologic fracture of lower arm

V54.23 Aftercare for healing pathologic fracture of hip

V54.24 Aftercare for healing pathologic fracture of leg, unspecified

V54.25 Aftercare for healing pathologic fracture of upper leg
Excludes *aftercare for healing pathologic fracture of hip (V54.23)*

V54.26 Aftercare for healing pathologic fracture of lower leg

V54.27 Aftercare for healing pathologic fracture of vertebrae

V54.29 Aftercare for healing pathologic fracture of other bone

4th **V54.8 Other orthopedic aftercare**

V54.81 Aftercare following joint replacement
Use additional code to identify joint replacement site (V43.60-V43.69)

V54.89 Other orthopedic aftercare
Aftercare for healing fracture NOS

V54.9 Unspecified orthopedic aftercare

4th **V55 Attention to artificial openings**
Includes adjustment or repositioning of catheter
closure
passage of sounds or bougies
reforming
removal or replacement of catheter
toilet or cleansing
Excludes *complications of external stoma (519.00-519.09, 569.60-569.69, 997.4, 997.5)*
status only, without need for care (V44.0-V44.9)

V55.0 Tracheostomy

V55.1 Gastrostomy

V55.2 Ileostomy

V55.3 Colostomy

V55.4 Other artificial opening of digestive tract

V55.5 Cystostomy

V55.6 Other artificial opening of urinary tract
Nephrostomy
Ureterostomy
Urethrostomy

V55.7 Artificial vagina

V55.8 Other specified artificial opening

V55.9 Unspecified artificial opening

4th **V56 Encounter for dialysis and dialysis catheter care**
Use additional code to identify the associated condition
Excludes *dialysis preparation – code to condition*

V56.0 Extracorporeal dialysis
Dialysis (renal) NOS
Excludes *dialysis status (V45.11)*

V53.59 – V56.0

V56.1 Fitting and adjustment of extracorporeal dialysis catheter
Removal or replacement of catheter
Toilet or cleansing
Use additional code for any concurrent extracorporeal dialysis (V56.0)

V56.2 Fitting and adjustment of peritoneal dialysis catheter
Use additional code for any concurrent peritoneal dialysis (V56.8)

5th **V56.3 Encounter for adequacy testing for dialysis**

V56.31 Encounter for adequacy testing for hemodialysis

V56.32 Encounter for adequacy testing for peritoneal dialysis
Peritoneal equilibration test

V56.8 Other dialysis
Peritoneal dialysis

4th **V57 Care involving use of rehabilitation procedures**
Use additional code to identify underlying condition

V57.0 Breathing exercises 1

V57.1 Other physical therapy 1
Z51.89 Encounter for other specified aftercare
Therapeutic and remedial exercises, except breathing

5th **V57.2 Occupational therapy and vocational rehabilitation**

V57.21 Encounter for occupational therapy 1

V57.22 Encounter for vocational therapy 1

▲**V57.3 Speech-language therapy** 1

V57.4 Orthoptic training 1

5th **V57.8 Other specified rehabilitation procedure**

V57.81 Orthotic training 1
Gait training in the use of artificial limbs

V57.89 Other 1
Z51.89 Encounter for other specified aftercare
Multiple training or therapy

V57.9 Unspecified rehabilitation procedure 1

4th **V58 Encounter for other and unspecified procedures and aftercare**
Excludes *convalescence and palliative care (V66.0-V66.9)*

V58.0 Radiotherapy 1
Encounter or admission for radiotherapy
Excludes *encounter for radioactive implant – code to condition*
radioactive iodine therapy – code to condition

5th **V58.1 Encounter for antineoplastic chemotherapy and immunotherapy**
Encounter or admission for chemotherapy
Excludes *chemotherapy and immunotherapy for nonneoplastic conditions – code to condition*

V58.11 Encounter for neoplastic chemotherapy 1
Z51.11 Encounter for antineoplastic chemotherapy

V58.12 Encounter for antineoplastic immunotherapy 1

V58.2 Blood transfusion, without reported diagnosis

5th **V58.3 Attention to dressings and sutures**
Change or removal of wound packing
Excludes *attention to drains (V58.49)*
planned postoperative wound closure (V58.41)

V58.30 Encounter for change or removal of nonsurgical wound dressing
Encounter for change or removal of wound dressing NOS

V58.31 Encounter for change or removal of surgical wound dressing

V58.32 Encounter for removal of sutures
Encounter for removal of staples

5th **V58.4 Other aftercare following surgery**
Note: *Codes from this subcategory should be used in conjunction with other aftercare codes to fully identify the reason for the aftercare encounter.*
Excludes *aftercare following sterilization reversal surgery (V26.22)*
attention to artificial openings (V55.0-V55.9)
orthopedic aftercare (V54.0-V54.9)

V58.41 Encounter for planned post-operative wound closure
Excludes *disruption of operative wound (998.31-998.32)*
encounter for dressings and suture aftercare (V58.30-V58.32)

V58.42 Aftercare following surgery for neoplasm
Conditions classifiable to 140-239

V58.43 Aftercare following surgery for injury and trauma
Conditions classifiable to 800-999
Excludes *aftercare for healing traumatic fracture (V54.10-V54.19)*

V58.44 Aftercare following organ transplant
Use additional code to identify the organ transplanted (V42.0-V42.9)

V58.49 Other specified aftercare following surgery
Change or removal of drains

V58.5 Orthodontics
Excludes *fitting and adjustment of orthodontic device (V53.4)*

5th **V58.6 Long-term (current) drug use**
Excludes *drug abuse (305.00-305.93)*
drug abuse and dependence complicating pregnancy (648.3-648.4)
drug dependence (304.00-304.93)
hormone replacement therapy (postmenopausal) (V07.4)
prophylactic use of agents affecting estrogen receptors and estrogen levels (V07.51-V07.59)

V58.61 Long-term (current) use of anticoagulants 2
Z79.01 Long term (current) use of anticoagulants
Excludes *long-term (current) use of antiplatelets/antithrombotics*

V58.62 Long-term (current) use of antibiotics 2

V58.63 Long-term (current) use of antiplatelets/antithrombotics 2
Excludes *long-term (current) use of aspirin (V58.66)*

V58.64 Long-term (current) use of non-steroidal anti-inflammatories (NSAID) 2
Excludes *long-term (current) use of aspirin (V58.66)*

V58.65 Long-term (current) use of steroids 2

V58.66 Long-term (current) use of aspirin 2

V58.67 Long-term (current) use of insulin 2

V58.69 Long-term (current) use of other medications 2
Z79.3 Long term (current) use of hormonal contraceptives
Z79.899 Other long-term (current) drug therapy
Long term current use of methadone
Long term current use of opiate analgesic
Other high-risk medications

5th **V58.7 Aftercare following surgery to specified body systems, not elsewhere classified**

Note: *Codes from this subcategory should be used in conjunction with other aftercare codes to fully identify the reason for the aftercare encounter.*

Excludes *aftercare following organ transplant (V58.44)*
aftercare following surgery for neoplasm (V58.42)

V58.71 Aftercare following surgery of the sense organs, NEC
Conditions classifiable to 360-379, 380-389

V58.72 Aftercare following surgery of the nervous system, NEC
Conditions classifiable to 320-359
Excludes *aftercare following surgery of the sense organs, NEC (V58.71)*

V58.73 Aftercare following surgery of the circulatory system, NEC
Conditions classifiable to 390-459

V58.74 Aftercare following surgery of the respiratory system, NEC
Conditions classifiable to 460-519

V58.75 Aftercare following surgery of the teeth, oral cavity and digestive system, NEC
Conditions classifiable to 520-579

V58.76 Aftercare following surgery of the genitourinary system, NEC
Conditions classifiable to 580-629
Excludes *aftercare following sterilization reversal (V26.22)*

V58.77 Aftercare following surgery of the skin and subcutaneous tissue, NEC
Conditions classifiable to 680-709

V58.78 Aftercare following surgery of the musculoskeletal system, NEC
Conditions classifiable to 710-739
Excludes *orthopedic aftercare (V54.01-V54.9)*

5th **V58.8 Other specified procedures and aftercare**

V58.81 Fitting and adjustment of vascular catheter
Z45.2 Encounter for adjustment and management of vascular access device
Removal or replacement of catheter
Toilet or cleansing
Excludes *complications of renal dialysis (996.73)*
complications of vascular catheter (996.74)
dialysis preparation – code to condition
encounter for dialysis (V56.0-V56.8)
fitting and adjustment of dialysis catheter (V56.1)

V58.82 Fitting and adjustment of non-vascular catheter NEC
Removal or replacement of catheter
Toilet or cleansing
Excludes *fitting and adjustment of peritoneal dialysis catheter (V56.2)*
fitting and adjustment of urinary catheter (V53.6)

V58.83 Encounter for therapeutic drug monitoring
Z51.81 Encounter for therapeutic drug level monitoring
Use additional code for any associated long-term (current) drug use (V58.61-V58.69)
Excludes *blood-drug testing for medicolegal reasons (V70.4)*

V58.89 Other specified aftercare

V58.9 Unspecified aftercare

4th **V59 Donors**

Excludes *examination of potential donor (V70.8)*
self-donation of organ or tissue-code to condition

ICD-9-CM Official Guidelines (Chapter 18):

d. Categories of V Codes

9) Donor

Category V59 is the donor codes. They are used for living individuals who are donating blood or other body tissue. These codes are only for individuals donating for others, not for self donations. They are not for use to identify cadaveric donations.

5th **V59.0 Blood**

V59.01 Whole blood I

V59.02 Stem cells I

V59.09 Other I

V59.1 Skin I

V59.2 Bone I

V59.3 Bone marrow I

V59.4 Kidney I

V59.5 Cornea I

V59.6 Liver I

5th **V59.7 Egg (oocyte)(ovum)**

V59.70 Egg (oocyte)(ovum) donor, unspecified ♀ I

V59.71 Egg (oocyte)(ovum) donor, under age 35, anonymous recipient ♀ I
Egg donor, under age 35 NOS

V59.72 Egg (oocyte)(ovum) donor, under age 35, designated recipient ♀ I

V59.73 Egg (oocyte)(ovum) donor, age 35 and over, anonymous recipient ♀ I
Egg donor, age 35 and over NOS

V59.74 Egg (oocyte)(ovum) donor, age 35 and over, designated recipient ♀ I

V59.8 Other specified organ or tissue I

V59.9 Unspecified organ or tissue I

PERSONS ENCOUNTERING HEALTH SERVICES IN OTHER CIRCUMSTANCES (V60-V69)

4th **V60 Housing, household, and economic circumstances**

V60.0 Lack of housing 2
Hobos
Social migrants
Tramps
Transients
Vagabonds

V60.1 Inadequate housing 2
Lack of heating
Restriction of space
Technical defects in home preventing adequate care

V60.2 Inadequate material resources 2
Economic problem
Poverty NOS

V60.3 Person living alone 2

V60.4 No other household member able to render care 2
Person requiring care (has) (is):
family member too handicapped, ill, or otherwise unsuited to render care
partner temporarily away from home
temporarily away from usual place of abode
Excludes *holiday relief care (V60.5)*

V60.5 Holiday relief care 2
Provision of health care facilities to a person normally cared for at home, to enable relatives to take a vacation

V60.6 Person living in residential institution 2
Boarding school resident

5th **V60.8 Other specified housing or economic circumstances** 2

● **V60.81 Foster care (status)** 2

● **V60.89 Other specified housing or economic circumstances** 2

V60.9 Unspecified housing or economic circumstance 2

4th **V61 Other family circumstances**

Includes when these circumstances or fear of them, affecting the person directly involved or others, are mentioned as the reason, justified or not, for seeking or receiving medical advice or care

5th **V61.0 Family disruption**

V61.01 Family disruption due to family member on military deployment
Individual or family affected by other family member being on deployment
Excludes *family disruption due to family member on non-military extended absence from home (V61.08)*

V61.02 Family disruption due to return of family member from military deployment
Individual or family affected by other family member having returned from deployment (current or past conflict)

V61.03 Family disruption due to divorce or legal separation

V61.04 Family disruption due to parent-child estrangement
Excludes *other family estrangement (V61.09)*

V61.05 Family disruption due to child in welfare custody

V61.06 Family disruption due to child in foster care or in care of non-parental family member

● **V61.07 Family disruption due to death of family member**
Excludes *bereavement (V62.82)*

Rationale: *Unfortunately in today's society, there are many circumstances that lead to disruption of the family. The specific circumstances can affect how the physician may have to deal with the patient and manage any ongoing medical problems. So that these circumstances can be more carefully monitored, the American Academy of Pediatrics (AAP) proposed an expansion of the V61.0 category, family disruption. Several codes (V61.0-V61.06 and V61.09) were added for 2009 and the addition of codes V61.07 and V61.08 continues this expansion.*

● **V61.08 Family disruption due to other extended absence of family member**
Excludes *family disruption due to family member on military deployment (V61.01)*

V61.09 Other family disruption
Family estrangement NOS

5th **V61.1 Counseling for marital and partner problems**
Excludes *problems related to:*
psychosexual disorders (302.0-302.9)
sexual function (V41.7)

V61.10 Counseling for marital and partner problems, unspecified
Marital conflict
Marital relationship problem
Partner conflict
Partner relationship problem

V61.11 Counseling for victim of spousal and partner abuse
Excludes *encounter for treatment of current injuries due to abuse (995.80-995.85)*

V61.12 Counseling for perpetrator of spousal and partner abuse

5th **V61.2 Parent–child problems**

V61.20 Counseling for parent–child problem, unspecified
Concern about behavior of child
Parent–child conflict
Parent–child relationship problem

V61.21 Counseling for victim of child abuse
Child battering
Child neglect
Excludes *current injuries due to abuse (995.50-995.59)*

V61.22 Counseling for perpetrator of parental child abuse
Excludes *counseling for non-parental abuser (V62.83)*

● **V61.23 Counseling for parent–biological child problem**
Concern about behavior of biological child
Parent–biological child conflict
Parent–biological child relationship problem

Rationale: *The AAP also raised concerns that problems between adopted children and parents, or foster children and parents should be able to be better monitored. To this end AAP proposed revisions to V61.2, "Parent-child problems," and that a code for foster care status be created.*

● **V61.24 Counseling for parent–adopted child problem**
Concern about behavior of adopted child
Parent–adopted child conflict
Parent–adopted child relationship problem

● **V61.25 Counseling for parent (guardian)–foster child problem**
Concern about behavior of foster child
Parent (guardian)–foster child conflict
Parent (guardian)–foster child relationship problem

▲ **V61.29 Other parent–child problems**
~~Problem concerning adopted or foster child~~

V61.3 Problems with aged parents or in-laws

5th **V61.4 Health problems within family**

V61.41 Alcoholism in family

● **V61.42 Substance abuse in family**

Rationale: *The use of illegal drugs or drug abuse by a family member can have an adverse effect on other members of the household. In order to better track the specific circumstances, new code V61.42 has been created for 2010.*

V61.49 Other
Care of sick or handicapped person in family or household
Presence of sick or handicapped person in family or household

V61.5 Multiparity

V61.6 Illegitimacy or illegitimate pregnancy M ♀

V61.7 Other unwanted pregnancy M ♀

V61.8 Other specified family circumstances
Problems with family members NEC
Sibling relationship problem

V61.9 Unspecified family circumstance

4th **V62 Other psychosocial circumstances**

Includes those circumstances or fear of them, affecting the person directly involved or others, mentioned as the reason, justified or not, for seeking or receiving medical advice or care

Excludes *previous psychological trauma (V15.41-V15.49)*

V62.0 Unemployment 2
Excludes *circumstances when main problem is economic inadequacy or poverty (V60.2)*

4th / 5th Fourth/Fifth Digit Required | ● New Code ▲ Revised Code | Unspecified Code Other Specified Code Manifestation Code ICD-10-CM xWalk
1 Principal Diagnosis only 2 Secondary Diagnosis only

V62.1 Adverse effects of work environment 2

5th V62.2 Other occupational circumstances or maladjustment

V62.21 Personal current military deployment status A 2

Individual (civilian or military) currently deployed in theater or in support of military war, peacekeeping and humanitarian operations

V62.22 Personal history of return from military deployment A 2

Individual (civilian or military) with past history of military war, peacekeeping and humanitarian deployment (current or past conflict)

V62.29 Other occupational circumstances or maladjustment A 2

Career choice problem
Dissatisfaction with employment
Occupational problem

V62.3 Educational circumstances 2

Academic problem
Dissatisfaction with school environment
Educational handicap

V62.4 Social maladjustment 2

Acculturation problem
Cultural deprivation
Political, religious, or sex discrimination
Social:
isolation
persecution

V62.5 Legal circumstances 2

Imprisonment
Legal investigation
Litigation
Prosecution

V62.6 Refusal of treatment for reasons of religion or conscience 2

5th V62.8 Other psychological or physical stress, not elsewhere classified

V62.81 Interpersonal problems, not elsewhere classified 2

Relational problem NOS

V62.82 Bereavement, uncomplicated 2

Excludes *bereavement as adjustment reaction (309.0)*
family disruption due to death of family member (V61.07)

V62.83 Counseling for perpetrator of physical/sexual abuse 2

Excludes *counseling for perpetrator of parental child abuse (V61.22)*
counseling for perpetrator of spousal and partner abuse (V61.12)

V62.84 Suicidal ideation

Excludes *suicidal tendencies (300.9)*

V62.89 Other 2

Borderline intellectual functioning
Life circumstance problems
Phase of life problems
Religious or spiritual problem

V62.9 Unspecified psychosocial circumstance 2

4th V63 Unavailability of other medical facilities for care

V63.0 Residence remote from hospital or other health care facility

V63.1 Medical services in home not available

Excludes *no other household member able to render care (V60.4)*

V63.2 Person awaiting admission to adequate facility elsewhere

V63.8 Other specified reasons for unavailability of medical facilities

Person on waiting list undergoing social agency investigation

V63.9 Unspecified reason for unavailability of medical facilities

4th V64 Persons encountering health services for specific procedures, not carried out

5th V64.0 Vaccination not carried out

V64.00 Vaccination not carried out, unspecified reason 2

V64.01 Vaccination not carried out because of acute illness 2

V64.02 Vaccination not carried out because of chronic illness or condition 2

V64.03 Vaccination not carried out because of immune compromised state 2

V64.04 Vaccination not carried out because of allergy to vaccine or component 2

V64.05 Vaccination not carried out because of caregiver refusal 2

Guardian refusal
Parent refusal

Excludes *vaccination not carried out because of caregiver refusal for religious reasons (V64.07)*

V64.06 Vaccination not carried out because of patient refusal 2

V64.07 Vaccination not carried out for religious reasons 2

V64.08 Vaccination not carried out because patient had disease being vaccinated against 2

V64.09 Vaccination not carried out for other reason 2

V64.1 Surgical or other procedure not carried out because of contraindication 2

V64.2 Surgical or other procedure not carried out because of patient's decision 2

V64.3 Procedure not carried out for other reasons 2

5th V64.4 Closed surgical procedure converted to open procedure

V64.41 Laparoscopic surgical procedure converted to open procedure 2

V64.42 Thoracoscopic surgical procedure converted to open procedure 2

V64.43 Arthroscopic surgical procedure converted to open procedure 2

4th V65 Other persons seeking consultation

V65.0 Healthy person accompanying sick person

Boarder

5th V65.1 Person consulting on behalf of another person

Advice or treatment for nonattending third party

Excludes *concern (normal) about sick person in family (V61.41-V61.49)*

▲ V65.11 Pediatric pre-birth visit for expectant parent(s) ~~mother~~

Pre-adoption visit for adoptive parent(s)

V65.19 Other person consulting on behalf of another person

V65.2 Person feigning illness

Malingerer
Peregrinating patient

V65.3 Dietary surveillance and counseling
Dietary surveillance and counseling (in):
NOS
colitis
diabetes mellitus
food allergies or intolerance
gastritis
hypercholesterolemia
hypoglycemia
obesity
Use additional code to identify Body Mass Index (BMI), if known (V85.0-V85.54)

5th **V65.4 Other counseling, not elsewhere classified**
Health:
advice
education
instruction
Excludes *counseling (for):*
contraception (V25.40-V25.49)
genetic (V26.31-V26.39)
on behalf of third party (V65.11, V65.19)
procreative management (V26.41-V26.49)

V65.40 Counseling NOS
V65.41 Exercise counseling
V65.42 Counseling on substance use and abuse
V65.43 Counseling on injury prevention
V65.44 Human immunodeficiency virus [HIV] counseling
V65.45 Counseling on other sexually transmitted diseases
V65.46 Encounter for insulin pump training
V65.49 Other specified counseling

V65.5 Person with feared complaint in whom no diagnosis was made
Feared condition not demonstrated
Problem was normal state
"Worried well"

V65.8 Other reasons for seeking consultation
Excludes *specified symptoms*

V65.9 Unspecified reason for consultation

4th **V66 Convalescence and palliative care**
V66.0 Following surgery 1
V66.1 Following radiotherapy 1
V66.2 Following chemotherapy 1
V66.3 Following psychotherapy and other treatment for mental disorder 1
V66.4 Following treatment of fracture 1
V66.5 Following other treatment 1
V66.6 Following combined treatment 1
V66.7 Encounter for palliative care 2
End-of-life care
Hospice care
Terminal care
Code first underlying disease
V66.9 Unspecified convalescence 1

4th **V67 Follow-up examination**
Includes surveillance only following completed treatment
Excludes *surveillance of contraception (V25.40-V25.49)*

ICD-9-CM Official Guidelines (Chapter 18):
d. Categories of V Codes
8) Follow-up
The follow-up codes are used to explain continuing surveillance following completed treatment of a disease, condition, or injury. They imply that the condition has been fully treated and no longer exists. They should not be confused with aftercare codes that explain current treatment for a healing condition or its sequelae. Follow-up codes may be used in conjunction with history codes to provide the full picture of the healed condition and its treatment. The follow-up code is sequenced first, followed by the history code.
A follow-up code may be used to explain repeated visits. Should a condition be found to have recurred on the follow-up visit, then the diagnosis code should be used in place of the follow-up code.

5th **V67.0 Following surgery**
V67.00 Following surgery, unspecified
V67.01 Follow-up vaginal pap smear ♀
Vaginal pap smear, status-post hysterectomy for malignant condition
Use additional code to identify:
acquired absence of uterus (V88.01-V88.03)
personal history of malignant neoplasm (V10.40-V10.44)
Excludes *vaginal pap smear status-post hysterectomy for non-malignant condition (V76.47)*
V67.09 Following other surgery
Excludes *sperm count following sterilization reversal (V26.22)*
sperm count for fertility testing (V26.21)

V67.1 Following radiotherapy
V67.2 Following chemotherapy
Cancer chemotherapy follow-up
V67.3 Following psychotherapy and other treatment for mental disorder
V67.4 Following treatment of healed fracture
Excludes *current (healing) fracture aftercare (V54.0-V54.9)*

5th **V67.5 Following other treatment**
V67.51 Following completed treatment with high-risk medication, not elsewhere classified
Z09 Encounter for follow-up examination after completed treatment for conditions other than malignant neoplasm
Excludes *long-term (current) drug use (V58.61-V58.69)*
V67.59 Other

V67.6 Following combined treatment
V67.9 Unspecified follow-up examination

4th **V68 Encounters for administrative purposes**
5th **V68.0 Issue of medical certificates**
Excludes *encounter for general medical examination (V70.0-V70.9)*
V68.01 Disability examination 1
Use additional code(s) to identify:
specific examination(s), screening and testing performed (V72.0-V82.9)
V68.09 Other issue of medical certificates 1

V68.1 Issue of repeat prescriptions 1
Issue of repeat prescription for:
appliance
glasses
medications
Excludes *repeat prescription for contraceptives (V25.41-V25.49)*

V68.2 Request for expert evidence 1

5th **V68.8 Other specified administrative purpose**
V68.81 Referral of patient without examination or treatment 1
V68.89 Other 1

V68.9 Unspecified administrative purpose 1

4th **V69 Problems related to lifestyle**

V69.0 Lack of physical exercise

V69.1 Inappropriate diet and eating habits

Excludes *anorexia nervosa (307.1)*
bulimia (783.6)
malnutrition and other nutritional deficiencies (260-269.9)
other and unspecified eating disorders (307.50-307.59)

V69.2 High-risk sexual behavior

V69.3 Gambling and betting

Excludes *pathological gambling (312.31)*

V69.4 Lack of adequate sleep

Sleep deprivation

Excludes *insomnia (780.52)*

V69.5 Behavioral insomnia of childhood P

V69.8 Other problems related to lifestyle

Self-damaging behavior

V69.9 Problem related to lifestyle, unspecified

PERSONS WITHOUT REPORTED DIAGNOSIS ENCOUNTERED DURING EXAMINATION AND INVESTIGATION OF INDIVIDUALS AND POPULATIONS (V70-V82)

Note: *Nonspecific abnormal findings disclosed at the time of these examinations are classifiable to categories 790-796.*

4th **V70 General medical examination**

Use additional code(s) to identify any special screening examination(s) performed (V73.0-V82.9)

ICD-9-CM Official Guidelines (Chapter 18):

d. Categories of V Codes

13) Routine and administrative examinations

The V codes allow for the description of encounters for routine examinations, such as, a general check-up, or, examinations for administrative purposes, such as, a pre-employment physical. The codes are not to be used if the examination is for diagnosis of a suspected condition or for treatment purposes. In such cases the diagnosis code is used. During a routine exam, should a diagnosis or condition be discovered, it should be coded as an additional code. Pre-existing and chronic conditions and history codes may also be included as additional codes as long as the examination is for administrative purposes and not focused on any particular condition.

Pre-operative examination V codes are for use only in those situations when a patient is being cleared for surgery and no treatment is given.

V70.0 Routine general medical examination at a health care facility I

Z00.00 Encounter for general adult medical examination without abnormal findings

Health checkup

Excludes *health checkup of infant or child over 28 days old (V20.2)*
health supervision of newborn 8 to 28 days old (V20.32)
health supervision of newborn under 8 days old (V20.31)
pre-procedural general physical examination (V72.83)

V70.1 General psychiatric examination, requested by the authority I

V70.2 General psychiatric examination, other and unspecified I

V70.3 Other medical examination for administrative purposes I

General medical examination for:
admission to old age home
adoption
camp
driving license
immigration and naturalization
insurance certification
marriage
prison
school admission
sports competition

Excludes *attendance for issue of medical certificates (V68.0)*
pre-employment screening (V70.5)

V70.4 Examination for medicolegal reasons I

Blood-alcohol tests
Blood-drug tests
Paternity testing

Excludes *examination and observation following:*
accidents (V71.3, V71.4)
assault (V71.6)
rape (V71.5)

V70.5 Health examination of defined subpopulations I

Armed forces personnel
Inhabitants of institutions
Occupational health examinations
Pre-employment screening
Preschool children
Prisoners
Prostitutes
Refugees
School children
Students

V70.6 Health examination in population surveys I

Excludes *special screening (V73.0-V82.9)*

V70.7 Examination of participant in clinical trial

Examination of participant or control in clinical research

V70.8 Other specified general medical examinations I

Examination of potential donor of organ or tissue

V70.9 Unspecified general medical examination I

4th **V71 Observation and evaluation for suspected conditions not found**

Note: *This category is to be used when persons without a diagnosis are suspected of having an abnormal condition, without signs or symptoms, which requires study, but after examination and observation, is found not to exist. This category is also for use for administrative and legal observation status.*

Excludes *suspected maternal and fetal conditions not found (V89.01-V89.09)*

ICD-9-CM Official Guidelines (Chapter 18d):

6) Observation

There are two observation V code categories. They are for use in very limited circumstances when a person is being observed for a suspected condition that is ruled out. The observation codes are not for use if an injury or illness or any signs or symptoms related to the suspected condition are present. In such cases the diagnosis/symptom code is used with the corresponding E code to identify any external cause.

The observation codes are to be used as principal diagnosis only. The only exception to this is when the principal diagnosis is required to be a code from the V30, Live born infant, category. Then the V29 observation code is sequenced after the V30 code. Additional codes may be used in addition to the observation code but only if they are unrelated to the suspected condition being observed.

5th **V71.0 Observation for suspected mental condition**

V71.01 Adult antisocial behavior A I

Dyssocial behavior or gang activity in adult without manifest psychiatric disorder

V69 – V71.01

V71.02 Childhood or adolescent antisocial behavior
Dyssocial behavior or gang activity in child or adolescent without manifest psychiatric disorder

V71.09 Other suspected mental condition

V71.1 Observation for suspected malignant neoplasm

V71.2 Observation for suspected tuberculosis

V71.3 Observation following accident at work

V71.4 Observation following other accident
Examination of individual involved in motor vehicle traffic accident

V71.5 Observation following alleged rape or seduction
Examination of victim or culprit

V71.6 Observation following other inflicted injury
Examination of victim or culprit

V71.7 Observation for suspected cardiovascular disease

5th V71.8 Observation and evaluation for other specified suspected conditions
Excludes *contact with and (suspected) exposure to (potentially) hazardous substances (V15.84-V15.86, V87.0-V87.31)*

V71.81 Abuse and neglect
Excludes *adult abuse and neglect (995.80-995.85)*
child abuse and neglect (995.50-995.59)

V71.82 Observation and evaluation for suspected exposure to anthrax

V71.83 Observation and evaluation for suspected exposure to other biological agent

V71.89 Other specified suspected conditions

V71.9 Observation for unspecified suspected condition

4th V72 Special investigations and examinations
Includes routine examination of specific system
Excludes *general medical examination (V70.0-70.4)*
general screening examination of defined populaiton groups (V70.5, V70.6, V70.7)
health supervision of newborn 8 to 28 days old (V20.32)
health supervision of newborn under 8 days old (V20.31)
routine examination of infant or child over 28 days old (V20.2)
Use additional code(s) to identify any special screening examination(s) performed (V73.0-V82.9)

ICD-9-CM Official Guidelines (Chapter 18):

d. Categories of V Codes

13) Routine and administrative examinations

The V codes allow for the description of encounters for routine examinations, such as, a general check-up, or, examinations for administrative purposes, such as, a pre-employment physical. The codes are not to be used if the examination is for diagnosis of a suspected condition or for treatment purposes. In such cases the diagnosis code is used. During a routine exam, should a diagnosis or condition be discovered, it should be coded as an additional code. Pre-existing and chronic conditions and history codes may also be included as additional codes as long as the examination is for administrative purposes and not focused on any particular condition.

Pre-operative examination V codes are for use only in those situations when a patient is being cleared for surgery and no treatment is given.

V72.0 Examination of eyes and vision

5th V72.1 Examination of ears and hearing

V72.11 Encounter for hearing examination following failed hearing screening

V72.12 Encounter for hearing conservation and treatment

V72.19 Other examination of ears and hearing

V72.2 Dental examination

5th V72.3 Gynecological examination
Excludes *cervical Papanicolaou smear without general gynecological examination (V76.2)*
routine examination in contraceptive management (V25.40-V25.49)

V72.31 Routine gynecological examination ♀
Z01.411 Encounter for gynecological examination (general) (routine) with abnormal findings
General gynecological examination with or without Papanicolaou cervical smear
Pelvic examination (annual) (periodic)
Use additional code to identify:
human papillomavirus (HPV) screening (V73.81)
routine vaginal Papanicolaou smear (V76.47)

V72.32 Encounter for Papanicolaou cervical smear to confirm findings of recent normal smear following initial abnormal smear ♀

5th V72.4 Pregnancy examination or test

V72.40 Pregnancy examination or test, pregnancy unconfirmed ♀
Possible pregnancy, not (yet) confirmed

V72.41 Pregnancy examintion or test, negative result ♀

V72.42 Pregnancy examination or test, positive result M ♀

V72.5 Radiological examination, not elsewhere classified
Routine chest x-ray
Excludes ~~*examination for suspected tuberculosis (V71.2)*~~
radiologic examinations as part of pre-procedural testing (V72.81-V72.84)

5th V72.6 Laboratory examination
Z01.89 Encounter for other specified special examinations
Encounters for blood and urine testing
~~**Excludes** *that for suspected disorder (V71.0-V71.9)*~~

Rationale: *It is now routine practice for patients to receive blood and radiology tests prior to certain treatments and procedures. These visits are generally done in an outpatient setting days before the treatment or procedure is scheduled. Prior to 2010, the ICD-9-CM already had codes for pre-procedural cardiovascular and respiratory evaluations, as well as a code for other pre-procedural examinations.*

It was requested that additional codes be created for certain types of pre-procedural exams, such as pre-chemotherapy ultrasounds. Because the V codes are reasons for encounter codes, not procedure codes, it would be inappropriate to create such codes. However, to advise coders that encounters for such exams should be assigned to code V72.83, "Other specified preoperative examination," it was decided that an inclusion term for examination prior to chemotherapy be added.

Additionally, prior to 2010 there was no way to identify encounters for laboratory tests as part of general physical exams, or for preparation for a procedure or treatment. As such, code V72.6, "Laboratory examination," has been expanded to provide codes for these different encounters. An excludes note was also added to exclude the pre-procedural codes from code V72.5 "Radiological examination," not elsewhere classified. Expanding V72.5 similarly to what is being proposed for V72.6 could also be considered in the future. The excludes notes under codes V72.5 and V72.6 were deleted as they are no longer applicable based on previous changes to the classification.

● V72.60 Laboratory examination, unspecified

● **V72.61 Antibody response examination**
Immunity status testing
Excludes *encounter for allergy testing (V72.7)*

Rationale: *Documentation of patient vaccinations helps ensure that persons in need of a vaccine receive it and that adequately vaccinated patients are not over immunized. However, vaccination providers frequently encounter persons who do not have adequate documentation (for example, international adoptees). Pre-vaccination serologic testing may be indicated to determine immunity as an alternative to unnecessary vaccinations for certain antigens (e.g., measles, mumps, rubella, varicella, tetanus, diphtheria, hepatitis A, hepatitis B, and poliovirus). Additionally, pre-vaccination serologic testing for susceptibility may be considered to reduce the cost of vaccinating adult populations that may have an expected high prevalence of a given disease (for example, hepatitis B infection).*

Post-vaccination testing for antibody response may be needed to help determine appropriate post exposure prophylaxis. For example post-vaccination testing may be indicated for health care workers who have received the hepatitis B vaccine but have blood or patient contact and are at ongoing risk for injuries with sharp instruments or needle sticks. Their medical management will depend on knowledge of their immune status. It may also be ordered to check whether or not adequate response has been achieved.

Previously there was no code specific for encounters for serologic antibody testing.

● **V72.62 Laboratory examination ordered as part of a routine general medical examination**
Blood tests for routine general physical examination

● **V72.63 Pre-procedural laboratory examination**
Blood tests prior to treatment or procedure
Pre-operative laboratory examination

● **V72.69 Other laboratory examination**

V72.7 Diagnostic skin and sensitization tests
Allergy tests
Skin tests for hypersensitivity
Excludes *diagnostic skin tests for bacterial diseases (V74.0-V74.9)*

5th **V72.8 Other specified examinations**
Excludes *pre-procedural laboratory examinations (V72.63)*

V72.81 Preoperative cardiovascular examination
Z01.810 Encounter for preprocedural cardiovascular examination
Pre-procedural cardiovascular examination

V72.82 Preoperative respiratory examination
Pre-procedural respiratory examination

V72.83 Other specified preoperative examination
Z01.818 Encounter for other preprocedural examination
Examination prior to chemotherapy
Other pre-procedural examination
Pre-procedural general physical
Excludes *routine general medical examination (V70.0)*

V72.84 Preoperative examination, unspecified
Z01.818 Encounter for other preprocedural examination
Pre-procedural examination, unspecified

V72.85 Other specified examination

V72.86 Encounter for blood typing

V72.9 Unspecified examination

ICD-9-CM Official Guidelines (Chapter 18):

d. Categories of V Codes

5) Screening

Screening is the testing for disease or disease precursors in seemingly well individuals so that early detection and treatment can be provided for those who test positive for the disease. Screenings that are recommended for many subgroups in a population include: routine mammograms for women over 40, a fecal occult blood test for everyone over 50, an amniocentesis to rule out a fetal anomaly for pregnant women over 35, because the incidence of breast cancer and colon cancer in these subgroups is higher than in the general population, as is the incidence of Down's syndrome in older mothers.

The testing of a person to rule out or confirm a suspected diagnosis because the patient has some sign or symptom is a diagnostic examination, not a screening. In these cases, the sign or symptom is used to explain the reason for the test.

A screening code may be a first listed code if the reason for the visit is specifically the screening exam. It may also be used as an additional code if the screening is done during an office visit for other health problems. A screening code is not necessary if the screening is inherent to a routine examination, such as a pap smear done during a routine pelvic examination.

Should a condition be discovered during the screening then the code for the condition may be assigned as an additional diagnosis.

The V code indicates that a screening exam is planned. A procedure code is required to confirm that the screening was performed.

4th **V73 Special screening examination for viral and chlamydial diseases**

V73.0 Poliomyelitis

V73.1 Smallpox

V73.2 Measles

V73.3 Rubella

V73.4 Yellow fever

V73.5 Other arthropod-borne viral diseases
Dengue fever
Hemorrhagic fever
Viral encephalitis:
mosquito-borne
tick-borne

V73.6 Trachoma

5th **V73.8 Other specified viral and chlamydial diseases**

V73.81 Human papillomavirus (HPV)

V73.88 Other specified chlamydial diseases

V73.89 Other specified viral diseases

5th **V73.9 Unspecified viral and chlamydial disease**

V73.98 Unspecified chlamydial disease

V73.99 Unspecified viral disease

4th **V74 Special screening examination for bacterial and spirochetal diseases**
Includes diagnostic skin tests for these diseases

V74.0 Cholera

V74.1 Pulmonary tuberculosis

V74.2 Leprosy [Hansen's disease]

V74.3 Diphtheria

V74.4 Bacterial conjunctivitis

V74.5 Venereal disease
Screening for bacterial and spirochetal sexually transmitted diseases
Screening for sexually transmitted diseases NOS
Excludes *special screening for nonbacterial sexually transmitted diseases (V73.81-V73.89, V75.4, V75.8)*

V74.6 Yaws

V74.8 Other specified bacterial and spirochetal diseases
Brucellosis
Leptospirosis
Plague
Tetanus
Whooping cough

V74.9 Unspecified bacterial and spirochetal disease

4th V75 Special screening examination for other infectious diseases

V75.0 Rickettsial diseases

V75.1 Malaria

V75.2 Leishmaniasis

V75.3 Trypanosomiasis
Chagas' disease
Sleeping sickness

V75.4 Mycotic infections

V75.5 Schistosomiasis

V75.6 Filariasis

V75.7 Intestinal helminthiasis

V75.8 Other specified parasitic infections

V75.9 Unspecified infectious disease

4th V76 Special screening for malignant neoplasms

V76.0 Respiratory organs

5th V76.1 Breast

V76.10 Breast screening, unspecified

V76.11 Screening mammogram for high-risk patient ♀ 1 4 6

V76.12 Other screening mammogram 1 4 6

Z12.31 Encounter for screening mammogram for malignant neoplasm of breast

V76.19 Other screening breast examination

V76.2 Cervix ♀

Z12.4 Encounter for screening for malignant neoplasm of cervix

Routine cervical Papanicolaou smear

Excludes *special screening for human papillomavirus (V73.81)*
that as part of a general gynecological examination (V72.31)

Layman's: *For Medicare, V15.89 is used in lieu of V76.2 for patients who meet the specified criteria as at high risk for cervical or vaginal cancer. Other carriers may follow different coding guidelines.*

V76.3 Bladder

5th V76.4 Other sites

V76.41 Rectum

Z12.12 Encounter for screening for malignant neoplasm of rectum

V76.42 Oral cavity

V76.43 Skin

V76.44 Prostate ♂

Z12.5 Encounter for screening for malignant neoplasm of prostate

V76.45 Testis ♂

V76.46 Ovary ♀

V76.47 Vagina ♀
Vaginal pap smear status-post hysterectomy for non-malignant condition
Use additional code to identify acquired absence of uterus (V88.01-V88.03)

Excludes *vaginal pap smear status-post hysterectomy for malignant condition (V67.01)*

V76.49 Other sites

5th V76.5 Intestine

V76.50 Intestine, unspecified

V76.51 Colon

Z12.11 Encounter for screening for malignant neoplasm of colon

Excludes *rectum (V76.41)*

V76.52 Small intestine

5th V76.8 Other neoplasm

V76.81 Nervous system

V76.89 Other neoplasm

V76.9 Unspecified

4th V77 Special screening for endocrine, nutritional, metabolic, and immunity disorders

V77.0 Thyroid disorders

V77.1 Diabetes mellitus

V77.2 Malnutrition

V77.3 Phenylketonuria [PKU]

V77.4 Galactosemia

V77.5 Gout

V77.6 Cystic fibrosis
Screening for mucoviscidosis

V77.7 Other inborn errors of metabolism

V77.8 Obesity

5th V77.9 Other and unspecified endocrine, nutritional, metabolic, and immunity disorders

V77.91 Screening for lipoid disorders
Screening cholesterol level
Screening for hypercholesterolemia
Screening for hyperlipidemia

V77.99 Other and unspecified endocrine, nutritional, metabolic, and immunity disorders

4th V78 Special screening for disorders of blood and blood-forming organs

V78.0 Iron deficiency anemia

V78.1 Other and unspecified deficiency anemia

V78.2 Sickle-cell disease or trait

V78.3 Other hemoglobinopathies

V78.8 Other disorders of blood and blood-forming organs

V78.9 Unspecified disorder of blood and blood-forming organs

4th V79 Special screening for mental disorders and developmental handicaps

V79.0 Depression

V79.1 Alcoholism

V79.2 Mental retardation

V79.3 Developmental handicaps in early childhood

V79.8 Other specified mental disorders and developmental handicaps

V79.9 Unspecified mental disorder and developmental handicap

4th V80 Special screening for neurological, eye, and ear diseases

5th V80.0 Neurological conditions

● V80.01 Traumatic brain injury

● V80.09 Other neurological conditions

V80.1 Glaucoma

V80.2 Other eye conditions
Screening for:
cataract
congenital anomaly of eye
senile macular lesions

Excludes *general vision examination (V72.0)*

V80.3 Ear diseases

Excludes *general hearing examination (V72.11-V72.19)*

4th V81 Special screening for cardiovascular, respiratory, and genitourinary diseases

V81.0 Ischemic heart disease

V81.1 Hypertension

V81.2 Other and unspecified cardiovascular conditions

V81.3 Chronic bronchitis and emphysema

V81.4 Other and unspecified respiratory conditions

Excludes *screening for:*
lung neoplasm (V76.0)
pulmonary tuberculosis (V74.1)

V81.5 Nephropathy

Screening for asymptomatic bacteriuria

V81.6 Other and unspecified genitourinary conditions

4th V82 Special screening for other conditions

V82.0 Skin conditions

V82.1 Rheumatoid arthritis

V82.2 Other rheumatic disorders

V82.3 Congenital dislocation of hip

V82.4 Maternal postnatal screening for chromosomal anomalies ♀

Excludes *antenatal screening by amniocentesis (V28.0)*

V82.5 Chemical poisoning and other contamination

Screening for:
heavy metal poisoning
ingestion of radioactive substance
poisoning from contaminated water supply
radiation exposure

V82.6 Multiphasic screening

5th V82.7 Genetic screening category

Excludes *genetic testing for procreative management (V26.31-V26.39)*

V82.71 Screening for genetic disease carrier status

V82.79 Other genetic screening

5th V82.8 Other specified conditions

V82.81 Osteoporosis

Use additional code to identify:
hormone replacement therapy (postmenopausal) status (V07.4)
postmenopausal (natural) status (V49.81)

V82.89 Other specified conditions

V82.9 Unspecified condition

GENETICS (V83-V84)

4th V83 Genetic carrier status

5th V83.0 Hemophilia A carrier

V83.01 Asymptomatic hemophilia A carrier

V83.02 Symptomatic hemophilia A carrier

5th V83.8 Other genetic carrier status

V83.81 Cystic fibrosis gene carrier

V83.89 Other genetic carrier status

4th V84 Genetic susceptibility to disease

Includes confirmed abnormal gene

Use additional code, if applicable, for any associated family history of the disease (V16-V19)

5th V84.0 Genetic susceptibility to malignant neoplasm

Code first, if applicable, any current malignant neoplasms (140.0-195.8, 200.0-208.9, 230.0-234.9)

Use additional code, if applicable, for any personal history of malignant neoplasm (V10.0-V10.9)

V84.01 Genetic susceptibility to malignant neoplasm of breast 2

V84.02 Genetic susceptibility to malignant neoplasm of ovary ♀ 2

V84.03 Genetic susceptibility to malignant neoplasm of prostate ♂ 2

V84.04 Genetic susceptibility to malignant neoplasm of endometrium ♀ 2

V84.09 Genetic susceptibility to other malignant neoplasm 2

V84.8 Genetic susceptibility to other disease

V84.81 Genetic susceptibility to multiple endocrine neoplasia [MEN] 2

V84.89 Genetic susceptibility to other disease 2

BODY MASS INDEX (V85)

4th V85 Body Mass Index [BMI]

Kilograms per meters squared

Note: *BMI adult codes are for use for persons over 20 years old*

V85.0 Body Mass Index less than 19, adult A 2

V85.1 Body Mass Index between 19-24, adult A 2

5th V85.2 Body Mass Index between 25-29, adult

V85.21 Body Mass Index 25.0-25.9, adult A 2

V85.22 Body Mass Index 26.0-26.9, adult A 2

V85.23 Body Mass Index 27.0-27.9, adult A 2

V85.24 Body Mass Index 28.0-28.9, adult A 2

V85.25 Body Mass Index 29.0-29.9, adult A 2

5th V85.3 Body Mass Index between 30-39, adult

V85.30 Body Mass Index 30.0-30.9, adult A 2

V85.31 Body Mass Index 31.0-31.9, adult A 2

V85.32 Body Mass Index 32.0-32.9, adult A 2

V85.33 Body Mass Index 33.0-33.9, adult A 2

V85.34 Body Mass Index 34.0-34.9, adult A 2

V85.35 Body Mass Index 35.0-35.9, adult A 2

V85.36 Body Mass Index 36.0-36.9, adult A 2

V85.37 Body Mass Index 37.0-37.9, adult A 2

V85.38 Body Mass Index 38.0-38.9, adult A 2

V85.39 Body Mass Index 39.0-39.9, adult A 2

V85.4 Body Mass Index 40 and over, adult A 2

5th V85.5 Body Mass Index, pediatric

Note: *BMI pediatric codes are for use for persons age 2-20 years old. These percentiles are based on the growth charts published by the Centers for Disease Control and Prevention (CDC)*

V85.51 Body Mass Index, pediatric, less than 5th percentile for age P 2

V85.52 Body Mass Index, pediatric, 5th percentile to less than 85th percentile for age P 2

V85.53 Body Mass Index, pediatric, 85th percentile to less than 95th percentile for age P 2

V85.54 Body Mass Index, pediatric, greater than or equal to 95th percentile for age P 2

ESTROGEN RECEPTOR STATUS (V86)

4th V86 Estrogen receptor status

Code first malignant neoplasm of breast (174.0-174.9, 175.0-175.9)

V86.0 Estrogen receptor positive status [ER+] 2

V86.1 Estrogen receptor negative status [ER-] 2

V80.3 – V86.1

OTHER SPECIFIED PERSONAL EXPOSURES AND HISTORY PRESENTING HAZARDS TO HEALTH (V87)

4th **V87 Other specified personal exposures and history presenting hazards to health**

5th **V87.0 Contact with and (suspected) exposure to hazardous metals**

Excludes *exposure to lead (V15.86)*
toxic effect of metals (984.0-985.9)

V87.01 Arsenic

V87.09 Other hazardous metals
Chromium compounds
Nickel dust

5th **V87.1 Contact with and (suspected) exposure to hazardous aromatic compounds**

Excludes *toxic effects of aromatic compounds (982.0, 983.0)*

V87.11 Aromatic amines

V87.12 Benzene

V87.19 Other hazardous aromatic compounds
Aromatic dyes NOS
Polycyclic aromatic hydrocarbons

V87.2 Contact with and (suspected) exposure to other potentially hazardous chemicals
Dyes NOS

Excludes *exposure to asbestos (V15.84)*
toxic effect of chemicals (980-989)

5th **V87.3 Contact with and (suspected) exposure to other potentially hazardous substances**

Excludes *contact with and (suspected) exposure to potentially hazardous body fluids (V15.85)*
toxic effect of substances (980-989)

V87.31 Exposure to mold

● **V87.32 Contact with and (suspected) exposure to algae bloom**

Rationale: *On October 1, 2007, a new external cause code E928.6, "Environmental exposure to harmful algae and toxins," was implemented for use to identify the external cause of the symptoms and conditions associated with algae blooms.*

A parallel V code is also necessary to identify the possible contact and exposure to an algae bloom for a person who may have been in the vicinity of the bloom and has not yet developed symptoms, or for a person who may have symptoms suspicious of being in the vicinity of an algae bloom, but a definitive cause has not been confirmed.

V87.39 Contact with and (suspected) exposure to other potentially hazardous substances

5th **V87.4 Personal history of drug therapy**

Excludes *long-term (current) drug use (V58.61-V58.69)*

Rationale: *Effective October 1, 2008 a new subcategory V87.4, "Personal history of drug therapy," became effective, as did codes for personal history of antineoplastic and monoclonal drug therapy. Comments received when this proposed new category was presented at the March 2008 meeting requested the creation of additional codes for other past drug therapies that may present hazards to health in the long term.*

V87.41 Personal history of antineoplastic chemotherapy 2

V87.42 Personal history of monoclonal drug therapy 2

● **V87.43 Personal history of estrogen therapy** 2

● **V87.44 Personal history of inhaled steroid therapy** 2

● **V87.45 Personal history of systemic steroid therapy** 2
Personal history of steroid therapy NOS

● **V87.46 Personal history of immunosuppression therapy** 2

Excludes *personal history of steroid therapy (V87.44, V87.45)*

V87.49 Personal history of other drug therapy 2

ACQUIRED ABSENCE OF OTHER ORGANS AND TISSUE (V88)

4th **V88 Acquired absence of other organs and tissue**

5th **V88.0 Acquired absence of cervix and uterus**

V88.01 Acquired absence of both cervix and uterus ♀ 2
Acquired absence of uterus NOS
Status post total hysterectomy

V88.02 Acquired absence of uterus with remaining cervical stump ♀ 2
Status post partial hysterectomy with remaining cervical stump

V88.03 Acquired absence of cervix with remaining uterus ♀ 2

OTHER SUSPECTED CONDITIONS NOT FOUND (V89)

ICD-9-CM Official Guidelines (Chapter 18)

d. Categories of V Codes

6) Observation

Codes from subcategory V89.0, Suspected maternal and fetal conditions not found, may either be used as a first listed or as an additional code assignment depending on the case. They are for use in very limited circumstances on a maternal record when an encounter is for a suspected maternal or fetal condition that is ruled out during that encounter (for example, a maternal or fetal condition may be suspected due to an abnormal test result). These codes should not be used when the condition is confirmed. In those cases, the confirmed condition should be coded. In addition, these codes are not for use if an illness or any signs or symptoms related to the suspected condition or problem are present. In such cases the diagnosis/symptom code is used.

Additional codes may be used in addition to the code from subcategory V89.0, but only if they are unrelated to the suspected condition being evaluated.

Codes from subcategory V89.0 may not be used for encounters for antenatal screening of mother. See Section I.C.18.d., Screening).

For encounters for suspected fetal condition that are inconclusive following testing and evaluation, assign the appropriate code from category 655, 656, 657 or 658.

4th **V89 Other suspected conditions not found**

5th **V89.0 Suspected maternal and fetal conditions not found**

Excludes *known or suspected fetal anomalies affecting management of mother, not ruled out (655.00-655.93, 656.00-656.93, 657.00-657.03, 658.00-658.93)*
newborn and perinatal conditions – code to condition

V89.01 Suspected problem with amniotic cavity and membrane not found M ♀
Suspected oligohydramnios not found
Suspected polyhydramnios not found

V89.02 Suspected placental problem not found M ♀

V89.03 Suspected fetal anomaly not found M ♀

V89.04 Suspected problem with fetal growth not found M ♀

V89.05 Suspected cervical shortening not found M ♀

V89.09 Other suspected maternal and fetal condition not found M ♀

19. SUPPLEMENTARY CLASSIFICATION OF EXTERNAL CAUSES OF INJURY AND POISONING (E000-E999)

This section is provided to permit the classification of environmental events, circumstances, and conditions as the cause of injury, poisoning, and other adverse effects. Where a code from this section is applicable, it is intended that it shall be used in addition to a code from one of the main chapters of ICD-9-CM, indicating the nature of the condition. Certain other conditions which may be stated to be due to external causes are classified in Chapters 1 to 16 of ICD-9-CM. For these, the "E" code classification should be used as an additional code for more detailed analysis.

Machinery accidents [other than those connected with transport] are classifiable to category E919, in which the fourth digit allows a broad classification of the type of machinery involved. ~~If a more detailed classification of type of machinery is required, it is suggested that the "Classification of Industrial Accidents according to Agency," prepared by the International Labor Office, be used in addition; it is included in this publication.~~

Categories for "late effects" of accidents and other external causes are to be found at E929, E959, E969, E977, E989, and E999.

ICD-9-CM Official Guidelines (Chapter 19):

Introduction: *These guidelines are provided for those who are currently collecting E codes in order that there will be standardization in the process. If your institution plans to begin collecting E codes, these guidelines are to be applied. The use of E codes is supplemental to the application of ICD-9-CM diagnosis codes. E codes are never to be recorded as principal diagnoses (first-listed in non-inpatient setting) and are not required for reporting to CMS.*

External causes of injury and poisoning codes (E codes) are intended to provide data for injury research and evaluation of injury prevention strategies. E codes capture how the injury or poisoning happened (cause), the intent (unintentional or accidental; or intentional, such as suicide or assault), and the place where the event occurred.

Some major categories of E codes include: transport accidents poisoning and adverse effects of drugs, medicinal substances and biologicals accidental falls accidents caused by fire and flames accidents due to natural and environmental factors late effects of accidents, assaults or self injury assaults or purposely inflicted injury suicide or self inflicted injury

These guidelines apply for the coding and collection of E codes from records in hospitals, outpatient clinics, emergency departments, other ambulatory care settings and provider offices, and nonacute care settings, except when other specific guidelines apply.

a. General E Code Coding Guidelines

1) Used with any code in the range of 001-V84.8

An E code may be used with any code in the range of 001-V84.8, which indicates an injury, poisoning, or adverse effect due to an external cause.

2) Assign the appropriate E code for all initial treatments

Assign the appropriate E code for the initial encounter of an injury, poisoning, or adverse effect of drugs, not for subsequent treatment.

External cause of injury codes (E-codes) may be assigned while the acute fracture codes are still applicable.

See Section I.C.17.b.1 for coding of acute fractures.

3) Use the full range of E codes

Use the full range of E codes to completely describe the cause, the intent and the place of occurrence, if applicable, for all injuries, poisonings, and adverse effects of drugs.

4) Assign as many E codes as necessary

Assign as many E codes as necessary to fully explain each cause. If only one E code can be recorded, assign the E code most related to the principal diagnosis.

5) The selection of the appropriate E code

The selection of the appropriate E code is guided by the Index to External Causes, which is located after the alphabetical index to diseases and by Inclusion and Exclusion notes in the Tabular List.

6) E code can never be a principal diagnosis

An E code can never be a principal (first listed) diagnosis.

7) External cause code(s) with systemic inflammatory response syndrome (SIRS)

An external cause code is not appropriate with a code from subcategory 995.9, unless the patient also has an injury, poisoning, or adverse effect of drugs.

b. Place of Occurrence Guideline

Use an additional code from category E849 to indicate the Place of Occurrence for injuries and poisonings. The Place of Occurrence describes the place where the event occurred and not the patient's activity at the time of the event.

Do not use E849.9 if the place of occurrence is not stated.

c. Adverse Effects of Drugs, Medicinal and Biological Substances Guidelines

1) Do not code directly from the Table of Drugs and Chemicals. Always refer back to the Tabular List.

2) Use as many codes as necessary to describe completely all drugs, medicinal or biological substances.

3) If the same E code would describe the causative agent for more than one adverse reaction, assign the code only once.

4) If two or more drugs, medicinal or biological substances are reported, code each individually unless the combination code is listed in the Table of Drugs and Chemicals. In that case, assign the E code for the combination.

5) When a reaction results from the interaction of a drug(s) and alcohol, use poisoning codes and E codes for both.

6) If the reporting format limits the number of E codes that can be used in reporting clinical data, code the one most related to the principal diagnosis. Include at least one from each category (cause, intent, place) if possible.

If there are different fourth digit codes in the same three digit category, use the code for "Other specified" of that category. If there is no "Other specified" code in that category, use the appropriate "Unspecified" code in that category.

If the codes are in different three digit categories, assign the appropriate E code for other multiple drugs and medicinal substances.

7) Codes from the E930-E949 series must be used to identify the causative substance for an adverse effect of drug, medicinal and biological substances, correctly prescribed and properly administered. The effect, such as tachycardia, delirium, gastrointestinal hemorrhaging, vomiting, hypokalemia, hepatitis, renal failure, or respiratory failure, is coded and followed by the appropriate code from the E930-E949 series.

d. Multiple Cause E Code Coding Guidelines

If two or more events cause separate injuries, an E code should be assigned for each cause. The first listed E code will be selected in the following order:

- *E codes for child and adult abuse take priority over all other E codes.*

  See Section I.C.19.e., Child and Adult abuse guidelines.
- *E codes for terrorism events take priority over all other E codes except child and adult abuse*
- *E codes for cataclysmic events take priority over all other E codes except child and adult abuse and terrorism.*
- *E codes for transport accidents take priority over all other E codes except cataclysmic events and child and adult abuse and terrorism.*

The first-listed E code should correspond to the cause of the most serious diagnosis due to an assault, accident, or self-harm, following the order of hierarchy listed above.

e. Child and Adult Abuse Guideline

1) Intentional injury

When the cause of an injury or neglect is intentional child or adult abuse, the first listed E code should be assigned

E Codes

from categories E960-E968, Homicide and injury purposely inflicted by other persons, (except category E967). An E code from category E967, Child and adult battering and other maltreatment, should be added as an additional code to identify the perpetrator, if known.

2) ***Accidental intent***

In cases of neglect when the intent is determined to be accidental E code E904.0, Abandonment or neglect of infant and helpless person, should be the first listed E code.

f. ***Unknown or Suspected Intent Guideline***

1) ***If the intent (accident, self-harm, assault) of the cause of an injury or poisoning is unknown***

If the intent (accident, self-harm, assault) of the cause of an injury or poisoning is unknown or unspecified, code the intent as undetermined E980-E989.

2) ***If the intent (accident, self-harm, assault) of the cause of an injury or poisoning is questionable***

If the intent (accident, self-harm, assault) of the cause of an injury or poisoning is questionable, probable or suspected, code the intent as undetermined E980-E989.

g. ***Undetermined Cause***

When the intent of an injury or poisoning is known, but the cause is unknown, use codes: E928.9, Unspecified accident, E958.9, Suicide and self-inflicted injury by unspecified means, and E968.9, Assault by unspecified means.

These E codes should rarely be used, as the documentation in the medical record, in both the inpatient outpatient and other settings, should normally provide sufficient detail to determine the cause of the injury.

h. ***Late Effects of External Cause Guidelines***

1) ***Late effect E codes***

Late effect E codes exist for injuries and poisonings but not for adverse effects of drugs, misadventures and surgical complications.

2) ***Late effect E codes (E929, E959, E969, E977, E989, or E999.1)***

A late effect E code (E929, E959, E969, E977, E989, or E999.1) should be used with any report of a late effect or sequela resulting from a previous injury or poisoning (905-909).

3) ***Late effect E code with a related current injury***

A late effect E code should never be used with a related current nature of injury code.

4) ***Use of late effect E codes for subsequent visits***

Use a late effect E code for subsequent visits when a late effect of the initial injury or poisoning is being treated. There is no late effect E code for adverse effects of drugs. Do not use a late effect E code for subsequent visits for follow-up care (e.g., to assess healing, to receive rehabilitative therapy) of the injury or poisoning when no late effect of the injury has been documented.

i. ***Misadventures and Complications of Care Guidelines***

1) ***Code range E870-E876***

Assign a code in the range of E870-E876 if misadventures are stated by the provider.

2) ***Code range E878-E879***

Assign a code in the range of E878-E879 if the provider attributes an abnormal reaction or later complication to a surgical or medical procedure, but does not mention misadventure at the time of the procedure as the cause of the reaction.

j. ***Terrorism Guidelines***

1) ***Cause of injury identified by the Federal Government (FBI) as terrorism***

When the cause of an injury is identified by the Federal Government (FBI) as terrorism, the first-listed E-code should be a code from category E979, Terrorism. The definition of terrorism employed by the FBI is found at the inclusion note at E979. The terrorism E-code is the only E-code that should be assigned. Additional E codes from the assault categories should not be assigned.

2) ***Cause of an injury is suspected to be the result of terrorism***

When the cause of an injury is suspected to be the result of terrorism a code from category E979 should not be assigned. Assign a code in the range of E codes based circumstances on the documentation of intent and mechanism.

3) ***Code E979.9, Terrorism, secondary effects***

Assign code E979.9, Terrorism, secondary effects, for conditions occurring subsequent to the terrorist event. This code should not be assigned for conditions that are due to the initial terrorist act.

4) ***Statistical tabulation of terrorism codes***

For statistical purposes these codes will be tabulated within the category for assault, expanding the current category from E960-E969 to include E979 and E999.1.

EXTERNAL CAUSE STATUS (E000)

Note: *A code from category E000 should be used in conjunction with the external cause code(s) assigned to a record to indicate the status of the person at the time the event occurred. A single code from category E000 should be assigned for an encounter.*

● 4th **E000 External cause status**

● **E000.0 Civilian activity done for income or pay**

Civilian activity done for financial or other compensation

Excludes *military activity (E000.1)*

● **E000.1 Military activity**

Excludes *activity of off duty military personnel (E000.8)*

● **E000.8 Other external cause status**

Activity NEC
Hobby not done for income
Leisure activity
Off-duty activity of military personnel
Recreation or sport not for income or while a student
Student activity
Volunteer activity

Excludes *civilian activity done for income or compensation (E000.0)*
military activity (E000.1)

● **E000.9 Unspecified external cause status**

ACTIVITY (E001-E030)

Note: *Categories E001 to E030 are provided for use to indicate the activity of the person seeking healthcare for an injury or health condition, such as a heart attack while shoveling snow, which resulted from, or was contributed to, by the activity. These codes are appropriate for use for both acute injuries, such as those from chapter 17, and conditions that are due to the long-term, cumulative effects of an activity, such as those from chapter 13. They are also appropriate for use with external cause codes for cause and intent if identifying the activity provides additional information on the event.*

These codes should be used in conjunction with other external cause codes for external cause status (E000) and place of occurrence (E849).

This section contains the following broad activity categories:

E001 Activities involving walking and running
E002 Activities involving water and water craft
E003 Activities involving ice and snow
E004 Activities involving climbing, rappelling, and jumping off
E005 Activities involving dancing and other rhythmic movement
E006 Activities involving other sports and athletics played individually
E007 Activities involving other sports and athletics played as a team or group
E008 Activities involving other specified sports and athletics
E009 Activity involving other cardiorespiratory exercise
E010 Activity involving other muscle strengthening exercises
E011 Activities involving computer technology and electronic devices
E012 Activities involving arts and handcrafts
E013 Activities involving personal hygiene and household maintenance
E014 Activities involving person providing caregiving
E015 Activities involving food preparation, cooking and grilling
E016 Activities involving property and land maintenance, building and construction
E017 Activities involving roller coasters and other types of external motion
E018 Activities involving playing musical instrument
E019 Activities involving animal care
E029 Other activity
E030 Unspecified activity

● 4th **E001 Activities involving walking and running**
Excludes *walking an animal (E019.0)*
walking or running on a treadmill (E009.0)

● **E001.0 Walking, marching and hiking**
Walking, marching and hiking on level or elevated terrain
Excludes *mountain climbing (E004.0)*

● **E001.1 Running**

● 4th **E002 Activities involving water and water craft**
Excludes *activities involving ice (E003.0-E003.9)*
boating and other watercraft transport accidents (E830-E838)

● **E002.0 Swimming**

● **E002.1 Springboard and platform diving**

● **E002.2 Water polo**

● **E002.3 Water aerobics and water exercise**

● **E002.4 Underwater diving and snorkeling**
SCUBA diving

● **E002.5 Rowing, canoeing, kayaking, rafting and tubing**
Canoeing, kayaking, rafting and tubing in calm and turbulent water

● **E002.6 Water skiing and wake boarding**

● **E002.7 Surfing, windsurfing and boogie boarding**

● **E002.8 Water sliding**

● **E002.9 Other activity involving water and watercraft**
Activity involving water NOS
Parasailing
Water survival training and testing

● 4th **E003 Activities involving ice and snow**
Excludes *shoveling ice and snow (E016.0)*

● **E003.0 Ice skating**
Figure skating (singles) (pairs)
Ice dancing
Excludes *ice hockey (E003.1)*

● **E003.1 Ice hockey**

● **E003.2 Snow (alpine) (downhill) skiing, snow boarding, sledding, tobogganing and snow tubing**
Excludes *cross country skiing (E003.3)*

● **E003.3 Cross country skiing**
Nordic skiing

● **E003.9 Other activity involving ice and snow**
Activity involving ice and snow NOS

● 4th **E004 Activities involving climbing, rappelling and jumping off**
Excludes *hiking on level or elevated terrain (E001.0)*
jumping rope (E006.5)
sky diving (E840-E844)
trampoline jumping (E005.3)

● **E004.0 Mountain climbing, rock climbing and wall climbing**

● **E004.1 Rappelling**

● **E004.2 BASE jumping**
Building, Antenna, Span, Earth jumping

● **E004.3 Bungee jumping**

● **E004.4 Hang gliding**

● **E004.9 Other activity involving climbing, rappelling and jumping off**

● 4th **E005 Activities involving dancing and other rhythmic movement**
Excludes *martial arts (E008.4)*

● **E005.0 Dancing**

● **E005.1 Yoga**

● **E005.2 Gymnastics**
Rhythmic gymnastics
Excludes *trampoline (E005.3)*

● **E005.3 Trampoline**

● **E005.4 Cheerleading**

● **E005.9 Other activity involving dancing and other rhythmic movements**

● 4th **E006 Activities involving other sports and athletics played individually**
Excludes *dancing (E005.0)*
gymnastic (E005.2)
trampoline (E005.3)
yoga (E005.1)

● **E006.0 Roller skating (inline) and skateboarding**

● **E006.1 Horseback riding**

● **E006.2 Golf**

● **E006.3 Bowling**

● **E006.4 Bike riding**
Excludes *transport accident involving bike riding (E800-E829)*

● **E006.5 Jumping rope**

● **E006.6 Non-running track and field events**
Excludes *running (any form) (E001.1)*

E001 – E006.6

● E006.9 Other activity involving other sports and athletics played individually
Excludes activities involving climbing, rappelling, and jumping (E004.0-E004.9)
activities involving ice and snow (E003.0-E003.9)
activities involving walking and running (E001.0-E001.9)
activities involving water and watercraft (E002.0-E002.9)

●4th E007 Activities involving other sports and athletics played as a team or group
Excludes ice hockey (E003.1)
water polo (E002.2)

● E007.0 American tackle football
Football NOS

● E007.1 American flag or touch football

● E007.2 Rugby

● E007.3 Baseball
Softball

● E007.4 Lacrosse and field hockey

● E007.5 Soccer

● E007.6 Basketball

● E007.7 Volleyball (beach) (court)

● E007.8 Physical games generally associated with school recess, summer camp and children
Capture the flag
Dodge ball
Four square
Kickball

● E007.9 Other activity involving other sports and athletics played as a team or group
Cricket

●4th E008 Activities involving other specified sports and athletics

● E008.0 Boxing

● E008.1 Wrestling

● E008.2 Racquet and hand sports
Handball
Racquetball
Squash
Tennis

● E008.3 Frisbee
Ultimate frisbee

● E008.4 Martial arts
Combatives

● E008.9 Other specified sports and athletics activity
Excludes sports and athletics activities specified in categories E001-E007

●4th E009 Activity involving other cardiorespiratory exercise
Activity involving physical training

● E009.0 Exercise machines primarily for cardiorespiratory conditioning
Elliptical and stepper machines
Stationary bike
Treadmill

● E009.1 Calisthenics
Jumping jacks
Warm up and cool down

● E009.2 Aerobic and step exercise

● E009.3 Circuit training

● E009.4 Obstacle course
Challenge course
Confidence course

● E009.5 Grass drills
Guerilla drills

● E009.9 Other activity involving other cardiorespiratory exercise
Excludes activities involving cardiorespiratory exercise specified in categories E001-E008

●4th E010 Activity involving other muscle strengthening exercises

● E010.0 Exercise machines primarily for muscle strengthening

● E010.1 Push-ups, pull-ups, sit-ups

● E010.2 Free weights
Barbells
Dumbbells

● E010.3 Pilates

● E010.9 Other activity involving other muscle strengthening exercises
Excludes activities involving muscle strengthening specified in categories E001-E009

●4th E011 Activities involving computer technology and electronic devices
Excludes electronic musical keyboard or instruments (E018.0)

● E011.0 Computer keyboarding
Electronic game playing using keyboard or other stationary device

● E011.1 Hand held interactive electronic device
Cellular telephone and communication device
Electronic game playing using interactive device
Excludes electronic game playing using keyboard or other stationary device (E011.0)

● E011.9 Other activity involving computer technology and electronic devices

●4th E012 Activities involving arts and handcrafts
Excludes activities involving playing musical instrument (E018.0-E018.3)

● E012.0 Knitting and crocheting

● E012.1 Sewing

● E012.2 Furniture building and finishing
Furniture repair

● E012.9 Activity involving other arts and handcrafts

●4th E013 Activities involving personal hygiene and household maintenance
Excludes activities involving cooking and grilling (E015.0-E015.9)
activities involving property and land maintenance, building and construction (E016.0-E016.9)
activity involving persons providing caregiving (E014.0-E014.9)
dishwashing (E015.0)
food preparation (E015.0)
gardening (E016.1)

● E013.0 Personal bathing and showering

● E013.1 Laundry

● E013.2 Vacuuming

● E013.3 Ironing

● E013.4 Floor mopping and cleaning

● E013.5 Residential relocation
Packing up and unpacking involved in moving to a new residence

● E013.8 Other personal hygiene activity

● E013.9 Other household maintenance

●4th E014 Activities involving person providing caregiving

● E014.0 Caregiving involving bathing

● E014.1 Caregiving involving lifting

● E014.9 Other activity involving person providing caregiving

●4th E015 Activities involving food preparation, cooking and grilling

● E015.0 Food preparation and clean up
Dishwashing

● E015.1 Grilling and smoking food

● E015.2 Cooking and baking
Use of stove, oven and microwave oven

● E015.9 Other activity involving cooking and grilling

●4th E016 Activities involving property and land maintenance, building and construction

● E016.0 Digging, shoveling and raking
Dirt digging
Raking leaves
Snow shoveling

● E016.1 Gardening and landscaping
Pruning, trimming shrubs, weeding

● E016.2 Building and construction

● E016.9 Other activity involving property and land maintenance, building and construction

●4th E017 Activities involving roller coasters and other types of external motion

● E017.0 Rollercoaster riding

● E017.9 Other activity involving external motion

●4th E018 Activities involving playing musical instrument
Activity involving playing electric musical instrument

● E018.0 Piano playing
Musical keyboard (electronic) playing

● E018.1 Drum and other percussion instrument playing

● E018.2 String instrument playing

● E018.3 Wind and brass instrument playing

●4th E019 Activities involving animal care
Excludes *horseback riding (E006.1)*

● E019.0 Walking an animal

● E019.1 Milking an animal

● E019.2 Grooming and shearing an animal

● E019.9 Other activity involving animal care

●4th E029 Other activity

● E029.0 Refereeing a sports activity

● E029.1 Spectator at an event

● E029.2 Rough housing and horseplay

● E029.9 Other activity

● E030 Unspecified activity

TRANSPORT ACCIDENTS (E800-E848)

Definitions and examples related to transport accidents

(a) A transport accident (E800-E848) is any accident involving a device designed primarily for, or being used at the time primarily for, conveying persons or goods from one place to another.

Includes accidents involving:
aircraft and spacecraft (E840-E845)
watercraft (E830-E838)
motor vehicle (E810-E825)
railway (E800-E807)
other road vehicles (E826-E829)

In classifying accidents which involve more than one kind of transport, the above order of precedence of transport accidents should be used.

Accidents involving agricultural and construction machines, such as tractors, cranes, and bulldozers, are regarded as transport accidents only when these vehicles are under their own power on a highway [otherwise the vehicles are regarded as machinery]. Vehicles which can travel on land or water, such as hovercraft and other amphibious vehicles, are regarded as watercraft when on the water, as motor vehicles when on the highway, and as off-road motor vehicles when on land, but off the highway.

Excludes *accidents:*
in sports which involve the use of transport but where the transport vehicle itself was not involved in the accident
involving vehicles which are part of industrial equipment used entirely on industrial premises
occurring during transportation but unrelated to the hazards associated with the means of transportation [e.g., injuries received in a fight on board ship; transport vehicle involved in a cataclysm such as an earthquake]
to persons engaged in the maintenance or repair of transport equipment or vehicle not in motion, unless injured by another vehicle in motion

(b) A railway accident is a transport accident involving a railway train or other railway vehicle operated on rails, whether in motion or not.

Excludes *accidents:*
in repair shops
in roundhouse or on turntable
on railway premises but not involving a train or other railway vehicle

(c) A railway train or railway vehicle is any device with or without cars coupled to it, designed for traffic on a railway.

Includes interurban:
electric car (operated chiefly on its own right-of-way, not open to other traffic)
streetcar (operated chiefly on its own right-of-way, not open to other traffic)
railway train, any power [diesel] [electric] [steam]
funicular
monorail or two-rail
subterranean or elevated
other vehicle designed to run on a railway track

Excludes *interurban electric cars [streetcars] specified to be operating on a right-of-way that forms part of the public street or highway [definition (n)]*

(d) A railway or railroad is a right-of-way designed for traffic on rails, which is used by carriages or wagons transporting passengers or freight, and by other rolling stock, and which is not open to other public vehicular traffic

(e) A **motor vehicle accident** is a transport accident involving a motor vehicle. It is defined as a motor vehicle traffic accident or as a motor vehicle nontraffic accident according to whether the accident occurs on a public highway or elsewhere.

Excludes *injury or damage due to cataclysm*
injury or damage while a motor vehicle, not under its own power, is being loaded on, or unloaded from, another conveyance

(f) A **motor vehicle traffic accident** is any motor vehicle accident occurring on a public highway [i.e., originating, terminating, or involving a vehicle partially on the highway]. A motor vehicle accident is assumed to have occurred on the highway unless another place is specified, except in the case of accidents involving only off-road motor vehicles which are classified as nontraffic accidents unless the contrary is stated.

(g) A **motor vehicle nontraffic accident** is any motor vehicle accident which occurs entirely in any place other than a public highway.

(h) A **public highway [trafficway]** or **street** is the entire width between property lines [or other boundary lines] of every way or place, of which any part is open to the use of the public for purposes of vehicular traffic as a matter of right or custom. A **roadway** is that part of the public highway designed, improved, and ordinarily used, for vehicular travel.

Includes approaches (public) to:
docks
public building
station

Excludes *driveway (private)*
parking lot
ramp
roads in:
airfield
farm
industrial premises
mine
private grounds
quarry

(i) A **motor vehicle** is any mechanically or electrically powered device, not operated on rails, upon which any person or property may be transported or drawn upon a highway. Any object such as a trailer, coaster, sled, or wagon being towed by a motor vehicle is considered a part of the motor vehicle.

Includes automobile [any type]
bus
construction machinery, farm and industrial machinery, steam roller, tractor, army tank, highway grader, or similar vehicle on wheels or treads, while in transport under own power
fire engine (motorized)
motorcycle
motorized bicycle [moped] or scooter
trolley bus not operating on rails
truck
van

Excludes *devices used solely to move persons or materials within the confines of a building and its premises, such as:*
building elevator
coal car in mine
electric baggage or mail truck used solely within a railroad station
electric truck used solely within an industrial plant
moving overhead crane

(j) A **motorcycle** is a two-wheeled motor vehicle having one or two riding saddles and sometimes having a third wheel for the support of a sidecar. The sidecar is considered part of the motorcycle.

Includes motorized:
bicycle [moped]
scooter
tricycle

(k) An **off-road motor vehicle** is a motor vehicle of special design, to enable it to negotiate rough or soft terrain or snow. Examples of special design are high construction, special wheels and tires, driven by treads, or support on a cushion of air.

Includes all terrain vehicle [ATV]
army tank
hovercraft, on land or swamp
snowmobile

(l) A **driver** of a motor vehicle is the occupant of the motor vehicle operating it or intending to operate it. A **motorcyclist** is the driver of a motorcycle. Other authorized occupants of a motor vehicle are **passengers**.

(m) An other road vehicle is any device, except a motor vehicle, in, on, or by which any person or property may be transported on a highway.

Includes animal carrying a person or goods
animal-drawn vehicle
animal harnessed to conveyance
bicycle [pedal cycle]
streetcar
tricycle (pedal)

Excludes *pedestrian conveyance [definition (q)]*

(n) A **streetcar** is a device designed and used primarily for transporting persons within a municipality, running on rails, usually subject to normal traffic control signals, and operated principally on a right-of-way that forms part of the traffic way. A trailer being towed by a streetcar is considered a part of the streetcar.

Includes interurban or intraurban electric or streetcar, when specified to be operating on a street or public highway
tram (car)
trolley (car)

(o) A **pedal cycle** is any road transport vehicle operated solely by pedals.

Includes bicycle
pedal cycle
tricycle

Excludes *motorized bicycle [definition (i)]*

(p) A **pedal cyclist** is any person riding on a pedal cycle or in a sidecar attached to such a vehicle.

(q) A **pedestrian conveyance** is any human powered device by which a pedestrian may move other than by walking or by which a walking person may move another pedestrian.

Includes baby carriage
coaster wagon
heelies
ice skates
perambulator
pushcart
pushchair
roller skates
scooter
skateboard
skis
sled
wheelchair
wheelies

(r) A **pedestrian** is any person involved in an accident who was not at the time of the accident riding in or on a motor vehicle, railroad train, streetcar, animal-drawn or other vehicle, or on a bicycle or animal.

Includes person:
changing tire of vehicle
in or operating a pedestrian conveyance
making adjustment to motor of vehicle
on foot

(s) A **watercraft** is any device for transporting passengers or goods on the water.

(t) A **small boat** is any watercraft propelled by paddle, oars, or small motor, with a passenger capacity of less than ten.

Includes boat NOS
canoe
coble
dinghy
punt
raft
rowboat
rowing shell
scull
skiff
small motorboat

Excludes *barge*
lifeboat (used after abandoning ship)
raft (anchored) being used as a diving platform
yacht

(u) An **aircraft** is any device for transporting passengers or goods in the air.

Includes airplane [any type]
balloon
bomber
dirigible
glider (hang)
military aircraft
parachute

(v) A **commercial transport aircraft** is any device for collective passenger or freight transportation by air, whether run on commercial lines for profit or by government authorities, with the exception of military craft.

RAILWAY ACCIDENTS (E800-E807)

Note: *For definitions of railway accident and related terms see definitions (a) to (d).*

Excludes *accidents involving railway train and:*
aircraft (E840.0-E845.9)
motor vehicle (E810.0-E825.9)
watercraft (E830.0-E838.9)

The following fourth-digit subdivisions are for use with categories E800-E807 to identify the injured person:

.0 Railway employee

Any person who by virtue of his employment in connection with a railway, whether by the railway company or not, is at increased risk of involvement in a railway accident, such as:
catering staff of train
driver
guard
porter
postal staff on train
railway fireman
shunter
sleeping car attendant

.1 Passenger on railway

Any authorized person traveling on a train, except a railway employee.

Excludes *intending passenger waiting at station (8)*
unauthorized rider on railway vehicle (8)

.2 Pedestrian

See definition (r)

.3 Pedal cyclist

See definition (p)

.8 Other specified person

Intending passenger or bystander waiting at station
Unauthorized rider on railway vehicle

.9 Unspecified person

4th **E800 Railway accident involving collision with rolling stock**
[.0-.3, .8-.9]

Requires fourth digit. See beginning of section E800-E807 for codes and definitions.

Includes collision between railway trains or railway vehicles, any kind
collision NOS on railway
derailment with antecedent collision with rolling stock or NOS

4th **E801 Railway accident involving collision with other object**
[.0-.3, .8-.9]

Requires fourth digit. See beginning of section E800-E807 for codes and definitions.

Includes collision of railway train with:
buffers
fallen tree on railway
gates
platform
rock on railway
streetcar
other nonmotor vehicle
other object

Excludes *collision with:*
aircraft (E840.0-E842.9)
motor vehicle (E810.0-E810.9, E820.0-E822.9)

4th **E802 Railway accident involving derailment without antecedent collision**
[.0-.3, .8-.9]

Requires fourth digit. See beginning of section E800-E807 for codes and definitions.

4th **E803 Railway accident involving explosion, fire, or burning**

[.0-.3, .8-.9]

Requires fourth digit. See beginning of section E800-E807 for codes and definitions.

Excludes *explosion or fire, with antecedent derailment (E802.0-E802.9)*
explosion or fire, with mention of antecedent collision (E800.0-E801.9)

4th **E804 Fall in, on, or from railway train**

[.0-.3, .8-.9]

Requires fourth digit. See beginning of section E800-E807 for codes and definitions.

Includes fall while alighting from or boarding railway train

Excludes *fall related to collision, derailment, or explosion of railway train (E800.0-E803.9)*

4th **E805 Hit by rolling stock**

[.0-.3, .8-.9]

Requires fourth digit. See beginning of section E800-E807 for codes and definitions.

Includes crushed by railway train or part
injured by railway train or part
killed by railway train or part
knocked down by railway train or part
run over by railway train or part

Excludes *pedestrian hit by object set in motion by railway train (E806.0-E806.9)*

4th **E806 Other specified railway accident**

[.0-.3, .8-.9]

Requires fourth digit. See beginning of section E800-E807 for codes and definitions.

Includes hit by object falling in railway train
injured by door or window on railway train
nonmotor road vehicle or pedestrian hit by object set in motion by railway train
railway train hit by falling:
earth NOS
rock
tree
other object

Excludes *railway accident due to cataclysm (E908-E909)*

4th **E807 Railway accident of unspecified nature**

[.0-.3, .8-.9]

Requires fourth digit. See beginning of section E800-E807 for codes and definitions.

Includes found dead on railway right-of-way NOS
injured on railway right-of-way NOS
railway accident NOS

MOTOR VEHICLE TRAFFIC ACCIDENTS (E810-E819)

Note: *For definitions of motor vehicle traffic accident, and related terms, see definitions (e) to (k).*

Excludes *accidents involving motor vehicle and aircraft (E840.0-E845.9)*

The following fourth-digit subdivisions are for use with categories E810-E819 to identify the injured person:

.0 Driver of motor vehicle other than motorcycle
See definition (l)

.1 Passenger in motor vehicle other than motorcycle
See definition (l)

.2 Motorcyclist
See definition (l)

.3 Passenger on motorcycle
See definition (l)

.4 Occupant of streetcar

.5 Rider of animal; occupant of animal-drawn vehicle

.6 Pedal cyclist
See definition (p)

.7 Pedestrian
See definition (r)

.8 Other specified person
Occupant of vehicle other than above
Person in railway train involved in accident
Unauthorized rider of motor vehicle

.9 Unspecified person

4th **E810 Motor vehicle traffic accident involving collision with train**

[.0-.9]

Requires fourth digit. See beginning of section E810-E819 for codes and definitions.

Excludes *motor vehicle collision with object set in motion by railway train (E815.0-E815.9)*
railway train hit by object set in motion by motor vehicle (E818.0-E818.9)

4th **E811 Motor vehicle traffic accident involving re-entrant collision with another motor vehicle**

[.0-.9]

Requires fourth digit. See beginning of section E810-E819 for codes and definitions.

Includes collision between motor vehicle which accidentally leaves the roadway then re-enters the same roadway, or the opposite roadway on a divided highway, and another motor vehicle

Excludes *collision on the same roadway when none of the motor vehicles involved have left and re-entered the roadway (E812.0-E812.9)*

4th **E812 Other motor vehicle traffic accident involving collision with motor vehicle**

[.0-.9]

Requires fourth digit. See beginning of section E810-E819 for codes and definitions.

Includes collision with another motor vehicle parked, stopped, stalled, disabled, or abandoned on the highway
motor vehicle collision NOS

Excludes *collision with object set in motion by another motor vehicle (E815.0-E815.9)*
re-entrant collision with another motor vehicle (E811.0-E811.9)

4th E813 Motor vehicle traffic accident involving collision with other vehicle

[.0-.9]

Requires fourth digit. See beginning of section E810-E819 for codes and definitions.

Includes collision between motor vehicle, any kind, and:
other road (nonmotor transport) vehicle, such as:
animal carrying a person
animal-drawn vehicle
pedal cycle
streetcar

Excludes *collision with:*
object set in motion by nonmotor road vehicle (E815.0-E815.9)
pedestrian (E814.0-E814.9)
nonmotor road vehicle hit by object set in motion by motor vehicle (E818.0-E818.9)

4th E814 Motor vehicle traffic accident involving collision with pedestrian

[.0-.9]

Requires fourth digit. See beginning of section E810-E819 for codes and definitions.

Includes collision between motor vehicle, any kind, and pedestrian
pedestrian dragged, hit, or run over by motor vehicle, any kind

Excludes *pedestrian hit by object set in motion by motor vehicle (E818.0-E818.9)*

4th E815 Other motor vehicle traffic accident involving collision on the highway

[.0-.9]

Requires fourth digit. See beginning of section E810-E819 for codes and definitions.

Includes collision (due to loss of control) (on highway) between motor vehicle, any kind, and:
abutment (bridge) (overpass)
animal (herded) (unattended)
fallen stone, traffic sign, tree, utility pole
guard rail or boundary fence
interhighway divider
landslide (not moving)
object set in motion by railway train or road vehicle (motor) (nonmotor)
object thrown in front of motor vehicle
safety island
temporary traffic sign or marker
wall of cut made for road
other object, fixed, movable, or moving

Excludes *collision with:*
any object off the highway (resulting from loss of control) (E816.0-E816.9)
any object which normally would have been off the highway and is not stated to have been on it (E816.0-E816.9)
motor vehicle hit by object:
set in motion by railway train or road vehicle (motor) (nonmotor) (E818.0-E818.9)
thrown into or on vehicle (E818.0-E818.9)
motor vehicle parked, stopped, stalled, disabled, or abandoned on highway (E812.0-E812.9)
moving landslide (E909.2)

4th E816 Motor vehicle traffic accident due to loss of control, without collision on the highway

[.0-.9]

Requires fourth digit. See beginning of section E810-E819 for codes and definitions.

Includes motor vehicle:
failing to make curve and:
colliding with object off the highway
overturning
stopping abruptly off the highway
going out of control (due to)
blowout and:
colliding with object off the highway
overturning
stopping abruptly off the highway
burst tire and:
colliding with object off the highway
overturning
stopping abruptly off the highway
driver falling asleep and:
colliding with object off the highway
overturning
stopping abruptly off the highway
driver inattention and:
colliding with object off the highway
overturning
stopping abruptly off the highway
excessive speed and:
colliding with object off the highway
overturning
stopping abruptly off the highway
failure of mechanical part and:
colliding with object off the highway
overturning
stopping abruptly off the highway

Excludes *collision on highway following loss of control (E810.0-E815.9)*
loss of control of motor vehicle following collision on the highway (E810.0-E815.9)

4th E817 Noncollision motor vehicle traffic accident while boarding or alighting

[.0-.9]

Requires fourth digit. See beginning of section E810-E819 for codes and definitions.

Includes fall down stairs of motor bus while boarding or alighting
fall from car in street while boarding or alighting
injured by moving part of the vehicle while boarding or alighting
trapped by door of motor bus boarding or alighting while boarding or alighting

E813 – E817

4th **E818 Other noncollision motor vehicle traffic accident**
[.0-.9]

Requires fourth digit. See beginning of section E810-E819 for codes and definitions.

Includes accidental poisoning from exhaust gas generated by motor vehicle while in motion
breakage of any part of motor vehicle while in motion
collision of railway train or road vehicle except motor vehicle, with object set in motion by motor vehicle
explosion of any part of motor vehicle while in motion
fall, jump, or being accidentally pushed from motor vehicle while in motion
fire starting in motor vehicle while in motion
hit by object thrown into or on motor vehicle while in motion
injured by being thrown against some part of, or object in motor vehicle while in motion
injury from moving part of motor vehicle while in motion
motor vehicle hit by object set in motion by railway train or road vehicle (motor) (nonmotor)
object falling in or on motor vehicle while in motion
object thrown on motor vehicle while in motion
pedestrian, railway train, or road vehicle (motor) (nonmotor) hit by object set in motion by motor vehicle

Excludes *collision between motor vehicle and:*
object set in motion by railway train or road vehicle (motor) (nonmotor) (E815.0-E815.9)
object thrown towards the motor vehicle (E815.0-E815.9)
person overcome by carbon monoxide generated by stationary motor vehicle off the roadway with motor running (E868.2)

4th **E819 Motor vehicle traffic accident of unspecified nature**
[.0-.9]

Requires fourth digit. See beginning of section E810-E819 for codes and definitions.

Includes motor vehicle traffic accident NOS
traffic accident NOS

MOTOR VEHICLE NONTRAFFIC ACCIDENTS (E820-E825)

Note: *For definitions of motor vehicle nontraffic accident and related terms see definition (a) to (k).*

Includes accidents involving motor vehicles being used in recreational or sporting activities off the highway
collision and noncollision motor vehicle accidents occurring entirely off the highway

Excludes *accidents involving motor vehicle and:*
aircraft (E840.0-E845.9)
watercraft (E830.0-E838.9)
accidents, not on the public highway, involving agricultural and construction machinery but not involving another motor vehicle (E919.0, E919.2, E919.7)

The following fourth-digit subdivisions are for use with categories E820-E825 to identify the injured person:

.0 Driver of motor vehicle other than motorcycle
See definition (l)

.1 Passenger in motor vehicle other than motorcycle
See definition (l)

.2 Motorcyclist
See definition (l)

.3 Passenger on motorcycle
See definition (l)

.4 Occupant of streetcar

.5 Rider of animal; occupant of animal-drawn vehicle

.6 Pedal cyclist
See definition (p)

.7 Pedestrian
See definition (r)

.8 Other specified person
Occupant of vehicle other than above
Person on railway train involved in accident
Unauthorized rider of motor vehicle

.9 Unspecified person

4th **E820 Nontraffic accident involving motor-driven snow vehicle**
[.0-.9]

Requires fourth digit. See beginning of section E820-E825 for codes and definitions.

Includes breakage of part of motor-driven snow vehicle (not on public highway)
collision of motor-driven snow vehicle with:
animal (being ridden) (-drawn vehicle)
another off-road motor vehicle
other motor vehicle, not on public highway
railway train
other object, fixed or movable
fall from motor-driven snow vehicle (not on public highway)
hit by motor-driven snow vehicle (not on public highway)
injury caused by rough landing of motor-driven snow vehicle (after leaving ground on rough terrain)
overturning of motor-driven snow vehicle (not on public highway)
run over or dragged by motor-driven snow vehicle (not on public highway)

Excludes *accident on the public highway involving motor driven snow vehicle (E810.0-E819.9)*

4th E821 Nontraffic accident involving other off-road motor vehicle
[.0-.9]

Requires fourth digit. See beginning of section E820-E825 for codes and definitions.

Includes breakage of part of off-road motor vehicle, except snow vehicle (not on public highway)
collision with:
animal (being ridden) (-drawn vehicle)
another off-road motor vehicle, except snow vehicle
other motor vehicle, not on public highway
other object, fixed or movable
fall from off-road motor vehicle, except snow vehicle (not on public highway)
hit by off-road motor vehicle, except snow vehicle (not on public highway)
overturning of off-road motor vehicle, except snow vehicle (not on public highway)
run over or dragged by off-road motor vehicle, except snow vehicle (not on public highway)
thrown against some part of or object in off-road motor vehicle, except snow vehicle (not on public highway)

Excludes *accident on public highway involving off-road motor vehicle (E810.0-E819.9)*
collision between motor driven snow vehicle and other off-road motor vehicle (E820.0-E820.9)
hovercraft accident on water (E830.0-E838.9)

4th E822 Other motor vehicle nontraffic accident involving collision with moving object
[.0-.9]

Requires fourth digit. See beginning of section E820-E825 for codes and definitions.

Includes collision, not on public highway, between motor vehicle, except off-road motor vehicle and:
animal
nonmotor vehicle
other motor vehicle, except off-road motor vehicle
pedestrian
railway train
other moving object

Excludes *collision with:*
motor-driven snow vehicle (E820.0-E820.9)
other off-road motor vehicle (E821.0-E821.9)

4th E823 Other motor vehicle nontraffic accident involving collision with stationary object
[.0-.9]

Requires fourth digit. See beginning of section E820-E825 for codes and definitions.

Includes collision, not on public highway, between motor vehicle, except off-road motor vehicle, and any object, fixed or movable, but not in motion

4th E824 Other motor vehicle nontraffic accident while boarding and alighting
[.0-.9]

Requires fourth digit. See beginning of section E820-E825 for codes and definitions.

Includes fall while boarding or alighting from motor vehicle except off-road motor vehicle, not on public highway
injury from moving part of motor vehicle while boarding or alighting from motor vehicle except off-road motor vehicle, not on public highway
trapped by door of motor vehicle while boarding or alighting from motor vehicle except off-road motor vehicle, not on public highway

4th E825 Other motor vehicle nontraffic accident of other and unspecified nature
[.0-.9]

Requires fourth digit. See beginning of section E820-E825 for codes and definitions.

Includes accidental poisoning from carbon monoxide generated by motor vehicle while in motion, not on public highway
breakage of any part of motor vehicle while in motion, not on public highway
explosion of any part of motor vehicle while in motion, not on public highway
fall, jump, or being accidentally pushed from motor vehicle while in motion, not on public highway
fire starting in motor vehicle while in motion, not on public highway
hit by object thrown into, towards, or on motor vehicle while in motion, not on public highway
injured by being thrown against some part of, or object in motor vehicle while in motion, not on public highway
injury from moving part of motor vehicle while in motion, not on public highway
motor vehicle nontraffic accident NOS
object falling in or on motor vehicle while in motion, not on public highway

Excludes *fall from or in stationary motor vehicle (E884.9, E885.9)*
overcome by carbon monoxide or exhaust gas generated by stationary motor vehicle off the roadway with motor running (E868.2)
struck by falling object from or in stationary motor vehicle (E916)

OTHER ROAD VEHICLE ACCIDENTS (E826-E829)

Note: *Other road vehicle accidents are transport accidents involving road vehicles other than motor vehicles. For definitions of other road vehicle and related terms see definitions (m) to (o).*

Includes accidents involving other road vehicles being used in recreational or sporting activities

Excludes *collision of other road vehicle [any] with:*
aircraft (E840.0-E845.9)
motor vehicle (E813.0-E813.9, E820.0-E822.9)
railway train (E801.0-E801.9)

The following fourth-digit subdivisions are for use with categories E826-E829 to identify the injured person:

.0 Pedestrian
See definition (r)

.1 Pedal cyclist
See definition (p)

.2 Rider of animal

.3 Occupant of animal-drawn vehicle

.4 Occupant of streetcar

.8 Other specified person

.9 Unspecified person

4th E826 Pedal cycle accident

[.0-.4, .8-.9]

Requires fourth digit. See beginning of section E826-E829 for codes and definitions.

Includes breakage of any part of pedal cycle
collision between pedal cycle and:
animal (being ridden) (herded) (unattended)
another pedal cycle
nonmotor road vehicle, any
pedestrian
other object, fixed, movable, or moving, not set in motion by motor vehicle, railway train, or aircraft
entanglement in wheel of pedal cycle
fall from pedal cycle
hit by object falling or thrown on the pedal cycle
pedal cycle accident NOS
pedal cycle overturned

4th E827 Animal-drawn vehicle accident

[.0, .2-.4, .8-.9]

Requires fourth digit. See beginning of section E826-E829 for codes and definitions.

Includes breakage of any part of vehicle
collision between animal-drawn vehicle and:
animal (being ridden) (herded) (unattended)
nonmotor road vehicle, except pedal cycle
pedestrian, pedestrian conveyance, or pedestrian vehicle
other object, fixed, movable, or moving, not set in motion by motor vehicle, railway train, or aircraft
fall from animal-drawn vehicle
knocked down by animal-drawn vehicle
overturning of animal-drawn vehicle
run over by animal-drawn vehicle
thrown from animal-drawn vehicle

Excludes *collision of animal-drawn vehicle with pedal cycle (E826.0-E826.9)*

4th E828 Accident involving animal being ridden

[.0, .2-.4, .8-.9]

Requires fourth digit. See beginning of section E826-E829 for codes and definitions.

Includes collision between animal being ridden and:
another animal
nonmotor road vehicle, except pedal cycle, and animal-drawn vehicle
pedestrian, pedestrian conveyance, or pedestrian vehicle
other object, fixed, movable, or moving, not set in motion by motor vehicle, railway train, or aircraft
fall from animal being ridden
knocked down by animal being ridden
ridden animal stumbled and fell
thrown from animal being ridden
trampled by animal being ridden

Excludes *collision of animal being ridden with:*
animal-drawn vehicle (E827.0-E827.9)
pedal cycle (E826.0-E826.9)

4th E829 Other road vehicle accidents

[.0, .4, .8, .9]

Requires fourth digit. See beginning of section E826-E829 for codes and definitions.

Includes accident while boarding or alighting from:
streetcar
nonmotor road vehicle not classifiable to E826-E828
blow from object in:
streetcar
nonmotor road vehicle not classifiable to E826-E828
breakage of any part of:
streetcar
nonmotor road vehicle not classifiable to E826-E828
caught in door of:
streetcar
nonmotor road vehicle not classifiable to E826-E828
collision between streetcar or nonmotor road vehicle, except as in E826-E828, and:
animal (not being ridden)
another nonmotor road vehicle not classifiable to E826-E828
pedestrian
other object, fixed, movable, or moving, not set in motion by motor vehicle, railway train, or aircraft
derailment of:
streetcar
nonmotor road vehicle not classifiable to E826-E828
fall in, on, or from:
streetcar
nonmotor road vehicle not classifiable to E826-E828
fire in:
streetcar
nonmotor road vehicle not classifiable to E826-E828
nonmotor road vehicle accident NOS
streetcar accident NOS

Excludes *collision with:*
animal being ridden (E828.0-E828.9)
animal-drawn vehicle (E827.0-E827.9)
pedal cycle (E826.0-E826.9)

E826 – E829

WATER TRANSPORT ACCIDENTS (E830-E838)

Note: *For definitions of water transport accident and related terms see definitions (a), (s), and (t).*

Includes watercraft accidents in the course of recreational activities

Excludes *accidents involving both aircraft, including objects set in motion by aircraft, and watercraft (E840.0-E845.9)*

The following fourth-digit subdivisions are for use with categories E830-E838 to identify the injured person:

.0 Occupant of small boat, unpowered

.1 Occupant of small boat, powered
See definition (t)
Excludes *water skier (4)*

.2 Occupant of other watercraft – crew
Persons:
engaged in operation of watercraft
providing passenger services [cabin attendants, ship's physician, catering personnel]
working on ship during voyage in other capacity [musician in band, operators of shops and beauty parlors]

.3 Occupant of other watercraft – other than crew
Passenger
Occupant of lifeboat, other than crew, after abandoning ship

.4 Water skier

.5 Swimmer

.6 Dockers, stevedores
Longshoreman employed on the dock in loading and unloading ships

● **.7 Occupant of military warcraft, any type**

.8 Other specified person
Immigration and custom officials on board ship
Person:
accompanying passenger or member of crew visiting boat
Pilot (guiding ship into port)

.9 Unspecified person

4th **E830 Accident to watercraft causing submersion**
[.0-.9]
Requires fourth digit. See beginning of section E830-E838 for codes and definitions.
Includes submersion and drowning due to:
boat overturning
boat submerging
falling or jumping from burning ship
falling or jumping from crushed watercraft
ship sinking
other accident to watercraft

4th **E831 Accident to watercraft causing other injury**
[.0-.9]
Requires fourth digit. See beginning of section E830-E838 for codes and definitions.
Includes any injury, except submersion and drowning, as a result of an accident to watercraft
burned while ship on fire
crushed between ships in collision
crushed by lifeboat after abandoning ship
fall due to collision or other accident to watercraft
hit by falling object due to accident to watercraft
injured in watercraft accident involving collision
struck by boat or part thereof after fall or jump from damaged boat
Excludes *burns from localized fire or explosion on board ship (E837.0-E837.9)*

4th **E832 Other accidental submersion or drowning in water transport accident**
[.0-.9]
Requires fourth digit. See beginning of section E830-E838 for codes and definitions.
Includes submersion or drowning as a result of an accident other than accident to the watercraft, such as:
fall:
from gangplank
from ship
overboard
thrown overboard by motion of ship
washed overboard
Excludes *submersion or drowning of swimmer or diver who voluntarily jumps from boat not involved in an accident (E910.0-E910.9)*

4th **E833 Fall on stairs or ladders in water transport**
[.0-.9]
Requires fourth digit. See beginning of section E830-E838 for codes and definitions.
Excludes *fall due to accident to watercraft (E831.0-E831.9)*

4th **E834 Other fall from one level to another in water transport**
[.0-.9]
Requires fourth digit. See beginning of section E830-E838 for codes and definitions.
Excludes *fall due to accident to watercraft (E831.0-E831.9)*

4th **E835 Other and unspecified fall in water transport**
[.0-.9]
Requires fourth digit. See beginning of section E830-E838 for codes and definitions.
Excludes *fall due to accident to watercraft (E831.0-E831.9)*

4th **E836 Machinery accident in water transport**
[.0-.9]
Requires fourth digit. See beginning of section E830-E838 for codes and definitions.
Includes injuries in water transport caused by:
deck machinery
engine room machinery
galley machinery
laundry machinery
loading machinery

4th **E837 Explosion, fire, or burning in watercraft**
[.0-.9]
Requires fourth digit. See beginning of section E830-E838 for codes and definitions.
Includes explosion of boiler on steamship
localized fire on ship
Excludes *burning ship (due to collision or explosion) resulting in:*
submersion or drowning (E830.0-E830.9)
other injury (E831.0-E831.9)

4th **E838 Other and unspecified water transport accident**
[.0-.9]
Requires fourth digit. See beginning of section E830-E838 for codes and definitions.
Includes accidental poisoning by gases or fumes on ship
atomic power plant malfunction in watercraft
crushed between ship and stationary object [wharf]
crushed between ships without accident to watercraft
crushed by falling object on ship or while loading or unloading
hit by boat while water skiing
struck by boat or part thereof (after fall from boat)
watercraft accident NOS

AIR AND SPACE TRANSPORT ACCIDENTS (E840-E845)

Note: *For definition of aircraft and related terms see definitions (u) and (v).*

The following fourth-digit subdivisions are for use with categories E840-E845 to identify the injured person:

.0 Occupant of spacecraft

.1 Occupant of military aircraft, any
Crew in military aircraft [air force] [army] [national guard] [navy]
Passenger (civilian) (military) in military aircraft [air force] [army] [national guard] [navy]
Troops in military aircraft [air force] [army] [national guard] [navy]
Excludes *occupants of aircraft operated under jurisdiction of police departments (5)*
parachutist (7)

.2 Crew of commercial aircraft (powered) in surface-to-surface transport

.3 Other occupant of commercial aircraft (powered) in surface-to-surface transport
Flight personnel:
not part of crew
on familiarization flight
Passenger on aircraft (powered) NOS

.4 Occupant of commercial aircraft (powered) in surface-to-air transport
Occupant [crew] [passenger] of aircraft (powered) engaged in activities, such as:
aerial spraying (crops) (fire retardants)
air drops of emergency supplies
air drops of parachutists, except from military craft
crop dusting
lowering of construction material [bridge or telephone pole]
sky writing

.5 Occupant of other powered aircraft
Occupant [crew] [passenger] of aircraft [powered] engaged in activities, such as:
aerobatic flying
aircraft racing
rescue operation
storm surveillance
traffic surveillance
Occupant of private plane NOS

.6 Occupant of unpowered aircraft, except parachutist
Occupant of aircraft classifiable to E842

.7 Parachutist (military) (other)
Person making voluntary descent
Excludes *person making descent after accident to aircraft (.1-.6)*

.8 Ground crew, airline employee
Persons employed at airfields (civil) (military) or launching pads, not occupants of aircraft

.9 Other person

4th E840 Accident to powered aircraft at takeoff or landing
[.0-.9]
Requires fourth digit. See beginning of section E840-E845 for codes and definitions.
Includes collision of aircraft with any object, fixed, movable, or moving while taking off or landing
crash while taking off or landing
explosion on aircraft while taking off or landing
fire on aircraft while taking off or landing
forced landing

4th E841 Accident to powered aircraft, other and unspecified
[.0-.9]
Requires fourth digit. See beginning of section E840-E845 for codes and definitions.
Includes aircraft accident NOS
aircraft crash or wreck NOS
any accident to powered aircraft while in transit or when not specified whether in transit, taking off, or landing
collision of aircraft with another aircraft, bird, or any object, while in transit
explosion on aircraft while in transit
fire on aircraft while in transit

4th E842 Accident to unpowered aircraft
[.6-.9]
Requires fourth digit. See beginning of section E840-E845 for codes and definitions.
Includes any accident, except collision with powered aircraft, to:
balloon
glider
hang glider
kite carrying a person
hit by object falling from unpowered aircraft

4th E843 Fall in, on, or from aircraft
[.0-.9]
Requires fourth digit. See beginning of section E840-E845 for codes and definitions.
Includes accident in boarding or alighting from aircraft, any kind
fall in, on, or from aircraft [any kind], while in transit, taking off, or landing, except when as a result of an accident to aircraft

4th E844 Other specified air transport accidents
[.0-.9]
Requires fourth digit. See beginning of section E840-E845 for codes and definitions.
Includes hit by aircraft without accident to aircraft
hit by object falling from aircraft without accident to aircraft
injury by or from machinery on aircraft without accident to aircraft
injury by or from rotating propeller without accident to aircraft
injury by or from voluntary parachute descent without accident to aircraft
poisoning by carbon monoxide from aircraft while in transit without accident to aircraft
sucked into jet without accident to aircraft
any accident involving other transport vehicle (motor) (nonmotor) due to being hit by object set in motion by aircraft (powered)
Excludes *air sickness (E903)*
effects of:
high altitude (E902.0-E902.1)
pressure change (E902.0-E902.1)
injury in parachute descent due to accident to aircraft (E840.0-E842.9)

4th E845 Accident involving spacecraft
[.0, .8, .9]
Requires fourth digit. See beginning of section E840-E845 for codes and definitions.
Includes launching pad accident
Excludes *effects of weightlessness in spacecraft (E928.0)*

E840 – E845

VEHICLE ACCIDENTS NOT ELSEWHERE CLASSIFIABLE (E846-E848)

E846 Accidents involving powered vehicles used solely within the buildings and premises of industrial or commercial establishment

Accident to, on, or involving:
- battery-powered airport passenger vehicle
- battery-powered trucks (baggage) (mail)
- coal car in mine
- logging car
- self-propelled truck, industrial
- station baggage truck (powered)
- tram, truck, or tub (powered) in mine or quarry

Breakage of any part of vehicle

Collision with:
- pedestrian
- other vehicle or object within premises

Explosion of powered vehicle, industrial or commercial

Fall from powered vehicle, industrial or commercial

Overturning of powered vehicle, industrial or commercial

Struck by powered vehicle, industrial or commercial

Excludes *accidental poisoning by exhaust gas from vehicle not elsewhere classifiable (E868.2)*
injury by crane, lift (fork), or elevator (E919.2)

E847 Accidents involving cable cars not running on rails

Accident to, on, or involving:
- cable car, not on rails
- ski chair-lift
- ski-lift with gondola
- téléférique

Breakage of cable

Caught or dragged by cable car, not on rails

Fall or jump from cable car, not on rails

Object thrown from or in cable car not on rails

E848 Accidents involving other vehicles, not elsewhere classifiable

Accident to, on, or involving:
- ice yacht
- land yacht
- nonmotor, nonroad vehicle NOS

PLACE OF OCCURENCE (849)

Note: *The following category is for use to denote the place where the injury or poisoning occurred.*

ICD-9-CM Official Guidelines (Chapter 19):

b. Place of Occurrence Guideline

Use an additional code from category E849 to indicate the Place of Occurrence for injuries and poisonings. The Place of Occurrence describes the place where the event occurred and not the patient's activity at the time of the event.

Do not use E849.9 if the place of occurrence is not stated.

4th **E849 Place of occurence**

E849.0 Home

Apartment

Boarding house

Farm house

Home premises

House (residential)

Noninstitutional place of residence

Private:
- driveway
- garage
- garden
- home
- walk

Swimming pool in private house or garden

Yard of home

Excludes *home under construction but not yet occupied (E849.3)*
institutional place of residence (E849.7)

E849.1 Farm

Buildings

Land under cultivation

Excludes *farm house and home premises of farm (E849.0)*

E849.2 Mine and quarry

Gravel pit

Sand pit

Tunnel under construction

E849.3 Industrial place and premises

Building under construction

Dockyard

Dry dock

Factory
- building
- premises

Garage (place of work)

Industrial yard

Loading platform (factory) (store)

Plant, industrial

Railway yard

Shop (place of work)

Warehouse

Workhouse

E849.4 Place for recreation and sport

Amusement park

Baseball field

Basketball court

Beach resort

Cricket ground

Fives court

Football field

Golf course

Gymnasium

Hockey field

Holiday camp

Ice palace

Lake resort

Mountain resort

Playground, including school playground

Public park

Racecourse

Resort NOS

Riding school

Rifle range

Seashore resort

Skating rink

Sports palace

Stadium

Swimming pool, public

Tennis court

Vacation resort

Excludes *that in private house or garden (E849.0)*

E849.5 Street and highway

E849.6 Public building

Building (including adjacent grounds) used by the general public or by a particular group of the public, such as:

airport
bank
cafe
casino
church
cinema
clubhouse
courthouse
dance hall
garage building (for car storage)
hotel
market (grocery or other commodity)
movie house
music hall
nightclub
office
office building
opera house
post office
public hall
radio broadcasting station
restaurant
school (state) (public) (private)
shop, commercial
station (bus) (railway)
store
theater

Excludes *home garage (E849.0)*
industrial building or workplace (E849.3)

E849.7 Residential institution

Children's home
Dormitory
Hospital
Jail
Old people's home
Orphanage
Prison
Reform School

E849.8 Other specified places

Beach NOS
Canal
Caravan site NOS
Derelict house
Desert
Dock
Forest
Harbor
Hill
Lake NOS
Mountain
Parking lot
Parking place
Pond or pool (natural)
Prairie
Public place NOS
Railway line
Reservoir
River
Sea
Seashore NOS
Stream
Swamp
Trailer court
Woods

E849.9 Unspecified place

ACCIDENTAL POISONING BY DRUGS, MEDICINAL SUBSTANCES, AND BIOLOGICALS (E850-E858)

Includes accidental overdose of drug, wrong drug given or taken in error, and drug taken inadvertently
accidents in the use of drugs and biologicals in medical and surgical procedures

Excludes *administration with suicidal or homicidal intent or intent to harm, or in circumstances classifiable to E980-E989 (E950.0-E950.5, E962.0, E980.0-E980.5)*
correct drug properly administered in therapeutic or prophylactic dosage, as the cause of adverse effect (E930.0-E949.9)

Note: *See Alphabetic Index for more complete list of specific drugs to be classified under the fourth-digit subdivisions. The American Hospital Formulary numbers can be used to classify new drugs listed by the American Hospital Formulary Service (AHFS). See Appendix C.*

4th **E850 Accidental poisoning by analgesics, antipyretics, and antirheumatics**

E850.0 Heroin

Diacetylmorphine

E850.1 Methadone

E850.2 Other opiates and related narcotics

Codeine [methylmorphine]
Meperidine [pethidine]
Morphine
Opium (alkaloids)

E850.3 Salicylates

Acetylsalicylic acid [aspirin]
Amino derivatives of salicylic acid
Salicylic acid salts

E850.4 Aromatic analgesics, not elsewhere classified

Acetanilid
Paracetamol [acetaminophen]
Phenacetin [acetophenetidin]

E850.5 Pyrazole derivatives

Aminophenazone [amidopyrine]
Phenylbutazone

E850.6 Antirheumatics [antiphlogistics]

Gold salts
Indomethacin

Excludes *salicylates (E850.3)*
steroids (E858.0)

E850.7 Other non-narcotic analgesics

Pyrabital

E850.8 Other specified analgesics and antipyretics

Pentazocine

E850.9 Unspecified analgesic or antipyretic

E851 Accidental poisoning by barbiturates

Amobarbital [amylobarbitone]
Barbital [barbitone]
Butabarbital [butabarbitone]
Pentobarbital [pentobarbitone]
Phenobarbital [phenobarbitone]
Secobarbital [quinalbarbitone]

Excludes *thiobarbiturates (E855.1)*

4th **E852 Accidental poisoning by other sedatives and hypnotics**

E852.0 Chloral hydrate group

E852.1 Paraldehyde

E852.2 Bromine compounds

Bromides
Carbromal (derivatives)

E852.3 Methaqualone compounds

E852.4 Glutethimide group

E852.5 Mixed sedatives, not elsewhere classified

E852.8 Other specified sedatives and hypnotics

E852.9 Unspecified sedative or hypnotic
Sleeping:
drug NOS
pill NOS
tablet NOS

4th E853 Accidental poisoning by tranquilizers

E853.0 Phenothiazine-based tranquilizers
Chlorpromazine
Fluphenazine
Prochlorperazine
Promazine

E853.1 Butyrophenone-based tranquilizers
Haloperidol
Spiperone
Trifluperidol

E853.2 Benzodiazepine-based tranquilizers
Chlordiazepoxide
Diazepam
Flurazepam
Lorazepam
Medazepam
Nitrazepam

E853.8 Other specified tranquilizers
Hydroxyzine
Meprobamate

E853.9 Unspecified tranquilizer

4th E854 Accidental poisoning by other psychotropic agents

E854.0 Antidepressants
Amitriptyline
Imipramine
Monoamine oxidase [MAO] inhibitors

E854.1 Psychodysleptics [hallucinogens]
Cannabis derivatives
Lysergide [LSD]
Marihuana (derivatives)
Mescaline
Psilocin
Psilocybin

E854.2 Psychostimulants
Amphetamine
Caffeine
Excludes *central appetite depressants (E858.8)*

E854.3 Central nervous system stimulants
Analeptics
Opiate antagonists

E854.8 Other psychotropic agents

4th E855 Accidental poisoning by other drugs acting on central and autonomic nervous system

E855.0 Anticonvulsant and anti-Parkinsonism drugs
Amantadine
Hydantoin derivatives
Levodopa [L-dopa]
Oxazolidine derivatives [paramethadione] [trimethadione]
Succinimides

E855.1 Other central nervous system depressants
Ether
Gaseous anesthetics
Halogenated hydrocarbon derivatives
Intravenous anesthetics
Thiobarbiturates, such as thiopental sodium

E855.2 Local anesthetics
Cocaine
Lidocaine [lignocaine]
Procaine
Tetracaine

E855.3 Parasympathomimetics [cholinergics]
Acetylcholine
Anticholinesterase:
organophosphorus
reversible
Pilocarpine

E855.4 Parasympatholytics [anticholinergics and antimuscarinics] and spasmolytics
Atropine
Homatropine
Hyoscine [scopolamine]
Quaternary ammonium derivatives

E855.5 Sympathomimetics [adrenergics]
Epinephrine [adrenalin]
Levarterenol [noradrenalin]

E855.6 Sympatholytics [antiadrenergics]
Phenoxybenzamine
Tolazoline hydrochloride

E855.8 Other specified drugs acting on central and autonomic nervous systems

E855.9 Unspecified drug acting on central and autonomic nervous systems

E856 Accidental poisoning by antibiotics

E857 Accidental poisoning by other anti-infectives

4th E858 Accidental poisoning by other drugs

E858.0 Hormones and synthetic substitutes

E858.1 Primarily systemic agents

E858.2 Agents primarily affecting blood constituents

E858.3 Agents primarily affecting cardiovascular system

E858.4 Agents primarily affecting gastrointestinal system

E858.5 Water, mineral, and uric acid metabolism drugs

E858.6 Agents primarily acting on the smooth and skeletal muscles and respiratory system

E858.7 Agents primarily affecting skin and mucous membrane, ophthalmological, otorhinolaryngological, and dental drugs

E858.8 Other specified drugs
Central appetite depressants

E858.9 Unspecified drug

ACCIDENTAL POISONING BY OTHER SOLID AND LIQUID SUBSTANCES, GASES, AND VAPORS (E860-E869)

Note: *Categories in this section are intended primarily to indicate the external cause of poisoning states classifiable to 980-989. They may also be used to indicate external causes of localized effects classifiable to 001-799.*

4th E860 Accidental poisoning by alcohol, not elsewhere classified

E860.0 Alcoholic beverages
Alcohol in preparations intended for consumption

E860.1 Other and unspecified ethyl alcohol and its products
Denatured alcohol
Ethanol NOS
Grain alcohol NOS
Methylated spirit

E860.2 Methyl alcohol
Methanol
Wood alcohol

E860.3 Isopropyl alcohol
Dimethyl carbinol
Isopropanol
Rubbing alcohol substitute
Secondary propyl alcohol

E860.4 Fusel oil
Alcohol:
amyl
butyl
propyl

E860.8 Other specified alcohols

E860.9 Unspecified alcohol

4th **E861 Accidental poisoning by cleansing and polishing agents, disinfectants, paints, and varnishes**

E861.0 Synthetic detergents and shampoos

E861.1 Soap products

E861.2 Polishes

E861.3 Other cleansing and polishing agents
Scouring powders

E861.4 Disinfectants
Household and other disinfectants not ordinarily used on the person
Excludes *carbolic acid or phenol (E864.0)*

E861.5 Lead paints

E861.6 Other paints and varnishes
Lacquers
Oil colors
Paints, other than lead
White washes

E861.9 Unspecified

4th **E862 Accidental poisoning by petroleum products, other solvents and their vapors, not elsewhere classified**

E862.0 Petroleum solvents
Petroleum:
ether
benzine
naphtha

E862.1 Petroleum fuels and cleaners
Antiknock additives to petroleum fuels
Gas oils
Gasoline or petrol
Kerosene
Excludes *kerosene insecticides (E863.4)*

E862.2 Lubricating oils

E862.3 Petroleum solids
Paraffin wax

E862.4 Other specified solvents
Benzene

E862.9 Unspecified solvent

4th **E863 Accidental poisoning by agricultural and horticultural chemical and pharmaceutical preparations other than plant foods and fertilizers**
Excludes *plant foods and fertilizers (E866.5)*

E863.0 Insecticides of organochlorine compounds
Benzene hexachloride
Chlordane
DDT
Dieldrin
Endrine
Toxaphene

E863.1 Insecticides of organophosphorus compounds
Demeton
Diazinon
Dichlorvos
Malathion
Methyl parathion
Parathion
Phenylsulphthion
Phorate
Phosdrin

E863.2 Carbamates
Aldicarb
Carbaryl
Propoxur

E863.3 Mixtures of insecticides

E863.4 Other and unspecified insecticides
Kerosene insecticides

E863.5 Herbicides
2,4-Dichlorophenoxyacetic acid [2, 4-D]
2,4,5-Trichlorophenoxyacetic acid [2, 4, 5-T]
Chlorates
Diquat
Mixtures of plant foods and fertilizers with herbicides
Paraquat

E863.6 Fungicides
Organic mercurials (used in seed dressing)
Pentachlorophenols

E863.7 Rodenticides
Fluoroacetates
Squill and derivatives
Thallium
Warfarin
Zinc phosphide

E863.8 Fumigants
Cyanides
Methyl bromide
Phosphine

E863.9 Other and unspecified

4th **E864 Accidental poisoning by corrosives and caustics, not elsewhere classified**
Excludes *those as components of disinfectants (E861.4)*

E864.0 Corrosive aromatics
Carbolic acid or phenol

E864.1 Acids
Acid:
hydrochloric
nitric
sulfuric

E864.2 Caustic alkalis
Lye

E864.3 Other specified corrosives and caustics

E864.4 Unspecified corrosives and caustics

4th **E865 Accidental poisoning from poisonous foodstuffs and poisonous plants**
Includes any meat, fish, or shellfish
plants, berries, and fungi eaten as, or in mistake for food, or by a child
Excludes *anaphlyactic shock due to adverse food reaction (995.60-995.69)*
food poisoning (bacterial) (005.0-005.9)
poisoning and toxic reactions to venomous plants (E905.6-E905.7)

E865.0 Meat

E865.1 Shellfish

E865.2 Other fish

E865.3 Berries and seeds

E865.4 Other specified plants

E865.5 Mushrooms and other fungi

E865.8 Other specified foods

E865.9 Unspecified foodstuff or poisonous plant

4th E866 Accidental poisoning by other and unspecified solid and liquid substances

Excludes *these substances as a component of:*
medicines (E850.0-E858.9)
paints (E861.5-E861.6)
pesticides (E863.0-E863.9)
petroleum fuels (E862.1)

E866.0 Lead and its compounds and fumes

E866.1 Mercury and its compounds and fumes

E866.2 Antimony and its compounds and fumes

E866.3 Arsenic and its compounds and fumes

E866.4 Other metals and their compounds and fumes
Beryllium (compounds)
Brass fumes
Cadmium (compounds)
Copper salts
Iron (compounds)
Manganese (compounds)
Nickel (compounds)
Thallium (compounds)

E866.5 Plant foods and fertilizers
Excludes *mixtures with herbicides (E863.5)*

E866.6 Glues and adhesives

E866.7 Cosmetics

E866.8 Other specified solid or liquid substances

E866.9 Unspecified solid or liquid substance

E867 Accidental poisoning by gas distributed by pipeline
Carbon monoxide from incomplete combustion of piped gas
Coal gas NOS
Liquefied petroleum gas distributed through pipes (pure or mixed with air)
Piped gas (natural) (manufactured)

4th **E868 Accidental poisoning by other utility gas and other carbon monoxide**

E868.0 Liquefied petroleum gas distributed in mobile containers
Butane or carbon monoxide from incomplete combustion of these gases
Liquefied hydrocarbon gas NOS or carbon monoxide from incomplete combustion of these gases
Propane or carbon monoxide from incomplete combustion of these gases

E868.1 Other and unspecified utility gas
Acetylene or carbon monoxide from incomplete combustion of these gases
Gas NOS used for lighting, heating, or cooking or carbon monoxide from incomplete combustion of these gases
Water gas or carbon monoxide from incomplete combustion of these gases

E868.2 Motor vehicle exhaust gas
Exhaust gas from:
farm tractor, not in transit
gas engine
motor pump
motor vehicle, not in transit
any type of combustion engine not in watercraft
Excludes *poisoning by carbon monoxide from:*
aircraft while in transit (E844.0-E844.9)
motor vehicle while in transit (E818.0-E818.9)
watercraft whether or not in transit (E838.0-E838.9)

E868.3 Carbon monoxide from incomplete combustion of other domestic fuels
Carbon monoxide from incomplete combustion of:
coal in domestic stove or fireplace
coke in domestic stove or fireplace
kerosene in domestic stove or fireplace
wood in domestic stove or fireplace
Excludes *carbon monoxide from smoke and fumes due to conflagration (E890.0-E893.9)*

E868.8 Carbon monoxide from other sources
Carbon monoxide from:
blast furnace gas
incomplete combustion of fuels in industrial use
kiln vapor

E868.9 Unspecified carbon monoxide

4th **E869 Accidental poisoning by other gases and vapors**
Excludes *effects of gases used as anesthetics (E855.1, E938.2)*
fumes from heavy metals (E866.0-E866.4)
smoke and fumes due to conflagration or explosion (E890.0-E899)

E869.0 Nitrogen oxides

E869.1 Sulfur dioxide

E869.2 Freon

E869.3 Lacrimogenic gas [tear gas]
Bromobenzyl cyanide
Chloroacetophenone
Ethyliodoacetate

E869.4 Second-hand tobacco smoke

E869.8 Other specified gases and vapors
Chlorine
Hydrocyanic acid gas

E869.9 Unspecified gases and vapors

MISADVENTURES TO PATIENTS DURING SURGICAL AND MEDICAL CARE (E870-E876)

Excludes *accidental overdose of drug and wrong drug given in error (E850.0-E858.9)*
surgical and medical procedures as the cause of abnormal reaction by the patient, without mention of misadventure at the time of procedure (E878.0-E879.9)

4th **E870 Accidental cut, puncture, perforation, or hemorrhage during medical care**

E870.0 Surgical operation

E870.1 Infusion or transfusion

E870.2 Kidney dialysis or other perfusion

E870.3 Injection or vaccination

E870.4 Endoscopic examination

E870.5 Aspiration of fluid or tissue, puncture, and catheterization
Abdominal paracentesis
Aspirating needle biopsy
Blood sampling
Lumbar puncture
Thoracentesis
Excludes *heart catheterization (E870.6)*

E870.6 Heart catheterization

E870.7 Administration of enema

E870.8 Other specified medical care

E870.9 Unspecified medical care

4th **E871 Foreign object left in body during procedure**

E871.0 Surgical operation

E871.1 Infusion or transfusion

E871.2 Kidney dialysis or other perfusion

E871.3 Injection or vaccination

E871.4 Endoscopic examination

E871.5 **Aspiration of fluid or tissue, puncture, and catheterization**
Abdominal paracentesis
Aspiration needle biopsy
Blood sampling
Lumbar puncture
Thoracentesis
Excludes *heart catheterization (E871.6)*

E871.6 **Heart catheterization**

E871.7 **Removal of catheter or packing**

E871.8 **Other specified procedures**

E871.9 **Unspecified procedure**

4th **E872 Failure of sterile precautions during procedure**

E872.0 **Surgical operation**

E872.1 **Infusion or transfusion**

E872.2 **Kidney dialysis and other perfusion**

E872.3 **Injection or vaccination**

E872.4 **Endoscopic examination**

E872.5 **Aspiration of fluid or tissue, puncture, and catheterization**
Abdominal paracentesis
Aspirating needle biopsy
Blood sampling
Lumbar puncture
Thoracentesis
Excludes *heart catheterization (E872.6)*

E872.6 **Heart catheterization**

E872.8 **Other specified procedures**

E872.9 **Unspecified procedure**

4th **E873 Failure in dosage**
Excludes *accidental overdose of drug, medicinal or biological substance (E850.0-E858.9)*

E873.0 **Excessive amount of blood or other fluid during transfusion or infusion**

E873.1 **Incorrect dilution of fluid during infusion**

E873.2 **Overdose of radiation in therapy**

E873.3 **Inadvertent exposure of patient to radiation during medical care**

E873.4 **Failure in dosage in electroshock or insulin-shock therapy**

E873.5 **Inappropriate [too hot or too cold] temperature in local application and packing**

E873.6 **Nonadministration of necessary drug or medicinal substance**

E873.8 **Other specified failure in dosage**

E873.9 **Unspecified failure in dosage**

4th **E874 Mechanical failure of instrument or apparatus during procedure**

E874.0 **Surgical operation**

E874.1 **Infusion and transfusion**
Air in system

E874.2 **Kidney dialysis and other perfusion**

E874.3 **Endoscopic examination**

E874.4 **Aspiration of fluid or tissue, puncture, and catheterization**
Abdominal paracentesis
Aspirating needle biopsy
Blood sampling
Lumbar puncture
Thoracentesis
Excludes *heart catheterization (E874.5)*

E874.5 **Heart catheterization**

E874.8 **Other specified procedures**

E874.9 **Unspecified procedure**

4th **E875 Contaminated or infected blood, other fluid, drug, or biological substance**
Includes presence of:
bacterial pyrogens
endotoxin-producing bacteria
serum hepatitis-producing agent

E875.0 **Contaminated substance transfused or infused**

E875.1 **Contaminated substance injected or used for vaccination**

E875.2 **Contaminated drug or biological substance administered by other means**

E875.8 **Other**

E875.9 **Unspecified**

4th **E876 Other and unspecified misadventures during medical care**

E876.0 **Mismatched blood in transfusion**

E876.1 **Wrong fluid in infusion**

E876.2 **Failure in suture and ligature during surgical operation**

E876.3 **Endotracheal tube wrongly placed during anesthetic procedure**

E876.4 **Failure to introduce or to remove other tube or instrument**
Excludes *foreign object left in body during procedure (E871.0-E871.9)*

▲ E876.5 **Performance of wrong ~~inappropriate~~ operation (procedure) on correct patient**
Excludes *correct operation (procedure) performed on wrong body part (E876.7)*

● E876.6 **Performance of operation (procedure) on patient not scheduled for surgery**
Performance of operation (procedure) intended for another patient
Performance of operation (procedure) on wrong patient

● E876.7 **Performance of correct operation (procedure) on wrong side/body part**
Performance of correct operation (procedure) on wrong side
Performance of correct operation (procedure) on wrong site

E876.8 **Other specified misadventures during medical care**
Performance of inappropriate treatment NEC

E876.9 **Unspecified misadventure during medical care**

SURGICAL AND MEDICAL PROCEDURES AS THE CAUSE OF ABNORMAL REACTION OF PATIENT OR LATER COMPLICATION, WITHOUT MENTION OF MISADVENTURE AT THE TIME OF PROCEDURE (E878-E879)

Includes procedures as the cause of abnormal reaction, such as:
displacement or malfunction of prosthetic device
hepatorenal failure, postoperative
malfunction of external stoma
postoperative intestinal obstruction
rejection of transplanted organ

Excludes *anesthetic management properly carried out as the cause of adverse effect (E937.0-E938.9)*
infusion and transfusion, without mention of misadventure in the technique of procedure (E930.0-E949.9)

ICD-9-CM Official Guidelines (Chapter 19):

i. Misadventures and Complications of Care Guidelines

1) Code range E870-E876

Assign a code in the range of E870-E876 if misadventures are stated by the provider.

2) Code range E878-E879

Assign a code in the range of E878-E879 if the provider attributes an abnormal reaction or later complication to a surgical or medical procedure, but does not mention misadventure at the time of the procedure as the cause of the reaction.

4th **E878 Surgical operation and other surgical procedures as the cause of abnormal reaction of patient, or of later complication, without mention of misadventure at the time of operation**

E878.0 Surgical operation with transplant of whole organ
Transplantation of:
heart
kidney
liver

E878.1 Surgical operation with implant of artificial internal device
Cardiac pacemaker
Electrodes implanted in brain
Heart valve prosthesis
Internal orthopedic device

E878.2 Surgical operation with anastomosis, bypass, or graft, with natural or artificial tissues used as implant
Anastomosis:
arteriovenous
gastrojejunal
Graft of blood vessel, tendon, or skin
Excludes *external stoma (E878.3)*

E878.3 Surgical operation with formation of external stoma
Colostomy
Cystostomy
Duodenostomy
Gastrostomy
Ureterostomy

E878.4 Other restorative surgery

E878.5 Amputation of limb(s)

E878.6 Removal of other organ (partial) (total)

E878.8 Other specified surgical operations and procedures

E878.9 Unspecified surgical operations and procedures

4th **E879 Other procedures, without mention of misadventure at the time of procedure, as the cause of abnormal reaction of patient, or of later complication**

E879.0 Cardiac catheterization

E879.1 Kidney dialysis

E879.2 Radiological procedure and radiotherapy
Excludes *radio-opaque dyes for diagnostic x-ray procedures (E947.8)*

E879.3 Shock therapy
Electroshock therapy
Insulin-shock therapy

E879.4 Aspiration of fluid
Lumbar puncture
Thoracentesis

E879.5 Insertion of gastric or duodenal sound

E879.6 Urinary catheterization

E879.7 Blood sampling

E879.8 Other specified procedures
Blood transfusion

E879.9 Unspecified procedure

ACCIDENTAL FALLS (E880-E888)

Excludes *falls (in or from):*
burning building (E890.8, E891.8)
into fire (E890.0-E899)
into water (with submersion or drowning) (E910.0-E910.9)
machinery (in operation) (E919.0-E919.9)
on edged, pointed, or sharp object (E920.0-E920.9)
transport vehicle (E800.0-E845.9)
vehicle not elsewhere classifiable (E846-E848)

4th **E880 Fall on or from stairs or steps**

E880.0 Escalator

E880.1 Fall on or from sidewalk curb
Excludes *fall from moving sidewalk (E885.9)*

E880.9 Other stairs or steps

4th **E881 Fall on or from ladders or scaffolding**

E881.0 Fall from ladder

E881.1 Fall from scaffolding

E882 Fall from or out of building or other structure
Fall from:
balcony
bridge
building
flagpole
tower
turret
viaduct
wall
window
Fall through roof
Excludes *collapse of a building or structure (E916)*
fall or jump from burning building (E890.8, E891.8)

4th **E883 Fall into hole or other opening in surface**
Includes fall into:
cavity
dock
hole
pit
quarry
shaft
swimming pool
tank
well
Excludes *fall into water NOS (E910.9)*
that resulting in drowning or submersion without mention of injury (E910.0-E910.9)

E883.0 Accident from diving or jumping into water [swimming pool]
Strike or hit:
against bottom when jumping or diving into water
wall or board of swimming pool
water surface
Excludes *diving with insufficient air supply (E913.2)*
effects of air pressure from diving (E902.2)

E883.1 Accidental fall into well

E883.2 Accidental fall into storm drain or manhole

E883.9 Fall into other hole or other opening in surface

4th E884 Other fall from one level to another

E884.0 Fall from playground equipment

Excludes *recreational machinery (E919.8)*

E884.1 Fall from cliff

E884.2 Fall from chair

E884.3 Fall from wheelchair

E884.4 Fall from bed

E884.5 Fall from other furniture

E884.6 Fall from commode

Toilet

E884.9 Other fall from one level to another

Fall from:
- embankment
- haystack
- stationary vehicle
- tree

4th E885 Fall on same level from slipping, tripping, or stumbling

E885.0 Fall from (nonmotorized) scooter

E885.1 Fall from roller skates

Heelies
In-line skates
Wheelies

E885.2 Fall from skateboard

E885.3 Fall from skis

E885.4 Fall from snowboard

E885.9 Fall from other slipping, tripping, or stumbling

Fall on moving sidewalk

4th E886 Fall on same level from collision, pushing, or shoving, by or with other person

Excludes *crushed or pushed by a crowd or human stampede (E917.1, E917.6)*

E886.0 In sports

Tackles in sports

Excludes *kicked, stepped on, struck by object, in sports (E917.0, E917.5)*

E886.9 Other and unspecified

Fall from collision of pedestrian (conveyance) with another pedestrian (conveyance)

E887 Fracture, cause unspecified

4th E888 Other and unspecified fall

Accidental fall NOS
Fall on same level NOS

E888.0 Fall resulting in striking against sharp object

Use additional external cause code to identify object (E920)

E888.1 Fall resulting in striking against other object

E888.8 Other fall

E888.9 Unspecified fall

Fall NOS

ACCIDENTS CAUSED BY FIRE AND FLAMES (E890-E899)

Includes asphyxia or poisoning due to conflagration or ignition
burning by fire
secondary fires resulting from explosion

Excludes *arson (E968.0)*
fire in or on:
- *machinery (in operation) (E919.0-E919.9)*
- *transport vehicle other than stationary vehicle (E800.0-E845.9)*
- *vehicle not elsewhere classifiable (E846-E848)*

4th E890 Conflagration in private dwelling

Includes conflagration in:
- apartment
- boarding house
- camping place
- caravan
- farmhouse
- house
- lodging house
- mobile home
- private garage
- rooming house
- tenement

conflagration originating from sources classifiable to E893-E898 in the above buildings

E890.0 Explosion caused by conflagration

E890.1 Fumes from combustion of polyvinylchloride [PVC] and similar material in conflagration

E890.2 Other smoke and fumes from conflagration

Carbon monoxide from conflagration in private building
Fumes NOS from conflagration in private building
Smoke NOS from conflagration in private building

E890.3 Burning caused by conflagration

E890.8 Other accident resulting from conflagration

Collapse of burning private building
Fall from burning private building
Hit by object falling from burning private building
Jump from burning private building

E890.9 Unspecified accident resulting from conflagration in private dwelling

4th E891 Conflagration in other and unspecified building or structure

Conflagration in:
- barn
- church
- convalescent and other residential home
- dormitory of educational institution
- factory
- farm outbuildings
- hospital
- hotel
- school
- store
- theater

Conflagration originating from sources classifiable to E893-E898, in the above buildings

E891.0 Explosion caused by conflagration

E891.1 Fumes from combustion of polyvinylchloride [PVC] and similar material in conflagration

E891.2 Other smoke and fumes from conflagration

Carbon monoxide from conflagration in building or structure
Fumes NOS from conflagration in building or structure
Smoke NOS from conflagration in building or structure

E891.3 Burning caused by conflagration

E891.8 Other accident resulting from conflagration
Collapse of burning building or structure
Fall from burning building or structure
Hit by object falling from burning building or structure
Jump from burning building or structure

E891.9 Unspecified accident resulting from conflagration of other and unspecified building or structure

E892 Conflagration not in building or structure
Fire (uncontrolled) (in) (of):
- forest
- grass
- hay
- lumber
- mine
- prairie
- transport vehicle [any], except while in transit
- tunnel

4th **E893 Accident caused by ignition of clothing**
Excludes *ignition of clothing:*
from highly inflammable material (E894)
with conflagration (E890.0-E892)

E893.0 From controlled fire in private dwelling
Ignition of clothing from:
normal fire (charcoal) (coal) (electric) (gas) (wood) in:
- brazier in private dwelling (as listed in E890)
- fireplace in private dwelling (as listed in E890)
- furnace in private dwelling (as listed in E890)
- stove in private dwelling (as listed in E890)

E893.1 From controlled fire in other building or structure
Ignition of clothing from:
normal fire (charcoal) (coal) (electric) (gas) (wood) in:
- brazier in other building or structure (as listed in E891)
- fireplace in other building or structure (as listed in E891)
- furnace in other building or structure (as listed in E891)
- stove in other building or structure (as listed in E891)

E893.2 From controlled fire not in building or structure
Ignition of clothing from:
- bonfire (controlled)
- brazier fire (controlled), not in building or structure
- trash fire (controlled)

Excludes *conflagration not in building (E892)*
trash fire out of control (E892)

E893.8 From other specified sources
Ignition of clothing from:
- blowlamp
- blowtorch
- burning bedspread
- candle
- cigar
- cigarette
- lighter
- matches
- pipe
- welding torch

E893.9 Unspecified source
Ignition of clothing (from controlled fire NOS) (in building NOS) NOS

E894 Ignition of highly inflammable material
Ignition of:
- benzine (with ignition of clothing)
- gasoline (with ignition of clothing)
- fat (with ignition of clothing)
- kerosene (with ignition of clothing)
- paraffin (with ignition of clothing)
- petrol (with ignition of clothing)

Excludes *ignition of highly inflammable material with:*
conflagration (E890.0-E892)
explosion (E923.0-E923.9)

E895 Accident caused by controlled fire in private dwelling
Burning by (flame of) normal fire (charcoal) (coal) (electric) (gas) (wood) in:
- brazier in private dwelling (as listed in E890)
- fireplace in private dwelling (as listed in E890)
- furnace in private dwelling (as listed in E890)
- stove in private dwelling (as listed in E890)

Excludes *burning by hot objects not producing fire or flames (E924.0-E924.9)*
ignition of clothing from these sources (E893.0)
poisoning by carbon monoxide from incomplete combustion of fuel (E867-E868.9)
that with conflagration (E890.0-E890.9)

E896 Accident caused by controlled fire in other and unspecified building or structure
Burning by (flame of) normal fire (charcoal) (coal) (electric) (gas) (wood) in:
- brazier in other building or structure (as listed in E891)
- fireplace in other building or structure (as listed in E891)
- furnace in other building or structure (as listed in E891)
- stove in other building or structure (as listed in E891)

Excludes *burning by hot objects not producing fire or flames (E924.0-E924.9)*
ignition of clothing from these sources (E893.1)
poisoning by carbon monoxide from incomplete combustion of fuel (E867-E868.9)
that with conflagration (E891.0-E891.9)

E897 Accident caused by controlled fire not in building or structure
Burns from flame of:
- bonfire (controlled)
- brazier fire (controlled), not in building or structure
- trash fire (controlled)

Excludes *ignition of clothing from these sources (E893.2)*
trash fire out of control (E892)
that with conflagration (E892)

4th **E898 Accident caused by other specified fire and flames**
Excludes *conflagration (E890.0-E892)*
that with ignition of:
clothing (E893.0-E893.9)
highly inflammable material (E894)

E898.0 Burning bedclothes
Bed set on fire NOS

E898.1 Other
Burning by:
- blowlamp
- blowtorch
- candle
- cigar
- cigarette
- fire in room NOS
- lamp
- lighter
- matches
- pipe
- welding torch

E899 Accident caused by unspecified fire
Burning NOS

E891.8 – E899

ACCIDENTS DUE TO NATURAL AND ENVIRONMENTAL FACTORS (E900-E909)

4th **E900 Excessive heat**

E900.0 Due to weather conditions

Excessive heat as the external cause of:
- ictus solaris
- siriasis
- sunstroke

E900.1 Of man-made origin

Heat (in):
- boiler room
- drying room
- factory
- furnace room
- generated in transport vehicle
- kitchen

E900.9 Of unspecified origin

4th **E901 Excessive cold**

E901.0 Due to weather conditions

Excessive cold as the cause of:
- chilblains NOS
- immersion foot

E901.1 Of man-made origin

Contact with or inhalation of:
- dry ice
- liquid air
- liquid hydrogen
- liquid nitrogen

Prolonged exposure in:
- deep freeze unit
- refrigerator

E901.8 Other specified origin

E901.9 Of unspecified origin

4th **E902 High and low air pressure and changes in air pressure**

E902.0 Residence or prolonged visit at high altitude

Residence or prolonged visit at high altitude as the cause of:
- Acosta syndrome
- Alpine sickness
- altitude sickness
- Andes disease
- anoxia, hypoxia
- barotitis, barodontalgia, barosinusitis, otitic barotrauma
- hypobarism, hypobaropathy
- mountain sickness
- range disease

E902.1 In aircraft

Sudden change in air pressure in aircraft during ascent or descent as the cause of:
- aeroneurosis
- aviators' disease

E902.2 Due to diving

High air pressure from rapid descent in water as the cause of:
- caisson disease
- divers' disease
- divers' palsy or paralysis

Reduction in atmospheric pressure while surfacing from deep water diving as the cause of:
- caisson disease
- divers' disease
- divers' palsy or paralysis

E902.8 Due to other specified causes

Reduction in atmospheric pressure while surfacing from underground

E902.9 Unspecified cause

E903 Travel and motion

4th **E904 Hunger, thirst, exposure, and neglect**

Excludes *any condition resulting from homicidal intent (E968.0-E968.9)*
hunger, thirst, and exposure resulting from accidents connected with transport (E800.0-E848)

E904.0 Abandonment or neglect of infants and helpless persons

Desertion of newborn
Exposure to weather conditions resulting from abandonment or neglect
Hunger or thirst resulting from abandonment or neglect
Inattention at or after birth
Lack of care (helpless person) (infant)

Excludes *criminal [purposeful] neglect (E968.4)*

E904.1 Lack of food

Lack of food as the cause of:
- inanition
- insufficient nourishment
- starvation

Excludes *hunger resulting from abandonment or neglect (E904.0)*

E904.2 Lack of water

Lack of water as the cause of:
- dehydration
- inanition

Excludes *dehydration due to acute fluid loss (276.51)*

E904.3 Exposure (to weather conditions), not elsewhere classifiable

Exposure NOS
Humidity
Struck by hailstones

Excludes *struck by lightning (E907)*

E904.9 Privation, unqualified

Destitution

4th **E905 Venomous animals and plants as the cause of poisoning and toxic reactions**

Includes chemical released by animal
insects
release of venom through fangs, hairs, spines, tentacles, and other venom apparatus

Excludes *eating of poisonous animals or plants (E865.0-E865.9)*

E905.0 Venomous snakes and lizards

Cobra
Copperhead snake
Coral snake
Fer de lance
Gila monster
Krait
Mamba
Rattlesnake
Sea snake
Snake (venomous)
Viper
Water moccasin

Excludes *bites of snakes and lizards known to be nonvenomous (E906.2)*

E905.1 Venomous spiders

Black widow spider
Brown spider
Tarantula (venomous)

E905.2 Scorpion

E905.3 Hornets, wasps, and bees

Yellow jacket

E905.4 Centipede and venomous millipede (tropical)

E905.5 Other venomous arthropods

Sting of:
- ant
- caterpillar

E905.6 Venomous marine animals and plants
Puncture by sea urchin spine
Sting of:
coral
jelly fish
nematocysts
sea anemone
sea cucumber
other marine animal or plant
Excludes *bites and other injuries caused by nonvenomous marine animal (E906.2-E906.8)*
bite of sea snake (venomous) (E905.0)

E905.7 Poisoning and toxic reactions caused by other plants
Injection of poisons or toxins into or through skin by plant thorns, spines, or other mechanisms
Excludes *puncture wound NOS by plant thorns or spines (E920.8)*

E905.8 Other specified

E905.9 Unspecified
Sting NOS
Venomous bite NOS

4th **E906 Other injury caused by animals**
Excludes *poisoning and toxic reactions caused by venomous animals and insects (E905.0-E905.9)*
road vehicle accident involving animals (E827.0-E828.9)
tripping or falling over an animal (E885.9)

E906.0 Dog bite

E906.1 Rat bite

E906.2 Bite of nonvenomous snakes and lizards

E906.3 Bite of other animal except arthropod
Cats
Moray eel
Rodents, except rats
Shark

E906.4 Bite of nonvenomous arthropod
Insect bite NOS

E906.5 Bite by unspecified animal
Animal bite NOS

E906.8 Other specified injury caused by animal
Butted by animal
Fallen on by horse or other animal, not being ridden
Gored by animal
Implantation of quills of porcupine
Pecked by bird
Run over by animal, not being ridden
Stepped on by animal, not being ridden
Excludes *injury by animal being ridden (E828.0-E828.9)*

E906.9 Unspecified injury caused by animal

E907 Lightning
Excludes *injury from:*
fall of tree or other object caused by lightning (E916)
fire caused by lightning (E890.0-E892)

4th **E908 Cataclysmic storms, and floods resulting from storms**
Excludes *collapse of dam or man-made structure causing flood (E909.3)*

E908.0 Hurricane
Storm surge
"Tidal wave" caused by storm action
Typhoon

E908.1 Tornado
Cyclone
Twisters

E908.2 Floods
Torrential rainfall
Flash flood
Excludes *collapse of dam or man-made structure causing flood (E909.3)*

E908.3 Blizzard (snow) (ice)

E908.4 Dust storm

E908.8 Other cataclysmic storms

E908.9 Unspecified cataclysmic storms, and floods resulting from storms
Storm NOS

4th **E909 Cataclysmic earth surface movements and eruptions**

E909.0 Earthquakes

E909.1 Volcanic eruptions
Burns from lava
Ash inhalation

E909.2 Avalanche, landslide, or mudslide

E909.3 Collapse of dam or man-made structure

E909.4 Tidalwave caused by earthquake
Tidalwave NOS
Tsunami
Excludes *tidalwave caused by tropical storm (E908.0)*

E909.8 Other cataclysmic earth surface movements and eruptions

E909.9 Unspecified cataclysmic earth surface movements and eruptions

ACCIDENTS CAUSED BY SUBMERSION, SUFFOCATION, AND FOREIGN BODIES (E910-E915)

4th **E910 Accidental drowning and submersion**
Includes immersion
swimmers' cramp
Excludes *diving accident (NOS) (resulting in injury except drowning) (E883.0)*
diving with insufficient air supply (E913.2)
drowning and submersion due to:
cataclysm (E908-E909)
effect of high and low air pressure (E902.2)
injury from striking against objects while in running water (E917.2)
machinery accident (E919.0-E919.9)
transport accident (E800.0-E845.9)

E910.0 While water-skiing
Fall from water skis with submersion or drowning
Excludes *accident to water-skier involving a watercraft and resulting in submersion or other injury (E830.4, E831.4)*

E910.1 While engaged in other sport or recreational activity with diving equipment
Scuba diving NOS
Skin diving NOS
Underwater spear fishing NOS

E910.2 While engaged in other sport or recreational activity without diving equipment
Fishing or hunting, except from boat or with diving equipment
Ice skating
Playing in water
Surfboarding
Swimming NOS
Voluntarily jumping from boat, not involved in accident, for swim NOS
Wading in water
Excludes *jumping into water to rescue another person (E910.3)*

E910.3 **While swimming or diving for purposes other than recreation or sport**
Marine salvage (with diving equipment)
Pearl diving (with diving equipment)
Placement of fishing nets (with diving equipment)
Rescue (attempt) of another person (with diving equipment)
Underwater construction or repairs (with diving equipment)

E910.4 **In bathtub**

E910.8 **Other accidental drowning or submersion**
Drowning in:
quenching tank
swimming pool

E910.9 **Unspecified accidental drowning or submersion**
Accidental fall into water NOS
Drowning NOS

E911 Inhalation and ingestion of food causing obstruction of respiratory tract or suffocation
Aspiration and inhalation of food [any] (into respiratory tract) NOS
Asphyxia by food [including bone, seed in food, regurgitated food]
Choked on food [including bone, seed in food, regurgitated food]
Compression of trachea by food lodged in esophagus
Interruption of respiration by food lodged in esophagus
Obstruction of respiration by food lodged in esophagus
Obstruction of pharynx by food (bolus)
Suffocation by food [including bone, seed in food, regurgitated food]
Excludes *injury, except asphyxia and obstruction of respiratory passage, caused by food (E915)*
obstruction of esophagus by food without mention of asphyxia or obstruction of respiratory passage (E915)

E912 Inhalation and ingestion of other object causing obstruction of respiratory tract or suffocation
Aspiration and inhalation of foreign body except food (into respiratory tract) NOS
Compression by foreign body in esophagus
Foreign object [bean] [marble] in nose
Interruption of respiration by foreign body in esophagus
Obstruction of pharynx by foreign body
Obstruction of respiration by foreign body in esophagus
Excludes *injury, except asphyxia and obstruction of respiratory passage, caused by foreign body (E915)*
obstruction of esophagus by foreign body without mention of asphyxia or obstruction in respiratory passage (E915)

4th **E913 Accidental mechanical suffocation**
Excludes *mechanical suffocation from or by:*
accidental inhalation or ingestion of:
food (E911)
foreign object (E912)
cataclysm (E908-E909)
explosion (E921.0-E921.9, E923.0-E923.9)
machinery accident (E919.0-E919.9)

E913.0 **In bed or cradle**
Excludes *suffocation by plastic bag (E913.1)*

E913.1 **By plastic bag**

E913.2 **Due to lack of air (in closed place)**
Accidentally closed up in refrigerator or other airtight enclosed space
Diving with insufficient air supply
Excludes *suffocation by plastic bag (E913.1)*

E913.3 **By falling earth or other substance**
Cave-in NOS
Excludes *cave-in caused by cataclysmic earth surface movements and eruptions (E909.8)*
struck by cave-in without asphyxiation or suffocation (E916)

E913.8 **Other specified means**
Accidental hanging, except in bed or cradle

E913.9 **Unspecified means**
Asphyxia, mechanical NOS
Strangulation NOS
Suffocation NOS

E914 Foreign body accidentally entering eye and adnexa
Excludes *corrosive liquid (E924.1)*

E915 Foreign body accidentally entering other orifice
Excludes *aspiration and inhalation of foreign body, any, (into respiratory tract) NOS (E911-E912)*

OTHER ACCIDENTS (E916-E928)

E916 Struck accidentally by falling object
Collapse of building, except on fire
Falling:
rock
snowslide NOS
stone
tree
Object falling from:
machine, not in operation
stationary vehicle

Code first:
collapse of building on fire (E890.0-E891.9)
falling object in:
cataclysm (E908-E909)
machinery accidents (E919.0-E919.9)
transport accidents (E800.0-E845.9)
vehicle accidents not elsewhere classifiable (E846-E848)
object set in motion by:
explosion (E921.0-E921.9, E923.0-E923.9)
firearm (E922.0-E922.9)
projected object (E917.0-E917.9)

E910.3 – E916

4th E917 Striking against or struck accidentally by objects or persons

Includes bumping into or against
object (moving) (projected) (stationary)
pedestrian conveyance
person
colliding with
object (moving) (projected) (stationary)
pedestrian conveyance
person
kicking against
object (moving) (projected) (stationary)
pedestrian conveyance
person
stepping on
object (moving) (projected) (stationary)
pedestrian conveyance
person
struck by
object (moving) (projected) (stationary)
pedestrian conveyance
person

Excludes *fall from:*
collision with another person, except when caused by a crowd (E886.0-E886.9)
stumbling over object (E885.9)
fall resulting in striking against object (E888.0-E888.1)
injury caused by:
assault (E960.0-E960.1, E967.0-E967.9)
cutting or piercing instrument (E920.0-E920.9)
explosion (E921.0-E921.9, E923.0-E923.9)
firearm (E922.0-E922.9)
machinery (E919.0-E919.9)
transport vehicle (E800.0-E845.9)
vehicle not elsewhere classifiable (E846-E848)

E917.0 In sports without subsequent fall
Kicked or stepped on during game (football) (rugby)
Struck by hit or thrown ball
Struck by hockey stick or puck

E917.1 Caused by a crowd, by collective fear or panic without subsequent fall
Crushed by crowd or human stampede
Pushed by crowd or human stampede
Stepped on by crowd or human stampede

E917.2 In running water without subsequent fall
Excludes *drowning or submersion (E910.0-E910.9)*
that in sports (E917.0, E917.5)

E917.3 Furniture without subsequent fall
Excludes *fall from furniture (E884.2, E884.4-E884.5)*

E917.4 Other stationary object without subsequent fall
Bath tub
Fence
Lamp-post

E917.5 Object in sports with subsequent fall
Knocked down while boxing

E917.6 Caused by a crowd, by collective fear or panic with subsequent fall

E917.7 Furniture with subsequent fall
Excludes *fall from furniture (E884.2, E884.4-E884.5)*

E917.8 Other stationary object with subsequent fall
Bath tub
Fence
Lamp-post

E917.9 Other striking against with or without subsequent fall

E918 Caught accidentally in or between objects
Caught, crushed, jammed, or pinched in or between moving or stationary objects, such as:
escalator
folding object
hand tools, appliances, or implements
sliding door and door frame
under packing crate
washing machine wringer

Excludes *injury caused by:*
cutting or piercing instrument (E920.0-E920.9)
machinery (E919.0-E919.9)
mechanism or component of firearm and air gun (E928.7)
transport vehicle (E800.0-E845.9)
vehicle not elsewhere classifiable (E846-E848)
struck accidentally by:
falling object (E916)
object (moving) (projected) (E917.0-E917.9)

4th E919 Accidents caused by machinery

Includes burned by machinery (accident)
caught between machinery and other object
caught in (moving parts of) machinery (accident)
collapse of machinery (accident)
crushed by machinery (accident)
cut or pierced by machinery (accident)
drowning or submersion caused by machinery (accident)
explosion of, on, in machinery (accident)
fall from or into moving part of machinery (accident)
fire starting in or on machinery (accident)
machinery accident NOS
mechanical suffocation caused by machinery (accident)
object falling from, on, in motion by machinery (accident)
overturning of machinery (accident)
pinned under machinery (accident)
run over by machinery (accident)
struck by machinery (accident)
thrown from machinery (accident)

Excludes *accidents involving machinery, not in operation (E884.9, E916-E918)*
injury caused by:
electric current in connection with machinery (E925.0-E925.9)
escalator (E880.0, E918)
explosion of pressure vessel in connection with machinery (E921.0-E921.9)
mechanism or component of firearm and air gun (E928.7)
moving sidewalk (E885.9)
powered hand tools, appliances, and implements (E916-E918, E920.0-E921.9, E923.0-E926.9)
transport vehicle accidents involving machinery (E800.0-E848)
poisoning by carbon monoxide generated by machine (E868.8)

E919.0 Agricultural machines
Animal-powered agricultural machine
Combine
Derrick, hay
Farm machinery NOS
Farm tractor
Harvester
Hay mower or rake
Reaper
Thresher

Excludes *that being towed by another vehicle on the highway (E810.0-E819.9, E827.0-E827.9, E829.0-E829.9)*
that in transport under own power on the highway (E810.0-E819.9)
that involved in accident classifiable to E820-E829 (E820.0-E829.9)

E919.1 Mining and earth-drilling machinery
Bore or drill (land) (seabed)
Shaft hoist
Shaft lift
Under-cutter
Excludes *coal car, tram, truck, and tub in mine (E846)*

E919.2 Lifting machines and appliances
Chain hoist except in agricultural or mining operations
Crane except in agricultural or mining operations
Derrick except in agricultural or mining operations
Elevator (building) (grain) except in agricultural or mining operations
Forklift truck except in agricultural or mining operations
Lift except in agricultural or mining operations
Pulley block except in agricultural or mining operations
Winch except in agricultural or mining operations
Excludes *that being towed by another vehicle on the highway (E810.0-E819.9, E827.0-E827.9, E829.0-E829.9)*
that in transport under own power on the highway (E810.0-E819.9)
that involved in accident classifiable to E820-E829 (E820.0-E829.9)

E919.3 Metalworking machines
Abrasive wheel
Forging machine
Lathe
Mechanical shears
Metal:
drilling machine
milling machine
power press
rolling-mill
sawing machine

E919.4 Woodworking and forming machines
Band saw
Bench saw
Circular saw
Molding machine
Overhead plane
Powered saw
Radial saw
Sander
Excludes *hand saw (E920.1)*

E919.5 Prime movers, except electrical motors
Gas turbine
Internal combustion engine
Steam engine
Water driven turbine
Excludes *that being towed by other vehicle on the highway (E810.0-E819.9, E827.0-E827.9, E829.0-E829.9)*
that in transport under own power on the highway (E810.0-E819.9)

E919.6 Transmission machinery
Transmission:
belt
cable
chain
gear
pinion
pulley
shaft

E919.7 Earth moving, scraping, and other excavating machines
Bulldozer
Road scraper
Steam shovel
Excludes *that being towed by other vehicle on the highway (E810.0-E819.9)*
that in transport under own power on the highway (E810.0-E819.9)

E919.8 Other specified machinery
Machines for manufacture of:
clothing
foodstuffs and beverages
paper
Printing machine
Recreational machinery
Spinning, weaving, and textile machines

E919.9 Unspecified machinery

4th **E920 Accidents caused by cutting and piercing instruments or objects**
Includes accidental injury (by) object:
edged
pointed
sharp
Excludes *injury caused by mechanism or component of firearm and airgun (E928.7)*

E920.0 Powered lawn mower

E920.1 Other powered hand tools
Any powered hand tool [compressed air] [electric] [explosive cartridge] [hydraulic power], such as:
drill
hand saw
hedge clipper
rivet gun
snow blower
staple gun
Excludes *band saw (E919.4)*
bench saw (E919.4)

E920.2 Powered household appliances and implements
Blender
Electric:
beater or mixer
can opener
fan
knife
sewing machine
Garbage disposal appliance

E920.3 Knives, swords, and daggers

E920.4 Other hand tools and implements
Axe
Can opener NOS
Chisel
Fork
Hand saw
Hoe
Ice pick
Needle (sewing)
Paper cutter
Pitchfork
Rake
Scissors
Screwdriver
Sewing machine, not powered
Shovel

E920.5 Hypodermic needle
Contaminated needle
Needle stick

E920.8 Other specified cutting and piercing instruments or objects
Arrow
Broken glass
Dart
Edge of stiff paper
Lathe turnings
Nail
Plant thorn
Splinter
Tin can lid
Excludes *animal spines or quills (E906.8)*
flying glass due to explosion (E921.0-E923.9)

E920.9 Unspecified cutting and piercing instrument or object

4th E921 Accident caused by explosion of pressure vessel
Includes accidental explosion of pressure vessels, whether or not part of machinery
Excludes *explosion of pressure vessel on transport vehicle (E800.0-E845.9)*

E921.0 Boilers

E921.1 Gas cylinders
Air tank
Pressure gas tank

E921.8 Other specified pressure vessels
Aerosol can
Automobile tire
Pressure cooker

E921.9 Unspecified pressure vessel

4th E922 Accident caused by firearm and air gun missile
Excludes *injury caused by mechanism or component of firearm and airgun (E928.7)*

E922.0 Handgun
Pistol
Revolver
Excludes *Verey pistol (E922.8)*

E922.1 Shotgun (automatic)

E922.2 Hunting rifle

E922.3 Military firearms
Army rifle
Machine gun

E922.4 Air gun
BB gun
Pellet gun

E922.5 Paintball gun

E922.8 Other specified firearm missile
Verey pistol [flare]

E922.9 Unspecified firearm missile
Gunshot wound NOS
Shot NOS

4th E923 Accident caused by explosive material
Includes flash burns and other injuries resulting from explosion of explosive material
ignition of highly explosive material with explosion
Excludes *explosion:*
in or on machinery (E919.0-E919.9)
on any transport vehicle, except stationary motor vehicle (E800.0-E848)
with conflagration (E890.0, E891.0, E892)
injury caused by mechanism or component of firearm and airgun (E928.7)
secondary fires resulting from explosion (E890.0-E899)

E923.0 Fireworks

E923.1 Blasting materials
Blasting cap
Detonator
Dynamite
Explosive [any] used in blasting operations

E923.2 Explosive gases
Acetylene
Butane
Coal gas
Explosion in mine NOS
Fire damp
Gasoline fumes
Methane
Propane

E923.8 Other explosive materials
Bomb
Explosion in munitions:
dump
factory
Explosive missile
Grenade
Mine
Shell
Torpedo

E923.9 Unspecified explosive material
Explosion NOS

4th E924 Accident caused by hot substance or object, caustic or corrosive material, and steam
Excludes *burning NOS (E899)*
chemical burn resulting from swallowing a corrosive substance (E860.0-E864.4)
fire caused by these substances and objects (E890.0-E894)
radiation burns (E926.0-E926.9)
therapeutic misadventures (E870.0-E876.9)

E924.0 Hot liquids and vapors, including steam
Burning or scalding by:
boiling water
hot or boiling liquids not primarily caustic or corrosive
liquid metal
steam
other hot vapor
Excludes *hot (boiling) tap water (E924.2)*

E924.1 Caustic and corrosive substances
Burning by:
acid [any kind]
ammonia
caustic oven cleaner or other substance
corrosive substance
lye
vitriol

E924.2 Hot (boiling) tap water

E924.8 Other
Burning by:
heat from electric heating appliance
hot object NOS
light bulb
steam pipe

E924.9 Unspecified

E920.8 – E924.9

4th **E925 Accident caused by electric current**

Includes electric current from exposed wire, faulty appliance, high voltage cable, live rail, or open electric socket as the cause of:
- burn
- cardiac fibrillation
- convulsion
- electric shock
- electrocution
- puncture wound
- respiratory paralysis

Excludes *burn by heat from electrical appliance (E924.8)*
lightning (E907)

E925.0 Domestic wiring and appliances

E925.1 Electric power generating plants, distribution stations, transmission lines
Broken power line

E925.2 Industrial wiring, appliances, and electrical machinery
Conductors
Control apparatus
Electrical equipment and machinery
Transformers

E925.8 Other electric current
Wiring and appliances in or on:
- farm [not farmhouse]
- outdoors
- public building
- residential institutions
- schools

E925.9 Unspecified electric current
Burns or other injury from electric current NOS
Electric shock NOS
Electrocution NOS

4th **E926 Exposure to radiation**

Excludes *abnormal reaction to or complication of treatment without mention of misadventure (E879.2)*
atomic power plant malfunction in water transport (E838.0-E838.9)
misadventure to patient in surgical and medical procedures (E873.2-E873.3)
use of radiation in war operations (E996-E997.9)

E926.0 Radiofrequency radiation
Overexposure to:
- microwave radiation from:
  - high-powered radio and television transmitters
  - industrial radiofrequency induction heaters
  - radar installations
- radar radiation from:
  - high-powered radio and television transmitters
  - industrial radiofrequency induction heaters
  - radar installations
- radiofrequency from:
  - high-powered radio and television transmitters
  - industrial radiofrequency induction heaters
  - radar installations
- radiofrequency radiation [any] from:
  - high-powered radio and television transmitters
  - industrial radiofrequency induction heaters
  - radar installations

E926.1 Infra-red heaters and lamps
Exposure to infra-red radiation from heaters and lamps as the cause of:
- blistering
- burning
- charring
- inflammatory change

Excludes *physical contact with heater or lamp (E924.8)*

E926.2 Visible and ultraviolet light sources
Arc lamps
Black light sources
Electrical welding arc
Oxygas welding torch
Sun rays
Tanning bed

Excludes *excessive heat from these sources (E900.1-E900.9)*

E926.3 X-rays and other electromagnetic ionizing radiation
Gamma rays
X-rays (hard) (soft)

E926.4 Lasers

E926.5 Radioactive isotopes
Radiobiologicals
Radiopharmaceuticals

E926.8 Other specified radiation
Artificially accelerated beams of ionized particles generated by:
- betatrons
- synchrotrons

E926.9 Unspecified radiation
Radiation NOS

4th **E927 Overexertion and strenuous and repetitive movements and loads**

Use additional code to identify activity (E001-E030)

E927.0 Overexertion from sudden strenuous movement
Sudden trauma from strenuous movement

E927.1 Overexertion from prolonged static position
Overexertion from maintaining prolonged positions, such as:
- holding
- sitting
- standing

E927.2 Excessive physical exertion from prolonged activity

E927.3 Cumulative trauma from repetitive motion
Cumulative trauma from repetitive movements

E927.4 Cumulative trauma from repetitive impact

E927.8 Other overexertion and strenuous and repetitive movements or loads

E927.9 Unspecified overexertion and strenuous and repetitive movements or loads

4th **E928 Other and unspecified environmental and accidental causes**

E928.0 Prolonged stay in weightless environment
Weightlessness in spacecraft (simulator)

E928.1 Exposure to noise
Noise (pollution)
Sound waves
Supersonic waves

E928.2 Vibration

E928.3 Human bite

E928.4 External constriction caused by hair

E928.5 External constriction caused by other object

E928.6 Environmental exposure to harmful algae and toxins
Algae bloom NOS
Blue-green algae bloom
Brown tide
Cyanobacteria bloom
Florida red tide
Harmful algae bloom
Pfiesteria piscicida
Red tide

● **E928.7 Mechanism or component of firearm and air gun**
Injury due to:
explosion of gun parts
recoil
Pierced, cut, crushed, or pinched by slide trigger mechanism, scope or other gun part
Powder burn from firearm or air gun
Excludes *accident caused by firearm and air gun missile (E922.0-E922.9)*

E928.8 Other

E928.9 Unspecified accident
Accident NOS stated as accidentally inflicted
Blow NOS stated as accidentally inflicted
Casualty (not due to war) stated as accidentally inflicted
Decapitation stated as accidentally inflicted
Injury [any part of body, or unspecified] stated as accidentally inflicted, but not otherwise specified
Killed stated as accidentally inflicted, but not otherwise specified
Knocked down stated as accidentally inflicted, but not otherwise specified
Mangled stated as accidentally inflicted, but not otherwise specified
Wound stated as accidentally inflicted, but not otherwise specified
Excludes *fracture, cause unspecified (E887)*
injuries undetermined whether accidentally or purposely inflicted (E980.0-E989)

LATE EFFECTS OF ACCIDENTAL INJURY (E929)

Note: *This category is to be used to indicate accidental injury as the cause of death or disability from late effects, which are themselves classifiable elsewhere. The "late effects" include conditions reported as such or as sequelae, which may occur at any time after the acute accidental injury.*

4th **E929 Late effects of accidental injury**
Excludes *late effects of:*
surgical and medical procedures (E870.0-E879.9)
therapeutic use of drugs and medicines (E930.0-E949.9)

E929.0 Late effects of motor vehicle accident
Late effects of accidents classifiable to E810-E825

E929.1 Late effects of other transport accident
Late effects of accidents classifiable to E800-E807, E826-E838, E840-E848

E929.2 Late effects of accidental poisoning
Late effects of accidents classifiable to E850-E858, E860-E869

E929.3 Late effects of accidental fall
Late effects of accidents classifiable to E880-E888

E929.4 Late effects of accident caused by fire
Late effects of accidents classifiable to E890-E899

E929.5 Late effects of accident due to natural and environmental factors
Late effects of accidents classifiable to E900-E909

E929.8 Late effects of other accidents
Late effects of accidents classifiable to E910-E928.8

E929.9 Late effects of unspecified accident
Late effects of accidents classifiable to E928.9

DRUGS, MEDICINAL AND BIOLOGICAL SUBSTANCES CAUSING ADVERSE EFFECTS IN THERAPEUTIC USE (E930-E949)

Includes correct drug properly administered in therapeutic or prophylactic dosage, as the cause of any adverse effect including allergic or hypersensitivity reactions

Excludes *accidental overdose of drug and wrong drug given or taken in error (E850.0-E858.9)*
accidents in the technique of administration of drug or biological substance such as accidental puncture during injection, or contamination of drug (E870.0-E876.9)
administration with suicidal or homicidal intent or intent to harm, or in circumstances classifiable to ~~E980-E989~~ (E950.0-E950.5, E962.0, E980.0-E980.5)

Note: *See Alphabetic Index for more complete list of specific drugs to be classified under the fourth-digit subdivisions. The American Hospital Formulary numbers can be used to classify new drugs listed by the American Hospital Formulary Service (AHFS). See Appendix C.*

ICD-9-CM Official Guidelines (Chapter 19):

c. ***Adverse Effects of Drugs, Medicinal and Biological Substances Guidelines***

1) *Do not code directly from the Table of Drugs and Chemicals. Always refer back to the Tabular List.*
2) *Use as many codes as necessary to describe completely all drugs, medicinal or biological substances.*
3) *If the same E code would describe the causative agent for more than one adverse reaction, assign the code only once.*
4) *If two or more drugs, medicinal or biological substances are reported, code each individually unless the combination code is listed in the Table of Drugs and Chemicals. In that case, assign the E code for the combination.*
5) *When a reaction results from the interaction of a drug(s) and alcohol, use poisoning codes and E codes for both.*
6) *If the reporting format limits the number of E codes that can be used in reporting clinical data, code the one most related to the principal diagnosis. Include at least one from each category (cause, intent, place) if possible.*
If there are different fourth digit codes in the same three digit category, use the code for "Other specified" of that category. If there is no "Other specified" code in that category, use the appropriate "Unspecified" code in that category. If the codes are in different three digit categories, assign the appropriate E code for other multiple drugs and medicinal substances.
7) *Codes from the E930-E949 series must be used to identify the causative substance for an adverse effect of drug, medicinal and biological substances, correctly prescribed and properly administered. The effect, such as tachycardia, delirium, gastrointestinal hemorrhaging, vomiting, hypokalemia, hepatitis, renal failure, or respiratory failure, is coded and followed by the appropriate code from the E930-E949 series.*

4th **E930 Antibiotics**
Excludes *that used as eye, ear, nose, and throat [ENT], and local anti-infectives (E946.0-E946.9)*

E930.0 Penicillins
Natural
Synthetic
Semisynthetic, such as:
ampicillin
cloxacillin
nafcillin
oxacillin

E930.1 Antifungal antibiotics
Amphotericin B
Griseofulvin
Hachimycin [trichomycin]
Nystatin

E928.7 – E930.1

E930.2 Chloramphenicol group
Chloramphenicol
Thiamphenicol

E930.3 Erythromycin and other macrolides
Oleandomycin
Spiramycin

E930.4 Tetracycline group
Doxycycline
Minocycline
Oxytetracycline

E930.5 Cephalosporin group
Cephalexin
Cephaloglycin
Cephaloridine
Cephalothin

E930.6 Antimycobacterial antibiotics
Cycloserine
Kanamycin
Rifampin
Streptomycin

E930.7 Antineoplastic antibiotics
Actinomycins, such as:
Bleomycin
Cactinomycin
Dactinomycin
Daunorubicin
Mitomycin
Excludes *other antineoplastic drugs (E933.1)*

E930.8 Other specified antibiotics

E930.9 Unspecified antibiotic

4th E931 Other anti-infectives
Excludes *ENT, and local anti-infectives (E946.0-E946.9)*

E931.0 Sulfonamides
Sulfadiazine
Sulfafurazole
Sulfamethoxazole

E931.1 Arsenical anti-infectives

E931.2 Heavy metal anti-infectives
Compounds of:
antimony
bismuth
lead
mercury
Excludes *mercurial diuretics (E944.0)*

E931.3 Quinoline and hydroxyquinoline derivatives
Chiniofon
Diiodohydroxyquin
Excludes *antimalarial drugs (E931.4)*

E931.4 Antimalarials and drugs acting on other blood protozoa
Chloroquine phosphate
Cycloguanil
Primaquine
Proguanil [chloroguanide]
Pyrimethamine
Quinine (sulphate)

E931.5 Other antiprotozoal drugs
Emetine

E931.6 Anthelmintics
Hexylresorcinol
Male fern oleoresin
Piperazine
Thiabendazole

E931.7 Antiviral drugs
Methisazone
Excludes *amantadine (E936.4)*
cytarabine (E933.1)
idoxuridine (E946.5)

E931.8 Other antimycobacterial drugs
Ethambutol
Ethionamide
Isoniazid
Para-aminosalicylic acid derivatives
Sulfones

E931.9 Other and unspecified anti-infectives
Flucytosine
Nitrofuran derivatives

4th E932 Hormones and synthetic substitutes

E932.0 Adrenal cortical steroids
Cortisone derivatives
Desoxycorticosterone derivatives
Fluorinated corticosteroids

E932.1 Androgens and anabolic congeners
Nandrolone phenpropionate
Oxymetholone
Testosterone and preparations

E932.2 Ovarian hormones and synthetic substitutes
Contraceptives, oral
Estrogens
Estrogens and progestogens combined
Progestogens

E932.3 Insulins and antidiabetic agents
Acetohexamide
Biguanide derivatives, oral
Chlorpropamide
Glucagon
Insulin
Phenformin
Sulfonylurea derivatives, oral
Tolbutamide
Excludes *adverse effect of insulin administered for shock therapy (E879.3)*

E932.4 Anterior pituitary hormones
Corticotropin
Gonadotropin
Somatotropin [growth hormone]

E932.5 Posterior pituitary hormones
Vasopressin
Excludes *oxytocic agents (E945.0)*

E932.6 Parathyroid and parathyroid derivatives

E932.7 Thyroid and thyroid derivatives
Dextrothyroxine
Levothyroxine sodium
Liothyronine
Thyroglobulin

E932.8 Antithyroid agents
Iodides
Thiouracil
Thiourea

E932.9 Other and unspecified hormones and synthetic substitutes

4th E933 Primarily systemic agents

E933.0 Antiallergic and antiemetic drugs
Antihistamines
Chlorpheniramine
Diphenhydramine
Diphenylpyraline
Thonzylamine
Tripelennamine
Excludes *phenothiazine-based tranquilizers (E939.1)*

E933.1 Antineoplastic and immunosuppressive drugs
Azathioprine
Busulfan
Chlorambucil
Cyclophosphamide
Cytarabine
Fluorouracil
Mechlorethamine hydrochloride
Mercaptopurine
Triethylenethiophosphoramide [thio-TEPA]
Excludes *antineoplastic antibiotics (E930.7)*

E933.2 Acidifying agents

E933.3 Alkalizing agents

E933.4 Enzymes, not elsewhere classified
Penicillinase

E933.5 Vitamins, not elsewhere classified
Vitamin A
Vitamin D
Excludes *nicotinic acid (E942.2)*
vitamin K (E934.3)

E933.6 Oral bisphosphonates

E933.7 Intravenous bisphosphonates

E933.8 Other systemic agents, not elsewhere classified
Heavy metal antagonists

E933.9 Unspecified systemic agent

4th E934 Agents primarily affecting blood constituents

E934.0 Iron and its compounds
Ferric salts
Ferrous sulphate and other ferrous salts

E934.1 Liver preparations and other antianemic agents
Folic acid

E934.2 Anticoagulants
Coumarin
Heparin
Phenindione
Prothrombin synthesis inhibitor
Warfarin sodium

E934.3 Vitamin K [phytonadione]

E934.4 Fibrinolysis-affecting drugs
Aminocaproic acid
Streptodornase
Streptokinase
Urokinase

E934.5 Anticoagulant antagonists and other coagulants
Hexadimethrine bromide
Protamine sulfate

E934.6 Gamma globulin

E934.7 Natural blood and blood products
Blood plasma
Human fibrinogen
Packed red cells
Whole blood

E934.8 Other agents affecting blood constituents
Macromolecular blood substitutes

E934.9 Unspecified agent affecting blood constituents

4th E935 Analgesics, antipyretics, and antirheumatics

E935.0 Heroin
Diacetylmorphine

E935.1 Methadone

E935.2 Other opiates and related narcotics
Codeine [methylmorphine]
Meperidine [pethidine]
Morphine
Opium (alkaloids)

E935.3 Salicylates
Acetylsalicylic acid [aspirin]
Amino derivatives of salicylic acid
Salicylic acid salts

E935.4 Aromatic analgesics, not elsewhere classified
Acetanilid
Paracetamol [acetaminophen]
Phenacetin [acetophenetidin]

E935.5 Pyrazole derivatives
Aminophenazone [aminopyrine]
Phenylbutazone

E935.6 Antirheumatics [antiphlogistics]
Gold salts
Indomethacin
Excludes *salicylates (E935.3)*
steroids (E932.0)

E935.7 Other non-narcotic analgesics
Pyrabital

E935.8 Other specified analgesics and antipyretics
Pentazocine

E935.9 Unspecified analgesic and antipyretic

4th E936 Anticonvulsants and anti-Parkinsonism drugs

E936.0 Oxazolidine derivatives
Paramethadione
Trimethadione

E936.1 Hydantoin derivatives
Phenytoin

E936.2 Succinimides
Ethosuximide
Phensuximide

E936.3 Other and unspecified anticonvulsants
Beclamide
Primidone

E936.4 Anti-Parkinsonism drugs
Amantadine
Ethopropazine [profenamine]
Levodopa [L-dopa]

4th E937 Sedatives and hypnotics

E937.0 Barbiturates
Amobarbital [amylobarbitone]
Barbital [barbitone]
Butabarbital [butabarbitone]
Pentobarbital [pentobarbitone]
Phenobarbital [phenobarbitone]
Secobarbital [quinalbarbitone]
Excludes *thiobarbiturates (E938.3)*

E937.1 Chloral hydrate group

E937.2 Paraldehyde

E937.3 Bromine compounds
Bromide
Carbromal (derivatives)

E937.4 Methaqualone compounds

E937.5 Glutethimide group

E937.6 Mixed sedatives, not elsewhere classified

E937.8 Other sedatives and hypnotics

E937.9 Unspecified
Sleeping:
- drug NOS
- pill NOS
- tablet NOS

4th E938 Other central nervous system depressants and anesthetics

E938.0 Central nervous system muscle-tone depressants
Chlorphenesin (carbamate)
Mephenesin
Methocarbamol

E938.1 **Halothane**

E938.2 **Other gaseous anesthetics**
- Ether
- Halogenated hydrocarbon derivatives, except halothane
- Nitrous oxide

E938.3 **Intravenous anesthetics**
- Ketamine
- Methohexital [methohexitone]
- Thiobarbiturates, such as thiopental sodium

E938.4 **Other and unspecified general anesthetics**

E938.5 **Surface and infiltration anesthetics**
- Cocaine
- Lidocaine [lignocaine]
- Procaine
- Tetracaine

E938.6 **Peripheral nerve- and plexus-blocking anesthetics**

E938.7 **Spinal anesthetics**

E938.9 **Other and unspecified local anesthetics**

4th **E939 Psychotropic agents**

E939.0 **Antidepressants**
- Amitriptyline
- Imipramine
- Monoamine oxidase [MAO] inhibitors

E939.1 **Phenothiazine-based tranquilizers**
- Chlorpromazine
- Fluphenazine
- Phenothiazine
- Prochlorperazine
- Promazine

E939.2 **Butyrophenone-based tranquilizers**
- Haloperidol
- Spiperone
- Trifluperidol

E939.3 **Other antipsychotics, neuroleptics, and major tranquilizers**

E939.4 **Benzodiazepine-based tranquilizers**
- Chlordiazepoxide
- Diazepam
- Flurazepam
- Lorazepam
- Medazepam
- Nitrazepam

E939.5 **Other tranquilizers**
- Hydroxyzine
- Meprobamate

E939.6 **Psychodysleptics [hallucinogens]**
- Cannabis (derivatives)
- Lysergide [LSD]
- Marihuana (derivatives)
- Mescaline
- Psilocin
- Psilocybin

E939.7 **Psychostimulants**
- Amphetamine
- Caffeine

Excludes *central appetite depressants (E947.0)*

E939.8 **Other psychotropic agents**

E939.9 **Unspecified psychotropic agent**

4th **E940 Central nervous system stimulants**

E940.0 **Analeptics**
- Lobeline
- Nikethamide

E940.1 **Opiate antagonists**
- Levallorphan
- Nalorphine
- Naloxone

E940.8 **Other specified central nervous system stimulants**

E940.9 **Unspecified central nervous system stimulant**

4th **E941 Drugs primarily affecting the autonomic nervous system**

E941.0 **Parasympathomimetics [cholinergics]**
- Acetylcholine
- Anticholinesterase:
  - organophosphorus
  - reversible
- Pilocarpine

E941.1 **Parasympatholytics [anticholinergics and antimuscarinics] and spasmolytics**
- Atropine
- Homatropine
- Hyoscine [scopolamine]
- Quaternary ammonium derivatives

Excludes *papaverine (E942.5)*

E941.2 **Sympathomimetics [adrenergics]**
- Epinephrine [adrenalin]
- Levarterenol [noradrenalin]

E941.3 **Sympatholytics [antiadrenergics]**
- Phenoxybenzamine
- Tolazoline hydrochloride

E941.9 **Unspecified drug primarily affecting the autonomic nervous system**

4th **E942 Agents primarily affecting the cardiovascular system**

E942.0 **Cardiac rhythm regulators**
- Practolol
- Procainamide
- Propranolol
- Quinidine

E942.1 **Cardiotonic glycosides and drugs of similar action**
- Digitalis glycosides
- Digoxin
- Strophanthins

E942.2 **Antilipemic and antiarteriosclerotic drugs**
- Cholestyramine
- Clofibrate
- Nicotinic acid derivatives
- Sitosterols

Excludes *dextrothyroxine (E932.7)*

E942.3 **Ganglion-blocking agents**
- Pentamethonium bromide

E942.4 **Coronary vasodilators**
- Dipyridamole
- Nitrates [nitroglycerin]
- Nitrites
- Prenylamine

E942.5 **Other vasodilators**
- Cyclandelate
- Diazoxide
- Hydralazine
- Papaverine

E942.6 **Other antihypertensive agents**
- Clonidine
- Guanethidine
- Rauwolfia alkaloids
- Reserpine

E942.7 **Antivaricose drugs, including sclerosing agents**
- Monoethanolamine
- Zinc salts

E942.8 **Capillary-active drugs**
- Adrenochrome derivatives
- Bioflavonoids
- Metaraminol

E942.9 **Other and unspecified agents primarily affecting the cardiovascular system**

4th E943 Agents primarily affecting gastrointestinal system

E943.0 Antacids and antigastric secretion drugs
Aluminum hydroxide
Magnesium trisilicate

E943.1 Irritant cathartics
Bisacodyl
Castor oil
Phenolphthalein

E943.2 Emollient cathartics
Sodium dioctyl sulfosuccinate

E943.3 Other cathartics, including intestinal atonia drugs
Magnesium sulfate

E943.4 Digestants
Pancreatin
Papain
Pepsin

E943.5 Antidiarrheal drugs
Bismuth subcarbonate
Kaolin
Pectin
Excludes *anti-infectives (E930.0-E931.9)*

E943.6 Emetics

E943.8 Other specified agents primarily affecting the gastrointestinal system

E943.9 Unspecified agent primarily affecting the gastrointestinal system

4th E944 Water, mineral, and uric acid metabolism drugs

E944.0 Mercurial diuretics
Chlormerodrin
Mercaptomerin
Mercurophylline
Mersalyl

E944.1 Purine derivative diuretics
Theobromine
Theophylline
Excludes *aminophylline [theophylline ethylenediamine] (E945.7)*

E944.2 Carbonic acid anhydrase inhibitors
Acetazolamide

E944.3 Saluretics
Benzothiadiazides
Chlorothiazide group

E944.4 Other diuretics
Ethacrynic acid
Furosemide

E944.5 Electrolytic, caloric, and water-balance agents

E944.6 Other mineral salts, not elsewhere classified

E944.7 Uric acid metabolism drugs
Cinchophen and congeners
Colchicine
Phenoquin
Probenecid

4th E945 Agents primarily acting on the smooth and skeletal muscles and respiratory system

E945.0 Oxytocic agents
Ergot alkaloids
Prostaglandins

E945.1 Smooth muscle relaxants
Adiphenine
Metaproterenol [orciprenaline]
Excludes *papaverine (E942.5)*

E945.2 Skeletal muscle relaxants
Alcuronium chloride
Suxamethonium chloride

E945.3 Other and unspecified drugs acting on muscles

E945.4 Antitussives
Dextromethorphan
Pipazethate hydrochloride

E945.5 Expectorants
Acetylcysteine
Cocillana
Guaifenesin [glyceryl guaiacolate]
Ipecacuanha
Terpin hydrate

E945.6 Anti-common cold drugs

E945.7 Antiasthmatics
Aminophylline [theophylline ethylenediamine]

E945.8 Other and unspecified respiratory drugs

4th E946 Agents primarily affecting skin and mucous membrane, ophthalmological, otorhinolaryngological, and dental drugs

E946.0 Local anti-infectives and anti-inflammatory drugs

E946.1 Antipruritics

E946.2 Local astringents and local detergents

E946.3 Emollients, demulcents, and protectants

E946.4 Keratolytics, keratoplastics, other hair treatment drugs and preparations

E946.5 Eye anti-infectives and other eye drugs
Idoxuridine

E946.6 Anti-infectives and other drugs and preparations for ear, nose, and throat

E946.7 Dental drugs topically applied

E946.8 Other agents primarily affecting skin and mucous membrane
Spermicides

E946.9 Unspecified agent primarily affecting skin and mucous membrane

4th E947 Other and unspecified drugs and medicinal substances

E947.0 Dietetics

E947.1 Lipotropic drugs

E947.2 Antidotes and chelating agents, not elsewhere classified

E947.3 Alcohol deterrents

E947.4 Pharmaceutical excipients

E947.8 Other drugs and medicinal substances
Contrast media used for diagnostic x-ray procedures
Diagnostic agents and kits

E947.9 Unspecified drug or medicinal substance

4th E948 Bacterial vaccines

E948.0 BCG vaccine

E948.1 Typhoid and paratyphoid

E948.2 Cholera

E948.3 Plague

E948.4 Tetanus

E948.5 Diphtheria

E948.6 Pertussis vaccine, including combinations with a pertussis component

E948.8 Other and unspecified bacterial vaccines

E948.9 Mixed bacterial vaccines, except combinations with a pertussis component

4th E949 Other vaccines and biological substances
Excludes *gamma globulin (E934.6)*

E949.0 Smallpox vaccine

E949.1 Rabies vaccine

E949.2 Typhus vaccine

E949.3 Yellow fever vaccine

E949.4 Measles vaccine

E949.5 Poliomyelitis vaccine

E949.6 Other and unspecified viral and rickettsial vaccines
Mumps vaccine

E949.7 Mixed viral-rickettsial and bacterial vaccines, except combinations with a pertussis component
Excludes *combinations with a pertussis component (E948.6)*

E949.9 Other and unspecified vaccines and biological substances

SUICIDE AND SELF-INFLICTED INJURY (E950-E959)

Includes injuries in suicide and attempted suicide
self-inflicted injuries specified as intentional

4th **E950 Suicide and self-inflicted poisoning by solid or liquid substances**
E950.0 Analgesics, antipyretics, and antirheumatics
E950.1 Barbiturates
E950.2 Other sedatives and hypnotics
E950.3 Tranquilizers and other psychotropic agents
E950.4 Other specified drugs and medicinal substances
E950.5 Unspecified drug or medicinal substance
E950.6 Agricultural and horticultural chemical and pharmaceutical preparations other than plant foods and fertilizers
E950.7 Corrosive and caustic substances
Suicide and self-inflicted poisoning by substances classifiable to E864
E950.8 Arsenic and its compounds
E950.9 Other and unspecified solid and liquid substances

4th **E951 Suicide and self-inflicted poisoning by gases in domestic use**
E951.0 Gas distributed by pipeline
E951.1 Liquefied petroleum gas distributed in mobile containers
E951.8 Other utility gas

4th **E952 Suicide and self-inflicted poisoning by other gases and vapors**
E952.0 Motor vehicle exhaust gas
E952.1 Other carbon monoxide
E952.8 Other specified gases and vapors
E952.9 Unspecified gases and vapors

4th **E953 Suicide and self-inflicted injury by hanging, strangulation, and suffocation**
E953.0 Hanging
E953.1 Suffocation by plastic bag
E953.8 Other specified means
E953.9 Unspecified means

E954 Suicide and self-inflicted injury by submersion [drowning]

4th **E955 Suicide and self-inflicted injury by firearms, air guns and explosives**
E955.0 Handgun
E955.1 Shotgun
E955.2 Hunting rifle
E955.3 Military firearms
E955.4 Other and unspecified firearm
Gunshot NOS
Shot NOS
E955.5 Explosives
E955.6 Air gun
BB gun
Pellet gun
E955.7 Paintball gun
E955.9 Unspecified

E956 Suicide and self-inflicted injury by cutting and piercing instrument

4th **E957 Suicide and self-inflicted injuries by jumping from high place**
E957.0 Residential premises
E957.1 Other man-made structures
E957.2 Natural sites
E957.9 Unspecified

4th **E958 Suicide and self-inflicted injury by other and unspecified means**
E958.0 Jumping or lying before moving object
E958.1 Burns, fire
E958.2 Scald
E958.3 Extremes of cold
E958.4 Electrocution
E958.5 Crashing of motor vehicle
E958.6 Crashing of aircraft
E958.7 Caustic substances, except poisoning
Excludes *poisoning by caustic substance (E950.7)*
E958.8 Other specified means
E958.9 Unspecified means

E959 Late effects of self-inflicted injury
Note: *This category is to be used to indicate circumstances classifiable to E950-E958 as the cause of death or disability from late effects, which are themselves classifiable elsewhere. The "late effects" include conditions reported as such or as sequelae which may occur at any time after the attempted suicide or self-inflicted injury.*

HOMICIDE AND INJURY PURPOSELY INFLICTED BY OTHER PERSONS (E960-E969)

Includes injuries inflicted by another person with intent to injure or kill, by any means

Excludes *injuries due to:*
legal intervention (E970-E978)
operations of war (E990-E999)
terrorism (E979)

ICD-9-CM Official Guidelines (Chapter 19):

e. Child and Adult Abuse Guideline

1) Intentional injury
When the cause of an injury or neglect is intentional child or adult abuse, the first listed E code should be assigned from categories E960-E968, Homicide and injury purposely inflicted by other persons, (except category E967). An E code from category E967, Child and adult battering and other maltreatment, should be added as an additional code to identify the perpetrator, if known.

2) Accidental intent
In cases of neglect when the intent is determined to be accidental E code E904.0, Abandonment or neglect of infant and helpless person, should be the first listed E code.

4th **E960 Fight, brawl, rape**
E960.0 Unarmed fight or brawl
Beatings NOS
Brawl or fight with hands, fists, feet
Injured or killed in fight NOS
Excludes *homicidal:*
injury by weapons (E965.0-E966, E969)
strangulation (E963)
submersion (E964)
E960.1 Rape

E961 Assault by corrosive or caustic substance, except poisoning
Injury or death purposely caused by corrosive or caustic substance, such as:
acid [any]
corrosive substance
vitriol
Excludes *burns from hot liquid (E968.3)*
chemical burns from swallowing a corrosive substance (E962.0-E962.9)

4th Fourth Digit Required | ● New Code | ▲ Revised Code | text New Text | ~~text~~ Deleted text

4th E962 **Assault by poisoning**

E962.0 **Drugs and medicinal substances**
Homicidal poisoning by any drug or medicinal substance

E962.1 **Other solid and liquid substances**

E962.2 **Other gases and vapors**

E962.9 **Unspecified poisoning**

E963 **Assault by hanging and strangulation**
Homicidal (attempt):
garrotting or ligature
hanging
strangulation
suffocation

E964 **Assault by submersion [drowning]**

4th E965 **Assault by firearms and explosives**

E965.0 **Handgun**
Pistol
Revolver

E965.1 **Shotgun**

E965.2 **Hunting rifle**

E965.3 **Military firearms**

E965.4 **Other and unspecified firearm**

E965.5 **Antipersonnel bomb**

E965.6 **Gasoline bomb**

E965.7 **Letter bomb**

E965.8 **Other specified explosive**
Bomb NOS (placed in):
car
house
Dynamite

E965.9 **Unspecified explosive**

E966 **Assault by cutting and piercing instrument**
Assassination (attempt), homicide (attempt) by any instrument classifiable under E920
Homicidal:
cut any part of body
puncture any part of body
stab any part of body
Stabbed any part of body

4th E967 **Perpetrator of child and adult abuse**
Note: *Selection of the correct perpetrator code is based on the relationship between the perpetrator and the victim.*

E967.0 **By father, stepfather, or boyfriend**
Male partner of child's parent or guardian

E967.1 **By other specified person**

E967.2 **By mother, stepmother, or girlfriend**
Female partner of child's parent or guardian

E967.3 **By spouse or partner**
Abuse of spouse or partner by ex-spouse or ex-partner

E967.4 **By child**

E967.5 **By sibling**

E967.6 **By grandparent**

E967.7 **By other relative**

E967.8 **By non-related caregiver**

E967.9 **By unspecified person**

4th E968 **Assault by other and unspecified means**

E968.0 **Fire**
Arson
Homicidal burns NOS
Excludes *burns from hot liquid (E968.3)*

E968.1 **Pushing from a high place**

E968.2 **Striking by blunt or thrown object**

E968.3 **Hot liquid**
Homicidal burns by scalding

E968.4 **Criminal neglect**
Abandonment of child, infant, or other helpless person with intent to injure or kill

E968.5 **Transport vehicle**
Being struck by other vehicle or run down with intent to injure
Pushed in front of, thrown from, or dragged by moving vehicle with intent to injure

E968.6 **Air gun**
BB gun
Pellet gun

E968.7 **Human bite**

E968.8 **Other specified means**

E968.9 **Unspecified means**
Assassination (attempt) NOS
Homicidal (attempt):
injury NOS
wound NOS
Manslaughter (nonaccidental)
Murder (attempt) NOS
Violence, non-accidental

E969 **Late effects of injury purposely inflicted by other person**
Note: *This category is to be used to indicate circumstances classifiable to E960-E968 as the cause of death or disability from late effects, which are themselves classifiable elsewhere. The "late effects" include conditions reported as such, or as sequelae which may occur at any time after the injury purposely inflicted by another person.*

LEGAL INTERVENTION (E970-E978)

Includes injuries inflicted by the police or other law-enforcing agents, including military on duty, in the course of arresting or attempting to arrest lawbreakers, suppressing disturbances, maintaining order, and other legal action
legal execution

Excludes *injuries caused by civil insurrections (E990.0-E999)*

E970 **Injury due to legal intervention by firearms**
Gunshot wound
Injury by:
machine gun
revolver
rifle pellet or rubber bullet
shot NOS

E971 **Injury due to legal intervention by explosives**
Injury by:
dynamite
explosive shell
grenade
motor bomb

E972 **Injury due to legal intervention by gas**
Asphyxiation by gas
Injury by tear gas
Poisoning by gas

E973 **Injury due to legal intervention by blunt object**
Hit, struck by:
baton (nightstick)
blunt object
stave

E974 **Injury due to legal intervention by cutting and piercing instrument**
Cut
Incised wound
Injured by bayonet
Stab wound

E975 **Injury due to legal intervention by other specified means**
Blow
Manhandling

E976 **Injury due to legal intervention by unspecified means**

E962 – E976

E977 Late effects of injuries due to legal intervention

Note: *This category is to be used to indicate circumstances classifiable to E970-E976 as the cause of death or disability from late effects, which are themselves classifiable elsewhere. The "late effects" include conditions reported as such, or as sequelae which may occur at any time after the injury due to legal intervention.*

E978 Legal execution

All executions performed at the behest of the judiciary or ruling authority [whether permanent or temporary] as:
- asphyxiation by gas
- beheading, decapitation (by guillotine)
- capital punishment
- electrocution
- hanging
- poisoning
- shooting
- other specified means

TERRORISM (E979)

ICD-9-CM Official Guidelines (Chapter 19):

j. Terrorism Guidelines

1) ***Cause of injury identified by the Federal Government (FBI) as terrorism***

When the cause of an injury is identified by the Federal Government (FBI) as terrorism, the first-listed E-code should be a code from category E979, Terrorism. The definition of terrorism employed by the FBI is found at the inclusion note at E979. The terrorism E-code is the only E-code that should be assigned. Additional E codes from the assault categories should not be assigned.

2) ***Cause of an injury is suspected to be the result of terrorism***

When the cause of an injury is suspected to be the result of terrorism a code from category E979 should not be assigned. Assign a code in the range of E codes based circumstances on the documentation of intent and mechanism.

3) ***Code E979.9, Terrorism, secondary effects***

Assign code E979.9, Terrorism, secondary effects, for conditions occurring subsequent to the terrorist event. This code should not be assigned for conditions that are due to the initial terrorist act.

4) ***Statistical tabulation of terrorism codes***

For statistical purposes these codes will be tabulated within the category for assault, expanding the current category from E960-E969 to include E979 and E999.1.

4th **E979 Terrorism**

Injuries resulting from the unlawful use of force or violence against persons or property to intimidate or coerce a Government, the civilian population, or any segment thereof, in furtherance of political or social objective

E979.0 Terrorism involving explosion of marine weapons
- Depth-charge
- Marine mine
- Mine NOS, at sea or in harbour
- Sea-based artillery shell
- Torpedo
- Underwater blast

E979.1 Terrorism involving destruction of aircraft
- Aircraft used as a weapon
- Aircraft:
  - burned
  - exploded
  - shot down
- Crushed by falling aircraft

E979.2 Terrorism involving other explosions and fragments
- Antipersonnel bomb (fragments)
- Blast NOS
- Explosion (of):
  - artillery shell
  - breech-block
  - cannon block
  - mortar bomb
  - munitions being used in terrorism
  - NOS
- Fragments from:
  - artillery shell
  - bomb
  - grenade
  - guided missile
  - land-mine
  - rocket
  - shell
  - shrapnel
- Mine NOS

E979.3 Terrorism involving fires, conflagration and hot substances
- Burning building or structure:
  - collapse of
  - fall from
  - hit by falling object in
  - jump from
- Conflagration NOS
- Fire (causing):
  - asphyxia
  - burns
  - NOS
  - other injury
- Melting of fittings and furniture in burning
- Petrol bomb
- Smouldering building or structure

E979.4 Terrorism involving firearms
- Bullet:
  - carbine
  - machine gun
  - pistol
  - rifle
  - rubber (rifle)
- Pellets (shotgun)

E979.5 Terrorism involving nuclear weapons
- Blast effects
- Exposure to ionizing radiation from nuclear weapon
- Fireball effects
- Heat from nuclear weapon
- Other direct and secondary effects of nuclear weapons

E979.6 Terrorism involving biological weapons
- Anthrax
- Cholera
- Smallpox

E979.7 Terrorism involving chemical weapons
- Gases, fumes, chemicals
- Hydrogen cyanide
- Phosgene
- Sarin

E979.8 Terrorism involving other means
- Drowning and submersion
- Lasers
- Piercing or stabbing instruments
- Terrorism NOS

E979.9 Terrorism, secondary effects

Note: *This code is for use to identify conditions occurring subsequent to a terrorist attack not those that are due to the initial terrorist attack*

Excludes *late effect of terrorist attack (E999.1)*

INJURY UNDETERMINED WHETHER ACCIDENTALLY OR PURPOSELY INFLICTED (E980-E989)

Note: *Categories E980-E989 are for use when it is unspecified or it cannot be determined whether the injuries are accidental (unintentional), suicide (attempted), or assault.*

ICD-9-CM Official Guidelines (Chapter 19):

f. Unknown or Suspected Intent Guideline

1) If the intent (accident, self-harm, assault) of the cause of an injury or poisoning is unknown

If the intent (accident, self-harm, assault) of the cause of an injury or poisoning is unknown or unspecified, code the intent as undetermined E980-E989.

2) If the intent (accident, self-harm, assault) of the cause of an injury or poisoning is questionable

If the intent (accident, self-harm, assault) of the cause of an injury or poisoning is questionable, probable or suspected, code the intent as undetermined E980-E989.

4th **E980 Poisoning by solid or liquid substances, undetermined whether accidentally or purposely inflicted**

E980.0 Analgesics, antipyretics, and antirheumatics

E980.1 Barbiturates

E980.2 Other sedatives and hypnotics

E980.3 Tranquilizers and other psychotropic agents

E980.4 Other specified drugs and medicinal substances

E980.5 Unspecified drug or medicinal substance

E980.6 Corrosive and caustic substances

Poisoning, undetermined whether accidental or purposeful, by substances classifiable to E864

E980.7 Agricultural and horticultural chemical and pharmaceutical preparations other than plant foods and fertilizers

E980.8 Arsenic and its compounds

E980.9 Other and unspecified solid and liquid substances

4th **E981 Poisoning by gases in domestic use, undetermined whether accidentally or purposely inflicted**

E981.0 Gas distributed by pipeline

E981.1 Liquefied petroleum gas distributed in mobile containers

E981.8 Other utility gas

4th **E982 Poisoning by other gases, undetermined whether accidentally or purposely inflicted**

E982.0 Motor vehicle exhaust gas

E982.1 Other carbon monoxide

E982.8 Other specified gases and vapors

E982.9 Unspecified gases and vapors

4th **E983 Hanging, strangulation, or suffocation, undetermined whether accidentally or purposely inflicted**

E983.0 Hanging

E983.1 Suffocation by plastic bag

E983.8 Other specified means

E983.9 Unspecified means

E984 Submersion [drowning], undetermined whether accidentally or purposely inflicted

4th **E985 Injury by firearms, air guns and explosives, undetermined whether accidentally or purposely inflicted**

E985.0 Handgun

E985.1 Shotgun

E985.2 Hunting rifle

E985.3 Military firearms

E985.4 Other and unspecified firearm

E985.5 Explosives

E985.6 Air gun

BB gun

Pellet gun

E985.7 Paintball gun

E986 Injury by cutting and piercing instruments, undetermined whether accidentally or purposely inflicted

4th **E987 Falling from high place, undetermined whether accidentally or purposely inflicted**

E987.0 Residential premises

E987.1 Other man-made structures

E987.2 Natural sites

E987.9 Unspecified site

4th **E988 Injury by other and unspecified means, undetermined whether accidentally or purposely inflicted**

E988.0 Jumping or lying before moving object

E988.1 Burns, fire

E988.2 Scald

E988.3 Extremes of cold

E988.4 Electrocution

E988.5 Crashing of motor vehicle

E988.6 Crashing of aircraft

E988.7 Caustic substances, except poisoning

E988.8 Other specified means

E988.9 Unspecified means

E989 Late effects of injury, undetermined whether accidentally or purposely inflicted

Note: *This category is to be used to indicate circumstances classifiable to E980-E988 as the cause of death or disability from late effects, which are themselves classifiable elsewhere. The "late effects" include conditions reported as such or as sequelae which may occur at any time after injury, undetermined whether accidentally or purposely inflicted.*

INJURY RESULTING FROM OPERATIONS OF WAR (E990-E999)

Includes injuries to military personnel and civilians caused by war and civil insurrections and occurring during the time of war and insurrection, and peacekeeping missions

Excludes *accidents during training of military personnel, manufacture of war material and transport, unless attributable to enemy action*

4th **E990 Injury due to war operations by fires and conflagrations**

Includes asphyxia, burns, or other injury originating from fire caused by a fire-producing device or indirectly by any conventional weapon

E990.0 From gasoline bomb

Incendiary bomb

● **E990.1 From flamethrower**

● **E990.2 From incendiary bullet**

● **E990.3 From fire caused indirectly from conventional weapon**

Excludes *fire aboard military aircraft (E994.3)*

E990.9 From other and unspecified source

4th **E991 Injury due to war operations by bullets and fragments**

Excludes *injury due to bullets and fragments due to war operations, but occurring after cessation of hostilities (E998.0)*

injury due to explosion of artillery shells and mortars (E993.2)

injury due to explosion of improvised explosive device [IED] (E993.3-E993.5)

injury due to sea-based artillery shell (E992.3)

E991.0 Rubber bullets (rifle)

E991.1 Pellets (rifle)

E991.2 Other bullets
- Bullet [any, except rubber bullets and pellets]
  - carbine
  - machine gun
  - pistol
  - rifle
  - shotgun

E991.3 Antipersonnel bomb (fragments)

● **E991.4 Fragments from munitions**
- Fragments from:
  - artillery shell
  - bombs, except antipersonnel
  - detonation of unexploded ordnance [UXO]
  - grenade
  - guided missile
  - land mine
  - rockets
  - shell

● **E991.5 Fragments from person-borne improvised explosive device [IED]**

● **E991.6 Fragments from vehicle-borne improvised explosive device [IED]**
- IED borne by land, air, or water transport vehicle

● **E991.7 Fragments from other improvised explosive device [IED]**
- Roadside IED

● **E991.8 Fragments from weapons**
- Fragments from:
  - artillery
  - autocannons
  - automatic grenade launchers
  - missile launchers
  - mortars
  - small arms

E991.9 Other and unspecified fragments
- ~~Fragments from:~~
  - ~~artillery shell~~
  - ~~bombs, except antipersonnel~~
  - ~~grenade~~
  - ~~guided missile~~
  - ~~land mine~~
  - ~~rockets~~
  - ~~shell~~
- Shrapnel NOS

4th **E992 Injury due to war operations by explosion of marine weapons**
- ~~Depth charge~~
- ~~Marine mines~~
- ~~Mine NOS, at sea or in harbor~~
- ~~Sea-based artillery shell~~
- ~~Torpedo~~
- ~~Underwater blast~~

● **E992.0 Torpedo**

● **E992.1 Depth charge**

● **E992.2 Marine mines**
- Marine mines at sea or in harbor

● **E992.3 Sea-based artillery shell**

● **E992.8 Other by other marine weapons**

● **E992.9 Unspecified marine weapon**
- Underwater blast NOS

4th **E993 Injury due to war operations by other explosion**
- ~~Accidental explosion of munitions being used in war~~
- ~~Accidental explosion of own weapons~~
- ~~Air blast NOS~~
- ~~Blast NOS~~
- ~~Explosion NOS~~
- ~~Explosion of:~~
  - ~~artillery shell~~
  - ~~breech block~~
  - ~~cannon block~~
  - ~~mortar bomb~~
- ~~Injury by weapon burst~~
- Injuries due to direct or indirect pressure or air blast of an explosion occurring during war operations

Excludes *injury due to fragments resulting from an explosion (E991.0-E991.9)*
injury due to detonation of unexploded ordnance but occurring after cessation of hostilities (E998.0-E998.9)
injury due to nuclear weapons (E996.0-E996.9)

● **E993.0 Aerial bomb**

● **E993.1 Guided missile**

● **E993.2 Mortar**
- Artillery shell

● **E993.3 Person-borne improvised explosive device [IED]**

● **E993.4 Vehicle-borne improvised explosive device [IED]**
- IED borne by land, air, or water transport vehicle

● **E993.5 Other improvised explosive device [IED]**
- Roadside IED

● **E993.6 Unintentional detonation of own munitions**
- Unintentional detonation of own ammunition (artillery) (mortars)

● **E993.7 Unintentional discharge of own munitions launch device**
- Unintentional explosion of own:
  - Autocannons
  - Automatic grenade launchers
  - Missile launchers
  - Small arms

● **E993.8 Other specified explosion**
- Bomb
- Grenade
- Land mine

● **E993.9 Unspecified explosion**
- Air blast NOS
- Blast NOS
- Blast wave NOS
- Blast wind NOS
- Explosion NOS

4th **E994 Injury due to war operations by destruction of aircraft**
- ~~Airplane:~~
  - ~~burned~~
  - ~~exploded~~
  - ~~shot down~~
- ~~Crushed by falling airplane~~

● **E994.0 Destruction of aircraft due to enemy fire or explosives**
- Air to air missile
- Explosive device placed on aircraft
- Rocket propelled grenade [RPG]
- Small arms fire
- Surface to air missile

● **E994.1 Unintentional destruction of aircraft due to own onboard explosives**

● **E994.2 Destruction of aircraft due to collision with other aircraft**

● **E994.3 Destruction of aircraft due to onboard fire**

● **E994.8 Other destruction of aircraft**

● **E994.9 Unspecified destruction of aircraft**

4th E995 Injury due to war operations by other and unspecified forms of conventional warfare
~~Battle wounds~~
~~Bayonet injury~~
~~Drowned in war operations~~

● E995.0 Unarmed hand-to-hand combat
Excludes *intentional restriction of airway (E995.3)*

● E995.1 Struck by blunt object
Baton (nightstick)
Stave

● E995.2 Piercing object
Bayonet
Knife
Sword

● E995.3 Intentional restriction of air and airway
Intentional submersion
Strangulation
Suffocation

● E995.4 Unintentional drowning due to inability to surface or obtain air
Submersion

● E995.8 Other forms of conventional warfare

● E995.9 Unspecified form of conventional warfare

4th E996 Injury due to war operations by nuclear weapons
~~Blast effects~~
Dirty bomb
~~Exposure to ionizing radiation from nuclear weapons~~
~~Fireball effects~~
~~Heat~~
~~Other direct and secondary effects of nuclear weapons~~
Excludes *late effects of injury due to nuclear weapons (E999.0, E999.1)*

● E996.0 Direct blast effect of nuclear weapon
Injury to bodily organs due to blast pressure

● E996.1 Indirect blast effect of nuclear weapon
Injury due to being thrown by blast
Injury due to being struck or crushed by blast debris

● E996.2 Thermal radiation effect of nuclear weapon
Burns due to thermal radiation
Fireball effects
Flash burns
Heat effects

● E996.3 Nuclear radiation effects
Acute radiation exposure
Beta burns
Fallout exposure
Radiation sickness
Secondary effects of nuclear weapons

● E996.8 Other effects of nuclear weapons

● E996.9 Unspecified effect of nuclear weapon

4th E997 Injury due to war operations by other forms of unconventional warfare

E997.0 Lasers

E997.1 Biological warfare

E997.2 Gases, fumes, and chemicals

● E997.3 Weapon of mass destruction [WMD], unspecified

E997.8 Other specified forms of unconventional warfare

E997.9 Unspecified form of unconventional warfare

4th E998 Injury due to war operations but occurring after cessation of hostilities
Injuries by explosion of bombs or mines placed in the course of operations of war, if the explosion occurred after cessation of hostilities
Injuries due to operations of war but occurring after cessation of hostilities by any means classifiable under E990-E997

● E998.0 Explosion of mines

● E998.1 Explosion of bombs

● E998.8 Injury due to other war operations but occurring after cessation of hostilities

● E998.9 Injury due to unspecified war operations but occurring after cessation of hostilities

4th E999 Late effect of injury due to war operations and terrorism
Note: *This category is to be used to indicate circumstances classifiable to E979, E990-E998 as the cause of death or disability from late effects, which are themselves classifiable elsewhere. The "late effects" include conditions reported as such or as sequelae which may occur at any time after injury resulting from operations of war or terrorism.*

E999.0 Late effect of injury due to war operations

E999.1 Late effect of injury due to terrorism

Official ICD-9-CM Government Appendices

Appendix A: Morphology of Neoplasms

The World Health Organization has published an adaptation of the International Classification of Diseases for Oncology (ICD-O). It contains a coded nomenclature for the morphology of neoplasms, which is reproduced here for those who wish to use it in conjunction with Chapter 2 of the *International Classification of Diseases, 9th Revision, Clinical Modification.*

The morphology code numbers consist of five digits; the first four identify the histological type of the neoplasm and the fifth indicates its behavior. The one-digit behavior code is as follows:

/0 **Benign**

/1 **Uncertain whether benign or malignant**
Borderline malignancy

/2 **Carcinoma in situ**
Intraepithelial
Noninfiltrating
Noninvasive

/3 **Malignant, primary site**

/6 **Malignant, metastatic site**
Secondary site

/9 **Malignant, uncertain whether primary or metastatic site**

In the nomenclature below, the morphology code numbers include the behavior code appropriate to the histological type of neoplasm, but this behavior code should be changed if other reported information makes this necessary. For example, "chordoma (M9370/3)" is assumed to be malignant; the term "benign chordoma" should be coded M9370/0. Similarly, "superficial spreading adenocarcinoma (M8143/3)" described as "noninvasive" should be coded M8143/2 and "melanoma (M8720/3)" described as "secondary" should be coded M8720/6.

The following table shows the correspondence between the morphology code and the different sections of Chapter 2:

Morphology Code /Behavior Code		ICD-9-CM Chapter 2	
Any	/0	210-229	Benign neoplasms
M8000–M8004	/1	239	Neoplasms of unspecified nature
M8010+	/1	235-238	Neoplasms of uncertain behavior
Any	/2	230-234	Carcinoma in situ
Any	/3	140-195 200-208	Malignant neoplasms, stated or presumed to be primary
Any	/6	196-198	Malignant neoplasms, stated or presumed to be secondary

The ICD-O behavior digit /9 is inapplicable in an ICD context, since all malignant neoplasms are presumed to be primary (/3) or secondary (/6) according to other information on the medical record.

Only the first-listed term of the full ICD-O morphology nomenclature appears against each code number in the list below. The ICD-9-CM Alphabetical Index (Volume 2), however, includes all the ICD-O synonyms as well as a number of other morphological names still likely to be encountered on medical records but omitted from ICD-O as outdated or otherwise undesirable.

A coding difficulty sometimes arises where a morphological diagnosis contains two qualifying adjectives that have different code numbers. An example is "transitional cell epidermoid carcinomas." "Transitional cell carcinoma NOS" is M8120/3 and "epidermoid carcinoma NOS" is M8070/3. In such circumstances, the higher number (M8120/3 in this example) should be used, as it is usually more specific.

CODED NOMENCLATURE FOR MORPHOLOGY OF NEOPLASMS

M800 Neoplasms NOS

M8000/0 Neoplasm, benign
M8000/1 Neoplasm, uncertain whether benign or malignant
M8000/3 Neoplasm, malignant
M8000/6 Neoplasm, metastatic
M8000/9 Neoplasm, malignant, uncertain whether primary or metastatic
M8001/0 Tumor cells, benign
M8001/1 Tumor cells, uncertain whether benign or malignant
M8001/3 Tumor cells, malignant
M8002/3 Malignant tumor, small cell type
M8003/3 Malignant tumor, giant cell type
M8004/3 Malignant tumor, fusiform cell type

M801-M804 Epithelial neoplasms NOS

M8010/0 Epithelial tumor, benign
M8010/2 Carcinoma in situ NOS
M8010/3 Carcinoma NOS
M8010/6 Carcinoma, metastatic NOS
M8010/9 Carcinomatosis
M8011/0 Epithelioma, benign
M8011/3 Epithelioma, malignant
M8012/3 Large cell carcinoma NOS
M8020/3 Carcinoma, undifferentiated type NOS
M8021/3 Carcinoma, anaplastic type NOS
M8022/3 Pleomorphic carcinoma
M8030/3 Giant cell and spindle cell carcinoma
M8031/3 Giant cell carcinoma
M8032/3 Spindle cell carcinoma
M8033/3 Pseudosarcomatous carcinoma
M8034/3 Polygonal cell carcinoma
M8035/3 Spheroidal cell carcinoma
M8040/1 Tumorlet
M8041/3 Small cell carcinoma NOS
M8042/3 Oat cell carcinoma
M8043/3 Small cell carcinoma, fusiform cell type

M805-M808 Papillary and squamous cell neoplasms

M8050/0 Papilloma NOS (except Papilloma of urinary bladder M8120/1)
M8050/2 Papillary carcinoma in situ
M8050/3 Papillary carcinoma NOS
M8051/0 Verrucous papilloma
M8051/3 Verrucous carcinoma NOS
M8052/0 Squamous cell papilloma
M8052/3 Papillary squamous cell carcinoma
M8053/0 Inverted papilloma
M8060/0 Papillomatosis NOS
M8070/2 Squamous cell carcinoma in situ NOS
M8070/3 Squamous cell carcinoma NOS
M8070/6 Squamous cell carcinoma, metastatic NOS
M8071/3 Squamous cell carcinoma, keratinizing type NOS
M8072/3 Squamous cell carcinoma, large cell, nonkeratinizing type
M8073/3 Squamous cell carcinoma, small cell, nonkeratinizing type
M8074/3 Squamous cell carcinoma, spindle cell type
M8075/3 Adenoid squamous cell carcinoma
M8076/2 Squamous cell carcinoma in situ with questionable stromal invasion
M8076/3 Squamous cell carcinoma, microinvasive
M8080/2 Queyrat's erythroplasia
M8081/2 Bowen's disease
M8082/3 Lymphoepithelial carcinoma

M809-M811 Basal cell neoplasms

M8090/1 Basal cell tumor
M8090/3 Basal cell carcinoma NOS
M8091/3 Multicentric basal cell carcinoma
M8092/3 Basal cell carcinoma, morphea type
M8093/3 Basal cell carcinoma, fibroepithelial type
M8094/3 Basosquamous carcinoma
M8095/3 Metatypical carcinoma
M8096/0 Intraepidermal epithelioma of Jadassohn
M8100/0 Trichoepithelioma
M8101/0 Trichofolliculoma
M8102/0 Tricholemmoma
M8110/0 Pilomatrixoma

M812-M813 Transitional cell papillomas and carcinomas

M8120/0 Transitional cell papilloma NOS
M8120/1 Urothelial papilloma
M8120/2 Transitional cell carcinoma in situ
M8120/3 Transitional cell carcinoma NOS
M8121/0 Schneiderian papilloma
M8121/1 Transitional cell papilloma, inverted type
M8121/3 Schneiderian carcinoma
M8122/3 Transitional cell carcinoma, spindle cell type
M8123/3 Basaloid carcinoma
M8124/3 Cloacogenic carcinoma
M8130/3 Papillary transitional cell carcinoma

M814-M838 Adenomas and adenocarcinomas

M8140/0 Adenoma NOS
M8140/1 Bronchial adenoma NOS
M8140/2 Adenocarcinoma in situ
M8140/3 Adenocarcinoma NOS
M8140/6 Adenocarcinoma, metastatic NOS
M8141/3 Scirrhous adenocarcinoma
M8142/3 Linitis plastica
M8143/3 Superficial spreading adenocarcinoma
M8144/3 Adenocarcinoma, intestinal type
M8145/3 Carcinoma, diffuse type
M8146/0 Monomorphic adenoma
M8147/0 Basal cell adenoma
M8150/0 Islet cell adenoma
M8150/3 Islet cell carcinoma
M8151/0 Insulinoma NOS
M8151/3 Insulinoma, malignant
M8152/0 Glucagonoma NOS
M8152/3 Glucagonoma, malignant
M8153/1 Gastrinoma NOS
M8153/3 Gastrinoma, malignant
M8154/3 Mixed islet cell and exocrine adenocarcinoma
M8160/0 Bile duct adenoma
M8160/3 Cholangiocarcinoma
M8161/0 Bile duct cystadenoma
M8161/3 Bile duct cystadenocarcinoma
M8170/0 Liver cell adenoma
M8170/3 Hepatocellular carcinoma NOS
M8180/0 Hepatocholangioma, benign
M8180/3 Combined hepatocellular carcinoma and cholangiocarcinoma
M8190/0 Trabecular adenoma
M8190/3 Trabecular adenocarcinoma
M8191/0 Embryonal adenoma
M8200/0 Eccrine dermal cylindroma
M8200/3 Adenoid cystic carcinoma
M8201/3 Cribriform carcinoma
M8210/0 Adenomatous polyp NOS
M8210/3 Adenocarcinoma in adenomatous polyp
M8211/0 Tubular adenoma NOS
M8211/3 Tubular adenocarcinoma
M8220/0 Adenomatous polyposis coli
M8220/3 Adenocarcinoma in adenomatous polyposis coli
M8221/0 Multiple adenomatous polyps
M8230/3 Solid carcinoma NOS
M8231/3 Carcinoma simplex
M8240/1 Carcinoid tumor NOS
M8240/3 Carcinoid tumor, malignant
M8241/1 Carcinoid tumor, argentaffin NOS
M8241/3 Carcinoid tumor, argentaffin, malignant

© 2009 MAG Mutual Healthcare Solutions, Inc.

M8242/1 Carcinoid tumor, nonargentaffin NOS
M8242/3 Carcinoid tumor, nonargentaffin, malignant
M8243/3 Mucocarcinoid tumor, malignant
M8244/3 Composite carcinoid
M8250/1 Pulmonary adenomatosis
M8250/3 Bronchiolo-alveolar adenocarcinoma
M8251/0 Alveolar adenoma
M8251/3 Alveolar adenocarcinoma
M8260/0 Papillary adenoma NOS
M8260/3 Papillary adenocarcinoma NOS
M8261/1 Villous adenoma NOS
M8261/3 Adenocarcinoma in villous adenoma
M8262/3 Villous adenocarcinoma
M8263/0 Tubulovillous adenoma
M8270/0 Chromophobe adenoma
M8270/3 Chromophobe carcinoma
M8280/0 Acidophil adenoma
M8280/3 Acidophil carcinoma
M8281/0 Mixed acidophil-basophil adenoma
M8281/3 Mixed acidophil-basophil carcinoma
M8290/0 Oxyphilic adenoma
M8290/3 Oxyphilic adenocarcinoma
M8300/0 Basophil adenoma
M8300/3 Basophil carcinoma
M8310/0 Clear cell adenoma
M8310/3 Clear cell adenocarcinoma NOS
M8311/1 Hypernephroid tumor
M8312/3 Renal cell carcinoma
M8313/0 Clear cell adenofibroma
M8320/3 Granular cell carcinoma
M8321/0 Chief cell adenoma
M8322/0 Water-clear cell adenoma
M8322/3 Water-clear cell adenocarcinoma
M8323/0 Mixed cell adenoma
M8323/3 Mixed cell adenocarcinoma
M8324/0 Lipoadenoma
M8330/0 Follicular adenoma
M8330/3 Follicular adenocarcinoma NOS
M8331/3 Follicular adenocarcinoma, well differentiated type
M8332/3 Follicular adenocarcinoma, trabecular type
M8333/0 Microfollicular adenoma
M8334/0 Macrofollicular adenoma
M8340/3 Papillary and follicular adenocarcinoma
M8350/3 Nonencapsulated sclerosing carcinoma
M8360/1 Multiple endocrine adenomas
M8361/1 Juxtaglomerular tumor
M8370/0 Adrenal cortical adenoma NOS
M8370/3 Adrenal cortical carcinoma
M8371/0 Adrenal cortical adenoma, compact cell type
M8372/0 Adrenal cortical adenoma, heavily pigmented variant
M8373/0 Adrenal cortical adenoma, clear cell type
M8374/0 Adrenal cortical adenoma, glomerulosa cell type
M8375/0 Adrenal cortical adenoma, mixed cell type
M8380/0 Endometrioid adenoma NOS
M8380/1 Endometrioid adenoma, borderline malignancy
M8380/3 Endometrioid carcinoma
M8381/0 Endometrioid adenofibroma NOS
M8381/1 Endometrioid adenofibroma, borderline malignancy
M8381/3 Endometrioid adenofibroma, malignant

M839-M842 Adnexal and skin appendage neoplasms

M8390/0 Skin appendage adenoma
M8390/3 Skin appendage carcinoma
M8400/0 Sweat gland adenoma
M8400/1 Sweat gland tumor NOS
M8400/3 Sweat gland adenocarcinoma
M8401/0 Apocrine adenoma
M8401/3 Apocrine adenocarcinoma
M8402/0 Eccrine acrospiroma
M8403/0 Eccrine spiradenoma
M8404/0 Hidrocystoma
M8405/0 Papillary hydradenoma
M8406/0 Papillary syringadenoma
M8407/0 Syringoma NOS
M8410/0 Sebaceous adenoma
M8410/3 Sebaceous adenocarcinoma
M8420/0 Ceruminous adenoma
M8420/3 Ceruminous adenocarcinoma

M843 Mucoepidermoid neoplasms

M8430/1 Mucoepidermoid tumor
M8430/3 Mucoepidermoid carcinoma

M844-M849 Cystic, mucinous, and serous neoplasms

M8440/0 Cystadenoma NOS
M8440/3 Cystadenocarcinoma NOS
M8441/0 Serous cystadenoma NOS
M8441/1 Serous cystadenoma, borderline malignancy
M8441/3 Serous cystadenocarcinoma NOS
M8450/0 Papillary cystadenoma NOS
M8450/1 Papillary cystadenoma, borderline malignancy
M8450/3 Papillary cystadenocarcinoma NOS
M8460/0 Papillary serous cystadenoma NOS
M8460/1 Papillary serous cystadenoma, borderline malignancy
M8460/3 Papillary serous cystadenocarcinoma
M8461/0 Serous surface papilloma NOS
M8461/1 Serous surface papilloma, borderline malignancy
M8461/3 Serous surface papillary carcinoma
M8470/0 Mucinous cystadenoma NOS
M8470/1 Mucinous cystadenoma, borderline malignancy
M8470/3 Mucinous cystadenocarcinoma NOS
M8471/0 Papillary mucinous cystadenoma NOS
M8471/1 Papillary mucinous cystadenoma, borderline malignancy
M8471/3 Papillary mucinous cystadenocarcinoma
M8480/0 Mucinous adenoma
M8480/3 Mucinous adenocarcinoma
M8480/6 Pseudomyxoma peritonei
M8481/3 Mucin-producing adenocarcinoma
M8490/3 Signet ring cell carcinoma
M8490/6 Metastatic signet ring cell carcinoma

M850-M854 Ductal, lobular, and medullary neoplasms

M8500/2 Intraductal carcinoma, noninfiltrating NOS
M8500/3 Infiltrating duct carcinoma
M8501/2 Comedocarcinoma, noninfiltrating
M8501/3 Comedocarcinoma NOS
M8502/3 Juvenile carcinoma of the breast
M8503/0 Intraductal papilloma
M8503/2 Noninfiltrating intraductal papillary adenocarcinoma
M8504/0 Intracystic papillary adenoma
M8504/2 Noninfiltrating intracystic carcinoma
M8505/0 Intraductal papillomatosis NOS
M8506/0 Subareolar duct papillomatosis
M8510/3 Medullary carcinoma NOS
M8511/3 Medullary carcinoma with amyloid stroma
M8512/3 Medullary carcinoma with lymphoid stroma
M8520/2 Lobular carcinoma in situ
M8520/3 Lobular carcinoma NOS
M8521/3 Infiltrating ductular carcinoma
M8530/3 Inflammatory carcinoma
M8540/3 Paget's disease, mammary
M8541/3 Paget's disease and infiltrating duct carcinoma of breast
M8542/3 Paget's disease, extramammary (except Paget's disease of bone)

M855 Acinar cell neoplasms

M8550/0 Acinar cell adenoma
M8550/1 Acinar cell tumor
M8550/3 Acinar cell carcinoma

M856-M858 Complex epithelial neoplasms

M8560/3 Adenosquamous carcinoma
M8561/0 Adenolymphoma
M8570/3 Adenocarcinoma with squamous metaplasia
M8571/3 Adenocarcinoma with cartilaginous and osseous metaplasia
M8572/3 Adenocarcinoma with spindle cell metaplasia
M8573/3 Adenocarcinoma with apocrine metaplasia
M8580/0 Thymoma, benign
M8580/3 Thymoma, malignant

M859-M867 Specialized gonadal neoplasms

M8590/1 Sex cord-stromal tumor
M8600/0 Thecoma NOS
M8600/3 Theca cell carcinoma
M8610/0 Luteoma NOS
M8620/1 Granulosa cell tumor NOS
M8620/3 Granulosa cell tumor, malignant
M8621/1 Granulosa cell-theca cell tumor
M8630/0 Androblastoma, benign
M8630/1 Androblastoma NOS
M8630/3 Androblastoma, malignant
M8631/0 Sertoli-Leydig cell tumor
M8632/1 Gynandroblastoma
M8640/0 Tubular androblastoma NOS
M8640/3 Sertoli cell carcinoma
M8641/0 Tubular androblastoma with lipid storage
M8650/0 Leydig cell tumor, benign
M8650/1 Leydig cell tumor NOS
M8650/3 Leydig cell tumor, malignant
M8660/0 Hilar cell tumor
M8670/0 Lipid cell tumor of ovary
M8671/0 Adrenal rest tumor

M868-M871 Paragangliomas and glomus tumors

M8680/1 Paraganglioma NOS
M8680/3 Paraganglioma, malignant
M8681/1 Sympathetic paraganglioma
M8682/1 Parasympathetic paraganglioma
M8690/1 Glomus jugulare tumor
M8691/1 Aortic body tumor
M8692/1 Carotid body tumor
M8693/1 Extra-adrenal paraganglioma NOS
M8693/3 Extra-adrenal paraganglioma, malignant
M8700/0 Pheochromocytoma NOS
M8700/3 Pheochromocytoma, malignant
M8710/3 Glomangiosarcoma
M8711/0 Glomus tumor
M8712/0 Glomangioma

M872-M879 Nevi and melanomas

M8720/0 Pigmented nevus NOS
M8720/3 Malignant melanoma NOS
M8721/3 Nodular melanoma
M8722/0 Balloon cell nevus
M8722/3 Balloon cell melanoma
M8723/0 Halo nevus
M8724/0 Fibrous papule of the nose
M8725/0 Neuronevus
M8726/0 Magnocellular nevus
M8730/0 Nonpigmented nevus
M8730/3 Amelanotic melanoma
M8740/0 Junctional nevus
M8740/3 Malignant melanoma in junctional nevus
M8741/2 Precancerous melanosis NOS
M8741/3 Malignant melanoma in precancerous melanosis
M8742/2 Hutchinson's melanotic freckle
M8742/3 Malignant melanoma in Hutchinson's melanotic freckle
M8743/3 Superficial spreading melanoma
M8750/0 Intradermal nevus
M8760/0 Compound nevus
M8761/1 Giant pigmented nevus
M8761/3 Malignant melanoma in giant pigmented nevus
M8770/0 Epithelioid and spindle cell nevus
M8771/3 Epithelioid cell melanoma
M8772/3 Spindle cell melanoma NOS
M8773/3 Spindle cell melanoma, type A
M8774/3 Spindle cell melanoma, type B
M8775/3 Mixed epithelioid and spindle cell melanoma
M8780/0 Blue nevus NOS
M8780/3 Blue nevus, malignant
M8790/0 Cellular blue nevus

M880 Soft tissue tumors and sarcomas NOS

M8800/0 Soft tissue tumor, benign
M8800/3 Sarcoma NOS
M8800/9 Sarcomatosis NOS
M8801/3 Spindle cell sarcoma
M8802/3 Giant cell sarcoma (except of bone M9250/3)

© 2009 MAG Mutual Healthcare Solutions, Inc.

M8803/3 Small cell sarcoma
M8804/3 Epithelioid cell sarcoma

M881-M883 Fibromatous neoplasms

M8810/0 Fibroma NOS
M8810/3 Fibrosarcoma NOS
M8811/0 Fibromyxoma
M8811/3 Fibromyxosarcoma
M8812/0 Periosteal fibroma
M8812/3 Periosteal fibrosarcoma
M8813/0 Fascial fibroma
M8813/3 Fascial fibrosarcoma
M8814/3 Infantile fibrosarcoma
M8820/0 Elastofibroma
M8821/1 Aggressive fibromatosis
M8822/1 Abdominal fibromatosis
M8823/1 Desmoplastic fibroma
M8830/0 Fibrous histiocytoma NOS
M8830/1 Atypical fibrous histiocytoma
M8830/3 Fibrous histiocytoma, malignant
M8831/0 Fibroxanthoma NOS
M8831/1 Atypical fibroxanthoma
M8831/3 Fibroxanthoma, malignant
M8832/0 Dermatofibroma NOS
M8832/1 Dermatofibroma protuberans
M8832/3 Dermatofibrosarcoma NOS

M884 Myxomatous neoplasms

M8840/0 Myxoma NOS
M8840/3 Myxosarcoma

M885-M888 Lipomatous neoplasms

M8850/0 Lipoma NOS
M8850/3 Liposarcoma NOS
M8851/0 Fibrolipoma
M8851/3 Liposarcoma, well differentiated type
M8852/0 Fibromyxolipoma
M8852/3 Myxoid liposarcoma
M8853/3 Round cell liposarcoma
M8854/3 Pleomorphic liposarcoma
M8855/3 Mixed type liposarcoma
M8856/0 Intramuscular lipoma
M8857/0 Spindle cell lipoma
M8860/0 Angiomyolipoma
M8860/3 Angiomyoliposarcoma
M8861/0 Angiolipoma NOS
M8861/1 Angiolipoma, infiltrating
M8870/0 Myelolipoma
M8880/0 Hibernoma
M8881/0 Lipoblastomatosis

M889-M892 Myomatous neoplasms

M8890/0 Leiomyoma NOS
M8890/1 Intravascular leiomyomatosis
M8890/3 Leiomyosarcoma NOS
M8891/1 Epithelioid leiomyoma
M8891/3 Epithelioid leiomyosarcoma
M8892/1 Cellular leiomyoma
M8893/0 Bizarre leiomyoma
M8894/0 Angiomyoma
M8894/3 Angiomyosarcoma
M8895/0 Myoma
M8895/3 Myosarcoma
M8900/0 Rhabdomyoma NOS
M8900/3 Rhabdomyosarcoma NOS
M8901/3 Pleomorphic rhabdomyosarcoma
M8902/3 Mixed type rhabdomyosarcoma
M8903/0 Fetal rhabdomyoma
M8904/0 Adult rhabdomyoma
M8910/3 Embryonal rhabdomyosarcoma
M8920/3 Alveolar rhabdomyosarcoma

M893-M899 Complex mixed and stromal neoplasms

M8930/3 Endometrial stromal sarcoma
M8931/1 Endolymphatic stromal myosis
M8932/0 Adenomyoma
M8940/0 Pleomorphic adenoma
M8940/3 Mixed tumor, malignant NOS
M8950/3 Mullerian mixed tumor
M8951/3 Mesodermal mixed tumor
M8960/1 Mesoblastic nephroma
M8960/3 Nephroblastoma NOS
M8961/3 Epithelial nephroblastoma
M8962/3 Mesenchymal nephroblastoma
M8970/3 Hepatoblastoma
M8980/3 Carcinosarcoma NOS
M8981/3 Carcinosarcoma, embryonal type
M8982/0 Myoepithelioma
M8990/0 Mesenchymoma, benign
M8990/1 Mesenchymoma NOS
M8990/3 Mesenchymoma, malignant
M8991/3 Embryonal sarcoma

M900-M903 Fibroepithelial neoplasms

M9000/0 Brenner tumor NOS
M9000/1 Brenner tumor, borderline malignancy
M9000/3 Brenner tumor, malignant
M9010/0 Fibroadenoma NOS
M9011/0 Intracanalicular fibroadenoma NOS
M9012/0 Pericanalicular fibroadenoma
M9013/0 Adenofibroma NOS
M9014/0 Serous adenofibroma
M9015/0 Mucinous adenofibroma
M9020/0 Cellular intracanalicular fibroadenoma
M9020/1 Cystosarcoma phyllodes NOS
M9020/3 Cystosarcoma phyllodes, malignant
M9030/0 Juvenile fibroadenoma

M904 Synovial neoplasms

M9040/0 Synovioma, benign
M9040/3 Synovial sarcoma NOS
M9041/3 Synovial sarcoma, spindle cell type
M9042/3 Synovial sarcoma, epithelioid cell type
M9043/3 Synovial sarcoma, biphasic type
M9044/3 Clear cell sarcoma of tendons and aponeuroses

M905 Mesothelial neoplasms

M9050/0 Mesothelioma, benign
M9050/3 Mesothelioma, malignant
M9051/0 Fibrous mesothelioma, benign
M9051/3 Fibrous mesothelioma, malignant
M9052/0 Epithelioid mesothelioma, benign
M9052/3 Epithelioid mesothelioma, malignant
M9053/0 Mesothelioma, biphasic type, benign
M9053/3 Mesothelioma, biphasic type, malignant
M9054/0 Adenomatoid tumor NOS

M906-M909 Germ cell neoplasms

M9060/3 Dysgerminoma
M9061/3 Seminoma NOS
M9062/3 Seminoma, anaplastic type
M9063/3 Spermatocytic seminoma
M9064/3 Germinoma
M9070/3 Embryonal carcinoma NOS
M9071/3 Endodermal sinus tumor
M9072/3 Polyembryoma
M9073/1 Gonadoblastoma
M9080/0 Teratoma, benign
M9080/1 Teratoma NOS
M9080/3 Teratoma, malignant NOS
M9081/3 Teratocarcinoma
M9082/3 Malignant teratoma, undifferentiated type
M9083/3 Malignant teratoma, intermediate type
M9084/0 Dermoid cyst
M9084/3 Dermoid cyst with malignant transformation
M9090/0 Struma ovarii NOS
M9090/3 Struma ovarii, malignant
M9091/1 Strumal carcinoid

M910 Trophoblastic neoplasms

M9100/0 Hydatidiform mole NOS
M9100/1 Invasive hydatidiform mole
M9100/3 Choriocarcinoma
M9101/3 Choriocarcinoma combined with teratoma
M9102/3 Malignant teratoma, trophoblastic

M911 Mesonephromas

M9110/0 Mesonephroma, benign
M9110/1 Mesonephric tumor
M9110/3 Mesonephroma, malignant
M9111/1 Endosalpingioma

M912-M916 Blood vessel tumors

M9120/0 Hemangioma NOS
M9120/3 Hemangiosarcoma
M9121/0 Cavernous hemangioma
M9122/0 Venous hemangioma
M9123/0 Racemose hemangioma
M9124/3 Kupffer cell sarcoma
M9130/0 Hemangioendothelioma, benign
M9130/1 Hemangioendothelioma NOS
M9130/3 Hemangioendothelioma, malignant
M9131/0 Capillary hemangioma
M9132/0 Intramuscular hemangioma
M9140/3 Kaposi's sarcoma
M9141/0 Angiokeratoma
M9142/0 Verrucous keratotic hemangioma
M9150/0 Hemangiopericytoma, benign
M9150/1 Hemangiopericytoma NOS
M9150/3 Hemangiopericytoma, malignant
M9160/0 Angiofibroma NOS
M9161/1 Hemangioblastoma

M917 Lymphatic vessel tumors

M9170/0 Lymphangioma NOS
M9170/3 Lymphangiosarcoma
M9171/0 Capillary lymphangioma
M9172/0 Cavernous lymphangioma
M9173/0 Cystic lymphangioma
M9174/0 Lymphangiomyoma
M9174/1 Lymphangiomyomatosis
M9175/0 Hemolymphangioma

M918-M920 Osteomas and osteosarcomas

M9180/0 Osteoma NOS
M9180/3 Osteosarcoma NOS
M9181/3 Chondroblastic osteosarcoma
M9182/3 Fibroblastic osteosarcoma
M9183/3 Telangiectatic osteosarcoma
M9184/3 Osteosarcoma in Paget's disease of bone
M9190/3 Juxtacortical osteosarcoma
M9191/0 Osteoid osteoma NOS
M9200/0 Osteoblastoma

M921-M924 Chondromatous neoplasms

M9210/0 Osteochondroma
M9210/1 Osteochondromatosis NOS
M9220/0 Chondroma NOS
M9220/1 Chondromatosis NOS
M9220/3 Chondrosarcoma NOS
M9221/0 Juxtacortical chondroma
M9221/3 Juxtacortical chondrosarcoma
M9230/0 Chondroblastoma NOS
M9230/3 Chondroblastoma, malignant
M9240/3 Mesenchymal chondrosarcoma
M9241/0 Chondromyxoid fibroma

M925 Giant cell tumors

M9250/1 Giant cell tumor of bone NOS
M9250/3 Giant cell tumor of bone, malignant
M9251/1 Giant cell tumor of soft parts NOS
M9251/3 Malignant giant cell tumor of soft parts

M926 Miscellaneous bone tumors

M9260/3 Ewing's sarcoma
M9261/3 Adamantinoma of long bones
M9262/0 Ossifying fibroma

M927-M934 Odontogenic tumors

M9270/0 Odontogenic tumor, benign
M9270/1 Odontogenic tumor NOS
M9270/3 Odontogenic tumor, malignant
M9271/0 Dentinoma
M9272/0 Cementoma NOS
M9273/0 Cementoblastoma, benign
M9274/0 Cementifying fibroma
M9275/0 Gigantiform cementoma
M9280/0 Odontoma NOS
M9281/0 Compound odontoma
M9282/0 Complex odontoma
M9290/0 Ameloblastic fibro-odontoma
M9290/3 Ameloblastic odontosarcoma
M9300/0 Adenomatoid odontogenic tumor
M9301/0 Calcifying odontogenic cyst
M9310/0 Ameloblastoma NOS
M9310/3 Ameloblastoma, malignant
M9311/0 Odontoameloblastoma
M9312/0 Squamous odontogenic tumor
M9320/0 Odontogenic myxoma
M9321/0 Odontogenic fibroma NOS
M9330/0 Ameloblastic fibroma
M9330/3 Ameloblastic fibrosarcoma
M9340/0 Calcifying epithelial odontogenic tumor

© 2009 MAG Mutual Healthcare Solutions, Inc.

M935-M937 Miscellaneous tumors
M9350/1 Craniopharyngioma
M9360/1 Pinealoma
M9361/1 Pineocytoma
M9362/3 Pineoblastoma
M9363/0 Melanotic neuroectodermal tumor
M9370/3 Chordoma

M938-M948 Gliomas
M9380/3 Glioma, malignant
M9381/3 Gliomatosis cerebri
M9382/3 Mixed glioma
M9383/1 Subependymal glioma
M9384/1 Subependymal giant cell astrocytoma
M9390/0 Choroid plexus papilloma NOS
M9390/3 Choroid plexus papilloma, malignant
M9391/3 Ependymoma NOS
M9392/3 Ependymoma, anaplastic type
M9393/1 Papillary ependymoma
M9394/1 Myxopapillary ependymoma
M9400/3 Astrocytoma NOS
M9401/3 Astrocytoma, anaplastic type
M9410/3 Protoplasmic astrocytoma
M9411/3 Gemistocytic astrocytoma
M9420/3 Fibrillary astrocytoma
M9421/3 Pilocytic astrocytoma
M9422/3 Spongioblastoma NOS
M9423/3 Spongioblastoma polare
M9430/3 Astroblastoma
M9440/3 Glioblastoma NOS
M9441/3 Giant cell glioblastoma
M9442/3 Glioblastoma with sarcomatous component
M9443/3 Primitive polar spongioblastoma
M9450/3 Oligodendroglioma NOS
M9451/3 Oligodendroglioma, anaplastic type
M9460/3 Oligodendroblastoma
M9470/3 Medulloblastoma NOS
M9471/3 Desmoplastic medulloblastoma
M9472/3 Medullomyoblastoma
M9480/3 Cerebellar sarcoma NOS
M9481/3 Monstrocellular sarcoma

M949-M952 Neuroepitheliomatous neoplasms
M9490/0 Ganglioneuroma
M9490/3 Ganglioneuroblastoma
M9491/0 Ganglioneuromatosis
M9500/3 Neuroblastoma NOS
M9501/3 Medulloepithelioma NOS
M9502/3 Teratoid medulloepithelioma
M9503/3 Neuroepithelioma NOS
M9504/3 Spongioneuroblastoma
M9505/1 Ganglioglioma
M9506/0 Neurocytoma
M9507/0 Pacinian tumor
M9510/3 Retinoblastoma NOS
M9511/3 Retinoblastoma, differentiated type
M9512/3 Retinoblastoma, undifferentiated type
M9520/3 Olfactory neurogenic tumor
M9521/3 Esthesioneurocytoma
M9522/3 Esthesioneuroblastoma
M9523/3 Esthesioneuroepithelioma

M953 Meningiomas
M9530/0 Meningioma NOS
M9530/1 Meningiomatosis NOS
M9530/3 Meningioma, malignant
M9531/0 Meningotheliomatous meningioma
M9532/0 Fibrous meningioma
M9533/0 Psammomatous meningioma
M9534/0 Angiomatous meningioma
M9535/0 Hemangioblastic meningioma
M9536/0 Hemangiopericytic meningioma
M9537/0 Transitional meningioma
M9538/1 Papillary meningioma
M9539/3 Meningeal sarcomatosis

M954-M957 Nerve sheath tumor
M9540/0 Neurofibroma NOS
M9540/1 Neurofibromatosis NOS
M9540/3 Neurofibrosarcoma
M9541/0 Melanotic neurofibroma
M9550/0 Plexiform neurofibroma
M9560/0 Neurilemmoma NOS
M9560/1 Neurinomatosis
M9560/3 Neurilemmoma, malignant
M9570/0 Neuroma NOS

M958 Granular cell tumors and alveolar soft part sarcoma
M9580/0 Granular cell tumor NOS
M9580/3 Granular cell tumor, malignant
M9581/3 Alveolar soft part sarcoma

M959-M963 Lymphomas, NOS or diffuse
M9590/0 Lymphomatous tumor, benign
M9590/3 Malignant lymphoma NOS
M9591/3 Malignant lymphoma, non Hodgkin's type
M9600/3 Malignant lymphoma, undifferentiated cell type NOS
M9601/3 Malignant lymphoma, stem cell type
M9602/3 Malignant lymphoma, convoluted cell type NOS
M9610/3 Lymphosarcoma NOS
M9611/3 Malignant lymphoma, lymphoplasmacytoid type
M9612/3 Malignant lymphoma, immunoblastic type
M9613/3 Malignant lymphoma, mixed lymphocytic-histiocytic NOS
M9614/3 Malignant lymphoma, centroblastic-centrocytic, diffuse
M9615/3 Malignant lymphoma, follicular center cell NOS
M9620/3 Malignant lymphoma, lymphocytic, well differentiated NOS
M9621/3 Malignant lymphoma, lymphocytic, intermediate differentiation NOS
M9622/3 Malignant lymphoma, centrocytic
M9623/3 Malignant lymphoma, follicular center cell, cleaved NOS
M9630/3 Malignant lymphoma, lymphocytic, poorly differentiated NOS
M9631/3 Prolymphocytic lymphosarcoma
M9632/3 Malignant lymphoma, centroblastic type NOS
M9633/3 Malignant lymphoma, follicular center cell, noncleaved NOS

M964 Reticulosarcomas
M9640/3 Reticulosarcoma NOS
M9641/3 Reticulosarcoma, pleomorphic cell type
M9642/3 Reticulosarcoma, nodular

M965-M966 Hodgkin's disease
M9650/3 Hodgkin's disease NOS
M9651/3 Hodgkin's disease, lymphocytic predominance
M9652/3 Hodgkin's disease, mixed cellularity
M9653/3 Hodgkin's disease, lymphocytic depletion NOS
M9654/3 Hodgkin's disease, lymphocytic depletion, diffuse fibrosis
M9655/3 Hodgkin's disease, lymphocytic depletion, reticular type
M9656/3 Hodgkin's disease, nodular sclerosis NOS
M9657/3 Hodgkin's disease, nodular sclerosis, cellular phase
M9660/3 Hodgkin's paragranuloma
M9661/3 Hodgkin's granuloma
M9662/3 Hodgkin's sarcoma

M969 Lymphomas, nodular or follicular
M9690/3 Malignant lymphoma, nodular NOS
M9691/3 Malignant lymphoma, mixed lymphocytic-histiocytic, nodular
M9692/3 Malignant lymphoma, centroblastic-centrocytic, follicular
M9693/3 Malignant lymphoma, lymphocytic, well differentiated, nodular
M9694/3 Malignant lymphoma, lymphocytic, intermediate differentiation, nodular
M9695/3 Malignant lymphoma, follicular center cell, cleaved, follicular
M9696/3 Malignant lymphoma, lymphocytic, poorly differentiated, nodular
M9697/3 Malignant lymphoma, centroblastic type, follicular
M9698/3 Malignant lymphoma, follicular center cell, noncleaved, follicular

M970 Mycosis fungoides
M9700/3 Mycosis fungoides
M9701/3 Sezary's disease

M971-M972 Miscellaneous reticuloendothelial neoplasms
M9710/3 Microglioma
M9720/3 Malignant histiocytosis
M9721/3 Histiocytic medullary reticulosis
M9722/3 Letterer-Siwe's disease

M973 Plasma cell tumors
M9730/3 Plasma cell myeloma
M9731/0 Plasma cell tumor, benign
M9731/1 Plasmacytoma NOS
M9731/3 Plasma cell tumor, malignant

M974 Mast cell tumors
M9740/1 Mastocytoma NOS
M9740/3 Mast cell sarcoma
M9741/3 Malignant mastocytosis

M975 Burkitt's tumor
M9750/3 Burkitt's tumor

M980 Leukemias NOS
M9800/3 Leukemia NOS
M9801/3 Acute leukemia NOS
M9802/3 Subacute leukemia NOS
M9803/3 Chronic leukemia NOS
M9804/3 Aleukemic leukemia NOS

M981 Compound leukemias
M9810/3 Compound leukemia

M982 Lymphoid leukemias
M9820/3 Lymphoid leukemia NOS
M9821/3 Acute lymphoid leukemia
M9822/3 Subacute lymphoid leukemia
M9823/3 Chronic lymphoid leukemia
M9824/3 Aleukemic lymphoid leukemia
M9825/3 Prolymphocytic leukemia

M983 Plasma cell leukemias
M9830/3 Plasma cell leukemia

M984 Erythroleukemias
M9840/3 Erythroleukemia
M9841/3 Acute erythremia
M9842/3 Chronic erythremia

M985 Lymphosarcoma cell leukemias
M9850/3 Lymphosarcoma cell leukemia

M986 Myeloid leukemias
M9860/3 Myeloid leukemia NOS
M9861/3 Acute myeloid leukemia
M9862/3 Subacute myeloid leukemia
M9863/3 Chronic myeloid leukemia
M9864/3 Aleukemic myeloid leukemia
M9865/3 Neutrophilic leukemia
M9866/3 Acute promyelocytic leukemia

M987 Basophilic leukemias
M9870/3 Basophilic leukemia

M988 Eosinophilic leukemias
M9880/3 Eosinophilic leukemia

M989 Monocytic leukemias
M9890/3 Monocytic leukemia NOS
M9891/3 Acute monocytic leukemia
M9892/3 Subacute monocytic leukemia
M9893/3 Chronic monocytic leukemia
M9894/3 Aleukemic monocytic leukemia

M990-M994 Miscellaneous leukemias
M9900/3 Mast cell leukemia
M9910/3 Megakaryocytic leukemia
M9920/3 Megakaryocytic myelosis
M9930/3 Myeloid sarcoma
M9940/3 Hairy cell leukemia

M995-M997 Miscellaneous myeloproliferative and lymphoproliferative disorders
M9950/1 Polycythemia vera
M9951/1 Acute panmyelosis
M9960/1 Chronic myeloproliferative disease
M9961/1 Myelosclerosis with myeloid metaplasia
M9962/1 Idiopathic thrombocythemia
M9970/1 Chronic lymphoproliferative disease

© 2009 MAG Mutual Healthcare Solutions, Inc.

Appendix C: Classification of Drugs by American Hospital Formulary Services List Number and their ICD-9-CM Equivalents

The coding of adverse effects of drugs is keyed to the continually revised Hospital Formulary of the American Hospital Formulary Service (AHFS) published under the direction of the American Society of Hospital Pharmacists.

The following section gives the ICD-9-CM diagnosis code for each AHFS list.

AHFS Pharmacologic/Therapeutic Classification		ICD-9 Code
4:00	ANTIHISTAMINE DRUGS	963.0
8:00	ANTI-INFECTIVE AGENTS	
8:04	Amebacides	961.5
	hydroxyquinoline derivatives	961.3
	arsenical anti-infectives	961.1
8:08	Anthelmintics	961.6
	quinoline derivatives	961.3
8:12.04	Antifungal Antibiotics	960.1
	nonantibiotics	961.9
8:12.06	Cephalosporins	960.5
8:12.08	Chloramphenicol	960.2
8:12.12	The Erythromycins	960.3
8:12.16	The Penicillins	960.0
8:12.20	The Streptomycins	960.6
8:12.24	The Tetracyclines	960.4
8:12.28	Other Antibiotics	960.8
	antimycobacterial antibiotics	960.6
	macrolides	960.3
8:16	Antituberculars	961.8
	antibiotics	960.6
8:18	Antivirals	961.7
8:20	Plasmodicides (antimalarials)	961.4
8:24	Sulfonamides	961.0
8:26	The Sulfones	961.8
8:28	Treponemicides	961.2
8:32	Trichomonacides	961.5
	hydroxyquinoline derivatives	961.3
	nitrofuran derivatives	961.9
8:36	Urinary Germicides	961.9
	quinoline derivatives	961.3
8:40	Other Anti-Infectives	961.9
10:00	ANTINEOPLASTIC AGENTS	963.1
	antibiotics	960.7
	progestogens	962.2
12:00	AUTONOMIC DRUGS	
12:04	Parasympathomimetic (Cholinergic) Agents	971.0
12:08	Parasympatholytic (Cholinergic Blocking) Agents	971.1
12:12	Sympathomimetic (Adrenergic) Agents	971.2
12:16	Sympatholytic (Adrenergic Blocking) Agents	971.3
12:20	Skeletal Muscle Relaxants	975.2
	central nervous system muscle-tone depressants	968.0
16:00	BLOOD DERIVATIVES	964.7
20:00	BLOOD FORMATION AND COAGULATION	
20:04	Antianemia Drugs	964.1
20:04.04	Iron Preparations	964.0
20:04.08	Liver and Stomach Preparations	964.1
20:12.04	Anticoagulants	964.2
20:12.08	Antiheparin agents	964.5
20:12.12	Coagulants	964.5
20.12.16	Hemostatics	964.5
	capillary-active drugs	972.8
	fibrinolysis-affecting agents	964.4
	natural products	964.7
24:00	CARDIOVASCULAR DRUGS	
24:04	Cardiac Drugs	972.9
	cardiotonic agents	972.1
	rhythm regulators	972.0
24:06	Antilipemic Agents	972.2
	thyroid derivatives	962.7
24:08	Hypotensive Agents	972.6
	adrenergic blocking agents	971.3
	ganglion-blocking agents	972.3
	vasodilators	972.5
24:12	Vasodilating Agents	972.5
	coronary	972.4
	nicotinic acid derivatives	972.2
24:16	Sclerosing Agents	972.7
28:00	CENTRAL NERVOUS SYSTEM DRUGS	
28:04	General Anesthetics	968.4
	gaseous anesthetics	968.2
	halothane	968.1
	intravenous anesthetics	968.3
28:08	Analgesics and Antipyretics	965.9
	antirheumatics	965.6
	aromatic analgesics	965.4
	non-narcotics NEC	965.7
	opium alkaloids	965.00
	heroin	965.01
	methadone	965.02
	specified type NEC	965.09
	pyrazole derivatives	965.5
	salicylates	965.1
	specified type NEC	965.8
28:10	Narcotic Antagonists	970.1
28:12	Anticonvulsants	966.3
	barbiturates	967.0
	benzodiazepine-based tranquilizers	969.4
	bromides	967.3
	hydantoin derivatives	966.1
	oxazolidine derivative	966.0
	succinimides	966.2
28:16.04	Antidepressants	969.0
28:16.08	Tranquilizers	969.5
	benzodiazepine-based	969.4
	butyrophenone-based	969.2
	major NEC	969.3
	phenothiazine-based	969.1
28:16.12	Other Psychotherapeutic Agents	969.8
28:20	Respiratory and Cerebral Stimulants	970.9
	analeptics	970.0
	anorexigenic agents	977.0
	psychostimulants	969.7
	specified type NEC	970.8
28:24	Sedatives and Hypnotics	967.9
	barbiturates	967.0
	benzodiazepine-based tranquilizers	969.4
	chloral hydrate group	967.1
	glutethimide group	967.5
	intravenous anesthetics	968.3
	methaqualone	967.4
	paraldehyde	967.2
	phenothiazine-based tranquilizers	969.1
	specified type NEC	967.8
	thiobarbiturates	968.3
	tranquilizer NEC	969.5
36:00	DIAGNOSTIC AGENTS	977.8
40:00	ELECTROLYTE, CALORIC, AND WATER BALANCE AGENTS NEC	974.5
40:04	Acidifying Agents	963.2
40:08	Alkalinizing Agents	963.3
40:10	Ammonia Detoxicants	974.5
40:12	Replacement Solutions NEC	974.5
	plasma volume expanders	964.8
40:16	Sodium-Removing Resins	974.5
40:18	Potassium-Removing Resins	974.5
40:20	Caloric Agents	974.5
40:24	Salt and Sugar Substitutes	974.5
40:28	Diuretics NEC	974.4
	carbonic acid anhydrase inhibitors	974.2
	mercurials	974.0
	purine derivatives	974.1
	saluretics	974.3
40:36	Irrigating Solutions	974.5
40:40	Uricosuric Agents	974.7
44:00	ENZYMES NEC	963.4
	fibrinolysis-affecting agents	964.4
	gastric agents	973.4
48:00	EXPECTORANTS AND COUGH PREPARATIONS	
	antihistamine agents	963.0
	antitussives	975.4
	codeine derivatives	965.09
	expectorants	975.5
	narcotic agents NEC	965.09
52:00	EYE, EAR, NOSE, AND THROAT PREPARATIONS	
52:04	Anti-Infectives	
	ENT	976.6
	ophthalmic	976.5
52:04.04	Antibiotics	
	ENT	976.6
	ophthalmic	976.5
52:04.06	Antivirals	
	ENT	976.6
	ophthalmic	976.5
52:04.08	Sulfonamides	
	ENT	976.6
	ophthalmic	976.5
52:04.12	Miscellaneous Anti-Infectives	
	ENT	976.6
	ophthalmic	976.5
52:08	Anti-Inflammatory Agents	
	ENT	976.6
	ophthalmic	976.5
52:10	Carbonic Anhydrase Inhibitors	974.2
52:12	Contact Lens Solutions	976.5
52:16	Local Anesthetics	968.5
52:20	Miotics	971.0
52:24	Mydriatics	
	adrenergics	971.2
	anticholinergics	971.1
	antimuscarinics	971.1
	parasympatholytics	971.1
	spasmolytics	971.1
	sympathomimetics	971.2
52:28	Mouth Washes and Gargles	976.6
52:32	Vasoconstrictors	971.2
52:36	Unclassified Agents	
	ENT	976.6
	ophthalmic	976.5
56:00	GASTROINTESTINAL DRUGS	
56:04	Antacids and Absorbents	973.0
56:08	Anti-Diarrhea Agents	973.5
56:10	Antiflatulents	973.8
56:12	Cathartics NEC	973.3
	emollients	973.2
	irritants	973.1
56:16	Digestants	973.4
56:20	Emetics and Antiemetics	
	antiemetics	963.0
	emetics	973.6
56:24	Lipotropic Agents	977.1
60:00	GOLD COMPOUNDS	965.6
64:00	HEAVY METAL ANTAGONISTS	963.8

© 2009 MAG Mutual Healthcare Solutions, Inc.

AHFS Pharmacologic/Therapeutic Classification		ICD-9 Code
68:00	HORMONES AND SYNTHETIC SUBSTITUTES	
68:04	Adrenals	962.0
68:08	Androgens	962.1
68:12	Contraceptives	962.2
68:16	Estrogens	962.2
68:18	Gonadotropins	962.4
68:20	Insulins and Antidiabetic Agents	962.3
68:20.08	Insulins	962.3
68:24	Parathyroid	962.6
68:28	Pituitary	
	anterior	962.4
	posterior	962.5
68:32	Progestogens	962.2
68:34	Other Corpus Luteum Hormones	962.2
68:36	Thyroid and Antithyroid	
	antithyroid	962.8
	thyroid	962.7
72:00	LOCAL ANESTHETICS NEC	968.9
	topical (surface) agents	968.5
	infiltrating agents (intradermal) (sub-cutaneous) (submucosal)	968.5
	nerve blocking agents (peripheral) (plexus) (regional)	968.6
	spinal	968.7
76:00	OXYTOCICS	975.0
78:00	RADIOACTIVE AGENTS	990

AHFS Pharmacologic/Therapeutic Classification		ICD-9 Code
80:00	SERUMS, TOXOIDS, AND VACCINES	
80:04	Serums	979.9
	immune globulin (gamma) (human)	964.6
80:08	Toxoids NEC	978.8
	diphtheria	978.5
	and tetanus	978.9
	with pertussis component	978.6
	tetanus	978.4
	and diphtheria	978.9
	with pertussis component	978.6
80:12	Vaccines NEC	979.9
	bacterial NEC	978.8
	with	
	other bacterial component	978.9
	pertussis component	978.6
	viral and rickettsial component	979.7
	rickettsial NEC	979.6
	with	
	bacterial component	979.7
	pertussis component	978.6
	viral component	979.7
	viral NEC	979.6
	with	
	bacterial component	979.7
	pertussis component	978.6
	rickettsial component	979.7

AHFS Pharmacologic/Therapeutic Classification		ICD-9 Code
84:00	SKIN AND MUCOUS MEMBRANE PREPARATIONS	
84:04	Anti-Infectives	976.0
84:04.04	Antibiotics	976.0
84:04.08	Fungicides	976.0
84:04.12	Scabicides and Pediculicides	976.0
84:04.16	Miscellaneous Local Anti-Infectives	976.0
84:06	Anti-Inflammatory Agents	976.0
84:08	Antipruritics and Local Anesthetics	
	antipruritics	976.1
	local anesthetics	968.5
84:12	Astringents	976.2
84:16	Cell Stimulants and Proliferants	976.8
84:20	Detergents	976.2
84:24	Emollients, Demulcents, and Protectants	976.3
84:28	Keratolytic Agents	976.4
84:32	Keratoplastic Agents	976.4
84:36	Miscellaneous Agents	976.8
86:00	SPASMOLYTIC AGENTS	975.1
	antiasthmatics	975.7
	papaverine	972.5
	theophyllin	974.1
88:00	VITAMINS	
88:04	Vitamin A	963.5
88:08	Vitamin B Complex	963.5
	hematopoietic vitamin	964.1
	nicotinic acid derivatives	972.2
88:12	Vitamin C	963.5
88:16	Vitamin D	963.5
88:20	Vitamin E	963.5
88:24	Vitamin K Activity	964.3
88:28	Multivitamin Preparations	963.5
92:00	UNCLASSIFIED THERAPEUTIC AGENTS	977.8

© 2009 MAG Mutual Healthcare Solutions, Inc.

Appendix D: Classification of Industrial Accidents According to Agency

Annex B to the Resolution concerning Statistics of Employment Injuries adopted by the Tenth International Conference of Labor Statisticians on 12 October 1962

1 MACHINES

11 Prime-Movers, except Electrical Motors

111 Steam engines

112 Internal combustion engines

119 Others

12 Transmission Machinery

121 Transmission shafts

122 Transmission belts, cables, pulleys, pinions, chains, gears

129 Others

13 Metalworking Machines

131 Power presses

132 Lathes

133 Milling machines

134 Abrasive wheels

135 Mechanical shears

136 Forging machines

137 Rolling-mills

139 Others

14 Wood and Assimilated Machines

141 Circular saws

142 Other saws

143 Molding machines

144 Overhand planes

149 Others

15 Agricultural Machines

151 Reapers (including combine reapers)

152 Threshers

159 Others

16 Mining Machinery

161 Under-cutters

169 Others

19 Other Machines Not Elsewhere Classified

191 Earth-moving machines, excavating and scraping machines, except means of transport

192 Spinning, weaving and other textile machines

193 Machines for the manufacture of foodstuffs and beverages

194 Machines for the manufacture of paper

195 Printing machines

199 Others

2 MEANS OF TRANSPORT AND LIFTING EQUIPMENT

21 Lifting Machines and Appliances

211 Cranes

212 Lifts and elevators

213 Winches

214 Pulley blocks

219 Others

2 MEANS OF TRANSPORT AND LIFTING EQUIPMENT – *continued*

22 Means of Rail Transport

221 Inter-urban railways

222 Rail transport in mines, tunnels, quarries, industrial establishments, docks, etc.

229 Others

23 Other Wheeled Means of Transport, Excluding Rail Transport

231 Tractors

232 Lorries

233 Trucks

234 Motor vehicles, not elsewhere classified

235 Animal-drawn vehicles

236 Hand-drawn vehicles

239 Others

24 Means of Air Transport

25 Means of Water Transport

251 Motorized means of water transport

252 Non-motorized means of water transport

26 Other Means of Transport

261 Cable-cars

262 Mechanical conveyors, except cable-cars

269 Others

3 OTHER EQUIPMENT

31 Pressure Vessels

311 Boilers

312 Pressurized containers

313 Pressurized piping and accessories

314 Gas cylinders

315 Caissons, diving equipment

319 Others

32 Furnaces, Ovens, Kilns

321 Blast furnaces

322 Refining furnaces

323 Other furnaces

324 Kilns

325 Ovens

33 Refrigerating Plants

34 Electrical Installations, Including Electric Motors, but Excluding Electric Hand Tools

341 Rotating machines

342 Conductors

343 Transformers

344 Control apparatus

349 Others

35 Electric Hand Tools

36 Tools, Implements, and Appliances, Except Electric Hand Tools

361 Power-driven hand tools, except electric hand tools

362 Hand tools, not power-driven

369 Others

37 Ladders, Mobile Ramps

38 Scaffolding

39 Other Equipment, Not Elsewhere Classified

4 MATERIALS, SUBSTANCES AND RADIATIONS

41 Explosives

42 Dusts, Gases, Liquids and Chemicals, Excluding Explosives

421 Dusts

422 Gases, vapors, fumes

423 Liquids, not elsewhere classified

424 Chemicals, not elsewhere classified

43 Flying Fragments

44 Radiations

441 Ionizing radiations

449 Others

49 Other Materials and Substances Not Elsewhere Classified

5 WORKING ENVIRONMENT

51 Outdoor

511 Weather

512 Traffic and working surfaces

513 Water

519 Others

52 Indoor

521 Floors

522 Confined quarters

523 Stairs

524 Other traffic and working surfaces

525 Floor openings and wall openings

526 Environmental factors (lighting, ventilation, temperature, noise, etc.)

529 Others

53 Underground

531 Roofs and faces of mine roads and tunnels, etc.

532 Floors of mine roads and tunnels, etc.

533 Working-faces of mines, tunnels, etc.

534 Mine shafts

535 Fire

536 Water

539 Others

6 OTHER AGENCIES, NOT ELSEWHERE CLASSIFIED

61 Animals

611 Live animals

612 Animals products

69 Other Agencies, Not Elsewhere Classified

7 AGENCIES NOT CLASSIFIED FOR LACK OF SUFFICIENT DATA

© 2009 MAG Mutual Healthcare Solutions, Inc.

Appendix E: List of Three-Digit Categories

1. INFECTIOUS AND PARASITIC DISEASES

Intestinal infectious diseases (001-009)

001 Cholera
002 Typhoid and paratyphoid fevers
003 Other salmonella infections
004 Shigellosis
005 Other food poisoning (bacterial)
006 Amebiasis
007 Other protozoal intestinal diseases
008 Intestinal infections due to other organisms
009 Ill-defined intestinal infections

Tuberculosis (010-018)

010 Primary tuberculous infection
011 Pulmonary tuberculosis
012 Other respiratory tuberculosis
013 Tuberculosis of meninges and central nervous system
014 Tuberculosis of intestines, peritoneum, and mesenteric glands
015 Tuberculosis of bones and joints
016 Tuberculosis of genitourinary system
017 Tuberculosis of other organs
018 Miliary tuberculosis

Zoonotic bacterial diseases (020-027)

020 Plague
021 Tularemia
022 Anthrax
023 Brucellosis
024 Glanders
025 Melioidosis
026 Rat-bite fever
027 Other zoonotic bacterial diseases

Other bacterial diseases (030-041)

030 Leprosy
031 Diseases due to other mycobacteria
032 Diphtheria
033 Whooping cough
034 Streptococcal sore throat and scarlet fever
035 Erysipelas
036 Meningococcal infection
037 Tetanus
038 Septicemia
039 Actinomycotic infections
040 Other bacterial diseases
041 Bacterial infection in conditions classified elsewhere and of unspecified site

Human immunodeficiency virus (042)

042 Human immunodeficiency virus [HIV] disease

Poliomyelitis and other non-arthropod-borne viral diseases of central nervous system (045-049)

045 Acute poliomyelitis
046 Slow virus infections and prion diseases of central nervous system
047 Meningitis due to enterovirus
048 Other enterovirus diseases of central nervous system
049 Other non-arthropod-borne viral diseases of central nervous system

Viral diseases accompanied by exanthem (050-059)

050 Smallpox
051 Cowpox and paravaccinia
052 Chickenpox
053 Herpes zoster
054 Herpes simplex
055 Measles
056 Rubella
057 Other viral exanthemata
058 Other human herpesvirus
059 Other poxvirus infections

Arthropod-borne viral diseases (060-066)

060 Yellow fever
061 Dengue
062 Mosquito-borne viral encephalitis
063 Tick-borne viral encephalitis
064 Viral encephalitis transmitted by other and unspecified arthropods
065 Arthropod-borne hemorrhagic fever
066 Other arthropod-borne viral diseases

Other diseases due to viruses and Chlamydiae (070-079)

070 Viral hepatitis
071 Rabies
072 Mumps
073 Ornithosis
074 Specific diseases due to Coxsackie virus
075 Infectious mononucleosis
076 Trachoma
077 Other diseases of conjunctiva due to viruses and Chlamydiae
078 Other diseases due to viruses and Chlamydiae
079 Viral infection in conditions classified elsewhere and of unspecified site

Rickettsioses and other arthropod-borne diseases (080-088)

080 Louse-borne [epidemic] typhus
081 Other typhus
082 Tick-borne rickettsioses
083 Other rickettsioses
084 Malaria
085 Leishmaniasis
086 Trypanosomiasis
087 Relapsing fever
088 Other arthropod-borne diseases

Syphilis and other venereal diseases (090-099)

090 Congenital syphilis
091 Early syphilis, symptomatic
092 Early syphilis, latent
093 Cardiovascular syphilis
094 Neurosyphilis
095 Other forms of late syphilis, with symptoms
096 Late syphilis, latent
097 Other and unspecified syphilis
098 Gonococcal infections
099 Other venereal diseases

Other spirochetal diseases (100-104)

100 Leptospirosis
101 Vincent's angina
102 Yaws
103 Pinta
104 Other spirochetal infection

Mycoses (110-118)

110 Dermatophytosis
111 Dermatomycosis, other and unspecified
112 Candidiasis
114 Coccidioidomycosis
115 Histoplasmosis
116 Blastomycotic infection
117 Other mycoses
118 Opportunistic mycoses

Helminthiases (120-129)

120 Schistosomiasis [bilharziasis]
121 Other trematode infections
122 Echinococcosis
123 Other cestode infection
124 Trichinosis
125 Filarial infection and dracontiasis
126 Ancylostomiasis and necatoriasis
127 Other intestinal helminthiases
128 Other and unspecified helminthiases
129 Intestinal parasitism, unspecified

Other infectious and parasitic diseases (130-136)

130 Toxoplasmosis
131 Trichomoniasis
132 Pediculosis and phthirus infestation
133 Acariasis
134 Other infestation
135 Sarcoidosis
136 Other and unspecified infectious and parasitic diseases

Late effects of infectious and parasitic diseases (137-139)

137 Late effects of tuberculosis
138 Late effects of acute poliomyelitis
139 Late effects of other infectious and parasitic diseases

2. NEOPLASMS

Malignant neoplasm of lip, oral cavity, and pharynx (140-149)

140 Malignant neoplasm of lip
141 Malignant neoplasm of tongue
142 Malignant neoplasm of major salivary glands
143 Malignant neoplasm of gum
144 Malignant neoplasm of floor of mouth
145 Malignant neoplasm of other and unspecified parts of mouth
146 Malignant neoplasm of oropharynx
147 Malignant neoplasm of nasopharynx
148 Malignant neoplasm of hypopharynx
149 Malignant neoplasm of other and ill-defined sites within the lip, oral cavity, and pharynx

Malignant neoplasm of digestive organs and peritoneum (150-159)

150 Malignant neoplasm of esophagus
151 Malignant neoplasm of stomach
152 Malignant neoplasm of small intestine, including duodenum
153 Malignant neoplasm of colon
154 Malignant neoplasm of rectum, rectosigmoid junction, and anus
155 Malignant neoplasm of liver and intrahepatic bile ducts
156 Malignant neoplasm of gallbladder and extrahepatic bile ducts
157 Malignant neoplasm of pancreas
158 Malignant neoplasm of retroperitoneum and peritoneum
159 Malignant neoplasm of other and ill-defined sites within the digestive organs and peritoneum

Malignant neoplasm of respiratory and intrathoracic organs (160-165)

160 Malignant neoplasm of nasal cavities, middle ear, and accessory sinuses
161 Malignant neoplasm of larynx
162 Malignant neoplasm of trachea, bronchus, and lung
163 Malignant neoplasm of pleura
164 Malignant neoplasm of thymus, heart, and mediastinum
165 Malignant neoplasm of other and ill-defined sites within the respiratory system and intrathoracic organs

Malignant neoplasm of bone, connective tissue, skin, and breast (170-176)

170 Malignant neoplasm of bone and articular cartilage
171 Malignant neoplasm of connective and other soft tissue
172 Malignant melanoma of skin
173 Other malignant neoplasm of skin
174 Malignant neoplasm of female breast
175 Malignant neoplasm of male breast

Kaposi's sarcoma (176)

176 Kaposi's sarcoma

Malignant neoplasm of genitourinary organs (179-189)

179 Malignant neoplasm of uterus, part unspecified
180 Malignant neoplasm of cervix uteri
181 Malignant neoplasm of placenta
182 Malignant neoplasm of body of uterus

© 2009 MAG Mutual Healthcare Solutions, Inc.

183 Malignant neoplasm of ovary and other uterine adnexa
184 Malignant neoplasm of other and unspecified female genital organs
185 Malignant neoplasm of prostate
186 Malignant neoplasm of testis
187 Malignant neoplasm of penis and other male genital organs
188 Malignant neoplasm of bladder
189 Malignant neoplasm of kidney and other and unspecified urinary organs

Malignant neoplasm of other and unspecified sites (190-199)

190 Malignant neoplasm of eye
191 Malignant neoplasm of brain
192 Malignant neoplasm of other and unspecified parts of nervous system
193 Malignant neoplasm of thyroid gland
194 Malignant neoplasm of other endocrine glands and related structures
195 Malignant neoplasm of other and ill-defined sites
196 Secondary and unspecified malignant neoplasm of lymph nodes
197 Secondary malignant neoplasm of respiratory and digestive systems
198 Secondary malignant neoplasm of other specified sites
199 Malignant neoplasm without specification of site

Malignant neoplasm of lymphatic and hematopoietic tissue (200-208)

200 Lymphosarcoma and reticulosarcoma
201 Hodgkin's disease
202 Other malignant neoplasm of lymphoid and histiocytic tissue
203 Multiple myeloma and immunoproliferative neoplasms
204 Lymphoid leukemia
205 Myeloid leukemia
206 Monocytic leukemia
207 Other specified leukemia
208 Leukemia of unspecified cell type

Neuroendocrine tumors (209)

209 Neuroendocrine tumors

Benign neoplasms (210-229)

210 Benign neoplasm of lip, oral cavity, and pharynx
211 Benign neoplasm of other parts of digestive system
212 Benign neoplasm of respiratory and intrathoracic organs
213 Benign neoplasm of bone and articular cartilage
214 Lipoma
215 Other benign neoplasm of connective and other soft tissue
216 Benign neoplasm of skin
217 Benign neoplasm of breast
218 Uterine leiomyoma
219 Other benign neoplasm of uterus
220 Benign neoplasm of ovary
221 Benign neoplasm of other female genital organs
222 Benign neoplasm of male genital organs
223 Benign neoplasm of kidney and other urinary organs
224 Benign neoplasm of eye
225 Benign neoplasm of brain and other parts of nervous system
226 Benign neoplasm of thyroid gland
227 Benign neoplasm of other endocrine glands and related structures
228 Hemangioma and lymphangioma, any site
229 Benign neoplasm of other and unspecified sites

Carcinoma in situ (230-234)

230 Carcinoma in situ of digestive organs
231 Carcinoma in situ of respiratory system
232 Carcinoma in situ of skin
233 Carcinoma in situ of breast and genitourinary system
234 Carcinoma in situ of other and unspecified sites

Neoplasms of uncertain behavior (235-238)

235 Neoplasm of uncertain behavior of digestive and respiratory systems
236 Neoplasm of uncertain behavior of genitourinary organs
237 Neoplasm of uncertain behavior of endocrine glands and nervous system
238 Neoplasm of uncertain behavior of other and unspecified sites and tissues

Neoplasms of unspecified nature (239)

239 Neoplasm of unspecified nature

3. ENDOCRINE, NUTRITIONAL AND METABOLIC DISEASES, AND IMMUNITY DISORDERS

Disorders of thyroid gland (240-246)

240 Simple and unspecified goiter
241 Nontoxic nodular goiter
242 Thyrotoxicosis with or without goiter
243 Congenital hypothyroidism
244 Acquired hypothyroidism
245 Thyroiditis
246 Other disorders of thyroid

Diseases of other endocrine glands (249-259)

249 Secondary diabetes mellitus
250 Diabetes mellitus
251 Other disorders of pancreatic internal secretion
252 Disorders of parathyroid gland
253 Disorders of the pituitary gland and its hypothalamic control
254 Diseases of thymus gland
255 Disorders of adrenal glands
256 Ovarian dysfunction
257 Testicular dysfunction
258 Polyglandular dysfunction and related disorders
259 Other endocrine disorders

Nutritional deficiencies (260-269)

260 Kwashiorkor
261 Nutritional marasmus
262 Other severe protein-calorie malnutrition
263 Other and unspecified protein-calorie malnutrition
264 Vitamin A deficiency
265 Thiamine and niacin deficiency states
266 Deficiency of B-complex components
267 Ascorbic acid deficiency
268 Vitamin D deficiency
269 Other nutritional deficiencies

Other metabolic disorders and immunity disorders (270-279)

270 Disorders of amino-acid transport and metabolism
271 Disorders of carbohydrate transport and metabolism
272 Disorders of lipoid metabolism
273 Disorders of plasma protein metabolism
274 Gout
275 Disorders of mineral metabolism
276 Disorders of fluid, electrolyte, and acid-base balance
277 Other and unspecified disorders of metabolism
278 Obesity and other hyperalimentation
279 Disorders involving the immune mechanism

4. DISEASES OF BLOOD AND BLOOD-FORMING ORGANS

Diseases of the blood and blood-forming organs (280-289)

280 Iron deficiency anemias
281 Other deficiency anemias
282 Hereditary hemolytic anemias
283 Acquired hemolytic anemias
284 Aplastic anemia
285 Other and unspecified anemias
286 Coagulation defects
287 Purpura and other hemorrhagic conditions
288 Diseases of white blood cells
289 Other diseases of blood and blood-forming organs

5. MENTAL DISORDERS

Organic psychotic conditions (290-294)

290 Senile and presenile organic psychotic conditions
291 Alcoholic psychoses
292 Drug psychoses
293 Transient organic psychotic conditions
294 Other organic psychotic conditions (chronic)

Other psychoses (295-299)

295 Schizophrenic psychoses
296 Affective psychoses
297 Paranoid states
298 Other nonorganic psychoses
299 Psychoses with origin specific to childhood

Neurotic disorders, personality disorders, and other nonpsychotic mental disorders (300-316)

300 Neurotic disorders
301 Personality disorders
302 Sexual deviations and disorders
303 Alcohol dependence syndrome
304 Drug dependence
305 Nondependent abuse of drugs
306 Physiological malfunction arising from mental factors
307 Special symptoms or syndromes, not elsewhere classified
308 Acute reaction to stress
309 Adjustment reaction
310 Specific nonpsychotic mental disorders following organic brain damage
311 Depressive disorder, not elsewhere classified
312 Disturbance of conduct, not elsewhere classified
313 Disturbance of emotions specific to childhood and adolescence
314 Hyperkinetic syndrome of childhood
315 Specific delays in development
316 Psychic factors associated with diseases classified elsewhere

Mental retardation (317-319)

317 Mild mental retardation
318 Other specified mental retardation
319 Unspecified mental retardation

6. DISEASES OF THE NERVOUS SYSTEM AND SENSE ORGANS

Inflammatory diseases of the central nervous system (320-326)

320 Bacterial meningitis
321 Meningitis due to other organisms
322 Meningitis of unspecified cause
323 Encephalitis, myelitis, and encephalomyelitis
324 Intracranial and intraspinal abscess
325 Phlebitis and thrombophlebitis of intracranial venous sinuses
326 Late effects of intracranial abscess or pyogenic infection
327 Organic sleep disorders

© 2009 MAG Mutual Healthcare Solutions, Inc.

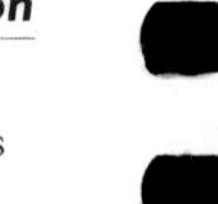
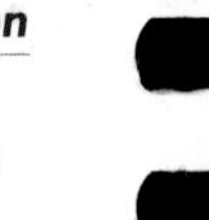
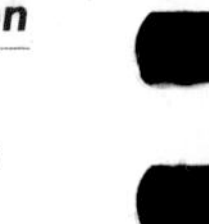
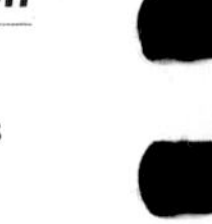

Hereditary and degenerative diseases of the central nervous system (330-337)

330 Cerebral degenerations usually manifest in childhood
331 Other cerebral degenerations
332 Parkinson's disease
333 Other extrapyramidal disease and abnormal movement disorders
334 Spinocerebellar disease
335 Anterior horn cell disease
336 Other diseases of spinal cord
337 Disorders of the autonomic nervous system

Pain (338)

338 Pain, not elsewhere classified

Other headache syndromes (339)

339 Other headache syndromes

Other disorders of the central nervous system (340-349)

340 Multiple sclerosis
341 Other demyelinating diseases of central nervous system
342 Hemiplegia and hemiparesis
343 Infantile cerebral palsy
344 Other paralytic syndromes
345 Epilepsy
346 Migraine
347 Cataplexy and narcolepsy
348 Other conditions of brain
349 Other and unspecified disorders of the nervous system

Disorders of the peripheral nervous system (350-359)

350 Trigeminal nerve disorders
351 Facial nerve disorders
352 Disorders of other cranial nerves
353 Nerve root and plexus disorders
354 Mononeuritis of upper limb and mononeuritis multiplex
355 Mononeuritis of lower limb
356 Hereditary and idiopathic peripheral neuropathy
357 Inflammatory and toxic neuropathy
358 Myoneural disorders
359 Muscular dystrophies and other myopathies

Disorders of the eye and adnexa (360-379)

360 Disorders of the globe
361 Retinal detachments and defects
362 Other retinal disorders
363 Chorioretinal inflammations and scars and other disorders of choroid
364 Disorders of iris and ciliary body
365 Glaucoma
366 Cataract
367 Disorders of refraction and accommodation
368 Visual disturbances
369 Blindness and low vision
370 Keratitis
371 Corneal opacity and other disorders of cornea
372 Disorders of conjunctiva
373 Inflammation of eyelids
374 Other disorders of eyelids
375 Disorders of lacrimal system
376 Disorders of the orbit
377 Disorders of optic nerve and visual pathways
378 Strabismus and other disorders of binocular eye movements
379 Other disorders of eye

Diseases of the ear and mastoid process (380-389)

380 Disorders of external ear
381 Nonsuppurative otitis media and Eustachian tube disorders
382 Suppurative and unspecified otitis media
383 Mastoiditis and related conditions
384 Other disorders of tympanic membrane
385 Other disorders of middle ear and mastoid
386 Vertiginous syndromes and other disorders of vestibular system
387 Otosclerosis
388 Other disorders of ear
389 Hearing loss

7. DISEASES OF THE CIRCULATORY SYSTEM

Acute rheumatic fever (390-392)

390 Rheumatic fever without mention of heart involvement
391 Rheumatic fever with heart involvement
392 Rheumatic chorea

Chronic rheumatic heart disease (393-398)

393 Chronic rheumatic pericarditis
394 Diseases of mitral valve
395 Diseases of aortic valve
396 Diseases of mitral and aortic valves
397 Diseases of other endocardial structures
398 Other rheumatic heart disease

Hypertensive disease (401-405)

401 Essential hypertension
402 Hypertensive heart disease
403 Hypertensive renal disease
404 Hypertensive heart and renal disease
405 Secondary hypertension

Ischemic heart disease (410-414)

410 Acute myocardial infarction
411 Other acute and subacute form of ischemic heart disease
412 Old myocardial infarction
413 Angina pectoris
414 Other forms of chronic ischemic heart disease

Diseases of pulmonary circulation (415-417)

415 Acute pulmonary heart disease
416 Chronic pulmonary heart disease
417 Other diseases of pulmonary circulation

Other forms of heart disease (420-429)

420 Acute pericarditis
421 Acute and subacute endocarditis
422 Acute myocarditis
423 Other diseases of pericardium
424 Other diseases of endocardium
425 Cardiomyopathy
426 Conduction disorders
427 Cardiac dysrhythmias
428 Heart failure
429 Ill-defined descriptions and complications of heart disease

Cerebrovascular disease (430-438)

430 Subarachnoid hemorrhage
431 Intracerebral hemorrhage
432 Other and unspecified intracranial hemorrhage
433 Occlusion and stenosis of precerebral arteries
434 Occlusion of cerebral arteries
435 Transcient cerebral ischemia
436 Acute but ill-defined cerebrovascular disease
437 Other and ill-defined cerebrovascular disease
438 Late effects of cerebrovascular disease

Diseases of arteries, arterioles, and capillaries (440-448)

440 Atherosclerosis
441 Aortic aneurysm and dissection
442 Other aneurysm
443 Other peripheral vascular disease
444 Arterial embolism and thrombosis
445 Atheroembolism
446 Polyarteritis nodosa and allied conditions
447 Other disorders of arteries and arterioles
448 Diseases of capillaries

Diseases of veins and lymphatics, and other diseases of circulatory system (451-459)

451 Phlebitis and thrombophlebitis
452 Portal vein thrombosis
453 Other venous embolism and thrombosis
454 Varicose veins of lower extremities
455 Hemorrhoids
456 Varicose veins of other sites
457 Noninfective disorders of lymphatic channels
458 Hypotension
459 Other disorders of circulatory system

8. DISEASES OF THE RESPIRATORY SYSTEM

Acute respiratory infections (460-466)

460 Acute nasopharyngitis [common cold]
461 Acute sinusitis
462 Acute pharyngitis
463 Acute tonsillitis
464 Acute laryngitis and tracheitis
465 Acute upper respiratory infections of multiple or unspecified sites
466 Acute bronchitis and bronchiolitis

Other diseases of upper respiratory tract (470-478)

470 Deviated nasal septum
471 Nasal polyps
472 Chronic pharyngitis and nasopharyngitis
473 Chronic sinusitis
474 Chronic disease of tonsils and adenoids
475 Peritonsillar abscess
476 Chronic laryngitis and laryngotracheitis
477 Allergic rhinitis
478 Other diseases of upper respiratory tract

Pneumonia and influenza (480-488)

480 Viral pneumonia
481 Pneumococcal pneumonia [Streptococcus pneumoniae pneumonia]
482 Other bacterial pneumonia
483 Pneumonia due to other specified organism
484 Pneumonia in infectious diseases classified elsewhere
485 Bronchopneumonia, organism unspecified
486 Pneumonia, organism unspecified
487 Influenza
488 Influenza due to certain identified influenza viruses

Chronic obstructive pulmonary disease and allied conditions (490-496)

490 Bronchitis, not specified as acute or chronic
491 Chronic bronchitis
492 Emphysema
493 Asthma
494 Bronchiectasis
495 Extrinsic allergic alveolitis
496 Chronic airways obstruction, not elsewhere classified

Pneumoconioses and other lung diseases due to external agents (500-508)

500 Coalworkers' pneumoconiosis
501 Asbestosis
502 Pneumoconiosis due to other silica or silicates
503 Pneumoconiosis due to other inorganic dust
504 Pneumopathy due to inhalation of other dust
505 Pneumoconiosis, unspecified
506 Respiratory conditions due to chemical fumes and vapors
507 Pneumonitis due to solids and liquids
508 Respiratory conditions due to other and unspecified external agents

Other diseases of respiratory system (510-519)

510 Empyema
511 Pleurisy
512 Pneumothorax
513 Abscess of lung and mediastinum
514 Pulmonary congestion and hypostasis
515 Postinflammatory pulmonary fibrosis
516 Other alveolar and parietoalveolar pneumopathy
517 Lung involvement in conditions classified elsewhere
518 Other diseases of lung
519 Other diseases of respiratory system

© 2009 MAG Mutual Healthcare Solutions, Inc.

9. DISEASES OF THE DIGESTIVE SYSTEM

Diseases of oral cavity, salivary glands, and jaws (520-529)

520 Disorders of tooth development and eruption
521 Diseases of hard tissues of teeth
522 Diseases of pulp and periapical tissues
523 Gingival and periodontal diseases
524 Dentofacial anomalies, including malocclusion
525 Other diseases and conditions of the teeth and supporting structures
526 Diseases of the jaws
527 Diseases of the salivary glands
528 Diseases of the oral soft tissues, excluding lesions specific for gingiva and tongue
529 Diseases and other conditions of the tongue

Diseases of esophagus, stomach, and duodenum (530-538)

530 Diseases of esophagus
531 Gastric ulcer
532 Duodenal ulcer
533 Peptic ulcer, site unspecified
534 Gastrojejunal ulcer
535 Gastritis and duodenitis
536 Disorders of function of stomach
537 Other disorders of stomach and duodenum
538 Gastrointestinal mucositis (ulcerative)

Appendicitis (540-543)

540 Acute appendicitis
541 Appendicitis, unqualified
542 Other appendicitis
543 Other diseases of appendix

Hernia of abdominal cavity (550-553)

550 Inguinal hernia
551 Other hernia of abdominal cavity, with gangrene
552 Other hernia of abdominal cavity, with obstruction, but without mention of gangrene
553 Other hernia of abdominal cavity without mention of obstruction or gangrene

Noninfective enteritis and colitis (555-558)

555 Regional enteritis
556 Ulcerative colitis
557 Vascular insufficiency of intestine
558 Other noninfective gastroenteritis and colitis

Other diseases of intestines and peritoneum (560-569)

560 Intestinal obstruction without mention of hernia
562 Diverticula of intestine
564 Functional digestive disorders, not elsewhere classified
565 Anal fissure and fistula
566 Abscess of anal and rectal regions
567 Peritonitis
568 Other disorders of peritoneum
569 Other disorders of intestine

Other diseases of digestive system (570-579)

570 Acute and subacute necrosis of liver
571 Chronic liver disease and cirrhosis
572 Liver abscess and sequelae of chronic liver disease
573 Other disorders of liver
574 Cholelithiasis
575 Other disorders of gallbladder
576 Other disorders of biliary tract
577 Diseases of pancreas
578 Gastrointestinal hemorrhage
579 Intestinal malabsorption

10. DISEASES OF THE GENITOURINARY SYSTEM

Nephritis, nephrotic syndrome, and nephrosis (580-589)

580 Acute glomerulonephritis
581 Nephrotic syndrome
582 Chronic glomerulonephritis
583 Nephritis and nephropathy, not specified as acute or chronic
584 Acute kidney failure
585 Chronic renal failure
586 Renal failure, unspecified
587 Renal sclerosis, unspecified
588 Disorders resulting from impaired renal function
589 Small kidney of unknown cause

Other diseases of urinary system (590-599)

590 Infections of kidney
591 Hydronephrosis
592 Calculus of kidney and ureter
593 Other disorders of kidney and ureter
594 Calculus of lower urinary tract
595 Cystitis
596 Other disorders of bladder
597 Urethritis, not sexually transmitted, and urethral syndrome
598 Urethral stricture
599 Other disorders of urethra and urinary tract

Diseases of male genital organs (600-608)

600 Hyperplasia of prostate
601 Inflammatory diseases of prostate
602 Other disorders of prostate
603 Hydrocele
604 Orchitis and epididymitis
605 Redundant prepuce and phimosis
606 Infertility, male
607 Disorders of penis
608 Other disorders of male genital organs

Disorders of breast (610-612)

610 Benign mammary dysplasias
611 Other disorders of breast
612 Deformity and disproportion of reconstructed breast

Inflammatory disease of female pelvic organs (614-616)

614 Inflammatory disease of ovary, fallopian tube, pelvic cellular tissue, and peritoneum
615 Inflammatory diseases of uterus, except cervix
616 Inflammatory disease of cervix, vagina, and vulva

Other disorders of female genital tract (617-629)

617 Endometriosis
618 Genital prolapse
619 Fistula involving female genital tract
620 Noninflammatory disorders of ovary, fallopian tube, and broad ligament
621 Disorders of uterus, not elsewhere classified
622 Noninflammatory disorders of cervix
623 Noninflammatory disorders of vagina
624 Noninflammatory disorders of vulva and perineum
625 Pain and other symptoms associated with female genital organs
626 Disorders of menstruation and other abnormal bleeding from female genital tract
627 Menopausal and postmenopausal disorders
628 Infertility, female
629 Other disorders of female genital organs

11. COMPLICATIONS OF PREGNANCY, CHILDBIRTH, AND THE PUERPERIUM

Ectopic and molar pregnancy and other pregnancy with abortive outcome (630-639)

630 Hydatidiform mole
631 Other abnormal product of conception
632 Missed abortion
633 Ectopic pregnancy
634 Spontaneous abortion
635 Legally induced abortion
636 Illegally induced abortion
637 Unspecified abortion
638 Failed attempted abortion
639 Complications following abortion and ectopic and molar pregnancies

Complications mainly related to pregnancy (640-649)

640 Hemorrhage in early pregnancy
641 Antepartum hemorrhage, abruptio placentae, and placenta previa
642 Hypertension complicating pregnancy, childbirth, and the puerperium
643 Excessive vomiting in pregnancy
644 Early or threatened labor
645 Prolonged pregnancy
646 Other complications of pregnancy, not elsewhere classified
647 Infective and parasitic conditions in the mother classifiable elsewhere but complicating pregnancy, childbirth, and the puerperium
648 Other current conditions in the mother classifiable elsewhere but complicating pregnancy, childbirth, and the puerperium
649 Other conditions or status of the mother complicating pregnancy, childbirth, or the puerperium

Normal delivery, and other indications for care in pregnancy, labor, and delivery (650-659)

650 Normal delivery
651 Multiple gestation
652 Malposition and malpresentation of fetus
653 Disproportion
654 Abnormality of organs and soft tissues of pelvis
655 Known or suspected fetal abnormality affecting management of mother
656 Other known or suspected fetal and placental problems affecting management of mother
657 Polyhydramnios
658 Other problems associated with amniotic cavity and membranes
659 Other indications for care or intervention related to labor and delivery and not elsewhere classified

Complications occurring mainly in the course of labor and delivery (660-669)

660 Obstructed labor
661 Abnormality of forces of labor
662 Long labor
663 Umbilical cord complications
664 Trauma to perineum and vulva during delivery
665 Other obstetrical trauma
666 Postpartum hemorrhage
667 Retained placenta or membranes, without hemorrhage
668 Complications of the administration of anesthetic or other sedation in labor and delivery
669 Other complications of labor and delivery, not elsewhere classified

Complications of the puerperium (670-677)

670 Major puerperal infection
671 Venous complications in pregnancy and the puerperium
672 Pyrexia of unknown origin during the puerperium
673 Obstetrical pulmonary embolism
674 Other and unspecified complications of the puerperium, not elsewhere classified
675 Infections of the breast and nipple associated with childbirth
676 Other disorders of the breast associated with childbirth, and disorders of lactation
677 Late effect of complication of pregnancy, childbirth, and the puerperium

Other maternal and fetal complications (678-679)

678 Other fetal conditions
679 Complications of in utero procedures

© 2009 MAG Mutual Healthcare Solutions, Inc.

12. DISEASES OF THE SKIN AND SUBCUTANEOUS TISSUE

Infections of skin and subcutaneous tissue (680-686)

680 Carbuncle and furuncle
681 Cellulitis and abscess of finger and toe
682 Other cellulitis and abscess
683 Acute lymphadenitis
684 Impetigo
685 Pilonidal cyst
686 Other local infections of skin and subcutaneous tissue

Other inflammatory conditions of skin and subcutaneous tissue (690-698)

690 Erythematosquamous dermatosis
691 Atopic dermatitis and related conditions
692 Contact dermatitis and other eczema
693 Dermatitis due to substances taken internally
694 Bullous dermatoses
695 Erythematous conditions
696 Psoriasis and similar disorders
697 Lichen
698 Pruritus and related conditions

Other diseases of skin and subcutaneous tissue (700-709)

700 Corns and callosities
701 Other hypertrophic and atrophic conditions of skin
702 Other dermatoses
703 Diseases of nail
704 Diseases of hair and hair follicles
705 Disorders of sweat glands
706 Diseases of sebaceous glands
707 Chronic ulcer of skin
708 Urticaria
709 Other disorders of skin and subcutaneous tissue

13. DISEASES OF THE MUSCULOSKELETAL SYSTEM AND CONNECTIVE TISSUE

Arthropathies and related disorders (710-719)

710 Diffuse diseases of connective tissue
711 Arthropathy associated with infections
712 Crystal arthropathies
713 Arthropathy associated with other disorders classified elsewhere
714 Rheumatoid arthritis and other inflammatory polyarthropathies
715 Osteoarthrosis and allied disorders
716 Other and unspecified arthropathies
717 Internal derangement of knee
718 Other derangement of joint
719 Other and unspecified disorder of joint

Dorsopathies (720-724)

720 Ankylosing spondylitis and other inflammatory spondylopathies
721 Spondylosis and allied disorders
722 Intervertebral disc disorders
723 Other disorders of cervical region
724 Other and unspecified disorders of back

Rheumatism, excluding the back (725-729)

725 Polymyalgia rheumatica
726 Peripheral enthesopathies and allied syndromes
727 Other disorders of synovium, tendon, and bursa
728 Disorders of muscle, ligament, and fascia
729 Other disorders of soft tissues

Osteopathies, chondropathies, and acquired musculoskeletal deformities (730-739)

730 Osteomyelitis, periostitis, and other infections involving bone
1 Osteitis deformans and osteopathies associated with other disorders classified elsewhere
Osteochondropathies
ther disorders of bone and cartilage
734 Flat foot
735 Acquired deformities of toe
736 Other acquired deformities of limbs
737 Curvature of spine
738 Other acquired deformity
739 Nonallopathic lesions, not elsewhere classified

14. CONGENITAL ANOMALIES

Congential anomalies (740-759)

740 Anencephalus and similar anomalies
741 Spina bifida
742 Other congenital anomalies of nervous system
743 Congenital anomalies of eye
744 Congenital anomalies of ear, face, and neck
745 Bulbus cordis anomalies and anomalies of cardiac septal closure
746 Other congenital anomalies of heart
747 Other congenital anomalies of circulatory system
748 Congenital anomalies of respiratory system
749 Cleft palate and cleft lip
750 Other congenital anomalies of upper alimentary tract
751 Other congenital anomalies of digestive system
752 Congenital anomalies of genital organs
753 Congenital anomalies of urinary system
754 Certain congenital musculoskeletal deformities
755 Other congenital anomalies of limbs
756 Other congenital musculoskeletal anomalies
757 Congenital anomalies of the integument
758 Chromosomal anomalies
759 Other and unspecified congenital anomalies

15. CERTAIN CONDITIONS ORIGINATING IN THE PERINATAL PERIOD

Maternal causes of perinatal morbidity and mortality (760-763)

760 Fetus or newborn affected by maternal conditions which may be unrelated to present pregnancy
761 Fetus or newborn affected by maternal complications of pregnancy
762 Fetus or newborn affected by complications of placenta, cord, and membranes
763 Fetus or newborn affected by other complications of labor and delivery

Other conditions originating in the perinatal period (764-779)

764 Slow fetal growth and fetal malnutrition
765 Disorders relating to short gestation and unspecified low birthweight
766 Disorders relating to long gestation and high birthweight
767 Birth trauma
768 Intrauterine hypoxia and birth asphyxia
769 Respiratory distress syndrome
770 Other respiratory conditions of fetus and newborn
771 Infections specific to the perinatal period
772 Fetal and neonatal hemorrhage
773 Hemolytic disease of fetus or newborn, due to isoimmunization
774 Other perinatal jaundice
775 Endocrine and metabolic disturbances specific to the fetus and newborn
776 Hematological disorders of newborn
777 Perinatal disorders of digestive system
778 Conditions involving the integument and temperature regulation of fetus and newborn
779 Other and ill-defined conditions originating in the perinatal period

16. SYMPTOMS, SIGNS, AND ILL-DEFINED CONDITIONS

Symptoms (780-789)

780 General symptoms
781 Symptoms involving nervous and musculoskeletal systems
782 Symptoms involving skin and other integumentary tissue
783 Symptoms concerning nutrition, metabolism, and development
784 Symptoms involving head and neck
785 Symptoms involving cardiovascular system
786 Symptoms involving respiratory system and other chest symptoms
787 Symptoms involving digestive system
788 Symptoms involving urinary system
789 Other symptoms involving abdomen and pelvis

Nonspecific abnormal findings (790-796)

790 Nonspecific findings on examination of blood
791 Nonspecific findings on examination of urine
792 Nonspecific abnormal findings in other body substances
793 Nonspecific (abnormal) findings on radiological and other examination of body structure
794 Nonspecific abnormal results of function studies
795 Nonspecific abnormal histological and immunological findings
796 Other nonspecific abnormal findings

Ill-defined and unknown causes of morbidity and mortality (797-799)

797 Senility without mention of psychosis
798 Sudden death, cause unknown
799 Other ill-defined and unknown causes of morbidity and mortality

17. INJURY AND POISONING

Fracture of skull (800-804)

800 Fracture of vault of skull
801 Fracture of base of skull
802 Fracture of face bones
803 Other and unqualified skull fractures
804 Multiple fractures involving skull or face with other bones

Fracture of spine and trunk (805-809)

805 Fracture of vertebral column without mention of spinal cord lesion
806 Fracture of vertebral column with spinal cord lesion
807 Fracture of rib(s), sternum, larynx, and trachea
808 Fracture of pelvis
809 Ill-defined fractures of bones of trunk

Fracture of upper limb (810-819)

810 Fracture of clavicle
811 Fracture of scapula
812 Fracture of humerus
813 Fracture of radius and ulna
814 Fracture of carpal bone(s)
815 Fracture of metacarpal bone(s)
816 Fracture of one or more phalanges of hand
817 Multiple fractures of hand bones
818 Ill-defined fractures of upper limb
819 Multiple fractures involving both upper limbs, and upper limb with rib(s) and sternum

Fracture of lower limb (820-829)

820 Fracture of neck of femur
821 Fracture of other and unspecified parts of femur
822 Fracture of patella
823 Fracture of tibia and fibula
824 Fracture of ankle
825 Fracture of one or more tarsal and metatarsal bones
826 Fracture of one or more phalanges of foot
827 Other, multiple, and ill-defined fractures of lower limb
828 Multiple fractures involving both lower limbs, lower with upper limb, and lower limb(s) with rib(s) and sternum
829 Fracture of unspecified bones

© 2009 MAG Mutual Healthcare Solutions, Inc.

Dislocation (830-839)
830 Dislocation of jaw
831 Dislocation of shoulder
832 Dislocation of elbow
833 Dislocation of wrist
834 Dislocation of finger
835 Dislocation of hip
836 Dislocation of knee
837 Dislocation of ankle
838 Dislocation of foot
839 Other, multiple, and ill-defined dislocations

Sprains and strains of joints and adjacent muscles (840-848)
840 Sprains and strains of shoulder and upper arm
841 Sprains and strains of elbow and forearm
842 Sprains and strains of wrist and hand
843 Sprains and strains of hip and thigh
844 Sprains and strains of knee and leg
845 Sprains and strains of ankle and foot
846 Sprains and strains of sacroiliac region
847 Sprains and strains of other and unspecified parts of back
848 Other and ill-defined sprains and strains

Intracranial injury, excluding those with skull fracture (850-854)
850 Concussion
851 Cerebral laceration and contusion
852 Subarachnoid, subdural, and extradural hemorrhage, following injury
853 Other and unspecified intracranial hemorrhage following injury
854 Intracranial injury of other and unspecified nature

Internal injury of chest, abdomen, and pelvis (860-869)
860 Traumatic pneumothorax and hemothorax
861 Injury to heart and lung
862 Injury to other and unspecified intrathoracic organs
863 Injury to gastrointestinal tract
864 Injury to liver
865 Injury to spleen
866 Injury to kidney
867 Injury to pelvic organs
868 Injury to other intra-abdominal organs
869 Internal injury to unspecified or ill-defined organs

Open wound of head, neck, and trunk (870-879)
870 Open wound of ocular adnexa
871 Open wound of eyeball
872 Open wound of ear
873 Other open wound of head
874 Open wound of neck
875 Open wound of chest (wall)
876 Open wound of back
877 Open wound of buttock
878 Open wound of genital organs (external), including traumatic amputation
879 Open wound of other and unspecified sites, except limbs

Open wound of upper limb (880-887)
880 Open wound of shoulder and upper arm
881 Open wound of elbow, forearm, and wrist
882 Open wound of hand except finger(s) alone
883 Open wound of finger(s)
884 Multiple and unspecified open wound of upper limb
885 Traumatic amputation of thumb (complete) (partial)
886 Traumatic amputation of other finger(s) (complete) (partial)
887 Traumatic amputation of arm and hand (complete) (partial)

Open wound of lower limb (890-897)
890 Open wound of hip and thigh
891 Open wound of knee, leg [except thigh], and ankle
892 Open wound of foot except toe(s) alone
893 Open wound of toe(s)
894 Multiple and unspecified open wound of lower limb
895 Traumatic amputation of toe(s) (complete) (partial)
896 Traumatic amputation of foot (complete) (partial)
897 Traumatic amputation of leg(s) (complete) (partial)

Injury to blood vessels (900-904)
900 Injury to blood vessels of head and neck
901 Injury to blood vessels of thorax
902 Injury to blood vessels of abdomen and pelvis
903 Injury to blood vessels of upper extremity
904 Injury to blood vessels of lower extremity and unspecified sites

Late effects of injuries, poisonings, toxic effects, and other external causes (905-909)
905 Late effects of musculoskeletal and connective tissue injuries
906 Late effects of injuries to skin and subcutaneous tissues
907 Late effects of injuries to the nervous system
908 Late effects of other and unspecified injuries
909 Late effects of other and unspecified external causes

Superficial injury (910-919)
910 Superficial injury of face, neck, and scalp except eye
911 Superficial injury of trunk
912 Superficial injury of shoulder and upper arm
913 Superficial injury of elbow, forearm, and wrist
914 Superficial injury of hand(s) except finger(s) alone
915 Superficial injury of finger(s)
916 Superficial injury of hip, thigh, leg, and ankle
917 Superficial injury of foot and toe(s)
918 Superficial injury of eye and adnexa
919 Superficial injury of other, multiple, and unspecified sites

Contusion with intact skin surface (920-924)
920 Contusion of face, scalp, and neck except eye(s)
921 Contusion of eye and adnexa
922 Contusion of trunk
923 Contusion of upper limb
924 Contusion of lower limb and of other and unspecified sites

Crushing injury (925-929)
925 Crushing injury of face, scalp, and neck
926 Crushing injury of trunk
927 Crushing injury of upper limb
928 Crushing injury of lower limb
929 Crushing injury of multiple and unspecified sites

Effects of foreign body entering through orifice (930-939)
930 Foreign body on external eye
931 Foreign body in ear
932 Foreign body in nose
933 Foreign body in pharynx and larynx
934 Foreign body in trachea, bronchus, and lung
935 Foreign body in mouth, esophagus, and stomach
936 Foreign body in intestine and colon
937 Foreign body in anus and rectum
938 Foreign body in digestive system, unspecified
939 Foreign body in genitourinary tract

Burns (940-949)
940 Burn confined to eye and adnexa
941 Burn of face, head, and neck
942 Burn of trunk
943 Burn of upper limb, except wrist and hand
944 Burn of wrist(s) and hand(s)
945 Burn of lower limb(s)
946 Burns of multiple specified sites
947 Burn of internal organs
948 Burns classified according to extent of body surface involved
949 Burn, unspecified

Injury to nerves and spinal cord (950-957)
950 Injury to optic nerve and pathways
951 Injury to other cranial nerve(s)
952 Spinal cord injury without evidence of spinal bone injury
953 Injury to nerve roots and spinal plexus
954 Injury to other nerve(s) of trunk excluding shoulder and pelvic girdles
955 Injury to peripheral nerve(s) of shoulder girdle and upper limb
956 Injury to peripheral nerve(s) of pelvic girdle and lower limb
957 Injury to other and unspecified nerves

Certain traumatic complications and unspecified injuries (958-959)
958 Certain early complications of trauma
959 Injury, other and unspecified

Poisoning by drugs, medicinals and biological substances (960-979)
960 Poisoning by antibiotics
961 Poisoning by other anti-infectives
962 Poisoning by hormones and synthetic substitutes
963 Poisoning by primarily systemic agents
964 Poisoning by agents primarily affecting blood constituents
965 Poisoning by analgesics, antipyretics, and antirheumatics
966 Poisoning by anticonvulsants and anti-Parkinsonism drugs
967 Poisoning by sedatives and hypnotics
968 Poisoning by other central nervous system depressants and anesthetics
969 Poisoning by psychotropic agents
970 Poisoning by central nervous system stimulants
971 Poisoning by drugs primarily affecting the autonomic nervous system
972 Poisoning by agents primarily affecting the cardiovascular system
973 Poisoning by agents primarily affecting the gastrointestinal system
974 Poisoning by water, mineral, and uric acid metabolism drugs
975 Poisoning by agents primarily acting on the smooth and skeletal muscles and respiratory system
976 Poisoning by agents primarily affecting skin and mucous membrane, ophthalmological, otorhinolaryngological, and dental drugs
977 Poisoning by other and unspecified drugs and medicinals
978 Poisoning by bacterial vaccines
979 Poisoning by other vaccines and biological substances

Toxic effects of substances chiefly nonmedicinal as to source (980-989)
980 Toxic effect of alcohol
981 Toxic effect of petroleum products
982 Toxic effect of solvents other than petroleum-based
983 Toxic effect of corrosive aromatics, acids, and caustic alkalis
984 Toxic effect of lead and its compounds (including fumes)
985 Toxic effect of other metals
986 Toxic effect of carbon monoxide
987 Toxic effect of other gases, fumes, or vapors

© 2009 MAG Mutual Healthcare Solutions, Inc.

988 Toxic effect of noxious substances eaten as food
989 Toxic effect of other substances, chiefly nonmedicinal as to source

Other and unspecified effects of external causes (990-995)

990 Effects of radiation, unspecified
991 Effects of reduced temperature
992 Effects of heat and light
993 Effects of air pressure
994 Effects of other external causes
995 Certain adverse effects, not elsewhere classified

Complications of surgical and medical care, not elsewhere classified (996-999)

996 Complications peculiar to certain specified procedures
997 Complications affecting specified body systems, not elsewhere classified
998 Other complications of procedures, not elsewhere classified
999 Complications of medical care, not elsewhere classified

18. SUPPLEMENTARY CLASSIFICATION OF FACTORS INFLUENCING HEALTH STATUS AND CONTACT WITH HEALTH SERVICES (V01-V89)

Persons with potential health hazards related to communicable diseases (V01-V09)

V01 Contact with or exposure to communicable diseases
V02 Carrier or suspected carrier of infectious diseases
V03 Need for prophylactic vaccination and inoculation against bacterial diseases
V04 Need for prophylactic vaccination and inoculation against certain viral diseases
V05 Need for other prophylactic vaccination and inoculation against single diseases
V06 Need for prophylactic vaccination and inoculation against combinations of diseases
V07 Need for isolation and other prophylactic measures
V08 Asymptomatic human immunodeficiency virus [HIV] infection status
V09 Infection with drug-resistant microorganisms

Persons with potential health hazards related to personal and family history (V10-V19)

V10 Personal history of malignant neoplasm
V11 Personal history of mental disorder
V12 Personal history of certain other diseases
V13 Personal history of other diseases
V14 Personal history of allergy to medicinal agents
V15 Other personal history presenting hazards to health
V16 Family history of malignant neoplasm
V17 Family history of certain chronic disabling diseases
V18 Family history of certain other specific conditions
V19 Family history of other conditions

Persons encountering health services in circumstances related to reproduction and development (V20-V29)

V20 Health supervision of infant or child
V21 Constitutional states in development
V22 Normal pregnancy
V23 Supervision of high-risk pregnancy
V24 Postpartum care and examination
V25 Encounter for contraceptive management
V26 Procreative management
V27 Outcome of delivery
V28 Antenatal screening
V29 Observation and evaluation of newborns and infants for suspected condition not found

Liveborn infants according to type of birth (V30-V39)

V30 Single liveborn
V31 Twin, mate liveborn
V32 Twin, mate stillborn
V33 Twin, unspecified
V34 Other multiple, mates all liveborn
V35 Other multiple, mates all stillborn
V36 Other multiple, mates live- and stillborn
V37 Other multiple, unspecified
V39 Unspecified

Persons with a condition influencing their health status (V40-V49)

V40 Mental and behavioral problems
V41 Problems with special senses and other special functions
V42 Organ or tissue replaced by transplant
V43 Organ or tissue replaced by other means
V44 Artificial opening status
V45 Other postsurgical states
V46 Other dependence on machines and devices
V47 Other problems with internal organs
V48 Problems with head, neck, and trunk
V49 Problems with limbs and other problems

Persons encountering health services for specific procedures and aftercare (V50-V59)

V50 Elective surgery for purposes other than remedying health states
V51 Aftercare involving the use of plastic surgery
V52 Fitting and adjustment of prosthetic device
V53 Fitting and adjustment of other device
V54 Other orthopedic aftercare
V55 Attention to artificial openings
V56 Encounter for dialysis and dialysis catheter care
V57 Care involving use of rehabilitation procedures
V58 Other and unspecified aftercare
V59 Donors

Persons encountering health services in other circumstances (V60-V69)

V60 Housing, household, and economic circumstances
V61 Other family circumstances
V62 Other psychosocial circumstances
V63 Unavailability of other medical facilities for care
V64 Persons encountering health services for specific procedures, not carried out
V65 Other persons seeking consultation without complaint or sickness
V66 Convalescence and palliative care
V67 Follow-up examination
V68 Encounters for administrative purposes
V69 Problems related to lifestyle

Persons without reported diagnosis encountered during examination and investigation of individuals and populations (V70-V82)

V70 General medical examination
V71 Observation and evaluation for suspected conditions
V72 Special investigations and examinations
V73 Special screening examination for viral and chlamydial diseases
V74 Special screening examination for bacterial and spirochetal diseases
V75 Special screening examination for other infectious diseases
V76 Special screening for malignant neoplasms
V77 Special screening for endocrine, nutritional, metabolic, and immunity disorders
V78 Special screening for disorders of blood and blood-forming organs
V79 Special screening for mental disorders and developmental handicaps
V80 Special screening for neurological, eye, and ear diseases
V81 Special screening for cardiovascular, respiratory, and genitourinary diseases
V82 Special screening for other conditions

Genetics (V83-V84)

V83 Genetic carrier status
V84 Genetic susceptibility to malignant neoplasm

Body Mass Index (V85)

V85 Body mass index

Estrogen Receptor Status (V86)

V86 Estrogen receptor status

Other specified personal exposures and history presenting hazards to health (V87)

V87 Other specified personal exposures and history presenting hazards to health

Acquired absence of other organs and tissue (V88)

V88 Acquired absence of other organs and tissue

Other suspected conditions not found (V89)

V89 Other suspected conditions not found

19. SUPPLEMENTARY CLASSIFICATION OF EXTERNAL CAUSES OF INJURY AND POISONING (E000-E999)

External Cause Status (E000)

E000 External Cause Status

Activity (E001-E030)

E001 Activities involving walking and running
E002 Activities involving water and water craft
E003 Activities involving ice and snow
E004 Activities involving climbing, rappelling, and jumping off
E005 Activities involving dancing and other rhythmic movement
E006 Activities involving other sports and athletics played individually
E007 Activities involving other sports and athletics played as a team or group
E008 Activities involving other specified sports and athletics
E009 Activity involving other cardiorespiratory exercise
E010 Activity involving other muscle strengthening exercises
E011 Activities involving computer technology and electronic devices
E012 Activities involving arts and handcrafts
E013 Activities involving personal hygiene and household maintenance
E014 Activities involving person providing caregiving
E015 Activities involving food preparation, cooking and grilling
E016 Activities involving property and land maintenance, building and construction
E017 Activities involving roller coasters and other types of external motion
E018 Activities involving playing musical instrument
E019 Activities involving animal care
E029 Other activity
E030 Unspecified activity

Railway accidents (E800-E807)

E800 Railway accident involving collision with rolling stock
E801 Railway accident involving collision with other object
E802 Railway accident involving derailment without antecedent collision
E803 Railway accident involving explosion, fire, or burning
E804 Fall in, on, or from railway train
E805 Hit by rolling stock
E806 Other specified railway accident
E807 Railway accident of unspecified nature

© 2009 MAG Mutual Healthcare Solutions, Inc.

Motor vehicle traffic accidents (E810-E819)
E810 Motor vehicle traffic accident involving collision with train
E811 Motor vehicle traffic accident involving re-entrant collision with another motor vehicle
E812 Other motor vehicle traffic accident involving collision with another motor vehicle
E813 Motor vehicle traffic accident involving collision with other vehicle
E814 Motor vehicle traffic accident involving collision with pedestrian
E815 Other motor vehicle traffic accident involving collision on the highway
E816 Motor vehicle traffic accident due to loss of control, without collision on the highway
E817 Noncollision motor vehicle traffic accident while boarding or alighting
E818 Other noncollision motor vehicle traffic accident
E819 Motor vehicle traffic accident of unspecified nature

Motor vehicle nontraffic accidents (E820-E825)
E820 Nontraffic accident involving motor-driven snow vehicle
E821 Nontraffic accident involving other off-road motor vehicle
E822 Other motor vehicle nontraffic accident involving collision with moving object
E823 Other motor vehicle nontraffic accident involving collision with stationary object
E824 Other motor vehicle nontraffic accident while boarding and alighting
E825 Other motor vehicle nontraffic accident of other and unspecified nature

Other road vehicle accidents (E826-E829)
E826 Pedal cycle accident
E827 Animal-drawn vehicle accident
E828 Accident involving animal being ridden
E829 Other road vehicle accidents

Water transport accidents (E830-E838)
E830 Accident to watercraft causing submersion
E831 Accident to watercraft causing other injury
E832 Other accidental submersion or drowning in water transport accident
E833 Fall on stairs or ladders in water transport
E834 Other fall from one level to another in water transport
E835 Other and unspecified fall in water transport
E836 Machinery accident in water transport
E837 Explosion, fire, or burning in watercraft
E838 Other and unspecified water transport accident

Air and space transport accidents (E840-E845)
E840 Accident to powered aircraft at takeoff or landing
E841 Accident to powered aircraft, other and unspecified
E842 Accident to unpowered aircraft
E843 Fall in, on, or from aircraft
E844 Other specified air transport accidents
E845 Accident involving spacecraft

Vehicle accidents, not elsewhere classifiable (E846-E849)
E846 Accidents involving powered vehicles used solely within the buildings and premises of an industrial or commercial establishment
E847 Accidents involving cable cars not running on rails
E848 Accidents involving other vehicles, not elsewhere classifiable
E849 Place of occurrence

Accidental poisoning by drugs, medicinal substances, and biologicals (E850-E858)
E850 Accidental poisoning by analgesics, antipyretics, and antirheumatics
E851 Accidental-poisoning by barbiturates
E852 Accidental poisoning by other sedatives and hypnotics
E853 Accidental poisoning by tranquilizers
E854 Accidental poisoning by other psychotropic agents
E855 Accidental poisoning by other drugs acting on central and autonomic nervous systems
E856 Accidental poisoning by antibiotics
E857 Accidental poisoning by anti-infectives
E858 Accidental poisoning by other drugs

Accidental poisoning by other solid and liquid substances, gases, and vapors (E860-E869)
E860 Accidental poisoning by alcohol, not elsewhere classified
E861 Accidental poisoning by cleansing and polishing agents, disinfectants, paints, and varnishes
E862 Accidental poisoning by petroleum products, other solvents and their vapors, not elsewhere classified
E863 Accidental poisoning by agricultural and horticultural chemical and pharmaceutical preparations other than plant foods and fertilizers
E864 Accidental poisoning by corrosives and caustics, not elsewhere classified
E865 Accidental poisoning from poisonous foodstuffs and poisonous plants
E866 Accidental poisoning by other and unspecified solid and liquid substances
E867 Accidental poisoning by gas distributed by pipeline
E868 Accidental poisoning by other utility gas and other carbon monoxide
E869 Accidental poisoning by other gases and vapors

Misadventures to patients during surgical and medical care (E870-E876)
E870 Accidental cut, puncture, perforation, or hemorrhage during medical care
E871 Foreign object left in body during procedure
E872 Failure of sterile precautions during procedure
E873 Failure in dosage
E874 Mechanical failure of instrument or apparatus during procedure
E875 Contaminated or infected blood, other fluid, drug, or biological substance
E876 Other and unspecified misadventures during medical care

Surgical and medical procedures as the cause of abnormal reaction of patient or later complication, without mention of misadventure at the time of procedure (E878-E879)
E878 Surgical operation and other surgical procedures as the cause of abnormal reaction of patient, or of later complication, without mention of misadventure at the time of operation
E879 Other procedures, without mention of misadventure at the time of procedure, as the cause of abnormal reaction of patient, or of later complication

Accidental falls (E880-E888)
E880 Fall on or from stairs or steps
E881 Fall on or from ladders or scaffolding
E882 Fall from or out of building or other structure
E883 Fall into hole or other opening in surface
E884 Other fall from one level to another
E885 Fall on same level from slipping, tripping, or stumbling
E886 Fall on same level from collision, pushing or shoving, by or with other person
E887 Fracture, cause unspecified
E888 Other and unspecified fall

Accidents caused by fire and flames (E890-E899)
E890 Conflagration in private dwelling
E891 Conflagration in other and unspecified building or structure
E892 Conflagration not in building or structure
E893 Accident caused by ignition of clothing
E894 Ignition of highly inflammable material
E895 Accident caused by controlled fire in private dwelling
E896 Accident caused by controlled fire in other and unspecified building or structure
E897 Accident caused by controlled fire not in building or structure
E898 Accident caused by other specified fire and flames
E899 Accident caused by unspecified fire

Accidents due to natural and environmental factors (E900-E909)
E900 Excessive heat
E901 Excessive cold
E902 High and low air pressure and changes in air pressure
E903 Travel and motion
E904 Hunger, thirst, exposure, and neglect
E905 Venomous animals and plants as the cause of poisoning and toxic reactions
E906 Other injury caused by animals
E907 Lightning
E908 Cataclysmic storms, and floods resulting from storms
E909 Cataclysmic earth surface movements and eruptions

Accidents caused by submersion, suffocation, and foreign bodies (E910-E915)
E910 Accidental drowning and submersion
E911 Inhalation and ingestion of food causing obstruction of respiratory tract or suffocation
E912 Inhalation and ingestion of other object causing obstruction of respiratory tract or suffocation
E913 Accidental mechanical suffocation
E914 Foreign body accidentally entering eye and adnexa
E915 Foreign body accidentally entering other orifice

Other accidents (E916-E928)
E916 Struck accidentally by falling object
E917 Striking against or struck accidentally by objects or persons
E918 Caught accidentally in or between objects
E919 Accidents caused by machinery
E920 Accidents caused by cutting and piercing instruments or objects
E921 Accident caused by explosion of pressure vessel
E922 Accident caused by firearm missile
E923 Accident caused by explosive material
E924 Accident caused by hot substance or object, caustic or corrosive material, and steam
E925 Accident caused by electric current
E926 Exposure to radiation
E927 Overexertion and strenuous and repetitive movements or loads
E928 Other and unspecified environmental and accidental causes

Late effects of accidental injury (E929)
E929 Late effects of accidental injury

Drugs, medicinal and biological substances causing adverse effects in therapeutic use (E930-E949)
E930 Antibiotics
E931 Other anti-infectives
E932 Hormones and synthetic substitutes
E933 Primarily systemic agents
E934 Agents primarily affecting blood constituents
E935 Analgesics, antipyretics, and antirheumatics

© 2009 MAG Mutual Healthcare Solutions, Inc.

E936 Anticonvulsants and anti-Parkinsonism drugs
E937 Sedatives and hypnotics
E938 Other central nervous system depressants and anesthetics
E939 Psychotropic agents
E940 Central nervous system stimulants
E941 Drugs primarily affecting the autonomic nervous system
E942 Agents primarily affecting the cardiovascular system
E943 Agents primarily affecting gastrointestinal system
E944 Water, mineral, and uric acid metabolism drugs
E945 Agents primarily acting on the smooth and skeletal muscles and respiratory system
E946 Agents primarily affecting skin and mucous membrane, ophthalmological, otorhinolaryngological, and dental drugs
E947 Other and unspecified drugs and medicinal substances
E948 Bacterial vaccines
E949 Other vaccines and biological substances

Suicide and self-inflicted injury (E950-E959)

E950 Suicide and self-inflicted poisoning by solid or liquid substances
E951 Suicide and self-inflicted poisoning by gases in domestic use
E952 Suicide and self-inflicted poisoning by other gases and vapors
E953 Suicide and self-inflicted injury by hanging, strangulation, and suffocation
E954 Suicide and self-inflicted injury by submersion [drowning]
E955 Suicide and self-inflicted injury by firearms and explosives
E956 Suicide and self-inflicted injury by cutting and piercing instruments
E957 Suicide and self-inflicted injuries by jumping from high place
E958 Suicide and self-inflicted injury by other and unspecified means
E959 Late effects of self-inflicted injury

Homicide and injury purposely inflicted by other persons (E960-E969)

E960 Fight, brawl, and rape
E961 Assault by corrosive or caustic substance, except poisoning
E962 Assault by poisoning
E963 Assault by hanging and strangulation
E964 Assault by submersion [drowning]
E965 Assault by firearms and explosives
E966 Assault by cutting and piercing instrument
E967 Child and adult battering and other maltreatment
E968 Assault by other and unspecified means
E969 Late effects of injury purposely inflicted by other person

Legal intervention (E970-E978)

E970 Injury due to legal intervention by firearms
E971 Injury due to legal intervention by explosives
E972 Injury due to legal intervention by gas
E973 Injury due to legal intervention by blunt object
E974 Injury due to legal intervention by cutting and piercing instruments
E975 Injury due to legal intervention by other specified means
E976 Injury due to legal intervention by unspecified means
E977 Late effects of injuries due to legal intervention
E978 Legal execution
E979 Terrorism

Injury undetermined whether accidentally or purposely inflicted (E980-E989)

E980 Poisoning by solid or liquid substances, undetermined whether accidentally or purposely inflicted
E981 Poisoning by gases in domestic use, undetermined whether accidentally or purposely inflicted
E982 Poisoning by other gases, undetermined whether accidentally or purposely inflicted
E983 Hanging, strangulation, or suffocation, undetermined whether accidentally or purposely inflicted
E984 Submersion [drowning], undetermined whether accidentally or purposely inflicted
E985 Injury by firearms and explosives, undetermined whether accidentally or purposely inflicted
E986 Injury by cutting and piercing instruments, undetermined whether accidentally or purposely inflicted
E987 Falling from high place, undetermined whether accidentally or purposely inflicted
E988 Injury by other and unspecified means, undetermined whether accidentally or purposely inflicted
E989 Late effects of injury, undetermined whether accidentally or purposely inflicted

Injury resulting from operations of war (E990-E999)

E990 Injury due to war operations by fires and conflagrations
E991 Injury due to war operations by bullets and fragments
E992 Injury due to war operations by explosion of marine weapons
E993 Injury due to war operations by other explosion
E994 Injury due to war operations by destruction of aircraft
E995 Injury due to war operations by other and unspecified forms of conventional warfare
E996 Injury due to war operations by nuclear weapons
E997 Injury due to war operations by other forms of unconventional warfare
E998 Injury due to war operations but occurring after cessation of hostilities
E999 Late effects of injury due to war operations

© 2009 MAG Mutual Healthcare Solutions, Inc.